Brief Table of Contents

Fundamentals of Nursing

Human Health and Function

EIGHTH EDITION

Fundamentals of Nursing

Human Health and Function

EIGHTH EDITION · **Ruth F. Craven, EdD, RN, FAAN**
Professor Emerita
Department of Biobehavioral Nursing and Health Systems
University of Washington School of Nursing
Seattle, Washington

Constance J. Hirnle, MN, RN-BC
Retired Faculty Member
Senior Lecturer
Department of Biobehavioral Nursing and Health Systems
University of Washington School of Nursing
Seattle, Washington

Christine M. Henshaw, EdD, RN-BC
Professional Development Specialist
Virginia Mason Medical Center
Seattle, Washington

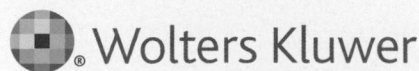. Wolters Kluwer

Philadelphia · Baltimore · New York · London
Buenos Aires · Hong Kong · Sydney · Tokyo

Executive Editor: Sherry Dickinson
Product Development Editor: Meredith Brittain
Production Project Manager: Marian Bellus
Editorial Assistant: Dan Reilly
Senior Book Designer: Joan Wendt
Art Director: Jennifer Clements
Manufacturing Coordinator: Karin Duffield
Prepress Vendor: SPi Global

Library of Congress Cataloging-in-Publication Data

Fundamentals of nursing (Craven)

Fundamentals of nursing : human health and function / editors, Ruth F. Craven, Constance J. Hirnle, Chris Henshaw. — Eighth edition.

   p. ; cm.

Includes bibliographical references and index.

  ISBN 978-1-4698-9860-5 (hardback)

I. Craven, Ruth F., editor. II. Hirnle, Constance J., editor. III. Henshaw, Chris, editor. IV. Title.

[DNLM: 1. Nursing Care. 2. Nursing Process. 3. Nursing. WY 100.1]

RT41

610.73—dc23

2015025654

DEDICATION

To Bill; Brent, Katie, and Lex; Judy, Shanyce, and Treven; Kyle and Carter Craven

Scott, Beth, Ethan, and Autumn; John Hirnle; Sarah, Peter, and Maddie Nimis;
Nancy Cassisk and Kathy Schaffer

David and Alex Henshaw

For their love, support, sacrifice, and encouragement that allowed us to make
this book a reality.

With sincere gratitude to all our students and colleagues who have helped shape
this book over its many editions and from whom we have learned and continue to learn.

CONTRIBUTORS TO THE EIGHTH EDITION

Dolly Alex-Wasielewski, MSN, RN
Perianesthesia Educator
UW Medicine/Valley Medical Center
Clinical Instructor
University of Washington School of
Nursing
Seattle, Washington
  PICO Displays

Marisa Gillaspie Aziz, MSN, RN, ACNS-BC
Heart Failure Specialist
St. Jude Medical
Seattle, Washington
  Chapter 24: Hygiene and Self-Care

Debra Beauchaine, MN, AGPCNP-BC,
CWOCN-AP
Nurse Practitioner
Cave Creek, Arizona
  *Chapter 30: Skin Integrity and Wound
  Healing*

Deanne A. Blach, MSN, RN
Nurse Educator—Professional
Conference Planner
DB Productions of NW AR, Inc.
Green Forest, Arkansas
  Concept Map Revisions

Doris M. Boutain, PhD, RN
Associate Professor
Psychosocial and Community Health
University of Washington School of
Nursing
Seattle, Washington
  Chapter 7: Values, Ethics, and Legal Issues

Terry F. Cicero, MN, CCRN
Senior Instructor
College of Nursing
Seattle University
Seattle, Washington
  Chapter 21: Intravenous Therapy

B. Jane Cornman, PhD, RN, QTTP/T,
HWC-BC
Senior Lecturer
University of Washington
Tacoma, Washington
  *Chapter 2: Health, Wellness, and
  Complimentary Medicine*

Tamara Cyhan Cunitz, MN, RN
Clinical Faculty
Department of Biobehavioral Nursing
and Health Systems
University of Washington School of
Nursing
Seattle, Washington
  Chapter 27: Cardiac Function

Jessica Dunn, MSN, BS, RN, CNL
Director, Ambulatory Care
Nursing
Virginia Mason Medical Center
Seattle, Washington
  *Chapter 10: Caring for the
  Older Adult*

Phyllis J. Eide, PhD, MPH, MN
Associate Professor of Nursing
Washington State University College
of Nursing
Spokane, Washington
  *Chapter 8: Nursing Research and
  Evidence-Based Care*

Marilyn J. Hammer, PhD, DC, RN
Assistant Professor
New York University College of
Nursing
New York, New York
  *Chapter 41: Stress, Coping, and
  Adaptation*

Kathryn Van Dyke Hayes,
PhD, RN, CNE
Professor and Director of Graduate
Nursing Programs
School of Nursing and Allied Health
Professions
Holy Family University
Philadelphia, Pennsylvania
  *Chapter 11: Foundations of Practice
  Chapter 12: Nursing Assessment
  Chapter 13: Nursing Diagnosis
  Chapter 14: Outcome Identification and
  Planning
  Chapter 15: Implementation and
  Planning*

Christine M. Henshaw, EdD, RN-BC
Professional Development
Specialist
Virginia Mason Medical Center
Seattle, Washington

Pavla Holman, RN
Nurse Manager, Inpatient
Orthopedics
Virginia Mason Medical Center
Seattle, Washington
  Chapter 25: Mobility

Sharon Jensen, MN, RN
Instructor
University of Hawaii, Manoa
Honolulu, Hawaii
  Chapter 17: Health Assessment

Deborah D. Kelly, MN, RN
Administrative Director, Clinical
Practice & Professional Development
Virginia Mason Medical Center
Seattle, Washington
  *Chapter 9: Patient Education and Health
  Promotion*

Beth Keyte, MSN, RN-BC
Professor, Psychiatric Nursing
Des Moines Area Community College
Ankeny, Iowa
  Chapter 6: Communication in the Nurse–
  Patient Relationship

Niki Kirby, MSN, RN
Professional Development Specialist
Virginia Mason Medical Center
Seattle, Washington
  Chapter 20: Medical Administration

Shirley Kopf-Klakken, MSN, RN
Professional Development Specialist
Virginia Mason Medical Center
Seattle, Washington
Chapter 32: Urinary Elimination

Carol Landis, PhD, RN, FAAN
Professor
University of Washington School of
Nursing
Seattle, Washington
  Chapter 34: Sleep and Rest

Lauren Valk Lawson, DNP, RN
Assistant Professor
Seattle University
Seattle, Washington
  Chapter 3: Healthcare in the Community
  and Home

Janet Lenart, MN, RN, MPH
Director for Online Education, School
of Nursing
Senior Lecturer, Biobehavioral Nursing
and Health Systems
University of Washington
Seattle, Washington
  Chapter 5: Culture and Diversity

Kim Leppert, MSN, RN, ACNS, CNOR, ONC
Clinical Supervisor-Perioperative
Services
Swedish Medical Center
Ballard, Washington
  Chapter 22: Perioperative Nursing

Patricia Lisk, MS, RN, DACCE
Professor/Dean of Nursing and Health
Technologies
Germanna Community College
Locust Grove, Virginia
  Chapter 43: Spiritual Health

Vanessa A. Makareiwicz, MN, RN-BC
Infection Control Operations Manager
Harborview Medical Center
Seattle, Washington
  Chapter 26: Respiratory Function

Heather A. Martin, MSN, RN, CNRN,
SCRN
Clinical Nurse Specialist—
Neuroscience
Virginia Mason Medical Center
Seattle, Washington
  Chapter 37: Cognitive Processes

Georgia L. Narsavage, PhD, APRN,
FAAN, FNAP
Director, Interprofessional Education
West Virginia Health Sciences Center
Professor, West Virginia School of
Nursing
West Virginia University
Morgantown, West Virginia
  Chapter 39: Families and Their
  Relationships

Ellen Noel, MN, RN, CPHQ
Faculty, Education Services
Virginia Mason Institute
Seattle, Washington
  Chapter 35: Pain

Mary Ann Osborne, DNP, FNP-C
Family Nurse Practitioner
Integrative Medicine Fellow
Institute for Integral Health
Colorado Springs, Colorado
  Chapter 2: Health, Wellness, and
  Complimentary Medicine

Anne P. Poppe, PhD, MN, RN
Jonas Scholar
Clinical Instructor
University of Washington School of
Nursing
Seattle, Washington
  Chapter 38: Self-Concept

Craig R. Sellers, PhD, RN, ANP-BC,
GNP-BC, FAANP
Professor of Clinical Nursing
University of Rochester School of
Nursing
Rochester, New York
  Chapter 40: Loss and Grieving

Judith L. St. Onge, PhD, RN, CNE
Assistant Professor
Troy University
Montgomery, Alabama
  Chapter 29: Nutrition

Susan A. Talbot, MN, RN, CGRN
Professional Development Specialist
Virginia Mason Medical Center
Seattle, Washington
  Chapter 33: Bowel Elimination

Ryan Townsend, MN, ARNP, BC
Director, Undergraduate Program
Washington State University College of
Nursing
Spokane, Washington
  Chapter 8: Nursing Research and Evidence-
  Based Care

Nancy Westvang, MS, RN
Professional Development Specialist
Virginia Mason Medical Center
Seattle, Washington
  Chapter 42: Human Sexuality

Jean Yockey, PhD, FNP-BC, CNE
Assistant Professor
The University of South Dakota
Vermillion, South Dakota
  Chapter 36: Sensory Perception

Jeri Yoder, MNHP, RN, CCRN, CNL, CLNC
Professional Development Specialist
Virginia Mason Medical Center
Seattle, Washington
  Chapter 31: Infection Prevention and
  Management

CONTRIBUTORS TO THE SEVENTH EDITION

Barbara Albertson, MN, RN-BC
Staff Development Specialist
University of Washington Medical
Center
Seattle, Washington
  Chapter 17: Vital Signs

Gail Armstrong, ND, RN, CNE
Assistant Professor
Denver College of Nursing
University of Colorado
Denver, Colorado
  Chapter 24: Mobility

Debra Beauchaine, MN, AGPCNP-BC,
CWOCN-AP
Nurse Practitioner
Cave Creek, Arizona
  *Chapter 29: Skin Integrity and Wound
  Healing*
  Chapter 31: Urinary Elimination

Eva Bookin, BSN, RN
Staff Nurse
Providence Regional Medical Center
Everett, Washington
  *Clinical Research Associate for Seventh
  Edition*

Doris M. Boutain, PhD, RN
Associate Professor
University of Washington
Seattle, Washington
  *Chapter 6: Values, Ethics, and
  Legal Issues*

Helen Teresa Buckland, PhD, MEd
Research Coordinator
Studies of IBS, School of Nursing
Clinical Assistant Professor
School of Nursing and School of Public
Health
University of Washington
Seattle, Washington
  *Chapter 5: Communication in the Nurse–
  Patient Relationship*

Terry F. Cicero, MN, CCRN
Instructor
College of Nursing
Seattle University
Seattle, Washington
  Chapter 20: Intravenous Therapy

B. Jane Cornman, PhD, RN, QTTP/T,
HWC-BC
Formerly Senior Lecturer
University of Washington School of
Nursing
Seattle, Washington
  *Chapter 2: Health, Wellness, and
  Complementary Medicine*

Lori Cray, PhD, RN
Instructor
College of Nursing
Seattle University
Seattle, Washington
  Chapter 25: Respiratory Function

Tamara Cyhan-Cunitz, MN, RN
Clinical Education Specialist
Virginia Mason Medical Center
Seattle, Washington
  Chapter 26: Cardiac Function

Phyllis J. Eide, PhD, MPH, MN
Associate Professor
Washington State University College of
Nursing
Spokane, Washington
  *Chapter 7: Nursing Research and Evidence-
  Based Care*

Noreen W. Esposito, EdD, WHNP-BC,
FNP-BC
Clinical Associate Professor
University of North Carolina
at Chapel Hill
Chapel Hill, North Carolina
  Chapter 41: Human Sexuality

Marisa Gillaspie Aziz, MSN, RN,
ACNS-BC
Clinical Nurse Specialist
St. Francis Hospital
Federal Way, Washington
  Chapter 23: Hygiene and Self-Care

Penny L. Gilliatt, MN, RN, CCRN
Education Specialist and CNE Planner
Virginia Mason Medical Center
Seattle, Washington
  Chapter 18: Asepsis
  *Chapter 30: Infection Prevention and
  Management*

Marilyn J. Hammer, PhD, DC, RN
Assistant Professor
College of Nursing
New York University
New York, New York
  Chapter 40: Stress, Coping, and Adaptation

Mary K. Haviland, MN, RN
Former Lecturer
Seattle University
Seattle, Washington
  *Chapter 27: Fluid, Electrolytes, and
  Acid–Base*

Kathryn Van Dyke Hayes, PhD, RN, CNE
Professor
Holy Family University
Philadelphia, Pennsylvania
  Chapter 11: Nursing Assessment
  Chapter 12: Nursing Diagnosis
  *Chapter 13: Outcome Identification and
  Planning*
  *Chapter 14: Implementation and
  Evaluation*

Christine M. Henshaw, EdD, RN-BC
Clinical Education Specialist
Virginia Mason Medical Center
Seattle, Washington
  Chapter 1: The Profession of Nursing

Deborah D. Kelly, MN, RN
Administrative Director
Clinical Education
Virginia Mason Medical Center
Seattle, Washington
  *Chapter 8: Patient Education and Health
  Promotion*

Carol Landis, PhD, RN, FAAN
Professor
University of Washington
Seattle, Washington
  Chapter 33: Sleep and Rest

Lauren Valk Lawson, DNP, RN
Instructor
College of Nursing
Seattle University
Seattle, Washington
  *Chapter 3: Healthcare in the Community
  and Home*

Janet Lenart, MN, MPH, RN
Senior Lecturer
University of Washington School of
Nursing
Seattle, Washington
Chapter 4: Culture and Diversity

**Sophia Lichenstein-Hill, DNP,
FNP-BC**
Adult Nurse Practitioner
Gastroenterology
Virginia Mason Medical Center
Seattle, Washington
Concept Maps

Patricia Lisk, MS, RN, DACCE
Professor of Nursing
Germanna Community College
Fredericksburg, Virginia
Chapter 42: Spiritual Health

Susan B. Matt, PhD, JD, RN
Assistant Professor
College of Nursing
Seattle University
Seattle, Washington
*Chapter 19: Medication
Administration*

Karen L. Moe, MEd, RN
Clinical Nurse Educator
University of Washington Medical
Center
Seattle, Washington
Chapter 21: Perioperative Nursing

**Georgia L. Narsavage, PhD, APRN,
FAAN, FNAP**
Dean and Professor
West Virginia School of Nursing
Morgantown, West Virginia
*Chapter 38: Families and Their
Relationships*

Ellen Noel, MN, RN, CPHQ
Faculty, Education Services
Virginia Mason Institute
Seattle, Washington
Chapter 34: Pain

Mary Ann Osborne, DNP, FNP-C
Integrative Family Nurse Practitioner
Clinical Faculty
University of Washington
Seattle, Washington
*Chapter 2: Health, Wellness, and
Complementary Medicine*

Anne Poppe, PhD, MN, RN
Research Nurse/Project Director
University of Washington School of
Nursing
Seattle, Washington
Chapter 37: Self-Concept

Alison Pyle, MN, MPH, RN
Clinical Director
Virginia Mason Medical Center
Seattle, Washington
NCLEX Questions

Shelia Sparks Ralph, PhD, RN, FAAN
Retired
Hamilton, Virginia
Chapter 11: Nursing Assessment
Chapter 12: Nursing Diagnosis
*Chapter 13: Outcome Identification and
Planning*
*Chapter 14: Implementation and
Evaluation*

**Craig R. Sellers, PhD, RN, ANP-BC,
GNP-BC, FAANP**
Associate Professor of Clinical Nursing
School of Nursing
University of Rochester
Rochester, New York
Chapter 39: Loss and Grieving

Mary Shelkey, PhD, ARNP
Adjunct Professor
Seattle University
Seattle, Washington
Chapter 9: Caring for the Older Adult

Judith L. St. Onge, PhD, RN, CNE
Assistant Professor
Troy University
Montgomery, Alabama
Chapter 28: Nutrition

Ryan Townsend, MN, ARNP, BC
Director of Professional Development
Washington State University College of
Nursing
Spokane, Washington
*Chapter 7: Nursing Research and Evidence-
Based Care*

Diana Twidwell, MS, RN
Associate Professor
Department of Nursing
University of South Dakota
Vermillion, South Dakota
Chapter 36: Cognitive Processes

Nancy Westvang, MS, RN
Clinical Education Specialist
Virginia Mason Medical Center
Seattle, Washington
Chapter 32: Bowel Elimination

Jean Yockey, PhD, FNP-BC, CNE
Associate Professor
University of South Dakota
Vermillion, South Dakota
Chapter 35: Sensory Perception

For a list of the contributors to the Student
and Instructor Resources accompanying this
book, please visit http://thepoint.lww.com/
Craven8e.

Terri Ades, DNP, FNP-BC, AOCN
Associate Professor, Clinical
Nell Hodgson Woodruff School of
Nursing
Emory University
Atlanta, Georgia

Earnest Ruth Agnew, DNP, RN
Associate Degree Nursing Instructor
Clinical Simulation Specialist
Itawamba Community College
Tupelo, Mississippi

Loretta Aller, MSN, RN
Nursing Faculty
Kent State University at Stark
North Canton, Ohio

Daria U. Amato, MSN, RN, CNE
Associate Professor for Nursing
Northern Virginia Community
College–MEC-Division of Nursing
Springfield, Virginia

Jane Bagley, MS, RN
Assistant Professor of Nursing
St. Cloud State University
St. Cloud, Minnesota

**Susan Barrett-Landau, EdD, MS, ANP/
FNP, RN-BC**
Assistant Professor
Farmingdale State College
Farmingdale, New York

Brenda Beshears, PhD, RN
President/Dean
Professor
Blessing-Rieman College of Nursing
Quincy, Illinois

**Carolanne Bianchi, DNP, MBA,
RN, ANP**
Assistant Professor of Clinical Nursing
University of Rochester School of
Nursing
Rochester, New York

Dana M. Botz, MSN, RN, CNE
Nursing Faculty
North Hennepin Community College
Brooklyn Park, Minnesota

Fara Bowler, MS, APN, ANP-C
Director Clinical Education Center &
Simulation
University of Colorado Denver,
Anschutz Medical Campus
Denver, Colorado

Joan Boyd, MS, RS
Professor of Nursing
Florida State College
Jacksonville, Florida

Nell Britton, MSN, RN, CNE, NHA
Education Site Visitor
SC Board of Nursing
Columbia, South Carolina

Patricia M. Burke, PhD, CNE, RNC
Associate Professor
Touro College
Brooklyn, New York

Erla Champ-Gibson, MDiv, RN, PhD(c)
Clinical Assistant Professor
Pacific Lutheran University
Tacoma, Washington

Joanna Commons, MSN, RN, NP-C
Nursing Instructor
Danville Area Community College
Danville, Illinois

Marianne Curia, PhD, MSN, RN
Assistant Professor
John and Cecily Leach College of
Nursing
University of St. Francis
Joliet, Illinois

Amber Davis, MSN, RN
Nursing Instructor
Northern Illinois University
DeKalb, Illinois

Hartensia Davis-Bailey, MSN, APRN
Instructor/Low-Fidelity Simulation
Coordinator
Winston-Salem State University
Winston-Salem, North Carolina

Doreen DeAngelis, MSN, RN
Nursing Instructor
Penn State Fayette, The Eberly Campus
Lemont Furnace, Pennsylvania

**Marci Dial, DNP, ARNP, NP-C, RN-BC,
CHSE, LNC**
Professor of Nursing
Valencia College
Orlando, Florida

Sonia Donaldson, MSN
Assistant Professor
Washington Adventist University
Takoma Park, Maryland

Donna Eberly, MSN, RN
Nursing Instructor
Western Iowa Tech Community
College
Sioux City, Iowa

Anita Fitzgerald, RN, PhD (c)
Lecturer
California State University, Long Beach
Long Beach, California

Kathleen Fraley, MSN, BSN, ADN, RN
Professor of Nursing
St. Clair County Community College
Port Huron, Michigan

Jennifer Gambal, MSN, RN
Instructor
DeSales University
Center Valley, Pennsylvania

Michelle Cafaro Gellar, MSN, RN, MPH
Assistant Professor
New York City College of Technology
Brooklyn, New York

Evalyn J. Gossett, MSN, RN
Clinical Assistant Professor
Indiana University Northwest
Gary, Indiana

Lori Hailey, MSN, RN, CHSE
Assistant Professor of Nursing
Arkansas State University
Jonesboro, Arkansas

Karla J. Hanson, MS, RN
Instructor
South Dakota State University
Brookings, South Dakota

Lori Hendrickx, EdD, RN, CCRN
Professor
South Dakota State University College
of Nursing
Brookings, South Dakota

Dinah R. Herrick, MSN/Ed, RN
Assistant Professor of Nursing
California Baptist University
Riverside, California

Belinda Higgins, MSN, RN
Associate Professor
Jackson State Community College
Jackson, Tennessee

Margo Hollenbach, MSN, RN
Instructor/Clinical Placement
Coordinator
Reading Hospital School of Health
Sciences
Reading, Pennsylvania

Susan Holt, MS
Professor and Staff Nurse
Grayson College
Denison, Texas

Jaime Huffman, PhD
Assistant Professor
Saginaw Valley State University
University Center, Michigan

Mary Kay Kasuba, MS, RN, CNE
Professor, Associate Degree Nursing
Berkshire Community College
Pittsfield, Massachusetts

Patricia T. Ketcham, MSN, RN
Director of Nursing Laboratories
Oakland University School of Nursing
Rochester, Michigan

Rosanina Ketchum, MSN, RN
Assistant Professor
Oklahoma Wesleyan University
Bartlesville, Oklahoma

Rebecca King, MSN, RN
Adjunct Professor
University of Arkansas Community
College at Batesville
Batesville, Arkansas

Tara J. Latto, MS, RN
Nursing Instructor
Morton College
Cicero, Illinois

Mary Beth Lukach, MSN, RN, CNS
Full Lecturer
College of Nursing
Kent State University
Kent, Ohio

Rosemary Macy, PhD, RN, CNE, CHSE
Associate Professor
School of Nursing
Boise State University
Boise, Idaho

Antoinette McCray, MSN, RNC, CNS, CNE
Instructor
Norfolk State University
Norfolk, Virginia

Jackie McMahon, RN, CNE
Nursing Educator
Cochran School of Nursing
Yonkers, New York

Jean Medor, MS
Science Instructional Specialist
New York University
New York, New York

Michelle Montpas, EdD, MSN, RN, CNE
Professor of Nursing
Mott Community College
Flint, Michigan

Lora J. Morris, MSN, RN
Associate Professor, Nursing
Kent State University Ashtabula
Ashtabula, Ohio

Jessica Naber, PhD, RN
Assistant Professor
Murray State University
Murray, Kentucky

Susan Kay Nelson, MSN, RN, FNP-BC
Master Faculty Specialist
Western Michigan University
Kalamazoo, Michigan

Jo Newman, MSN, RN, FNP, CHSE
Clinical Assistant Professor
Indiana University Northwest
Gary, Indiana

Susan L. Olson, PhD, MSN, RN
Associate Degree Nursing
McLennan Community College
Waco, Texas

Rebecca Otten, EdD, RN
Associate Professor
California State University, Fullerton
Fullerton, California

Jennifer Douglas Pearce, MSN, RN, CNE
Professor of Nursing
University of Cincinnati Blue Ash
College
Associate Degree Program in Nursing
Blue Ash, Ohio

Deidra Pennington, MSN, RN
Assistant Professor of Nursing
Jefferson College of Health Sciences
Roanoke, Virginia

Barbara Jeanne Pinchera, DNP,
ANP-NC
Professor
Curry College
Milton, Massachusetts

Patricia Poirier, PhD, RN, AOCN
Associate Professor
University of Maine
Orono, Maine

Lillian Rafeldt, MA, RN, CNE
Professor of Nursing
Three Rivers Community College—
CT-CCNP
Norwich, Connecticut

Susan M. Randol, MSN, RN, CNE
Semester Coordinator and Master
Instructor
College of Nursing and Allied Health
Professions
University of Louisiana at Lafayette
Lafayette, Louisiana

Carol Della Ratta, PhD, RN, CCRN
Clinical Assistant Professor
Stony Brook University School of
Nursing
Stony Brook, New York

Kim Resanovich, MSN, RN-BC
Lecturer/Simulation Lab Coordinator
Ohio University
Athens, Ohio

Marty Richardson, MSN, RN
Nursing Professor
Grayson College
Denison, Texas

Laura M. Robbins-Frank, MSN, RNC, APN
Instructor
Marcella Niehoff School of Nursing
Loyola University Chicago
Chicago, Illinois

Deborah Roberts, EdD, MSN, BSN
Professor and Chair Department of
Nursing
Sonoma State University
Rohnert Park, California

Tina M. Rosetti, MSN, RN
Assistant Professor
Aquinas College
Nashville, Tennessee

Allyson Saary, MSN Ed., RN
Assistant Professor
Purdue University (North Central)
Westville, Indiana

Sally Schultz, MSN, RN
Nursing Instructor
Fox Valley Technical College
Appleton, Wisconsin

Craig R. Sellers, PhD, RN, ANP-BC,
GNP-BC, FAANP
Professor of Clinical Nursing
University of Rochester School of
Nursing
Rochester, New York

Eileen Shah, MA, RN, CNE
Assistant Professor
Molloy College
Rockville Centre, New York

Lynnie Skeen, PhD, RN
Assistant Professor
Langston University
Langston, Oklahoma

Julie Slack, MSN, RN
Associate Professor
Eastern Michigan University
Ypsilanti, Michigan

Laura C. Starrett, MSN, RN, CPNP
Associate Professor of Nursing
Piedmont College
Demorest, Georgia

Milena P. Staykova, EdD, APRN, FNP-BC
RN-BSN Program Director
Jefferson College of Health Sciences
Roanoke, Virginia

Nancy Stell, MSN, RN, CPN
Nursing Instructor
Loyola University Chicago
Chicago, Illinois

Tracey Stephen, BScN, MN, RN
Faculty Lecturer
Faculty of Nursing
University of Alberta
Edmonton, Alberta, Canada

Charlotte D. Strahm, DNSc, RN, CNS
Associate Professor
Colorado Mountain College
Glenwood Springs, Colorado

Christine Sump, MSN, RN, CNE
Senior Lecturer
Old Dominion University
Norfolk, Virginia

Nanci A. Swan, MSN, RN, CCRN
Nursing Instructor
University of Alabama at Birmingham
Birmingham, Alabama

Linda M. Tate, PhD, APRN-bc
Assistant Professor of Nursing
Arkansas State University
Jonesboro, Arkansas

Angela Trawick, MSN, RN
Professor of Nursing
Florida SouthWestern State College
Ft. Myers, Florida

Debbie Treloar, PhD
Associate Degree Nursing Faculty
East Mississippi Community
College
Mayhew, Mississippi

Jean M. Truman, DNP, RN, CNE
ASN Program Coordinator & Associate
Professor of Nursing
University of Pittsburgh at Bradford
Bradford, Pennsylvania

Virginia Tufano, EdD, MSN, RN
Associate Professor of Nursing
Director of MSN Program
College of Saint Mary
Omaha, Nebraska

Suzanne W. Van Orden, MSN,
MSEd, RN
Senior Lecturer
Old Dominion University
Norfolk, Virginia

Patricia Voelpel, MS, RN, ANP, CCRN
Clinical Assistant Professor
Stony Brook University
Stony Brook, New York

Patricia Vuolo, MS Nursing, RN
Instructor
Nursing Department
State University of New York–Orange
County (SUNY Orange)
Middletown, New York

Mary Welhaven, PhD, RN
Professor
Winona State University Rochester
Rochester, Minnesota

Terri Wenzig, MSN, RN
Nursing Faculty
Chemeketa Community College
Salem, Oregon

Danielle L. White, MSN, RN
Associate Professor
Austin Peay State University
Clarksville, Tennessee

Kiersten Kielwasser Withrow, MSN,
RNC-OB, CBE
Assistant Professor of Nursing
DeSales University
Center Valley, Pennsylvania

For a list of the reviewers of the Test
Generator questions accompanying this
book, please visit http://thepoint.lww.com/
Craven8e.

WHY THIS BOOK?

We are witnessing an era of seismic change in the nursing world. In this new landscape, the nurse's role is expanding dramatically, bringing new demands and challenges. Even the focus of nursing practice is shifting: although always important, patient safety, communication, and critical thinking have become paramount. It is vital to have a textbook that can keep pace.

The first duty of a professional nurse is to support or restore patients to health so that they can function independently and safely in various settings. Because hospital stays are shorter—and patient loads often high—nurses are under pressure to make judgments on the spot. In short order, they need to (a) accurately assess a patient's health status, (b) diagnose problems or challenges in the case, (c) help the patient understand what kinds of outcomes he or she can expect, and (d) plan for and arrange for appropriate interventions. Additionally, nurses have to monitor and evaluate each patient's progress along the way.

For today's nursing students, building a foundation of up-to-the-minute nursing knowledge and clinical skills is essential but no longer enough. You must also develop critical thinking skills and learn how to apply them in a clinical setting. With that in mind, this book takes a big-picture approach to prepare you for a challenging and dynamic nursing practice.

MAKING KNOWLEDGE WORK FOR YOU

The healthcare system is growing more complex, and the pool of nursing candidates is becoming more diverse. You and your fellow students come with different skill sets and represent a wide range of backgrounds. To keep up, nursing schools are expanding various courses in their curricula and adding new teaching methods and media to accommodate different learning styles.

Still, all nursing students have one thing in common: the need for a framework—a system for acquiring knowledge and putting it to work. The right framework simplifies the whole process of clinical thinking. It helps you prioritize information so that you do not feel overwhelmed. The right framework lets you work in a logical sequence and process data calmly and efficiently. It teaches you to think about each case in a meaningful, systematic way, and it builds intuition, so you can instantly grasp the kinds of problems you are up against. Most important, working within a proven framework helps you protect your patients' safety and ensure the best possible outcomes for those under your care.

That is why the system we have devised for this book is so important. We are still teaching the basics—how to promote health, differentiate between normal function and dysfunction, use scientific rationales, and follow the approved nursing process. But each chapter has also been designed for the clinical environment, with input from nurses who are currently practicing in a range of settings and situations. Our aim is to help you ease the transition from school to your first nursing job. This book will give you a mastery of critical healthcare knowledge as well as something just as valuable: an understanding of how successful nurses think and act.

It is important to remember that, today more than ever, a nurse is a player in a collaborative process. To provide the best care for patients and their families, you must hone your communication skills, learn how to use reputable healthcare databases for evidence, and know how to put your research into practice.

WHAT MAKES THIS EDITION UNIQUE?

This is our most ambitious edition to date. It does more than provide healthcare knowledge. This edition breathes life into theoretical principles. It puts you in the mindset of a successful nurse and gives you a framework for tackling real-life challenges in a clinical setting. It is organized in an innovative way that ties together all the different elements of the nursing practice, revealing them as a dynamic whole.

Patients respond differently to health problems—it is that variation that makes being a nurse so meaningful and challenging. This book has been thoughtfully designed to help you practice with confidence and offer the best care for your patients right from the start.

HOW THIS BOOK IS STRUCTURED

The content is presented in four parts, with the most important information clearly highlighted.

Unit 1: Conceptual Foundations of Nursing

This section introduces vital concepts that weave their way through all of the chapters in the book. Safety, life span, culture, evidence-based care, communication, patient education, and scope of care are all addressed. Together, this material forms the basis for professional nursing practice.

Unit 2: Nursing Process

In this section, you will be introduced to a way of thinking—a framework for acquiring and processing information—that provides the basis for nursing practice. The framework allows you to stay on track while customizing care for each patient. You will learn to identify normal function, assess risk for dysfunction, envision potential outcomes, plan and provide for interventions, and evaluate the effectiveness of care.

Unit 3: Clinical Nursing Therapies

In this section, you will learn a broad set of skills vital to many aspects of nursing care. Topics include health assessment, asepsis, medication administration, intravenous therapy, and perioperative care. The information you will learn here forms an essential part of a nurse's toolkit, teaching you how to offer safe, individualized care in various clinical settings.

Unit 4: Clinical Nursing Care

This section is clearly organized by areas of human function, from physical to psychological, including how they overlap. It covers mobility, respiratory and cardiac health, and nutrition and elimination. You will also learn about sleep, pain, sensory and cognitive issues, self-concept, coping, sexuality, and spiritual health.

NEW AND IMPROVED IN THE EIGHTH EDITION

- **A timely new chapter**—Chapter 4, The Nurse's Role in Healthcare Quality and Patient Safety—responds to multiple imperatives in today's healthcare focusing on safety and quality. The chapter helps students understand systems that promote exceptional care in a complex environment. The topic of safety as it applies to the individual patient is further explored in Chapter 23.
- **New, richly illustrated concept maps**, ideal for visual learners, apply the nursing process and critical thinking to the case scenarios that begin each chapter.
- **PICO (patient/problem, intervention, comparison, outcome) displays** illustrate examples of a structured, evidence-based way to find an answer to a clinical question related to the chapter-opening scenario.
- **Concept Mastery Alerts** clarify fundamental nursing concepts to improve the reader's understanding of potentially confusing topics, as identified by Misconception Alerts in Lippincott's Adaptive Learning Powered by prepU. Data from thousands of actual students using this program in courses across the United States identified common misconceptions to be clarified in this new feature.
- **Photos** have been updated in some of the procedures, and **new procedures** have been added—for example, end-tidal

carbon dioxide monitoring ($EtCO_2$; capnography) and sputum specimen collection.
- **Apply Your Critical Thinking** features appear in nearly every chapter that guide students to explore concepts and situations more deeply. Answers provided in Appendix B allow students to check their thinking.

SPECIAL FEATURES

Many features appear throughout the text to help students grasp the important content. Refer to the "How to Use This Book" section immediately following this preface to learn more about them.

A FULLY INTEGRATED COURSE EXPERIENCE

We are delighted to introduce an expanded suite of digital solutions and ancillaries to support instructors and students using *Fundamentals of Nursing: Human Health and Function, Eighth Edition*. To learn more about any solution, please contact your local Wolters Kluwer representative.

Lippincott CoursePoint+
Lippincott CoursePoint+

Lippincott CoursePoint+ is an integrated digital learning solution designed for the way students learn. It is the only nursing education solution that integrates:

- **Leading content in context:** Content provided in the context of the student learning path engages students and encourages interaction and learning on a deeper level.
- **Powerful tools to maximize class performance:** Course-specific tools, such as adaptive learning powered by prepU, provide a personalized learning experience for every student.
- **Real-time data to measure students' progress:** Student performance data provided in an intuitive display lets you quickly spot which students are having difficulty or which concepts the class as a whole is struggling to grasp.
- **Preparation for practice:** Integrated virtual simulation and evidence-based resources improve student competence, confidence, and success in transitioning to practice.
  - *vSim for Nursing:* Co-developed by Laerdal Medical and Wolters Kluwer, *vSim for Nursing* simulates real nursing scenarios and allows students to interact with virtual patients in a safe, online environment.
  - *Lippincott Advisor for Education:* With over 8,500 entries covering the latest evidence-based content and drug information, *Lippincott Advisor for Education* provides students with the most up-to-date information possible, while giving them valuable experience with the same point-of-care content they will encounter in practice.

- **Training services and personalized support:** To ensure your success, our dedicated educational consultants and training coaches will provide expert guidance every step of the way.

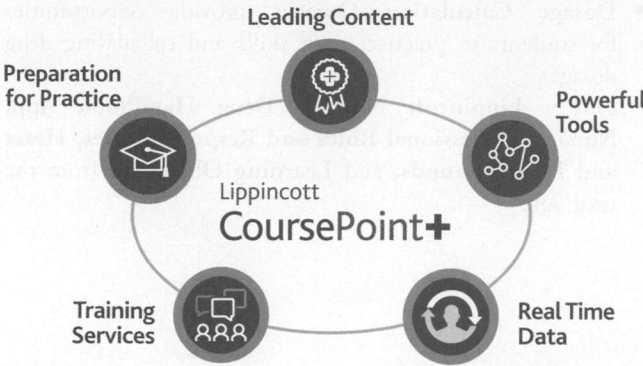

vSim for Nursing
Simulation and Other Resources

- **vSim for Nursing | Fundamentals, a new virtual simulation platform** (*available via thePoint*). Co-developed by Laerdal Medical and Wolters Kluwer, *vSim for Nursing | Fundamentals* helps students develop clinical competence and decision-making skills as they interact with virtual patients in a safe, realistic environment. *vSim for Nursing* records and assesses student decisions throughout the simulation, then provides a personalized feedback log highlighting areas needing improvement.
- **DocuCare Lippincott DocuCare** (available via thePoint). Lippincott DocuCare combines web-based electronic health record simulation software with clinical case scenarios that relate to content in *Fundamentals of Nursing: Human Health and Function*. Lippincott DocuCare's nonlinear solution works well in the classroom, simulation lab, and clinical practice.

TEACHING/LEARNING PACKAGE

A comprehensive teaching/learning package has been developed to assist faculty and students.

Resources for Instructors

Tools to assist you with teaching your course are available upon adoption of this text at http://thepoint.lww.com/Craven8e.

- An **e-Book** on thePoint gives you access to the book's full text and images online.
- The **Test Generator** lets you put together exclusive new tests from a bank containing more than 1,000 questions to help you in assessing your students' understanding of the material. Test questions link to chapter learning objectives.
- An extensive collection of materials is provided for each book chapter:
  - **Prelecture Quizzes** (and answers) are quick, knowledge-based assessments that allow you to check students' reading.
  - **PowerPoint Presentations** provide an easy way for you to integrate the textbook with your students' classroom experience, either via slide shows or handouts. Multiple choice and true/false questions are integrated into the presentations to promote class participation and allow you to use i-clicker technology.
  - **Guided Lecture Notes** walk you through the chapters, objective by objective, and provide you with corresponding PowerPoint slide numbers.
  - **Discussion Topics** (and suggested answers) can be used as conversation starters or in online discussion boards.
  - **Assignments** (and suggested answers) include group, written, clinical, and web assignments.
  - **Case Studies** with related questions (and suggested answers) give students an opportunity to apply their knowledge to a patient case similar to one they might encounter in practice.
- Two **Image Banks**—one that includes all the images in the book, and one made up of all the book's concept maps—let you use the photographs and illustrations from this textbook in your PowerPoint slides or as you see fit in your course.
- A sample **Syllabus** provides guidance for structuring your nursing fundamentals course.
- **Journal Articles,** updated for the new edition, offer access to current research available in Wolters Kluwer journals.
- Adaptable **Procedure Checklists** walk through procedures from the book step by step and can be used to help you evaluate your students' mastery of skills.
- **Master Checklist for Skills Competency** provides a list of all skills in the book to help you track your students' progress in achieving skill competency.
- **Learning Management System cartridges**.
- **Strategies for Effective Teaching** offer creative approaches.

Contact your sales representative or check out LWW.com/Nursing for more details and ordering information.

RESOURCES FOR STUDENTS

An exciting set of free resources is available to help students review material and become even more familiar with vital concepts. Students can access all these resources at http://thePoint.lww.com/Craven8e using the codes printed in the front of their textbooks.

- **NCLEX-Style Review Questions** for each chapter help students review important concepts and practice for NCLEX. Over 850 questions are included.

- **Multimedia Resources** appeal to various learning styles. Icons in the text direct readers to relevant resources:
  - **Watch & Learn Video Clips** reinforce skills from the textbook and appeal to visual and auditory learners.
  - **Practice & Learn Activities** present case scenarios and offer interactive exercises and questions to help students apply what they have learned.
  - **Concepts in Action Animations** bring physiologic and pathophysiologic concepts to life and enhance student comprehension.
- **Procedure Checklists** walk through skills from the book step by step and can be used to help evaluate your mastery of skills.
- A table of **Medical Terminology: Prefixes, Roots, and Suffixes** provides clues to deciphering many medical terms students will encounter.

- A **Spanish–English Audio Glossary** provides helpful terms and phrases for communicating with patients who speak Spanish.
- **Journal Articles** offer access to current research available in Wolters Kluwer journals.
- **Dosage Calculation Quizzes** provide opportunities for students to practice math skills and calculating drug dosages.
- Plus a **Lippincott Nursing Drug Handbook App, Nursing Professional Roles and Responsibilities, Heart and Breath Sounds,** and **Learning Objectives** from the textbook.

Fundamentals of Nursing: Human Health and Function, Eighth Edition includes many features to help you gain and apply the knowledge that you'll need to meet the challenges of today's nursing profession.

FEATURES THAT SET THE STAGE FOR THE REST OF THE CHAPTER

- **Key Terms** listed at the beginning of each chapter and bolded in text highlight important vocabulary. A glossary provides definitions of all the key terms in the book.

- **Learning Objectives** help readers identify important chapter content and focus their reading.

LEARNING OBJECTIVES

Upon completion of this chapter, you will be able to do the following:

1. Identify benefits of sleep sufficiency and consequences of sleep deficiency.
2. Describe normal patterns of sleep and of NREM and REM sleep stages throughout the life span.
3. Identify factors that affect quality sleep and rest.
4. Conduct an assessment interview regarding normal sleep patterns, risk for disturbance, and actual sleep problems.
5. Develop a daily schedule with a patient, incorporating his or her unique needs and patterns for sleep and rest.
6. Discuss interventions to promote sleep health.
7. Develop a nursing plan of care for a patient with sleep disturbance.

KEY TERMS

circadian rhythms
enuresis
fatigue
hypnotics
hypopnea
insomnia
narcolepsy
parasomnias
polysomnography
rest
sleep
sleep deficiency
sleep-disordered breathing (SDB)
sleep health
sleepiness
sleep latency
sleep loss
somnambulism
sleep sufficiency

FEATURES THAT STRENGTHEN CRITICAL THINKING

- **Apply Your Critical Thinking** features, which have been renamed since the last edition to more accurately reflect their content, and which now appear in nearly every chapter, guide students to explore concepts and situations more deeply. Answers provided in Appendix B allow students to check their thinking.

 APPLY YOUR CRITICAL THINKING

Esther Bennet, 79, comes to the clinic for a follow-up of her bladder infection, which was originally diagnosed and treated 1 week ago. Her husband tells you that the bladder infection seems much improved, but his wife has watery diarrhea and a severely inflamed perineum. He is frustrated and his wife is in pain, not wanting to sit up.

What assessment data do you need to obtain at this point? How will you assist the patient in managing the diarrhea and the perineal skin problem?

Check your answers in Appendix B.

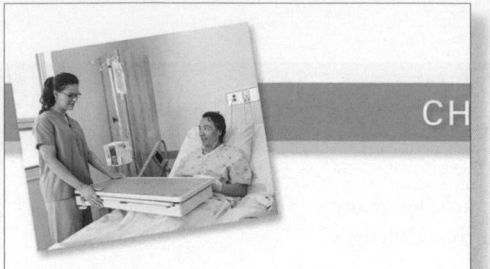

Hygiene and Self-Care

Marisa Gillaspie Aziz

Case Scenario

You are caring for a 37-year-old bachelor who is recovering from urologic surgery. He lived with his mother until her death a few years ago. He works independently as an accountant. This is your patient's first surgery, and although the pathology reports are not back, there is concern that your patient may have bladder cancer. After your morning assessment, you tell your patient that you will help him wash. He states that he does not want to wash and just wants to be left alone. Your assessment reveals dirt under his fingernails, which are untrimmed and jagged; body odor and halitosis, which is easily detected; and dirty tissues all over his bed.

Once you have completed this chapter and have incorporated self-care and hygiene into your knowledge base, review the above scenario and reflect on the following areas of Critical Thinking:

1. Identify factors that might make your patient reluctant to participate in morning care.
2. Discuss the reasons why you as a nurse believe that the patient should participate in morning care.
3. Reflect on your own feelings as you encounter this situation.
4. Identify two or three conclusions that you might draw before obtaining more information from the patient.
5. Predict positive and negative potential consequences of directly approaching this patient and "forcing" him to wash.

FEATURES THAT STRENGTHEN CRITICAL THINKING (continued)

- **Case scenarios** that open each chapter show nurses thinking holistically and reflecting on critical thinking questions.

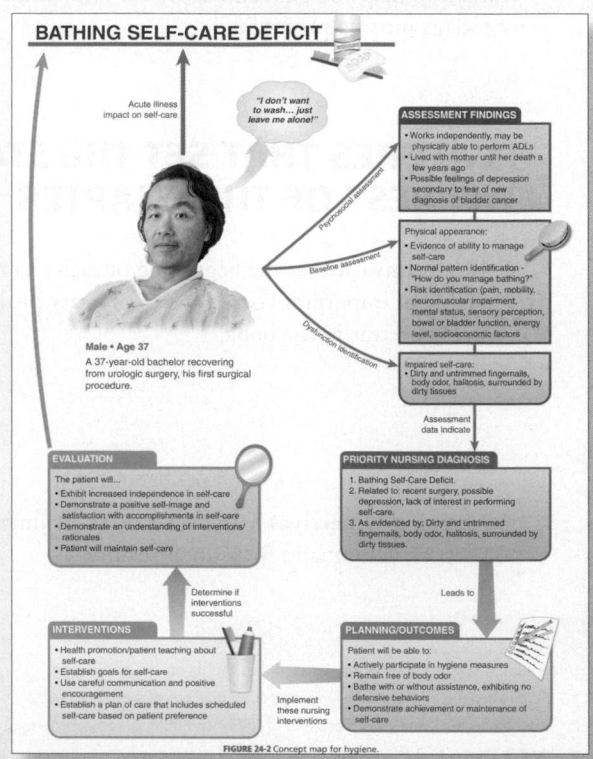

FIGURE 24-2 Concept map for hygiene.

- **New, richly illustrated concept maps**, ideal for visual learners, apply the nursing process and critical thinking to the case scenarios that begin each chapter.

Feature That Focuses on Evidence-Based Practice as Well as Critical Thinking

- **PICO (patient/problem, intervention, comparison, outcome) displays**, new to the eighth edition, illustrate examples of a structured, evidence-based way to find an answer to a clinical question related to the chapter-opening scenario.

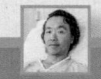

Hygiene and Self-Care PICO

You are the nurse taking care of the patient from the chapter-opening case scenario. He is finally showing some interest in his self-care. As you are setting him up to brush his teeth, he asks you if there is *really* a big difference between using a regular toothbrush and a powered one. In hopes of keeping up his interest in oral hygiene, you tell him that you will look to see if there is any evidence pointing to powered versus manual toothbrushes. You conduct your search by formulating a PICO statement: *Does using a powered toothbrush (compared to regular toothbrush) improve oral hygiene in adults?*

Population = Adults
Intervention = Using powered toothbrush
Comparison = Regular toothbrush
Outcome   = Improve oral hygiene

You discover a meta-analysis study that included 56 studies of randomized controlled trials with 5,068 participants. The evidence looked at both short-term and long-term effects on plaque and gingivitis. The results indicated that in the first 3 months alone, there was an 11% decrease in plaque when using a powered toothbrush. After the 3 months, the results continued to improve with showing a 21% reduction. Gingivitis improved by 6% within the first 3 months and jumped to an 11% after the 3 months.

   After you share the results, your patient considers switching to a powered toothbrush when he gets home.

REFERENCE:

Yaacob, M., Worthington, H.V., Deacon, S.A., Deery, C., Walmsley, A.D., Robinson, P.G., & Glenny, A.M. (2014). Powered versus manual toothbrushing for oral health. *Cochrane Database of Systematic Reviews*, 6, CD002281. doi: 10.1002/14651858.CD002281.pub3.

FEATURES THAT STRENGTHEN CRITICAL THINKING (continued)

Feature That Incorporates an Understanding of Ethical–Legal Issues as Well as Critical Thinking

- **Ethical–Legal Issues**, which are included in many chapters, incorporate critical thinking questions to help students think about complex situations in nursing.

 ETHICAL/LEGAL ISSUE

DELEGATION OF CARE TO UNLICENSED PERSONNEL

You are the registered nurse at a long-term care facility, supervising care for over 30 residents. You have one licensed practical nurse (LPN) and three nursing assistants working with you. When you are passing medications, you enter a room where a nursing assistant and the LPN are bathing a comatose patient. They are discussing their boyfriends and their social plans for the upcoming weekend. The patient is completely uncovered and appears cold. At no time do you observe them talking with the patient. They appear rough in the way they move and position him.

CRITICAL THINKING CHALLENGE

- Reflect on your own feelings as you encounter this situation, trying to identify those elements that make you feel uncomfortable.
- Identify underlying assumptions you have concerning what you think is ethically appropriate behavior.
- Refer to the Patient's Bill of Rights in Chapter 7. Do you believe this situation illustrates a breach of this contract?
- Think about three different ways to respond to this situation. Identify a possible approach that might bring about long-term changes in behavior that would improve the quality of care.

 COLLABORATING WITH THE HEALTH CARE TEAM
Calling the Physician Concerning a Patient's Increased Agitation

Mrs. Latapie, age 67 years, has had cognitive changes over the 3 hours that you have been caring for her. She has gone from being oriented to time, place, and person to being acutely agitated and hallucinating.

SITUATION: Mrs. Latapie has demonstrated rapid cognitive changes over a short period of time. She is acutely agitated about the "bugs" she thinks she sees in her bed and on the walls.

BACKGROUND: Mrs. Latapie, age 67 years, was admitted yesterday following an accident in which she tripped over an electric cord in her home. She was admitted for repair of a fractured hip, which is scheduled for tomorrow morning.

ASSESSMENT: The family were here briefly but have now gone. They think that maybe Mrs. Latapie may have been drinking more over the past month and that may be why she tripped. I am concerned that her change in agitation and hallucinations might indicate alcohol withdrawal.

RECOMMENDATION: Could you come and evaluate Mrs. Latapie within the next hour and provide orders for controlling the agitation and the hallucinating and determining whether she should go to surgery tomorrow?

CRITICAL THINKING CHALLENGE

- Discuss the rationale for requesting that the physician come and evaluate Mrs. Latapie rather than just provide orders over the phone.
- Are there other data you could collect to support your assessment that Mrs. Latapie may be experiencing alcohol withdrawal?
- Would you try to contact the family for more data about Mrs. Latapie and their comment about her increased alcohol consumption?
- Would you want to consider using restraints? What would be your decision-making process?

Features That Focus on Communication as Well as Critical Thinking

- **Collaborating with the Healthcare Team** demonstrates examples of effective communication using the SBAR technique. These allow students to more effectively communicate information accurately and safely.

- **Therapeutic Dialogues** offer side-by-side comparisons of communication with patients. Although most communication with patients is adequate, close listening and a few well-chosen questions can enhance communication, providing important information for the nurse while supporting and acknowledging the patient.

THERAPEUTIC DIALOGUE: URINARY INCONTINENCE

SCENE FOR THOUGHT

Mrs. Clements is a 55-year-old woman who has been referred for complaints of incontinence of urine for 3 months. The nurse is scheduled to perform a history and physical.

LESS EFFECTIVE		MORE EFFECTIVE	
Nurse:	Good morning, Mrs. Clements. How are you today? Please sit down so I can ask you about your history. (*Asks about age, address, number of children, and other items on assessment sheet.*)	Nurse:	Good morning, Mrs. Clements. Please sit down so we can talk a while before I do your physical. (*Acknowledges Mrs. Clements, gives simple directions.*) What can I do for you this morning? (*Asks open-ended question.*)
Mrs. Clements:	(*Answers all questions quietly.*)	Mrs. Clements:	You can help me stop wetting myself. (*Looks down at her lap.*)
Nurse:	I understand that you have an incontinence problem. Many women your age have that kind of difficulty, and I'm sure we can fix you up so you'll be just fine.	Nurse:	You look worried about that. (*Observes behavior accurately.*)
Mrs. Clements:	My mother's doctor told her that years ago, but she never got better. (*Looks down at her lap.*)	Mrs. Clements:	Yes, I am. (*Looks relieved.*) Before my mother died last year, she had to wear adult diapers; she always smelled and had bladder infections, and it was awful for her and for everyone else. I don't want to get that way.
Nurse:	Well, we'll just see what we can do for you here. Could you undress and put on this gown? I'll be back in a minute to do your physical. (*Leaves room, closing the door quietly.*)	Nurse:	So what you would like for me to help you figure out a way to deal with the wetting problem so you don't have to live the way your mother did. Is that right? (*States understanding of what Mrs. Clements wants and clarifies with her.*)
		Mrs. Clements:	Yes! That would be great.
		Nurse:	Okay. Why don't we start with some questions and then I'll do a physical and we can go from there. (*Gives Mrs. Clements some idea of planning.*)

CRITICAL THINKING CHALLENGE

- Critique what the nurse did that was effective in the second scene.
- Determine what was less effective about the first scene.
- Consider how you think Mrs. Clements felt in both scenes.
- Although each nurse spent the same amount of time with Mrs. Clements, analyze how the first nurse could have been more effective.

USING THE NURSING PROCESS TO INDIVIDUALIZE PATIENT CARE

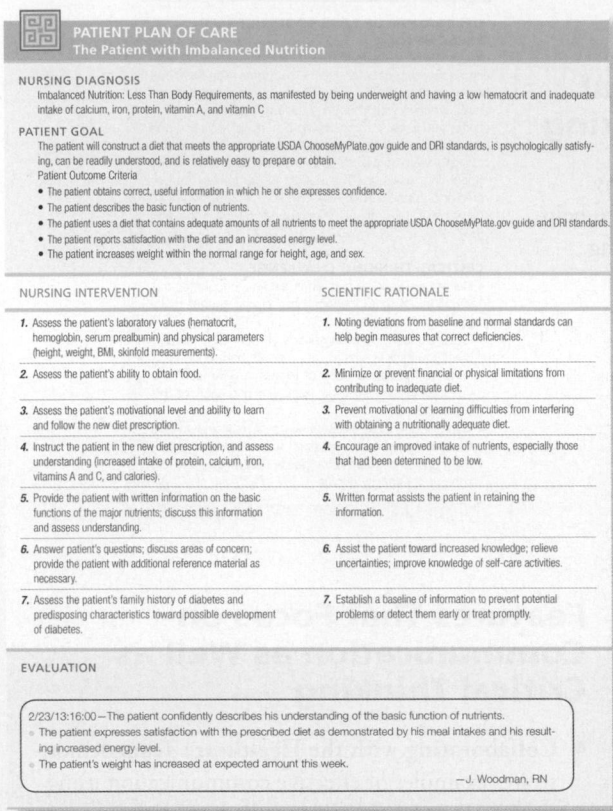

PATIENT PLAN OF CARE
The Patient with Imbalanced Nutrition

NURSING DIAGNOSIS
Imbalanced Nutrition: Less Than Body Requirements, as manifested by being underweight and having a low hematocrit and inadequate intake of calcium, iron, protein, vitamin A, and vitamin C

PATIENT GOAL
The patient will construct a diet that meets the appropriate USDA ChooseMyPlate.gov guide and DRI standards, is psychologically satisfying, can be readily understood, and is relatively easy to prepare or obtain.
Patient Outcome Criteria
• The patient obtains correct, useful information in which he or she expresses confidence.
• The patient describes the basic function of nutrients.
• The patient uses a diet that contains adequate amounts of all nutrients to meet the appropriate USDA ChooseMyPlate.gov guide and DRI standards.
• The patient reports satisfaction with the diet and an increased energy level.
• The patient increases weight within the normal range for height, age, and sex.

NURSING INTERVENTION	SCIENTIFIC RATIONALE
1. Assess the patient's laboratory values (hematocrit, hemoglobin, serum prealbumin) and physical parameters (height, weight, BMI, skinfold measurements).	1. Noting deviations from baseline and normal standards can help begin measures that correct deficiencies.
2. Assess the patient's ability to obtain food.	2. Minimize or prevent financial or physical limitations from contributing to inadequate diet.
3. Assess the patient's motivational level and ability to learn and follow the new diet prescription.	3. Prevent motivational or learning difficulties from interfering with obtaining a nutritionally adequate diet.
4. Instruct the patient in the new diet prescription, and assess understanding (increased intake of protein, calcium, iron, vitamins A and C, and calories).	4. Encourage an improved intake of nutrients, especially those that had been determined to be low.
5. Provide the patient with written information on the basic functions of the major nutrients; discuss this information and assess understanding.	5. Written format assists the patient in retaining the information.
6. Answer patient's questions; discuss areas of concern; provide the patient with additional reference material as necessary.	6. Assist the patient toward increased knowledge; relieve uncertainties; improve knowledge of self-care activities.
7. Assess the patient's family history of diabetes and predisposing characteristics toward possible development of diabetes.	7. Establish a baseline of information to prevent potential problems or detect them early or treat promptly.

EVALUATION

2/23/13:16:00 — The patient confidently describes his understanding of the basic function of nutrients.
• The patient expresses satisfaction with the prescribed diet as demonstrated by his meal intakes and his resulting increased energy level.
• The patient's weight has increased at expected amount this week.

—J. Woodman, RN

• **Plan of Care** features "put it all together" for students. Scientific rationales are included to build knowledge.

OUTCOME-BASED TEACHING PLANS

When Mr. Lyman, a recent widower, comes to the clinic for a routine checkup, data reveal that he has lost 15 lb since his wife's death 6 months ago. He is 6 feet tall and currently weighs 160 lb. During your assessment, you discover that he usually eats cereal for breakfast, a sandwich for lunch, and skips dinner or has some soup. He states, "My wife always took care of the cooking. Since she died, nothing tastes good anymore." He has one son who lives 300 miles away and lots of friends in the area, but he doesn't feel comfortable hinting for dinner invitations. He asks you to help him develop a plan that he feels inclined and motivated to follow.

• Discuss possible community agencies that could support his efforts (e.g., Meals on Wheels; senior program at the community center).
• Discuss foods that are dense in calories and protein.
• Suggest protein supplements between meals to boost caloric intake.
• Discuss easy-to-prepare frozen dinners that can be microwaved.
• Provide home health follow-up to assess and provide encouragement for weight gain and good nutrition.
• Refer Mr. Lyman to a nutritionist if he continues to lose weight despite the above efforts.

OUTCOME
Mr. Lyman will verbalize a realistic plan to increase food intake, which will permit him to maintain his present weight.

STRATEGIES
• Explore Mr. Lyman's feelings about his recent weight loss and desire to reverse weight loss trend.
• If Mr. Lyman is motivated to maintain or gain weight, discuss his eating pattern before his wife's death, including food likes and dislikes.
• Have Mr. Lyman keep a food diary.

EVALUATION

2/23/13: 16:30 — Examples of progress toward his goal as evidenced by:
• Mr. Lyman has identified a list of favorite foods to begin his program to gain weight.
• Mr. Lyman's food diary indicates that he has increased his protein and calorie intake to levels recommended by his physician for weight gain.
• Mr. Lyman reports increased mealtime pleasure since joining the local senior meal program.
• Mr. Lyman has gained 3 lb in the past month.

—J. Woodman, RN

• **Outcome-Based Teaching Plans** provide clear examples of patient teaching. Focusing on the outcome of the teaching facilitates clear evaluation of learning that occurred.

NANDA Table 37-4 SELECTED NANDA-I NURSING DIAGNOSES INVOLVING COGNITION

Nursing Dx	Related Factors	Dx Statement	NOC*	NIC†
Acute Confusion—abrupt onset of a cluster of global, transient changes and disturbances in attention, cognition, psychomotor activity, level of consciousness, and/or sleep–wake cycle	Age older than 70 y, alcohol abuse, abuse, cognitive impairment, uncontrolled pain, multiple comorbidities, medications, dehydration, infection, sensory deficit, and compromised ADLs	**Acute Confusion** R/T medications, dehydration, infection AEB fluctuation in cognition, sleep–wake cycle, level of consciousness, and in agitation or restlessness	Cognitive Orientation Distorted Thought Self-Control Electrolyte and Acid/Base Balance Fall Prevention Behavior Fluid Balance Neurologic Status: Consciousness	Cognitive Restructuring Neurologic Status: Consciousness Delirium Management Fall Prevention Memory Training Neurologic Monitoring Reality Orientation
Chronic Confusion—irreversible, long-standing, and/or progressive deterioration of intellect and personality characterized by decreased ability to interpret environmental stimuli and decreased capacity for intellectual thought processes, and manifested by disturbances of memory, orientation, and behavior	Multi-infarct dementia; Korsakoff psychosis; and brain injury, Alzheimer disease, and related dementias	**Chronic Confusion** R/T Alzheimer disease AEB altered interpretation and/ or response to stimuli, altered personality, impaired memory (short and long term), impaired socialization, and decreased ability to participate in self-care	Patient Satisfaction: Safety Cognitive Orientation Distorted Thought Self-Control Fall Prevention Behavior Identity Safe Home Environment Sleep	Neurologic Status: Consciousness Dementia Management Fall Prevention Memory Training Reality Orientation

Dx, diagnosis; R/T, related to; AEB, as evidenced by.
*From: Moorhead, S., Johnson, M., Maas, M., & Swanson, E. (2013). *Iowa Outcomes Project: Nursing Outcomes Classification (NOC)* (5th ed.). St. Louis, MO: C. V. Mosby.
†From: Bulechek, G., Butcher, H., Dochterman, J., & Wagner, C. (2013). *Iowa Intervention Project: Nursing Interventions Classification (NIC)* (6th ed.). St. Louis, MO: C. V. Mosby.
From: North American Nursing Diagnosis Association International (NANDA-I). (2014). *Nursing diagnoses: Definitions and classification, 2015–2017.* West Sussex, England: Wiley-Blackwell.

• **NANDA-I Tables** clearly outline the relationship between nursing diagnosis, outcomes, and interventions. Rather than viewing each process in isolation, students can instantly grasp how they flow together.

FEATURES THAT FOCUS ON SAFETY

> **⚠ SAFETY ALERT**
> Teach patients never to ignore chest pain or discomfort and to report such unrelieved symptoms to medical personnel immediately.

- **Safety Alerts** are small boxes that appear close to related text issues and address specific safety concerns for students.

- **Evidence-Based Bundles to Improve Patient Care boxes** focus on bundles, which are structured methods of improving patient care. For a specific problem, a bundle recommends a set of evidenced-base practices, which when performed collectively and reliably improve patient outcomes.

EVIDENCE-BASED BUNDLES TO IMPROVE PATIENT CARE
Prevention of Catheter-Associated Urinary Tract Infections (CAUTI)

BACKGROUND
UTIs account for approximately 40% of all hospital-acquired infections annually, and fully 80% of these can be attributed to indwelling urethral catheters. In the United States, up to 5 million urinary catheters are placed annually. Between 12% and 25% of all hospitalized patients will receive a urinary catheter during their hospital stay, and up to half of these do not have an appropriate indication.

It is well established that the duration of catheterization is directly related to risk for developing a UTI. With a catheter in place, the daily risk of developing a UTI ranges from 3% to 7%. When a catheter remains in place for up to a week, the risk increases to 25%; at 1 month, this risk is nearly 100%.

RISK FACTORS
- Prolonged catheterization greater than 6 days
- Female gender
- Catheter insertion outside operating room
- Other active sites of infection
- Diabetes
- Malnutrition
- Azotemia (creatinine greater than 2.0 mg per deciliter)
- Ureteral stent
- Catheter in place solely for monitoring of urine output
- Drainage tube below level of bladder and above collection bag
- Antimicrobial drug therapy

KEY RECOMMENDATIONS
1. **Avoid unnecessary urinary catheters.**

   NURSING IMPLICATIONS
   - Catheters are appropriate in patients with acute urinary retention or bladder outlet obstruction or in patients undergoing prolonged surgeries or are anticipated to receive large-volume infusions or diuretics during surgery. Catheters are also indicated for patients with stage 3 to 4 decubitus ulcers with incontinence or for patients receiving palliative care if they request an indwelling catheter.
   - Catheters are *inappropriate* if used as a substitute for nursing care of the patient with incontinence, as a means of collecting serial urine specimens, or for prolonged postoperative duration without appropriate indications (which include structural repair of urethra or other contiguous structures or prolonged effect of epidural anesthesia).

2. **Insert necessary catheters using aseptic technique.**

   NURSING IMPLICATIONS
   - Perform hand hygiene immediately before and after insertion or any manipulation of the catheter device or site.
   - Ensure that only properly trained persons who know the correct technique of aseptic catheter insertion and

---

FEATURES THAT TEACH SKILLS AND CONCEPTS

- **Procedures** in the clinical chapters use clear descriptions, rationales, and pictures to assist students in learning important nursing care skills. Each procedure focuses on patient safety and comfort and includes the latest evidence-based practice and technology.

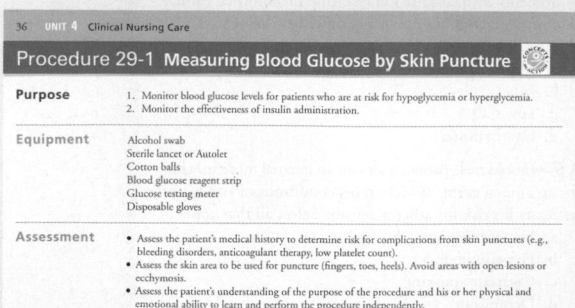

36   UNIT 4   Clinical Nursing Care

Procedure 29-1 Measuring Blood Glucose by Skin Puncture

Purpose	1. Monitor blood glucose levels for patients who are at risk for hypoglycemia or hyperglycemia. 2. Monitor the effectiveness of insulin administration.
Equipment	Alcohol swab Sterile lancet or Autolet Cotton balls Blood glucose reagent strip Glucose testing meter Disposable gloves
Assessment	• Assess the patient's medical history to determine risk for complications from skin punctures (e.g., bleeding disorders, anticoagulant therapy, low platelet count). • Assess the skin area to be used for puncture (fingers, toes, heels). Avoid areas with open lesions or ecchymosis. • Assess the patient's understanding of the purpose of the procedure and his or her physical and emotional ability to learn and perform the procedure independently.

Procedure

1. Review the provider's orders to determine the type and frequency of glucose monitoring. (*Note:* The procedure should be performed before meals because carbohydrate ingestion alters blood glucose levels.)
   Rationale: Prevents errors.
2. Perform hand hygiene.
   Rationale: Reduces microbe transmission.
3. Identify the patient.
   Rationale: Ensures correct patient receives proper assessment or treatment and reduces errors.
4. Close door or bed curtains and explain the procedure to the patient.
   Rationale: Ensures patient privacy, increases patient compliance, reduces patient anxiety, and promotes learning.
5. Have the patient wash hands with soap and warm water.
   Rationale: The fingertips are the most common skin puncture sites in adults. Washing not only decreases the chances of infection but, due to the warm water, promotes vasodilation of the puncture site.
6. Position the patient comfortably.
   Rationale: Ensures the patient's comfort during the procedure.
7. Remove the test strip from the container and handle according to the manufacturer's instructions.
   Rationale: The glucose meter may need recalibration or "re-zeroing."

8. Place the test strip with test pad up on a dry surface.
   Rationale: Moisture on the test pad could alter the final test results.
9. Don gloves.
   Rationale: Part of Standard Precautions against transfer of microorganisms.
10. Choose the finger to be punctured, massage gently, and hold in a dependent position (Fig. 1).

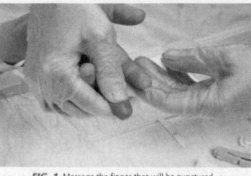

FIG. 1 Massage the finger that will be punctured.

Rationale: The dependent position and stimulation will help increase circulation to the puncture site.

- **Videos, activities, and animations** are indicated by icons in the text. All of these free accompanying video clips (Watch and Learn icon), activities (Practice and Learn icon), and animations (Concepts in Action icon) are available at http://thepoint.lww.com/Craven8e.

FEATURES THAT PREPARE STUDENTS FOR THE NCLEX

- New to the eighth edition, **Concept Mastery Alerts** clarify fundamental nursing concepts to improve the reader's understanding of potentially confusing topics, as identified by Misconception Alerts in Lippincott's Adaptive Learning Powered by prepU. Data from thousands of actual students using this program in courses across the United States identified common misconceptions to be clarified in this new feature.

 Concept Mastery Alert

It is difficult to simultaneously assess a patient's physical status and perform the detailed interview that forms the basis of the nursing history. In many cases, it is beneficial to obtain the nursing history first in order to provide context for the physical assessment.

- **NCLEX review questions**, the kind you can expect to see on your licensing examination, are included in each chapter. Appendix A provides answers, with rationales for correct and incorrect answers. These allow you to test your clinical thinking skills and can jumpstart discussions with your instructors.

PRACTICING FOR THE NCLEX
CHECK YOUR ANSWERS IN APPENDIX A.

1. A patient with renal failure is found to have an elevated potassium of 6.0 mEq/L. The effect of the high potassium is problems with conduction resulting in abnormal cardiac rhythm. Which of the following describes this type of abnormality?
   a. Mitral regurgitation
   b. MI
   c. Low CO
   d. Dysrhythmia

2. A 65-year-old male patient is seen in an internal medicine clinic for an annual exam. Which of his conditions or risk factors increases his risk for atherosclerosis? Select all that apply:
   a. Hypertension
   b. Hyperlipidemia
   c. Cigarette smoking
   d. Depression

Lippincott CoursePoint+
LIPPINCOTT COURSEPOINT+

Lippincott CoursePoint+ is an integrated digital learning solution designed for the way students learn. It is the only nursing education solution that integrates leading content in context, powerful tools to maximize class performance, real-time data to measure students' progress, preparation for practice, and training services and personalized support. Please see the preface for more information.

Acknowledgments

Sincere appreciation and warmest thanks are extended to the many people who supported us and contributed to the production of this edition.

The contributors, who worked diligently to provide up-to-date information in their specialty areas and were patient with our many requests that were always quickly addressed.

Our students, who have taught us much and continue to keep our feet planted in the real clinical world.

The Wolters Kluwer team who ensured that the eighth edition meets the needs of the nursing market and remains the highest quality possible: Sherry Dickinson, Meredith Brittain, Dean Karampelas, Marian Bellus, and Dan Reilly.

Lastly, but most importantly, we acknowledge with love and gratitude the constant support and encouragement of family, friends, students, and colleagues throughout this major revision.

Ruth F. Craven, EdD, RN, FAAN

Constance J. Hirnle, MN, RN-BC

Christine M. Henshaw, EdD, RN-BC

Acknowledgments

Sincere appreciation and warmest thanks are extended to the many people who supported us and contributed to the production of this edition.

The contributors who worked diligently to provide up-to-date information on their specialty areas and were patient with our many requests that ultimately aided [address].

Our students, who have taught us much and continue to keep our feet planted in the real clinical world.

The Wolters Kluwer team who ensured that the eighth edition meets the needs of the nursing market and sustains the highest quality possible: [illegible names].

Last, but not least, we acknowledge with love and gratitude the support and encouragement of family, friends, students, and colleagues throughout this major revision.

Contents

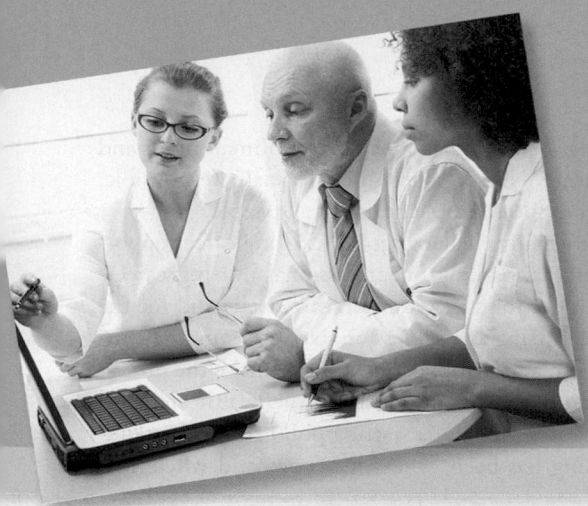

UNIT 1
Conceptual Foundations of Nursing

CHAPTER 1

The Profession of Nursing

Christine M. Henshaw

Case Scenario

You are a student beginning your nursing program. As you complete your first week of classes, you notice that your instructors have focused on several consistent themes. They are stressing such concepts as community-based care, the need for consumer participation in healthcare, and the influence of technologic advances. They are asking for your opinions on financial, ethical, and legal concerns. Many of your fellow classmates are returning to school after several years away. They mention to you how many responsibilities they are juggling and the hopes that they have for success. You feel both excited and slightly scared but are eager to better understand the many ideas you and your fellow students are encountering.

Once you have completed this chapter, return to the above scenario and reflect on the following areas of Critical Thinking:

1. Describe how you anticipate that current trends in nursing will affect the way you practice, your relationships with patients, and your relationships with coworkers.
2. Discuss ways that technologic advancements help patients and ways they might put patients at risk.
3. Explore possibilities for learning more about community-based healthcare delivery, technologic developments, and financial considerations.
4. Based on the information in this chapter, how would you expect nurses to practice 50 years from now?

KEY TERMS

advanced practice nursing
American Nurses Association
clinical nurse specialist
conceptual framework
environment
functional health patterns
general systems theory
health
human needs
licensed practical nurse
Maslow's hierarchy of human needs
National League for Nursing
nurse administrator
nurse anesthetist
nurse educator
nurse midwife
nurse practice act
nurse practitioner
nurse researcher
nursing
nursing theory
person
professional nurse
self-actualization
socialization

LEARNING OBJECTIVES

Upon completion of this chapter, the student will be able to do the following:

1. Discuss how nurses have developed more independent practice during the last 50 years.
2. Discuss the influence of nursing's historical development on contemporary views of professional nursing.
3. Identify distinct pathways for entrance into and continuation of professional nursing practice.
4. Identify roles and responsibilities of professional nurses within the healthcare delivery system.
5. Describe the purpose and function of professional nursing organizations.
6. Recognize major nursing theories and their relevance to nursing practice.
7. Identify the four major concepts of nursing theories.
8. Explain the relationship of functional health pattern typology to nursing.

As you turn the pages of this textbook, you are preparing for a career in nursing. In this journey, you will master many scientific, physiologic, psychosocial, and fundamental facts. You will learn many things: how to touch people, assess for health, and observe for pain. You will learn to see physical clues that a person is suffering from inadequate oxygenation or cardiac insufficiency. You will learn to hear how the heart sounds and how to listen for changes in the breathing of one who is dying. You will see the power of the human body as you witness the processes of labor and birth. You will experience the incredible abilities of technology to extend and improve human life.

In the midst of such experiences, you will develop critical thinking skills that will enable you to place multiple factors into complex equations and arrive at appropriate conclusions. You will learn the importance of knowing yourself, your values, and how you arrive at decisions. You will need to consider the problems of today's society and issues involving healthcare allocation, the extent and use of technology, the treatment for disease, and the promotion of **health**. The word **nursing** calls to mind many ideas and images. For some, these images are from traditional and perhaps outdated sources, including white uniforms, nursing caps, needles, and bedpans. For others, images of nursing include kindness, skill, compassion, and intelligence. Modern nursing practice involves many such images and also encompasses new and perhaps unique perspectives on what the profession involves.

Many factors have affected the way the public, nursing professionals and their colleagues, and those beginning their nursing careers perceive nursing. History, especially the social, political, and cultural events of the 20th century, has influenced today's practice. Evolving roles of women, portrayals of nursing in the media, and issues involving educational preparation have had a considerable impact on the image of nursing today. The roles and responsibilities of nurses are changing along with the evolving healthcare environment, and the profession must be prepared to face the challenges of the 21st century.

Nursing is caring, commitment, and dedication to meeting the health needs of all people. Nurses direct care to promote, maintain, and restore health in various settings. They are prepared to identify and to assist with the healthcare needs of individuals, families, communities, and populations. As technology advances, society's healthcare needs increase in complexity, and the demands of the healthcare system change. At the same time, nurses provide a point of human contact in the face of this complexity. The need for educated nurses who are committed to maintaining expertise in the theory, art, and practice of professional nursing will continue to grow in response to such developments.

Nursing care provided in settings other than hospitals, such as in the homes of patients or in ambulatory clinics, is now common. While 60% of nurses work in hospitals (Health Resources and Services Administration, 2008), changes in reimbursement for healthcare services and cost-containment measures have moved nursing practice to areas beyond such settings. Nursing means caring for communities and populations of people, such as the homeless, and addressing issues with far-reaching social implications, such as human rights and access to healthcare. Nursing means being socially responsible, involved, and committed to the health of all people.

Nursing offers many challenging and exciting career opportunities. Students embarking on professional nursing careers accept responsibility for society's healthcare needs and for the advancement of nursing as a profession. Never in nursing's history has there been a more opportune time to move the profession forward and to make a difference in the healthcare of all people. This chapter provides a starting point for understanding where nursing has been, where it is now, and where it is headed.

HIGHLIGHTS OF THE HISTORICAL EVOLUTION OF PROFESSIONAL NURSING

Although nursing in some form has probably existed throughout history, documentation of the profession as we know it today has only been available for the last 150 years (Nightingale, 1860). Nursing probably began as women intuitively identified and provided for their families' healthcare needs. As certain individuals emerged with the desire and ability to nurture others and provide care for them, the profession of nursing began. This section highlights critical events that have shaped nursing's history and have influenced issues affecting today's profession. An overview of this historical evolution provides the background necessary to understanding current nursing practice (Table 1-1). For more in-depth discussions of nursing's historical evolution, examine textbooks dedicated solely to this topic.

Ancient History

Ancient history makes few references to nursing as its own discipline; any discussions of nursing are blurred with those of medicine. Brief accounts of men and women engaging in practices that may be associated with nursing have been found. Around the world, women have long served as midwives. In ancient Babylonia, Egypt, and Samaria, rich families were the primary recipients of nursing care. If and when nursing care was available outside wealthy homes, nurses were primarily servants. Early hospitals were often founded by religious groups. The Greeks made significant contributions to the care of the sick and, to an extent, to the nursing profession. Hippocrates, the "father of medicine," made a major advance in medicine by rejecting the belief that diseases had supernatural causes. He has been credited with developing assessment standards for patients, establishing overall medical standards, and recognizing a need for nurses. In western civilization, nursing grew with the continuing spread of Christianity, which had positive effects on cultural values and institutions. Christianity's influence also improved the status of nursing by attracting intelligent individuals from respected families. The Crusades

TABLE 1-1   THEN AND NOW—A SELECTION OF SIGNIFICANT EVENTS IN THE HISTORY OF NURSING

Date	Then	Now
Approximately AD 1–500	Nursing care primarily involves meeting the hygiene and comfort needs of individuals and families. Christians working in close association with an organized church primarily provide care.	Nursing care today involves a high degree of technical skill and includes responsibilities above and beyond hygiene and comfort measures, although these components of care continue to be important. Today's nurse must be highly skilled and up-to-date with technologic advances, be computer literate, and have a strong foundation in the sciences and humanities. Responsibilities are complex and require critical thinking skills. Nursing is no longer tied to the church, and nurses are educated in colleges and universities.
1836	Theodor Fliedner opens a small hospital and training school in Kaiserworth, Germany, where Florence Nightingale, "the founder of modern nursing," receives her nursing education.	Hospital-based schools of nursing continue to exist, but these programs have been declining in number as the profession moves forward and requires education in academic settings.
1854–1860	Florence Nightingale makes major contributions to modern nursing, is named Superintendent of Nursing, cares for soldiers in the Crimean War, opens a training school at St. Thomas Hospital in London, and publishes *Notes on Nursing: What It Is, and What It Is Not*.	Nightingale's many contributions to nursing continue to influence the profession. The components of her theory apply even today, and nurses around the world recognize the courage, dedication, and work of this early professional leader.
1861–1865	Dorothea Dix establishes the Nurse Corps of the United States Army during the Civil War. Dix was not a nurse but an advocate for the mentally ill.	Nurses continue to choose careers in the armed services where opportunities for exciting and rewarding careers are offered.
1872	America's first trained nurse, Linda Richards, graduates from the New England Hospital for Women in Boston.	Nursing continues to prepare educated, competent individuals to provide nursing care in institutions of higher education.
1873	Three nursing schools patterned after the Nightingale plan develop in the United States: Bellevue Training School, Connecticut Training School, and Boston Training School.	New nursing programs continue to develop. The profession now offers several routes to a career in nursing, including diploma, associate degree, baccalaureate degree, graduate entry, and doctoral programs.
1882	Clara Barton organizes the American National Red Cross.	The Red Cross continues to exist today, offering care to victims of disasters, maintaining the nation's blood supply, and educating about AIDS.
1893	Lillian Wald and Mary Brewster found the Henry Street Settlement, the first home visiting nurse organization in the United States. The Henry Street Settlement can still be visited in New York City.	Visiting nurse associations have grown and become essential healthcare components in society. Cost containment and healthcare reform concerns have moved nursing from the hospital setting to the community once again.
1897	The American Society of Superintendents of Training Schools of the United States is organized. It is renamed the American Nurses Association (ANA) in 1911.	The ANA continues to function as nursing's professional organization.
1898	The Volunteer Nurse Corps is established.	Became the Army Nursing Corps.
1899	The International Council of Nurses is established.	The ICN continues to represent and speak to international nursing concerns.
1900	The *American Journal of Nursing*—the first nursing journal to be owned, operated, and published by nurses—is developed.	The *American Journal of Nursing* continues to be a major reference for clinical nursing practice.
1923	The Goldmark report of the Rockefeller Foundation is published, advocating financial support of university-based schools of nursing.	There is a decline in available financial support to incoming students of nursing. However, nursing organizations and leaders are working to improve financial assistance to students.
1940	World War II results in another nursing shortage. Esther Lucille Brown completes the Brown report on nursing education, advocating that education for nursing belongs in colleges and universities, not in hospitals.	Although hospital-based schools of nursing continue to exist, they are declining in number, and students are more frequently choosing college and university educations.
1953	The National Students Nurses' Association (NSNA) is established.	The NSNA continues to encourage students of nursing to become involved in professional issues. Students are given opportunities to hold leadership positions at state and national levels.

Continued

TABLE 1-1 THEN AND NOW—A SELECTION OF SIGNIFICANT EVENTS IN THE HISTORY OF NURSING *(Continued)*

Date	Then	Now
1965	The ANA issues its first "position paper on nursing education," calling for all nursing education to take place in institutions of higher education and stipulating the baccalaureate as minimum preparation for professional nursing and the associate degree for technical nursing practice.	The entry-level debate has not been completely resolved. Preparation of nurses for the future continues to be one of professional nursing's concerns.
1985	The National Center for Nursing Research is established at the National Institutes of Health in Bethesda, Maryland.	1993—The National Center for Nursing Research is upgraded by President Clinton to Institute status.
1994	Healthcare reform is a discussion that permeates professional circles. Cost-containment measures, access to healthcare, and the need for health promotion are integral components of the issues.	Healthcare reform will continue to be an integral issue to the nursing profession. Nurses will continue to explore options for advanced practice nurses to maintain nursing's role and move it forward in this environment of change.
1999		Managed care, cost, reimbursement issues, and complex technologic advances continue to affect healthcare. Advanced practice roles for nurses are increasing as issues related to access to healthcare and the need for health promotion programs become central.
2007		Redesigning and downsizing of the workforce and the changes in patient profiles have numerous effects on nursing. Healthcare is facing the implications of the changing supply and demand of nurses.
2011	The Institute of Medicine and the Robert Wood Johnson Foundation release their report, The Future of Nursing: Leading Change, Advancing Health.	The report recognizes the contribution nurses make to the health care system and calls on nursing to advance the profession through education, collaboration, and workforce planning and development.

resulted in the establishment of military nursing orders and the recruitment of men into nursing, which was well organized during this time.

Florence Nightingale and the Crimean War

Florence Nightingale (Fig. 1-1) has been called the founder of modern nursing. Stubborn and unyielding, Nightingale improved health laws, reformed hospitals, reorganized military medical services, and established nursing as a profession with two missions: sick nursing and health nursing. Nightingale viewed "sick nursing" as helping patients use their own reparative processes to get well and "health nursing" as preventing illness.

Nightingale was born in 1820 in Florence, Italy, to a wealthy English family. She was educated in languages, philosophy, and the liberal arts. She entered the nursing profession against the wishes of her parents. Nightingale was the superintendent of nurses at King's College Hospital until she left to care for soldiers during the Crimean War. Her efforts during this war were credited with decreasing the mortality rate by half, and she soon became known as "the lady with the lamp" because of her midnight rounds to the soldiers. In 1859, Nightingale published *Notes on Nursing* and started the Nightingale Training

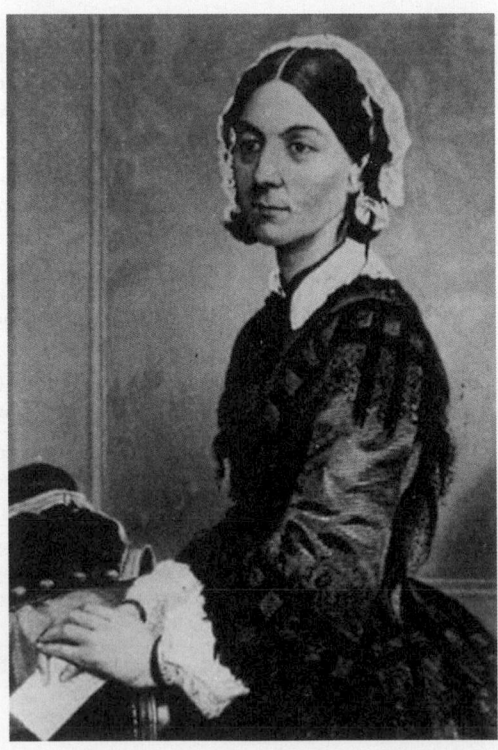

FIGURE 1-1 Florence Nightingale. (Photo courtesy of the Center for the Study of the History of Nursing.)

School for Nurses. Nightingale was gracious and hardworking, and her many contributions to nursing continue to influence the profession.

Development of American Nursing

During the American Civil War (1861–1865), more hospitals and better-prepared nurses were needed. Although she was not a nurse, Dorothea Dix established the Nurse Corps of the United States Army, further expanding nursing's role. Another early nursing leader, Clara Barton, practiced nursing on Civil War battlefields. Barton founded the American Red Cross, an organization that continues to contribute significantly to contemporary healthcare needs.

Military influences on nursing and nursing education in the 20th century have been numerous. During the Spanish American War, the Volunteer Nurse Corps (1898) was established and, in 1901, became the Army Nurse Corps. In 1908, the U.S. Congress authorized the Navy Nurse Corps. During World War I, nurses were transported to war areas in Europe and the Far East to care for the sick and wounded.

The casualties of World War II brought a critical nursing shortage, prompting quick solutions to increase the number of nurses and causing a setback in the move toward university-based nursing education. During World War II, black nurses were first admitted to the nursing service.

The Vietnam War saw many nurses involved in the Army and Navy Nurse Corps caring for the wounded. In addition, Air Force nurses were assigned to Vietnam. Conflicts in the Persian Gulf involved mobilization of nurses to Iraq, Afghanistan, and Saudi Arabia. The harsh environments in war-torn areas present challenges for patients and nurses (Fig. 1-2).

In the early 20th century, professional organizations such as the American Nurses Association (ANA), the **National League for Nursing** (NLN), and the American Association of Colleges of Nursing (AACN) emerged. Nursing journals were developed, and research was conducted into the need for higher education in nursing. The *American Journal of Nursing* (*AJN*), first published in 1900, was the first nursing journal to be owned, operated, and published by nurses. Rapid scientific advances and increasingly complex technology marked the latter part of the 20th century. Longer life spans, increased incidence of chronic illness, and new family structures dramatically affected where and how nurses practiced. Despite such changes, nurses continued to focus on delivery of care that was safe, comprehensive, and effective.

Nursing in the 21st Century

Nursing's history has influenced today's educational requirements, practice settings, and roles. Likewise, when, how, and why the profession evolves will directly relate to the contributions of present and future nursing professionals. Social forces can be expected to influence future definitions of nursing, just as these forces have shaped nursing practice to date.

Today's nurses must be knowledgeable, flexible, and innovative. Nurses care for patients in a wide range of settings and must adapt to the needs of diverse patients. Technology allows nurses to connect to patients in new ways, but it also provides new challenges such as maintaining patient privacy and developing human connections with patients we may never see face-to-face.

SOCIALIZATION TO PROFESSIONAL NURSING

Socialization is a process that involves learning theory and skills and internalizing an identity appropriate to a specific role. Internalizing a specific role allows one to participate as a member of a group.

Professions generally have a specific body of knowledge, a set of values, and skills that differentiate them from one another. Professional nursing curricula teach foundations of the discipline. Theoretical and clinical instruction facilitates the development of a professional identity and prepares students to function as beginning nurses. Beyond this initial socialization, continuing socialization occurs as nurses gain experience in the workplace and perhaps pursue advanced education.

In *From Novice to Expert*, Patricia Benner (1984) discussed socialization and skill acquisition in nursing (Table 1-2). A nurse passes through five levels of proficiency when acquiring and developing nursing skill: novice, advanced beginner, competent, proficient, and expert. Differences in each level reflect changes in three areas of skill performance. In the first area, the nurse moves from relying on abstract principles to using concrete experiences. The second area involves a change from seeing situations in parts to seeing them more conceptually, or as a whole. Finally, in the third area, the nurse is no longer outside the situation observing but is directly involved. This process takes 5 to 10 years after graduation.

Nursing and Professionalism Defined

Because definitions of nursing reflect society's values and influences, the profession is subject to misinterpretation. One common misconception is that nurses are inferior to physicians,

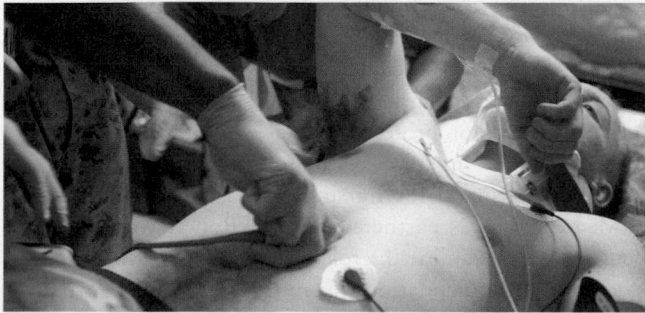

FIGURE 1-2 Military nurses examining soldier prior to medical evacuation. (Reprinted with permission from Cosby, K. S., & Kendall, J. L. (2014). *Practical guide to emergency ultrasound.* Philadelphia, PA: Wolters Kluwer.)

TABLE 1-2 NOVICE TO EXPERT

Level of Proficiency	Summary Description
Novice	A beginning nursing student or any nurse entering a situation in which he or she has had no previous experience. Behavior is governed by established rules and is limited and inflexible.
Advanced beginner	The advanced beginner can demonstrate marginally acceptable performance. He or she has had enough experience in actual situations to identify meaningful aspects or global characteristics that can be identified only through prior experience.
Competent	Competence is reflected by the nurse who has been on the same job for 2 or 3 years and who consciously and deliberately plans nursing care in terms of long-range goals.
Proficient	The proficient nurse perceives situations as a whole rather than in terms of aspects and manages nursing care rather than performing tasks.
Expert	The expert nurse no longer relies on rules or guidelines to connect understanding of a situation to an appropriate action. The expert nurse, with an enormous background of experience, has an intuitive grasp of the situation and zeroes in on the problem.

The five levels of proficiency listed in the left column were developed by Stuart Dreyfuss and Hubert Dreyfuss. The second column reflects the author's summary of a discussion by Patricia Benner in *From novice to expert: Excellence and power in clinical nursing practice.* San Francisco, CA: Addison-Wesley, 1984.

simply following their orders. Instead, nurses have their own scope of practice and provide care within the scope of nursing practice. Beginning nursing professionals must develop a clear, accurate understanding of professional practice if other members of the healthcare team and the public are to share this precise interpretation.

Nursing is a multifaceted profession and, as such, has been defined in many ways. Florence Nightingale defined nursing as "the act of utilizing the environment of the patient to assist him in his recovery" (Nightingale, 1859/1992). The ANA developed the following definition of nursing: "Nursing is the protection, promotion, and optimization of health and abilities, prevention of illness and injury, facilitation of healing, alleviation of suffering through the diagnosis and treatment of human response, and advocacy in the care of individuals, families, groups, communities, and populations" (ANA, 2015, p. 1).

Despite the many definitions, common themes are evident. Holism, caring, teaching, advocacy, and supporting, promoting, maintaining, and restoring health are all components of nursing practice. Nursing care involves creativity, sensitivity, and applications based on evidence. All of these components are essential to the practice, but nurses should not limit themselves to these themes.

Educational Preparation

Nursing has a long history of debating over the educational preparation for its profession. This is continuing, as there is a scope of practice that ranges from a practical nurse program to the doctorate of nursing practice. There are many levels between these as well as many specialties.

PRACTICAL NURSING

In the United States, people interested in a practical nursing career attend 1-year programs that prepare them to perform technical skills under the supervision of registered nurses (RNs). Students successfully completing the program

requirements may sit for the National Council Licensure Exam-Practical Nursing (NCLEX-PN) to become a **licensed practical nurse** (LPN) or licensed vocational nurse. LPNs are employed in hospitals, long-term care facilities, and rehabilitation centers and by healthcare providers such as physicians. LPNs differ from RNs in two areas: educational preparation and scope of practice. LPNs always practice under the supervision of an RN. Practical nursing was established to prepare healthcare providers for patient care and to assist professional nurses with routine technical procedures.

REGISTERED NURSING

Nursing in the United States continues to have three major routes leading to RN licensure. Educational preparation may be at the diploma, associate degree, or baccalaureate degree level. Programs are now emerging that have the master's degree or doctorate as entry-level preparation. The issue of educational preparation for entry into practice has been debated since the 1930s and 1940s, when the Brown and Goldmark reports recommended two levels of nursing preparation. In 1965, the ANA adopted a resolution proposing that minimum preparation for beginning professional practice should be a baccalaureate degree in nursing and that minimum preparation for technical practice should be an associate degree in nursing. The debate over entry-level preparation continues to influence many critical issues. Included in this debate are the competencies of new nursing graduates, the public view of nursing roles, the need for professional status within the healthcare community, the organization of nursing education, and the supply and demand for nursing professionals. The Institute of Medicine (2011) partnered with the Robert Wood Johnson Foundation to examine the role of nursing in the future. They made five recommendations for nursing (Box 1-1). As part of the second recommendation—that nurses achieve higher levels of education—the task force recommended that 80% of RNs be educated at the baccalaureate level or higher. Leaving open the issue of minimum education for entry into the profession, they focused on the educational level of practicing nurses. This approach acknowledges the benefit of diploma and associate degree programs in providing opportunities for those unable to access a baccalaureate program.

Diploma Nursing

Diploma nursing schools were the first type of educational preparation available for RNs. In the United States, diploma programs usually require 3 years of study. Students earn some college credit, but college credit is not awarded for nursing courses. Clinical experience is extensive, which is an advantage of this route. Students successfully completing diploma programs take the National Council Licensure Examination-RN (NCLEX-RN). Graduates of diploma programs work as beginning practitioners in acute, intermediate, long-term, and ambulatory healthcare facilities. Graduates demonstrate competency in the assessment, planning, implementation, and evaluation phases of the nursing process. The number of diploma programs has declined as nursing education moves into institutions of higher learning. This decline is also related to efforts to achieve professional status and control over nursing practice.

Associate Degree Nursing

Associate degree nursing (ADN) initially was developed in the 1950s in response to a nursing shortage, and it continues to thrive today. Students pursuing this degree attend a community or junior college for 2 years or more, receiving college credit for all courses and clinical experiences in nursing. Students successfully completing the requirements of an ADN program also take the NCLEX-RN. As providers of nursing care, ADNs use the nursing process to formulate and maintain individualized patient plans of care. They also teach patients who need information or support to maintain health.

Baccalaureate Degree Nursing

The baccalaureate degree in nursing (or bachelor of science in nursing [BSN]) offers students a full college or university education with a background in liberal arts. The programs are rigorous and provide students with credits for nursing courses and clinical experiences in all areas of nursing practice. Baccalaureate degree programs in nursing emphasize community health, research, leadership, and management. Students successfully completing the baccalaureate degree in nursing take the NCLEX-RN. Nurses are prepared as generalists to provide comprehensive services that assess, promote, and maintain the health of individuals, families, communities, and groups.

Graduate Entry Programs

Graduate entry programs are generally designed for people with baccalaureate degrees in fields of study other than nursing. The pre-licensure nursing portion of the program is often at an accelerated pace; students may be able to sit for the NCLEX-RN after 12-18 months of study. Students then track directly into a master of science in nursing or a doctoral program. Students completing these programs have advanced clinical capabilities and some opportunity for clinical concentration in a nursing specialty.

ADVANCING EDUCATION

Continuing Education

Some states require nurses to obtain continuing education hours for ongoing licensure. Courses range from an hour to days to weeks in length and may be offered by the nurse's employer, by local colleges or universities, or by independent companies offering continuing education. Courses may also be offered through nursing journals or online. Nurses must check their licensure renewal requirements to determine the exact number of hours of education required and the types of courses accepted by the licensing board.

RN to BSN

Graduates of diploma and ADN programs often elect to advance their education by earning a baccalaureate degree in nursing. Many colleges and universities offer these degree-completion programs. In some programs, the RNs may be integrated with traditional undergraduate students, taking some or all of the coursework required for the traditional students. In other programs, the RNs may be in completely separate tracks designed just for them, usually focused on those areas of study emphasized in baccalaureate programs. Once coursework is completed, students are awarded a BSN.

Master's Degree in Nursing

Nurses interested in attaining advanced education in specialties may complete graduate programs in their specific area of interest. Graduate education prepares nurses for advanced, independent practice with continued emphasis on research. Graduate education requires independent critical thinking, and nurses pursuing graduate education must have solid scholastic abilities. A BSN usually is required for entry into these programs. Some programs admit diploma or ADN students if those RNs hold a bachelor's degree in another field. Although currently advanced clinical practice pathways such as nurse practitioner (NP), clinical nurse specialist (CNS), nurse anesthetist, and nurse midwife are offered at the master's level, the profession is moving toward requiring doctorate-level preparation for those pathways. Nurse educators, nurse administrators, and clinical nurse leaders will likely continue to be prepared at the master's level. Although people in those pathways may ultimately decide to pursue doctoral-level education, it will likely not be a requirement for certification or practice.

Doctor of Nursing Practice

The increased complexity of care, changing patient demographics, and shifting healthcare delivery systems are necessitating a transformation of graduate and advanced practice. The doctor of nursing practice (DNP) is proposed to replace the advanced practice master's degree. The DNP focuses on preparing NPs, the CNS, nurse anesthetists, and nurse midwives as expert clinicians with enhanced leadership and research skills (American Association of Colleges of Nursing, 2014).

Research Doctoral Degrees

Students may earn a doctor of philosophy (PhD), doctor of education (EdD), or doctor of nursing science (DNS) degree. People interested in careers as nurse researchers or nurse educators usually must obtain doctoral degrees. Doctoral education has become more available to nurses, and the number of nurses earning doctoral degrees continues to increase. Nurses usually obtain doctoral education after completing master's programs. Many PhD programs incorporate the master's degree for students who enter directly from BSN programs without first earning a master's degree.

CERTIFICATION

Nurses can choose to become certified in a nursing specialty. The American Nurses Credentialing Center (ANCC, 2014) states that certification validates nursing specialty knowledge. Also, it builds confidence in nurses as professionals, demonstrating that they meet nationally recognized standards in the specialty. Certification is a voluntary process to provide professional recognition of the knowledge, skills, and abilities of certified nurses.

EXPANDED NURSING ROLES

Accelerated changes in healthcare with an emphasis on primary care have intensified interest in **advanced practice nursing**. An example of an advanced practice nurse is the NP. Regulation of advanced practice nursing is done by statute or by certification. Regulation by statute involves modification of the state nurse practice act to regulate advanced nursing practice and involves issuance of a second license. Regulation by certification involves a process whereby professional boards validate an individual nurse's advanced qualifications in a particular area of nursing.

Many additional opportunities for career development and advancement are available for RNs. These opportunities, some of which require advanced education, lead to new and varied roles and exciting challenges. Some expanded nursing

roles include NP, CNS, nurse midwife, nurse anesthetist, nurse researcher, nurse administrator, and nurse educator. The educational level of NPs, the CNS, nurse midwives, and nurse anesthetists is changing. While some continue to be prepared at the master's level, many more of these advanced-level practitioners have education at the doctoral level, most commonly in DNP programs.

Nurse Practitioner

A **nurse practitioner** is a nurse with advanced education who has graduated from an NP program. NPs function with more independence and autonomy than do other nurses and are highly skilled at doing nursing assessments, performing physical examinations, counseling, teaching, and treating health problems. NPs have a specialty, such as obstetrics, pediatrics, geriatrics, or family care. The NP's scope of practice is determined by the practice act of the state in which the NP works; NPs in some states have a broad scope of practice that includes ability to prescribe medications.

Clinical Nurse Specialist

A **clinical nurse specialist** has advanced experience and expertise in a specialized area of practice such as gerontology, pediatrics, critical care, or pulmonary disease. The CNS works in various settings, depending on his or her specialty. Roles of the CNS include clinician, educator, manager, consultant, and researcher.

Nurse Midwife

A **nurse midwife** has advanced education in nursing and midwifery and, in the United States, is certified by the American College of Nurse Midwives. Nurse midwives provide independent care for women during normal pregnancy, labor, and delivery. They practice in conjunction with specific healthcare agencies from which medical services are available in the event a patient develops complications. Nurse midwives also may perform routine Papanicolaou (Pap) smears and breast examinations and assist patients with family planning.

Nurse Anesthetist

A **nurse anesthetist** provides general anesthesia for patients undergoing surgery. Nurse anesthetists are RNs with advanced education in anesthesiology. They work in hospitals and outpatient surgery settings.

Nurse Researcher

A **nurse researcher** is responsible for the continued development and refinement of nursing knowledge and practice through the investigation of nursing problems. Nurse researchers have advanced education, usually at the doctoral level. They tend to work in large teaching hospitals and research centers or in academic settings. All nurses have a responsibility to be involved in research and to use evidence-based findings to improve nursing care and to practice from a research basis. Even nurses without advanced preparation in research can work with individuals who have such training.

Nurse Administrator

A **nurse administrator** manages and controls patient care. Nurse administrators may be responsible for specific nursing units or may serve as the chief nursing executive for an organization Nurse administrators typically are required to hold at least a master's degree.

Nurse Educator

The **nurse educator** role can be developed in many settings, including schools of nursing and hospital staff development departments. Clinically based educators and faculty teaching in practical nursing and associate degree RN programs usually need a master's degree; faculty in baccalaureate, master's, or doctoral programs usually need a doctoral degree. Nurse educators generally have specific clinical specialties and advanced clinical experience. People in this career role must continue to maintain expertise in the practice setting, develop expert knowledge of theory, perfect classroom teaching methods, and have in-depth knowledge of curriculum development and higher education.

PROFESSIONAL NURSING PRACTICE

Standards of Practice

As nursing became an independent profession, it began to develop its own standards of practice. Standards of practice are essential because they serve as guidelines for providing and evaluating nursing care. They help to ensure high-quality care and serve as criteria in legal questions of whether adequate care was provided. Standards of practice appear in Box 1-2.

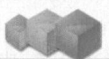

Concept Mastery Alert

It is important to differentiate between scope of practice and standards of practice. Standards of practice are the minimum acceptable levels of professional behavior that are expected of nurses. In contrast, a nurse's scope of practice is the legislation describing what nurses are legally authorized to do.

The ANA's standards include two lists: standards of care and standards of professional performance. Measurement criteria are printed in the ANA book *Nursing: Scope and Standards of Practice* (2015). The standards of care list designate professional nursing responsibilities such as assessment, diagnosis, outcome identification, planning, implementation, and evaluation. These responsibilities are inherent in the nursing process and are discussed throughout this text. Standards of professional

---

BOX 1-2	ANA Standards of Professional Nursing Practice

Standards of Practice

ASSESSMENT. The RN collects comprehensive data pertinent to the patient's health or situation.

DIAGNOSIS. The RN analyzes the assessment data to determine the diagnoses or issues.

OUTCOMES IDENTIFICATION. The RN identifies expected outcomes for a plan individualized to the patient or the situation.

PLANNING. The RN develops a plan that prescribes strategies and alternatives to attain expected outcomes.

IMPLEMENTATION. The RN implements the identified plan. This includes coordination of care, health teaching and health promotion, consultation, and prescriptive authority and treatment.

EVALUATION. The RN evaluates progress toward attainment of outcomes.

Revised Standards of Professional Performance

ETHICS. The RN practices using ethical principles.

CULTURALLY CONGRUENT PRACTICE. The RN practices in a manner that is congruent with cultural diversity and inclusion principles.

COMMUNICATION. The RN communicates effectively in all areas of practice.

COLLABORATION. The RN collaborates with the patient and key stakeholders.

LEADERSHIP. The RN demonstrates leadership in the practice setting and the profession.

EDUCATION. The RN attains knowledge and competency that reflects current nursing practice and promotes futuristic thinking.

EVIDENCE-BASED PRACTICE AND RESEARCH. The RN integrates evidence and research findings into practice.

QUALITY OF PRACTICE. The RN contributes to quality nursing practice.

PROFESSIONAL PRACTICE EVALUATION. The RN evaluates one's own and others' nursing practice.

RESOURCE UTILIZATION. The RN utilizes appropriate resources to plan, provide, and sustain evidence-based nursing services that are safe, effective, and fiscally responsible.

ENVIRONMENTAL HEALTH. The RN practices in an environmentally safe and health manner.

Reprinted with permission from: American Nurses Association. (2015). *Nursing: Scope and standards of practice* (3rd ed.). Silver Spring, MD: Author. (Measurement criteria for these standards are listed in their publication.)

performance include culturally congruent practice, collaboration, leadership, evidence-based practice and research, and quality of practice. All of these performance standards are integrated into this text under related discussions.

Nurse Practice Acts

The **nurse practice act** of each state defines the practice of nursing within that area. The board of nursing in each state sets requirements for licensure. New graduates must take and pass the NCLEX to qualify for a nursing license. Once licensed in one state, the nurse can gain licensure in another state through reciprocity. Reciprocity involves meeting the licensure requirements in the new state. As long as the nurse maintains licensure, the licensure exam does not need to be retaken. The Nurse Licensure Compact allows nurses licensed in a compact state to practice in other compact states without obtaining licensure in the new state. Twenty-four states are members of the compact. With the emergence of more autonomous and expanded roles for nurses, many states have started to revise their nurse practice acts to reflect the greater responsibilities associated with current nursing practice.

Nursing Program Accreditation

Although all nursing programs must be approved by the state in which they operate, nursing program accreditation is a voluntary process that demonstrates achievement of national standards of excellence. Three organizations are accredited by the US Department of Education to accredit nursing programs. Some nursing programs are accredited by more than one organization.

COMMISSION FOR NURSING EDUCATION ACCREDITATION

The Commission for Nursing Education Accreditation (CNEA) is a subsidiary of the NLN. The NLN was the first national nursing organization in the United States. The main purpose of the NLN is to support nursing education with the goal of producing a well-prepared and diverse nursing workforce (NLN, 2013). Members of the NLN include nurses and other members of the health team, lay people, and agencies concerned with nursing education and service. The NLN works within the community and in association with individuals and groups outside nursing. The CNEA accredits practical nursing programs; associate degree, diploma, and baccalaureate-level registered nursing programs; and master's and doctoral programs in nursing.

COMMISSION ON COLLEGIATE NURSING EDUCATION

The Commission on Collegiate Nursing Education (CCNE) is an autonomous accrediting agency established by the AACN. The AACN is focused on baccalaureate and higher degree programs in nursing. This organization sets standards and publishes essential components of baccalaureate, master's, and doctoral education in nursing. Accreditation by the CCNE is a nongovernmental peer review process that uses nationally recognized standards to evaluate the integrity of nursing programs and to foster continued improvement in nursing education programs and in professional practice.

ACCREDITATION COMMISSION FOR EDUCATION IN NURSING

The Accreditation Commission for Education in Nursing (ACEN) is a third organization that provides accreditation services for nursing programs. Like CNEA, ACEN accredits nursing programs at all levels of education.

Nursing Organizations

As the nursing profession has developed and advanced, organizations integral to the profession have increased. The number of associations continues to grow at local, state, and national levels. Nursing organizations may be related to a specialty, or they may encompass all areas of nursing. The organizations that involve most nurses or nursing students are the ANA, Sigma Theta Tau International, and the National Student Nurses' Association (NSNA).

AMERICAN NURSES ASSOCIATION

The **American Nurses Association** is nursing's professional organization in the United States. Membership in state constituents of the ANA is open only to RNs. The ANA is important because it sets the standards of practice for nurses (ANA, 2015) and makes decisions about the functions, activities, and goals of the nursing profession. The organization is a voice for nurses because it acts on issues and wishes expressed by its membership. The ANA's functions and activities have been adapted or expanded in accordance with the changing needs of the profession and public. Its goals, as stated in the current bylaws, are to work for the improvement of health standards and the availability of healthcare services for all, to foster high standards of nursing, and to stimulate and promote the professional development of nurses and advance their economic and general welfare.

SIGMA THETA TAU INTERNATIONAL, HONOR SOCIETY OF NURSING

Sigma Theta Tau International, the honor society of nursing, was founded in 1922 and is headquartered in Indianapolis, Indiana. The six nurse founders named the organization from the Greek words *Storgé*, *Tharsos*, and *Timé*, meaning "love," "courage," and "honor." Sigma Theta Tau International provides leadership and scholarship in practice, education, and research to enhance the health of all people. Membership is by invitation to students who demonstrate excellence in scholarship and to nurses in the community who demonstrate excellence in leadership.

NATIONAL STUDENT NURSES ASSOCIATION

The NSNA, established in 1953, is the national organization for nursing students in the United States. Its goals are to contribute to nursing education to provide for the highest quality of healthcare; to provide programs representative of fundamental and current professional interests and concerns; and to aid in the development of the whole person, his or her professional role, and his or her responsibility for the healthcare of people in all walks of life. The NSNA is autonomous, student financed, and student run. It serves as the voice of nursing students, speaking out on issues of concern to the entire profession.

 APPLY YOUR CRITICAL THINKING

You are considering joining a nursing professional organization but aren't sure what direction to take. What are some of the benefits of joining an organization? How will you decide which organization to join among the many organizations available? What might you consider in making your decision? What resources might help you decide?

Check your answers in Appendix B.

NURSING RESPONSIBILITIES

Historically, the nurse's sole duty was to provide care and comfort to the sick. Advances in technology, knowledge, health promotion, and prevention have expanded the functions of today's nurses. Nursing functions include activities that nurses perform independently or collaboratively. For instance, nurses may initiate activities, such as turning or positioning bed patients every 2 hours, which are nurse-prescribed interventions. On the other hand, when physicians delegate actions (physician-prescribed interventions) that require nurses to use their own judgment, nurses are addressing collaborative problems. For example, although physicians must prescribe medications, they rely on the judgment of nurses for proper administration. Nurses must thoroughly understand medications, observe for side effects, and teach patients about medications. Nurse- and physician-prescribed interventions are discussed further in Unit 2.

In addition to these roles, the profession has many other requirements, including assertiveness; a sound knowledge base in the sciences, humanities, and arts; the ability to make safe judgments; the ability to communicate the healthcare needs of patients in written and oral form; and a spirit of collegiality with other members of the healthcare team. **Professional nurse**s are autonomous and assume the responsibilities of caregivers, patient advocates, educators, decision makers, managers and coordinators of healthcare needs, and communicators.

Caregiver

As providers of care, nurses assume responsibility for helping patients promote, restore, and maintain health and wellness. Nurses view each patient as unique and consider the whole person in the caring process. Nurses address not only physiologic concerns but also spiritual, emotional, and social needs. They must set priorities for care and assist patients in meeting all needs in the safest, most timely and cost-effective manner possible, while ensuring excellence.

Patient Advocate

Nurses act as patient advocates in many situations; examples include communicating the needs and concerns of patients and ensuring that patients understand their treatments. Nurses must promote safe environments that facilitate the restoration of health. They are responsible for thoroughly understanding their patients' health problems, histories, and potential problems. They consistently take responsibility for protecting patients and helping them assert their legal rights.

Educator

Health promotion and disease prevention are a growing concern and focus of the healthcare delivery system. Educating patients about diseases, prevention, nutrition, and healthy behaviors is essential. Nurses must explain treatments and procedures for which they are responsible, answer any questions patients have, and evaluate the progress of patients toward health. Education is involved in all nursing activities.

Decision Maker

Nurses are continually identifying obstacles or difficulties in the promotion, restoration, and maintenance of health. Problem resolution requires the ability to make sound judgments and decisions. Nurses must choose the best approaches to patient care, help patients participate in decision making, and use safe and effective judgments when providing care. They also are responsible for involving other members of the healthcare team and the families of patients in decision making to ensure that sound choices are made (Fig. 1-3).

Manager and Coordinator

Promoting, restoring, and maintaining health involves coordinating the services of various healthcare professionals. In addition to managing their own time, nurses also must coordinate all activities or treatments that involve patients. The goal of their role as manager and coordinator is to complete patient care effectively, efficiently, and in a manner that benefits the patient.

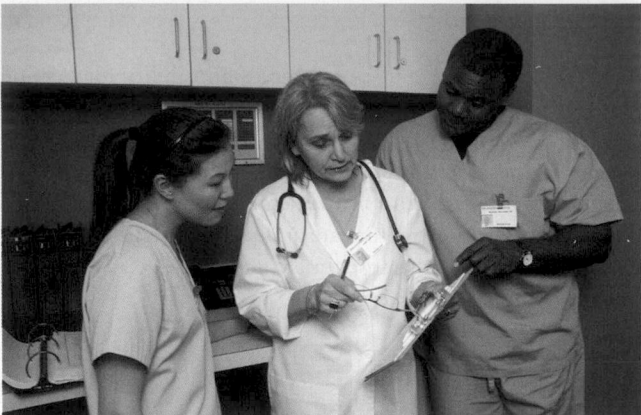

FIGURE 1-3 Nurses are responsible for involving other members of the healthcare team in decision making.

Communicator

Central to all other roles is the role of communicator. Because nurses usually are the healthcare professionals who spend the most time with patients, they have the best opportunity for observing, communicating, and identifying problems or improvements in the plan of care. Nurses are responsible for communicating findings to the healthcare team in oral and written form. The quality of this communication is critical to helping patients meet their healthcare needs; nurses must be knowledgeable, articulate, and capable of effective written and verbal expression.

NURSING COMPETENCIES

The Quality and Safety Education for Nurses (QSEN, 2014) initiative has identified key quality and safety competencies for nurses: patient-centered care, teamwork and collaboration, evidence-based practice, quality improvement, safety, and informatics. These competencies support the responsibilities defined previously. Providing care focused on patients requires the nurse to balance patient advocacy with safety. Effective management and coordination of care requires teamwork and collaboration. Evidence-based practice leads to safe and effective care. Nurses must continually evaluate and improve the quality of care. Competence in informatics allows nurses to use the latest technology in the provision, documentation, and evaluation of care. Nurses who achieve these competencies are able to improve the quality and safety of patient care wherever they work.

NURSING THEORY

A **conceptual framework** describes ideas about individuals, groups, situations, and events. The framework is a set of concepts and the propositions that integrate them. The four central concepts in nursing practice are the person, environment, health, and nursing (Parker & Smith, 2010).

In a broad sense, the concept of **person** refers to all human beings. People are the recipients of nursing care; they include individuals, families, communities, and groups. **Environment** includes factors that affect individuals internally and externally. It means not only everyday surroundings but also settings where nursing care is provided. Health generally addresses the person's state of well-being. The concept of nursing is central to all nursing theories. Definitions of nursing describe what nursing is, what nurses do, and how nurses interact with patients. Most nursing theories address each of the four central concepts implicitly or explicitly. Propositions show the relationship of these four concepts. The concepts and propositions of a conceptual framework are highly abstract and general.

Nursing theory provides the foundation for nursing knowledge and gives direction to nursing practice. Theories go a step beyond conceptual frameworks. They are a way to relate concepts and the significant relationships between them. The concepts and propositions of a theory are much more specific than are those of a conceptual framework.

Nursing theory should guide the development and future direction of nursing research. Table 1-3 lists each major nursing theorist, the central purpose of each theory, and each theorist's definitions of the four major concepts. Each theory defines, relates, and emphasizes these concepts differently.

NON-NURSING THEORIES USED IN NURSING

General Systems Theory

The general systems theory, or a systems framework, provides an approach for studying individuals in their environments and is used by many disciplines. **General systems theory** includes purpose, content, and process, breaking down the "whole" and analyzing the parts. The relationships between the parts of the whole are examined to learn how they work together.

General systems theory assumes the following (Von Bertalanffy, 1969, 1976):

- All systems must be goal directed.
- A system is more than the sum of its parts.
- A system is ever changing, and any change in one part affects the whole.
- Boundaries are implicit, and human systems are open and dynamic.

Examples of nursing theories that have used the systems approach to patient care include Roy's (1970) adaptation model, Neuman's (1972) healthcare systems model, Johnson's (1980) behavioral model, and Parse's (1981) theory for nursing.

Human Needs Theory: Maslow's Hierarchy of Human Needs

Human needs are any physiologic or psychological factors necessary for a healthy existence. The most prominent theorist to focus on human needs has been Abraham Maslow.

TABLE 1-3 OVERVIEW OF MAJOR NURSING THEORISTS

Theorist	Purpose	Views of Components
Florence Nightingale (1860), *Notes on Nursing: What It Is, and What It Is Not*	To help individuals responsible for caring for the sick to "think how to nurse." Theory addresses fundamental needs of the sick and basic principles of good healthcare.	*Person*: An individual with vital reparative processes to deal with disease. *Environment*: External conditions that affect life and the individual's development. Focus is on ventilation, warmth, odors, and light. *Health*: Focus is on the reparative process of getting well. *Nursing*: Goal is to place the individual in the best condition for good healthcare.
Hildegard E. Peplau (1952), *Interpersonal Relations in Nursing*	To develop an interpersonal interaction between patient and nurse	*Person*: An organism striving to reduce tension generated by needs. *Environment*: Implicitly defined; the interpersonal process is always included, and the psychodynamic milieu receives attention, with emphasis on the patient's culture and mores. *Health*: Ongoing human process that implies forward movement of personality and other ongoing human processes in the direction of creative, constructive, productive, personal, and community living. *Nursing*: Interpersonal therapeutic process that "functions cooperatively with other human processes that make health possible for individuals in communities. Nursing is an educative instrument, a maturing force that aims to promote forward movement of personality."
Virginia Henderson (1955), *The Nature of Nursing*	To assist the patient in gaining independence as rapidly as possible	*Person*: Individual requiring assistance to achieve health and independence or a peaceful death. Mind and body are inseparable. *Environment*: All external conditions and influences that affect life and development. *Health*: Equated with independence, viewed in terms of the patient's ability to perform 14 components of nursing care unaided: breathing, eating, drinking, maintaining comfort, sleeping, resting, clothing, maintaining body temperature, ensuring safety, communicating, worshiping, working, recreation, and continuing development. *Nursing*: Assists and supports the individual in life activities and the attainment of independence.
Martha E. Rogers (1970), *Theoretical Basis of Nursing*	To assist the patient in achieving a maximum level of wellness	*Person*: Unitary man, a four-dimensional energy field. *Environment*: Encompasses all that is outside any given human field. Person exchanging matter and energy. *Health*: Not specifically addressed, but emerges out of interaction between human and environment, moves forward, and maximizes human potential. *Nursing*: A learned profession that is both science and art. The professional practice of nursing is creative and imaginative and exists to serve people.
Dorothea E. Orem (1971), *Nursing: Concepts of Practice*	To provide care and to assist the patient to attain self-care	*Person*: Biopsychosocial being capable of self-care. Includes physical, psychological, interpersonal, and social aspects of human functioning. *Environment*: Internal and external stimuli. Requisites for self-care have their origins in human beings and the environment. *Health*: State of wholeness or integrity of human beings, including physical, mental, and social well-being. *Nursing*: A creative effort of one human being to help another human being. Consists of three nursing systems: wholly compensatory, partially compensatory, and supportive/educative.
Betty Neuman (1972), *The Neuman Systems Model: Application to Nursing Education and Practice*	To address the effects of stress and reactions to it on the development and maintenance of health	*Person*: A patient system that is composed of physiologic, psychological, sociocultural, and environmental variables. *Environment*: Internal and external forces surrounding humans at any time. *Health*: Health or wellness exists if all parts and subparts are in harmony with the whole person. *Nursing*: A unique profession concerned with all variables affecting an individual's response to stressors.
Sister Callista Roy (1970)	To identify the types of demands placed on a patient and the patient's adaptation to the demands	*Person*: A biopsychosocial being and the recipient of nursing care. *Environment*: All conditions, circumstances, and influences surrounding and affecting the development of an organism or groups of organisms. *Health*: The person encounters adaptation problems in changing environments. *Nursing*: A theoretical system of knowledge that prescribes a process of analysis and action related to the care of the ill or potentially ill person.
Jean Watson (1979), *Nursing: The Philosophy and Science of Caring*	To focus on curative factors derived from a humanistic perspective and from scientific knowledge	*Person*: A valued being to be cared for, respected, nurtured, understood, and assisted; a fully functional, integrated self. *Environment*: Social environment, caring, and the culture of caring affect health. *Health*: Physical, mental, and social well-being. *Nursing*: A human science of people and human health; illness experiences that are mediated by professional, personal, scientific, aesthetic, and ethical human care transactions.

Maslow's hierarchy of human needs (1970) states that all humans are born with instinctive needs. These needs, grouped into five categories, are arranged in order of importance from those essential for physical survival to those necessary to develop a person's fullest potential. Maslow's hierarchy provides a framework for recognizing and prioritizing basic human needs. This hierarchy is constructed as a pyramid (Fig. 1-4). From the pyramid's base to its apex, people must meet lower-level needs to some degree before they can address higher-level needs. A person is not motivated by all five categories of human needs at the same time. The category most relevant to the person's circumstances at a particular time is the primary motivator. Meeting needs is a dynamic process that involves continual resolution of, progression beyond, and return to any given category of needs.

Human needs are motivational forces. Culture, socioeconomic factors, personal values, and health influence the motivational strength for and manner of expression of these needs. All people develop behaviors that help them meet their needs. They can learn to delay meeting their needs and modify the specific behaviors that satisfy needs, depending on each need's motivational strength. If a need goes unmet, physical illness, psychological disequilibrium, or death can occur.

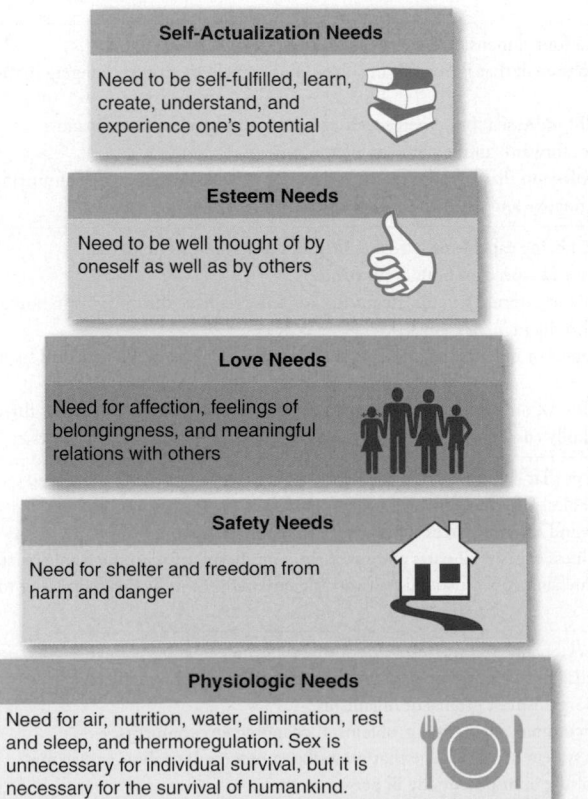

FIGURE 1-4 A pyramid represents Maslow's hierarchy of human needs. According to Maslow, basic physiologic needs, such as nutrition and water, must be met before the person can move on to higher-level needs. Nursing helps people meet needs they cannot meet by themselves.

PHYSIOLOGIC NEEDS

Physiologic needs are fundamental motivating forces and provide the base for Maslow's pyramid. Oxygen, food, water, elimination, activity, rest, temperature maintenance, and sexuality are essential for existence. Nurses assess each patient's ability to meet his or her physiologic needs and identify the nature and degree of nursing interventions necessary to enable the person to satisfy these needs.

SAFETY NEEDS

After meeting basic physiologic needs, the person must address safety needs. Humans need to be physically safe and free from the fear and anxiety that result from a lack of security and protection. Safety is often a dominant motivator. For example, in a country at war, safety becomes a primary force as long as physiologic needs are minimally satisfied. The same is true during natural disasters, such as floods or tornadoes. Such events cause major disruptions in personal, family, and societal routines and can lead to chaos. According to Maslow (1970), an essential aspect of safety is the need for predictability and routine (see Chapter 23). The Institute of Medicine and The Joint Commission are organizations that focus on safety, especially in relation to medication errors, patient falls, and skin breakdown.

LOVE NEEDS

The need for love and belonging is the next tier on Maslow's pyramid. After a sense of safety is achieved, people need to feel that they belong and are loved to avoid loneliness and isolation. To meet this need, a person must give and receive love.

ESTEEM NEEDS

According to Maslow (1970), there are two types of esteem needs: esteem derived from others and self-esteem. People need to know that others think well of, admire, and respect them. Self-esteem is a person's sense of his or her own adequacy and worth. To be genuine, it must be firmly grounded in a realistic appraisal of one's strengths and weaknesses. If esteem needs go unmet, the person faces a life characterized by self-doubt and feelings of helplessness and worthlessness. What others value in a person and what that person values in himself or herself may differ, and these evaluations are influenced by cultural, social, and psychological variables (see Chapter 4).

SELF-ACTUALIZATION NEEDS

According to Maslow (1970), the need for **self-actualization** is the innate need to realize fully all of one's abilities and qualities—that is, to maximize one's potential. Maslow sees this process as never ending. Although early life experiences affect self-actualization, people have the capacity to change and to reach a state of optimal psychological health as they strive for it.

NURSING THEORISTS' PERCEPTIONS OF HUMAN NEEDS

Through the years, nursing theories have incorporated ideas from human needs theory. Typically, nurses identify a patient's needs, using them as a basis for planning and implementing care. Human needs theory has led to the development of nursing models and frameworks for holistic nursing.

Change Theory

People grow and change throughout their lives. This growth and change are evident in the dynamic nature of basic human needs and how they are met. Change happens daily. It is subtle, continuous, and manifested in both everyday occurrences and more disruptive life events. Reactions to change are grounded in the basic human needs for self-esteem, safety, and security.

Change involves a modification or alteration. It may be planned or unplanned. Although various change theories exist, Kurt Lewin (1962) developed the classic theory of change, which identifies the following six components:

1. Recognition of the area where change is needed
2. Analysis of a situation to determine what forces exist to maintain the situation and what forces are working to change it
3. Identification of methods by which change can occur
4. Recognition of the influence of group mores or customs on change
5. Identification of the methods that the reference group uses to bring about change
6. The actual process of change

Lewin (1962) identified three states of change: unfreezing, movement, and refreezing. *Unfreezing* is the recognition of the need for change and the dissolution of previously held patterns of behavior. *Movement* is the shift of behavior toward a new and more healthful pattern. Movement marks the initiation of change. *Refreezing* is the long-term solidification of the new pattern of behavior.

The healthcare delivery system and the practice of professional nursing continually evolve. Nurses must recognize the dynamic nature of change and assist individuals and groups to adapt. The impact of change on basic human needs is constant and should be recognized to best use this framework to organize nursing care.

Change theory offers insight into expected behaviors when significant change occurs within an environment. Nurse theorists have incorporated various aspects of change theory. For example, Peplau's (1952) use of the nursing process applies aspects of change theory as patient needs are assessed and necessary alterations in specific patterns of behavior are determined.

FUNCTIONAL HEALTH PATTERNS AS A FRAMEWORK FOR NURSING

Nurses deal with the whole person, examining the physical, psychological, interpersonal, and spiritual aspects of each patient's life. The whole person concept emphasizes a holistic approach to professional nursing. Holistic practice also considers the patient's family and community, which is especially important now that the community is a common location for healthcare delivery.

Nursing faculty and clinicians have struggled to organize information in a way that is focused on the nursing domain rather than the medical domain. In addition to using specific nursing theories, another way to organize nursing information in a holistic way is to use Marjory Gordon's (2002) concept of **functional health patterns**. These patterns delineate the human needs of the person, family, community, and group. The patterns, which focus on behaviors that occur with time, present a total picture of the patient rather than just a small part of his or her life. Functional health patterns represent basic health needs that develop as people strive to meet those needs. These patterns are unique because they are interrelated: One pattern often provides answers to another. No pattern can be studied as a separate category.

Gordon's patterns, which are consistent with the human needs philosophy and general systems theory, can provide a framework for holistic nursing assessment (Fig. 1-5). Gordon provides a comprehensive discussion of patient needs; Maslow's hierarchy offers a rationale for determining the order in which to address those needs; and systems theory requires an analysis of relationships, purposes, reasons, and tasks.

Health Perception and Health Management

The health perception–health management pattern is the first in a series of 11 patterns that Gordon (2002) addressed. This pattern focuses on health values and beliefs and the resources in the community that are available to meet health needs. It is based on the awareness that although promoting health is a primary nursing function, patients actually manage their own health. Success in meeting human needs in this pattern relies heavily on culture, societal beliefs, personal expectations, and one's own health. The patient's family may play an important part in this function because one family member may make major health decisions for the entire group.

Activity and Exercise

Energy required to meet human needs is examined in the activity and exercise pattern. Patients must be evaluated for their ability to engage in self-care activities to meet basic physiologic needs. Another aspect involves determining how much energy is available to ensure the safety of their environment. For example, energy requirements for an older person who lives alone differ vastly from those of a young adult who lives in an intact family. The relationship of activity–exercise to health perception–health management is evident because the nurse must learn the importance the patient places on the person, family, or community. The community may not have adequate transportation for its members to engage in exercise or activity. Problems meeting needs in this category may affect other needs, such as human companionship and nutritional concerns.

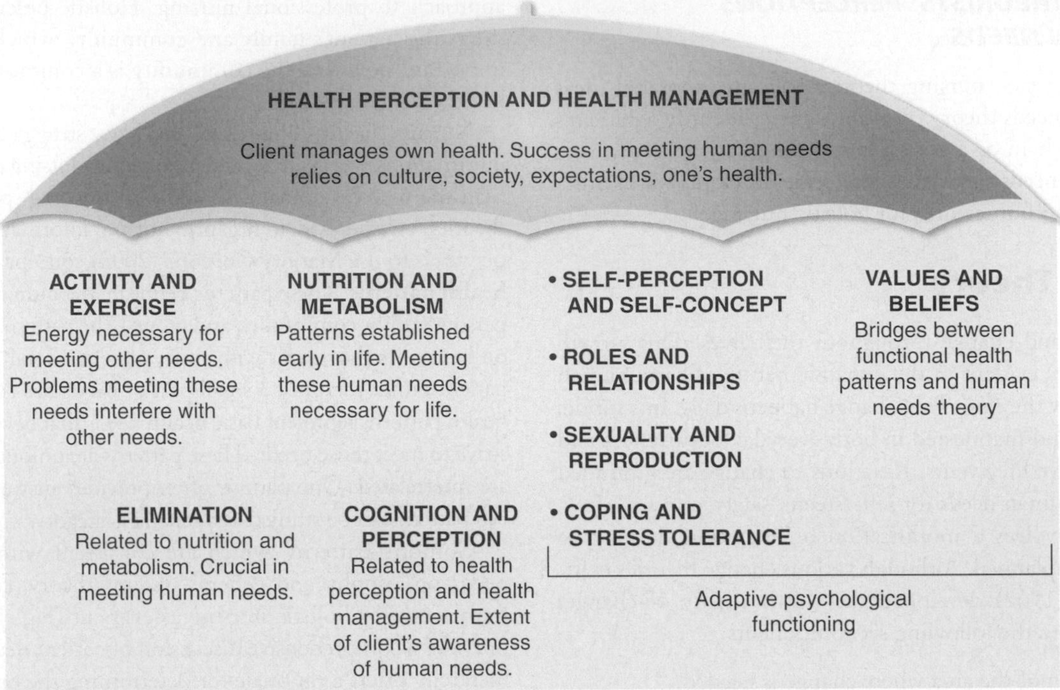

HEALTH PERCEPTION AND HEALTH MANAGEMENT

Client manages own health. Success in meeting human needs relies on culture, society, expectations, one's health.

ACTIVITY AND EXERCISE
Energy necessary for meeting other needs. Problems meeting these needs interfere with other needs.

NUTRITION AND METABOLISM
Patterns established early in life. Meeting these human needs necessary for life.

- **SELF-PERCEPTION AND SELF-CONCEPT**
- **ROLES AND RELATIONSHIPS**
- **SEXUALITY AND REPRODUCTION**

VALUES AND BELIEFS
Bridges between functional health patterns and human needs theory

ELIMINATION
Related to nutrition and metabolism. Crucial in meeting human needs.

COGNITION AND PERCEPTION
Related to health perception and health management. Extent of client's awareness of human needs.

- **COPING AND STRESS TOLERANCE**

Adaptive psychological functioning

FIGURE 1-5 Relationship of functional health patterns, human needs theory, and delivery of nursing care. The first function, health perception and health management, forms an umbrella for the remaining 10 patterns.

Nutrition and Metabolism

Life cannot be sustained without meeting human needs in the category of nutrition and metabolism. People establish patterns for meeting these needs early in life, and many such behaviors are learned in the family. This pattern does not deal simply with eating. It encompasses food knowledge, food preparation, financial resources and limits, and cultural ideas and beliefs. The community is important here because of the resources it can offer.

Elimination

Elimination is closely related to nutrition and metabolism. Often, these areas can be assessed simultaneously. Both are crucial to understanding the patient's needs. Problems with elimination may lead to issues in such patterns as roles and relationships and self-perception and self-concept.

Sleep and Rest

Sleep and rest are primary human needs. Patterns begin to develop at birth and change throughout life. Newborns, for example, spend much time sleeping. Parents can reveal the amount of time and how an infant sleeps, thus showing a pattern. The person's environment may help or hinder this category of needs.

Cognition and Perception

The cognitive–perceptual pattern examines the extent of the patient's awareness of human needs, which ties in with the first pattern, health perception–health management. Life span considerations are important when evaluating this pattern.

Other Patterns

The remaining patterns—self-perception and self-concept, roles and relationships, coping and stress tolerance, sexuality and reproduction, and values and beliefs—involve a complex group of needs that are intimately related to the person's level of adaptive psychological functioning. Adequate examination of these patterns requires assessment of the patient's interpersonal functioning, which means looking at the patient in relation to self, family, significant others, and community. Values and beliefs provide the bridge to connect functional health patterns, human needs, and other theories. Understanding the patient's value and belief system is crucial to learning about the importance of each human need as a motivating factor in the patient's life, as a community member, and in relationships in his or her family.

ISSUES AND TRENDS IN CURRENT NURSING

During the past 50 years, nursing has undergone dynamic changes in its scope of practice. Nurses have moved from simply observing and giving prescribed medications to coordinating clinical information for the entire healthcare team. This coordination allows the design of the best possible plans of care. In many instances, nurses are the healthcare professionals who physically assess patients, consult with various team members (e.g., physicians, physical therapists, social workers, pharmacists), design plans of care, and implement plans with patients.

Many changes in the healthcare industry have led to the broadening scope of nursing practice. Settings for healthcare have shifted from hospitals and other institution-based settings to community-based settings. Community-based settings for healthcare are discussed here and in detail in Chapter 3. The shift to community-based care is related to "rising consumerism," or the public's desire to participate more actively in healthcare decisions, issues, and choices. Technologic advances have increased the public's knowledge of healthcare and greatly broadened the possibilities of what healthcare can do for people. Related to all these issues are concerns about healthcare costs and the need for all people to be able to access the healthcare resources they need.

Influence of Today's Healthcare Settings

A person seeking healthcare today faces a tremendous array of settings in which care is provided. Some suggest that this maze is so complex that the average person needs an advocate to help him or her move through it. Services vary—some concentrate on health promotion and disease prevention; others focus on diagnosis and treatment, rehabilitation, or supportive care. Because of the recent increases in the number and variety of agencies that provide healthcare, any attempt to categorize them would be incomplete.

Until recently, hospitals and medical centers were the largest and most organized of healthcare agencies. Because of rising costs, more procedures and treatments are being performed on an outpatient, ambulatory basis. Patients come to an ambulatory care facility and usually do not stay overnight. A hallmark of good ambulatory care is thorough family and patient education. The role of nurses in an ambulatory center can vary considerably, depending on their education and the center's management.

Community healthcare agencies offer care to a neighborhood or community. Many care facilities, such as day care centers and ambulatory care centers, also are community based. Many have come into existence as a result of federal legislation. Because hospital stays are shorter, care provided in the community has expanded (Fig. 1-6). The following stories illustrate how this shift has influenced nursing practice.

Technologic Advances

Advances in technology have drastically changed healthcare and significantly altered the profile of the hospitalized patient. Less invasive diagnostic tools can assist in identifying conditions at an early stage, while they are still treatable. People with cancer can receive high doses of chemotherapy that destroy the malignant cells. Damaged immune systems can be replaced with transplantations of bone marrow from other people. Premature newborns can be saved with the use of hi-tech computerized monitoring systems and critical care interventions (Fig. 1-7). Nurses translate the newest findings of research, science, and technology into care for their patients.

Many previously incurable diseases can now be treated. Life can now be maintained mechanically long after biologic systems have stopped functioning. Heart, lung, and liver transplantations,

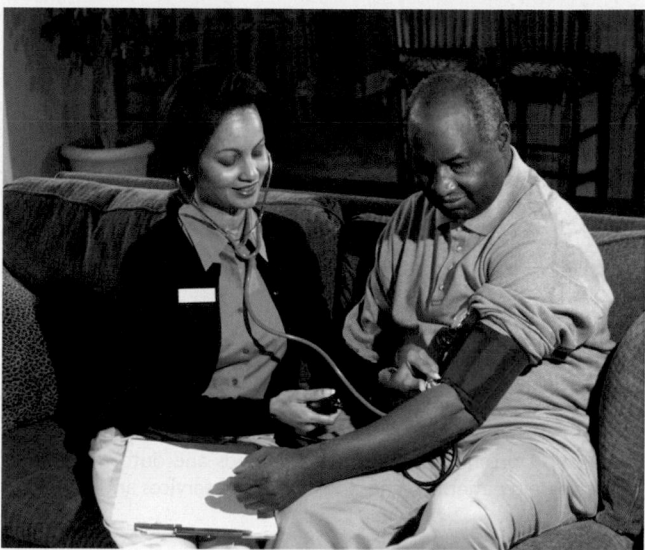

FIGURE 1-6 Community-based healthcare services have expanded due to shorter hospital stays, rising consumerism, and advances in technology. Home health nurses provide nursing care services in the comfort of the patient's home.

unheard of three decades ago, are common. New technology, however, is expensive, and some advances raise formidable questions. For example, should insurance plans cover expensive transplantations? How do we decide when to remove a person from life-support equipment? Who decides to whom organs should be given?

Access to Healthcare and Financial Resources

Historically, the poor either had to be satisfied with a decreased quality of care or do without healthcare entirely. Today, many citizens view equal access to healthcare as everyone's right. An ongoing debate centers on who should pay for this care. Healthcare costs in the United States are an ongoing concern. The government and the healthcare industry have adopted several measures to offset some costs. For example, healthcare delivery through organizations such as

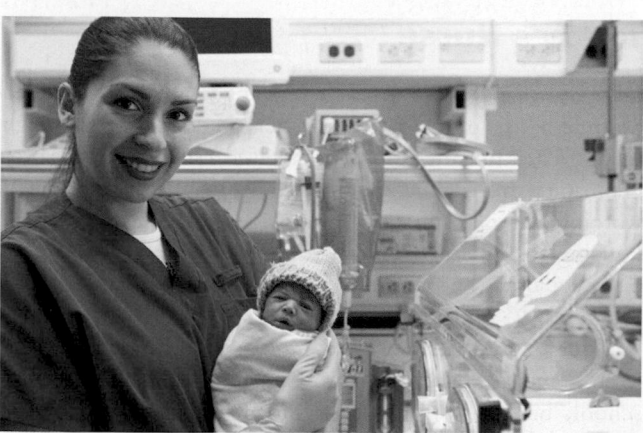

FIGURE 1-7 Today's nurses face a new set of opportunities and challenges due to ongoing advances in technology.

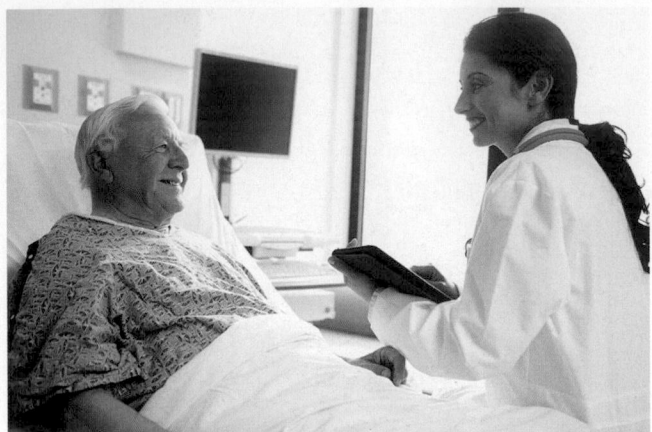

FIGURE 1-8 Documentation of patient needs and outcomes allows nurses to help patients secure the healthcare services and resources they need.

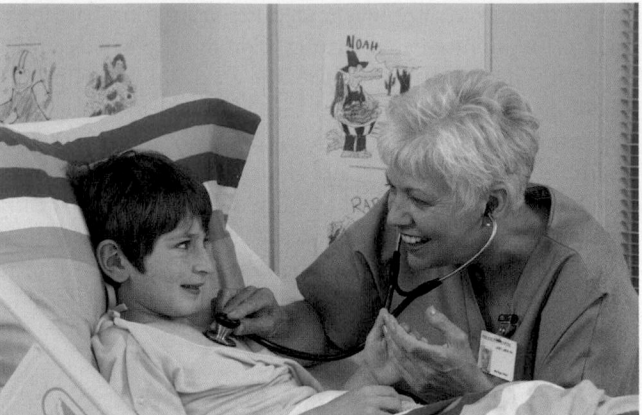

FIGURE 1-9 Many individuals are looking to nursing as a second career opportunity.

managed care organizations has expanded, and the government has established prospective payment for Medicare. As the availability of resources has decreased, however, several issues have emerged. With limited resources, the question of healthcare rationing must be addressed. The change to lower-cost providers by hospitals and clinics has created job security concerns for many nurses. All healthcare providers are being asked to put a dollar value on their services and to relate these costs to patient outcomes (Fig. 1-8). Finally, quality-of-life versus quantity-of-life questions are being debated at all levels.

Access to healthcare services refers to a person's ability to find and receive care from a healthcare provider. Access has been a public health issue for many years. Although more people are involved in the healthcare system than ever before, some areas of the United States still lack adequate healthcare resources. Research has suggested that access varies depending on an individual's income, race, and geographic location. Rural and remote areas with sparse populations cannot support the levels of specialization and technology that are available in large urban centers. Numerous plans have been attempted to solve the access issue. The need for solutions is a continuing concern.

Today's Nurse

Fifty years ago, most nurses were young women who entered hospital-based programs right after graduation from high school. Their nursing education involved a strict academic program and a strong clinical component of mandatory time spent working at the hospital with which the school was affiliated. Nursing students had to adhere to dress codes and curfews. They could not be married and had to observe all rules of their programs.

Today's students reflect a much more diverse population. Some still enter their programs immediately after high school, but many more have pursued other paths before choosing nursing as a career. Consequently, nursing students must find ways to balance the demands of being an adult learner with the responsibilities of adult life. Many have children, partners, and other employment demands. These learners must balance family, finances, and career development (Fig. 1-9).

FUTURE TRENDS IN NURSING PRACTICE

Professional nursing changes to reflect society's values. Examples of issues that are affecting today's profession include healthcare cost containment, scientific and technologic advances, and social issues. Current trends in nursing practice include the development of nursing centers, wellness promotion programs, care of older adults, birthing centers, and home and community healthcare. As nursing practice changes, so too must the preparation of its practitioners.

Given the limits on resources, cost containment has become imperative. Patients enter the healthcare system acutely ill and leave much sooner than they did in the past, increasing the demand on nurses to ensure high-quality, comprehensive care before discharge. The healthcare system must place increasing emphasis on such areas as illness prevention, nutrition, and healthy lifestyles. Science and technology continue to affect the nursing profession. In the past, nurses relied on their experience, observation, and tradition to make decisions. Today, the profession has defined a specific body of knowledge that continues to develop through research and practice. Contemporary nurses work in a more technical and more controversial healthcare delivery system that demands a high degree of skill. New ethical dilemmas and questions continue to arise in the process of providing healthcare. Social issues and concerns are intimately linked to the provision of healthcare. Just as past issues have affected today's nursing practice, those of today will influence what happens in the future. The profession must remain dynamic in its attempts to meet society's healthcare needs. You will develop the expertise and experience to provide care at an excellent level, beginning with this first foundational course!

KEY CONCEPTS

- Critical thinking is a key skill in nursing; it is the tool that enables development of one's own concept of nursing.

- Nursing's history has shaped the profession's educational requirements, roles, and practice settings.

- Educational preparation and career opportunities in nursing are numerous. Diploma, associate, baccalaureate, master's, and doctoral degrees are available to those seeking a career in nursing.

- Nurses function as caregivers, patient advocates, educators, decision makers, managers and coordinators, and communicators.

- The ANA's standards of practice guide and direct the practice of nursing in the United States, designating nursing responsibilities that include collecting data, making nursing diagnoses, planning and implementing care, and evaluating outcomes of patient care.

- Nursing theories use definitions of significant relationships between concepts to describe nursing. Common to all nursing theories are four major concepts: person, environment, health, and nursing.

- General systems theory requires analysis of the parts of a system; the relationships among those parts; and the purposes, reasons, and tasks of the system.

- Maslow's theory of human needs presents a hierarchical ordering of human needs: physiologic needs, safety needs, love needs, esteem needs, and self-actualization needs.

- Change theory recognizes the dynamic nature of growth and the need for constant reevaluation of nursing practice.

- Use of functional health patterns offers a holistic approach to nursing. Patterns delineate the human needs of the patient, family, and community. Functional health patterns provide for a comprehensive discussion of patient needs by incorporating other nursing and non-nursing theories into a pattern design and description.

- Because of advances in technology and science, the population requiring healthcare is now more complex with regard to injury and disease acuteness, mandating more critical evaluation and intervention and a higher level of nursing.

PRACTICING FOR THE NCLEX

CHECK YOUR ANSWERS IN APPENDIX A.

1. According to Patricia Benner's *From Novice to Expert*, there are five distinct levels of proficiency. Micah is a nurse with 3 years of experience who is now able to analyze his patient's heart failure as conceptually related to the renal failure and anemia that are present rather than as separate issues. Which level most appropriately describes his proficiency?
   a. Competent
   b. Expert
   c. Novice
   d. Advanced beginner

2. Marcy is aware that nursing responsibilities are related to standards of professional performance. Which are included in these standards? Select all that apply:
   a. Collaboration
   b. Performances appraisal
   c. Outcomes identification
   d. Quality of practice

3. A nurse is found guilty of performing procedures outside her scope of practice. Identify which element is true related to nursing scope of practice.
   a. Scope of practice is defined by each state's nurse practice act.
   b. The ANA sets requirements for licensure.
   c. Scope of practice is defined by CNEA-accredited school curricula.
   d. Reciprocity explains the relationship between scope of practice and state licensure.

4. An antibiotic is ordered that the patient has had an allergic reaction to in the past. Which would be an appropriate nursing action as determined by the professional nursing role? Select all that apply.
   a. Identify that the antibiotic is inappropriate.
   b. Document the allergy and call the physician.
   c. Administer the drug as ordered.
   d. Complain to other nurses about the physician's poor judgment.

5. A patient reports frustration that she has been unable to sleep while in the hospital and that she is exhausted. The nurse also notes that the patient has an unreliable social support network, has poor confidence in her ability to care for herself after discharge, and is a fall risk. Which of these issues would take priority according to Maslow's hierarchy of human needs?
   a. Sleep
   b. Fall risk
   c. Social support
   d. Doubt related to self-care

REFERENCES

American Association of Colleges of Nursing. (2014). *DNP talking points*. Retrieved from http://www.aacn.nche.edu/dnp/about/talking-points

American Nurses Association. (2015). *Nursing: Scope and standards of practice* (3rd ed.). Silver Spring, MD: Author.

American Nurses Credentialing Center. (2014). *About ANCC*. Retrieved from http://www.nursecredentialing.org/FunctionalCategory/AboutANCC

Benner, P. (1984). *From novice to expert: Excellence and power in clinical nursing practice*. San Francisco, CA: Addison-Wesley.

Gordon, M. (2002). *Nursing diagnosis, process and application* (10th ed.). St. Louis, MO: Elsevier.

Health Resources and Services Administration. (2008). *Registered nurse population: Findings from the 2008 National Sample Survey of registered nurses*. Washington, DC: Department of Health and Human Services. Retrieved from http://bhpr.hrsa.gov/healthworkforce/rnsurveys/rnsurvey-final.pdf

Henderson, V. (1955). *The nature of nursing*. New York: Macmillan.

Institute of Medicine. (2011). *The future of nursing: Leading change, advancing health*. Washington, DC: National Academies Press.

Johnson, D. E. (1980). The behavioral system model for nursing. In J. P. Riehl & C. Roy (Eds.), *Conceptual models for nursing practice* (3rd ed.). New York, NY: Appleton-Century-Crofts.

Lewin, K. (1962). Quasi-stationary social equilibria and the problem of permanent changes. In G. W. Bennis, K. D. Bennee, & R. Chin (Eds.), *The planning of change*. New York, NY: Holt, Rinehart, & Winston.

Maslow, A. H. (1970). *Motivation and personality* (2nd ed.). New York, NY: Harper & Row.

National League for Nursing. (2013). *Mission/goals/core values*. Retrieved from http://www.nln.org/aboutnln/ourmission.htm

Neuman, B. (1972). *The Neuman systems model: Application to nursing education and practice*. New York, NY: Appleton-Century-Crofts.

Nightingale, F. (1860). *Notes on nursing: What it is, and what it is not*. New York, NY: D. Appleton (First American Edition). Retrieved from http://digital.library.upenn.edu/women/nightingale/nursing/nursing.html

Nightingale, F. N. (1992). *Notes on nursing: What it is and what it is not*. Philadelphia, PA: J. B. Lippincott. (Original work published 1859.)

Orem, D. E. (1971). *Nursing: Concepts of practice* (3rd ed.). New York, NY: McGraw-Hill.

Parker, M. E., & Smith, M. C. (2010). *Nursing theories and nursing practice* (3rd ed.). Philadelphia, PA: F. A. Davis.

Parse, R. R. (1981). *Man–living–health: Theory of nursing*. New York, NY: John Wiley & Sons.

Peplau, H. E. (1952). *Interpersonal relations in nursing*. New York, NY: Putnam.

Quality and Safety Education for Nurses. (2014). *Quality and safety competencies*. Retrieved from http://qsen.org/competencies/pre-licensure-ksas/

Rogers, M. E. (1970). *Theoretical basis of nursing*. Philadelphia, PA: F. A. Davis.

Roy, C. (1970). Adaptation: A conceptual framework for nursing. *Nursing Outlook*, 18, 42–45.

Von Bertalanffy, L. (1969). *General system theory*. New York, NY: George Braziller.

Von Bertalanffy, L. (1976). *Perspectives on general system theory: Scientific-philosophical studies*. New York, NY: George Braziller.

Watson, J. (1979). The nature and development of conceptual frameworks. In F. S. Donws, & J. W. Fleming (Eds.), *Issues in nursing research*. New York, NY: Appleton-Century-Crofts.

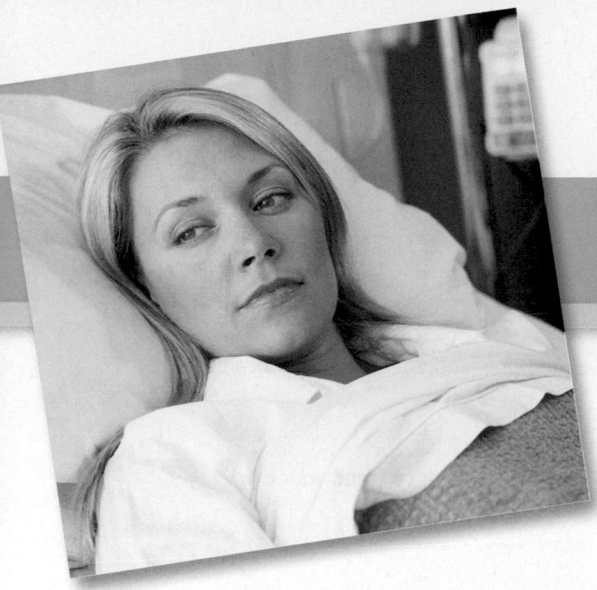

CHAPTER 2

Health, Wellness, and Integrative Healthcare

B. Jane Cornman and Mary Ann Osborne

Case Scenario

Emma Rose is 25 years old and independent. Yesterday, she had unexpected surgery after a skiing injury that resulted in a compound fracture of her left femur. She has never been in a hospital. This morning, she overheard the physician on rounds refer to her as "the surgery in Room 304." Being in a hospital bed and overhearing this comment make Emma Rose feel like a piece of furniture one minute and a child the next. No one seems interested in how this operation has affected her. She has always taken her health for granted. Now she feels sick and disabled.

During the last half of the 20th century, healthcare professionals changed their perspectives about health. The concept of holism is at the forefront of current thinking. This chapter will help you understand various definitions of health and concepts related to wellness. Once you have completed this chapter and have incorporated health, wellness, and integrative healthcare into your knowledge base, review the above scenario and reflect on the following areas of Critical Thinking:

1. Examine models of care that complement allopathic healthcare.
2. List the key concepts of integrated healthcare. What is required of you and your patient to practice in an integrated or holistic fashion?
3. Reflect on the physical, emotional, and spiritual dimensions of your patient's care.
4. Examine your current or future nurse career setting. Is there an opportunity for an integrated philosophy? From a medical–legal viewpoint, can you not inform patients of all their options, such as complementary and integrative health.

KEY TERMS

acupuncture
allopathic medicine
botanicals
complementary and alternative medicine
concentrative meditation
disease
environments
expressive meditation
health
health and wellness coaching
health promotion
herbs
high-level wellness
holism
holistic healthcare
holistic interventions
homeostasis
iatrogenic illness
illness
integrative healthcare
integrative medicine
meditation
psychosomatic
qi
receptive meditation
reflective meditation
self-awareness
self-care deficit
Therapeutic Touch
traditional Chinese medicine
wellness
yang
yin

Upon completion of this chapter, you will be able to do the following:

1. Define *wellness, holism,* and *health promotion.*
2. Compare and contrast selected models of the concept of health.
3. Identify the connections among mind, body, spirit, and symptoms.
4. Explain the differences among allopathic medicine, complementary and alternative medicine, and integrative healthcare.
5. Explain the role of holistic healthcare in nursing.
6. Give examples of some commonly used holistic interventions.
7. Reflect on how you will incorporate wellness, health, and integrative healthcare into your patients' care and your own.

HEALTH AND WELLNESS

Since 1948, the World Health Organization (WHO) has defined **health** as "a state of complete physical, mental, and social well-being, not merely the absence of disease or infirmity" (World Health Organization, 1948).

This definition has remained unchanged since 1948 and is a dramatic departure from the conventional Western view, which considered a person to be healthy if he or she were merely symptom free.

The WHO's definition of health is a useful starting point because it considers all dimensions of the person (functioning physically, psychologically, and socially) as essential to a state of health and **wellness**. In the 21st century, the most notable change in the concept of health is that of the necessity of global solutions. Given the shrinking of our world due to technology such as the Internet sites such as, Twitter, Facebook, YouTube, and televised coverage of events around the globe, and economic globalization, our awareness of the connection of all health for all peoples has been raised. Although we consider individual health in our own experience and that of our patients, we are reminded of the wider context of family health, school health, healthy cities, and of course, healthy **environments** including social, familial, and even the air, water, and the earth we require to exist (https://www.youtube.com/watch?v=1H2iCibm8hs from WHO 2008).

HEALTH MODELS

Various models of the concept of health exist. Some models are based narrowly on the presence or absence of definable **illness**. Others are based more conceptually on health beliefs, wellness, and **holism**.

CLINICAL MODEL

The clinical model interprets health narrowly as the absence of signs and symptoms of disease or injury; therefore, the opposite of health is disease. Dunn (1961) defines *health* in this model as "a relatively passive state of freedom from illness... a condition of relative homeostasis" (p. 2). Illness, therefore, is something that happens to a person. Many healthcare providers focus on relieving signs and symptoms of disease and conclude that when these findings are no longer present, the person is healthy.

This model may not consider a patient's health beliefs or the lifestyle factors that continue to place the patient at high risk for disease. Relieving obvious signs and symptoms may not address larger issues in the person's life that affect his or her health. For example, a person who persists in smoking cigarettes and living a sedentary life is likely to eventually experience signs and symptoms that relate to these lifestyle patterns, regardless of whether those signs and symptoms are apparent now.

HEALTH BELIEF MODEL

In the health belief model, a relationship exists between a person's beliefs and actions (Fig. 2-1). Factors that influence those beliefs include the following:

- Perceived benefits
- Perceived barriers
- Cues to action
- Definition
- Beliefs about the effectiveness of taking action to reduce risk or seriousness
- Beliefs about the material and psychological costs of taking action

Factors that activate "readiness to change" include the following:

- Personal expectations in relation to health and illness, for example, beliefs about susceptibility, self-efficacy, seriousness of condition
- Earlier experiences with health and illness
- Factors that activate a person's readiness to change
- Sociocultural context
- Age and developmental state

According to this model, someone who expects to have a cold at the same time every year may find that those expectations

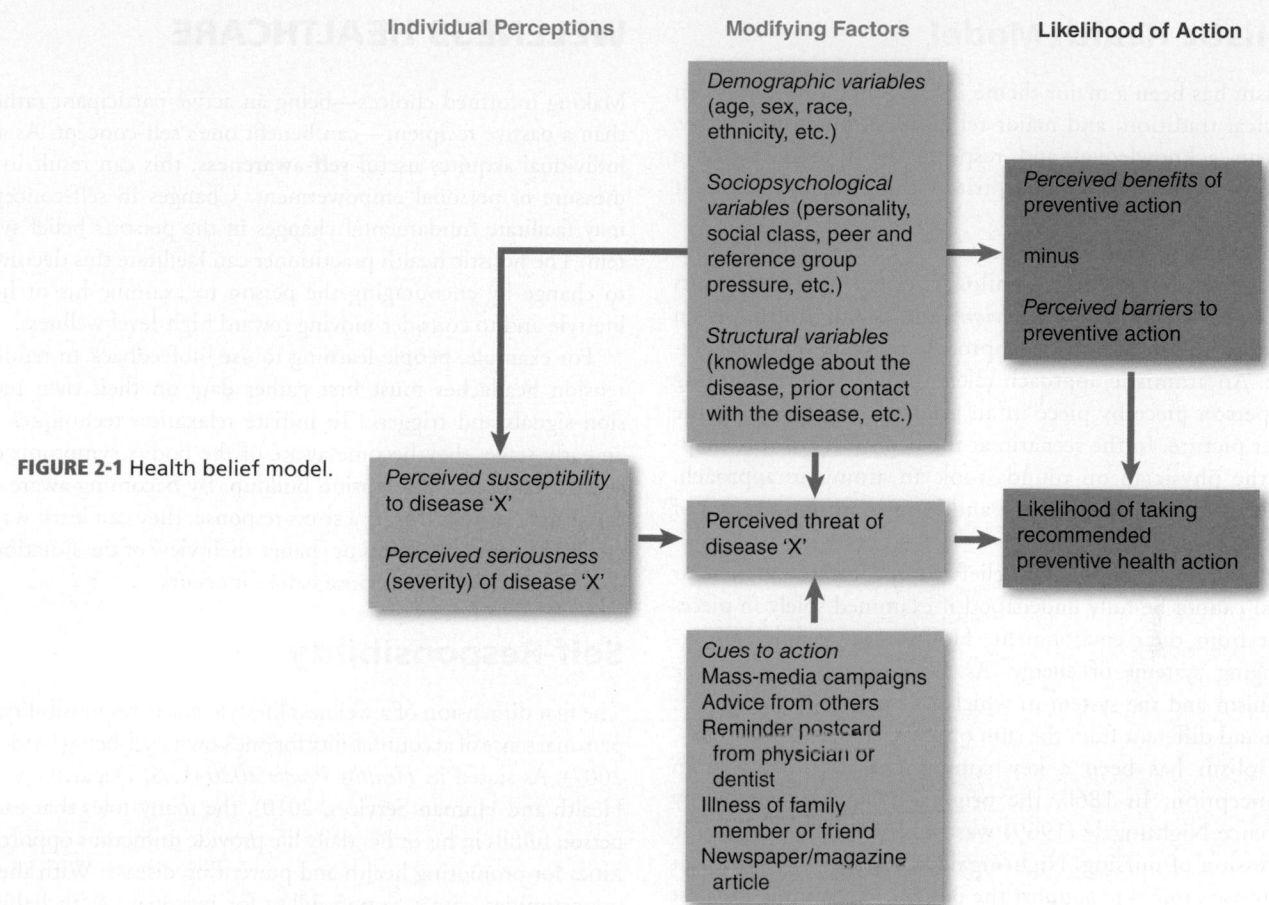

FIGURE 2-1 Health belief model.

Individual Perceptions

Perceived susceptibility to disease 'X'

Perceived seriousness (severity) of disease 'X'

Modifying Factors

Demographic variables (age, sex, race, ethnicity, etc.)

Sociopsychological variables (personality, social class, peer and reference group pressure, etc.)

Structural variables (knowledge about the disease, prior contact with the disease, etc.)

Perceived threat of disease 'X'

Cues to action
Mass-media campaigns
Advice from others
Reminder postcard from physician or dentist
Illness of family member or friend
Newspaper/magazine article

Likelihood of Action

Perceived benefits of preventive action

minus

Perceived barriers to preventive action

Likelihood of taking recommended preventive health action

come true. Conversely, positive, health-oriented expectations might keep the person from developing an illness. Previous experience with an illness has a major influence on how the person reacts to subsequent challenges; previous pain experiences, for example, shape future pain experiences.

Peer influence, personality characteristics, ethnicity, and socioeconomic factors may affect a person's response to illness. Someone who gets sick but whose experience is similar to that of his or her peers or socioeconomic group may not consider that he or she is in "poor health." Group values influence the health beliefs of each person.

Age and developmental stage are important considerations in the health belief model. For example, an older adult may be more tolerant of a particular illness or disability than a younger person because of perceived greater susceptibility to poor health. Infants and very young children do not differentiate illness from health because they have not developed a conscious memory of one state compared with the other.

The health belief model provides insight into the connection between the way a person sees his or her state of health and that person's response to health, illness, and treatment.

High-Level Wellness Model

Dunn (1961) introduced the term **high-level wellness**, recognizing health as an ongoing process toward a person's highest

potential of functioning. This process involves the person, the family, and the community. Dunn describes high-level wellness as "the experience of a person alive with the glow of good health, alive to the tips of their fingers with energy to burn, tingling with vitality—at times like this the world is a glorious place." Ardell (2007) believes that achieving high-level wellness requires first the choice to assume responsibility for the quality of one's life. This begins with the conscious decision to choose a healthy lifestyle leading to high levels of well-being and life satisfaction. A person's lifestyle is a dynamic process that involves beliefs, needs, and values. Choices in life become opportunities to move toward wellness, using methods such as self-responsibility, nutritional awareness, stress management, physical fitness, spiritual growth, and environmental sensitivity.

The wellness–illness continuum (Travis & Ryan, 1988) is a visual comparison of high-level wellness and traditional medicine's view of wellness. At the neutral point, no signs or symptoms of disease appear. A person moving toward the left experiences a worsening state of health. Someone with wellness-oriented goals wants to move beyond the neutral point (mere absence of disease) to the right (toward high-level wellness). This person evaluates the current conduct of his or her life, learns about available options, and grows toward self-actualization by trying out options in the search for high-level wellness.

Holistic Health Model

Holism has been a major theme in the humanities, Western political tradition, and major religions throughout history. Holism acknowledges and respects the interaction of a person's mind, body, and spirit within the environment (Fig. 2-2).

Holism, derived from the Greek *holos* ("whole"), was first used by South African philosopher Jan Christian Smuts (1926) in *Holism and Evolution*. Smuts saw holism as an antidote to the atomistic approach of contemporary science. An atomistic approach takes things apart, examining the person piece by piece in an attempt to understand the larger picture. In the scenario at the beginning of this chapter, the physician on rounds took an atomistic approach, concentrating on the surgery and ignoring other aspects of the patient's life.

Holism is based on the belief that people (or even their parts) cannot be fully understood if examined solely in pieces apart from their environment. Holism sees people as ever-changing systems of energy. As Figure 2-2 illustrates, the organism and the system in which it lives are seen as greater than and different from the sum of their parts.

Holism has been a key component in nursing from its inception. In 1860, the original *Notes on Nursing* by Florence Nightingale (1969) was published and shaped the profession of nursing. Nightingale expressed her belief that the nurse's role is to support the patient in attaining the best possible condition so that nature could act and self-healing could occur. In the current healthcare system, nurses are incorporating many ideas and practices from various traditions and cultures to support patients in self-healing. To better understand the progression toward this **integrative healthcare** (IHC) model, nurses must examine the terms used, the motivation for change, and the implications for practice.

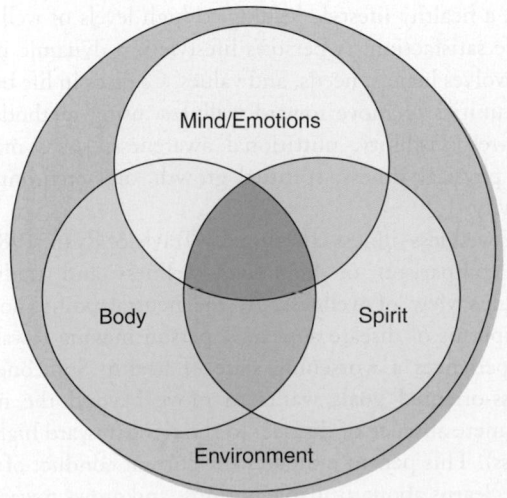

FIGURE 2-2 Schematic representation of holism. The system is greater than and different from the sum of the parts.

WELLNESS HEALTHCARE

Making informed choices—being an active participant rather than a passive recipient—can benefit one's self-concept. As an individual acquires useful **self-awareness**, this can result in a measure of personal empowerment. Changes in self-concept may facilitate fundamental changes in the person's belief system. The holistic health practitioner can facilitate this decision to change by encouraging the person to examine his or her lifestyle and to consider moving toward high-level wellness.

For example, people learning to use biofeedback to reduce tension headaches must first gather data on their own tension signals and triggers. To initiate relaxation techniques at an early stage, they become aware of the body's symptoms or signals that warn of a tension buildup. By becoming aware of the situations that trigger a stress response, they can learn ways to change those situations or change their view of the situations to prevent the stress response before it occurs.

Self-Responsibility

The first dimension of a wellness lifestyle is self-responsibility, a personal sense of accountability for one's own well-being (Ardell, 2007). As stated in *Healthy People 2020* (U.S. Department of Health and Human Services, 2010), the many roles that each person fulfills in his or her daily life provide numerous opportunities for promoting health and preventing disease. With these opportunities comes responsibility for personal health habits. To make informed choices, the patient must first be self-aware. Self-awareness means knowing and caring for oneself and recognizing one's strengths and limitations. Holistic health practices add to this self-knowledge on all levels (physical, psychological, social, and spiritual), enabling the person to identify his or her state of being and decide the priorities of service required. Self-knowing is likely to be the first step toward self-caring.

Self-Worth

Self-respect and self-worth are developed in the process of caring for oneself. The standards of holistic nursing practice affirm that "as active partners in the healing process, people are empowered when they take some control of their own lives, health, and well-being" (Mariano, 2013, p. 59). Participating in self-care gives the patient a greater feeling of independence and control. The altered concept of self as an active agent can help the person move toward high-level wellness. The concept of self as an active health agent extends across the wellness–illness continuum and applies to people at all developmental levels.

Meaning of Disease, Illness, and Self-Care Deficit

DISEASE

Because health is a state of harmony, **disease** is a state of disharmony of mind, body, emotions, and spirit. Allopathic or conventional medicine often equates disease with failure, either of medicine or of the person. Even language, such as "chief complaint," may convey a negative message. When going to see the school nurse, a child is often asked: "What's wrong?"

A disease's course and manifestations depend on how the patient integrates the experience into his or her life. The school nurse can ask the child, "How are things going for you today?" Disease can be transformed into an experience of personal value and growth.

ILLNESS

Illness is a product of the disharmonious interaction (disease) among mind, body, emotions, and spirit. Claude Bernard, a 17th-century French physiologist, developed the concept of **homeostasis**, the organism's attempt to restore balance. With self-regulatory mechanisms, the human body responds to constant challenges from the external environment in an effort to maintain equilibrium or health. Illness is the body's way of signaling that a person has exceeded the natural capacity to mediate between the internal and external environments. Illness can be an opportunity to discover meaning in life and to heal, identifying areas of disharmony and determining how best to move toward a natural state of harmony.

Illness can be a signal that a person's important needs are not being met. It can be an invitation from within to look at the balance between activity and rest or between self- and other-oriented care.

SELF-CARE DEFICIT

Self-care deficit is an impaired ability to perform or complete activities of daily living (Carpenito Moyet, 2012). This can generate therapeutic concern on the part of the patient, family, or friends and the nurse.

Therapeutic interventions for self-care deficits are directed at contributing factors. Interventions for potential self-care deficits are directed at prevention by reducing risk factors. Resources are identified that are useful in optimizing the autonomy and independence of the patient. A disease orientation leads to a disability orientation whereas focusing on health leads to an ability orientation (Schell, Gillen, & Scaffa, 2014). A positive association has been reported between a self-reported "health-conscious" or "health-active" orientation and engaging in wellness information-seeking behavior (Weaver, May, Hopkins, Eroglu, & Bernhardt, 2010).

Therefore, the person with altered function is not necessarily disabled but should be able to adapt strengths toward being an able person. This transformation is evident in the lives of famous individuals whose illnesses did not limit their potential, such as Helen Keller and Franklin D. Roosevelt.

NURSING IN WELLNESS

Nursing has traditionally been focused on wellness, with nursing theorists promoting aspects of wellness and self-care. Self-responsibility is paramount in Dorothea Orem's nursing theory

(Sparks & Taylor, 2014), which focuses on self-care so that the person can maintain life, health, and well-being. According to Martha Rogers (1990), the primary purpose of nursing is to help people achieve their maximum health potential. By promoting high-level wellness and preventing illness whenever possible, the nurse uses an approach that minimizes risk and empowers the patient.

Illness Prevention

Preventing illness is one aspect of wellness care that focuses on detection or prevention of disease. Primary prevention focuses on the health of a person or population, with the goal of preventing a disease or illness. Immunizations are prime examples of primary prevention, as are educational programs, such as nutritional instruction for children and their parents, which improve the health and general well-being of communities.

Secondary prevention includes screening for those at risk for developing an illness or those who could have disease diagnosed early in the process for prompt treatment. Recommending annual skin evaluation in someone with a history of sunburn or recurrent use of tanning bed to screen for early cancer detection is an example of secondary prevention.

Tertiary prevention occurs when diagnosis of a long-term disease or disability has already been made. The goal is to minimize complications and maximize function in any way possible for these patients. A rehabilitation or long-term care facility provides tertiary preventive care.

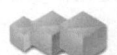 **Concept Mastery Alert**

Nurses must be careful to avoid confusing primary prevention and secondary prevention. Primary prevention is a proactive intervention that aims to reduce an individual's future likelihood of developing an illness. Secondary prevention involves identifying people who are at particular risk of developing a health problem or those who may unknowingly have a health problem. To examine the difference, let's look at the example of cholesterol screening. Teaching people about the consequences of hypercholesterolemia and presenting strategies for reducing blood cholesterol demonstrates primary prevention. Measuring individuals' cholesterol levels or identifying those at high risk of developing this health problem demonstrates secondary prevention.

Health Promotion

Health promotion focuses on lifestyle choices to prevent illness and strives toward high-level wellness (Fitzpatrick, 2007). Many preventive measures either protect the person's health (e.g., car seats for children) or prevent loss of health (e.g., regular dental checkups). Pender, Murdaugh, and Parsons's (2010) health promotion model includes an assessment of the multiple factors that can determine how people interact with their environments in ways that affect their health. A baseline measure of body, mind, and spiritual variables includes health attitudes as well as cultural beliefs and practices. Physical measures include current states of nutrition, rest and sleep, elimination, exercise, and hygiene. Psychosocial variables include coping, interactions, self-concept, significant relationships, and cultural practices and recreation. Spiritual assessment includes beliefs and values. "The desired outcomes of health assessment are to: (1) identify health assets; (2) identify health-related lifestyle strengths; (3) determine key health-related beliefs; (4) identify health beliefs and health behaviors that put the patient at risk; and (5) determine how the patient wants to change to improve the quality of life" (Pender et al., 2010).

The Nurse as Health and Wellness Coach

Given the financially unsustainable and ineffective healthcare system in the United States, particularly in the face of the epidemic prevalence of chronic diseases, a new role for nurses has emerged.

Eight health behaviors were identified by the 2010 World Economic Forum (WEF) as major contributors to fifteen most costly chronic conditions. These behaviors include: smoking, physical inactivity, poor diet, alcohol consumption levels, poor standard-of-care compliance, poor stress management, insufficient sleep, and lack of health screening.

Integrative **Health and wellness coaching** is a collaborative partnership between the nurse as a professional coach and the patient/healing partner to assist the patient to identify their own health goals and how to best achieve them. Prevention across the wellness–illness continuum, healthy lifestyle, and integrative modalities merge with coaching individuals/groups to support optimal mind/body/spirit health.

Fundamental aspects of the coaching relationship include creating an effective partnership, exploring the patient's current readiness for change, and facilitating the patient's identification of SMART goals and facilitating the development of a wellness plan evolved from the patient's vision of their best life possible and their motivation to achieve these healthy changes while concurrently supporting the patient's vision and motivation to make healthy changes (Arloski, 2014).

Health coaching is found in various settings with many different delivery methods (May & Russel, 2013). Whether the patients are identified in a primary care setting as an individual or diagnostic group, or as part of an employee wellness program, they can work with a coach on a one-to-one or group basis in person, online, or telephonically.

Effect of Stress

Healthcare practitioners recognize that life stresses affect how and when an illness is manifested. Any change, even a positive one, results in a certain amount of stress. Psychosocial stress, such as the death of a spouse or being diagnosed with a progressively deteriorating illness, can lead to depression, anger, and despair, all of which harm the immune system. A cluster of events that requires life adjustment is associated with the onset of illness. Underlying cardiovascular disease and cancer, the two leading causes of disability and death in North America, are prolonged states of sympathetic nervous system activity mediated through the hormonal pathways. They are the body's response to prolonged stress reactivity (National Cancer Institute, 2012).

The Burden of Stress in America survey (2014) revealed that 49% of respondents admitted to a stressful event in the past year, with 43% reporting that the stressful event was related to a health issue. Women were more likely to be stressed by a family member's illness than men. The report confirmed that poor health was a major stressor along with financial problems and too many life responsibilities, such as managing various schedules within the family.

Stress is not always a negative event and to a certain degree can be beneficial to performance. The Yerkes–Dobson principle demonstrates that when stress or arousal is too low, performance may also be low; however, once stress or arousal exceeds maximum performance, the individual moves into distress, and their performance and/or health declines. This theory supports the idea that some stress is necessary; however, continuing to push yourself beyond an optimal level has a negative effect on performance and health (Seaward, 2013).

Your perception of stress as negative or positive may also be a factor in how stress affects your health. Keller et al. (2012) discovered that people with high levels of stress who perceived that the stress was detrimental to their health increased their risk of premature death.

Healthcare practitioners recognize that the mind–body connection is strong, and the impact of stress on health can be significant. Therefore, teaching skills to notice stress and/or shift your perception of the impact when possible could be helpful. See the Mind–Body Interventions section for more information on stress.

Lifestyle Modification

Nurses who are focused on wellness advocate the use of lifestyle modification skills that alleviate stress and promote a state less susceptible to disease. These skills increase an individual's energy level rather than reduce awareness of tension. Programs have been developed to teach the patient methods of self-care, including exercise, nutrition, and cognitive restructuring, as well as a spiritual component (e.g., **meditation**, yoga, other relaxation methods) and other approaches. Evidence of the paradigm shift from illness care to wellness care and prevention is the coverage by some insurance companies of lifestyle modification programs that include mind–body interventions. Notable examples are Benson and Stuart's medical symptoms reduction programs, Gordon's Center for Mind-Body Medicine, Kabat-Zinn's Stress Reduction Program, the UCLA Mindful Awareness Research Center and Ornish's Program for Reversing Heart Disease. These programs (Box 2-1), increasingly considered mainstream, combine a vast array of therapies that require the patient's willingness to change.

Helping patients to change behaviors and make more life-affirming choices requires knowledge of the change process. Prochaska, Diclemente, and Norcross (1992) have classically identified a six-stage process that patients move through in their search for effective wellness behaviors. These stages have

- Benson-Henry Institute for Mind Body Medicine (www.massgeneral.org/bhi/)
- The Center for Mind-Body Medicine (www.cmbm.org)
- Center for Mindfulness in Medicine, Health Care, and Society (www.umassmed.edu/cfm/index.aspx)
- Preventive Medicine Research Institute (www.pmri.org/dean_ornish.html)

been used to measure specific changes related to health (Lam, Wiley, Siu, & Emmett, 2010). The following stages of change are listed with characteristic behaviors to help both patients and providers identify their place in the cycle:

1. *Precontemplation:* Denial/demoralized
2. *Contemplation:* Stuck/stalling
3. *Preparation:* Planning, going public means telling friends and family about desire to change
4. *Action:* Begin to modify behavior
5. *Maintenance:* Struggle to prevent lapses; work to consolidate gains
6. *Termination:* Complete confidence; cycle of change completed

Some think that the last stage is misnamed. Given that a person often finds that this process is nonlinear, the final stage may actually be "permanent maintenance."

People can "relapse" at any point. For example, the average several attempts to stop smoking is nine before most people successfully maintain their nonsmoking state. The authors suggest that patients see this set of stages as a spiral and reassure themselves that most successful changers go through various stages three or four times before accomplishing a real change.

HOLISTIC HEALTHCARE AND NURSING

The healthcare community for centuries thought of body and mind as distinct entities. An illness-labeled **psychosomatic** (*psyche,* "mind," and *soma,* "body") was considered a mental health problem best dealt with by mental health practitioners. The general approach was an atomistic, newtonian model in which the parts seemed more important than the whole person.

In her examination of the historical roots of "holistic practice," Lowenberg (1992) relates the practice to several movements that were influential in the 1960s, including feminism, counterculturalism, environmentalism, and civil rights. These movements coincided with a crisis in healthcare in the 1970s. With accelerating costs and limited resources, the healthcare system faced growing dissatisfaction from the public, who wanted to be active participants in their own care, working as a partner with their healthcare provider.

The holistic framework that emerged respected the mind, body, and spirit of each person. It recognized each person as a bio-psycho-social-spiritual being within a family unit and community. Today, the holistic movement continues to struggle as technology has placed a barrier between the patient and the healthcare provider, leading to care that lacks personal relationships while costs continue to rise (Weil, 2009).

Health and wellness became valued goals within the holistic framework. Health is a dynamic state in which the person constantly adapts to changes in the internal and external environments. Each person defines health in relation to personal expectations and values. The concept of health must allow for this individual variability, and a holistic framework accommodates this view. For example, a person may see him- or herself as healthy while experiencing a respiratory infection. Someone who has a temporary disability related to mobility may consider him- or herself "not healthy," but a person with a permanent disability may consider such a condition a "normal" state and define health differently.

The concept of wellness also allows for individual variability. Wellness can be thought of as a dynamic balance among the physical, psychological, social, and spiritual aspects of a person's life. As with health, each person defines wellness in relation to personal expectations. Wellness behaviors promote healthy functioning and help prevent illness. Examples of wellness behaviors include stress management, nutritional awareness, and physical fitness. Chapter 9 discusses wellness behaviors in greater detail.

Holistic healthcare emphasizes humanism, choices, self-care activities, and a peer relationship between the healthcare provider and patient. **Holistic interventions** focus on the interrelated needs of body, mind, emotions, and spirit. Holistic practitioners use the term *psychosomatic* to mean not simply that the mind or emotions cause illness but also that the mind and body are so interrelated that they act on each other intimately, directly, and inseparably. Therefore, holistic health practitioners acknowledge the interactive processes of mind, body, and spirit.

Nursing is returning to its historical roots while simultaneously responding to ever-evolving technology, cost containment, and consumer demands. Nurses are challenged to retain the human aspect, including the spiritual aspect of nursing that values the meaning and purpose of life and death.

Many nurses recognize the complementary nature of what Dossey (2013) referred to as "doing" and "being" therapies. "Doing" therapies, such as giving medications, altering diets, and changing dressings, have measurable, linear outcomes. "Being" therapies recognize the less measurable effects of consciousness both within the person and as a bridge between individuals. Meditation, imagery, and prayer are some examples of "being" therapies.

Holistic nurses also recognize a duty to provide the healthiest environment for themselves and generations to come. The American Holistic Nurses Association (AHNA), formed in 1980, states in their *Holistic Nursing: Scope & Standards of Practice,* "Practicing holistic nursing requires nurses to integrate self-care, self-responsibility, spirituality, and reflection in their lives" (Mariano, 2013, p. 60). These standards reflect the nurse as a member of the global community. Nurses can become nationally certified in the specialty of holistic nursing through the American Holistic Nurses Certification Corporation. Additional information is available at their website (www.ahncc.org).

CAM THERAPIES AND INTEGRATIVE HEALTHCARE

NCCAM has had a name change recently to the National Center for Complementary and Integrative Health (NCCIH). Integrative health care is defined as "a comprehensive, often interdisciplinary approach to treatment, prevention and health promotion that brings together complementary and conventional therapies." "NCCIH's mission is to define, through rigorous scientific investigation, the usefulness and safety of complementary and integrative health approaches and their roles in improving health and health care." Federal funding of complementary and integrative health research and education has increased from $2 million in 1992 to $124.1 million in 2015 (NCCIH, 2014). NCCAM describes complementary therapies as therapies and systems of whole medicine that would be used in addition to conventional Western medicine; whereas alternative therapies would be used instead of conventional medicine (Barnes, Bloom, & Nahin, 2008). Traditional medicine refers to ancient systems of medicine such as Traditional Chinese Medicine or Native American medicine.

Holistic and Integrative Health practitioners do not want to abandon the established successes of **allopathic medicine**, which is conventional Western medicine. They recognize the incredible advances that conventional medicine has made, including antibiotics and trauma surgery. They are especially mindful of the risk of **iatrogenic illness**, or illness that results from treatment and may be traced to overuse and adverse responses to medication, in addition to abuse of prescription medications. Integrative Health practitioners try to combine the proven successes of Western conventional medicine and a wide range of therapies considered CAM. CAM was introduced in 1996 and generally refers to a group of diverse medical and healthcare systems, practices, and products that are **not** generally considered as part of conventional allopathic medicine. Integrative Health is more than CAM therapies added to allopathic medicine; there's a strong focus on nutrition, exercise, and stress reduction all of which is anchored in Lifestyle Medicine.

 APPLY YOUR CRITICAL THINKING

Sue Hornsby has just been told that she has breast cancer and needs to undergo surgery, chemotherapy, and radiation. She wonders if she needs to have all of these treatments or if she could just use naturopathy or perhaps an Integrative Health approach. She turns to you for advice. Knowing that Integrative Health is more than allopathic medicine and CAM therapies, what are some important data that you need from Sue? What data do you think would be helpful for her? What are the resources to whom she can turn for additional input? What is most important about your relationship with Sue?

Check your answer in Appendix B.

Consumer Use of CAM

In the seminal study by Eisenberg et al. (1993), 34% of U.S. adults surveyed reported using some form of CAM. In 2007, the estimate was placed at 38.3% of adults and 11.8% of children and adolescents (Nahin, Barnes, & Cohen, 2009). The National Health Statistics Survey in 2007 is the most recent survey examining the prevalence of CAM use nationally. This survey showed that adults spent $33.9 billion on CAM, with two thirds ($22 billion) spent on self-care products (Nahin et al., 2009; NCCAM Strategic Plan 2011–2015).

Studies have shown that more women than men are likely to use CAM therapies, both in the United States and in other countries. In a study by Upchurch, Dye, Chyu, Gold, and Greendale (2010), using data from the National Health Interview Survey (NHIS), women in midlife (ages 40 to 59 years) were found to be the highest users of CAM. **Herbs** and natural products, massage, relaxation, yoga, and chiropractic care were found to be the top five therapies in use. A study in 2013 (Goertz et al.) showed that military members used CAM at a higher rate than civilian populations. Stress reduction therapies were used more frequently (2 to 7.5 times higher) in military respondents than civilian survey respondents.

According to Weeks (2014) "the 2010 Patient Protection and Affordable Care Act (ACA), a.k.a. Obamacare, has brought unprecedented inclusion for Integrative Health concepts and practitioners. Now it's 2014 and the Act is officially the law of the land." The intent is that any plan within the ACA "offering group or individual health insurance coverage shall not discriminate with respect to participation under the plan or coverage against any health care provider who is acting within the scope of that provider's license or certification under applicable State law" (Patient Protection and Affordable Healthcare Act [HR3590]). The Patient-Centered Outcomes Research Institute (PCORI) authorized by the ACA 2010, is "a nonprofit organization that funds research aimed at providing patients, caregivers, and clinicians with information to make better health care decisions" (PCORI, 2010). Given the focus on comparative effectiveness research, conducted in typical patients and care delivery settings, PCORI could fund studies that compare conventional to complementary approaches.

As use, education, and research increase in the area of CAM, the terminology used to describe this method of care also is evolving, changing, and broadening.

Evolution of Integrative Healthcare

Many people use the terms *CAM* and **integrative medicine** (IM) synonymously. Nevertheless, there is a difference. Although all the modalities listed in the NCCAM classification system are holistic in philosophy and conceptual basis, CAM consists of various individual modalities with specific guidelines, approaches, and foundations. IHC is larger than allopathic plus CAM and includes all areas of lifestyle, body, mind, and spirit as well as partnering with the patient and focusing on health promotion and disease prevention (http://integrativemedicine.arizona.edu/about/definition.html).

In 1994, Dr. Andrew Weil and leaders across the nation founded the first fellowship training in PIM—the Program in Integrative Medicine (Weil, 1994). This program recently celebrated its 20th year and has grown to include residency programs in Integrative Family Medicine, Oncology, Pediatrics, and the Integrative Health and Lifestyle Program for Registered Nurses and other health professionals (ACIM, 2014). There are many formal definitions of IM; however, the PIM offers the following definition of IM:

"Integrative medicine is healing-oriented medicine that takes account of the whole person (body, mind, spirit and community), including all aspects of lifestyle. It emphasizes the therapeutic relationship and makes use of all appropriate therapies, both conventional and alternative." (Lemly, 2014, pp. 2–14)

In addition to this definition, several principles encompass the basic goals of IM:

- Establish a partnership between patient and practitioner.
- Facilitate the body's innate healing abilities.
- Neither rejects allopathic medicine nor embraces CAM practices uncritically.
- Effective interventions that are natural and less invasive should be used whenever possible.
- Realize that good medicine is grounded in good science and open to new paradigms.
- Focus on promoting health and preventing illness as well as treating disease.
- Practitioners of IM should exemplify its principles and commit themselves to self-exploration and self-development.

The term *integrative* truly captures the evolving model of healthcare. Nursing leaders at the Gillette Nursing Summit (Kreitzer & Disch, 2003) proposed that rather than labeling the practice strictly as medicine, the term IHC more accurately reflects the cross-disciplinary reality and progressive acceptance of a broader aspect of care. This is demonstrated as allopathic providers become knowledgeable of CAM practices, learn to communicate with CAM practitioners, partner with patients on decisions about the use of CAM modalities, focus on promoting health, and strive to be role models of health. IHC is increasing with the evidence base supporting it; more academic institutions are making a commitment to education in IHC (Booth-Laforce et al., 2010).

Another key difference between CAM and IHC is the incorporation of nursing principles. IHC incorporates these principles within its foundation, whereas CAM consists of various individual modalities. Many of these modalities are easily incorporated into nursing practice when appropriate and safe; however, IHC is connected to nursing by including such principles as relying on the therapeutic relationship, accounting for the whole person (body, mind, spirit, and community), including all aspects of lifestyle, and focusing on healing versus curing.

According to Jean Watson (2012), there is an emerging model that transcends nursing and has an integrative, expanded perspective. This new model requires an authentic presence and has the ability to center on healing and wholeness and not just focus on disease and pathology. This new paradigm is called *integral healthcare,* which proposes to incorporate all dimensions of healing.

The theory of integral nursing was developed by Barbara Dossey and based on the work of philosopher Ken Wilber. According to Dossey (2013), *integral nursing* is defined as a comprehensive integral worldview and process plus holistic theories and other paradigms, which indicates holistic nursing practice is included and transcended. It encourages the nurse to view nursing from four perspectives: (1) the individual interior (personal, intentional); (2) individual exterior (physiologic, behavioral); (3) collective interior (shared, cultural); and (4) collective exterior (systems, structures).

Integral nursing is a philosophy more than a therapeutic approach and incorporates all aspects of healing to include challenging healthcare providers to reflect on their own personal self-care. It is a model that encourages the complex multidimensional aspects of human experience. According to Dossey (2013), an integral awareness and worldview allows us to become more aware of our wholeness and healing, and strengthen our personal and professional capacities to more fully open to the mysteries of life's journey and the wondrous stages of discovery with self and others. See Box 2-2 for an example of integral nursing.

Nursing's Relationship to the Integrative Health Continuum

Given the consumer desire to access Integrative Health, nurses are responsible for responding appropriately. Not every nurse desires to or should become a CAM practitioner. Within a continuum of involvement with CAM, however, all nurses can be held accountable for the following skills:

- Starting with the initial contact with a patient, the nurse includes a basic assessment of his or her use of CAM in any intake interview. The nurse asks about vitamins and supplements as well as any healing practices. An Integrative Health assessment requires presence and deep listening skills and is not performed by following a checklist of questions.
- When reviewing a patient's current drug regimen, the nurse queries about the use of vitamins, supplements, and herbal teas and dosages used. Many consumers take herbs with some degree of risk because the U.S. Food and Drug Administration does not regulate these substances. In addition, some patients may mistakenly believe that something "natural," such as herbs, is never harmful. In fact, some herbs, just like drugs, affect heart rate and blood pressure while others affect liver function, posing risks for patients. It is important to note that overall herbs are safer and slower acting than drugs and many drugs have interactions as well with foods, herbs, and other drugs. It is important to be knowledgeable of how all three act when combined so as not to scare or offend the patient when discussing this topic.

BOX 2-2   Exploring Alternative Treatments

Trey is a nurse in the office of a busy endocrinology practice. Most days, he interacts closely with physicians and nurse practitioners (NP) who examine patients referred from primary care practices and focus on chronic disease such as type 2 diabetes mellitus. Once a week, Trey assists with diabetic education classes. He enjoys the diversity his job offers and learns a great deal in the educational classes offered to patients.

Trey has been at his job for 2 years and thinks he is ready for a new project. Last week, he met with a NP about a proposal for expanding the care provided. Trey has suggested implementing a patient education initiative to specifically address Integrative Health for patients with type 2 diabetes. He has noticed more patients coming to the office with questions about Integrative Health. Until now, the office has had no formal education for patients regarding these treatments and no accepted procedure for physicians and nurses to review the wealth of emerging evidence in this area. Trey feels that he has a professional, legal, and ethical responsibility to better educate himself on Integrative Health.

The NP has approved Trey's proposal and has put him in charge of implementing this education project. Although it is a big undertaking, Trey is genuinely excited about the effects a standardized and thorough program can have on the care provided to patients. The NP suggests that Trey start by picking one topic, researching available evidence, and then reporting a description of his findings. Trey decides to investigate a topic that he has heard a lot about not only from

patients but also from various anecdotal news reports—the use of antioxidants from multi-vitamins and supplements.

Trey begins his search on the Cochrane database. He has used this database in the past and knows that it is an excellent source of current literature available on a particular topic. Trey finds a Cochrane review on this topic. The review includes randomized trials comparing antioxidant supplements in type 2 diabetic patients and evaluation of their endothelial function. The review looks specifically at supplementation of Vitamin E and Vitamin C and their effect on endothelial function. He was surprised that there was an inverse relationship in the effect being improved for less obese patients. Trey feels this information could be important for the patients in the clinic education class as he's aware that type 2 diabetes increases the risk of vascular disease.

Trey plans to investigate more closely but this gives him a great start. He now plans to look at a few of the individual research articles that were included in the Cochrane review. He's even curious about the type of supplements used, whether they were the same brand or dosage and whether natural or synthetic Vitamin E was used in each clinical trial. The Cochrane database has proven to be a valuable resource in Trey's new project.

Source: Montero, D., Walther, G., Sthouwer, C. D. A., Houben, A. J. M., Beckman, J. A., & Vinet, A. (2014). Effective antioxidant vitamin supplementation on endothelial function in Type 2 Diabetes Mellitus: A systematic review and meta-analysis of randomized controlled trials. *Obesity Reviews, 15*(2), 107–116.

- When discussing current dietary habits and preferences, the nurse asks if the patient has been following any particular plan, such as a vegetarian, macrobiotic, or other specific nutritional regimen (e.g., the Paleo diet).
- When asking how a patient's condition has been treated to date, the nurse inquires if the patient ascribes to any CAM therapies or healing practices other than or in addition to what a physician has recommended. These might include culturally diverse practices such as seeking advice from lay "healers," receiving care from CAM providers such as naturopathic or Ayurvedic physicians or chiropractors, or participating in stress management/self-care practices such as yoga or meditation. Asking "what has helped you in the past?" can be an effective way of allowing patients to open up about these topics. Integrative Health requires cultural competence when assessing patients in any setting.

Conveying an open and nonjudgmental attitude is a key to accurate collection of this information. In a study of older adults, 70% did not discuss their use of CAM with their physician (Crute, 2008). This same study found that patients did not tell of their use because they did not have confidence that the allopathic provider was knowledgeable of the CAM modality or did not ask. This finding has critical ramifications for how nurses communicate with patients and devise methods to gain their confidence.

For nurses who want to move beyond the basic level of involvement with CAM, the next step includes familiarity with CAM literature. At first, this may mean simply building knowledge of where to look for information. For example, if a nurse is unsure about a patient's use of **acupuncture** or Integrative treatment in patients with depression, knowing where to access reliable information such as the NCCAM position on acupuncture research (http://nccam.nih.gov/health/acupuncture) would be useful. Accessing information on an integrative approach to depression would benefit patients and possibly decrease the amount of medications required for treatment (Arvidsdotter & Marklund, 2013; Arvidsdotter, Marklund, & Taft, 2014). A nurse may then want to explore the Integrative Health literature to educate him- or herself about a particular modality.

The next step on the continuum is to actively consult with a CAM practitioner. Being familiar with the more popular CAM practices and the current research enables nurses to better understand the total healthcare delivery system available to patients.

Common CAM Modalities

The NCCAM identifies five major domains of CAM practices:

- Whole medical systems
- Mind–body interventions
- Biologically based therapies

BOX 2-3 NCCAM Domains of Complementary and Alternative Practices

1. **Alternative Medical Systems:** Complete systems of theory and practice that evolved independent of the biomedical approach.
   Examples: Oriental medicine (methods include acupuncture, herbal medicine, Oriental massage, and **qi** gong). Ayurvedic medicine (methods include diet, exercise, meditation, and herbs). Other medical systems developed by Native American, Aboriginal, African, Middle-Eastern, Tibetan, and Central and South American cultures. Homeopathy and naturopathic medicine.
2. **Mind–Body Interventions:** These interventions use various techniques to facilitate the positive influence of the mind and body's intimate connections.
   Examples: Meditation,* certain uses of hypnosis, dance, music,* art therapy, prayer,* and imagery.*
3. **Biologically Based Therapies:** Practices, products, and interventions that are natural and biologically based.

Examples: Use of herbs;* special diet therapies such as those of Drs. Atkins, Ornish, Pritikin, and Weil;* orthomolecular therapies;* and biologic therapies such as the use of laetrile, shark cartilage, or bee pollen.
4. **Manipulative and Body-Based Methods:** Methods that involve manipulation or movement of the body.
   Examples: Chiropractic treatments, osteopathy, and massage.*
5. **Energy Therapies:** These practices focus on energy originating within or around the body.
   Examples: Qi gong, reiki,* Therapeutic Touch,* and the use of magnets.

*Complementary therapy commonly used in nursing.
Adapted from: NCCAM Report, 2008. Retrieved July 10, 2011, from http://nccam.nih.gov/news/2008/nhsr12.pdf

---

- Manipulative and body-based methods
- Energy medicine

Koithan (2014) posits that advanced practice nurses are uniquely positioned to use therapeutic strategies now identified as CAM practices by NCCAM in the current IHC environment. Nursing research of the 1970s and 1980s examined the effects of mind–body therapies (guided imagery, breathing and relaxation techniques on pain, anxiety and depression). Nursing textbooks from the same era identified energetic (therapeutic/healing touch) and manipulative and body-based therapies (massage) as independent nursing interventions. Examples of CAM therapies are marked with an asterisk in Box 2-3. In this section, five of the most common are discussed in more depth: mind–body interventions, meditation, **traditional Chinese medicine** (TCM), **botanicals**, and **Therapeutic Touch** (TT).

MIND–BODY INTERVENTIONS

Our culture has been diagnosed with the new pandemic "super stress" (Lee, 2010). Between 60% and 90% of all visits to primary care providers are related to stress. The primary programs mentioned under lifestyle modification developed in response to this stress epidemic recognize the powerful effect/response that can be evoked by teaching patients mind–body interventions for self-care. Patients referred to these programs have conditions as varied as hypertension, diabetes, gastrointestinal (GI) distress, cancer, chronic pain, posttraumatic stress disorder, insomnia, anxiety, and depression, to name a few.

Mind–body interventions, such as hypnosis, meditation, biofeedback, imagery, progressive muscle relaxation, yoga, and tai chi, have demonstrated effects on a range of physical parameters such as cardiovascular function and glucose tolerance as well as immune and inflammatory responses (Taylor et al., 2010). All of these interventions provide "lines of communication

between the mind/brain and the body" (p. 31). These therapies are effective and efficient and can be used as primary or adjunctive treatments to increase the effectiveness of other treatments (Guarneri, Horrigan, & Perhura, 2010).

MEDITATION

Meditation, deep personal thought and reflection, may be one of the most basic and powerful self-care activities that people can incorporate into their lives. It stills the chattering mind and sharpens understanding of the internal and external worlds. Meditation is a way to tune and train the mind, leading to greater efficiency in everyday life. It helps decrease anxiety and assists the person to handle stress. Those who meditate may find increased ability to withstand life changes and fewer illnesses. Box 2-4 provides guidelines for meditation.

Although meditation seems like a simple tool, it can have powerful results. It is considered the cornerstone of the lifestyle modification programs mentioned previously. The goal of meditation is twofold, according to Drs. Joel and Michelle Levey (2014): (1) conscious cultivation of mental qualities that enhance understanding, power, and love, and (2) intentional transformation or lessening of those mind states that block these qualities.

Many types of meditation fall into the following categories: concentrative, receptive, reflective, and expressive. These types of meditation are not mutually exclusive. Yoga, for example, can be considered a type of **concentrative meditation**. The important component for all types is that the patient takes time to focus the mind in a way that develops his or her ability to live each moment to its fullness.

Concentrative Meditation

Concentrative meditation is probably the most familiar to most people. The person focuses on a specific object. The object can be internal, such as a prayer, a chant, a repetitive

BOX 2-4   General Guidelines for Meditation

- Have a particular place to do meditative practice. Arrange that space in a way that supports the qualities you nurture through meditation. You may have objects or pictures that speak to that peaceful state you are nurturing. Having a particular place makes it easier to return to that focused state when you return to that place each time.
- Providing a quiet space of respect means turning off pagers, telephones, and the myriad technologic interruptions that can be distracting.
- Straighten your spine, and relax your body. Lying down may cause you to fall asleep, so sitting upright is recommended.
- A daily practice of 20 minutes morning and evening usually is recommended. At first, you may try 5 to 10 minutes and discover that the benefits are so pervasive that you will allow your practice to extend for longer periods.
- Scheduling will take a commitment. Try various strategies, such as marking this time in your daily planner, setting your morning alarm a bit earlier, or settling into a bedtime ritual that includes your meditation time. Eventually, the practice will become self-reinforcing.
- Quiet the chattering mind. Focus your attention. The handiest focus of all is one's own breath. Here are two methods that can assist in this process:
  - Count silently on inhalation, 1 to 4… and then 4 to 1 as you exhale.
  - Consciously "belly breathe"; that is, have your abdomen visibly expand on the inhalation and deflate on the exhalation. Most of us breathe very shallow breaths that only involve the upper chest. If thoughts intrude, acknowledge them by saying "thinking, thinking," and let them go as if watching small, white, fluffy clouds gently crossing the clear blue sky of your mind.

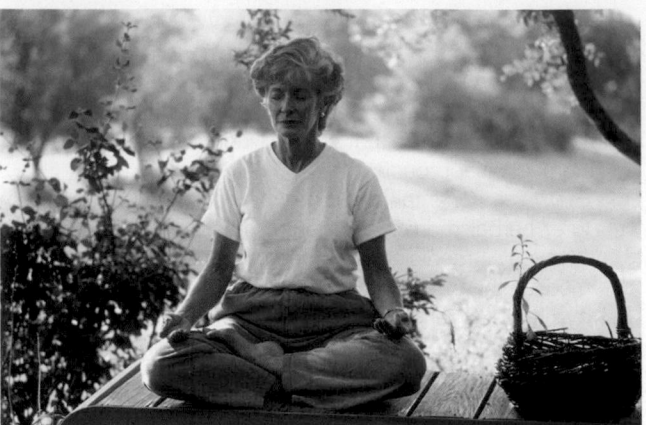

FIGURE 2-3 Concentrative meditation. Focusing one's attention and stilling the mind allows greater awareness and clarity to emerge.

word or phrase, or even an image or visualization, or it can be an external object, such as music or a candle flame (Fig. 2-3).

Receptive Meditation

Receptive meditation focuses on the deep interconnection between the mind and body. Vipassana and mindfulness meditation are within this category. Being mindful involves an awareness of this present moment and being nonjudgmentally and fully open to that moment with all senses engaged fully (Sharma & Rush, 2014).

Reflective Meditation

In **reflective meditation**, the person chooses a theme, question, or topic of reflection to gain insight into significant questions or concepts related to philosophy or spirituality. The focus is on the person's query; he or she returns to it as the object of attention.

Expressive Meditation

Expressive meditation usually includes movement or expression with the concentrative methods of whirling, shaking, or dancing.

TRADITIONAL CHINESE MEDICINE

Traditional Chinese medicine (TCM) is a complete healing system and includes acupuncture, massage, herbal treatments, nutrition, moxibustion, movement such as qi gong, and meditation. At the core of TCM is the concept of a vital energy source or life force known as qi (pronounced *chee*). Qi does not translate well into English because qi is a small reflection of a much greater whole. It comprises all forces of nature: spirit, energy, and life itself. Therefore, it may be difficult for Westerners to completely understand TCM (Gao, 2013).

TCM evolved more than 4,000 years ago from Taoist philosophy. The physical body that conventional allopathic medicine believes in treating is just a small portion of healing in TCM. According to TCM, humans are not only physical beings but also part of the energetic workings of nature. Thoughts and emotions are major factors in physical health. Therefore, TCM views disease in varying degrees based on how out of balance a person is with the fundamental laws of nature. Balance and harmony play a major role in health (Gao, 2013).

Yin and **yang** are two equal and opposite aspects of qi. These concepts are critical expressions of the philosophy of TCM and yet are not as simple as they first appear. Both are forces of qi, yet each is unique. Yang is symbolic of the forces of heaven and is considered more active, dynamic, and representative of male energy. Yin represents the qi of the earth and is considered more foundational and female. Neither force is superior to the other, and neither one can stand alone. Each must contain a small portion of the other dynamic force at all times.

Diagnosis via TCM requires a firm understanding of yin and yang. There are two diagnostic models: the Eight Principle and the Five Element. Each model is a complete system and yet is flexible enough to complement the other. The Eight Principle model includes four pairs of polarity: interior/exterior, hot/cold, deficiency/excess, and yin/yang. The Five Element model consists of the energetic qualities of all things: wood, fire, earth, metal, and water. Each element is symbolic and represents related qualities. For instance, in spring, wood is growing or increasing; therefore, wood qi represents these qualities (Gao, 2013).

Meridians are the channels in which energy or qi flows throughout the body. The meridian system unifies all parts of the body and is essential for maintaining its balance. The many major and minor meridians correspond to each of the five yin and six yang organs. In addition, TCM considers the pericardium a separate organ. This is another area that can be hard for Westerners to conceptualize because the organ meridian system does not directly correlate to the actual biomedical organ system.

Acupuncture is one component of TCM that has become quite popular in the United States. It is based on the basic principle of inserting very fine needles into various areas of the body to stimulate the meridians and promote harmony within the system. Depending on the treatment, the needle stimulates the increase or decrease of qi flowing through the meridians. Moxibustion, the act of heating a point on the skin using the herb mugwort, is thought to work on the same theory (Gao, 2013).

Several different types of acupuncture are available in the United States: Korean, Japanese, French, Vietnamese, English, and American. They are also based on the theory of correcting energy disharmony.

Acupuncture can be used to correct disharmony or prevent disharmony from developing. Most Western patients primarily use acupuncture to decrease pain or treat specific diseases (Garcia, et al., 2013). A Cochrane review determined that acupuncture is effective for the prophylaxis of migraine headaches (Linde et al., 2009). Studies have shown that acupuncture is safe and effective, particularly helpful in primary care with osteoarthritis of the knee, low back pain, chronic neck pain,

and headaches (Mao & Kapur, 2010). A systematic review of randomized controlled clinical trials of acupuncture for postoperative pain demonstrated that acupuncture had clear value and that it decreased pain intensity and lowered opioid side effects (Edwards et al., 2013; Sun, Gan, Dubose, & Habib, 2008). Recently, the American Pain Society and the American College of Physicians published new clinical treatment guidelines for persistent back pain that now include acupuncture as a treatment option (Hutchinson, Ball, Andrews, & Jones, 2012; Strauss, 2008).

Most states require that practitioners of acupuncture or TCM graduate from an accredited program pass a national certification examination and meet other state guidelines. Nevertheless, some practitioners who were trained in other countries, such as China, or who successfully completed a preceptorship have been "grandfathered" into licensing.

DIETARY SUPPLEMENTS AND BOTANICALS

The terms botanicals and herbs are interchangeable and represent plant species with medicinal properties. Every culture has used botanical medicine for thousands of years and the West is seeing an increase in use. As Western allopathic medicine shifts its focus toward self-care and more people look for ways to stay young and healthy, the use of botanical and dietary supplement products has surged. Such use poses many challenges and underscores the need for nurses at every level to become knowledgeable of herbal medicine and micronutrient supplements to ensure safe and effective practice (Table 2-1). The botanical and dietary supplement market is surging. Since the passage of

TABLE 2-1 SELECTED HERBS, MINERALS, AND VITAMINS FOR MENTAL HEALTH USE

Herbs, Minerals, and Vitamins	Uses	Actions and Precautions	Dose
California poppy, yellow and orange	Relieves pain Acts as a sedative Relieves mild anxiety	Poppy contains mild alkaloids similar to codeine and morphine. Do not use with monoamine oxidase inhibitors (MAOIs).	1 teaspoon/cup tea 2–3 times daily
Ginkgo biloba	Reduces senility Reduces short-term memory loss in normal older adults Improves peripheral circulation	Use as a circulatory aid and antioxidant. Fruit or seed should not be handled or eaten. May enhance papaverine. Possible side effects include GI distress, headache, and allergic reaction. Cautious use is recommended if taking aspirin or other blood-thinning drugs.	60 mg BID Alzheimer—240 mg divided 2–3 times daily
Ginseng (Asian and American)	Reduces stress and fatigue Improves physical and mental function, especially with elderly patients Assists smoking cessation efforts	Use the root. Use may raise blood pressure and serum glucose levels and can increase the growth of estrogen-dependent cancer.	American—0.03% ginsenoside, 1–2 g fresh root Asian—1.5% ginseng, 1–2 g fresh root For both, 200–600 mg liquid extract daily
Butterbur	Treatment of migraine headache and allergic rhinitis	Raw unprocessed Butterbur contains pyrrolizidine alkaloids (PAs) which can cause liver damage. PA–free are considered safe for children and adolescents for up to 12–16 wk.	50–100 mg BID with meals. Dosage varies by product

Continued

TABLE 2-1 SELECTED HERBS, MINERALS, AND VITAMINS FOR MENTAL HEALTH USE (*Continued*)

Herbs, Minerals, and Vitamins	Uses	Actions and Precautions	Dose
Hops	Has a sedative effect Reduces anxiety	Forms include tea, extract, or capsule. The active ingredient is in glandular hairs on its scaly, conelike fruits.	1 teaspoon/cup tea 2–3 times daily or 30–40 drops tincture
Kava kava	Reduces stress and anxiety Reduces insomnia	It comes from the root of the pepper tree family. It has a soothing effect on the amygdala (alarm center of the brain). Do not use with tranquilizers, sedatives, or alcohol. Large doses can produce an intoxicating effect. Long-term use can lead to dry, scaly skin. Recent research has linked kava to at least 25 cases of liver toxicity, including hepatitis, cirrhosis, and liver failure; people with liver disease or liver problems or those who are taking drugs that affect the liver should talk with their healthcare provider before using kava (NCCAM Report, 2002). Toxicity may be linked to acetone used during extraction.	2–4 g as decoction TID for 4–12 wk 1 teaspoon with 70–85 mg kava lactones
Passion flower	Causes mild hypnosis Reduces insomnia Reduces nervousness, restlessness, and agitation	Depresses the central nervous system (CNS) for mild sedative effect. Forms include tea, capsules, and extracts.	Infusion of 2–5 g (1 teaspoon) dried herb TID
Rosemary and other mints	Normalizes nerve impulses Acts as an antioxidant Relieves headache Acts as a sedative Helps improve memory and prevent dementia	Slows/inhibits action of acetylcholinesterase to acetylcholine, which stays in synapse longer. Antioxidant is carnosic acid that is concentrated in young growing leaves, peaks in the summer, lessens in older leaves, and is hardly present in old wood stems. Forms include whole essential oils for external use.	Tincture (1:5) 2–4 mL TID
St. John's wort	Treats mild to moderate depression, loss of interest, anorexia, fatigue, chronic fatigue immune dysfunction syndrome, and anxiety	Leaves or flowering tips can be used; hypericin is the active ingredient. May interfere with HIV drugs. Use may cause light sensitivity. Use with other drugs can be dangerous; do not take with other psychoactive medications (i.e., selective serotonin reuptake inhibitors [SSRIs], tricyclics, and MAOIs). Has fewer side effects compared with antidepressants. May lower activity of nonsedating antihistamines, oral contraceptives, antiepileptics, calcium channel blockers, cyclosporins, macrolides, and some antifungals.	300–500 mg TID with meals for 4–6 wk 0.5 mg hypericin per capsule
SAMe (S-adenosylmethionine)	Treats mild to moderate depression and arthritis, protects the liver, eases fibromyalgia	SAMe is a naturally occurring compound that regulates action of serotonin and dopamine. Approved as a prescription drug in Italy, Germany, Spain, and Russia. Takes effect in 10 d, faster than prescription drugs. Use enteric-coated tablets with 96% pure product. Do not use for bipolar disorder. Must take 800 µg folic acid and 1,000 µg vitamin B_{12} daily; the herb will not work if these vitamin levels are low.	200–800 or 1,600 mg BID 1 h before breakfast and lunch For arthritis, 400–800 mg/d For fibromyalgia, 800 mg/d
Valerian	Relieves anxiety and insomnia	Forms include a tea (2–3 g dried root several times daily) or capsules. Herb is nonaddictive. Do not take with tranquilizers, sedatives, or alcohol. Possible side effects include blurred vision, excitability, and changes in heartbeat if taken in large doses or for more than 2 wk.	300–400 mg 1–2 times daily
5-Hydroxytryptophan (5-HTP)	Treats bipolar disorder in conjunction with lithium Reduces depression Relieves insomnia	This amino acid is a precursor of serotonin. Taken from *Griffonia simplicifolia* seed.	Bipolar disorder—200 mg; depression—150–300 mg; insomnia—200–600 mg

the Dietary Supplement Health Education Act (DSHEA) an increase in sales from approximately 4,000 products to over 29,000 products are available (Tsouronunis & Bent, 2010, p. 147–149). Due to this rise, it is critically important that nurses increase their knowledge of botanicals and supplements. Reputable courses are available through Universities or the American Botanical Council.

History

In 1897, aspirin was developed by Friedrich Bayer as the first synthetic drug. Prior to this, botanicals and natural products were used for medicinal purposes and are the foundation for modern pharmaceutical products. However, as the market place abounds with choices, nurses should be aware that many product bear little resemblance to its original crude plan preparation and misinformation is easily spread on the Internet.

Today, the WHO estimates that 80% of the world population use herbal medicine. This occurs mostly because of a lack of availability of conventional practitioners and pharmaceuticals in many nations (WHO, 2010). In the United States, herbs and supplements are the most commonly used CAM choice among patients with GI conditions (Dossett et al., 2014).

Safety

Just as a patient must use caution when taking multiple prescription medications, he or she also must use caution when taking herbs complementarily and concurrently with prescription and over-the-counter medications. Nursing assessment should include evaluating the use of such medications as well as the patient's dietary intake and use of herbal teas. Because of the lack of human studies on herb–drug interactions, suspected interactions usually are evaluated by case reports or animal and in vitro herb pharmacology studies (Braun, 2007). However, herbs are less likely to cause side effects and generally are safer than pharmaceutical drugs (Braun & Cohen, 2007).

Nurses should ensure that each assessment includes a discussion of the use of herbs, vitamins, supplements, and teas. They also should discuss why the patient feels a need to take the complementary product. Nurses should become familiar with contraindications and adverse effects and keep reputable resources available. A nonjudgmental attitude encourages an atmosphere that promotes open discussion and sharing of information.

Standardization Issues

Standardization is the attempt by herbal manufacturers to produce a consistent, measured amount of product per unit dose. Generally, one or more constituents are chosen and thought to produce the therapeutic activity. For example, St. John's wort is standardized to hypericin. Although standardization is useful, it is also limited because not all the compounds or the required levels are known (Ribnicky, Pouley, Schmidt, Cefalu, & Raskin, 2008).

Regulatory Issues

In 1994, the Dietary Supplement Health and Education Act (DSHEA) set new guidelines for supplements regarding quality, labeling, packaging, and marketing. Herbal products cannot make therapeutic and prevention claims but are allowed to make "structure and function claims." An example is that the label on St. John's wort might state it "optimizes mood"; however, it cannot state that it is a "natural antidepressant."

Quality control is another important issue to consider when evaluating the use of herbal products. Consumers would like to be reassured that the product contains the ingredients and quantities on the label and that purity is maintained. It is recommended that patients purchase products from companies with a U.S. Pharmacopoeia (USP) or National Sanitation Foundation (NSF) quality seal, a Good Manufacturing Practices (GMP) seal, or those that have passed tests by Consumer Labs or have been clinically tested.

Credentialing Issues

In the United States, the American Herbalists Guild (AMG) is the only peer-reviewed organization for professional herbalists specializing in herbal medicine. There is no current licensing body for herbalists; however, the AMG is working toward standardizing educational requirements, creating national tests, and possibly establishing licensing parameters. Naturopaths and acupuncturists may use herbal therapies under their individual license.

THERAPEUTIC TOUCH

Therapeutic Touch® (TT), a holistic, evidence-based therapy that incorporates the intentional and compassionate use of universal energy to promote balance and well-being, was developed more than 30 years ago by Dora Kunz (a healer) and Dolores Krieger (Krieger, 1993; Wager, 1996). TT is a holistic, evidence-based therapy that incorporates the compassionate use of universal energy to promote balance and well-being (Therapeutic Touch International Association, 2014). In some ways, the terminology involved is confusing because the practitioner does not have to physically touch the patient for a beneficial effect. This technique always involves making contact with the recipient's energy field. A review of the theories upon which TT is based will help explain the underlying premise of this modality.

Both Rogers's (1990) science of unitary human beings and Kunz and Peper's (1995) human energy field model view energy fields as fundamental units of all beings and their environments. This view is consistent with many Eastern philosophies, which emphasize that the universe is composed of interacting systems of energy, derived from a unified source. Human beings are open and complex systems of energy in constant flux as they interact with the environment of energy that surrounds them. In this view, the essence of human beings does not end with the body but extends beyond mere physical boundaries. Physical health, as well as thoughts and feelings, affect each person's energy field. Because these systems of energy interact, they can affect and are affected by others' energy fields. Thus, practitioners of TT recognize the interconnectedness of all energy systems, including those of the nurse and patient, acknowledging a universal energy with order and wholeness (Kunz, 1995; Quinn, 2009).

When a person is healthy, life energy flows in a balanced, harmonious way (Kunz, 1995). Disease or illness means that

BOX 2-5   Steps in Therapeutic Touch

Centering
First phase: The practitioner brings his or her attention inward to a quiet, still, peaceful state of consciousness.

Assessment
Second phase: While remaining centered, the practitioner moves his or her hands 2 to 6 inches from the patient's skin surface to gather information about the patient's energy fields.

Treatment
Third phase: Using assessment information, the goal is to direct or modulate the energy and restore balance.

Indications for Therapeutic Touch
Promoting relaxation
Altering pain perception
Decreasing anxiety
Accelerating healing
Promoting comfort in dying

Potential Outcomes
Reduced respiratory rate
Facial flushing
Increased temperature of extremities
Relief of pain
Relaxation
Reduced anxiety

a patient's energy is imbalanced; the pattern and organization are disrupted. Yet organisms do have an intrinsic movement toward balance, order, and healing. In TT, the practitioner attempts to find areas of imbalance in a person's energy field. By using his or her hands as a focal point, the TT practitioner rebalances that energy to facilitate the field's natural movement toward harmony (Monzillo & Gronowicz, 2011). Box 2-5 provides an overview of the steps in TT, indications for its use, and potential outcomes; however, a crucial component is the practitioner's training and practice with a skilled TT practitioner.

Legal Issues and CAM

As discussed previously, more nurses are incorporating Integrative Health into their practice; therefore, the legal issues surrounding practice must be considered. Issues include investigating whether the nurse will use CAM modalities and if they fit within the nurse practice act of their particular state. Nurses should be knowledgeable of which modalities require individual licensing (i.e., massage) and which are covered under other practice acts (Radzyminski, 2007). Currently, registered nurses officially can include some CAM in their practice in many states, and other states are evaluating this issue (California Board of Nursing, 2014). Nurses should become familiar with their particular state nurse practice act and remain knowledgeable of the policies and guidelines that govern their practice. It is likely that within a short time, nurses and other healthcare providers will be held liable for not being knowledgeable of CAM and IHC practices (D. Bass, *personal communication*, April 2002; Cohen, 1998).

The concepts of health, wellness, and IHC have always been a part of nursing models of care. While the American healthcare system has been slow to make changes, the current discussion of healthcare reform provides nursing the opportunity to lead the way by modeling and providing care that is holistic, caring, and integrative.

KEY CONCEPTS

- Nurses are incorporating a wide range of ideas and practices from various traditions and cultures to support patients in their self-healing. Cultural competence is essential in today's healthcare setting.
- Patients who wanted to be treated as whole persons, not just a disease, challenged Western medicine and sought holistic healthcare.
- Nursing has had a tradition of holistic care and now are uniquely positioned to assist in the transition to Integrative Health.
- CAM was first introduced in 1996; the movement was driven by consumers wanting a more integrated model of healthcare.
- IM takes into account the whole person, emphasizing the relationship and use of all appropriate therapies, both conventional and alternative.
- TCM is a complete healing system and includes acupuncture, massage, herbal treatments, nutrition, moxibustion, movement such as qi gong, and meditation.
- Herbs and botanicals have been used for thousands of years in every culture.
- TT involves making contact with the energy field of the recipient.
- CAM will continue to be integrated with more allopathic medicine and nursing therapies.
- Integrative Health requires presence and deep listening and is larger than just adding CAM to allopathic medicine.

PRACTICING FOR THE NCLEX

CHECK YOUR ANSWERS IN APPENDIX A.

1. A patient is seen in the emergency department related to complaints of fatigue and weakness. Upon further questioning, the nurse finds that the patient has recently lost his job after 35 years and reports no appetite since he was let go 2 weeks ago. Which model of health and well-being best describes this patient's belief system?
   a. Holism
   b. High-level wellness
   c. Clinical model
   d. Health belief model

2. A nurse is working with a patient who recently received a mastectomy to prevent breast cancer due to a high rate of breast cancer in her family. The patient seems unengaged in the wound care and complains about nurses "doing stuff to her all of the time." Which of the following statements would be appropriate for the nurse to make to increase this patient's engagement and self-worth? Select all that apply.

  a. You have taken a great step in safeguarding your health by having this surgery.

  b. I'd like to show you how to change the dressing and what I am assessing when I look at your incision site so that you can do it at home.

  c. What do you think the hardest part of discharge care is going to be for you?

  d. You need to be responsible for your wound care once you leave. Here are some written instructions to tell you what you need to do.

3. A community health nurse is working with a smoking cessation group. One member states, "I had quit for a year and now I'm back to smoking with all this stress at work lately. I'll never be able to maintain it!" Which phase of change best describes this statement?

  a. Precontemplation

  b. Contemplation

  c. Preparation

  d. Termination

4. A nurse is admitting an elderly patient and is inquiring about her current health conditions and treatments. The patient states that she uses melatonin for frequent insomnia. Which of the following nursing actions are most appropriate to detail the use of CAM therapies? Select all that apply:

  a. Ask if there are any prescriptions taken for insomnia and document appropriately.

  b. Ask if the patient uses any other CAM therapies in addition to this supplement.

  c. Document the use of melatonin along with other vitamins, prescription, and nonprescription medications.

  d. Ask if the patient uses any other "non–evidence-based" therapies.

5. A patient is receiving acupuncture treatments in addition to chemotherapy to increase her energy and "keep her blood counts up." The nurse caring for this patient is not familiar with acupuncture in cancer care. Which of the following actions would improve her understanding of this type of CAM therapy? Select all that apply:

  a. Knowing where to access reliable information (e.g., NCCAM)

  b. Educating herself on acupuncture modality and history

  c. Actively referring to acupuncturists and developing a relationship

  d. Researching qualifications and credentials of practitioners

REFERENCES

Ardell, D. B. (2007). *Aging beyond belief: 69 Tips for REAL wellness*. Duluth, MN: Whole Person Associates.

Arloski, M. (2014). *Wellness coaching for lasting lifestyle change* (2nd ed.). Duluth, MN: Whole Person Associates, Inc.

Arvidsdotter, T., Marklund, B., & Taft, C. (2014). Six month effects of integrative treatment, therapeutic acupuncture and conventional treatment in alleviating psychological distress in primary care patients—follow up from an open, pragmatic randomized controlled trial. *BMC Complement and Alternative Medicine, 14*:210.

Barnes, P. M., Bloom, B., & Nahin, R. (2008). *Complementary and alternative medicine use among adults and children: United States, 2007 (National Health Statistics Rep. No. 12)*. Hyattsville, MD: National Center for Health Statistics.

Booth-Laforce, C., Scott, C. S., Heitkemper, M. M., Cornman, J., Lan, M., Bond, E. F., et al. (2010). Complementary and alternative medicine (CAM) attitudes and competencies of nursing students and faculty: Results of integrating CAM into the nursing curriculum. *Journal of Professional Nursing, 26*(5), 293–300.

California Board of Nursing. (2014). *Complementary and alternative therapies in registered nursing practice*. Retrieved December 4, 2014, from http://www.rn.ca.gov/pdfs/regulations/npr-b-28.pdf

Carpenito-Moyet, L. J. (2012). *Handbook of nursing diagnosis* (13th ed.) Philadelphia, PA: Lippincott Williams & Wilkins.

Crute, S. (2008). The best medicine. *AARP Magazine*, March/April, 58–64.

Dossett, M. L., Davis, R. B., Lembo, A. L., Yeh, G. Y. (2014). Complementary and alternative medicine use by US adults with gastrointestinal conditions: Results from the 2012 National Health Interview Survey. *The American Journal of Gastroenterology*. DOI:10.1038/ajg.2014.108

Dossey, B. M. (2013). A theory of integral nursing. In B. M. Dossey, & L. Keegan (Eds.), *Holistic nursing: A handbook for practice* (6th ed.). Burlington, MA: Jones & Bartlett Publishing.

Dunn, H. L. (1961). *High-level wellness*. Arlington, VA: R. W. Beatty.

Edwards, E., Belard, J. L., Glowa, J., Khalsa, P., Weber, W., Huntley, K. (2013). DoD-NCCAM/NIH workshop on acupuncture for treatment of acute pain. *Journal of Alternative and Complementary Medicine, 19*(3): 266–279. DOI: 10.1089/acm.2012.9229.dod. Epub 2012 Sep 28.

Fitzpatrick, J. J. (2007). Research on health promotion. *Applied Nursing Research, 20*(2), 55.

Gao, D. (2013). *Traditional Chinese medicine: The complete guide to acupressure, acupuncture, Chinese herbal medicine, food cures and Qi Gong*. London: Carlton Books.

Garcia, M. K., McQuade, J., Haddad, R., Patel, S., Lee, R., Yang, P., et al. (2013). Systematic review of acupuncture in cancer care: A synthesis of the evidence. *Journal of Clinical Oncology, 31*(7):952–960.

Guarneri, E., Horrigan, B. J., & Perhura, C. M. (2010). The efficacy and coast effectiveness of Integrative Medicine: A review of the medical and corporate literature. *Explore, 6*(5):308–312.

Hutchinson, A. J., Ball, S., Andrews, J. C., & Jones, G. G. (2012). The effectiveness of acupuncture in treating chronic non-specific low back pain: A systematic review of the literature *Journal of Orthopedic Surgical Research, 7*:36. DOI: 10.1186/1749-799X-7-36

Koithan, M. (2014). Concepts and principles of integrative nursing. In M. J. Kreitzer, & M. Koithan (Eds.), *Integrative Nursing* (1st ed.). New York: Oxford University Press.

Krieger, D. (1993). *Accepting your power to heal: The personal practice of therapeutic touch*. Santa Fe, NM: Bear & Co. Publishing.

Kunz, D. (Ed.) (1995). *Spiritual healing*. Wheaton, IL: Theosophical Publishing House.

Lam, C. S., Wiley, A. H., Siu, A., & Emmett J. (2010). Assessing readiness to work from a stages of change perspective: Implications for return to work. *Work, 37*(3), 321–329.

Lee, R. (2010). The new pandemic: SuperStress. *Explore, 6*(1), 7–10.

Lemly, B. (2014). *Balanced Living. Weil.com News.* Retrieved December 4, 2014, from http://www.drweil.com/drw/u/ART02054/Andrew-Weil-Integrative-Medicine.html

Levey, J., & Levey, M. (2014). *Living in balance: A mindful guide for thriving in a complex world.* Studio City, CA: Divine Arts.

Mao, J. J., & Kapur, R. (2010). Acupuncture in primary care. *Primary Care, 37*(1), 105–117.

Mariano, C. (2013). Holistic nursing: Scope and standards of practice. In B. M. Dossey & L. Keegan (Eds.), *Holistic nursing: A handbook for practice* (pp. 47–74). Sudbury, MA: Jones & Bartlett.

May, C. S., & Russell, C. S. (2013). Health coaching: Adding value in health-care reform. *Global Advances in Health and Medicine, 2*(3), 92–94.

Montero, D., Walther, G., Stehouwer, C. D., Houben, A. J., Beckman, J. A., & Vinet, A. (2014). Effect of antioxidant vitamin supplementation on endothelial function in type 2 diabetes mellitus: A systematic review and meta-analysis of randomized controlled trials. *Obesity Reviews, 15*(2), 107–116.

Monzillo, E., & Gronowicz, G. (2011). New insights on therapeutic touch: A discussion of experimental methodology and design that resulted in significant effects on normal human cells and osteosarcoma. *Explore: The Journal of Science and Healing, 7*(1), 44–51.

National Cancer Institute. (2012). *Theory at a glance: A guide for health promotion practice.* US Department of Health and Human Services, Public Health Service, National Institutes of Health, National Cancer Institute. NCCAM (2013). Retrieved August 15, 2014, from http:/nccam.nih.gov/sites/nccam.nih.gov/about/nccam/2013febmin.pdf

National Center for Complementary and Integrative Health (NCCIH) (2014). https://nccih.nih.gov/news/press/12172014 (accessed June 19, 2015).

Nightingale, F. (1969). *Notes on nursing: What it is and what it is not.* New York, NY: Dover Publications. (Unabridged republication of the first American edition, as published in 1860 by D. Appleton & Company.)

Patient Centered Outcomes Research Institute. (2010). Retrieved August 15, 2014, from http://www.pcori.org/assets/{CORI-Authorizing-Legislation-032310.pdf

Pender, N. J., Murdaugh, C. L., & Parsons, M. A. (2010). *Health promotion in nursing practice* (6th ed.). Upper Saddle River, NJ: Prentice Hall.

Quinn, J. (2009). Transpersonal human caring and healing. In B. M. Dossey & L. Keegan (Eds.), *Holistic nursing* (5th ed., pp. 91–99). Sudbury, MA: Jones & Bartlett.

Radzyminski, S. (2007). Legal parameters of alternative-complementary modalities in nursing practice. *Nursing Clinics of North America, 42*(2), 189–212.

Rogers, M. (1990). *An introduction to the theoretical basis of nursing.* Philadelphia, PA: F. A. Davis.

Rosenstock, I. (1974). Historical origin of the health belief model. *Health Education Monographs, 2*, 334.

Schell, B., Gillen, G., & Scaffa, M. (2014). *Willard and Spackman's occupational therapy.* Philadelphia, PA: Lippincott Williams & Wilkins.

Sharma, M., & Rush, S. E. (2014). Mindfulness-based stress reduction as a stress management intervention for healthy individuals: A systemized review. *Journal of Evidenced Based Complementary and Alternative Medicine, 19*(4), 271–286. DOI: 2156587214543143

Smuts, J. C. (1926). *Holism and evolution.* New York, NY: Macmillan.

Sparks, S. M. & Taylor, C. M. (2014). *Nursing diagnosis reference manual* (9th ed.). Philadelphia, PA: Lippincott Williams & Wilkins.

Strauss, S. E. (2008). *NCCAM Strategic Plan, 2005–2009. A message from the director.* Retrieved December 4, 2014, from http://nccam.nih.gov/about/ATAGLANCE

Sun, Y., Gan, T. J., Dubose, J. W., & Habib, A. S. (2008). Acupuncture and related techniques for postoperative pain: A systematic review of randomized controlled trials. *British Journal of Anaesthesia, 101*(2), 151–160.

Taylor, A. G., Goehler, L. E., Galper, D. I., Innes, K. E., & Bourguignon, C. (2010). Top-down and bottom-up mechanisms in mind-body medicine: Development of an integrative framework for psychophysiological research. *Explore, 6*(1), 29–41.

Therapeutic Touch International Association. (2014). Retrieved August 10, 2014, from http://therapeutic-touch.org

Travis, J. W., & Ryan, R. S. (1988). *Wellness workbook.* Berkeley, CA: Ten Speed Press.

Tsouronunis, C., & Bent, S. (2010). Why change is needed in research examining dietary supplements. *Clinical Pharmacology and Therapeutics, 87*(2), 14709.

Upchurch, D. M., Dye, C. E., Chyu, E., Gold, E. B., & Greendale, G. E. (2010). Demographic, behavioral, and health correlates of complementary and alternative medicine and prayer use among midlife women: 2002. *Journal of Women's Health, 19*(1), 23–30.

US Department of Health and Human Services, Public Health Service. (2010). *Healthy people 2020.* Washington, DC: U.S. Government Printing Office.

Wager, S. (1996). *A doctor's guide to therapeutic touch.* New York, NY: Berkeley Publishing Group.

Weaver, J. B., May, D., Hopkins, G. L., Eroglu, D. & Bernhardt, J. M (2010). Health information: Seeking behaviors, health indicators, and health risks. *American Journal of Public Health, 100*(8), 1520–1525.

Weeks, J. (2014). *Integrative medicine, complementary and alternative medicine and health round-up #81.* Retrieved August 14, 2014, from http://theintegratorblog.com/index.php?option=view&id=Itemid=93

Weil, A. (1994). *Healthy aging.* Retrieved December 4, 2014, from http://www.drweil.com/drw/u/ART02011/healthy-aging

Weil, A. (2009). *Why our health matters. A vision of medicine that can transform our future.* New York, NY: Hudson Street Press.

World Health Organization. (1948). *Preamble to the Constitution of the World Health Organization as adopted by the International Health Conference*, New York, NY, June 19–22, 1946. Retrieved December 4, 2014, from www.who.int/about/definition/en/print.html

CHAPTER 3

Healthcare in the Community and Home

Lauren Valk Lawson

Case Scenario

You are employed as a clinic nurse at an Indian Health Service (IHS) facility serving a population of 4,300 tribal members on a reservation. You identify that the incidence and severity of diabetes problems are escalating dramatically for tribal members. You note that there is a high rate of missed appointments in the diabetes clinic. You find it difficult to follow up with patients because many have no telephones. Patients tell you that some of their difficulties getting to clinic are due to lack of reliable transportation to the clinic and the long distance they need to travel to get there. Some patients say they don't feel they are respected when they do make it to the clinic. In addition, you learn that many grandparents and great-grandparents may be unable to leave home because of child care responsibilities for extended family members. The nearest hospital and dialysis facility is over 100 miles away at another IHS unit. You decide to consult with the community health nurses who work for the Tribal Health Department to assist you in developing a plan that will lead to more effectively meeting the health needs of the people you serve with the resources available regionally.

Once you have completed this chapter and have incorporated healthcare in the community and home into your knowledge base, review the above scenario and reflect on the following areas of Critical Thinking:

1. Describe the work skills and knowledge base you will need to function effectively in community-based nursing practice.
2. Explain the importance of continuity of care and discharge planning in the emerging healthcare system.
3. Propose how nurses will work with various sectors of the community and healthcare professionals.
4. Predict the opportunities for the nursing profession within the changing healthcare system.
5. Calculate what will happen to hospitals in the future.

KEY TERMS
advocacy
aesthetics/spirituality
case management
community-based healthcare
community-based nursing care
community resources
continuity of care
coordination
discharge planning
facilitator
health determinants
healthy communities/healthy cities
home healthcare
hospice
levels of healthcare
nursing competencies for community-based care patient education

LEARNING OBJECTIVES

Upon completion of this chapter, the student will be able to do the following:

1. Discuss what is meant by community-based healthcare.
2. Identify three levels of healthcare and the services under each level.
3. Identify the role of various settings for community-based healthcare.
4. Explain how social, professional, and financial considerations have influenced the growth of community-based healthcare.
5. Determine the focus of nursing care in all settings and situations.
6. Discuss forms of community-based nursing practice, both traditional and more recent.
7. Identify the importance of continuity of care and discharge planning.
8. Describe the management of healthcare needs in the home from a systems perspective.
9. Identify factors that influence the patient's ability to manage healthcare within the home.
10. Explain the major areas requiring assessment by a home care nurse.
11. Describe nursing roles and responsibilities in home care.
12. Identify the importance of community resources in the care of patients receiving home care services.

The *Patient Protection and Affordable Health Care Act* (ACA), which was passed in 2010, seeks to make healthcare more affordable, create competitive insurance plans, provide greater accountability, end discrimination, and make the budget and economy more stable (White House, 2014). As the various components of the ACA are phased in (see Box 3-1), opportunities will exist for nurses to play an influential role in the implementation of new health policy. For example, as the focus of healthcare moves away from the acute care setting into community-based services, nurses provide the ideal prospective for the case management required in transitional care (Vincent & Reed, 2014).

Most legislative discussions about national healthcare share two key strategies: primary healthcare measures and the public health concepts of health promotion/disease prevention services. Primary care is defined as the provision of health services to individuals within the context of the community in which they live. As hospital stays are shortened, care provided in the community has expanded. Community-based care becomes more significant than institution-based care as emphasis moves to primary healthcare. With the integration of the public health concepts of health promotion and disease prevention, primary care services can partner with individuals to help them obtain their optimal level of health (Institute of Medicine, 2012).

The nurse's essential role includes collaborating with individuals to manage their healthcare needs in the home setting and using community resources to support patients in this effort. The management of healthcare needs in the home setting involves not only the patient but also family members, friends, and other sources of support. The goals are to allow people to regain or maintain optimal health, to function within their limitations, and to remain in the home environment. A key to successful care management is the quality of the nurse–patient relationship in the context of the patient's family and community. In partnership with patients, the nurse facilitates individuals' abilities to accomplish health and self-care goals.

BOX 3-1 **Major Provisions of the Affordable Care Act**

- Requires all US citizens and legal residents to have healthcare; those without coverage pay tax penalties
- Creates state-based healthcare exchanges through which individuals may purchase healthcare
- Requires employers with 50 or more employees to offer healthcare coverage
- Expands Medicaid to cover individuals with incomes up to 133% of the federal poverty level
- Provides coverage for children up to 26 years of age
- Prohibits annual and lifetime dollar amount limits
- Prohibits exclusion from coverage for children based on preexisting medical condition

- Creates a value-based purchasing program within Medicare that pays hospitals based on performance measures
- Eliminates co-payments for preventive services recommended by the U.S. Preventive Services Task Force
- Provides Medicaid coverage for smoking cessation services for pregnant women
- Narrows the coverage gap for prescription drugs in Medicare Part D
- Increases primary care physician training positions
- Increases support and training for healthcare professionals in primary care and in underserved areas

People have a perception of themselves in relation to the world and their ability to maintain independence. Independence is often linked to the ability to manage and care for oneself at home, within their family and community. It involves the ability to meet basic needs and to manage the complex activities necessary for self-care and independent functioning in society.

As a patient moves or is moved from one environment to another, nurses must consider the patient's ability to carry out activities of daily living (ADLs). Understanding the patient in relation to the living environment, their home, their family, and their community is important in developing plans for care that maximize the person's ability to maintain independence safely.

LEVELS OF HEALTHCARE

The U.S. Department of Health and Human Services Division of Nursing has analyzed current nursing practice and education in relation to population healthcare needs. **Levels of healthcare** are categorized as primary, secondary, and tertiary (Fig. 3-1). Most current resources, services, nursing practice, and nursing education exist within the category of secondary healthcare: emergency care, acute and critical care, diagnosis, and treatment. The population's needs, however, fall mostly within the categories of primary healthcare (health promotion, education, protection, and screening) and tertiary healthcare (rehabilitation, long-term care, support services, and hospice care).

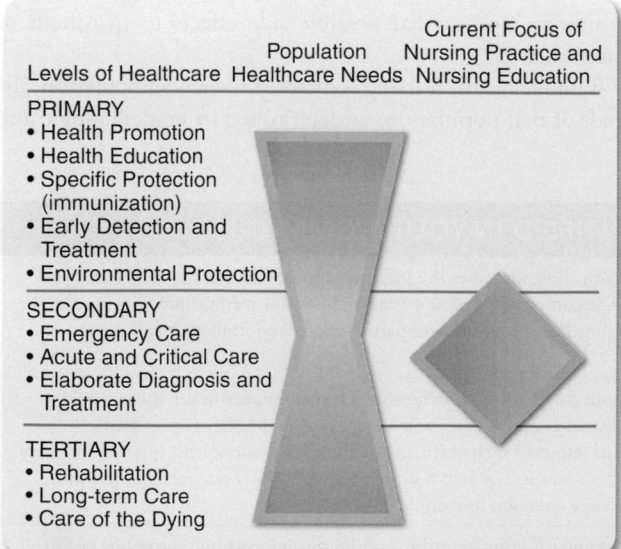

FIGURE 3-1 Levels of healthcare need. Whereas the population's needs are clustered at the primary and tertiary levels, nursing practice and education concentrate at the secondary level. (Developed by the Nursing Practice Branch, Department of Health and Human Services.)

Community-Based Healthcare Trends and the Determinants of Health

People believe "quality of life" to be synonymous with a healthy community. There is growing recognition that to achieve the goals of *Healthy People 2020: Understanding and Improving Health*, a model inclusive of multiple **health determinants** is needed. Clinical care has typically focused on diagnosing and treating symptoms. Understanding health in relation to personal behaviors, social factors, and other determinants provides a holistic context. As an example, it is important to know an individual's access to a grocery store with fresh fruits and vegetables to comprehend his or her nutritional needs (U.S. Department of Health and Human Services, 2014). To affect social, economic, political, and educational health determinants, health initiatives are more effective if they are based in the community and incorporate community collaboration.

Community-Based Healthcare

Community-based healthcare is the design, delivery, and evaluation of healthcare services developed in partnership with communities. *Community* is broadly defined and may be a workplace, school district attendance area, enrollees of a managed care insurance provider, a geographically defined area, or a group or place identified by a categorical or medical need. Community-based healthcare is found where people are—where they work, recreate, and go to school and church—and is developed within the context of a given community (e.g., its unique needs and strengths). Partnerships assume equity in contributions, participation, commitment to common interests, and close association. Respect, appreciation, and cooperation characterize successful partnerships. The nature of the nurse–patient relationship in community-based care is one of partnership.

Primary care providers, hospitals, retirement communities, pharmacies, rehabilitation centers, and other types of providers from a large geographic area will be connected formally. For example, the ACA provided for establishment of accountable care organizations (ACOs). These ACOs consist of a network of hospitals and providers that are responsible for collaborating to provide efficient and quality care to assigned patients. Key to these services is the premise that ACOs will need to demonstrate adequate management of chronic illnesses and prevention of costly hospital readmissions (National Council of State Boards of Nursing, 2014).

Nursing's Agenda for Health Care Reform (American Nurses Association [ANA], 2008) is the US nursing community's proactive position on how, where, and by whom healthcare should be delivered. It promotes an approach in which healthcare is taken to the consumer who, in turn, will be an increasingly informed participant in decisions affecting his or her care. Healthcare services will be delivered in such places as the place of employment or school-based clinics. Hospitals and other institutions will remain significant components of the healthcare system, but they will no longer be the central focus or dominant influence. The consumer will assume a more dominant position. The ACA makes strides toward nursing's vision of healthcare focused on health promotion, delivered where the individual needs it, and focused on wellness rather than disease management, but there is much work still to be done as the effects of the ACA become known.

Community-Based Nursing

Community-based nursing care can be defined as nursing care directed toward individuals of a specific group or population within the context of the community where they live. Examples of community-based nursing care are clinics in schools or home healthcare. Community-based care is generally secondary or tertiary care, addressing the acute and chronic health issues commonly seen in a population. Case management is an important tool of a community-based nurse; it includes skills such as coordination of care, health education, and **advocacy** (Stanhope & Lancaster, 2012). Community-based nursing presents a special opportunity for nurses to apply the nursing process and knowledge, in partnership with patients.

There are three defined roles in which nurses work in the community: community-based nursing, community health nursing, and public health nursing. As healthcare reform moves services away from tertiary care with more provision of care in the community, these roles may overlap and the difference can be confusing. Though all three specialties function in the community, the key difference is the relationship. Community-based nursing provides acute or chronic care services to the individual within the context of the individual's community. A community health nurse provides services to individuals, families, and groups identified by the risk factors of the community. Services of the community health nurse focus on prevention and health promotion. In public health nursing, the community is the patient with the focus of practice on primary prevention (Stanhope & Lancaster, 2012; ANA, 2013, 2014). Table 3-1 provides an example of the different scopes of practice for the diagnosis of asthma. The spectrum of care between community-based, community health, and public health nursing demonstrates the versatility and opportunity that community care provides.

FOCUS OF NURSING CARE

Although the setting for care and the type of intervention may change, the nursing focus is always the same, the holistic care of an individual. Wherever he or she practices, the nurse's concern is to provide for healthcare that focuses not only the physiologic needs but also the psychosocial and spiritual needs of the person in relation to the environment.

In nursing practice in the hospital, physical and mental stabilization is a primary goal for most patients. Needs include physiologic monitoring, complete or partial personal care, exercise, nutritional support, pain management, treatment and medication administration, anticipatory guidance, counseling, and teaching. Care needs are complex. Because of the trend toward shorter lengths of stay, the patient may be discharged before counseling and teaching are finished.

In settings outside the hospital, the nurse's activities change. If nursing care is directed toward an individual—for example, in home healthcare—the physiologic crisis is resolving, but care needs may remain intense. Assessment of the home and involvement of family/significant others in direct care are essential. Planning and intervention focus on using individual, family, and community resources to assist in restoring a patient's health to maximum possible functioning while continuing to monitor for possible side effects to treatment or complications.

If public health nursing is directed toward a population, the needs of that population, as determined by epidemiologic and

TABLE 3-1 A CURRENT HEALTH CONCERN IS IDENTIFIED IN YOUR COMMUNITY	
Community-based nurse	A community-based nurse at the local community health clinic identifies the patients at the clinic that have children in the identified age range with the diagnosis of asthma. The community-based nurse would review medications with the family, assure they know the signs and symptoms requiring medical attention, and participate in a clinical case management review.
Community health nurse	A community health nurse would provide follow-up with the family at a home visit. The community health nurse would educate the parents regarding preventive methods; would assess for deterrents to access of healthcare, such as medical insurance; and would refer the family to other needed resources such as for an environmental assessment. Information from the home visit will assist the nurse in developing other resources, such as a support group for parents with children with asthma or written material that outlines ways to decrease common household allergens.
Public health nurse	A public health nurse would monitor the statistics regarding ER visits for asthma. From this information, the public health nurse may identify that most of the children admitted to hospitals with complications secondary to their asthma have inadequate health insurance. A subsequent intervention would be for the public health nurse to advocate for the availability of low-cost healthcare for the at-risk children or develop a program linking elementary schools with an asthma prevention program.

There is a documented increase in asthma-related emergency room admission among children at a local elementary school.

demographic data and input from the population, help to set priorities. For example, work site healthcare services are individualized to the industry involved (factory workers vs. white-collar workers).

COMMUNITY-BASED NURSING PRACTICE IN TRANSITION

Many state health departments focus on patient contact during clinic visits for maternity and child services, infectious diseases, and primary care. Other common community-based settings for nursing practice include schools (school nursing), the workplace (occupational health nursing), and homes (hospice and home healthcare nursing). School nurses focus on the health of children attending their schools. Health screening, education, counseling, crisis intervention, and first aid or chronic care management are some functions within school nursing practice. Occupational health nurses focus on worker populations; they stress the promotion, protection, and restoration of workers' health within the context of a safe and healthy work environment. Hospice nurses focus on the dying. Palliative care within a multidisciplinary team and family support are essential elements of hospice practice.

Currently, the focus of nursing care in home healthcare (see Fig. 3-2) is on complex chronic health situations (e.g., multiple medications, patient confusion, or poor social support) or acute care assistance (e.g., fetal monitoring or home intravenous antibiotic therapy). This focus is largely determined by care covered by the healthcare system and may not meet all patient needs.

Many nurses working in community settings provide services in the home by making home visits. Home visits reveal information that the nurse cannot gather in other ways. Safe sleeping environments and other household risks are examples of information gathered through observations during home visits. By focusing on the whole person within his or her environment, the nurse will be able to determine optimal interventions not otherwise apparent.

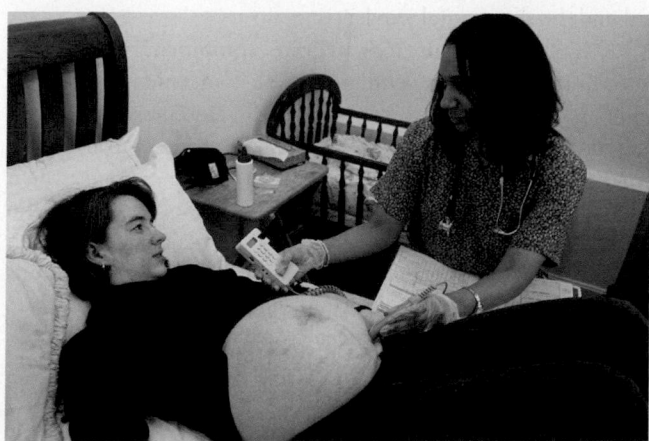

FIGURE 3-2 Home health nurses provide holistic care to patients with complex chronic health situations or acute care needs.

HOME HEALTHCARE

Home healthcare is characterized by a range of health issues and related services. Such services are delivered to persons at home who are recovering from illness, are disabled, or are chronically or terminally ill and need various services to progress, maintain function, or perform their ADLs. Services to manage healthcare needs at home can involve a team of interdisciplinary professionals, including social workers; physical, occupational, and speech therapists; and home health aides. Home care nursing is the provision of nursing care to acute, chronically ill, and well patients of all ages in their homes. It integrates community health nursing principles that focus on health promotion and on environmental, psychosocial, economic, cultural, and personal health factors affecting an individual's and family's health status.

Trends Affecting Home Healthcare

One aspect of the changing healthcare system is the increasing role of home management. A major reason for this growth has been earlier discharge of people from hospital to home and a growing demand for home-based services from patients and their families. This trend has been further enhanced through the expansion of payments for community- and home-based services in the ACA (Harrington, Ng, La Plante, & Kaye, 2012).

In addition, prospective payment has been introduced in home healthcare. Home health agencies are now required by Medicare to collect and report standardized information: the Outcome and Assessment Information Set (OASIS). OASIS provides standardized guidelines for admission and care as well as a national database for evaluation, reimbursement, and quality improvement (Marrelli, 2012).

Home as Healthcare Setting

A person's environment comprises his or her physical, psychological, and social surroundings. An important aspect of this environment is that it is where a person turns for support, intimacy, relaxation, sustenance, and protection from the outside world. For most people, this place is called "home." Living in one's own home is usually linked to the ability to manage and care for oneself.

Optimal management in the home occurs when a person can independently maintain a growth-promoting environment (Fig. 3-3). The home is comfortable and safe, and the person performs self-care and hygiene tasks, interacts with others, meets financial obligations, and engages in activities that are satisfying and worthwhile. Although some people may have deficits, they can adjust to their situation through their own resourcefulness or with assistance from others.

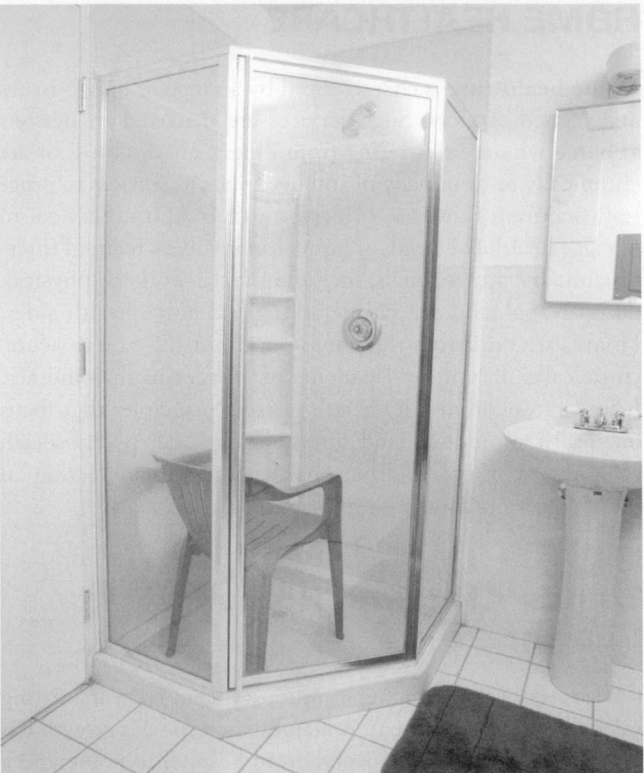

FIGURE 3-3 Safety features such as guardrails and helpful equipment such as a shower chair can assist patients to manage their healthcare independently.

Home Care Versus Acute Care

An essential difference in home care versus acute care is that the home care nurse is a "guest" in the patient's home and on the patient's turf. In the home, patients and families retain the power and control that they give to providers in other settings. Nurses in the home usually work as members of a therapeutic team. In addition, home care nurses usually have a caseload of patients of varying ages and with a range of health concerns. Therefore, a generalist background and focus are useful. The home management of many healthcare needs also requires broad assessment skills and a knowledge base to provide patients with appropriate teaching to help them remain as independent as possible. Because of the increased independent role in home management, the nurse must know resources within the agency and community to support care at home and must have basic knowledge of payors and their regulations. Support and education of lay caregivers such as family or friends require that the nurse in the home collaborate closely with them.

Role of Family and Community: A Systems View

The home management of a person's healthcare needs usually occurs within the context of family, friends, and community. A systems view suggests that the individual, family, and

community continually interact and influence one another by exchanging information and energy. This interaction and influence occur within all environments: physical, social, behavioral, economic, and political. What affects a person can also affect his or her family and the community in which they all live. For example, if a person has a communicable disease, this disease may spread to the family as well as friends and neighbors. Community resources such as the local health department may then provide services to the individual and family.

Factors Affecting Home Healthcare Management

Altered ability to manage healthcare needs independently may result from decreased functional abilities, insufficient family or social supports, or insufficient community resources. Physical deficits or chronic debilitating diseases that decrease the patient's ability to perform ADLs can lead to difficulty in maintaining independence. Such factors include the medical diagnosis of a chronic debilitating or limiting condition, the medical prognosis for the condition, and the need for treatments and complex medication regimens (Carpenito-Moyet, 2013). In addition, deficits in social support or community resources may compromise a family's capacity for independence in all ADLs. The Blaylock Risk Assessment Screening Score (BRASS) helps identify patients who may need assistance at discharge from the hospital. The evidence-based screening tool has also been shown to be predictive of extended length of hospital stay (Cunic, Lacombe, Mohajer, Grant, & Wood, 2014).

FUNCTIONAL ABILITIES

Developmental Stage

The patient's developmental stage necessitates specific home care needs. The patient requires physical care, but the nurse also needs to address developmental needs. An advanced understanding of the many challenges of various developmental levels is imperative if the nurse is to meet the patient's physical and developmental needs.

A high-risk infant may require equipment to monitor breathing or to assist ventilation that is intimidating to parents. That infant, however, still needs closeness and bonding with parents. The nurse supports the parents to meet the infant's physical and emotional needs and encourages them to strengthen the parent–child bond. A school-age child who requires home care for either an acute or a chronic condition needs support for normal socialization and peer relationships and for continuity in education. The needs that home care nursing can immediately meet are only part of this child's overall needs.

The adolescent who is in need of long-term home care has a unique combination of support needs. In addition to the physical needs that necessitated home care, the adolescent may be struggling with issues related to independence, maintaining peer relationships while unable to participate in activities, and keeping up with educational demands. The home care nurse can assist in coordinating care needs and encouraging family, teachers, schoolmates, and friends to understand the patient's struggles and help support his or her needs.

Patients at the end of their lives will need support beyond meeting health needs. Encouragement to complete a life review, education for family and friends about what to expect during the dying process, and assisting with funeral arrangements may all be part of the home care nurse's role description.

Health Promotion and Safety Deficits

Injury potential, altered health maintenance, and knowledge deficit regarding self-care procedures are important considerations in home management. Injury potential is an issue if any person's safety is threatened; an example is a stairway without railings on which children could fall and hurt themselves. Altered health maintenance due to health beliefs, change in financial situation, or lack of supervision can also impair a person's ability to live at home independently or safely. If a patient cannot learn to manage necessary diets or treatments, the ability to promote health at home is impaired. People living alone who have decreased functional abilities may manifest the following:

- Decreased ability for self-care or care of family members
- Decreased maintenance of safe and clean living space
- Decreased maintenance of economic obligations
- Decreased cognitive functioning and ability to respond appropriately to environmental stimuli

Cognitive and Sensory Deficits

Sensory loss, especially blindness, can hinder the ability to manage independently. Loss of sight can decrease independent functioning and increase the risk of injury. Severe pain can also decrease a person's ability to carry out daily activities and functions. An alteration in thought processes, if not responsive to treatment, can profoundly affect the ability to manage at home. Dementia is a progressive condition in which memory loss and confusion greatly affect the patient's functional abilities. The severely confused person cannot live independently and may be unable to live safely with the family because of the care demand. Mental illness, such as schizophrenia and substance abuse, also may impair a person's ability to manage at home with or without significant support from family or community resources.

Decreased Mobility

Many medical problems (e.g., arthritis, neurologic impairments, fractures, respiratory disease, cardiovascular disease, cancer) can impair a patient's mobility and alter self-care abilities. Minor mobility problems may make housework or home repairs difficult; limited mobility may also hinder the patient's ability to leave the house safely in case of fire or emergency. The inability to do grooming, toileting, and personal hygiene tasks may impair the person's ability to live independently. The inability to maintain home hygiene and cleanliness may pose health and safety risks.

Altered Elimination

Inability to control bowel or bladder function affects the ability to manage independently in a home setting. Often, such impairment occurs with other dysfunction, such as mobility problems after a stroke, neurologic insult, or decreasing cognitive function.

Altered Nutrition

The inability to provide adequate nutrition impairs the patient's ability to manage independently. Buying and cooking food and cleaning up require energy. Depression can decrease the desire to eat properly, especially when the person lives alone or a specialized diet is required. Lack of financial resources may also hinder proper nutrition. Physical changes affecting chewing and swallowing also contribute to the potential for impaired home management.

Family and Social Supports

Family and social supports can compensate for functional deficits, and the extent to which family members and friends are interested or able to help is a crucial factor in keeping a person with healthcare needs in the home. The family and friends' coping abilities and reserves, commitment and ability to be caregivers, and personal health are factors in the amount of support that can be given. Busy adults may need their energy for their own home and family; they may not have time to meet the needs of an older person or a person with special needs. Family members of the person with functional health deficits may show signs of not being able to maintain the patient or themselves at home. Caregivers responsible for around-the-clock supervision of the patient may show signs of stress, reduced ability to cope, alterations in functional abilities, and financial loss. Physical or verbal abuse may signal severe family stress. Those individuals classified as "baby boomers" (usually classified as born between 1946 and 1964) are often caring for older parents while still raising children. This has resulted in this group being called the "sandwich generation" because they are in the middle of meeting the needs of older and younger family members dependent on them for care.

People with decreased family, social, or community resources and decreased internal resources may manifest altered or impaired home management in any of the following ways:

- Decreased ability or availability of caregivers to assist with or perform self-care activities
- Decreased assistance in meeting financial obligations
- Inability to reach available resources
- Unavailability of community resources or services specific to the patient's needs

COMMUNITY RESOURCES

Community and service deficits (lack of community agencies that provide supportive health and social services to assist the patient) affect a patient's ability to manage in the home.

TABLE 3-2 WEBSITES FOR COMMUNITY-BASED INITIATIVES

Website Address	Website Name/Description
www.ncl.org	National Civic League, Healthy Communities Program
www.healthycommunities.org	Association for Community Health Improvement
www.hmhb.org	National Healthy Mothers, Healthy Babies Coalition
www.sustainable.org	Sustainable Communities Online
www.paho.org	Pan American Health Organization
www.globalhealthaction.org	Global Health Action
www.nursemanifest.com/manifesto.htm	NurseManifest: A Call to Conscience and Action
www.compact.org	Coalition of campuses to support students and faculty in community partnership efforts
www.faithbasedcommunityinitiatives.org	White House Office of Faith and Community-Based initiatives

Some chronically mentally ill and developmentally disabled people cannot manage their finances or maintain hygienic living conditions without community assistance. Their environmental conditions may be stable, but without daily supervision from professionals or family, they would be evicted and could become homeless.

Unhealthy or unsanitary living conditions indicate impaired home management. Unsanitary conditions, rodent infestation, or environmental hazards are visual cues to an unhealthy environment. Lack of running water, electricity, heat, or proper storage facilities for food also are seen in poor living conditions. Many websites highlight community resources available (Table 3-2).

COMMUNITY-BASED HEALTHCARE ISSUES

Fragmentation of Service

Explosive growth of knowledge in healthcare has led to specialization throughout the healthcare system. The price for this specialization is fragmented care. For example, a surgical patient with diabetes receives care from a surgeon and an endocrinologist or internist. If that same patient has heart problems during surgery, a cardiologist is called. The patient may spend time in surgery, the recovery room, the intensive or coronary care unit, a step-down unit, and a medical or surgical unit. After discharge, this fragmentation may continue as different specialists prescribe different medications and require follow-up visits. This can confuse and upset the patient and family. It can also compound the patient's health problems.

Of equal importance is the fragmentation that often results as patients move from one system of care to the next or when a government agency or program is not able to address community needs because the issues are so complex. For example, to address a community issue such as domestic violence, professionals in law enforcement, the judicial system, social services,

and health services may be required to work together when no such collaborations have been established. Without systematic partnership building and coordination of services and communication, individuals, families, and communities continue to suffer and problems go unaddressed. Fragmented services not only result in poor healthcare outcomes but also excessive healthcare costs valued in the billions (Center for Health Research & Transformation, 2014).

Complementary and Alternative Healthcare Services

Complementary and alternative healthcare is care composed of treatments outside Western medicine. These treatments may include acupuncture, acupressure, therapeutic touch, herbal treatments, hypnosis, imagery, homeopathy, and chiropractic. The Office of Alternative Medicine is a part of the National Institutes of Health (NIH) whose role it is to examine these treatments and their effects on patient outcomes. Reflecting the increasing significance and impact of these practices, the office was recently upgraded to an NIH "Center," with the subsequent name change to the National Center for Complementary and Alternative Medicine (NCCAM; http://nccam.nih.gov).

Self-Care

Self-care is a concept whose time has come, as evidenced by several trends. Prior to 2014, more than 41 million nonelderly Americans were without health insurance (Centers for Disease Control and Prevention, 2013). By necessity, self-care becomes important and highly valued. Consumers are no longer passive regarding their health; they understand the relationships of lifestyle, attitudes, and behaviors to well-being. Many healthcare providers and services are promoting self-care as a strategy to reduce consumption of expensive medical services. Nurses are in a significant position to encourage individuals, families, communities, and organizations to build on inherent strengths, capacities, and self-care abilities.

Discharge Planning

Continuity of care is provision of health services without disruption, regardless of movement between settings. Continuity of care is a concern across the healthcare continuum. All models of community-based nursing address it. An organizational structure must be in place to ensure continuity of care from one healthcare setting to the next and among health professionals and community systems.

As part of the Affordable Care Act, hospitals may accrue penalties for readmissions of patients with certain diagnoses within 30 days of discharge. To improve patient outcomes and avoid penalties, care transitions are being implemented to improve the continuity of services from hospital to home and to reduce readmissions (Center for Health Research & Transformation, 2014). A collaborative discharge plan that includes the patient's primary care services as well as any home care is essential for transitional care to be successful.

Discharge planning prepares a patient to move from one level of care to another within or outside the current healthcare facility. Traditionally, this process involved discharge from the hospital to the home. In the current healthcare system, discharge planning occurs from all settings, including ambulatory surgical centers, rehabilitation units, drug treatment centers, and childbirth centers. Discharge can also occur within a facility as a patient moves from one unit to another (e.g., a patient with a cerebrovascular accident moves from a medical–surgical unit to the rehabilitation unit). Discharge planning is also important for patients returning to the home, with arrangement for services as needed.

Discharge planning is most successful when it is done in collaboration with the patient and family, not for them. The discharge planner is the health or social services professional who is responsible for coordinating the transition and serving as a link between the discharging facility and the community. Often, the discharge planner is a nurse who cares for the patient. Frequently, the discharge planner may be a specialized role filled by a nurse or social worker who works collaboratively with the healthcare team, patient, and family to assist with more complex needs. Discharge planning does not solve all problems, but it can reduce readmissions, minimize residual effects of the health condition through continuity of care, and improve patient and family satisfaction with the healthcare system.

DISCHARGE PLANNING ELEMENTS FOR THE PATIENT

Goal Setting

The nurse should develop goal setting in the areas of education, advocacy, and case management in collaboration with the patient and family/caregiver. Outcomes for each identified health goal should be stated in realistic, clear, measurable, and time-oriented terms. Factors to consider in setting goals should include the following:

- Patient's level of functioning and independence to achieve or maintain goals
- Extent of family/caregiver involvement
- Availability of community resources and the patient's and family/caregiver's motivation to use those resources

An example of a goal is "Mr. Jones will be able to walk 20 steps with his walker in his home within 7 days of discharge from the hospital."

Transition. When people undergo transitions, their assumptions about themselves change, and they develop new assumptions that allow them to adapt. Issues involving transition are particularly obvious when a patient moves between settings, such as from the hospital to home or from home to a long-term care facility. The physical move is only one type of transition the patient makes. Other related changes may involve self-concept, role performance, mobility, self-care, or communication with family members. For example, a mother with terminal cancer may experience the transition from her role as caregiver for her children to the role of care recipient.

Continuity of Care. Continuity of care is both an ideal and a necessity. Continuity of care is the provision of health services without disruption, regardless of the patient's movement between settings. From the patient's perspective, it involves having a home health nurse visit within 24 hours of hospital discharge or having the physician's office contact the local pharmacy about the patient's medication needs. When health services are disrupted, the patient may experience a relapse and require additional healthcare or hospitalization. Thus, continuity of care helps to maintain the patient's health status and reduces healthcare costs.

Organizational policy and financial realities can work against continuity. Communication between health professionals about a patient's needs may not occur. Starting discharge plans at admission can help ensure continuity of care by identifying needs early; planning ahead allows for expedient referrals to community services and agencies.

Discharge Planning Elements for the Nurse. The nurse is responsible for ensuring that the patient is prepared for discharge and that the family or caregiver has received necessary information and assistance. Safety is a key factor in planning for the patient to return home. For the nurse, the key elements of discharge planning are coordination, facilitation, and negotiation.

Collaboration. Collaboration is the act of assembling and directing activities to provide services harmoniously. The result of coordination is a team working together with a unified purpose

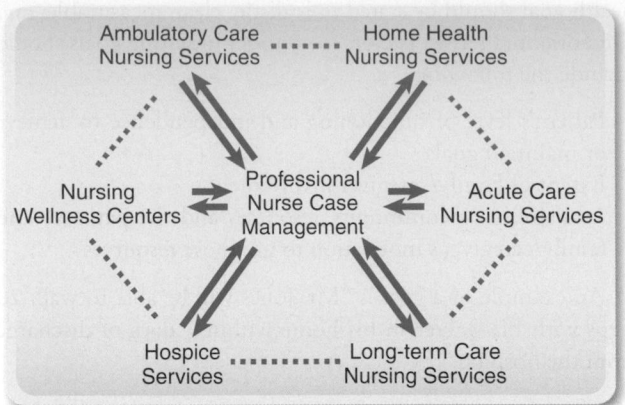

FIGURE 3-4 Coordination among healthcare team members is vital to the success of a patient's discharge planning.

(Fig. 3-4). Payment based on diagnosis-related groups (DRGs) has led to shorter US hospital stays; as a result, nurses must coordinate health and social services for patients' needs after discharge. One way to coordinate services is to initiate and conduct team and family conferences, preferably before the patient is discharged. Otherwise, the patient's problems may become unnecessarily complex. At a team conference, the discussion should focus on individualizing the patient's care. For example, the nurse can bring to the team's awareness any special considerations regarding the patient's home setting or other circumstances. At a family conference, professionals and the family gather to discuss family issues related to the patient. For example, concern may exist about the availability of family members to assist with care, their understanding of care required, or other issues. Both types of conferences provide an opportunity to plan care and set goals. If patients require special equipment (e.g., oxygen, walking aids) in the home, the nurse may be responsible for securing the appropriate orders or authorizations, contacting the vendor, and arranging for delivery.

Facilitation. Facilitation means making something easier and smoother by eliminating problems and barriers. To facilitate the patient's transition, the discharge planner must anticipate needs and plan ahead. For example, the patient may be overwhelmed by just thinking about going home, let alone planning for transportation from hospital to home. The nurse may be able to reduce the patient's anxiety by anticipating and planning for transportation. Anticipation of discharge needs begins at admission and continues through the patient's stay. The nurse must consider the different settings, the patient's needs, and available resources.

Negotiation. Negotiation is the process by which the patient, nurse, and family determine goals. The most elaborate plan of care is doomed if the patient, family, or healthcare professional hampers attempts to achieve the goals. Negotiation may be formal or informal; it must involve dialogue with the patient and family to help articulate desires, values, and feelings about their views of a realistic plan of care. For example, the home care priorities of a young mother with a respirator-dependent

infant may differ from those of the nurse. Negotiating with the mother about which goals and objectives take priority has two effects: The mother will be more willing to work with the nurse to attain goals, and the mother will feel more in control of the situation.

At times, clarification is a priority, so a more formal process involving contracts is necessary. A contract is a written agreement between the nurse and patient that delineates each person's roles and responsibilities. A contract regarding care clarifies expectations of the nurse, patient, and family members. It provides a concrete reference for all parties to access should issues arise.

Contracts help to limit the helplessness, stress, or disempowerment that patients and families may feel. The sense of control and empowerment achieved through the contract enhances the patient's internal resources—specifically, motivation and commitment. The nurse and the patient or caregiver discuss who is responsible for what, and all participants reach a consensus. The consensus on responsibilities is written, and then each person receives a copy so every participant can see clearly who is accountable for which responsibilities.

Levels of Discharge Planning

Discharge plans vary depending on the patient's needs and the nursing interventions required to assist the patient after discharge. All patient goals and nursing interventions should be developed from the perspective that human responses to health and illness occur regardless of setting. Discharge planning is needed, for example, when a child is discharged from a day surgery center after a tonsillectomy, an older woman leaves a clinic requiring additional diagnostic tests to exclude a diagnosis of cancer, or a young man with a long history of substance abuse is discharged from a drug rehabilitation center. The level of discharge planning increases depending on the complexity of healthcare required and the complexity of the patient's transition. The three levels of discharge planning are summarized in Table 3-3.

Basic Discharge Plan. The least complicated and most common discharge plan is teaching the patient about self-care for the illness. Patient teaching may include instruction about medications, treatments, community resources, or energy conservation techniques. The teaching should anticipate problems the patient may experience at home. For instance, when discharging a

TABLE 3-3 LEVELS OF DISCHARGE PLANNING

Discharge Plan Level	Nursing Interventions	People Involved
Basic, universal	Self-care and illness teaching	Nurse, patient, caregiver
Simple referral	Refer to community resources	Nurse, patient, caregiver
Complex referral	Refer to discharge planner	Nurse, discharge planner, family

newborn with an apnea monitor to a home with three other small children, the nurse should teach the parents to check the monitor frequently to ensure that the other children have not inadvertently changed the monitor's parameters.

Simple Referral. The second type of discharge plan involves referring the patient to community resources (e.g., a smoker to a smoking cessation clinic, a high-risk mother to the local health department, a caregiver to a respite service). A referral is a request for a service outside the referring professional's scope. The nurse acts as the discharge planner and must know both the community resources and the patient's ability to reach those resources. Knowledge of the community resources is based on the community assessment and on personal knowledge.

Complex Referral. The third and most complex type of discharge plan involves referring the patient to the discharge planner. The nurse may choose to involve the discharge planner because the patient's situation is complex, so planning and making referrals to appropriate community resources would be too time-consuming or beyond the nurse's knowledge level or ability. This type of discharge planning is particularly appropriate for patients who are considered high risk.

This level of discharge plan involves interdisciplinary collaboration and coordination. The discharge planner takes responsibility for coordinating the activities necessary to transfer the patient from one setting to another. However, referring the patient to a discharge planner does not absolve the nurse of responsibility. The nurse must follow up to ensure that the discharge planner has acted and must evaluate to learn if the patient is satisfied with the discharge plan. The nurse may need to reinforce plans.

A referral to the discharge planner is appropriate for coordinating placement of the patient in a skilled nursing facility or a long-term care facility. The discharge planner can also coordinate and initiate services the patient will need if discharged to home (e.g., a visiting nurse). Table 3-4 provides a list of healthcare providers often used as referrals during discharge planning.

 APPLY YOUR CRITICAL THINKING

Mrs. Ellis has been hospitalized for 3 days with pneumonia. She is recovering but still requires oxygen by nasal cannula to maintain her oxygen saturation level. Prior to this admission, Mrs. Ellis lived independently in her own home. She has a strong support network through her church, and her adult daughter and son-in-law live nearby, although they both work 40 to 50 hours per week. Mrs. Ellis has no stairs to navigate in the home and previously had bathroom handrails installed. Mrs. Ellis is alert and oriented, but she is occasionally forgetful. She has a good appetite and has been progressing well with physical therapy. She has limited financial resources and is worried about paying for prescribed medications.

What resources are available in the hospital for discharge planning? What resources might be available in the community? What strengths does Mrs. Ellis have in this situation? What elements in her background cause concern? What is a likely discharge plan for Mrs. Ellis?

Check your answer in Appendix B.

STANDARDS OF HOME HEALTH NURSING PRACTICE

The American Nurses Association (2014) described standards of home health nursing practice that have two parts: standards of care (following steps of the nursing process) and standards of professional performance, which are shown in Box 3-2. These standards can guide the home care nurse in his or her collaborative role with the patient and family (caregiver) to identify the healthcare needs for management in the home setting.

PHASES OF THE HOME NURSING VISIT

Stanhope and Lancaster (2012) suggested five phases of the home visit. First, the *initiation phase* includes clarifying the source of referral and the purpose of the visit and initial

TABLE 3-4 HEALTHCARE PROVIDERS USED IN DISCHARGE REFERRALS

Healthcare Provider	Role
Home health nurse	Provides assessments; directs care, patient teaching, and support; coordinates services; evaluates outcomes
Home health aide	Provides hygiene care, cooking, supervision, and companionship
Social worker	Assists in finding and connecting with community resources or financial resources, provides counseling and support
Physical therapist	Assists with restoring mobility, strengthens muscle groups, teaches ambulation with new devices
Occupational therapist	Helps patients adjust to limitations by teaching new vocational skills and better ways to perform activities of daily living
Nutritionist	Teaches patients about meal planning and diet restrictions
Speech therapist	Assists patients to communicate better and works with patients who have swallowing problems
Respiratory therapist	Provides home follow-up for patients with respiratory problems including assessment, oxygen administration, and home ventilator care

BOX 3-2   Home Health Nursing Standards of Practice and Professional Performance

Standards of Practice

Standard 1—Assessment
The home health registered nurse collects comprehensive data pertinent to the patient's health and/or the situation.

Standard 2—Diagnosis
The home health registered nurse analyzes the assessment data to determine the diagnoses, needs, or issues.

Standard 3—Outcome Identification
The home health registered nurse identifies expected outcomes for a plan individualized to the patient, family, other caregivers, and caregiving situation.

Standard 4—Planning
The home health registered nurse develops a plan that prescribes strategies and alternatives to attain expected outcomes.

Standard 5—Implementation
The home health registered nurse implements the individualized patient plan of care.

Standard 6—Evaluation
The home health registered nurse evaluates progress toward attainment of outcomes.

Standards of Professional Performance

Standard 7— Ethics
The home health registered nurse practices ethically.

Standard 8—Education
The home health registered nurse attains knowledge and competence that reflect current nursing practice.

Standard 9—Evidence-Based Practice and Research
The home health registered nurse integrates evidence and research findings into practice.

Standard 10—Quality of Practice
The home health registered nurse contributes to quality nursing practice.

Standard 11—Communication
The home health registered nurse communicates effectively in a variety of formats in all areas of practice.

Standard 12—Leadership
The home health registered nurse demonstrates leadership in the professional practice setting and the profession.

Standard 13—Collaboration
The home health registered nurse collaborates with patients, families, caregivers, interprofessional healthcare team, and others in the conduct of nursing practice.

Standard 14—Professional Practice Evaluation
The home health registered nurse evaluates one's own nursing practice in relation to professional practice standards and guidelines, relevant statutes, rules, and regulations.

Standard 15—Resource Utilization
The home health registered nurse uses appropriate resources to plan and provide nursing services that are safe, effective, and financially responsible.

Standard 16—Environmental Health
The home health registered nurse practices in an environmentally safe and healthy manner.

From: American Nurses Association. (2014). *Home health nursing: Scope and standards of practice* (2nd ed.). Silver Spring, MD: NursesBooks.org

---

contact with the family. The *previsit phase* includes establishing an understanding with the family for the purpose of the visit, scheduling the visit, and reviewing pertinent records and information. The *in-home phase* involves establishing the professional therapeutic relationship and implementing the nursing process. Social interactions help to establish rapport in this phase of home visiting. In the *termination phase* of the home visit, the nurse and family summarize accomplishments of the visit and make plans for future visits. Finally, the *postvisit phase* includes recording findings and carrying out activities necessary to plan for the next visit.

ASSESSMENT

Assessment should encompass the functional abilities, strengths, and assets of the patient, family, home, and community. The nurse collects subjective information to assess how the person normally manages at home, what the home is like, and what family and community support is available. The nurse must explore the patient's beliefs and culture, competencies, capabilities, concerns, deficits, and limitations to understand how the patient manages at home and what he or

she desires. Box 3-3 provides key questions that can be used to elicit this information.

Assessing the Individual

Interviewing the patient provides valuable information about his or her ability to manage at home, risk factors contributing to decreased ability, and identification of actual problems. Assessment starts by asking the patient to describe his or her ability to manage self-care tasks such as bathing, dressing, grooming, and eating. Document the patient's ability to carry out household chores independently or with assistance from others. The patient can describe how he or she handles functional limitations at home and whether management has been satisfactory. Determine whether the patient needs aids such as walkers, oxygen equipment, assistive feeding devices, or a hospital bed. Assess medications and treatments and the patient's ability to manage self-care (Fig. 3-5).

Assessing the Family

Assess family support to determine how well a person can function at home. Family assessment can be done with questionnaires covering a broad range of topics. The most significant

BOX 3-3   Key Questions for Assessing Home Management

Patient

- What goals do you have for yourself?
- What will help you achieve these goals?
- How will you manage at home on a day-to-day basis?
- What treatments will you be doing at home?
- What medications will you be taking at home?
- Is there anything within yourself or your home that you would like to change?
- What do you need to make these changes?
- What do you want it to be like at home?
- What kinds of problems do you think you will have at home?
- How have you dealt with challenges in the past?

Family and Social Support

- Have you ever needed help and support in the past?
- How much can you rely on friends and relatives?
- What kind of help and support do you need now?
- What help will you have at home?
- How much do you think your friends and relatives understand your health and medical problems?
- Whom would you like me to talk to about your health and medical problems?
- How do you think your spouse and friends will handle or cope with your being home?

factors to assess are strengths of family members and barriers to ability of family members to provide care.

Assessing family support focuses on characteristics that show decreased family involvement with or support for the patient. To assess family involvement with the patient, ask directly how much support family members are willing and able to provide. Observe for evidence of family visits. Look for evidence of family concern, such as cards and presents. Observe family communication patterns and dynamics. Families differ in their reactions to a member's illness. The prognosis and sever-

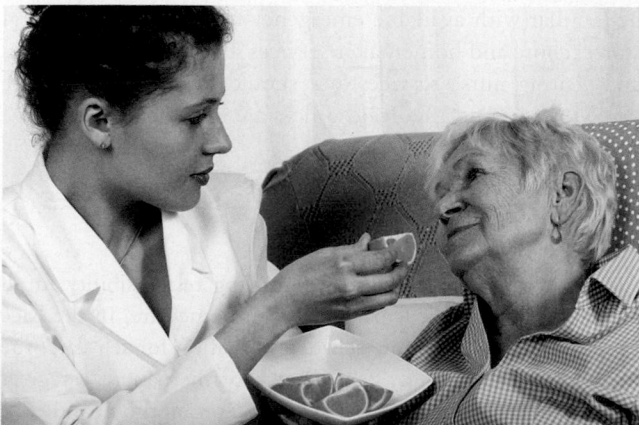

FIGURE 3-5 Assisting with meals provides opportunities for assessment.

ity of the illness can affect family interactions and subsequent involvement with the patient. Chronic illness can lead to rejection of the patient and can impair family dynamics.

Assess the caregiver's ability and willingness to perform, or to help the patient perform, any therapeutic treatments. Caregiving often consists of bathing, dressing, toileting, transferring, feeding, housekeeping, shopping, preparing meals, managing finances, and providing transportation. Therefore, assess caregivers for their ability and willingness to carry out these activities and for the emotional and physical strains of providing care or an overload of responsibility. Wound dressing changes, ostomy care, home parenteral therapy, and physical therapy may require additional time and energy (see Chapters 21 and 30).

Assessing Risk

Currently, the basis for most reimbursable home healthcare services is acute illness or exacerbations of a chronic problem that require skilled care. Rarely is a single factor the basis for home care. The relationship between functional impairments and available internal and external supports determines the risk of impaired ability to manage at home: The greater the functional impairment, the greater the risk, and the fewer available supports, the greater the risk. Common risk factors associated with the need for home care include the following:

- Multiple or catastrophic illnesses
- Limited social, mental, or physical functioning
- Repeated hospital admissions within 6 months
- Age older than 80 years, especially for women
- Age older than 70 years with a disability
- Lack of social or family support and living alone
- Complex medical treatment regimen and multiple medications

These risk factors do not automatically indicate a problem; the importance of the risk factors for each patient must be determined. During the entire assessment, be continually aware of cues that would indicate cognitive impairments, such as repeating the same question or giving vague answers that are not consistent. People with cognitive impairments often are unable to manage in the home and rarely are able to realistically identify their own limitations.

Community deficits also can contribute to decreased ability to manage at home. The incidence of unsuccessful health management is greater in the following situations:

- Unsafe neighborhoods
- Inadequate housing for the disabled
- Refusal of agencies to accept difficult patients
- Inadequate home health services
- Lack of volunteer programs
- Long waiting lists for services (especially long-term care facilities)
- Lack of affordable housing

A dysfunctional pattern can be identified when the patient or family verbalizes the inability to perform daily tasks and manage at home. People have a deficit when they cannot perform self-care and hygiene tasks, do not engage in activities and interactions with others, and do not do things from which they would otherwise derive enjoyment and a sense of worth.

Assessing the Home

Although its assessment is often performed at the same time as the patient and family assessment, the patient's living area is important enough to be considered a separate assessment element. A comprehensive home assessment includes safety, sanitation, mobility, temperature, and personal space. Box 3-4 summarizes home assessment (see also Chapter 23). Before discharging a patient to the home setting, ensure a safe environment:

- Learn whether the house is rented or owned, as this determines whether modifications are feasible.
- Look for smoke or fire alarms, adequate lighting, flat door sills, and adequate security.
- Determine whether the house is clean and free from insect or rodent infestation.
- Ask about sewer and garbage services.
- Determine the source of water and the condition of the plumbing.
- Assess for adequate and safe cooking and food storage equipment, including running water and working electricity. Although rural and urban areas differ in the types of sanitation measures, sanitation should not be a source of disease.
- Assess for easy access throughout the house.

BOX 3-4   Assessment of Home Conditions

From Patient
- *Ownership:* Rent hotel room, apartment, or house; own; live with others
- *Access:* Ground floor and stairs
- *Condition*
- *Utilities:* Heat, water, telephone, and electricity
- *Hygiene:* Housekeeping habits
- *Sanitation:* Rodents, sewer, and infestations
- *Safety:* Handrails

From Home Visit
- *Neighborhood:* Crime potential, located near environmental hazards
- *Access:* Ground floor, condition of stairs and sidewalk, proximity to public transportation
- *Utilities:* Type of utilities available and in service, cooking arrangements
- *Hygiene:* Odors, facilities for cleaning, appropriateness of food storage
- *Sanitation:* Presence or evidence of vermin or rodents
- *Safety:* Short electrical cords, handrails, fire alarms, stable rugs
- *Telephone:* Private phone, accessibility, answering machine

---

- Look for handrails on tubs and staircases, wide doorways for wheelchair access, and flat and even floors that contribute to easy mobility. There should not be any scatter rugs, and halls should be uncluttered.
- Determine the adequacy of heating and cooling systems. Inadequate temperature control can lead to hypothermia or hyperthermia.

Do not overlook the home's personal aspects. Having mementos, pictures, or religious items in a home reflects self-image. A garden, sewing equipment, or a workshop provides additional information on the person's values and avocations. A person may be unable to continue such self-actualizing activities in the face of health challenges. Being aware of the patient's past gives the nurse a more complete understanding of the patient and how the current health condition has changed his or her way of living. For example, an active 80-year-old man who gardens daily may interpret a broken hip as devastating, but a sedentary man who enjoys watching television and doing crossword puzzles may find the same situation less devastating.

The nurse may recommend changes in the home based on home assessment. Common physical changes include installing ramps and handrails, moving furniture to make room for a rented hospital bed, or providing space for equipment such as oxygen tanks and suction machines. If a severely disabled patient is expected to return home, a home visit should ideally be made before discharge.

Assessing Community Resources

The purpose of community assessment is to identify resources that people needing assistance at home can use. A comprehensive community assessment is not needed to diagnose impairments, but being familiar with **community resources** allows the nurse to develop a more realistic and individualized nursing plan of care for the patient. The nurse needs information about the community's economic stability, the patient's neighborhood, the social and health resources available in the community, and the community's cultural norms. The presence of services as recorded in service directories is one way to validate objectively what the patient describes. Nurses should be familiar with available emergency care, equipment rental stores, chore and homemaker services, home-delivered meals, and visiting nurse services and should know where welfare and Medicare and Medicaid offices are located.

CARE MANAGEMENT AND RESPONSIBILITIES IN HOME CARE

Although care management is a nursing responsibility in all settings of practice, it is paramount in home care. In the Rice (2006) model of dynamic self-determination for self-care, the home care nurse acts as a **facilitator** of the patient/caregiver system through education, advocacy, communion, and case management. Key to the facilitator role is the development of mutual goals with the patient.

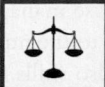

ETHICAL/LEGAL ISSUE

DECISION MAKING FOR FAMILY MEMBERS

You have been assigned to care for Mr. Connelly, an 82-year-old man with diabetes and chronic heart disease. His reaction times are slowing, and his vision, although satisfactory during the daytime, is failing at dusk and in poor weather. He has had several mild accidents in the car, but insists on continuing to drive. Mrs. Connelly is very concerned, and their two adult children are pressuring her to take away his car keys. Mrs. Connelly calls you and asks you to tell her husband he can no longer drive.

CRITICAL THINKING CHALLENGE

- What might explain Mr. Connelly's insistence on continuing to drive?
- What concerns do you have about the situation?
- What is the nurse's role in this situation?
- What resources might be available to help the decision-making process?
- Identify possible approaches that might be used to assist the family in this situation.

Patient Education

Patient education is an interactive, collaborative process between the nurse and patient to progress toward the patient's goal of assuming responsibility for his or her health and self-care (Fig. 3-6). The education process includes several steps. First, nurses assess. They gather information about the readiness of patient and family to learn and target their learning needs and priorities. They interpret their findings to arrive at a nursing diagnosis for education needs.

Second, nurses negotiate the learning objectives and anticipated outcomes with the patient and family. Well-written behavioral objectives are characterized as measurable, related to assessment data, developed collaboratively, and oriented to

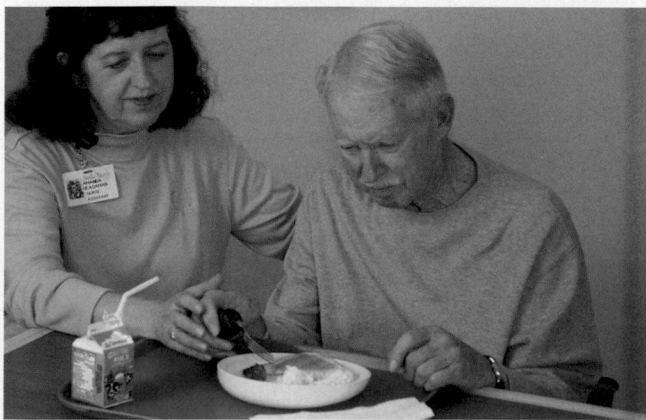

FIGURE 3-6 Patient education is an important aspect of home healthcare.

the learner. They contain the elements of performance, conditions, and criteria. Objectives can be classified as cognitive (knowledge based), affective (values, feelings), or psychomotor (motor skills) (Stanhope & Lancaster, 2012) (see Chapter 14).

Third, nurses and the patient and family develop and implement a teaching plan. The teaching plan includes objectives and outcomes, a content outline, teaching format (e.g., group discussion with patient and family), teaching tools (e.g., handouts, videos, return demonstration, role-play), and use of a teaching–learning contract with mutually developed objectives to achieve outcomes.

Finally, nurses evaluate patient education. Such an evaluation can be done continuously during home visits. In the evaluation, nurses include a measurement of the achievement of the objectives, analyze the barriers and facilitators to learning, summarize the results with the patient and family, provide and receive constructive feedback, and continuously reinforce the patient's and family's learning.

General areas for teaching to manage healthcare needs at home include information specific to a diagnosis of altered health status (e.g., signs and symptoms, diet, rest, activity, spirituality, self-image, developmental tasks, role transitions, medications, equipment, technical procedure), ways to cope or adapt to limits and restrictions related to the health issue, relevant community resources to support the patient and family, and source of payment for healthcare at home (e.g., Medicare). The home care nurse is challenged by the wide range of information needed for patient and family education.

Advocacy

The **American Nurses Association** (ANA, 2010) defines advocacy as "the protection, promotion, and optimization of health and abilities, prevention of illness and injury, alleviation of suffering through the diagnosis and treatment of human response, and advocacy in the care of individuals, families, communities, and populations" (p. 8). A patient advocate model suggests that nurses are responsible for promoting patient autonomy and self-actualization. Nurses make decisions with patients and caregivers to assist patients to achieve the best possible health outcomes and to access appropriate health services. Advocacy develops from ongoing, caring relationships with patients and families. In a three-step advocacy process, nurses initially explore personal values and beliefs and then begin the informing process (Stanhope & Lancaster, 2012). To inform, nurses engage patients and family about the nature, content, and consequences of their choices. Informing is not merely exchanging information, but viewing information in light of a patient's values and understanding. Supporting is the second step of advocacy—that is, nurses uphold the patient's right to make and act on a choice and help the patient and family to access and communicate with a range of resources and other providers. In affirming, the third step in advocacy, nurses validate with the patient and family that choices are consistent with their values and goals. Home care nurses recognize that the needs of patients and their families are dynamic and may vary; therefore, ongoing evaluation of choices is needed to promote self-determination.

At different stages of patients' independent functioning, the nurse's role as advocate may change. Areas in which nurses may act as advocates include helping the patient and family to clarify and prioritize their choices, promote optimal functioning at home, or communicate with other family members, friends, or professional services (e.g., healthcare providers, third-party payors) to access information or services in the home setting.

Holistic Care

To acknowledge the holistic nature of patients (and caregivers), an important aspect of care management within the nurse's role as facilitator is what Rice (2006) terms **aesthetics/spirituality**. The nurse works with families to:

- Know health through the arts
- Explore alternative and complementary therapies
- Experience self-awareness, faith, hope, and love

For care management to be balanced, the nurse's approach must include strategies that engage the whole person: body, mind, and spirit. Communion of the nature described allows (facilitates) meeting needs within the patient/caregiver in the domain of larger meaning, which can lead to greater self-knowledge, self-reverence, self-healing, and self-care processes. Often, this type of relationship is facilitated through aesthetic expression (e.g., drawings, stories, music, poetry) and the use of alternative or complementary health modalities.

Care/Case Management

Case management is a term with numerous definitions (Stanhope & Lancaster, 2012). Case management focuses on the whole person, not just health-related issues. The holistic approach requires the case manager to be a generalist with a range of skills and knowledge. The case manager should have "nursing expertise, but he or she also needs counseling skills, knowledge of community resources, vocational expertise, mental health expertise, sensitivity to multicultural issues, proficiency in evidence based practice and a high level of problem-solving abilities." The components of the case management process include the following:

- Assessment
- Planning
- Coordinating
- Making referrals
- Monitoring medical progress
- Filing and completing paperwork
- Monitoring outcomes and the plan's effectiveness
- Determining case closure
- Transferring the case at closure

These steps do not necessarily occur in sequence; sometimes, they may happen simultaneously.

For home care nurses who may be the patient's and family's most direct contact with the healthcare system, these skills are necessary to promote the patient's health and function. Thus,

nursing care management is integrally related to case management. The complex array of skills has been likened to the nursing process (Stanhope & Lancaster, 2012). (See also skills for discharge planning described in Chapter 2.)

Coordination of care for a patient and family requires development of plans of care that maximize the person's ability to remain in a safe environment, and often that environment is the patient's home. Nurses work collaboratively with many healthcare professionals in planning, implementing, and evaluating the patient's care, including physicians; social workers; physical, occupational, and speech therapists; and home health aides. Nurses integrate their understanding of community-based nursing with their abilities to collaborate, coordinate, provide, and evaluate care within many settings.

If the patient requires special equipment, the home care nurse needs to know how to obtain the equipment and to whom it will be charged. Once such equipment is in the patient's home, the nurse needs to know how to operate it, how to handle common malfunctions, and how to assist the patient and family with learning to use it.

In the role of coordinating services, the home care nurse may work with a case manager from a managed care system or other third-party payor. Although both persons provide care for the patient, they have slightly different concerns. The case manager may focus more on the aspects of reimbursable care to limit the insurer's financial liability. The home care nurse may focus on objective documentation of the patient's care needs to convince the healthcare provider and the insurer of the need for continued home health services. In this function, the home care nurse acts as the patient's advocate.

Accessing Community Resources

As mentioned, the home care nurse may need to access and coordinate the procurement of needed equipment for patients. This activity may be as simple as obtaining a prescription from a local pharmacy or as complex as arranging for reimbursement and delivery of large pieces of equipment from a durable medical supply house.

In today's healthcare environment, changes in funding for home services, especially through Medicare and managed care regulations, affect their availability. The challenge for home care nurses is to plan creatively with individuals and families to meet their needs. As a result, home care nurses must stay aware of community resources to assist individuals and families in the home.

Agencies may provide services at no cost or across a range of fees. The United Way funds many types of community services and programs. Churches and social service agencies may also support or provide direct services to individuals and families. For older adults, nurses should contact any agency that has "older," "aging," or "senior" in its title. Local senior centers may be a source of information. Often, a community has an umbrella agency that supports or organizes services for particular groups, such as older adults, low-income families, or selected ethnic or racial groups. Local government agencies (city, county, and state) may also be sources of information.

Some agencies have toll-free numbers. Organizations focusing on health issues also offer information; for example, local chapters of the national heart, lung, diabetes, or Alzheimer associations often provide support groups, printed materials, and other information. Professional colleagues are frequently excellent resources. With the increased use of technology, online sources are more accessible to patients and families.

HOSPICE

Hospices, run by public or private agencies, are designed to care for terminally ill patients and their families by providing supportive, palliative services. The focus of hospice is that each of us has the right to die pain-free and with dignity and that our friends and family will receive the necessary support to allow us to do so (Matzo & Sherman, 2014). Many patients receiving these services have cancer, AIDS, multiple sclerosis, congestive heart failure, or end-stage renal disease. Nurses play a major role in hospice care; a team approach also usually involves physicians, therapists, trained volunteers, and clergy members. Nurses focus on managing pain, treating symptoms, and helping patients live life to the fullest until death. They work with family members to assist in bereavement and reorganizing their lives. Hospice care was initially provided in the home and still is. More recently, hospital- and community-based units also have developed hospice programs.

KEY CONCEPTS

- The goal of home care is to allow people to regain or maintain optimal health and to function within their limitations in the home environment.
- The home management of a person's healthcare needs usually occurs within the context of family, friends, and community.
- Altered ability to manage healthcare needs independently may result from decreased functional abilities, insufficient family or social supports, or insufficient community resources.
- Key components of the Rice model for home care include motivational factors of the patient and family and the nurse as facilitator of home independence in the roles of educator, advocate, aesthetic/spiritual communer, and case manager.
- The central issue of today's healthcare industry is how to deliver cost-effective and quality healthcare that is accessible to and results in positive health outcomes for everyone.
- Levels of healthcare are categorized as primary, secondary, and tertiary. Most current sources and services are in secondary healthcare, but the population's needs fall within the categories of primary and tertiary healthcare.
- Care once considered safe only within the hospital now is delivered routinely in community-based settings.

- Common to all community-based programs is the need for nurses to have greater individual authority, accountability, responsibility, and allegiance to patients while relying less on institutional authority and policies. At the same time, nurses have a greater need to collaborate effectively as members of interdisciplinary teams.
- Although the site and circumstances of nursing care may change, the focus is always the nurse's concern for health of the whole person in relation to that person's environment.
- Community nursing centers deliver primary healthcare to a specific population, are managed and staffed by nurses, and have physician backup and consultation as needed.
- An organizational structure must be in place to ensure continuity of care from one healthcare setting to another and among healthcare professionals.

PRACTICING FOR THE NCLEX

CHECK YOUR ANSWERS IN APPENDIX A.

1. Among Pima Indians, 50% of adults have diabetes and 95% of those are overweight. Diabetes and obesity are directly correlated with rerouting of waterways, which impacted traditional farming and subsequent dietary supplementation with processed commercial foods. Which health determinants are implicated in this scenario? Select all that apply:
   a. Educational
   b. Economic
   c. Political
   d. Healthcare services

2. A nurse is providing care on an acute care unit to a patient admitted for cellulitis of the right leg, with a history of bipolar disorder and intravenous drug use. She appropriately plans for discharge in order to address mobility issues, safety risk, and continued drug rehabilitation. Such interventions illustrate which type of nursing care?
   a. Community-based healthcare
   b. Community-based nursing care
   c. Primary care
   d. Secondary prevention

3. A patient is discharged following a triple coronary artery bypass graft and is seen for follow-up by his cardiologist, his surgeon at the hospital, his primary care physician, and the anticoagulation clinic. He is also seen for diabetes management and renal failure by two other specialists. This patient is at risk for what problem with this healthcare coordination?
   a. Discontinuity
   b. Schism of care
   c. Fragmentation
   d. Decentralization

4. A patient who has recently begun hemodialysis for kidney failure is discharging home from the hospital. Which of the following elements of discharge planning are integral in order to meet this patient's healthcare needs? Select all that apply:

    a. A team meeting is planned between the physician, social worker, nurse, and family.
    b. Discharge planner establishes a dialysis schedule at a facility near the patient's home.
    c. The nurse provides discharge paperwork as the patient is leaving.
    d. A tolerable renal diet is discussed between the dietician and the patient.

5. A nurse is performing a safety assessment at the home of an elderly man who lives independently. He is returning home following hospitalization for a below-the-knee amputation and will have a wheelchair as needed for several weeks. Which of the following issues should be noted by the nurse? Select all that apply:

    a. The surrounding neighborhood has a high crime rate
    b. Infrequent home health service availability in the area
    c. Wide doorways and handrails on stairs
    d. A well-kept garden in the backyard

REFERENCES

American Nurses Association. (2008). *ANA Health Systems Reform Agenda.* Silver Springs, MD: ANA. Retrieved from http://www.nursingworld.org/content/healthcareandpolicyissues/agenda/anashealthsystemreformagenda.pdf

American Nurses Association. (2010). *Nursing's Social Policy Statement* (2nd ed.). Silver Spring, MD: NursesBooks.org.

American Nurses Association. (2013). *Public Health Nursing: Scope and Standards of Practice.* (2nd ed.). Silver Springs, MD: ANA. NursesBooks.org

American Nurses Association. (2014). *Home Health Nursing: Scope and Standards of Practice.* (2nd ed.). Silver Springs, MD: ANA. NursesBooks.org

Carpenito-Moyet, L. J. (2013). *Nursing diagnosis: Application to clinical practice* (14th ed.). Philadelphia, PA: Lippincott Williams & Wilkins.

Center for Healthcare Research & Transformation. (2014). Care transitions: Best practices and evidence-based programs. *Home Health Nurse, 32*(5), 309–316.

Centers for Disease Control and Prevention. (2013). *The medically uninsured.* Retrieved from http://www.cdc.gov/healthcommunication/toolstemplates/entertainmented/tips/medicallyuninsured.html

Cunic, D., Lacombe, S., Mohajer, K., Grant, H., & Wood, G. (2014). Can the Blaylock Risk Assessment Screening Score (BRASS) predict length of hospital stay and need for comprehensive discharge planning for patients following hip and knee replacement surgery? Predicting arthroplasty planning and stay using the BRASS. *Canadian Journal of Surgery, 57*(6), 391–397.

Harrington, C., Ng, T., La Plante, M., & Kaye, H. S. (2012). Medicare home- and community-based services: Impact of the Affordable Care Act. *Journal of Aging & Social Policy, 24,* 169–187.

Institute of Medicine. (2012). *Primary care and public health: Exploring integration to improve population health.* Retrieved from http://www.iom.edu/~/media/Files/Report%20Files/2012/Primary-Care-and-Public-Health/Primary%20Care%20and%20Public%20Health_Revised%20RB_FINAL.pdf

Marrelli, T. M. (2012). *Handbook of home health standards and documentation guidelines for reimbursement.* St. Louis, MO: Mosby.

Matzo, M., & Sherman, D. W. (2014). *Palliative care in nursing: Quality care to the end of life* (4th ed.). New York, NY: Springer.

National Council of State Boards of Nursing. (2014). Implications of the Affordable Care Act on nursing regulation and practice. *Journal of Nursing Regulation, 5*(1), 26–34.

Rice, R. (2006). *Home health nursing practice: Concepts and application* (4th ed.). St. Louis, MO: Mosby–Year Book.

Stanhope, M., & Lancaster, J. (2012). *Community and public health nursing* (8th ed.). St. Louis, MO: Mosby.

U.S. Department of Health and Human Services. (2014). *Office of Disease Prevention and Health Promotion. Healthy People 2020.* Washington, DC, Available at www.healthypeople.gov/2020/default.aspx

Vincent, D., & Reed, P. G. (2014). Affordable Care Act: Overview and implications for advancing nursing. *Nursing Science Quarterly, 27*(3), 254–259.

White House. (2014). *Health reform.* Retrieved from http://www.whitehouse.gov/healthreform/healthcare-overview

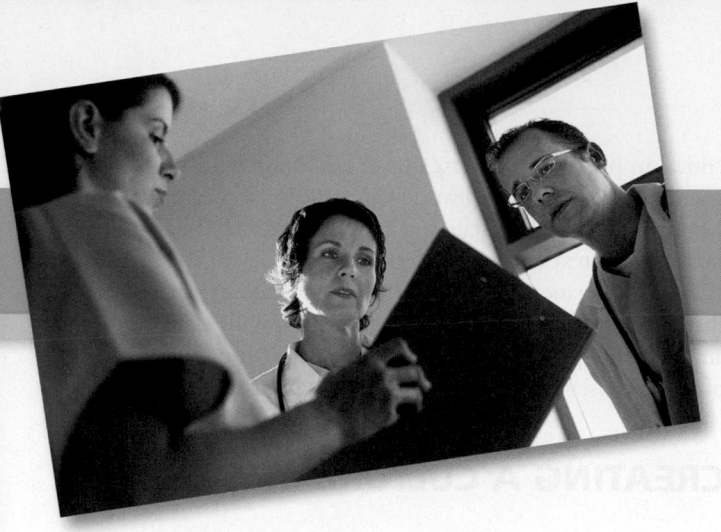

CHAPTER 4

The Nurse's Role in Healthcare Quality and Patient Safety

Christine M. Henshaw

Case Scenario

During morning huddle, your nurse manager asks every nurse to pay attention to nurse-sensitive quality indicators. The rate of falls per patient day has been decreasing, and the unit is focused on getting to zero falls. In the meantime, hospital-acquired pressure ulcer rates have risen slightly, and nurses are encouraged to be diligent in using the pressure ulcer prevention bundle to protect patients. The manager reminds staff that nurses play an important role in achieving good patient outcomes and keeping patients safe. The hospital is on track to receive increased reimbursement from the Centers for Medicare and Medicaid Services (CMS) if quality and safety targets are met.

Once you have completed this chapter and have incorporated quality and safety science into your knowledge base, review the above scenario and reflect on the following areas of Critical Thinking:

1. What is the appropriate number of "defects" in patient care?
2. Whose responsibility is it to keep patients safe?
3. How do cost containment and the emphasis on quality and safety potentially conflict?

KEY TERMS

bundle

Centers for Medicare and Medicaid Services

incident report

Institute for Healthcare Improvement

Institute of Medicine

just culture

quality

Quality and Safety Education for Nurses

root cause analysis

safety

safety science

sentinel event

LEARNING OBJECTIVES

Upon completion of this chapter, you will be able to do the following:

1. Describe the elements of safety science.
2. Discuss aspects of patient care for which nurses have primary responsibility.
3. Identify agencies involved in measuring quality care and patient safety.
4. Identify national organizations that focus on safety concerns of patients and healthcare workers.
5. Describe how safety and quality affect hospital reimbursement practices.

The concepts of **quality** and **safety** are closely interrelated. Quality refers to the excellence or superiority of something. Quality is often viewed on a continuum, from poor quality to high quality. Safety is the avoidance or prevention of adverse outcomes for patients. Quality healthcare must be safe; unsafe care is not quality healthcare. However, quality is more than just safety. The Institute of Medicine, Committee on Quality of Health Care in America (2001), identified six aims of 21st century healthcare: that all healthcare should be safe, effective, patient centered, timely, efficient, and equitable. Taken together, these characteristics define quality healthcare.

In this chapter, we will explore the concepts of safe healthcare and quality healthcare. The focus will be primarily on hospital and other institutional settings and on personal safety for nurses. Additional safety concepts, specifically related to safety risks for individuals outside of healthcare settings, will be described in Chapter 23.

SAFETY CRISIS IN HEALTHCARE

Research suggests that 400,000 people die in U.S. hospitals every year from preventable healthcare errors (James, 2013), making errors the third leading cause of death after heart disease and cancer (Hoyert & Xu, 2012; Table 4-1).

In every healthcare setting, keeping patients safe is a primary role of nurses. As the largest component of the healthcare workforce, nurses have a direct role in patient safety. Assessment and monitoring of patients is referred to as "surveillance" and is the cornerstone of protecting patients from harm. Regular assessment and early detection of changes in the patient's status are

TABLE 4-1	LEADING CAUSES OF DEATH IN HOSPITALS IN THE UNITED STATES (2011 DATA)
Cause of Death	Number of Deaths
Heart disease	596,339
Cancer	575,313
Preventable medical errors	400,000
Chronic lower respiratory diseases	143,382
Cerebrovascular diseases	128,931
Accidents (unintentional injuries)	122,777
Alzheimer disease	84,691
Diabetes	73,282
Influenza and pneumonia	53,667
Nephritis, nephrotic syndrome, and nephrosis	45,731
Intentional self-harm (suicide)	38,285

Adapted from Hoyert, D., & Xu, J. (2012). Deaths: Preliminary data for 2011. *National Vital Statistics Report, 61*(6), 1–51. Retrieved from http://www.cdc.gov/nchs/data/nvsr/nvsr61/nvsr61_06.pdf

critical in preventing adverse outcomes. Safety is an individual, community, national, and worldwide concern. In healthcare, the scope of safety in hospitals and healthcare agencies has shifted from the context of a single nurse concerned with the physical safety of the patient assigned to his or her care to a realization that safety is a far greater concept with responsibilities distributed among many professionals. **Safety science** examines the nature of safety, causes of errors, and systems to keep patients safe.

CREATING A CULTURE OF SAFETY

Healthcare organizations are striving to create a **culture of safety** in which every member of the organization contributes to the safety of patients and employees. In the past, staff were often disciplined or their employment terminated for errors. In that kind of environment, staff may feel they must hide errors to avoid punishment. Even errors due to system deficits may go unreported or underreported. In an organization with a strong culture of safety, staff are empowered to report errors and **near misses** to alert organizational leaders to system issues. Near misses are events where an error was likely to occur if the situation had not been corrected.

Having a taxonomy of errors and understanding the **root causes** of errors helps to create a culture where errors can be openly discussed and addressed. Errors may be classified as active or latent. Active errors are those caused by the actions of frontline staff, usually with immediate result. Latent errors may be due to equipment design issues, faulty maintenance, or poor organizational structure (Kohn, Corrigan, & Donaldson, 1999). For example, administration of the wrong drug may be viewed as an active error. Further **root cause analysis** (RCA) of the error, however, may reveal that the correct drug in the situation and the drug administered have similar names and come in similar vials. This realization may lead to the conclusion that the error was a latent one. Focusing on the active aspect of the error might result in disciplining of the staff member who administered the incorrect drug. Focusing on the latent nature of the error may result in a change in the drug name or a change in the packaging of the drug with a different vial size or label, preventing future errors of the same kind.

RCA is a process used to determine the underlying cause of an event. One tool used in RCA is asking the question "why" five times. As an example, let's consider a patient who doesn't receive an ordered medication prior to surgery. Figure 4-1 lists a series of "why" questions that might be asked to get at the root cause of the problem, along with possible answers. Each answer suggests the following question. Although this is often referred to as "asking 'why' five times," the question "why" would be asked until the root cause is identified. Suggesting that it be asked five times simply encourages the investigator not to stop after one or two rounds of questioning. In addition, the questions aren't necessarily asked of the person who made the error, although that person should be interviewed for information; often, it is the "system" being asked the questions, through interviewing managers, looking at processes, or asking other workers in similar positions.

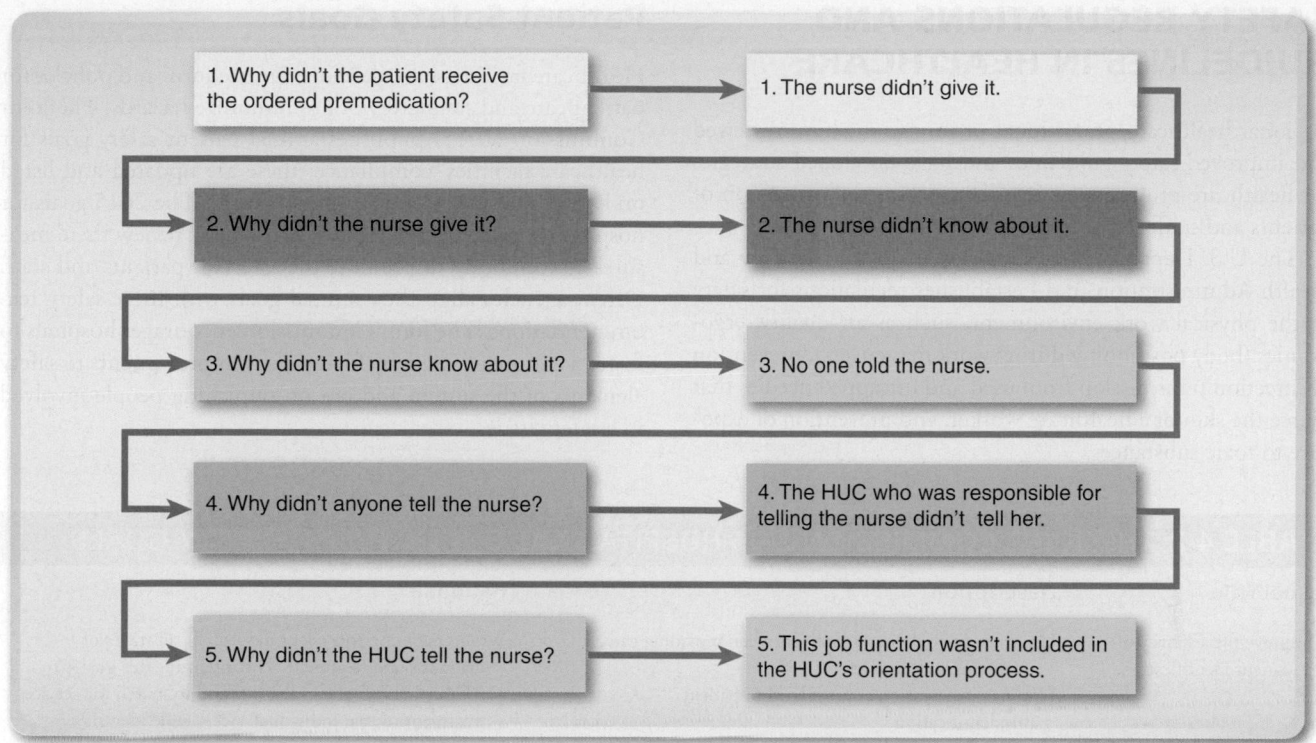

FIGURE 4-1 Root cause analysis: Asking "Why" five times. The question "why" should be asked until the root cause is identified. In this case, the root cause may have been a deficit in the orientation of this specific health unit coordinator (HUC) or unit secretary, or a deficit with the orientation system in general. Additional investigation may even reveal that relying on the HUC to relay the message is not the most reliable or effective system of notification for the nurse, so a different system needs to be used or developed.

It is important to note that errors are rarely either solely active or solely latent. An overemphasis of the active nature of the error by blaming the person who committed the error rarely resolves the issue, as latent factors still remain. Unless the system issues are addressed, a high likelihood exists that the error will occur again. Overemphasizing the latent nature of errors removes personal responsibility from the equation.

Just culture is an approach to error evaluation that examines the nature of the error to assist in determining the appropriate response to the individual who made the error. In evaluating the error, attention is paid to whether the error represented human error, at-risk behavior, or reckless behavior (Marx, 2012).

As human beings, healthcare personnel will make errors. A one-time medication error is typically a human error that will happen in the complex healthcare world. A nurse who makes a human error should be consoled and perhaps asked to review his or her practice to see what he or she could learn from it. A pattern of human errors requires further evaluation.

At-risk behavior may occur when a nurse is not aware of or does not appreciate the risky nature of a behavior. For example, a nurse who predocuments medication administration may be doing so in an effort to be timely. However, this may lead to miscommunication or errors if a medication is not actually administered, but the record is not changed to reflect this. Coaching of the nurse may include education about safe practices and consequences of not following accepted standards.

A nurse who does not change behavior may be at risk for discipline.

Intentional reckless behavior is rare in healthcare. Most staff want to do what is best for patients. Falsifying records to conceal errors and failing to assist a patient not assigned to the nurse are examples of reckless behavior that put patients at substantial risk. Reckless behavior is grounds for discipline. In each situation, several questions can help evaluate whether the error was due to human error, at-risk behavior, or reckless behavior (see Box 4-1), which can in turn help direct the response to the issue.

BOX 4-1   **Questions to Help Evaluate Why an Error Was Made**

- Was this a one-time incident or a pattern of behavior?
- Is there a low or a high risk of patient harm?
- Does the nurse have the knowledge and skill to perform the task correctly?
- Have policies and standards been enforced in other similar situations?
- Did the nurse self-identify the issue and report it, or did the nurse cover up an error?

Source: North Carolina Board of Nursing. (2011). Complaint Evaluation Tool. Retrieved from http://www.ncbon.com/myfiles/downloads/ce-tool.pdf

SAFETY REGULATIONS AND GUIDELINES IN HEALTHCARE

National healthcare professional organizations have reviewed and improved safety guidelines and have developed strategies for healthcare professionals to adhere to for the protection of patients and staff.

The U.S. Department of Labor's Occupational Safety and Health Administration (n.d.) establishes regulations for safety in the physical work environment, such as air quality, ergonomics (body positioning during work maneuvers), prevention of infection transmission from used and uncapped needles that pierce the skin of a healthcare worker, and prevention of exposure to toxic substances.

Patient Safety Goals

Healthcare facilities have developed procedures and policies for patient care and standard work to minimize hazards. The Joint Commission (2015) publishes annual patient safety goals for healthcare facilities' compliance; these are updated and listed on its website (www.jointcommission.org). The 2015 goals for hospitals are outlined in Table 4-2. Facilities review these measures continuously to promote the safety of patients and staff. Often, agencies align their annual goals with these safety recommendations. The Joint Commission encourages hospitals to foster a culture of safety by focusing on improvements to safety elements of the system and not on punishing people involved in a safety issue.

TABLE 4-2 THE JOINT COMMISSION 2015 HOSPITAL NATIONAL PATIENT SAFETY GOALS

Goal Title	Description	Rationale
Improve the accuracy of patient identification.	Use at least two patient identifiers when providing care, treatment, and services. Eliminate transfusion errors related to patient misidentification.	Wrong-patient errors occur in virtually all stages of diagnosis and treatment. The intent for this goal is to reliably identify the individual and to match the service/treatment to that individual. Acceptable identifiers may be the patient's name, an assigned identification number, telephone number, or other person-specific identifier.
Improve the effectiveness of communication among caregivers.	Report critical results of tests and diagnostic procedures on a timely basis.	Critical results that fall outside the normal range may indicate a life-threatening situation.
Improve the safety of using medications.	Label all medications, medication containers, and other solutions on and off the sterile field in perioperative and other procedural settings. Reduce the likelihood of patient harm associated with the use of anticoagulant therapy. Maintain and communicate accurate patient medication information.	Medications or other solutions in unlabeled containers are unidentifiable. Anticoagulation therapy can be used as a therapeutic treatment for several conditions. It is important to note that anticoagulation medications are more likely than are others to cause harm due to errors in monitoring and administration. Medication discrepancies can affect patient outcomes. Medication reconciliation is intended to identify and resolve discrepancies.
Reduce the harm associated with clinical alarm systems.	Improve the safety of clinical alarm systems.	Clinical alarm systems are intended to alert caregivers of potential patient problems, but if they are not properly managed, they can compromise patient safety.
Reduce the risk of healthcare-associated infections (HAIs).	Comply with either the current CDC hand hygiene guidelines or the World Health Organization (WHO) hand hygiene guidelines. Implement EBPs to prevent HAIs due to multidrug-resistant organisms in acute care hospitals. Implement EBP to prevent HAIs due to multidrug-resistant organisms in acute care hospitals. Implement EBP to prevent central line–associated bloodstream infections. Implement EBP for preventing surgical site infections. Implement EBP to prevent indwelling catheter–associated urinary tract infections (CAUTI).	According to the CDC, each year, millions of people acquire an infection while receiving care, treatment, and services in a healthcare organization. One of the most important ways to address HAIs is by improving the hand hygiene of healthcare staff. Patients continue to acquire HAIs at an alarming rate. Prevention and control strategies must be tailored to the specific needs of each hospital based on its risk assessment.
The hospital identifies safety risks inherent in its patient population.	Identify patients at risk for suicide.	Suicide of a patient while in a staffed, around-the-clock setting is a frequently reported type of sentinel event.

CDC, Centers for Disease Control and Prevention; EBP, Evidence-based practices.

Source: Joint Commission. (2015). *National patient safety goals*. Retrieved from http://www.jointcommission.org/standards_information/npsgs.aspx

Reporting Sentinel Events

Hospitals are required to report serious safety events to regulatory agencies such as the Joint Commission and to state health agencies. Safety errors that result in death or serious injury are called **sentinel events**. Teams at a hospital analyze the environment and the factors that contribute to a sentinel event and develop solutions to eliminate the possibility of that safety issue occurring again. The solutions are reported to regulatory agencies, which then monitor that changes are enforced (Joint Commission, 2014b). Nursing assessment of factors that put patients at risk for injuries should help identify safety concerns and the precautions necessary to minimize risks.

QUALITY AND SAFETY EDUCATION FOR NURSES

The **Quality and Safety Education for Nurses** (QSEN) project has been designed to provide a framework for the knowledge, skills, and attitudes necessary for future nurses.

Using the **Institute of Medicine's** (IOM) competencies, QSEN has defined quality and safety competencies for nursing that are essential for entry into practice (QSEN Institute, 2014). The six competencies are:

- Patient-centered care
- Teamwork and collaboration
- Evidence-based practice (EBP)
- Quality improvement (QI)
- Safety
- Informatics

Within each competency, QSEN defines the knowledge, skills, and attitudes needed to achieve that competency. The competencies are leveled for prelicensure and graduate education. Table 4-3 lists each competency and its definition. The safety competency will be discussed in this chapter. Refer to the appropriate chapter for the other competencies.

Safety is an important component of your nursing education from the first to the last quarter. You will see a wide range of practices in the clinical setting, including safety checks, smart pumps, and evidence-based practice. In the beginning, you will build knowledge and skills related to safety. These include using communication techniques such as SBAR, practicing with alarms and alerts, and integrating national standards with practice in the clinical setting. At the end of your education, you will learn to value the importance of safety practices in the clinical setting and your own role in preventing errors. Table 4-4 includes the QSEN knowledge, skills, and attitudes related to your learning about safety.

SAFETY ISSUES IN HEALTHCARE

Many types of issues create the potential for safety defects in healthcare settings. Problems with equipment, procedural errors, and impairment of patients may cause adverse patient outcomes. Examples of equipment problems include a wheelchair with nonlocking wheels, which can cause a fall when the patient attempts to sit in it, or a malfunctioning heating pad unit, which can cause a fire. The use of faulty or ungrounded electrical equipment increases the risk of electrical shock. The frequent use of oxygen in patient care areas increases the risk of fire; therefore, smoking is prohibited, and healthcare sites have adopted totally smoke-free environments to promote safety and health. Procedural errors, such as failure to check patient identification bands before administering medications or not monitoring intravenous (IV) infusion rates, can harm patients. Patients can experience falls or burns because they are impaired by medication, blindness, or hearing loss; decreased mobility because of language or other communication barriers; or confusion.

An accident or injury occurring in the hospital necessitates the filing of a report known by different names (e.g., **incident report**, quality assurance memo, patient safety alert). This document remains confidential and is not part of the patient's med-

TABLE 4-3 DEFINITIONS OF QSEN COMPETENCIES

Competency	Definition
Patient-centered care	Recognize the patient or designee as the source of control and full partner in providing compassionate and coordinated care based on respect for patient's preferences, values, and needs.
Teamwork and collaboration	Function effectively within nursing and interprofessional teams, fostering open communication, mutual respect, and shared decision making to achieve quality patient care.
EBP	Integrate best current evidence with clinical expertise and patient/family preferences and values for delivery of optimal healthcare.
QI	Use data to monitor the outcomes of care processes and use improvement methods to design and test changes to continuously improve the quality and safety of healthcare systems.
Safety	Minimize risk of harm to patients and providers through both system effectiveness and individual performance.
Informatics	Use information and technology to communicate, manage knowledge, mitigate error, and support decision making.

TABLE 4-4 QSEN SAFETY COMPETENCIES

Knowledge	Skills	Attitudes
Examine human factors and other basic safety design principles as well as commonly used unsafe practices (e.g., work-arounds and dangerous abbreviations). Describe the benefits and limitations of selected safety-enhancing technologies (e.g., bar codes, computerized provider order entry, medication pumps, and automatic alerts/alarms). Discuss effective strategies to reduce reliance on memory.	Demonstrate effective use of technology and standardized practices that support safety and quality. Demonstrate effective use of strategies to reduce risk of harm to self or others. Use appropriate strategies to reduce reliance on memory (e.g., forcing functions, checklists).	Value the contributions of standardization/reliability to safety. Appreciate the cognitive and physical limits of human performance.
Delineate general categories of errors and hazards in care. Describe factors that create a culture of safety (e.g., open communication strategies and organizational error reporting systems).	Communicate observations or concerns related to hazards and errors to patients, families, and the healthcare team. Use organizational error reporting systems for near miss and error reporting.	Value own role in preventing errors.
Describe processes used in understanding causes of error and allocation of responsibility and accountability (e.g., RCA and failure mode effects analysis).	Participate appropriately in analyzing errors and designing system improvements. Engage in RCA rather than blaming when errors or near misses occur.	Value vigilance and monitoring (even of own performance of care activities) by patients, families, and other members of the healthcare team.
Discuss potential and actual impact of national patient safety resources, initiatives, and regulations.	Use national patient safety resources for own professional development and to focus attention on safety in care settings.	Value relationship between national safety campaigns and implementation in local practices and practice settings.

Reprinted with permission from: *Nursing Outlook,* Volume 55, Issue 3, May–June 2007, Pages 122–131, Special Issue: Quality and Safety Education. Reprinted with permission from Elsevier.

ical record. It completely describes all aspects of the event that occurred. Specifically, the report should include the accident, patient assessment, and interventions provided for the patient. The report is used for internal review to improve the system to prevent similar errors. Internal quality documents such as an error report usually cannot be used against the facility or nurse.

 APPLY YOUR CRITICAL THINKING

A coworker who is a good friend of yours tells you about a medication error he made. He shares that he did not file an incident report about this. You encourage him to do so, but he says, "Nothing happened to the patient, and I don't want to get in trouble for the mistake." You know the nurse is always very careful and hasn't made errors before. What are the priorities in this situation?

Check your answer in Appendix B.

Medication Safety

Medication administration is a common activity for nurses in many settings. Safe medication administration requires the nurse to be knowledgeable, attentive, and careful at all times. Several factors contribute to medication errors. Failure to follow any of the six rights of medication administration as described in Chapter 20 may lead to an error. But what

causes that failure? Any number of factors, such as nurse fatigue, deficient staffing, or emergency situations, may lead to a failure to follow the six rights. A major contributor to medication errors is interruptions during the medication administration process (Cloete, 2015). Many hospitals have implemented "no interruption" zones around medication-dispensing cabinets (see Fig. 4-2); some have nurses wear special vests or covers while they are administering medications to signal no interruptions.

Medications with similar names may lead to administration errors. The Institute for Safe Medication Practices (ISMP) has advocated a system of using capitalized letters within a drug name to differentiate drugs with similar names. This system is called "Tall Man Letters" (ISMP, 2011; see Fig. 4-3). For example, the drugs dopamine and dobutamine have similar sounding and looking names. The FDA-approved Tall Man Letters for those drugs is DOPamine and DOBUTamine. Using the capital letters draws attention to the fact that these drugs have similar names and might be confused for each other. The full list of Tall Man Letter drug names is available at http://www.ismp.org/tools/tallmanletters.pdf.

Bar code medication administration helps reduce medication errors. Bar code scanning of medications and patient wristbands matches the drug being administered to the patient, reducing the incidence of wrong-patient/wrong-drug errors (see Fig. 4-4). Bar code scanning can also reduce the incidence of administration of the wrong dose of medication. For example, if the order is for two tablets and the nurse scans only one tablet, the computer system will signal

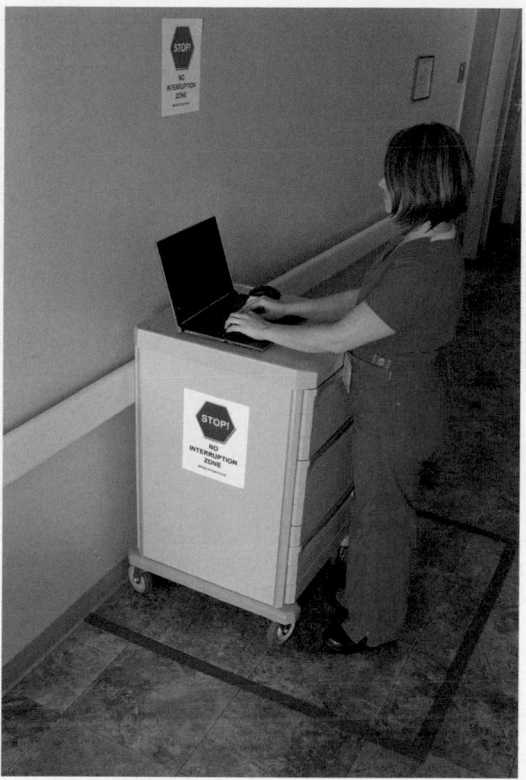

FIGURE 4-2 A "No Interruption Zone" alerts other staff that medication administration is in process and the nurse should not be interrupted.

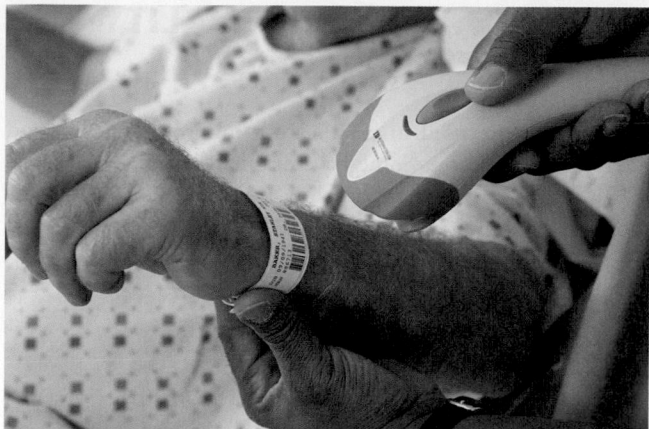

FIGURE 4-4 Bar code scanning of the patient and the medication helps reduce errors.

a wrong dose is being administered. As with all systems and procedures, it is usually possible to work around the system to continue the task despite error messages. Such work-arounds are to be avoided as they bypass safety systems put in place to avoid errors. If an error message is received during medication administration, the nurse must be diligent in determining the reason for the message and correcting whatever is causing the error.

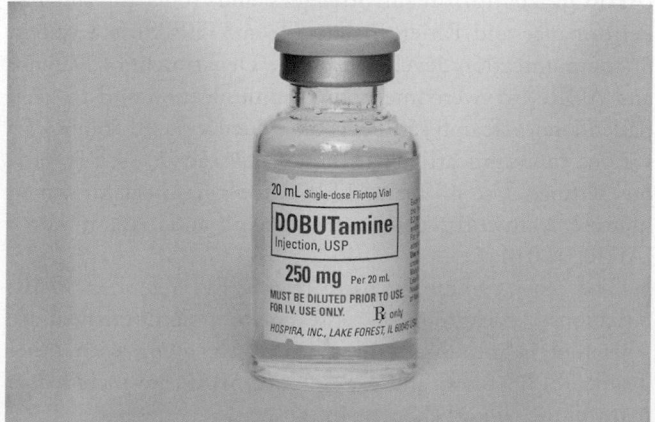

FIGURE 4-3 The ISMP's Tall Man Letters system helps differentiate medications with similar names.

Healthcare Worker Risks

Healthcare workers must also be aware of risks to their own safety in any healthcare environment. Common risks include exposure to blood-borne pathogens from puncture injuries from sharps such as needles or scalpels; back injuries caused by lifting heavy objects, including patients; and potential adverse reproductive outcomes as a result of overexposure to antineoplastic medications. Threats of violence and assaults from patients and visitors have also emerged in recent years as a serious hazard for healthcare workers. Safety habits ensure an optimal therapeutic environment and promote health for workers.

All hazardous exposures or conditions require some type of intervention to protect workers. Training regarding strategies for prevention is essential. Use of needleless devices can prevent needlesticks. Proper lifting devices can prevent back injuries. Chemical exposures often require the use of some type of personal protective equipment and special handling procedures. Controls to prevent violence in the healthcare setting can include use of alarms, increased security measures, improved lighting, and increased staffing.

Environmental Safety

Increasingly, nursing is facing critical issues related to environmental health and safety in the workplace. As a result, many agencies are creating "green teams" to identify areas of polluting waste and to do secondary recovery of many items that had previously been considered trash. For example, the chemical components of commonly used fluid and medication delivery systems are being reexamined to prevent unintentional leaching of chemicals from plastic or polyvinyl materials into the recipient. A healthcare green team will become progressively more important in terms of patient, healthcare workers, and community health as well as modifying the waste stream (Meija & Sattler, 2009).

TOOLS TO IMPROVE QUALITY AND SAFETY

Several tools are used in healthcare to improved quality and safety of patient care. Some have originated in the healthcare arena and some come from other industries. A few of these tools will be highlighted here.

General Tools for Quality and Safety Improvement

As professionals, nurses are responsible for their actions and must make every effort to provide safe, evidence-based care. Several system tools are available to help reduce the risk of errors and to enhance the likelihood that quality care is provided. Some examples of general principles to reduce errors include mistake-proofing, checklists, and building in redundancies or successive checks.

An example of mistake-proofing is the creation of tubing connections that are not interchangeable. For example, enteral feeding tube should not physically be able to connect with IV tubing. As patient care becomes more and more complex, the potential for error increases. While nurses should be diligent in tracing lines prior to connecting anything, making unsafe connections impossible moves the burden of responsibility away from the fallible nurse who may make a human error to a system that is potentially more reliable in preventing errors. If the tubing won't connect, the nonsterile tube feeding solution can't be accidentally infused into a vein.

Checklists provide opportunities to keep patients safe and to ensure quality care. An early example of checklist use in healthcare is the Universal Protocol for surgical procedures (Joint Commission, 2014a). This standardized checklist facilitates operating room and procedural area staff completing a "time-out" that allows all present to confirm the patient, the procedure to be done, and the site. Additional information about the Universal Protocol (sometimes called a "time-out") is provided in Chapter 22. Another example of checklist use is to guide care that is provided. For example, a checklist may be completed while a central venous catheter is inserted to ensure all safety points are followed. A checklist might be used at the time of discharge of a patient with diabetes to ensure all required teaching was completed. A checklist may be used as an internal quality control document (i.e., not part of the patient record) to ensure that all required care is completed and documented.

Successive checks for certain high-risk procedures or events add needed safety redundancy. For example, two registered nurses check the information about the patient and about a blood product about to be administered to ensure the blood product is the right one and is safe for the patient (Fig. 4-5). Certain medications may require checking by two nurses prior to administration. New medication orders go through several successive checks: they may be checked by a health unit coordinator, a registered nurse, a pharmacy technician, a pharmacist,

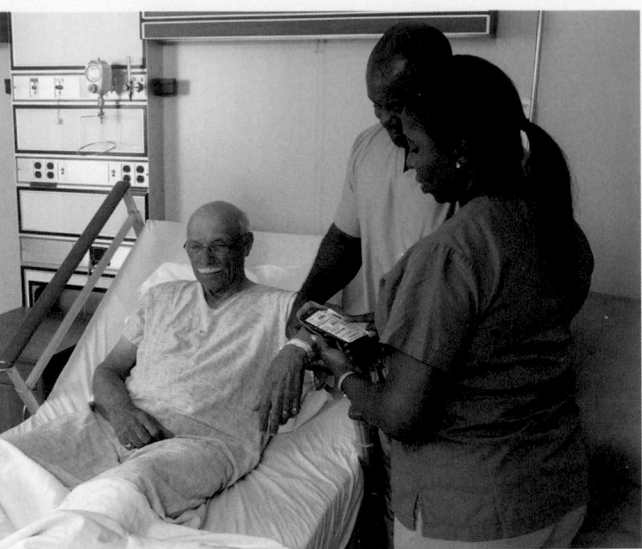

FIGURE 4-5 High-risk tasks, such as blood administration, require two nurses to ensure accuracy and safety of the procedure.

and a registered nurse prior to administration. While avoidance of "overwork" is important, certain high-risk or complex situations may require built-in double-checking to ensure safety.

Communication

Humans are in communication with each other throughout the day. In healthcare settings, communication is key to ensuring safe and quality care: communication with the patient and communication among healthcare workers. Chapter 6 discusses basic principles of communication and focuses on communication with the patient.

Because communication within healthcare is continuous and essential, it must be clear, accurate, and concise. Communication that is unclear, inaccurate, or untimely leads to quality defects and errors. Evidence suggests that poor communication contributes to approximately 66% of healthcare errors (Agency for Healthcare Research and Quality [AHRQ], 2014b). Team Strategies and Tools to Enhance Performance and Patient Safety (TeamSTEPPS) is a system of communication developed by the Department of Defense and AHRQ to overcome poor communication and to keep patients safe. TeamSTEPPS is an evidence-based toolbox of various communication techniques that can be used in various settings. Use of TeamSTEPPS tools has been shown to increase teamwork, team effectiveness, and patient safety (AHRQ, 2014a).

The most commonly used TeamSTEPPS tool is SBAR: *Situation, Background, Assessment, Recommendation*. This tool is introduced in Chapter 16, along with other TeamSTEPPS tools, and examples of SBAR are included in many of the clinical chapters in this text.

Other commonly used TeamSTEPPS tools include huddles and debriefs. Huddles are often held at the beginning of shift to highlight important issues to pay attention to during the shift.

Huddles may also be used to introduce new equipment or processes being implemented or to recognize staff for a job well done. Debriefs typically are held after an event, for example, an emergency code. Common issues discussed during a debrief are what went well, what didn't go well, and what should be done differently next time. Learnings from the debrief can be shared with other staff to improve processes and procedures.

Care Bundles

Research has demonstrated that combining patient care elements into **bundles** and consistently implementing those bundles of care can reduce harm to patients. The **Institute for Healthcare Improvement** has developed several bundles of care that help keep patients safe. Other organizations, such as specialty nursing or medical groups, have developed other bundles of care that serve as the standard of practice.

One example of a bundle is the central line–associated bloodstream infection (CLABSI). The presence of an IV catheter in a vein, especially a centrally located vein, increases the risk for infection. The central line bundle elements are designed to reduce the risk of CLABSI. The five elements of the bundle are (IHI, 2012):

* Hand hygiene
* Maximal barrier precautions during insertion of the line (sterile gown and gloves, cap, face shield, sterile drape)
* Preparation of skin at insertion site with chlorhexidine
* Optimal catheter site selection, avoiding the femoral vein site in adults
* Daily review of line necessity with prompt removal when no longer needed

The bundle is a short, focused list that is not intended to replace any other procedures or care already in place. For example, the components of the central line dressing and daily site care are addressed by other standards of care, for example, from the Centers for Disease Control and Prevention (CDC, 2011).

Measuring Quality and Safety Outcomes

It has been noted by many authors that "What gets measured, gets done." When organizations that pay for healthcare, such as the **Centers for Medicare and Medicaid Services** (CMS), started tracking healthcare outcomes, improvement in outcomes was seen. For example, tracking CLABSI rates has been associated with a reduction in CLABSI. Since 2003, hospitals have voluntarily reported compliance with various process measures, such as whether aspirin was prescribed at discharge to patients who had experienced myocardial infarction. It is not always known whether such process measures improve short- or long-term outcomes for patients. More recently, outcome measures have been added to the reporting process, such as infection rates, hospital readmission rates, and mortality rates.

Included in the Patient Protection and Affordable Care Act (ACA), which passed into law in 2010, was the value-based purchasing (VBP) program. This program allows CMS to withhold a small percentage of reimbursement to hospitals that do not meet the national standards on these core process and outcome measures. Those hospitals that exceed standards receive extra reimbursement.

A portion of VBP is also based on patient's responses to satisfaction surveys. For hospitals, this survey is the Hospital Consumer Assessment of Healthcare Providers and Systems, usually abbreviated HCAHPS and pronounced "H-CAPS." Questions on the HCAHPS survey ask about effectiveness of communication between providers and patients, including both physicians and nurses; management of pain; cleanliness of the facility; and how quiet it was at night. While there is some concern that such patient satisfaction questions do not equate with the quality of the care provided, clearly, patients who feel they were not treated with respect and who were not able to sleep due to noise or pain were not receiving the best quality care.

Results of these core measures are reported to both CMS and the Joint Commission. Results of many of the measures are published on CMS's Hospital Compare website, http://www.medicare.gov/hospitalcompare/search.html. On this site, consumers are able to compare, for example, infection rates among area hospitals. A similar website allows comparisons of long-term care facilities, http://www.medicare.gov/nursinghomecompare/search.html.

CMS has identified several incidents or events that are called "never events." These are events that should never happen in healthcare. Never events include such things as falls, development of pressure ulcers, and certain hospital-acquired infections. If these events occur while a patient is hospitalized, the cost of the care associated with that event will not be paid by CMS but will be borne by the hospital. After CMS implemented this regulation, private insurance companies quickly followed suit. In addition to being the standard of care, this lack of reimbursement provides a strong financial incentive to hospitals to ensure that patients do not experience these never events while hospitalized.

KEY CONCEPTS

■ Safety of patients is the responsibility of all healthcare providers, including nurses.

■ While safe care contributes to quality care, quality is more than just safety.

■ Effective communication is essential to safe, quality care.

■ Use of evidence-based communication strategies improves teamwork and patient care.

■ Use of evidence-based bundles of care improves patient outcomes.

■ Healthcare providers should strive to prevent "never events."

■ Reimbursement of hospitals depends on achieving good outcomes.

PRACTICING FOR THE NCLEX

CHECK YOUR ANSWERS IN APPENDIX A.

1. Your nurse manager informs you he is using the tool "Asking Why 5 Times" to investigate medication error in which you were involved. What was the nurse manager doing?
    a. Conducting root cause analysis
    b. Applying concepts of just culture
    c. Assessing outcomes for CMS
    d. Using bundles of care

2. Which description of value-based purchasing is most accurate?
    a. Ensuring "never events" never occur
    b. Conducting a thorough investigation to analyzing the root cause of all errors
    c. Adjusting reimbursement based on measurement of processes, outcomes, and patient satisfaction
    d. Determining the actual cost of care to calculate reimbursement

3. Which statement is correct about patient safety?
    a. Physicians have sole responsibility for patient safety.
    b. Safe patient care is the same as quality care.
    c. High scores on HCAHPS surveys indicate patient safety.
    d. Nurses play an important role in keeping patients safe.

4. You have been asked to participate in a committee writing a policy for the care of a patient with an indwelling catheter. What is most important to include?
    a. Information retrieved from a website directed toward the lay public
    b. The nationally recognized catheter-associated urinary tract infection prevention bundle
    c. The policy from a well-respected nearby hospital
    d. Information from a nursing textbook that is more than 10 years old

5. Which statement is true about latent errors?
    a. They are errors whose effects are not known for a long time.
    b. Latent errors cause minimal effects to patients.
    c. Latent errors are traceable to a particular individual.
    d. They are errors that are due to system issues.

REFERENCES

Agency for Healthcare Research and Quality. (2014a). *TeamSTEPPS fundamentals course: Module 3, Communication, Classroom Slides*. Retrieved from http://www.jointcommission.org/standards_information/up.aspx

Agency for Healthcare Research and Quality. (2014b). *TeamSTEPPS fundamentals course: Module 1, Introduction*. Retrieved from http://www.ahrq.gov/professionals/education/curriculum-tools/teamstepps/instructor/fundamentals/module1/m1evidencebase.html

Centers for Disease Control and Prevention, Healthcare Infection Control Practices Advisory Committee. (2011). *Guidelines for the prevention of intravascular catheter-related infections, 2011*. Retrieved from http://www.cdc.gov/hicpac/pdf/guidelines/bsi-guidelines-2011.pdf

Cloete, L. (2015). Reducing medication errors in nursing practice. *Nursing Standard, 29*(20). doi: 10.7748/ns.29.20.50.e9507

Hoyert, D., & Xu, J. (2012). Deaths: Preliminary data for 2011. *National Vital Statistics Report, 61*(6), 1–51. Retrieved from http://www.cdc.gov/nchs/data/nvsr/nvsr61/nvsr61_06.pdf

Institute for Healthcare Improvement. (2012). *How-to guide: Prevent central line-associated bloodstream infection (CLABSI)*. Cambridge, MA: Author. Retrieved from http://www.ihi.org/resources/Pages/Tools/HowtoGuidePreventCentralLineAssociatedBloodstreamInfection.aspx

Institute of Medicine, Committee on Quality of Health Care in America. (2001). *Crossing the quality chasm: A new health system for the 21st century*. Washington, DC: National Academies Press.

Institute of Safe Medication Practices. (2011). FDA and ISMP lists of look-alike drug names with recommended tall man letters. Retrieved from http://www.ismp.org/tools/tallmanletters.pdf

James, J. (2013). A new, evidence-based estimate of patient harms associate with hospital care. *Journal of Patient Safety, 9*(3), 122–128. doi: 10.1097/PTS.9b913e3182948a69

Joint Commission. (2014a). *Facts about the Universal Protocol*. Retrieved from http://www.jointcommission.org/standards_information/up.aspx

Joint Commission. (2014b). *Sentinel events: Statistics*. Retrieved from http://www.jointcommission.org/Sentinel_Event_Policy_and_Procedures/

Joint Commission. (2015). *National patient safety goals*. Retrieved from http://www.jointcommission.org/standards_information/npsgs.aspx

Kohn, L., Corrigan, J., & Donaldson, M. (Eds.); Institute of Medicine, Committee on Quality of Health Care in America. (1999). *To err is human: Building as safer health care system*. Washington, DC: National Academies Press.

Marx, D. (2012). *Just culture algorithm v3.2 for employers*. Plano, TX: Outcome Engenuity (http://www.justculture.org)

Mejia, E. A., & Sattler, B. (2009). Starting a health care system green team. *Association of Operating Room Nurses Journal, 90*(1), 33–40.

Occupational Safety & Health Administration. (n.d.). *About OSHA*. Retrieved from www.osha.gov

QSEN Institute. (2014). *QSEN*. Retrieved from http://qsen.org/competencies/pre-licensure-ksas/

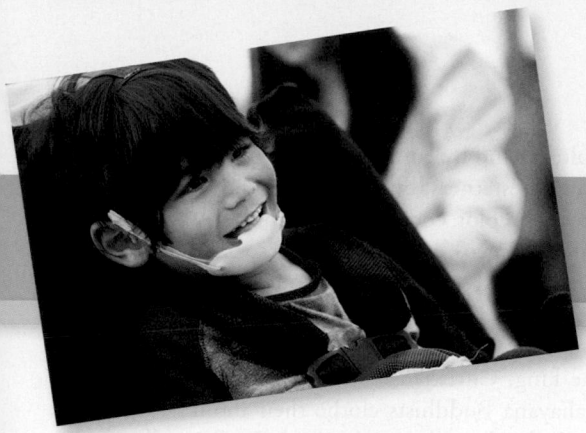

CHAPTER 5

Culture and Diversity

Janet Lenart

Case Scenario

You work in a rehabilitation facility where you are the primary nurse for 6-year-old Spencer. When Spencer was 3 years old, he was in a motor vehicle incident in which his neck was broken at the fourth cervical vertebra. He is alert and intelligent, but he is immobile from the neck down and requires total care. His parents are Samoan. They have stated that Spencer will come home for future care. Staff members think it is more appropriate that he go to another long-term care facility. How will these two different opinions be resolved?

Once you have completed this chapter and have incorporated culture and diversity into your knowledge base, review the above scenario and reflect on the following areas of Critical Thinking:

1. Determine the major problems that Spencer's parents would face if they cared for Spencer at home. Explore how the family's cultural beliefs might affect Spencer's care.
2. Considering your own cultural background, analyze how you would feel if you were Spencer's parent and indicate how you would respond in this situation.
3. Analyze how your cultural background affected your thinking when you originally read about the family and after you studied the chapter.

KEY TERMS
cultural diversity
cultural relativity
culturally competent nursing
culture
culture shock
ethnicity or ethnic identity
ethnocentrism
health disparity
health equity
implicit bias
key informants
minority
race
racism
rituals
stereotypes
subculture
transcultural nursing

LEARNING OBJECTIVES

Upon completion of this chapter, you will be able to do the following:

1. Discuss characteristics of culture.
2. Define concepts related to culture.
3. Build an understanding of people by observing human responses in a cultural context.
4. Identify patterns of one's own and others' behavior that reflect stereotypical thinking and ethnocentric assumptions.
5. Communicate effectively with people of diverse cultures.
6. Demonstrate an increased awareness of one's own culture and its influence on one's own nursing practice.
7. Conduct an ethnographic interview.

Nursing is concerned with human responses to actual or potential health problems (American Nurses Association [ANA], 2010). In the Case Scenario, you are asked to think about how family responses might be affected by the **culture** of patients, families, and healthcare professionals. Understanding culture and ethnicity helps improve the quality of nursing care by doing the following:

- Increasing the diversity of people with whom nurses communicate effectively
- Enabling nurses to attend more accurately to the integrity of the patient as a socially and culturally connected person
- Preventing nurses from imposing, however unintentionally, their own culturally shaped assumptions, values, and bias on patients and peers

The first part of this chapter examines the theoretical interpretations of culture and related concepts such as **culture change**, ethnicity or ethnic identity, **minority**, **ethnocentrism**, **race**, **racism**, **ritual**, **subculture**, and **stereotype**. The second part of the chapter discusses the relationship of culture and ethnicity to nursing care. Nursing assessment and intervention are emphasized.

WHAT IS CULTURE?

In nursing, the concept of culture and methods for studying it are derived from anthropology. Most classic anthropologists would agree that "culture controls behavior in deep and persisting ways, many of which are outside of awareness and therefore beyond conscious control of the individual" (Hall, 1959). The following definition of culture is used in this chapter:

> Culture is a learned, patterned behavioral response acquired over time that includes implicit versus explicit beliefs, attitudes, values, customs, norms, taboos, arts, and life ways accepted by a community of individuals. Culture is primarily learned and transmitted in the family and other social organizations, is shared by the majority of the group, includes an individualized worldview, guides decision making, and facilitates self-worth and self-esteem (Giger, 2013, p. 2).

It is important to note that cultural characteristics pertain more to groups than to individuals; individual members of the same group may adhere to different, even conflicting, cultural beliefs and behaviors. Stereotyping, discussed later in this chapter, occurs when notions about culture that pertain to a cluster of people are uniformly applied to all persons in that cluster, thereby ignoring cultural and individual variability. For example, research to understand **health disparities** revealed that people from ethnic minority groups were more likely to have fatalistic views of cancer compared to White non-Hispanic populations. Yet, it would be a mistake to assume this is true for all individuals in these groups (Ramírez, Rutten, Oh, Vengoechea, Moser, et al., 2013).

Culture is communicated through language, behavior, and symbols. Almost anything can carry symbolic meaning. Colors, for example, tend to do so universally, but their meaning varies across cultures and by context. Black signifies death and mourning among Westerners, but white does the same for the Chinese. Westerners color code gender (pink and blue) and movement (red and green), but not time or social status. The Thai color code time and social status, but not gender or movement. They designate a specific color as auspicious for each day of the week and reserve blue for royalty and yellow–gold for monks and the king. Christians clothe their priests in black and white; Mahayana Buddhists clothe their monks in gray; and the Mien clothe their shamans in red. Traditionally, the white of hospital nurses' uniforms has symbolized the cleanliness and purity of nursing. Physicians also wear white jackets or coats that convey the same symbolic meaning but with dark pants or skirts, the dark color signifying authority.

According to the National Center for Cultural Competence (2014a):

> Culture is the learned and shared knowledge that specific groups use to generate their behavior and interpret their experience of the world. It comprises beliefs about reality, how people should interact with each other, what they know about the world, and how they should respond to the social and material environments in which they find themselves. It is reflected in their religions, morals, customs, technologies, and survival strategies. It affects how they work, parent, love, marry, and understand health, mental health, wellness, illness, disability, and death.

In most Western societies, for example, spitting in public is considered dirty and aggressive, but exposing the nude body for physical examination by nurses or physicians is a generally accepted protocol. In contrast, in Muslim societies, spitting during ritual ablutions is understood as a religious act of cleansing, whereas exposure of the bare body, particularly to people of the opposite sex, is highly embarrassing and offensive because it violates strong cultural mores associated with intimacy. Such different interpretations of the same behaviors indicate that culture is learned and taught within a society. Culture is the accumulated "common sense" that members of a group share and generate. It provides solutions to common problems of living that have been handed down through generations (Gray & Thomas, 2006).

Culture is dynamic and changes over time. For example, in Western societies, spitting was not disparaged for centuries. Spitting became an unattractive behavior in the West only when public health science changed understanding by showing that bacteria cause disease and that sputum carries bacteria. What triggered the reversal of Westerners' attitude toward spitting was the association of spitting with tuberculosis, which in the late 19th century was highly prevalent and feared. This example shows that culture is created by people, often unconsciously, when their old common sense does not work, such as when they attempt to deal with new knowledge, situations, challenges, or threats.

Nurses need to understand how culture affects behavior and what functions it serves because nurses are accountable for observing and assessing patients' responses, which are influenced by culture (Douglas, Pacquiao, Callister, Hattar-Pollara, Lauderdate, et al., 2014). Culture is an integral component of nursing's knowledge base. Transcultural nursing refers to nursing practice that is patient-centered, evidence-based and considers culture (Giger, 2013, p. 5). Communication among people who share the same culture is often highly efficient, but communication among people of diverse cultures can be confusing and difficult. Culture enables people of similar cultural heritage to understand the meanings of each other's communication as part of the particular context in which they are expressed; to read each other's nonverbal behavior fairly accurately (Hall, 1959); and to communicate through words, symbols, and silence.

At least two thirds of the meaning of a social interaction is estimated to be communicated nonverbally—that is, in gestures, in vocalizations (e.g., sighs, throat clearing, laughter, grunts, whistling), and in the use of space and distance. Even when a nurse and patient share the same language, if they do not understand each other's cultures, they may misconstrue at least two thirds of each other's messages or information (Douglas et al., 2014).

Characteristics of Culture

Characteristics of culture are discussed in the following paragraphs. They are also summarized in Box 5-1.

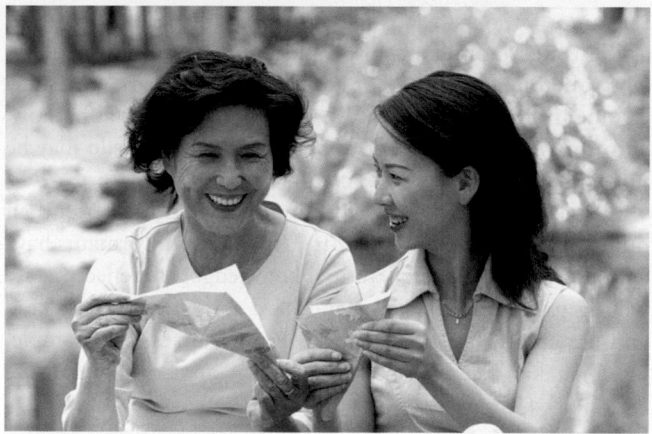

FIGURE 5-1 Artwork is a form of culture that is often passed down from one generation to the next.

BOX 5-1   Characteristics of Culture

Culture Is
- *Learned from other people,* not innate
- *Learned over a period of time*
- *Shared* by people who communicate with each other over time
- *Shared unequally by its members:* Some learn and use more of it than others do, and some have and access to it or to other cultures than others do.
- *Dynamic:* It is always changing at variable rates.
- *Diverse:* It increases ideas and opinions.
- *Reasonable* from the perspective of the members of the culture; it makes good sense to them
- *Implicit:* It is habit and habituated assumptions.
- *Not easily described by its own members*
- *Stabilizing:* It makes human responses generally predictable.
- *Ethnocentric:* It uses one's own culture as the correct standard.
- *Relative* to socioecologic context
- *Pervasive and holistic*
- *Ritualistic*
- *Recognizable* in patterns at many levels

Culture Is Not
- Predictable at the level of the individual
- Necessarily logical or reasonable to the outside observer
- A set of traits

Culture Functions to
- *Guide behavior* by providing a "blueprint" for action
- *Interpret or give meaning to experience*
- *Explain what is otherwise unknowable:* Why we are born; why we are born into the families we are; why we suffer our afflictions, dream our dreams, die our deaths, and have experiences different from those of others

---

CULTURE IS LEARNED

Culture is learned through sustained contact between groups and repeated observations of and participation in a group (Fig. 5-1). It takes time to learn a culture. Some learning is purposeful, and some is absorbed without awareness. When the culture one has learned differs from the culture in one's environment, a person can become disoriented and stressed. The acute experience of not comprehending the culture in which one is situated is called **culture shock** (Oberg, 1954). Culture shock is a stress syndrome that normally progresses through a series of recognizable stages (honeymoon, disenchantment, beginning resolution, and effective function) to its resolution. Patients from other cultures or countries where healthcare systems are not as technologically complex as in North America may experience culture shock if they are suddenly hospitalized here. Resolution of culture shock requires time, opportunity to observe and participate in the new setting, and careful anticipatory guidance that introduces people and explains behaviors and events of the new environment.

Similarly, nurses who work in cultures they are not familiar with may experience culture shock, which can provide an impetus to reflect on their own culture and increase their cultural competency. Through self-reflection, a nurse may reach the final stage of culture shock, referred to as effective function, in which the individual is increasingly aware of the strengths and weaknesses or his or her own culture and the new culture (Egenes, 2012).

CULTURE IS SHARED UNEQUALLY BY ITS MEMBERS

Not all members of the same culture act and think alike—culture is unequally shared by its members. Knowing a cultural norm does not enable one to predict a person's response. Generalizing about cultural norms in contemporary societies is inappropriate because people belong to more than one subcultural group and are influenced uniquely by multiple and diverse groups. Exceptions to cultural norms always exist. For example, many people from the United States pride themselves on being generous and altruistic and admire others who are the same. Yet, our society does not always reflect this altruism, as illustrated by millions of people and families with children who are homeless or do not get basic healthcare because they cannot afford it. Americans also think of themselves as friendly, and Americans who do not readily smile and say hello may be judged harshly based on the cultural norm.

People who know certain aspects of their culture better than others are called **key informants**. Usually, key informants have an especially rich base of cultural knowledge, are reflective, are willing to share their views, and have consciously considered and are able to articulate their culture. Nurses, for example, often make excellent key informants on hospital culture (Kennedy, Groom, Evans, & Fasano, 2010).

CULTURE IS DYNAMIC

Culture is dynamic: It changes as people come into contact with new beliefs and ideas. Termed culture change, this dynamic is much more rapid now than ever before because of the vast reduction in the time it takes to travel the globe and the ease of communication between distant places. Immigrants and refugees from developing countries who resettle in North America often change their cultures quickly. Consciously or not, they revise their cultures, often by trial and error, by blending elements from their original culture with new behaviors, attitudes, or beliefs that they find work and make life easier for them. Simultaneously, the introduction of cultural ideas from refugees, immigrants, foreign business persons, and media personnel from abroad changes North American society. For example, consumer demand for and use of Chinese acupuncture in healthcare has risen, and the popularity across the country of "ethnic" foods, restaurants, clothes, and music has surged.

CULTURE IS DIVERSE

The **cultural diversity** of a population increases the plurality of ideas and options for behavior, adding to the texture and complexity of the society and increasing the potential for well-being and achievement as well as for tension and conflict. Variety and diversity occur both within groups and across groups. In the United States, about 5.6% of the 2.6 million registered nurses are educated overseas (Sherwood & Shaffer, 2014). Several internationally educated nurses are not simply a response to the nursing shortage. It also reflects an increase in the size of the foreign-born population in the United States of about 9 million between the censuses of 2000 and 2010, such that by 2010, 12.9% of the total population were born abroad (U.S. Census Bureau, 2014a). Perhaps because of this rapid increase in cultural pluralism within a hitherto culturally homogeneous group (of middle-class White American women working within the male-dominated hierarchical healthcare system), racism (see discussion below) is prevalent within nursing (Hall & Fields, 2013). For example, Hispanic nurses report bias in the workplace that includes being discounted or belittled and needing to prove their capability to patients who refused care from them (Moceri, 2014).

It is important to understand that a society benefits from diversity when the playing field is level—when equal opportunity exists for various cultural perspectives and groups. When most culture overpowers the other cultures, inequity impacts all areas of daily life. Such situations can be highly stressful and, as with slavery and the historic treatment of Native Americans, can have lasting disempowering effects (Palacios & Portillo, 2009). Power differences in a society result in inequities in many areas of life and disparities in health outcomes (Braveman, Kumanyika, Fielding, Laveist, Borrell, et al., 2011). In today's society, we must meet the challenge of reducing inequity that is often based on race, ethnicity, and educational level. If we fail to meet this challenge, the outcomes are predictable: stigmatization and disempowerment of those perceived as not like "me" and the spread of seeds of mistrust, dislike, miscommunication, oppression, and denial of human rights (U.S. Department of Health and Human Services, National Partnership for Action, 2014c).

CULTURE IS REASONABLE FROM THE PERSPECTIVE OF ITS MEMBERS

Members of any given culture find their own culture reasonable, even though it has internal contradictions (such as to value the family but to ignore spousal abuse as a societal and health issue) and might seem illogical, counterproductive, or insensitive to outsiders. People such as spouses in cross-cultural marriages, resettled refugees, patients who come from abroad for specialized healthcare, and those who for whatever reasons move quickly from one culture to another tend to act according to the rules of their culture of origin. When those rules do not reasonably fit with cultural rules in their new setting, they are culturally stressed and may experience culture shock. Ways in which culturally competent nurses can minimize this stress are discussed later in the chapter.

CULTURE IS NOT EASILY DESCRIBED BY ITS MEMBERS

Much of culture is implicit—a combination of habit and assumptions about the world. Habits are enacted without reflection in the daily course of living and are thus not easily described by its members. Thus, before asking patients about their cultural beliefs, for example, "What do you believe about prenatal care?," it is helpful to read about a cultural group or talk with a key informant. Then, a more specific question can be posed, such as "Some women believe they should rest for 10 days following birth; what are your expectations or traditions following delivery?" Cultural models that illustrate implicit culture are described in other resources (see Sager, 2011).

Implicit bias is an extension of implicit cultural perspectives. According to Blair, Havranek, Price, Hanratty, Fairclough, et al. (2013, p. 92), bias is "the negative evaluation of one group and its members relative to another." Implicit bias is frequent and long-lasting, functioning at an unconscious level and impacting one's views, conduct, and recall of events. Blair et al. (2013) found that primary care providers demonstrated a strong implicit bias against Latinos and African Americans compared to Whites. Implicit bias may negatively impact the care that nurses provide to many groups, for example, people who are overweight. Waller, Lampman, and Lupfer-Johnson (2012) found that nursing students demonstrated a statistically significant implicit bias against overweight people.

Culture imbues people with assumptions, or ways of behaving and believing, that are learned through socialization and participation in various subcultures. Cultural habituation has some advantages. It reduces the extent to which people must take environmental cues into account—allowing them to respond to routines almost without thinking. This is also a key element in expertise. Benner, Sutphen, Leonard, and Day (2010) differentiate the expert nurse from the novice nurse on the basis of being able to take in several cues rapidly; to scan, assess, and prioritize them; and to respond appropriately and effectively in unusually short order. To the extent that culture is shared with others in the community, cultural habituation makes the world familiar, stable, and predictable. A predictable environment and being able to perceive the world as coherent are essential for human functioning. However, assumptions may result in unconscious stereotypes and ethnocentrism.

CULTURE IS ETHNOCENTRIC

Because many aspects of culture are learned from authority figures (e.g., parents, clergy, healthcare providers, or celebrities), cultural beliefs usually are held as truths. Ethnocentrism is viewing one's own culture as the only correct standard by which to view people of other cultures. It may reflect a fear of difference from one's belief system and consequent derision or disqualification of people and practices that do not conform to one's own view. Because cultural habituation makes people unaware of many of their cultural assumptions, they are not always aware of their cultural biases. For example, some Whites have difficulty accepting the charge of White supremacy that may be leveled against them by blacks. Some men have trouble understanding charges of male chauvinism made by women. In addition, some healthcare providers assume they know better than their patients what will help their patients. Another way of thinking about ethnocentrism in nursing is that it can reflect an individual, group, or agency's cultural blindness, or lack of capacity to reach out effectively to minorities or culturally stigmatized groups (Capell, 2008). After conducting content analysis of the concept of ethnocentrism, Sutherland (2002) proposed the following operational definition:

Ethnocentrism is a way of looking at the world through a personal lens that has been influenced by personality, genetics, family/relationships, and media. In its mildest form, ethnocentrism presents as subconscious disregard for cultural differences; in its most severe form, it presents as authoritarian dominance over groups different from one's own (p. 280).

An effective approach to eliminating ethnocentrism by healthcare professionals is to request that the population of interest take the lead in planning healthcare services and resources. An example is the *Model of Values for Teaching and Learning of Cancer-Related Information by American Indian and Alaska Native People* in which a symbol that is sacred to the population is used. Other values such as connections across generations, storytelling, and learning by experience are incorporated (Vogel, Cowens-Alvarado, Eschiti, Samos, Wiener, et al., 2013).

CULTURE IS RELATIVE

The earlier example of the variation in the meanings of colors across cultures demonstrates the principle of **cultural relativity**, which is the understanding that cultures relate in different manners to the same given situations. For example, consider the handshake. Westerners attribute trust and agreement to the handshake and view it as a positive social act. Some Asians avoid shaking hands because the act involves touching a stranger or hands that may be dirty. A cultural interpretation of the difference is that the handshake by itself is meaningless. When carried out by Westerners, it is invested with one meaning. When enacted by Asians, it has another meaning. At the extreme, the principle of cultural relativity would assume that no absolutes exist, nothing has meaning by itself, and the meaning or significance of any act or symbol is simply that created and assigned by human groups. Theorists have argued that such an extreme position is untenable because it is amoral. Most nurses accept the principle of cultural relativity only to a certain (but variable and debatable) degree to preserve moral standards. For example, nursing practice does not condone wife abuse even when a minority group, including the abused woman, defends it as a culturally appropriate practice. Another example is female genital cutting, which is a cultural–religious tradition in some countries that causes lifelong harm and is considered child abuse in most of the world (Goldenstein, 2014). Nurses frequently are in patient care situations that raise the question, "Where is the line between ethical behavior and cultural integrity?" Issues related to this question require open discussion among staff, a bioethicist, and the patients concerned to determine the best among possible decisions. The best decisions are grounded in ethical principles that are widely used in nursing and medical practice: fairness; respect for persons, families, and communities; and benefit outweighing harm or risk. *The Code of Ethics for Nurses* (American Nurses Association, 2014) guides nurses when confronting ethical dilemmas.

CULTURE IS PERVASIVE AND HOLISTIC

A culture is a learned systematic way of interacting and interpreting behaviors and events holistically. The holistic nature of culture is compatible with holistic, individualized, and safe nursing care. Both the cultural and nursing approaches regard people in their entire humanity and direct attention to the total context of a person or group (Leininger, 1970). Culture links various behaviors and events uniquely. For example, for Western nurses, autopsy is culturally linked to medical beliefs (i.e., that the cause of death can be discovered or validated by examination of the internal organs and tissues and that by learning the organic cause of death in one person, the deaths of others can be postponed or prevented), to the belief in the separation of the body and soul, and to the Judeo–Christian belief that the body ultimately decomposes into "dust" or generic organic matter. People of other cultural heritages may link autopsy with other belief systems and practices. For example, Hmong[1] who have not converted to Christianity tend to link autopsy to their recent experience of genocide in Laos and to their beliefs in reincarnation, multiple souls, and the inseparability of body and spirit. They tend to interpret autopsy as preventing the continuation of their society by preventing the union of a person's soul with its body after death, thereby making its rebirth impossible and condemning the deceased to floundering forever in distress in purgatory.

CULTURE IS OBSERVABLE IN RITUALS

Rituals are common and observable expressions of culture in hospitals, clinics, homes, schools, and work settings. Patients and their families practice rituals that are intimately important to them, particularly during illness and hospitalization. Observance of rituals in times of stress and uncertainty helps restore a sense of control, competence, and familiarity, and to that extent, it is a desirable adjunct to nursing care.

Generally, most people think of rituals as events such as thanksgiving dinner, weddings, funerals, and parades. However, there are also nursing rituals, such as report, hand washing, gowning, nursing rounds, and annual professional meetings. Nurses' observance of professional rituals helps standardize practice and ensure efficiency. Nurse–patient misunderstanding, however, may arise unintentionally when the nurse's rituals are incompatible with those of the patient. For example, a common home remedy for fever among Southeast Asians is to keep the body well covered with clothes or blankets to keep it warm. This secular ritual of caring conflicts with Western nurses' rituals or procedures of caring for febrile patients, which are designed to cool, rather than to warm, the body. In a metaethnographic analysis of 22 studies, Higginbottom, Hadziabdic, Yohani, and Paton (2014) found that during inpatient maternity care, numerous barriers caused neglect of the patient's cultural traditions and rituals.

CULTURE IS RECOGNIZABLE AT MANY LEVELS

The easiest level of culture to recognize is material—in artwork, drama, tools, clothes, food, buildings, and rituals (Fig. 5-2). Values and beliefs are harder to recognize. Sometimes, they can be accessed by asking about items of material culture. For

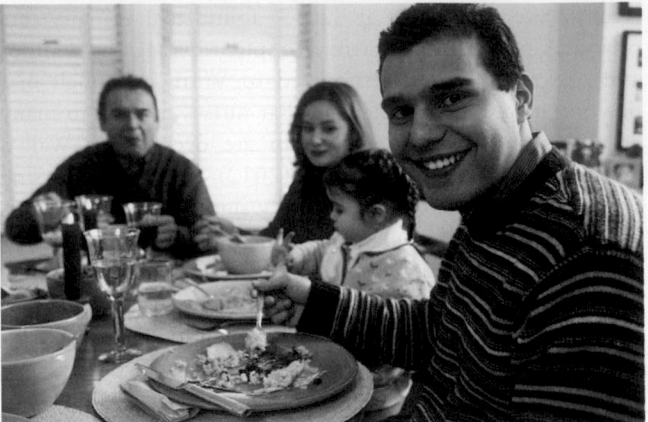

FIGURE 5-2 Culture is reflected through traditional holiday meals.

example, interested, nonjudgmental inquiry about a tattoo on a patient's arm could lead to explanations about the person's religious background, belief in magic, or occupational history. Understanding people's values and beliefs may require long-term contact, with careful observation and inquiry about patterns in behavior, although there are interview frameworks that assist nurses in learning about culture from the patient (for more information on this topic, see the section "Nursing Assessments Based on the Patient's Perspective" later in this chapter).

Concepts Related to Culture

ETHNICITY OR ETHNIC IDENTITY

Ethnicity or **ethnic identity** refers to a self-conscious, past-oriented form of identity based on a notion of shared cultural and perhaps ancestral heritage and current position within the larger society. Whites in North America, for example, have an ethnic identity that is grounded in a sense of common European heritage and the associated migrations to the land where they were free to practice their religions, govern themselves, and develop frontiers. Their ethnic identity may also be influenced by the shame of their ancestor's oppression of Native Americans and enslavement of African Americans. The ethnicity of African Americans in North America is linked to common descent from African peoples and a history of having been brought from Africa against their wills as slaves to a land dominated by Whites. However, the meaning of an ethnic label varies depending upon who uses it. For example, Africans and Blacks from the Caribbean who voluntarily immigrated to the United States and whose forebears were not slaves tend to identify themselves as African Americans and be so identified in medical records, but African Americans who are descendants of slaves might not see them as belonging to the same ethnic group.

Differences in ethnic identity have emerged between Native Americans in the United States and the First Nations People of Canada even though at one time they all freely moved back and forth across what have become national boundaries. The term *aboriginal* in Canada refers to anyone who is First Nations, Inuit, or Metis.

---

[1]The Hmong resettled in Western countries as refugees from the Vietnam War. For a sensitive account of cultural clashes between Hmong in the United States and healthcare providers and institutions, see Fadiman (1997).

What distinguishes ethnic identity from culture is that ethnic identity is self-conscious about select symbolic elements that are taken as the emblem of group social identity. In one context, an ethnic group might use native language to distinguish itself from other ethnic groups. In another context, the group might draw on other ethnic indicators, such as style of dress (as when Hmong of one tribe encounter Hmong of another tribe) or religion (as when animist Hmong exclude Christian Hmong from the ranks of "true" Hmong) to stress within-group differences.

Ethnicity is a cluster of ways for people to define themselves and be defined by others. It involves the selection of certain shared cultural characteristics as symbols of a common group origin, history, or descent. That selection may be made by the ethnic group or by the larger society to which it is subordinate.

Ethnicity is dynamic, as is culture. In a multicultural society, lines of ethnicity become blurred as parents and children represent different ethnic groups through adoption or marriage.

MINORITY

The term minority refers to a group of people within a society whose members have different ethnic, racial, national, religious, sexual, political, linguistic, or other characteristics from most of society. Being of a minority group often results in having less power and being disadvantaged in a society.

The concepts of minority, disadvantaged, and less powerful are key to understanding and correcting health disparities. According to the National Partnership for Action to End Health Disparities (2014), a disparity is

[a] particular type of *health difference* that is closely linked with social or economic disadvantage. Health disparities adversely affect groups of people who have systematically experienced greater social and/or economic obstacles to health and/or a clean environment based on their racial or ethnic group; religion; socioeconomic status; gender; age; mental health; cognitive, sensory, or physical disability; sexual orientation; geographic location; or other characteristics historically linked to discrimination or exclusion. It is the responsibility for Nurses to act at the local, State and National level to attain health equity, which is defined by the National Partnership for Action as "attainment of the highest level of health for all people." Achieving health equity requires valuing everyone equally with focused and ongoing societal efforts to address avoidable inequalities, historical and contemporary injustices, and the elimination of health and healthcare disparities.

The term *majority* refers to the ethnic group that represents more than 50% of the US population, which currently are White non-Hispanics. By 2043, no single group will represent more than 50% of the US population, therefore rendering the terms *minority* and *majority* meaningless in the context of ethnic group demographics.

RACE

Although the terms *race* and *ethnic group* sometimes refer to the same people, race takes biologic characteristics as the markers of separate social status, and *ethnic group* takes social characteristics (such as language, religious tenets, shared beliefs of origin) as markers of cultural identity. However, there are no true or readily identifiable physiologic boundaries between races. In fact, there is more variation in supposedly "racial" characteristics *within* than across groups. Race is a social construct—that is, a set of categories created by society. The categories were based on physical appearance or place of origin. We now know that there is no biologic basis for this social construct (Hall & Fields, 2013). Race or ethnicity cannot be defined by biologic or genetic methods and, therefore, in clinical and research settings, is identified based on physical characteristics or self-definition that are inconsistent and unreliable. Because race cannot be defined, the U.S. Census Bureau asks each person to identify his or her own race or racial mix. People may self-identify as more than one race and as Hispanic or non-Hispanic, according to the U.S. Census Bureau (2014b).

RACISM

For centuries, European expansion occurred at the expense of people of color including Native Americans, African Americans, Asians, and Mexicans. As a result, skin color became the symbol of social status, power, and cultural difference. Racism uses skin color as the primary indicator of social value. In Euro-American society, racism perpetuates dominance by those with white skin and penalizes others by minimizing their value. This form of racism defines peoples with darker skin as inferior. *Racism* may be defined as an ideology that gives White people power and dominance resulting in oppression and exploitation of peoples of different skin color, or racism may be described as any negative belief or action that stereotypes another person on the basis of skin color. Racism is implicated in disparities in health outcomes and healthcare services (Nadimpalli & Hutchinson, 2012).

There are numerous egregious examples of racism in US healthcare research, including the Tuskegee project. The researchers purposefully subjected black prisoners to syphilis without treatment to study the natural course of the disease. That is, for the sake of medical knowledge, the researchers consciously caused the study participants decades of suffering that led to their deaths. Other examples of unethical catastrophic practices include the sterilization of Native American women and girls without their knowledge. The legacy of these atrocities is seen today in mistrust of healthcare services and research by some populations (Hodge, 2012).

Institutionalized racism contributes to racial and ethnic health disparities. Williams (2012) explains that an institution's organizational structures, policies, and practices may be discriminatory despite the best intentions to make them equitable. He describes research that identifies racial or ethnic discrimination that is associated with numerous poor health outcomes including lower screening rates for cancer, high blood pressure, high body mass index, smoking, and mental health disorders.

SUBCULTURES

A subculture is "an ethnic, regional, economic, or social group exhibiting characteristic patterns of behavior sufficient to distinguish it from others" (Merriam-Webster Dictionary Online, 2014). Therefore, a subculture could be based on any common interest or identity—for example, sexual preference, gender, age, hobby, profession, and so on. Identity with a subculture may be stronger or more meaningful than with one's original or historical culture.

Nursing is considered a middle-class subculture of Western society, particularly of Western medicine, that epitomizes the valued role of nurturers and caregivers. The RN Workforce composition is different than the general population; 90% are female and 83% classify themselves as non-Hispanic White (Hart & Mareno, 2013). Nurses reflect many values of the dominant group:

- They generally adhere to the work ethic, with work viewed as a reward independent of other compensation.
- They spend much talent and time on planning for the future.
- They are keenly sensitive to use of time.

Nurses also are recognizable as a subgroup in numerous ways, such as the following:

- Their legally sanctioned authoritative stance vis-à-vis patients and the general public
- Their manner of dress
- Their language ("nurse-ese" includes a large vocabulary of acronyms specific to healthcare professions as well as its own subcultural lingo)
- The rituals and ritualized behaviors into which nurses are socialized as nurses

Nurses who are aware of their own subcultural values and behaviors can see how their own cultural makeup might distance, confine, or threaten persons from other cultural backgrounds.

Subcultural identity, like ethnic identity, can be a source of social support or a target for stigma and exploitation. For example, in the 1960s, the work of Oscar Lewis (1966) spread the misleading notion that poverty is a subculture. He thought that family disorganization made people poor. The theory that culture accounts for poverty blames the poor for being poor, implying that if people were not fatalistic and if they pulled themselves up by their bootstraps, they would not be poor. Critics disproved this theory by demonstrating that societal mechanisms and early life experiences (e.g., the lack of adequate day care for children of working parents, overcrowding in inner-city schools, and lack of access to healthcare) keep people in poverty (Juon et al., 2014). They noted that early life experiences—such as foster care experience, educational opportunities, and childhood illness—are characteristic of poverty, not of culture. Informed professionals no longer adhere to the notion of a subculture of poverty.

The lesbian, gay, bisexual, and transgender (LGBT) community is an example of a group where social support may be strong and where stigma and discrimination is perpetuated by people from outside the group. Discriminatory behavior by healthcare professionals is experienced by about 50% of LGBT people (Kane-Lee & Bayer, 2012). Healthy People 2020 objectives and recommendations for improving healthcare services for this community have reached a wide audience (Lesbian, Gay, Bisexual and Transgender Health, 2014).

STEREOTYPES

Assigning people to specific categories because of their culture, race, or ethnicity is stereotypical thinking. Stereotypes are preconceived and untested beliefs about people. They are exaggerated descriptors of character or behavior that are commonly reiterated in mass media, idiomatic expressions, and folklore. They may be demeaning ("People on welfare are lazy, just living off handouts") or idealizing ("Vietnamese are the valedictorians"; "Nurses are patient people"). Either way, they mislead and deny the individuality of the person.

The use of stereotypes in nursing results in incorrect assessments and, consequently, inappropriate and potentially harmful and unethical interventions or lack of action. For example, acting on the stereotype that "Asians are stoic" could result in a nurse's failure to assess pain and institute measures to alleviate it. It is imperative that nurses examine their own stereotypes; otherwise, they may be expressed in unconscious behavior and thereby demean the people they aim to help (Hall & Fields, 2013).

CONCEPTS OF CULTURE IN NURSING CARE

Culture shapes, but does not determine, all learned human responses. Culture is most evident at the levels of the group, society, or population because at these levels, individual variation is less apparent and patterns of similar cultural behaviors become more apparent. One can observe culture in various ways, including in *patterned group behavior* (such as ways of tending to personal hygiene, preventing disease, relating to the opposite sex, expressing pain, or performing rituals associated with important life events such as pregnancy, birth, coming of age, illness, marriage, and death), in *texts* (such as what a group considers its classical literature, songs, media, and official records), and in *architecture* (such as the use and placement of asylums, hospitals, palaces, prisons, schools, or temples).

Although individuals reflect the influence of their cultures, they do not share the same culture equally (Douglas et al., 2014). For example, spectator sports are a cultural characteristic of life in the United States, but many people in the United States pay little attention to them while still considering themselves culturally American. Similarly, because the public image of nursing in North America is still viewed as a female profession, some patients show surprise when receiving care from a male nurse.

Culturally Competent Nursing

Patients have the right to receive care that is individualized and culturally acceptable to them and that builds on the support and healing that cultural ties may provide. Because nursing focuses on human responses to actual or threatened health problems, nurses increase the quality and safety of their care by considering cultural influences on their own responses as well as on those of the patient, family, or community to health, illness, disease, and injury. Care that assures quality and safety relies heavily on **culturally competent nursing** (American Association of Colleges in Nursing, 2014). *Cultural competence is the "attitudes, knowledge, and skills necessary for providing quality care to diverse populations" (American Association of Colleges of Nursing, 2014, p. 1).* Cultural competency is an integral component of the knowledge and practice base of nursing and is continually improved through a lifelong learning process and commitment to **health equity**. Transcultural nursing refers to nursing practice that is patient-centered, evidence-based and considers culture (Giger, 2013, p. 5).

Standards of practice for culturally competent nursing care continue to be refined and are driven by the principles of social justice and health equity with the aim of reducing health disparities (Douglas et al., 2014). *The Essential Guide to Nursing Practice: Applying ANA's Scope and Standards in Practice and Education* (White & O'Sullivan, 2012) highlights the importance of culture in nursing practice, education, research, and health policy.

> The registered nurse develops in partnership with the person, family and others an individualized plan considering the person's characteristics or situation, including but not limited to, values, beliefs, spiritual and health practices, preferences, choices, developmental level, coping style, culture and environment and available technology (American Nurses Association, 2010, p. 31).

> The registered nurse uses health promotion and health teaching methods appropriate to the situation and the patient's values, beliefs, health practices, developmental level, learning needs, readiness and ability to learn, language preference, spirituality, culture, and socioeconomic status (American Nurses Association, 2010, p. 36).

Other standards and resources include *The National Standards for Culturally and Linguistically Appropriate Services in Health and Health Care* (U.S. Department of Health and Human Services, Office of Minority Health, 2014a) and *Culturally Competent Nursing Care: A Cornerstone of Caring* (U.S. Department of Health and Human Services, Office of Minority Health, 2014b) and *Cultural Competency in Baccalaureate Nursing Education* (American Association of Colleges in Nursing, 2014).

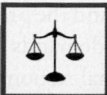

ETHICAL/LEGAL ISSUE

REFUSAL OF TREATMENT BASED ON PREJUDICE

As you begin to work in the clinic, you overhear the medical assistant and receptionist talking about a patient who has come into the waiting room. The patient is coughing and appears flushed.

"There he is again. He comes into the clinic over the most minor things and takes up so much of our time. I'm sure he is an illegal alien."

"I know. It isn't right that my tax dollars are spent on noncitizens!"

"Well, just tell him that there are no appointments available."

CRITICAL THINKING CHALLENGE

Explore your own feelings about this interaction and appropriate actions to take.

• Identify your personal values and beliefs in this situation.
• Think about ways in which you can respond to this situation.
• Identify a possible approach that might bring about changes in behavior and would improve the quality of patient care.

The emphasis of culturally competent nursing is the need for the nurse to understand the culture of the patient. However, that is only part of the process of therapeutic nursing interactions. Another component is the nurse's recognition of her or his own culture and biases *and* the culture of the biomedical healthcare system. Prejudices and bias were among the top three barriers to culturally competent care in a study of 374 nurses in the United States (Hart & Mareno, 2013). Critical reflection, feedback from colleagues, and self-assessment are ways to explore one's own culture, biases, and perspectives. Our own culture tends to be invisible to us and therefore requires a specific effort to explore it (National Center for Cultural Competence, 2014b).

Culturally sensitive nurses adapt care to respect each patient's cultural characteristics in order to create a collaborative, patient-centered relationship and ensure safe care. Cultural assessment is ongoing and increases the nurse's understanding of the patient. This process may require the assistance of a trained interpreter or cultural mediator.

Culturally competent care minimizes culture shock for the patient who suddenly finds herself or himself in the subculture of a hospital or healthcare agency. The collaborative and patient-centered relationship reinforces the patient's sense of competency, thereby promoting learning of self-care.

Changes in society, such as the AIDS pandemic and the practice of early discharge from hospitals, place added demands on nurses' cultural sensitivity. The stigma and emotional responses attached to HIV infection and AIDS require that nurses be skilled in eliciting what the illness means to the patient and what the patient's support system is. The shift in site of nursing care away from hospitals to the community (homes, worksites, schools, ambulatory care settings) has changed the nurse–patient power balance in favor of patients. In hospital settings, patients are guests or visitors in the nurse's domain; outside hospitals, nurses are guests of patients, and their patients are better supported by their cultural traditions, requiring that the nurse be skilled in providing culturally competent assessments and care.

Health Behaviors and Traditions

It is important for nurses to learn about patients' health-related behaviors and cultural traditions, including seeking information about the patient's ethnic group when planning a nursing assessment. Although the information found may not represent the patient's behaviors or traditions, it may facilitate the assessment. For example, such prior research might allow the nurse to ask questions such as "I understand that some people from your country often eat rice and beans in the evening; is that your practice?" It is essential that the nurse learn from the patient. Evidence-based resources such as www.ethnomed.org provide cultural information related to issues such as children's growth, nutrition, personal care traditions, breastfeeding, concepts of time and space, decision making, and end of life. Caution in applying culture-specific information to individuals is advised; however, background information about the population may improve nursing assessments and interventions (Giger, 2013).

Nursing Assessments Based on the Patient's Perspective

Accurate nursing assessments require minimizing the nurse's bias and ethnocentric tendencies and maximizing cultural sensitivity. Cultural assessments identify the patients' (or the families') views of themselves, their health, their patterns of daily living, demands that are made on them, their resources, and their values and goals. When gathering cultural information, the interviewee is the expert. In the domain of nursing, gathering, and recording subjective data—including information about the patient's life, experience, responses, resources, and world as he or she sees them—without adulterating, it is critical.

There are several ways to obtain an understanding of the patient's perspective. Usually, combining several methods over time yields more complete and accurate results than relying on any single approach. The most effective methods are open-ended interviewing, variants of which are the ethnographic interview and the explanatory model, the key informant technique, and observation over time.

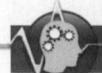 **APPLY YOUR CRITICAL THINKING**

You discover that Mrs. R., a recent refugee from Afghanistan, has been taking her asthma medications haphazardly. While discussing this with Mrs. R. and her husband via an interpreter, they recount their experiences in a refugee camp where few medications were available. You observe their discomfort with notes being taken, and they show you an unlabeled bottle of liquid they report helps wheezing. How would you seek to understand cultural issues that pertain to this visit? How would you organize your interview, and what interviewing approaches would be helpful?

Check your answer in Appendix B.

OPEN-ENDED INTERVIEWING

A positive provider–patient relationship based on effective communication is associated with improved survival and quality of life among cancer patients (Mead, Doorenbos, Javid, Haozous, Arviso Alvord, et al., 2013). Various techniques are used in open-ended interviewing to elicit responses from the interviewee that are as free from influence by the interviewer's comments as possible. Open-ended questions require that the respondent use his or her own words to answer. Silent pauses are sometimes useful because they give the respondent time to think about more things to say. Prompts such as "Could you tell me more about… ?" encourage the patient to elaborate on a point of interest to the nurse.

The Ethnographic Interview

The ethnographic interview is a structured way to elicit the respondent's concepts and understandings. The nurse interviewer asks questions, the patient answers, and the nurse interviewer asks for clarification of the patient's responses, if needed. Highly skilled nurse interviewers conduct ethnographic interviews that sound so much like friendly conversations that respondents do not feel they are being interviewed. In effect, nurse interviewers guide patients to teach about the subject at hand by expressing interest in the topic, incorporating the patients' own words, and using hypothetical examples. Asking patients to clarify words reveals their culture-based meaning. The interviewer follows the lead of the patient and encourages him or her to be a teacher (Kwan-Gett, 2014).

There are three parts to an ethnographic interview:

1. It begins with an open-ended, general question such as "How have you been feeling since I saw you yesterday?" or "I'm wondering about your family…."
2. From the patient's response, the nurse selects some key terms and asks for clarification. For example, "You felt 'hot in your throat'? I'm not sure what you mean; would you tell me more?" or "You said your 'absent father'—what did you mean by that?" Note that the nurse repeats exactly the

words and phrases that the patient used. The terms are clues to what is important to the patient, so the nurse asks the patient to talk more about them.

3. The last part of the ethnographic interview is documentation. Information on the patient's view of himself or herself or of the issue discussed should be recorded as soon as possible after the interview so that it can be retained as accurately and completely as possible.

The Explanatory Model

The explanatory model is similar to the ethnographic interview. Given that the patient is the expert on his or her own multicultural identity, questions are posed by the nurse in order to understand the patient's beliefs about his or her health or the patient's explanation for his or her condition (Kleinman & Benson, 2006). It is essential that the nurse understand his or her own explanatory model. For example, many people in the United States have a view of mental illness that is influenced by the cultural values of self-reliance and independence. Therefore, depression, anxiety, grief, and stress are viewed as conditions that require intervention, whereas other cultures view these as part of life and not as mental illness (Gholizadeh, Davidson, Heydari & Salamonson, 2014).

KEY INFORMANT TECHNIQUE

The key informant technique is a method in which the interviewer looks for, locates, and interviews people who have expert or native knowledge about a culture that the interviewer needs to know. A willingness to discuss this knowledge and rapport with the interviewer are critical. The optimal key informant about a patient is the patient himself, but medically or culturally compromised patients (i.e., those who are unable to function optimally in the culture) might not be able to fill the role. Direct, regular, and ubiquitous contact (in the hospital, clinic, home, school, or workplace) of nurses with their patients enables them to observe and assess patient behaviors, social support systems, and environmental constraints and resources. But without an understanding of the cultural meaning of what is observed, the nurses' observations have little value.

For most patients with limited English-speaking ability, the most useful key informants in the hospital or clinic situation may be bilingual, bicultural, trained interpreters, or family and friends. The role of religious figures in health, including as key informant, is important because people often interpret life–death and health–illness issues in terms of their cultural heritage or religious beliefs.

Language Differences Between the Patient and the Nurse

A deliberate search for the meaning behind patient responses enables the nurse to plan and provide safe and individualized patient care. Language differences between the patient and the nurse compound cultural differences and can keep the nurse from understanding the patient's point of view (U.S. Department of Health and Human Services, Office of Minority Health, 2014a). When the patient does not speak the same language or does so only to a limited extent, the nurse may decide to act in the patient's best interests—without actually knowing what the patient believes those interests to be. For example, when a patient from an ethnic minority is alert but not talkative or responds only with affirmatives, healthcare providers might conclude that the patient does not understand English. If no interpreter is at hand, the healthcare providers might do what they think is best or necessary for the patient even if they do not have the subjective data normally required to guide clinical decision making. The result can be tragic in terms of the patient's welfare and loss of trust with a subcultural community.

For example, a patient with limited English proficiency underwent major surgery and recuperated without complications in the intensive care unit (ICU) of a tertiary care hospital. Prior to surgery, his behavior was engaged and appropriate. After he was transferred to a regular care unit, his behavior changed dramatically. He exhibited anxious and paranoid behavior. When a psychiatric nurse and an interpreter were consulted, they became the first healthcare providers to attempt to understand the patient's point of view. They found that the transfer from the ICU to a regular unit did not signify recuperation to the patient at all. In fact, he interpreted it as meaning the hospital had given up on him because they thought he was so sick that he was no longer worth caring for. In his view, he had been moved from an environment of expert care and the best of technologic assistance into an old part of the hospital that was practically devoid of technologic props and limited in staff. The healthcare team's belief that the transfer was a self-explanatory demonstration of recuperation is a classic example of medical/nursing ethnocentrism because they neglected to assess the patient's perspective.

In the example above, the patient's confusion, fear, and isolation were all preventable. They could be considered *iatrogenic* (i.e., caused by hospitalization). Cases such as this one could be defined as negligent in today's healthcare system because an interpreter must be arranged to explain to the patient the facility's plans for him *before* the patient is admitted to the hospital. Hospitals are required to provide trained language interpreters for "the patient who does not speak or understand the predominant language of the community" (The Joint Commission, 2014). Furthermore, hospitals that receive Medicare or Medicaid reimbursement are subject to Title VI of the Civil Rights Act, which prohibits recipients of federal funds from discriminating or denying benefits on the basis of race, color, or national origin. According to the *The National Standards for Culturally and Linguistically Appropriate Services,* hospitals that fail to provide trained interpreters for people who speak no or only limited English, or for deaf people who use sign language, are in violation of the law. Therefore, nurses who are frustrated in their efforts to communicate with a patient because of language differences or impaired hearing or speech, and who are unable to provide the quality of care deemed appropriate, have the legal recourse to urge the hospital to provide a trained interpreter to resolve the language situation (U.S. Department of Health and Human Services, Office of Minority Health, 2014a).

Obtaining trained interpreters rather than bilingual members of the patient's family or friends, however well intentioned or convenient the latter might be, is important because interpretation of behavior goes beyond translation of words. Much medical vocabulary and terminology is difficult to translate into other languages. For example, the phrase "the lab tech dialed the wrong number" could not be translated into the language of a culture that did not have telephones or scientific laboratories. Furthermore, if the patient's condition deteriorates, the emotional burden of responsibility could be overwhelming on someone close to the patient. In addition, the patient's right to privacy and confidentiality is essential.

For example, a Vietnamese woman was hospitalized with cancer. Her 20-year-old daughter was in a long-term care facility with leukemia. The husband/father spoke little English. The hospital staff relied on the 12-year-old daughter/sister to act as interpreter. First, the sister with leukemia died and then the mother. The 12-year-old, suffering from a sense of complicity in their deaths because of her influence on care owing to her role as translator, had an acute psychotic episode for which she needed to be institutionalized. The use of a professional interpreter instead may have prevented this tragic outcome.

Numerous resources are available to assure availability of interpreters through 24-hour phone services (U.S. Department of Health and Human Services, Office of Minority Health, 2014a). It is essential to establish a person's need for an interpreter at first contact with the healthcare agency. Provide an interpreter whenever it is requested and definitely at any time when plans for the patient are being made or a change in procedure is being proposed. Occasions for involving an interpreter include during admission, for consent for treatment, during treatments, for discharge planning, and for patient education. Tips for communicating through an interpreter are given in Box 5-2.

Increased Effectiveness of Patient Education

Culturally sensitive nurses make nonjudgmental observations and seek to understand the beliefs and perspectives behind the behaviors. . If a behavior is practiced by many people in a group, it may represent a tradition that pertains to their identity and beliefs. When refugees from rural and mountainous areas of Southeast Asia first arrived in the United States, healthcare and social service providers observed behaviors they were not familiar with. A culturally sensitive nurse would communicate with the patient in order to

---

BOX 5-2   Communicating Through an Interpreter

Meet with the interpreter *before* you and the interpreter meet with the patient. Tell the interpreter what you want to learn from the patient and what messages you want to convey to the patient. Also, discuss your concerns about how to communicate with the patient, and ask for feedback on how to help the interpreter succeed in reaching mutual understanding with the patient.

- Speak to the *patient* rather than to the interpreter: This enables the patient to "read" your nonverbal language.
- *Watch* the verbal and nonverbal interactions between the interpreter and patient: "Read" their nonverbal language.
- *Speak slowly.*
- Use *simple* sentences.
- Rephrase a question in different words or ask it indirectly if the answer that you received is inappropriate or inconsistent with other indications.
- Avoid using metaphors (e.g., "Have you been feeling down?" "Once in a blue moon" "Does it feel like pins and needles?"); they are difficult to translate.
- Expect that it might take an interpreter longer to say or explain something in another language than in English. This is especially true when the concept is a medical one for which there is no equivalent in the other language or culture or when the topic is considered taboo or embarrassing in the other culture.
- When unsure how to broach a delicate subject, ask the interpreter for advice: *Use the interpreter as a key informant* on the culture of the patient.
- Try to work consistently with the same interpreter; with practice, you and the interpreter can learn to communicate better with each other.
- Relate to the interpreter as a professional colleague; your nursing care depends on the interpreter's skill.

---

understand the beliefs that contributed to the behaviors. An understanding of the patient's health beliefs and behaviors is essential to create patient-centered communication, complete an assessment, and plan and implement care and education. Examples of behaviors that indicate the need for a culturally competent interview include the following:

- When women who were taking birth control pills forgot to take a pill, they either took two pills the next day or gave the extra pill to their husbands.
- Several newborns in families of non–English-speaking refugees were brought into the emergency room with dehydration.
- Many refugee households with newborns put the heat on in their apartments even during the hot summer, and they swaddled infants and toddlers who had fevers in layers of clothing.

By using the ethnographic interview, consulting key informants, and making observations in patients' homes, the following rationales for the refugee behaviors may be discovered:

- The women who forgot to take a birth control pill were trying to compensate for its omission. Because they did not know the principles on which the pills work, they made legitimate guesses about how to overcome their oversight. Also, their cultural heritage had taught them not to ask questions of authority figures, lest they be considered rude and offensive.
- The mothers of dehydrated babies had followed feeding instructions that they had received in the postpartum unit. A hospital nurse who researched the problem discovered that the mothers had learned their lesson well. The problem was that the method they were taught was correct only for the ready-to-use formula that the hospital gave out as free samples. Once those samples were used up, the women began using formula from the Women, Infants, and Children (WIC) Program. However, the WIC milk used was a dry powder. Because the women could not read the English language directions on the labels, they guessed how to mix the dry formula. Many guessed wrong, resulting in dehydrated babies.
- The households that turned up the heat and overdressed children with fevers were exercising their belief in the humoral theory of physiology that is prevalent in Southeast Asia (Muecke, 1976). According to this theory, blood is hot, and because women lose blood during delivery, they lose heat. To keep them from getting sick, this theory advocates that their bodies be kept so warm that they regain the heat they have lost. Similarly, children, who tend to have higher fevers than adults, are thought to lose heat when they have a fever. Dressing them warmly is thought to prevent heat from leaving their bodies.

Culturally sensitive nursing assessments resulted in improved communication and planning for care. The health education that resulted from these assessments increased the patients' and their ethnic communities' trust of nurses and of healthcare agencies.

THERAPEUTIC DIALOGUE: CULTURE

SCENE FOR THOUGHT

Spencer, whose situation was described at the beginning of this chapter, is being prepared for discharge. Plans are being made for the next step in Spencer's care. A discharge planner at the hospital is having difficulty discussing Spencer's future care with his parents, who are Samoan. The discharge planner asks the primary nurse to speak with them.

LESS EFFECTIVE	
Nurse:	Hello again. Thank you for coming in this morning. I wanted to talk to you about where to place Spencer after he gets discharged next month. I understand that you want to care for him at home, is that right?
Mr. Lewis:	Yes (*He looks miserable, and his wife stares straight ahead with her teeth clenched.*).
Nurse:	Do you really think that's a good idea? He cannot feed himself, needs to be exercised with the standing board, and needs to be turned all the time so his skin stays healthy. Complications can occur at any time. Do you think you can handle that?
Mr. Lewis:	Yes (*His wife is crying quietly beside him and he looks as though he's going to cry, too.*).
Nurse:	(*Tries not to act exasperated.*) Okay, if that's your decision, we'll be happy to work with you on that. When do you want to come here to start

MORE EFFECTIVE	
Nurse:	Hello, Mr. and Mrs. Lewis. I appreciate your coming in today. It seems that there has been some difficulty determining where Spencer will go to be cared for next month after his discharge from here. Could you tell me more about why you'd prefer to care for him at home?
Mr. Lewis:	We can't let him go to another hospital (*Looks at his hands in his lap. His wife stares straight ahead, her teeth clenched.*).
Nurse:	You don't seem very comfortable about that decision. Could you tell me more? (*Uses a relaxed manner, seeks more information.*)
Mr. Lewis:	It isn't my decision to make. It doesn't matter what we think (*He looks ashamed, and his wife's eyes fill with tears.*).
Nurse:	(*Tries not to look surprised.*) I don't understand. Could you explain that to me?

(continued)

THERAPEUTIC DIALOGUE: CULTURE (Continued)

learning how to take care of him? I think we can do it in a week and then have you practice for a couple of weeks before we send him home with you (*Mr. and Mrs. Lewis take deep breaths and start to arrange for each of them to come in and learn about Spencer's care.*).

Mrs. Lewis: (*Breathlessly interrupts.*) We don't want you to think we're bad parents. We think he should go to another hospital. He needs so much care and we don't know how... ! (*Cries.*)

Mr. Lewis: It's because my father is in charge of our family and he makes the decisions for all of us, especially for Spencer, because I was driving the car when Spencer got hurt, and my father thinks I was at fault and shouldn't make decisions for him. He thinks we should take care of him at home (*Looks miserable.*).

Nurse: (*Remains nonjudgmental.*) Thank you for telling me. I understand better now. I have an idea on how we might work this out, but you need to tell me if this will work with your father (*Shows consideration for both the parents' feelings and the cultural conventions.*). Suppose we ask him to come to a special team meeting with the doctor and me and all the others who care for Spencer and show him what we do with him all day. Perhaps, we can then ask his advice about Spencer's placement. What do you think? (*Mr. and Mrs. Lewis talk this over together and decide that Mr. Lewis Senior would feel important and included. They decide it would be a good idea. They look hopeful.*)

CRITICAL THINKING CHALLENGE

- Describe the tone each nurse sets at the beginning of the discussion.
- Determine who did most of the talking in each of the examples.
- Judge if either nurse knew anything about the Samoan culture, and give a reason for your answer.
- Examine the method the second nurse used to determine how this particular family operates.
- Propose places you could learn about the family structure of the various South Pacific cultures.

KEY CONCEPTS

- Culture is defined as a belief system that the members of the culture hold, consciously or unconsciously, as absolute truth. This belief system guides everyday behavior and makes it routine; provides answers to the unanswerable questions of life, sickness, and death; and makes the world make sense. Because culture is unequally shared by its members, culture is more evident in groups or societies than it is in individuals.
- Culture enables a person to behave reasonably in contexts that the person shares with members of the same culture.
- Culture is an integral component of nursing's knowledge base.
- Accurate nursing assessments require that the nurse minimize his or her ethnocentric tendencies and maximize cultural sensitivity.
- Patient assessments that consider the patient's perspective are most likely to yield diagnoses and interventions appropriate to the patient.

- Methods to gain the patient's perspective include open-ended interviewing, a variant of which is the ethnographic interview; the use of key informants; observation over time; and use of the patient's language.

PRACTICING FOR THE NCLEX
CHECK YOUR ANSWERS IN APPENDIX A.

1. Which of the following are characteristics of culture? Select all that apply:
    a. Learned
    b. Dynamic
    c. Ethnocentric
    d. Relative to context
    e. Logical
    f. A set of traits

2. Nursing care may be influenced by the culture of both the patient and nurse. Which of the following techniques will assist nurses in performing culturally competent care? Select all that apply:
   a. Minimize ethnocentric tendencies
   b. Knowledge of biocultural variation
   c. Use family as bilingual interpreters
   d. Consider patient perspective
   e. Assign to specific category based on culture

3. Shared culture is most accurately seen among people with which of the same traits?
   a. Ethnicity
   b. Skin color
   c. Rituals
   d. Language

4. When language differences exist between the nurse and patient, the nurse should do which of the following first?
   a. Act in the patient's best interest
   b. Use a bilingual family member to facilitate assessment/care
   c. Establish whether a trained interpreter is needed
   d. Obtain a key informant to navigate patient's cultural cues

5. Examples of subcultures include which of the following communities? Select all that apply:
   a. Deaf or hearing impaired
   b. Lesbian, gay, bisexual, transgender, queer (LGBTQ)
   c. HIV/AIDs
   d. Truck drivers
   e. Impoverished

REFERENCES

American Association of Colleges in Nursing. (2014). *Cultural Competency in Baccalaureate Nursing Education*. Retrieved May 30, 2014, from http://www.aacn.nche.edu/education-resources/cultural-competency

American Nurses Association. (2010). *Scope and standards of practice*. Washington, DC: American Nurses Association

American Nurses Association. (2014). *ANA nursing code of ethics*. Retrieved June 1, 2014, from http://www.nursingworld.org/mobile/code-of-ethics

Benner, P., Sutphen, M., Leonard, V., & Day, L. (2010). *Educating nurses: A call for radical transformation*. San Francisco, CA: Jossey-Bass.

Blair, I. V., Havranek, E. P., Price, D. W., Hanratty, R., Fairclough, D. L., Farley, T., et al. (2013). Assessment of biases against Latinos and African Americans among Primary Care Providers and community members. *American Journal of Public Health*, 103(1), 92–98.

Braveman, P. A., Kumanyika, S., Fielding, J., Laveist, T., Borrell, L. N., Manderscheid, R., et al. (2011). Health disparities and health equity: The issue is justice. *American Journal of Public Health*, 101(Suppl 1), S149–S155. doi: 10.2105/AJPH.2010.300062

Capell, J., Dean, E., & Veenstra, G. (2008). The relationship between cultural competence and ethnocentrism of health care professionals. *Journal of Transcultural Nursing*, 19, 121–125.

Douglas, M. K., Rosenkoetter, M., Pacquiao, D. F., Callister, L. C., Hattar-Pollara, M., Lauderdate, J, Milstead, J., et al. (2014). Guidelines for implementing culturally competent nursing care. *Journal of Transcultural Nursing*, 25, 109–121. doi: 10.1177/1043659614520998

Egenes, K. J. (2012). Health care delivery through a different lens: The lived experience of culture shock while participating in an international educational program. *Nurse Education Today*, 32(7), 760–764.

Fadiman, A. (1997). *The spirit catches you and you fall down*. New York: The Noonday Press.

Gholizadeh, L., Davidson, P. M., Heydari, M., & Salamonson, Y. (2014). Heart disease and depression: Is culture a factor? *Journal of Transcultural Nursing*, 25(3):290–295. doi: 10.1177/1043659614523453

Giger, J. (2013). *Transcultural nursing: Assessment and intervention* (6th ed.). St. Louis, MO: Elsevier/Mosby, Inc.

Goldenstein, R. A. (2014). Female genital cutting: Nursing implications. *Journal of Transcultural Nursing*, 25, 95–101. doi: 10.1177/1043659613493441

Gray, D. P., & Thomas, D. J. (2006). Critical reflections on culture in nursing. *Journal of Cultural Diversity*, 13(2), 76–82.

Hall, E. T. (1959). *The silent language* (p. 35). Greenwich, CT: Fawcett Premier.

Hall, J. M., & Fields, B. (2013). Continuing the conversation in nursing on race and racism. *Nursing Outlook*, 61(3), 164–173. http://dx.doi.org/10.1016/j.outlook.2012.11.006

Hart, P. L., & Mareno, N. (2013). Cultural challenges and barriers through the voices of nurses. *Journal of Clinical Nursing*, 23(15-16):2223–2232. doi: http://dx.doi.org/10.1111/jocn.12500

Higginbottom, G. M. A., Hadziabdic, E., Yohani, S., & Paton, P. (2014). Immigrant women's experience of maternity services in Canada: A meta-ethnography. *Midwifery*, 30(5), 544–559.

Hodge, F. (2012). No meaningful apology for American Indian Unethical Research Abuses. *Ethics & Behavior*, 22(6), 431–444. doi: 10.1080/10508422.2012.730788

Juon, H. S., Evans-Polce, R. J., & Ensminger, M. (2014). Early life conditions of overall and cause-specific mortality among inner-city African Americans. *American Journal of Public Health*, 04(3), 548–554. doi: 10.2105/AJPH.2013.301228

Kane-Lee, E., & Bayer, C. R. (2012). Meeting the needs of LGBT patients and families. *Nursing Management*, 43(2), 42–46. doi: 10.1097/01.NUMA.0000410866.26051.ff

Kennedy, A., Groom, H., Evans, V., & Fasano, N. (2010). A qualitative analysis of immunization programs with sustained high coverage, 2000–2005. *Journal of Public Health Management and Practice*, 16(1), E9–E17.

Kleinman, A., & Benson, P. (2006). Anthropology in the clinic: The problem of cultural competency and how to fix it. *PLoS Medicine*, 3(10), 1673–1676.

Kwan-Gett, T. (2014). *Collecting ethnographic data: The ethnographic interview*. Retrieved May 30, 2014, from http://ethnomed.org/about/contribute/collecting-ethnographic-data-the-ethnographic-interview/?searchterm=ethnographic%20interview

Leininger, M. (1970). *Nursing and anthropology: Two worlds to blend*. New York: John Wiley & Sons.

Lesbian, Gay, Bisexual and Transgender Health. (2014). Retrieved June 1, 2014, from http://www.healthypeople.gov/2020/topicsobjectives2020/overview.aspx?topicid=25

Lewis, O. (1966). The culture of poverty. *Scientific American*, 215(4), 19–25.

Mead, E. L., Doorenbos, A. Z., Javid, S. H., Haozous, E. A., Arviso Alvord, L., Flum, D. R., et al. (2013). Shared decision-making for cancer care among racial and ethnic minorities: A systematic review. *American Journal of Public Health*, 103, e15–e29. doi: 10.2105/AJPH.2013.301631

Merriam-Webster Dictionary Online. (2014). *Subculture*. Retrieved May 30, 2014, from http://www.merriam-webster.com/dictionary/subculture

Moceri, J. T. (2014). Hispanic nurses' experiences of bias in the Workplace. *Journal of Transcultural Nursing*, 25, 15–22. doi: 10.1177/1043659613504109

Muecke, M. A. (1976). Health care systems as socializing agents: Childbearing the North Thai and Western ways. *Social Science and Medicine*, 10, 377–383.

Nadimpalli, S. B., & Hutchinson, M. (2012). An integrative review of relationships between discrimination and Asian American Health. *Journal of Nursing Scholarship*, 44(2), 127–135. doi: 10.1111/j.1547-5069.2012.01448.x

National Center for Cultural Competence. (2014a). *Cultural awareness: What is culture?* Retrieved May 27, 2014, from www.nccccurricula.info/awareness/C4.html

National Center for Cultural Competence. (2014b). *Self-assessments*. Retrieved May 27, 2014, from http://nccc.georgetown.edu/resources/assessments.html

National Partnership for Action to End Health Disparities. (2014). *Health equity & disparities*. Retrieved May 27, 2014, from http://minorityhealth.hhs.gov/npa/templates/browse.aspx?lvl=1&lvlid=34

Oberg, K. (1954). Culture shock. Indianapolis, IN: Bobbs-Merrill.

Palacios, J. F., & Portillo, C. J. (2009). Understanding native women's health: Historical legacies. *Journal of Transcultural Nursing, 20*, 15–27.

Ramírez, A. S., Rutten, L. J., Oh, A., Vengoechea, B. L., Moser, R. P., Vanderpool, R. C., et al. (2013). Perceptions of cancer controllability and cancer risk knowledge: The moderating role of race, ethnicity, and acculturation. *Journal of Cancer Education, 28*(2), 254–261. doi: 10.1007/s13187-013-0450-8

Sager, P. L. (2011). *Transcultural nursing theory and models: Application in nursing education, practice and administration*. New York: Springer Publishing Company, LLC.

Sherwood, G. D., & Shaffer, F. A. (2014). The role of internationally educated nurses in a quality, safe workforce. *Nursing Outlook, 62*(1), 46–52. http://dx.doi.org/10.1016/j.outlook.2013.11.001

Sutherland, L. L. (2002). Ethnocentrism in a pluralistic society: A concept analysis. *Journal of Transcultural Nursing, 13*(4), 274–281.

The Joint Commission. (2014). *Advancing effective communication, cultural competence, and patient- and family-centered care*. Retrieved June 1, 2014, from http://www.jointcommission.org/Advancing_Effective_Communication//

U.S. Census Bureau. (2014a). *America's foreign born in the last 50 years*. Retrieved May 27, 2014, from http://www.census.gov/how/infographics/foreign_born.html

U.S. Census Bureau. (2014b). *U.S. Census Bureau Projections Show a Slower Growing, Older, More Diverse Nation a Half Century from Now.*

Retrieved June 1, 2014, from http://www.census.gov/newsroom/releases/archives/population/cb12-243.html

U.S. Department of Health and Human Services, Office of Minority Health. (2014a). *The National Standards for Culturally and Linguistically Appropriate Services in Health and Health Care*. Retrieved from https://www.thinkculturalhealth.hhs.gov/Content/clas.asp#clas_standards

U.S. Department of Health and Human Services, Office of Minority Health. (2014b). *Culturally competent nursing care: A cornerstone of caring*. Retrieved from https://ccnm.thinkculturalhealth.hhs.gov/default.asp

U.S. Department of Health and Human Services, National Partnership for Action. (2014c). *National Partnership for Action to End Health Disparities: Toolkit for Community Action*. Retrieved from http://www.minorityhealth.hhs.gov/npa/files/Plans/Toolkit/NPA_Toolkit.pdf

Vogel, O., Cowens-Alvarado, R., Eschiti, V., Samos, M., Wiener, D., Ohlander, K., et al. (2013). Circle of life cancer education: Giving voice to American Indian and Alaska Native communities. *Journal of Cancer Education: The Official Journal of the American Association for Cancer Education, 28*(3), 565–572.

Waller, T., Lampman, C., & Lupfer-Johnson, G. (2012). Assessing bias against overweight individuals among nursing and psychology students: An implicit association test. *Journal of Clinical Nursing, 21*(23/24), 3504–3512. doi: 10.1111/j.1365-2702.2012.04226.x

White, K. M., & O'Sullivan, A. (Eds.) (2012). *The essential guide to nursing practice: Applying ANA's scope and standards in practice and education*. Washington, DC: American Nurses Association.

Williams, D. R. (2012). Miles to go before we sleep: Racial inequities in health. *Journal of Health and Social Behavior, 53*(3):279–295. doi: 10.1177/0022146512455804

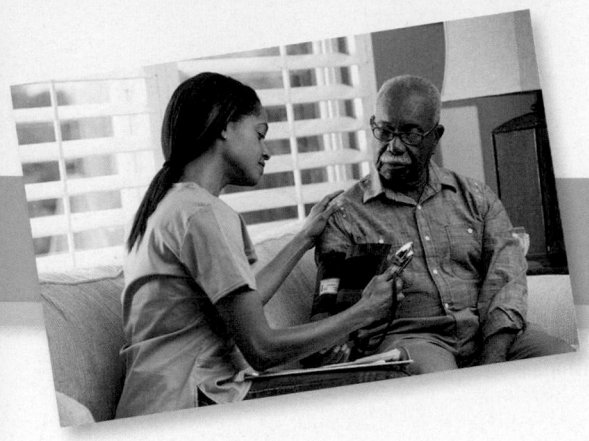

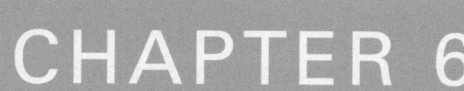

Communication in the Nurse–Patient Relationship

Beth Keyte

Case Scenario

While you are visiting your patient in his retirement apartment, you begin to discuss his recent hospitalization and the fall that occurred during his recovery period. Your concern is for his safety and for preventing further falls. When you ask him why he thinks the fall occurred, you notice that his posture changes. He becomes more erect, and his facial expression is guarded and resolute. He tells you curtly that he simply "lost [his] balance and fell." He goes on to remind you that he used to be a banker. He continues, "I still advise family and friends, and I am very capable." He does not need "bars" on his bed or little "alarms" to wear like they put on him in the hospital. "Thank you for inquiring, but I understand how to be safe and how to protect myself." You feel that he has no further interest in discussing what you believe is a significant problem.

Once you have completed this chapter and have incorporated therapeutic communication into your knowledge base, review the above scenario and reflect on the following areas of Critical Thinking:

1. Analyze what might have triggered your patient's response to your inquiry, and identify how you as the sender of the message might have contributed to his response.
2. Outline the threats that your patient may perceive from this interaction.
3. Assess the incongruencies between verbal and nonverbal communication in this visit.
4. Based on your analysis of the above responses, identify the blocks to communication that may be occurring.
5. Construct some options for how you might proceed to improve communication and accomplish your plan of care.

KEY TERMS

advocacy
circle of confidentiality
cognitive reframing
communication channel
compassion fatigue
decode
empathy
encoding
feedback
metacommunication
nonverbal communication
reflection
restatement
self-awareness
therapeutic communication
verbal communication
written communication

Upon completion of this chapter, you will be able to do the following:

1. Define the four major types of communication.
2. Discuss the elements of the communication process and their relevance to nursing.
3. Describe how language and experience affect the communication process.
4. Explain the importance of self-awareness in the therapeutic nurse–patient relationship.
5. Assess personal qualities and values.
6. Explain the nature of the nurse–patient relationship.
7. Distinguish between a professional and a social relationship.
8. Name the elements of an informal nurse–patient contract.
9. Discuss three key ingredients of therapeutic communication.
10. Name two professional self-care safety nets.
11. Identify important assessment areas to address when communicating with patients.
12. Give an example for each type of therapeutic communication technique.
13. Identify three key nontherapeutic responses, explaining how each interferes with therapeutic communication.
14. Describe two special situations that affect communication.

Nursing is an art and science. Nurses artistically apply scientific knowledge, gained through formal training and experience, to affect health outcomes. The artistic skill resides in the nurse's ability to understand and respond effectively to the patient's need for help and support. To do so, the nurse uses tools of communication. This chapter explores the concepts and principles of communication that are the foundations of interactions between the nurse and patient as they affect health, healing, and recovery.

Nurses play many roles, including teacher, patient advocate, administrator, and researcher. However, their fundamental roles are to promote health, prevent illness, restore health, and alleviate suffering (International Council of Nurses, 2014). Because of rapidly changing demands placed upon nurses due to healthcare reform and technologic advances, confidence that he or she can fulfill such roles with skill establishes a nurse's professional identity, autonomy, and ability to practice in a holistic manner. The nurse–patient relationship is the cornerstone of all nursing practice. The relationship is built on interpersonal or person-to-person communication that occurs in a specific setting. Effective communication between the nurse and patient is not so much a natural process as a learned skill. It is a way of being helpful to patients that differs from the way a clerk in a grocery store is helpful or the way friends are helpful to each other. For example, when the grocery clerk gives a courteous answer to a question about a product, the result is a satisfied customer. In a conversation between two friends who are sharing their problems, each friend feels cared for and understood. Although nurse–patient communication may include some of the elements in these examples, it differs considerably.

In the nurse–patient relationship, the patient and his or her experiences, problems, and issues are the main subject of communication. The goals are directed toward increasing understanding and improving coping skills related to the patient's health status and well-being. Thus, **therapeutic communication** facilitates interactions focused on the patient and the patient's concerns. The patient expresses and works through feelings and problems related to his or her situation, goals, treatments, and care.

What kind of a process is therapeutic communication, and how does it fit into the context of nursing practice? The following things happen during the communication process:

- The nurse and patient work together to solve problems centered on the patient's healthcare needs.
- The patient feels cared for and understood.
- The family or significant others are included in the care.
- Health teaching is conducted.
- Health promotion and preventive care are delivered.

Hildegard Peplau (1997), a psychiatric nurse and nurse theorist, emphasized in her classic work on theory of interpersonal relations that interpersonal competencies of nurses are key to helping patients regain health and well-being. On a broader scale, health communication can promote self-care behaviors among patients through customized approaches based on skilled assessment of patient characteristics (Myers, 2010). In short, communication is at the heart of all nursing.

To understand therapeutic communication, the nurse must gain an understanding of the communication process, including the important roles of language, experience, and **reflection**. Specific ingredients and techniques of communication also are important, as is knowledge about the nurse–patient relationship, contract setting, **advocacy**, confidentiality, and developmental issues related to communication.

THE COMMUNICATION PROCESS

Many definitions of communication exist. To communicate means to impart information, to exchange ideas, and to express one's self in such a way as to be understood. Communication can be defined as a system of sending and receiving messages, forming a connection between the sender and the receiver (Fig. 6-1). It is a process for giving and receiving information, a form of interaction or transaction.

Communication is a continuous human function, much like breathing or cardiac functioning. The process goes on all the time. In many ways, the statement "One cannot *not* communicate" is true. For example, when a person decides not to share information, or one person stops talking to another person because of hurt or anger, communication has still taken place.

Communication is basic and essential to human life. Through communication, people relate to their environment and to each other. Without it, people would be unable to learn, to direct their lives, or to work together cooperatively in families, organizations, and communities. Communication is basic to human feeling and intellect; without it, the human race could not survive.

Types of Communication

People communicate in various ways. Written, verbal, nonverbal, and **metacommunication** are all forms of communication. Words, associated gestures, and actions of the nurse convey power, authority, and knowledge that are laden with social, cultural, and political meaning. Styles of communication can vary from discipline to discipline. For example, nurses have historically been trained to be detailed and physicians to be brief; these differences can lead to difficulty in maintaining interdisciplinary communication, leading to poorer patient outcomes (Pope, Rodzen, & Spross, 2008). On a daily basis, nurses are responsible for conveying to other health professionals information that informs patient care, and any breakdown in this communication process will compromise patient safety (Mascioli, Laskowski-Jones, Urban, & Moran, 2009). Nurses use communication to lay the foundation for therapeutic relationships and influence behavior leading to improved patient outcomes (Stuart, 2012). Thus, the development of skill in communication of all types should be one of utmost importance to the nurse. Box 6-1 provides some examples of various types of communication.

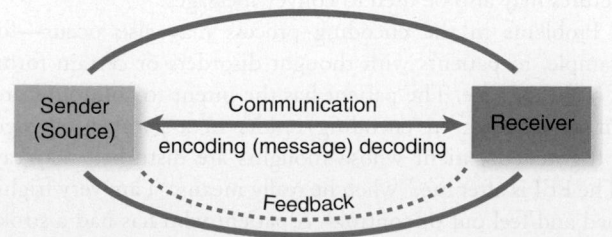

FIGURE 6-1 Communication is a process in which information is sent and received. It is a form of interaction that is continuous and ever changing.

BOX 6-1	Examples of Types of Communication

Written/Verbal	Nonverbal
Written	Touch
Spoken	Eye contact
Television and radio	Facial expression
Movies	Body posture
Magazines	Gestures
Books	Physical appearance
Computers	Voice tone
Posters	Rate of speech
Brochures	Neatness
Written handoffs and SBAR	Movement

WRITTEN COMMUNICATION

Written communication is a means to document and convey information to others. The writer selects and organizes words in a way that is legible and comprehensible to the reader. This is an important component in nursing practice because documentation in the patient's records informs treatment and care. More information on written communication and interdisciplinary communication is covered in Chapter 16 of this text.

VERBAL COMMUNICATION

Verbal communication involves the spoken word. It is an exchange using the elements of language. The significance of written and verbal communications cannot be underestimated. The specific use of words and jargon in nursing is particularly powerful because it defines the perceptions and realities of people's experiences. An important role of the nurse is motivating patients to make behavior changes that lead to improved health. Words of education, persuasion, and sometimes coercion have been common strategies with questionable success rates; changing the verbal strategies to those of encouragement, support, and timely **feedback** allows patients to build on individual strengths and resources, moving in the direction of their goals (Hayes & Kalmakis, 2007; Colineau & Paris, 2011).

NONVERBAL COMMUNICATION

Equally important is **nonverbal communication**. A person communicates by gestures, facial expressions, posture, space, appearance, body movement, touch, voice tone and volume, and rate of speech. Silence is a form of nonverbal communication that the nurse needs to become comfortable using. Patients who are ill may require longer than average periods of time to process information and formulate a response. When the nurse accompanies silence by other nonverbal methods such as eye contact and nodding, the patient can be assured the nurse is attentive.

METACOMMUNICATION

Another kind of communication, metacommunication, is communication about the communication or lack thereof. This form of communication means different things at different levels. It can be verbal or nonverbal and is information that is constantly available during the process of communication, giving context and clues for ways in which messages are to be interpreted (Kelman & Branco, 2009). It includes anything that is taken into account when interpreting what is happening, such as the role of the communicator, the nonverbal messages sent, and the context of the communication taking place.

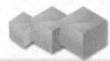 **Concept Mastery Alert**

Nursing documentation is an example of nonverbal communication. Although it is true that documentation and other forms of writing are not audible, these are considered to be forms of verbal communication because they use words and numbers as the medium for conveying a message.

RELATIONSHIPS AMONG TYPES OF COMMUNICATION

The relationships among the different types of communication (written, verbal, nonverbal, and metacommunication) are important. The way they fit together (are congruent) or do not fit together (are incongruent) reflects the complexity of communication. The following two examples illustrate this concept.

Congruent Relationship

A nurse makes rounds on assigned patients at the beginning of the shift. She explains her role to each patient, confers with them about their nursing care needs, and schedules with them the care tasks to be done on that shift. The nurse is dressed in a professional manner and wears a name tag and hospital identification badge. He or she speaks in a well-modulated voice and listens carefully to what each patient says.

In this example, each kind of communication conveys messages that are congruent. The messages say, "I am your professional nurse. We will work together to meet your nursing care needs. I respect you." There is a "good fit" among verbal communication, nonverbal communication, and metacommunication.

Incongruent Relationship

A patient and a nurse have been working together on diabetic teaching. After the teaching session is completed, the patient says to the nurse, "Yes, I understand my diabetic diet and how to take my insulin." On the surface, this seems to be a straightforward communication indicating that the patient understands the components of care needed to deal successfully with diabetes. If, however, the words of the message are said with an irritated facial expression and a harsh tone of voice, the nonverbal and metacommunication aspects of the message do not "fit" with the verbal message; they are incongruent.

The metacommunication in this example may be conveying, "I am tired of being told how to run my life. I am angry about having a chronic illness." Furthermore, if the patient is later seen having a candy bar, this nonverbal communication may convey the message that the patient has not yet fully accepted his or her condition. In this example, recognizing incongruence between kinds of communication informs the nurse about the patient's experience.

Elements of the Communication Process

As shown in Figure 6-1, communication is a continuous, dynamic, ongoing, and ever-changing operation. Although it is somewhat artificial to break down communication into components, doing so can be useful. Knowing the individual elements of a process can be helpful in identifying where in the process a problem is occurring. The elements of the model presented here are based on the classic work of David Berlo (1960), a communication theorist.

All communication has a sender (a person or group with a purpose for the communication). The sender's purpose must be translated into a code. This is done with language or nonverbal signals, such as gestures, facial expressions, or body cues. The process of getting the purpose translated into the code is called **encoding**. Encoding results in a message.

Another element in the communication process is the **communication channel**, the medium or carrier of the message. For example, television is a channel, the voice or written word is a channel, and touch can be a channel.

If the communication process were to stop at this element, no communication would take place because there must be someone at the other end of the channel—the receiver. The receiver is the target of the communication and must be able to understand or **decode** the message. Once messages are decoded and received, feedback occurs. Feedback means that the sender and the receiver use one another's reactions to produce further messages.

Understanding the elements of the communication process is useful because sometimes specific difficulties in communication can be traced to one or more of these elements. A basic example is the patient who speaks a different language from the nurse. In this case, the nurse needs to attend to the communication channel. An interpreter may be needed to help carry the message or help the patient decode the nurse's messages. Pictures may also be used to convey messages.

Problems in the encoding process may also occur—for example, in patients with thought disorders or certain forms of brain damage. The patient has the intent to communicate, but impairment in encoding results in a garbled message. A frightened patient whose thoughts are disturbed may say, "The FBI is after me," when he really means, "I am very frightened and feel out of control." A patient who has had a stroke may be able to understand a communication directed at her but not be able to encode a returning message because of brain damage.

Difficulty in the nurse–patient encounter is often attributed to the patient. A small but significant and heterogeneous subgroup of patients can shake nurses' confidence, challenge their authority, or reduce them to tears. The goal of this chapter is to begin to prepare the reader to care for such patients, who, for lack of a better phrase, are referred to as **difficult patients**. Some nurses may object to the use of this phrase, feeling that it may be labeling people unfairly.

Another way to view this terminology is to speak of "difficult behaviors" or "challenging patients." When patients display any of the following, productive interactions are more limited (Hull & Broquet, 2007; Forrest, 2012):

- Defensive, angry, frightened, or resistant behavior
- Impulsive and manipulative behaviors
- Somatizing behavior (vague or exaggerated symptoms)
- Grief
- Frequent visits to healthcare providers

These behaviors can be addressed through targeted application of critical communication skills such as reflective statements, sincere apologies, listening to understand patient expectations, validating emotional experiences, and sharing expressions of compassion.

Difficult behaviors can also be attributed to the healthcare provider or situational factors. In Hull and Broquet's (2007) and Forrest's (2012) reviews of strategies to manage difficult patient encounters, anger and defensiveness, fatigue and lack of time, and overemphasis on personal beliefs and emotions of the healthcare provider are cited as problematic contributions to difficult encounters. In addition, they also implicate language and literacy issues, multiple people in exam rooms, having to break bad news, and environmental factors that are not conducive to good communication (noise, chaos, lack of privacy). Taking time to reflect on one's own triggers, as well as environmental triggers, leads to reduction of difficulties.

A second way to look at the issue is through the lens of "difficult encounters." Macdonald (2007) and Zolnierek (2014) explored the origins of difficulty in nurse–patient encounters and found six key elements that contributed to reduction in difficult encounters: knowing the patient, knowing families, collaborative relationships with other staff while at work, availability of supplies and equipment, and care space changes (changes in the patient's care environment, often focused on medical needs having to be met too quickly related to rapid discharge). Each of these elements has communication at its core. If time is taken to establish relationships—with patients, their families, and staff—many of these difficult encounters can be prevented.

Importance of Language and Experience

Language, culture, and experience are crucial to the process of communication. Language is used to communicate and develop a person's view of life and the world. Thus, language and experience are closely related. Bandler and Grinder (1975) suggest in their early and now classic work on neurolinguistic programming that a person's view of the world is developed through several kinds of filters.

One such filter consists of the neurologic receptor systems: sight, hearing, touch, taste, and smell. Stimuli processed through these receptor systems enable the person to experience the outside world. Through language, such experiences can be compared with the experiences of others. Alterations in sensory perceptions can change the person's view of the world. For example, a person with altered hearing or vision may experience the world differently.

Another filter is the particular language system into which the person is socialized. As discussed previously, words and sentences give meaning to things and events. Language allows us to conceptualize the world. For example, a person whose language has only three words for all the possible visible color distinctions would conceptualize colors differently from someone whose language offered more choices. Someone with a limited vocabulary may have more difficulty describing experiences than someone with a rich, diverse vocabulary. In fact, limitations in language skills may actually limit a person's choices in life.

A third filter is the person's unique history. Factors such as cultural background, family relationships, place in the sibling ranking, type of parenting received, and genetic makeup all enter into the personal history.

The nurse and the patient bring their backgrounds into the communication. Some aspects of their background are shared, and some are different. Consider, for example, the image of "a nurse" brought to a nurse–patient situation. Some patients may view nursing as a female profession, invoking certain stereotypes about female behaviors and roles. In some societies, women are defined as subservient to men, and their work is devalued. Often, the "caring" image of nursing overshadows the knowledge, decision-making abilities, and technical skills of the nurse. The physical appearance and dress of the nurse reflect not only society's view of the nurse but also the nurse's view of self. The image created in first impressions easily becomes the reality to the patient; the attire a nurse appears in communicates that image and influences the relationship and nature of communication that follows (Clavell, Goodwin, & Tivas, 2013).

The nurse–patient interaction is productive when communication is aimed toward a common understanding. To communicate effectively, the nurse understands and appreciates his or her own background while at the same time acknowledging different perspectives held by the patient.

In the clinical setting, the extent of successful exchange of information between patient and nurse is affected by the degree to which their realities are mutually compatible. The typical nursing work environment, which often involves the use of technical language, produces barriers to communication. The inability of many patients to understand technical language intimidates them, possibly preventing them from asking questions on their own behalf. Other barriers include talking about the patient in front of him or her, withholding information from the patient, and being too busy to spend time with the patient.

Stereotypes are common in relationships, particularly those involving professionals and those they serve. These stereotypes come from both the professional and the patient perspective. Examples include stereotypes about ethnicity, sexual orientation, social class, age, and psychiatric or medical diagnoses. Examining one's own preconceptions is important to prevent them from interfering with a therapeutic nurse–patient relationship.

 APPLY YOUR CRITICAL THINKING

You are working with William Snyder, 76, on a rehabilitation unit. You have been told that he has had a stroke and is aphasic. He can still think and respond with nonverbal gestures but not with verbal communication. You begin planning your care for him by thinking about an effective way to communicate. Establishing an effective communication system with Mr. Snyder is central to providing good nursing care. How will you assess the best way to approach him? What indicators might you use to determine if you are effective? How will you collaborate with speech therapy?

Check your answers in Appendix B.

THE NURSE–PATIENT RELATIONSHIP: A HELPING RELATIONSHIP

The nurse–patient relationship differs from a social or intimate relationship. Table 6-1 compares the nurse–patient relationship with a social relationship. Within the nurse–patient relationship, the nurse assumes the roles of a professional and a helper. The patient is the one seeking help. The nurse–patient relationship focuses on the patient, is goal directed, and has defined parameters. In the professional relationship, the nurse also assesses how his or her own role, communication skills, personal history, and values may be affecting the interactions.

Note that Table 6-1 also helps us understand the difference between **empathy** and sympathy. Whereas sympathy is common in social or intimate relationships, empathy is therapeutic and professional. In sympathetic interactions, one tends to feel sorry for the other person, but in empathetic interactions, the nurse recognizes how the patient is feeling and attempts to find out how to best support the patient.

Phases

The nurse–patient relationship can be thought of in terms of three phases: orientation, working, and termination. The orientation phase consists of introductions and an agreement between nurse and patient about their mutual roles and responsibilities. The first few moments shared by the nurse and patient are critical. What they see, hear, touch, and smell of each other during initial engagement sets the tone for how subsequent interactions will unfold. In the psychiatric setting, the orientation phase of the relationship represents the first phase of therapeutic work. The goal of this phase is to establish trust and rapport so that a realistic understanding of the patient's problems and plan of action can be negotiated. As the nurse and patient get to know each other, the initial anxiety of meeting a stranger subsides and trust increases, paving the way for a comprehensive assessment.

Because healthcare delivery occurs within an increasingly compressed time frame, it is critical that the nurse brings focus and quality to brief patient interactions. The use of therapeutic communication skills facilitates empathetic and effective communication and saves time. In addition, the professional nurse is often in the role of supervisor or delegator, needing to deliver nursing care and to manage effective communication through licensed and unlicensed assistive personnel. This requires organization proficiency that includes clear and concise communication by the professional nurse.

During the working phase, the nurse and patient explore and develop solutions that are enacted and evaluated in subsequent interactions. The nurse functions as a coach and advocate while attending to the patient's physical and emotional healthcare needs.

TABLE 6-1 COMPARISON OF PROFESSIONAL WITH SOCIAL RELATIONSHIP		
	Nurse–Patient	Social
Key Focus	Patient	Both participants
Goals	Meeting patient's needs. Help patient identify feelings and concerns; solve problems, cope, and adapt in relation to healthcare situation	Meeting own needs. Mutual companionship, enjoyment, and interaction. May lead to intimacy and commitment
Parameters	Limited primarily to the needs incurred by the healthcare situation. Nurse self-discloses only what is appropriate for the patient's benefit. Relationship is terminated when goals are met and service no longer is needed.	Sharing of life's events, activities, or other aspects of self. May stay superficial or lead to long-term relationship. Relationship may be terminated when own needs are no longer met.
Self-Assessment	Nurse assesses own role, communication skills, values, and so forth and how these affect the professional relationship.	Each person assesses how own needs for enjoyment, affection, and sharing, or love and intimacy, are met in the relationship.

Termination is the closure of the relationship. The nurse and patient review health changes and how the patient has dealt with physical and emotional responses. Discharge planning is a key component in the termination process. Termination can take various forms. For example, the nurse–patient relationship can end when the patient is discharged or the nurse is reassigned. Be clear about termination. Continued contact beyond professional responsibilities usually is not advisable and may violate professional and ethical codes of conduct.

During all phases, the nurse solicits feedback from the patient so that the nurse can adjust subsequent encounters to maximize care. This can be accomplished by simply asking the patient, "How was this for you?" or "What worked and didn't work?"

Contract Setting

The nurse–patient relationship is based, in general, on an informal contractual model. In the contractual relationship, patients are seen as having control over the significant decisions that affect their own bodies. Patients are given information necessary for making decisions, and patients choose among options, including acceptance, refusal, or termination of treatment. Aspects of care, goals of treatment, and necessary adaptations are discussed with the patient. The nurse takes no major action without consulting the patient or a family member representing the patient. The nurse discusses his or her role, the patient's condition, treatment, and nursing care with the patient. Decisions about nursing and healthcare are made collaboratively and are based on the patient's values and preferences.

The contractual relationship between nurse and patient is an informal one that is verbal and is assumed by both parties. Box 6-2 summarizes the elements of an informal contract between nurse and patient. In the area of psychiatric nursing practice, contracts usually are more formal, sometimes written. Often, they are used as a therapeutic tool to help a patient develop more insight and control over his or her own behavior.

The usual way for a nurse to establish an informal contract with a patient is to make a verbal agreement about how they are to work together. A nurse might approach a patient as follows: "I will be your nurse while you are a patient here. This means I'm responsible for planning your care. I'll be here every day this week but will be off on the weekend and nights. Other nurses will care for you according to the plan we decide on together. Do you have any questions or concerns about your care?"

| **BOX 6-2** | **Elements of an Informal Nurse–Patient Contract** |

- Nurse and patient know each other's names.
- Roles and responsibilities are clarified.
- Parameters of the professional relationship are clear.
- Mutual expectations are agreed on.
- Circle of confidentiality is respected.

An important advantage to the informal contractual relationship involves values and rights. The nurse maintains his or her own rights while respecting those of the patient. Consider, for instance, a nurse who disagrees with abortion and a patient is considering having one. The nurse can contract with the patient to provide the information but need not participate in the procedure. The nurse must respect the patient's rights. Because abortion is a legal procedure, the nurse cannot restrain the patient from having one. Furthermore, the nurse is obligated to provide the patient with information so that the patient can make an informed decision. However, this does not deny the nurse's personal right to oppose legalized abortion and to choose not to work for an institution that performs abortions.

Advocacy

Advocacy, or taking the patient's side, is the basis for communication with patients. Advocacy supports the patient's right to the information necessary to make his or her own decisions about treatment options and nursing care. Patients need information about their health status and the course of illness so that they can make the necessary adjustments in their lives. Sharing information reduces anxiety and is an integral aspect of therapeutic communication.

Engaging in collaborative relationships with patients in order to help them negotiate decisions in their healthcare is an attitude that requires mindful attention if patient participation is truly valued (Johns, 2013). This type of partnership between nurse and patient does not happen without having adequate time to address concerns, questions, values, and patient perspectives. Once attention to patient involvement has been prioritized, communicating meaningful information about a person's care and treatment through the use of narrative will ensure effective identification and recoding of important issues for the patient (Johns, 2013).

The interaction of increased consumerism and managed care has had an effect on nursing advocacy and communication. With advocacy, nurses focus on the knowledge patients need and want to make their own decisions about their health and healthcare. Being an advocate for the patient means avoiding an authoritarian approach, which assumes that the professional will make decisions for the patient. Inducing guilt or blame is also to be avoided.

An example of inducing guilt is a mother telling her child, "I cooked this dinner especially for you, and now you aren't going to eat it." The underlying message is, "Because you did not eat the dinner, mother is hurt and you are selfish." Whether it is used in childrearing situations or in the nurse–patient relationship, inducing guilt is inappropriate and manipulative. Table 6-2 compares the authoritarian, guilt inducement, and advocacy approaches.

Patient advocacy sometimes conflicts with the physician's viewpoint. To keep the patient's best interest in the forefront, the nurse needs to develop a collaborative working relationship with the physician. Helping the patients express their views and concerns with physicians also is a positive approach.

For instance, a patient may confide to the nurse that she believes she is not receiving enough information about her condition.

TABLE 6-2 COMPARISON OF AUTHORITARIAN, GUILT INDUCEMENT, AND ADVOCACY APPROACHES

Clinical example: Surgery has been recommended, but the patient is reluctant to have the operation.

	Authoritarian	Guilt Inducement	Advocacy
Approach	No choice	Choice based on consequences of actions	Choice based on information and examination of alternatives
Response	"Surgery is your only choice. You need this operation."	"If you don't have the surgery, you may not live to see your grandchildren. Your family needs you."	"Whether or not you have the surgery is your choice. It is your body. What is your understanding of the situation?"
Underlying Message	The professional knows best and should make the decisions for you.	If you don't do what the professional recommends, you and others will get hurt.	The professional is here to help you make informed choices about your health and well-being.

The patient complains that the physician does not spend enough time with her, and she feels left out of the decisions made about treatment. If the nurse provides the information to the patient without conferring with the physician, the nurse has intruded into the physician–patient relationship because the patient's perception is that more information is needed from the physician.

In this instance, several options are appropriate. The nurse can discuss the problem with the patient and help the patient assert herself through such means as writing a list of questions to ask the physician. With the patient's permission, the nurse can seek out the physician and share the patient's perceptions with him or her. With such actions, the nurse is acting on the patient's behalf without interfering in the physician–patient relationship, thereby practicing true advocacy.

However, there may be times when the nurse, in the role as advocate, will need to engage in limit setting for the patient. This condition exists when imminent harm may result if the patient's wishes, despite information presented for making decisions, are counter to their personal safety. For example, a nurse may prohibit the patient from walking down stairs because of the danger of falling or may refuse to give a morphine injection before it is due.

Circle of Confidentiality

Every patient has a right to privacy. However, depending on legal restrictions, certain patient information must be shared with other professionals involved in a patient's care. This can be thought of as a **circle of confidentiality**, and it includes all the people in a nursing unit who have responsibility for the patient. It usually includes the family unless the patient objects.

It is important to clarify with the patient that he or she is part of a team. Consider, for example, a nurse who has been caring for a patient with a serious prognosis. The patient says to the nurse, "If I tell you something, will you promise to keep it in the strictest confidence? Don't tell anyone else, not even my family." The nurse agrees. Then, the patient says that he plans to kill himself after he is discharged, stating that he has a loaded gun at home.

The nurse in this example failed to adhere to the concept of the circle of confidentiality. The proper response would have been to tell the patient that the nurse is part of the healthcare team and that clinically relevant information is shared with the team. This protects both the nurse and patient and clearly defines the limits of patient confidentiality.

Transmission of information beyond the nursing unit is rarely indicated and must be carefully considered. In this era of electronic record keeping, health information is readily available. Because of this, use of e-mail, cell phones, and other communication technology needs to be carefully monitored to ensure the patient's right to privacy. For example, a patient may not want others to know about his or her hospitalization or the nature of his or her illness. This is especially true in cases associated with stigma, such as AIDS, substance addiction, and psychiatric illness. Always consider patient confidentiality even in such mundane situations as talking at lunch or at home. To further understand how to avoid violations of the Health Insurance Portability and Accountability Act (HIPAA), see Chapter 7.

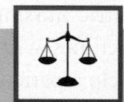

ETHICAL/LEGAL ISSUES

RESPECTING PATIENT CONFIDENTIALITY
You are a nursing student and are entering the classroom. You hear your classmates talking about their patients by name and laughing about information related to their patients that your classmates obtained from the patients and their medical records.

CRITICAL THINKING CHALLENGE
- Reflect on your feelings in this situation and identify them.
- Identify concerns you may have about ethically appropriate behavior.
- Refer to the Patients' Bill of Rights in Chapter 7. Think about whether this situation demonstrates a violation of this contract.
- Identify possible approaches to your classmates that may alter their behavior yet not impair your communication with them.

INGREDIENTS OF THERAPEUTIC COMMUNICATION

What makes communication therapeutic, and in what ways is it different from other forms of communication? Carl Rogers (1961), a founding father of psychotherapy research, studied the process of therapeutic communication, believing that a person cannot be separated from the techniques of communication he or she uses. Based on his research, the characteristics of a therapeutic, "helpful" person were identified. Empathy, positive regard, and a comfortable sense of self were among the key ingredients.

Empathy

Empathy encompasses the ability to look at things from another's perspective, to walk in his or her shoes, and to be able to share the essence of that understanding through verbal and nonverbal communication (Shives, 2012; Varcarolis & Halter, 2014). Varcarolis and Halter (2014) point out the importance of maintaining objectivity in order to assist a patient through therapeutic communication. In order to maintain empathy, the nurse must keep the patient's needs and concerns primary, not allowing personal feelings and experiences to lead them away from focusing on the patients (Fig. 6-2). This is done through the process of reflective or "active" listening (see later discussion under Implementation).

Empathy is a complex process. The nurse must:

- Have enough knowledge and experience to perceive the patient's perspective accurately
- Feel secure enough not to be intimidated if the patient experiences a situation differently
- Feel comfortable enough to be able to imagine what a situation might be like for someone else, while remaining outside that situation to maintain objectivity
- Convey to the patient that the nurse perceives the patient's feelings, thoughts, and experiences accurately

Empathy is a strong component of therapeutic relationships. However, it is not necessarily appropriate to use the entire empathic process (described above) in every clinical situation. Simple actions such as touch, kindness, attentiveness, and information sharing also signify empathy. As discussed previously in this chapter and Table 6-1, the nurse must take care not to confuse empathy with sympathy. Whereas social relationships are characterized by sympathetic interactions, the professional relationship is based on empathy of the nurse for the patient. Sympathy is not appropriate in professional relationships with patients and may signal boundary violations by the nurse.

Positive Regard

Positive regard refers to warmth, caring, interest, and respect for the person, seeing the person unconditionally or nonjudgmentally (Fig. 6-3). Respect for the person does not depend on his or her behavior; instead, the person is regarded as worthwhile simply for being human.

How can this work? What if, for example, the nurse is caring for a person who has been convicted of a serious crime? Does positive regard mean that the nurse condones the things this person has done?

Positive regard does not mean that the nurse accepts all aspects of a person's behavior. The nurse does not condone or encourage behavior that is socially inappropriate or abusive. However, the nurse must separate that behavior from the person. The underlying assumption is that the person is worthwhile and has value and dignity.

Positive regard also means that the professional avoids unnecessary labeling of patients. The focus of healthcare professionals on disease tends to label the patient as an object (e.g., a diabetic, an amputee, an alcoholic). As a result, the patient is seen as someone who is defective. Also, viewing a patient as his or her disease, rather than as someone who has that disease, can interfere with seeing the person behind the label. This viewpoint tends to come through in the communication process. Ignoring the person makes it more difficult to

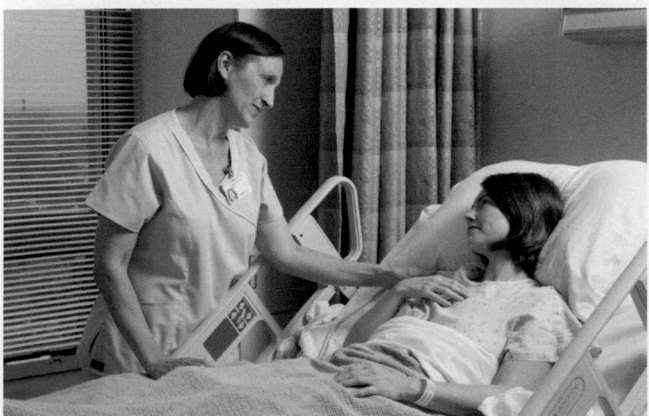

FIGURE 6-2 Empathy is the ability to identify with another person's feelings and interpret his or her attached meanings.

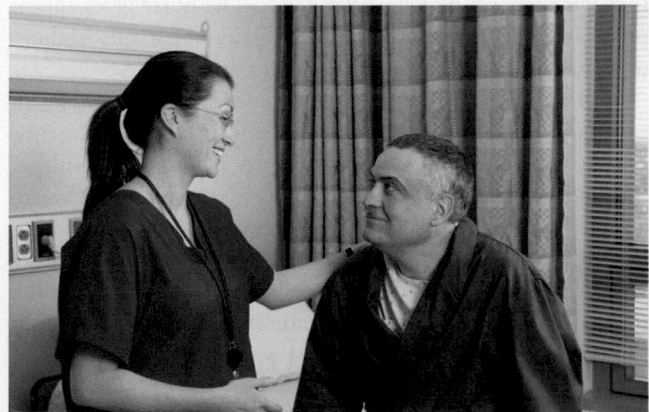

FIGURE 6-3 A nurse expressing positive regard sees patients nonjudgmentally.

know and understand his or her response to health and illness and to use the patient's strengths and potential.

Self-Awareness and Self-Reflection

Before a nurse can communicate therapeutically, a comfortable sense of self, such as being aware of one's own personality, values, cultural background, and style of communication, is necessary. A person's sense of self comprises a collection of characteristics. For example, a nurse may be a professional, a parent, and a sibling and may be overweight, tall, or athletic. How the nurse experiences these characteristics influences how he or she sees others.

The nurse with a comfortable sense of self can evaluate his or her strengths and weaknesses. For example, one nurse may say, "I work well with postoperative patients, but I have less aptitude for working with rehabilitation patients because I like things to happen more quickly." Another nurse might enjoy working with psychiatric patients because he or she finds working on interpersonal goals rewarding.

Self-evaluation also means taking responsibility for one's actions as a professional. For example, a nurse might think, "I could have said something more supportive," or "I should have included the family in the planning phase." Through this process, the nurse grows in professional competency.

A person with a comfortable sense of self is open to experiences and is aware of his or her feelings and attitudes. This allows the person to take a more flexible view of life. For example, the nurse may notice that not all patients respond the same way to a similar surgical procedure and that not all people in a given culture fit the stereotypes of that culture. The differences between the nurse and the patient can be seen as interesting or challenging rather than threatening or "bad."

The professional with a comfortable sense of self feels separate from but connected to others—an important aspect of being therapeutic. Because it is easy for a nurse to over identify with patients, clear interpersonal boundaries need to be maintained. A nurse who becomes too involved in the suffering of patients soon becomes emotionally and physically exhausted, lacking the objectivity it takes to be therapeutic. Also, the ability to separate prevents the nurse from seeking gratification through excessive patient dependence. The nurse gives appropriate support and care but has confidence in patients' abilities to make choices about their health and lives.

Self-awareness is one of the most important steps in communicating therapeutically and effectively with patients. Nurses cannot really understand and help others without self-understanding. With self-awareness, nurses can relate to and better understand the experiences of others. According to Peplau (1997), nurses need to understand themselves in order to promote growth in their patients. Self-awareness enables nurses to avoid limiting patient choices to those that the nurse values.

In their literature review, Caldwell and Grobbel (2013) found that self-reflection on one's practice is essential. In order for self-reflection to be effective, open-mindedness, courage, and a willingness to accept and act on criticism must be present (Bulman, Lathlean, & Gobbi, 2012). Students in their study reported that self-reflection was responsible for "changing and improving" their practice by shifting their thinking and actions. Self-reflection is a skill to be developed. It was only by participation in the process that students became more confident in practicing the skill. The process of self-reflection not only helps the nurse to make needed changes but also allows one to reflect on achievements and celebrate good practice.

THE JOHARI WINDOW

One useful tool for helping to develop self-awareness is the Johari window (Luft, 1970), shown in Figure 6-4. The Johari window helps individuals reflect on and explore areas of ourselves that we might not normally consider. Videbeck (2014) invites us to carefully consider our values, our strengths, behaviors, accomplishments, needs, desires, thoughts, and feelings. According to Videbeck, we become more independent and effective when we understand which qualities or values we choose regularly over others. By taking time to reflect on the qualities we value most in ourselves and others, we can become conscious and aware of their influence in our lives.

The Johari window can be used to make a "word portrait" of a person in four areas. The first pane of the Johari window is where qualities that one presents to others are listed. Because these qualities are known by others, this pane is often referred to as the open and public self. The open pane includes qualities that one is comfortable sharing with others. It may also include false qualities or values that are presented to others. These "masks" that we present to others, which we may also believe ourselves, can prevent us from developing self-awareness and can erect barriers to interpersonal intimacy. Often, these "masks" are presented because of one's need for approval from others.

The first step in using the Johari window is to identify and list your personal qualities and values (for ideas, consult the

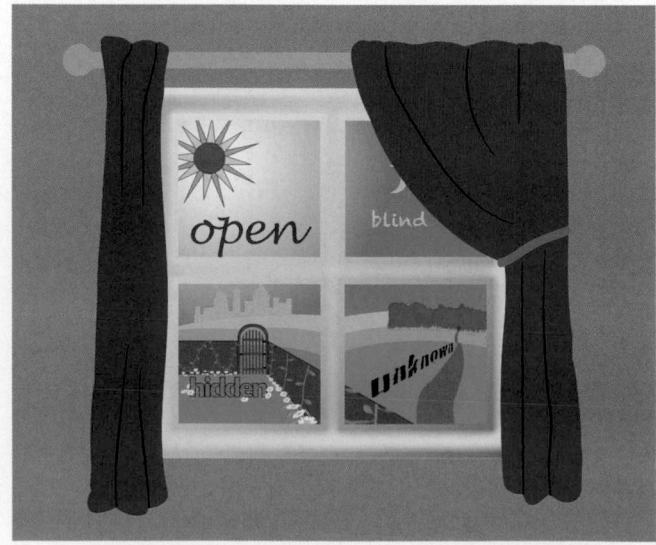

FIGURE 6-4 Johari window. (Artist: Melinda Keyte.)

| BOX 6-3 | Descriptors of Personal Qualities and Values |

- Introvert, Extrovert, Ambivert
- Confident, Competitive, Self-conscious, Modest, Proud, Secure, Comfortable, Seek Approval, Impartial
- Optimistic, Pessimistic, Cheerful, Happy, Silly, Serious
- Idealistic, Pragmatic, Logical, Sensible
- Dependable, Organized, Able, Trustworthy, Honest, Spontaneous, Independent, Dependent, Focused, Thorough, Loyal
- Caring, Loving, Accepting, Kind, Sentimental, Sensitive, Romantic, Sensual, Sympathetic, Empathetic, Warm, Giving, Helpful, Spiritual, Purposeful,
- Flexible, Adaptable, Rigid, Concrete, Abstract
- Calm, Patient, Tense, Relaxed, Nervous,
- Observant, Reflective, Curious, Task Oriented,
- Bold, Powerful, Shy, Courageous, Risk-Taker
- Aggressive, Self-Assertive, Passive
- Intelligent, Clever, Knowledgeable, Ingenious, Smart, Wise, Theoretical, Analytical, Inventive, Creative
- Mature, Dignified, Complex
- Energetic, Responsive, Congenial, Hardworking, Playful, Charming, Popular, Productive, Busy, Bored,
- Healthy, Fit, Attractive, Neat, Feeling Safe, Financial Security

- The patient who has become frightened or upset because of something specific
- The chronically angry or easy-to-anger patient who is otherwise cognitively intact
- The delirious, agitated patient; although a specific incident may lead to the anger, fear and anger are inherent in many types of delirium
- The intoxicated patient or patient in alcohol or drug withdrawal
- The patient with a major psychiatric disorder (e.g., bipolar disorder, schizophrenia, Alzheimer disease, antisocial personality disorder)

Naturally, the plan of care depends on the cause of the patient's anger. Because most expressions of anger are legitimate and honest manifestations of distress, listening to the patient may be a tool in assessment and a therapeutic intervention.

The nurse's emotional response is key to identifying when anger may escalate to violence. Nurses must listen to their gut feelings and heed their own fears. Because the same neurochemistry underlies both anger and fear, they are often referred to as flip sides of the same coin. They are distinguished by a person's perception of the situation.

Professional Self-Care Safety Nets

Because nursing involves intense emotional work, it is not without risks. The circumstances around which people experience illness, distress, and suffering can challenge and overwhelm the nurse's sense of self, safety, and meaning in the world. Patients' stories of violence, abuse, neglect, despair, and loneliness are common. The nurse, as an empathic listener, can begin to experience the patient's trauma secondarily. This phenomenon leading to stress and burnout is known as **compassion fatigue** and results when nurses continue to care for their patients, in addition to their families and significant others, but become unable to care for themselves (Shives, 2012). Nurses who have been living under stress for lengthy periods may not even recognize that they are stressed. Some nurses cope emotionally by shutting down, distancing themselves, or becoming callous. Others may be prone to boundary violations with patients by becoming overly involved with patients and seeking to have their own needs met by the patient. Although these responses may protect the nurse, they generally are not helpful to the patient. In severe cases of compassion, fatigue nurses may struggle with depression, anxiety, substance abuse (including diversion of patient medications for self-administration), or suicidal ideation.

Several strategies have been found to reduce work stress. As described throughout the chapter, self-awareness is key. Keeping a written journal of personal feelings and reactions that develop through interpersonal work helps the nurse decide what emotions are acceptable or unacceptable or of concern. Videbeck (2014) recommends reading books on topics that support strengths and help to develop areas of weakness that are identified during journaling. Reflections about thoughts,

examples in Box 6-3). Identify your personal qualities and values, and then place them in the order you think they influence you, from most to least influential.

Pane two of the Johari window is the blind area. This pane contains qualities we are not aware of but that others notice and know about us. We can learn about this area by asking others for feedback. It is important to be open to both positive and negative qualities identified by others. Being open to how others see us can enhance personal growth. Encouraging others to be honest with us without fear of reprisal will give us a clear picture of how others see us. After adding the qualities observed by others to your list, place each quality in the appropriate pane of the Johari window.

Pane three is the hidden self and contains qualities that are known only to oneself. These are qualities that we do not feel comfortable sharing with others.

The fourth pane is the unknown pane. This pane symbolizes qualities that are unknown or not yet discovered by oneself or others.

During the process of self-reflection and personal growth, the location of qualities will move from one pane to another. Pane one will expand as we develop greater self-awareness, and pane four will decrease in size. This process of growth and change will allow the nurse to experience greater interpersonal intimacy.

The Angry Patient

Many things can cause a sick or hospitalized patient to become angry. When assessing an angry patient, it helps to consider some broad categories, as each type requires a different response (Forrest, 2012):

feelings, and responses also provide the nurse with an opportunity to analyze and consider alternative thoughts and actions. The perception of an event can vary greatly from individual to individual. Although one person may view an event as an overwhelming problem, another may view the same event as an exciting challenge. There are many events in life that cannot be controlled, but how we choose to respond to an event is one thing that we can learn to control. Nurses who learn to cognitively reframe stressful thoughts into more helpful thinking and to acknowledge what they have control over and what they do not fare better are less likely to suffer from compassion fatigue. They also demonstrate more resilient ways of responding to stress. **Cognitive reframing** is a coping skill that helps one to alter or reframe one's perception of an event and helps us overcome catastrophic thinking about an event. For example, a student who is anxious about an upcoming exam can disrupt their anxiety by using cognitive reframing and thinking about their thinking (metacognition). A thought such as "What if I fail this exam?" can be changed or reframed to helpful thoughts such as "I am studying the notes from class and I have read the book. I will ask questions about anything that I do not understand. I will study and learn the material for the exam." In this example, the reframing of the original question "What if I fail this exam?" prevents increasing anxiety from problem magnification and feelings of helplessness and resignation. Circular thinking that might occur in the above example can be disrupted as well. Here is an example of circular thinking: "What if I fail this exam? If I fail this exam I will not pass nursing school. If I don't pass this class I will not meet my goal to become a nurse. If I do not meet my goal, I will be a failure. I feel terrible when I am anxious. Because I feel terrible, anxiety is terrible." Cognitive reframing allows us to refocus on problem solving.

Positive self-talk about what nurses bring to the workplace is another important step in self-care and building resilience (Laskowski-Jones, 2011). The culture of a workplace can add to the stress of nurses. Focusing on our contributions and problem solving rather than focusing on negative thoughts is a step that can strengthen self-efficacy, build resilience, increase positive patient outcomes, and increase the nurse's sense of job satisfaction.

Healthy lifestyle choices also support resilience. Adequate sleep, rest, and breaks away from responsibilities while at work are restorative. Nutritious food and taking time for a full meal break away from the routine renews stamina. Exercise and play build both mental and physical endurance. Building satisfying relationships with friends, cultivating attitudes of openness to new knowledge, love of learning, and a sense of humor promote self-growth and resilience. A self-care plan that is referred to at regular intervals can help us accomplish goals. Development of stress reducing self-care skills helps to counter the stress response and lower stress hormone levels. If left unchecked, these hormones can contribute to negative health effects such as metabolic syndrome. Relaxation skills such as deep breathing, guided imagery, progressive relaxation, meditation, and massage are good examples of stress-reducing skills.

Chapter 41 gives more specifics on stress-reducing self-care skills. Learn to utilize what you teach patients about self-care in your own self-care.

Another strategy is clinical supervision, a mechanism through which the nurse can examine, process, and learn from interpersonal challenges. Clinical supervision is defined as a regular protected time for facilitated in-depth reflection of clinical practice as guided by an expert or peer. Its aim is to improve nurse effectiveness by clarifying, extending, or validating one's efforts in the clinical setting. Clinical supervision can increase job satisfaction and improve patient care. Although there are many models of one-to-one or group supervision, a structured program may not always be available to nurses. For that reason, an alternative opportunity for reflection might require initiative on the part of the nurse, such as asking for and listening to feedback from colleagues about one's relationships with patients. Seeking out internships and preceptorships can provide opportunities as well.

Laskowski-Jones (2011) suggests that support for one another in the work setting by committing to teamwork, mutual trust and caring for one another, and intolerance for horizontal violence can inspire resilience in the workplace.

COMMUNICATION AND THE NURSING PROCESS

The nurse–patient relationship and therapeutic communication are instruments used to implement the nursing process. The nursing process can also be applied to the communication that takes place between nurse and patient—the nurse assesses the patient's communication and uses specific therapeutic communication techniques appropriate for the patient's stage of development during nursing interventions.

Assessment

THE NURSE–PATIENT RELATIONSHIP

Because therapeutic communication takes place within the nurse–patient relationship, the goals of the relationship must be determined. These goals vary depending on the patient's needs, the area of nursing practice, and the specific role of the nurse in each particular clinical situation. Consider the following two examples.

One nurse works on a postpartum unit where the average length of stay is only 2 days. Each nurse cares for an average of eight patients per shift. The nurse's role is primarily to assist with care of the mother's physical needs, to facilitate mother–infant bonding, and to assess and conduct whatever teaching is necessary to help the family care for and adjust to the newborn. In this situation, the nurse–patient relationship is short term and focused. The nurse renders little direct physical care, working instead as an adviser and health teacher. The nurse and patient move through each phase of the nurse–patient relationship quickly.

In contrast, another nurse works for a hospice program providing care to terminally ill patients in their homes. The nurse spends 2 hours three times weekly with the patient and family. Her role is to give direct physical care, to support the patient and family, and to teach the family how to care for the patient. This relationship is intense and demanding. During the orientation phase, the nurse establishes a working relationship with the family and the patient, discussing how the patient and family will communicate and work together, thus establishing a verbal contract. In this situation, the nurse works as a direct caregiver, teacher, and therapeutic counselor.

During the initial phase of the relationship, the nurse assesses the patient's communication, using the theoretical base presented earlier in this chapter. Some key assessments about communication include the following:

- What patient impairments influence communication? Does the sender or receiver have sensory deficits or loss of function that could impair communication?
- What message variables for nonverbal and verbal communication influence the patient's communication? How do nonverbal variables such as facial expression, gestures, body movement, tone of voice, affect, posture, eye contact, and voice volume, quality, and pitch impact communication? How do verbal variables such as rate of speech, patterns of speech (stammering, excessive, tangential, silence, blocking), volume of speech, and content of the message affect communication?
- What communication skills does the patient exhibit? These can include openness, use of clarification, requests for feedback, tolerance of silence, and acceptance of confrontation.
- How does the setting (inpatient vs. community setting) influence patient communication?
- Is there a need for any media (communication boards, pictures, auditory or visual supports) to assist patient communication? If so, what would that include and what impact does that have on communication?
- When the nurse sends messages, how does the patient return feedback about the nurse's communication? Is the feedback positive, negative, goal directed, pertinent, and organized?
- How does the environment influence patient communication? Are there external influences such as temperature, lighting, noise level, and the physical arrangement of the room that would influence the patient's comfort and ability to concentrate and participate actively in communication? What are the patient's beliefs, experiences, thoughts, and attitudes that would influence communication?
- How does culture influence patient communication? What health practices, religious beliefs, language barriers, and preferences influence the patient's communication?
- What emotions and themes are present in the patient's communication? What emotions such as fear, confidence, anxiety, anger, sadness, or guilt does the patient display? What subjects and concerns does the patient focus on?
- Are the patient's verbal and nonverbal communications congruent?

THE ENVIRONMENT

Assessing the environment in which communication takes place is also important. The external environment must be conducive to communication. For example, how are the nurse and patient positioned in relation to each other? How far apart are they?

Noise and privacy are other facets of the environment that are important to consider. Telephones, televisions, radios, and machines such as ventilators, cardiac monitors, and suctioning equipment can be distracting. Other patients and employees can interfere with comfortable communication.

The patient's internal environment, made up of his or her cultural background, beliefs, and experiences, also may affect nurse–patient communication. For example, do the patient's religious beliefs pervade all aspects of his or her life and decision making? If so, this will affect communication, especially if the nurse has a different belief system. Language and cultural practices also should be assessed.

OTHER FACTORS

Shives (2012) points out additional factors that influence communication between the nurse and patient: interpersonal perceptions, attitudes, past experiences, knowledge of subject matter, and ability to relate to others. Although Shives focuses on these factors from the perspective of the nurse's ability to communicate, considering the implications of each of these from the patient perspective is illuminating as well. Interpersonal perception allows people to take the information they get through emotions, senses, and intellect and to use it to make sense of others and what they think. Inquiring into the understanding of the patient's perceptions about their health issues may reveal important information. Attitudes, formed through past life experiences, make a dramatic difference in the patient's ability to be accepting and open-minded, responsive to the nurse's attention. Knowledge of the health condition directly affects the patient's ability to effectively take control of his or her care and treatment and work collaboratively with care providers. There is a vast difference in the progress the nurse can make with a patient depending upon whether the patient is uncertain and tentative versus well educated and inquisitive. And finally, the patient's ability to relate to others—whether introverted or extroverted, careful and thoughtful, or reckless and impulsive—influences communication.

Not only do these factors pertain to the patient, but they pertain to the nurse as well. How do each of these factors make a difference in terms of *your* ability to be fully present to the patient? Take time to mentally review how these same factors might influence your ability to meet the patient's needs. Consider your own voice tone, quality, and pitch, body language, facial expressions, and verbal fluency, and know how anxiety may affect these factors. Communication is a two-way street; time spent assessing the patient's communication and the nurse's communication is worthwhile. They are partners in care. Anything undertaken to increase the success of that partnership is a good investment.

Implementation

Once communication has been assessed, how does the nurse use communication as a therapeutic intervention? Table 6-3 summarizes specific techniques to facilitate therapeutic communication. The therapeutic communication skills highlighted in this section are considered basic to any therapeutic relationship. More advanced skills are usually studied in psychiatric nursing.

HELPING THE PATIENT GET STARTED

Nurses are generally involved in informal therapeutic relationships, which can be important to the patient. In the acute care setting, the nurse often combines physical care with a discussion about the patient's concerns. The nurse can encourage a patient to express concerns by sitting down; often, patients are reluctant to express themselves to someone

TABLE 6-3 THERAPEUTIC COMMUNICATION TECHNIQUES

Technique	Definition	Examples of What the Nurse Might Say to an Adult, Adolescent, or Child
Offering self	Making oneself available to listen to the patient	To adult: "I will walk with you for a while." To adolescent: "We can sit together here. I'm interested in what has been on your mind." To child: "I have time to play with you now. What would you like to tell me about yourself?"
Open-ended questions	Asking neutral questions that encourage the patient to express concerns	To adult: "I'm interested in hearing about issues of concern to you." To adolescent: "How do you feel about that?" To child: "What would you like to talk about today?"
Opening remarks	Using general statements based on observations and assessments about the patient	To adult: "Where would you like to begin?" To adolescent: "I notice you are going through some important changes." To child: "You seem to be feeling better today."
Restatement	Repeating to the patient the main content of his or her communication	**Nurse dialogue with adult:** Adult: "I was up and down all night." Nurse: "You had difficulty sleeping last night." **Nurse dialogue with adolescent:** Adolescent: "I could not get my homework done. I kept thinking about other things." Nurse: "You are having difficulty concentrating." **Nurse dialogue with child:** Child: Tearfully states, "My tummy hurt and my food all came up." Nurse: "You do not feel well and you are upset."
Reflection	Identifying the main emotional themes contained in a communication and directing these back to the patient	**Nurse dialogue with adult:** Adult: "What do you think I should do about this problem?" Nurse: "What do *you* think you should do?" **Nurse dialogue with adolescent:** Adolescent: "My older brother keeps getting into trouble. My parents think that I will do the same things." Nurse: "You feel angry with your brother and your parents?" **Nurse dialogue with child:** Child: "This tasted icky!" Nurse: "You do not like the way the medicine tastes?"
Focusing	Asking goal-directed questions to help the patient focus on key concerns	**Nurse dialogue with adult:** Adult: "I have three children. One from my girlfriend and two from my wife." Nurse: "Tell me a little about your children." **Nurse dialogue with adolescent:** Adolescent: "Everything is going wrong!" Nurse: "Give me an example of what you mean." **Nurse dialogue with child:** Child: "I hate all the people in my house." Nurse: "Tell me about Mary first."
Encouraging elaboration	Helping the patient to describe more fully the concerns or problems under discussion	**Nurse dialogue with adult:** Adult: "I am going to be fired, I hate my boss!" Nurse: "Can you tell me a little about your boss?" **Nurse dialogue with adolescent:** Adolescent: "I can't stand it anymore." Nurse: "Tell me about what is upsetting you." **Nurse dialogue with child:** Child: "There was a crotcheter in the basement." Nurse: "A crotcheter? Tell me about that."

TABLE 6-3 THERAPEUTIC COMMUNICATION TECHNIQUES (*Continued*)

Technique	Definition	Examples of What the Nurse Might Say to an Adult, Adolescent, or Child
Seeking clarification	Helping the patient put into words unclear thoughts or ideas	**Nurse dialogue with adult:** Adult: "My son does not realize that his wife is ruining them!" Nurse: "I am not sure I understand what you are saying. Please tell me more about that." **Nurse dialogue with adolescent:** Adolescent: "We were standing on the corner. It was an armpit!" Nurse: "I did not understand what you meant. An armpit?" **Nurse dialogue with child:** Child: "I got buzzed!" Nurse: "You told me you got buzzed. Tell me what you mean."
Giving information	Sharing with the patient relevant information for his or her healthcare and well-being	To adult: "My purpose in being here is…" To adolescent: "Many people have problems remembering to take their medication. We could talk about some strategies for remembering to take your medicine." To child: "My name is… I will check to make sure you are okay all day."
Looking at alternatives	Helping the patient see options and participate in the decision-making process related to his or her healthcare and well-being	To adult: "Perhaps we can talk about your anger and discover what triggers your anger." To adolescent: "If this situation occurs again, what are options that you have?" To child: "What will you need to do differently next time you feel sad?"
Silence	Allowing for a pause in communication that permits the nurse and patient time to think about what has taken place	To adult: "Take your time to answer, I have time and I am interested in your thoughts and feelings about this." To adolescent: "I heard you say [insert appropriate information here]… I am thinking about what you said." To child: Do not speak; sit quietly and attentively using good eye contact and remain silent.
Summarizing	Highlighting the important points of a conversation by condensing what was said	To adult: "Today we have talked about your plans after discharge. They include [insert appropriate information here]…." To adolescent: "Let's review what we've talked about today." To child: "We talked about what to do if you feel mad today. Tell me three things that you can choose to do."

who is always in a hurry or seems too busy. Draw the curtain between beds, and focus the patient's attention away from any roommates and toward the nurse. Call the patient by name, asking whether he or she prefers to be called by the first or last name. Many adults find it intrusive or rude to be called

by their first name. Convey interest and readiness to listen. By leaning toward the patient, making eye contact, and assuming a relaxed, open posture, the nurse offers himself or herself to the patient. Box 6-4 lists general guidelines for facilitating communication.

BOX 6-4   Guidelines for Facilitating Communication

- Speak in a normal tone.
- Do not raise your voice or shout.
- Realize that speaking more loudly does not increase comprehension.
- Speak to the patient on an adult level.
- Remember that impaired communication does not indicate impaired intelligence.
- Avoid carrying on more than one conversation at a time.
- Ask simple questions that require simple answers.
- Keep the atmosphere quiet and relaxed.
- Reduce or eliminate environmental noises.

- Make sure you have the patient's attention before you speak.
- Maintain eye contact with the patient throughout the conversation.
- Assume patients can understand you. Do not discuss their cases or other inappropriate topics in front of them.
- Do not rush the patient. Give the patient adequate time to respond.
- Do not correct mistakes.
- If you do not understand, ask the patient to repeat what he or she said.
- Praise patients for their attempts at speech.

Open-Ended Questions

An open-ended question is one that elicits more than a "yes" or "no" answer. Such questions ask how, what, where, or when. Examples of appropriate questions include "How are things going for you at this point?" and "What have your experiences been like?"

Opening Remarks

Other ways to help a patient get started include opening remarks based on observations and assessment about the patient. For example, assessment-based statements such as "You've been having a pretty rough time," "I notice you're going through some important changes," or "You seem to be feeling better" provide the patient with the opportunity to respond.

These questions and statements must be neutral and tentative, not probing or interrogating. "Why" questions usually are not considered therapeutic because they are too intrusive; newspaper reporters and schoolteachers ask "why" questions. For example, asking patients why they are upset is more threatening than asking what is going on or just noting that they seem to be upset.

Active Listening

Listening is essential to understanding what the patient perceives, thinks, and feels (Stuart, 2012). Listening actively involves the ability to focus on the patient and the content of the patient's messages, conveying back to the patient an accurate picture of what he or she is expressing (Fig. 6-5). Thinking about what you will say next instead of actively listening to the patient is a common mistake in beginning students. Keep your focus on what the patient is saying and, if needed, use nonverbal eye contact and nodding as you pause and think about what you want to say that will be most helpful for the patient. It is acceptable to state "I am thinking about what you just said" and to pause if needed. Work on not letting your potential anxiety early in relationships get in the way of relationship building with your patient.

Active listening also involves constant decoding of the content and feeling of the messages sent by the listener. The content part of the message includes thoughts, words, opinions, and ideas. The feeling part refers to the patient's emotions.

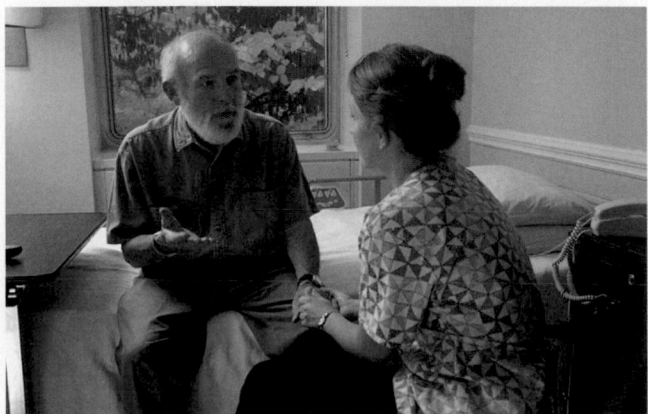

FIGURE 6-5 Active listening provides vital information about patient needs.

Emotions may be described verbally, but usually, they are manifested more accurately through nonverbal means, such as facial expression, body posture, laughter, or crying. Note congruence or incongruence among these messages to help understand how patients are experiencing the things they are discussing.

Also, observe what is behind the message sent by the patient. For example, is the patient conveying an attitude of helplessness, rejection, or aggression toward the nurse?

While decoding the conversation, listen actively by using two important techniques: **restatement** and reflection. These key techniques are used to help a patient feel listened to and understood.

Restatement and Reflection

Restatement refers mainly to the content portion of the communication. After listening carefully to the patient, repeat the content of the message back to the patient in order to verify understanding with the patient. When the content is restated, the patient has the opportunity to hear himself or herself and to gain understanding of his or her own communication.

Reflection means identifying the main emotional themes contained in a communication and directing them back to the patient. The purpose is to verify and check the feelings that are being heard. Listen for the underlying feeling that a patient is conveying; then, repeat this understanding in a neutral, open manner. With this technique, the patient gains a clearer understanding of the feelings he or she is experiencing.

These two techniques do not involve exact repetition of the patient's statements. Rather, the nurse picks up on the content or feeling, rephrases it, and then states it back to the patient. The following example shows how these techniques might be used in an informal therapeutic relationship:

Patient: I can't sleep. It's too hot in here and the noise is bothering me.

Nurse: You can't sleep because it's uncomfortable in here. *(Restatement.)*

Patient: That's right. All I can think about is having that operation in the morning. *(Sounds irritable, looks anxious.)*

Nurse: The thought of having surgery is keeping you awake. *(Reflection.)*

Patient: Yes. I'm really scared.

In this situation, the nurse listened carefully and found that it was not really the environment but the anxiety about having surgery that was keeping the patient awake. By communicating back to the patient in a careful way the things being heard, the nurse opened up an opportunity to clarify concerns and misperceptions about the impending surgery.

EXPLORING

Exploring is a way of communicating therapeutically without giving direct advice. Instead, the nurse helps patients express their concerns and solve their own problems by investigating the situation, how the patient feels about it, and what some alternatives might be.

Focusing

Focusing involves asking goal-directed questions to help the patient stay on the topic and talk more about it. The questions, still open ended, are directed toward the patient's key concerns. An example of focusing is, "We were talking about how people will respond to your mastectomy. Can you say more about that?"

Asking focused questions helps the patient discuss the main issues of concern. It keeps the conversation on target without changing the subject or becoming too generalized, conveying the message that the nurse will stay with the patient and help explore concerns.

Sometimes, helping a patient to express things of importance can be frightening. The nurse encounters suffering when working with ill and dying patients. To be therapeutic, maturity and a sense of perspective about life, which takes time and experience, are crucial.

Encouraging Elaboration

Encouraging elaboration is a technique used to help the patient describe more fully the concerns or problems being discussed. Nodding one's head, using an attentive demeanor, and making comments such as "Go on" or "I see" encourage the patient to keep talking and express himself or herself more thoroughly. This provides additional information about the patient's emotional state, coping abilities, and view of the situation.

Seeking Clarification

Seeking clarification means helping the patient put into words unclear thoughts or ideas. It can also be used to clarify events by putting them in a time sequence. Examples include "I'm not sure I understand what you mean," "What else happened?," and "What happened then?" Such questions help the patient to order his or her thoughts, put events into context, and place things in a more manageable perspective. By clarifying the problem or event being discussed, the patient gains new insight into his or her situation.

Giving Information

Giving information involves sharing information about the patient's health and well-being in a timely manner and based on what is currently known about the patient's condition. Giving information can mean sharing what is known about a patient's illness, treatment, and recovery. It can also mean correcting misperceptions.

For example, a young woman is brought to the emergency room after being raped. After medical care has been completed, police reports filled out, and the patient's family notified, the nurse sits with the patient for a few minutes while she waits for a family member to come. The patient says, "I should have been more careful. I was wearing a short skirt. Maybe that caused the rape." Based on what the nurse knows about rape victims' perceptions, a timely intervention might be for the nurse to say, "When people are raped, it is normal for them to look for the cause within themselves. But the rape is not your fault. You are the victim in this situation." This information is based on research showing that rape victims commonly assume that they provoked the rape. In addition to giving this information, the nurse might also refer the patient to a rape counseling center in the community.

Giving information is a skill commonly used in health teaching, often done while giving physical care. Information must be distinguished from suggestions or advice. A typical way to give advice is to start by saying, "Why don't you …" or "You should …" Such giving of advice reinforces the patient's dependence on the nurse. A more useful strategy is giving the information the patient needs to be able to make a decision.

Looking at Alternatives

Looking at alternatives means exploring options for the patient's consideration. When more options are identified, the patient's perceived choices are increased. The nurse does not always need to present the alternatives; the patient can be asked for them instead. Examples of questions to use include the following:

- What are some of your ideas about how to handle this?
- Have you thought about [alternative courses of action]?
- What else could you do?
- If you met someone in the same situation as you, what would you advise him or her to do?
- What are some advantages (or disadvantages) of the alternatives we have just discussed?

Alternatives should not be discussed too early or before the patient has a clear understanding of the current situation. Sometimes, a patient must first express feelings such as grief or anger before he or she can explore how to deal with the situation. Avoid the trap that beginning students commonly fall into of attempting to help the patient by "fixing" the situation.

Using Silence

Another useful therapeutic technique is using silence, a pause in communication that allows the nurse and patient to reflect on what has taken place. By waiting quietly and attentively, the nurse encourages the patient to initiate and maintain conversation. Keep in mind that hospitalized or ill patients may need more time than usual to process information. Silence is sometimes difficult for nurses who are used to more active forms of communicating. However, it is important to recognize when silence is appropriate.

Summarizing

Summarizing means highlighting the important points of a conversation by condensing what has been said. This is useful toward the end of a therapeutic conversation. Summarizing helps both the nurse and patient review the main themes of the conversation and gives a sense of closure. It also enables the nurse and patient to think about what else needs to be considered or discussed in the future. It emphasizes the progress made toward self-understanding and problem solving. Examples of summarizing include "Today, it seems that you've thought about …" and "Let's review what we've talked about today."

DEVELOPING COMMUNICATION SKILLS

Communication between the nurse and patient in the clinical setting is based on patient needs, not on personal or social interests. When the nurse has a professional approach and is patient centered, a focus on the patient's health and well-being is maintained.

Time and experience are needed to become skilled at using therapeutic communication. One way to develop this skill is to study one's interactions, either by recording a therapeutic conversation (after obtaining the patient's permission) or by recreating the conversation from memory. After making a transcript of the conversation, analyze it by reviewing the techniques used, their timing and appropriateness, and how the patient responded to the nurse. The nurse's own thoughts and feelings also are noted because these affect how he or she responds to the patient. An example of how to use a process recording to enhance communication skills is shown in Table 6-4.

NONTHERAPEUTIC RESPONSES

Nontherapeutic responses interfere with or block therapeutic communication. Often, such responses are the more natural responses that people make in social situations. Nontherapeutic responses may prevent nurses from functioning as professionals and therapeutic agents in the care of patients.

Nurses must meet their own needs outside the therapeutic context. For example, some nurses might become overly involved with patients because they have not developed social lives in ways that meet their needs. Other nurses might be uncomfortable with patients who express feelings

---

TABLE 6-4 HOW TO USE A PROCESS RECORDING TO ENHANCE COMMUNICATION SKILLS

The purpose of a process recording is to help the nurse analyze verbal and nonverbal communication with patients with the goal of identifying helpful techniques and areas for improvement. Consider the following situation:

The patient is a 35-year-old man who sustained burns on his face and upper body in a car accident. He was transferred from the burn unit to the rehabilitation unit 2 days ago.

Verbal and Nonverbal Interaction	Analysis
Less Effective	
Nurse: How are you doing today? *(Standing next to door.)*	Open-ended question invites response, but nonverbal communication (i.e., standing next to door) indicates nurse may be busy and needs to move on.
Patient: It's been a rough 2 days.	Patient makes a general statement.
Nurse: Do you need any pain medication?	Nurse makes assumption that patient is referring to physical discomfort. Nurse's request is narrowly focused and limits patient's options in responding.
Patient: No, I think I'm OK for now. *(Looks down at floor.)*	
Nurse: Well, let me know if you need anything.	Nurse ends interaction without exploring other reasons for patient's distress.
Patient: OK, thanks.	Patient does not feel invited to discuss what is really bothering him.
More Effective	
Nurse: When I left you yesterday, things weren't going very well for you. How are you doing today? *(Nurse sits down, facing patient.)*	Opening remark establishes that nurse remembers events from previous day. Indicates working phase of relationship. Open-ended question helps patient get started. Nurse offers self.
Patient: It's been a rough 2 days.	Patient makes a general statement.
[SILENCE.]	Nurse allows silence so patient can collect his thoughts.
Patient: I've come to the realization that I'm not going to look the same as I did …	Patient begins to clarify what he means.
Nurse: … and … ? *(Remains attentive.)*	Nurse encourages elaboration.
Patient: It's hard. *(Becomes tearful.)*	Patient showing feelings nonverbally.
Nurse: *(Gently.)* It is upsetting to deal with the after effects of your burns.	Reflection—the nurse reflects patient's feelings so he can own them.
Patient: I shouldn't cry. *(Appears embarrassed.)*	Nurse assesses that patient's past experiences and personal history have led him to the conclusion that men should not cry.
Nurse: You think men shouldn't cry when they have a really difficult adjustment to make?	Reflection of metacommunication (embarrassment about crying). The nurse shows patient what he feels about his feelings.
Patient: *(Laughs slightly.)* I guess it's OK for me to cry. My situation isn't easy to deal with.	Patient gains understanding of his feelings and his metacommunication.
[SILENCE.]	
Patient: *(Looks sad. Remains thoughtful.)*	
Nurse: Some of what you are experiencing is a natural grieving process that people in your situation go through. You have lost part of your former self, and that is a painful experience.	Giving information—nurse, experienced and well read in the rehabilitation of burn patients, shares this information in a timely manner. Nurse realizes there is no easy solution for this patient's problem. She provides support.

Table developed by Laina Gerace, PhD, RN, associate professor, University of Illinois at Chicago, College of Nursing.

because they have never been able to express their own. Engage in self-evaluation to determine your own strengths and weaknesses.

Inexperienced healthcare workers may believe that serious problems can be solved easily. On television, dire problems are solved in half an hour, but in real life, this is not always the case. Presenting quick solutions and unwarranted cheerfulness blocks the therapeutic process. Some people have terminal illnesses. Others must adapt to situations for which there are no quick or simple answers. Through experience, nurses learn that they can help but cannot always provide perfect solutions. Maintain a supportive presence and provide competent care while patients struggle with their difficulties.

Rescue Feelings

Rescue feelings occur when a nurse feels essential to the patient's welfare. The nurse thinks that he or she has exceptional abilities to help the patient, and the nurse's expectations for the patient will be high.

Some rescue feelings are useful because having confidence in one's ability to be helpful is part of being therapeutic. Strong rescue feelings, however, impede the therapeutic process. The nurse may believe that only he or she can meet the patient's needs, alienating himself or herself from the healthcare team. These feelings should be a warning to the nurse and the nurse's colleagues that the boundaries of the professional relationship are being breached. The nurse may also raise the patient's expectations too high. When these expectations are not met, the patient is disappointed.

False Reassurance

False reassurance means giving reassurance that is not based on the real situation. It is a way of minimizing the patient's situation. For example, saying "Don't worry, everything will be fine" minimizes the patient's concerns. Other forms of false reassurance include telling a patient not to dwell on his or her problems and saying that an injection will not hurt. Giving false reassurance violates the patient's trust. If the nurse tells a patient not to worry when the patient actually is worried or that something does not hurt when it does hurt, how can the patient have confidence in the nurse? Instead, supply any needed information and give reassurances based on actuality.

Real reassurance must be based on fact. For example, telling a patient that there will be postoperative pain and how it will be controlled is much more reassuring than saying "There's nothing to this operation. We do it all the time." A procedure may seem routine to the nurse, but to the patient, it is a major event. The patient will feel much more supported if allowed to express anxiety and ask questions.

Giving Advice

Giving advice is another common nontherapeutic response. Doing so focuses exclusively on the nurse's experiences and opinions. Examples of giving advice include statements that begin, "I think you should …," "Why don't you …," and "The same thing happened to me and I …" Giving advice diminishes the patient's responsibilities and choices and tends to be controlling. Patients may believe they must do what the nurse says, even though the advice might not work well for them.

Giving advice is different from giving a suggestion, an alternative idea for the patient's consideration. If carefully done, giving a suggestion increases the patient's perceived options. Usually, however, it is better if the patient comes up with his or her own ideas. A helpful way to give a suggestion is to frame it tentatively, such as "I wonder if you have thought about [an alternative course of action]."

Changing the Subject

Changing the subject is a nontherapeutic response that usually indicates anxiety on the nurse's part. It is a way of resisting hearing about a patient's distress, sadness, and difficulties. Changing the subject might be an attempt to cheer up the patient or to distract the patient from painful thoughts. However, changing the subject can be a way to avoid listening to what the patient has to say. The patient is left with the feeling that his or her feelings have been discounted.

Being Moralistic

Being moralistic means seeing a situation as good or bad or right or wrong. It is a judgmental approach. The nurse must become aware of how he or she uses the word *should*. Talking to patients in terms of "shoulds" infers a preconceived idea about the "right" thing to do. For instance, saying to an unwed mother "I think you should keep the baby" is being moralistic. Many factors go into making a decision of this magnitude. What works for one person might not work for another.

Another way of being moralistic is to give approval or disapproval by judging the patient's actions as good or bad. Everyone has moral attitudes, and being moral is part of being human. Nurses have a right to their own values. However, in the clinical situation, they must transcend them and view their patients in more objective terms. The nurse can communicate the value and worth of each patient even though he or she may not agree with a patient's behavior.

Nonprofessional Involvement

Nonprofessional involvement occurs at a time when the nurse goes outside the boundaries of the therapeutic relationship and establishes a social, economic, or personal relationship with the patient (Stuart, 2009). Although appropriate at times (e.g., chatting briefly about the weather or a major news event), too much socializing points to a nonprofessional relationship. Nurses who talk too much with patients about themselves and their own goals and problems are being nonprofessional. The purpose of a professional relationship is to meet the patient's needs, not the nurse's. The nurse should use self-disclosure— the act of revealing personal information within the context of a professional relationship—judiciously. Self-disclosure should be brief and used only for the benefit of the patient.

Sexual boundary violation is another example of nonprofessional involvement. Sexual boundary transgression occurs at a time when the nurse expresses romantic or sexual feelings toward a patient (Stuart, 2012). Sexual contact of any kind is not acceptable within the therapeutic nurse–patient relationship.

The nurse is responsible for defining and maintaining professional boundaries, even if the patient behaves sexually toward the nurse.

Nontherapeutic involvement has pitfalls for both nurse and patient. The patient is receiving nursing care because of a need for professional services and wants to feel confident that a professional is in charge of nursing care. The nurse must maintain a professional attitude to remain objective in clinical decision making. Becoming a friend to the patient abdicates the professional role.

SPECIAL SITUATIONS

Not all communication techniques are effective with all patients. Certain situations call for particular communication techniques or modifications, depending on the patient's developmental stage or environment.

Children and Adolescents

Children and adolescents present unique challenges to effective communication. Persons in these age groups are undergoing many changes that make clear communication more difficult.

Children are responsive to nonverbal communication, such as body movements, voice tone, and eye contact. Talking to children at eye level can help to minimize intimidation (Fig. 6-6). Speaking gently and calmly and using quiet body movements engenders greater trust.

When children first learn words, they sometimes have difficulty understanding what they mean. The way words are combined does not always convey the exact meaning intended. Clarify meanings with children until they can understand the message by using restatement and clarification. Consider the following example:

Child: Baby socks.
Nurse: You have little socks?
Child: *(No response.)*
Nurse: You have socks?
Child: *(Shakes head to indicate no.)*
Nurse: You want your socks?
Child: *(Smiles and nods head to indicate yes.)*

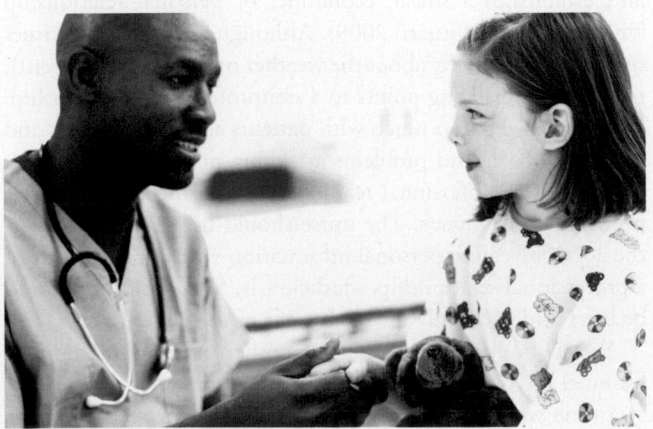

FIGURE 6-6 Communicating at eye level is important for all patients, including children.

Young children are more attentive to simplified speech. Use language that children can understand. When speaking to children who do not respond, rephrase the communication. For example:

Nurse: It's time for your dinner now.
Child: *(No response.)*
Nurse: Time to eat now.
Child: *(Takes nurse's hand to go to dining area.)*

Use play to help children deal with the stress of hospitalization. For example, having children play with dolls representing physicians and nurses can help them act out their fears appropriately. By participating in such play, children can develop feelings of mastery over the situation. Many hospitals caring for young children provide structured play to help patients deal with their illnesses and treatments. By observing play, nurses can identify children's concerns.

Hospitalization for physical problems in this age group produces anxiety. Children and adolescents often feel embarrassed about their bodies and vulnerable to the control of adults. Therefore, be considerate of personal space, and do not be too intrusive. Use touch judiciously, and maintain modesty. Adolescents are particularly conscious of the need for privacy and modesty in communication situations with health professionals.

Provide information about procedures and treatments in a straightforward manner without giving false reassurance. For example, if a procedure might be painful, it is best to share this information in a matter-of-fact way.

To work effectively with children and adolescents, a sense of give and take is needed. Although the approach may be a little less formal than with adults, some professional distance is still maintained. Limit setting is a key factor in working effectively with children and adolescents. To set limits, the nurse must be seen as authoritative by the young patient. Being authoritative means being in charge but permitting freedom within reasonable, closely established behavioral limits that elicit participation in their reinforcement. This is different from being authoritarian, which means exerting power over another person.

Adults and Older Adults

Specifying communication strategies for any phase of development is difficult, and this is especially true for adulthood. Adulthood is an ongoing developmental period. As people grow and age, they must constantly adapt to many changes. Less is known about adulthood than about any other phase of development.

Hospitalization can create a period of transition in which adults question the progress of their lives, their goals, and even life's meaning. When illness disrupts their responsibilities, feelings of vulnerability may overwhelm them. Active, achieving adults may find it difficult to suddenly need assistance from nurses. As such, adults may sometimes behave in ways that are difficult to manage.

Nurses also may experience a range of feelings in relation to various adult patients. For example, an older male patient may remind the nurse of his or her grandfather. The nurse may then relate to the patient as if to the grandfather. Or the nurse may treat the patient as if he were helpless and unable to make any decisions. If the patient is a physician or a wealthy or well-known person, feelings of intimidation may arise on the nurse's part. Numerous complex situations come into play when communicating therapeutically with adults. Recognizing feelings and sharing them with fellow professionals is important because these feelings affect the way in which communication takes place.

For older adults, normal age-related changes further challenge communication skills. Age-related changes in hearing and vision often add barriers and additional obstacles to effective communication. Decreased hearing and impaired vision diminish the ability of some older adults to participate comfortably in some areas of communication. These patients may require additional communication skills to help them compensate for these changes.

Communication strategies with adults draw on all the concepts discussed in this chapter. The contractual approach provides an opportunity to establish with the patient how communication will take place. For example, discuss whether to call an adult by his or her first or last name at the outset. Remember that all human beings—no matter what their job, social status, or income—at some point in their lives are vulnerable and suffer anxiety and worry. The use of therapeutic communication skills will facilitate expression and problem solving with any adult.

Cross-Cultural Communication

The population of the United States is becoming increasingly diverse. Nurses must be prepared to communicate with patients from various cultural and ethnic groups. It is helpful if the nurse is aware of which ethnic groups live in the community and is familiar with common beliefs and practices of those groups related to healthcare, but this may be unrealistic in urban centers with multiple ethnic communities. Fortunately, there are numerous books, journals, and Web-based resources to assist healthcare professionals to provide culturally competent care.

When working with patients who have limited English-speaking ability, it is important to remember that the patient has a language barrier, not a hearing problem (unless one exists). Speak clearly and distinctly in a normal tone of voice, using hand motions, pictures, and demonstrations when appropriate. Even with the most careful efforts, misunderstandings may occur, and in healthcare, it is particularly important to avoid them. Language interpreters should be used whenever possible. Skillful interpreters can provide insight into cultural meanings and nuances of the language and the related culture that may have a bearing on the patient's healthcare needs. Family members, particularly children, should not be used as interpreters. Box 6-5 summarizes guidelines for working with language interpreters in healthcare settings.

The nurse should also be aware of cultural differences in nonverbal communication. For example, direct eye contact in some cultures is considered rude or threatening. Touching a patient's head, except when clinically indicated, is prohibited in some cultures, as is touching a person of the opposite gender. Cultural norms may also determine which family members should be addressed and who makes decisions for the family. It is unrealistic to expect nurses to know the cultural beliefs

---

BOX 6-5	Guidelines for Interpreter-Dependent Communication

- Take time to meet with the interpreter before meeting with the patient.
- Allow sufficient time—working with an interpreter may take twice as long as a meeting in which a common language is spoken.
- Speak directly to the patient.
- Speak in short sentences, and allow the interpreter to interpret.
- Develop alternatives to direct questions.
- Avoid ambiguous language, abstractions, and technical jargon.
- Speak slowly and clearly; use repetition as needed.
- Be aware of nonverbal messages that may require interpretation just as verbal messages do.
- Avoid using family members as interpreters.

Source: Hadziabdic, E., & Hjelm, K. (2013). Working with interpreters: practical advice for use of an interpreter in healthcare. *International Journal of Evidence Based Healthcare, 11*(1), 69–76. doi: 10.1111/1744-1609.12005

---

and practices of all of the patients with whom they will work. However, sensitivity and a willingness to learn enhance the nurse's ability to communicate effectively in various cultural contexts.

The Patient in the Intensive Care Unit

The intensive care unit (ICU) is an environment designed to help maintain the lives of seriously ill patients. Unfamiliar sounds and noises, artificial lighting, and undefined colors characterize the ICU. Being admitted to the ICU is stressful. The patient fears the diagnosis and the extent of the injury and may be unable to communicate. Communication is hindered further if the patient does not know or understand the severity of the illness, feels a lack of control over what is happening, does not know the reason for therapies, receives care from several different providers, or loses contact with the outside world, including a sense of day and time.

Getting caught up in the complexities and technology of the ICU is easy. As a result, minimal communication may occur with the patient. Be constantly aware that the patient in this life-threatening situation is a person for whom communication is more important than ever. Even when the patient cannot answer (because of decreased level of consciousness, intubation, or other reasons), assume that the patient can hear. Talk to the patient about what you are doing, just as you would with any other patient. Nonverbal communication (e.g., touch, facial expressions) is especially meaningful for ICU patients.

To give cues about day and time, provide clocks and calendars where the patient can see them. For patients who can use their hands but cannot speak, notepads or magic slates aid in communication. Call bells within easy reach help patients to communicate their needs.

Once the patient has been stabilized, help him or her understand the illness and the reason for various therapies. Explanations must be clear, direct, and simply stated. Because of the patient's state, expect to repeat the explanations. If the patient is able, discussing his or her perceptions and understanding enhances the patient's sense of control and decreases stress.

KEY CONCEPTS

- Effective communication within the nurse–patient relationship focuses on the patient and the patient's experiences and results in improved health status and well-being.
- Communication is a system of sending and receiving messages that forms a connection between the sender and the receiver.
- Verbal communication involves language; nonverbal communication includes gestures, facial expressions, body posture, body movement, voice tone, rate of speech, and dress.
- The elements of communication are the source (sender), the message, and the receiver; the processes are encoding, decoding, and feedback.
- The nurse–patient relationship is focused on the patient and is goal directed with defined parameters.
- The three phases in the nurse–patient relationship are orientation, working, and termination.
- Empathy, positive regard, and a comfortable sense of self are among the key ingredients of the nurse–patient relationship.
- Self-awareness and reflective practice are essential components to growth in expertise of therapeutic communication skills.
- The nurse–patient relationship and therapeutic communication are instruments used to implement the nursing process.
- Skillful use of therapeutic responses is essential for accurate assessment and interventions.
- Nontherapeutic responses, such as rescue feelings, false reassurance, giving advice, changing the subject, being moralistic, and nonprofessional involvement, block communication.
- Communication techniques may need to be modified when dealing with children, adolescents, older adults, persons who speak a foreign language, or persons admitted to the ICU.

PRACTICING FOR THE NCLEX

CHECK YOUR ANSWERS IN APPENDIX A.

1. Nontherapeutic communication may interfere with professional nursing care by hindering the patient–nurse relationship. Which of the following are examples of nontherapeutic communication? Select all that apply:
   a. A nurse provides education on smoking cessation: "The same thing happened to me and I was able to quit."
   b. A nurse attempts to distract a patient at the end of their life: "Let's focus on your walking for the day, not your worries about death."
   c. A nurse states during report that "the patient should not get an abortion because it is wrong."
   d. A nurse is sending a pediatric patient for cardiac surgery. As he leaves she states "Don't worry, everything will be fine!"
   e. A nurse is discussing care options with the family of a patient: "What have your experiences been like with home healthcare in the past?"

2. A previously healthy and active 31-year-old patient with a radical mastectomy snaps at the nurse and asks her to leave her alone. In analyzing this, the nurse is able to attribute the behavior to:
   a. Empathy
   b. Comfortable sense of self
   c. Developmental stage of intimacy versus isolation
   d. Vulnerability of illness

3. In communicating with a developmentally delayed adult patient, which of the following would be the best techniques for the nurse to use?
   a. Silence
   b. Providing reassurance at all times
   c. Setting clear limits while allowing participation
   d. Establishing a contract including values and rights

4. A patient's sister expresses her dissatisfaction to the nurse regarding the discharge care coordination between the physician and cardiology team. In order to practice patient advocacy, what should the nurse do first?
   a. Call the social worker to coordinate the discharge care.
   b. Call the physician immediately to request a visit with the patient's sister.
   c. Assist the patient's sister in compiling a list of questions related to discharge.
   d. Admit to the patient's sister that there are problems with the discharge system and resolve to correct these oversights.

5. The circle of confidentiality is essential in maintaining sensitive information among appropriate professionals. A nurse overhears a conversation about an unknown patient's care in the elevator. The best immediate response would be:
   a. "Clinically relevant information should be shared with the healthcare team, thanks for your report."
   b. "I'm concerned to hear discussions like this in nonprivate areas, let's be mindful of patient privacy."
   c. An incident report describing the event with the names of those employees involved.
   d. Interjections with suggestions for the patient's care plan considering his or her current situation.

REFERENCES

Bandler, R., & Grinder, J. (1975). *The structure of magic: A book about language and therapy.* Palo Alto, CA: Science & Behavior Books.

Berlo, D. K. (1960). *The process of communication: An introduction to therapy and practice.* New York: Holt, Rinehart, & Winston.

Bulman, C., Lathlean, J., & Gobbi, M. (2013). The process of teaching and learning about reflection: research insights from professional nurse education. Studies in Higher Education http://www.tandfonline.com/doi/abs/10.1080/03075079.2013.777413

Caldwell, L., Grobbel, C. (2013). The importance of reflective practice in nursing. *International Journal of Caring Sciences, 6*(3).

Colineau, N., & Paris, C. (2011). Motivating reflection about health within the family: The use of setting and tailored feedback. *User Modeling and User–Adapted Interaction, 21*(4–5), 341–376. doi: http://dx.doi.org/10.1007/s11257-010-9089-x

Forrest, C. (2012). Working with 'difficult' patients. *Primary Health Care, 22*(8), 20–22. Retrieved from http://search.proquest.com/docview/1114855076?accountid=458

Hayes, E., & Kalmakis, K. A. (2007). From the sidelines: Coaching as a nurse practitioner strategy for improving health outcomes. *Journal of the American Academy of Nurse Practitioners, 19*, 555–562.

Hull, S. K., & Broquet, K. (2007). How to manage difficult patient encounters. *Family Practice Management, 14*(6), 30–34.

International Council of Nurses. (2014). ICNP Translations, *Geneva, Switzerland.* Retrieved August 15, 2014, from www.icn.ch/pillarsprograms/icnpr-translati

Johns, C. (2013). *Becoming a reflective practitioner* (4th ed.). West Sussex, UK: John Wiley & Sons Ltd.

Kelman, C. A., & Branco, A. U. (2009). (Meta)communication strategies in inclusive classes for deaf students. *American Annals of the Deaf, 154*(4), 371–381.

Luft, J. (1970). *Group processed: An introduction in group dynamics.* Palo Alto, CA: National Press Books.

Macdonald, M. (2007). Origins of difficulty in the nurse-patient encounter. *Nurse Ethics, 14*(4), 510–521.

Mascioli, S., Laskowski-Jones, L., Urban, S., & Moran, S. (2009). Improving handoff communication. *Nursing, 39*(2), 52–55.

Myers, R. E. (2010). Promoting healthy behaviors: How do we get the message across? *International Journal of Nursing Studies, 47*(4), 500–512.

Peplau, H. E. (1997). *Interpersonal relations in nursing.* New York: G. P. Putnam's Sons.

Pope, B. B., Rodzen, L., & Spross, G. (2008). Raising the SBAR: How better communication improves patient outcomes. *Nursing, 38*(3), 41–43.

Rogers, C. (1961). *On becoming a person.* Boston, MA: Houghton Mifflin.

Shives, L. R. (2012). *Basic concepts of mental health nursing* (8th ed.). Philadelphia, PA: Lippincott Williams & Wilkins.

Stuart, G. (2012). Therapeutic nurse–patient relationship. In G. Stuart (Ed.), *Principles and practice of psychiatric nursing* (10th ed.). St. Louis, MO: Elsevier Mosby.

Varcarolis, E. M., & Halter, M. J. (2014). *Varcarolis' foundations of psychiatric mental health nursing: A clinical approach* (7th ed.). St. Louis, MO: Saunders.

Videbeck, S. (2014). *Psychiatric mental health nursing* (6th ed.). Philadelphia, PA: Lippincott, Williams & Wilkins.

Zolnierek, C. D. (2014). An Integrative Review of Knowing the Patient. *Journal of Nursing Scholarship, 46*(1), 3–10.

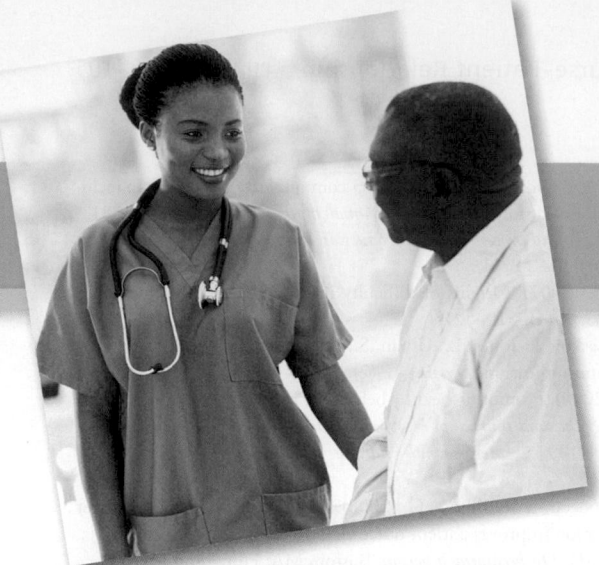

Values, Ethics, and Legal Issues

Doris M. Boutain

Case Scenario

As a home health nurse, you are working with a patient who is 59 years old, lives alone, and has two adult children living nearby. The children rotate transporting the patient to clinic appointments for chronic restrictive pulmonary disease treatments. In recent visits, the patient seemed weak and fatigued, struggled with shortness of breath, and had lost approximately 10 lb in the last month. These issues resulted in a hospitalization for 4 days. The children mentioned concerns about the worsening respiratory condition and the increasing clinic visits. You know that patients with this disease deteriorate over time and usually require ventilator support when they no longer have the strength to breathe independently.

Once you have completed this chapter and have incorporated the concepts about values, ethics, and legal issues into your knowledge base, review the above scenario and reflect on the following areas of Critical Thinking:

1. Develop a plan for gathering information about the patient's and the family's values, the comprehension of the patient and family, expectations of the patient's health, your professional values as a nurse, and your legal obligations to the patient.
2. Based on the information collected, identify value conflicts that may arise for you personally and professionally.
3. Describe appropriate strategies that will assist the patient and family in the context of their value system and your legal responsibilities as a nurse to plan for realistic health and healthcare possibilities.
4. Describe the value conflicts, ethical conflicts, and legal conflicts that you may encounter in your role as a nurse.

KEY TERMS

active euthanasia
advance directives
assault
assisted suicide
attitude
autonomy
battery
behaviors
beliefs
beneficence
brain death
capacity
civil law
community-based no code order
confidentiality
crime
criminal law
do not resuscitate (DNR) orders
durable power of attorney for healthcare
ethics
fidelity
justice
laws
liability
libel
living will
malpractice
morality
moral courage
negligence
no code order
nonmaleficence
personal values
privacy
professional ethics
proxy directive
res ipsa loquitur
respondeat superior
resuscitation
slander
standards of care
surrogate decision maker
terminal sedation
tort
values
value system
veracity
worldview

Upon completion of this chapter, you will be able to do the following:

1. Distinguish between personal values and professional values.
2. Explain how behaviors relate to values.
3. Apply cultural and developmental perspectives when identifying values.
4. Examine value conflicts and resolutions in nursing care situations.
5. Differentiate law and institutional policies from professional values.
6. Identify principles of healthcare ethics.
7. Describe a systematic approach for resolving ethical dilemmas.
8. Distinguish among licensure, a standard of care, a crime, and a tort.
9. Define four elements of negligence.
10. Describe legal protections for nurses and cite measures to take.

Nurses are at a pivotal point in history with the passage of the Health Care and Education Reconciliation Act of 2010 and the development of accountable care organizations in 2012 (DeCamp et al., 2014). These overarching changes are the most comprehensive healthcare delivery reforms in a generation. Nurses are poised for increased participation in the health and healthcare decisions within organizations. Nursing involvement will demand multidisciplinary systems thinking and care coordination as well as ethical leadership on the part of every nurse (Gallagher & Tschudin, 2010).

New nurses will encounter situations which will challenge their personal viewpoints of what is right and wrong in order to provide professional ethical care to patients. Nurses frequently encounter difficult situations involving discussions about how health is viewed and valued, how healthcare is organized, and how patients are treated. Those circumstances require nurses to exhibit moral courage in the workplace.

Moral courage is the ability to surmount fear and act to protect patient's rights (Whittington & Mack, 2010) and values. Moral courage helps nurses provide both ethical and legal patient care. Using ethical thinking to make decisions about care promotes ethical nursing practice. Legal nursing practice is based on standards of care and the applicable nurse practice act within a nurse's state or territory of licensure. Nurses achieve personal and professional success by identifying ethical and legal clinical practice problems and by using their knowledge and skills to achieve resolution. This chapter highlights the critical considerations needed for new nurses to begin to engage in discussions about values, ethics, and legal issues in nursing care.

VALUES

Values, implicit and explicit, are mental maps for decision making that endure for a significant time in one's life (Hofstede, 2001). Values are ideas used to determine what is right or wrong. That is, values guide what is important or what should be important in life. Consider the words *truth* and *honesty*.

These words are often thought of as values. Yet, everyone does not define those words the same or ascribe significance to them in a way that will guide their actions. The degree to which a word becomes a value depends upon the degree to which someone uses it for decision making and life choices.

Values are embedded within a value system. A **value system** is a learned set of principles and rules (Hofstede, 2001). When choosing between alternatives and making decisions, value systems help people decide which values are most important.

Suppose a nurse is confronted with the following situation:

A patient undergoes a series of diagnostic tests that reveal the early stages of a particular cancer. The doctor explains that this cancer typically progresses rapidly but has an excellent prognosis if treated aggressively with radiation and surgery. Later that day, the patient informs you of the intention to self-treat the cancer with herbal and other natural remedies for a few months before considering the doctor's recommendations.

A nurse who does not share the same value system as the patient may be unsure how to respond to the patient's decision. The nurse will need to understand his/her own values *and* the patient's values. Some values the nurse may have, for example in this case, can include medical intervention, responsibility, and immediate action. Conversely, the patient's value system may reflect a desire for natural remedies, responsibility, and reflective time. The situation might be further complicated if the nurse knows that the patient's family or other healthcare team members have different values.

Attitudes, beliefs, and behaviors are often linked with values but are not the same as values (Hofstede, 2001). An **attitude** is one's disposition toward an object or a situation. An attitude can be a mental or emotional mind-set, and it can be positive, negative, or neutral. **Beliefs** are ideas that one accepts as true; they may be expressed by such things as decisions, opinions, and creeds. **Behaviors** are actions that can be perceived or noticed (Hofstede, 2001). A nurse's behaviors demonstrate the values that hold priority. Behaviors are value indicators. As nurses take time to reflect on their behaviors, those behaviors can help illuminate their values and value systems.

LEARNING AND COMMUNICATING VALUES

Values are learned. They are communicated through behaviors that occur when interacting with others. Values are codified in social systems such as family, school, and religious interactions. These social systems enable people to develop culturally and over their life span.

How values are adopted, adapted, or dismissed is influenced by culture and society as well as a person's age and stage of development. Most people's values change or are refined by their various life experiences within social systems. Table 7-1 illustrates some generalized values during different life stages, combining Erikson's (1982) and Hall's theories of development (1982).

Socializing Influences

FAMILY INTERACTIONS

Children learn cultural values in several ways. Parent and family caregivers are the first teachers of cultural values (Hofstede, 2001). Caregivers reward and punish behavior, use language to influence thinking and perception, and model behavior. At the most basic level, infants begin value development with the establishment of trust and **autonomy**. Caregivers, as influenced by social values and prior family values, teach cultural values to children.

Caregivers are also influenced by the worldview they learned and are socialized within daily. **Worldview** is an unquestioned framework or predominant set of assumptions through which people view life; it is a perspective, an outlook. It is an idea originating from German philosophy. A worldview determines values which guide actions. For example, one culture's worldview may be more easily captured in a story or a phrase that explains how the people came to be and how they should live. The phrase "American dream" encompasses a whole range of values, such as individualism, equality, freedom, privacy, change, progress, achievement, and materialism. Behaviors that may result include living apart from family members (because of the values of individualism and privacy) and speaking for or against some topics openly (because of the values of freedom or change).

Children are taught cultural worldviews and value orientations early in life (Hofstede, 2001). Many published theories of value development generalize about how values are developed across the life span, so most of this chapter presents common principles of development more than differences. For toddlers, value development begins as they identify behaviors that elicit reward, punishment, or neutrality. Preschoolers learn that rules are imposed by parents and other adults. In this later stage of development, children recognize and accept fairness and cooperation, although their self-interest and self-will limit the capacity to do so. Children are concerned when the situation seems *unfair* to them yet do not have enough maturity to project that same sense of fairness to their peers.

TABLE 7-1 VALUES AND LIFE STAGES

Developmental Stage	Erikson's Values	Hall's Phases of Consciousness and Associated Values
Infant	Hope	**Phase I** Security
Toddler	Will	Survival Wonder
Preschool	Purpose	Awe
School age	Competence	**Phase II** Belonging Work
Adolescence	Loyalty	Self-competence Self-worth
Young adulthood	Love	**Phase III** Independence Service/vocation
Middle adulthood	Care	Creation Being self
Older adulthood	Wisdom	**Phase IV** Harmony Interdependence Intimacy Esthetics

Source: Erikson, E. (1982). *The life cycle completed*. New York, NY: W. W. Norton & Co. Extended Version edition (June 17, 1998);
Hall, B. (1982). *The personal discernment inventory*. New York, NY: Paulist Press.

SCHOOL INTERACTIONS

Interactions in school also teach cultural values through peer and supervisory adult behaviors, and day-to-day procedural norms. Schools range from day care facilities to higher education institutions like universities. School provides a central opportunity for peer value sharing and interaction.

The attitudes, beliefs, and behaviors that develop within peer group relationships are powerful (Fig. 7-1). Peer groups define themselves by common interests, needs, and problems. Out of these similar interests and bonds, the group clarifies its values.

Supervisory adults like teachers and tutors help children learn values about learning and social rules. School-age children are industrious, recognizing the need for social rules. Younger children in this age group maintain a strict understanding and application of the rules, seeing things in clearly dichotomous ways (i.e., right or wrong). As children grow into preadolescence, they become more flexible. The threat of discipline becomes less important than social expectations.

For adolescents, the influence of peer identification reaches its greatest persuasiveness and often occurs through school-based interactions. Although this period of development is often characterized by rebellion, adolescents have a high level of moral judgment with a law-and-order orientation. Adolescents understand that **morality** derives from principles of conscience and that rules are cooperative agreements that can be modified. As youth reach late adolescence, they begin to move away from strong peer influence according to their individual principles, and peer group values decrease in importance.

During adolescence and young adulthood, people are likely to encounter various values and become more aware of differences. The process of value refinement may be a result of a planned, self-conscious discovery process, or it may be a matter of living and dealing with life situations as they arise. Adolescents and young adulthood begin to test their reasoning and ascribe values to their decisions.

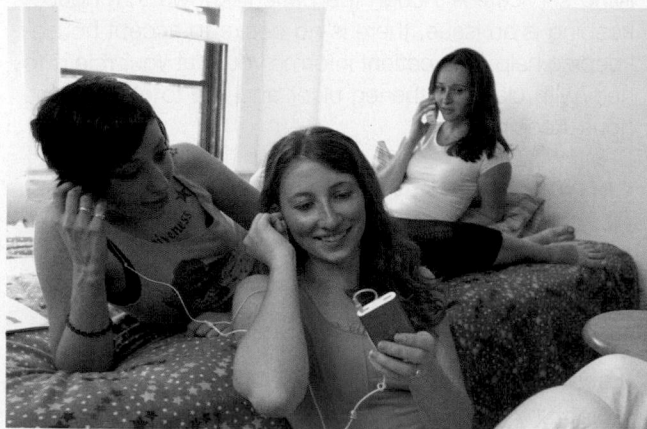

FIGURE 7-1 Peer relationships can have a significant influence on an individual's values.

RELIGIOUS INTERACTIONS

Religious institutions form communities of belonging anchored in faith traditions that shape a person's sense of values. Religious institutions often codify and ritualize values into their various activities. Institutions teach faith principles deemed important for decision making in daily living. Religion-based and faith-based value systems are often embedded in a patient's decision making about health. Value conflicts are most notably seen when someone is diagnosed with an illness, is considering treatment options, or is in need of end-of-life care.

WORKPLACE AND SERVICE INTERACTIONS

In workplace and service interactions, adults learn and exhibit values. Institutional values in the workplace are noted in how workplaces are operated, managed, and evaluated. Adults may or may not ascribe to workplace values. Primary value challenges relate to workplace expectations, workplace processes, and workplace interactions. Adults prioritize values to interact effectively in various settings, and balance work, personal and service obligations. Values that adults learned and developed in childhood usually evolve into what they will accept as guiding principles for life.

As people get older, although they may retire from formal work, informal service to others arises through volunteering opportunities. Many older adults use the values and knowledge they have accumulated over a lifetime by sharing with others in service activities. Older adults are able to recognize their own values and can clearly note the differing values of others.

VALUES CLARIFICATION METHODS

Values clarification methods are approaches used to help providers or patients understand what is important when given an option or attributes of options in a decision-making situation in order to identify preferences (Pignone et al., 2012). There are multiple values clarification methods. Some of the common methods include a pros and cons list approach, a rating and ranking task approach, a rating sheet approach using a scale (e.g., 0 = not important at all to 5 = very important), and a values check-off approach (Pignone et al., 2012). These methods do not evaluate values as such but help people identify their own values when provided with a specific decision. People can use values clarification in several ways:

- To examine past situations and decisions
- To reflect on current options and future decisions
- To explore how they spend their time by listing activities in a typical 24-hour period

Whatever the vehicle for examination of values, certain assumptions underlie the process. First, those participating must feel comfortable openly identifying and sharing values. The person must have the freedom to not need to agree or disagree with others. Time is also important to allow for reflection on the questions as values are so deeply engrained that they can take time to identify.

VALUES INQUIRY

Values inquiry is a method of examining social issues and the values that motivate human choices. Case study incidents provide ways to facilitate the value inquiry process. Using a viewpoint lens to understand values can help nurses see how values differ depending on one's viewpoint. As an example, a nurse has a conflict and wishes to understand the values underlying the conflict. Consider asking the following questions:

- What are the facts from the viewpoint of the patient? What are the facts from the viewpoint of the nurse? What are the facts from the viewpoint of the family?
- What values are represented in each of the viewpoints of the facts?
- What is the cultural worldview and orientation system that helps to define the facts?
- What are the possible solutions from the point of view of the patient, family, and nurse?
- What are the advantages and disadvantages of each possible solution?

Unlike values clarification, which can be an individual or a group experience, values inquiry lends itself more exclusively to group discussion (Fig. 7-2). The process increases understanding of values based on the value perspective of another, and it can enable clarity of personal values. As people talk in safe environment, personal values and patient values can be identified.

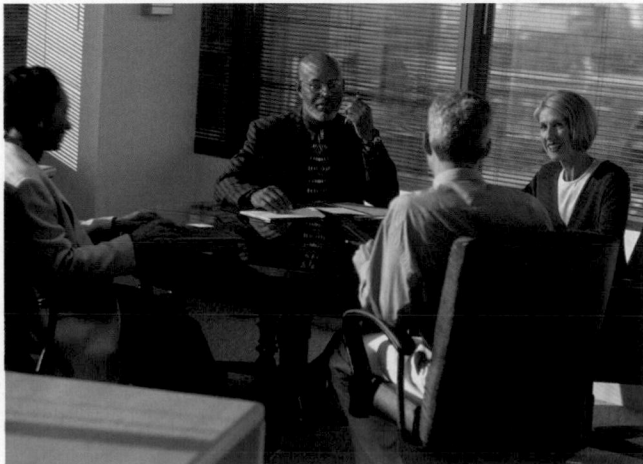

FIGURE 7-2 Values inquiry uses group discussion to examine social issues and values that motivate human choice.

VALUE CONFLICTS

Whenever there is human interaction, value conflicts are likely to occur. These conflicts can be resolved if nurses are aware of their own values and the values of others. Resolving such conflicts may entail using values clarification and values inquiry activities.

Family Conflicts

Value conflicts between family members arise from differences in developmental stages, experiences, and personal value preferences. One fairly common example is when one partner in a relationship does not wish to have a health checkup. One person may say that the person is *refusing care*, while another may say the person is *advocating for self-care*. Both phrases are embedded with value judgments. Depending on how a person experienced the healthcare system in early life, the person not wishing care may hold the values of self-control, independence, and fate in higher regard than the value of regular healthcare visits. These values may reflect an underlying struggle with the values of the other partner, such as security, safety, and protection. The nurse's role might be to help the partners explore their personal health history and

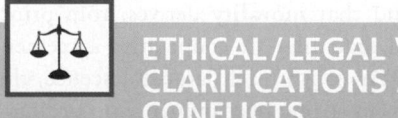

ETHICAL/LEGAL VALUE CLARIFICATIONS AND CONFLICTS

CARE, HOUSING, AND HEALTH
You are working as a home care nurse. You are assigned to a 74-year-old patient who has no living relatives and lives alone in an older home in a historical neighborhood. The house is cold as you enter. A strong odor is in the air from spoiled food in the sink, and there is dust on most surfaces. The toilet has not been flushed recently. The patient's clothes are soiled. You offer to contact agencies to help with the housekeeping tasks and with assisted living services. Although the patient knows that housekeeping is an issue, there is no desire to accept housekeeping help. The patient informs you that your role is to help with cleaning the leg ulcer and not to observe the housekeeping.

CRITICAL THINKING CHALLENGE
- List the feelings you have after reading this situation.
- Next to each feeling, write the value upon which that feeling is based.
- Write the values you believe the patient holds.
- Which values are similar and which values are different between you and the patient?
- Recognizing the patient's right to make choices, define what you see as your ethically appropriate behavior.

needs rather than continuing the argument about the health checkup. Ideally, the nurse could assist each partner in setting some attainable personal health goals and help each share how value conflicts are influencing their conversations about the health check-up topic.

Healthcare Conflicts

Areas of conflict between patients and healthcare providers can center on knowledge differences, developmental differences, or cultural value system differences. For example, there may be a case of a family in which a grandparent died. Parents may prefer that young children not enter the hospice room, believing that children do not understand death and that it might be difficult for them. Realizing that death is a traumatic event for the survivors and that the parents' protection of the children is really a protection of their own feelings, the nurse might explore ways in which to assess (and meet, if needed) the children's grief and loss needs (see Chapter 40). Depending on the children's ages, possibilities other than attending the funeral might include telling stories and drawing pictures about the grandparent (Dunlop, 2008). These strategies can be used with appropriate agreement from the parents.

Resolving Value Conflicts in the Healthcare System

Three main issues arise regarding resolution of value conflicts: (1) the perception of conflict, (2) the meaning of resolution, and (3) the values underlying the resolution process. Nurses encountering value conflicts usually examine their own values regarding conflict (see the "Clarifying Values" section). It is critical for nurses to explore how patients perceive the conflict, how patients define resolution, and what values underlie the process of resolution. Nurses are there to support the patient's value system in the context of providing safe, ethical care.

A nurse who views conflict as negative might feel threatened because his or her own values of self-competence, duty, success, authority, and esteem may be questioned. However, a nurse who views conflict as positive might find the values of respect, communication, care, equilibrium, harmony, service, and creativity enhanced. These two views of conflict are based on the nurse's life experiences and values. Therefore, one of the first goals for the nurse is to assist the patient in exploring and defining the relevant issues and values from the patient's point of view. This clarification or explanation may be the resolution, or it may be the first step in a resolution process.

Another step is to investigate healthcare system policies as a guide for practice. *Institutional policies* are guidelines developed by organizations or agencies to direct professional practice. Hospitals, long-term care facilities, and other organizations that employ nurses may have policies concerning some ethical issues such as use of substances, providing abortion services, and do not resuscitate (DNR) orders. Institutional policies are often developed by consulting legal guidelines and professional standards but also may reflect an institution's religious affiliation. For example, some long-term care facilities do not permit artificially provided nutrition and hydration to be withdrawn because of religious teachings, even though stopping such medical therapy is legally permissible in appropriate situations. Nurses need to be aware of institutional policies, but these policies are not the same as professional values. See more information in the next section.

ETHICS

It is important to distinguish among several key terms related to ethics. **Ethics** is a branch of philosophy with emphasis on morality. *Morality* focuses on intentions and actions that are viewed as good or right compared to those which are viewed as bad or wrong (Hunt & Carnevale, 2011). *Morality* is the set of beliefs about the standards of right and wrong that help a person determine the correct or permissible action in a given situation. Contemporary approaches to morality focus on what is most important to people as individual patients, as family members, or as community members. There is an emphasis on understanding cultural meanings, social experiences, and inner emotions (Hunt & Carnevale, 2011).

Personal values are beliefs a person considers highly important and are learned through interactions with social systems as described previously. Life choices and healthcare decisions vary according to what people value as morally right or wrong and important. **Professional ethics** are values held by a disciplinary group (like nursing association, dental associations, or medical associations) deemed as having generalizable standards of conduct to be upheld in all situations. In professional ethical practice, nurses avoid allowing personal values to distort their treatment for patients. For example, a particular nurse may value candor in family relationships but, as a nurse, should abide by the professional ethics obligation to maintain patient **confidentiality**.

Although no set of absolute guidelines provides answers for all problems (Fairchild, 2010), professional values are articulated into professional guidelines. *Professional values* are set forth by national and international nursing organizations. In the United States, the American Nurses Association (ANA, 2015) *Code of Ethics for Nurses* is a professional guideline delineating the conduct and responsibilities expected of all nurses in nursing practice (Box 7-1). Nurses are responsible for knowing and complying with the standards of ethical practice and ensuring that other nurses also comply. Interpretive statements have been developed that explain how each item in the code is manifested in nursing practice. The complete document can be obtained from the ANA. The International Council of Nurses (ICN) also has

BOX 7-1   The Code of Ethics for Nurses

The ANA developed The Code of Ethics for Nurses. It is a guide for nurses to ensure quality and ethical care. It consists of nine ethical obligations with interpretive statements.

1. The nurse practices with compassion and respect for the inherent dignity, worth, and unique attributes of every person.
2. The nurse's primary commitment is to the patient, whether an individual, family, group, community, or population.
3. The nurse promotes, advocates for, and protects the rights, health, and safety of the patient.
4. The nurse has authority, accountability, and responsibility for nursing practice; makes decisions; and takes action consistent with the obligation to promote health and to provide optimal care.
5. The nurse owes the same duties to self as to others, including the responsibility to promote health and safety, preserve wholeness of character and integrity, maintain competence, and continue personal and professional growth.
6. The nurse, through individual and collective effort, establishes, maintains, and improves the ethical environment of the work setting and conditions of employment that are conducive to the safe, quality healthcare.
7. The nurse, in all roles and settings, advances the profession through research and scholarly inquiry, professional standards development, and the generation of both nursing and health policy.
8. The nurse collaborates with other health professionals and the public to protect human rights, promote health diplomacy, and reduce health disparities.
9. The profession of nursing, collectively through its professional organizations, must articulate nursing values, maintain the integrity of the profession, and integrate principles of social justice into nursing and health policy.

Reprinted with permission from American Nurses Association. (2015). *Code of Ethics with Interpretative Statements.* Retrieved April 27, 2015, from http://www.nursingworld.org/MainMenuCategories/EthicsStandards/CodeofEthicsforNurses/Code-of-Ethics-For-Nurses.html

published a code of ethics that reflects tenets of nursing practice (Box 7-2). These standards represent ethical principles for nurses deemed professionally important across multiple countries.

Principles of Healthcare Ethics

Principlist approaches are common in healthcare ethics. This is an ethical framework that assesses situations as right and wrong by outlining and defining major tenets of ethical care.

The major principles of healthcare ethics important to uphold in all situations includes, respect for persons, beneficence, non-maleficence, and justice. These principles serve as the basis for rules that govern the relationships between healthcare providers and patients.

DEFINITIONS OF PRINCIPLES

Respect For Persons

Respect for persons means that individuals are treated as autonomous agents and that persons who have limited autonomy are protected (Beauchamp & Childress, 2012). Autonomy means creating the conditions in which patients can make their own decisions (Erlen, 2010). In the U.S. healthcare system, patients are entitled to make decisions about what will happen to them and their bodies. Informed consent protects the patient's right for healthcare decision making. A sample of an informed consent form is shown in Chapter 8.

Since informed consent is based on patient preferences, providers must uphold patient autonomy by respecting cultural diversity (Council on Community Pediatrics and Committee on Native American Child Health, 2010; Hoye & Severinsson, 2010). Some cultures, for example, prefer to withhold information about severe or terminal illness from patients. In these situations, the healthcare team should strive to have an open discussion with the patient about whom he or she wishes to involve in treatment decisions, including who should receive bad news (i.e., the patient alone, the patient and specified family members, or specified family members). Ideally, this discussion occurs at the initiation of the professional relationship and is revisited at critical junctures. Some cultures, such as the Navajo, view talking about possible risks in an informed consent discussion as ill intended and even malicious because of their belief that speaking ill causes ill. In these situations, discussing risks and side effects using a hypothetical third person may be appropriate (Carrese & Rhodes, 2000). Consulting with cultural or spiritual experts early can help healthcare providers act sensitively and respectfully.

Adults with the **capacity** (mental or physical ability) to make healthcare decisions have the right to consent to or refuse treatment. Even if healthcare providers do not agree with a patient's decision, they must respect the patient's wishes (Beauchamp & Childress, 2012). Infants, young children, people who are severely mentally handicapped or incapacitated, and people in a persistent vegetative state or coma are judged not to have the capacity to participate in healthcare decision making (Philipsen, Murray, Wood, Bell-Hawkins, & Setlow, 2013). For such groups, a **surrogate decision maker** must be identified to act on their behalf.

Patients communicate their wishes to healthcare providers by verbally participating in healthcare decision making and by employing written documents called **advance directives**

BOX 7-2 The ICN Code of Ethics for Nurses

The ICN adopted an international code of ethics for nurses in 1953. The organization has revised and reaffirmed this material at various times, with the recent revision completed in 2012. See http://www.icn.ch/images/stories/documents/about/icncode_english.pdf

Preamble

Nurses have four fundamental responsibilities: to promote health, to prevent illness, to restore health, and to alleviate suffering. The need for nursing is universal.

Inherent in nursing is respect for human rights, including cultural rights, the right to life and choice, to dignity and to be treated with respect. Nursing care is respectful of and unrestricted by considerations of age, color, creed, culture, disability or illness, gender, sexual orientation, nationality, politics, race, or social status.

Nurses render health services to the individual, the family, and the community and coordinate their services with those of related groups.

The *ICN Code of Ethics for Nurses* has four principal elements that outline the standards of ethical conduct.

Elements of the Code

1. Nurses and people

The nurse's primary professional responsibility is to people requiring nursing care. In providing care, the nurse promotes an environment in which the human rights, values, customs, and spiritual beliefs of the individual, family, and community are respected.

The nurse ensures that the individual receives accurate, sufficient, and timely information in a culturally appropriate manner on which to base consent for care and related treatment.

The nurse holds in confidence personal information and uses judgment in sharing this information. The nurse shares with society the responsibility for initiating and supporting action to meet the health and social needs of the public, in particular those of vulnerable populations.

The nurse advocates for equity and social justice in resource allocation, access to healthcare, and other social and economic services. The nurse demonstrates professional values such as respectfulness, responsiveness, compassion, trustworthiness, and integrity.

2. Nurses and practice

The nurse carries personal responsibility and accountability for nursing practice and for maintaining competence by continual learning. The nurse maintains a standard of personal health such that the ability to provide care is not compromised. The nurse uses judgment regarding individual competence when accepting and delegating responsibility. The nurse at all times maintains standards of personal conduct that reflect well on the profession and enhance its image and public confidence.

The nurse, in providing care, ensures that use of technology and scientific advances are compatible with the safety, dignity, and rights of people. The nurse strives to foster and maintain a practice culture promoting ethical behavior and open dialogue.

3. Nurses and the profession

The nurse assumes the major role in determining and implementing acceptable standards of clinical nursing practice, management, research, and education. The nurse is active in developing a core of research-based professional knowledge that supports evidence-based practice.

The nurse is active in developing and sustaining a core of professional values.

The nurse, acting through the professional organization, participates in creating a positive practice environment and maintaining safe, equitable social and economic working conditions in nursing. The nurse practices to sustain and protect the natural environment and is aware of its consequences on health. The nurse contributes to an ethical organizational environment and challenges unethical practices and settings.

4. Nurses and coworkers

The nurse sustains a collaborative and respectful relationship with coworkers in nursing and other fields. The nurse takes appropriate action to safeguard individuals, families, and communities when their health is endangered by a coworker or any other person. The nurse takes appropriate action to support and guide coworkers to advance ethical conduct.

Reprinted with permission from International Council of Nurses. (2012). International Council of Nurses Code of Ethics for Nurses. Geneva, Switzerland. Retrieved October 25, 2014, from http://www.icn.ch/images/stories/documents/about/icncode_english.pdf

(Fig. 7-3). These directives specify what interventions patients would or would not want if they became terminally ill or sustained an injury or illness that impeded their ability to make or communicate decisions and whom they would wish to act as their surrogate decision maker. A **living will** is an advance directive that specifies the types of medical treatment patients do and do not want to receive should they become unable to speak for themselves in a terminal or permanently unconscious condition. Living wills often include instructions about resuscitation, drugs, blood transfusions, tube feedings, and mechanical ventilation. A second type of advance directive is a **proxy directive**, sometimes referred to as a **durable power of attorney for healthcare**. This advance directive allows patients to designate another person to make decisions if they become incapacitated and cannot make decisions independently. The surrogate decision maker would then act on a patient's behalf.

DECLARATION

I, _Mildred Jones_, being of sound mind, willfully and voluntarily make this declaration to be followed if I become incompetent. This declaration reflects my firm and settled commitment to refuse life-sustaining treatment under the circumstances indicated below.

I direct my attending physician to withhold or withdraw life-sustaining treatment that serves only to prolong the process of my dying, if I should be in a terminal condition or in a state of permanent unconsciousness.

I direct that treatment be limited to measures to keep me comfortable and to relieve pain, including any pain that might occur by withholding or withdrawing life-sustaining treatment.

In addition, if I am in the condition described above, I feel especially strongly about the following forms of treatment. **I realize that if I do not specifically indicate my preference regarding any of the forms of treatment listed above, I may receive that form of treatment.**

- Cardiac resuscitation: I do want (x)   I do not want ( )
- Mechanical respiration: I do want ( )   I do not want (x)
- Tube feeding or any other artificial or invasive form of nutrition (food)   I do want ( )   I do not want (x)
- Any artificial or invasive form of hydration (water):   I do want ( )   I do not want (x)
- Blood or blood products: I do want ( )   I do not want (x)
- Any invasive diagnostic tests: I do want ( )   I do not want (x)
- Any form of surgery: I do want ( )   I do not want (x)
- Kidney dialysis: I do want ( )   I do not want (x)
- Antibiotics: I do want (x)   I do not want ( )

Other instructions:

I (x) do ( ) do not want to designate another person as my surrogate to make medical treatment decisions for me if I should be incompetent and in a terminal condition or in a state of permanent unconsciousness.

Name and address of surrogate (if applicable):

Jonathan Jones

423 Main Street

Crossroads SC

Name and address of substitute surrogate (if surrogate designated above is unable to serve):

Trudy Conover

619 Wyoming Drive

Crossroads SC

I made this declaration on the _21_ day of _10/95_ (month, year).

Declarant's signature: _Mildred Jones_   Declarant's address: _423 Main Street, Crossroads SC_

The declarant, or the person on behalf of and at the direction of the declarant, knowingly and voluntarily signed this writing by signature or mark in my presence.

1. Witness's signature: _Mary Martin_   Witness's address: _818 Hill Drive, Bayside GA_

2. Witness's signature: _Rosa Díaz_   Witness's address: _1043 River Road, Summit SC_

FIGURE 7-3 Sample of an advance directive.

Beneficence and Nonmaleficence

Beneficence means doing or promoting good to help others (Beauchamp & Childress, 2012). Nurses, physicians, and all other healthcare practitioners work to accomplish good for patients by promoting their best interests and striving to achieve optimal outcomes. Nurses take beneficent actions when they act on behalf of patients to do good as defined by patients. For example, administering pain medication, performing dressing changes to promote wound healing, and providing emotional support to patients who are anxious or depressed as desired by patients are acts of goodness.

The principle of **nonmaleficence** means to avoid doing harm, to remove from harm, and to prevent harm. It is a strong proactive duty for all healthcare professionals. Upholding the principle of nonmaleficence is evidenced by actions, such as providing medication to prevent patients from additional suffering, protecting patients from a chemically impaired practitioner, or reporting suspected child abuse to prevent additional victimization.

Doing good and avoiding harm seem fairly simple but in many cases are complex. For example, bone marrow transplantation often saves lives; however, patients undergoing the procedure may experience a great deal of pain and suffering to achieve the desired benefit. Confronting a colleague's substance abuse may lead that person to obtain therapeutic help but also may result in that person being suspended temporarily from employment.

Nurses are often the first to learn about changes a patient is contemplating. The nurse must then document the patient's wishes and notify the patient's physician and other involved professionals so the plan of care is altered to reflect these changes.

Justice

Justice is a concept involving making decisions about resource allocations for societies or groups. On an individual patient level, nurses are called to ensure that they are providing equitable time, service, and care to each person with dignity and respect. Nurses mostly assess intentional and unintentional biases that may reduce the time and care to patients under their care. Consider this example:

A nurse provides the necessary medications to a patient who is married to a person of the same sex. The nurse often walks quickly into the room, avoids eye contact with the patient and the patient's partner, provides the medications, and exits promptly. Upon discharge, the patient asks no questions about future care at home because of the perceived discomfort of the nurse.

In this example, the patient and family are not receiving the benefits of full nursing care. However, the mandatory care of medication provision is provided. The conditions of care provision (rushed, no eye contact, etc.) is promoting unjust service delivery.

Nurses commonly face issues of justice in clinical practice. Nurses are called to be advocates for just healthcare systems and policies (Kagan, Smith, & Chinn, 2014) to ensure they can provide direct patient care effectively. For example, in the United States, there are wide and significant disparities between adults with above-average incomes and those with below-average incomes relative to healthcare service provision. These differences persist even after controlling for insurance coverage and population demographic characteristics (Schoen & Doty, 2004). Nurses are called to be active in understanding how institutional policies or procedures may impact their quality, duration, or appropriateness of care. Nurses must also engage in understanding health policy and legislation that affects healthcare access to groups with less social power, resources, or funds. When nurses encounter patients like this in practice, it is also important for nurses to identify government and community resources for assistance. Nurses also work at the policy level to advocate for equitable benefits for vulnerable patients. Most people agree that a just healthcare system provides care on the basis of medical need and the degree of need rather than by ability to pay, social status, racial identity, or gender (Beauchamp & Childress, 2012).

Rights and Ethical Rules of Professional–Patient Relationships

The American Hospital Association (AHA) created a brochure with six basic rights for patients and families during hospitalization (Box 7-3). In addition to these rights, there are ethical values and legal rules that guide the behavior of healthcare

---

BOX 7-3	**The Patient Care Partnership (formerly "A Patient's Bill of Rights")**

The AHA has a brochure that informs patients of their rights and responsibilities. This brochure is available in eight languages from the AHA website. The new brochure covers six areas described as the basics that patients and their families can expect in their treatment during their hospital stay.

What to Expect During Your Hospital Stay
1. High-quality hospital care.
2. A clean and safe environment.
3. Involvement in your care.
   - Discussing your medical condition and information about medically appropriate treatment choices.
   - Discussing your treatment plan.
   - Getting information from you.
   - Understanding your healthcare goals and values.
   - Understanding who should make decisions when you cannot.
4. Protection of your privacy.
5. Help when leaving the hospital.
6. Help with your billing claims.

Reprinted with permission from American Hospital Association. *The patient care partnership: Understanding expectations, rights and responsibilities.* Retrieved October 25, 2014, from http://www.aha.org/advocacy-issues/communicatingpts/pt-care-partnership.shtml

professionals toward patients and their families. These include veracity, fidelity, privacy, and confidentiality (Beauchamp & Childress, 2012). Although some circumstances create exceptions to the rules, for the most part nurses are required to adhere to these obligations.

VERACITY

Veracity means telling the truth. Healthcare professionals are obliged to be honest with patients. The right to self-determination becomes meaningless if the patient does not receive accurate, unbiased, and understandable information (Beauchamp & Childress, 2012).

In general, truth telling has become an accepted healthcare practice in North America, particularly as related to the disclosure of a patient's diagnosis, prognosis, and treatment options. Nevertheless, several issues regarding honesty continue to present challenges. First, preferences for honesty vary significantly according to culture, particularly those related to sensitive issues such as disclosing a cancer diagnosis (Finset, Heyn, & Ruland, 2013). Second, specific areas present unique challenges to honesty, such as disclosing a diagnosis of dementia (Mitchell, McCollum, & Monaghan, 2013) or errors to patients (Jeffs et al., 2011). Finally, to communicate honestly, yet compassionately, requires specific communication skills and techniques that all providers must develop (Reinke, Shannon, Engleberg, Young, & Curtis, 2010).

Patients and families frequently disclose questions and concerns to nurses. Nurses can assist them to obtain information and understand how it applies to their situation by arranging discussions among the patient, family, and physician, and by providing emotional support for these difficult conversations (Mitchell, McCollum, & Monaghan, 2013).

FIDELITY

Fidelity means being faithful to one's commitments or promises. Nurses' commitments to patients include providing safe care and maintaining competence in nursing practice. Fidelity can also be thought of as the social contract that exists between a patient and any nurse who cares for that patient—that is, what does the patient have a right to expect from any nurse, regardless of the individual nurse's age, ethnic or religious background, or personal values?

In some instances, nurses make promises to patients in an overt way. For example, in psychiatric day treatment programs, detailed patient care contracts are made between patients and the team. If a nurse agrees to be the resource to a patient during crisis, the nurse must fulfill this commitment. If the nurse cannot be available, the ethical action is to discuss this with the patient and to arrange a substitute when needed. Making promises to patients requires good judgment. Being responsive to a patient's request is important, but the nurse must evaluate whether or not he or she can uphold agreements. Consider this example:

A nurse admitted a patient with a history of alcohol abuse. The patient asked for assurance that leather restraints would not be used under any circumstances. In an attempt to calm the patient, the nurse agreed to this request. After surgery, the patient grew agitated, delirious, and combative. Although restraints were indicated to preserve the patient's safety, the nurse opposed the use of restraints because of the promise.

This promise was not safe. Ethical practice in this case would have incorporated the patient's concerns and an explanation of circumstances in which restraints would be applied. Especially in cases of agitation, nurses must take special care not to compromise care.

PRIVACY

Privacy involves appropriately using patient information. A loss of privacy occurs if others inappropriately use their access to a person. Nurses have access to information recorded in the medical record, information shared or observed through care or interactions with friends and family, and through access to the patient's physical body. Nurses protect the patient's privacy by ensuring that the patient's body is appropriately covered. Nurses cannot discuss medically irrelevant physical features (such as tattoos, piercings, or cosmetic surgery results). Nurses cannot post pictures or comments about patients on social media outlets, even if initials are used and faces cannot be seen. Nurses should also avoid discussing intimate details about patients unless necessary for the provision of good care. Consider this example:

A patient had surgery at the same hospital where patient worked. A coworker noticed the patient in the room and asked the nurse for information about the patient to send a get well card. The nurse accessed the patient's record and talked to the coworker about the patient.

The nurse coworker violated the patient's privacy. Although nurses have access to health information, this access is limited to patient care–related reasons. Nurses need to establish a culture of privacy and not access medical information unless necessary for patient care.

CONFIDENTIALITY

The principle of confidentiality requires that information about a patient be kept private. Confidentiality is a professional duty and a legal obligation. What is documented in the patient's record is accessible only to those providing care to that patient. No one else is entitled to that information unless the patient has signed a consent for release of information that identifies what information can be shared, with whom, and for what purpose. Discussing patients outside the clinical setting, telling friends or family about patients, or even discussing patients in the elevator with other workers violates patient confidentiality and must be avoided (Ulrich et al., 2010). For example:

A patient was hospitalized for nearly 1 month. The patient's recovery was complicated by compromised pulmonary function caused by a 50-year history of smoking cigarettes. Once transferred from the intensive care unit (ICU), the patient requested an escort to the smoking area. The patient directed the nursing staff to not inform family members about the smoking.

In this situation, the nurse is obligated to protect the patient's confidentiality and not to give the family information about the patient's smoking. One approach the nurse can take is to talk with the patient about reasons for smoking, smoking cessation resources, and strategies for discussing the issue with family members. If asked directly by the family, the nurse should explain that patient confidentiality requires the nurse to not reveal patient information unless permitted by the patient. In situations in which the nurse is tempted to break confidentiality, he or she should consult with a supervisor, ethics consultant, and possibly legal counsel to confirm that the breach in confidentiality is legally and ethically justified. Information can only be shared if the benefit outweighs the risk of harm resulting from a breach of confidentiality (McMullen, Howie, Howie, & Philipsen, 2013).

Resolving Ethical Dilemmas

Ethical dilemmas in healthcare involve issues surrounding professional actions and patient care decisions. They can lead to discomfort and conflict among the members of the healthcare team; between providers and the patient and family; or among the provider, nurses, and healthcare organization. Dilemmas can take many forms.

A dilemma is a situation in which:

- Two or more choices are available.
- It is difficult to determine which choice is best.
- Available alternatives cannot solve the needs of all those involved.
- Each alternative in a dilemma may have both favorable and unfavorable features.

 APPLY YOUR CRITICAL THINKING

Your patient, Mr. Washington, 67, is receiving home care for his disability caused by chronic obstructive pulmonary disease. He is on disability and on low-flow oxygen at night and during the day when needed. On a home care visit to Mr. Washington, you observe that he has been smoking. When you ask about his smoking, he tells you that he smokes only when the oxygen is off. He asks you to promise not to tell his physician or his daughter.

You know that smoking is contraindicated for his diagnosis. He is asking you to withhold important clinical information from his care provider. How will you respond? What factors do you need to consider? Is there a breach of confidentiality by sharing your concerns? What are the ethical principles involved? Is your obligation solely to Mr. Washington?

Check your answer in Appendix B.

STRATEGIES

The strategies that follow may be used to prevent and resolve ethical dilemmas (Wocial, Bledsoe, Helft, & Everett, 2010):

Validate Feelings

Validation is a way of acknowledging and identifying feelings as credible. When a person is validated, he or she feels accepted. Acceptance promotes communication necessary for well-coordinated healthcare. Because conflict may erupt in situations involving ethical dilemmas, conflict resolution strategies such as clarifying misunderstanding, validating, consensus building, and collaborating also contribute to resolution of the ethical dilemmas.

Conduct a Case Analysis

Case analysis is one method for values inquiry. Using the model also prompts consideration of values that are underlying the difficult decision. A case analysis can be done by those directly involved in the case.

For example, the people involved in a case fulfill different roles. The physician contributes facts about the patient's medical condition and prognosis. Nurses describe the patient's responses to illness and treatment, and share information about health resources. A physical therapist describes how physical capabilities will affect quality of life. Social workers provide information about neighborhood or social service resources. Family and friends provide information about the patient's prior healthcare preferences and values. Assistance also may be requested from a member of the organizational ethics committee or ethics consultation service. Compiling case information helps clarify problems and weigh solutions.

Identify Outcomes

Planning care according to outcomes provides focus and consistency to a treatment plan. Many times, ethical conflicts arise because the parties involved hold different values underlying the goals for treatment or those concerning treatment options. Once information in all the categories has been considered, realistic outcomes can be formulated.

Identify Short- and Long-Term Goals

Outcomes for the care and treatment for a terminally ill patient may include goals such as planning for pain relief, setting up hospice care, identifying a surrogate decision maker, and determining whether or not the patient will be resuscitated if cardiac arrest occurs. Clarifying what will be done with each of these concerns promotes the patient's sense of well-being.

Clarify Accountabilities

Different people may be accountable for carrying out actions identified as part of the plan. For instance, if the team has received information that an incompetent patient had completed a living will, a nurse or social worker can take responsibility for contacting the family and requesting that they bring in a copy of this document for review and consideration of the patient's wishes. If questions remain about whether or not a medical condition would respond to treatment, the physicians may need to pursue additional tests or request consultation. If patient preference is unclear, a psychosocial clinical nurse specialist may be designated to work with the patient to assess what he or she wants or hopes from treatment. In cases when a decision is made to withhold medically futile care, the physician is accountable to communicate this to the family.

Follow Through

Once a plan has been established, participants are ethically bound to uphold their accountabilities and professional responsibilities by following through or using professional fidelity. Failing to do so breaks the implicit contract between nurse and patient, possibly jeopardizing the patient's health, safety, or well-being. It also undermines the integrity of the nursing profession and healthcare system as well as violates trust the public has in nurses.

Resolve Reactions and Evaluate Impact

Healthcare decisions are complex and can have dramatic consequences. The existence of an ethical dilemma can make a situation more vexing, which adds to the emotional reactions of those involved. Working through the reactions to a particularly significant event is an important step for learning from the experience and preventing residual feelings from hampering one's ability to work through similar situations in the future. Discussing feelings and reactions among the team, with peers, or a supervisor is an important step to promote resolution. This type of discussion can lead to planning care for future patients in a way that avoids repeating the same problems.

ETHICS COMMITTEES

Organizational ethics committees, required by the Joint Commission, are important vehicles for working through ethical issues in practice. The AHA encourages the development of these committees as interdisciplinary vehicles for identifying and addressing ethical issues. These committees have three primary functions: policy development, education, and consultation (Elliott & Hunter, 2008). As part of the education and consultative functions, regular case reviews can promote ethical practice by assisting staff to recognize the ethical implications in practice and to develop strategies for resolution (Elliott & Hunter, 2008).

LAWS AND NURSING

Nurses today should be more aware than ever of the laws for nursing practice. **Laws** are rules or standards of human conduct established by legislative bodies and interpreted by courts to protect the rights of citizens. Professional liability cases are brought against all healthcare providers, including nurses, and the case outcomes affect the way that healthcare is delivered. In addition, issues such as consent to and refusal of treatment, which used to be handled privately among the patient, nurse, physician, and family, are, today, often the subject of legislation and court actions. Nurses must be aware of the legal guidelines that govern their particular area of practice, and also recognize that myths abound (Ganzini, Volicer, Nelson, Fox, & Derse, 2004).

Sources of Law

The legal system in most of the United States has its foundation in the English common law system. The primary sources of law are constitutions, legislative statutes, and common law (Fig. 7-4).

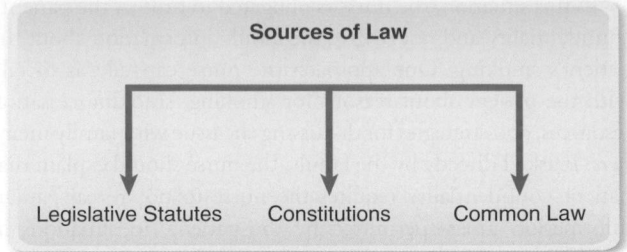

FIGURE 7-4 Sources of law.

Constitutions are the foundation of the system of justice. In the U.S. Constitution is a supreme constitutional law that establishes the organization of the federal government and grants power. Legislative statutes are laws derived from a legislative body. Nurse practice acts and adult or child abuse laws are examples of legislative statutes. Common law evolves from decisions of courts. These decisions are ones that cannot be supported by statutory or constitutional law alone.

As a society changes its values, laws generally evolve to correspond with current thinking and societal values. At any time, societal and patient values may not conform to law. As a result, the law alone may not provide specific answers to difficult healthcare dilemmas. Nurses have a responsibility to understand the current legal and ethical guidelines that govern patient care.

Types of Laws

Laws can be classified as civil or criminal (Fig. 7-5). **Civil law** is also referred to as private law. It is the body of law that deals with relationships between private individuals. Civil law can be subdivided into contract law and tort law. **Criminal law** is a type of public law that deals with the public's safety and welfare. Criminal law is divided into felonies and misdemeanors. Examples include homicide, manslaughter, and theft.

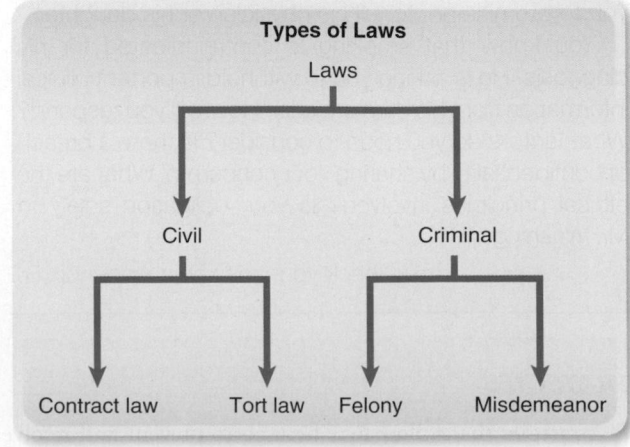

FIGURE 7-5 Types of laws.

Nursing Licensure

Licensure is mandatory for nursing. That is, to practice as a nurse, a person must be licensed as a nurse in a specific state or territory. Licensure is the legal ability to practice as a nurse. Each state, province, or territory has a nurse practice act, although the language of each act is different. Generally, nurse practice acts define nursing, describe the scope and expectations of nursing practice, detail how nursing will be governed, and outline the criteria for nursing education. In all states, there are exceptions for those who provide uncompensated nursing care to ill friends or family members. Almost all states and provinces recognize advanced registered nurse practitioners, most of whom have prescriptive authority.

Liability for licensing arises in several areas. Care given below nursing standards can result in liability to the Board of Nursing for malpractice. In addition, the Board of Nursing is concerned with nurses practicing beyond the scope of their license, even when the practice meets quality standards. For example, a nurse without an advanced practice license who decides to suture wounds or prescribe medicine may be liable for practice beyond his or her scope in accordance with the nurse practice act. Drug diversion or abuse gives rise to several licensing actions, although many states provide an alternative program that promotes treatment and rehabilitation rather than discipline.

Unfortunately, patient abuse and sexual contact with patients constitute an increasing area of liability in licensing cases. Sex with a current patient is never acceptable. Particularly in psychiatric nursing, sexual contact with former patients will undoubtedly violate disciplinary standards. Violation of other statutes or regulations may give rise to licensing action.

Standards of Care

Standards of care, which constitute the expected level of performance or practice as established by guidelines, authority, or custom, are important in malpractice and licensing cases. Each nurse practice act provides one set of guidelines for the standard that nursing care should meet. These guidelines vary as to how specifically they govern practice. The ANA and other specialty organizations define standards of care on the national level. The Joint Commission accredits healthcare facilities and sets nursing standards for some aspects of care, such as documentation.

Institutions or agencies usually have their own policies and procedures that define their standards for nursing care. Standardized nursing plans of care or protocols also may reflect the care expected for a specific patient group. The care provided by each nurse also is measured against the expected behavior of a nurse with a similar level of expertise and experience. Standards that an agency sets should be updated frequently to reflect technologic changes. Nurses must familiarize themselves with the standards. When circumstances prevent compliance with standards, nurses should document the reasons for deviation.

Torts and Crimes

Torts and crimes are legal wrongs committed against a person or property. A **tort** is subject to action in a civil court. A **crime** is a violation punishable by the state. Types of torts and crimes and their differences are listed in Box 7-4.

A tort is a private wrong for which the law provides a remedy. In these cases, the plaintiff (usually the patient or legal representative) sues the defendants (hospital, nurse, physician, or physical therapist). Tort actions compensate for damages. Successful tort actions result in money damages paid to the victim. Torts may be intentional or unintentional (discussed below).

A crime is any wrong punishable by the state. Two elements are necessary: evil intent and a criminal act. Crimes may exist, however, in which intent is not absolutely clear (e.g., reckless driving). Crimes are prosecuted in the criminal justice system and classified as felonies (e.g., rape, murder) or misdemeanors.

INTENTIONAL TORTS

Assault and Battery

Assault and battery may result in criminal trials. Assault is the threat of touching another person without his or her consent.

BOX 7-4   **Differences Between Crimes and Torts**

Crime
Results in prison term, fine, or short jail sentence to punish offender

Felony
Premeditated killing (first-degree murder)
Impulsive or unintentional killing (second-degree murder; manslaughter, rape, arson, treason, kidnapping, burglary, bribery, child abuse, drug trafficking, fraud, and terrorism)

Misdemeanor
An offense punishable by imprisonment of less than 1 year or a fine of less than $1,000. Does not amount to a felony.

Tort
Results in civil trial to assess compensation for plaintiff

Intentional
Assault and battery
Defamation of character
Fraud
Invasion of privacy
False imprisonment

Unintentional
Negligence—mistake or failure to be prudent
Malpractice—negligence in the practice of a profession (e.g., failure to assess a significant change in condition, failure to act appropriately in treating a patient, error in sponge counts, causing a burn, failure to use aseptic technique, falls, medical errors, misadministration of blood)

Battery is the actual carrying out of such a threat (i.e., the unlawful touching of a person's body). A nurse may be sued for battery if he or she fails to obtain consent for a procedure. A patient in radiology sued for battery when the nurse intentionally gave a sedative that the patient had specifically refused and the patient experienced a severe allergic reaction *(Duncan v. Scottsdale Medical Imaging, Ltd., 2003)*. Sexual assaults by staff or other patients can result in liability on the part of the agency as well as the nurse *(Duggan v. Board of Registration in Nursing, 2010)*.

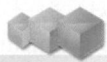 **Concept Mastery Alert**

Under the law, assault is defined as a threat to make bodily contact with another person without that person's consent. Battery takes place when the individual acts on this threat by touching the other person.

Defamation of Character

Defamation of character includes false communication that results in injury to a person's reputation by means of print (**libel**) or spoken word (**slander**). The nurse is permitted to make statements about patients only as part of his or her nursing practice and only within the limits provided by law. For example, disclosure of a false AIDS diagnosis may constitute defamation of character.

Fraud

Fraud is willful. It is a purposeful misrepresentation of self or an act that may cause harm to a person or property. A nurse who misrepresents his or her qualifications or bills for care not given may be committing a fraud.

Invasion of Privacy

The nurse is bound to limit discussion about a patient to appropriate parties. Disclosing confidential information to an inappropriate third party subjects the nurse to liability for invasion of privacy, even if the information is true. The nurse should discuss the patient with others only when the discussion is necessary for treatment and care or when the patient consents to disclosure. Congress passed the Health Insurance Portability and Accountability Act (HIPAA) in 1996. The Department of Health and Human Services promulgated the final privacy rule in late 2000. Hospitals and other agencies have developed policies to meet strict provisions regarding the handling of medical records and healthcare information. Nurses should carefully review and follow agency policy.

False Imprisonment

Prevention of movement or unjustified retention of a person without consent may be false imprisonment. Nurses must use restraints only in accordance with agency policies and usually with a physician's order. A patient cannot be forced to remain in the healthcare facility against his or her will (assuming that the patient is mentally alert, oriented, and capable of participating in care decisions). If the patient refuses to remain in the facility, the agency will have the patient sign a release stating that he or she left without medical approval. Those with mental impairments may be committed involuntarily in accordance with court proceedings if they are dangerous to themselves or others.

UNINTENTIONAL TORTS

Negligence

Negligence may be an act of omission (neglecting to do something that a reasonably prudent person would do) or commission (doing something that a reasonably prudent person would not do). **Malpractice** is negligence on the professional's part. Intent to harm is *not* an element of a malpractice suit. To prove nursing malpractice, a lawyer must prove that a deviation from the standard of care occurred that resulted in damage to a patient. In a malpractice case, violations of the standard of care are generally proved or disproved by expert testimony. A nurse expert in a given field of nursing will be called to testify about the standard of practice as it relates to the particular case.

To prove malpractice, four elements are necessary:

- A duty to the plaintiff
- A failure to meet the standard of care, or a breach of duty, which may be an act of omission
- Causation (i.e., that the breach of duty produced the injury in a natural and continuous sequence)
- Damages, which require a physical, emotional, financial, or other injury to the patient

Duty. Duty describes the relationship between the plaintiff (the person bringing suit) and the defendant (the person being sued). Nurses have a duty to care for their patients. The existence of a duty is rarely an issue in a malpractice suit.

Hospitals have a legal duty to treat patients who come to their emergency rooms; nurses, as hospital employees, have a duty to treat patients the hospital admits. In some cases, patients were denied emergency treatment because they could not pay hospital fees. A nurse who refuses care to a patient can be held liable for injuries resulting from such refusal. In addition, the federal government may impose a fine on the hospital for such refusal.

Breach of Duty. Breach of duty is the failure to conform to the standard of practice, thus creating a risk for a person that a reasonable person would have foreseen. Breach of duty may be charged when a nurse fails to meet published standards of any relevant professional organization or the agency in which the nurse is employed. The nurse may be accused of breach of duty whenever reasonably accepted standards of nursing care are not met. Failure to observe and monitor a patient's condition and behavior is a breach of duty (Weld & Garmon Bibb, 2009). Failure to make a proper nursing assessment or nursing diagnosis is a breach of the standard of care. As nurses assume more responsibility for patient care, the amount of independent patient diagnosis judgment afforded nurses surely will increase. Failure to communicate relevant information about the patient to the physician or other healthcare provider is a breach of duty (*Sewell v. King County Hospital District, 2004*). Failure to follow physicians' orders is a breach of duty unless the nurse knows or should know that executing an order would pose a clear risk of patient harm. In those cases, the nurse is obliged to clarify the order or to use independent judgment in calling on others to intervene. Increasingly, the law sets specific standards. In some states, legislation governs patient care ratios in acute care settings by licensure type (Buerhaus, Donelan, DesRoches, & Hess, 2009).

Proximate Cause. Causation must be proven for the courts to find negligence. A nurse's carelessness might not result in injury. Or injury may occur without the nurse's carelessness as its proximate cause. For example, nurses might be alleged to have failed to communicate signs of bladder perforation after surgery, but no liability would adhere because there was no evidence of causation (*Sewell v. King County Hospital District No. 2, 2004*). A nurse or hospital may not be liable for damage to a patient, even if the nurse is negligent, when the negligence does not cause the plaintiff's injury.

Courts frequently use foreseeability as a criterion for determining whether a cause is considered proximate. The question focuses on whether a reasonable person should have foreseen that injury would result from a failure to conform to the standard of care (Weld & Garmon Bibb, 2009). More commonly, plaintiffs can establish proximate cause between a breach of duty and damages. When it is obvious that the patient's injury resulted from someone's negligence but it is impossible to prove who was at fault, the doctrine of **res ipsa loquitur** ("the thing speaks for itself") may be invoked. Retained surgical sponges or instruments are typical res ipsa loquitur cases. Three elements must be proven (*Powell v. Methodist Healthcare—Jackson Hospitals, 2004*):

- The defendant or defendants (e.g., nurse, physician, or hospital) must have control of the instrumentality causing the injury.
- The injury must be such that it would not normally occur in the absence of negligence.
- The plaintiff (patient) did not voluntarily create the injury.

Damages. For a plaintiff to prevail in a malpractice suit, the plaintiff must have suffered damages. The purpose of the suit is to compensate for these damages. General damages include pain and suffering, disfigurement, and disability. Special damages are for losses and expenses related to the injury, such as medical expenses and lost wages. Punitive damages, rarely seen in nursing cases, are imposed when there is reckless, indifferent, or malicious conduct (Weld & Garmon Bibb, 2009).

Trends in Nursing Malpractice

In the past, nurses generally were not named in malpractice suits because it was considered better to sue the person or institution with the most money or insurance. Today, however, nurses are increasingly named in malpractice litigation because of the availability of insurance and because of their increasing autonomy. Patients still sue nurses for medication errors, falls, and retained sponges. In *Bailey v. Cooper Green Hospital et al. (2000)*, the patient reported pain after abdominal surgery. Later, it was determined that she had a retained foreign body. She sued the surgical nurses and was awarded $78,000 in damages.

During the past few decades, medical care has seen dramatic advances in knowledge about how to support health and prevent disease, how to treat disease processes, and how to use technology for diagnosis and treatment for illnesses. The number of malpractice suits has increased as a result of these highly complex and advanced methods of supporting health and delivering healthcare. The result has been higher standards of care for nurses.

Nurses may also experience pressure to delegate professional functions. In *Singleton v. AAA Home Health, Inc. (2000)*, a home health patient sued the agency when a nurse allegedly delegated wound care to an unqualified aide without direct supervision. The original deep packing was left in the hip wound, and only the outer dressing was changed. The court awarded more than $100,000 for delayed healing of more than a year.

Nurses rushing to perform technical tasks correctly may forget to really listen to their patients. In one case, nurses who were giving chemotherapy apparently did not listen to a patient's reports of burning on administration, and they did not communicate with the physician about the patient's continuing problems. A court awarded $500,000 for damages that included multiple surgeries and skin grafting (*Iacano v. St. Peter's Medical Center, 2000*).

LIABILITY

Liability denotes legal responsibility to pay damages. When the four elements of negligence are proven (i.e., when the nurse's breach of a duty owed to the patient was the proximate cause of injury to the patient), the nurse can be found liable. The hospital, clinic, or community nurse service may be held responsible for a nurse's negligence under the doctrine of **respondeat superior** ("let the master answer"). This notion of vicarious liability, or liability assigned to an employer by way of the terms of employment, can be applied whenever the nurse is acting within the scope of employment. Rarely, the employer may attempt to prove that the nurse was not acting within the scope of employment when the negligent act occurred. This is one reason individual liability insurance is recommended. Nurses are generally covered by vicarious liability when they are acting under their employer's control. It is important to remember that this means *both* the employer and the nurse are responsible. The employer cannot make the nurse immune from liability. General areas of liability are summarized in Table 7-2.

Legally Sensitive Areas of Nursing Practice

There are many legally sensitive areas of nursing practice. Some areas include the following:

- *Payment for Enhanced Care Services and Technology Use.* Some healthcare consumers are currently requested to pay annual membership fees for expanded services, which often involve current technology. For example, these expanded

TABLE 7-2 GENERAL AREAS OF LIABILITY

	To Whom Is the Healthcare Provider Responsible?	Patient Injury Necessary?	Result if Successful
Malpractice or Negligence	Patient	Yes	Money paid to patient by healthcare provider
Administrative/Licensing	Board of Nursing	No	Loss of license or keeping license on certain conditions; fine
Criminal	State represented by prosecutors	No	Jail or fine

services sometimes include access to medical records via mobile devices, e-communications with providers, and an opportunity to have an e-visit (Abner, 2014). These fees may create a two-tier healthcare access system for those who are able to pay versus those who are not able to pay or do not have the technology to benefit from the services.

- *Use of Online Communication Technologies.* Ethical challenges will increase with the use of social media by nurses. Many nurses use social networking sites as a way to share information with family and friends. At the same time, postings of pictures and events related to work show the blurring between personal and professional values. An evaluation of 124 nurses' social media pages in the United Kingdom and Italy showed, in some cases, pictures of nurses at work preparing drugs or injections, being with patients at workplace events, or engaging in unhealthy behaviors (Levati, 2014). Nurses are challenged to demonstrate patient privacy and ethical conduct while working or presenting oneself as a nurse online.

- *Controlled substances.* In 1970, the Comprehensive Drug Abuse Prevention and Control Act was passed in the United States. In most states, nurses may administer controlled substances (opioids, depressants, stimulants, and hallucinogens) only under the direction of a physician or other authorized provider, unless the substances are authorized under advanced practice licenses. The safekeeping of controlled substances continues is important.

- *Death and dying.* Death occurs either when there is irreversible cessation of heart and lung functions or an irreversible loss of all functions of the entire brain. It is the nurse's duty to recognize cardiovascular death. In most states, the physician has the legal responsibility of pronouncing the person dead. Diagnosing **brain death** in patients with mechanical ventilators is a medical determination requiring specific tests and examinations (John, Reyes, Thachil, Flaherty, & Emmett, 2007).

- *Assisted suicide.* **Assisted suicide** is defined as providing the patient with the means to end his or her life but not providing the direct action to cause the death. It is important for nurses to know what care they are to provide to patients requesting assisted suicide. Physician- or nurse-caused death (**active euthanasia**) is defined as deliberately hastening a person's death and is considered murder in all states and almost all countries. Actions that constitute deliberate hastening of death include injecting a bolus of potassium or overdose of insulin. Actions that *do not* constitute hastening death include extubating a mechanically ventilated

patient with the informed consent of the patient or surrogate and a physician's order.

- *Terminal sedation.* **Terminal sedation** is not considered euthanasia. Rather, it is an infrequently used method of pain management provided in response to a dying patient's persistent and unremitting pain and suffering. In these cases, it is considered legally and ethically permissible to provide analgesia to a level that produces light sedation, even though this is likely to hasten death somewhat secondary to resulting immobility. Terminal sedation is considered an option of last resort for ensuring that patients can die comfortably and with dignity (Randall & Downie, 2010).

- *Advance directives.* In 1990, the federal legislature passed the Patient Self-Determination Act. The act requires that each hospital, long-term care facility, visiting nurse agency, hospice, or health maintenance organization that provides care to patients receiving Medicare or Medicaid funding must develop written policies concerning advance directives. Nurses must become familiar with statutes in their states and provinces regarding the execution of living wills or directives to physicians and proxy directives that specify surrogate decision makers.

- *Resuscitation.* Nurses must always know the code status of their patients regarding **resuscitation**, verify the code status on the patient's order sheet, and follow agency policy. Orders not to provide resuscitation in the event of a cardiopulmonary arrest are frequently referred to as **no code order** or **do not resuscitate** (DNR) orders. Most recently, some experts are calling for a new name—allow natural death (AND) orders—to focus on what is being done rather than on what is not being done. When nurses are unaware and encounter a patient in cardiac arrest, they should resuscitate the patient pending confirmation of the code status. If there is a no code order, resuscitation may be stopped once initiated.

Patients not in acute care settings also may wish to avoid resuscitation should they experience a cardiopulmonary arrest. Many states have addressed this need by providing a means to obtain a **community-based no code order**. These forms have various names, including EMS-No CPR orders, portable no code orders, and community-based DNR orders. They generally require the signatures of the primary physician or nurse practitioner and the patient or legal surrogate. Unlike advance directives, these orders must be obtained through a healthcare provider. A community-based no code order allows emergency medical personnel, if called, to provide care and support to the patient and family without attempting resuscitation.

TABLE 7-3 MALPRACTICE POLICY QUESTIONS TO ASK BEFORE PURCHASING

	Questions
Coverage Inclusions	What does the policy cover?
	Does the policy cover what I am doing in my clinical practice?
Coverage Exclusions	What is excluded from coverage?
Policy Limits	What are the policy limits?
Type of Policy Coverage	Is the policy offered based on claims made or occurrence? Occurrence is best.
Financial Stability	Is policy used by others in my type of clinical practice? What is the financial stability rating of the policy or company authoring the policy?

Adapted with permission from Buppert, C. (2011). Three frequently asked questions about malpractice insurance. *The Journal of Nurse Practitioners, 7*(1), 16–17.

- *Good Samaritan laws.* Good Samaritan laws offer legal immunity for healthcare professionals who assist in an emergency and render reasonable care under such circumstances. Because most states and provinces do not require nurses or citizens to aid the distressed, such assistance becomes an ethical, rather than legal, duty. Although these laws limit liability for the nurse, he or she may be liable for gross negligence. A nurse who helps is obligated to remain until additional assistance is obtained. The nurse should then relinquish care to official rescue personnel unless asked to remain. Because emergency assistance is generally outside the scope of the nurse's employment, the employer's malpractice insurance will not provide coverage. This is another reason for nurses to carry their own insurance (Table 7-3).

Protecting Yourself Legally

Nurses may minimize the risk of legal problems, including malpractice, in several ways. First, nurses should keep current with advances in practice. Continuing education is absolutely essential to stay knowledgeable about general and specialized care. Likewise, nurses should be familiar with regulations governing nursing practice.

PROFESSIONAL PRACTICE

Nurses involved in the development of policies, procedures, protocols, or standardized nursing plans of care should be sure to make them realistic for their own practices, for an agency, or both. Such standards should be evidence based and practicable with the resources available. Staffing and equipment to conform to these guidelines must be available at all times. Those who develop standards to apply to various practice settings should keep in mind the differences in resources and facilities of different sizes, acuity, and geographic area. Those involved in

policy making need to continue to update policies in a timely and sensible manner in accordance with nursing's demands. New knowledge must be applied. Policies, procedures, and protocols must be followed. Propounding unrealistic policies and procedures and then not following them is an invitation to malpractice suits.

The patient's condition must be monitored, and observations must be documented. Whether the patient is in a hospital recovering from surgery, in home care coping with a chronic illness, or in a setting where direct observation is limited (e.g., as a telephone triage nurse), assessment of the patient must be recorded. Significant changes in the patient's condition need to be reported to a physician or other professional in a timely manner. The report to the physician also must be documented. When physicians do not follow up with assessment or intervention, the nurse needs to challenge the physician's care. Hospitals and nurses may be liable when nurses do not challenge physicians in the face of obvious negligence. In *Reinen v. Northern Arizona Orthopedics, LTD* (2000), the nurse allegedly failed to follow the chain of command when a patient with diabetes experienced deterioration in condition after trauma surgery. The appellate court held that the nurse could be found negligent when she did not get a physician to follow up on abnormal laboratory values and to treat his critical condition. She did not seek the assistance of her supervisor, which the court clearly expected.

PROFESSIONAL LIABILITY INSURANCE

Malpractice claims are on the rise against all healthcare professionals. Because a nurse may be sued for some act related to nursing but outside the limits of her or his employment, each nurse also should have her or his own insurance. Nursing students generally are covered for their student clinical experiences as long as they are registered students and are practicing under appropriate supervision. To obtain information about nursing malpractice insurance carriers, visit your state's association of long-term care facilities page or search the Internet. There are some questions to ask about professional liability insurance prior to purchasing the insurance (Buppert, 2011).

DOCUMENTATION

Documentation should be accurate, complete, and contemporaneous with care given. Avoid precharting or documenting events before they occur; this is the easiest way for nurses to put themselves at risk for lawsuits (Singh, 2010). Two issues associated with electronic health records are: (1) pasting copied information from one health record to another and (2) excessive documentation of private health information (Rose, 2014). Each patient record requires individualized documentation relevant to that patient in the format approved by the agency. Assess and record vital signs in accordance with the agency's policy and the patient's condition. When critical events occur, note the precise time and event in the records. Documentation should be objective. Criticisms and negative comments about other providers, patients, or family members have no place in the medical record. Chart errors correctly using the standard

THERAPEUTIC DIALOGUE: ETHICAL ISSUES

SCENE FOR THOUGHT

A patient who has been unconscious since major abdominal surgery for metastatic cancer has been in the ICU for 3 weeks. The adult child of the patient meets with the physician and the nurse. The purpose of this meeting is to re-explain the plan of care and its rationale. There is confusion about the diagnosis by the adult child.

LESS EFFECTIVE

Physician: We need to talk again about why we're decreasing the IVs and oxygen.

Daughter: I thought you were taking the oxygen and IVs away because you saw improvement. I was expecting discharge papers soon. I don't understand what you're doing. (*Cries and looks angry.*)

Nurse: I thought you understood that your mother isn't getting any better and that, in fact, she probably won't come out of her coma at all. (*Said softly but firmly.*)

Daughter: No, I didn't get that! How is this possible? How is death possible? How can you take away life?

Nurse: I know it's hard for you to understand. I think it would be a good thing if you called your minister and the rest of your family so you can talk it over and decide what to do.

Daughter: I think I'll call our family lawyer, too. There's something funny going on here! (*Crying and reaching for a cell phone.*)

MORE EFFECTIVE

Physician: We need to talk again about why we're decreasing the IVs and oxygen.

Daughter: I thought you were taking the oxygen and IVs away because you saw improvement. I was expecting discharge papers soon. I don't understand what you're doing. (*Cries and looks angry.*)

Physician: I really thought you understood. I'm sorry you're upset about this.

Nurse: Could you tell us what you see when you go into the room for your visits? (*Assesses her viewpoint before making any assumptions.*)

Daughter: I see quiet rest periods. I see a lot of sleeping. (*Still cries quietly, face set in a stiff frown.*)

Nurse: The physician and I have noticed some changes over the last few weeks. Have you? (*Assesses her perceptions.*)

Daughter: Well… I've noticed less movement, even when you do something to her. I suppose you think that means something! (*Looks frightened and angry at the same time.*)

Nurse: Yes, the physician and I think it means that the coma is deeper. There may be little chance of that changing. (*Nurse and physician further explain coma and its relationship to the cancer.*)

Daughter: (*Puts her head in her hands and cries quietly. The room is quiet. She looks up.*) I knew this. The doctor said that before. I didn't want to believe it.

Nurse: I know it's difficult to "give up" on someone you love. I want to reassure you that we are still working to provide care. The goals have changed from hoping for a recovery to allowing a natural and comfortable death. It might be helpful to talk some more about what to expect over the next few days and how we can be helpful to you. Would that be good for you?

Daughter: Yes, that would be helpful. I hope you don't mind if I cry, though. I expected better news.

Nurse: That's very understandable. I won't mind. (*The discussion continues. Support is suggested from clergy or other family members. A family meeting is arranged the next day to include all persons.*)

CRITICAL THINKING CHALLENGE

- What is the main difference between the first and second communication examples?
- In the second communication example, which items of the ANA Code of Ethics were demonstrated in the nurse's communication?
- In the second communication example, who are the recipients of nursing care?
- After reading the AHA's brochure for patients, *What to Expect During Your Hospital Stay*, which issues are particularly relevant to the family's situation?

agency protocols. If a specific incident, such as a fall or medication error, occurs, follow these principles:

- *Maintain rapport with the patient.* Do not avoid communication with the patient who is experiencing stress and uncertainty. Offer simple explanations if you can do so honestly, calmly, and without blaming anyone.
- *Document the incident on the appropriate forms of your institution.* Incident reports are useful to remind you of the events surrounding the incident. They are useful to enhance continuous quality improvement.

Nursing students must perform duties only within the scope of their professional training to date. These acts are performed with the same degree of competence that a registered nurse would exhibit. Under the auspices of a clinical supervisor, nursing students may carry out assignments. Nursing students assume liability for their negligent or wrong acts. The clinical supervisor or school also may be held liable.

KEY CONCEPTS

- Values are standards for decision making that endure for a significant time in one's life.
- To understand ethics as it pertains to nurses or other clinicians, it is important to distinguish among personal values, professional ethics, institutional policies, or legal obligations.
- The major principles of healthcare ethics that are important to uphold include respect for persons and autonomy, beneficence, nonmaleficence, and justice.
- Rights and ethical rules of professional–client relationships include veracity, fidelity, privacy, and confidentiality.
- Individual state, provincial, or territorial nurse practice acts provide some guidance for standards of nursing. Following the current standard of nursing care as evidenced in statutes and regulations, standards of professional organizations, and current literature helps to minimize the risk of legal problems.
- The four elements of negligence are duty, breach of duty, proximate cause, and damage.
- Nurses need to obtain professional liability insurance to protect their best interests should their practice be called into question through legal action.
- Clear, accurate documentation using the procedures of the institution will substantiate care provided to patients.

PRACTICING FOR THE NCLEX

CHECK YOUR ANSWERS IN APPENDIX A.

1. A nurse is working in an organization that prescribes and supports Plan B ("the morning after pill") as a form of contraception. In analyzing her role and moral values, the nurse should consider which of the following? Select all that apply:
   a. Is she affirming the patient's desires?
   b. Is she upholding the ethics of the profession?
   c. What are the nurse's beliefs/biases related to this medication?
   d. What are the consequences and alternatives of giving or not giving this medication?

2. A patient with esophageal cancer is no longer able to consume foods by mouth and is now fed via a gastric feeding tube. The patient is withdrawn and states, "My family used to have big dinners with friends, family, lots of laughter, and loud conversation." Which of the patient's values are apparent and best describe the behavior? Select all that apply:
   a. Independence and individuality
   b. Family role
   c. Socialization
   d. Human nature

3. A nurse is caring for a patient with necrosing leg ulcers. The nurse assesses that these are related to venous stasis, but when asked, the patient reports that there is a someone "shooting lasers through the floor" in the apartment. In order to progress with wound treatment, what must the nurse understand about resolving value conflicts? Select all that apply:
   a. It is necessary to establish common ground about therapy goals.
   b. Further exploration of the patient's belief system may be needed to identify beliefs related to care.
   c. The nurse may need to answer patient questions related to care.
   d. The nurse may need to examine personal values related to mental health and care.

4. A nurse in the transplant ICU is caring for a teenager following a liver transplant as a result of a Tylenol overdose. The patient also superseded another ICU patient (reformed alcoholic) who subsequently died without the transplant. The patient does not want treatment and states: "I just want to die." The nurse questions the principles of healthcare ethics in this case. Which principle would be most in question?
   a. Beneficence
   b. Nonmaleficence
   c. Autonomy
   d. Justice

5. A nurse fails to observe and document a patient's change in neurologic status, ultimately resulting in the patient's death from a stroke. Which type of malpractice is most relevant?
   a. Fraud
   b. Breach of duty
   c. Negligence by commission
   d. Battery

REFERENCES

Abner, C. (2014). Two classes of care: The ethical dilemma of providing access to electronic health data and resources. *Nurse Leader, 12*(4), 74–77.

American Nurses Association. (2015). *Code of ethics with interpretative statements.* Retrieved April 27, 2015, from http://www.nursingworld.org/MainMenuCategories/EthicsStandards/CodeofEthicsforNurses/Code-of-Ethics-For-Nurses.html

American Hospital Association. *The patient care partnership: Understanding expectations, rights and responsibilities.* Retrieved October 25, 2014, from http://www.aha.org/advocacy-issues/communicatingpts/pt-care-partnership.shtml

Beauchamp, T. L., & Childress, J. F. (2012). *Principles of biomedical ethics* (7th ed.). New York, NY: Oxford University Press.

Buerhaus, P. I., Donelan, K., DesRoches, C., & Hess, R. (2009). Registered nurses' perceptions of nursing staffing ratios and new hospital payment regulations. *Nursing Economics, 27*(6), 372–376.

Buppert, C. (2011). Three frequently asked questions about malpractice insurance. *The Journal of Nurse Practitioners, 7*(1), 16–17.

Carrese, J. A., & Rhodes, L. A. (2000). Bridging cultural differences in medical practice: The case of discussing negative information with Navajo patients. *Journal of General Internal Medicine, 15*(2), 92–96.

Council on Community Pediatrics and Committee on Native American Child Health. (2010). Policy statement—health equity and children's rights. *Pediatrics, 125*(4), 838–849. Epub 2010 Mar 29.

DeCamp, M., Farber, N., Torke, A., George, M., Berger, Z., Keirns, C., et al. (2014). Ethical challenges for accountable care organizations: A structured review. *Journal of General Internal Medicine, 29*(10), 1392–1399.

Dunlop, S. (2008). The dying child: Should we tell the truth? *Paediatric Nursing, 20*(6), 28–31.

Elliott, L., & Hunter, D. (2008). The experiences of ethics committee members: Contradictions between individuals and committees. *Journal of Medical Ethics, 34*(6), 489–494.

Erikson, E. (1982). *The life cycle completed.* New York, NY: W. W. Norton & Co.

Erlen, J. A. (2010). Informed consent: Revisiting the issues. *Orthopedic Nursing, 29*(4), 276–280.

Fairchild, R. M. (2010). Practical ethical theory for nurses responding to complexity in care. *Nursing Ethics, 17*(3), 353–362.

Finset, A., Heyn, L., & Ruland, C. (2013). Patterns in clinicians' responses to patient emotion in cancer care. *Patient Education & Counseling, 93*(1): 80–85.

Gallagher, A., & Tschudin, V. (2010). Educating for ethical leadership. *Nurse Education Today, 30,* 224–227.

Ganzini, L., Volicer, L., Nelson, W. A., Fox, E., & Derse, A. R. (2004). Ten myths about decision-making capacity. *Journal of the American Medical Directors Association, 5*(4), 263–267.

Hall, B., Kalven, J., Rosen, L., & Taylor, B. (1982). *Readings in value development.* Ramsey, NJ: Paulist Press.

Høye, S., & Severinsson, E. (2010). Professional and cultural conflicts for intensive care nurses. *Journal of Advanced Nursing, 66*(4), 858–867.

Hofstede, G. (2001). *Culture's consequences: Comparing values, behaviors, institutions, and organizations across nations.* Thousand Oaks, CA: Sage.

Hunt, M., & Carnevale, F. (2011). Moral experience: A framework for bioethics research. *Journal of Medical Ethics, 37,* 658–662.

International Council of Nurses. (2012). *International Council of Nurses Code of Ethics for Nurses.* Geneva, Switzerland:. Retrieved October 25, 2014, from http://www.icn.ch/images/stories/documents/about/icncode_english.pdf

Jeffs, L., Espin, S., Rorabeck, L., Shannon, S., Robins, L., Levinson, W., et al. (2011). Not overstepping professional boundaries: The challenging role of nurses in simulated error disclosures. *Journal of Nursing Care Quality, 26*(4), 320–327.

John, K., Reyes, B. J., Thachil, R., Flaherty, S., & Emmett, M. (2007). Brain death: A challenging diagnosis in trauma patients. *West Virginia Medical Journal, 103*(3), 13–16.

Kagan, P., Smith, M., & Chinn, P. (2014). *Philosophies and Practices of Emancipatory Nursing: Social Justice as Praxis.* New York, NY: Routledge.

Levati, S. (2014). Professional conduct among registered nurses in the use of online social networking sites. *Journal of Advanced Nursing, 70*(1), 2284–2292.

McMullen, P., Howie, B., Howie, W., & Philipsen, N. (2013). Caring for the dangerous patient: Legal and ethical considerations. *Journal for Nurse Practitioners, 9*(9), 568–575.

Mitchell, G., McCollum, P., & Monaghan, C. (2013). Disclosing a diagnosis of dementia: A background to the phenomenon. *Nursing Older People, 25*(10), 16–21.

Philipsen, N., Murray, T., Wood, C., Bell-Hawkins, A., & Setlow, P. (2013). Surrogate decision making: How to promote best outcomes in difficult times. *Journal for Nurse Practitioners, 9*(9), 581–587.

Pignone, M., Fagerlin, A., Abhyankar, P., Col, N., Feldman-Stewart, D., Gavaruzzi, T., et al. (2012). Clarifying and expressing values. In R. Volk & H. Llewellyn-Thomas (Eds.). *2012 Update of the International Patient Decision Aids Standards (IPDAS) Collaboration's Background Document.* Chapter D. Accessed 10/26/14 from http://ipdas.ohri.ca/resources.html

Randall, F., & Downie, R. (2010). Assisted suicide and voluntary euthanasia: Role contradictions for physicians. *Clinical Medicine, 10*(4), 323–325.

Reinke, L., Shannon, S., Engelberg, R., Young, J., and Curtis, J. (2010). Supporting hope and prognostic information: Nurses' perspectives on their role when patients have life-limiting prognosis. *Journal of Pain and Symptom Management, 39*(6), 982–992.

Rose, R. (2014). Five ways to avoid noncompliance with privacy laws. *Healthcare Financial Management, 68*(2), 40.

Schoen, C., & Doty, M. M. (2004). Inequities in access to medical care in five countries: Findings from the 2001 Commonwealth Fund International Health Policy Survey. *Health Policy, 67*(3), 309–322.

Singh, T. (2010). Avoid malpractice & protect your license: Never pre-chart! *Nevada RN Formation, 19*(2), 12.

Ulrich, C. M., Taylor, C., Soeken, K., O'Donnell, P., Farrar, A., Danis, M., et al. (2010). Everyday ethics: Ethical issues and stress in nursing practice. *Journal of Advanced Nursing, 66*(11), 2510–2519. Epub 2010 Aug 23.

Weld, K. K., & Garmon Bibb, S. C. (2009). Concept analysis: Malpractice and modern-day nursing practice. *Nursing Forum, 44*(1), 2–10.

Whittington, A., & Mack, E. (2010). Inspiring courage in girls: An evaluation of practices and outcomes. *Journal of Experiential Education, 33*(2), 166–180. DOI:10.5193/JEE33.2.166

Wocial, L. D., Bledsoe, P., Helft, P. R., & Everett, L. Q. (2010). Nurse ethicist: Innovative resource for nurses. *Journal of Professional Nursing, 26*(5), 287–292.

Legal Case References

Bailey v. Cooper Green Hospital et al., Ala. S. Ct., 2000 Ala. LEXIS 550 (2000).

Duggan v. Board of Registration in Nursing, 456 Mass. 666, N.E.2d, 2010 WL 1797114 (2010).

Duncan v. Scottsdale Medical Imaging, Ltd., 205 Ariz. 306; 70 P.3d 435; Ariz. LEXIS 82; 415 Ariz. Adv. Rep. (2003).

Iacano v. St. Peter's Medical Center, 760 A.2d 348 N.J. Super. Ct. App. Div. (2000).

Powell v. Methodist Healthcare—Jackson Hospitals, 876 So.2d 347; Miss. LEXIS 779 (2004).

Reinen v. Northern Arizona Orthopedics, LTD, 991 P.2d 242, 2000; Ariz. LEXIS 1 (2000).

Sewell v. King County Hospital District, No. 2, Wash. App. LEXIS 968 (2004).

Singleton v. AAA Home Health, Inc., 772 So.2d 346 La. App. (2000).

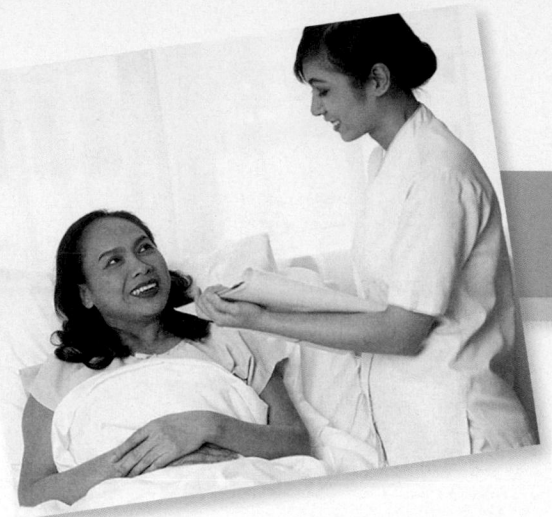

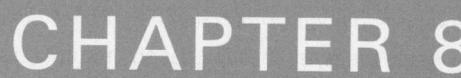

CHAPTER 8

Nursing Research and Evidence-Based Care

Phyllis J. Eide and Ryan Townsend

Case Scenario

You are a nurse working in a rehabilitation unit of a large medical center. As you enter a patient's room to conduct a follow-up assessment, you find the patient engrossed in a conversation with a woman in a lab coat who introduces herself as a graduate nursing student from the university affiliated with the medical center. The student says that she is conducting research for her master's thesis. You know that no arrangements have been made for this patient to be a participant in a research study to evaluate nursing care, and you had no knowledge that this student might collect data in this setting. You reviewed the patient's records at the beginning of your shift and know that the patient did not sign a consent form to participate in any study. The student states that she was only interviewing the patient, not providing any treatment, and was not putting the patient at any risk. Therefore, she does not think that she needed to obtain consent.

Once you have completed this chapter and have incorporated nursing research and evidence-based care into your knowledge base, review the above scenario and reflect on the following areas of Critical Thinking:

1. Critique the graduate student's actions in light of how you understand the protection of patient rights in research.
2. Based on your understanding of patient rights, describe your reaction to the graduate student's response.
3. Now that you have clarified your understanding and considered the graduate student's response, identify how you will proceed.

KEY TERMS

anonymity
Cochrane Database of Systematic Reviews
confidentiality
comparative effectiveness research
dependent variable
evidence-based practice
foreground questions
hypothesis
independent variable
literature review
meta-analyses
mixed methods
networking
nursing research
problem statement
qualitative research
quantitative research
research design
systematic reviews
theory
variables

Biomedical, environmental, psychological, and sociologic research has resulted in monumental advances in modern healthcare. One example of such an advance is in the intersecting areas of information and technology (including biotechnology), as they impact health. Christensen and Petrie (2012) have identified this intersection of technologies, along with Web 2.0's ability to rapidly expand the global village's access to information, as key to accelerating advances in mental healthcare.

A major reason for conducting research is to expand a profession's knowledge base. Currently, research focusing on outcomes, or evidence-based research, has molded clinicians' practice in the hope of improving health outcomes for recipients. This type of "translational" research forms the bridge between theory and practice and is sometimes referred to as a "bench-side (as in lab bench) to bedside" process. It also flows the other way when clinical observations are transferred to the laboratory (Memorial Sloan-Kettering Cancer Center, 2010).

One of the goals of this textbook is to emphasize the pivotal role of research in everyday nursing practice. Throughout the text, there are "PICO" displays that highlight the focus of each chapter. Take an opportunity to read, contemplate, and perhaps apply the research information as you learn about the concepts in that chapter.

Nursing practice and patient outcomes are enhanced when professional nurses choose to use treatment methods that are based on research. Untested treatments may seemingly improve or alter the outcome a patient experiences, but no confirmation exists that choosing the same treatment a second time would similarly improve outcome. Research-based nursing practice leads to improved care.

The science of nursing draws heavily on other sciences, in particular the biopsychosocial fields, such as physiology, pharmacology, psychology, and sociology. Nurses must be able to discriminate "good" research from "poor" research to know what to use in clinical practice. Therefore, they must have a working knowledge of research methods and a beginning ability to read for application and to critique research. This chapter helps nursing students understand the research process and, in particular, the application of research to the practice of nursing. Research use forms the underpinnings of all nursing practice, continuing throughout the nurse's career and improving outcomes for patients.

RESEARCH AND NURSING

For the purposes of this chapter, research is defined as a formalized process of systematic investigation designed to test a research question or **hypothesis** and draw conclusions from collected data. Many similarities are found between the formalized research process and the nursing process format that is an integral part of nursing education.

Nursing research is defined as a systematic inquiry into the problems encountered in nursing practice and into the modalities of patient care, such as support and comfort, prevention of trauma, promotion of recovery, health education, health appraisal, and coordination of healthcare (Gortner, 1975, Polit & Beck, 2011; LoBiondo-Wood & Haber, 2013). Nursing research concerns nursing and things that nurses do that are different from the actions of other disciplines. The purpose of research may be to learn about a specific problem (e.g., "Why do residents not use the exercise facilities?") or to understand a situation ("I wonder what is the experience of…?") (Richards & Morse, 2012). Clinical nursing research is designed to guide nursing practice and typically begins with questions arising from practice problems (Polit & Beck, 2014; LoBiondo-Wood & Haber, 2013).

Evidence-based practice (EBP) is an approach to healthcare that realizes that pathophysiologic reasoning and personal experience are necessary, but not sufficient, for making decisions. This technique emphasizes decision making based on the best available evidence (usually from research conducted by nurses and other healthcare professionals) and the use of outcome studies to guide decisions (Polit & Beck, 2011). The concept of EBP has been evolving for the last 35 years (Polit & Beck, 2011). Many recent journal articles and textbooks have focused on identifying the steps involved in the process of EBP. Medical decisions should be based, as much as possible, on a firm foundation of high-grade scientific evidence rather than on experience or opinion, and should integrate individual clinical expertise with the best available external clinical evidence from systematic research (Leape, Berwick, & Bates, 2002; The Cochrane Collaboration, 2015). (See Box 8-1.) Utilization of the results of scientific studies is referred to in the nursing literature as evidence-based nursing (LoBiondo-Wood & Haber, 2013; Cullum, Ciliska, Haynes & Marks, 2008).

BOX 8-1	Evidence-Based Clinical Practice: Introduction to Systematic Reviews

Healthcare professionals base patient care decisions on many factors. These include education, experience, consultation with peers, and current research. In all disciplines within the healthcare arena, an emphasis is placed on EBP.

Evidence-based clinical practice is an approach to healthcare in which the clinician uses current research to help guide patient care decisions. The practice of evidence-based care means integrating individual clinical expertise with the best available external clinical evidence from systematic research.

Nurses use EBP in many ways. For example, it can be used to write institution-wide policies and procedures on culturally appropriate care (Douglas, Rosenkoetter, Pacquiano, Callister, Hattar-Pollara, et al., 2014), contribute to the standardization of central venous catheter practices in neonatal units (Taylor, McDonald, & Tan, 2014), or to help determine nurse–patient staffing ratios on a particular unit. In all cases, it is used to answer this question: What does the research say on how we can do this better?

One problem with research is the sheer volume of studies published on any one topic. The use of **systematic reviews** is one way to look at a body of research literature on a specific topic. Systematic reviews use explicit methods to identify, select, and critically evaluate relevant research. Systematic reviews minimize the possibility of bias by using explicit criteria for inclusion. **Meta-analyses** are systematic reviews that combine the results of several studies using qualitative statistics.

You can locate systematic reviews by using databases of systematic reviews. The Cochrane Collaboration (http://www.cochrane.org/) is an international not-for-profit organization dedicated to preparing, maintaining, and promoting the accessibility of systematic reviews of the effects of healthcare. The Collaboration defines evidence-based healthcare as the "conscientious use of current best evidence in making decisions about the care of individual patients or the delivery of health services." A key element of the Collaboration is the **Cochrane Database of Systematic Reviews** (CDSR), located at the Cochrane Collection (http://www.cochrane.org/). The CDSR is a full test database containing systematic reviews and protocols (reviews still in progress) of the effects of healthcare interventions. Most of the reviews available on the CDSR are randomized controlled trials, the gold standard of high-quality, systematic reviews.

Nursing research is identical to that of any other discipline in which practitioners are interested in seeking the truth. Nurses interested in improving the health of their patients engage in systematic inquiry designed to develop trustworthy evidence, which forms the basis for EBP (Polit & Beck, 2011). The patterns exposed through predictive modeling and research can predict future nursing outcomes and yield knowledge that is essential for healthcare practice (Crockett, 2013). Nurses engaged in holistic care must possess complex knowledge that encompasses both subjective and objective forms of knowing, which coupled with reflection comprise the "whole" of nursing knowledge (Mantzoukas & Jasper, 2008) (Table 8-1).

Research affects the clinical practice of nurses in all areas, particularly in relation to the goals of nursing (Fig. 8-1). The American Nurses Association (ANA) Research Agenda (2011) advocates for quality outcomes for patient care, which requires the use of research for evidence-based practice. Evidence areas identified by ANA as relevant to quality include patient safety, improvements in nursing efficiency, population health, and workforce mix to meet the needs of the population. Some examples of relevant research that may be of interest to nurses working in specialty units include evidence-based best practices for treatment for burn blisters (Murphy & Amblum, 2014), cancer pain management (Choi, Kim, Chung, Ahn, Yoo, et al., 2014), and oral care for ICU patients (Ganz, Ofra, Khalaila, Levy, Arad, et al., 2013). Nurses working with older patients might benefit from review of articles on prevention of falls (Lang, 2014) or the effects of guided imagery on pain, pain disability, and depression (Lewandowski & Jacobson, 2013).

Observational data on cases of measles, collected by the Centers for Disease Control and Prevention (CDC) during the 1980s, led to the conclusion that measles outbreaks in school-aged and teen populations were related to vaccine failure of the initial immunization. This conclusion had direct effects on public health nursing practice because a second measles, mumps, and

TABLE 8-1 CONCEPTUALIZATIONS OF KNOWLEDGE USED IN NURSING PRACTICE

Type of Knowledge	Description
Descriptive Rule-Based Knowledge	Early nursing knowledge was guided by descriptive rules in providing appropriate nursing care, which lacked explanatory ability and was authoritative in nature (e.g., doctors and nurse managers).
Development of Theoretical Knowledge	Knowledge acquired through formal nursing education providing quantifiable and measurable information about nursing practice. Exemplified by pioneering nursing theorists such as Peplau, Orem, and Roy
Development of Reflective Practice Knowledge	Subjective and contextual-based knowledge
Development of EBP Knowledge	Objective and acontextual-based knowledge
Movement Toward Consilience	Complex; focus is on combining forms of knowledge to produce a "whole" of nursing knowledge.

Source: Mantzoukas, S., & Jasper, M. (2008). Types of nursing knowledge used to guide care of hospitalized patients. *Journal of Advanced Nursing*, *62*(3), 318–326.

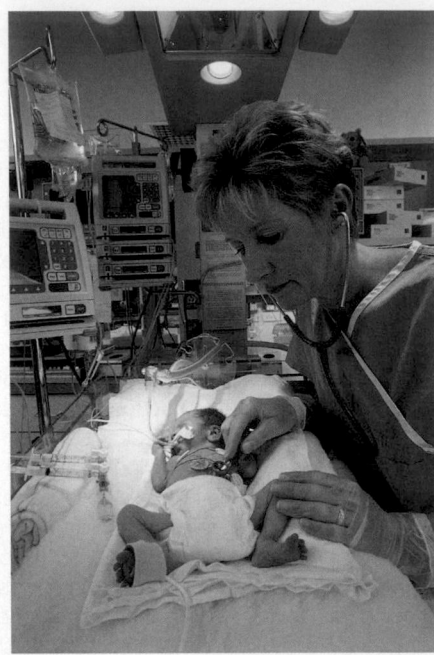

FIGURE 8-1 Clinical research defines nursing practice and raises the standards of nursing care. Research findings about newborn thermoregulation help promote evidence-based nursing care during the newborn period.

rubella (MMR) immunization was instituted for children at entry into grade school or middle school (Centers for Disease Control and Prevention, 1999; Immunization of adolescents, 1996). An ongoing source of data to inform practice related to measles can be found at the CDC's site (http://www.cdc.gov/measles/).

Specialists become familiar with research related to their disciplines by paying attention to reviews of research or through the use of expert or consensus panels relevant to their areas. The change in focus from pure research to outcomes research is changing the way that practitioners view their profession.

Although many problems that nurses encounter in clinical practice affect people of all ages, some problems are age or person specific. One nurse may be interested in the health benefits of aerobic exercise for a healthy geriatric population; another may be interested in the effect of positioning on the oxygen saturation of patients who have undergone coronary artery bypass surgery. Cardiac care can also be informed by application of Kolcaba's comfort theory, which can guide both research and practice (Krinsky, Murillo, & Johnson, 2014). Commitment to healthcare improvement at the corporate level can be found in Kaiser Permanente's Community Health Initiatives. Their ambitious goal for their 40+ participating communities is to create "population-level" improvements on such health outcomes as increased physical activity, healthier diets, and reductions in obesity (and related improvements in high blood pressure and diabetes). Kaiser Permanente has set out to "use data to improve, not just to prove" (Kaiser Permanente, 2014).

The focus of nursing research must be on generating fundamental knowledge to guide nursing practice (LoBiondo-Wood & Haber, 2013). With the widespread use of the Internet, nurses, like all others, have an enhanced ability to seek, find, and apply information about healthcare. The availability of electronic media information alters the depth and breadth of information available to all, thereby changing the way in which fundamental knowledge is disseminated and used.

In addition to generating practice-specific results, nurse researchers are expanding the overall sum of nursing knowledge. For example, research can yield economic benefits when analyzing nursing workforce issues such as appropriate staffing mix or key elements contributing to nursing shortages (Auerbach et al., 2013). Research on Medicaid's cost and quality challenges is another area of inquiry with potential economic benefits and is the focus of the Agency for Health Care Policy and Research, sited within the Agency for Healthcare Research and Quality (Agency for Healthcare Research and Quality, 2014).

Scientific Process and Nursing Research

In general, research means the search for a valid answer to a question. How the question is raised and by whom often is critical to solving the problem. The scientific method, the problem-solving method, and the nursing process all use research methods. The problem-solving method and the nursing process are compared in Chapter 10. In this section, the scientific process is compared with nursing practice.

Ways of seeking and finding answers and acquiring knowledge in any field include formal and informal classes, clinical experiences, discussions with classmates or expert panels, scientific problem solving, continuing education courses, and research studies relevant to the area of interest. These methods of seeking knowledge have the following common characteristics:

- Identifying what one needs to know or is curious about
- Deciding the approach to seeking the answer
- Devising a plan
- Implementing the plan
- Assessing the evidence

The first step for the practicing nurse is to assess a problem; for the researcher, the first step is to recognize the general problem area. The next step for the practicing nurse is to make a nursing diagnosis, and defining the specific problem is the second step in the research process. The clinical nurse then proceeds with planning and intervention, whereas the researcher proposes hypotheses, tests these hypotheses through experimental and nonexperimental approaches, and manages data. In the final step, the clinician evaluates outcomes; the researcher analyzes the data collected and disseminates the findings in relation to the patterns uncovered.

Nurses can become involved in research and research use in several ways. As "research users," staff nurses can use the nursing process framework to begin to formulate and answer questions they encounter in clinical settings and to seek out research-based information that is relevant to their practice. Such behavior encourages the nurse and others to improve the nursing care delivered, with the presumed outcome of improved patient care. Another way to become involved in research is to be a research subject or a data collector for another person's research project. As "research creators," nurses can conduct research in their practice area by actively designing and implementing research studies, with guidance from others skilled in research methods (LoBiondo-Wood & Haber, 2013).

Historical Appreciation of Nursing Research

Appreciation of the place of research in professional nursing has grown significantly. Nursing research has been an integral part of the profession since Florence Nightingale documented the care of soldiers in the Crimean War. Her careful statistical records are a model for nurses and social scientists alike (Nies & McEwen, 2014).

LoBiondo-Wood and Haber (2013), Nieswiadomy (2011), and Polit and Beck (2011) identified several historical events that have been key to developments in nursing research. Between 1900 and 1940, research in nursing centered on education, methods of teaching, and methods of evaluating how nurses learned. During and after World War II, research interest turned to supply and demand for nurses as the need for nurses to serve in both the military and civilian sectors increased.

More master's programs in nursing emerged in the 1950s. True to the emerging scientific focus, most programs included courses on research methods. Increased federal funding enabled nurses to continue these studies. Publications of nursing research became more common. The journal *Nursing Research* began publishing the results of studies by individuals and schools of nursing. At about the same time, a 5-year research project sponsored by the ANA focused on nurses' activities and functions.

Federal funding for graduate study and research expanded in the 1960s, enabling many baccalaureate-prepared nurses to continue with graduate education. At that time, the federally funded Nurse Scientist Training Program provided support for nurses to obtain doctorates (PhDs) in allied fields such as anthropology and psychology because few nursing PhD programs existed at that time (Abhdellah, 1969; Hutchinson, 2001; Murphy, 1981). Dr. Madeleine Leininger was a leading example of a noted nurse scholar who received such a doctoral degree (anthropology) during that era (Cameron & Luna, 2005).

The nursing profession was strengthened with the development of conceptual frameworks (early stages of theory development wherein interrelated concepts help shape the proposed research) and the use of the scientific method in nursing practice. Nursing organizations established priorities for research investigations. Such research endeavors led to improvements in the quality and specificity of nursing care.

With the base of nurses prepared at the master's level, rapid growth in nursing research continued during the 1970s and 1980s. In 1969, Dr. Moyra Allen of McGill University started the first Canadian nursing research journal, titled *Nursing Papers* (later renamed the *Canadian Journal of Nursing Research*). Three more journals of nursing research were born in the 1970s: *Advances in Nursing Science*, *Research in Nursing and Health*, and *Western Journal of Nursing Research*. In 1981, the ANA Commission on Nursing Research recommended further research in areas of health promotion, illness prevention, cost-effective healthcare, and nursing care for high-risk

patients. Researchers also examined the conceptual frameworks that were offered in the 1960s and 1970s.

In a 1983 study, the Institute of Medicine (IOM) urged the federal government to increase the level of funding for nursing research. As a result, the National Institute of Nursing Research (NINR) was established under the National Institutes of Health (NIH). The institute's purpose was to place nursing securely in the sphere of scientific investigation and to support research and training in patient care, health promotion, and disease prevention as well as the mitigation of effects of acute and chronic disabilities. The NINR has continued to fund and support nursing research and is instrumental in the support and dissemination of seminal work in nursing (National Institute of Nursing Research, 2006).

Groups began to establish priorities in nursing research during the 1980s (Polit & Beck, 2011). In 1985, the American Nurses Association Cabinet on Nursing Research identified 11 priorities for nursing research (Box 8-2) (American Nurses Association Cabinet on Nursing Research, 1985). *Applied*

BOX 8-2   Eleven Priorities for Nursing Research

1. Promote health, well-being, and ability to care for one-self among all age, social, and cultural groups.
2. Minimize or prevent behaviorally and environmentally induced health problems that compromise the quality of life and reduce productivity.
3. Minimize the negative effects of new health technologies on the adaptive abilities of individuals and families experiencing acute or chronic health problems.
4. Ensure that the care needs of particularly vulnerable groups, such as the elderly, children with congenital health problems, individuals from diverse cultures, those who are mentally ill, and the poor, are met in effective and acceptable ways.
5. Classify nursing practice phenomena.
6. Ensure that principles of ethics guide nursing research.
7. Develop instruments to measure nursing outcomes.
8. Develop integrative methodologies for the holistic study of human beings as they relate to their families and lifestyles.
9. Design and evaluate alternative models for delivering healthcare and for administering healthcare systems so that nurses will be able to balance high quality and cost-effectiveness when meeting the nursing needs of identified populations.
10. Evaluate the effectiveness of alternative approaches to nursing education for the kind of practice that requires broad knowledge and a wide repertoire of skills and for the kind of practice that requires specialized knowledge and a focused set of skills.
11. Identify and analyze historical and contemporary factors that influence the shaping of nursing professionals' involvement in national health policy development.

From American Nurses Association Cabinet on Nursing Research. (1985). *Directions for nursing research: Toward the twenty-first century*. Kansas City, MO: American Nurses Association, with permission.

Nursing Research, a journal with studies related to the practice of nursing, was established in 1988. The various nursing theories developed in the 1970s and 1980s offered different lenses for critiquing and interpreting the different kinds of evidence necessary for theory-guided, evidence-based holistic nursing practice (Fawcett, Watson, Neuman, Walker, & Fitzpatrick, 2001).

In the early years of the 21st century, a heightened focus on EBP has developed, which relies on research findings to inform nursing practice (Polit & Beck, 2011). An outstanding resource for evidence-based practice reports that are pertinent to nursing practice is the database maintained by the US government's Agency for Healthcare Research and Quality (AHRQ), which can be accessed at this link: http://www.ahrq.gov/research/findings/evidence-based-reports/a-z/index.html. This type of inquiry implementation into practice, also referred to as "translational research," will be explored in greater depth later in this chapter.

Characteristics of Nursing Research

Traditionally, nursing has been concerned with the whole person, not just the individual "parts." This style has its proponents and detractors. When nurses conduct research, they tend to focus on the physiologic, psychological, sociologic, cultural, and economic factors that affect a person. They view the situation from a nursing perspective and ask questions about what they see. Diers (1979) listed four properties of nursing research and how to maintain a holistic perspective:

1. The focus of nursing research must be on a variance that makes a difference in improving patient care.
2. Nursing research has the potential for contributing to the development of theory and the body of scientific nursing knowledge.

3. A research problem is a nursing research problem when nurses have access to and control over the phenomena being studied.
4. A nurse interested in research must have an inquisitive, curious, and questioning mind.

Methods of Nursing Research

There are three main methods of research. Two broad approaches to research are quantitative and **qualitative research**. A third approach, **mixed methods**, uses both quantitative and qualitative approaches to research inquiry. Key to the combination is integrating the two forms of data collected to illuminate research findings. The assumption in this approach is by examining two sets of data, the results will yield a more complex level of understanding (Clark & Creswell, 2011).

Quantitative research involves the systematic collection of measurable numeric data, usually under conditions of considerable control, and the analysis of that information using statistical procedures. This type of research seeks to test theories and hypotheses.

Qualitative research involves the systematic collection and analysis of more subjective narrative data, using procedures in which there tends to be a minimum of researcher-imposed control (Polit & Beck, 2011). In general, these data can be observed but not measured. Some types of qualitative research, such as grounded theory, explore social processes, and the data that are generated lead to the development of midrange theory rather than testing existing theory (Richards & Morse, 2012). Quantitative researchers tend to use deductive reasoning, logic, and measurable attributes of human experience, whereas qualitative researchers tend to use dynamic, descriptive individual aspects of the human experience in a holistic approach (Table 8-2). Both methods have strengths and weaknesses and specific applications.

TABLE 8-2 COMPARISON OF QUANTITATIVE AND QUALITATIVE RESEARCH

	Quantitative Research	Qualitative Research
Focus	Focuses on few specific concepts in order to elucidate cause-and-effect relationships.	Tends to be holistic; striving for an understanding of the whole.
Initial Concept	Begins with concepts that are fairly well developed, about which there is an existing body of literature and reliable methods of measurement that have been (or can be) developed.	Begins with intent to thoroughly describe and explain a phenomenon, often because some aspect is poorly understood.
Method	Guided by research hypotheses; uses formal protocols to collect data.	Requires the researcher to become the instrument; data are collected in real-world, naturalistic settings.
Controls	Confounding subject characteristics need to be controlled for findings to be interpretable.	Researcher rarely controls or manipulates any aspect of the people or environment under study.
Objectivity Versus Subjectivity	Values objectivity and attempts to hold personal beliefs and biases in check in order to avoid contaminating the phenomena under study.	Sees reality not as a fixed entity but as existing in a context and that many constructions of this reality are possible. Subjective interactions are viewed as the primary way to access understanding of the phenomena.
Analysis	Uses statistical procedures to organize, interpret, and communicate numerical information.	Using creativity and intuition, researchers put together an array of data from many sources to arrive a holistic understanding on a phenomenon.

Source: Polit, D. F., & Beck, C. T. (2011). *Nursing research: Principles and Methods* (9th ed.). Philadelphia, PA: Wolters Kluwer/Lippincott Williams & Wilkins.

THE RESEARCH PROCESS

An understanding of the process that researchers use is essential for beginning practitioners and users of nursing or evidence-based research. Understanding the process helps nurses judge the appropriateness of the research presented and allows them to apply the findings to clinical situations. The process of research forms the underpinnings of the nursing profession and will be used throughout one's professional career. The steps summarized here are universal for all professions that use research as their base.

Problem Area Identification

Practical experience, scientific literature, and untested theories or theories with limited testing influence the development of a research idea. Clinical practice can provide numerous opportunities to piece together observations that may lead to a problem for research. Every day, the practical experience and puzzlement of nurses can lead to questions that need to be solved. The nurses note the differences in methods and speculate about other factors that might contribute to the ultimate adoption of the current protocol.

The PICO model is a widely used mnemonic in EBP that will help you formulate good clinical **foreground questions** (Box 8-3). Foreground questions are those that are specific to a particular patient. PICO will also help you determine key words that can help narrow your literature search and find the information you need. First, you must identify the clinical question of concern in the care of a given patient. Next, you must locate in the nursing literature all relevant evidence supporting an answer to the question. As mentioned earlier in this chapter, PICO will be featured in this eighth edition.

For example, Federwisch, Ramos, and Adams (2014) evaluated the application of an aviation industry rule (the "sterile cockpit" approach that forbids nonessential conversation and activities during takeoff, landing, and taxiing) to medication administration, with the intent of reducing medication errors. Nursing concerns for patient safety, and reimbursement implications of zero tolerance of certain critical errors, can spur this type of research (Sack, 2008).

Evidence-based studies of "how we think, feel and behave profoundly influence the onset of some diseases, the progression of many and the management of nearly all" (Institute for the Future, 2003, p. 194). Taking the opportunity to question and investigate can lead to problem identification and research-based practice. For example, when investigating feelings and behaviors, Schuster, Bornovalova, and Hunt (2012) found relationships among comorbid depression, risky sexual behaviors, and HIV progression.

Nurses can work together to design and implement different methods for investigating such problems. Every day can be a revelation of problem area identification if the nurse is constantly questioning and linking events and observations.

BOX 8-3   PICO

P—stands for the *patient* or problem and its delineation
I—signifies the *intervention* considered
C—denotes *comparison* if appropriate, or it may be optional
O—represents the *outcome* of interest or relevant outcomes

Example

Your patient is a 72-year-old woman with osteoarthritis of the knees and moderate hypertension. She is accompanied by her daughter, a lab tech from the hospital. The daughter wants you to give her mother a prescription for one of the new cyclooxygenase-2 (COX-2) inhibitors for her osteoarthritis. She has heard that they cause less gastrointestinal (GI) bleeding. Her mother is concerned that the new drugs will mean more out-of-pocket costs each month.

	P	I	C	O
	72-year-old woman with osteoarthritis of the knee and moderate hypertension	COX-2 inhibitor	Other NSAIDs	Less GI bleeding; pain control
Key words/phrases for search terms include the following:	Adult Osteoarthritis Older adults	COX-2	NSAIDs	More effective in reducing osteoarthritis pain
Formulating your question:	*Background question:* What are effective pain medications given to osteoarthritis patients? *Foreground question:* In a 72-year-old woman with osteoarthritis of the knee, can COX-2 inhibitor use decrease the risk of GI bleeding compared with other NSAIDs?			

Source: Evidence Based Practice, University of Washington. (2014). *PICO.* Retrieved February 5, 2015 from http://libguides.hsl.washington.edu/content.php?pid=231619&sid=1931590; *and* Formulating answerable research questions. Retrieved June 17, 2014 from http://ktclearinghouse.ca/cebm/practise/formulate/

Review of Scientific Literature

Literature review is the process of selecting published materials that have relevance to the potential research. Doing such a review helps the researcher find out what is already known about the subject and prevents duplication of effort if the subject is already well studied. In addition, it helps illuminate what gaps in knowledge exist in the subject area and can point the way for new research directions. These materials can be research or evidence based, or they may be anecdotal (short, written experiences and impressions that convey a greater understanding of a problem but are not considered research literature). Such materials contribute to and substantiate a summary of the concepts to be studied.

Untested theories are good starts for nursing research. A classic example is Haase's (1987) study of critically ill adolescents using a "courage" theory. The study gave insight into this special population and served to further develop a knowledge base surrounding adolescent care. Research interviews can help researchers understand people's responses to illness or a particular diagnosis because it allows the participant to tell his or her story with minimal interruption by the researcher (Richards & Morse, 2012). The work of Majumdar, Browne, Roberts, and Carpio (2004) that investigated patient satisfaction with care provided by nurses who had cultural sensitivity training may lead other nurses to examine their desire to increase their own cultural awareness.

Critical appraisal of the scientific literature may lead nurses to speculate about a problem area, particularly if the literature is in conflict or is inconsistent with their own practice. For example, a nurse working in coronary care may read two articles on postoperative pain management after cardiac surgery that suggests two different protocols. The nurse may wonder which of the protocols is more valid. Because of the conflict in the literature, an evaluation of this area may provide the answer.

Literature review must be systematic and exhaustive. Researchers must take a critical, almost dubious, approach to the available material. Research builds on previous work, so an extensive literature review, properly executed, allows researchers to place current ideas in the context of previous work. A complete review also helps develop the conceptual frame of reference for the study. It gives clues on how to study the problem (the **methods**) and suggests instruments that might help.

The literature search can seem overwhelming. Indispensible skills include the ability to identify, locate, and organize pertinent documentation on a particular topic and to critically evaluate the merits of specific research designs (Vance, Talley, Azuero, Pearce, & Christian, 2013). To start, students must know which library sources to use. Books and indexes of journals, reports, the Internet, and abstracts are places to start. Books provide overviews of topics or deal with a specific detailed topic, although they become dated almost as soon as they are published. Bibliographies in books and references lists in articles are valuable because they provide sources for original articles.

Indexes are the gateway to the enormous volume of literature in the health sciences. Indexes such as the *Cumulative Index to Nursing and Allied Health Literature* (CINAHL), *PubMed/Medline, Cochrane Library, Thomson Reuters Web of Science*, and *Google Scholar* are valuable. Such data sources are primarily available online through university libraries and may be available in print; consult a librarian for details.

Continuously growing as a resource for nursing research is the Internet, a global directory of commercial, educational, and governmental agencies. The Internet has developed into a sophisticated tool in information retrieval and research for the public and for nursing and health professionals. As of June 2014, the Google search terms "nursing sites" returned 115 million "hits" on the Internet. Because of this overwhelming amount of data, researchers need to apply critical thinking skills to evaluate content found on the Internet because not all sources are reliable. Box 8-4 summarizes guidelines commonly provided to university students and research scholars on how to determine if website content is valid, accurate, and reliable. Researchers can narrow their focus to find specific information from online databases such as CINAHL.

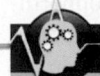

APPLY YOUR CRITICAL THINKING

You are asked to write a sample PICO for your clinical instructor. The patient you have been seeing in your community health rotation has experienced chronic constipation, and during the last visit, she asked you if biofeedback might help and decrease her need for laxatives. You develop the following PICO question to help you establish your search strategy.

Patient / Problem: chronic constipation, female, age 46
Intervention: biofeedback program
Comparison (if any): standard medical care with laxatives at prescribed intervals
Outcome: Patient will achieve satisfactory bowel emptying

Now you are ready to begin your search. What databases will you explore, and how will you limit your search criteria? How will you share this information with your patient after you have researched her problem?

Check your answer in Appendix B.

Theoretical Framework

Nursing science and theory development are being refined. As discussed in Chapter 1, a **theory** is a set of interrelated constructs or propositions that attempts to present or explain some phenomenon systematically. Several nursing theorists have developed models and theories that continue to offer opportunities for testing. The evolving nature of models and theories gives researchers an opportunity to use the work of a nursing theorist to test concepts from that theory for practice application. An example might be a nurse who wants to study Orem's self-care model for patients undergoing ambulatory surgical procedures. The nurse might design a study to investigate factors influencing self-care abilities before and after surgery or self-care practices of homeless children.

The nursing model or theory should be a guide to identify and study systematically the logical relationships between **variables**.

BOX 8-4   Criteria for Evaluating Websites

Authority
- Is the author clearly identified?
- Are the author's credentials listed?
- Is there an institutional affiliation?
- Does the author have standing in the field?
- Can you easily contact the author for clarification of information?
- Is there a non-Web version of the material that might allow you to verify its legitimacy?
- Does the site have an editorial board? Is the information reviewed before it is posted?

Accuracy
- Is the information accurate?
- Does the site offer a selected list of resources that can be consulted to verify accuracy of the document?
- Is the source of information clearly stated?
- Is there an explanation of the research method used to gather data?

Objectivity
- Is the purpose of the site clearly stated?
- Is the information impartially presented?
- Is sponsorship acknowledged? Is there a statement or other evidence to suggest that the document has official approval of a sponsoring institution?
- Does the author's affiliation with this institution suggest any bias?

Coverage
- Who is the intended audience for this document?
- What does the purpose of the article seem to be (e.g., inform, persuade, entertain, etc.)?
- Does the site satisfy the needs of its intended audience?
- Is the subject coverage comprehensive?
- Does the site offer extra features not available in other formats?

Currency
- Is the site current?
- Was the site updated recently?
- Are the links kept up-to-date?

Design
- Is the site clearly organized?
- What is the document's domain (e.g., .com, .edu, .gov, .mil, .net, .org)?
- Is there an internal search engine?
- Is the site user friendly?
- Can the site be accessed reliably?
- Do visual effects enhance the resource?
- Are there options for text only and nonframes views?
- Can the site be accessed without additional viewers or plug-ins?

Source: MedlinePlus. *MedlinePlus guide to healthy web surfing.* Retrieved June 12, 2014 from www.nlm.nih.gov/medlineplus/healthywebsurfing.html

---

Each nursing model depends on the individual researcher's philosophy of human behavior and how that philosophy meshes with other ways of looking at science.

Often, a theoretical framework is likened to an architectural blueprint. These renderings, although not exact models of vision, help the user move from vision to reality. They help nurses further construct theories and distinguish nursing from other disciplines.

Formulation of a Problem Statement

The **problem statement**, a key step in the research process, identifies the direction that a research project will take. As beginning consumers of research literature, nursing students are in a position to evaluate whether the study is a logical extension of the problem. Sometimes, the problem area is not clearly stated and the reader is unsure of the study's direction. The problem statement should be clear and unambiguous, express a relationship between two or more variables, identify the population to be studied, and encourage empiric testing.

The problem statement is introduced early in the research and should reflect a well-defined, specific focus. Stating the problem requires specifying the population to be studied. The researcher states who will be the focus in the problem statement. For instance, the problem statement "Is there a relationship between fathers who have been abused as children and their school-age sons' emergency room records for suspicious injury?" suggests that the populations to be studied are fathers and sons.

The focus is best viewed when the problem has significance for nursing, either directly as with evidence-based research or as a foundation for the development of further research. Research applicable to nursing practice, education, or administration is highly useful to a practice-based profession. That is, the outcomes have the potential for altering nursing practice or protocol and benefiting patients, other nurses, or students. Research that is theoretically relevant is also more useful.

Questions about judgments, ethics, morals, or values are not as amenable to a scientific research process without changing the question. For example, the question "Is it better to tell patients about their diagnosis of terminal cancer or let them discover it themselves?" is impossible to answer. What is meant by "better"? Whose value system is being considered? The study of values has no right answer. If the question were framed differently, it could be researched through clinical inquiry. For instance, a nurse interested in determining how often each method is used could investigate attitudes toward each method.

Proposed Research Questions or Hypotheses

In the problem statement, the relationship is expressed between two or more variables or operationalized concepts. Variables, or properties that vary from each other, are the focus of the study. For example, a researcher studying postoperative patients might be interested in preoperative preparation in relation to the outcome of respiratory function. Variables can be dependent or independent, according to their role in a particular study.

An **independent variable** has the presumed effect on the **dependent variable**. It may be manipulated if the researcher is doing an experimental study; in a nonexperimental study, it is assumed to have occurred naturally before or during the study. The dependent variable is what you believe might be influenced or modified by the independent variable or is the consequence or presumed effect that varies as changes occur in the independent variable. The dependent variable is the one that the researcher is interested in understanding and explaining. For example, a nurse may study the problem that cardiac output measurement (the dependent variable) varies with the temperature of the injectate solution (the independent variable). In this case, the researcher would try to explain the effects of temperature on the measurements (Polit & Beck, 2011).

The final consideration when evaluating a research problem is testability. The problem must be measurable by qualitative or quantitative methods. If the question is posed in such a way that there is a relationship between an independent and a dependent variable and that relationship can be measured, it is likely that the question can be researched.

Data Management: Research Design

Research design is the overall plan for the collection and analysis of the data. The study's design is crucial. If the design can limit the number of research problems before the study, the outcome may be more useful. If an instrument is to be used in a study or a new instrument needs to be developed, a consultant in methods (a methodologist) can alleviate some reliability and validity problems by helping the novice researcher select or develop the instrument.

Because most nursing research occurs outside laboratory settings, researchers must consider the institution's policies, parameters, and constraints. Researchers also must consider the costs of the facility, equipment, and personnel time (Fig. 8-2).

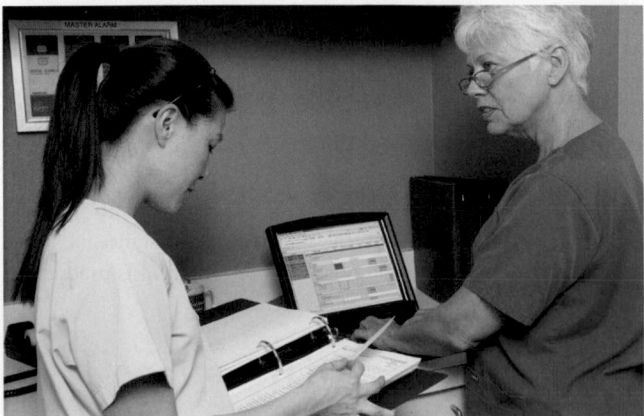

FIGURE 8-2 Nursing research can be time consuming for personnel, and the value of research must be weighed against the cost.

Sometimes, researchers cannot conduct a study because the costs outweigh the benefits. Research involving human subjects also needs approval by institutional review boards (IRBs) before implementation. It is not unusual for more than one IRB to be involved in the research approval process (e.g., a university IRB and a hospital IRB). IRB discussion occurs in more detail later in the chapter.

Analysis of Results

Data are not the final results. They are a raw form of the answer. Reviewers put the data through various types of analysis and interpretation and manage them in an orderly, planned manner. Researchers look for patterns of information. They may analyze this information objectively or subjectively (see Table 8-2) by quantitative or qualitative analysis.

The results must make sense and be consistent with the data; this is part of the responsibility of researchers in interpretation. The implications are examined. The following question is asked: "How do these implications apply in the broader context?" Researchers return to their original question or problem statement and should be able to answer it with the analysis and interpretation of the results. Even findings that yield insignificant results are valuable in that they prompt the researcher to continue to search for the factors that are of significance.

Dissemination of Results

Once the results of a study are determined, the findings must be disseminated so that clinical application or research replication by other nurses can occur. Conclusions are strengthened and validated by similar findings in more than one research study.

Findings can be disseminated by oral and poster presentations at research meetings or in print through research and clinical journals. Presentations and publication of the results of studies allow other nurses interested in improving nursing practice to act on the findings. Nurses may adopt the findings for their clinical practice. A nurse acquainted with the original research may choose to do the same study but with a different group of study subjects or subjects in another clinical area. Others may extend the same study or stop using a clinical procedure or therapy that has shown little or no merit.

A bonus of presenting the results at meetings or publishing them may be that the researcher will meet other nurses with similar interests. This practice, called **networking**, is a good way to disseminate and expand one's knowledge. Examples of research meetings that allow networking opportunities and dissemination of scholarly findings include the annual Western Institute of Nursing (WIN), held at rotating sites in the western United States, and the Sigma Theta Tau State of the Science Congress on Nursing Research. Nurses from all educational backgrounds and experience benefit from attendance at these types of meetings.

Translation to Practice

As stated previously in this chapter, translational research is the bridge between theory and practice. It forms the foundation for evidence-based protocols and interventions that increase the quality of nursing care and improve patient outcomes. As an example of the value of this type of research, Lin (2013) describes how these methods are the key in greatly reducing the many decades that it can take to implement interventions in healthcare by distilling knowledge gained in practice-based research through translational methods. Furthermore, Christian (2012) points out that excellence in nursing care is created by the translation of research evidence into clinical best practice guidelines. EBP is an outcome of translational research. The goal of EBP is to provide patients with the highest quality individualized care based upon thorough assessment and history taking, sound research evidence, clinical proficiency, and information from the patient on values and care preference to ensure favorable outcomes (Melnyk & Fineout-Overholt, 2015). A relevant example would be the unfortunate news that a loved one at a recent checkup was discovered to have cancer. In this case, the family members would certainly want the care provider for this person to base clinical decisions on the best supporting evidence for treatment options.

Nurses must critique evidence and integrate the best evidence into the care of the patient. Articles on evidence assessment to assist in the critiquing process include the American Association of Critical-Care Nurses' levels of evidence model to guide adoption of best evidence for practice (Peterson, Barnason, Donnelly, Hill, Miley, et al., 2014) and the Association of periOperative Registered Nurses (AORN)'s model for evidence rating (Spruce, Van Wicklin, Hicks, Conner, & Dunn, 2014). The last step in the process is the evaluation of the care decision based on data gathered from this best evidence (Melnyk & Fineout-Overholt, 2015). Although the concept of EBP is still evolving, all facets of the healthcare team should make strides toward implementation of this process into patient care, with the goal of ensuring optimal patient care outcomes (Steinberg & Luce, 2005).

ETHICAL AND LEGAL ISSUES

Ethical and legal issues related to the research process continually arise. The primary issue is that of "human rights" or "subject rights." In the past, research has been conducted without proper consent or any consent from the participants. There has been an evolution of ethical principles in nursing, as in all research projects. The five rights outlined in 1985 by the ANA human rights guidelines—self-determinism, privacy and dignity, anonymity and confidentiality, fair treatment, and protection from discomfort and harm—apply to all people involved in research projects and continue to be the standard today.

Institutional Review Boards

The passing of the 1974 National Research Act required any agency applying for funding for any project involving biomedical or behavioral research on humans to submit assurances that it had an IRB to look over the research and protect the rights of human subjects. This act resulted from Senate hearings on the Tuskegee Syphilis Study, in which unknowing, infected, and relatively powerless research subjects (who had been recruited by deceptive means) were deliberately denied treatment for 40 years to allow researchers to study the effects of the disease (Emanuel & Grady, 2007; Polit & Beck, 2011). At agencies where the government has not awarded federal money, a review mechanism, similar to the IRB, usually is present.

Nurse researchers need to apply to the appropriate IRB for approval before starting their research. The application includes a detailed plan for data collection, secure storage and analysis, and the proposed consent form. Full board review is required if the target population is deemed particularly vulnerable, such as with children and cognitively impaired prisoners (Miser, 2005).

ETHICAL/LEGAL ISSUES

RESEARCH STUDIES ON HUMAN SUBJECTS

Three years ago, Michael Thomas, a 29-year-old accountant, received a diagnosis of HIV infection. Over the past few months, his diagnosis has progressed into AIDS, with the appearance of some related cancers. He has been admitted to the hospital to participate in a research program that is studying new drugs to treat AIDS-related cancers. His partner is trying to talk him out of participating, knowing that this type of drug trial is a "double-blind" study, in which Michael may receive a placebo rather than the drug. The research team is encouraging Michael to participate in the study.

When you enter the room to check on Michael, he appears distraught and upset. He says to you, "I don't know what to do. I know this drug trial may be my best chance of living, but I don't want to upset my partner. Can you help me be sure that I get selected for the trial drug and not the placebo?"

REFLECTION

- Review Chapter 7 about informed consent and information in this chapter about the protection of human subjects. What information might apply to the above scenario?
- Reflect on your feelings in this situation and identify them.
- Articulate your role as a nurse providing care and as a nurse assisting in a research project.
- Think about the ways in which you might respond to this situation. Identify possible approaches.

BOX 8-5   Articles of the Nuremberg Tribunal Related to Ethical, Moral, and Legal
Concepts for the Conduct of Experiments

- The voluntary consent of the human subject is absolutely essential.
- The experiment should be such as to yield fruitful results for the good of society, unprocurable by other means of study, and not random and unnecessary in nature.
- The experiment should be so designed and based on the results of animal experimentation and knowledge of the natural history of the disease or other problems under study that the anticipated results will justify the performance of the experiment.
- The experiment should be conducted to avoid all unnecessary physical and mental suffering and injury.
- No experiment should be conducted where there is a prior reason to believe that death or disabling injury will occur.
- The degree of risk to be taken should never exceed that determined by the humanitarian importance of the problem to be solved by the experiment.

- Proper preparations should be made and adequate facilities provided to protect the subject against injury, disability, or death.
- The experiment should be conducted only by scientifically qualified persons.
- The human subject should be at liberty to bring the experiment to an end.
- During the experiment, the scientist, if he or she has probable cause to believe that a continuation of the experiment is likely to result in injury, disability, or death to the experiment subject, will bring it to a close.

Reprinted with permission from Shuster, E. (1997). Fifty years later: The significance of the nuremberg code. *The New England Journal of Medicine, 337*, 1436–1440. DOI: 10.1056/NEJM199711133372006

Why are IRBs necessary? After World War II, the Nuremberg military tribunal was charged with prosecuting Nazis who had performed biomedical research on concentration camp prisoners. Because the tribunal had no measures against which to test the defendants, a set of basic principles of ethical, moral, and legal concepts for the conduct of acceptable experiments had to be written (Trials of war criminals before the Nuremberg military tribunals under Control Council Law No. 10, 1949–1953). The articles of the Nuremberg tribunal are listed in Box 8-5.

Subject Rights

The first statement of the Nuremberg Code, developed in 1949, addresses the rights of research subjects. Voluntary consent; the right to withdraw from investigations at any time without penalty; the protection from physical and mental suffering, injury, disability, and death; and a balance between benefits and risks are paramount. Nursing researchers must provide the following information to human subjects (Commission on Nursing Research, 1981; Polit & Beck, 2011):

- An explanation of the study in lay language rather than technical terms
- A clear distinction between research activities and treatment activities
- A description of what type of data will be collected
- The procedures to be followed and their purposes
- Information on the nature of the commitment, such as estimated time commitment and number of contacts
- Information on who is sponsoring or funding the research and if the research is part of an academic commitment
- A discussion of how prospective participants were chosen for recruitment (this is known as "inclusion criteria")
- Discussion of potential risks and benefits
- Alternatives for prospective participants, such as alternative treatments or procedures to the ones included in the study

- Compensation, if stipends or reimbursements are to be paid
- A clear statement that participation in the study is strictly voluntary and that the failure to volunteer will not result in loss of benefits or penalty
- The right to withdraw at any time and the right to refuse to provide specific pieces of information, even after the consenting process
- A clear description of physical and mental discomforts, any invasion of privacy, and any threat to dignity
- The methods used to protect anonymity and ensure confidentiality
- Contact information on who can be contacted by the participant in the event of comments, complaints, or questions

These provisions may seem obvious, but before 1974, several human research studies were conducted in the United States that probably would not be allowed today. During that era, the judgment of the caring and compassionate researcher, it was argued, was more important than informed consent—a position founded on the assumption that researchers were concerned about the participants' well-being and wished to protect them (Emanuel & Grady, 2007). However, subjects of some studies underwent unethical experimental procedures, including sterilization, euthanasia, injection with live cancer cells, and the withholding of treatment for syphilis (Diers, 1979; LoBiondo-Wood & Haber, 2013). The ethical principles of autonomy, beneficence, and justice serve as guides in maintaining the rights of research participants when the specific goals of research projects are determined (Polit & Beck, 2011).

Patients involved in research must be assured that their privacy is being protected. Privacy is protected in two general ways. **Anonymity** is the protection of the subject so that not even the researcher can link the subject to the information provided. **Confidentiality** ensures that the subjects' identities will not be linked with the information they provide and will not be publicly divulged.

Furthermore, in 1996, the US federal government enacted the Health Insurance Portability and Accountability Act (HIPAA). A key federal regulation covered under HIPAA is the Privacy Rule that outlines the handling of protected health information (PHI) by certain healthcare groups. The Privacy Rule pertains to those who conduct research in that it outlines the rules for the usage and access to PHI when conducting research (NIH, 2007). Nursing researchers must familiarize themselves with HIPAA and the Privacy Rule to ensure that they are following federal guidelines and must include with their IRB application the HIPAA form authorizing sharing of information. Similarly, in Canada, federal and provincial regulations have been established to control access to personal health information.

Although students may have few opportunities to seek or to obtain informed consent from people selected as potential subjects of research, students may have a role in data collection or may provide medications or treatments in a research study. The role that nurses or students are to play in research studies must be clarified with involved faculty members and the research team. Any educational institution will have an IRB for their faculty and student projects involving human subjects. Ask your research faculty or research dean about how your school's IRB works.

RESEARCH AND THE PROFESSIONAL NURSE

Levels of Nursing Participation

Some nurses may think mistakenly that they have little to contribute to research. Nurses actually have a great deal to contribute by observing patient responses to treatments and techniques. A nurse with several years of clinical experience in a particular unit may generate many unanswered questions. He or she would be in a position to initiate research with a skilled researcher or would be valuable in assisting with patient management or data collection in someone else's research project.

The education of nurses who are in advanced practice usually emphasizes clinically relevant research. In the practice arena, they can do their own research, act as consultants to novice researchers, and collaborate with other healthcare professionals on more complex patient situations. For example, a clinical specialist in oncology may collaborate with a clinical psychologist to study stressors of pain or side effects related to therapy.

The ANA's Commission on Nursing Education has developed guidelines for the investigative function of nurses (Box 8-6).

BOX 8-6   Guidelines for Investigative Function of Nurses

Associate Degree in Nursing
The nurse:
- Demonstrates awareness of the value or relevance of research in nursing
- Assists in identifying problem areas in nursing practice
- Assists in collection of data within an established, structured format

Baccalaureate Degree in Nursing
The nurse:
- Reads, interprets, and evaluates research for applicability to nursing practice
- Identifies nursing problems that need to be investigated and participates in implementation of scientific studies
- Uses nursing practice as a means of gathering data for refining and extending practice
- Applies established findings of nursing and other health-related research to nursing practice
- Shares research finding with colleagues

Master's Degree in Nursing
The nurse:
- Analyzes and reformulates nursing practice problems so that scientific knowledge and scientific methods can be used to find solutions
- Enhances the quality and clinical relevance of nursing research by providing expertise in clinical problems and by providing knowledge about the way in which these clinical services are delivered
- Facilitates investigation of problems in clinical settings through such activities as contributing to a climate supportive of investigative activities, collaborating with others in investigations, and enhancing nursing's access to patients and data
- Conducts investigations for the purpose of monitoring the quality of the practice of nursing in a clinical setting
- Assists others to apply scientific knowledge in nursing practice

Doctoral Degree in Nursing or Related Discipline
The graduate of a practice-oriented doctoral program:
- Provides leadership for the integration of scientific knowledge with other sources of knowledge for the advancement of practice
- Conducts investigations to evaluate the contribution of nursing activities to the well-being of patients
- Develops methods to monitor the quality of the practice of nursing in a clinical setting and to evaluate contributions of nursing activities to the well-being of patients

The graduate of a research-oriented doctoral program:
- Develops theoretical explanations of phenomena relevant to nursing by empirical research and analytical processes
- Uses analytic and empirical methods to discover ways to modify or extend existing scientific knowledge so it is relevant to nursing
- Develops methods for scientific inquiry of phenomena relevant to nursing

  This language was developed as a part of the work of the ANA Commission on Nursing Education and was included in the report of that commission to the 1980 ANA House of Delegates.

Source: Commission on Nursing Research. (1981). *Guidelines for the investigative function of nurses.* Kansas City, MO: Author.

These standards give information about how different educational levels may enhance the research contributions that nurses can make.

Clinical Nursing Practice

CLINICAL RESEARCH

The problem-solving methods that nurses use can help practicing nurses translate clinical problems into research projects. Nurses in clinical areas regularly raise questions that could be considered researchable. Because of daily interactions with patients, nurses have the opportunity to solve problems but, in the strict sense, do not research nursing questions.

Patient care informed by research findings allows nurses to define and seek solutions to various problems. Nurses interested in research, use of observation skills, discussions with colleagues, and personal clinical experience can learn to organize priorities and offer patients the most efficient and timely care. One example of using research in this way is for psychiatric nurses to be aware of the advances in drug therapy, such as the use of aripiprazole, and incorporate this knowledge into patient education and advocacy (Berman et al., 2007).

Nurse researchers use techniques similar to those they developed first as students and then refined as skilled clinicians. Nurse researchers broaden the area of study and try to discover various conditions (variables) that affect the situation. For example, a nurse in the neonatal unit might be concerned with the temperature balance of newborns receiving phototherapy for physiologic jaundice. The researcher recognizes that to study this problem, the related fields of physical thermodynamics and developmental physiology must be investigated. The researcher also needs to investigate the placement of temperature probes, site selection, nurse technique, and the soundness of previous research.

Nurse researchers recognize the need to consult other experts and to consider other organizational patterns. Recruitment of research team members who are skilled in particular areas, such as statisticians, ensures that the results will be more useful and gives the design and statistical analysis more merit.

Multidisciplinary Clinical Research

No one discipline can provide the breadth of evidence needed for EBP. The Agency for Health Care Policy and Research (AHCPR) was established in December 1989 under Public Law 101–239 (Omnibus Budget Reconciliation Act of 1989) and was reauthorized on December 6, 1999, as the Agency for Healthcare Research and Quality (AHRQ). The AHRQ, a part of the U.S. Department of Health and Human Services, functions as the lead agency charged with supporting research designed to improve the quality, safety, efficiency, and effectiveness of healthcare for all Americans (National Archives, 2014). The AHRQ's broad programs of research, including nursing research, bring practical, science-based information to healthcare practitioners and to consumers and other healthcare purchasers. The findings of studies across disciplines are combined to pro-

vide guidelines for clinical care, including guidelines for therapies for practitioners, as well as education guides for patients.

AHRQ is playing a leading role in tracking health care cost savings and reduction in mortality in areas related to patient safety. For example, from 2010 to 2013, AHRQ determined that efforts on the part of U.S. hospitals to reduce hospital-acquired conditions (HAC's) resulted in approximately 50,000 fewer deaths in the hospital, and saved approximately $12 billion in healthcare costs (Agency for Health Care Research and Quality, 2014).

An interesting approach to evaluating health care costs is the association between place of residence and utilization rates, as discussed by Gawande (2011) and mapped by such states as Massachusetts (Prevention and Wellness Advisory Board: An overview of health care costs for chronic conditions in Massachusetts, 2013). Analysis of these correlations allows for targeted implementation of services to reduce utilization rates of such costly services as emergency rooms and inpatient care. This blending of the science of geography and the science of health care allows for new knowledge and interventions connected to chronic health care to emerge.

Applying Research to Practice

Direct research, except in the role of data collection or administration of medications and treatments as a protocol in a research project, usually does not involve student nurses and novice nurses. Even with limited direct participation in research, novice nurses should be consumers of research. They can read research literature applicable to the practice setting and attempt to evaluate it or use it in clinical practice after collaboration with more expert practitioners. For novice nurses, the ability to read articles carefully and critically is important. Coughlin, Cronin, and Ryan (2007) offer a checklist designed to help nurses with varying skills critique reported quantitative research studies.

Through the teaching and learning process in basic nursing education, new nurses can be exposed to evidence-based nursing care practice. Analysis of the material learned does not necessarily mean finding flaws and faults. It is the conscious decision to undertake an objective and careful evaluation of the research project in light of how practicing nurses, working directly with patients or a patient population, would be able to use this knowledge. Knowing that the "answers" are not always known, the nurse is wise to keep learning and being aware that every day, new practices could be employed with knowledge gained through research and new evidence. The thrust to use more EBP should lead to better outcomes for all consumers (Polit & Beck, 2011). Practitioners need skills and resources to appraise, synthesize, and use the best evidence for nursing care (Melnyk & Fineout-Overholt, 2015).

After a study or research project has been evaluated, the findings might be used in clinical practice. However, nurses should not assume that just because something has been published, it is appropriate for clinical practice. On the contrary, nurses should view the contents of published studies with some degree of skepticism before adopting them to the clinical setting in which they function, as the research may not be directly applicable to their situation.

Applying research findings to clinical practice has utility. Nurses need to narrow the gap between research and application by selecting useful studies to put into place. The expanding use of community-based nursing and family-centered care offers a completely new area of research. Collaboration between researchers and practitioners will enhance diffusion of EBP (Melnyk & Fineout-Overholt, 2015).

An area of expanding interest in the application of findings to clinical practice is **comparative effectiveness research** (CER). CER is a systematic research design comparing the effectiveness of different interventions. The goal is finding an intervention that is the best for a given patient with specific circumstances. CER must be highly comprehensive and diverse to provide results with such specificity (National Institutes of Health, 2014).

In conjunction with research findings, a planned program of evaluation and implementation will help nurses find appropriate approaches to patient care situations. For example, the journal *Focus on Critical Care* has a column "Research Review" that helps critical care nurses apply relevant research to their practice. Other journals provide similar information.

KEY CONCEPTS

- Expanding nursing's knowledge base is an important goal of nursing research.

- Nursing research is the systematic inquiry into clinical practice problems, modes of patient care, nursing education, and nursing administration.

- The scientific method of research and the nursing process are similar.

- Research is a step-by-step process of defining ideas, reviewing literature, developing a theoretical framework, formulating a problem statement, proceeding with the study, and disseminating findings.

- Nursing research results must be disseminated so that the profession can evaluate and apply the findings.

- Legal and ethical considerations, including the rights of human subjects, anonymity, and confidentiality, are central to any research study.

- Practicing nurses encounter many questions that may be bases for research studies.

PRACTICING FOR THE NCLEX

CHECK YOUR ANSWERS IN APPENDIX A.

1. A nurse is evaluating the medical center's approach to mobilizing secretions in patients with tracheotomies. Which would be the benefit to using EBP? Select all that apply:
    a. EBP is evaluated based on outcome studies.
    b. Practitioner knowledge and personal experience are insufficient.
    c. EBP integrates clinical expertise with external evidence.
    d. Hospitals can utilize experts in their facility.
    e. Provide cost-saving, quality care.

2. Which of the following are ethical and legal issues related to the research process that are evaluated by IRBs? Select all that apply:
    a. Blinded participation
    b. Privacy and dignity
    c. Balance between benefits and risk
    d. Protection from mental and physical suffering

3. Nursing research includes systematic inquiry into which of the following?
    a. Clinical practice
    b. Education
    c. Administration
    d. All of the above

4. Bundling findings to improve care is now a nursing standard in the care of congestive heart failure and has been shown to reduce readmission rates. This is one example of which of the following research aspects?
    a. Qualitative and quantitative data collection
    b. Disseminating research results
    c. Classifying nursing phenomena
    d. Translation of research to practice

5. A nurse is conducting a research study of postoperative pain medications. What should be done first?
    a. Develop a theoretical framework.
    b. Define a hypothesis.
    c. Review the literature.
    d. Gather participants.

REFERENCES

Abhdellah, F. (1969). The nature of nursing science. *Nursing Research, 18*(5), 390–392.

Agency for Health Care Research and Quality. (2014). The role of AHCPR Research. Retrieved June 9, 2014, from http://www.archives.gov/research/guide-fed-records/groups/510.html#510.1

Agency for Healthcare Research and Quality. (2013). Interim update on 2013 annual hospital-acquired condition rate and estimates of cost savings and deaths averted from 2010 to 2013. Retrieved June 17, 2015, from http://www.ahrq.gov/professionals/quality-patient-safety/pfp/interimhacrate2013.pdf

Agency for Healthcare Research and Quality. (2014). AHRQ Profile: Advancing excellence in health care. Retrieved June 17, 2015, from http://www.ahrq.gov/cpi/about/profile/index.html

American Nurses Association Cabinet on Nursing Research. (1985). *Directions for nursing research: Toward the twenty-first century.* Kansas City, MO: American Nurses Association

Auerbach, D. I., Staiger, D. O., Muench, U., & Buerhaus, P. I. (2013). The nursing workforce in an era of health care reform. *New England Journal of Medicine, 368*(16), 1470–1472.

Berman R. M., Marcus R. N., Swanink R., McQuade, R. D., Carson, W. H., Corey-Lisle, P. K., et al. (2007). The efficacy and safety of aripiprazole as adjunctive therapy in major depressive disorder: A multicenter, randomized, double-blind, placebo-controlled study. *Journal of Clinical Psychiatry, 68*(6), 843–853.

Cameron, C., & Luna, L. (2005). Leininger's transcultural nursing. In J. Fitzpatrick & A. Whall (Eds.), *Conceptual models of nursing: Analysis and application* (4th ed., pp. 177–193). Upper Saddle River, NJ: Pearson Prentice Hall.

Centers for Disease Control and Prevention. Epidemiology of measles—United States, 1998. (1999). *MMWR Morbidity and Mortality Weekly Report, 48*, 749–753.

Centers for Disease Control and Prevention. Measles (Rubeola). Retrieved February 5, 2015, from http://www.cdc.gov/measles

Choi, M., Kim, H., Chung, S., Ahn, M., Yoo, J., Park, O., et al. (2014). Evidence-based practice for pain management for cancer patients in an acute care setting. *International Journal of Nursing Practice, 20*, 60–69. DOI: 10.1111-ijn.12122

Christensen, H., & Petrie, K. (2012). Information technology as the key to accelerating advances in mental health care. *Australian & New Zealand Journal of Psychiatry, 47*(2), 114–116.

Christian, B. (2012). Translating research into everyday practice—The essential role of pediatric nurses. *Journal of Pediatric Nursing, 27*(2), 184–185.

Clark, V. L. P., & Creswell, J. W. (2011). *Designing and conducting mixed methods research.* (2nd. ed.). Thousand Oaks, CA: Sage.

The Cochrane Collaboration. (2015). Retrieved June 16, 2015, from http://www.cochrane.org

Commission on Nursing Research. (1981). *Guidelines for the investigative function of nurses.* Kansas City, MO: Author.

Coughlan, M., Cronin, P., & Ryan, F. (2007). Step-by-step guide to critiquing research. Part 1: quantitative research. *British journal of nursing, 16*(11), 658–663.

Crockett, D. (2013). Four essential lessons for adopting predictive analytics in health care. *Health Catalyst.* Retrieved June 9, 2014, from http://www.healthcatalyst.com/predictive-analytics-healthcare-lessons

Diers, D. (1979). *Research in nursing practice.* Philadelphia, PA: J. B. Lippincott.

Douglas, M., Rosenkoetter, M., Pacquiano, D., Callister, L., Hattar-Pollara, M., Lauderdale, J., et al. (2014). Guidelines for implementing culturally competent nursing care. *Journal of Transcultural Nursing, 25*(2):109–121. DOI: 10.1177/1043659614520998. Retrieved June 6, 2014 from http://tcn.sagepub.com/content/early/2014/02/14/1043659614520998

Emanuel, E. J., & Grady, C. (2007). Four paradigms of clinical research and research oversight. *Cambridge quarterly of healthcare ethics, 16*(1), 82–96.

Fawcett, J., Watson, J., Neuman, B., Walker, P. H., & Fitzpatrick, J. J. (2001). On nursing theories and evidence. *Journal of Nursing Scholarship, 33*(2), 115–120.

Federwisch, M., Ramos, H., & Adams, S. (2014). The sterile cockpit: An effective approach to reducing medication errors? *American Journal of Nursing, 114*(2), 47–55.

Ganz, F., Ofra, R, Khalaila, R., Levy, H., Arad, D., Kolpak, O., et al. (2013). Translation of oral care practice guidelines into clinical practice by intensive care nurses. *Journal of Nursing Scholarship, 45*(4), 355–362.

Gawande, A. (2011). *The hot spotters.* The New Yorker. Retrieved June 17, 2015, from http://www.newyorker.com/magazine/2011/01/24/the-hot-spotters

Gortner, S. (1975). Research for a practice profession. *Nursing Research, 24*(6), 193–197.

Haase, J. (1987). The components of courage in chronically ill adolescents. *ANS—Advances in Nursing Science, 9*(2), 64–80.

Immunization of adolescents. Recommendations of the Advisory Committee on Immunization Practices, the American Academy of Pediatrics, the American Academy of Family Physicians, and the American Medical Association. (1996). *MMWR Recommendations and Reports, 45*(RR-13), 1–16.

Institute for the Future. (2003). *Health and health care 2010: The forecast, the challenge* (2nd ed.). Menlo Park, CA: Author.

Kaiser Permanente. (2014). Taking action: Community health initiatives. Retrieved June 9, 2014 from http://share.kaiserpermanente.org/article/evaluation-and-learning/

Krinsky, R., Murillo, I., & Johnson, J. (2014). A practical application of Katharine Kolcaba's comfort theory to cardiac patients. *Applied Nursing Research, 27*(2), 147–150.

Lang, C. (2014). Do sitters prevent falls? A review of the literature. *Journal of Gerontological Nursing, 40*(5), 24–33.

Leape, L., Berwick, D., & Bates, D. (2002). What practices will most improve safety? Evidence-based medicine meets patient safety. *Journal of the American Medical Association, 288*, 501–507.

Lewandowski, W., & Jacobson, A. (2013). Bridging the gap between mind and body: A biobehavioral model of the effects of guided imagery on pain, pain disability, and depression. *Pain Management Nursing, 14*(4), 368–378.

Lin, C. (2013). Why does translational research matter to cancer nursing researchers? *Cancer Nursing, 36*(4), 337–338.LoBiondo-Wood, G., & Haber, J. (2013). *Nursing research: Methods and critical appraisal for evidence-based practice* (8th ed.). St. Louis, MO: Mosby.

Majumdar, B., Browne, G., Roberts, J., & Carpio, B. (2004). Effects of cultural sensitivity training on health care provider attitudes and patient outcomes. *Journal of Nursing Scholarship, 36*(2), 161–166.

Mantzoukas, S., & Jasper, M. (2008). Types of nursing knowledge used to guide care of hospitalized patients. *Journal of Advanced Nursing, 62*(3), 318–326.

Melnyk, B. M., & Fineout-Overholt, E. (2015). *Evidence-based practice in nursing and healthcare* (3rd ed.). Philadelphia, PA: Lippincott Williams & Wilkins.

Memorial Sloan-Kettering Cancer Center. (2010). *Memorial Hospital Research.* Retrieved June 17, 2014, from http://www.mskcc.org/mskcc/html/65977.cfm

Miser, W. (2005). Educational research—to IRB or not to IRB? *Family Medicine, 37*(3), 168–173.

Murphy, F., & Amblum, J. (2014). Treatment of burn blisters: Debride or leave intact? *Emergency Nurse, 22*(2), 24–27.

Murphy, J. (1981). Doctoral education in, of, and for nursing: An historical analysis. *Nursing Outlook, 29*(11), 645–649.

National Archives. (2014). Records of the Agency for Health Care Policy and Research. Retrieved June 9, 2014, from http://www.archives.gov/research/guide-fed-records/groups/510.html#510.1

National Institutes of Health. (2014). Comparative effectiveness research (CER). Retrieved June 13, 2014, from http://www.nlm.nih.gov/hsrinfo/cer.html

National Institutes of Health. (2007). Protecting personal health information in research: Understanding the HIPAA Privacy Rule. Retrieved February 5, 2015, from http://privacyruleandresearch.nih.gov/

National Institute of Nursing Research. (2006). Mission & strategic plan. Retrieved February 5, 2015, from http://www.ninr.nih.gov/aboutninr/ninr-mission-and-strategic-plan#.VNJefPldVu4

Nies, M., & McEwen, M. (2014). *Community/Public health nursing: Promoting the health of populations* (6th ed.). Philadelphia, PA: Saunders.

Nieswiadomy, R. M. (2011). *Foundations in nursing research* (6th ed.). Upper Saddle River, NJ: Pearson Education.

Peterson, M., Barnason, S., Donnelly, B., Hill, K., Miley, H., Riggs, L., et al. (2014). Choosing the best evidence to guide clinical practice: Application of AACN levels of evidence. *Critical Care Nurse, 34*(2), 58–68.

Polit, D. F., & Beck, C. T. (2011). *Nursing research: Principle and methods* (9th ed.). Philadelphia, PA: Wolters Kluwer/Lippincott Williams & Wilkins.

Polit, D. F., & Beck, C. T. (2014). *Essentials of nursing research: Appraising evidence for nursing practice* (4th ed.). Philadelphia, PA: Lippincott Williams & Wilkins.

Richards, M., & Morse, J. (2012). *README FIRST for a user's guide to qualitative methods* (3rd ed.). Thousand Oaks, CA: Sage Publications.

Sack, K. (2008). Medicare won't pay for medical errors. *New York Times.* Retrieved June 17, 2014, from www.nonprofithealthcare.org/archives/Medicare_001.pdf

Schuster, R., Bornovalova, M. & Hunt, E. (2011). The influence of depression on the progression of HIV: Direct and indirect effects. *Behavior Modification, 36*(2), 123–145.

Shuster, E., (1997). Fifty years later: The significance of the nuremberg code. *The New England Journal of Medicine, 337*, 1436–1440. DOI: 10.1056/NEJM199711133372006

Spruce, L. Van Wicklin, S., Hicks, R., Conner, R., & Dunn, D. (2014). Introducing AORN's new model for evidence rating. *AORN Journal, 99*(2), 243–255. DOI: 10.1016/j.aorn.2013.11.014

Taylor, J., McDonald, S., & Tan, K. (2014). A survey of central venous catheter practices in Australian and New Zealand tertiary neonatal units. *Australian Critical Care, 27*(1), 36–42.

Trials of war criminals before the Nuremberg military tribunals under Control Council Law No. 10. (1949–1953). Washington, DC: U.S. Government Printing Office.

Vance, D., Talley, M., Azuero, A., Pearce, P., & Christian, B. (2013). Conducting an article critique for a quantitative research study: Perspectives for doctoral students and other novice readers. *Nursing: Research and Reviews, 3*, 67–75.

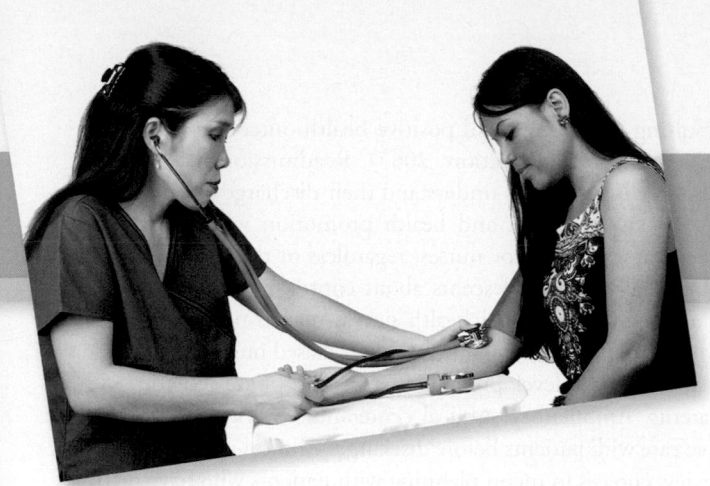

CHAPTER 9

Patient Education and Health Promotion

Deborah D. Kelly

Case Scenario

Mrs. Hussein, accompanied by her husband, comes to the clinic for a blood pressure check. As they enter the office, you hear the husband speaking rapidly in a foreign language. He appears upset. The wife does not respond but looks down and appears to withdraw. Because her blood pressure is elevated for the second consecutive visit, the physician decides to prescribe a blood pressure medication and a low-sodium diet. As the office nurse, you have 15 minutes to teach the couple about hypertension and its management.

Once you have completed this chapter and have incorporated patient education and health promotion into your knowledge base, review the above scenario, and reflect on the following areas of Critical Thinking:

1. Prioritize important assessment data to collect from the couple so you can determine their readiness to learn and individualize your health promotion teaching.
2. Describe factors that might hinder or facilitate the couple's learning.
3. Role-play how you might individualize teaching, focusing on three realistic goals.
4. Identify how you will evaluate learning and use your findings to revise future teaching.

KEY TERMS
adherence
affective
cognitive
compliance
disease prevention activities
health literacy
health promotion
health promotion activities
health protection activities
learning
motivation
motivational interviewing
noncompliance
psychomotor
return demonstration
role-playing
simulation
teach-back
telehealth

LEARNING OBJECTIVES

Upon completion of this chapter, the student will be able to do the following:

1. Describe important qualities of a teaching–learning relationship.
2. Explain the domains of knowledge and how learning relates to each.
3. Identify four purposes of patient education.
4. Define factors that inhibit and facilitate learning.
5. Discuss important assessment data used to individualize patient teaching.
6. Describe individualized teaching methods and evaluation strategies for patients of different ages or abilities.
7. Give examples of health promotion and disease prevention behaviors.
8. Recognize major factors that affect motivation and health maintenance.

Patient education has been an important function of nursing practice since the days of Florence Nightingale. Empowering patients and their families with knowledge about their health improves clinical outcomes and health. Patient education is aimed at assisting patients to gain skills and knowledge to promote and maintain their health. The focus of, and activities related to, patient education have changed over time. Historically, healthcare professionals viewed patients as passive receivers of care, where education meant telling patients what to do. Patient education has moved beyond this approach; the current mind-set is that it is essential to involve patients in decisions about their health to develop a plan that fits with the patient's values and healthcare goals. Patient education plans are individualized to align with the abilities, preferences, and life circumstances of each person. Today's patients are more likely to be active participants in the decision making about their care and treatment. Patients and their families work collaboratively with healthcare professionals to achieve their healthcare goals. This collaborative teaching–learning process empowers patients to achieve increased wellness through health promotion activities or to manage specific healthcare needs. Nurses are often the primary teachers, as well as coordinators of information from other healthcare professionals, for patients.

Patient and family education is an integral part of any comprehensive healthcare delivery system. The American Hospital Association created a plain language brochure for patients, The Patient Care Partnership, Understanding Expectations, Rights and Responsibilities (2003), to emphasize that patients have not only the right to high-quality hospital care but also the right of involvement in care decisions about diagnosis, treatment, and prognosis (American Hospital Association, 2003). The American Nurses Association Nursing: Scope and Standards of Practice includes a standard of practice that describes a competent level of nursing care for health teaching and health promotion, "The registered nurse employs strategies to promote health and a safe environment" (ANA, 2010). Educating patients about their illness, treatment, health promotion, or self-care activities is essential to improve their health and contributes to changing healthcare from a culture of illness to a culture of health (HRET, 2014). The Joint Commission, a healthcare accreditation organization, has established a comprehensive guide for healthcare organizations that outlines the keys strategies to create a healthcare delivery system that advances patient and family-centered care (TJC, 2010).

Today, the cost of healthcare remains a continuing concern and is driving healthcare reform. The Affordable Care Act, federal legislation enacted in 2011, says that health promotion is an integral part of needed healthcare reform (HHS, 2011). Healthcare facilities are now discharging patients more quickly. Both The Joint Commission and the federal government require healthcare organizations to provide patients with discharge plans. According to the National Patient Safety Foundation, "The challenge and complexity of patient education today involves providing clear communication and creating effective teaching–learning partnerships so that patients and their families can obtain, process, and understand health information resulting in safe care and positive health outcomes" (National Patient Safety Foundation, 2007). Readmissions can be prevented when patients understand their discharge plan.

Patient education and health promotion will continue to be a primary focus for nurses, regardless of the setting. School nurses talk with adolescents about contraception and safe sex practices. Occupational health nurses may conduct classes on workplace safety. Ambulatory or clinic-based nurses discuss normal childhood development and age-appropriate activities with parents. Ambulatory surgical center nurses discuss postoperative care with patients before discharge. Clinical nurse specialists review choices in menu planning with patients who have diabetes. Nurse practitioners, when prescribing drugs for treatment, describe medication side effects to patients. Public health nurses stress the importance of current immunizations to prevent the spread of illness. Nursing educational programs are creating innovative partnerships to provide students the opportunity to practice in community-based settings. By doing so, nursing students have exposure to health promotion nursing activities in nontraditional educational settings (Carter et al., 2013).

Although nurses can influence and promote positive healthcare outcomes, they cannot control their patients through education. Despite the best intentions, patients will not always follow the recommendations. Gaining knowledge and changing behaviors are voluntary actions; however, nurses can act as health coaches to effect positive behavior changes based on patients' motivation and readiness for change. Nurses can coach and encourage patients to improve their health status, but no matter how important a nurse believes certain actions and attitudes to be, the choice is always that of the patients.

Patient education is seldom the formal process that most people experienced in school. Much patient teaching occurs informally during nursing care. During any patient care activity, a patient or family member may ask questions. This curiosity indicates a degree of motivation that nurses can act on. During these teachable moments, patient education can be extremely effective. Simply being knowledgeable about the patient's health status and care, however, is not enough. To take advantage of these spontaneous opportunities for teaching, nurses must know the teaching and learning processes, possess teaching skills, be able to define the patient's learning needs quickly and accurately, and know how best to include the patient's family in the process. Part of this understanding is realizing that patient education consists of more than handouts, pamphlets, and videotapes. It requires a therapeutic relationship in which the nurse empowers the patient and family toward autonomy and self-care.

PURPOSES OF PATIENT EDUCATION

Patient education has long been considered an independent role for nurses, so it is important for nurses to gain not only subject matter knowledge but also specific knowledge and skills for patient education. Nursing students must be prepared to

TABLE 9-1 THREE LEVELS OF DISEASE PREVENTION

Level	Description	Examples
Primary prevention	Seeks to prevent a disease or condition at a prepathologic state; to stop something from ever happening	Immunizations, fluoride supplements, car seat restraints, oral contraceptives, education in elementary schools about drug addiction
Secondary prevention	Seeks to identify specific illnesses or conditions at an early stage with prompt intervention to prevent or limit disability; to prevent catastrophic effects that could occur if proper attention and treatment are not provided	Physical assessments, developmental screening, vision screening, breast and testicular self-examinations, pregnancy testing
Tertiary prevention	Occurs after a disease or disability has occurred and the recovery process has begun; intent is to halt the disease or injury process and assist the person in obtaining an optimal health status	Rehabilitation for handicapped children, support groups such as Reach for Recovery and Alcoholics Anonymous, cardiac rehabilitation, health education for a patient with newly diagnosed diabetes

teach health promotion concepts to patients and families, with a focus on prevention of illness and maintenance of health (Samawi et al., 2012). The goals of patient education are to promote health/wellness (primary prevention), prevent or diagnose illness early (secondary prevention), restore optimal health and function if illness has occurred (tertiary prevention), and assist patients and families to cope with alterations in health status. Levels of disease prevention are outlined in Table 9-1. Patient teaching at each level encompasses all areas of function, as reflected in Table 9-2.

Nurses have a professional, ethical, and social responsibility to assist individuals, families, and communities to maintain and improve health. Nursing interventions should focus on enhancing the abilities of patients and families to engage in safe, effective, and efficient health behaviors.

Health Promotion

The importance of health promotion is an essential element of healthcare reform in the United States, Canada, internationally,

and globally. **Health promotion**, as defined by the World Health Organization (WHO), "is the process of enabling people to increase control, and to improve, their health. It moves beyond a focus on individual behavior towards a wide range of social and environmental interventions" (WHO, 2014a, 2014b). There are many factors that, combined, affect the health of individuals, families, and communities. The state of health for an individual or family is determined by social and economic environment, physical environment, and the person's individual characteristics and behaviors (WHO, 2014a, 2014b). Nurses who are knowledgeable about the determinants of health enable all people to achieve their fullest health potential.

Health promotion activities seek to expand the potential for health and are often associated with lifestyle choices, increasing the level of wellness. Put simply, people use health promotion activities to feel better. Health promotion behaviors enhance overall well-being. **Disease prevention activities** involve efforts to avoid or prevent specific diseases or conditions. Both health promotion and disease prevention share the

TABLE 9-2 EXAMPLES OF HEALTH PROMOTION AND PATIENT EDUCATION

Health Pattern	Example of Possible Teaching
Health perception–health management	Breast self-examination, importance of regular physical examinations and immunizations
Activity–exercise	Importance of regular exercise, how to use ambulation devices (e.g., crutches, walker), deep breathing and coughing, leg exercises
Nutrition–Metabolic	Healthy diet, dietary restrictions, wound care, how to monitor temperature, total parenteral nutrition at home
Elimination	How to maintain regular bowel function, Kegel exercises to decrease stress incontinence, self-catheterization
Sleep–rest–cognition–perception–cognitive–perceptual	Importance of getting adequate rest, aids to promote sleep
Self-perception–self-concept	Normal body changes, methods of promoting self-esteem
Roles–relationships	Assertiveness training, parenting classes
Coping–stress tolerance	Biofeedback, relaxation techniques
Sexuality–reproductive	Prenatal classes, contraception
Value–belief	Patient rights, "do not resuscitate" options

goal of improving health. A difference between them is that health promotion activities may be more general and concern improving someone's overall well-being.

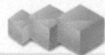 **Concept Mastery Alert**

Disease prevention (illness prevention) activities address ways of reducing the risk of a particular health problem. Health promotion often has a more general focus, including strategies for enhancing overall wellness and quality of life.

 APPLY YOUR CRITICAL THINKING

Patricia returns to the clinic 1 week after your teaching session with her. She shows you the following diary of activity and food intake. Below, you will find a sample of 1 day.

Breakfast:
Orange juice
Large chocolate chip muffin
Coffee

Lunch:
Ham and Swiss cheese on rye with mayo
Potato chips
Pickles
Salad with blue cheese dressing
Donut

Dinner:
Hamburger
French fries
Salad with blue cheese dressing
Ice cream

Exercise:
Walking with a friend in the neighborhood

Identify healthy aspects of Patricia's diet and exercise pattern to provide positive feedback? What are some important changes that can promote optimal health? What further teaching measures would you indicate for Patricia?

Check your answers in Appendix B.

Disease prevention concentrates prevention efforts on one specific illness. Another distinction is that health promotion activities may be more inclusive of community, seeking the input of others about health concerns and their priority in a community. Disease prevention is more likely to stem from outside information that suggests a significant health need in a community, such as rates of a particular disease as collected by a local health department. Together, health promotion and disease prevention efforts can improve and maintain the health of people in a community.

Health protection activities are environmental or regulatory measures that seek to protect the health of a community or large population. Examples of health protection activities include air and water quality regulations and food and drug regulations enforced by federal, state, and local governments.

Focus on health promotion has gained much momentum in recent decades. Nurses, regardless of their practice arena, are involved in patient education to promote optimum health and function. Knowledge and values are important when determining choices people make daily. Such things as food, rest, coping abilities, and hygiene and safety practices may influence optimal wellness. People may lack the motivation to change comfortable, unhealthy habits when they are feeling well. Nurses often aim health promotion at young people to prevent bad habits from developing.

Behavior change and breaking long-established habits are required for health promotion. The Stages of Change model developed by Prochaska and DiClemente describes the five phases that are necessary for health-related behavior change. The model is based on the belief that most people experience similar stages as they attempt to change health behavior over time (Table 9-3) (Shaffer, 2013). It is important for nurses to understand the Stages of Change model to support and coach patients through the change process.

HEALTHY PEOPLE 2020

In the United States, Healthy People 2020 is a national health promotion and disease prevention initiative. The goal of the initiative is to bring together many individuals and agencies to improve the health of all Americans, eliminate disparities, and improve the health of all people.

The four goals of (*Healthy People 2020*) are to assist the people of the United States to do the following (*Healthy People 2020 Framework*):

- Attain high-quality, longer lives free of preventable disease, disability, injury, and premature death.
- Achieve health equity, eliminate disparities, and improve the health of all groups.
- Create social and physical environments that promote good health for all.
- Promote quality of life, healthy development, and healthy behaviors across all life stages.

TABLE 9-3 STAGES OF CHANGE

Stages	Time Frame
Precontemplation	Not thinking about change in the next 6 mo
Contemplation	Seriously thinking about change in the next 6 mo
Preparation	Actively planning change
Action	Overtly making changes
Maintenance	Taking steps to sustain change and resist temptation to relapse

INTERNATIONALS AND GLOBAL CONCERNS

Key to addressing health promotion is action not only on a local level but also at an international and global level. This will require an integrated approach to health promotion. The World Health Organization has outlined four key commitments to health for all people. The commitments are central to the global development agenda, a core responsibility for all government, a key focus of communities and society, and a requirement for good corporate practice (WHO, 2009). The increasing emphasis on community partnerships places responsibilities on nurses to work cooperatively with all levels of government, college programs, community and business organizations, and neighborhoods to improve the health of groups as well as individuals.

Disease Prevention

Patient education also focuses on teaching patients the knowledge and skills for early detection or prevention of disease and disability. As research increases, the understanding of risk factors for disease improves. For example, studies have demonstrated the link between some types of cancer and a high-fat diet. This knowledge enables nurses to focus on dietary teaching to help decrease cancer risk. Studies also have proven the importance of early detection and support the teaching of regular screening. Research has better identified people at risk for specific illnesses, so resources and teaching programs can be directed at high-risk groups. For example, diabetic patients are at risk for cardiovascular problems, so frequent blood pressure and cholesterol screening with appropriate prescribed medication can prevent myocardial infarction or stroke.

Restoration of Health or Function

When illness or dysfunction occurs, patient education is important to help limit disability or restore function. In the home, community, and rehabilitation center, much teaching focuses on helping people deal with chronic health problems such as heart disease or diabetes (Fig. 9-1). In the acute care facility, teaching also focuses on restoring health. Patients who are admitted for

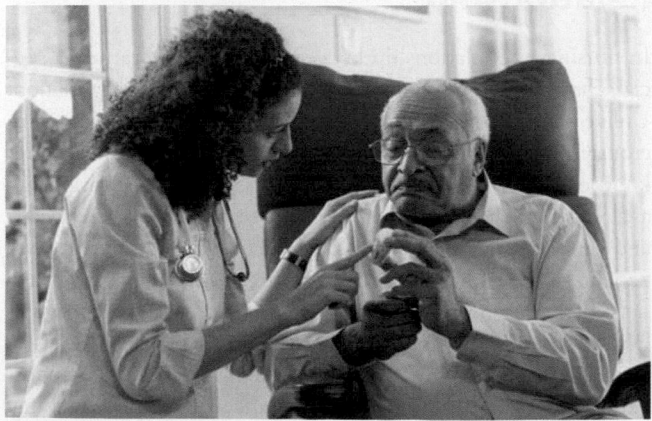

FIGURE 9-1 The nurse teaches the patient about medications so that the patient can manage chronic health problems.

TABLE 9-4 IMPORTANT TEACHING OPPORTUNITIES	
Opportunity	Possible Learning Need
Clinic visit	Immunization record, routine screening, weight reduction and diet, medications
Hospital admission	Unit policies, how to work call light and bed, specific treatments that have been ordered and why
Beginning of each shift	Review plan of care; explain any new treatments, tests, or medications
New medication	Action of drug, possible side effects, frequency, and any special considerations
Diagnostic procedure	Necessary preparations, what will be experienced during the procedure, any restrictions or special considerations after the procedure
Surgery	Preoperative preparation, postoperative protocols (e.g., deep breathing, leg exercises), pain control, how to get out of bed and turn easily
Discharge	Limitations on activity or diet, procedures such as wound care, when to call the physician

surgery receive instruction during the preoperative and postoperative periods to help prevent complications and to ensure optimal recovery. In the ambulatory care setting, nurses explain medications or diagnostic procedures to patients to reduce anxiety and to assist them in making informed healthcare decisions. Important patient teaching opportunities are outlined in Table 9-4.

Promotion of Coping

Patient education is important for individuals and families who must cope with new and frightening procedures or adjust and continue to live with chronic illness or disability. Providing patient-specific information rather than general information has been found to increase knowledge, decrease anxiety, and increase satisfaction for patients (Friedman et al., 2011). Adjusting to a loss of function can be difficult for patients and their families. Teaching may assist people to adapt to using new devices (e.g., a walker to assist with ambulation) or to alter diet or activity. Some teaching assists with changes in body image or role expectations. Teaching may be necessary to prepare caregivers for the technical and psychological challenges of caring for loved ones who have impaired function. Patient education also is important for helping patients and families deal with grief, loss, and eventual death.

TEACHING–LEARNING PROCESS

Learning is the acquisition of a skill or knowledge by practice, study, or instruction. Learning theory has changed over the centuries. According to an early, teacher-centered theory, learning required a disciplined mind, and the goal was to memorize many facts. Later, student-centered theorists believed that learning could be completely intuitive; by encouraging self-direction, an active unfolding of knowledge would occur. Still others claimed that learning must build on prior knowledge and experience, with the teacher actively imparting new ideas and the learner passively associating them with related ideas to grasp principles. Different conceptual models of the learning process also viewed the teacher's role differently: director, designer, programmer, or producer. More recent views suggest that the core of effective teaching is to produce capable self-learners, who continue their learning well past the teaching–learning encounters. Nursing students have experienced all of these theories at work. For example, to learn anatomy, one must memorize facts. Dealing with people, especially patients, always requires an intuitive component. Pharmacology builds on the student's previous knowledge of pathophysiology, chemistry, anatomy, physiology, and mathematics.

Adult learning theory helps us to understand how adults learn best. Malcolm Knowles developed a theory that explains how adults learn. Adults need to know why they are learning something; they need to know the reason and rationale. Adults learn by doing and practicing skills. Effective instruction involves adults in problem-solving situations that are relevant to them (TEAL, 2011).

Domains of Learning

Learning can be acquired in three different domains: cognitive, affective, and psychomotor (Bloom, 1956). Although the following section discusses each domain separately, the nurse should remember that learning does not occur in one domain without affecting other domains and frequently involves interdependent processes that include all three domains.

COGNITIVE

The word **cognitive** refers to rational thought, what one generally considers "thinking." Cognitive learning may involve learning facts, reaching conclusions, solving problems, making decisions, or using critical thinking skills. Nurses frequently participate in teaching–learning experiences in which patients must use new information to promote optimal health. Moving from the simple to the complex is likely to yield the best results during a cognitive teaching session. Depending on the patient, starting with basic facts and concepts and moving to discuss how they relate seems to work best. As patients learn to apply the material correctly in various situations, the nurse can add more information and offer in-depth explanations when the patient or family asks questions. Short, specific learning sessions and limiting teaching to essential information allow for patients to learn effectively.

Teaching a new mother the physiology of the breast and its role in milk production is an example of cognitive learning. After the mother understands the physiology of her milk supply, the letdown reflex, and how these two factors work together, she has demonstrated cognitive knowledge.

AFFECTIVE

Affective learning refers to emotions or feelings. Affective learning changes beliefs, attitudes, or values. Sensitivity and emotional climate influence all types of learning but are especially important in the affective domain. Affective learning is more difficult to measure than is cognitive or psychomotor learning because it focuses on thoughts and feelings. When working with patients to change beliefs, values, or attitudes, the nurse must understand his or her own feelings and emotions related to the topics being discussed; create an atmosphere in which patients can honestly and freely discuss their feelings and emotions; and situate the changes within the reality of the patients' lifestyle environment. Finally, for affective learning to occur, the nurse must allow sufficient time for exploration of feelings and emotions within a nonjudgmental environment. An example of affective learning is helping a new mother explore the possible benefits of breast-feeding for the health of her baby.

PSYCHOMOTOR

Psychomotor refers to the muscular movements learned to perform new skills and procedures. This type of knowledge is easiest to measure because it can be physically demonstrated. Teaching a new mother to breast-feed is an example of psychomotor learning. When the mother can successfully and independently breast-feed her infant to the physical satisfaction of both, she has demonstrated psychomotor learning.

Nurses are frequently responsible for teaching patients to perform certain skills independently (e.g., effective hand hygiene, good body mechanics). Nurses teach principles and demonstrate skills, patients practice these skills, and nurses answer any questions and identify further resources.

An important consideration in the psychomotor domain is that patients demonstrate the dexterity to manipulate the body parts, tools, or objects needed to perform the skill or procedure. A **return demonstration**, by which the nurse observes the patient performing the new skill, is critical for evaluating psychomotor learning.

Qualities of a Teaching–Learning Relationship

In nursing, the relationship between teacher and learner is special, characterized by mutual sharing, advocacy, and negotiation. Unlike some traditional views, nurses are not experts who generously bestow knowledge upon patients, nor do nurses barter knowledge for compliance. Both images represent the relationship as a power imbalance in which nurses, because of their knowledge and expertise, control the situation. Effective learning occurs when patients and healthcare professionals are equal participants/partners in the teaching–learning process. This requires that nurses explore the types of learning strategies that best help patients to learn during any teaching–learning situation. Developing rapport with the patient and family is important prior to any teaching. Often, teaching may best be delayed until the patient demonstrates readiness to learn and actively participate.

PATIENT FOCUS

Patient education is a therapeutic relationship that should focus on the patient's specific needs. Patient educational needs can differ; educational needs change with acute or chronic conditions, short- or long-term health conditions, or ones that will require temporary or long-term adjustments to patient lifestyles (Scruggs, 2009).

Patients also have unique values, beliefs, cognitive abilities, and preferential ways of learning that affect involvement and educational outcomes. Allowing patients to share their beliefs and preferences enables nurses to understand better this uniqueness and to individualize teaching to the patient's needs.

HOLISM

The teaching–learning relationship should consider the whole person rather than focusing on the specific content. Assessment data permit nurses to determine the "big picture," which provides broad contextual meaning. Nurses also use their own experiential knowledge. For example, a nurse teaching insulin injections to a patient with newly diagnosed diabetes anticipates problems or questions based on those that past patients have had; thus, the nurse anticipates the impact of diabetes on all areas of functioning.

NEGOTIATION

Together, nurses and patients determine what is already known and what is important to learn. Decision making is a shared process and a plan is developed with input from both parties. Sometimes, negotiation is a more formalized process with a written contract that guides the learning experience, such as when changes in attitude or behavior are needed. More often, the process is informal and ongoing, with continual checking and validating to guide the learning process.

INTERACTIVE

The teaching–learning relationship is a dynamic, interactive process that involves active participation from both the nurse and patient. Nurses learn from patients, and patients learn from nurses as they discuss content, clarify and revisit specific points, or determine new needs. This interactive, nonlinear model differs from the simplistic model that many texts describe: presentation of content, learning, and evaluation of learning.

ASSESSMENT FOR LEARNING

Assessing Learning Needs

The educational assessment begins with determining what the patient needs to know or do to function more independently. It is important to know the purpose of the teaching and to identify the expected result (patient outcome or goal). New knowledge or skill acquisition may need to occur before a patient leaves a clinic or is discharged from the hospital or home care. For example, parents must demonstrate the ability to feed their infant with a new feeding tube before the infant can be discharged home.

BASELINE KNOWLEDGE

Many times, patients articulate specifically what learning is important to them and why. Other times, requests for knowledge are less direct. For example, a patient may say, "I'm just not sure about all these new medications." Compare the patient's knowledge, attitudes, and skills with those necessary for independent functioning. "Tell me what you know about (relevant topic)" is a useful opener. Finding out what a patient already knows and finding out about previous patient education experiences may give a nurse some indication about where to begin his or her teaching. Determining additional factors that may impede learning is an important part of this assessment.

CULTURAL AND LANGUAGE NEEDS

Culture, values, and beliefs influence health maintenance practices, including preventive care, diet, childbearing and child-rearing customs, self-medication, and alternate therapies. To improve individual health and build healthy communities, healthcare providers need to recognize and address the unique culture, language, and health literacy of diverse consumers and communities. Assess the patient's ability to understand and speak English. If there are deficits, an interpreter (other than a family member) will need to be arranged for any significant teaching session. Both in person and electronic or virtual interpreters are available in many healthcare settings.

Nurses also need to consider components of diversity such as race/ethnicity, religion, health beliefs, language, and sex role beliefs when planning patient education. In general, the more the nurse educator can learn about the patient, including lifestyle, occupation, affiliations, and where the patient gets his or her health information, the more likely it is that educational interventions will be successful.

Spiritual beliefs and personal or family values also affect health maintenance. Some people place great value on physical health to achieve spiritual health. Others may have religious beliefs that prohibit certain medical practices and treatments or any medical treatment at all (e.g., Christian Scientists and Jehovah's Witnesses). Not all groups share certain "mainstream" healthcare norms and values. For instance, Jehovah's Witnesses do not accept blood transfusions; most Islamic sects do not donate or receive organs, and many Native American and Chinese people practice and trust folk medicine beliefs. Those who do not speak English require an interpreter.

If a patient from a different culture needs to be educated about nutrition, a registered dietitian may be able to help. Registered dietitians often are familiar with cultural food beliefs and can tailor a plan for individual patient needs. In many cultures, women are the only ones to prepare food or care for the sick. Therefore, identify and include these women in any dietary or health teaching for male patients.

ETHICAL/LEGAL ISSUE

LITERACY

The physician writes discharge orders for Mrs. Gonzales. They include a complex medication regimen and self-management of an indwelling catheter. Mrs. Gonzales speaks very little English. Her daughter is at work, and when you call for a interpreter, one is not available until tomorrow. You realize the physician will be upset if Mrs. Gonzales is not discharged today since her insurance coverage will not pay for a longer stay.

CRITICAL THINKING CHALLENGE

- Legally, must you provide a interpreter for Mrs. Gonzales during the teaching session?
- Role-play how you might respond to the upset physician in this situation.
- Brainstorm other alternatives to help provide Mrs. Gonzales with the teaching she requires for safe discharge.

PRIORITIES

Patients usually have many learning needs; therefore, nurses, the patient, and involved family members must set priorities to help ensure that teaching will prove effective. Priority setting may involve teaching patients the basic skills in the hospital and arranging home nursing visits for follow-up teaching. It is important to begin assessment and priority setting early in the patient–nurse interaction because time for teaching may be limited. Hospital lengths of stay are often 3 days or less, while in other settings, appointment times are brief. The National Patient Safety Foundation (2007) is promoting a campaign, *Ask Me 3*, for patients to better understand their health and obtain key information that is important for each patient to know. The three questions can serve as a standard guide for teaching when time is limited. The questions are as follows:

1. What is my main problem?
2. What do I need to know?
3. Why is it important for me to do this?

Ask patients to identify their learning needs; assess what is important to them. Patients may perceive learning needs when they wish to learn more to maintain or promote health or to fix a perceived problem that has occurred. For example, a routine physical examination may reveal an elevated cholesterol level. This information can increase a patient's need and desire to learn about lifestyle changes that can prevent heart disease. Teaching should occur when learning is a high priority for the patient. "Seizing teachable moments" when patients and their families are invested in learning enables them to be active participants. Sometimes, the perceived need for health teaching comes from a patient's personal reflection (e.g., a desire to exercise more and to lose weight after the holidays).

In many situations, nurses will discuss with patients knowledge or skills that are important to include in the teaching plan. For example, after listening to a patient who comes to the clinic for treatment for a urinary tract infection, the nurse provides information to prevent future infections and provides information about the ordered medication.

REALISTIC APPROACH

Nurses who take a realistic approach set priorities and try not to teach too much in any one teaching session. Consider the following:

- *The patient's energy/comfort level*: Physical weakness, pain, discomfort, and fatigue can affect attention span and decrease learning.
- *The patient's age*: Educational goals for children, adolescents, and adults differ, and patients require different teaching styles at different ages.
- *The patient's emotional state*: Patients may be too anxious or depressed to learn. It is not uncommon for those who have received a new diagnosis, suffered a loss, or experienced trauma to have difficulty learning.
- *The patient's cognitive abilities*: Patients with dementia, short-term memory deficits, or altered mental status may be unable to retain information or learn new skills. It may be necessary to identify another person (caregiver/family member) to include in the teaching.

Assessing Learning Readiness

MOTIVATION

Motivation provides the incentive for learning. Often, nurses associate noncompliance or lack of adherence to a treatment plan as an indication that patients lack motivation. The notion that a patient sufficiently motivated will "comply" with physician or nurse instructions belies the complexity of motivating factors and incentives. Motivation for learning starts with the patient's recognition of the need to know. Financial problems, inconvenience, denial, lack of social support, nonacceptance of the disease, anxiety, fear, shame, and negative self-concept can affect motivation. Motivating factors can seem to change daily. Attitudes and beliefs also influence motivation. For instance, a middle-aged man who has started taking antihypertensive medications to control blood pressure may show less motivation to continue taking the medications and learn more about his treatment options if a close friend confides that he experienced erectile dysfunction when taking a similar medication.

Because motivation is complex, often involving several different incentives (or disincentives), discovering factors that promote adhering to healthcare regimens and those that create barriers to achieving success may be difficult. Often, patients are not aware of all the motivating factors involved in their actions. There may be verbal cues (e.g., a patient who says, "My wife takes care of all that") or nonverbal cues (lack of attention, missed appointments) that point to decreased motivation to learn. An important part of assessing what motivates any

TABLE 9-5 MOTIVATIONAL INTERVIEWING STRATEGIES

Strategy	Main Components
Elicit-Provide-Elicit (E-P-E)	• *Elicit*: Find out what the patient already knows by asking. • *Provide*: Fill in missing information and/or correct any misconceptions. • *Elicit*: Find out what this information means to the patient.
Assessing importance	• The patient rates importance of health behavior on a scale of 0–10. • Ask why he or she rates this level of importance instead of a lower score. • Find out what would increase the score. • Summarize the discussion.
Evoking change talk	• Ask the patient open-ended questions to elicit desire, ability, or reasons or need to change.

Source: Butterworth, S. (2010). Health-coaching strategies to improve patient-centered outcomes. *Journal of the American Osteopathic Association, 110*(4 Suppl. 5), eS12–eS14.

patient is to learn what the patient values and, especially, what has resulted in past successes. Patients who associate healthcare goals with something they already value probably will be more motivated to adhere to healthcare regimens.

Motivational interviewing is a technique where the goal is to involve the patient in developing his or her own plan through strategies as outlined in Table 9-5. Motivational interviewing can be used as a tool to determine the patient's readiness for change and where they are in the Stages of Change model. One of the guiding principles of motivational interviewing is to have the patient voice the arguments for change (Miller, 2009). Motivational interviewing is a collaborative conversation to strengthen a person's own motivation for and commitment to change.

Motivational interviewing has four guiding principles (Tillman, 2013):

- Express empathy to understand and show acceptance of the patient experience including ambivalence for change.
- Assist the patient to develop an awareness of discrepancy that highlights the mismatch between "where they are" and "where they want to be."
- Roll with resistance and don't directly oppose new perspectives to leave little for the patient to resist.
- Support self-efficacy by expressing a belief in the patient's capabilities to change successfully.

Nurses can assess patient readiness for change by listening for statements made by patients that reveal their consideration of, motivation for, or commitment to change; the more someone talks about change, the more likely it is to occur (Tillman, 2013).

Different types of change talk can be described using the mnemonic DARN-CAT:

- **D**esire (I want to change)
- **A**bility (I can change)

- **R**eason (It's important to change)
- **N**eed (I should change)

And most predictive of positive change:

- **C**ommitment (I will make changes)
- **A**ctivation (I am ready, prepared, willing to change)
- **T**aking steps (I am taking specific actions to change)

COMPLIANCE VS. ADHERENCE

Issues of **compliance** or **noncompliance** (i.e., following or not following the recommended plan) are losing favor as authoritarian and rigid terms to describe why patients do or do not follow healthcare regimens. In the past, compliance implied that the nurse dictated what the patient must do and that the patient had to follow through or risk being labeled "noncompliant," or unwilling or unable to follow the recommendations. **Adherence**, or "the extent to which health behavior reflects a health plan constructed and agreed to by the patient as a partner" (Gould & Mitty, 2010), is an alternate perspective. The original intention of judging (and labeling) patients negatively when they do not follow a healthcare provider's medical advice conflicts with the prevailing view of developing partnerships with patients for optimal healthcare success. Instead, a more collaborative patient–nurse relationship involving respect, trust, mutuality of goals, and, most importantly, an understanding of the complexities involved in changing health behaviors and promoting adherence is suggested.

It is important for nurses to realize that following even mutually agreed-upon goals and recommendations may be difficult when patients are experiencing pain, anxiety, financial constraints, social isolation, and loss of independence. Identifying the reasons for nonadherence, either purposeful or unintentional, is important (Gould & Mitty, 2010). Understanding that the process of change will involve backsliding and failures, nurses working for and with patients can help to identify the obstacles to following treatment goals and develop strategies to achieve success. For instance, asking supportive, open-ended questions such as "People often find it hard to take blood pressure pills twice a day, every day. Has this ever been a problem for you?" is a useful lead when assessing a patient's ability to follow treatment guidelines. Giving patients an agenda ("As I listen to you, it sounds as if we need to talk about wound care and diet. What do you think?") may also be useful. Suggesting follow-up with support groups to continue success with smoking cessation, healthy eating, or regular exercise can help promote long-term compliance. People may decide not to follow conventional medical advice for various reasons. This is often frustrating to nurses and other healthcare providers, but the choice to follow advice is, in the end, that of the patient, and the nurse must respect it as such.

SENSORY AND PHYSICAL STATE

The patient's sensory abilities and physical state affect learning readiness, and the teaching plan must be modified accordingly. For example, patients with poor vision or compromised fine motor skills may be unable to give themselves subcutaneous injections safely. Patients who receive pain medication postoperatively may have difficulty concentrating. A woman who has just given birth may be too tired to participate actively in the learning session.

LITERACY LEVEL

One major barrier to optimal healthcare outcomes and successful patient education is literacy, especially involving minority and disparate populations. Literacy is the ability to read and write; the ability to use language, numbers, and images to understand the written and spoken word. Poor literacy causes individuals to have trouble finding pieces of information or numbers in a lengthy text, integrating multiple pieces of information in a document, or finding two or more numbers in a chart and performing a calculation. Patients and families with poorer reading skills are believed to have greater difficulty navigating the healthcare system and to be at risk for experiencing poorer health outcomes.

Low levels of literacy also affect patients' abilities to understand oral communication provided by nurses and physicians, further complicating the ability of patients to follow healthcare regimens, navigate healthcare systems, and follow healthcare instructions. It is possible to find people with low literacy in every occupation, among all races, at all ages, and at all socioeconomic levels. Appearance and use of spoken language do not indicate a person's literacy. Many people with low literacy levels are of average or above average intelligence and speak articulately. A roughly dressed laborer may be able to read well, but a professionally dressed person may be unable to read at a functional level. Educational level gives only a rough estimate of literacy. A correlation between literacy and the number of grades completed in school does not always exist. Some adults may not understand written directions, videotapes, or even some audiotapes. Because most patient education materials are aimed at people who read at a high school level or above, this material confuses a huge segment of the population who may be too ashamed to admit their inability to read and understand. The ability to interpret clocks and calendars is not universal, and this can contribute to the inability to follow instructions and keep appointments.

Tools to determine literacy level include reading tests, such as the Wide Range Achievement Test (WRAT) and Rapid Estimate at Adult Literacy in Medicine (REALM). Direct testing is the most accurate way to assess literacy, but it is often impractical in the clinical setting. Some "red flags" can cue you to limited literacy, as outlined in Box 9-1. Here are some less accurate, but expedient, methods:

- Check the level of the patient's pleasure reading. This will present a measure of literacy level but not of functional health literacy (ability to read and understand healthcare information).
- Give the patient something to read, and later request a description of the contents in his or her own words.
- If possible, offer the patient several options (reading, watching, or listening) for learning.

BOX 9-1 Behaviors and Responses that May Indicate Limited Literacy

Behaviors
- Incompletely or inaccurately filled out forms
- Frequently missed appointments
- Lack of follow-through with instructions

Responses to Written Information
- "I forgot my glasses. I'll read this when I get home."
- "I forgot my glasses. Can you read this to me?"
- "Let me bring this home so I can talk to my son/daughter about this."

Responses to Questions About Medications
- Unable to name medications
- Unable to explain what medication are for

Source: Weiss, B. (2007). *Health literacy and patient safety: Help patients understand. Manual for clinicians* (2nd ed., p. 17). Chicago, IL: American Medical Association Foundation.

- When in doubt and when time may be limited, use the lowest grade literacy information material available. Even with high functional literacy ability, when patients are stressed by illness and teaching, it is better to start with simpler material and add complexity later.

It may seem that these kinds of assessments take too much time. Nevertheless, nurses have an ethical and legal responsibility to make sure that the patient receives information in a manner that he or she understands (The Joint Commission, 2010).

HEALTH LITERACY LEVEL

Compounding the dilemma of low literacy is the need to consider health literacy levels. **Health literacy** is the ability to obtain, process, and understand basic health information and services needed to make appropriate health decisions and follow instructions for treatment (Weiss, 2007). Without fully understanding health information, it may be difficult for patients to act on directions or instructions. Many complex factors such as cultural values, beliefs, and customs can contribute to an individual's understanding of health and illness (Hulme, 2010). The problem of health literacy is a national focus in healthcare today because many studies have shown that patients do not often understand the information given to them. In fact, health literacy is considered the sixth vital sign or "newest vital sign" (Dunn, 2010).

There are many instruments to assess health literacy skills, and they are often impractical to use in the clinical setting because of the amount of time that they require to complete. The easy-to-use Brief Health Literacy Screen (BHLS), a three-item screening tool, can be used by nurses as a health literacy

TABLE 9-6 BRIEF HEALTH LITERACY SCREEN (BHLS)

Item	Response options				
How confident are you filling out medical forms by yourself?	Extremely	Quite a bit	Somewhat	A little bit	Not at all
How often do you have someone help you read hospital materials?	All of the time	Most of the time	Some of the time	A little of the time	None of the time
How often do you have problems learning about your medical condition because of difficulty understanding written materials?	All of the time	Most of the time	Some of the time	A little of the time	None of the time

Reprinted with permission from Wallston, K., Cawthon, C., McNaughton, C., Rothman, R., Osborn, C., & Kripalani, S. (2013). Psychometric properties of the brief health literacy screen in clinical practice. *Journal of General Internal Medicine,* 29(1), 119–126.

measure (Wallston et al., 2013). Scores on the tool can range from 3 to 15, with higher scores indicating better health literacy (see Table 9-6).

 APPLY YOUR CRITICAL THINKING

Mrs. Babbitt, an 84-year-old woman with chronic heart problems, is being discharged with three new heart medications, a stool softener, and a PRN pain medication for her arthritis. She is very compliant, always patting your hand and saying, "Oh, you are so smart. I will try my best to follow all your instructions." She lives alone, but her son visits weekly and calls often.

What additional information should you collect to individualize Mrs. Babbitt's teaching?

Describe some principles that might guide your teaching with Mrs. Babbitt.

How might you evaluate Mrs. Babbitt's learning?

Check your answers in Appendix B.

NURSING DIAGNOSES

Selected nursing diagnoses associated with health promotion and patient teaching include Ineffective Health Management (Individual or Family), Ineffective Health Maintenance, and Deficient Knowledge; these are summarized in Table 9-7. The table also includes associated Nursing Outcomes Classification (NOC) and Nursing Interventions Classification (NIC).

OUTCOME IDENTIFICATION AND PLANNING

The planning phase of patient education involves working with patients to develop a teaching plan, identifying appropriate teaching strategies, and developing a written plan to coordinate teaching among healthcare team members. Factors to consider in planning include the patient's assessed learning need and motivation level, learning style preference, language translation needs, literacy level, health literacy level, inclusion of family member or support persons, timing, and the appropriate amount of information to cover.

Outcome Identification

Patient-centered, patient-involved goals are most effective. Including patients in the planning process helps show clearly what patients are willing or unwilling to do, clarifying goals.

Be brief and realistic when writing goals and outcome criteria. Do not promise overly optimistic outcomes. Create measurable goals with a time frame. A possible form for writing patient outcomes is as follows:

$$Who + Does + What + How + When = Goal$$

For example:

$$Patient + will\,demonstrate + dressing\,change +$$
$$without\,cueing + before\,discharge = to\,achieve\,goal$$

Evaluate and revise learning goals as necessary. If learning has been successful, new learning goals may be formulated. If outcomes have not been met, the time frame may be changed or, based on additional assessment data, the outcomes may be revised.

Planning Teaching Strategies and Methods of Delivery

Availability of resources, learning style preference, literacy level, and health literacy level affect planning of effective teaching strategies. Teaching sessions can be individual, small group, or large group sessions. One-to-one teaching can be individualized, so it is usually most effective, but it also is most expensive in terms of money and time. Box 9-2 lists key points to remember for various teaching sessions. There are many methods to deliver patient information to patients and families.

Choosing the right strategy or method for patient education can make the experience more enjoyable for both nurse and patient. If possible, use several strategies to enhance learning and retention. Combining modalities such as seeing, hearing, and touching promotes better learning than does using only one modality. The use of electronic teaching materials such as computer-assisted programs, videos, and Internet-based tools can enhance learning.

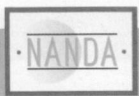

Table 9-7 SELECTED NANDA-I NURSING DIAGNOSES INVOLVING PATIENT EDUCATION AND HEALTH PROMOTION

Nursing Dx	Related Factors	Statement of Dx	NOC*	NIC†
Ineffective Therapeutic Regime Management (Individual or Family)—Difficulty effectively integrating a treatment program into daily activities to meet health goals	Complex regime, financial concerns, lack of motivation, side effects of treatment	Ineffective Therapeutic Regime Management R/T complex new medications and their side effects, lack of insurance coverage and money AEB unfilled prescriptions and continued high blood pressure	Adherence Behavior, Knowledge: Health Resources, Knowledge: Medication, Health-Seeking Behavior	Financial Resource Assistance, Medication Management, Teaching: Prescribed Medication
Ineffective Health Maintenance—Inability to identify, manage, and/or seek help to maintain health	Cognitive impairment, ineffective coping, insufficient resources, inability to make appropriate judgments	Ineffective Health Maintenance R/T poor coping after wife's death and financial stress AEB missing appointments and verbalization that he can't deal with the insurance details	Coping, Health Promoting Behavior, Motivation, Compliance Behavior	Coping Enhancement, Counseling, Health System Guidance, Support System Enhancement
Deficient Knowledge—Absence of cognitive information related to a specific topic	Cognitive limitations, information misinterpretation, lack of exposure to information, unfamiliarity with resources	Deficient Knowledge of infant care R/T first-time mom, no prior child care experience AEB verbalization of lack of knowledge and fear of ability to care for baby after discharge	Personal and infant well-being, Psychosocial Adjustment: Life Change, Safe Home Environment, Coping	Anticipatory Guidance, Family Involvement, Promotion, Sleep Enhancement

Dx, diagnosis; R/T, related to; AEB, as evidenced by.

*From: Moorhead, S., Johnson, M., Maas, M., & Swanson, E. (2013). *Iowa Outcomes Project: Nursing Outcomes Classification (NOC)* (5th ed.). St. Louis, MO: C. V. Mosby.

†From: Bulecheck, G., Butcher, H., Dochterman, J., and Wagner, C. (2013). *Iowa Intervention Project: Nursing Interventions Classification (NIC)* (5th ed.). St. Louis, MO: Elsevier Mosby.

From: NANDA-International (NANDA-I. 2014). *Nursing diagnoses: Definitions and classification, 2015–2017.* West Sussex, England: Wiley-Blackwell.

DEMONSTRATION

Demonstrations are particularly useful for psychomotor learning. Explaining a skill while slowly demonstrating it leads to talking patients through the procedure for the first few times. Videotapes or audiotapes can be used, but human contact is almost always preferable. Repeated practice can help patients move toward independent functioning. Return demonstrations help nurses evaluate learning. Reinforcement in the form of praise ("Nice job there"), correction ("Try leaning a bit more on the cane as you walk"), or constructive feedback ("I see you've figured out how to use your glucometer for glucose testing") is particularly important for identifying and continuing appropriate actions and behaviors.

BOX 9-2 Key Points for Teaching Sessions

- Focus on the patient's perspective—what he or she needs to know. Avoid general background information.
- Emphasize behaviors or actions. Focus on what to do and why, *not* what to know.
- Avoid medical terminology whenever possible. If you must use it, limit the amount and find a comparable everyday word to substitute (e.g., shortness of breath for dyspnea).
- Keep it simple:
  - Offer small, yet vital, bits of information *one* at a time.
  - Keep to the main objectives.
  - Add information *only* when you have determined that the previous information was thoroughly understood.
  - Use short sentences in concrete language. For example, "Take your water pill at dinner time. This gives you time to pee before bedtime. You can then sleep through the night" versus "Make sure to take your diuretic at least 2 hours before you go to bed to ensure that you do not get up during the night to urinate."

- Use words without double meanings. For example, "positive" can mean good (in form of praise) or bad (disease finding as in positive for cancer).
- Repeat and emphasize main topic points at the end of each session as a summary (remember: *not* too many).
- Ask patient to restate what you have said or what he or she has read or heard.
- Highlight specific phrases of information if using print materials.
- Give educational materials that promote patient's active involvement, such as short quizzes, checklists, questionnaires, diaries, or medication records.
- Use photos and graphics that enhance the message, *not* compete with it.
- Use positive words, phrases, and messages. Avoid scare tactics.
- Evaluate and test the message and materials for effectiveness (such as focus groups).

DISCUSSION AND VERBAL TEACHING

Discussion and verbal teaching is an opportunity for patients to focus learning through exchange of ideas by sharing information, clarifying feelings, or asking questions. It can be useful with individual patients or groups. Discussion involves learners more deeply in the process because it requires participation. This strategy can enhance cognitive and affective learning. During the discussions, your role is to be a facilitator. Use positive comments and open-ended questions to promote further discussion, clarification, and understanding. For instance, "Mrs. Dodge, your point about how to deal with losing your hair during chemotherapy is important. Please tell us more about what you found that worked." Discussion works best when it is combined with written information (Friedman et al., 2011).

WRITTEN INFORMATION

Access to written materials can assist nurses in planning teaching–learning sessions. Agencies such as the American Cancer Society, Canadian Cancer Society, American Heart Association, American Diabetes Association, and other health-related groups frequently prepare written materials. Some are prepared within agencies by clinical nurse specialists or other nurses with a specialized teaching role. Being familiar with available written resources is important. Material should pertain to the patient's concern and be written clearly, with up-to-date information. Written material and verbal information must be consistent. Written information that includes illustrations has been shown to be more effective than written information alone (Friedman et al., 2011).

The reading level of any written material must be screened for appropriateness for the individual patient. Recommendations suggest that educational pamphlets containing healthcare information are written at or below the sixth grade reading level to ensure comprehension and understanding. It is important to use one- or two-syllable words and to keep the information limited to only the essential content (Weiss, 2007). When evaluating educational material for the person of low literacy, look for materials that contain short sentences and words with few syllables. Large print is important for patients with visual impairment.

Frequently, nurses provide written materials in advance of a teaching session to give patients time to assimilate information and formulate questions or concerns. Whenever possible, encourage patients to make use of such materials immediately by circling or highlighting important information to review before the teaching session. It is best to select a few well-written materials rather than to overwhelm patients with dozens of pamphlets (Fig. 9-2).

ROLE-PLAYING

Role-playing, or acting out feelings or knowledge, is especially useful for teaching effective behavior to adults or children. Most children and adults enjoy role-playing sessions as a form of education. Role-playing can be helpful in decreasing anxiety

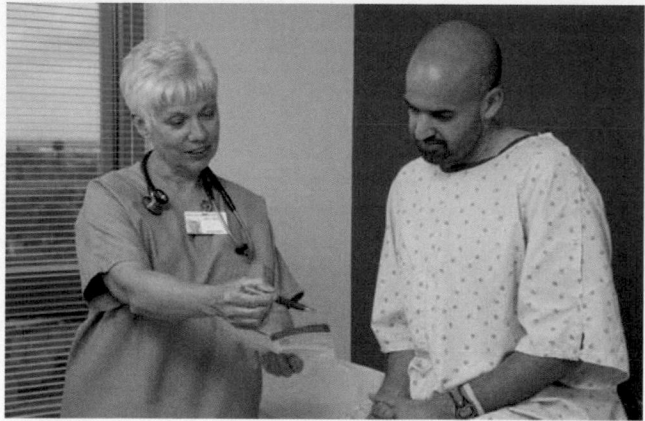

FIGURE 9-2 The nurse provides an instructive, well-written pamphlet to the patient to support teaching regarding asthma management.

during learning. It can be used to work through past, present, or anticipated feelings or new situations. Patients react based on their experiences, while nurses offer guidance and feedback. Dolls can be used, especially with children. For example, a child may be asked to demonstrate how his or her mother's illness has affected the family by using dolls to represent each family member.

LECTURES

A lecture is a formal presentation of information by a teacher to a group of learners. This format is most effective when communicating facts (cognitive learning), but it can be used for psychomotor or affective learning. A simple lecture (a one-way communication from teacher to learner) is much more effective when combined with discussion, question-and-answer sessions, or both. A lecture may stifle learners who are eager to contribute. Determine whether patients appear bored, anxious, or easily distracted. Limit how much information you give verbally; have supportive printed materials that include additional information. Informational overload is very common when using the lecture method. A rule of thumb to avoid information overload is to type exactly what you are planning to say, cut it in half, and then cut it in half again. Allow at least half the time scheduled for the lecture session for questions and discussion. Always take a break after 40 minutes.

Teaching Aids and Resources

Teaching aids assist learning but are not substitutes for human contact. They are best used to supplement or reinforce face-to-face teaching.

AUDIOVISUAL AIDS

Videotapes, CDs, audiotapes, slide-tape programs, and computer-assisted instruction can be useful for subjects taught often, such as insulin injections or breast-feeding. Visual aids often increase learning during formal lectures. Audiotapes can be especially useful for instructing patients with low literacy

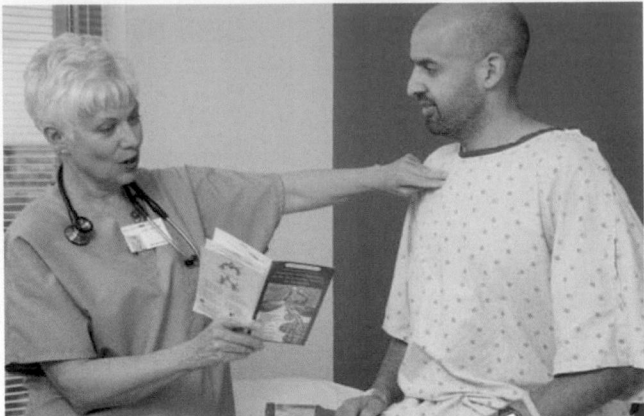

FIGURE 9-3 Combining audiovisual aids with discussion and patient participation will lead to more effective learning.

skills, reducing anxiety in learning situations by allowing for later review of health information, counseling, teaching relaxation techniques, and increasing satisfaction with healthcare outcomes and can be created in multiple languages (Zirwas & Holder, 2009). Some healthcare facilities have a special television channel with programming to provide health education on various topics. Let patients decide which aid might be helpful if more than one form is available. Do not use audiovisual aids in isolation, but combine them with discussion or one-on-one teaching (Fig. 9-3). The most effective audiovisual education materials are short in duration, no more than 15 minutes total.

THE INTERNET

The Internet has become an extremely broad and valuable source of information and advice for patients. Access to computers (at home, the office, and libraries) is common in today's society. Learning via the Internet encompasses learning primarily in the cognitive and affective domains. It is entertaining, informative, and accessible at any time; is relatively anonymous; and offers much diversity and variety of available information. For instance, Internet message boards offer counseling and support, allowing patients to connect with other individuals to share information and experiences to gain insight. For patients who are homebound, the Internet offers ways to communicate, relieve boredom, and elevate mood. Evaluation by various researchers regarding the quality of information retrieved from the Internet found the following:

- Although many healthcare educational materials were available, most were above the recommended reading level for patients with low literacy skills.
- Few health information sites provided evaluative information regarding their materials.
- Problems with keeping sites current and up-to-date were reported.
- Multifocused sites, such as those targeting audiences, including care providers, professions (including nurses), and patients/patients, were less individualized and made it difficult to generalize to any given person accessing the site.

- Lack of stability for site continuation or locations created confusion and frustration, and good sites sometimes were discontinued or lost.

Despite these challenges, researchers recommended the Internet as an important and growing medium for healthcare educational materials and supporting optimal health and well-being, suggesting that healthcare professionals mediate for patients by identifying and recommending reliable sites with truthful and reliable healthcare information rather than leaving them to search on their own (Zirwas & Holder, 2009).

Another use of the Internet is by using telehealth strategies for education and patient care management. **Telehealth** is an interactive system that allows communication to happen simultaneously between a patient's home and the clinical medical setting (Everett & Kerr, 2010). Telehealth phone links are being established, often with 24-hour nursing coverage, to provide health education, address patient questions, and help patients determine what level of healthcare they may require. Such links are of particular importance in rural areas where families may live an hour or more from the nearest hospital.

EQUIPMENT AND MODELS

In order to promote learning, create situations for patients to see and practice on equipment. Whenever possible, obtain the equipment that a patient will *actually* use for practice. For instance, when teaching glucose monitoring to a patient with diabetes, use the type of monitor that the patient will use in the future. Models can be used to simulate actual conditions. For example, models of breasts have been developed to assist in teaching breast self-examination, permitting patients to palpate what a lump would feel like. When using models of the human body, be sensitive to cultural considerations. Some patients are more comfortable using and handling these materials with only the nurse present, even without family members. It is important to be sensitive to these possibilities and to ask patients their preferences *before* models are taken out and displayed.

Patients and families must, in some situations, learn technically complex self-care skills while coping with the onset or an exacerbation of serious illness. Coordinated programs such as those for management of patients with heart failure include telephone calls, postdischarge return appointments within a week, and the use of patient-friendly materials to track weight.

Use of Interpreters and Translators

If a patient, family member, or caregiver cannot speak English, an interpreter is necessary during the teaching session. A 2000 law requires all federally run programs to make accommodations for people with limited English proficiency. The Joint Commission (2010) requirements for patient rights include language that states, "The hospital provides interpreting and translation services, as necessary." Medical interpreters receive special training in the use of medical language and terms and are certified to provide translation services. When the nurse needs a medical interpreter, the teaching session will take longer because each message must be repeated twice. In addition

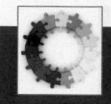

COLLABORATING WITH THE HEALTHCARE TEAM
Making a Referral for an Interpreter

Your teaching session with Mrs. Hussein, the patient in the opening scenario, was unsuccessful due to limited time and a language barrier. You did get her and her husband to agree to return next week for a follow-up so that more teaching can be done. Since communication was challenging, you put in a consult for an interpreter providing the following SBAR report.

S*ITUATION:* Mrs. Hussein, an Iranian-speaking woman, has recently been diagnosed with hypertension and started on blood pressure medication and a low-sodium diet.

B*ACKGROUND:* I attempted to do medication and diet teaching, but Mr. Hussein was upset and said "no more." Mrs. Hussein sat quietly and did not maintain eye contact. They talked rapidly in a dialect I did not understand. I did get them to agree to return on Monday for a follow-up visit and more teaching.

A*SSESSMENT:* For my teaching session to be effective, I will need an interpreter. I think it would be helpful if the interpreter was male because Mr. Hussein seems to relate better with the male staff here at the clinic. He is important in managing his wife's care and the primary family decision maker.

R*ECOMMENDATION:* Please let me know if an interpreter speaking Iranian languages is available next Monday at 0900 for 1 hour to interpret.

CRITICAL THINKING CHALLENGE
* Did the nurse provide essential information in this referral for the interpreter?
* Is an SBAR report necessary when requesting a consult?
* Does it make a difference whether the interpreter is male or female?
* What might you discuss with the actual interpreter before the session with the Husseins? Refer to Box 5-2 after you have answered this question for additional ideas.

---

to speaking the language, the interpreter must be aware of the culture and able to interpret medical information clearly and objectively. Doing so is difficult, especially when a family member or friend acts as interpreter. Better choices for interpreters are bilingual staff members or professionals (who may be available in large medical centers). Female interpreters may be able to communicate more freely with female patients without encountering cultural prohibitions. Return to the opening scenario and see the SBAR in the "Collaborating with the Healthcare Team" box, which the nurse uses for making a referral to an interpreter.

When using an interpreter, remember to continue to talk to and look at the patient. Keep information simple and direct. Instruct the interpreter to translate word for word as much as possible. Keep the name and phone number of the interpreter in the patient's record. A nod or "Yes" from the patient does not always indicate understanding because some people agree just to avoid "losing face." Be sure to also provide written translated material. See Box 5-2 for more detailed information about communicating through an interpreter.

Many telephone companies now offer a Language Line service whereby the patient and healthcare provider talk on the telephone with a bilingual operator who provides translation. This service is cost-effective and provides 24-hour coverage in most languages. It is valuable for small agencies and for agencies located in rural areas. One disadvantage is the inability to see nonverbal communication. Many smart phones also have the ability to translate selected languages.

Another option for interpretation is the use of computer technology. Using a computer that is equipped with cameras allows the interpreter and patient to interact "face to face." Using this emerging technology gives the ability to see both verbal and nonverbal communication.

Timing and Amount of Information

When planning a teaching session, consider factors such as the amount of time available and the amount of material that needs to be covered. The time when patients are very receptive to teaching is often referred to as a "teachable moment." For example, if the patient asks questions when you administer medications, take a few minutes to explain each newly ordered medication and its possible side effects. Reinforce this informal teaching whenever the medication is administered until the patient can verbalize this information to you. When a more formal teaching session is necessary, planning the best time can help ensure teaching effectiveness. Consider the following principles when planning a good time to teach:

* The patient should not be tired.
* The patient should be comfortable.
* Family members or caregivers may be present.
* Uninterrupted time must be available so that meals or necessary treatments do not interrupt the teaching session.
* Teaching should not occur just before an event (e.g., discharge, surgery).

Hospital teaching sessions should be limited to no more than 20 to 30 minutes to avoid tiring patients. Approximately half the session time should be allotted for the nurse to "give out" information; the other half should be allotted for the patient to "take in" information (i.e., ask questions and give comments). Warn patients about any time restraints. Saying "I have 20 minutes to talk" communicates clearly the nurse's time limit, minimizing the chance that patients will feel slighted when the nurse has to leave.

Hospitalization is not the best time for teaching. Plan to cover essential material, but do not expect patients to learn all that is necessary while anxiety or pain is present. Combining the teaching session with one or two informational pamphlets with highlighted portions for later review helps to ensure that the patient can remember and use information later. Outpatient education is usually more effective than is inpatient education for several reasons. Patients are usually less stressed and therefore better able to learn when they are no longer in the hospital. Following hospital discharge, they have lived at home with the condition and bring practical, everyday questions to the session. Simply attending an outpatient education session indicates a willingness to learn, and motivation is a strong indicator of educational success.

Appropriate Family and Friend Involvement

Whenever possible, with the patient's permission, plan to include family members and friends in patient education. Their support strongly affects patient success. A statement such as "I'm here because my wife made me come" may indicate denial on the patient's part and tells the nurse about the wife's attitudes and influence. Never assume that because someone is a blood relative, he or she automatically wants to participate in patient education or care. Friends are often as supportive as family members. When a family member or friend assumes the caregiver role, it may be necessary for that person to attend teaching sessions and demonstrate mastery of important skills and knowledge (Fig. 9-4).

Written Teaching Plan

The written teaching plan guides the teaching process and coordinates teaching among members of the healthcare team. Without a written plan, teaching is likely to be haphazard and ineffective. A written plan clearly stating expected outcomes also serves as a useful reference for evaluation and fosters communication with other professionals so that they may participate. A written teaching plan may be incorporated into critical pathways, indicating at what point specific teaching should occur. The Fracture Recovery Pathway developed at Virginia Mason Medical Center (Fig. 9-5) illustrates a patient-focused pathway that can be used for patient teaching. Box 9-3 shows the format for an outcome-based teaching plan, examples of which are provided in each clinical chapter in this text.

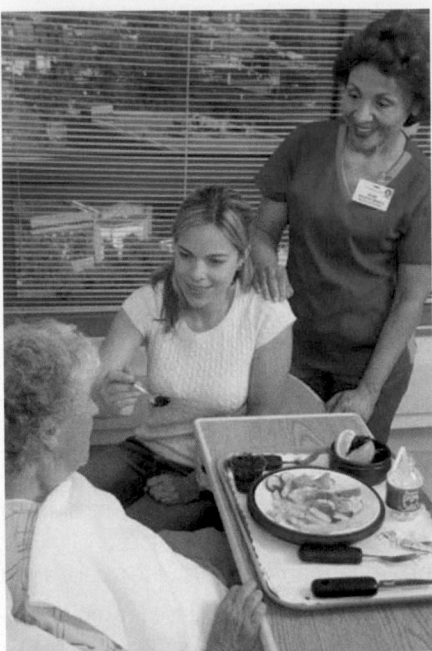

FIGURE 9-4 Involving family members in patient education helps improve outcomes after discharge.

IMPLEMENTATION OF PATIENT TEACHING

Meeting Priority Needs First

Before any teaching, the patient should be comfortable. Easing acute symptoms, such as pain, hunger, thirst, nausea, or dyspnea, allows the patient to focus on learning. Give the patient a chance to use the toilet. Offer pain medication, and determine whether the patient is comfortable. Ask, "Is this a good time for us to talk?"

Anger, fear, anxiety, worry, grief, and guilt block learning. Nurses who are sensitive to distress can modify the plan accordingly. Supportive body language and statements are useful. No matter how thorough planning has been, last-minute changes may be needed.

Comfortable Environment

Anyone who has tried to study in a room that was too hot, cold, dim, bright, noisy, or distracting knows that the environment affects learning. During patient education sessions, try to make the environment conducive to learning. If necessary, send uninvolved visitors away temporarily. Privacy is important; closing the curtains in a semiprivate room, sitting near the patient, and speaking quietly, slowly, and facing the patient all contribute to a greater sense of privacy.

Individualized Teaching Sessions

Trying to teach too much at once can block learning. Slowing down, using plain language, showing or drawing pictures, limiting the amount of information you provide, using the

Fracture Recovery Pathway

My Fracture		Before Surgery	Day of Surgery	After Surgery	Checklist for Discharge
	My Recovery Plan	My Care Team will help prepare me for surgery, including blood work, x-rays, heart testing and other tests as needed.	My nurses will do my pre surgery checks, both in my room and in the pre-op room. I will have blood tests done and will have my vitals monitored.	My vital signs are stable. My medical team will manage my medical conditions. My surgical team will see me every day.	☐ I am medically stable. ☐ My pain is controlled with oral medications. ☐ My family and I understand my medications. ☐ I understand my activity limitations. ☐ My family and I understand where I am going next. ☐ My family and I know my follow-up plan. ☐ All of our questions and concerns have been addressed
	What About My Pain?	I will be seen by the Pain Team about pain management, including pills, shots and possibly a procedure to block my pain.	My Pain Team will manage my pain during surgery. After surgery, I will take pain medication by mouth but may still need I.V. pain medication. I may still have my pain block in place.	I may still have some pain, but I will be taking medication to manage it so I can get out of bed.	
	When Can I Eat?	I cannot eat after midnight before my surgery.	After surgery, I can start to eat and drink as I am able.	I can eat what I want within my diet guidelines.	
	When Can I Get Up?	For safety, I cannot get out of bed, but my nurses will help turn me for comfort.	After surgery, with help, I am able to sit on the edge of bed. My nurses will help turn me so I don't get sore.	I will be seen by physical and occupational therapy to help me get back on my feet. Nursing will help me get up to the bathroom.	
	What Happens Next?	I will meet briefly with a social worker to start talking about what will happen after I leave the hospital.	My urinary catheter is removed as soon as possible after surgery. I may have an I.V. line for fluids and medications.	The social worker will help my family and I finalize my discharge plan.	

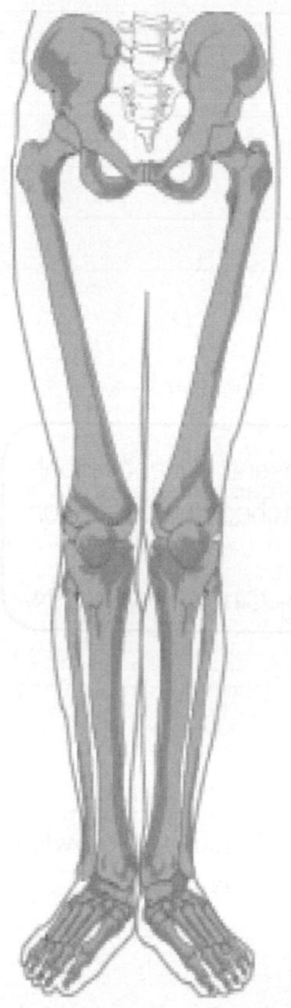

FIGURE 9-5 The Fracture Recovery Pathway is a patient-focused pathway that can be used for patient teaching. (©2014 Virginia Mason Medical Center)

"teach-back" technique, and creating an environment that makes patients feel comfortable enhance patient learning (Weiss, 2007). Listening to the patient's response gives excellent feedback about his or her progress. Always allow time for patient questions.

People have different learning styles. Some prefer to do, and others prefer to watch. When teaching a psychomotor skill, be sensitive to those who like to do. A demonstration may have been planned, but if the patient reaches out to touch the materials, consider talking the patient through the skill instead. Children learn through play and are usually energetic and eager doers. However, if a child prefers to watch, a demonstration instead of instructive play may be best.

Communication

Good communication is necessary for effective patient teaching. Chapter 6 discusses communication in the nurse–patient relationship in more detail. Active listening requires the nonverbal communication techniques of silence, attending, and observing. If a patient is comfortable and believes that he or she has the nurse's undivided attention, learning is greatly enhanced. If rapport between the nurse and the patient is not established before the teaching session, learning is negatively impacted.

Participation is the best measure of involvement. Getting a person to participate can occur by leading—making a pointed, specific statement. The patient who rambles may need to be focused.

BOX 9-3   Example of an Outcome-Based Teaching Plan

Outcome/Deadlines: Patient will demonstrate blood glucose testing independently by discharge

Teaching Plan	RN Initials	Date/Time
Assess patient's fears and readiness to learn.	CH	7/15/16
Assess patient's preferred learning style.	CH	7/15/16
Assess what patient knows about blood glucose testing.	CH	7/15/16
Verbalize steps in procedure as it is performed by nurse.	CH	7/15/16
Ask if patient has any questions and/or feels comfortable trying procedure.	CH	7/15/16
Verbally cue patient as she completes blood glucose testing.		
Include family and significant others.		
Have patient practice and demonstrate glucose testing three times or until she verbalizes comfort.		

Documentation

7/15/17 13:00: Blood glucose testing teaching session in patient's room without family members present. Patient verbalizes nervousness about needles and sticking herself but started to read pamphlet she was handed. Watched demonstration and asked questions. Stated she wanted to wait until mother arrived for return demonstration.

—Cindy Howles, RN

To clarify understanding, repeat what you hear the patient saying and ask whether it is accurate. Reflecting or restating (repeating the patient's words) also can be a valuable communication tool.

Repetition

The realities of today's healthcare system—short hospital stays, limited home care opportunities, and very ill patients—provide less time for patient teaching. Setting priorities and repeating information are imperative. When cognitive or psychomotor learning is the goal, try repeating the information in various ways. For example, if the patient has been learning a therapeutic diet, ask about appropriate food choices in different restaurants, on a picnic, or at a party. Have patients repeat information several times. Ask patients how new learning will affect their daily routines, and check to see whether they are integrating new routines into activities of daily activities. Ask patients to practice and demonstrate psychomotor skills several times before discharge. Repetition may point out deficits in learning that would not be evident in a single session.

Because discharge instructions can be overwhelming, clarify important concepts, provide written instructions, review factual information, and have patients repeat the knowledge and practice the skills. Most healthcare agencies have discharge forms that are printed, so nurses can give a copy of the specific discharge teaching to patients as they document it. These forms also help alert nurses to essential information that they must provide before discharge.

Teaching Methods

Methods of teaching differ in the three domains of knowledge. Principal teaching methods are listed in Box 9-4.

COGNITIVE

Because the cognitive domain of learning involves expanding knowledge, the material must be organized from the simple to the complex. Introduce patients to the basic concepts, and give

BOX 9-4   Principal Teaching Methods

Cognitive (Knowledge)
1. Lecture
2. Discussion (factual questions and answers)
3. Stimulation (application of knowledge in different contexts)
4. Independent study

Affective (Values)
1. Discussion and values clarification
2. Role-playing
3. Simulation
4. Discussion

Psychomotor (Skill)
1. Skill demonstration
2. Talking the learner through the skill
3. Repeated practice

definitions. Then help patients integrate these concepts into something meaningful and beneficial to health. People do not learn isolated facts well. Learning is enhanced when information builds on previous knowledge and the reason and rationale are included. The most common error is trying to teach too much in a single session. It is better to teach some basic ideas well than to overload patients with many hard-to-remember facts.

AFFECTIVE

When trying to modify an attitude or emotional response, keep a nonjudgmental, nonthreatening attitude. Acknowledging the patient's ability to accept or reject the material can empower the patient and lead to more healthy decision making. The nurse who states emphatically the rightness of his or her position and the wrongness of the patient's position loses all credibility and influence. Listen carefully to what the patient values, and work from there. For example, a nurse is trying to encourage a depressed, noncompliant paraplegic to join a support group. The patient is too depressed to be involved in self-care but does seem to have a strong sense of contributing as a family member. The nurse gently approaches the patient with the idea that better physical and mental health would enable him to contribute better to his family's well-being. The patient may begin to assign a higher value to health when it is tied to better family functioning.

PSYCHOMOTOR

Psychomotor methods involve the muscular motions needed to learn a skill. Assemble the appropriate equipment (e.g., dressings, syringes); having the necessary supplies at hand can save time and prevent interruptions. Written material, providing a step-by-step guide, acts as a reference during the session and as a reminder to patients the first few times they practice the skill independently. Allow patients to ask questions and make comments. Many adults are intimidated by learning a new skill, so encouragement and praise almost always improve performance. Comments such as "Lots of people have that same concern" or "I've had many patients with that same problem" help patients feel less isolated. Positive corrective feedback such as "You've just about figured out how to give yourself an injection; now, angle the syringe a little more this way" acknowledges and reinforces learning accomplishments but at the same time provides significant correction to facilitate a better performance.

EVALUATION OF LEARNING

Evaluation of learning is most effective when it is systematic, practical, and ongoing. Measurable, clearly stated outcomes streamline evaluation. When patients actively participate in outcome formation, they can likely do much of the evaluation.

This final phase depends heavily on what has preceded it. If evaluation becomes unclear, review the outcomes. Were they realistic for the patient's abilities, time frame, and resources? Were they clearly stated and measurable? Elicit the patient's feedback in this process at each step.

Evaluation occurs continually as teaching proceeds rather than after teaching is completed. In this way, the teaching session can be continually adjusted to meet the patient's needs. Feedback from nurse to patient is most effective when it enhances the patient's self-concept and motivates the patient to higher learning. Asking patients to repeat or demonstrate what they have learned to family members is one way to accomplish this, especially with children. Remind patients of the progress they have made rather than what still needs to be done. Evaluation can take several forms, including written tests and questionnaires, oral tests, "teach-back" techniques, return demonstration, check-off lists, and simulations.

"Teach-Back"

An effective strategy to evaluate learning is to use the **teach-back** technique. This technique is one where the patient teaches back to you the information that he or she has learned and closes the communication loop to insure that the content delivered was heard and understood. Using this technique is a quick way to evaluate the effectiveness of your instruction. The National Patient Safety Foundation recommends and strongly advocates for the use of the teach-back technique. The technique utilizes open-ended questions or statements to elicit responses from patients and their families. For example, "I want to be sure that I've explained everything correctly to you. Will you please explain to me how you will take your medication?" Closed-ended questions, or ones that require a yes or no answer, are ineffective to assess learning, and experience shows that patients often answer yes to questions even when they don't understand (Weiss, 2007). If a patient is unable to "teach back," then assume you haven't provided the information in a way that is most useful to the patient. Adjust your approach and try again.

Return Demonstration

The return demonstration is a way of testing skill performance. A patient's degree of accuracy and independence in performing a skill is almost always a clear indication of learning. Psychomotor skills can be evaluated with this method. Give feedback about parts done well, along with areas for improvement. Figure 9-6 shows how nurses use return demonstration to evaluate the patient's skill in using a metered-dose inhaler.

Check-off Lists

Check-off lists have the advantage of highlighting accomplishments while showing whether the patient has performed each step in a particular learning process. For instance, check-off lists work well when documenting whether a patient can perform activities of daily living or identifying gaps in organizational skills. Most patients find check-off lists helpful and achieve a sense of pride and fulfillment when they complete one. Patients also can use check-off lists effectively with psychomotor evaluation, such as return demonstrations.

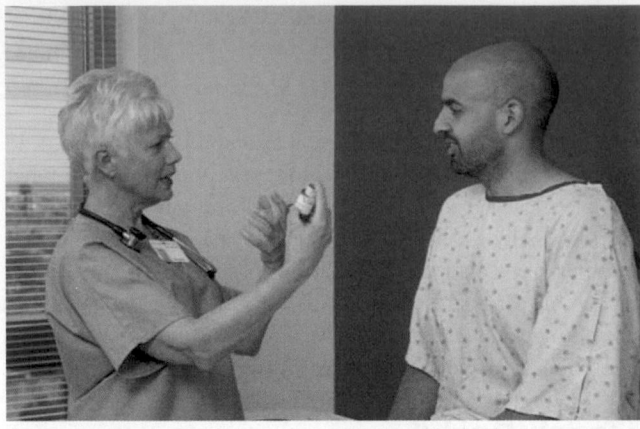

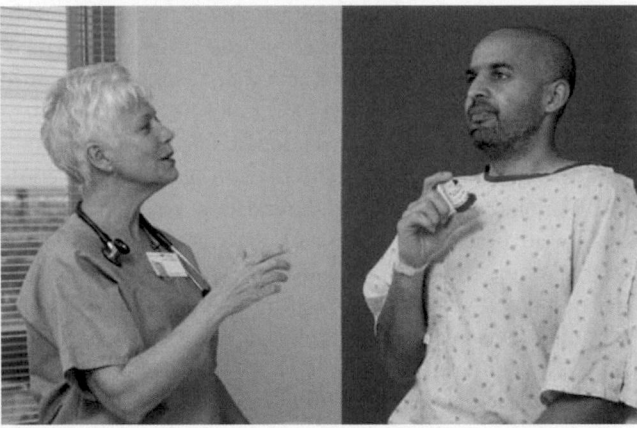

FIGURE 9-6 A. The nurse teaches the patient how to use a metered-dose inhaler. **B.** In the return demonstration, the patient demonstrates his skill performance.

Simulation

Simulation evaluates whether the patient can apply learning in different situations. Offer a scenario to the patient, and ask what the best choice or choices would be. For example, the nurse could evaluate dietary learning by asking the patient about the best choices in various restaurants, or the nurse could evaluate diabetic sick-day care by posing various sick-day scenarios.

Written Tests and Questionnaires

Written tests are time-consuming, intimidating, and not always specific to the patient. They are useful only in the following situations:

- The patient is literate (do not take this for granted).
- Clear educational objectives have been mutually decided.
- It is necessary to measure a broad sample of factual information.
- A skilled test writer has prepared the test.
- The test has been beta-tested with a subset of patients to determine effectiveness.

As in the classroom, written tests are most useful for evaluating cognitive learning. Affective learning cannot be tested this way because no answer is right or wrong. Written test questions may be useful as assessment tools (pretests) or as evaluation tools to check a patient's progress. A questionnaire may be used to evaluate how helpful an educational program has been for a group of learners so that positive changes can be made if the program is offered again.

Oral Tests

Oral tests are usually more expedient and less intimidating than are written ones. Questions can be informally phrased, and patients usually give immediate, specific, and useful feedback. Stay as casual as possible because the greater the patient's anxiety about being tested, the less likely it is that the evaluation will be accurate. Evaluation of the patient's verbal response can be useful in testing cognitive learning, but affective learning in the form of an attitude change is more difficult to measure.

Documentation of Learning

Documenting patient education is as important as documenting any other aspect of patient care. Documentation of patient education serves several purposes:

- It communicates the plan and progress to other healthcare professionals.
- It fulfills the nursing job description as delineated by local, state, and national licensing agencies.
- It provides a legal record.
- It may be required for financial reimbursement of care

Documentation must contain the subject matter, the patient's response to teaching, and any necessary break in the process (e.g., if, after evaluation, the nurse found it necessary to return to the planning stage). Well-documented patient education is a record of methods that did or did not work, and it can give some indication of patient accomplishments and adherence to healthcare regimens over time.

Documenting the patient's response to teaching should include statements like:

1. Patient able to verbalize understanding by repeating back information about his or her medications
2. Patient able to demonstrate skills for wound care by following instructions for irrigation and dressing application

LIFE SPAN CONSIDERATIONS

Newborn and Infant

Newborns and infants learn by interacting with their environment. During this period of rapid development, infants learn a great deal (e.g., how to recognize their mothers, how to follow objects as they move, how to hold toys). Encourage an environment rich in appropriate stimuli to foster normal cognitive development.

During this stage, infants are not ready for formalized teaching; instead, direct any necessary teaching at parents and caregivers. Health promotion teaching for the caregiver may include providing information about immunizations, normal growth and development, and car seat safety. Teaching about various aspects of child care, demonstrating capabilities of newborns and infants, and modeling appropriate and effective interactions help support and promote positive parent–child relationships.

Toddler and Preschooler

Because toddlers and preschoolers are accustomed to learning from and communicating with their parents, the parents are usually the most effective teachers. Teaching parents about safety practices, well-child visits, and proper sleep and nutrition are important for health promotion of this age group (Fig. 9-7). Children learn through play, so using dolls or toys as models can enhance learning.

Children 2 to 5 years old like to be addressed with their parents listening. Trust is vital. If you tell a preschooler that a procedure will not hurt but it does, you have lost credibility with the child and learning is hindered. Children of these ages are likely to have many questions and may ask the same ones many times. Answer their questions immediately, directly, and in language they can understand. Sometimes, this means checking with a parent or caregiver about words that a child uses to describe body functions or important things. Preschoolers are generally energetic and restless, so try to limit the session to 5 to 10 minutes. Let children handle machines or supplies as soon as possible. Children of this age can understand some anatomy, so when possible, use models and correct anatomic names.

Evaluate learning frequently to ensure that children understand. Preschoolers usually enjoy displaying new knowledge, giving nurses the chance to praise them repeatedly and to offer rewards such as stickers, picture books, or rubber stamps.

School-Age Child and Adolescent

School-age children are usually eager to learn. Including health promotion teaching about proper nutrition, sleep, exercise, safety, and learning how to deal with stress and frustration assists in their understanding of their role in maintaining their own health.

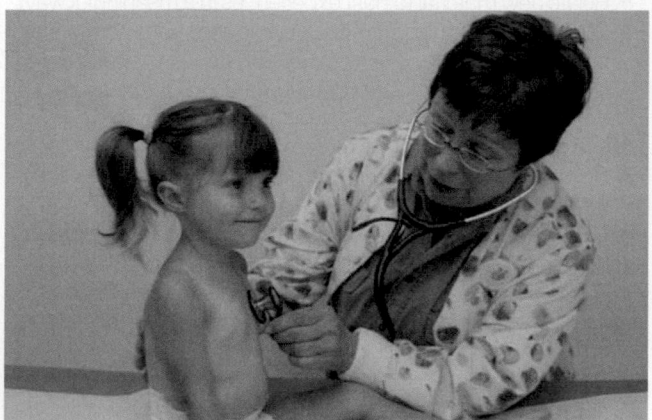

FIGURE 9-7 Routine checkups help protect the child's health and ensure continued growth and development.

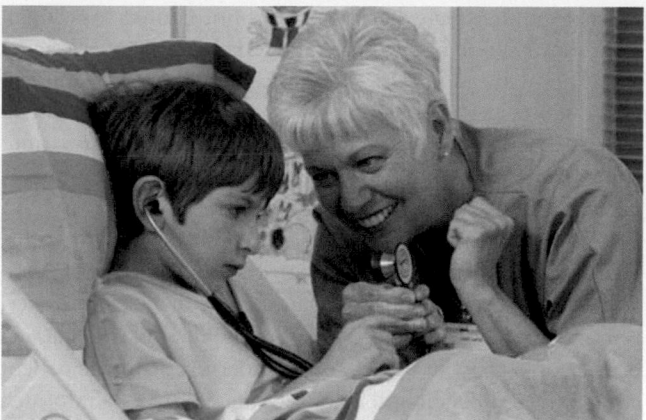

FIGURE 9-8 Allowing the child to participate and handle equipment to demonstrate procedures are effective methods for educating children about healthcare.

Development of concrete thinking, an increased understanding of their bodies, and continuing curiosity about how things work contribute to the school-age child's understanding of the healthcare experience (Fig. 9-8). They can understand cause and effect ("If I don't stay off my leg, it won't heal as quickly, and it'll be longer before I can play outside at recess"). Include children in educational planning, allowing them to help set goals. Being accustomed to a classroom atmosphere, they understand the scheduling of work and play.

Answer all questions quickly and truthfully. Trust is vital to learning and to establishing a relationship in which children feel comfortable enough to express fears and concerns.

Educational content can be more sophisticated for this group than for preschoolers. Coloring books for teaching anatomy work well. Written material is fine at the proper reading level. Keep in mind that hospitalized children may regress. Explain procedures directly to these children with the parents in the background. Sessions should be no longer than 20 minutes.

"Winning" is important for school-age children, so they usually value success highly. Use of charts with stickers to mark progress is an effective motivating tool with this group.

Adolescents usually appreciate complete, open, and honest explanations to their questions. Their peers are usually more influential than are parents, teachers, or nurses. If given permission, it is fine to include peers in a teaching session; in fact, general healthcare information may be included for the benefit of these visitors. Take the opportunity to include health promotion education when possible. Adolescence is a time for experimenting, so providing information about smoking, safe driving, preventing sexually transmitted infections, and avoiding drugs and alcohol may influence their choices. A sensitive, caring attitude is essential to educate adolescents effectively. In order to maintain the adolescent's trust, keep confidences; if a confidence must be broken, explain to the patient whom you must tell and why.

Include adolescents in any educational planning, because their struggle for independence makes them averse to having anything imposed on them. They are more likely to comply when provided with alternatives and consequences. It is also helpful when working with adolescents to give them the reason and rationale behind your information. Ask them what they need to know. Find out the value system a teenager associates with an illness, and work from his or her point of view. Adolescents are generally sophisticated learners, able to understand broad concepts and assimilate much information. They frequently access and get information from the internet. They are oriented to the present, however, and are more in tune with immediate advantages than with long-term results.

This age group is accustomed to teaching sessions of 45 to 50 minutes in school, but this is unrealistic in a healthcare setting. It may be better not to include parents (unless requested by the adolescent) in the session in order to encourage patient autonomy and heighten self-concept; parents can be informed later. Literature and audiovisual and computer-related educational materials to review between sessions can be useful with this group.

Adult and Older Adult

Adults tend to be motivated by activities that enhance or maintain their self-esteem. Self-direction and achievement generally boost self-esteem; dependence and error generally decrease it. Adults tend to take errors personally, thinking poorly of themselves if they believe they are taking too long to grasp a concept.

Adult learners respond well to a straightforward teaching approach and can apply knowledge immediately. Try to provide a comfortable, informal, friendly learning environment where the patient can feel appreciated. Adults may become at risk for lifestyle-related chronic conditions, so, when possible, incorporate health promotion behaviors such as exercise, nutrition, self-examinations, health screening, stress management, and reduction or cessation of smoking and alcohol consumption.

Young adults usually have plenty of energy and take good health for granted. Learning must be practical because these people usually lead busy lives. When setting educational goals with patients from this group, take a practical approach, if possible, explaining how the change will improve daily life. Young adults are often motivated by the thought of maintaining their functioning to care for their children.

In general, middle-aged adults are more aware of health problems and do not take good health for granted the way younger adults do. People in this age group sometimes lack the self-confidence to try something new. Middle-aged adults should be involved in all aspects of the teaching plan because they are usually familiar with the concepts of goal setting and achievement. These people have a broad base of life experience, and teaching goals will more likely be met if they are given time to assimilate new knowledge into old. Approach learning directly, and explain all rationales fully. Try to keep sessions to less than 45 minutes, and allow time for patients to practice skills in private. Middle-aged people also enjoy praise. Evaluate patients in a supportive atmosphere, stressing how much progress they have made. Gently correct misconceptions and be sensitive to fears and anxieties.

Older adults are the fastest-growing segment of our population. General adult learning principles apply to this group;

however, some special considerations are required. Motivation to learn may be decreased if patients believe life is near its end. Two motivational strategies may be tried:

- Show patients how new knowledge will improve their quality of life, regardless of its length.
- Show how the new knowledge could improve the patient's independence.

Physiologic changes that normally occur with aging may hinder learning. Vision may decrease because of cataracts; smaller, less-reactive pupils; or a decrease in color perception. The ability to hear high-pitch sounds usually decreases, although low-pitch hearing may be intact. Rapid speech may become unintelligible because older adults often take longer to process what they hear. Hearing loss can be a source of shame and frustration for the older learner, causing withdrawal and worsening feelings of isolation.

Older adults may suffer from short-term memory loss. Do not assume that memory loss exists, but be sensitive to it. When it does exist, it is usually associated with meaningless learning, complex learning, or new information that has required a reassessment of old learning.

The older learner has large stores of information, so scanning for recall may take longer. Generally, older learners need more time to learn psychomotor skills. Often, they compensate by putting a great deal of effort into accuracy.

Box 9-5 lists guidelines for assisting older adults with learning.

BOX 9-5 | Teaching the Older Learner

Teaching Tips
- Use a brightly lit, glare-free room.
- Use visual aids with large, well-spaced letters and primary colors.
- Eliminate extraneous noise.
- Face the learner.
- Speak in low, slow tones.
- Limit sessions to 20 to 30 minutes.
- Watch for cues indicating inadequate hearing, such as leaning forward, cupping an ear, frowning when trying to hear, or starting a separate conversation.
- Relate new material to past experiences in a meaningful way.
- Supply one idea at a time. Use frequent summaries and positive feedback.
- Provide a written or recorded summary of the session.

Medication Teaching
- Be sure that the patient is the one who manages their medications.
- Be sure the patient knows what each medication does, how many pills to take, and when.
- Discuss what to do if the patient misses a dose. (Containers that hold a week's worth of medications improve accuracy and consistency.)
- Be sure the patient has written medication instructions in appropriate size, form, and language.

THERAPEUTIC DIALOGUE: PATIENT TEACHING

SCENE FOR THOUGHT

Jennifer Cohan is 14 years old and has a diagnosis of diabetes mellitus. She wants to learn to give herself insulin injections. The diabetes nurse specialist comes to the clinic to talk to her.

LESS EFFECTIVE

Nurse: Hi, Jennifer. I'm Laurel Mandrake, the diabetes nurse. I'm here to teach you how to give yourself your shots.

Jennifer: *(Looks doubtfully at the equipment but doesn't say anything.)*

Nurse: I see you're looking at the equipment I brought. It's okay to be nervous. I'll show you how to do it and then you can ask me questions.

Jennifer: Can I see it first? I know I need this insulin stuff so I don't get sick like I did at school. That was so embarrassing! But I hate shots, so I don't know how good I'll be at this. *(Begins to take out syringes, alcohol swabs, vials, etc.)*

Nurse: It will be easier if you just let me show you what to do. I have to cover a lot of information. I'll give you some pamphlets to take home after you are done. I'll go over all this stuff with your mom, too, so she'll be able to help you.

Jennifer: Okay. *(Mumbles the word. Bites her lip to keep from crying.)*

MORE EFFECTIVE

Nurse: Hi, Jennifer. I'm Lorraine Morris, the diabetes nurse. Your doctor told me you wanted to learn how to give yourself your shots. Is that right? *(Makes sure information is accurate.)*

Jennifer: Yeah, I told him that, but I don't know now. *(Looks doubtfully at the equipment.)*

Nurse: It's okay to be unsure. I see you're looking at the equipment I brought. Do you want to see it or talk about it first? *(Assesses Jennifer's learning readiness and gives choices.)*

Jennifer: Can I see it first? I know I need this insulin stuff so I don't get sick like I did at school. That was so embarrassing! But I hate shots, so I don't know how good I'll be at this. *(Begins to take out syringes, alcohol swabs, vials, etc.)*

Nurse: *(Sits and watches Jennifer explore.)*

Jennifer: Look at those needles. They're so little!

Nurse: They do look small, don't they?

Jennifer: Do we have to do this today? *(Looks pleadingly.)*

Nurse: I have a suggestion. How about if we go over the equipment today, and I'll give you a few pamphlets to take home and read. We can reschedule the actual teaching next week. How does that sound?

Jennifer: I like that better. Maybe if I read this for a week I'll get more courage. *(Looks relieved.)*

Nurse: That means your Mom will have to give you the insulin until next week. Is that okay with you?

Jennifer: Yeah, if it's okay with Mom. She hates shots, too! *(Laughs. Lorraine and Jennifer look at the equipment together and make plans for next week. Jennifer's mother comes in and learns how to give insulin as Jennifer watches.)*

CRITICAL THINKING CHALLENGE

- Determine how many of the three domains of learning Jennifer will use to acquire knowledge.
- Evaluate from the above information what kind of learner Jennifer might be.
- Examine how the first nurse approached Jennifer's learning style. What actions contributed to a less effective teaching session?
- Detect what the second nurse did that makes you think she knew the principles of teaching adolescents.
- Develop additional options the nurse might consider for teaching Jennifer.

KEY CONCEPTS

- Patient education is a dynamic process used to empower the patient toward autonomy and high-level wellness.

- In patient education, the nurse can influence but cannot control. Education must be patient centered.

- Individualize teaching strategies and evaluation methods for each type of learning (cognitive, affective, or psychomotor).

- Knowing the patient's literacy level and ability to comprehend oral and written English is important in choosing methods and content.

- Patient education is a process that considers the patient's health literacy as well as his or her literacy level.

- The nurse, in collaboration with the patient, assesses the patient's learning needs and readiness to learn; he or she then forms a teaching plan. The plan is implemented, the learning is evaluated, and the process is documented.

- People have varying learning styles, and different age groups require different approaches.

PRACTICING FOR THE NCLEX

CHECK YOUR ANSWERS IN APPENDIX A.

1. A nurse is teaching a postoperative patient how to change his leg bag prior to discharge. This skill demonstration by the patient displays which type of learning?
   a. Cognitive
   b. Affective
   c. Psychomotor
   d. All of the above

2. A nurse is assisting a postoperative patient with effective use of the incentive spirometer (IS). The nurse states that using the IS 10 times every hour while awake will help prevent atelectasis, enabling the patient to regain her baseline health and return home sooner to be with her children. Together, the patient and nurse develop a practice schedule that allows the patient to take a break for visitors in the afternoon. Then, the patient verbalizes to the nurse what she has learned and demonstrates her skill with the IS. Which patient education practices are evident in this scenario? Select all that apply:
   a. Developing patient rapport
   b. Individualizing education to patient
   c. Negotiation of plan of care
   d. Interactive education technique

3. A patient has just received a new cancer diagnosis after being hospitalized for fatigue and anemia (low red blood cell levels). The nurse has information about how to improve red blood cell counts through appropriate nutrition. What is the most important thing that the nurse should know prior to conducting this education?
   a. Patient's current level of fatigue
   b. Patient's age
   c. Patient's cognitive status
   d. Patient's emotional state

4. During shift handoff, a patient is described as being noncompliant to her diabetes management. Her past medical history includes bipolar disorder, depression, chronic back pain, and renal failure with hemodialysis. Upon talking to the patient, the nurse learns that the patient is from the Philippines, has no family locally, and has high levels of chronic pain. Which statement by the nurse is the most appropriate?
   a. "No wonder she is depressed, she's ruining her life by not following medical advice."
   b. "I get so frustrated with noncompliant patients; we treat them and they just come right back."
   c. "It seems that she has a lot of issues that may be related to her psychological state and may be impacting her ability to be adherent."
   d. "I think there may be some cultural issues that are leading her to be noncompliant."

5. A nurse sees a patient in the cardiology office for coronary artery disease and congestive heart failure. It has been recommended that the patient eat a diet low in sodium, but he confesses that he has not consistently modified his diet, though he does understand that sodium intake increases fluid retention. Which of the following nursing diagnoses is most appropriate for this patient?
   a. Health-Seeking Behavior
   b. Ineffective Therapeutic Regime Management
   c. Ineffective Health Maintenance
   d. Deficient Knowledge

REFERENCES

American Hospital Association. (2003). *The patient care partnership: Understanding expectations, rights and responsibilities.* Chicago, IL: Author.

American Nurses Association. (2010). *Nursing: Scope and standards of practice.* Silver Springs, MD: Nursesbooks.org

Bloom, B. (1956). *Taxonomy of educational objectives: The classification of educational goals.* New York, NY: David McKay.

Building Healthier Communities by Investing in Prevention (2011). U.S. Department of Health and Human Services. Retrieved from http://www.hhs.gov/healthcare/facts/factsheet/2011/09/prevention02092011.html

Butterworth, S. (2010). Health-coaching strategies to improve patient-centered outcomes. *Journal of the American Osteopathic Association, 110*(4 Suppl. 5), eS12–e14.

Carter, M., Kelly, R., Montgomery, M., & Chesire, M. (2013). An innovative approach to health promotion experiences in community health nursing: A university collaborative partnership. *Journal of Nursing Education, 51*(2), 109–111.

Dunn, D. J. (2010). The sixth vital sign: Health literacy assessment. *Florida Nurse, 59*(2), 12.

Everett, J., & Kerr, D. (2010). Telehealth as adjunctive therapy in insulin pump treated patients: A pilot study. *Practical Diabetes International, 27*(1), 9–11.

Friedman, A., Cosby, R., Boyko, S., Hatton-Bauer, J., & Turnbull, G. (2011). Effective teaching strategies and methods of delivery for patient education: A systematic review and practice guidelines recommendations. *Journal of Cancer Education, 26*, 12–21.

Gould, E., & Mitty, E. (2010). Medication adherence is a partnership, medication compliance is not. *Geriatric Nursing, 31*(4), 290–298.

Health Research & Educational Trust. (2014). *Hospital-based strategies for creating a culture of health.* Chicago, IL: Health Research & Educational Trust.

Healthy People 2020 Framework. Retrieved November 13, 2010, from www.healthypeople.gov/2020/consortium/HP2020Framework.pdf

Hulme, P. (2010). Cultural considerations in evidence-based practice. *Journal of Transcultural Nursing, 21*(3), 271–290.

Miller, W. R., & Rollnick, S. (2009). Ten things that motivational interviewing is not. *Behavioral Cognitive Psychotherapy, 37*(2), 129–140.

National Patient Safety Foundation. (2007). *Ask Me 3.* Retrieved January 19, 2015, from www.npsf.org/askme3

Samawi, Z., Haras, M., & Miller, T. (2012). Age appropriate health promotion education: Roots firmly established in baccalaureate nursing pediatric rotation. *Journal of Pediatric Nursing, 27*, 44–49.

Scruggs, B. (2009). Chronic health care, it is so much different than acute health care-or it should be. *Home Health Care Management Practice, 22*(1), 43–48.

Shaffer, J. A. (2013). Stages-of-change model. In: *Encyclopedia of behavioral medicine.* New York: Springer-Verlag. 1971–1974.

Teaching Excellence in Adult Literacy (TEAL). (2011). *Teal fact sheet no. 11: Adult learning theories (2011).* U.S. Department of Education. Retrieved from https://teal.ed.gov/resources

The Joint Commission. (2010). *Advancing effective communication, cultural competence, and patient- and family-centered care: A roadmap for hospitals.* Oakbrook Terrace, IL: The Joint Commission.

Tillman, J. Patient engagement and activation: Motivational interviewing for busy healthcare settings. *Presentation, Nurse Educators Conference,* Seattle, WA, 2013.

Wallston, K., Cawthon, C., McNaughton, C., Rothman, R., Osborn, C., & Kripalani, S. (2013). Psychometric properties of the brief health literacy screen in clinical practice. *Journal of General Internal Medicine, 29*(1), 119–126.

Weiss, B. (2007). *Health literacy and patient safety: Help patients understand. Manual for clinicians* (2nd ed.). Chicago, IL: American Medical Association Foundation.

World Health Organization. (2009). *Milestones in Health Promotion, Statements from Global Conferences.* Retrieved from http://www.who.int/healthpromotion/milestones/en

World Health Organization. (2014a). *Health Impact Assessment (HIA).* Retrieved from http://www.who.int/hia/evidence/doh/en/

World Health Organization. (2014b). *Health promotion.* Retrieved January 22, 2015, from www.who.int/topics/health-promotion/en/

Zirwas, M. J., & Holder, J. L. (2009). Patient education strategies in dermatology, Part 2: Methods. *Journal of Clinical Aesthetic Dermatology, 2*(121), 29–34.

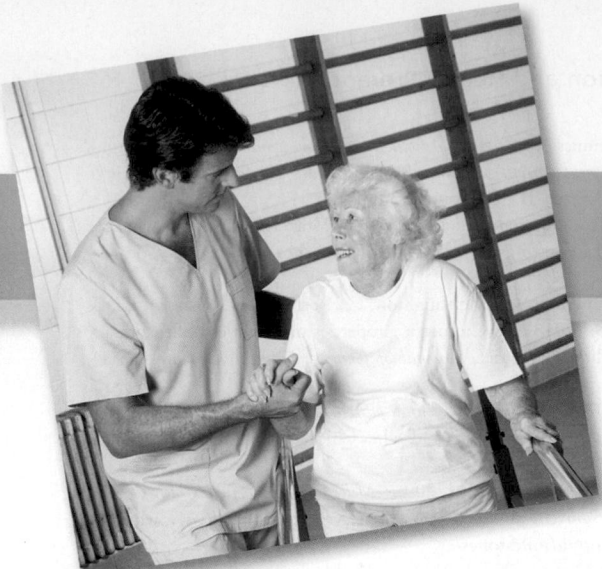

CHAPTER 10

Caring for the Older Adult

Jessica Dunn

Case Scenario

You are a nursing student assigned to do your first clinical rotation in a nearby skilled nursing facility. Many of your classmates comment that they are not looking forward to working with "old people." You have had positive experiences with the older adults in your family; however, you are a little anxious about having to care for older, frail adults. You have heard that nursing facilities have only older people who are confused, lonely, and need help with all of their activities of daily living (ADLs).

On the rehab unit, you see a resident who is actively participating in physical therapy after she tripped and fell during her daily walk with her dog, fracturing her hip. Mary, the 86-year-old resident, lives alone, enjoys gardening, and is very active in her community. She spent a week in the hospital recuperating postsurgery and is working hard with therapy so she may return to her prior living situation. She is happy to see you and can't wait to learn all about your nursing school as well as sharing her story with you.

Previous life experience greatly affects our thoughts, feelings, and behaviors in facing new situations. This tendency prevails in our interactions with specific groups, such as the older population. This chapter explores various aspects of aging as well as some of the common syndromes of aging. Syndromes are an association of several clinically recognizable features, signs, symptoms, phenomena, or characteristics that often occur together. Specific characteristics of today's older population and misconceptions of aging will be discussed. Many of the details of aging considerations are explored further in other chapters to which the reader will be referred. Once you have completed this chapter and have incorporated caring for the older adult into your knowledge base, review the above scenario and reflect on the following areas of Critical Thinking:

1. Describe your initial reaction to thoughts of caring for older adults.
2. Identify some assumptions that you had about older adults prior to reading this chapter.
3. Identify areas of new information that you will now be able to use in your clinical practice.
4. Construct a care plan that would best fit the specific needs of the woman described in the above scenario.

KEY TERMS

chronic illness

cognition

communication

elder abuse and mistreatment

health promotion

immunity

infections

loneliness

mobility

mood

pain management

rest

self-care

sexuality

skin integrity

sleep

spirituality

Upon completion of this chapter, you will be able to do the following:

1. Describe the demographics of older adults in North America.
2. Discuss a comprehensive knowledge base that can help nurses display commitment to providing humane and dignified care.
3. Identify health promotion and health maintenance strategies that can give older adults advantages in maintaining optimal health.
4. Explain functional and physiologic changes that place older adults at greater risk for declines in health and quality of life.

Older adults are a very diverse group. Most of them agree, however, that they prefer to be referred to as older adults or seniors, not as elderly. Myriad differences in lifestyle, experience, and health make it difficult to generalize about this group, especially because their age differences span four decades. Older adults (people aged 65 years or older) are considered one of the fastest growing age groups. The first "baby boomers" turned 65 in 2011 (Healthy People 2020). As adults age, they are more likely to experience chronic health disorders that impair function and adversely affect quality of life, and many older adults have multiple health conditions that exacerbate one another. Approximately 60% of older adults will experience one chronic condition by 2030, which usually include diabetes mellitus, arthritis, heart failure, or dementia (Healthy People 2020). These health conditions interact based on physiology, environment, and the person's unique health profile; however, new technology and an emphasis on **health promotion** and preventative health services have enabled this population to thrive.

This chapter discusses the importance of health promotion in this population and illustrates ways older adults can stay healthy and maintain independence. This chapter also examines health conditions that often coincide in older adults. Subsequent chapters explore these health conditions in more detail. Beginning with Chapter 23, many chapters describe special considerations for people throughout the life span, including older adults. Some chapters focus on functional changes in the older adult that may be more problematic, such as **mobility**, self-care, and **cognition** (which refers to mental functioning). The actual pathophysiology and medical treatments are beyond the scope of this text. The syndromes or conditions discussed in this chapter are not necessarily always found together. In fact, older adults may experience different health conditions in concert at various times. It is critical to keep in mind that as people age, the complex interplay of their health conditions may affect their function, well-being, and quality of life.

DEMOGRAPHICS

It is estimated that in this country every 6 seconds, someone is turning 50, and every 8 seconds someone is turning 65. In the United States and worldwide, the number of older adults has grown exponentially. Since 1900, the percentage of Americans 65 years or older has tripled, from 4.1% in 1900 to 13.7% in 2012 (see Fig. 10-1), and the number has increased over 13 times, from 3.1 million to 43.1 million (which is 13.7% of the U.S. population, or about 1 in every 7 Americans). The older adult population is expected to grow to 21% of the population by 2040.

The older population itself is older than it has been in the past. In 2012, the 65 to 74 age range was more than 10 times larger than in 1900; however, in contrast, the 75- to 84-year age group was 17 times larger, and the age group of 85 years or older was 48 times larger. The 85+ population is projected to triple from 2012 to 2040, going from 5.9 million to 14.1 million. There were about 3.6 million people celebrating their 65th birthday in 2012 and approximately 62,000 people were 100 years old or older; this is a 93% increase from the 1980 figure of approximately 32,000 (Administration on Aging [AOA], 2013).

Life expectancy has increased for both men and women. In 1900, life expectancy was 47 years. A child born in 2011 could expect to live 78.7 years, about 30 years longer than a child born in 1900. This increase in life expectancy is attributed to reduced death rates for children and young adults.

Geographic distribution varies across North America (see Fig. 10-2), with some states experiencing a far greater growth in their older population as compared to others. The figures below are estimates produced by the U.S. Census Bureau representing this distribution. Many older adults live in metropolitan areas (approximately 81%) (AOA, 2013).

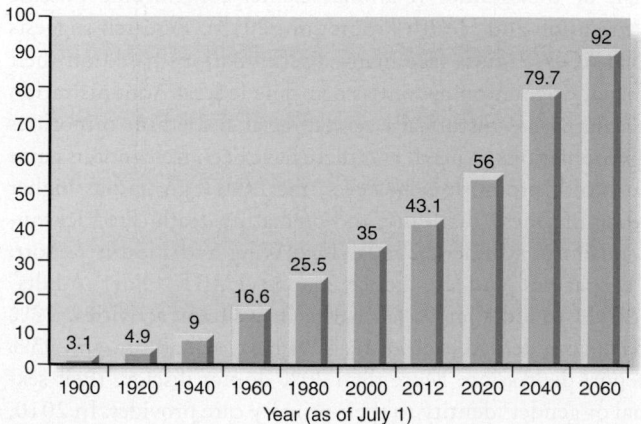

FIGURE 10-1 Number of persons 65 years or older (numbers in millions), 1900–2060. (From the U.S. Department of Health and Human Services, Administration on Aging; From the US Census Bureau, 2012 & Population Estimates and Projections.)

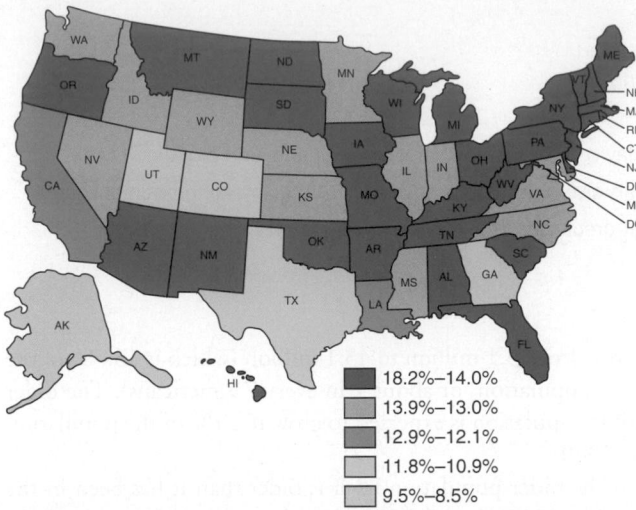

FIGURE 10-2 Persons 65 years and older as a percentage of the total population in 2012. (From the US Census Bureau, 2012 & Population Estimates.)

18.2%–14.0%
13.9%–13.0%
12.9%–12.1%
11.8%–10.9%
9.5%–8.5%

Diversity

In 2012, 21% of people 65 and over were members of racial or ethnic minority populations. Racial and ethnic minority groups have increased from 6.1 million in 2002 (17% of the older population) to 8.9 million in 2012 (21% of the older population) and are projected to increase to 20.2 million in 2030 (28% of the older population). Between 2012 and 2030, the white non-Hispanic population 65 years or older is projected to increase by 54% compared with 123.5% for older racial and ethnic minorities, including Hispanics (155%), African Americans (104%), American Indian and Native Alaskans (116%), and Asians (119%) (AOA, 2013).

We are also witnessing the aging of lesbian, gay, bisexual, and transgender (LGBT) older people and the first generation of people to age with HIV/AIDS (National Resource Center on LGBT Aging, 2014). It is estimated that up to 4 million older Americans identify themselves as gay, lesbian, bisexual, or transgender (National Center for Chronic Disease Prevention and Health Promotion, 2013). Research suggests that LGBT adults face many discriminations based on their sexual orientation as well as age. The federal Administration on Aging has historically served racial and ethnic minorities as populations of need, and there have been tremendous gains in health promotion; however, the LGBT group has higher levels of illness, disability, and premature death (Fredrickson-Godson & Muraco, 2010). The Aging and Health Report: "Disparities and Resilience among LGBT Older Adults" (2011) found that 91% engage in wellness activities, 13% have been denied healthcare, 50% have a disability, and 33% report depression. More than 20% do not disclose their sexual or gender identity to their primary care provider. In 2010, Services and Advocacy for GLBT Elders (SAGE) was funded to create a national resource center on LGBT aging; it can be found at www.lgbtagingcenter.org.

Marital Status and Living Arrangements

In 2013, older men were much more likely to be married than were older women—71% of men and 45% of women. Widows accounted for 36% of all older women in 2013. There were over three times as many widows (8.7 million) as widowers (2.3 million) (Fig. 10-3) (AOA, 2013).

Divorced and separated (including married/spouse absent) older persons represented only 13% of all older persons in 2013. However, this percentage has increased since 1980, when approximately 5.3% of the older population were divorced or separated/spouse absent (AOA, 2013).

Living arrangements vary widely based on gender (Fig. 10-4). In 2013, more than half of noninstitutionalized older adults lived with a spouse (71% of older men and 45% of older women). The proportion living with their spouse decreased with age, especially for women. Only 32% of women 75 years or older lived with a spouse (AOA, 2013).

Approximately 28% (12.1 million) of all noninstitutionalized older adults in 2013 lived alone (8.4 million women and 3.7 million men). In 2013, the percentage of living alone increased with age; for example, half of the women 75 years or older lived alone. In 2012, over 500,000 grandparents over 65 years old were primarily responsible for their grandchildren, and about 2.1 million older adults lived with a grandchild.

Although a relatively small number (1.5 million) and percentage (3.5%) of the 65 years or older population in 2012 lived in institutional settings such as long-term care facilities, the percentage increases dramatically with age, ranging from 1% for persons 65 to 74 years to 3% for persons 75 to 84 years to 10% for persons 85 years or older. In addition, approximately 2.7% of older adults lived in senior housing with at least one supportive service available (AOA, 2013).

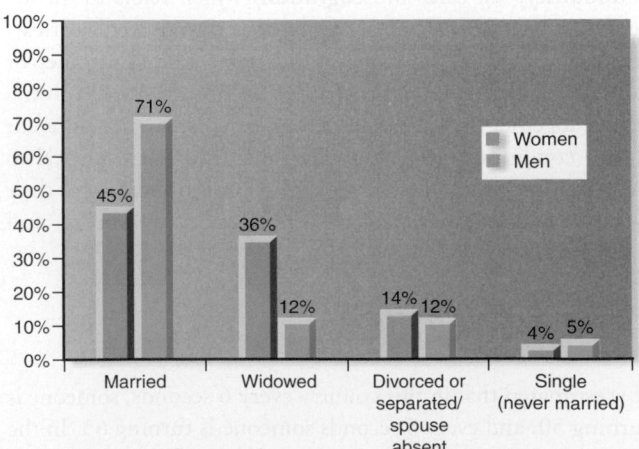

FIGURE 10-3 Marital status of persons 65 years or older, 2013. (From the US Census Bureau, Current Population Survey, Annual Social and Economic Supplement, 2013.)

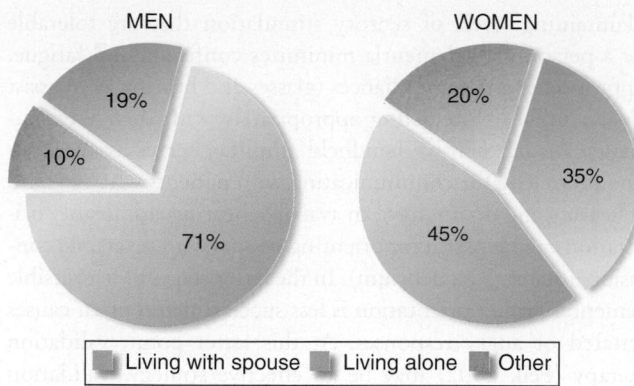

FIGURE 10-4 Living arrangements for men and women 65 years or older, 2013. (From the US Census Bureau, Current Population Survey, Annual Social and Economic Supplement, 2013.)

Income

Financial situations vary. The median income of older persons in 2012 had increased from 2008 by $27,612 for males and $16,040 for females. Households containing families headed by persons 65 years or older reported a median income in 2012 of $48,957 ($50,701 for non-Hispanic Whites; $33,913 for Hispanics; $40,348 for African Americans; and $56,378 for Asian Americans) (AOA, 2013) (see also Fig. 10-5).

For all older adults reporting income in 2012 (41.8 million), 9.1% were below poverty level, which is statistically worse than 2011 at 8.7% (AOA, 2013). Another 5.5% were classified as "near poor" (income between the poverty level and 125% of this level). Of older Whites (non-Hispanic), 6.8% were poor in 2012 compared to 18.2% of African Americans, 12.3% of Asians, and 20.6% of Hispanics. Higher than average poverty rates were found in 2012 for older persons who lived in principal cities (12.5%) and in the South (10.2%).

Older women had a higher poverty rate (11%) than did older men (6.6%) in 2012. Conversely, there is a higher percentage of older women and men living above poverty (89% and 93.4%, respectfully). Older persons living alone were much more likely to be poor (16.8%) than were older persons living with families (5.4%). The highest poverty rates were experienced among Hispanic women (41.6%) who lived alone and also by older African American women (33%) who lived alone (AOA, 2013).

In 2013, 18.7% of older Americans (65 years or more) were working or actively seeking work and constituted 5% of the U.S. labor force. This trend has been increasing gradually since 2000, especially with older women ages 65 to 69 (AOA, 2013).

Health and Healthcare

From 2010 to 2012, 42% of noninstitutionalized older adults assessed their health as excellent or very good (compared to 55% of people ages 45 to 64). There is not much of a difference in terms of gender; however, racial and ethnic minorities assess themselves much lower. Most older adults have at least one chronic condition, and many have multiple conditions. The most frequent occurring conditions for older adults from 2010 to 2012 were arthritis, heart disease, cancer, diabetes, and hypertension (50%, 30%, 24%, 20%, 72%, respectfully). In 2012, 93% of noninstitutionalized people 65 years and over were covered by Medicare, and approximately 56% also had some type of private insurance (Fig. 10-6) (AOA, 2013).

In 2010, President Obama signed the Affordable Care Act. In 2014, all Americans had access to affordable health insurance options, and the Medicaid program expanded to help cover more low-income Americans. All Americans who were previously uninsured, including older American adults, now have coverage (US Department of Health and Human Services, 2014).

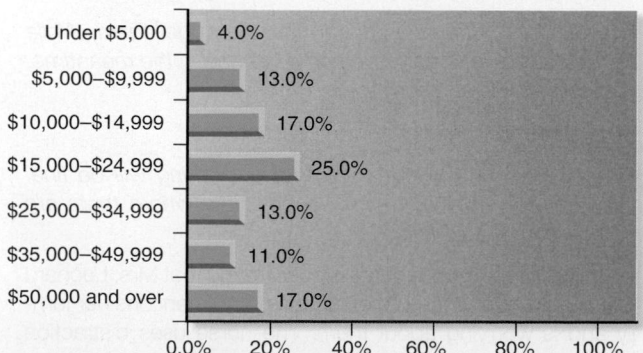

FIGURE 10-5 Income for persons 65 years or older reporting income, 2012. (From the US Census Bureau, Current Population Survey, Annual Social and Economic Supplement, 2013.)

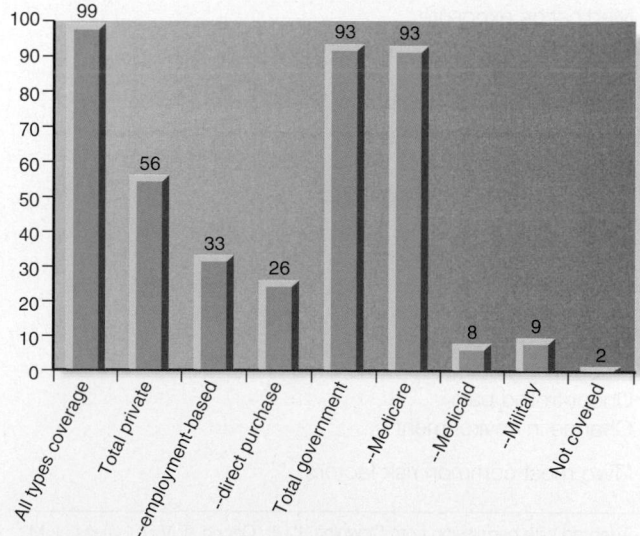

FIGURE 10-6 Type of health insurance coverage for people 65 years or older, 2012. (From the US Census Bureau, Current Population Survey, Annual Social and Economic Supplement, 2013.)

COGNITION AND COMMUNICATION, MOOD, AND SELF-CARE

Cognition and Communication

Many older adults retain full cognitive (thinking) function into advanced age. Although not a normal part of aging, the incidence of dementia (irreversible loss of intellectual function), such as Alzheimer disease, is rising in line with the aging population. In fact, the prevalence of Alzheimer disease doubles every 5 years beyond age 65 (Alzheimer's Association, 2014). In addition, older adults experience higher rates of delirium (reversible acute change in thinking and/or function usually caused by a medical condition) as compared to younger adults (Box 10-1). These conditions disrupt thinking and function in many ways. Some people exhibit losses in attention span or short-term memory. Judgment and insight may be impaired, and language deficits may occur. These cognitive and language deficits, in conjunction with any sensory deficits, impair effective **communication** (exchange of information).

Several strategies allow the nurse to facilitate communication and minimize the adverse consequences of confused thinking.

Maintaining levels of sensory stimulation that are tolerable for a person with dementia minimizes confusion and fatigue. Appropriate sensory appliances (glasses and hearing aids) assist older adults in interacting appropriately with their environments. An inexpensive handheld amplifier serves as an excellent alternative for communicating with patients who are hard of hearing and do not have an available hearing aid. Reality orientation can be useful for orienting people with reversible confusional states (e.g., delirium). In the latter stages of irreversible dementia, reality orientation is less successful and often causes agitated or angry responses. At this latter point, validation therapy (Feil, 2002) may be an effective strategy. Validation therapy is a type of interpersonal interaction in which the caregiver attempts to understand and validate the person's reality (Box 10-2). People with dementia have increased difficulty expressing their thoughts and emotions and trouble understanding others. For example, they may invent new words to describe familiar objects, lose their train of thought, use familiar words repeatedly, or revert back to their native language (Alzheimer's Association, 2014); see Box 10-3. However, there are many respectful communication strategies that can be used to effectively communicate with those who have

---

BOX 10-1 Delirium

Definition of delirium: An acute disturbance of consciousness with reduced ability to focus, sustain, or shift attention. A change in cognition or the development of perceptual disturbance that is not better accounted for by a preexisting, established, or evolving dementia.

　　Risk factors: (usually more than one is contributing)

*Advanced age
*Preexisting cognitive impairment
Medication exposure
Trauma (i.e., fall, surgery, head injury)
Severe illness
Immobility
Metabolic abnormalities
Poor nutrition
Sensory deprivation or overload
Sleep deprivation
Dehydration and anemia
Constipation
Urinary retention
Infection
Alcohol or medication withdrawal
Uncontrolled pain
Change in environment

*Two most common risk factors.

Adapted with permission from Downing, L. J., Caprio, T. V., & Lyness, J. M. (2013). Geriatric psychiatry review: Differential diagnosis and treatment of the 3 D's - delirium, dementia, and depression. *Current Psychiatry Report*, 15(365), 1–10. http://dx.doi.org/10.1007/s11920-013-0365-4

BOX 10-2 Validation Therapy

Mrs. Leonard is living in a long-term care facility. She encounters one of the nursing caregivers in the hall outside her room. She appears very upset and tearful.

Nurse: *"Mrs. Leonard, is everything all right? You seem very upset."*

Mrs. Leonard: *"I need to go and get my children who will be getting out of school soon. I don't know where my husband is either."*

　　The nurse knows that Mrs. Leonard's children are adults and that her husband died several years ago. She does not, however, confront Mrs. Leonard with any of these facts, knowing that Mrs. Leonard has had a negative reaction to that approach in the past. The nurse knows that Mrs. Leonard has Alzheimer disease and that reassurance and distraction will be more successful strategies.

Nurse: *"It is still a little early to leave and get them. While we're waiting, let's go make some tea and in the meantime, you can tell me all about them."*

Mrs. Leonard: *"All right, but I can't be late."*

Nurse: *"I know. I assure you that everything will be fine. Let's go get the tea. I think I even know where there are some delicious cookies."*

　　In this scenario, the nurse is considering that Mrs. Leonard is anxious for any number of reasons. She mentions her family and is worrying about them. The nurse uses distraction (using Mrs. Leonard's short-term memory deficit to her benefit) and a reassuring social interaction to allay Mrs. Leonard's anxieties while continuing to validate her experience.

BOX 10-3	Adverse Dementia Behavioral Symptoms

Asking questions repeatedly
Anxiety
Emotional lability (rapid mood fluctuations)
Hoarding
Irritability
Misplacing things
Physical aggressiveness
Socially/sexually inappropriate behavior
Suspiciousness/paranoia
Undressing in public
Verbal aggressiveness
Wandering

cognitive impairment (see Box 10-4). Environmental modifications, socialization strategies, and family support are other interventions for people with cognitive disorders and language difficulties (see Chapter 37).

Antidepressant or antipsychotic medications are used commonly to treat depression or adverse behavioral symptoms associated with dementia. Antipsychotics, however, have adverse side effects (including increased confusion, falls, and increased risk of adverse cardiovascular events) and should be used judiciously with careful monitoring. Their use should be reserved for situations in which behavioral strategies and environmental strategies

have failed or the patient poses a threat to self or others (Box 10-4). Antipsychotic medications are typically prescribed only when the patient displays psychotic behavior, and these medications are meant only for short-term use.

Mood

Mood disorders (especially depression) are often unrecognized or misdiagnosed in older adults partly due to the false belief that depression is a natural reaction to illness, advanced age, or life changes that occur with age and is therefore not viewed as something that needs to be treated. Furthermore, symptoms of depression may include poor cognitive performance, sleep problems, and lack of initiative—symptoms commonly seen in people with multiple chronic comorbidities such as diabetes or heart failure and in patients with dementia or delirium, causing it to be unrecognized (Chapter 37). Although depression is not a normal part of aging, older adults are at an increased risk of experiencing depression due to **chronic illness** and other age-related changes, and it is associated with functional decline, increased mortality, and poor outcomes and decreased quality of life. The older population is also less likely to report symptoms due to the stigma attached (Tanner, Martinez, & Harris, 2014). Suicide is the most serious consequence of depression. Currently, older white men have the highest rate of suicide in the United States.

The good news is that most older adults are not depressed, and depression can be treated. The use of a standardized screening tool, such as the Yesavage Geriatric Depression Scale (Box 10-5)

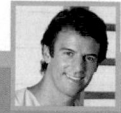

Caring for the Older Adult PICO

The student nurse from the chapter-opening scenario is asked by the clinical instructor to write about the activities used in the Alzheimer's care unit. The student decides to interview some of his patients to see what they liked about the activities that were offered in the facility. Several of his patients say that they liked going for their daily exercise. The student wonders if exercise had any benefits for patients suffering from dementia, turning to the Cochrane library for evidence to help with the assignment. The PICO question the student uses is: *In patients with dementia, how does exercise compared to no exercise affect cognition and mood?*

P = patients with dementia
I = exercise
C = no exercise
O = affect, cognition, and mood

The student finds several studies relating to this topic. One systematic review in particular questioned how exercise programs affected many factors including cognition, behavior, and depression. The review evaluated 16 randomized controlled trials, which comprised 937 patients. The studies showed that patients were more able to perform the ADL with exercise. Some of the results even seemed to indicate an improvement on cognition. However, there were unexplained variations in the study outcomes, which would benefit from further research. Unfortunately, the studies did not prove that exercise had a statistical difference with mood or behavior. With the information gathered from the research and the interviews, the student concludes that exercise provided some benefit for people suffering from dementia.

REFERENCE:

Forbes, D., Thiessen, E. J., Blake, C. M., Forbes, S. C., & Forbes S. (2013). Exercise programs for people with dementia. *Cochrane Database of Systematic Reviews*, (12), Art. No.: CD006489. DOI: 10.1002/14651858.CD006489.pub3

BOX 10-4 — Communication Strategies for Those with Cognitive Impairment

Behavioral
- Identify yourself with every interaction.
- Call the person by name.
- Treat the person with dignity and respect.
- Use short, simple words and sentences.
- Speak slowly (not loudly) and calmly.
- Wait for a response; don't be rushed.
- Rephrase questions when needed; be clear.
- Turn questions into answers (i.e., *"the bathroom is right here" instead of "do you have to use the bathroom"*).
- Avoid confusing and vague statements; simplify tasks.
- Give visual cues.
- Write things down.
- Be patient and supportive and offer comfort and reassurance.
- Avoid criticizing, correcting, or arguing.

- Offer a guess if the person is having trouble word finding.
- Limit distractions and focus on feelings and behaviors.

Environmental
- Use clear signage.
- Use enclosed bulletin boards.
- Reduce the amount of unnecessary noise.
- Encourage geriatric-friendly furniture (solid base with arm rests).
- Promote life-enhancing art that is conducive to the level of cognitive impairment.
- Recommend nonglare flooring.
- Ensure ready access to music and snack foods.
- Use sound-absorbing wall and ceiling materials.

Source: Alz.org

BOX 10-5 — Short Form: Yesavage Geriatric Depression Scale

NAME _____ AGE _____ SEX _____ DATE _____

WING _____ ROOM _____ PHYSICIAN _____ ASSESSOR _____

Scoring System
Answers indicating depression are bolded. Each **BOLDFACE** answer counts one (1) point.

1. Are you basically satisfied with your life?	YES/**NO**
2. Have you dropped any of your activities and interests?	**YES**/NO
3. Do you feel that your life is empty?	**YES**/NO
4. Do you often get bored?	**YES**/NO
5. Are you in good spirits most of the time?	YES/**NO**
6. Are you afraid that something bad is going to happen to you?	**YES**/NO
7. Do you feel happy most of the time?	YES/**NO**
8. Do you often feel helpless?	**YES**/NO
9. Do you prefer to stay in your room/facility rather than going out and doing new things?	**YES**/NO
10. Do you feel you have more problems with memory than most?	**YES**/NO
11. Do you think it is wonderful to be alive?	YES/**NO**
12. Do you feel worthless the way you are now?	**YES**/NO
13. Do you feel full of energy?	YES/**NO**
14. Do you feel that your situation is hopeless?	**YES**/NO
15. Do you think that most people are better off than you?	**YES**/NO

Score greater than 5 Probable Depression   **SCORE** _____

Notes/Current Medications: _____
_____
_____

Instructions for Use
1. The same certified nursing assistant (CNA) caregiver should administer this test each time.
2. Choose a quiet place, preferably the same location each time the test is administered.
3. The administration of this test should not be immediately after some mental trauma or unsteady period.
4. Speak in a soft, pleasant tone.
5. Answer all questions by circling the answer (Yes or No) to the question.
6. Add the total number of **BOLDFACE** answers circled, and record that number in the **SCORE** box.
7. Scores totaling five (5) points or more indicate probable depression.

A 30-item version of the Geriatric Depression Scale is also available. Address inquiries regarding this scale to Jerome A. Yesavage, M.D., Director, Psychiatric ICU, Veterans Administration Medical Center, 3801, Miranda Avenue, Palo Alto, CA, 94304. Reprinted with permission.

TABLE 10-1 PSYCHIATRIC DISORDERS

Disorder	Characteristics
Major depression	Persistent depressed mood (every day for 2 wk) or loss of interest and other symptoms such as significant change in weight or appetite; problems sleeping; psychomotor retardation or agitation; fatigue; feelings of worthlessness or inappropriate guilt; diminished ability to think or concentrate, or indecisiveness; and recurring thoughts of death or suicidal ideation. Symptoms cause significant distress or impairment in daily functioning and cannot be the result of medications or medical conditions.
Bipolar disorder	Mood swings that progress from symptoms of depression to symptoms of mania. Mania is characterized by a distinct period of abnormally and persistently elevated, expansive, or irritable mood lasting at least 1 wk. Other symptoms include inflated self-esteem or grandiosity, decreased need for sleep, pressured speech, racing thoughts, distractibility, increase in goal-directed activities, and excessive involvement in pleasurable activities with high potential for painful results.
Generalized anxiety disorder	Excessive anxiety and worry about several events or activities, occurring more days than not for at least 6 mo. Other symptoms include restlessness, being easily fatigued, difficulty concentrating or mind going blank, irritability, muscle tension, and sleep disturbance. These symptoms cause significant impairment in functioning, cannot be due to a medication or medical condition, and do not occur exclusively during a mood or psychotic disorder.
Schizophrenia	A psychotic illness characterized by disturbances in many areas of mental functioning. Thinking, perception, behavior, motivation, and emotional life are all affected. The illness impairs functioning in work, relationships, and self-care. Delusions (usually persecutory) are present.
Delusional disorder	Relatively uncommon disorder characterized by a persistent, usually well-organized delusion, often persecutory. Hallucinations are not prominent. There is less impairment in the person's functioning as compared with schizophrenia.

or the Patient Health Questionnaire (PHQ9) (www.phqscreeners .com/pdfs/02_PHQ-9/English.pdf), assists the nurse to identify an older person with depression (Yesavage & Brink, 1983; Kroenke, Spitzer, & Williams, 2001). Knowledge of these risk factors, signs, and symptoms and careful assessment of older adults allow the nurse to provide support, counseling, and appropriate and timely referral to a health provider for pharmacologic or psychotherapeutic interventions, therefore improving overall function and quality of life.

Less common psychiatric disorders, such as delusional disorder, bipolar disorder, anxiety disorder, and schizophrenia, may occur alone or coexist in older patients (Table 10-1). Psychotic symptoms (delusions and hallucinations) may result from delirium, dementia, mood, or psychiatric disorders. These disorders negatively affect the person's function and ability to communicate. Most of these disorders, when recognized and treated, respond to treatment. Antipsychotic medications typically are used to treat adverse delusions (fixed beliefs that contradict reality) and hallucinations (false perceptions such as sounds, smells, visions that have no relation to reality). Nonpharmacologic therapies (e.g., individual therapy, family therapy, peer support groups) are also used in treatment. These psychiatric disorders are severe and persistent, requiring treatment throughout the person's lifetime, and are not specific to the older adult.

Self-Care

Medications or medical conditions may cause or obscure psychotic symptoms. Conditions that mimic dementia or depression present distinct challenges because they impair thinking, mood, and communication. Such conditions also affect the older adult's ability to manage **self-care**. Activities such as shopping, managing finances, and cooking are usually affected first. As the number or severity of impairments increases, the older adult will lose his or her ability to bathe, feed, and ambulate (Chapter 24). The older adult often requires extensive care at this point. Families are the main providers of care to older adults (National Family Caregivers Association, 2010). In the absence of family or friends, or when the older adult's needs are greater than the family's ability to provide help, institutionalization (i.e., placement in a nursing facility) may be required. When personal care needs become as extensive as to require institutionalization, the older adult's independence is increasingly compromised.

Nurses frequently encounter older adults and their families in various healthcare settings (e.g., emergency rooms, acute care, clinics, nursing facilities). Numerous community agencies are available to provide necessary assistance (meals, transportation, visiting healthcare providers, home helpers) to the older adult or family. The nurse who is aware of the patient's needs and appropriate referral sources may serve as the healthcare provider best situated to link patient and families to appropriate services.

MOBILITY, ELIMINATION, AND SKIN INTEGRITY

Mobility

Physical activity is good for all people including the older adult. Being physically active (1) lowers the risk of heart disease, stroke, and diabetes, (2) reduces depression symptoms, and (3) improves thinking (Healthy People 2020). Staying active will increase or maintain strength and balance, allowing for continued independence and the prevention of injuries.

Some chronic conditions can negatively affect aspects of mobility such as walking, driving, shopping, and exercise. Arthritis, gait and balance disorders (caused by musculoskeletal or neurologic conditions), and cataracts are among the many health conditions that cause mobility problems. As a result, older adults may experience one or several impairments, including hemiparesis (weakness on one side of the body), ataxia (impaired muscular coordination), spasticity (stiff or awkward muscle movements), and coordination or balance problems. For people older than 65 years, falls are the leading cause of both fatal and nonfatal injuries, with hip fractures resulting in significant morbidity and mortality (Centers for Disease Control and Prevention [CDC], 2014a). Multiple factors place the older adult at risk for falls, including the use of medications affecting balance, thinking, memory, and elimination; impaired vision; environmental hazards (i.e., slippery floors, throw rugs, poor lighting); decreased strength; loss of bone mass; and neurologic and musculoskeletal problems (Chang & Cassio, 2010). Many older adults often experience chronic health conditions that require treatment with multiple medications that may have unwanted side effects. Some people are more sensitive to these side effects, and many of the prescribed medications can contribute to falls and other adverse complications. In 2000, Beers and Berkow developed criteria for potentially inappropriate medication use in older adults based on the risk–benefit definition of appropriateness—that is, that the use of a medication has benefits that outweigh the risks. In 2012, the Beers' list was updated (see Table 10-2).

TABLE 10-2 2012 AGS BEERS CRITERIA FOR POTENTIALLY INAPPROPRIATE MEDICATION USE IN OLDER ADULTS

Organ System/Therapeutic Category/Drug(s)	Rationale	Recommendation	Quality of Evidence	Strength of Recommendation
First-generation antihistamines (as single agent or as part of combination products) Brompheniramine Carbinoxamine Chlorpheniramine Clemastine Cyproheptadine Dexbrompheniramine Dexchlorpheniramine Diphenhydramine (oral) Doxylamine Hydroxyzine Promethazine Triprolidine	• Highly anticholinergic • Clearance reduced with advanced age • Tolerance develops when used as hypnotic • Increased risk of confusion, dry mouth, constipation, and other anticholinergic effects/toxicity *Use of diphenhydramine in special situations such as acute treatment of severe allergic reaction may be appropriate.	Avoid	Hydroxyzine and promethazine: high. All others: moderate	Strong
Antiparkinson agents				
Benztropine (oral) Trihexyphenidyl	• Not recommended for prevention of extrapyramidal symptoms with antipsychotics • More effective agents available for treatment of Parkinson disease	Avoid	Moderate	Strong
Antispasmodics Belladonna alkaloids				
Clidinium–chlordiazepoxide Dicyclomine Hyoscyamine Propantheline Scopolamine	• Highly anticholinergic • Uncertain effectiveness	Avoid **except** in short-term palliative care to decrease oral secretions	Moderate	Strong
Antithrombotics				
Dipyridamole, oral short acting* (does not apply to the extended-release combination with aspirin)	• May cause orthostatic hypotension • More effective alternatives available • IV form acceptable for use in cardiac stress testing	Avoid	Moderate	Strong
Ticlopidine*	• Safer, effective alternatives available	Avoid	Moderate	Strong

TABLE 10-2 2012 AGS BEERS CRITERIA FOR POTENTIALLY INAPPROPRIATE MEDICATION USE IN OLDER ADULTS (Continued)

Organ System/Therapeutic Category/Drug(s)	Rationale	Recommendation	Quality of Evidence	Strength of Recommendation
Anti-infective				
Nitrofurantoin	• Potential for pulmonary toxicity • Safer alternatives	Avoid for long-term suppression	Moderate	Strong
Cardiovascular				
Alpha1 blockers Doxazosin Prazosin Terazosin	• High risk of orthostatic Hypotension • Not recommended as routine treatment for hypertension • Alternative agents have superior risk–benefit profile	Avoid use as an antihypertensive	Moderate	Strong
Alpha agonists, central				
Clonidine Guanabenz* Guanfacine* Methyldopa* Reserpine (>0.1 mg/d)*	• High risk of adverse CNS effects may cause bradycardia and orthostatic hypotension. • Not recommended as routine treatment for hypertension	Avoid clonidine as a first-line antihypertensive. Avoid others as listed	Low	Strong
Antiarrhythmic drugs (class la, lc, III)				
Amiodarone Dofetilide Dronedarone Flecainide Ibutilide Procainamide Propafenone Quinidine Sotalol	• Data suggest that rate control yields better balance of benefits and harms than rhythm control for most older adults • Amiodarone is associated with multiple toxicities, including thyroid disease, pulmonary disorders, and QT interval prolongation	Avoid antiarrhythmic drugs as first-line treatment of atrial fibrillation	High	Strong
Disopyramide	• Disopyramide is a potent negative inotrope and therefore may induce heart failure in older adults • Strongly anticholinergic • Otherantiarrhythmic drugs preferred	Avoid	Low	Strong
Dronedarone	• Worse outcomes have been reported in patients taking dronedarone who have permanent atrial fibrillation or heart failure • In general, rate control is preferred over rhythm control for atrial fibrillation	Avoid in patients with permanent atrial fibrillation or heart failure	Moderate	Strong
Digoxin > 0.125 mg/d	• In heart failure, higher dosages associated with no additional benefit and may increase risk of toxicity • Slow renal clearance maylead to risk of toxic effects	Avoid	Moderate	Strong
Nifedipine, immediate release	• Potential for hypotension • Risk of precipitating myocardial ischemia	Avoid	High	Strong

(Continued)

TABLE 10-2 2012 AGS BEERS CRITERIA FOR POTENTIALLY INAPPROPRIATE MEDICATION USE IN OLDER ADULTS (*Continued*)

Organ System/Therapeutic Category/Drug(s)	Rationale	Recommendation	Quality of Evidence	Strength of Recommendation
Spironolactone > 25 mg/d	• In heart failure, the risk of hyperkalemia is higher in older adults especially if taking > 25 mg/d or taking concomitant NSAID, angiotensin-converting enzyme inhibitor, angiotensin receptor blocker, or potassium supplement	Avoid in patients with heart failure or with a CrCl < 30 mL/min.	Moderate	Strong
Central Nervous System				
Tertiary TCAs, alone or in combination: Amitriptyline Chlordiazepoxide–amitriptyline Clomipramine Doxepin > 6 mg/d Imipramine Perphenazine–amitriptyline Trimipramine	• Highly anticholinergic and sedating and cause orthostatic hypotension • Safety profile of low-dose doxepin (≤6 mg/d) is comparable with that of placebo.	Avoid	High	Strong
Antipsychotics First (conventional) and second (atypical) generation	• Increased risk of cerebrovascular accident (stroke) and mortality in persons with dementia	Avoid use for behavioral problems of dementia unless nonpharmacologic options have failed and patient is threat to self or others	Moderate	Strong
Thioridazine Mesoridazine	Highly anticholinergic and risk of QT-interval prolongation	Avoid	Moderate	Strong
Barbiturates				
Amobarbital Butabarbital Butalbital Mephobarbital Pentobarbital Phenobarbital Secobarbital	• High rate of physical dependence • Tolerance to sleep benefits • Risk of overdose at low dosages	Avoid	High	Strong
Benzodiazepines				
Short and intermediate acting: Alprazolam Estazolam Lorazepam Oxazepam Temazepam Triazolam *Long acting:* Clorazepate Chlordiazepoxide Chlordiazepoxide–amitriptyline Clidinium–chlordiazepoxide Clonazepam Diazepam Flurazepam Quazepam	• Older adults have increased sensitivity to benzodiazepines and slower metabolism of long-acting agents • In general, all benzodiazepines increase risk of cognitive impairment, delirium, falls, fractures, and motor vehicle accidents in older adults • May be appropriate for seizure disorders, rapid eye movement sleep disorders, benzodiazepine withdrawal, ethanol withdrawal, severe generalized anxiety disorder, periprocedural anesthesia, end-of-life care	Avoid benzodiazepines (any type) for treatment of insomnia, agitation, or delirium	High	Strong
Chloral hydrate	• Tolerance occurs within 10 d, and risks outweigh benefits in light of overdose with doses only 3 times the recommended dose	Avoid	Low	Strong

TABLE 10-2 2012 AGS BEERS CRITERIA FOR POTENTIALLY INAPPROPRIATE MEDICATION USE IN OLDER ADULTS (*Continued*)

Organ System/Therapeutic Category/Drug(s)	Rationale	Recommendation	Quality of Evidence	Strength of Recommendation
Nonbenzodiazepine hypnotics				
Eszopiclone Zolpidem Zaleplon	• Benzodiazepine receptor agonists that have adverse events similar to those of benzodiazepines in older adults (e.g., delirium, falls, fractures) • Minimal improvement in sleep latency and duration	Avoid chronic use (>90 d)	Moderate	Strong
Ergot mesylates* Isoxsuprine*	• Lack of efficacy	Avoid	High	Strong
Endocrine androgens				
Methyltestosterone* Testosterone	Potential for cardiac problems and contraindicated in men with prostate cancer	Avoid unless indicated for moderate to severe hypogonadism	Moderate	Weak
Desiccated thyroid	• Concerns about cardiac effects • Safer alternatives available	Avoid	Low	Strong
Estrogens with or without progestins	• Evidence of carcinogenic potential (breast and endometrium); lack of cardioprotective effect and cognitive protection in older women Evidence that vaginal estrogens for treatment of vaginal dryness is safe and effective in women with breast cancer, especially at dosages of estradiol < 25 mcg twice weekly	• Avoid oral and topical patch. Topical vaginal cream: acceptable to use low-dose intravaginal estrogen for the management of dyspareunia, lower urinary tract infections, and other vaginal symptoms	Oral and patch: high Topical: moderate	Oral and patch: strong Topical: weak
Growth hormone	Effect on body composition is small and associated with edema, arthralgia, carpal tunnel syndrome, gynecomastia, and impaired fasting glucose	Avoid, except as hormone replacement after pituitary gland removal	High	Strong
Insulin, sliding scale	Higher risk of hypoglycemia without improvement in hyperglycemia management regardless of care setting	Avoid	Moderate	Strong
Megestrol	Minimal effect on weight; increases risk of thrombotic events and possibly death in older adults	Avoid	Moderate	Strong
Sulfonylureas, long duration Chlorpropamide Glyburide	Chlorpropamide: prolonged half-life in older adults; can cause prolonged hypoglycemia; causes syndrome of inappropriate antidiuretic hormone secretion. Glyburide: greater risk of severe prolonged hypoglycemia in older adults	Avoid	High	Strong
Gastrointestinal				
Metoclopramide	Can cause extrapyramidal effects including tardive dyskinesia; risk may be even greater in frail older adults	Avoid, unless for gastroparesis	Moderate	Strong
Mineral oil, oral	Potential for aspiration and adverse effects; safer alternatives available	Avoid	Moderate	Strong
Trimethobenzamide	One of the least effective antiemetic drugs; can cause extrapyramidal adverse effects	Avoid	Moderate	Strong

(*Continued*)

TABLE 10-2 2012 AGS BEERS CRITERIA FOR POTENTIALLY INAPPROPRIATE MEDICATION USE IN OLDER ADULTS (*Continued*)

Organ System/Therapeutic Category/Drug(s)	Rationale	Recommendation	Quality of Evidence	Strength of Recommendation
Non–COX-selective NSAIDs				
Aspirin > 325 mg/d Diclofenac Diflunisal Etodolac Fenoprofen Ibuprofen Ketoprofen Meclofenamate Mefenamic acid Meloxicam Nabumetone Naproxen Oxaprozin Piroxicam Sulindac Tolmetin	Increases risk of GI bleeding and peptic ulcer disease in high-risk groups, including those aged > 75 or taking oral or parenteral corticosteroids, anticoagulants, or antiplatelet agents. Use of proton pump inhibitor or misoprostol reduces but does not eliminate risk. Upper GI ulcers, gross bleeding, or perforation caused by NSAIDs occurs in approximately 1% of patients treated for 3–6 mo and in approximately 2%–4% of patients treated for 1 y. These trends continue with longer duration of use.	Avoid chronic use unless other alternatives are not effective and patient can take gastroprotective agent (proton pump inhibitor or misoprostol)	Moderate	Strong
Indomethacin Ketorolac, includes parenteral	Increases risk of GI bleeding and peptic ulcer disease in high-risk groups. (See above Non–COX-selective NSAIDs.) Of all the NSAIDs, indomethacin has most adverse effects.	Avoid	Indomethacin: moderate Ketorolac: high	Strong
Pentazocine	Opioid analgesic that causes CNS adverse effects, including confusion and hallucinations, more commonly than other narcotic drugs; is also a mixed agonist and antagonist; safer alternatives available	Avoid	Low	Strong
Skeletal muscle relaxants				
Carisoprodol Chlorzoxazone Cyclobenzaprine Metaxalone Methocarbamol Orphenadrine	Most muscle relaxants are poorly tolerated by older adults because of anticholinergic adverse effects, sedation, and risk of fracture; effectiveness at dosages tolerated by older adults is questionable	Avoid	Moderate	Strong

Note: The criteria in this table apply to all elderly patients, not just nursing facility residents.
*Infrequently used drugs.
Reprinted with permission from American Geriatrics Society 2012 Beers Criteria Update Expert Panel (2012).

The tension between fear of falling and striving for independence is a daily challenge for many older adults. Instituting appropriate interventions relies on a thorough assessment of the person's mobility impairments (Chapter 25). Interventions may include muscle strengthening, range-of-motion exercises, gait and balance training, medication review (especially for medications that cause postural hypotension), and assistive device (canes, walkers) training. Other interventions include routine eye examinations, improved lighting, and reducing environmental hazards (CDC, 2014c).

Elimination

Approximately 10 million Americans experience urinary incontinence (involuntary loss of urine). Although it is common among older adults, it is not considered a normal part of aging. Urinary incontinence can present significant financial and emotional burden on older adults and impact their quality of life (US Department of Health and Human Services, 2014). Bladder incontinence is associated with many factors such as normal age-related changes, chronic conditions, diabetes, stroke, mobility and cognitive impairments, and infection. Incontinence can be a predictor of functional limitations and be associated with decreasing mental health or depression (US Department of Health and Human Services, 2014). There are different types of incontinence, which are listed below, but in general, incontinence is referred to the involuntary loss of bladder or bowel control. Both *urge incontinence* (caused by an overactive detrusor muscle causing involuntary bladder contraction) and *stress incontinence* (caused by pelvic floor muscle weakness or urethral hypermobility) may cause older adults to rush to a toilet, resulting in a fall. *Overflow incontinence* (occurring when the bladder muscle distends and urine is forced out) and *functional incontinence* (occurring when a physical or psychological impairment impedes continence despite a competent urinary system) are other types of urinary incontinence. *Acute* or *temporary incontinence* is easily reversible and may be caused by medication side effects, urinary tract **infections**, or limited mobility. The incidence of urinary incontinence in older women is approximately twice that in men, occurring particularly in those who have had several pregnancies (Ruby et al., 2010).

Interventions are specific to the type of incontinence. Strategies most frequently used include bladder training, external catheters, avoiding medications that may contribute to incontinence, exercise, weight loss, and protective pants. Careful assessment of the effects of incontinence on the person's quality of life is also very important, along with the development of an individualized care plan to improve or maintain dignity and quality of life.

Skin Integrity

Although older adults experience age-related skin changes that may put them at risk for disruptions in **skin integrity**, most adults maintain intact skin and healthy skin integrity well into their older adulthood. An injury from a fall, malnutrition, dehydration, immobility, or incontinence (bladder or bowel) without proper skin care can result in skin breakdown. A pressure ulcer—also known as "pressure sore," "decubitus ulcer," or "bed sore"—is defined as an injury to the skin or tissue caused by prolonged, unrelieved pressure, usually over a bony prominence (Langer & Fink, 2014). Many factors predispose an individual to have pressure ulcers. Factors can be physical (local infections, malnutrition), functional (impaired mobility, incontinence), and psychosocial (poor adherence to treatment, impaired cognition). Several scales, such as the Braden Scale, have been developed to assess the person's risk for pressure ulcers (see Box 30-2). Prevention of pressure ulcers relies on the prevention of sustained pressure to a body surface area. Using standardized scales, nurses are able to identify persons at risk for pressure ulcers and institute preventive strategies (e.g., pressure-relieving mattresses, turning and positioning schedules). For an existing pressure ulcer, based on the stage of the pressure ulcer, various wound treatments (dressings, removal of dead tissue) are available. In all age groups, proper skin care (e.g., proper cleansing, lubrication) and maintenance of skin integrity are critical in maintaining optimal health and comfort (see Chapter 30).

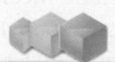 **Concept Mastery Alert**

The skin plays an important role in thermoregulation, but impaired thermoregulation is not the most serious risk faced by a patient who has skin that is thin and dry. Thin, dry skin is much more susceptible to shearing, abrasion, and other forms of physical injury than to impaired thermoregulation.

 APPLY YOUR CRITICAL THINKING

Esther Bennet, 79, comes to the clinic for a follow-up of her bladder infection, which was originally diagnosed and treated 1 week ago. Her husband tells you that the bladder infection seems much improved, but his wife has watery diarrhea and a severely inflamed perineum. He is frustrated and his wife is in pain, not wanting to sit up.

What assessment data do you need to obtain at this point? How will you assist the patient in managing the diarrhea and the perineal skin problem?

Check your answers in Appendix B.

NUTRITION AND HEALTH MAINTENANCE

Lower income adversely affects nutritional status. Close to 4 million older adults lived at or below poverty in 2012. Older women had a higher poverty rate (11%) as compared to men (6.6%), and those living alone were much more likely to live in poverty (AOA, 2013). Conversely, the median household income for people 65 years and older in 2012 was $48,957 with 29% of households making $75,000 (AOA, 2013).

Other causes affect nutritional status including physiologic age-related changes, poor dentition, medication side effects, depression, and chronic illness. As people age, changes in the gastrointestinal tract can affect nutrition. For example, a decrease in the number of taste buds and saliva production can decrease taste sensation and appetite. Dental problems (e.g., poorly fitting dentures, difficulty chewing, and broken teeth) make effective eating difficult. Medications may adversely affect appetite or cause a decrease in saliva or a change in taste. Several medical conditions—such as chronic obstructive pulmonary disease, dementia, chronic pain, and depression—contribute to poor appetite. In addition, psychosocial aspects, such as eating alone after the death of a spouse, also cause problems in maintaining adequate nutrition.

Careful nutritional assessment using a tool like the Mini Nutritional Assessment (MNA) to assess for risk of malnutrition (www.mna-elderly.com/forms/mini/mna_mini_english.pdf) and patient-specific interventions are necessary in helping the older adult maintain optimal health. At a basic level, simply eating and digesting food may be difficult for some older adults; helpful aids include over-the-counter products that increase saliva so eating is more pleasant for the patient and food is easier to digest. Prompt and aggressive treatment of health disorders, such as dental problems, depression, or chronic pain, may reverse adverse nutritional consequences. Community agencies are available to deliver meals to homebound adults (e.g., Meals on Wheels). Many seniors participate in meals and activities at senior centers; these shared experiences further enhance the psychosocial aspects of nutrition.

The National Health and Nutrition Examination Survey (NHANES), which uses body measurements for accurate prevalence rates, states that 34.6% of older adults are obese. The adverse effects of being obese in middle age are well documented, and the environment plays a huge role in fighting the obesity epidemic for a person of any age. The health consequences of being overweight in old age (having a body mass index [BMI] between 25 and 29.9 kg/m²) or obese (BMI greater than or equal to 30 kg/m²) are not well understood.

However, body weight is not the only indicator of nutritional health (sufficient intake and utilization of food/nutrients). Although only 1% of older adults who are independent and healthy are malnourished, the NHANES data indicate that 16% of community-dwelling Americans older than 65 years consumed fewer than 1,000 calories per day—a statistic that would place these persons at high risk for undernutrition. The nutritional risk of malnutrition increases in the community-dwelling seniors who are sick, poor, and homebound and have limited access to medical care. When not directly attributable to underlying disease, weight loss in the institutionalized older adult is most commonly due to depression, use of anorexigenic drugs, and dependency on staff to assist with meals (U.S. Department of Health and Human Services, 2014).

Consensus is lacking about the optimal nutritional health requirements for older persons as they age. There are very few large research studies to rely on; there is a shortage of long-range studies, and there are problems related to researching older adults with multiple medical disorders. Researchers generally agree, however, that food intake declines with aging. Various physiologic age-related processes appear to explain this, including decreased thirst and smell, alterations in taste, early satiation (feeling full), and anorexia. Decreased dietary intake is also associated with a decline in physical activity that further limits the intake of essential micronutrients (Institute of Medicine, 2010).

In recent decades, research exploring the role of nutrition has looked at the role of weight, longevity, and antioxidants in slowing the aging process. Clear evidence is still lacking about the most efficacious strategies for older adults. Good management of chronic illnesses and good nutrition, exercise, and health promotion strategies (e.g., immunizations, reduction of stress) have been found to contribute to healthy immune functioning and an increased quality of life (see Chapters 29 and 31).

CHRONIC ILLNESS, INFECTIONS, AND IMMUNITY

Chronic Illness

Approximately 33% of older Americans have multiple chronic conditions, and 66% of healthcare costs for older adults are for treating chronic illnesses (US Department of Health and Human Services, 2010). Many people with chronic diseases may also have other health problems such as substance abuse or addiction disorders, mental illness, disabilities, or cognitive impairments.

Functional and cognitive decline and death associated with chronic illnesses are often preventable or can be delayed. Although the risk of developing chronic disease increases as we age, the root cause usually happens earlier in life (CDC, 2014b). Engaging in health activity including smoking cessation, exercise, and proper nutrition are ways to eliminate or delay risk of developing diseases such as diabetes, heart disease, and cancer.

Infections and Immunity

As people age, their immune systems become less efficient. Humoral **immunity** declines because of changes in T-cell function, and older adults have lower antibody response to microorganisms that cause influenza and pneumonia (Frasca et al., 2010). Inadequate nutrition and chronic illnesses adversely affect the immune system and the ability to ward off infection. Without proper nutrients, basic body functions lack the necessary vitamins, minerals, and food substances (proteins, carbohydrates, and fats) to maintain optimal functioning.

Routine health examinations and screening assist in uncovering health problems early and preventing later, more serious complications. The Centers for Disease Control and Prevention (CDC) recommend routine screening for breast cancer, colorectal cancer, diabetes, lipid disorders, and osteoporosis. Furthermore, annual influenza vaccinations and pneumococcal vaccinations every 5 years are strongly recommended for prevention of illness in this age group (CDC, 2014c). Prevention of health problems and careful monitoring and treatment of coexisting problems are especially important for older adults with compromised immune function (see Chapter 31 for further discussion of immune function and infection).

SLEEP AND REST

Sufficient **rest** and good **sleep** are essential in all age groups for optimal functioning. Sleep difficulties may become more prevalent and increase in severity with age. Sleep disturbances can mean anything from difficulty falling or staying asleep, early morning awakening, or too much sleep. A healthy older adult may wake up close to four times during the night (Williams, Kay, & McCrae, 2013). Normal sleep changes that occur in older persons include an increase in stage 1 sleep and a decrease in deep sleep (Venugopal & Susman, 2000). These changes lead to more frequent nighttime awakenings and less restful sleep. In addition, older persons experience many pathologic processes that further impair good sleep and rest (see Chapter 34). Many of these impairments include medications (antipsychotics, beta-blockers, and decongestants), restless legs syndrome (an uncomfortable sensation in legs relieved by moving or rubbing them), sleep apnea, pain, and cardiovascular and pulmonary disorders. Some other causes include Alzheimer disease, alcohol, caffeine, inactivity, nocturia (urination at night), and pain. Sleep disturbances often impair the person's daytime functioning and have a negative effect on health.

BOX 10-6	Good Sleep Habits

- Avoid alcohol, nicotine, and caffeine.
- Avoid exercise 3 to 4 hours before bedtime.
- Avoid frequent napping during the day.
- Avoid large meals and excitement before bedtime.
- Avoid technology before bed (i.e., television, cell phones, computers).
- Maintain a routine; go to bed and get up at the same time each night.
- Sleep in a cool, quiet environment.
- Upon awakening, get up and avoid watching the clock.
- Use the bed for sleeping (or intimacy or sex) only.

Source: Bloom, H. G., et al. (2009). Evidence-based recommendations for the assessment and management of sleep disorders in older persons. *Journal of American Geriatric Society, 57,* 761–789; National Institute of Health, 2014.

BOX 10-7	Strategies for Treating Pain in Older Adults

- Distraction techniques such as listening to music, watching television, and storytelling
- Participating in regular individualized physical activity
- Acupuncture
- Counseling/psychotherapy
- Massage or warm applications
- Meditation/imagery
- Sensory stimulation such as pet therapy or folding warm towels
- Pharmacologic
- Psychosocial (socialization, recreational therapies)
- Transcutaneous electrical nerve stimulation (TENS)

Many sleep disturbances can be prevented or treated. A thorough assessment by a healthcare provider is essential in determining cause for sleep disturbances and preparing a treatment plan. Good sleep habits may improve sleep initiation and maintenance (Box 10-6). These strategies, in addition to treatment of any coexisting medical conditions, may increase the person's effective sleep. Sleep medications may be used, but these drugs are most effective when limited to short-term use (7 to 14 days); otherwise, the medications may actually interfere with sleep and cause other adverse outcomes such as falls, confusion, and constipation. Persistent, excessive daytime sleepiness may be indicative of a serious sleep disturbance and needs to be evaluated by a sleep specialist.

PAIN MANAGEMENT

Pain is common in older adults and is a major cause of sleep impairment, depression, functional decline, increased healthcare utilization, and disability (Chapters 34 and 35). Pain is unique to each individual and depends on biologic, social, and psychological characteristics. Approximately 100 million Americans report having chronic pain (Institute of Medicine 2011a, 2011b).

Chronic pain is most commonly caused by osteoarthritis. Other conditions causing chronic pain include neuropathic pain (chronic pain resulting from an injury to the nervous system), central or neuropathic pain after stroke, postherpetic neuralgia (result of damage to nerve fibers caused by the herpes zoster virus, commonly known as shingles), and phantom limb pain after amputation. Cognitive impairments limit an older adult's ability to report pain and may account for sleep disturbances and many of dementia's adverse behavioral symptoms. Barriers to adequate **pain management** in older persons include misconceptions about addiction, lack of knowledge about dose management and tolerance (especially to opioids),

belief that older adults experience less pain, and failure to assess and treat pain in cognitively impaired persons (National Pain Foundation, 2010).

Strategies to identify older adults in pain and assist in choosing appropriate therapies include education for healthcare providers, patients, and families, recognition of risk factors (e.g., depression, multiple health problems, immobility), and careful initial assessment and ongoing reassessment (Box 10-7). Inadequate pain management has many negative consequences for older adults; those consequences include decreased quality of life, depression, decreased socialization, suicidal ideation, decreased appetite, increased healthcare utilization, and increased costs. Providing good pain palliation is one of the most valuable ways nurses can maximize quality of life for older adults.

LOSS AND GRIEF, LONELINESS, ELDER ABUSE/NEGLECT, AND COPING AND STRESS

Loss and Grief

Older adults face numerous potential and immediate losses as they continue to age. Typically, they experience losses related to health, significant others (spouses, family, friends, pets), finances, geography (e.g., moves to assisted living or long-term care facilities), and leisure activities. Loss of a spouse (or significant other) is highly substantial and may be a critical threat to self-concept and sense of wholeness. In fact, death, including death from suicide, is most likely to occur during the first year of widowhood. In 2013, 36% of women were widowed by age 65 years, compared with 12% of men. Of women 65 years or older, only 45% lived with a spouse compared to 71% of men (AOA, 2013). Often, these older adults are forced to face many losses simultaneously; as a result, their remaining resources are very low.

People who experience losses of any type are expected to grieve (Chapter 40). Initial grief reactions include shock, disbelief, anger, or denial of the loss. The severity and length of the grieving (or bereavement) vary with the individual and the type of loss. Social support, therapy, and religious faith are sources of adaptive coping. Maladaptive coping strategies include using alcohol or drugs to blunt the pain (Siegel & Anderman, 2004). Nursing interventions, which assist the older adult in using adaptive strategies to cope with loss, decrease the risk of prolonged or pathologic grief reactions.

Loneliness

Loss of important relationships places an older person at risk for **loneliness**. Loneliness refers to a subjective emotional state of being alone, and there is a relationship between loneliness and health outcomes (Ivbijaro, 2013). Sensory losses may make it difficult for an older adult to communicate with others and can contribute to loneliness and depression. Depression may cause the person to become more socially isolated or physically separated from other people such as living alone (Ivbijaro, 2013). Cognitive disorders, such as dementia, diminish the capacity to interact meaningfully or appropriately in social situations. Cultural differences and language barriers make communication difficult and exacerbate loneliness.

In healthcare settings, nursing staff may focus strongly on tasks while overlooking the older adult's need to maintain her or his integrity and dignity. Often, older adults who are dying are isolated further, due in part to the staff's inability to deal with their own feelings and fear of death. Loneliness can predispose a person to poor health outcomes (e.g., increased health utilization, increased medication usage). The nurse, in spending time with the older adult, may uncover reasons for the patient's loneliness or even discover ways to decrease loneliness (e.g., pet therapy, reminiscence). Older adults may have musical or art talents to share with others. Many older adults have the occupational and educational skills to serve as mentors or tutors for children and younger adults. Encouraging the older adult to remain active and socially engaged may have many positive physical and psychological effects.

Elder Abuse and Neglect

Social isolation is one of the risk factors for older adults becoming victims of mistreatment. Types of abuse include physical, emotional, sexual, exploitation, neglect, or abandonment (Box 10-8) (NCEA, 2014). Dementia and frailty also predispose an elder to mistreatment. The problem of elder mistreatment is a predominantly hidden and growing problem; consequently, it is hard to know how many people are suffering from abuse. It is estimated that in the United States, more than 500,000 older adults are abused or neglected each year (National Center on Elder Abuse [NCEA], 2014), with females experiencing more abuse than males and incidence increasing with age. The good news is that recent data from Adult Protective Services (APS) show an increasing trend in reporting of abuse, although there is still much work to be done to increase awareness and reporting (NCEA, 2014).

BOX 10-8   Types of Abuse and Mistreatment

- Physical: Inflicting or threatening to inflict pain or injury on a vulnerable older adult; depriving them of basic needs
- Emotional/psychological: Verbally or nonverbally causing mental pain, anguish, or distress on an older adult
- Sexual: Nonconsensual sexual contact of any kind; coercing an older adult to witness sexual behaviors
- Exploitation: Illegally taking or misusing funds, property, or assets of a vulnerable older adult
- Neglect: Refusing or failure by those responsible to provide food, shelter, protection, or healthcare for a vulnerable older adult.
- Abandonment: Desertion of a vulnerable older adult by anyone who has assumed responsibility for their care

Source: National Center on Elder Abuse: Administration on Aging. (2014). Statistics and data on elder abuse. Retrieved on July 20, 2014, from http://www.ncea.aoa.gov/Library/Data/index.aspx#problem

---

Nurses can perform an Elder Mistreatment Assessment (consultgerirn.org/uploads/File/trythis/try_this_15.pdf) to determine if the older adult has evidence of abuse/neglect (Fulmer & Cahill, 1984). The many types of abuse (Box 10-8) and warning signs nurses should be aware of include but are not limited to unexplained bruises, abrasions, pressure sores, sudden changes in mood or financial situations, unattended medical needs, poor hygiene, strained or tense relationships, and withdrawal (NCEA, 2014). Neglect can be self-inflicted as well, and if suspected should be investigated. Examples of signs to look for include hoarding, failure to thrive, refusal of services or medications, poor hygiene, inappropriate attire for weather, confusion, or leaving a burning stove on unattended.

It is the obligation of nurses and other healthcare providers to report any suspicion of abuse or neglect in a *vulnerable* adult. A vulnerable adult is a person 60 years or older who lacks the functional, physical, or mental ability to care for himself or herself; an adult with disability or one with a legal guardian; or an adult in a long-term care facility or living in his or her own home receiving services from an agency or individual provider (Department of Social and Health Services [DSHS], 2014). It is important to be alert to changes, because many times, abuse and neglect are hidden and silent.

Coping and Stress

Older adults are faced with adapting to multiple stressors (e.g., physiologic, psychological, sociocultural, or environmental stresses). Coping is how people deal with difficulties in their lives. Having efficient coping skills helps enhance individual self-control and direction (Bazrafshan, Jahangir, Mansouri, & Kashfi, 2014). Several theories exist about how individuals manage stress (Chapter 41). In one of the most frequently used stress/coping models, Lazarus and Folkman

(1984) initially described two major categories of coping strategies: emotion-focused and problem-focused. In emotion-focused coping, the individual attempts to change the way he or she thinks about or appraises a stressful situation rather than changing the situation itself. For example, crying, sleeping, or talking about the stressful situation helps improve the individual's feeling about the stressor but doesn't reduce the root cause. Problem-focused or action-based coping, which involves attempts to reduce stress by changing the stressful situation, is considered the better of the two approaches. An example of this type of coping would be finding a job if in financial distress (Bazrafshan et al., 2014).

How older adults adapt to stress varies tremendously based on many factors, including previous coping styles and current resources (see Chapter 41 for further discussion). Older adults vary dramatically in their perceptions of, as well as their reactions to, stressors in their environment. Interventions are most effective when tailored to maximize the older adult's unique goals, strengths, and available resources.

SEXUALITY, ROLES AND RELATIONSHIPS, AND SELF-PERCEPTION

Sexuality

Human beings are never too old to enjoy a healthy and satisfying sex life. Human touch and healthy sexual activity do increase joy, affection, intimacy, and romance throughout one's life. Despite this, many people, old and young, find it hard to believe that sexual activity can continue through later adulthood. One belief is that sexual desire or activity diminishes with age. As persons age, the reproductive system loses efficacy; physiologically, both men and women experience changes that affect certain aspects of **sexuality** (e.g., arousal and orgasm). Certain medical conditions (e.g., cardiac problems, diabetes, neurologic problems, arthritis) and medications (antidepressants, antihypertensives, antipsychotics) make the expression of sexuality difficult (Greenberg, 2001). Despite these changes, research has demonstrated that older persons continue to engage in and enjoy sexual experiences, even into their 90s. Expressions of sexuality extend beyond overt sexual acts and include a yearning for intimacy (psychosocial and physical), security, and belonging. Touch remains an important aspect of sexual expression and an integral part of human well-being.

Unfortunately, older adults who are alone or institutionalized are often deprived of this important sensory input. Often, older persons lack the privacy necessary to initiate or develop new relationships. In institutional settings, the older person may be subjected to the staff's moral interpretation or restriction of behavior considered to be unacceptable (e.g., same-sex relationships, extramarital relationships). Older gays and lesbians (approximately 4 million older adults) experience unique issues (AOA, 2013). It wasn't until 1973 that the American Psychiatric Association (2013) removed homosexuality from its list of mental illnesses. Currently, many states continue to have laws prohibiting homosexuals from consensual intimate relations or marriage.

It is important to keep in mind that numerous individual preferences and differences in sexual behavior exist. In one study by DeLamater and Moorman (2007), men and women expressed differences in describing a satisfying sexual relationship: Older men preferred erotic reading materials/movies, sexual daydreams, physical intimacy, oral sex, and masturbation; older women preferred talking, sitting, making themselves attractive, and saying loving words. For all older adults, however, sexuality is one of the important aspects in which they view their role in society. Sexuality continues to impact their relationships in later life.

To maintain an open, nonjudgmental stance in exploring older adults' sexuality, nurses need to understand their own cultural and moral belief systems. Nurses are often reluctant to inquire about sexual behavior; their reluctance is based, in part, on the societal norm that considers discussions of sexuality and sexual behavior to be private. Such discussions are crucial, however, in evaluating the older adult's overall health. Older adults surveyed about ways in which healthcare providers may assist them in dealing with sexual questions suggested the following: Spend time with the older adult; use clear, easy-to-understand language; help the patient feel more comfortable talking about sex; be open-minded and talk openly; listen; encourage discussion; give advice or suggestions as needed; and understand that "sex is not just for the young" (DeLamater & Moorman, 2007).

There is very little accurate, easily accessible information for older adults about their sexuality. As in other healthcare situations, nurses have a unique opportunity to provide support, education, and appropriate referral to their older patients (Chapter 42).

Roles and Relationships

Many other factors impact the older adult's roles and relationships throughout aging. Family structures have changed due to increases in life span. Older adults divorce, or their spouses die. Children divorce and may return to the family home. The numbers of four- and even five-generation families have increased. Grandparents and great grandparents play several roles, depending on a multitude of factors, including health, geographic proximity, and cultural expectations. Caregiving often becomes an issue as parents or spouses become very old or ill. Relationships with family, friends, neighbors, and service providers are as unique and complex as the older individuals themselves.

Caregiving for ill children, spouses, or aging parents usually spans several years; sometimes, caregiving spans decades. Successful nursing strategies include careful assessment of physical and psychological health, referral to appropriate healthcare providers, and assistance in accessing agencies that provide help to caregivers (respite care, day centers, caregiver support groups). For information about services in their community, persons may access the U.S. Administration on Aging website www.aoa.gov.

Self-Perception

The older adult's multiple evolving roles define his or her self-concept. The individual's sense of self incorporates many aspects, including physical functioning, cognition, social relationships, and life experiences (Chapter 38). The older adult attempts to maintain her or his self-esteem despite numerous changes in physiologic and psychological attributes. These changes with aging can be viewed as negative or positive, impacting quality of life. In their interactions with older adults, nurses form part of their patients' social network, and it is important to understand how the older adult is responding to life events and age-related changes. Dignified and humane nursing care is essential in positively reinforcing a person's self-esteem and sense of self. In maintaining a high level of quality care, nurses serve as advocates for older adults, especially those who are frail or disadvantaged.

VALUES, BELIEFS, AND SPIRITUALITY

Most older adults retain good function and quality of life into advanced age. **Spirituality** remains a source of health and healing power (Chapter 43) for some, but not all, adults as they age (Manning, Leek, & Radina, 2012) It is important for nurses to understand how the older adult views spirituality in terms of health and well-being. The FICA Spiritual History Tool (FICA) (consultgerirn.org/uploads/File/trythis/try_this_sp5.pdf), developed as a quick guide to help clinicians conduct a spiritual assessment, should be incorporated into a holistic patient health history (Borneman, Ferrel, & Puchalski, 2010) (Box 10-12). As persons age, they approach death—a stage that has been called the last developmental stage. Older adults react in numerous and diverse ways to the experience of dying: Some feel fright, anger, and resignation; others experience acceptance and equanimity. For many, advancing age provides the opportunity for transcendence or gerotranscendence (a shift in perspective from the material world to the cosmic and an increase in life satisfaction) (Tornstam, 2005). Throughout the dying process, persons need to have their physical, psychosocial, and spiritual needs met. Caring for these older adults requires that nurses provide competent palliation and compassionate end-of-life care. End-of-life care can happen in any setting such as hospitals, nursing facilities, and homes.

Today, educational opportunities about providing effective palliative care are commonplace. One great resource is ELNEC (End-of-Life Nursing Education Consortium). This is a national initiative to improve training in palliative care. There is more information about this initiative on the American Association of Colleges of Nursing website (www.aacn.nche.edu).

Effective pain management remains an ongoing and primary aspect of care. Hospice provides care for terminally ill older patients and their families. Multiple disciplines (nurses, physicians, clergy, pain specialists, complementary providers, legal/financial advisors) are required to provide the holistic care necessary at this life stage.

Dealing with matters of dying is sometimes uncomfortable for the older adult, her or his family, and the nurses providing care. For others, death is considered to be a natural part of life's journey. Many nurses who accompany these older adults on their final journeys find those experiences to be some of the most rewarding and meaningful of their professional careers.

KEY CONCEPTS

- Providing excellence in nursing care to older adults depends on a comprehensive knowledge base and a commitment to providing humane and dignified care.

- Older adults, even into advanced age, demonstrate remarkable resilience.

- Physiologic changes and an increased incidence of chronic illnesses place older adults at greater risk for declines in health and quality of life. Health promotion strategies (good lifestyle habits) and health maintenance (disease prevention and treatment) afford even the oldest adult an advantage in maintaining optimal health.

- Medications or medical conditions may cause or obscure psychotic symptoms. Conditions that mimic dementia or depression present distinct challenges because they impair thinking, mood, and communication. Such conditions also affect the older adult's ability to manage. Activities such as shopping, managing finances, and cooking are usually affected first. As the number or severity of impairments increases, the older adult will lose his or her ability to bathe, feed, and ambulate (Chapters 23 to 25 and 29). The older adult often requires extensive care at this point. Families are the main providers of care to older adults (National Family Caregivers Association, 2010; Healthy People 2020).

- Nursing as a discipline has always been concerned with the multiple domains of the person, family, and community. Nurses are educated to act as providers, advocates, educators, and resource persons for their patients. In caring for older adults, all of those roles are required.

- Some older adults are at risk for abuse and neglect. Nurses play a vital role in detecting abuse and neglect and ensure appropriate interventions take place. It is the obligation of nurses to report to APS any suspicion of abuse or neglect in vulnerable adults.

- As the number of persons growing older increases, the task of maintaining excellent nursing care may appear to be daunting. However, our commitment to this task is not entirely selfless. The quality of our nursing care does not only assist our older patients. As a result of our efforts, we participate in creating a future for ourselves and for the generations to follow.

PRACTICING FOR THE NCLEX

CHECK YOUR ANSWERS IN APPENDIX A.

1. Which of the following demographic factors are true of older adults? Select all that apply:
   a. The number of adults over age 65 years is static.
   b. Most household incomes are under $35,000.
   c. Older adults are the first generation to age with HIV/AIDS.
   d. Half of women older than 75 live alone.

2. The nurse is working with a patient with severe dementia. Which of the following interventions would be appropriate to facilitate communication?

a. Reality orientation
b. Rephrasing questions when needed
c. Using short, simple words and sentences
d. Validation therapy

3. An older adult is admitted, and the nurse recognizes that there may be an increased risk for fall and injury. Which of the following would be risk factors unique to this population? Select all that apply:

a. History of falls
b. Impaired mobility
c. Environmental hazards
d. Use of benzodiazepine medications

4. The nurse is scoring a patient's risk for skin breakdown using the Braden Scale. He determines a score of 13, indicating high risk. Which interventions would be appropriate to minimize this risk? Select all that apply:

a. Turning every 2 hours
b. Toileting every 2 hours and as needed
c. Ordering a specialty bed to reduce pressure on bony prominences
d. Increasing protein intake

5. A nurse is identifying nursing diagnoses that would be appropriate for an older adult with failure to thrive after the loss of a spouse. Which of the following would be most appropriate?

a. Ineffective Coping
b. Loneliness
c. Impaired Sleep Pattern
d. Impaired Self-Perception

REFERENCES

Administration on Aging (AOA). (2013). *A profile of older Americans: 2013.* Washington, DC: U.S. Department of Health and Human Services.

Alzheimer's Association. (2014). Retrieved July 7, 2014, from www.alz.org

American Geriatrics Society 2012 Beers Criteria Update Expert Panel. (2012). American Geriatrics Society updated Beers criteria for potentially inappropriate medication use in older adults. *Journal of the American Geriatrics Society, 60,* 616–631. doi: 10.1111/j.1532-5415.2012.03923

American Psychiatric Association. (2013). *Diagnostic and statistical manual of mental disorders* (5th ed., text revision). Washington, DC: Author.

Bazrafshan, M. R.., Jahangir, F., Mansouri, A., & Kashfi, S. H. (2014). Coping strategies in people attempting suicide. *International Journal of High Risk Behavior Addiction, 3*(1).

Bloom, H. G., Ahmed I., Alessi C. A., Ancoli-Israel S, Buysse D. J., Kryger M. H., et al. (2009). Evidence-based recommendations for the assessment and management of sleep disorders in older persons. *Journal of American Geriatric Society, 57,* 761–789.

Borneman, T., Ferrel, B., & Puchalski, C. (2010). Evaluation of the FICA tool for spiritual assessment. *Journal of Pain and Symptom Management, 40*(2), 163–173. Retrieved from www.consultgeriRN.org

Centers for Disease Control and Prevention. (2014a). *Falls among older adults: An overview.* Retrieved July 1, 2014, from http://www.cdc.gov/HomeandRecreationalSafety/Falls/adultfalls.html

Centers for Disease Control and Prevention. (2014b). *Chronic disease prevention and health promotion.* Retrieved July 18, 2014, from http://www.cdc.gov/chronicdisease/overview/index.htm

Centers for Disease Control and Prevention. (2014c). *Aging services: Clinical preventive services.* Retrieved on July 18, 2014, from http://www.cdc.gov/features/olderamericansmonth/index.html

Chang, H. J., & Cassio, L. (2010). Falls and Older Adults. *The Journal of the American Medical Association, 303*(3), 288.

DeLamater, J., & Moorman, S. M. (2007). Sexual behavior in later life. *Journal of Aging and Health, 19*(6), 921–945.

Department of Health and Social Services (DSHS). (2014). *Adult abuse and prevention.* Retrieved on July 26, 2014, from http://www.altsa.dshs.wa.gov/APS/

Downing, L. J., Caprio, T. V., & Lyness, J. M. (2013). Geriatric psychiatry review: Differential diagnosis and treatment of the 3 D's - delirium, dementia, and depression. *Current Psyciatry Report, 15*(365), 1–10. http://dx.doi.org/10.1007/s11920-013-0365-4

Feil, N. (2002). *Validation breakthrough: Simple techniques for communicating with people with Alzheimer's type dementia* (2nd ed.). Baltimore, MD: Health Professions Press.

Flicker, L., McCaul K. A., Hankey G. J., Jamrozik K., Brown W. J., Byles J. E., et al. (2010). Body mass index and survival in men and women aged 70–75. *Journal of the American Geriatrics Society, 58*(2), 234–241.

Frasca, D., Diaz, A., Romero, M., Landin, A. M., & Blomberg, B. B. (2010). Age effects on B cells and humoral immunity in humans. *Ageing Research Reviews,* 2010 August 20 [Epub ahead of print].

Fulmer, T., & Cahill, V. M. (1984). Assessing elder abuse: A study. *Journal of Gerontological Nursing, 10*(12), 16–20. Retrieved on July 20, 2014, from http://consultgerirn.org/uploads/File/trythis/try_this_15.pdf

Greenberg, S. A. (2001). Sexual health. In M. D. Mezey (Ed.), *The encyclopedia of elder care* (pp. 589–592). New York, NY: Springer Publishing.

Healthy People 2020. *Older Adults.* Retrieved July 1, 2014, from http://www.healthypeople.gov/2020/topicsobjectives2020/overview.aspx?topicId=31

Institute of Medicine. (2010). *Dietary reference intakes.* Retrieved September 27, 2010, from www.iom.edu/Activities/Nutrition/SummaryDRIs/~/media/Files/Activity%20Files/Nutrition/DRIs/DRI_Macronutrients.aspx

Institute of Medicine. (2011a). *The health of lesbian, gay, bisexual, and transgender people: Building a foundation for better understanding.* Washington, DC: The National Academies Press.

Institute of Medicine. (2011b). Relieving pain in America: A blueprint for transforming prevention, care, education and research. Retrieved July 18, 2014, from http://iom.edu/Reports/2011/Relieving-Pain-in-America-A-Blueprint-for-Transforming-Prevention-Care-Education-Research.aspx

Ivbijaro, G. (2013). Loneliness and the elderly: opportunities for health promotion. *Mental Health in Family Medicine, 10,* 1–2.

Kroenke, K., Spitzer, R. L., & Williams, J. B. (2001). The PHQ-9: Validity of a brief depression severity measure. *Journal of General Internal Medicine, 16*(9), 606–613.

Langer, G., & Fink, A. (2014). Nutritional interventions for preventing and treating pressure ulcers. Retrieved July 8, 2014, from Cochrane Library.

Lazarus, R. S., & Folkman, S. (1984). *Stress, appraisal, and coping.* New York, NY: Springer Publishing.

Manning, L. K., Leek, J. A., & Radina, M. E. (2012). Making sense of extreme longevity: Explorations into the spiritual lives of centenarians. *Journal of Religion and Spiritual Aging, 24*(4), 345–349.

National Center for Chronic Disease Prevention and Health Promotion: Division of Population health. (2013). *The State of Aging and Health in America, 2013.* Retrieved July 1, 2014, from http://www.cdc.gov/aging/help/dph-aging/state-aging-health.html

National Center on Elder Abuse: Administration on Aging. (2014). Statistics and data on elder abuse. Retrieved on July 20, 2014, from http://www.ncea.aoa.gov/Library/Data/index.aspx#problem

National Family Caregivers Association. (2010). Who are America's family caregivers? Retrieved June 10, 2010, from www.nfcacares.org/who_are_family_caregivers/

National Pain Foundation. (2010). Pain causes among older adults. Retrieved June 10, 2010, from www.nationalpainfoundation.org/articles/245/pain-causes-among-older-adults

National Resource Center on LGBT Aging. (2014). Retrieved July 1, 2014, from http://www.lgbtagingcenter.org/resources/index.cfm?s=9999

Ruby, C. M., Hanlon J. T., Boudreau, R. M., Newman, A. B., Simonsick, E. M., Shorr, R. I., et al. (2010). The effect of medication use on urinary incontinence in community-dwelling elderly women. *Journal of the American Geriatrics Society, 58*(9), 1715–1720.

Siegel, K., & Anderman, S. J. (2004). Bereavement. In M. D. Mezey (Ed.), *The encyclopedia of elder care* (pp. 92–95). New York: Springer Publishing.

Tanner, E. K., Martinez, I. L., & Harris, M. (2014). Examining functional and social determinants of depression in community-dwelling older adults: implications for practice. *Geriatric Nursing, 35*, 236–240.

The Aging and Health Report: Disparities and Resilience among Lesbian, Gay, Bisexual, and Transgender Older Adults. (2011). Retrieved July 8, 2014, from http://www.lgbtagingcenter.org/resources/resource.cfm?r=419

The U.S. Department of Health and Human Services. (2014). *Affordable Care Act.* Retrieved June 24, 2014, from http://www.hhs.gov/healthcare/rights/index.html

Tornstam, L. (2005). *Gerotranscendence: A Developmental theory of positive aging.* New York, NY: Springer Publishing Company.

US Department of Health and Human Services. (2010). *Multiple chronic conditions: A strategic framework optimum health and quality of life for individuals with multiple chronic conditions.* Washington, DC: US Dept of Health and Human Services. http://www.hhs.gov/ash/initiatives/mcc/mcc_framework.pdf

US Department of Health and Human Services. (2014). Prevalence of incontinence among older Americans. *Vital Health Statistics, 3*(36), 1–33.

Venugopal, M., & Susman, J. L. (2000). Insomnia in the elderly: Toward a good night's sleep. *Consultant: Consultations in Primary Care, 40*(7), 1234–1247.

Williams, J. M., Kay, D. B., & McCrae, C. S. (2013). Sleep discrepancy, sleep complaint, and poor sleep among older adults. *The Journal of Gerontology, 68*(5), 712–720.

Yesavage, J., & Brink, T. L. (1983). Development and validation of the geriatric depression screening scale: A preliminary report. *Journal of Psychiatry Research, 17*, 37–49.

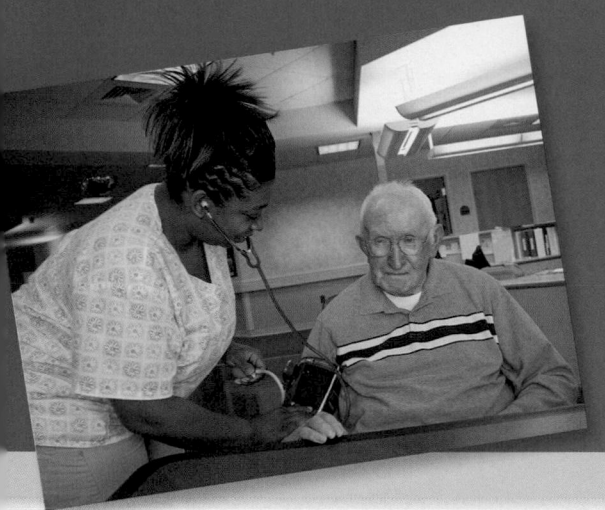

CHAPTER 11

Critical Thinking and the Nursing Process: Foundations for Practice

Kathryn Van Dyke Hayes

Case Scenario

You are a nursing student beginning your clinical nursing program. The nursing courses are different from those you have taken previously, and you are finding it difficult to know how to study. This week will be your first time taking care of a patient at a long-term care facility. You receive your assignment and find that you will be caring for an older man who has heart disease. He has 5 other medical problems and takes 11 medications. His plan of care includes 12 nursing diagnoses. Your previous experience with long-term care facilities is limited, and most of what you have heard and read about them is negative.

This situation is one that nursing students commonly encounter. Although some details may differ, most beginners worry about being capable of handling clinical situations with a limited knowledge base and little experience. This chapter, the other courses you are taking, your life experiences, and later chapters in this text will help you build a solid foundation for learning.

Once you have completed this chapter and have incorporated critical thinking and the nursing process into your knowledge base, review the above scenario and reflect on the following areas of Critical Thinking:

1. What factors influence your ability to think critically about this patient?
2. How do your values and experience influence your ability to provide nursing care?
3. How can you use critical thinking as you prepare for his care?
4. How do you use clinical reasoning to make nursing judgments as you care for him in the long-term care facility?
5. How will you build your knowledge base about this patient's care in the long-term care facility?

KEY TERMS

advanced beginner
clinical experience
clinical reasoning
competence
critical thinking
diagnostic reasoning
diagnostic reasoning process
expert
human patient simulator
learning styles
novice
nursing judgment
nursing process
primary source
proficient
reflection
secondary sources

Upon completion of this chapter, you will be able to do the following:

1. Identify the components of the nursing process.
2. Discuss the requirements for effective use of the nursing process.
3. Explain how critical thinking is used in nursing.
4. Distinguish the relationships among knowledge, experience, critical thinking, reflection, clinical reasoning, and nursing judgment.
5. Explore ways to enhance and develop critical thinking skills, especially as they apply to nursing.

The foundation of the nursing profession is **nursing process**. Skill in using the nursing process is necessary for the clinical application of knowledge and theory in nursing practice. Concepts related to nursing process continue to evolve. This textbook uses the six-step nursing process of assessment, diagnosis, outcome identification, planning, implementation, and evaluation (ADOPIE). It summarizes each phase and gives a brief review of the theoretical foundations of the nursing process.

This chapter defines and explains **critical thinking** concepts within the nursing context. A conceptual model illustrates how critical thinking, **reflection**, and **clinical reasoning** relate to **nursing judgment**. It provides an opportunity for learning how to develop further critical thinking skills.

COMPONENTS OF THE NURSING PROCESS

Definition

The nursing process is a systematic problem-solving approach toward giving individualized nursing care. Note the similarities among the definitions shown in Box 11-1. Regardless of the definition, nurses use the nursing process as a problem-solving method in all settings with patients of all ages to identify and treat human responses to potential or actual health problems. By incorporating each patient's unique aspects, the nursing process facilitates the development of individualized care. The nursing process is also used to identify and treat potential or actual health problems of families and communities. In the chapters on nursing process in this book, the term *patient* refers to an individual, family, or community. The nursing process complements the current role of consumers in healthcare—that is, patients play an active role in decisions affecting their health, no longer passively accepting the decisions that healthcare professionals make (American Association of Colleges of Nursing [AACN], 2008).

The nursing process serves as a guide for professional nursing practice. It has the following characteristics:

- It is a framework for providing specific nursing care to individuals, families, and communities.
- It is orderly and systematic.
- It is interdependent.
- It is patient centered, using the patient's strengths.
- It is appropriate for use throughout the life span.
- It can be used in all settings.

BOX 11-1 Definitions of Nursing Process

Marjory Gordon
"Nursing process is a method of problem identification and problem solving. Although derived from the supposedly objective scientific method, nursing process is not applied in an objective, value-free way. Human values influence both problem identification and problem solving. The components of nursing process discussed in textbooks vary but generally include assessment and diagnosis. These are the problem-identification components. Outcome projection, intervention, and outcome evaluation are the problem-solving components" (Gordon, 1994, pp. 9–10).

Ralph and Taylor
"The nursing process is a key systematic method for taking independent nursing action. Steps in the nursing process include:

- Assessing the patient's problems.
- Forming a diagnostic statement.
- Identifying expected outcomes.
- Creating a plan to achieve expected outcomes and solve the patient's problems.
- Implementing the plan or assigning others to implement it.
- Evaluating the plan's effectiveness.

These phases of the nursing process—assessment, nursing diagnosis formation, outcome identification, care planning, implementation, and evaluation—are dynamic and flexible; they commonly overlap" (Ralph & Taylor, 2014, p. x).

Alfaro-LeFevre
"The nursing process consists of six interrelated steps—Assessment, Diagnosis, Outcome, Planning, Implementation, and Evaluation—which is designed to help you:

1. Organize and prioritize patient care.
2. Keep the focus on what's important—the patient's health status and quality of life.
3. Form thinking habits that help you gain confidence and skills you need to think critically in the clinical setting.

The nursing process serves as a critical thinking model for nursing" (Alfaro-LeFevre, 2014).

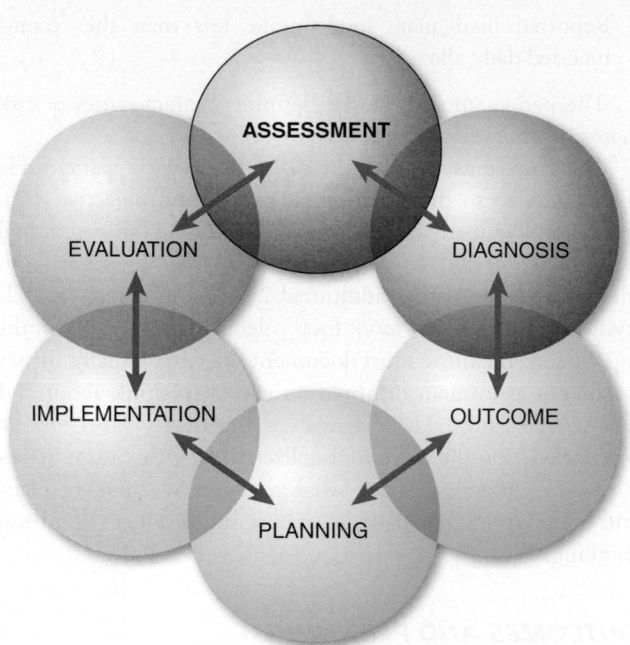

FIGURE 11-1 Six phases of the nursing process.

Phases

The six phases of the nursing process are assessment, diagnosis, outcome identification, planning, implementation, and evaluation. Figure 11-1 illustrates these phases. "Critical thinking underlies each step of the nursing process, problem-solving and decision-making. The nursing process is cyclical and dynamic, interpersonal and collaborative, and universally applicable" (American Nurses Association [ANA], 2010, p. 5).

ASSESSMENT

Assessment commonly refers to evaluation or appraisal of a patient's health state. In nursing, assessment is the systematic collection of subjective and objective data. During assessment, the nurse appraises the patient's total situation by considering the physical, psychological, emotional, sociocultural, and spiritual factors that may affect the patient's health status.

The nurse must gather all relevant information about a patient's present, past, or potential problems to develop a complete database. Data collection takes place during every nurse–patient interaction and from many other available sources (Jensen, 2015). The patient is the **primary source** of information for assessment. **Secondary sources** include family members, significant others, other healthcare professionals, health records, and literature review.

Gathering of assessment data takes place through observing, interviewing, and examining the patient and interpreting laboratory data and diagnostic tests. Observation begins with the first patient encounter and is ongoing. The nursing interview allows for the systematic assessment of functional health, including the patient's perception and interpretation of problems (Jensen, 2015). During the physical examination, nurses use techniques of inspection, percussion, palpation,

and auscultation to obtain further data. Objective information from health records, including laboratory and diagnostic data, completes the database.

An in-depth nursing history and physical assessment are usually required at admission to a hospital or long-term care facility or during the first visit by a community or home health nurse. This initial database becomes the reference point for all further nursing assessments. Thorough assessment data provide the foundation for nursing diagnoses.

DIAGNOSIS

Diagnosing human responses to actual or potential health problems is the second phase of the nursing process. Diagnosis is the clinical act of identifying problems. It also is the term given to the patient's problem. To diagnose means to analyze assessment information and derive meaning from this analysis.

Registered nurses are educated and licensed to make nursing diagnoses just as physicians are licensed to make medical diagnoses. NANDA-International (Herdman, 2014) defines *nursing diagnosis* as "a clinical judgment concerning a human response to health conditions/life processes, or a vulnerability for that response, by an individual, family, group, or community" (p. 464). A medical diagnosis describes a disease, whereas a nursing diagnosis describes an individual, family, or group response to an actual or potential health problem. A nursing diagnosis provides the basis for selection of nursing interventions to achieve positive patient outcomes (Herdman, 2014). Registered nurses are responsible for identifying nursing diagnoses for patients under their care.

Nursing diagnoses are separate and different from medical diagnoses. The patient is a partner with the nurse in the diagnostic process. For example, the patient may be at risk for infection because of poor nutrition, so the nurse might direct interventions at improving nutrition. The physician may treat the infection with antibiotics. In a patient with diabetes, the physician might prescribe insulin. The nurse may give the insulin and observe the effect on blood sugar but focus the care on improving the patient's knowledge base by teaching. Thus, nurses and physicians both provide interventions but in slightly different ways.

The nursing diagnostic process uses cue clustering, cluster interpretation, and diagnostic validation to ensure accuracy in the selection of the correct diagnoses. Formulating the diagnostic statement requires knowledge of the differences among actual, risk, possible, and health promotion nursing diagnoses.

The **diagnostic reasoning process** is used to make accurate clinical diagnoses about patient problems. It is a complex process that is composed of several interrelated steps and is affected by variables such as the background of the diagnostician and the patient. The diagnosis requires that the practitioners have **competence** in intellectual, interpersonal, and technical domains and develop personal strengths of tolerance for ambiguity and use of reflective practice (Herdman, 2014). Although the steps are discussed sequentially, in practice, there is much overlap until the diagnosis is made and confirmed. **Diagnostic reasoning** is the process of gathering and clustering data to draw inferences and propose diagnoses. NANDA-I

(Herdman, 2014) has formulated five steps of diagnostic reasoning: organizing the existence of cues, generating possible diagnoses, comparing cues to possible diagnoses, conducting a focused data collection, and validating diagnoses. A comparison of diagnostic reasoning to the nursing process is shown in Table 11-1.

Nurses make judgments at each step of the nursing process. Judgments lead to effective care planning, interventions, and intervention revisions based on evaluation of the care. Protocols, plans of care, and care maps are ways that nurses use the nursing process to plan care. Nurses base such care on judgments for a common problem; however, every patient's care must be individualized. Thus, nurses use protocols within the context of critical thinking. They draw upon the individual's assessment and analysis to adapt guidelines to a patient.

As beginners, you must realize that you have only small numbers of experiences on which to base your clinical judgment. As you gain experience, you will begin to notice common concepts among situations. Identifying these key concepts and ideas is essential. Thinking critically about each case will help you avoid applying inaccurate knowledge from one situation to another.

Students also must continuously revise ways to state the concepts that might have slightly different meanings. For example, a nurse might have cared for patients with infections, such as a new mother with a postcesarean wound infection, a teenager with a sexually transmitted infection, and a patient with a urinary tract infection in hospice care. How are the concepts related to infection similar? How do they differ?

NANDA-I (Herdman, 2014) has a list of diagnoses with defining characteristics that nurses use to make the diagnoses (see Chapter 13). The nurse can make the diagnosis based on assessment data that are present and that cluster together. The nurse should not use a diagnosis if the defining characteristics are unmet. A different diagnosis may be better. An example might be diagnosing if the patient were at risk for imbalanced nutrition. Some defining characteristics for Imbalanced Nutrition: Less Than Body Requirements are as follows:

- Body weight 20% or more under ideal
- Loss of weight with adequate food intake

TABLE 11-1 DIAGNOSTIC REASONING COMPARED TO NURSING PROCESS

Diagnostic Reasoning	Nursing Process
Recognize the existence of cues	Assessment
Generate possible diagnoses	Diagnosis
Compare cues to possible diagnoses	Assessment and diagnosis
Conduct a focused data collection	Assessment
Validate diagnoses	Diagnosis

- Reported inadequate food intake less than the recommended daily allowance

The patient must have the defining characteristics or risk factors for the nursing diagnosis to apply.

The nurse must confirm the diagnosis with the patient. He or she can do so by gathering subjective and objective data. For example, the nurse might ask the patient about abdominal pain, appetite, and satiety immediately after ingesting food. He or she could gather additional information, such as ability to chew or swallow food, food tolerance, nausea, or vomiting. Finally, the nurse must document the data. Usually, nurses document assessment information and then think about and analyze the issues. The diagnosis is the nurse's label for the problem. Using the pattern of collected data, the nurse makes a nursing judgment about what to do next. Nursing plans and interventions for patient care are the products of critical thinking.

OUTCOMES AND PLANNING

According to the ANA (2010) *Nursing: Scope and Standards of Practice* (2nd ed.), outcome identification refers to formulating and documenting measurable, realistic, patient-focused goals. Identification of outcomes, including patient goals and outcome criteria, is an integral part of the nursing process.

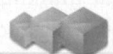 **Concept Mastery Alert**

Within the nursing process, outcomes are rooted in the nursing diagnoses that have been identified following assessment, not in medical diagnoses or procedures.

After determining nursing diagnoses, establishing priorities, and writing expected outcomes, nurses begin the planning phase. Nurses work together with patients to identify goals and intervention strategies that will reduce identified problems. The planning phase involves preparing a patient plan of care, which directs the activities of the nursing staff in the provision of patient care.

The patient plan of care is a written summary of the care that a patient is to receive. The Joint Commission requires a written plan of care for each patient. The plans of care may be handwritten notes, electronic records, preprinted forms, care paths or maps, individualized preprinted plans of care, or standards of practice (Keenan, Yakel, Tschannon, & Mandeville, 2008). Although many institutions have developed standardized plans of care, all plans must be individualized. Chapter 14 discusses patient plans of care in more depth. The skills involved in planning include establishing patient goals and outcome criteria and determining nursing interventions.

Because the plan of care remains a permanent part of the record, the beginning practitioner may collaborate with more experienced nurses or ask the nursing instructor questions to confirm the individualized plan. As nurses develop their skill in writing plans and begin to recognize their responsibility to carry out other nurses' plans of care, their independence increases. Once the plan of care is written, it must be implemented on the patient's behalf.

Nurses write outcomes for patients so that as they provide care, they know if that care is making a difference. In the patient with Imbalanced Nutrition: Less Than Body Requirements, the nurse may write an outcome such as, "Patient will maintain weight at 55 kg within the next week" (Moorhead, Johnson, Maas, & Swanson, 2013). The outcomes must be specific to the patient, realistic, and measurable. This requires critical thinking as the nurse individualizes care. Where it may be unreasonable for the patient to gain weight, the goal is set for the patient to maintain weight. The nurse also must identify a time during which the behavior will be seen, which in this case is within the next week. Outcomes help nurses know if their interventions are working.

IMPLEMENTATION

Implementation is the action phase of the nursing process. It is the actual initiation of the plan, evaluation of response to the plan, and recording of nursing actions and patient response to these actions. To implement means to carry out, to perform, to intervene, or to do something. Implementation may include delegating or coordinating interventions within the plan of care. This phase also may include designating the patient, significant others, or healthcare providers to implement the preestablished plan of care. Nursing actions are goal directed, assisting the patient to reach maximum functional health. Because nursing care is provided to assist in meeting patient goals, nurses must focus on their actions, making sure that each action they undertake is necessary and required.

The components of implementation include reassessment, initiation of the plan, evaluation of the response, and recording of actions taken. Nursing actions focus on resolving or improving a patient's problems.

Implementation requires the use of intellectual, interpersonal, and technical skills. Developing expertise in each of these areas is required for professional nursing practice. Once nurses have provided the care, they evaluate it.

Although outcomes focus on the patient, interventions focus on what the nurse will do (Bulechek, Butcher, Dochterman, & Wagner, 2013). For the patient with Imbalanced Nutrition: Less Than Body Requirements, one intervention includes ascertaining the patient's food preferences. Another more specific intervention might be, "Contact patient's family to bring in home-cooked meal."

When designing interventions, nurses must be aware not only of positive consequences but also unintended or negative consequences. For example, if a home-cooked meal is low in calories or nutrition, the nurse may need to revise the intervention as follows: "Contact dietitian to advise family on highly nutritious food choices that can be brought from home." Clinical reasoning has implications and consequences that nurses can anticipate by using critical thinking. They determine the effectiveness of the care performed when evaluating the nursing process.

EVALUATION

Evaluation commonly refers to rating, grading, and judging. In the evaluation phase, nurses discover why the patient plan of care was a success or failure (Alfaro-LeFevre, 2014). They determine the patient's reaction to nursing interventions and judge whether the goals of the plan of care were achieved. The plan of care provides the basis for evaluation. Reassessing patients provides new information for changing or eliminating nursing diagnoses, goals, or interventions. Determining goal achievement is a joint decision between the patient and the nurse. This is similar to the evaluation between the student and the instructor.

Evaluation focuses on individual patients and groups of patients. Quality assurance monitors provide input for development and refinement of standards of care for groups of similar patients. Although evaluation is a separate and distinct phase, it also is an ongoing and continuous process performed throughout all phases of the nursing process. Judgments in previous phases of the nursing process result in prompt reassessment, rediagnosing, and replanning. The evaluation phase involves a detailed reassessment of the entire plan of care. An in-depth, comprehensive judgment about patient goal attainment and fulfillment of outcome criteria takes place in this phase.

The process of evaluation requires various skills. These skills include knowledge of standards of care, normal patient responses, and conceptual models of nursing; the ability to monitor the effectiveness of nursing interventions; and awareness of clinical research.

When evaluating care, nurses compare the patient assessment after the interventions to the patient outcomes written earlier. For example, the nurse would weigh the patient in the previously discussed example 1 week later to see if he still weighed 55 kg. If the outcomes were met, the nurse may continue the intervention. He or she also may decide to change the outcome. The next patient outcome might be, "Increase weight to 58 kg by next month." Not all outcomes are met, however. In such cases, the nurse may decide to change the interventions. For example, a new intervention might be, "Encourage 100 mL of nutritional supplement between meals and at bedtime." By evaluating if the outcomes were met, the nurse can appropriately continue or revise the interventions, outcomes, or both. He or she uses critical thinking to make these judgments.

THERAPEUTIC DIALOGUE: NURSING PROCESS

SCENE FOR THOUGHT

Linda Castro, a 34-year-old mother of two, is scheduled for a course of chemotherapy for leukemia. She has been in the oncology outpatient clinic for this treatment twice before and is known to the staff. She is sitting in the treatment chair.

LESS EFFECTIVE

Nurse (Carol):	Is it good to see a familiar face? (*Checking out the patient's perception.*)
Linda:	Yes. I was worried that there would be a lot of changes since I was here last.
Nurse:	How have you been since we last saw each other? (*Assessment of coping outside the hospital.*)
Linda:	Not too bad. The kids are a handful, but my husband helps most of the time, and I manage. Then I get so tired that I can't do anything. The bruising is back again, too. (*Shows several large bruises on her arms and legs.*)
Nurse:	Yes, I see. Well, that's to be expected. (*Turns away from patient to get chart.*)
Linda:	When do the treatments start?
Nurse:	(*Looks at patient's chart; hears phone ring. Looks away and doesn't hear patient's question.*)
Linda:	Can you tell me when the treatments start?
Nurse:	In about an hour, I think. The lab results have to come up. Then we can get started.
Linda:	I'm wondering if I'll have the same problem with my veins as the last time. (*Looks worried.*)
Nurse:	I doubt it. Don't worry. We'll take care of it.

MORE EFFECTIVE

Nurse (Lesley):	Is it good to see a familiar face? (*Checking out the patient's perception.*)
Linda:	Yes. I was worried that there would be a lot of changes since I was here last.
Nurse:	How have you been since we last saw each other? (*Assessment of coping outside the hospital.*)
Linda:	Not too bad. The kids are a handful, but my husband helps most of the time, and I manage. Then I get so tired that I can't do anything. The bruising is back again, too. (*Shows several large bruises on her arms and legs.*)
Nurse:	I see. They look painful. You look tired. Is there something I can help you with or get you? (*Assessment of immediate needs.*)
Linda:	I'd love it if you could adjust the footrest for me. I can't seem to move today.
Nurse:	Sure. Is that okay? (*Evaluation of intervention.*)
Linda:	That's good. When do the treatments start?
Nurse:	In about an hour, I think. The lab results have to come up. Then we can get started. Are you concerned? (*Assessment.*)
Linda:	Well, I'm wondering if I'll have the same problem with my veins as the last time. (*Looks worried.*)
Nurse:	Let me check your old chart. I think we did some magic with warm compresses that seemed to work last time; remember? (*Evaluation of prior intervention.*)
Linda:	Oh yeah. That worked great. I'm glad you remembered.
Nurse:	Anything else you need before I see to those labs?
Linda:	Yes could you get me a laxative order? I've been too tired to eat or drink much, so I guess I'm a little out of whack right now. (*Laughs, a little embarrassed.*)
Nurse:	Not a problem. Perhaps we could talk about some foods that will help keep you regular. I will bring you some water. We'll work on it together. (*Planning with the patient.*)

CRITICAL THINKING CHALLENGE

- Identify all the phases of the nursing process that you see the nurse, Lesley, use.
- Analyze whether it was an orderly progression or she skipped phases and then returned to them.
- Describe how the less effective interaction by Carol the nurse affected the interaction. Discuss alternative responses that Carol could have used.

NURSING PRACTICE AND THE NURSING PROCESS

Nursing practice is interactive and involves individualizing care for the patient. Nurses use their thinking to focus their care.

Interactive Nature of Each Phase

Each phase of the nursing process interacts with and is influenced by the other phases. For example, a nurse collecting assessment information may implement some aspects of care at the same time. In a similar manner, as the nurse evaluates nursing care, he or she makes and implements new plans. During an emergency, a nurse may carry out all phases of the nursing process with no apparent divisions among them.

As the patient's condition changes, the nurse gathers and incorporates new data into the plan of care. When care is provided, evaluation of the patient's response may indicate a need for immediate revision of the plan or for the identification of new nursing diagnoses.

Professional Relevance

The nursing process is a systematic, organized way of providing nursing care for any patient in any situation. Its adaptability and practicality contribute to high-quality nursing care. Because a concise patient plan of care is written, continuity of care is facilitated and communication among nurses is enhanced.

The nursing process focuses on the patient's unique problems. The patient or family members are involved in setting priorities, developing goals and outcome criteria, and selecting nursing interventions. Because of this involvement, they play an important role in decisions that directly affect patient care. The patient's responses to nursing interventions are continually assessed and evaluated, which fosters individualized nursing care.

Legally, the nursing process is recognized as the standard for nursing practice. Nurses are held accountable to practice according to legal statutes and the nurse practice act of the state. Most states use the term *nursing process* when describing the act of nursing.

Professionally, the nursing process is recognized as the method of practicing nursing. It is the model on which professional nursing standards are based. Although it sometimes is criticized for not being adaptable to the changing healthcare environment, the nursing process remains the almost universally accepted method for providing nursing care.

IMPORTANCE OF CRITICAL THINKING IN NURSING

The enormous amount of information available in healthcare changes continually. Simple memorization-style thinking is insufficient to complement the nurse's tasks of sorting, organizing, and identifying relevant information for efficient, effective use. The growing complexity of healthcare demands the use of critical thinking for effective, creative, and efficient nursing care.

Critical thinking helps nurses to choose solutions or identify options for patient care situations. Nurses are required to think critically in all settings, including home, school, ambulatory care, critical care units, and community centers. Nurses must work from a broad knowledge base that individualizes care for each patient and setting. A nurse's ability to think critically will be one of his or her most important skills.

Conceptual Development of Critical Thinking

Dictionaries describe *critical thinking* as self-guided, self-disciplined thinking that attempts to reason at the highest level of quality in a fair-minded way (Paul & Elder, 2007). Critical thinking, then, assumes a turning point because of a thought process. The definitions of critical thinking are summarized in Box 11-2. From this review, it is easy to see that a critical thinker has many characteristics.

There are similarities between the process of thinking described above and nursing process. Nursing school provides experiences, reflection, communication, and observations in various classroom and clinical settings to promote development of these critical thinking skills.

BOX 11-2   Selected Definitions of Critical Thinking

AACN (2008, p. 36)
"All or part of the process of questioning, analysis, synthesis, interpretation, inference, inductive and deductive reasoning, intuition, application, and creativity (AACN, 2008). Critical thinking underlies independent and interdependent decision making."

Alfaro-LeFevre (2014)
Purposeful thinking that aims to make judgments based on evidence.

Healsip (2008)
"In nursing, critical thinking for clinical decision-making is the ability to think in a systematic and logical manner with openness to question and reflect on the reasoning process used to ensure safe nursing practice and quality care."

NLN (2011)
Critical thinking in nursing practice is a discipline-specific, reflective reasoning process that guides a nurse in generating, implementing, and evaluating approaches for dealing with patient care and professional concerns.

LEARNING STYLES AFFECTING CRITICAL THINKING

Each nursing student learns in different ways. The nursing student who knows how to use many styles is at an advantage. A student will benefit from practicing various **learning styles** so that he or she can adapt strategies that best fit the situation. Learning in the clinical setting may be more active, kinesthetic, and random, whereas the classroom setting is more sequential, reflective, and competitive. These different ways of learning can complement one another.

Alfaro-LeFevre (2014) has developed many materials on critical thinking for both the instructor and the student. A model of critical thinking includes technical skills, interpersonal skills, theoretical and experiential knowledge, and critical thinking attitudes and behaviors. Technical skills and experiential knowledge are gained in nursing school in the laboratory and clinical setting. Interpersonal skills are gained in the communication courses, group work, and the clinical setting during work with the patient, instructor, and other healthcare professionals. Theoretical knowledge is acquired by active reading, writing, and studying for nursing courses. The critical thinking characteristics can be developed in all domains. Some things that can be done to promote critical thinking are as follows (Alfaro-LeFevre, 2014):

- Anticipate questions that others might ask (e.g., the instructor), such as "What's the most important problem?" or "Tell me the rationale for this intervention."
- Anticipate what's next, such as "What if my patient gets short of breath?" or "If I give this medication, what do I expect will happen?"
- Look for ways to improve, such as "Does my paper match the assignment?" and "How can I deepen or broaden my knowledge?"
- Ask someone else to look for flaws in your thinking. Get a second opinion.
- Replace "I don't know" and "I'm not sure" with "Let's find out."
- Turn errors into learning opportunities.
- Raise the bar! Expect more of yourself.

SKILLS IN PROVIDING CARE

Listening

Active listening implies that nurses are responsive to the cues that patients are sending. Patients who are anxious or preoccupied may respond to questions with short or inappropriate answers. Astute nurses listen to what the patient says to follow up on misconceptions and misunderstandings or to correct misinformation.

Being an active listener involves paying attention to nonverbal cues and spoken responses. Patients may hesitate to give certain information. Although respecting patients and not prying are important, nurses need to gather information that is essential for good patient care. As interviewing skills develop, nurses learn how to phrase certain questions and approach personal matters. Often, the way in which questions are asked can make the difference between complete and superficial responses.

Collaborating

Effective collaboration with all members of the healthcare team is vital to the development of an individualized plan of care for the patient. The foundations of collaborative practice are positive professional relationships built on trust and respect for the unique contribution of each healthcare team member. Scheduling regular time (e.g., handoffs or team rounds) for team members to discuss each patient's progress is essential, as is the inclusion of the patient in the discussion.

Communicating

Writing skills are necessary to communicate information on the patient's health record and other agency forms. Writing enables others to develop a picture of the patient at the time of the assessment. Often, written records are the only way to discover historical information about the progression of a disease and the patient's response to it. Writing skillfully requires the ability to summarize information while maintaining comprehensiveness and accuracy. Succinct descriptive terms are useful for providing an accurate, detailed written report. Documentation of findings in medical terms is a challenging but important task.

Increasing numbers of institutions and agencies use computerized records. Therefore, nurses need a working knowledge of computers to effectively function in today's healthcare system. Internet access is becoming increasingly important in obtaining healthcare information for developing the plan of care or for using databases for research.

Clinical Reasoning

When nurses encounter health and illness in individuals, families, and communities, they experience rich opportunities for critical thinking and reflection. It is important that you learn, review, and remember knowledge gained from previous courses to apply in clinical settings. When encountering real patients, nurses need to integrate that academic knowledge into a complete view. Using critical thinking, they can see how all preexisting knowledge and current information fit together to create new, higher-level thinking. Critical thinking occurs within an existing knowledge base and is paralleled by **clinical experience**.

For example, consider the patient in the long-term care facility at the beginning of this chapter. One of his medical diagnoses is congestive heart failure. To deal with the patient's problem appropriately, the student nurse will need to use his or her knowledge base from previous classes. From an assessment course, the student nurse will know how to listen to the patient's heart and lungs. He or she will use knowledge from anatomy, physiology, and pathophysiology courses to understand the disease. As the student nurse reviews the medication list, he or she will know the purpose, side effects, and nursing care related to his medications from pharmacology classes. From nutrition classes, the student nurse will understand the rationale for a cardiac diet and be able to teach it. The student nurse will be able to communicate and develop a relationship with the patient, as well as provide help with bathing, transfers, and ambulation, based on knowledge from foundational nursing courses. In this way, the student nurse will apply critical thinking, which integrates knowledge that until this point had been theoretical, to an actual patient scenario. This is called *clinical reasoning*.

You must become actively involved in your learning by taking advantage of every opportunity to learn more. When you think that you have all the answers, you should ask yourself more questions. It is often said that it is better to have the right question than the right answer. Nursing practice highly values the pattern of inquisitiveness. This habit will assist you to become **expert** nurses more quickly. Critical thinking helps to solve problems.

SKILLS IN LEARNING

Critical thinking and nursing process are linked together both in clinical practice and in the courses that you take. Nursing is a practice profession, and you will learn about knowledge that is applied to an individual patient's care. Each patient is unique, and nursing process is used to gather this information and what you will do with it.

Using Critical Thinking Skills

As you develop within your nursing role, you will build critical thinking skills and apply them to real healthcare situations. A commitment to think critically often and at a high level will benefit a nurse's ability to care for patients most effectively. Critical thinking requires conscious, deliberate effort. With repetition, critical thinking will become a habit, and you will become an expert nurse with time.

Critical thinking has many facets to analyze and examine. The nurse may develop some aspects of thinking but may have to improve other aspects. By looking at the parts of critical thinking, the nurse can see skills that he or she needs to develop.

Analyze what problems are most important. Priority setting is an essential nursing skill. To help decide priorities, consider the following: the severity of the problem (e.g., life threatening would always be first), amount of time spent on the problem (nursing and medical care), which problems are related, and what the patient views as most important. As you gain experience, nursing priority-setting skills will improve. When nurses gather and analyze data, priority setting leads to important diagnoses and issues. In this case, the use of critical thinking and clinical reasoning leads to identification of the top priorities.

All parts of the nursing process require clinical reasoning: assessment, diagnosis, outcome identification, planning, implementation, and evaluation. The National League for Nursing

---

BOX 11-3   Critical Thinking Behaviors

Application of critical thinking to nursing practice is demonstrated by the ability to:

A: Interpret
Ask relevant questions and explore ideas.
Validate data.
Recognize issues and concerns.

D: Analyze
Interpret evidence.
Consider viewpoints and recognize assumptions.
Identify missing information.

O: Outcome
Results that are measurable and observable

P: Evaluate
Detect bias.
Consider legal/ethical standards.
Use reflective skepticism.
Examine alternatives.
Judge worth of evidence.

I: Infer
Predict consequences.
Apply deductive/inductive reasoning.
Support conclusions with evidence.
Set priorities.
Plan approaches.
Modify/individualize interventions.
Apply research in practice.

E: Explain
Determine outcome attainment.
Revise plans.
Identify patient's perception of results.

Source: National League for Nursing. (2011). *Critical thinking in clinical nursing practice/RN examination.* Retrieved December 7, 2010, from http://dev.nln.org/testproducts/pdf/CTinfobulletin.pdf; American Nurses Association. (2010). *Nursing: Scope and standards of practice* (2nd ed.). Silver Spring, MD: Author.

(NLN, 2011) describes behaviors that show critical thinking use at each stage of the nursing process (Box 11-3). As nurses think about assessment, they ask relevant questions and validate data. During analysis, they consider other viewpoints and recognize assumptions. To increase skills in critical reasoning, nurses must consider how well they are using the described behaviors. They also need to take time to develop their less used skills.

Taking Examinations

The exams that you are taking in nursing school may be very different from other exams that you have taken before. These critical thinking questions require more than one step in the

<table>
<tr><td>

BOX 11-4

</td><td>

NCSBN Categories of Questions for the NCLEX-RN

</td></tr>
</table>

Safe and Effective Care Environment
   Coordinated Care (16% to 22%)
   Safety and Infection Control (10% to 16%)
Heath Promotion and Maintenance (7% to 13%)
Psychosocial Integrity (8% to 14%)
Physiological Integrity
   Basic Care and Comfort (7% to 13%)
   Pharmacological Therapies (11% to 17%)
   Reduction of Risk Potential (10% to 16%)
   Physiological Adaptation (7% to 13%)

Reprinted with permission from National Council of State Boards of Nursing (2014). *2014 NCLEX-RN detailed test plan, candidate version.* Retrieved September 29, 2015 from https://www.ncsbn.org/testplans.htm

thinking process; other exams may be focused on foundational knowledge with facts that can be recalled from a book. These new behaviors can be learned. They will require you to analyze new information and examine alternative solutions. You must identify the need for additional data and suggest the highest priority findings. You will be asked to make inferences based upon the available data, prioritize nursing interventions, and revise a plan based upon your evaluation (Assessment Technologies Institute, 2010). Priority-setting items test your ability to make decisions and select the patient with the highest level of need and those problems at greatest risk for the patient, identify a patient with a chronic or emergency need, and select the primary intervention.

Frameworks for setting priorities include Maslow's hierarchy of needs, ABCs (airway, breathing, and circulation), safety and risk reduction, acute versus chronic conditions, nursing process (assess before implement), least to most invasive, and least to most likely to survive. You will need to use your knowledge base to select the best multiple-choice answer, select all of the answers that are correct, fill in the blank, or identify items from a drawing. The NCLEX-RN licensing exam may have as few as 75 questions, based upon your performance. You can see that the items need to be challenging to test your knowledge and thinking for all that you have learned. Instructors will help with your learning by providing exam items that are similar to this way of thinking. Take advantage of the learning opportunities and how to be a good critical thinker—these skills will help you not only on test taking but also in the clinical area (National Council of State Boards of Nursing [NCSBN], 2014). See Box 11-4 for categories of questions that appear on the NCLEX.

Practicing Reflection

Elder and Paul (1996) have developed a spectrum of universal standards by which to judge thinking including attributes such as clarity, accuracy, precision, relevance, depth, breadth, logic and fairness. These standards provide the language by which a student or a nurse can expand his or her abilities. As you write papers, prepare for examinations, and participate in nursing care planning, you may use these standards to improve thinking. Critical thinking and clinical reasoning develop with time if a person makes the effort to improve.

Reflection is defined as "those intellectual and affective activities in which individuals engage to explore their experiences in order to lead to new understandings and appreciations" (Boud, Keogh, & Walker, 1985). As with the other skills, reflection takes time and attention to develop. Two types of reflection are reflection-in-action, which occurs in clinical practice, and reflection-on-action, which occurs after the event. Because nursing is a practice profession, nurses practice reflection-in-action every clinical day. When practicing reflection-on-action, nurses need deliberate time and effort to think about what has happened.

Reflection at the most basic level begins with descriptions of events. It is helpful to identify a positive or negative situation to think about further, one that might be resurfacing at times (Mezirow, 2000). Think about the situation, the people, and the environment, and then recall what happened. Recall the sequence of events, think about both positive and negative feelings, and pay attention to those feelings. Think about the context of the situation and the relationships involved. At higher levels of reflection, ask what perceptions, judgments, and thoughts occurred. What values were placed on the experience? What assumptions were made that may have been true or false? As the event is explored, new issues can be identified. In reflection, the experience is reevaluated in light of behavior, ideas, feelings, and values surrounding the event.

Highest learning occurs at the point of critical reflectivity or "becoming aware of our awareness and critiquing it" (Mezirow, 2000). It is when a person questions judgments and considers other ways of thinking about the situation. For example, ask why an event was important. What meaning does it have for the person or student or nurse? Consider values and beliefs that are different and what these differences mean. New meanings and alternative explanations may be more useful than old ones.

Nursing values the ability to look at issues from different points of view. Different perspectives allow nurses to recognize more broadly and inclusively the meanings of life experiences. What are some other ways of looking at the issue? How has one's perspective changed? How is a person different because of this experience? Asking these questions helps you prepare to care for patients with different views. Questioning develops skills in understanding, which leads to valuing each person and her or his unique life experience. By avoiding judgments and recognizing assumptions, nurses can provide more competent care to an increasingly diverse group of patients.

Recognize assumptions and consider different viewpoints without making judgments. The NLN (2010) has outlined critical thinking behaviors that nurses can practice in relation to these issues. This means admitting that a person may take for granted something not based on facts. Television stories about neglect and abuse in long-term care facilities might lead one to assume that these are places to avoid. By gathering facts, a student may learn that the skilled nursing facility where he or she has been placed for training has many patient resources. For example, the facility has activities with schoolchildren, holds reminiscing sessions, and takes van trips to the countryside. The residents say that they enjoy the environment, and the facility delivers high-quality care. This example illustrates the importance of taking time to gather facts and be open to new viewpoints.

Understand the position from which something is observed. Consider how to think about the situation differently. A student in long-term care might think about the losses that his or her patient has experienced. Examples would include the loss of function, loss of independent living, or loss of a spouse. The patient's perspective might be different. For example, the patient may have struggled through life, working and caring for family with minimal economic resources. The long-term care experience may be the first time the patient has had help from others, food prepared for him or her, and activities for enjoyment. You must take time to talk with patients about their points of view. That process involves asking open-ended, nonjudgmental questions and listening carefully to patients' responses.

Adopt an attitude of doubt toward supposed truths. The NLN (2010) describes the use of reflective skepticism. For example, you might assume that a person in a skilled nursing facility has a family that doesn't care about her or him. The facts might be that the family cares deeply but does not have the economic or physical resources to care for the elder in their home.

Evaluate the worth of evidence that is present. If the nurse works only day shift, recognize that the nurse knows only what happens during the workday. Consider that the family may be making evening visits. When bias is detected, find out if unreasoned judgments have been made. You or the nurse might assume that family members do not participate in care, when in fact they participate but at a different time of day. Take the effort to correct these misperceptions by communicating this information to other shifts.

Simulation

As the complexity and acuity of patient care has increased dramatically, it has become difficult to find appropriate clinical experiences that allow nurses to develop safe clinical judgment and decision-making skills. Many schools of nursing and hospitals are using simulation laboratories to develop and evaluate clinical skills and competence (Bremner, Aduddell, Bennett, & VanGeest, 2006). The **human patient simulator**, a life-sized mannequin with a sophisticated computer interface, presents you with clinical scenarios that evolve based on decisions that you make. Sessions often include the presentation of a patient situation where a group of learners discuss and decide on a plan of action, experiencing positive and negative consequences of decisions made. Organization, prioritization, communication, and collaboration are important skills necessary to achieve a

positive outcome for the simulated situation. The simulation lab is especially important in that it provides experience with high-risk situations that may never be encountered. Debriefing sessions allow you to reflect on and share insight with other students.

Developing Expertise

As you progress through your nursing career, you will use critical thinking processes to develop skills. Achieving a high level of expertise, however, takes time. As a beginner, you need to practice and problem solve. This involves learning to use these processes, finding out what works and what does not, and adapting the processes to themselves as individuals and nurses.

Benner (2000) has developed a model of skill acquisition that outlines the stages of increasing expertise. The first stage is **novice**, in which learners use rules to guide practice. Examples of such rules include information and skills that you learn from instructors, practice in laboratory, and read in books. **Advanced beginner** is the next stage. After more experience in clinical situations, nurses learn to consider more facts and complex rules. If an intervention is unsuccessful, the nurse may question the rule that was followed. At **competence**, nurses devise new rules and reasoning procedures. They feel responsible for the outcomes and may question rules. Nurses gain competence through more experience. As situations become complex, nurses assimilate experiences and implement plans. As nurses become **proficient**, they realize that the events, context, and patient situation are as important as the nurse's individual resources. Based on the evaluation, nurses develop and implement future actions. The actions become easier. The outcomes become more important than the interventions. Thinking is more flexible and intuitive rather than planned and deliberate. The last stage is **expert**. The expert knows the goal to achieve and how to achieve it. The best experts think before they act. They intuitively use sound theoretical thinking to reflect on the goal and decide on the seemingly appropriate action. They avoid getting caught in one perspective. The expert can link theory, practice, and intuition. This is the goal. As beginners, you must be patient, because this level of expertise takes years after nursing school to develop.

APPLYING CRITICAL THINKING TO LEARNING ACTIVITIES

This textbook will serve as an important tool for you to learn the fundamentals of nursing practice. It presents many critical thinking opportunities. At the beginning of each chapter is a Case Scenario that describes a brief situation and then asks questions to help you apply what you have learned. As you begin reading, you consider the guidelines for critical reading. You need to integrate new information into your existing knowledge base. You ask yourself questions about how things fit together and take the time to apply the information to your own experience. You also see how critical thinking and clinical reasoning are evident as the text progresses throughout the phases of nursing process: assessment, diagnosis, outcomes planning, implementation, and evaluating.

You will benefit from reading the highlighted boxes that provide opportunities for critical thinking. The Apply Your Critical Thinking boxes give clinical vignettes related to the chapter's topic. In addition, you can compare your responses against suggested guidelines at the end of the book. The Outcome-Based Teaching Plans have situations with outcomes and strategies to meet those outcomes. You can use clinical reasoning to arrive at nursing judgments about the best way to approach the situation. The Ethical/Legal Issue boxes have situations that ask nurses to synthesize information and arrive at conclusions; many different answers are possible. The boxes provide reflection questions, and nurses can use skills in critical reflection. There is an opportunity for thinking about which answer is best. Key concepts are summarized at the end of each chapter. There are also opportunities for practicing the NCLEX-style questions at the end of each chapter.

Thus, you can build your existing knowledge base by reading this book. You can incorporate this knowledge into your clinical experiences in nursing school. You will have opportunities to use the critical thinking and reflection skills. You will use clinical reasoning as you make nursing judgments. By putting time and effort into developing these skills, you will ultimately provide more individualized and appropriate nursing care.

KEY CONCEPTS

- The nursing process is the systematic, problem-solving approach to providing nursing care to individuals, families, and communities.

- The nursing process has evolved during the last 50 years to consist of six phases: assessment, diagnosis, outcome identification, planning, implementation, and evaluation.

- The nursing process is used in all settings with patients of all ages to identify actual and potential health problems and to design strategies to resolve them.

- Critical thinking and clinical reasoning process are the theoretical foundations for the nursing process.

- Many authors have defined critical thinking. Each definition differs slightly, but all view critical thinking as a positive process that helps people make decisions and take action.

- Critical thinking is essential for use in the nursing process and is an important element in effective nursing practice.

- A sound knowledge base and clinical experience provide the foundation for clinical reasoning to make nursing judgments.

- Critical thinking is important in all nurse–patient interactions.

- You can develop critical thinking skills through self-reflection, building on existing skills, optimizing thinking, expressing thinking verbally and in writing, reading about and discussing critical thinking, listening carefully, and practicing critical thinking.

PRACTICING FOR THE NCLEX
CHECK YOUR ANSWERS IN APPENDIX A.

1. A nurse is conducting an admission assessment on a confused patient brought in by his son. Which of the following would be included in primary sources for information? Select all that apply:
   a. Physical assessment
   b. Health history per the patient's son
   c. Clinical notes in the computer system from a past admission
   d. Patient's report of physical symptoms

2. A nurse receives a patient at handoff who is experiencing acute changes in neurologic status. Which nursing action should be done first?
   a. Call the physician.
   b. Perform an in-depth neurologic assessment.
   c. Administer an antihypertensive medication stat.
   d. Move the patient back to bed.

3. A nurse is revising a plan of care for a patient with dysphagia (difficulty swallowing) related to an esophageal mass. The patient's goal was to eat more than 50% of a blenderized diet, but he is reporting 8/10 pain and shortness of breath when eating. Which phase of the nursing process is impacted when the nurse develops an intermediate goal of pain less than 4/10 while eating?
   a. Assessment
   b. Outcomes/planning
   c. Implementation
   d. Evaluation

4. A patient is scheduled to receive metoprolol for blood pressure control at 09:00. The order reads: "for SBP > 90, 25 mg PO daily." Prior to administration, the nurse rechecks the blood pressure and finds it to be 90/50 with a heart rate of 68. This is an example of using what type of nursing skill?
   a. The nursing process
   b. Critical thinking
   c. The Nurse Practice Act
   d. Medical simulation

5. A new nurse is caring for four patients for the first time. One patient is admitted with respiratory distress, reports no shortness of breath, SpO_2 is 95% on 2LNC, RR is 18. The other patient is admitted for a laparoscopic prostatectomy, complains of 6/10 pain, and has new onset of hematuria in the Foley catheter. The third is an IV drug user with abscess and pain 3/10 and wants to go outside to smoke. The final patient is an elderly confused patient admitted with a urinary tract infection and is determined to be a fall risk. Which patient should be the nurse's priority?
   a. Patient 1
   b. Patient 2
   c. Patient 3
   d. Patient 4

REFERENCES

Alfaro-LeFevre, R. (2014). *Applying nursing process: The foundation for clinical reasoning* (8th ed.). Philadelphia, PA: Wolters Kluwer Health/Lippincott Williams & Wilkins.

American Association of Colleges of Nursing. (2008). *The essentials of baccalaureate education for professional nursing practice.* Washington, DC: Author.

American Nurses Association. (2010). *Nursing: Scope and standards of practice* (2nd ed.). Silver Spring, MD: Author.

Assessment Technologies Institute. (2010). *ATI 2010 item writing workshop.* Kansas City, MO.

Benner, P. (2000). *From novice to expert: Excellence and power in clinical nursing practice* (Commemorative ed.). Englewood Cliffs, NJ: Prentice Hall.

Boud, D., Keogh, R., & Walker, D. (1985). *Promoting reflection in learning: A model. In reflection: Turning experience into learning.* London, UK: Kogan Page.

Bremner, M. N., Aduddell, K., Bennett, D. N., & VanGeest, J. B. (2006). *The use of human patient simulators: Best practices with novice nursing students.* Retrieved July 11, 2014, from www.laerdal.com/us/Research/42408228/The-Use-of-Human-Patient-Simulators-Best-Practices-with-Novice-Nursing-Students

Bulecheck, G. M., Butcher, H. K., Dochterman, J. M., & Wagner, C. M. (2013). *Nursing interventions classification (NIC)* (6th ed.). St. Louis, MO: Elsevier Mosby.

Elder, L., & Paul, R. (1996). *Universal intellectual standards.* Retrieved December 7, 2010, from www.criticalthinking.org/articles/universal-intellectual-standards.cfm

Foundation for Critical Thinking. (2013). The analysis and assessment of thinking. Retrieved July 27, 2015 from http://www.criticalthinking.org/pages/the-analysis-amp-assessment-of-thinking/497

Gordon, M. (1994). *Nursing diagnosis: Process and application* (2nd ed.). New York, NY: McGraw-Hill.

Healsip, P. (2008). *Critical thinking: To think like a nurse.* Retrieved December 9, 2010, from www.criticalthinking.org/resources/HE/ctandnursing.cfm

Herdman, T. H & Kamitsuru, S. (Ed.) (2014). *NANDA International. Nursing Q9 diagnoses: Definitions and classifications 2015–2017.* West Sussex, UK: Wiley-Blackwell.

Jensen, S. (2015). *Nursing health assessment: A best practice approach* (2nd ed.). Philadelphia, PA: Lippincott Williams & Wilkins.

Keenan, G. M., Yakel, E., Tschannon, D., & Mandeville, M. (2008). Chapter 49: Documentation and the nurse care planning process. In R. G. Hughes (Ed.), *Patient safety and quality: An evidenced-based handbook for nurses* (Vol. 2). Retrieved July 4, 2014 from www.ncbi.nlm.nih.gov/books/NBK2674/

Mezirow, J. (2000). *Learning as transformation: Critical perspectives on a theory in progress.* San Francisco, CA: Jossey-Bass.

Moorhead, S., Johnson, M., Maas, M., & Swanson, E. (2013). *Nursing Outcomes Classification (NOC): Measurement of health-outcomes* (5th ed.). St. Louis, MO: Elsevier Mosby.

National Council of State Boards of Nursing (2014). *2014 NCLEX-RN detailed test plan, candidate version.* Retrieved September 29, 2015 from https://www.ncsbn.org/testplans.htm

National League for Nursing. (2011). *Critical thinking in clinical nursing practice/RN examination.* Retrieved December 7, 2010, from http://dev.nln.org/testproducts/pdf/CTinfobulletin.pdf

Herdman, T. H. (Ed.) (2012). *North American Nursing Diagnosis Association International (NANDA-I). Nursing diagnoses: Definitions and classification 2012–2014.* West Sussex, UK: Wiley-Blackwell.

Paul, R., & Elder, L. (2007). *Defining critical thinking.* Retrieved December 7, 2010, from www.criticalthinking.org/aboutCT/define_critical_thinking.cfm

Ralph, S. S., & Taylor, C. M. (2014). *Sparks and Taylor's nursing diagnosis reference manual* (9th ed.). Philadelphia, PA: Wolters Kluwer Health/Lippincott Williams & Wilkins.

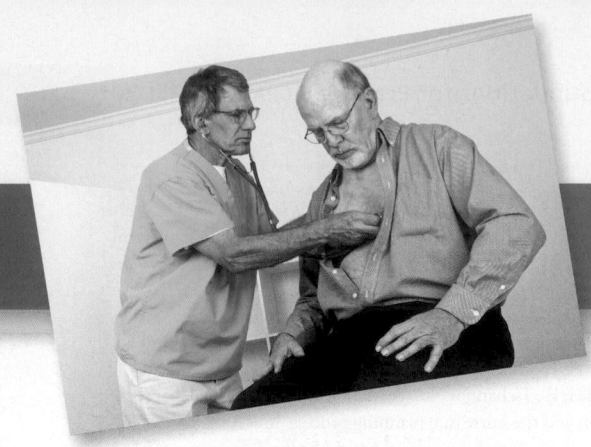

CHAPTER 12

Nursing Assessment

Kathryn Van Dyke Hayes

Case Scenario

You are a nurse working in a busy medical clinic attached to a large medical center. An older man comes alone to the health clinic. You are asked to make an initial health assessment. His major complaint is generalized abdominal pain and decreased appetite. His wife of 51 years died 2 months ago. He moves slowly but appears steady on his feet. He is able to answer questions but does not look directly at you and mumbles his responses. You have 15 minutes to complete your health assessment.

Once you have completed this chapter and have incorporated nursing assessment into your knowledge base, review the above scenario and reflect on the following areas of Critical Thinking:

1. Measure the importance of rapport in this assessment, and propose methods you would use to establish rapport.

2. From the limited information provided, detect possibilities of what might be wrong with this patient, supporting these informed guesses with data from the situation.

3. Summarize subjective and objective data collection, and plan techniques or questions you will use to obtain additional data.

4. Given your limited time for assessment, determine how you will prioritize collection of essential information.

KEY TERMS

assessment
auscultation
confidentiality
cues
inspection
interviewing
objective data
observation
palpation
percussion
physical examination
subjective data
validation

LEARNING OBJECTIVES

Upon completion of this chapter, you will be able to do the following:

1. Describe the assessment phase of the nursing process.

2. Discuss the purpose of assessment in nursing practice.

3. Identify the skills required for nursing assessment.

4. Differentiate the three major activities involved in nursing assessment.

5. Describe the process of data collection.

6. Explain the rationale for data validation.

7. Discuss the frameworks used to organize assessment data.

The first phase of the nursing process, called **assessment**, is the collection of data for nursing purposes. Information is collected using the skills of observation, interviewing, physical examination, and intuition and from many sources, including patients, their family members or significant others, health records, other health team members, and literature review. Figure 12-1 shows the assessment phase in relation to the other phases in the nursing process. Interpretation or analysis of the data takes place in the diagnosis phase of the nursing process. Assessment is the phase of the nursing process during which data are gathered for the purpose of identifying actual or potential health problems. Accurate assessment information is essential for the provision of high-quality nursing care.

Although overlap in the collection of some data by other members of the healthcare team may occur, the specific way in which the data are used differs from one profession to another. Physicians collect assessment data to make a medical diagnosis or evaluate the patient's response to medical interventions. Nursing assessment focuses on the gathering of data about a patient's state of wellness, functional ability, physical status, strengths, and responses to actual and potential health problems.

The purpose of nursing assessment is to gather data about the patient (individual, family, or community) that can be used in diagnosing, identifying outcomes, planning, and implementing care. This promotes individualized patient care. Assessment is done for the following reasons:

- To establish baseline information on the patient
- To determine the patient's normal function
- To determine the patient's risk of dysfunction
- To determine the presence or absence of dysfunction
- To determine the patient's strengths
- To provide data for the diagnosis phase

The following activities make up the assessment phase:

- Collection of data
- Validation of data
- Organization of data

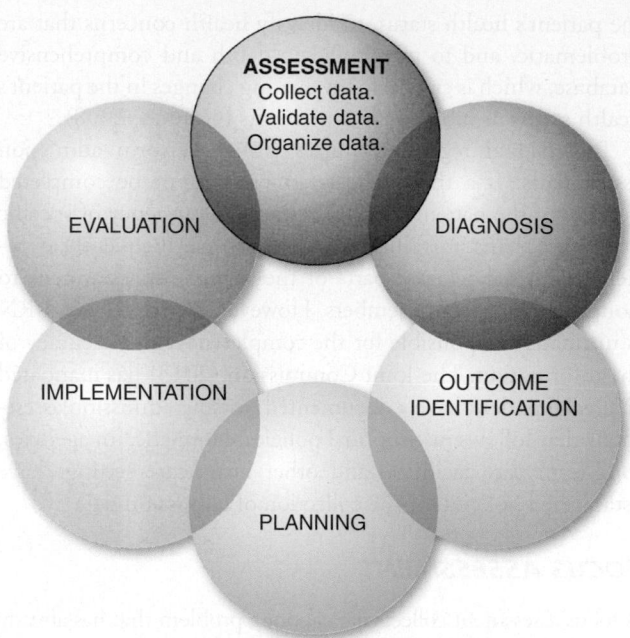

FIGURE 12-1 American Nurses Association Standard I states: "The nurse collects patient health data." This illustration shows activities used in the assessment phase and also the relationship of assessment to the other phases of the nursing process.

PREPARING FOR ASSESSMENT

Types of Assessment

Assessment takes many forms, depending on the clinical situation, patient status, time available, and purpose of data collection. The types of assessment are the admission assessment, focus assessment, time-lapse reassessment, and emergency assessment (Table 12-1).

ADMISSION ASSESSMENT

An admission assessment, also referred to as an initial assessment, is performed when the patient enters a healthcare facility, receives care from a home health agency, or is seen for the first time in an outpatient clinic. The purposes are to evaluate

TABLE 12-1 TYPES, AIMS, AND TIME FRAME FOR ASSESSMENT

Type	Aim	Time Frame
Admission assessment	Initial identification of normal function, functional status, and collection of data concerning actual or potential dysfunction. Baseline for reference and future comparison	Within the specified time frame after admission to a hospital, skilled nursing facility, ambulatory healthcare center, or home healthcare setting
Focus assessment	Status determination of a specific problem identified during previous assessment	Ongoing process; integrated with nursing care; a few minutes to a few hours between assessments
Time-lapse reassessment	Comparison of patient's current status to baseline obtained previously; detection of changes in all functional areas after an extended period of time has passed	Several months (3, 6, or 9 mo or more) between assessments
Emergency assessment	Identification of life-threatening situation	Any time a physiologic, psychological, or emotional crisis occurs

the patient's health status, to identify health concerns that are problematic, and to provide an in-depth and comprehensive database, which is critical for evaluating changes in the patient's health status in subsequent assessments (Gordon, 2008).

Professional registered nurses (RNs) perform admission assessments. If a thorough assessment cannot be completed because of the patient's health status or the urgency of specific health problems, it is finished at a later time. Frequently, experienced nurses delegate parts of the admission assessment to nonprofessional staff members. However, the professional RN is ultimately responsible for the completeness and accuracy of the information. The Joint Commission (2013) has mandated that each patient have a documented nursing admission assessment that follows institutional policies. Home health agencies, long-term care facilities, and other healthcare settings have established policies for the collection of admission data.

FOCUS ASSESSMENT

A focus assessment collects data about a problem that has already been identified. This type of assessment has a narrower scope and a shorter time frame than does the admission assessment. The nurse applies methods relevant to assessing the previously targeted problem (Bickley & Szilagyi, 2013). In focus assessments, nurses determine whether the problem still exists and whether the status of the problem has changed (i.e., improved, worsened, or resolved). This assessment also includes the appraisal of any new, overlooked, or misdiagnosed problems. In intensive care units, nurses may perform focus assessments every few minutes; on medical–surgical units, focus assessments are completed every shift.

Often, nurses assess patients for specific problems and provide nursing care at the same time. For example, while bathing a patient with weakness in the lower extremities, the nurse can assess the patient's skin, muscular strength, and ability to perform self-care activities.

TIME-LAPSE REASSESSMENT

Time-lapse reassessment, another type of assessment, takes place after the initial assessment to evaluate any changes in the patient's health. Nurses perform time-lapse reassessments when substantial periods of time have elapsed between assessments (e.g., periodic outpatient clinic visits, home health visits, health and developmental screenings). Like the focus assessment, the time-lapse reassessment determines the status of problems already identified. Because of the varying time interval between reassessments (e.g., 3 to 12 months), a complete review of all health areas is carried out. For example, several weeks or months may elapse between reassessments of a patient in an ambulatory setting. Time-lapse reassessment is usually less comprehensive than the initial assessment (Gordon, 2008).

EMERGENCY ASSESSMENT

Emergency assessment takes place in life-threatening situations in which the preservation of life is the top priority. Time is of the essence for rapid identification of and intervention for the patient's health problems. Often, the patient's difficulties involve airway, breathing, and circulatory problems (the ABCs). Usually, 2 to 7 seconds are taken to evaluate the heart, lung, and neurologic status (Gordon, 2008). Abrupt changes in self-concept (suicidal thoughts) or roles or relationships (social conflict leading to violent acts) can also initiate an emergency. Emergency assessment is not comprehensive because taking time to collect this information could delay treatment and pose serious risks for the patient. Once the patient's condition is stable, the nurse conducts a more comprehensive assessment.

Setting and Environment

Assessment can take place in any setting where nurses care for patients and their family members: in the patient's home, at a clinic, in a hospital room, at a health fair, or at the patient's workplace. The patient's physical comfort helps facilitate data collection. Therefore, if possible, the assessment should be scheduled at an appropriate time of the day so that the patient is not tired, hungry, or in pain.

An assessment is best performed in a quiet, private setting that lends itself to the discussion of sensitive, personal, and confidential information. The setting must be restricted or secluded to prevent undue embarrassment of the patient during the interview and physical examination. Visitors and family members may need to leave the room temporarily. Distractions such as a television or radio, announcements over the intercom, and interruptions by other healthcare personnel should be minimized. Closing the door, pulling the curtains, adjusting the heat, or moving the patient to another place may be necessary if the environment cannot be modified.

ASSESSMENT SKILLS

To obtain comprehensive data, nurses use various skills as they assess patients and their family members. Reading about various skills is helpful, but actual clinical experience and repeated use of these skills develop proficiency in nursing assessment.

Assessment involves recognizing and collecting **cues**, pieces of information about a patient's health status. Cues may be objective (signs) or subjective (symptoms). Examples of objective cues are a description of an incision site ("reddened, small amount bloody drainage on dressing") or a blood pressure measurement ("180/100"). An example of a subjective cue is the patient's statement, "I have a sharp pain in my shoulder." In the diagnosis phase, these cues are interpreted, clustered, and analyzed.

Nurses use the clinical skills of observation, interviewing, physical examination, and intuition to assess patients across the lifespan in various settings. Nurses use these skills simultaneously when assessing patients. For example, during the patient interview, the nurse asks questions, observes the patient, listens to the patient's answers, and mentally stores information for further exploration during the physical examination. Table 12-2 summarizes the clinical skills used in assessment.

TABLE 12-2 CLINICAL SKILLS USED IN ASSESSMENT

Type	Definition
Observation	The act of noticing patient cues
Interviewing	Interaction and communication process for gathering data by questioning and information exchange
Physical examination	Analysis of bodily functioning using the techniques of inspection, palpation, percussion, and auscultation

Nurses come in contact with patients of all ages and abilities, so assessment techniques may need to be modified according to each patient's developmental stage, abilities, and characteristics. For example, the assessment of a child often involves parental assistance. The parent or other caregiver may hold the child on his or her lap to facilitate examination. Distraction techniques, such as flashing a light or moving an object, are helpful to divert an infant's attention during assessment—for example, when examining the ear (Bickley & Szilagyi, 2013). When assessing an obese patient, a larger blood pressure cuff may be needed. Speaking more slowly and distinctly may be required when examining an older adult with degenerative hearing loss. A patient with joint problems or muscular weakness may require additional time to change positions during the physical examination.

Observation

Observation lays the groundwork for collecting assessment data. As assessment proceeds, nurses anticipate the type of information that will be necessary or appropriate to obtain for a particular patient. **Observation** involves using all the senses to collect data; nurses use the senses of smell, hearing, touch, and, rarely, the sense of taste (Jarvis, 2012; Weber & Kelley, 2014).

Observation begins the moment the nurse meets the patient. As the patient walks into the room, gets out of the wheelchair, or is assisted into bed, the nurse is constantly observing, using all of the appropriate sensory modalities. Observation includes looking, watching, examining, scrutinizing, surveying, scanning, and appraising. Using knowledge of nursing care, physical assessment, basic sciences, social sciences, and pathophysiology, nurses observe patients in a sophisticated manner. Intellectual skills also come into play as nurses decide what data they need to complete the assessment.

VISION

The sense of vision is used in a specialized manner. The nurse's ability to survey how the patient "looks" is key. Does the patient show signs of distress or discomfort, such as grimacing, scowling, or frowning, and guarding or holding a body part? Is the patient sitting upright in a chair with arms resting comfortably at the sides or curled up in bed? What is the patient's body size and nutritional status? Is the patient overweight, obese, normal weight, or undernourished and emaciated? What is the patient's preferred posture? Can he or she walk? Are there any abnormal movements?

How is the patient groomed and dressed? Is the patient's clothing clean, excessively worn, or inappropriate for the season or weather? If a patient's appearance and clothing are disheveled, further information is needed to determine possible contributing factors to self-neglect. Comparing the patient's appearance to the probable norm for the patient and taking into account the patient's lifestyle, occupation, age, and socioeconomic group are key components of this visual appraisal of the patient (Bickley & Szilagyi, 2013).

Nonverbal behavior is noted during every interaction with the patient. The patient's nonverbal demeanor yields information about feelings toward the nurse, staff, and family (Varcarolis & Halter, 2014). Does the patient show any signs of anger, suspicion, anxiety, or hostility? For example, the patient may deny any anxiety or apprehension about health problems but may have an anxious facial expression or tear-filled eyes. The patient may be argumentative and hostile with family members but cooperative and friendly with staff.

SMELL

A keen sense of smell is used when observing the patient. Any body or breath odors may indicate an underlying physical condition. For example, foul-smelling breath may signify an oral or pulmonary infection. A fruity breath odor may indicate a metabolic disorder such as ketosis in diabetes mellitus. Alcohol on the patient's breath can mean that alcohol intake is one explanation for mental and physical findings (Bickley & Szilagyi, 2013). Body odors indicate sweat and sebaceous gland function and the patient's overall cleanliness. A homeless person may have body odors related to lifestyle circumstances and the inability to bathe.

HEARING

Observation includes the nurse's ability to listen to and hear what the patient says. The skill of active listening involves activities such as restating and clarifying what the patient has said. For example, a patient may state: "I feel woozy when I take my pain medication." The nurse needs to ask what the patient means by the term *woozy*. The nurse would ask the patient about light-headedness or dizziness. The patient's level of consciousness and awareness of surroundings are noted. The patient's ability to state his or her name, location, and date accurately is determined when asking questions and observing how the patient answers. The ability to initiate conversation or to respond only when spoken to provides clues about the patient's mental and physical condition. If the patient is confused, the validity of the information obtained should be questioned. Family members or significant others, if available, can provide information for a patient who is confused or incapacitated.

TOUCH

General observations continue through the use of touch. Touch is used to greet the patient (a handshake), to provide nonverbal communication and reassurance, and to perform a preliminary appraisal of skin temperature and moisture. Observe for perspiration, warmth or coldness, and strength of the patient's handshake. A gentle touch on the arm or hand may reassure the patient and, at the same time, reveal dry, scaly skin indicative of dehydration or a thyroid problem. A specialized kind of touching called palpation is performed during the physical examination.

Always consider the patient's sociocultural background when using touch. In some cultures, the use of touch must be modified to minimize the patient's sense that privacy has been invaded. For example, patients of Chinese heritage are very modest about having their bodies touched and may find it difficult to perform self-examinations for their own health promotion (i.e., breast self-examinations) (Tsai, 2013). Patients from some cultures may interpret touching as a hostile action. Patients of Chinese heritage may believe that painful procedures such as drawing blood for laboratory tests deplete the body's energy, which cannot be regenerated (Tsai, 2013). Other cultural groups use touch in other ways. For example, patients of Mexican heritage demonstrate touch to signify closeness in relationships. By shaking the hand of a Mexican American patient, the healthcare provider shows respect and support for his or her cultural background (Zoucha & Zamarripa, 2013).

Interviewing

To obtain accurate information, nurses must be effective communicators. Among the factors affecting an interview's quality and comprehensiveness are the nurse's skill and experience and the patient's willingness to share information. The admission assessment is often the patient's first encounter with the nurse. As you assess the patient, the patient assesses you, the nurse, with thoughts such as the following: Do you care about me and my current health situation? Are you organized and competent? Can I trust you? It is important for the nurse to be professional, concerned, and attentive throughout the interview.

Several techniques facilitate communication between nurses and patients. These techniques establish rapport, help nurses elicit thoughts and feelings of patients, encourage conversation, and ensure mutual understanding (Townsend, 2014; Varcarolis & Halter, 2014). Barriers that hinder interaction have the opposite effect on communication (Carpenito-Moyet, 2013; Townsend, 2014; Varcarolis & Halter, 2014). Table 12-3 summarizes the techniques that facilitate and hinder effective communication. Chapter 6 discusses communication techniques in detail.

TABLE 12-3 TECHNIQUES THAT FACILITATE AND BLOCK COMMUNICATION DURING AN INTERVIEW

Facilitators of Communication	Barriers to Communication
Using broad opening statements	Making stereotyped comments
Giving general leads	Giving advice or stating your opinion
Listening	Agreeing with the patient
Acknowledging the patient's feelings	Defending
Using silence	Giving approval
Giving information	Using reassuring clichés
Reflecting or repeating the patient's words	Requesting an explanation
Sharing observations	Expressing disapproval
Clarifying	Belittling the patient's feelings
Summarizing	Changing the subject
Validating	Disagreeing with the patient
Verbalizing implied thoughts or feelings	Appearing inattentive, impatient, or distracted

Interviewing, an essential skill for obtaining information for the nursing history, consists of asking questions designed to elicit subjective data from the patient or family members. The nursing history focuses on the patient's account of the actual or potential health problems and their impact on his or her health status. The nursing history helps the nurse do the following:

- Clarify and verify the patient's perception of his or her health status
- Compare the patient's present and past health status, lifestyle behaviors, and coping abilities
- Identify actual and potential nursing diagnoses
- Develop the patient plan of care
- Implement nursing interventions to support the patient's adaptive responses

Healthcare institutions usually have a form for the systematic collection and documentation of the nursing history. Such documentation improves communication among nursing staff and other health team members.

A nursing history can take 30 to 60 minutes to perform. Although it is usually completed in one session, several sessions may be required. If the patient's condition (e.g., severe pain, breathing difficulties) or the setting (e.g., excessive noise, lack of privacy) makes data collection difficult, information about urgent problems should be collected and other questions deferred until a more suitable time.

An interview can be divided into four phases: preparatory, introductory, maintenance, and concluding.

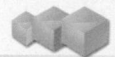

Concept Mastery Alert

It is difficult to simultaneously assess a patient's physical status and perform the detailed interview that forms the basis of the nursing history. In many cases, it is beneficial to obtain the nursing history first in order to provide context for the physical assessment.

PREPARATORY PHASE

The preparatory or preinteraction phase occurs before the nurse meets the patient. Actions taken in this phase help ensure that the interview will be as productive as possible. The nurse's attention is directed toward preparing for the first nurse–patient interaction. During this phase, do the following (Varcarolis & Halter, 2014):

- Review as much information as possible about the patient.
- Decide what data are needed and what type of data collection form will be used.
- Review the literature pertinent to the patient's developmental age, psychosocial aspects, and pathophysiologic considerations, if needed.
- Assess your own feelings or reactions to previous patients that might interfere with the nurse–patient relationship.
- Seek assistance from more experienced nurses, mentors, or supervisors if concerned about how to carry out the interview.
- Plan for a private, quiet setting for the interview; schedule a mutually convenient time of day; and determine the length of time needed for data collection.
- Modify the environment to facilitate the interview.

INTRODUCTORY PHASE

The second phase of an interview is referred to as the introductory phase or orientation phase. It begins when the nurse and patient meet. Actions in this phase assist in establishing rapport, clarifying roles, and alleviating anxiety. The nurse and patient are actively involved in asking questions, getting acquainted, and exchanging their expectations for the interview and health assessment. During this phase, do the following (Varcarolis & Halter, 2014):

- Introduce yourself by name and position, and explain the purpose and content of the interview.
- Begin to establish rapport with the patient by conveying a caring, interested attitude; rapport is essential for a trusting, helpful nurse–patient relationship.
- Observe the patient's behavior, and listen attentively to determine the patient's self-perceptions and how the patient views his or her health problems; validate the patient's perceptions as the interview progresses.
- Let the patient know how long the interview is expected to last.
- Inform the patient how the information collected will be used and that confidentiality will be maintained.

- Start with nonthreatening, specific questions and proceed to open-ended questions.
- Establish a verbal contract with the patient, incorporating the goals of the interview.

MAINTENANCE PHASE

The maintenance phase, or working phase, is the third phase of an interview. The nurse and patient work toward achieving the specific task or goal agreed on in the introductory phase. Both participants maintain the interaction for the purpose of getting the "work" done, but it is the nurse's responsibility to ensure that the goals are met. The goals may be mutually revised by the patient and nurse. In this phase, do the following (Varcarolis & Halter, 2014):

- Keep focused on the tasks or goals to ensure that needed data are obtained and goals are achieved.
- Encourage the patient to express his or her feelings, concerns, and questions.
- Use techniques that facilitate communication between the nurse and patient (e.g., silence, general leads, validation).
- Observe the nonverbal behavior that accompanies verbal responses (e.g., a patient may say she is not nervous, worried, or anxious while biting her fingernails or moving constantly).
- Assess the patient's ability to continue the interview (e.g., grimace of pain, shortness of breath, fatigue).
- Facilitate goal attainment by moving to the next topic of discussion after needed data are collected.

CONCLUDING PHASE

In the concluding or termination phase, the interview is completed. Actions taken in this phase can help ensure that the termination will be a positive experience for both participants. The focus is on reviewing goals or tasks attained and expressing concerns related to this phase. In this phase, do the following (Varcarolis & Halter, 2014):

- Review goal or task attainment; such a review can foster a sense of achievement in the patient and nurse.
- Summarize the highlights of the interview and its meaning to the nurse and the patient.
- Encourage the patient to express and share his or her feelings regarding the termination of the interview.
- Use language congruent with the patient's cultural background and local custom (e.g., "goodbye" may mean a final farewell in some cultures; promises to contact the patient in the future may be taken literally).

Physical Examination Techniques

The **physical examination** is a systematic data collection method that uses the senses of sight, hearing, smell, and touch to detect health problems. Four techniques are used: inspection, palpation, percussion, and auscultation. Usually, the nursing interview is completed before the physical examination is performed (Fig. 12-2).

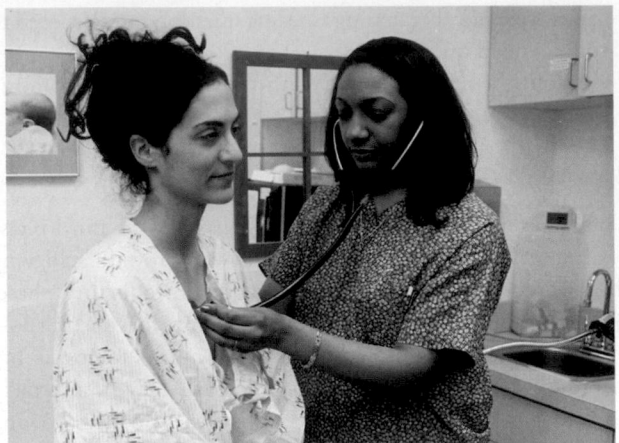

FIGURE 12-2 The physical examination is used to verify the data gathered during the nursing interview.

INSPECTION

Inspection is a visual examination of the patient that is done in a methodical and deliberate manner. Beginning with the first patient contact, it is conducted intentionally and continuously to avoid omitting data. Not haphazard or passive, inspection is an important first step in the physical examination process. During inspection, the patient's anatomic structures are considered and any abnormalities that may be present are identified. Factors such as color, shape, symmetry, movement, pulsations, and texture of the involved body part are noted (Bickley & Szilagyi, 2013).

Inspection is carried out during the interview and subsequent physical examination. For example, an enlarged thyroid or growth in the neck may be visible during the interview with the patient. Detailed inspection of the neck would take place after the interview.

PALPATION

Palpation is the specialized use of touch for data collection that augments the inspection process. The nurse uses the fingertips and palms of the hand to determine the size, shape, and configuration of underlying body structures. Using palpation, a nurse can detect the pulsations of blood vessels; the outlines of organs such as the thyroid, spleen, or liver; the size, shape, and mobility of masses; the temperature of the skin; the vibration or movement of blood in a blood vessel; and the tenderness or sensitivity of a body part.

PERCUSSION

Percussion is a technique in which one or both hands are used to strike the body surface in a precise manner to produce a sound called a *percussion note*. Underlying body structures have characteristic percussion notes that indicate their denseness or hollowness. Percussion is used to discover the location and level of organs (liver, heart, diaphragm), the consistency of body structures (fluid filled, air filled, or solid), tenderness (over the kidneys or near the spine), and the identification of masses or tumors.

AUSCULTATION

Auscultation is the technique of listening to body sounds with a stethoscope placed on the body surface to amplify normal and abnormal sounds. It yields information by amplifying the movement of air or fluid in the body. Mastery of auscultation lies in practice and the ability to interpret the findings. A novice nurse may consult with a more experienced nurse to verify auscultation findings, often to verify and confirm abnormal sounds.

Various body systems, including the respiratory, cardiovascular, and gastrointestinal systems, may be auscultated for characteristic sounds. Bowel sounds, breath sounds, heart sounds, and the sound of blood moving through a narrowed or twisted blood vessel (known as a bruit) are heard through auscultation.

ASSESSMENT ACTIVITIES

During the assessment phase, nurses collect, validate, and organize data. Because these activities are so closely related, shifting from one to another often occurs. For example, collecting and organizing of data may occur at the same time. Nurses may choose to validate information as they collect it rather than at the completion of data collection. As they organize data, they may discover ambiguous cues that require further clarification and validation.

Collect Data

Data collection, the process of compiling information about the patient, begins with the first patient contact. Nurses use observation, interviewing, and physical examination. Usually, they collect data using a systematic format that ensures comprehensive, accurate information.

TYPES OF DATA

Subjective and objective data—integral parts of assessment—are obtained during data collection. Table 12-4 shows the differences in the methods of obtaining subjective and objective data and provides examples of each type.

Subjective data, also known as symptoms, include the patient's feelings and statements about his or her health problems. Patients supply subjective data. Often, attempts to validate, confirm, or substantiate subjective data through other sources are not feasible. Subjective data are obtained through the interview and are best recorded as direct quotations from the patient, such as:

"I haven't felt good for the last couple of months."
"I get a sharp pain in my stomach after I eat."
"Every time I move, I feel nauseated."

Objective data, also known as signs, are observable, perceptible, and measurable. Other data can validate or verify objective data. Examples include bowel sounds, temperature readings, peripheral pulses, distended neck vessels, and skin rashes. Objective data may be obtained by the senses (e.g., vision, touch, smell) or by measuring devices or equipment (e.g., thermometer,

Nursing Assessment CHAPTER 12   209

TABLE 12-4 COMPARISON OF SUBJECTIVE AND OBJECTIVE DATA

	Subjective Data (Symptoms)	Objective Data (Signs)
Method of Obtaining Data	Interview	Techniques of inspection, palpation, percussion, and auscultation Measurement devices Health record Laboratory studies, radiologic tests, diagnostic procedures
Examples	Symptoms Values Perceptions Feelings Attitudes Sensations Beliefs	Physical examination findings: heart sounds, palpable tumor, discolored skin Blood pressure, temperature Written reports of other healthcare team members on health record Complete blood count results; chest radiography results

sphygmomanometer), laboratory studies (e.g., complete blood count), or diagnostic procedures (e.g., colonoscopy).

SOURCES OF DATA

Two major sources of data exist for the collection of information about the patient. The patient is considered the primary source of data because only he or she can give a firsthand description of the health problem and its effects on his or her lifestyle. All other sources, including family members, significant others, other members of the healthcare team, laboratory tests, and literature review, are considered secondary sources.

 APPLY YOUR CRITICAL THINKING

You have collected the following data for your assigned patient:

- Complete blood count
- Patient's health history: "I haven't felt good for the last 2 weeks. I think it's the flu." History of diabetes for 5 years; no complaints of pain.
- Physical examination: Afebrile; pulse—72; respirations—22; blood pressure—122/64. Abdomen soft and nontender. Bowel sounds present in all four quadrants.
- Family member's description of how the patient has reacted to his or her illness
- Patient's perception of ability to cope with life stressors
- Chest radiology results
- Consultation report from physical therapy

Which data are considered primary sources, and which are considered secondary sources?

Check your answer in Appendix B.

Primary Source

The patient is the primary source of data, and the information collected from the patient is considered to be the most reliable, unless circumstances such as altered level of consciousness, severe pain, impending surgery, acute illness, or age make data collection impossible. The patient is deemed unreliable if he or she is confused or suffering from physical or mental conditions that alter thinking, judgment, or memory. In these situations, secondary sources help provide the necessary assessment information.

Secondary Sources

Secondary sources provide data that supplement, clarify, and validate information obtained from the patient.

Family members or significant others supplement and verify information obtained from the patient, often providing information that the patient forgets to mention or is unwilling to reveal. They may be the only source of data for children or for confused, unresponsive, or severely ill patients. Data provided by family members and significant others include a description of how the patient reacts to illness, the patient's perceptions of changes in health status, the patient's ability to cope with life stressors, and information about the patient's home situation.

Usually, the patient's permission is obtained before information is sought from family members or significant others. All people involved must understand the confidential nature of the information they provide. The patient's permission must also be obtained to divulge any information (e.g., diagnosis of cancer, positive HIV status, pregnancy) to family members or significant others.

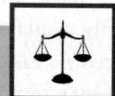 **ETHICAL/LEGAL ISSUE**

CONFIDENTIALITY OF ASSESSMENT FINDINGS

Mr. Jones, a 51-year-old patient, recently was given a diagnosis of advanced colon cancer with metastasis. Due to a large bowel obstruction, Mr. Jones had a bowel resection 6 days ago and is recovering at home. Your assessment reveals that the patient lives alone and has been estranged from his wife for the past 2 years. He states, "We really don't talk much." During your home visit, Mr. Jones's wife arrives and asks you to tell her what is wrong with her husband. How would you handle this situation? What information would you give Mrs. Jones?

CRITICAL THINKING CHALLENGE

- Consider your responsibilities to the patient. Consider your responsibilities to his wife.
- How does the Health Insurance Portability and Accountability Act (HIPAA) impact your legal and ethical responsibility in this situation?
- Identify additional information you would need to assess before proceeding.
- Propose possible strategies for handling this situation.

Past and current health records (e.g., consultation reports, medical and nursing histories, physical examination findings) contain a wealth of information about the patient and are helpful in completing assessment data. Facts about the patient's previous illnesses, hospitalizations, function, and dysfunction are obtained. The health record may also reveal data not expressed by the patient or picked up by the nurse. Reviewing health records can also reduce the number of times a patient is asked the same questions by various health team members.

Laboratory tests and diagnostic procedures, another secondary source of data for completing the database, supplement and verify findings from the interview and physical examination. Laboratory test results are always interpreted in relation to the patient's underlying health problems and treatment modalities. These results can also identify actual or potential health problems not disclosed by the patient or explored by the nurse. Sometimes, laboratory tests and diagnostic procedures are used to judge the effectiveness of nursing interventions or medical treatment.

Written and verbal reports from other health team members are another source of assessment data. Health team members include nurses, social workers, physical therapists, physicians, clergy, respiratory therapists, and assistive personnel such as certified nursing assistants. Take advantage of the expertise of other colleagues who are caring for the patient. All of them are valuable sources of information about the patient's current and past health status. Consulting other health team members helps verify and supplement the assessment data.

Reviewing the literature helps complete the patient's database. Pertinent literature includes textbooks, journals, and online resources. Web-based data sources are readily available at the point of care, so using these resources has become easier and a common practice in care delivery. The patient's health status must be viewed in relation to current knowledge and theory. A thorough review of the literature provides information on recent developments in nursing and medical practice.

RECORDING DATA

Using a framework or outline, assessment data are systematically recorded and become a permanent part of the medical record. Institutions usually have a specific form for recording data and facilitating its use by other nurses who are caring for the patient. Baseline assessment data are referred to periodically to reaffirm assessment findings and to compare the patient's current status with his or her initial condition. Two methods can be used: the traditional written assessment record and the computerized assessment record. **Confidentiality**, or keeping information private, applies to all information entered in the patient's medical record. Information is discussed or shared only with healthcare professionals directly involved in providing care for the patient. Chapter 16 discusses documentation of patient assessment in detail.

VALIDATE DATA

Validation, commonly referred to as double-checking the information at hand, is the process of confirming the accuracy

of assessment data collected. As data are collected, multiple cues are identified. Inferences are made about the cues (i.e., a meaning or interpretation is attached to the cue). One or more inferences can be made about a particular cue or group of cues (Alfaro-LeFevre, 2014), as seen in the examples provided in Box 12-1.

Validation assists in verifying and clarifying cues and inferences, thus increasing the likelihood that cues and inferences are accurate, free from bias, and interpreted correctly (Alfaro-LeFevre, 2014). Incorrect cues and inferences lead to the development of inappropriate nursing diagnoses and patient plans of care. Figure 12-3 illustrates the connection between cues and inferences and methods for data validation.

BOX 12-1   Examples of Cues and Inferences

Example 1
Group of Patient Cues
- Blurry vision or visual defect
- Headache
- Tingling and numbness in extremities
- Dizziness

Possible Inferences
- Patient has a brain tumor.
- Patient is having warning signals of a stroke.
- Patient may be diabetic.
- Patient is anxious.

Example 2
Cue
Mr. Spencer has dry, flaky skin.

Possible Inferences
1. Mr. Spencer may be dehydrated.
2. Mr. Spencer has hypothyroidism.
3. Mr. Spencer has some type of dermatitis.

Example 3
Cue
Patient has frequency and burning on urination.

Inference
Patient has a urinary tract infection.

Example 4
Cue
Mrs. Smith's blood sugar is 55 mg/dL.

Inference
Mrs. Smith is having a hypoglycemic reaction.

Example 5
Cue
Patient states, "I just can't seem to shake this pain in my joints."

Inference
Patient has inadequate pain management.

DATA VALIDATION

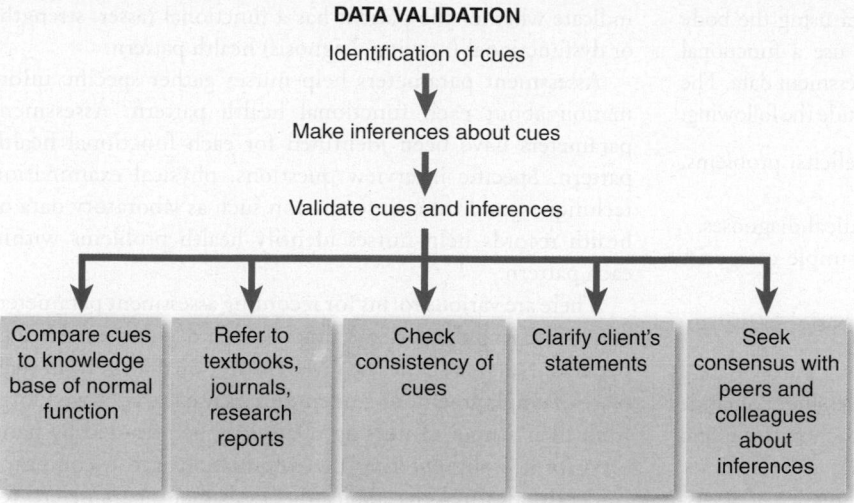

FIGURE 12-3 Methods for the validation of cues and inferences.

Identification of relevant cues and correct inferences depends on the nurse's clinical nursing knowledge, assessment skills, personal values, and past experience (Alfaro-LeFevre, 2014). Inferences must be validated before cues are clustered and analyzed for identification of nursing diagnoses.

Methods of validating data include (Alfaro-LeFevre, 2014):

- *Comparing cues to normal function.* For example, Mr. Jones is a professional athlete and has a resting pulse of 50 beats per minute; the nurse knows that physiologic heart changes in physically fit people can result in a slower pulse rate (bradycardia).
- *Referring to textbooks, journals, and research reports.* For example, the nurse may consider brown macules or "liver spots" on the hands and forearms of an elderly patient to be abnormal. After checking a textbook on physical changes that occur with aging, the nurse learns that they are common in older adults.
- *Checking consistency of cues.* Data can be checked, for example, by retaking the patient's temperature or blood pressure or by using another piece of equipment. Subjective and objective data can be compared. For example, the patient may state "I feel hot," but his or her temperature is 37°C, or the patient may state "I can't get my breath," but respirations are 20 and lung sounds are clear.
- *Clarifying the patient's statements.* Ask specific questions to collect additional information, share observations with the patient and family members, clarify ambiguous or vague statements, and verify inferences. For example, a patient who is asked whether he or she has any allergies to foods, medicines, or pollutants may respond, "I am allergic to antibiotics." If questioned further about the medication bottle labeled "penicillin" the patient brought from home, he or she may state, "Oh, I'm not allergic to all antibiotics, just erythromycin."
- *Seeking consensus with colleagues about inferences.* This is usually done after the data have been validated using the methods already described. If peers or colleagues independently reach the same conclusion as the nurse did, and if

that conclusion is based on valid data, the nurse's inferences are supported. If colleagues present an alternative view, it assists the nurse in questioning the validity of his or her own inferences.

Organize Data

Various frameworks exist for the orderly collection and recording of assessment data. Frameworks serve as guides during the nursing interview and physical examination, help prevent the omission of pertinent information, and foster data analysis in the diagnosis phase. Frameworks may be modified based on the patient's physical status and the nurse's personal preference.

Nursing conceptual models provide one such framework. Institutions, nursing schools, and individual nurses use one or more of these frameworks to guide their nursing practice. Each conceptual framework has a frame of reference for carrying out nursing care. Some examples are Orem's self-care model, Roy's adaptation model, Neuman's systems model, and Johnson's behavioral model (Fawcett & DeSanto-Madeya, 2013). When using one of these frameworks, refer to specific texts that describe these models in detail. See also Chapter 1 for more information.

FUNCTIONAL HEALTH APPROACH

The patient's strengths, talents, and functional health status are an integral part of the assessment data. This information occasionally is obscured or forgotten in some assessment frameworks. An assessment of functional health focuses on the patient's normal function and his or her altered function or risk of altered function. Because the information gathered using the 11 functional health patterns is basic to nursing, it is applicable to all conceptual models or theories of nursing practice (Gordon, 2008). Functional health assessment can be used for patients of all ages and in all specialty areas, and it is relevant for the assessment of the person, family, or community.

Some nurses collect physical assessment data using the body systems model or the head-to-toe model but use a functional health framework to organize and document assessment data. The advantages of a functional health framework include the following:

- Patient strengths and assets (not merely deficits, problems, or limitations) can be identified.
- The focus is on nursing diagnoses, not medical diagnoses.
- Clustering is easier to do because of the simple categories and concise typology.
- It may contribute to the delineation of basic assessment areas relevant for all patients.

The components of functional health assessment include the pattern label, assessment parameters for each pattern, and recording of assessment data.

The pattern label is the name given to a category of assessment data. Gordon (2008; 2010) identified 11 categories of assessment data, called *functional health patterns*. Pattern labels indicate whether the patient has a functional (asset, strength) or dysfunctional (nursing diagnosis) health pattern.

Assessment parameters help nurses gather specific information about each functional health pattern. Assessment parameters have been identified for each functional health pattern. Specific interview questions, physical examination techniques, and other information such as laboratory data or health records help nurses identify health problems within each pattern.

There are various forms for recording assessment parameters and identifying the patient's functional or dysfunctional health patterns. Nurses use the approved institutional form from their place of employment, or student nurses use the approved form from their school of nursing. Data may be recorded by hand on a form or by entering the information into a computer. In-depth information about the assessment parameters for each functional health pattern is described in Chapter 17 and highlighted in Table 12-5.

TABLE 12-5 FUNCTIONAL HEALTH PATTERNS AND ASSESSMENT PARAMETERS

Functional Health Pattern	Assessment Parameters
Health perception and health management	General survey of the patient's health status Usual health behaviors
Activity and Exercise	Mobility Status Cardiovascular status Respiratory status Exercise routine Leisure activities
Nutrition and metabolism	Eating habits Appraisal of appetite Weight loss or gain Changes in skin, hair, or nails
Elimination—excretory function (bowel, bladder, and skin)	Usual bowel and bladder elimination habits, last bowel movement Laxative use Excretory function of the skin (e.g., excessive perspiration)
Sleep and rest	Regular sleep habits and routine
Cognition and perception	Changes in cognitive function Ability to hear, see, and speak Pain, numbness, or other sensations
Self-perception and self-concept	Descriptions of self Physical appearance Effects of illness Major life accomplishments
Roles and relationships	Patient's perceptions of key relationships Observations of interactions with others
Coping and stress tolerance	Current stress level Coping ability Ability to endure life stressors Physiologic responses to stress (e.g., blood pressure, heart rate)
Sexuality and reproduction	Patient's appraisal of his or her sexual role and sexual health
Values and beliefs	Identification of valued people and possessions Sources of support Religious practices

HEAD-TO-TOE MODEL

Using the head-to-toe framework for assessment, nurses systematically examine every part of the body starting from the head and progressing down to the toes. Similar to most assessment models, the head-to-toe method first assesses the patient's general state of health. Vital signs may be taken before the physical examination begins. Chapter 17 presents the order of physical assessment using a head-to toe framework. Modifications can be used for young children to ensure that invasive techniques, such as examining the ears with an otoscope, are done last.

BODY SYSTEMS MODEL

The body systems model (also referred to as the medical model or review of systems) focuses on the patient's major anatomic systems. This framework allows nurses to collect data about the past and present condition of each organ or body system and to examine thoroughly all body systems for actual and potential problems. This review often reveals information that the patient did not consider important or neglected to mention. It starts with an assessment of the patient's general state of health, followed by systematic assessment of each body system (neurologic, cardiovascular, respiratory, gastrointestinal, and so on) until all systems have been assessed. Chapter 17 describes the order of the physical assessment as performed by the staff nurse using a body systems framework.

KEY CONCEPTS

- Assessment is the collection of subjective and objective data from the patient and other sources for the purpose of describing health problems.

- Types of assessment vary depending on the clinical situation, the patient's health status, the time available, and the purpose of data collection.

- An in-depth, comprehensive appraisal of a patient's health at the time of entry into a healthcare facility or at the time of the first home health visit or outpatient clinic visit is called an *admission assessment*.

- Environmental factors can facilitate or hinder collection of assessment data.

- Observation helps the nurse anticipate appropriate data to be collected during the nursing interview and physical examination.

- Proficient interviewing skills are necessary for obtaining comprehensive assessment data.

- The physical examination is a systematic analysis in which inspection, palpation, percussion, and auscultation are used.

- The patient, family and significant others, health team members, and health records are sources of assessment data.

- Assessment data are recorded and become a permanent part of the health record.

- The functional health pattern assessment provides a framework for collecting and organizing patient data, providing a foundation for the development of nursing diagnoses.

PRACTICING FOR THE NCLEX

CHECK YOUR ANSWERS IN APPENDIX A.

1. A nurse is conducting a focus assessment of a hospitalized patient who is a fall risk. Which of the following would be most appropriate?
   a. "Do you have many stairs that you need to navigate at home?"
   b. "Are you more unsteady on your feet when you are out of bed today?"
   c. "Are you feeling any pain in your abdomen?"
   d. "What is your usual or baseline diet at home?"

2. A nurse is admitting a patient with congestive heart failure. Which of the following describe appropriate aspects of assessment?
   a. Define patient goals for increasing ability for self-care.
   b. Evaluate current therapeutic regimen at home.
   c. Identify activities that exacerbate symptoms.
   d. Apply oxygen therapy via nasal cannula.

3. In conducting an assessment of a patient with gastrointestinal bleeding, the nurse uses which of the following pieces of subjective data? Select all that apply:
   a. Hematocrit 20%
   b. Appearance of stool
   c. Spouse's statement of symptoms
   d. Health record description of signs

4. The nurse has admitted a single mother with nausea and vomiting for the last 3 days and upper left quadrant abdominal pain. Which of the statements below indicate that the nurse is using the functional health patterns model of assessment? Select all that apply:
   a. "Please describe your appetite over the last week."
   b. "What kind of help have you had from your family since this started?"
   c. "Have you been able to sleep or rest lately as usual?"
   d. "Have you had symptoms like this in the past?"
   e. "Your blood pressure is 94/48; heart rate is 122."

5. Which of the following are true about the introductory phase of interviewing? Select all that apply:
   a. The introductory phase is the first phase of the interviewing process.
   b. Introduce yourself by name and position.
   c. Focus on goals and move to the next topic after data are collected.
   d. Observe behavior and patient's self-perceptions.

REFERENCES

Alfaro-LeFevre, R. (2014). *Applying nursing process: The foundation for clinical reasoning* (8th ed.). Philadelphia, PA: Wolters Kluwer Health/Lippincott Williams & Wilkins.

Bickley, L. S., & Szilagyi, P. G. (2013). *Bates' guide to physical examination and history taking* (12th ed.). Philadelphia, PA: Wolters Kluwer Health/ Lippincott Williams & Wilkins.

Carpenito-Moyet, L. J. (2013). *Nursing diagnosis: Application to clinical practice* (14th ed.). Philadelphia, PA: Wolters Kluwer Health/Lippincott Williams & Wilkins.

Fawcett, J., & DeSanto-Madeya, S. (2013). *Contemporary nursing knowledge: Analysis and evaluation of nursing models and theories* (3rd ed.). Philadelphia, PA: F. A. Davis.

Gordon, M. (2008). *Assess notes: Nursing assessment and diagnostic reasoning.* Philadelphia, PA: F. A. Davis.

Gordon, M. (2010). *Manual of nursing diagnosis* (12th ed.). Sudbury, MA: Jones & Bartlett.

Jarvis, C. (2012). *Physical examination and health assessment* (6th ed.). St. Louis, MO: Elsevier Saunders.

The Joint Commission. (2013). *2014 hospital accreditation standards.* Oakbrook Terrace, IL: Joint Commission Resources.

Townsend, M. C. (2014). *Psychiatric mental health nursing: Concepts of care in evidence-based practice* (8th ed.). Philadelphia, PA: F. A. Davis.

Tsai, H.-M. (2013). People of Chinese heritage. In L. D. Purnell (Ed.), *Transcultural health care: A culturally competent approach* (4th ed., pp. 178–196). Philadelphia, PA: F. A. Davis.

Varcarolis, E. M., & Halter, M. J. (2014). *Varcarolis' foundations of psychiatric mental health nursing: A clinical approach* (7th ed.). St. Louis, MO: Saunders Elsevier.

Weber, J. R., & Kelley, J. H. (2014). *Health assessment in nursing* (5th ed.). Philadelphia, PA: Lippincott Williams & Wilkins.

Zoucha, R., & Zamarripa, C. A. (2013). People of Mexican heritage. In L. D. Purnell & B. J. Paulanka (Ed.), *Transcultural health care: A culturally competent approach* (4th ed., pp. 374–390). Philadelphia, PA: F. A. Davis.

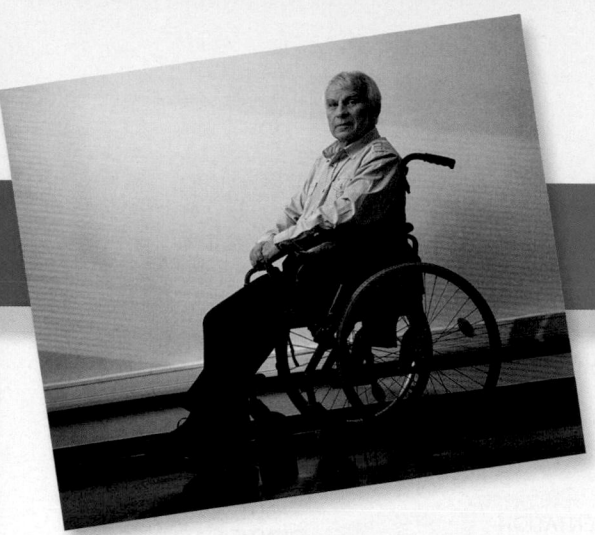

CHAPTER 13

Nursing Diagnosis

Kathryn Van Dyke Hayes

Case Scenario

Jake Mason, a middle-aged former carpenter, comes to the health clinic with a temperature of 101°F. He has paralysis of all four extremities and has been wheelchair dependent for 6 months since he was injured in a construction accident. He is not working but still considers himself to be the provider for his wife and two children. He displays anger that his wife has to work to pay the bills and that she also has the responsibility of disciplining the children. You are the nurse caring for him.

Once you have completed this chapter and have incorporated information about nursing diagnoses into your knowledge base, review the above scenario and reflect on the following areas of Critical Thinking:

1. Cluster the data provided in this situation under various nursing diagnoses, and provide justification for your decisions regarding placement. (Note: Some data may fit under several diagnoses.)
2. Evaluate patterns in data clustering that provide adequate support for identifying a nursing diagnosis.
3. Validate with the patient and the NANDA-I taxonomy whether the data collected are sufficient to confirm possible nursing diagnoses.
4. Formulate nursing diagnostic statements that could be added to the plan of care.
5. Role-play how you will discuss the identified problems with the patient and family.

KEY TERMS
actual nursing diagnosis
cluster
collaborative health problems
medical diagnosis
nursing diagnosis
possible nursing diagnosis
premature closure
risk nursing diagnosis
taxonomy
validation

LEARNING OBJECTIVES

Upon completion of this chapter, the student will be able to do the following:

1. Define *diagnosis* in relation to the nursing process.
2. Describe the components of a nursing diagnosis.
3. Discuss the significance of nursing diagnosis for nursing practice.
4. Differentiate between a nursing diagnosis and collaborative problems.
5. Identify the clinical skills needed to make nursing diagnoses.
6. Formulate nursing diagnoses for a patient situation.
7. Discuss the categorization of nursing diagnoses by functional health patterns.

Diagnosing human responses to actual or potential health problems is the second phase of the nursing process. After collecting relevant information about patients, nurses need to analyze and interpret the data. The result of this interpretation is the nursing diagnosis (Fig. 13-1). Registered nurses (RNs) are educated and licensed to make nursing diagnoses. As such, they have a duty to identify and plan care for patients based on them.

NANDA-International (Herdman & Kamitsuru, 2014) defines **nursing diagnosis** as follows:

> A clinical judgment about individual, family, or community responses to actual or potential health problems/life processes. A nursing diagnosis provides the basis for selection of nursing interventions to achieve outcomes for which the nurse is accountable. (p. 465)

The term *nursing diagnosis* serves as both the label for and the action of describing a patient's health problems. Its purpose is to identify problems and synthesize the information gathered during the nursing assessment by doing the following:

- Analyzing collected data
- Identifying the patient's strengths
- Identifying the patient's normal functional level and indicators of actual or potential dysfunction
- Formulating a diagnostic statement in relation to this synthesis

In the diagnosis phase, the nurse does the following:

- Identifies patterns
- Validates the diagnosis
- Formulates the nursing diagnosis statement

Figure 13-2 shows the diagnosis phase in relation to the other phases of the nursing process.

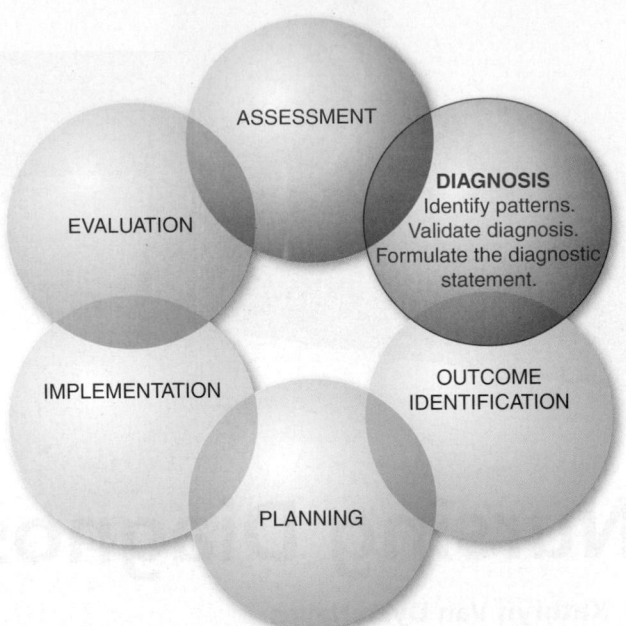

FIGURE 13-2 American Nurses Association Standard II states that the nurse analyzes the assessment data in determining diagnoses. This illustration shows activities used in the nursing diagnosis phase and also the relationship of nursing diagnosis to the other phases of the nursing process.

NURSING DIAGNOSIS TAXONOMY

Professions require a sound scientific base; the nursing process is nursing's scientific base. To achieve this scientific foundation, nursing requires a **taxonomy**, or classification system, to provide a structure for nursing practice. The NANDA-I taxonomy has three levels: domains, classes, and nursing diagnosis (Herdman & Kamitsuru, 2014). A classification system for nursing diagnoses involves knowledge of nursing practice, theoretical frameworks, and the characteristics of taxonomies.

NANDA-I's goal has been to develop a nursing diagnosis taxonomy. In 1973, at the first conference, 86 nursing diagnoses were listed alphabetically and published for use and development by RNs (Gebbie & Lavin, 1975). There was no claim as to the validity of the diagnoses, nor was the list considered final. No classification system was selected.

Through the first six conferences, the listing of nursing diagnoses remained alphabetical, but attention was focusing on selecting a classification system. Involved with the classification from the outset, nursing theorists in 1977 were formally asked to participate in the development of the classification system.

As of 2014, NANDA-I has accepted 241 nursing diagnoses for clinical use and testing (Herdman & Kamitsuru). NANDA-I is reviewing and staging additional diagnoses (Herdman & Kamitsuru, 2012). Psychiatric nurses requested inclusion of their nursing diagnoses at the 11th biennial conference, and their labels were accepted for development (NANDA, 2009).

The complete NANDA-I Taxonomy II (Herdman & Kamitsuru, 2014) is presented in Appendix E. Taxonomy II was approved at the 14th biennial NANDA conference. It uses a multiaxial format to aid in adding new diagnoses or modifying existing ones.

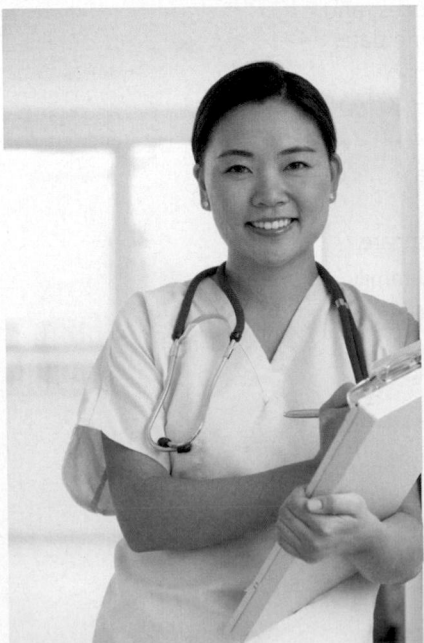

FIGURE 13-1 After collecting relevant data, the nurse identifies, validates, and formulates the nursing diagnosis. The patient's individualized nursing care is based on these nursing diagnoses.

New or revised nursing diagnoses may be submitted to NANDA-I for review and staging. To obtain new guidelines for submission and an abstract form, visit the NANDA-I website (www.nanda.org).

NURSING DIAGNOSES AND OTHER HEALTHCARE PROBLEMS

Nursing diagnoses must be distinguished from medical diagnoses. A **medical diagnosis** describes a disease or pathology of specific organs or body systems. Medical diagnoses convey information about the signs and symptoms of disease processes and provide a convenient means for communicating treatment requirements. The physician focuses on treating the underlying pathology.

In contrast, a nursing diagnosis describes an actual, risk, or wellness human response to a health problem that nurses are responsible for treating independently. Nursing diagnoses describe the patient's response to the disease process, developmental stage, or life process and provide a convenient way to communicate nursing therapies or interventions.

Nursing diagnoses carry legal ramifications. Only healthcare problems within the scope of nursing practice can be identified as nursing diagnoses. A nurse cannot diagnose a medical disease and is not licensed to independently treat such a problem. RNs must take care to identify patient problems within their scope, practice abilities, and education.

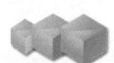 **Concept Mastery Alert**

Nurses must be careful to avoid confusing medical diagnoses with nursing diagnoses. Disease processes and their associated signs and symptoms are the essence of medical diagnoses. Nursing diagnoses are statements that describe the way that a patient responds to a health problem or life process.

When identifying problems from assessment data, nurses determine whether they can address such problems legally and independently. If so, the problems can receive nursing diagnoses. If such problems require both physician- and nurse-prescribed actions, however, they are **collaborative health problems**. Collaborative problems refer to actual or potential physiologic complications that can result from disease, trauma, treatment, or diagnostic studies for which nurses intervene in collaboration with personnel of other disciplines (Carpenito-Moyet, 2013). Table 13-1 compares nursing diagnoses with collaborative and medical diagnoses, and Figure 13-3 shows how a nurse makes these determinations. Procedures, medical terminology, symptoms, patient needs, and treatments are often confused with nursing diagnoses. For example, if the nurse writes "Foley catheter," this is a treatment, not the response the patient may have to the treatment. Other examples include "Need for oxygen" or "Dyspnea," terms that describe symptoms and do not provide enough information to validate a nursing diagnosis. Another common mistake is to write "Lack of adequate nutrition" as the nursing diagnosis. This phrase describes a patient need, but it is not a nursing diagnosis. The nursing diagnosis, in this case, would be Imbalanced Nutrition: Less Than Body Requirements.

The following list shows the proper use of various terms for a patient with a specific breathing problem. These terms are often confused:

- *Medical diagnosis*: Pneumonia
- *Nursing diagnosis*: Ineffective Airway Clearance related to thick tracheobronchial secretions
- *Patient need*: Oxygenation
- *Procedure*: Bronchoscopy
- *Treatment*: Oxygen therapy

Formulating an accurate nursing diagnosis is a clinical judgment, but nursing diagnoses should not be written judgmentally. For example, it is incorrect to write "Failure to carry out medical regimen related to drug use." The reasons for the patient's noncompliance with the regimen should be explored and analyzed to avoid labeling or stereotyping a patient's behavior based on insufficient evidence.

TABLE 13-1 COMPARISON OF NURSING DIAGNOSES WITH COLLABORATIVE PROBLEMS AND MEDICAL DIAGNOSES

	Nursing Diagnoses	Collaborative Problems and Medical Diagnoses
Focus of Assessment Activities	Main focus is on monitoring human responses to actual and potential health problems.	Main focus is on monitoring for pathophysiologic response of body organs or systems.
Problem Identification	Nurse identifies and validates independently that problem exists and can be treated legally by nursing staff.	Nurse may identify problem but is required to refer to physician for validation that problem exists (may require additional diagnostic studies to label problem). Nurse may not be qualified to diagnose exact nature of problem but refers abnormal data to physician.
Treatment	Nurse legally initiates actions for treatment.	Nurse collaborates with physician to initiate interventions for treatment. Nurse may have standing orders from physician or institution (delegated authority) to initiate diagnostic studies or treatment interventions for problem without physician's orders.

Source: Alfaro-LeFevre, R. (2014). *Applying nursing process: The foundation for clinical reasoning* (8th ed.). Philadelphia, PA: Wolters Kluwer/Lippincott Williams & Wilkins.

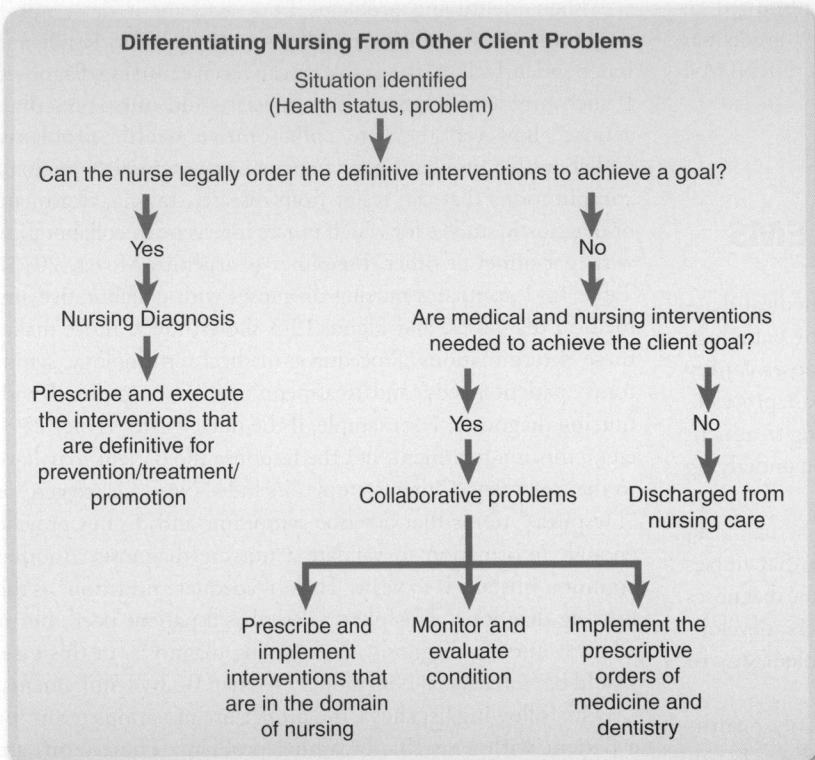

FIGURE 13-3 Differentiating a nursing diagnosis from other patient problems. (Adapted with permission from Carpenito, L. J. (2013). *Nursing diagnosis: Application to clinical practice* (14th ed.). Philadelphia, PA: Wolters Kluwer Health/Lippincott Williams & Wilkins.)

COMPONENTS OF A NURSING DIAGNOSIS

Diagnostic Label

The diagnostic label is the name of the nursing diagnosis as listed in the taxonomy. It describes the essence of the problem using as few words as possible. Some examples include Stress Urinary Incontinence, Anxiety, and Feeding Self-Care Deficit. Each nursing diagnosis represents a pattern of related patient cues.

Descriptors

Descriptors or modifiers are words used to give additional meaning to a nursing diagnosis. They describe changes in condition, state of the patient, or some qualification of the specific nursing diagnosis. They accompany the labels in Appendix E. Examples of descriptors used by NANDA-I (Herdman & Kamitsuru, 2014) include the following:

- *Compromised*: Made vulnerable to threat
- *Decreased*: Lessened; lesser in size, amount, or degree
- *Deficient/Deficit*: Inadequate in amount, quality, or degree; not sufficient; incomplete
- *Delayed*: Postponed, impeded, and retarded
- *Disproportionate*: Not consistent with a standard or norm
- *Disabled*: Limited; incapacitated; handicapped
- *Disorganized*: Not properly arranged or positioned
- *Disturbed*: Agitated or interrupted, interfered with

- *Dysfunctional*: Abnormal, incomplete functioning
- *Effective*: Producing the intended or expected effect
- *Excess*: Characterized by an amount or quantity that is greater than that necessary, desirable, or useful

Definition

Each nursing diagnosis that NANDA-I approves for clinical use and testing has a definition that describes the characteristics of the human response under consideration. For example, the definition of the diagnostic label of Hypothermia is "body temperature below normal diurnal range due to failure of thermoregulation" (Herdman & Kamitsuru, 2014, p. 428).

Defining Characteristics

Defining characteristics are the "observable cues/inferences that cluster as manifestations of a problem-focused, health promotion diagnosis or syndrome" (Herdman & Kamitsuru, 2014, p. 468). Each piece of patient information is considered a clinical cue; a set of clinical cues forms a cluster that is present if the diagnosis is accurate.

Related Factors

Related factors describe the conditions, circumstances, or etiologies that contribute to the problem. Although there is usually not a direct causal relationship between the nursing diagnosis and the related factors, some relationships can be described. Terms that can be used are *associated with*, *related to*, or *contributing to*. Identifying related factors helps nurses develop specific interventions to resolve the health problem. For example, nurses would use different nursing interventions when caring for a patient with Stress Incontinence related to high intra-abdominal pressure than for a patient with Stress Incontinence related to overdistention between voidings.

Risk Factors

The term *risk factor* is used to describe clinical cues in risk nursing diagnoses and is not used for actual nursing diagnoses. They are "environmental factors and physiological, psychological, genetic, or chemical elements that increase the vulnerability of an individual, family, or community to an unhealthful event" (Herdman & Kamitsuru, 2014, p. 468). Examples of risk factors for the nursing diagnosis Risk for Deficient Fluid Volume include extremes of age, physical immobility, and medication (e.g., diuretics). If the risk factors are not addressed, a potential problem may become an actual problem.

DIAGNOSIS ACTIVITIES

Identify Pattern

After completing the patient assessment, nurses analyze the data they obtained to identify specific patient problems. The data, both subjective symptoms and objective signs, form cues, or pieces of information collected during the nursing assessment. But not all data examined will be grouped to identify problems. Significant cues to be clustered involve subjective and objective data that deviate from standards or from what is considered normal. Several cues form a **cluster**, which is then interpreted and validated. The result is a nursing diagnostic label that accurately reflects the specific patient problem. Because clustering, interpreting, and validating patient cues are integral to nursing practice, each step is described separately. However, this process is cyclical—that is, as new information is obtained, new cue patterns may emerge and cue clusters may change. As nurses develop skill in making clinical judgments, they evaluate individual pieces of data for their clarity, relevance, and validity (Alfaro-LeFevre, 2014). This activity leads to clustering of diagnostic cues.

CUE CLUSTERING

As cues are collected, some data organization takes place. Typically, nurses use a standardized assessment form (see Chapter 17) that automatically puts information into categories or systems. Clustering goes beyond systems. Cue clustering brings together cues that, if viewed separately, would not convey the same meaning. The purpose of cue clustering is to take individual cues and group them to derive meaning.

Cue clustering can be compared with piecing together a puzzle. All of the puzzle pieces form one picture (the patient problem), and each piece is a cue. Figure 13-4 illustrates the

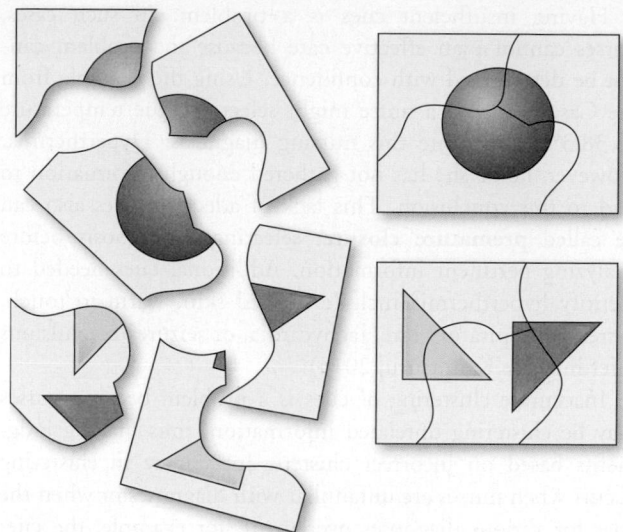

FIGURE 13-4 Collecting the puzzle pieces is assessment. Pieces that are similar form a cluster. Identifying the pattern and putting the puzzle together is nursing diagnosis. Other parts of the puzzle (e.g., a star) would form another diagnosis.

puzzle concept. The puzzle shows a circle and two triangles. All the pieces of the puzzle with the circle form a cluster, as do all the pieces for the triangles. Placing the circle pieces into a cluster helps identify the pattern of the puzzle (the diagnosis). A separate and distinct cue cluster forms each nursing diagnosis.

During cue clustering, critical thinking is used to analyze and synthesize the cues. Each cue is analyzed for its fit into a particular problem. The cues are then put together to form meaningful clusters that describe specific patient problems.

To see how this process works, refer to the patient in the scenario at the beginning of the chapter. Review the situation of the former carpenter and then see which cues belong together when describing a particular problem.

Although the first tendency is to identify Hyperthermia as a nursing diagnosis, look at other cues the patient has given. For the purpose of illustration, one nursing diagnosis has been selected here. The relevant cues follow:

- Not currently working
- Recent change from active, mobile individual to wheelchair-dependent, quadriplegic person
- Considers self to be provider
- Angry at wife for carrying out role of breadwinner

Taken together, these cues fit the defining characteristics of a specific nursing diagnosis. Recognizing this cue cluster leads to the next step—cluster interpretation. First, however, some problems that can occur in cue clustering must be described.

Problems in Cue Clustering

The major problems in cue clustering are insufficient, inaccurate, and inconsistent cues. Skill in cue clustering comes with experience and practice. Expect to use various reference materials to develop these skills.

Having insufficient cues is a problem. In such cases, nurses cannot plan effective care because the problem cannot be determined with confidence. Using the example from the Case Scenario, a nurse might select the cue temperature of 38.3°C and write this nursing diagnosis: Hyperthermia. However, he or she has not gathered enough information to lead to this conclusion. This lack of adequate cues also can be called **premature closure**: selecting a diagnosis before analyzing pertinent information. Additional cues needed to identify hyperthermia include flushed skin, warm to touch, increased respiratory rate, tachycardia, or seizures/convulsions (Herdman & Kamitsuru, 2014).

Inaccurate clustering of cues is a problem because nurses may be clustering unrelated information, thus making judgments based on incorrect clusters. Inaccuracy in clustering occurs when nurses are unfamiliar with diagnoses or when the cues for various diagnoses overlap. If, for example, the cues (wheelchair-dependent quadriplegic, not working, and anger) are clustered and the nursing diagnosis of Impaired Physical Mobility related to dependency is made, nursing interventions will be geared toward resolving the impaired mobility, which is not possible. It does not focus on properly identifying the anger and dependency, which are important concerns for the patient.

Inconsistent cues are a problem because the meaning attached to one cue may be altered based on another cue. For example, one patient may say that she cannot eat a regular diet, but later, she is seen eating a steak and potatoes. Because the cues do not match, further information is needed to validate the problem and the cues.

CLUSTER INTERPRETATION

Cluster interpretation means synthesizing the cue clusters. This intellectual activity requires nurses to see the whole picture and to attach meaning to the cluster, looking at the pattern the cluster suggests. It is the ability to derive the meaning and implications of the human response for a patient.

A specific cue cluster was presented in the opening scenario. Review it now, and think of possible nursing diagnoses. The following nursing diagnoses are listed as possible choices:

- Ineffective Coping related to dependency. *Cues*: anger, wheelchair-dependent quadriplegic.
- Impaired Adjustment related to disability requiring change in lifestyle. *Cues*: wheelchair-dependent quadriplegic for 6 months, not working.
- Ineffective Role Performance related to recent change. *Cues*: not working; angry at wife for carrying out breadwinner role; perceives self as provider; recent change from active, mobile person to wheelchair-dependent quadriplegic.

Analyzing these suggested nursing diagnostic statements would involve reviewing each definition and associated defining characteristics.

The first two possible nursing diagnoses cannot be supported by clinical cues. Ineffective Coping relies on two cues that are not defining characteristics of this diagnosis. This diagnosis requires evidence of a patient's verbalization of the inability to cope or to ask for help or the inability to solve problems. More information is needed to support the use of this diagnosis. The second diagnosis, Impaired Adjustment, may or may not describe this patient. The nurse has assumed that by becoming a wheelchair-dependent quadriplegic, this patient has not made a satisfactory adjustment to his new lifestyle. Additional defining characteristics are needed to evaluate this problem.

In the third diagnosis, Ineffective Role Performance, all the cues supporting the defining characteristics for the diagnosis are present. The patient had a change in the perception of his role, in his physical capacity to resume a previous role, and in his usual patterns of responsibility. There is evidence of conflict, as shown by his anger toward his wife. The nurse can make this diagnosis with confidence and plan nursing interventions to assist the patient in resolving this problem.

Problems in Cluster Interpretation

Analysis of cue clusters can be impeded by incorrect clustering of data and misinterpretation of cue clusters. If the cues are not clustered correctly, nurses cannot make accurate clinical judgments. For example, if the cues (malnourished, feeds self, and dependent in mobility) are clustered, the nurse may arrive at the erroneous diagnosis of Feeding Self-Care Deficit related to inadequate intake. However, there is no information here about the daily intake of food. The fact that the patient feeds himself does not explain the cue of dependent in mobility. Does the patient use assistive devices? What is the state of malnourishment? Are supplemental feedings being given? By forming this particular cue cluster, the nurse has neglected other important areas for analysis. In this example, these include defining characteristics for the nursing diagnoses of Imbalanced Nutrition: Less Than Body Requirements and Impaired Physical Mobility.

Misinterpretation of cue clusters occurs when the nurse fails to recognize the correct pattern. This can happen if the nurse is unfamiliar with the nursing diagnosis or is inexperienced in relating how these particular cues fit together. If the defining characteristics for the diagnosis under consideration are complex and require extensive analysis for correct interpretation, ask an experienced clinician to assist with interpreting the cues.

Validate Diagnosis

After selecting a nursing diagnosis (Ineffective Role Performance, in the clinical example), the nurse should validate it with the patient. **Validation** legitimizes the diagnosis and helps to discover its significance for the patient. The patient may deny that a problem exists, may not want to deal with it, or may acknowledge it but want to deal with it later. These are acceptable reasons for not dealing with an identified diagnosis,

TABLE 13-2 TYPES OF DIAGNOSTIC STATEMENTS

Type	Construction	Example
Actual nursing diagnosis	Three-part statement includes diagnostic label, related factors, and defining characteristics.	Acute Pain related to surgical trauma and inflammations evidenced by grimacing and verbal reports of pain
Risk nursing diagnosis	Two-part statement includes diagnostic label and risk factors.	Risk for Infection related to surgery and immunosuppression
Possible nursing diagnosis	Two-part statement includes diagnostic label and related factors (unknown).	Possible Self-Esteem Disturbance related to unknown etiology
Health Promotion Diagnosis	One-part statement includes diagnostic label.	Readiness for Enhanced family processes

but the problem and its status should be documented. For most problems, the patient will agree that there is a problem that can be resolved with nursing assistance.

Diagnostic validation occurs in two stages. In the first stage, the cue clusters that have been interpreted are compared with norms for the patient and for patients in general. In the second stage, the specific nursing diagnosis is evaluated for its nursing research base. This research base is different for each diagnosis.

In the clinical example, these diagnoses may be made if additional data collection identifies cues to support them:

- Ineffective Coping
- Impaired Adjustment
- Hyperthermia

For each diagnosis, the nurse should discuss with the patient the significance of the problem, determine the patient's perception of the reason for the problem, and ask whether the patient desires help to resolve or diminish the problem. Some patients are not ready or motivated to seek help even when a problem clearly exists.

PROBLEMS IN DIAGNOSTIC VALIDATION

Problems can occur in diagnostic validation because of a nurse's limited experience, lack of a knowledge base about the nursing diagnosis, or insufficient characteristics of a diagnosis.

If the nurse has limited clinical experience, exposure to various patients under the guidance of an instructor, mentor, or expert practitioner can provide an opportunity to practice these skills. Each nursing diagnosis and defining characteristic should be discussed and errors corrected. A nonthreatening environment, patience, and understanding are required for both parties. It is helpful to trace the steps taken to arrive at a particular problem; errors in logic or missing steps in the process can sometimes be identified and suggestions made for avoiding them.

Formulate the Diagnostic Statement

Formulating the nursing diagnostic statement involves writing the label of the actual, risk, wellness, or **possible nursing diagnosis** that has been made through the nursing diagnostic process. The correct way of stating these diagnoses is described

in the following section and illustrated in Table 13-2 and Figure 13-5. Accurate and inaccurate examples also are given in the text and in Table 13-3.

ACTUAL NURSING DIAGNOSES

An **actual nursing diagnosis** describes a human response to a health problem that is being manifested. It is written as a three-part statement: diagnostic label, defining characteristics, and related factors. Patient cues supporting the existence of the problem can be found in the documented assessment data. In the nursing diagnosis statement, cues are identified by "as manifested by" or "as evidenced by." Problems sometimes occur when nurses invert the label and the "related to" phrase. To avoid this problem, determine the main focus of the problem (the diagnostic label) and the factor that is contributing to the patient's inability to resolve it (related factor).

Accurate: Impaired Physical Mobility related to pain

Inaccurate: Ineffective Movement related to arthritis, which causes pain when moving. (The nurse has selected an incorrect descriptor, has not used an approved diagnostic label, has repeated the problem in the "related to" phrase, and has used a medical diagnosis in the statement.)

RISK NURSING DIAGNOSES

NANDA-I replaced the term *potential* with the term *risk* because it was believed that the latter term is more descriptive of some patients' particular vulnerability to health problems. For example, all patients admitted to a hospital are at risk for infection, but some people, such as those with compromised immune systems, are at higher risk than others. This terminology also could assist in third-party reimbursement for nursing care and is the term used in the ICD-10 list of nursing diagnoses. A **risk nursing diagnosis**, as defined by NANDA-I (Herdman & Kamitsuru, 2014), a clinical judgment concerning the vulnerability of an individual, family, group, or community for developing an undesirable human response to health conditions/life processes" (p. 464). Problems in identifying risk nursing diagnoses include lack of knowledge of a patient's risk factor profile and the particular risks involved in care and treatment for the underlying health problem. Risk nursing diagnoses are two-part statements because they do not include defining characteristics.

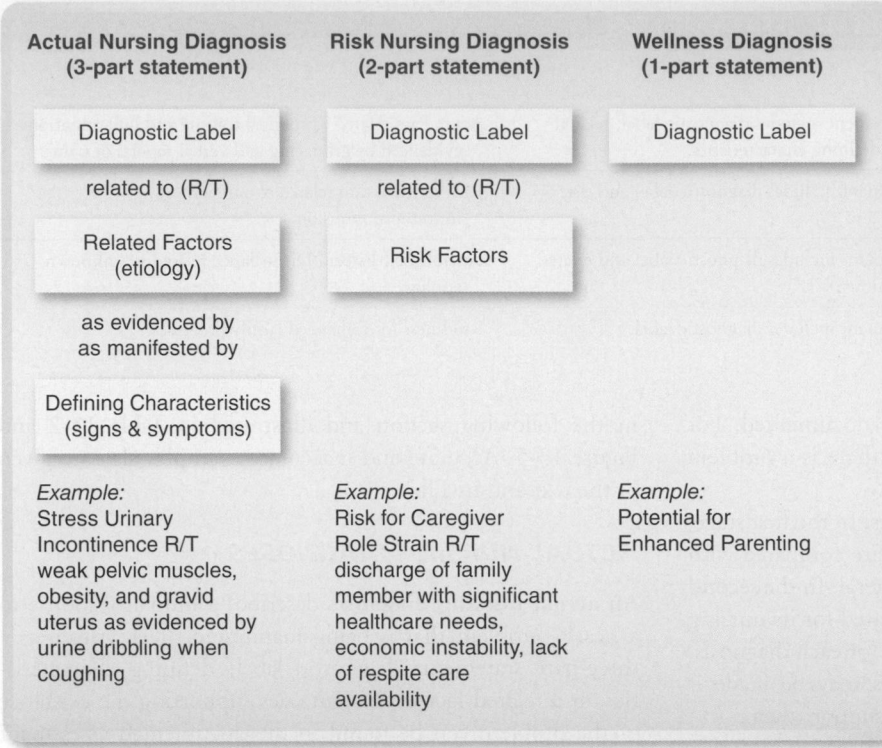

Actual Nursing Diagnosis
(3-part statement)

Diagnostic Label

related to (R/T)

Related Factors
(etiology)

as evidenced by
as manifested by

Defining Characteristics
(signs & symptoms)

Example:
Stress Urinary
Incontinence R/T
weak pelvic muscles,
obesity, and gravid
uterus as evidenced by
urine dribbling when
coughing

Risk Nursing Diagnosis
(2-part statement)

Diagnostic Label

related to (R/T)

Risk Factors

Example:
Risk for Caregiver
Role Strain R/T
discharge of family
member with significant
healthcare needs,
economic instability, lack
of respite care
availability

Wellness Diagnosis
(1-part statement)

Diagnostic Label

Example:
Potential for
Enhanced Parenting

FIGURE 13-5 Examples of a three-part actual nursing diagnostic statement, a two-part risk nursing diagnostic statement, and a one-part wellness nursing diagnostic statement.

Accurate: Risk for Aspiration related to reduced level of consciousness

Inaccurate: Risk for Secretions entering the airway from impaired swallowing. (The nurse has listed part of the definition and one of the at-risk factors in the label.)

HEALTH PROMOTION DIAGNOSES

A health promotion diagnosis is a diagnostic statement that is a "clinical judgment concerning motivation and desire to increase well-being and to actualize human health potential" (Herdman & Kamitsuru, 2014, p. 22).

TABLE 13-3 EXAMPLES OF ACCURATE VERSUS INACCURATE STATEMENT OF NURSING DIAGNOSES

Type	Accurate Statement	Rationale	Inaccurate Statement	Rationale
Actual nursing diagnosis	Constipation related to decreased activity and fluids as manifested by small, hard, formed stool every 4 days	Properly stated using three-part statement, including diagnostic label (constipation), related factors (decreased activity), and defining characteristics (small, hard, formed stool every 4 days)	Altered Bowel Function related to production of hard stool	Incorrect diagnostic label; altered bowel function is nonspecific and not accepted by NANDA-I. Only a two-part statement; related factors are omitted, and defining characteristics (hard stool) are substituted.
Risk nursing diagnosis	Risk for Activity Intolerance related to prolonged bed rest	"Risk" is used rather than "potential." Risk diagnoses use risk factors. Defining characteristics should not be included.	Activity Intolerance, Potential	"Potential" is used rather than "risk." Diagnostic label is reversed. No risk factors are provided.
Possible nursing diagnosis	Possible Impaired Adjustment related to unknown etiology	Unknown etiology used until more data can be collected to validate diagnosis.	Adjustment impaired, possibly due to recent car accident that resulted in quadriplegia	Diagnostic label is reversed, and cues are included in "related to" without validation.
Health promotion nursing diagnosis	Readiness for Enhanced Family Coping	Health promotion diagnoses are one-part statements without risk factors or defining characteristics.	Family coping potential due to desire for better health	Diagnostic statement is reversed, and more information than just the diagnostic label is provided.

APPLY YOUR CRITICAL THINKING

You are the nursing student assigned to care for Mr. Mason, the patient in the opening scenario. You have reviewed Mr. Mason's record and met him briefly yesterday. One of the nursing diagnoses on Mr. Mason's plan of care is Ineffective Role Performance R/T new wheelchair-bound status and inability to work after accident AEB anger at wife for paying the bills and caring for the children. You are comfortable dealing with nursing diagnoses such as constipation or impaired physical mobility but do not feel comfortable with this nursing diagnosis. You think that Mr. Mason may become defensive and not welcome any interventions. How can you be sure this is a valid concern for Mr. Mason?

Check your answer in Appendix B.

NURSING PRACTICE AND NURSING DIAGNOSES

Applying Nursing Diagnosis in the Clinical Setting

This chapter has provided information regarding the process of identifying a nursing diagnosis from assessment data. It is a complex skill and requires practice to become proficient. To help you develop your skill, refer back to the Case Scenario and answer the questions posed. Box 13-1 illustrates how the entire process fits together.

Significance of Nursing Diagnosis

Nursing diagnoses provide a means of communicating nursing requirements for patient care to other nurses, the healthcare

---

BOX 13-1   Putting It All Together—Applying Nursing Diagnosis in the Clinical Setting

1. Collect assessment data

Mr. Ellis, a 69-year-old retired carpenter with a 10-year history of chronic obstructive pulmonary disease, is admitted to your medical floor with pneumonia.

He states he hasn't been feeling well for 3 days, complaining of increasing dyspnea, fatigue, and a cough with moderate tan sputum production. He reports he hasn't slept in 2 nights and is mostly eating soup but has little appetite. His wife died 6 months ago, and in addition to having no appetite, his cooking skills are limited. He was brought in by ambulance because his three children live out of town. He is irritable and states, "Why are you asking me all these stupid questions when I feel so sick?" Your physical assessment reveals the following: blood pressure 164/90, pulse 104, respirations 26 (using accessory muscles), temperature 38.3°C, oxygen saturation 86%, lung sounds diminished with crackles bilaterally and expiratory wheezing. You defer any extensive questioning because he is very short of breath as he attempts to answer your questions and is growing more agitated. Oxygen is ordered and administered at 2 L/min via cannula, a nebulizer treatment with albuterol is given, and intravenous antibiotics are started.

2. Cluster the data

- *Health perception–health management:* 10-year history of COPD and feeling ill for last 3 days
- *Nutrition–metabolic:* Febrile, temperature 38.3°C, no appetite, eating soup, limited cooking skills
- *Activity–exercise:* Respiration tachypneic at 26 with increased work of breathing as he is using accessory muscles; oxygen saturation is decreased; supplemental oxygen and nebulizer treatments are given; dyspnea is significant even when sitting and talking; lung sounds indicate airway constriction (wheezing) and diminished gas exchanges (crackles); fatigue is present; blood pressure elevated at 164/90 and pulse tachycardic at 104
- *Elimination:* No data available
- *Cognitive–perceptual:* Alert but irritable and restless

- *Coping–stress:* Lost wife 6 months ago, children live out of town, came into hospital unaccompanied in an ambulance

3. Identify possible nursing diagnoses

Possible nursing diagnoses for Mr. Ellis include the following: Imbalanced Nutrition: Less Than Body Requirements, Impaired Gas Exchange, Ineffective Airway Clearance, Ineffective Health Maintenance, Complicated Grieving, Readiness for Enhanced Self-Care, and Activity Intolerance. Note that pneumonia is not included because it is a medical diagnosis or collaborative problem.

4. Validate selected diagnoses

Validate with Mr. Ellis or with the NANDA-I taxonomy whether the data are sufficient to confirm each possible diagnosis. Look at defining characteristics for each diagnosis to see if the selected nursing diagnosis is supported. At times, more data need to be collected to validate a specific nursing diagnosis. For Mr. Ellis, enough data exist to confirm Impaired Gas Exchange (low oxygen saturation, high respiratory rate, and abnormal breath sounds) and Imbalanced Nutrition: Less Than Body Requirements (caloric intake has been poor and his metabolic requirements have increased because of the infection). More data need to be collected to validate the other possible nursing diagnoses. When Mr. Ellis's respiratory condition stabilizes, you can interview him and collect the additional needed information.

5. Add correct nursing diagnosis statements to plan of care

- Impaired Gas Exchange *related to* lung infection, obstructive lung condition *as evidenced by* dyspnea, oxygen saturation of 86%, respiratory rate of 26, wheezes, crackles, and use of accessory muscles
- Imbalanced Nutrition: Less than Body Requirements *related to* anorexia, increased metabolic requirements *as evidenced by* limited food intake for 3 days

6. Discuss plan with patient/family

team, and the public. Nursing continues to change rapidly around the world, and our concepts, language, and terms must provide the communication tools needed. Nursing diagnostic labels can serve as shorthand for specific patient problems.

Although many nursing diagnoses need further research to be clinically useful, all have suggested lists of defining characteristics or risk factors that validate the existence of the problem. Making accurate nursing diagnoses helps to ensure that patients receive quality nursing care.

By focusing attention on the actual or potential health needs of patients, nursing diagnoses increase the specificity of nursing interventions for each patient. This specificity can be measured and monitored to make sure that effective interventions are acknowledged for their contribution to resolving healthcare problems. Coding of nursing diagnoses in computerized systems allows direct reimbursement for nurses. Acknowledging nursing's specific contribution in resolving health problems advances professional nursing practice.

Studies of specific nursing diagnoses improve understanding of the nursing diagnostic process and contribute to examination of the nurse's role in healthcare. As research supports nursing diagnoses, a clear description of the scope of nursing practice will emerge. The development and publication of a taxonomy of nursing diagnoses should significantly affect practice, education, research, legislation, and nursing as a profession. A nursing diagnosis taxonomy will help to bridge the gap between knowledge and practice and will articulate the scope of nursing practice, which is essential to developing nursing's professional role in healthcare.

Each nurse will decide the usefulness of the nursing diagnosis taxonomy. As the profession develops, the taxonomy will be critically reviewed, revised, and tested. For today's practitioner, the taxonomy meets the need for organization of nursing diagnoses.

The limitations of NANDA-I Taxonomy II do not mean that it cannot or should not be used in clinical practice. Nursing process and nursing diagnosis taxonomy continue to evolve with the addition of new nursing diagnoses and revisions of existing diagnoses. All nurses have the opportunity and responsibility to use the taxonomy in practice. The challenge for each practitioner is to learn the concepts and skills required to assist patients by accurately diagnosing, planning, and implementing nursing care.

Functional Approach to Nursing Diagnosis

Gordon (2008, 2010) has suggested a framework for organizing nursing diagnoses based on functional health, thus offering a convenient way to cluster similar diagnoses. Because this book focuses on function, and data collected during assessment are discussed and organized in this fashion, it is useful to organize nursing diagnoses in the same manner. The complete list of nursing diagnoses organized by function is shown in Box 13-2.

Reviewing function and nursing diagnoses for each pattern ensures that nurses have considered all actual, possible, or risk nursing diagnoses, therefore ensuring that physiologic problems do not overshadow the patient's emotional, social, or spiritual needs.

BOX 13-2   **Nursing Diagnoses Organized by Functional Health Patterns**

Health Perception–Health Management
Deficient Community Health
Risk-Prone Health Behavior
Ineffective Health Maintenance
Ineffective Health Management
Readiness for Enhanced Health Management
Ineffective Therapeutic Regimen Management
Risk for Ineffective Therapeutic Regimen Management
Ineffective Family Health Management
Noncompliance
Contamination
Risk for Contamination
Readiness for Enhanced Immunization Status
Risk for Dry Eye
Risk for Injury
Risk for Thermal Injury
Risk for Vascular Trauma
Risk for Bleeding
Risk for Falls
Risk for Perioperative Positioning Injury
Risk for Poisoning
Risk for Suffocation
Ineffective Protection

Activity–Exercise
Activity Intolerance
Risk for Activity Intolerance
Sedentary Lifestyle
Fatigue
Deficient Diversional Activity
Impaired Physical Mobility
Impaired Bed Mobility
Impaired Transfer Ability
Impaired Wheelchair Mobility
Impaired Walking
Wandering
Risk for Disuse Syndrome
Self-Neglect
Bathing–Hygiene Self-Care Deficit
Dressing–Grooming Self-Care Deficit
Feeding Self-Care Deficit
Toileting Self-Care Deficit
Readiness for Enhanced Self-Care
Delayed Surgical Recovery
Risk for Delayed Development
Risk for Disproportionate Growth
Impaired Home Maintenance

Activity–Exercise (Continued)

Dysfunctional Ventilatory Weaning Response
Impaired Spontaneous Ventilation
Ineffective Airway Clearance
Ineffective Breathing Pattern
Impaired Gas Exchange
Decreased Cardiac Output
Risk for Shock
Ineffective Peripheral Tissue Perfusion
Risk for Ineffective Peripheral Tissue Perfusion
Risk for Decreased Cardiac Tissue Perfusion
Risk for Ineffective Gastrointestinal Perfusion
Ineffective Renal Perfusion
Risk for Ineffective Cerebral Tissue Perfusion
Autonomic Dysreflexia
Risk for Autonomic Dysreflexia
Risk for Sudden Infant Death Syndrome
Disorganized Infant Behavior
Risk for Disorganized Infant Behavior
Readiness for Enhanced Organized Infant Behavior
Risk for Peripheral Neurovascular Dysfunction
Decreased Intracranial Adaptive Capacity

Nutritional–Metabolic

Overweight Obesity
Risk for Overweight
Imbalanced Nutrition: Less Than Body Requirements
Readiness for Enhanced Nutrition
Frail Elderly Syndrome
Ineffective Breast-Feeding
Interrupted Breast-Feeding
Readiness for Enhanced Breast-Feeding
Ineffective Infant Feeding Pattern
Insufficient Breast Milk
Neonatal Jaundice
Risk for Neonatal Jaundice
Impaired Swallowing
Nausea
Risk for Aspiration
Impaired Oral Mucous Membrane
Impaired Dentition
Deficient Fluid Volume
Risk for Deficient Fluid Volume
Excess Fluid Volume
Risk for Imbalanced Fluid Volume
Readiness for Enhanced Fluid Balance
Risk for Electrolyte Imbalance
Impaired Skin Integrity
Risk for Impaired Skin Integrity
Impaired Tissue Integrity
Risk for Allergy Response
Latex Allergy Response
Risk for Latex Allergy Response
Ineffective Thermoregulation
Hyperthermia
Hypothermia
Risk for Imbalanced Body Temperature
Risk for Impaired Liver Function
Risk for Unstable Blood Glucose Level

Elimination

Bowel Incontinence
Constipation
Perceived Constipation
Risk for Constipation
Diarrhea
Dysfunctional Gastrointestinal Motility
Risk for Dysfunctional Gastrointestinal Motility
Functional Urinary Incontinence
Overflow Urinary Incontinence
Reflex Urinary Incontinence
Stress Urinary Incontinence
Urge Urinary Incontinence
Risk for Urge Urinary Incontinence
Impaired Urinary Elimination
Readiness for Enhanced Urinary Elimination
Urinary Retention

Sleep–Rest

Insomnia
Sleep Deprivation
Disturbed Sleep Pattern
Readiness for Enhanced Sleep

Cognitive–Perceptual

Acute Pain
Chronic Pain
Impaired Comfort
Readiness for Enhanced Comfort
Unilateral Neglect
Deficient Knowledge
Readiness for Enhanced Knowledge
Ineffective Activity Planning
Acute Confusion
Risk for Acute Confusion
Chronic Confusion
Ineffective Impulse Control
Impaired Environmental Interpretation Syndrome
Impaired Memory
Readiness for Enhanced Decision Making
Decisional Conflict

Self-Perception

Anxiety
Death Anxiety
Fear
Risk for Loneliness
Hopelessness
Readiness for Enhanced Hope
Powerlessness
Risk for Powerlessness
Readiness for Enhanced Power
Risk for Compromised Human Dignity
Situational Low Self-Esteem
Risk for Situational Low Self-Esteem
Chronic Low Self-Esteem
Risk for Chronic Low Self-Esteem
Readiness for Enhanced Self-Concept
Disturbed Body Image

Continued

BOX 13-2 Nursing Diagnoses Organized by Functional Health Patterns *(Continued)*

Self-Perception *(Continued)*
Disturbed Personal Identity
Risk for Disturbed Personal Identity
Risk for Self-Directed Violence

Role–Relationship
Grieving
Complicated Grieving
Risk for Complicated Grieving
Chronic Sorrow
Ineffective Role Performance
Social Isolation
Impaired Social Interaction
Relocation Stress Syndrome
Risk for Relocation Stress Syndrome
Ineffective Relationship
Readiness for Enhanced Relationship
Risk for Ineffective Relationship
Interrupted Family Processes
Dysfunctional Family Processes
Readiness for Enhanced Family Processes
Impaired Parenting
Risk for Impaired Parenting
Parental Role Conflict
Risk for Impaired Attachment
Readiness for Enhanced Parenting
Caregiver Role Strain
Risk for Caregiver Role Strain
Impaired Verbal Communication
Readiness for Enhanced Communication
Risk for Other-Directed Violence

Coping–Stress Tolerance
Ineffective Activity Planning
Ineffective Coping
Readiness for Enhanced Coping

Defensive Coping
Ineffective Denial
Impaired Resilience
Risk for Impaired Resilience
Risk for Compromised Resilience
Readiness for Enhanced Resilience
Compromised Family Coping
Disabled Family Coping
Readiness for Enhanced Family Coping
Ineffective Community Coping
Readiness for Enhanced Community Coping
Post-Trauma Syndrome
Risk for Post-Trauma Syndrome
Risk for Suicide
Stress Overload
Self-Mutilation
Risk for Self-Mutilation

Sexuality–Reproductive
Ineffective Sexuality Patterns
Sexual Dysfunction
Rape Trauma Syndrome
Ineffective Childbearing Process
Readiness for Enhanced Childbearing Process Risk for
    Ineffective Childbearing Process
Risk for Disturbed Maternal–Fetal Dyad

Value–Belief
Moral Distress
Spiritual Distress
Risk for Spiritual Distress
Readiness for Enhanced Spiritual Well-Being
Impaired Religiosity
Risk for Impaired Religiosity
Readiness for Enhanced Religiosity

KEY CONCEPTS

- Collection of assessment data provides the basis for identifying nursing diagnoses.
- RNs are educated and licensed to make nursing diagnoses.
- A nursing diagnosis is a clinical judgment about individual, family, or community responses to actual or potential health problems and life processes.
- Activities of nursing diagnoses include pattern identification, diagnostic validation, and formulation of the nursing diagnosis statement.
- NANDA-I–accepted nursing diagnoses are organized using Taxonomy II, which has three levels: domains, classes, and nursing diagnoses.
- A nursing diagnosis must address a problem within the scope and education of RNs, and RNs must be able to intervene legally and independent of physician-prescribed actions.

- The nurse is responsible and accountable to identify and treat collaborative problems, which focus on pathophysiologic responses, in cooperation with the physician.
- A nursing diagnosis consists of the diagnostic label, definition, defining characteristics, risk factors, related factors, and descriptors.
- A cue is a piece of information (subjective or objective) collected during the nursing assessment.
- Cluster interpretation involves synthesis of the cue clusters. It is an intellectual activity requiring the ability to see the whole picture, attach meaning to the cluster, and discern the pattern the cluster suggests.
- Diagnostic validation occurs in two stages: comparing the clusters with norms and evaluating the specific nursing diagnosis for its particular nursing research base.
- Formulating the nursing diagnostic statement involves writing the actual, risk, wellness, or possible nursing diagnoses.

PRACTICING FOR THE NCLEX

CHECK YOUR ANSWER IN APPENDIX A.

1. Which of the following are true related to nursing diagnoses? Select all that apply:
   a. Describes a disease or pathology of body systems
   b. Describes human response to a health problem
   c. Actual or potential physiologic complications related to disease or treatment
   d. Include descriptors and risk factors
   e. Relates contributing factors or relationships to identified health problem
   f. There are not associated legal ramifications

2. The nurse is developing nursing diagnoses for a patient with chronic pain related to bone cancer. Which of the following would be most correct?
   a. Constipation related to impaired mobility as evidenced by daily, soft bowel movements
   b. Activity Intolerance related to chronic pain as evidenced by patient stating pain 10/10 with movement
   c. Effective Management of Therapeutic Regimen as evidenced by normal cell counts
   d. Ineffective Coping related to terminal cancer diagnosis

3. A patient is admitted with renal failure and oliguria. Which should be done first in formulating a nursing diagnosis?
   a. Synthesize data including urine output, color of urine, and potassium levels.
   b. Compare data with physiologic norms and norms for this patient.
   c. Assign diagnosis of Impaired Urinary Elimination.
   d. Validate diagnosis using research of the health problem and management.

4. A nurse is formulating a nursing diagnosis for a hospitalized patient with acute mental status changes and urinary tract infection (UTI). Which nursing diagnoses are appropriate? Select all that apply:
   a. Total Incontinence related to UTI as evidenced by patient's spontaneous urination and inability to recognize urge
   b. Acute Confusion related to UTI as evidenced by patient's statement that she is at home
   c. Situational Low Self-Esteem related to incontinence as evidenced by patient crying
   d. Ineffective Health Maintenance related to acute mental status changes as evidenced by UTI

5. Which of the following statements is an accurate nursing diagnosis?
   a. Poor Parenting Abilities related to lack of sleep
   b. Disturbed Body Image, Possibly related to recent childbirth
   c. Risk for Ineffective Breastfeeding related to poor infant latch
   d. Sleep Deprivation, Potential related to frequent infant feeding schedule

REFERENCES

Alfaro-LeFevre, R. (2014). *Applying nursing process: The foundation for clinical reasoning a tool for critical thinking* (8th ed.). Philadelphia, PA: Wolters Kluwer Health/Lippincott Williams & Wilkins.

Carpenito-Moyet, L. J. (2013). *Nursing diagnosis: Application to clinical practice* (14th ed.). Philadelphia, PA: Wolters Kluwer Health/Lippincott Williams & Wilkins.

Gebbie, K., & Lavin, M. (1975). *Classification of nursing diagnoses: Proceedings from the first national conference.* St. Louis, MO: C. V. Mosby.

Gordon, M. (2008). *Assess notes: Nursing assessment and diagnostic reasoning.* Philadelphia, PA: F. A. Davis.

Gordon, M. (2010). *Manual of nursing diagnosis* (12th ed.). Sudbury, MA: Jones & Bartlett.

Herdman, T. H. (Ed.) (2012). *NANDA International Nursing Diagnoses: Definitions and classification 2012–2014.* West Sussex, UK: Wiley-Blackwell.

Herdman, T. H & Kamitsuru, S. (Ed.) (2014). *NANDA International. Nursing diagnoses: Definitions and classifications 2015–2017.* West Sussex, UK: Wiley-Blackwell.

North American Nursing Diagnosis Association International. (2009). *Nursing diagnoses: Definitions and classification, 2009–2011.* West Sussex, England: Wiley-Blackwell.

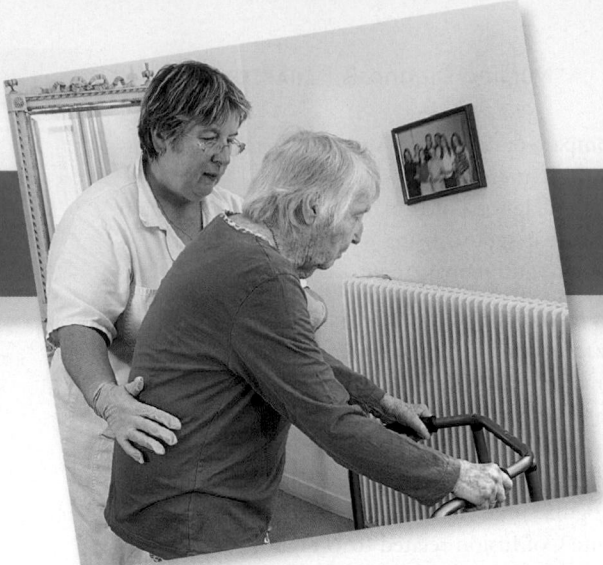

CHAPTER 14

Outcome Identification and Planning

Kathryn Van Dyke Hayes

Case Scenario

You are working as a nurse in a skilled nursing facility. You admit a patient from the community hospital who had a total hip replacement 1 week ago. Your admission assessment reveals the following:

- Patient states: "They sent me here until I could walk better because my daughter isn't willing to take me like this! I can't even get up to go to the bathroom by myself."
- Medical history includes arthritis controlled with nonsteroidal anti-inflammatory drugs (NSAIDs) and irregular heart rhythm controlled with digoxin (Lanoxin); vital signs stable, incision healing well; fair appetite, no swallowing difficulties; hard, painful BM every 2 or 3 days (often needs laxative); physical therapy twice a day to work on ambulating with a walker and increasing muscle strength and endurance.

From these data, you identify the following nursing diagnoses:

- Impaired physical mobility related to inability to ambulate or transfer independently and decreased muscle strength and endurance
- Constipation related to decreased physical mobility and inability to perform toileting tasks

Once you have completed this chapter and have incorporated outcome identification and planning into your knowledge base, review the above scenario and reflect on the following areas of Critical Thinking:

1. Analyze how you would prioritize the nursing diagnoses for this patient, and suggest additional information you may need to collect.

2. State possible outcomes for each diagnosis that should be met before the patient's discharge to the home.

3. Construct possible methods to work with the patient to individualize the plan of care and develop realistic outcomes.

4. Develop a hypothetical written plan of care for one of the above nursing diagnoses, indicating what additional information is needed.

KEY TERMS

concept map
evaluation
goal
nursing interventions
Nursing Interventions Classification (NIC)
Nursing Outcome Classification (NOC)
outcome
outcome criteria
outcome identification
planning
priority
qualifier
scientific rationale
variances

Upon completion of this chapter, you will be able to do the following:

1. Define outcome identification and planning.
2. Explain the purposes of outcome identification and planning.
3. Discuss the Nursing Outcome Classification and the Nursing Interventions Classification projects.
4. Describe the components of the patient plan of care.
5. Formulate a patient plan of care for a patient given a nursing assessment database.

After collecting and analyzing assessment data and identifying and validating nursing diagnoses, nurses are ready to begin planning care with patients. Nursing is a practice discipline involving application of theoretical knowledge to actual patient situations. Nurses and patients set realistic goals in what the nursing process calls outcome identification. A plan specifies interventions to meet patient goals.

OUTCOME IDENTIFICATION

Outcome identification is the formulation of goals and measurable outcomes that provide the basis for evaluating nursing diagnoses. Outcome identification is the most recent addition to the nursing process, as described in the current American Nurses Association (ANA, 2014) *Nursing: Scope and Standards of Practice* (2nd ed.). The ANA describes seven measurement criteria for outcome identification, which include specifying intermediate and long-term outcomes that focus on health promotion, health maintenance, or health restoration.

Outcome identification serves the following purposes:

- Providing individualized care
- Promoting patient participation
- Planning care that is realistic and measurable
- Allowing for involvement of support people

The following are activities performed in this phase:

- Establish priorities.
- Establish patient goals and outcome criteria.

Outcome identification in relation to other phases of the nursing process is shown in Figure 14-1.

Nursing-Sensitive Patient Outcomes

Nurses must demonstrate to the public how they achieve patient outcomes. To meet this need, a research team at the University of Iowa College of Nursing has been conducting nursing-sensitive patient outcomes research (Moorhead, Johnson, Maas, & Swanson, 2013). The research is aimed at identifying, validating, and classifying nursing-sensitive patient outcomes and indicators, field testing the outcomes, and testing measurement procedures for the outcomes and indicators.

Nursing Outcome Classification

The nursing-sensitive outcomes classification system is organized according to categories, classes, labels, outcome indicators, and measurement activities for outcomes. In electronic health records, **Nursing Outcome Classification (NOC)** can be used in standardized care plans and critical pathways to set expected goals and compare individual patients or groups of patients to determine effectiveness of nursing interventions (Moorhead et al., 2013). Each nursing-sensitive outcome has a definition, a measurement scale, and associated indicators and measures. A taxonomy of nursing-sensitive patient outcomes is available from the research team at the University of Iowa. The current classification consists of 490 outcomes for individuals, families, communities, or caregivers (Box 14-1).

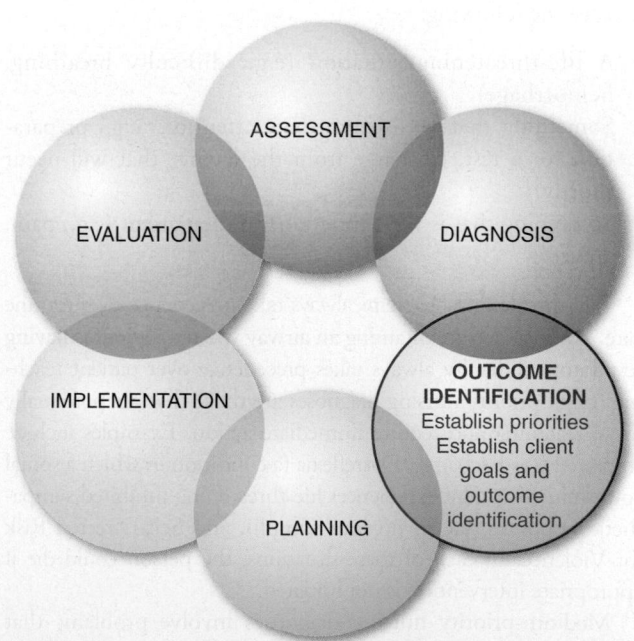

FIGURE 14-1 ANA Standard III states: "The nurse identifies expected outcomes individualized to the patient." This illustration shows activities used in the outcome identification phase and also the relationship of outcome identification to the other phases of the nursing process.

BOX 14-1 Nursing Outcome
Classification System Example

MOBILITY LEVEL. Domain Functional Health (I) Class-Mobility
(c) Definition: Ability to move purposely. Mobility Level:
1. Severely compromised
2. Substantially compromised
3. Moderately compromised
4. Mildly compromised
5. Not compromised
Indicators: Ambulation: walking 1 2 3 4 5.

Reprinted with permission from Moorhead, S., Johnson, M., Maas, M., &
Swanson, E. (2013). *Nursing Outcomes Classification (NOC)* (5th ed.).
St. Louis, MO: Elsevier.

OUTCOME IDENTIFICATION ACTIVITIES

Establish Priorities

A **priority** is a choice that comes first over other possible options. This choice is often based on urgency or importance. Priority setting is a decision-making process that ranks the order of nursing diagnoses in terms of importance to the patient. Priorities constantly change as the patient's situation and condition change. Nurses use assessment skills and data collection, clinical experience, and evidence-based practice to determine priorities. High priorities for patients usually involve the following:

- A life-threatening situation (e.g., difficulty breathing, hemorrhage)
- Something that needs immediate attention (e.g., preparation for a test, discharge from the facility that will occur shortly)
- Something that is very important to the patient (e.g., pain, anxiety)

Life-threatening problems always take precedence over routine care. For instance, maintaining an airway when a patient is having respiratory difficulty always takes precedence over patient teaching. High-priority nursing diagnoses are those that are potentially life threatening and require immediate action. Examples include Impaired Gas Exchange, Dysreflexia (a condition in which a spinal cord–injured patient experiences life-threatening inhibited sympathetic responses due to noxious stimuli), and Self-Directed Risk for Violence. In each of these situations, the person could die if appropriate intervention is not initiated.

Medium-priority nursing diagnoses involve problems that could result in unhealthy consequences, such as physical or emotional impairment, but are not likely to threaten life. Examples include Fatigue, Stress Incontinence, or Dysfunctional Grieving. Assessment data obtained from the patient determine the significance of each nursing diagnosis and what priority it is assigned.

Often, the patient's physical condition is more stable and determining priorities is more subtle. Low-priority nursing diagnoses involve problems that usually can be resolved easily with minimal interventions and have little potential to cause significant dysfunction. The low-priority status often is based on the significance for the patient and the high likelihood that the problem will be easily resolved. For example, Pain might be a nursing diagnosis for a patient after minor surgery, but because the pain is moderate and probably will last only a short time, the diagnosis is not the highest priority.

Sometimes, patients and nurses disagree on the priority given to problems. For example, a postoperative patient may view pain as the most important problem and try to avoid moving or ambulating so that pain will decrease. The nurse might view Ineffective Breathing Pattern as much more significant. Through dialogue, the nurse and patient are able to share their opinions, experiences, and values so that they can determine an agreeable plan. After listening to the patient, the nurse may say, "I understand that you are in pain, but it is important to walk so that you do not develop respiratory complications. How about planning to get you up 30 minutes after you get your pain medication so your pain is well controlled?" During shift handoff, patient goals and progress can be shared with other staff to promote continuity of care.

Nurses use priorities to plan care and determine the order in which interventions are carried out. For example, if the patient is receiving care in the home, establishing priorities might include determining what to teach a patient with newly diagnosed diabetes during a 60-minute home visit. Sometimes, availability limits whether all desirable interventions can actually be carried out. For example, a nurse may want to wash a patient's hair to promote self-esteem, but time may not allow this intervention if the patient is scheduled for a diagnostic test or two other patients are scheduled for surgery

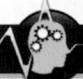 **APPLY YOUR CRITICAL THINKING**

Refer to the patient in the opening scenario. Given the 2 nursing diagnoses—Impaired Physical Mobility and Constipation—which has the highest priority? State your rationale for your prioritization. Are there any missing nursing diagnoses that should be explored?

Check your answer in Appendix B.

Establish Patient Outcomes and Outcome Criteria

The terms *goals, objectives,* and *outcomes* are used interchangeably because they are statements of expectations. For this reason, nurses should be familiar with the specific use of terms in the clinical setting in which they work. A distinction is made in this textbook: Patient goals and outcome criteria are not interchangeable. Their definitions and use are described in the following sections.

PATIENT OUTCOMES

A patient **outcome** is an educated guess, made as a broad statement, about what the patient's state will be after the nursing intervention is completed. It directly addresses the problem stated in the nursing diagnosis. Using clinical knowledge and experience, the nurse, in collaboration with the patient, determines appropriate outcomes.

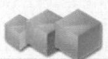 **Concept Mastery Alert**

Nurses must be careful to avoid confusing nursing interventions with nursing outcomes. A nursing outcome states a measurable, time-dependent goal by which to evaluate a nursing intervention. The intervention states what the nurse will do; the outcome provides a point of reference for determining whether the intervention is appropriate and effective.

Behavioral outcomes, written to indicate a desired state, contain an action verb and a qualifier that indicate the level of performance that needs to be achieved. Some commonly used behavioral verbs are presented in Box 14-2. The **qualifier** is a description of the parameter for achieving the outcome. For instance, "Walks" would not be a specific patient outcome. Restating this patient outcome as "Ambulates safely with one-person assistance" clarifies this outcome statement.

Outcomes may be short term or long term. A short-term outcome can be met in a relatively short period (within days or less than 1 week). A long-term outcome requires more time (perhaps several weeks or months). A long-term outcome also may indicate ongoing activity. Long-term outcomes usually describe expected benefits or results that are seen after the plan of care has been implemented (Alfaro-LeFevre, 2014).

The nurse needs to revise outcomes if the patient's situation or medical condition changes. For example, let's say a nurse is working in the home with a patient who has mobility deficits from multiple sclerosis. During the home visit, the nurse and the patient decide that an outcome should state, "Ambulates safely with a quad cane." Two weeks later, during another home visit, the nurse notices increased mobility problems caused by an exacerbation of multiple sclerosis. The nurse did not expect this change in the patient's medical condition, and the change was outside the nurse's control. An appropriate revision of this outcome might state, "Transfers safely to a chair, with one-person assistance." As this patient's mobility status improves or deteriorates, the nurse will need to revise mobility outcomes.

OUTCOME CRITERIA

Outcome criteria are specific, measurable, realistic statements of goal attainment. They may restate the goal, but they also present information that will guide the evaluation phase of the nursing process. To be specific and measurable, certain requirements must be met when writing outcome criteria. Outcome criteria answer the questions who, what actions, under what circumstances, how well, and when. According to Alfaro-LeFevre (2014), requirements include the following:

- *Subject*: Who is the person expected to achieve the goal?
- *Verb*: What actions must the person do to achieve the goal?
- *Condition*: Under what circumstances is the person to perform the action?
- *Criteria*: How well is the person to perform the action?
- *Specific time*: When is the person expected to perform the action?

An example of an outcome criterion would be, "The patient [who] verbalizes [what action] three dietary modifications of a low-salt diet to his wife [under what circumstances] accurately [how well] after the teaching session [when]."

PLANNING

Planning, the fourth phase of the nursing process, refers to the development of nursing strategies designed to ameliorate patient problems. A plan of care is developed to direct nursing care activities related to the person for whom the goals and outcome criteria were developed. A written plan of care directs the activities of the nursing staff in the provision of patient care.

Purposes of planning include the following:

- Direct patient care activities.
- Promote continuity of care.
- Focus charting requirements.
- Allow for delegation of specific activities.

Activities of the planning phase involve the following:

- Planning nursing interventions
- Writing the patient plan of care

Planning in relation to other phases of the nursing process is illustrated in Figure 14-2.

BOX 14-2	**Behavioral Verbs Used in Patient Goals**	
Calculate	Distinguish	Practice
Classify	Draw	Recall
Communicate	Explain	Recite
Compare	Express	Record
Construct	Identify	Stand
Contrast	List	State
Define	Maintain	Use
Demonstrate	Name	Verbalize
Describe	Participate	Walk
Discuss	Perform	

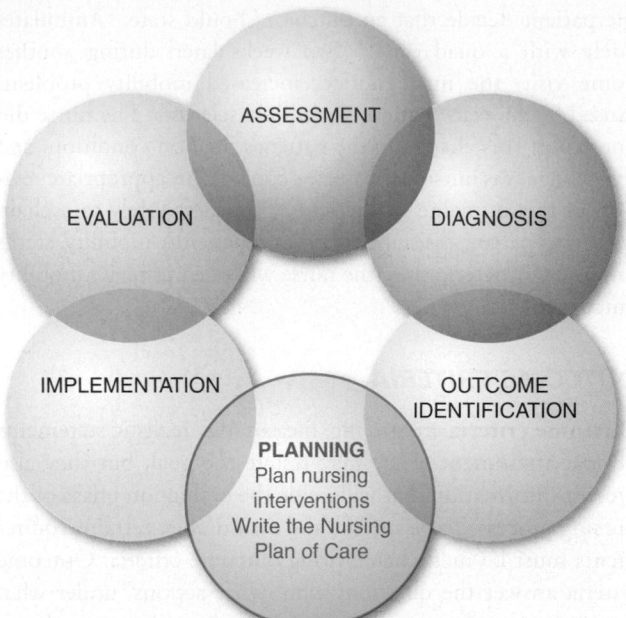

FIGURE 14-2 ANA Standard IV states: "The nurse develops a plan of care that prescribes interventions to attain expected outcomes." This illustration shows activities used in the planning phase and also the relationship of planning to the other phases of the nursing process.

Nursing Interventions Classification (NIC)

Since 1987, a research team at the University of Iowa College of Nursing has been engaged in constructing, validating, and implementing nursing interventions (Bulecheck, Butcher, Dochterman, & Wagner, 2013). The interventions are organized in a three-level taxonomy consisting of domains, classes, and interventions. Interventions can be direct or indirect care activities; they include nurse-initiated interventions as well as treatments initiated by the physician or other provider.

At the most abstract level, the taxonomy includes seven domains:

- Physiologic: Basic
- Physiologic: Complex
- Behavioral
- Safety
- Family
- Health system
- Community

Each domain group contains classes, which are groups of interventions that are then broken down into individual interventions. The domains, classes, and interventions are coded numerically to permit computerization. Each intervention consists of a definition and a list of activities that describe the nursing actions that need to be performed. There are 542 interventions included in the **Nursing Interventions Classification** (Bulecheck et al., 2013) (Box 14-3).

BOX 14-3	Nursing Interventions Classification System Example

DOMAIN 1. Physiologic: Basic CLASS A. Activity and Exercise Management INTERVENTION 0140 Body Mechanics Promotion

Reprinted with permission from Bulecheck, G., Butcher, H., Dochterman, J., Wagner, C. M. (2013). *Nursing Interventions Classification (NIC)* (6th ed.). St Louis, MO: Elsevier Mosby.

Planning Activities

PLANNING NURSING INTERVENTIONS

Selecting appropriate nursing interventions directs activities to be carried out in the implementation phase. **Nursing interventions** are "any treatment, based upon clinical judgment and knowledge, that a nurse performs to enhance patient/client outcomes" (Bulecheck et al., 2013, p. xv). Alfaro-LeFevre (2014) states that nursing interventions are used to monitor health status; prevent, resolve, or control a problem; assist with activities of daily living (ADLs); or promote optimum health and independence. Interventions are written as specific activities on the plan of care.

Determining appropriate nursing interventions for a specific patient requires clinical knowledge and practice. In general, interventions can be grouped to describe the activity being suggested. Types of interventions include the following:

- Psychomotor (positioning, inserting, applying)
- Psychosocial (supporting, exploring, encouraging)
- Educational (demonstrating, teaching, observing return demonstrations)
- Maintenance (skin care, hygiene)
- Surveillance (detecting changes)
- Supervisory (other healthcare providers)
- Sociocultural (spending time, incorporating cultural differences into care regimen)

WRITING A PATIENT PLAN OF CARE

A patient plan of care documents the problem-solving process. The ability to create the patient plan of care has become a standard expected of every nurse. The plan is a critical element in focusing nursing activity. To serve as evaluation criteria and meet the standards of The Joint Commission (2013), the plan must be developed by a registered nurse, it must be documented in the patient's health record, and it must reflect the standards of care established by the institution and the profession. Medicare and Medicaid standards and some third-party reimbursement plans require patient plans of care for each patient.

Two important concepts guide a patient plan of care:

- The plan of care is patient centered.
- The plan of care is a step-by-step process.

A step-by-step process is evidenced by the following:

- Sufficient data are collected to substantiate nursing diagnoses.
- At least one goal must be stated for each nursing diagnosis.
- Outcome criteria must be identified for each goal.
- Nursing interventions must be specifically designed to meet the identified goal.
- Each intervention should be supported by a scientific rationale.
- Evaluation must address whether each goal was completely met, partially met, or completely unmet.

TYPES OF PATIENT PLANS OF CARE

The patient plan of care can be written in various ways. Institutions may use a written or a computerized care plan design. Despite these design differences, the plan of care usually contains three key elements: the nursing diagnosis (patient problem), patient goals, and nursing interventions (nursing orders, nursing actions). The plan of care can be written for the individual patient, standardized for a patient population, generic for a specific problem, or computer generated from assessment data. Students learning to write plans use the instructional patient plan of care format as a learning exercise. In practice settings, nurses use the clinical patient plan of care format to individualize patient care.

Instructional Patient Plans of Care

Instructional patient plans of care, or student care plans, allow students to demonstrate their knowledge of various patient problems and apply the processes nurses use to solve them. Scientific rationales from nursing literature are given as references for the information and to illustrate the nurse's decision-making process. Specific recommendations for completing this type of plan of care are given using each step of the nursing process.

Usually, student nurses are required to complete some form of an instructional patient plan of care to demonstrate in a written format an understanding of the problem-solving process used in assisting patients to maintain or regain a higher level of function. Components of instructional patient plans of care usually include nursing diagnoses, patient goals, outcome criteria, nursing interventions, scientific rationale, and evaluation.

The patient plans of care used in later clinical chapters of this text illustrate this format and include one nursing diagnosis, one or more patient goals, several patient outcome criteria, nursing interventions, scientific rationale, and evaluation. These plans are based on the sample format given in the Sample Patient Plan of Care shown here, along with what to include in each section of the plan. For assistance in learning how to correctly state nursing diagnoses, patient goals, outcome criteria, nursing interventions, scientific rationale, and evaluation, refer to Table 14-1.

PATIENT PLAN OF CARE:
Sample Patient Plan of Care

NURSING DIAGNOSIS

(Use the NANDA-I–accepted list of nursing diagnoses. List in priority order. Use the diagnostic label and "related to" [related factor], followed by "manifested by" [supporting defining characteristics].)

PATIENT GOAL

(One or more patient goals established from nursing diagnosis. A broadly stated objective that indicates an overall picture of the state of the patient if the problem is resolved.)

PATIENT OUTCOME CRITERIA

(Specific, measurable, realistic statements that can be evaluated to judge goal attainment. Stated as behavioral objectives, they include a verb, a short phrase describing the specific measure to be accomplished, and a time reference.)

NURSING INTERVENTION	SCIENTIFIC RATIONALE
(Write interventions [nursing orders] that are specific and relate to the goal. The "related to" phrase of the nursing diagnostic statement directs choice of nursing interventions. Interventions include who, what, when, and how the order is to be carried out.)	(Gives justification for carrying out the intervention. Demonstrates synthesis of physiologic, psychological, and pathophysiologic concepts.)

EVALUATION

5/1/17: 08:45—The degree to which the patient outcomes have been met and appropriate revision of the plan if needed.

—S. Zoe, RN

TABLE 14-1 CORRECT AND INCORRECT PLAN OF CARE ENTRIES

Entry	Rationale
Nursing Diagnoses **Correct** Feeding Self-care Deficit related to right-sided weakness manifested by inability to pick up spoon, lack of attention to food on tray, and inability to open containers	Correct statement of actual nursing diagnosis using three-part statement, including diagnostic label, related factors, and defining characteristics
Incorrect Self-care Deficit, Feeding: due to left cerebrovascular accident, manifested by not eating	Incorrect statement of actual diagnosis. Diagnostic label is inverted, a medical diagnosis is used for the causative agent, and defining characteristics are not provided for validation of the diagnosis
Patient Goal **Correct** Patient demonstrates correct skin care regimen	Correctly stated patient goal: general statement of overall picture of patient if problem is resolved and is realistic
Incorrect Patient's skin is free of eczema	Incorrect statement of patient goal. The goal is not achievable through nursing interventions and may be unrealistic even with medical treatment
Patient Outcome Criteria **Correct** Ambulates 30 feet with walker before discharge	Correctly stated patient outcome: specific, measurable, and realistic
Incorrect Walks in the hall	Incorrectly stated outcome criterion because it is not specific and does not include qualifiers for the outcome
Nursing Interventions **Correct** Staff will perform passive range-of-motion exercises to all extremities during morning care and evening care	Correctly stated nursing intervention, including who, what, when, and how nursing order will be carried out
Incorrect Encourage joint mobility	Incorrectly stated nursing intervention because time frame, type of exercise, and who will perform the exercise are not specified
Scientific Rationale **Correct** Small shifts in body weight promote circulation and help to prevent skin breakdown (Craven, Hirnle & Henshaw, 2016).	Correctly stated rationale: tells scientific basis for nursing action and correctly cites source
Incorrect Changes position every 2 h	Incorrectly stated scientific rationale: restates a nursing intervention without documenting why it is an appropriate nursing intervention, and no source is cited
Evaluation **Correct** Unable to complete passive range of motion to right upper extremity after morning care because of reported pain when arm is elevated above shoulder level. Physician notified, and patient instructed to rest arm.	Correctly stated evaluation because it indicates that goal was not met, with specific documentation providing the data for revision
Incorrect Range of motion discontinued due to pain	Incorrect evaluation statement: statement does not contain patient's response or follow-up on the problem

Nursing Diagnosis. The nursing diagnostic statement is recorded in the space labeled "Nursing Diagnosis," using NANDA-International (NANDA-I) terminology if possible. All identified nursing diagnoses for a patient should be listed in order of priority for patient care. Use of a functional approach helps nurses focus on real or potential functional problems rather than on disease pathology.

Patient Goals. One or more patient goals are established for each nursing diagnosis. Some examples of goal statements are "Maintains present weight," "Demonstrates no evidence of infection," and "Administers insulin correctly." The goal describes a patient outcome in broad terms.

The patient **goal** reflects resolution or correction of the identified problem.

Patient Outcome Criteria. Patient outcome criteria are specific, measurable, realistic statements that can be evaluated to judge goal attainment. Examples include the following:

- Accurately draws up correct dosage of insulin at next teaching session
- Demonstrates deep breathing and coughing exercises following instruction

Nursing Interventions. An intervention is a treatment performed to enhance patient outcomes. An intervention is

TABLE 14-2 EXAMPLES OF NURSING INTERVENTIONS TO SUPPORT THE MEDICAL REGIMEN

Medical Order	Nursing Intervention
Weight qd, report loss >5#	Bedscale weight every day at 6 AM; report weight >(specify #) to physician.
Increase caloric intake	Provide between-meal snack at 10 AM, 2 PM, and 10 PM. Request consultation with dietitian (done 10/19). Transfer patient to chair for each meal and snack.

considered direct when it is performed through interaction with the patient. Indirect interventions are treatments performed away from the patient in order to support the effectiveness of direct care interventions. Sometimes called *nursing orders,* nursing interventions are written in specific terms that relate to the goals. The statements should be comprehensive but brief; nurses may refer to procedures, protocols, or standing policies for further information. In some cases, nursing interventions include specific measures needed to carry out the medical regimen and are not directed at a nursing diagnosis. Examples are shown in Table 14-2.

Scientific Rationale. The **scientific rationale** is the justification or reason for carrying out the intervention. It often synthesizes psychological and pathophysiologic concepts. The rationale—the "why" of the intervention—describes a research-based reason for performing the intervention. Usually, student nurses are required to supply scientific rationales to show understanding of the basic reasons for carrying out specific nursing interventions. A reference for each scientific rationale may be given, citing the author, year, title, and page of the article or book used. In clinical practice settings, nurses may use rationales to illustrate new research findings or support controversial approaches to problems, but these are not routinely written in the plan of care. Sometimes, nurses think that interventions are based on common sense, but this is not so: many nursing interventions previously thought to be sensible have turned out to be unsafe, impractical, or unnecessary. For example, massaging bony prominences was once thought to promote skin integrity, but research has shown that this practice may cause tissue damage and should not be performed. Asking why certain nursing interventions are performed aids in the scientific development of nursing practice.

Evaluation. The **evaluation** of a nursing intervention is a written statement that determines the patient's status in relation to the outcome criteria at a particular time. Evaluation focuses on patient progress, not on how well the student or nurse carried out nursing interventions. The evaluation stage answers the question, Was the outcome achieved? It provides the necessary feedback to guide revision of the plan of care or resolution of the problem. Changes may be needed in the time frame for goal achievement or to facilitate new skill development in the patient. In some cases, the student will state what would have been evaluated if nursing care had been provided during additional clinical experiences.

Evaluation of care usually is recorded in the nursing progress note (see Chapter 16) and includes the patient's response to the intervention and the objective clinical findings. Each intervention is evaluated for effectiveness, modified if needed, and deleted if not necessary.

Instructional Concept Maps

Concept maps can also be assigned for students to demonstrate their understanding and application of the nursing process. A **concept map** is a graphical tool for organizing and representing knowledge. It includes concepts (usually within boxes or circles) with words on lines connecting the boxes or circles demonstrating relationships (Novak & Canas, 2008). Concept maps can improve critical thinking by helping students organize and categorize information and see the relationship between concepts. Specific patient information is organized and filled in by the student. Examples of concept maps, using the nursing process as a framework, are included in all clinical chapters of this text.

Clinical Plans of Care

The clinical plan of care used in practice is different from the required instructional plan of care done by students. The nursing process is used, but the plan is organized in a practical, concise format for daily use. Usually, there is less specific detail, and rationales are not documented. The focus is to individualize the plan of care for each patient using findings from the nursing assessment and identified nursing diagnoses. The various forms of clinical patient plans of care are highlighted in Box 14-4.

The focus of the clinical plan of care is the patient. To promote better communication among all members of the healthcare team, the clinical plan of care should be multidisciplinary. Often, nurses take primary responsibility for developing and updating the clinical plan of care, but all members of the team are encouraged to read and add to the plan of care. Nurses continually refine the process of writing plans of care and actively using them in implementing daily care as they gain experience. A well-written, continually updated plan of care is an invaluable tool.

Assessment and Data Collection. The history and physical assessment are guidelines for the initial plan. Data are gathered in each subsequent meeting with the patient to revise the plan.

Nursing Diagnosis or Problem List. The nursing diagnosis in a working plan of care is written using the guidelines in Chapter 13. Multidisciplinary plans of care may use a problem list that identifies current patient problems. The clinical plan of care focuses on individual patient needs and priority patient problems.

Outcome Identification. Patient goals and outcome criteria are often seen in the same statement. The goals are specific to meeting the patient problems identified in the nursing diagnoses.

Interventions. Appropriate actions specific to each patient's needs are documented. The healthcare person responsible for performing the nursing intervention is identified. This action may be most appropriately completed by the nurse. In some

BOX 14-4   Plans of Care Used in Clinical Practice

Individual Plan of Care

Individual plans of care are written for each patient by a registered nurse. The nursing diagnoses are listed, along with specific goals and interventions to resolve the problem. This method is ideal, but it is time consuming.

Standardized Plan of Care

Standardized plans of care are written by a group of nurses who are experts in a given area of practice (e.g., obstetrics, rehabilitation, or orthopedics). The plans are written for a patient population with a specific medical diagnosis (e.g., total hip replacement, pressure ulcer, vaginal delivery, coronary artery bypass surgery). These experts identify the most common nursing diagnoses for this patient population and write the goals and interventions usually necessary to resolve the problem. Each time a standardized plan of care is used, it must be individualized for a specific patient. This method assures the nurse that the plan is correct for the patient. The danger of a standardized plan of care lies in the fact that it may not fit a specific patient. Nurses must make judgments as to the degree to which standardized plans should be modified or whether they should not be used in individual cases.

Generic Plan of Care

Generic plans of care usually are written for a specific nursing diagnosis. They contain the goals and interventions most commonly seen when that particular nursing diagnosis is identified. Again, the generic plan of care must be individualized for a specific patient. Because generic plans are written by experts in a particular diagnostic area, they may serve as a learning tool for the inexperienced nurse who is unfamiliar with the content.

Computerized Plan of Care

Computerized plans of care are generated from assessment data entered into a computer about a specific patient. The plan is written by experts in the area, and the content is similar to that of the standardized or generic plan of care. Once the plan is on the computer screen, the nurse has an opportunity to customize it for the patient. Because these plans are linked to assessment data, it is critical that all pertinent information be collected and entered into the system. The generated plan of care is only as good as the data on which it is based.

---

instances, it is performed by other members of the healthcare team or delegated to auxiliary nursing personnel. This leads to better communication and use of plans for daily assignments.

Rationale. Although the scientific rationale is not documented in the clinical plan, it is no less important than in the instructional plan. Nurses and other members of the healthcare team must know the rationale behind the intervention or must question and review the rationale before performing the action. This professional responsibility is expected of all members of the healthcare team to ensure safe patient care.

Evaluation. Evaluation is ongoing from initial care through resolution of the problem. Healthcare professionals base evaluation on specific observations made of patient's progress toward the outcome criteria. The plan is updated and changed—minute by minute in critical care, shift by shift in acute care, and weekly or monthly in long-term or home healthcare.

COLLABORATIVE CARE PLAN: CRITICAL PATHWAYS

Critical pathways (paths) are the commonly used standard guidelines for patient care in many hospitals. The focus on outcome management, controlling costs, and continuous quality improvement has been the driving force for most organizations as they convert to critical paths and case management as a system for care delivery (Moorhead et al., 2013). Various terms for critical paths are used: clinical paths, collaborative care plans, care maps, multidisciplinary care plan, and case management plans. A standardized plan or critical path is acceptable to The Joint Commission (2013).

The critical path is a grid that describes a patient's problems with intermediate outcomes and multidisciplinary staff actions along a timeline. The critical path tool can be designed for patients with a particular illness, diagnostic-related grouping (DRG), procedure, or condition. Timelines can be developed for a continuum of care in the hospital in terms of hours, days, and months, across geographic care units (e.g., emergency room, critical care unit, telemetry), or for a continuum of care in the community (see Fig. 14-3 for an example of a critical pathway for a patient having a total joint replacement).

Some agencies use other plans of care in combination with critical paths for patients who have additional problems that are not addressed on the critical path. Information on the critical path is based on evidenced-based research and the most cost-efficient practice patterns for a particular diagnosis or procedure. This method addresses key events in the treatment process that must be accomplished to achieve predetermined outcomes at a minimal cost. The staff nurse is responsible for initiating, maintaining, and completing the critical path, including documentation of variances (deviations from expected outcomes). Some hospitals are developing a version of the critical path for patients and families to help increase understanding of and participation in the plan of care. Figure 14-3 demonstrates how a critical pathway can be developed and used as a teaching tool for patients and families, providing a clear outline for expected care when recovering from a fracture.

Most critical paths incorporate quality indicators and discharge criteria to measure the quality of care provided. The patient's progress at the time of discharge is measured against established criteria. The paths reflect the criteria of the Centers for Medicare and Medicaid Service. Patients who do not meet the discharge criteria and are discharged must be monitored for readmissions and premature discharges. Theorists have proposed that the adaptation of pathways, especially in inpatient healthcare facilities, may ensure the delivery of quality care and reduce the occurrence of medical errors.

VIRGINIA MASON MEDICAL CENTER/GROUP HEALTH
Clinical Pathway: Total Joint Replacement (Hip/Knee/Shoulder)

Clinical Pathway

Discharge Outcomes	Day of Surgery	PHASE 1 acute	PHASE 2 pre discharge
☐ Baseline mental status ☐ Vital sign stable/ temperature normal ☐ Adequate oral intake ☐ Oral analgesics for adequate pain control ☐ No signs of infection/nor ☐ Deep Vein Thrombosis ☐ All ambulation/mobility goals met ☐ Independent or baseline with activity of daily living (ADL) skills ☐ Coumadin teaching completed ☐ Transfer/fall/dislocation precautions able to be repeated by patient/family. **Estimated length of stay 2 days** **Please record date all criteria are met:** _____	Date: **Staff INTERVENTION:** ☐ Follow Patient Care Standard for *Total Hip/Knee/Shoulder Replacement* and individualize *Daily Pt. Care* section per MD orders. ☐ Assess post-op teaching needs and review as needed. ☐ Review hip/knee/shoulder precautions often with patient/family/caregiver. ☐ Discharge plan in place (see pre-operative note) ☐ RN Initiate mobilization within 3 hrs of pt's arrival (sit edge of bed, stand if tolerated) ☐ Pain Management for Total Knees – adductor canal block (ambi pump)	Date: **Staff INTERVENTION:** ☐ Remove Foley catheter (POD 1) once patient is able to get OOB, with assistance and ambulate ☐ Switch IV to saline lock once patient has taken 500 CC PO ☐ Discontinue Pt Controlled Analgesia (PCA)/Initiate oral analgesic ☐ Physical Therapy (PT) eval (POD 1) ☐ Out of bed with assist @ least 3 times a day (per Physical Therapy [PT] exercise protocol) ☐ Advance diet as tolerated ☐ Occupational Therapy (OT) eval (POD 1 for total shoulder replacement). ☐ Review "Steps to Going Home" ☐ Pain Management for Total Knees and ORIFs: At 2100 bolus through femoral catheter (see MD order details) then discontinue Femoral nerve catheter ☐ Pain Management for Total Shoulders: Remove interscalene catheter at 1600 POD 1 unless otherwise specified.	Date: **Staff INTERVENTION:** ☐ Discontinue saline lock ☐ Change dressing PRN ☐ Out of bed @ least TID/ambulate twice a day in hall with standby assistance ☐ Occupational Therapy (OT) final visit ☐ Physical Therapy (PT) f/u visits ☐ Review appropriateness of discharge plan. ☐ Equipment needs and/or transitional care placement needs met. ☐ If not progressing as planned by PT visit #3 (notify Social Services/Worker [SW]). ☐ Review all discharge instructions ☐ Coumadin teaching ☐ Patient views TV/video if on Coumadin tx
	Pt. OUTCOME: ☐ VS stable/circulation, movement & sensation normal ☐ Pain relief with PCA/other ☐ Tolerating oral fluids or if nausea/vomiting relief achieved with antiemetic medication ☐ Understands and complies with total hip/shoulder precautions	**Pt. OUTCOME:** ☐ Pain relief with oral meds ☐ Oral fluids > 500 cc's ☐ IV fluids discontinued ☐ Tolerating solid food ☐ Able to void urine 6–8 hours after foley removal ☐ Knows weight bearing status ☐ Ambulates at bedside/within room with assist ☐ HCT within normal limits	**Pt. OUTCOME:** ☐ Ambulating in hall twice a day with standby assistance ☐ Up in chair for meals ☐ ADL's with minimal assist ☐ OT eval complete ☐ All mobility outcomes met (see PT pathway for TJR in chart) ☐ SW notified of any changes in status re: discharge planning ☐ All discharge teaching goals met ☐ Safe discharge/transition plan in place ☐ Follow-up appointment and or plan in place

	Day of Surg			POD1			POD 2			POD 3		
RNs Initial - Record Signature on back of sheet. 3 If outcomes met.	Noc	Day	Eve	Noc	Day	Eve	Noc	Day	Eve	Noc	Day	Eve
* If outcomes NOT met and chart variations (pt specific issues/delays/rapid move thru pathway) in progress notes.										Noc	POD 4+ Day	Eve

PATIENT NAME & ID #

VIRGINIA MASON MEDICAL CENTER
Total Joint Replacement (TJR) Pathway/Plan of Care

TREATMENT GOALS

Early and frequent mobilization helps prevent post operative complications and speeds recovery. Patient's care includes progressive mobility support by nursing and includes scheduled ambulation and out of bed activities as tolerated. Functional comfort is supported by pre-emptive pain medication delivery, adequate rest periods and discussion of daily goals with patient and family.

Prevention of hip dislocation: (anterior and posterior approach precautions integrated)
- Pillow between knees
- Maintain hip flexion to less than 70 degrees
- Operated leg must not cross midline
- Keep knees apart at all times
- No external rotation >30 degrees

Prevention of venous thromboembolism:
Venous thromboembolism is a common and potentially serious condition of total joint surgery of the lower extremity. Antithrombotics, sequential compression devices (SCD's) and ambulation significantly reduces this risk. Keep SCD's on patient at all times while in bed.

Prevention of atelectasis & pneumonia:
Adequate pain management facilitates respiratory health post op. Encourage active cough & deep breathe & frequent position changes in bed. Incentive spirometry Q 1 hour while awake.

RN Initials	Nurse Signature	RN Initials	Nurse Signature

FIGURE 14-3 Example of a collaborative care plan/critical pathway (© 2014 Virginia Mason Medical Center).

Some hospitals use critical paths as a guideline for patient care of most of the hospital's population. Care managers can use clinical pathways to coordinate care for patients with complex health problems, complications, or need for follow-up or referral.

A criterion for success of the critical path is consistency in healthcare delivery. Lack of consistency in care delivery usually results in a variance from the critical path. **Variances** result when a deviation occurs in the path that alters an expected outcome or the date of discharge. Patient, staff, and system variances can occur. Some hospitals also include variances in the community. Variances are monitored concurrently and retrospectively for continuous quality improvement. Data mining, the extraction of hidden predictive information from large databases, is a powerful new technology with great potential to help companies focus on the most important information in their data warehouses (Thearling, 2009). Variance measurement has the potential for identifying patient problems and complications early in hospitalization, variations in practice patterns, and system problems.

The critical path includes documentation as a permanent part of the patient's health record. Incorporating documentation in the design of the critical path eliminates much of the redundancy in charting. Critical path documentation consists of writing the provider's initials next to the outcome and intervention or indicating whether a variance has occurred. Some hospitals place a "V" next to the outcome or intervention if a variance occurs. Documentation of patient variance is written in the nurse's progress notes. Staff document variances on a separate variance sheet so that they can monitor data for continuous quality improvement.

Critical paths that function as comprehensive multidisciplinary care plans allow for the evaluation of the nursing process, documentation of that process, and monitoring for continuous quality improvement. Integration of the nursing process within the critical path framework is essential to ensure an outcome-based, accountability-driven system. By including a documentation section next to each outcome and intervention, evaluation of the nursing process is possible, ensuring accountability for the critical path.

Nurses in hospital and community settings will be expected to function as case managers and to develop and use critical paths in their case management role. Nurses are responsible for evaluating care variances in standardized plans to maximize patient outcomes, thus ensuring quality care (Alfaro-LeFevre, 2014).

KEY CONCEPTS

- Outcome identification is crucial for selecting and evaluating nursing interventions.
- Patient goals are stated as behavioral objectives and indicate the desired state of the patient if the problem has been resolved.
- Outcome criteria are specific, measurable, realistic statements of goal attainment.
- The patient plan of care is designed to direct patient care activities, promote continuity of care, focus charting requirements, and specify who is to carry out the nursing actions.

- The key elements of the patient plan of care are the nursing diagnosis or problem list, patient goals and outcome criteria, and nursing interventions.
- Nursing interventions are independent, dependent, and interdependent activities that nurses carry out to provide patient care.
- The use of critical pathways (paths) is helpful in standardizing evidence-based care to improve quality and control costs. They provide a collaborative plan of care.

PRACTICING FOR THE NCLEX

CHECK YOUR ANSWERS IN APPENDIX A.

1. Outcome identification serves which of the following purposes? Select all that apply:
   a. Providing individualized care
   b. Identifying potential health problems
   c. Planning care that is realistic and measurable
   d. Eliminating the need for the involvement of support people

2. A day 1 postoperative patient has the following abnormal assessment findings: pain 7/10, diminished lung sounds, hypoactive bowel sounds, and a saturated bloody abdominal dressing and bedsheets. Which would be the nursing priority?
   a. Pain
   b. Lung sounds
   c. Bowel sounds
   d. Wound care

3. A nurse is developing patient goals for a patient following abdominal surgery. Which of the following are appropriate goals? Select all that apply:
   a. "Ambulates in the hall prior to discharge"
   b. "Demonstrates deep breathing and splinting of incision "
   c. "Reports pain level at 4/10 with movement"
   d. "Incentive spirometry every 2 hours"

4. A nurse is developing outcome criteria for a patient following abdominal surgery. Which of the following is most appropriate?
   a. "Patient ambulates by time of discharge"
   b. "Identify two techniques to safely rise out of bed"
   c. "Patient reports pain less than 6/10"
   d. "Patient ambulates safely in hall twice on post-op day 2"

5. The nurse is establishing a plan of care for a patient with dyspnea and pneumonia. Which of the following is an appropriate nursing diagnosis for this patient?
   a. Impaired mobility related to dyspnea as evidenced by shortness of breath with position change
   b. Patient reports no shortness of breath after ambulating to bathroom by time of discharge
   c. Ambulates frequently
   d. Clinical pathway for pneumonia including anticipated length of stay
   e. No shortness of breath with incentive spirometry therapy

REFERENCES

Alfaro-LeFevre, R. (2014). *Applying nursing process: The foundation for clinical reasoning* (8th ed.). Philadelphia, PA: Wolters Kluwer Health/Lippincott Williams & Wilkins.

American Nurses Association. (2014). *Nursing: Scope and standards of practice* (2nd ed.). Silver Spring, MD: Author.

Bulecheck, G., Butcher, H., Dochterman, J., & Wagner, C. M. (2013). *Nursing Interventions Classification (NIC)* (6th ed.). St. Louis, MO: Elsevier Mosby.

Moorhead, S., Johnson, M., Maas, M., & Swanson, E. (2013). *Nursing Outcomes Classification (NOC)* (5th ed.). St. Louis, MO: C. V. Mosby.

Novak, J., & Canas, A. (2008). *The theory underlining concept maps and how to construct them.* Retrieved June 14, 2011 from http://cmap.ihmc.us/publications/researchpapers/theorycmaps/theoryunderlyingconceptmaps.htm

Thearling, K. (2009). *An introduction to data mining: Discovering hidden value in your data warehouse.* Retrieved June 14, 2011, from www.thearling.com/text/dmwhite/dmwhite.htm

The Joint Commission. (2013). *2014 Hospital Accreditation Standards.* Oakbrook Terrace, IL: Joint Commission Resources.

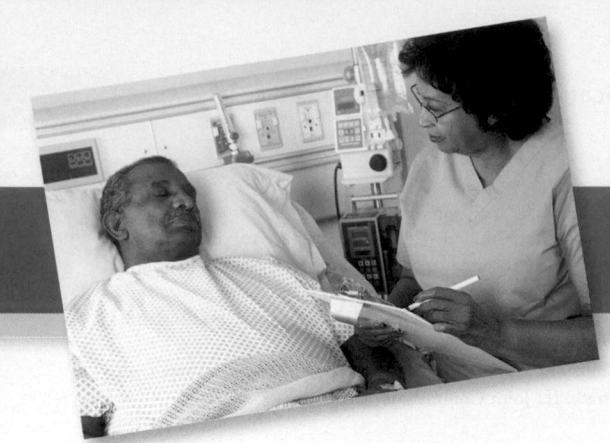

CHAPTER 15

Implementation and Evaluation

Kathryn Van Dyke Hayes

Case Scenario

You are assigned to care for a 68-year-old patient who has just returned to your nursing unit after abdominal surgery with general anesthesia. He has a history of arthritis for which he takes nonsteroidal anti-inflammatory agents (NSAIDs) and uses a cane to ambulate. He lives alone in a large two-story home. His postoperative assessment reveals the following: skin pale, warm, and dry; abdominal dressing dry and intact; temperature, 97.2°F (36.2°C); pulse, 78 beats/min and regular; respirations, 16 per minute; blood pressure, 136/74 mm Hg; responsive but sleepy; reluctant to cough, deep breathe, and turn because of pain.

The plan of care identifies the following nursing diagnoses and goals for this patient:

- Risk for Aspiration related to effects of anesthesia and decreased level of consciousness; patient will maintain a patent airway and remain free from signs and symptoms of aspiration.
- Pain related to surgical trauma; patient will report that postoperative pain is well controlled.
- Impaired Physical Mobility related to pain and underlying arthritis; patient will maintain optimal state of mobility, progressively increasing activities daily.
- Risk for Disuse Syndrome related to effects of anesthesia and surgery and underlying arthritis; patient will remain free from complications of immobility, achieving optimal level of functioning.

Once you have completed this chapter and have incorporated implementation and evaluation into your knowledge base, review the above scenario and reflect on the following areas of Critical Thinking:

1. Analyze how you would set priorities for your care for this patient. Suggest additional data you would need to collect, and propose possible additional nursing diagnoses and goals that might be appropriate.
2. Reflect on the intellectual, interpersonal, and technical skills you would need to care for this patient.
3. Propose possible interventions to carry out for this patient. Classify each action proposed as cognitive, interpersonal, or technical.
4. Explore how you would evaluate this patient's goal achievement. Suggest possible factors that might facilitate or interfere with his goal attainment.

KEY TERMS

delegation

evaluation

implementation

Nursing Interventions Classification (NIC)

nursing audit

peer review

quality improvement programs

standards of care

After the nurse and patient identify problems and strengths, they plan together methods of helping the patient maintain or return to healthy function. Outcome criteria are set for goals, and a plan of care is developed. Now they are ready for the implementation phase of the nursing process, the activity that provides planned care, and the evaluation phase, in which the patient's status is measured in response to the nursing care provided.

IMPLEMENTATION

Implementation refers to the action phase of the nursing process in which nursing care is provided. It is the actual initiation of the plan and recording of nursing actions. Its purpose is to provide technical and therapeutic nursing care required to help the patient achieve an optimal level of health.

Competence in intellectual, interpersonal, and technical skills is required to carry out the implementation phase. Nurses can delegate parts of the plan of care to other members of the healthcare team, but the registered nurse (RN) maintains accountability for the supervision and evaluation of these people. Figure 15-1 illustrates the activities of implementation, which include the following:

- Reassess
- Set priorities
- Perform nursing interventions
- Record nursing actions

Implementation Skills

INTELLECTUAL SKILLS

The intellectual skills used in implementation include problem solving, decision making, and teaching. To solve problems, nurses ask patients pertinent questions, discuss alternatives, and are open to new ideas. To enrich the decision-making abilities of patients, nurses give them opportunities to choose which treatments are performed, when, and in what sequence. Teaching requires knowledge about teaching–learning principles and information to convey.

INTERPERSONAL SKILLS

The ability to work with others to accomplish goals is critical to nursing. Nurses use communication skills to carry out planned nursing interventions. Skill at verbal and nonverbal communication is refined through practice. Chapter 6 gives more details on communication.

TECHNICAL SKILLS

Technical skills are used to carry out treatments and procedures. Nurses learn the specific skills through clinical practice. Technical competence means being able to use equipment, machines, and supplies in a particular specialty. For example, nurses working in delivery rooms must be familiar with fetal monitoring, positioning on the delivery room table, and neonatal resuscitation equipment. On the other hand, nurses

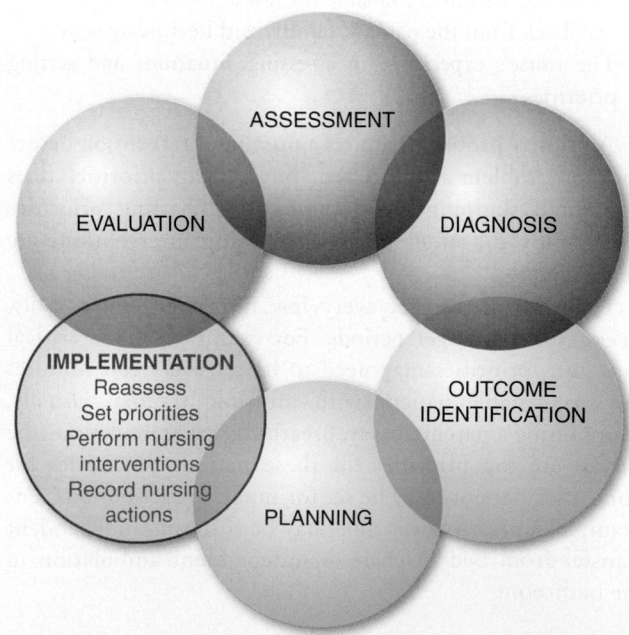

FIGURE 15-1 ANA Standard V states: "The registered nurse Implements the identified plan." This illustration shows activities used by nurses in the implementation phase and the relationship of implementation to the other phases of the nursing process.

working on medical units may need technical competence in using intravenous infusion pumps, therapeutic beds, or feeding pumps. Home health nurses must be familiar with adaptive equipment, patient-controlled analgesia pumps, and wound dressing supplies. Nurses also use technical skills to retrieve and record patient information on a computer.

Implementation Activities

REASSESS

During each encounter with patients, nurses assess function, ensuring prompt attention to emerging problems. Because a patient's condition can change quickly, astute nurses remain alert to subtle cues and inferences. For example, the patient who is experiencing pain may become quiet and withdraw from external stimuli. Recognizing such a change, nurses can intervene, validate, and assist the patient to become more comfortable. A patient who is demanding and irritable may be masking anxiety about a surgical procedure or fear about the results of a diagnostic test. As they initiate the plan of care, nurses must ensure that the planned interventions are still relevant.

SET PRIORITIES

Because a person's condition changes, priorities also may change. Priorities are based on information collected during reassessment. When setting priorities, nurses rank nursing problems in order of importance based on several factors (Fig. 15-2):

- The patient's condition
- New information from reassessment
- Time and resources available for nursing interventions
- Feedback from the patient, family, and healthcare staff
- The nurse's experience in assessing situations and setting priorities

A priority problem requires a nursing intervention before another problem is addressed, but setting priorities does not entail skipping any interventions. Setting priorities affects only the order in which nursing interventions are performed.

Priorities can be set every few minutes, hourly, daily, weekly, or for longer periods. For example, in the critical care unit, priorities may need to be set every few minutes for an unstable patient with multiple trauma. Usually, maintaining a patent airway, breathing, and circulation (the ABCs) are top priorities for these patients. Priorities for home care patients may be set for much longer periods. For example, a priority over time may be fostering independent transfer from bed to chair or independent ambulation to the bathroom.

PERFORM NURSING INTERVENTIONS

Nurses (or designees) carry out the nursing interventions listed on the patient plan of care. If a nurse is caring for several

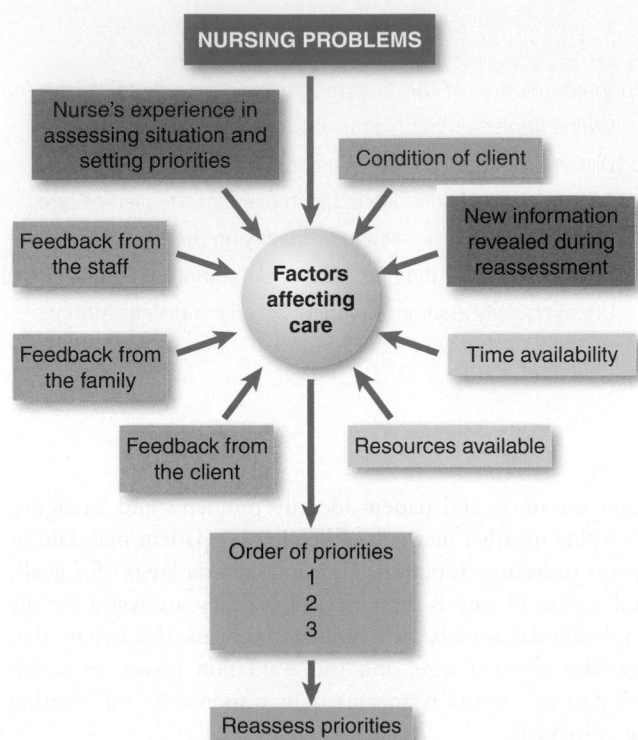

FIGURE 15-2 Nurses set priorities (position of prominence) by considering factors that affect care.

patients, he or she develops a schedule so that all patients are cared for in a timely fashion.

Intervention for Collaborative Problems

Nurses manage collaborative problems using both nurse- and physician-prescribed interventions to reduce risk of complications (Carpenito, 2012). Nursing diagnoses are determined, in part, when nurses ask, "Is this a problem that a nurse can legally treat without an order from a physician (or licensed provider)?" Interventions based on such diagnoses are nurse-prescribed actions. When nurses cannot legally make treatment decisions but have to follow physician's orders, the action is physician prescribed. Both types of interventions involve nursing judgment because both require legal mandates. The problem is a collaborative problem (Alfaro-LeFevre, 2014) when nurses use both nurse- and physician-prescribed interventions to give nursing care. For instance, the physician prescribes pain medication, but the nurse makes decisions as to when the medication is given. The nurse also may use alternative methods for pain relief.

Collaborative functioning within the healthcare team is essential to quality patient care. The nurse is actively involved in team rounds and team conferences where the plan for specific collaborative problems is revised and then discussed with the patient and family. The nurse is often responsible for reinforcing key points of the discussion and providing answers to the patient's questions. The nurse may make referrals to other healthcare providers (e.g., physical therapy, respiratory therapy, pain specialists, social work, etc.) to assist with collaborative problems. At times, a physician's order is required for selected referrals to assure payment by insurance, but some referrals are within the scope of independent nursing practice.

RECORD ACTIONS

After carrying out nursing interventions, nurses record them in the patient's health record. Each healthcare agency determines the specific requirements for documentation and should prepare written guidelines for the use of all forms. Chapter 16 discusses the recording of information.

Types of Nursing Interventions

The **Nursing Interventions Classification (NIC)** assists in defining the role of the professional nurse by listing direct and indirect treatments performed within the nursing role. Similar to the nursing diagnoses taxonomy of the NANDA-International (NANDA-I), the NIC provides a label or name for each intervention, a definition of the intervention, and a set of defining activities or actions that a nurse performs to implement the intervention (Bulechek, Dochterman, & Wagner, 2013). The NIC has identified 554 interventions and continues to evolve. Interventions will continue to be added and refined.

Possible advantages of the NIC include the following (Bulechek et al., 2013):

- Creation of a standardized language that promotes better understanding and communication of nursing interventions
- Expansion of knowledge about similarities and differences across nursing diagnoses
- Exploration of nursing care information systems
- Assistance in determining cost of services that nurses provide
- Demonstration of the impact nurses have within the healthcare system

Nursing interventions fall within three major categories: those using cognitive skills, those using interpersonal skills, and those using technical skills (Table 15-1). Selection of the

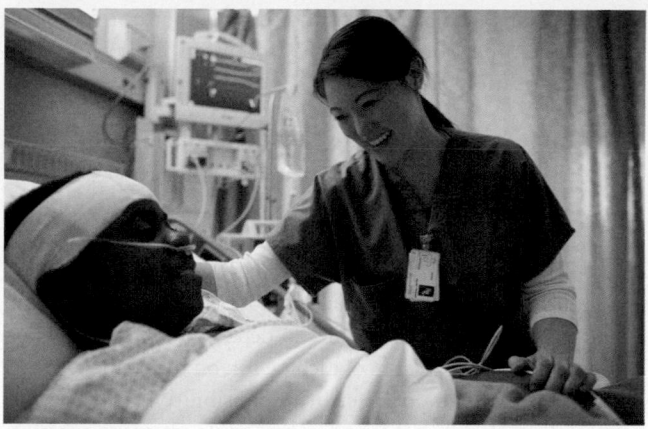

FIGURE 15-3 Nursing is an art—one that relies equally on cognitive, interpersonal, and technical skills.

type of nursing intervention to be used in patient situations depends on the patient's dysfunction and functional requirements and the best available evidence. (See Fig. 15-3.)

COGNITIVE INTERVENTIONS

Educational Interventions

Nurses carry out educational nursing interventions by applying general principles about the teaching and learning process. They develop teaching plans and provide instruction about health promotion or specific healthcare problems and their management. The ability to teach patients requires knowledge of normal anatomy and physiology, pharmacology, usual patterns of patient response to health changes, and pathophysiology of the disease process. A careful assessment of the patient yields information about his or her level of motivation, level of knowledge, willingness to follow the health regimen, and physical and psychological abilities to carry out the plan. Once a nurse is aware of the patient's readiness for learning, he or she can implement outcome-based

TABLE 15-1 TYPES OF NURSING INTERVENTIONS

Cognitive	Interpersonal	Technical
Teach/educate.	Coordinate activities.	Provide basic hygiene, skin care.
Relate knowledge to activities of daily living (ADLs).	Provide caregiving.	Perform routine nursing activities.
Provide feedback.	Use therapeutic communication.	Detect change from baseline data.
Create strategies for patients with dysfunctional communication.	Provide a personal presence.	Reorganize abnormal responses.
Delegate to UAP.	Set limits.	Provide independent and dependent treatment.
Supervise nursing team.	Provide opportunity to examine values and attitudes.	Assist with ADLs.
Supervise patient in performance.	Explore and legitimize feelings.	Provide appropriate sensory stimulation.
Supervise family in performance.	Provide spiritual support.	Mobilize equipment.
Alter the environment as needed.	Use humor.	Maintain equipment.
	Provide individual therapy.	Use special abilities or talents.
	Provide group therapy.	
	Become patient's advocate.	
	Support patient and family plans.	
	Make referrals for follow-up.	
	Serve as a role model.	

teaching plans, using instruction methods that optimize successful outcomes. See Chapter 9 for more information on patient education.

Delegation and Supervisory Interventions

The term *supervisory interventions* is applied in the context of overseeing a patient's overall care. Supervisory nursing interventions include ensuring that other members of the nursing team carry out specified aspects of the plan of care and that those involved with the patient or family show return demonstration of skills. Supervision of nursing team members requires in-depth knowledge of the job descriptions and capabilities of each person on the team.

Delegation is the transfer of responsibility for the performance of a task to another individual while retaining accountability for the outcome. In many health care settings especially in the last few decades, the use of unlicensed assistive personnel (UAP) has increased. The RN often delegates to LPN/LVN or UAPs to provide care for a group of patients in a cost-effective manner. This requires the nurse to understand the principles of delegation, which are outlined in Box 15-1. "The art and science of nursing is complex and knowledge based, thus the nursing process in its entirety cannot be delegated" (NCSBN, 2005, p. 14). Nurses may delegate specific aspects of care to nonprofessional staff, but RNs are held accountable for selecting appropriate nursing care measures for these personnel to perform. RNs cannot delegate the practice-pervasive functions of assessment, planning, diagnosis, evaluation, and nursing judgment (NCSBN, 2005).

RNs may delegate technical activities (i.e., feeding, ambulating) or provision of amenities (i.e., hospitality services, including making beds, setting up meals, cleaning the care environment), but the activities must not require critical thinking or professional judgment (American Nurses Association [ANA], 2012). For example, when a nurse obtains a patient's vital signs, it is considered assessment, because the nurse obtains the measurement but also evaluates the significance of the data based on trends over the last 24 hours and the patient's diagnosis. Assistive nursing personnel can monitor vital signs and report readings to the nurse, but assistive personnel do not have the knowledge or training to interpret the results or make care decisions based on the vital signs obtained.

Nurses also maintain responsibility to ensure that nursing care measures have been carried out correctly. Important information about the patient's response to the care is communicated verbally and in written form to the nurse responsible for the patient.

When supervising the patient or family in skill performance, it is important to provide encouragement, give feedback about correct and incorrect performance, and facilitate introduction of new skills to be learned. Patients and their families often are unfamiliar with nursing care regimens, equipment, and supplies. They need ample opportunity to carry out interventions under supervision. Nurses include patients and family members in planning and implementing initial care. They help patients and families begin to assume responsibility for self-management. Skills are built with practice. Doing an activity once usually is not sufficient for a patient or family member to achieve proficiency.

BOX 15-1 Principles of Delegation to UAP

Delegation—The transfer of responsibility for the performance of a task to another staff while retaining accountability for the outcome. A licensed RN will delegate tasks to unlicensed assistive personnel (UAP).

1. Right Person
   - The task is within the scope of the UAP's duties.
   - The individual has been trained and has the skill to perform the task.
   - The individual is willing to accept the responsibility for performing the task.
2. Right Task
   - The task is permitted by the state board of nursing and your institution's policies.
   - The task is commonly performed by UAP.
   - The task is performed according to an established sequence of steps.
   - The task involves little or no modification from one patient to another.
   - The task involves minimal risk.
   - The task does not involve assessment or clinical judgment.
   - The nursing process, including assessment, may not be delegated.
   - Patient teaching cannot be delegated to UAP.
3. Right Circumstance
   - Assess the patient to be sure his or her condition remains stable and delegation is appropriate.
   - Match complexity of the activity with the competency level of the UAP.
   - Be sure appropriate supervision is possible.
4. Right Communication
   - Identify tasks and expectations for patient assignment.
   - Provide clear report, including unique patient requirements and expected observations to report and record.
   - Assess UAP understanding of expectations, welcome questions, and provide clarification if needed.
5. Right Evaluation
   - Check in with the UAP to assess need for additional supervision or a revision in the plan.
   - Assess if the delegated task was performed correctly and documented.
   - Ask if the UAP has any information about the patient he or she would like to share.
   - Provide feedback to the UAP regarding what was done well and if there are areas for improvement.

INTERPERSONAL INTERVENTIONS

Coordinating Interventions

Coordinating patient activities serves many purposes. Coordination involves acting as a patient advocate, making referrals for follow-up care, collaborating with other healthcare team members, and ensuring that the patient's schedule is therapeutic.

For some patients, speaking for the patient or encouraging the patient to ask questions fulfills the advocacy role. For example, a patient may need help in refusing a suggested

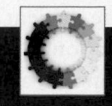

COLLABORATING WITH THE HEALTHCARE TEAM:
Delegating to a UAP

You are working with Bob, a nursing assistant on a medical unit. Together, the two of you are caring for a group of 4 patients. You update Bob on the care required for Mr. Jimmez, an 86-year-old patient who was admitted last evening with pneumonia.

SITUATION: Let's take a few minutes to review Mr. Jimmez's plan of care before we get to work.

BACKGROUND: Mr. Jimmez was admitted last evening from his assisted care facility with pneumonia. He was started on oxygen and antibiotics, and the doctor is worried that he may be developing sepsis. He has mild dementia and needs help getting up and ambulating with oxygen.

ASSESSMENT: We need to monitor him closely to promptly recognize signs of sepsis.

RECOMMENDATION: Could you monitor and record his vital signs every 2 hours. Notify me if his temperature is above 37.6°C, blood pressure is less than 110/70, or pulse is above 100. Also make sure he keeps his oxygen on and let me know if his O$_2$ sats are less than 90% or his respiration rate is above 22 or more labored. Increased confusion can be a sign of sepsis in the elderly even if their vital signs are normal, so let me know if he seems more confused. Please let me know if you need help. Bob, do you have any questions about Mr. Jimmez's care?

CRITICAL THINKING CHALLENGES
- Describe what principles of delegation this nurse used in communication with Bob about Mr. Jimmez.
- Were the delegated tasks within the scope for a nursing assistant or UAP?
- Was the SBAR communication respectful, and will it foster teamwork?
- What follow-up will be needed during the day as you work with Bob?

treatment or requesting a second opinion about surgery. In the advocacy role, the nurse presents the patient's point of view and suggests ways in which the patient's requests can be met.

Nurses are in a position to know what type of nursing follow-up patients need. They make referrals to home health agencies, visiting nurse associations, or other healthcare providers to facilitate return of optimal function. Many self-help groups and community services are available to provide assistance to patients with health-related problems; creativity in matching patients with these services can help ensure continued monitoring of the patient's health status, minimizing the risk of relapses.

Supportive Interventions

Supportive nursing interventions emphasize the use of communication skills, relief of spiritual distress, and caring behaviors. A combination of good communication and caring provides comfort and promotes a healthy response to health problems. Being supportive means recognizing the need for encouragement, unconditional acceptance of behaviors, and the positive effects of "being there" for patients during stress or crises. For example, the nurse may sit with a patient who is anxious, listen to a patient's experience grieving for the loss of a loved one, or touch the forehead of a patient with a spinal cord injury. Such interventions are referred to as "therapeutic use of self."

Nurses provide spiritual support by giving patients time to carry out religious practices, meditate, or read. Respecting the patient's privacy during these times conveys acceptance and understanding. If the patient wants to talk, the nurse listens to assess spiritual distress without being judgmental. If the

patient asks for a spiritual support person, the nurse contacts the patient's minister, rabbi, or priest or the hospital chaplain.

Psychosocial Interventions

Psychosocial nursing interventions focus on resolving emotional, psychological, or social problems. Humor, individual or group therapy, role-modeling social skills, and exploring feelings are all ways of carrying out psychosocial nursing interventions.

Some patients and families respond to stress by joking, teasing, or laughing about it. They may use humor as a way to relieve stress. A patient may say jokingly, "Gee, my arm must be target practice for everyone learning how to draw blood." Pick up on this cue and find out how many times the patient has been "stuck," determine why there was such a problem, and instruct the patient to speak up and request special consideration for future blood-drawing attempts.

Providing individual and group therapy is the nurse's responsibility in various settings. Individual therapy, used as a means of resolving psychological problems, usually requires additional training or certification. Group therapy is often used to provide support and guidance for patients and their support people with similar needs or problems. Recognizing the need for individual or group therapy, nurses make referrals to healthcare providers with the required expertise. In some settings, nurses hold group meetings with families of patients with Alzheimer disease or families of children with cancer. Most group therapy sessions have a stated purpose and schedule of activities. Group members rely on their own experiences and gain new ways of dealing with problems from others who have experienced the same problems. The nurse therapist serves as the group facilitator and assists group members to share feelings, advice, and helpful hints with one another.

The role modeling of social skills is used for patients who have not acquired them because of lack of exposure or lengthy illness. In some long-term care settings, patients have grown to depend on the staff to make all of their decisions. In other cases, patients have never practiced acceptable social behaviors. Treating patients with respect and using appropriate language and social behaviors (e.g., saying "please" and "thank you" and not interrupting) can help such patients become more socially adept.

Exploring feelings is a way to provide psychosocial intervention. Many patients with chronic or life-threatening illnesses need an opportunity to express their feelings in a nonjudgmental setting. Nurses are in a ideal position to help these patients ventilate their feelings and relieve fears and anxiety.

TECHNICAL INTERVENTIONS

Maintenance Interventions

Maintenance nursing interventions help patients retain a certain state of health, preventing deterioration of physical or psychological functioning and preserving independence. Maintenance interventions include basic hygiene, skin care, and other routine nursing activities. Maintenance nursing interventions are sometimes undervalued or considered insignificant, but they allow patients to preserve function and reduce the chance of developing complications.

Surveillance or Monitoring Interventions

Surveillance or monitoring nursing interventions includes detecting changes from baseline data and recognizing abnormal responses. This activity also can be categorized as observation, inspection, or vigilance. Nurses rely on the senses to detect changes: observing the appearance and characteristics of patients; hearing by auscultation, pitch, and tone; detecting odors and comparing them with past experience and knowledge of specific problems; and using touch to assess body temperature, skin condition, clamminess, or diaphoresis. Nurses use all of these surveillance or monitoring activities to determine the current status of patients and changes from previous states. Nurses often detect subtle changes in a patient's condition and communicate them to the physician to minimize problems. Expert nurse clinicians develop skill in detecting and preventing complications. For example, a patient who returns to the medical–surgical unit after a cardiac catheterization, an invasive test involving a catheter insertion in the femoral area, needs close monitoring. Monitoring activities may include frequent checking of vital signs, assessment of pedal pulses, and observation of the femoral area for possible bleeding.

Psychomotor Interventions

Psychomotor nursing interventions—those requiring technical expertise—include inserting, removing, changing, applying, administering, cleansing, or any other activity that requires a psychomotor action. For example, a nurse may regularly assess the lungs of a patient with a tracheostomy to ensure a patent airway. When needed, the nurse will suction the patient's airway to remove secretions and facilitate oxygenation. The management and care of equipment, supplies, treatments, and procedures also falls into this category of nursing interventions. Nurses gain psychomotor competence through practice.

EVALUATION

Evaluation, the sixth phase of the nursing process, follows implementation of the plan of care. **Evaluation** is defined as the judgment of the effectiveness of nursing care to meet patient goals based on the patient's behavioral responses. This phase involves a thorough, systematic review of the effectiveness of nursing interventions and a determination of patient goal achievement. Nurses use various skills to judge the effectiveness of nursing care. These skills include knowledge of standards of care, normal patient responses, and conceptual models and theories of nursing; ability to monitor the effectiveness of nursing interventions; and awareness of clinical research. Critical appraisal of goal attainment is determined jointly by the nurse, patient, and members of the healthcare team.

Although a separate and distinct phase, evaluation also is ongoing throughout the nursing process (Alfaro-LeFevre, 2014). Judgments made in previous phases usually result in prompt reassessment, rediagnosis, and replanning. Nurses continually assess responses of patients to particular nursing interventions, establish different priorities for nursing diagnoses, and alter plans of care as necessary.

The plan of care is the foundation for evaluation. The identified nursing diagnoses, patient goals, outcome criteria, and nursing interventions are the guides. Through this process, nurses determine the appropriateness, accuracy, and relevance of these nursing care components. Evaluation also helps nurses discover any errors that may have occurred in previous steps of the nursing process. Nurses always consider evaluation in light of how the patient responded or reacted to the planned course of action. Figure 15-4 illustrates the relationship of the activities of the evaluation phase to the other phases of the nursing process.

There are several purposes for carrying out evaluation (Alfaro-LeFevre, 2014; Carpenito, 2012):

- To examine the patient's behavioral responses to nursing interventions
- To compare the patient's behavioral responses with predetermined outcome criteria
- To appraise the extent to which patient goals were attained or problems resolved
- To appraise involvement and collaboration of the patient, family members, nurses, and healthcare team members in healthcare decisions
- To provide a basis for the revision of the plan of care
- To collect subjective and objective data to make judgments about nursing care delivered
- To monitor the quality of nursing care and its effect on the patient's health status

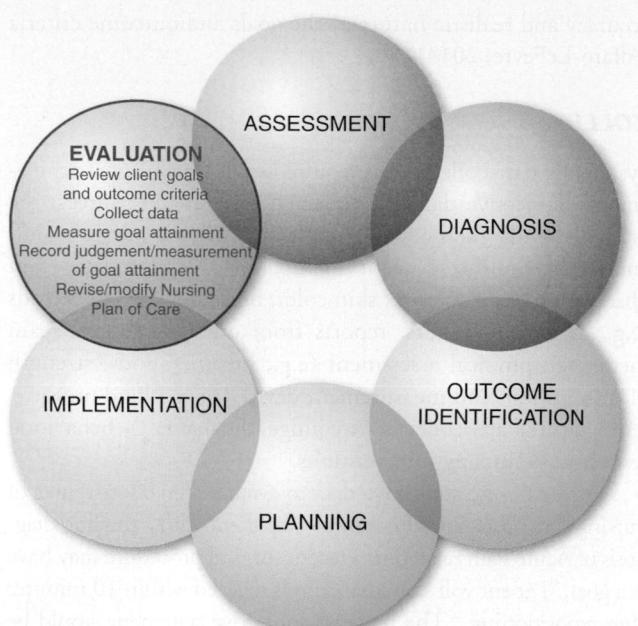

FIGURE 15-4 ANA Standard VI states: "The nurse evaluates the patient's progress toward attainment of outcomes." This illustration shows activities used in the evaluation phase and also the relationship of evaluation to the other phases of the nursing process.

Specific activities during this phase include the following:

- Review patient goals and outcome criteria
- Collect data
- Measure goal attainment
- Record judgments or measurements of goal attainment
- Revise or modify the patient's plan of care

Evaluation Skills

KNOWLEDGE OF STANDARDS OF CARE

Standards of care are authoritative statements made by nursing organizations (e.g., American and Canadian Associations of Neuroscience Nurses), external review boards (e.g., The Joint Commission, 2013), or healthcare institutions (e.g., your employer) that describe the responsibilities of the nursing profession, against which its practitioners are held accountable (ANA, 2010). Knowledge of the current standards of care proposed by nursing organizations, external review boards, and one's own healthcare institution (e.g., policies and procedures) is necessary to evaluate nursing care. Standards of care guide professional practice and serve as the framework for the evaluation of practice (ANA, 2010).

KNOWLEDGE OF NORMAL PATIENT RESPONSE

The nurse's knowledge of many subjects, such as physiology, pathophysiology, biochemistry, psychology, sociology, and pharmacology, comes into play when evaluating normal patient responses. Nurses obtain a tremendous knowledge base about patient responses during their basic nursing education. They acquire additional knowledge and updating of information

through formal and informal continuing education. Obtaining college credits in nursing is an example of formal continuing education. Attendance at nursing conferences and seminars is an example of informal continuing education. Nurses also sharpen skills and update knowledge about patient responses through clinical experience, guidance and assistance from mentors, and reading textbooks and journal articles.

ABILITY TO MONITOR THE EFFECTIVENESS OF NURSING INTERVENTIONS

Many intellectual and technical skills are necessary to monitor the effectiveness of nursing interventions. Nurses need interviewing techniques and physical assessment skills to obtain subjective and objective data from patients and their family members. Knowledge of interviewing techniques, such as types of questions, interview phases, and the appropriate environment for interviewing, facilitates the collection of subjective data for evaluation of the plan of care.

Physical and functional assessment skills are necessary to monitor the effectiveness of nursing interventions. The ability to inspect, palpate, percuss, and auscultate proficiently provides objective data about the effectiveness of nursing interventions. For example, if a patient has impaired gas exchange related to shallow breathing and congestion, auscultation of breath sounds will yield information about the effectiveness of nursing interventions.

Knowledge and skill when using measurement devices yield further information about the effectiveness of nursing interventions. Many technologic advances in medicine and nursing make it mandatory for nurses to have knowledge and skill in the use of multiple measurement devices. Nurses use devices such as blood pressure cuffs, thermometers, blood glucose meters, arterial lines, and intracranial pressure monitors, depending on the practice setting. Measurement devices provide objective information for the evaluation of patient outcomes.

Nursing also requires knowledge and skill in interpreting laboratory data. Laboratory studies, such as complete blood counts, arterial blood gas determinations, and routine urinalysis tests, provide data for evaluation of patient outcomes. For example, in the same patient with Impaired Gas Exchange related to shallow breathing and congestion, arterial blood gas measurements help nurses determine the patient's oxygenation, respiratory status, metabolic status, and the need for suctioning.

AWARENESS OF CLINICAL RESEARCH

The nursing profession uses research findings to develop innovative methods to sharpen assessment and diagnostic skills; establish future standards for developing patient goals, patient outcomes, and nursing interventions in the planning stage; and provide the latest knowledge to enhance nursing practice. Reviews of clinical research also provide a basis for best practice guidelines and serve as another excellent resource for nurses in evaluating care. The Institute for Healthcare Improvement (IHI) is an independent not-for-profit organization that has partnered with many healthcare organizations to improve the quality and safety of care delivery while decreasing cost and inefficiency. Among IHI's many programs are IHI bundles, which present evidence-based practices (three to five interventions) that have been demonstrated to significantly improve care when all elements in the bundle are collectively and consistently practiced. IHI bundles are highlighted in many clinical chapters throughout this text.

Types of Evaluation

STRUCTURE EVALUATION

Structure evaluation focuses on the attributes of the setting or surroundings where healthcare is provided. It deals with the environmental aspects that directly or indirectly influence the quality of care provided. Availability of equipment, layout of physical facilities, nurse–patient ratios, administrative support, and maintenance of nursing staff competence are some areas of concern for structure evaluation.

PROCESS EVALUATION

Process evaluation focuses on the nurse's performance and whether the nursing care provided was appropriate and competent. The phases of the nursing process are used as the framework for the evaluation of nursing care. Areas of concern for this type of evaluation include the type of information obtained by interview and physical assessment, the validity of the nursing diagnostic statements, and the nurse's technical competence.

OUTCOME EVALUATION

Outcome evaluation, which focuses on the patient and the patient's function, is currently receiving a great deal of emphasis. Outcome evaluation determines the extent to which the patient's behavioral response to nursing intervention reflects the desired patient goal and outcome criteria. Outcome evaluation can take place only after standards have been developed. An example of an outcome evaluation is to establish standards of care for a specific diagnosis and then compare actual patient outcomes with that standard.

Evaluation Activities

REVIEW PATIENT GOALS AND OUTCOME CRITERIA

Measuring goal attainment starts by reviewing the patient goals and outcome criteria, written in measurable terms, developed for each problem or nursing diagnosis. Nurses review expected patient behaviors by examining the time frames and methods for measurement of goal fulfillment. They evaluate patient goals and outcome criteria in various ways, including observing patient behaviors, using documentation of the patient's responses to interventions, and receiving feedback from the patient, family members, and other healthcare providers, if appropriate. This review helps nurses focus on data they need to assess the accuracy and realistic nature of the goals and outcome criteria (Alfaro-LeFevre, 2014).

COLLECT DATA

Systematic data collection is required to determine goal achievement. Subjective data are collected from many sources: the patient, family members or significant others, nursing staff, and other healthcare team members. Objective data from observation (e.g., posture, skin color, behavior), health records (e.g., laboratory results, reports from other healthcare team members), physical assessment (e.g., breath sounds, strength of extremities), and measurement devices (e.g., blood pressure, temperature) are collected to judge the patient's behavioral responses to nursing interventions.

Nurses also use subjective data to evaluate the effectiveness of nursing care provided. For example, a patient with a nursing diagnosis of Acute Pain related to a recent surgical procedure may have as a goal, "Patient will state that pain is relieved within 10 minutes after repositioning." The patient's subjective statement would be needed to judge whether this goal has been achieved.

MEASURE GOAL/OUTCOME ACHIEVEMENT

After collecting data, nurses form a comprehensive picture of the patient's behavioral responses. The next activity is to make a judgment about goal attainment by comparing the patient's actual behavioral responses to the predicted responses or predetermined outcome criteria developed in the planning phase. When possible, the patient is involved.

The four possible judgments that may be made are as follows (Alfaro-LeFevre, 2014):

- The goal was completely met.
- The goal was partially met.
- The goal was completely unmet.
- New problems or nursing diagnoses have developed.

The fourth judgment can exist simultaneously with any of the first three. Table 15-2 provides some examples of a completely met goal, a partially met goal, and a completely unmet goal. Once the judgment about the attainment or lack of attainment of the outcome criteria is made, the plan of care is revised. (See the Revise or Modify the Plan of Care section presented later in this chapter.)

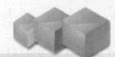 **Concept Mastery Alert**

If the nurse determines that the expected outcomes of the patient's plan of care are unrealistic or inappropriate, there are other options apart from creating a completely new plan of care. This could include adjusting the timing of outcomes, amending them so that they are more readily achievable, or changing the interventions with the goal of facilitating the patient's progress. Amending the plan of care is usually preferable to discarding it.

TABLE 15-2 CLINICAL EXAMPLES OF EVALUATION OF GOAL ATTAINMENT

Nursing Diagnosis	Patient Goal	Subjective Data Collected	Objective Data Collected	Goal Judgment
Impaired Swallowing related to neuromuscular impairment	Patient will demonstrate correct eating techniques to maximize safe swallowing.	Patient states, "I sit up in a chair for a half hour after I eat."	Patient wears dentures when eating; performs return demonstration of facial exercises; bends head forward when eating; checks mouth for any remaining food particles; remains in Fowler's position for at least 30 min after eating; lies on side while lying in bed.	Goal completely met.
Chronic Low Self-Esteem	Patient interacts verbally in group therapy session.	Patient states, "I feel uncomfortable when speaking in front of others."	Patient observed sitting in group session, looking at floor, and participating minimally.	Goal partially met.
Impaired Physical Mobility related to neuromuscular impairment	Patient will carry out prescribed mobility regimen.	Patient states, "I can't do anything by myself. I need a lot of help with everything."	Patient unable to perform active range-of-motion exercises independently; unable to transfer from bed to wheelchair; unable to dress and groom independently.	Goal completely unmet.

Assess Facilitators of Goal Attainment

Patients, family members, significant others, and other healthcare team members are invaluable in facilitating or helping with goal attainment. Occasionally, only those closest to the patient can identify the subtle or elusive factors that helped (or hindered) goal achievement. Examples of other resources that facilitate goal attainment include audiovisual materials, written handouts, repetition of material, and easily accessible and interested nursing staff.

Assess Barriers to Goal Attainment

Several barriers to goal attainment have been identified. Barriers may involve the patient, family members or significant others, and the nurse or other healthcare team members. Examples of how goal attainment may be blocked include providing incorrect information, withholding information, poor communication between team members, having an unexpected reaction to treatment (e.g., allergic response), possessing inadequate coping ability, and experiencing a worsened underlying pathologic condition.

Family members also may act as barriers to goal achievement in many ways. For example, their lack of understanding of the plan of care, lack of interest in the patient, or failure to realize that the patient actually has a problem can impede movement toward a goal.

Nurses may unwittingly block goal achievement, for instance, by neglecting to collect pertinent assessment data, assigning an inappropriate priority rating to nursing diagnoses, or delegating nursing care to inappropriate nursing staff members. Nurses may fail to include patients in the planning step, neglect to incorporate facets of the medical regimen when developing the plan of care, or forget to share critical information with other members of the healthcare team.

Other healthcare team members also may be barriers. They may lack communication among themselves, be unable to work together as a team, or fail to coordinate the activities of all healthcare team members. When healthcare team members do not share information among themselves, continuity in the planning and implementation of care is hampered. The evaluation phase identifies the barriers that are interfering with the patient's advancement toward goal achievement.

RECORD JUDGMENT OR MEASUREMENT OF GOAL ATTAINMENT

Written documentation of the subjective and objective data gathered and the judgment made about goal attainment is required on the patient's health record. Judgments about goal attainment are written clearly and concisely. Avoid ambiguous terminology, such as "inadequate," "good," or "extremely well," which can be interpreted differently by different people.

REVISE OR MODIFY THE PLAN OF CARE

Revision or modification of the plan of care is part of the evaluation phase. It provides a feedback mechanism that starts the entire chain of events again. Figure 15-5 illustrates the feedback mechanism and the cyclic nature of the nursing process, starting with a complete reassessment of the patient.

Nursing diagnoses that are resolved require no further nursing intervention and may be removed from the plan of care.

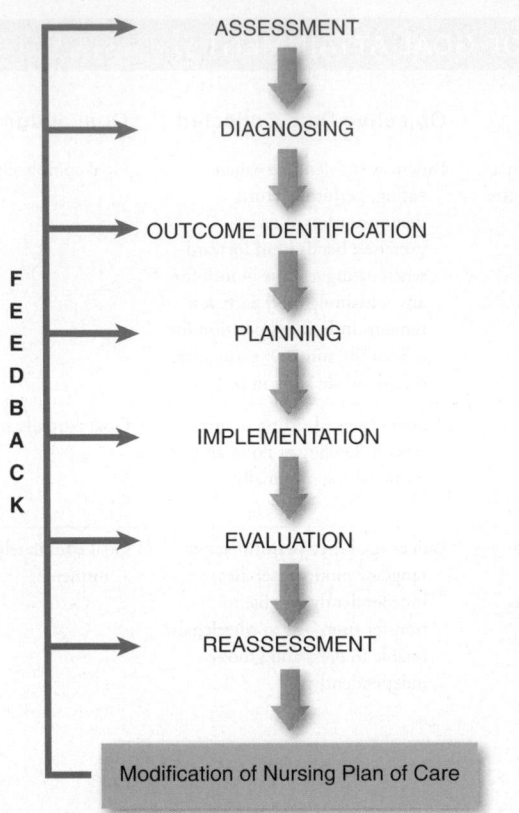

FIGURE 15-5 Feedback mechanism and cyclic nature of the nursing process.

To maintain the patient's "problem-free status," a plan of care may be developed that incorporates potential for wellness and other health-promoting nursing diagnoses and focuses nursing actions toward maximal functioning. The level of functioning and changes in health status are periodically reassessed to determine whether new problems or nursing diagnoses have developed.

Some patient goals are partially met or completely unmet. Modification begins with a complete patient reassessment. Changes in patient goals, patient outcome criteria, and nursing interventions are required. If new problems have arisen, new nursing diagnoses must be identified and a patient plan of care written. Figure 15-6 illustrates the steps taken after judging goal attainment and needed revisions of the plan of care.

QUALITY IMPROVEMENT PROGRAMS

Evaluation can also focus on the quality of nursing care provided to groups of patients with similar problems or nursing diagnoses. **Quality improvement programs** are mechanisms for healthcare organizations to assess and improve care (Ellis & Hartley, 2012). Formerly referred to as quality assurance monitors, total quality management (TQM), total quality improvement (TQI), or continuous quality improvement (CQI), these programs ensure that

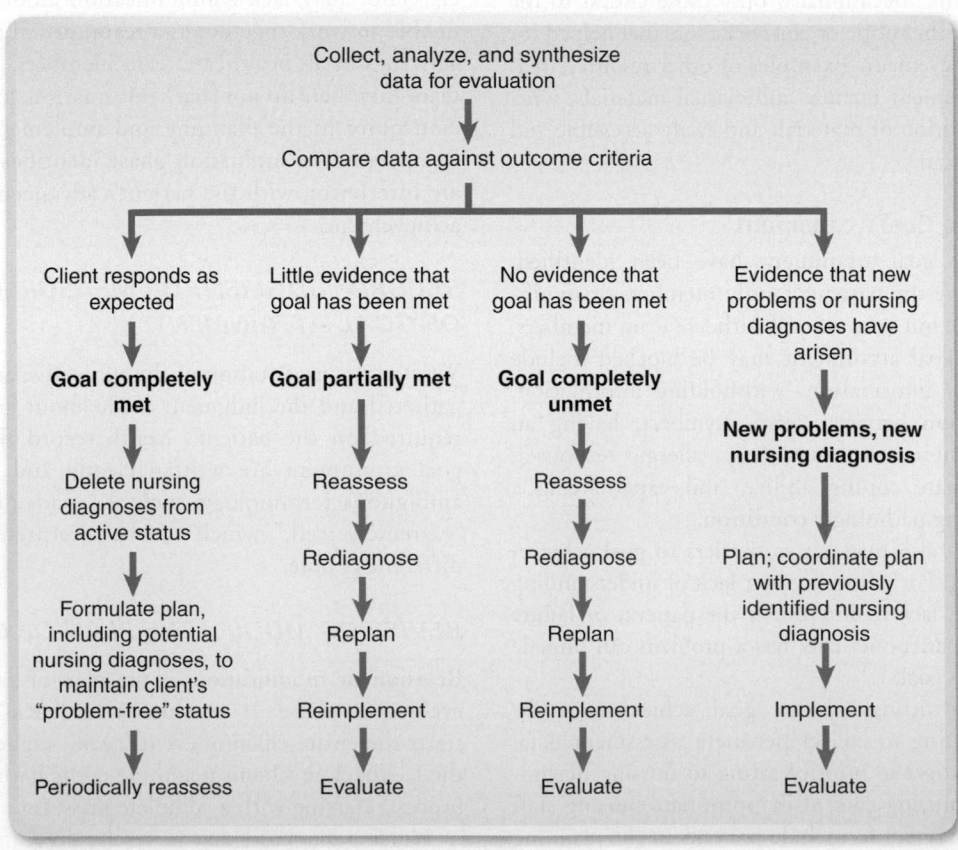

FIGURE 15-6 Flowchart to identify actions taken after judgment of goal achievement.

quality patient care is provided and standards are upheld. They provide input for the development and refinement of standards of care for groups of similar patients. Standards provide the basis for quality monitors because they express nursing's professional accountability to the public and provide a framework for the evaluation of nursing practice (ANA, 2010).

Quality improvement involves measuring the extent to which standards have been achieved. Focus on quality improvement is the combined result of consumer demands for high-caliber health services and soaring healthcare costs. Also, governmental agencies, accreditation groups, and regulatory bodies have pressured the nursing profession to respond to quality improvement issues. Standards of care have been proposed by the ANA, the Joint Commission, the IHI, specialty nursing organizations, and individual healthcare institutions.

American Nurses Association

The ANA first established the *Standards of Nursing Practice* in 1973. In 2004, the ANA published *Nursing: Scope and Standards of Practice*, which included "standards of practice" and "standards of professional performance." In the 2010 edition, an expansion of measurement criteria and the addition of a leadership standard were included. Based on a nursing process framework, standards of practice are composed of six nursing standards for providing nursing care to all patients in any setting. The behaviors and roles of professional nurses are described in the nine standards of professional performance. In the 2010 edition, an additional standard of professional performance, "environmental health," was added that outlined key aspects of environmentally safe and healthy nursing practice. Both sets of standards include measurement criteria for evaluating nursing care and performance.

Some specialty nursing groups, in conjunction with the ANA, have developed processes and outcome criteria for several nursing diagnoses. For example, the Association of Rehabilitation Nurses and the American Association of Neuroscience Nurses have set standards based on nursing diagnoses applied to their specialty.

Joint Commission

The Joint Commission (2013) is an external review board that establishes standards for institutions to ensure that the institution functions within specified guidelines. The hospital standards for nursing care are applicable to all patients in every setting where nursing care is provided. Recent changes in the guidelines require the continuous monitoring and evaluation of the quality of nursing care provided by the department of nursing. The guidelines are general, and each institution develops a specific quality improvement program suited to its organizational structure.

Peer Review

Peer review is the evaluation and judgment of a nurse's performance by other nurses. It is another mechanism for evaluating and monitoring the nursing care provided. The two types of peer review are nursing monitors and individual peer review.

NURSING AUDIT

The **nursing audit**, sometimes referred to as a nursing monitor, is any review completed by a nurse of a patient's care or records to evaluate whether established standards were met. Nursing audit committees generally establish the standards against which observed data are measured. Although nursing departments develop their own standards for particular nursing care settings, the ANA's (2010) *Nursing: Scope and Standards of Practice* (2nd ed.) is often used as a model in generating unique standards for a particular setting or institution. Members of the audit committee may review a nurse's documentation of care in the health record, or they may determine the patient's health status through observation.

INDIVIDUAL PEER REVIEW

The second type of peer review is individual peer review, which focuses on the nurse. An individual nurse's performance is evaluated and judged by other nurses with similar education and experience. This type of review also is based on pre-established standards and may be part of a nurse's annual performance evaluation.

 APPLY YOUR CRITICAL THINKING

Your nurse manager asks you to participate in a pain audit. You are asked to review 100 patient records, on your surgical unit, to evaluate whether each patient's pain rating was documented before and 30 minutes after pain medication was administered. You have never participated in an audit before but are pleased that your nurse manager has confidence in you. How will such an audit benefit you, the unit, and the patients who receive care?

Check your answer in Appendix B.

KEY CONCEPTS

- Nurse-prescribed actions are based on patient interventions that nurses can legally perform without a physician's order. Collaborative problems are those in which nurses use both physician- and nurse-prescribed interventions to give care.
- Implementing the plan of care requires intellectual, interpersonal, and technical skills.
- Evaluation is a process for determining to what degree patient outcomes and goals have been met. It occurs throughout all steps of the nursing process but also is a distinct, separate step.
- An in-depth, comprehensive judgment about patient goal attainment and fulfillment and degree that outcomes have been met is performed during the evaluation step of the nursing process.
- The patient's plan of care forms the foundation for evaluation. The nurse and patient determine goal attainment.
- The nurse, patient, family members, significant others, and other healthcare team members may help or hinder goal attainment.

- Revising the plan of care involves reassessment, rediagnosis, and replanning.
- Evaluation determines the reasons the plan of care was a success or failure.
- Quality improvement involves the monitoring (audits) and evaluating of nursing care against standards of nursing practice.

PRACTICING FOR THE NCLEX

CHECK YOUR ANSWERS IN APPENDIX A.

1. What are important factors in setting nursing priorities? Select all that apply:
   a. Patient condition
   b. Reassessment data
   c. Modification of the plan of care
   d. Feedback from the family and healthcare team

2. A nurse is caring for a patient with anorexia. Which of the following would be an example of interpersonal nursing interventions?
   a. Provide basic dental hygiene
   b. Educate on minimal dietary requirements
   c. Supervise patient's oral intake
   d. Provide opportunity to examine values

3. A nurse is developing medication safety protocols for the hospital and is looking at the appropriate delivery of crushed medications via gastric tubes. This is an example of what type of evaluation?
   a. Structure evaluation
   b. Process evaluation
   c. Outcome evaluation
   d. Functional evaluation

4. The nurse is caring for a patient after gastric bypass surgery. The goal is for the patient to be able to feed herself appropriately. The patient correctly states, "I should only drink 30 cc of juice an hour." The patient struggles to demonstrate measuring and monitoring of intake frequency, as she is having frequent vomiting. How would the nurse evaluate the attainment of this goal?
   a. Goal completely met
   b. Goal partially met
   c. Goal completely unmet
   d. Modification of plan of care needed

5. Evaluation of nursing quality may be directly done by which of the following? Select all that apply.
   a. Peer review
   b. Management audit
   c. The ANA
   d. The Joint Commission

REFERENCES

Alfaro-LeFevre, R. (2014). *Applying nursing process: The foundation for clinical reasoning* (8th ed.). Philadelphia, PA: Wolters Kluwer Health/Lippincott Williams & Wilkins.

American Nurses Association. (2010). *Nursing: Scope and standards of practice* (2nd ed.). Silver Spring, MD: Author.

American Nurses Association. (2012). *Principles for delegation by registered nurses to unlicensed assistive personnel (UAP)*. Silver Spring, MD: Author.

Bulechek, G. M., Butcher, H. K., Dochterman, J. M. & Wagner, C. M. (2013). *Nursing interventions classification (NIC)* (6th ed.). St. Louis, MO: Elsevier Mosby.

Carpenito, L. J. (2012). *Nursing diagnosis: Application to clinical practice* (14th ed.). Philadelphia, PA: Wolters Kluwer Health/Lippincott Williams & Wilkins.

Ellis, J. R., & Hartley, C. L. (2012). *Nursing in today's world: Trends, issues, and management* (10th ed.). Philadelphia, PA: Wolters Kluwer Health/Lippincott Williams & Wilkins.

National Council of State Boards of Nursing. (2005). *Working with others: A position paper*. Chicago, IL: Author. Retrieved July 11, 2015, from https://www.ncsbn.org/Working_with_Others.pdf

The Joint Commission. (2013). *2014 hospital accreditation standards*. Oakbrook Terrace, IL: Joint Commission Resources.

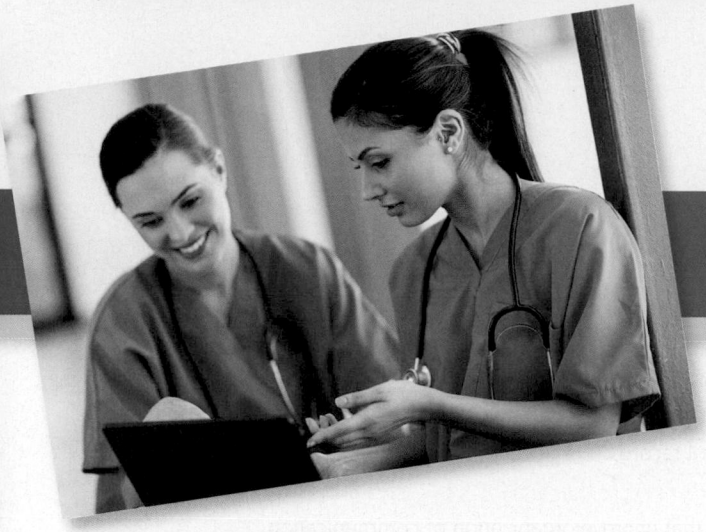

CHAPTER 16

Documentation and Communication in the Healthcare Team

Constance Hirnle

Case Scenario

You arrive for work at 7:00 AM and receive a report from the night shift nurse. The following information was documented in the electronic health record (EHR) and related to you verbally at handoff:

- Mrs. Smith had a terrible night. She was bloated and very nauseated. Bowel sounds present in all quadrants. She complained that her doctor never came in to see her, and when he did, he didn't seem very interested in how she felt.
- Vital signs: BP 176/74, P 92, R 18, oxygen saturation 95%.
- Complaining of incisional pain; morphine sulfate given. She was also upset about her family.

Once you have completed this chapter and have incorporated documentation and communication in the healthcare team into your knowledge base, review the above scenario and reflect on the following areas of Critical Thinking:

1. Identify missing information that you need to safely assume care for Mrs. Smith.
2. Identify some positive qualities in the charting. Then identify at least five weaknesses in this charting and why you see them as problematic.
3. Assume you are the registered nurse (RN) giving the report. Construct RN to RN verbal handoff for this patient using SBAR and written documentation using SOAP, PIE, and FOCUS formats. Add hypothetical data as necessary to reflect information that would be important to chart. Compare and contrast charting using these different methods.
4. Reflect on possible legal or ethical problems with the chart entries as written originally.

KEY TERMS

audit
batch charting
charting by exception (CBE)
clinical pathways
computer-based personal record (CPR)
Computerized Physician (Provider) Order Entry (CPOE)
confidentiality
consults
documentation
electronic medication administration record (eMAR)
flow sheets
FOCUS system
handoff
Health Insurance Portability and Accountability Act (HIPAA)
incident
meaningful use
Never Events
Outcome and Assessment Information Set (OASIS)
PIE charting
plan of care
point of care documentation (POC)
quality assurance memos
reporting
Resident Assessment Instrument (RAI)
SBAR
SOAP note
TeamSTEPPS™
variance

Upon completion of this chapter, you will be able to do the following:

1. Describe the importance of timely, accurate communication in healthcare.
2. Describe the purposes of the patient record.
3. List key principles of charting.
4. Discuss the relevance of electronic records in documentation.
5. Properly create nursing progress notes by SOAP, PIE, FOCUS, or narrative format.
6. Identify flow sheets, plans of care, and critical pathways used in patient records.
7. Identify critical components for safe patient handoff.
8. Describe communication tools in TeamSTEPPS™ (such as SBAR, CUS) that improve organization of communication.
9. Discuss the importance of confidentiality and the RN's legal responsibility in documenting and reporting.

Ongoing, effective communication among all members of the healthcare team assures that patients receive care that is safe, timely, and responsive to patient needs. Nurses are integral to this process as they coordinate care and apply their knowledge and skill using the nursing process to deliver care. The nursing process is communicated in writing and verbally. Inaccurate, absent, or delayed communication can subject the patient to serious risks or delayed recovery. The Joint Commission identified critical communication failure as one of the most common root causes responsible for sentinel events during 2004–2014 (Joint Commission, 2014).

Handwritten or typed communication, or documentation, serves as a permanent record of patient information and care. The patient record is a repository for documentation of each encounter and resides in an electronic record or paper chart. It provides information during the current visit or admission and may be consulted in the future to review the patient's history or for educational, research, and legal purposes. Reporting takes place when two or more people share information about patient care, either face-to-face (as in a team meeting or handoff), by audiotape or voice mail, or by telephone (e.g., as in reports to a case manager or physician from a nurse making home visits).

Nurses are responsible for accurate, complete, and timely documentation and reporting. As an instrument of continuous patient care and as a legal document, the patient record should contain all pertinent assessments, planning, interventions, and evaluations for that patient.

Documentation and reporting of the patient's condition require adherence to the highest standards of confidentiality. At all times, nurses must be aware that what is written and spoken about patients is of a personal nature and should reflect consideration for each person's basic human dignity. Patients expect that information about them will be shared only with those who need to know and who will be contributing to their care.

PATIENT MEDICAL RECORD

Clear, accurate, and up-to-date patient documentation is a cornerstone for safe care delivery providing flow of information between providers of care. The record of a patient's progress and the care provided is a compilation of health-related data. Management of these data—their organization, input, and retrieval—forms the basis for interdisciplinary communication. The manner in which each member of the healthcare team accesses and contributes to the record may differ. Each piece of data, however, is crucial in forming an actual picture of the patient, his or her health status, and the care he or she has received. The patient record promotes a coherent plan of care, communication of common and individual goals, and progress of the patient toward those goals. An accurate and complete record must be accessible to members of the healthcare team who care for the patient. If a patient record or portions of it are unavailable or inaccurate, a vital line of communication is blocked.

Documentation of the nursing process within this record provides essential data related to assessment, interventions, and goals. Nurses' entries on the patient record are important because they show medical and nursing orders carried out, independent assessments and interventions performed, the exact dates and times of care delivered, and evaluation of care provided. Documented patient responses to nursing interventions allow revision of the plan to assist the patient in meeting goals and obtaining optimal health and function.

The specific manner in which nursing documentation occurs reflects the philosophy and goals of the agency in which a nurse works. These, in turn, are affected by larger system issues, such as standards of care and documentation established by accrediting bodies, reimbursement requirements, changes in healthcare systems toward multisite and multiagency coordination, and the movement toward a universal computer-based patient record.

Purposes of the Medical Record

COMMUNICATION

Clearly documented information on the patient record communicates the plan of care and the patient's progress to all members of the healthcare team. Team members who interact with the patient at different times and in different ways get a clear picture of what took place in their absence. This communication helps ensure continuity of care and provides essential data for revision or continuation of care.

ASSESSMENT

Nurses and other team members gather assessment data from the patient record. By reading about the patient's history and initial assessment and comparing these data with additional subjective and objective information that has been obtained, current health status and progress toward goals can be determined. Progressive assessments of lung sounds, for example, might alert the nurse to a developing infection or indicate that fluid is accumulating in the lungs of a postoperative patient.

CARE PLANNING

Formulation of a plan of care flows from assessment data in the patient record. The nurse considers all data on the patient record when developing problems, goals, outcome criteria, interventions, and evaluation criteria for and with patients. An individualized plan of care is essential for each patient and becomes part of the permanent patient record. The exact written form can vary, depending on the agency, setting, and specialty in which care is delivered.

LEGAL DOCUMENT

The patient record serves as a legal document of the patient's health status and care received. It may be used in court to prove or disprove injuries a patient incurred unintentionally or to implicate or absolve a healthcare professional with regard to improper care. Legal cases have been argued with the principle that "if it was not documented, it was not done." For this reason, it is important to document normal as well as abnormal findings. Because nurses and other healthcare team members cannot remember specific assessments or interventions involving a patient years after the fact, accurate and complete documentation at the time of care is essential. The care may have been excellent, but the documentation must prove it.

QUALITY ASSURANCE

An **audit** is a review of records. Audits of patient records serve a dual purpose: quality assurance and reimbursement. Auditing is done for quality assurance when records are randomly selected to determine whether certain standards of care were met and documented. Results of an audit may then lead to changes in the manner in which care is provided. The goal is to review continually to improve the quality of nursing care provided. For example, a review of charts in a hospice setting may explain patterns of use of round-the-clock professional care for symptom management. As a result, the agency may provide additional training in symptom management to staff or to family members, or it may establish new policies regarding the use of 24-hour care. The Joint Commission audits patient records regularly and requires that institutions set up ongoing quality assurance programs as part of accreditation requirements. If deficiencies are detected, educational programs can be designed to improve outcomes in those areas. Additionally, the Joint Commission sets documentation standards to which institutions must adhere to maintain accreditation. These standards can change, so institutions must stay aware of current recommendations.

REIMBURSEMENT

Documentation of patient care provides the basis for decisions regarding care and subsequent reimbursement to the agency. Medicare, Medicaid, workers' compensation insurance, and third-party insurance companies usually require specific criteria to be met to cover specific health-related expenses. Documentation may support a diagnostic-related group (DRG) classification or identify interventions that were actually performed for the patient.

Several examples illustrate this point. To obtain reimbursement when a wound culture is done, documentation would indicate that appropriate assessment data were gathered and that the test was ordered by a provider and carried out by the laboratory. Administration of medication or the use of supplies may then be verified with additional documentation. Patients must meet "homebound" eligibility requirements for agencies to receive Medicare reimbursement for home care services; therefore, homebound status becomes an essential documentation component in the admission and ongoing assessment. Hospice beneficiaries generally receive care limited to their admitting diagnosis and must also meet standards for eligibility, such as consent to seek palliative care instead of curative treatments. Nurses must be familiar with the criteria for reimbursement in each setting and knowledgeable about obtaining authorization for care. Often, consulting other members of a care team, such as social workers and case managers, is helpful. Documentation must show that nurses have adhered to these guidelines in establishing and providing care.

In 2008, Medicare and Medicaid stopped reimbursement for some hospital-acquired complications that were deemed reasonably preventable through the use of evidence-based guidelines. These complications, including foreign objects left in the body after surgery, air emboli, infusion of incompatible blood, falls resulting in trauma, catheter-associated urinary tract infections, certain infusion-associated infections, and pressure ulcers, have been referred to as **Never Events** since they should never occur (Rosenthal, 2007). Documentation of preexisting conditions and assessments is essential in these situations to qualify for reimbursement when the record is reviewed.

The Health Information Technology for Economic and Clinical Health (HITECH) Act was established in 2009 to create incentives for professionals and agencies to receive financial payment for the **meaningful use** of technology to improve patient care. This act has encouraged healthcare agencies to computerize the patient record and use the data from these records to report on clinical quality measures (CQMs). CQMs include many aspects of patient care such as patient safety, care coordination, and patient engagement, and they become the basis for incentive payments from the Centers for Medicare and Medicaid Services (CMS). Meaningful use allows agencies to demonstrate the ability to electronically transfer clinical information as the patient moves from one care provider to another. Meaningful use also includes incentives to increases patients' access to their own medical records (Wilson, Murphy, & Newhouse, 2012) and to use data in the EHR to make appropriate clinical decisions about patient care. For example, computer programs can be written for the EHR to search data for early signs of sepsis. When identified, an alert would appear for the nurse or provider to further assess the patient for indicators of sepsis.

RESEARCH

Nursing and healthcare research is often carried out by studying patient records. Accurate documentation helps assure that research outcomes are valid and reliable. When information from patient records is obtained for nursing or medical research, strict guidelines must be followed to protect the privacy and rights of individual patients. Prior approval from the agency's institutional review board (IRB) must be obtained before proceeding with any research study. Data may be gathered from groups of records to determine significant similarities in disease presentation, to identify contributing factors, or to determine the effectiveness of therapies.

At times, data are collected without IRB approval for studies that are limited to internal quality improvement. In these cases, the data can never be reported to or used by any outside group. For example, a hospital nurse epidemiologist may review the records of patients who have had methicillin-resistant *Staphylococcus aureus* (MRSA) to determine patterns of hospital-acquired or drug-resistant infections. This information might be used to evaluate infection control measures and to plan more effective prevention strategies.

EDUCATION

Members of the healthcare team, including students of nursing, medicine, and other disciplines, use the patient record as an educational tool. It contains valuable information about signs and symptoms of disease, diagnostic tests, treatment modalities, and patient responses to the disease and to treatment. For example, a nursing student may read the record of a patient experiencing a stroke to learn the signs and symptoms the patient initially experienced, the results of the computed axial tomography scan, the effects of medications given to minimize brain injury, and the contribution of physical therapy to help the patient reach rehabilitation goals.

Electronic Health Records

Most clinical agencies have computerized part or all of the patient's record. Software programs allow nurses to enter assessment data quickly, usually by checking boxes and adding free text when appropriate. The **electronic medication administration record (eMAR)** interfaces medication orders with pharmacy dispensing and allows direct computer charting of medication administration. **Computerized physician (provider) order entry (CPOE)** allows authorized providers to enter all orders directly into the computer, electronically communicating orders to the laboratory, pharmacy, and nursing personnel. Appropriate staff members receive a computerized communication ("task") when treatments and medications are due during their assigned shift. They also receive a message when the patient requires reassessment (e.g., assessment of the effectiveness of the pain medication 15 minutes after administration) (Arditi, Rege-Walther, Wyatt, Durieux, & Burnand, 2012).

Although implementing an EHR is expensive and requires much planning and education, such systems significantly increase patient safety. They allow several health team members to view the patient record simultaneously. Those with special clearance may view the EHR off-site to note changes in patient condition or to order necessary laboratory tests, diagnostic studies, or medications. Computerization ensures that all entries are legible and time dated. It enables the graphing of trends in vital signs or assessment data. It minimizes compliance issues because programs will not let nurses enter data until they have completed all required fields. This ensures a more complete assessment. Some programs create plans of care from entered assessment data. Clinical agencies have protocols in place in the event of power loss or computer upgrades when documentation is completed on paper and later transferred to the EHR.

A confidential access code or password is provided to identify the nurse or other healthcare worker accessing the EHR; the access code allows the employee to sign on to the system and identifies entries as being made by that person, much as a handwritten signature does.

 SAFETY ALERT

To prevent unauthorized access to patient records, it is essential that employees not share access codes or passwords.

The nurse may record information about patient progress, using separate standard nursing formats, such as a plan of care or progress note (see later discussion). The system may rely on keyboard entry for progress notes, or it may use mouse-driven commands to access appropriate screens from which interventions may be selected as completed. The nurse may use the computer to review previous nursing assessments and interventions, print a current plan of care, or retrieve data from other disciplines.

UNIVERSAL COMPUTER-BASED PATIENT RECORD

In response to a federally initiated goal to have a single record for each citizen, much conversation regarding electronically maintained records now focuses on the **computer-based personal record (CPR)** (Kahn, Aulak, & Bosworth, 2009). Centralization of the patient record lends itself to increased accessibility beyond the primary institution. Healthcare practitioners within large and geographically dispersed healthcare organizations can have uniform access to a single patient record, allowing greater accuracy and improved care. The goal with the universal CPR is to have these benefits extend beyond specific care providers, allowing patients to share complete health information with any practitioner, regardless of institutional affiliation or time and place when care was originally provided. With the CPR, practitioners might, for example, have access to a listing of the patient's current medications and a thorough cardiac history at the time of an emergency. Patients with cancer could share reports between specialists and the primary care team with ease. People who are traveling would know that records of previous illnesses and conditions can be accessed readily.

An individual could have all or selected information from office appointments, hospital visits, laboratory tests, or prescriptions downloaded into their record. Standardization of technology is important to permit information from all sources to be easily scanned and downloaded, so these systems are in early development and testing. These systems also allow individuals to get medical information, find doctors and providers, make appointments, and communicate online with care providers.

CLINICAL SURVEILLANCE TOOLS

Computerization of the medical record also permits the use of automated clinical surveillance tools to scan in real time the medical record of all patients to detect assessment data indicating problems. One such tool, the Risk Assessment Report, provides risk scores on sepsis, pressure ulcers, falls, abnormal laboratory reports, and other criteria of interest (Whittington, White, Haig, & Slock, 2007). This permits early intervention and saves lives. An effective surveillance system depends on timely input of assessment data so the system can promptly detect problems (Jones, 2013). Frequently, patients show clinical signs of deterioration, but healthcare providers fail to respond for 24 hours before a critical adverse event. Many systems color code risk so that a nurse can monitor warnings from the surveillance system for a group of patients and intervene for patients with high-risk scores.

HANDHELD DEVICES

Smartphones and tablet computers are used by many staff in the clinical setting to quickly access information. Programs and applications are downloaded on these devices that can provide medical terminology, drug information, assessment tools, calculations, conversion tables, immunization guidelines, language translation, and medical sign language. Handheld devices can provide up-to-date information to teams on infection control or intravenous (IV) therapy, to enhance evidence-based clinical decisions. In some hospitals, these devices can scan a patient's identification band prior to medication administration. Benefits include improved patient outcomes and increased patient safety, including decreased medication errors.

> **SAFETY ALERT**
>
> Care must be taken to protect the confidentiality of any patient information stored on the device and to ensure protection when submitting patient information during a synchronization or wireless transaction.

STANDARDIZED VOCABULARY

The advent of electronic documentation has given impetus to the use of standardized medical and nursing vocabularies in the patient record. The American Nurses Association (ANA) endorses the development of nursing databases to support clinical practice. These databases, using standardized vocabularies, can assist in describing the practice of nursing, supporting research, and identifying the cost and effectiveness of nursing interventions. These can then be incorporated into nursing information systems to facilitate nursing practice and documentation. The ability to enhance consistency of data through standardization of language also makes retrieval of information easier. The ANA Steering Committee on Databases to Support Clinical Nursing Practice approves specific vocabularies as appropriate for nursing practice. At this time, these vocabularies include Omaha, Nursing Interventions Classification (NIC), Nursing Outcomes Classification (NOC), Home Health Care Classification (HHCC), NANDA-I, and Ozbolt's Patient Care Data Set (PCDS). The clinical chapters of this text present tables that include nursing diagnoses along with NIC and NOC criteria.

Principles of Documentation

Principles of good documentation are easier to accept and adopt if nurses keep in mind the purposes of the record. Remember that any entry made serves as communication within the healthcare team but also may be scrutinized carefully by students, lawyers, reimbursement agents, and researchers. The EHR has improved the quality of nursing documentation in some areas but poses challenges in other areas.

CONFIDENTIAL

Nurses are required legally and ethically to keep all information in the patient record confidential. The **Health Insurance Portability and Accountability Act (HIPAA)** that gives patients greater control over their medical records became effective in 2003. HIPAA regulates all areas of information management, including reimbursement, coding, and security of records. The HIPAA Privacy Rule requires an agency to make reasonable efforts to limit use of, disclosure of, and requests for protected health information to the minimum necessary to accomplish the intended purpose. Most agencies require students and employees to complete HIPAA training. HIPAA also provides for patient education on privacy protection, patient access to medical records, patient consent prior to disclosing information from the record, and patient recourse if privacy protections are violated.

> **SAFETY ALERT**
>
> Healthcare providers who violate HIPAA may face fines of up to $250,000 or even jail time (HIPAA, 1996). Employees have been fired for breaching HIPAA laws concerning confidentiality.

Confidentiality means keeping information private. This principle applies to computerized and written medical records and any information pertaining to the patient's health status or care received. All patient information is confidential and discussed only with other healthcare professionals directly involved in the patient's care. Do not discuss patient information with family members, friends, clergy, or nurses or physicians who are friends of the family without permission from the patient. Nurses should never discuss patients (with or without names) and their situations in public places such as elevators, hallways, or the cafeteria. People who hear conversations can misinterpret information, leading to anxiety or fear. Additional methods of protecting confidentiality include never sharing computer passwords and never leaving a computer with patient information unattended. Information from the patient's chart should not be removed from the patient care area.

> **SAFETY ALERT**
>
> Students must be careful to deidentify any patient information in written assignments to be HIPAA compliant. Never take forms from the agency even if patient identifiers (medical record number, age, birth date, agency name) have been removed. Instead, copy information into a notebook with all patient identifiers removed.

Do not send patient information over email, unless it has been encrypted to protect unauthorized access.

In recent years, social media sites provide an avenue for people to communicate, maintain friendships, and share information and pictures. Patient information, even without patient identifiers, should not be shared on social media. It is important for employees and students to be aware of school and agency policies regarding the appropriate use of social media.

> **SAFETY ALERT**
>
> Breach of patient confidentiality or noncompliance with policies can result in job termination, or dismissal or suspension from nursing school.

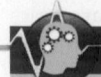

APPLY YOUR CRITICAL THINKING

You are working in a walk-in medical clinic. You see your cousin's boyfriend sitting in the waiting room. After his appointment, you look through his chart and discover that he was diagnosed and treated for a sexually transmitted infection (STI). You worry about the risk this poses to your cousin. What should you do?

Check your answer in Appendix B.

ACCURATE

Entries must be accurate. Nurses must chart only observations that they have seen, heard, smelled, or felt. An observation made by another health professional must be clearly identified as such. Precise measurements and times must be used whenever possible. For example, a wound should be described as "3 cm by 0.5 cm," rather than "small." If words are not adequate to describe the shape and color of a wound, documentation can also include photographs to depict the actual state of the wound on a given day. Correct spelling and correct use of medical terms are important. Proofreading of notes also helps to ensure readability. To avoid confusion, make certain that the names of physicians or other professionals mentioned are correct.

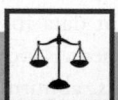

ETHICAL/LEGAL ISSUE

ACCURACY OF RECORDS

You are working on a busy medical unit where your responsibilities include administering medications to your patients. In preparing morning medications for a patient, you notice that an important cardiac medication that should have been given at 6:00 AM was not signed off as given in the medication record. You consult with another nurse, and she states, "The night nurse probably gave the medication and forgot to sign it off. I will just initial the medication so that she doesn't get in trouble with our charge nurse."

CRITICAL THINKING CHALLENGE

- Identify possible consequences of this situation for:
  - The patient
  - The nurse signing off the medication
  - The nurse who did not chart the medication
  - You, who witnessed the act
- How might you respond if you were witnessing this situation?
- Would your views on the situation differ if the medication was a laxative?

When information is charted in error, the patient record must be corrected. The EHR has systems that enter the corrected data, but all information that was charted remains in the patient record and can be retrieved and viewed at any time. Erasure is not permissible when documenting in a paper system. You must make a notation about the error.

Draw a single line through the error, and place your initials above it. Some institutions require an explanation of the error, such as "Charted for wrong patient." The computerized medical record provides a drop-down menu that includes "charted in error," allowing the nurse to reenter correct information yet keeping all previous entries.

Accuracy can be enhanced through **point of care documentation**, which is discussed later in this chapter. This may be as simple as recording data by hand onto the chart during an admission interview with a patient or as sophisticated as using a handheld electronic device that downloads the information into a system wide database.

CONCISE AND COMPLETE

Good charting is concise and brief, yet complete. Most EHR do not let nurses enter data until all required fields have been completed. In narratives, use partial sentences and phrases; drop the patient's name and terms referring to the patient. Use abbreviations but only those that are commonly accepted and approved by your facility. Common medical abbreviations are found in Appendix C. Table 16-1 lists abbreviations not endorsed for use by the Joint Commission and the Institute for Safe Medication Practices (ISMP) because they have been linked with increased risk for errors. Unnecessary elaboration confuses important issues. Being concise also is helpful in time management because nurses can spend less time charting and more time with patients.

Checklists have been used as tools to help organize and ensure that important tasks are completed and documented. Research conducted on teams using checklists has demonstrated a significant reduction in postoperative complications and resulted in cost savings (Semel et al., 2010). A simple checklist of four to five critical elements could be developed for various clinical situations. Developing standard tools, including simple checklists based on evidence, will help nurses consistently deliver safe and effective care to patients.

OBJECTIVE

When charting subjective findings, make every effort to identify the source and context for the finding. This point is particularly important when recording information about psychosocial and mental health issues. Directly quoting statements made by the patient can help maintain objectivity. For example, charting that a patient "States he misses the company of friends and is upset that they are no longer visiting" is more objective than is charting "Patient lonely and frustrated."

TABLE 16-1 ISMP LIST OF ERROR-PRONE ABBREVIATIONS, SYMBOLS, AND DOSE DESIGNATIONS

The 2004 Joint Commission on National Patient Safety Goals calls for organizational compliance with a list of prohibited "dangerous" abbreviations, acronyms, and symbols. To assist with this effort, we have updated our list of error-prone abbreviations, symbols, and dose designations, many of which have resulted in patient harm after being misinterpreted. As such, these items should be avoided with handwritten, preprinted, and electronic forms of communication. Since the Joint Commission has specified that certain abbreviations must appear on the organization's list, we have highlighted these items with a double asterisk (**). As of April 1, 2004, each organization must also include at least three additional items on its list. Selections can be made from below; however, we hope you will consider others beyond this minimum requirement.

Abbreviations	Intended Meaning	Misinterpretation	Correction
µg	Microgram	Mistaken as "mg"	Use "mcg"
AD, AS, AU	Right ear, left ear, each ear	Mistaken as OD, OS, OU (right eye, left eye, each eye)	Use "right ear," "left ear," or "each ear"
OD, OS, OU	Right eye, left eye, each eye	Mistaken as AD, AS, AU (right ear, left ear, each ear)	Use "right eye," "left eye," or "each eye"
BT	Bedtime	Mistaken as "BID" (twice daily)	Use "bedtime"
cc	Cubic centimeters	Mistaken as "u" (units)	Use "mL"
D/C	Discharge or discontinue	Premature discontinuation of medications if D/C (intended to mean "discharge") has been misinterpreted as "discontinued" when followed by a list of discharge medications.	Use "discharge" and "discontinue"
IJ	Injection	Mistaken as "IV" or "intrajugular"	Use "injection"
IN	Intranasal	Mistaken as "IM" or "IV"	Use "intranasal" or "NAS"
HS	Half-strength	Mistaken as bedtime	Use "half strength" or "bedtime"
hs	At bedtime, hours of sleep	Mistaken as half strength	
IU*	International unit	Mistaken as IV (intravenous) or 10 (ten)	Use "units"

Continued

TABLE 16-1 ISMP LIST OF ERROR-PRONE ABBREVIATIONS, SYMBOLS, AND DOSE DESIGNATIONS (*Continued*)

Abbreviations	Intended Meaning	Misinterpretation	Correction
q.d. or QD	Once daily	Mistaken as "right eye" (OD—oculus dexter), leading to oral liquid medications administered in the eye	Use "daily"
OJ	Orange juice	Mistaken as OD or OS (right or left eye); drugs meant to be diluted in orange juice may be given in the eye	Use "orange juice"
Per os	By mouth, orally	The "os" can be mistaken as "left eye" (OS—oculus sinister)	Use "PO," "by mouth," or "orally"
q.d. or QD˙	Every day	Mistaken as q.i.d., especially if the period after the "q" or the tail of the "q" is misunderstood as an "i"	Use "daily"
qhs	Nightly at bedtime	Mistaken as "qhr" or every hour	Use "nightly"
qn	Nightly or at bedtime	Mistaken as "qh" (every hour)	Use "nightly" or "at bedtime"
q.o.d. or QOD˙	Every other day	Mistaken as "q.d." (daily) or "q.i.d." (four times daily) if the "o" is poorly written	Use "every other day"
q1d	Daily	Mistaken as q.i.d. (four times daily)	Use "daily"
q6pm, etc.	Every evening at 6 PM	Mistaken as every 6 hours	Use "6 PM nightly" or "6 PM daily"
SC, SQ, sub q	Subcutaneous	SC mistaken as SL (sublingual); SQ mistaken as "5 every"; the "q" in "sub q" has been mistaken as "every" (e.g., a heparin dose ordered "sub q 2 hours before surgery" misunderstood as every 2 hours before surgery)	Use "subcut" or "subcutaneously"
ss	Sliding scale (insulin) or 12 (apothecary)	Mistaken as "55"	Spell out "sliding scale;" use "one half" or "½"
SSRI	Sliding scale regular insulin	Mistaken as selective serotonin reuptake inhibitor	Spell out "sliding scale (insulin)"
SSI	Sliding scale insulin	Mistaken as Strong Solution of Iodine (Lugol's)	
1/d	One daily	Mistaken as "tid"	Use "1 daily"
TIW or tiw	3 times a week	Mistaken as "3 times a day" or "twice in a week"	Use "3 times weekly"
U or u˙	Unit	Mistaken as the number 0 or 4, causing a 10-fold overdose or greater (e.g., 4U seen as "40" or 4u seen as "44"); mistaken as "cc" so dose given in volume instead of units (e.g., 4u seen as 4cc)	Use "unit"
Trailing zero after decimal point (e.g., 1.0 mg)˙	1 mg	Mistaken as 10 mg if the decimal point is not seen	Do not use trailing zeros for doses expressed in whole numbers
No leading zero before a decimal dose (e.g., .5 mg)˙	0.5 mg	Mistaken as 5 mg if the decimal point is not seen	Use zero before a decimal point when the dose is less than a whole unit

˙Identified abbreviations above are also included on the Joint Commission's "minimum list" of dangerous abbreviations, acronyms, and symbols that must be included on an organization's "Do Not Use" list, effective January 1, 2004. An updated list of frequently asked questions about this Joint Commission requirement can be found on their website at www.joint commission.org.

When documenting observations of patient behavior, the nurse must maintain objectivity by describing the actual behaviors rather than attempting to interpret the behaviors. For example, the nurse should chart that a patient is withdrawn and answers questions with one- or two-word answers. The nurse should not describe that patient as depressed or angry. Often, an EHR allows the nurse to type (free text) these observations in addition to checking boxes.

ORGANIZED AND TIMELY

Each entry must clearly show a logical and systematic grouping of important information by problem or occurrence. Computerized charting provides templates that organize data entry and required fields to ensure that important information is not omitted.

There must be a chronologic flow of information about patient care according to time and procedures completed, with

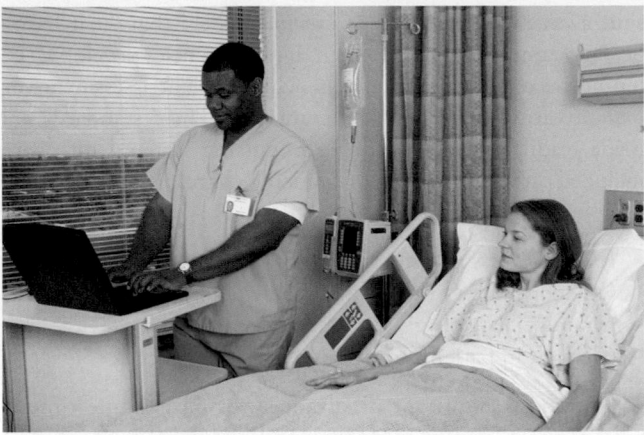

FIGURE 16-1 Portable computers allow for POC documentation.

- Falsifying patient records
- Failure to record changes in patient's condition
- Failure to document that physician was notified when patient's condition changed
- Inadequate admission assessment
- Failure to document completely
- Failure to follow agency's standards or policies on documentation
- Charting in advance

the patient's reaction documented. Recording as the events of the day unfold can prevent out-of-sequence or fragmented entries that may cause confusion.

Documentation that takes place as care occurs is referred to as point of care (POC) documentation (Fig. 16-1). With the goal of promoting efficiency, accuracy, and timeliness, POC documentation has become increasingly common. Nurses may carry handheld devices or portable computers that allow them to document care as they provide it to patients. In inpatient settings, terminals may be mobile or located at patients' bedsides. Information may then be downloaded via secured telecommunication links to the home agency or central computer server. As the field of telehealth develops, POC documentation can become interactive and include multimedia access. For example, homebound patients may be given monitoring equipment that reports vital signs to a remote hookup and alerts nursing staff to the need for follow-up.

Documentation in a timely manner can help avoid errors. Record all medications at the time they are given and procedures, treatments, and assessments as soon as possible after their completion. When charting electronically, make sure that your time signature coincides accurately with the time of the documented action. Timely documentation is especially important when the patient's status changes rapidly or frequent assessments are made. Document those changes as soon as possible. In inpatient and ambulatory settings, do not leave the unit for breaks or other long periods until important information is recorded. General statements regarding the patient's condition may require completion of the shift or visit before their entry into the record to maximize organization and conciseness of the report.

Most agencies and all EHR require documentation using a 24-hour clock (also known as military time) to avoid possible errors. Initiation of POC documentation in many settings is another strategy used to maximize accuracy and timeliness of entries. For example, a hospital may maintain assessment records at the bedside, or a home health agency may provide a handheld computer for nurses who make home visits.

Timeliness also helps avoid forgetting important information. Waiting until the end of the shift to record events on several patients, known as **batch charting**, may cause a nurse to omit important data or enter inaccurate information. If litigation occurs, lawyers use charted documentation to reconstruct time

sequences. Recording events in sequence provides support to demonstrate that appropriate responses were identified and reported. Doing so can be essential for protection from negligence or malpractice claims. See Box 16-1 for a list of high-risk errors in documentation. As all institutions move toward computerized documentation, timeliness becomes more important. The patient record must be complete and current so that care decisions can be made based on all information currently known. Care providers can access the records from many settings and may not even be on site when writing orders.

Nursing Entries in the Patient Record

PATIENT CARE SUMMARY OR KARDEX

The patient care summary or patient profile is a document that provides current patient information. The EHR continually updates orders into the patient care summary so that a nurse can get an overview of the treatments that are required. Historically, this information was entered and updated by a unit secretary onto a card usually kept in a portable file, thus the term *kardex*. Agencies that have not yet computerized the patient record may still use the kardex. The kardex is not part of the patient's record. Entries are made in pencil so that they can be erased when updating is needed.

Information commonly found on either the patient care summary or the kardex includes the following:

- Pertinent demographic information such as name, medical record number, emergency contacts, physician, admission date, allergies, diagnosis, surgery, or diagnostic procedures
- Code status
- Safety precautions for infection, falls, or skin breakdown
- Basic care needs such as activity status, diet, and hygiene
- Treatments and procedures (vital signs, dressings, catheters, respiratory therapy)
- IV therapy and blood transfusions
- Diagnostic and laboratory tests

ADMISSION ENTRIES

When a patient enters the healthcare system, a nursing history is completed. Nutrition, activity, sleep, and coping patterns are assessed and documented, as are the pertinent medical history and the history relating to the reason for current care. A complete physical assessment is performed and documented, usually within 24 hours. This information, which is entered on the nursing admission history and physical assessment sheet, provides a baseline for comparison when future assessments are done (see Chapter 17 for a full description of nursing history and physical assessment).

FLOW SHEETS

Flow sheets are tables that have vertical and horizontal columns that allow nurses to document routine assessments and procedures. In the EHR, the information documented in a table can be reformatted as a graph that can provide a visual picture of trends. Vital signs, intake and output, and routine assessments are often documented this way. In the critical care area, flow sheets are often more complex. Some flow sheets provide a form on which the nurse can indicate, usually by making a check mark, that assessment findings and care fall within the agency's standards. Standards require periodic assessments and notations, such as once per shift or weekly, so it is easy to note changes in patient status. More comprehensive documentation is required any time the patient's status changes significantly. Additional documentation is required when any deviation from standards is detected.

CHARTING BY EXCEPTION

Charting by exception (CBE) permits the nurse to document only those findings that fall outside the standard of care and norms that have been developed by the institution. CBE is a shift away from the concept previously held that "if it hasn't been documented, it hasn't been done." Agencies develop written norms and standards against which patient assessments or patient care activities can be compared. These standards are made readily available within the nursing site and often are included on the form or in the patient's chart for easy reference. CBE has some advantages:

- It requires less nursing time.
- Guidelines about expected outcomes and normal assessment parameters are clear.
- Changes in patient status can readily be detected.

The most significant disadvantage of CBE is the time it takes for each agency to develop and maintain standards and flow sheets; also, some agencies worry about legal challenges. CBE seems to work best in agencies or with conditions for which routine care can be anticipated.

NURSING PROGRESS NOTES

Nursing progress notes are recorded for all patients but vary in format depending on the agency and setting. Progress notes reflect a specific problem being addressed or the care provided over a specific period. Narrative notes, SOAP (Subjective, Objective, Assessment, Plan) notes, DAR (Data, Action, Response) notes, and PIE (Problem, Intervention, Evaluation) notes are all descriptive forms of documentation that summarize nursing assessments, interventions, and patient responses. Table 16-2 compares various formats for writing nursing

TABLE 16-2 COMPARING DOCUMENTATION NOTES

	Format	Advantages	Disadvantages
Narrative	Information provided in written sentences or phrases; usually time sequenced	Easy to learn; easy to adjust length as needed; can explain in detail	Time-consuming; difficult to retrieve information; irrelevant information often included; possibly unfocused and disorganized
SOAP	S—subjective data O—objective data A—assessment P—plan	All charting focuses on identified patient problems; interdisciplinary—all team members can chart on the same progress notes; easy to track progress for identified problem; steps in the nursing process are mirrored.	Difficult to master. Specific focus makes it difficult to chart general information without identifying a problem; lengthy and time-consuming; assessment identification difficult for nurses and confusing, because assessment data are provided in S and O.
PIE	P—problem I—intervention E—evaluation	Plan of care incorporated into progress notes; outcomes included, which increases quality assurance; daily review to determine progress; less redundancy; easily adapted to automated charting	Must read progress notes to determine plan of care; if problem has not been identified, difficult to chart; not multidisciplinary
FOCUS	D—data A—action R—response	Broad view permitting charting on any significant area, not just problems; concise, flexible; works well in long-term or ambulatory care	Not multidisciplinary; difficult to identify chronologic order; progress notes may not relate to the care plan.
Charting by exception (CBE)	Standards met—sign or check off; standards not met—write narrative or SOAP note	Efficient; use of flow sheets permitting rapid detection of changes in condition; outline normal assessments; can take the place of plan of care	Expensive to institute; in-servicing of staff is needed; not prevention focused; not appropriate for long-term or ambulatory care

progress notes. Because variations exist within each format, you must be familiar with your agency's guidelines to ensure complete documentation of patient care.

Regardless of the format used, the progress note is an evaluative statement summarizing significant problems or improvements. Flow sheets record collected data, whereas progress notes allow nurses to use critical thinking to document and communicate priority issues to other health team members. In the EHR, templates (SOAP, PIE, or DAR) can be provided in which the nurse can enter data using free texting.

Narrative Notes

This type of documentation is a method for recording relevant patient and nursing activities throughout a shift or during a single visit. It is commonly found in inpatient settings where records are organized according to the discipline charting or have a specially designated area for narrative notes by all disciplines. The note includes the date and time of the entry, identification of the role of the person writing the note, and specific activities accomplished (Fig. 16-2).

Many settings combine flow sheets with narrative notes to shorten recording time and reduce redundancy. Routine assessments (e.g., vital signs) or routine activities (e.g., IV care, dressing changes, bowel elimination) are recorded on flow sheets. They are then documented as they are completed throughout the day.

A form of the narrative note also may be used in home care settings, but it usually focuses on the problem or problems for which the patient is being seen. The nurse records assessment data, interventions performed, and responses noticed in a narrative format. Each individual visit report also may have a designated area that addresses routine issues covered—such as vital signs, communication with other disciplines, evaluation of care delegated to assisting personnel, or medications reordered.

A disadvantage of narrative notes is that they are time-consuming to write and that much reading can be required to learn about a specific problem. Narrative notes may necessitate checking various places within the chart to identify all activities that have occurred or to follow assessment data. The narrative form of charting increases the difficulty of performing audits

or chart reviews for quality assurance and is used infrequently now that most agencies are using an electronic medical record.

SOAP Notes

The SOAP note is a progress note that relates to only one health problem. All healthcare team members use the same format. The left-hand column or first line of the SOAP note identifies the problem being addressed from the master problem list. With this method, the patient's progress on that particular problem can be assessed without sorting through the whole chart. The team member need only read down the left-hand column of the interdisciplinary progress notes and read the notes of all disciplines that relate to that numbered problem.

After documenting the problem to be addressed, the next step is organizing the information in the SOAP note format. The "S" stands for *subjective* and refers to data or symptoms the patient expresses. Quotation marks are often used to document the patient's specific statements. If the patient cannot give information or gave none relevant to this problem, the "S" may be omitted or noted as "None."

"O" refers to *objective* findings and includes data collected by the nurse that are relevant to the problem. Objective data include what the nurse can see, feel, smell, or hear and relevant laboratory data, diagnostic tests, and vital signs.

"A" stands for *assessment*, which represents a diagnosis, an impression, or a condition change. This assessment is made after analyzing the data from the subjective and objective portions and must be supported by those data. If assessment cannot be made from the data gathered, write "Further data gathering necessary" or a statement such as "Abdominal pain, unknown etiology" under the "A" portion of the SOAP note.

"P" stands for *plan*. This portion deals with nursing interventions specifically related to the identified problem. The plan section may simply state, "Continue present regimen" if the assessment shows that the patient is progressing adequately using the plan already outlined. The plan also can specify revisions of the present nursing interventions as need are determined. Figure 16-3 provides an example of SOAP nursing progress notes.

3/15/2016	07:30—Client awake, alert, denies complaints, sitting up in bed watching TV, VS taken, IV infusing without difficulty, IV site right hand without redness, left hip drsg dry and intact. 08:30—100% of full liquid breakfast taken. 09:00—Partial bath at bedside, pt tolerated sitting in chair X 30 min without fatigue. 09:30—Change drsg to left hip approx 50 cc pink drng, sutures intact, no redness or edema at incision line, pt tol without pain. 10:15—1,000 cc D5 1/2 NS added to present IV to run at 125 cc/hr. pt resting. 11:00—To x-ray via stretcher. 11:45—Returned from x-ray, back to bed for rest. 12:00—Reg lunch taken 100% —M. S. Gorski, RN

FIGURE 16-2 Example of narrative nursing progress notes.

Problem #3	6/1/16 09:00	**"S"** My head hurts right in the back of my eyes. Patient describes pain worse bending over, like sinus headaches in past. **"O"** Eyes closed, lights dim, hesitant to move head when questioned. HR80 R20 P140/90 T98.6 **"A"** HA probable 2° sinus pressure. **"P"** 1. Decongestant prn as ordered 2. Warm wash cloth to eyes 3. Monitor temp q 4° 4. Assess pain after med and contact physician as indicated —M. S. Gorski, RN

FIGURE 16-3 Example of SOAP nursing progress notes.

Some agencies use the "SOAPIER" format of recording, which adds "I" for *intervention*, "E" for *evaluation*, and "R" for *revision*. This format allows the team member to record interventions, the patient's response to the plan, and any revisions needed to the plan. Remember that all information recorded under the SOAP or SOAPIER headings must pertain to the same problem.

In some circumstances, a full SOAP note may be unnecessary. Routine care may be documented on a flow sheet. Routine nursing assessments need not be written as a SOAP note if they are not specifically related to a problem (e.g., routine temperature and blood pressure in a patient who has had no problem with fever and has stable blood pressure).

PIE Notes

The **PIE charting** system simplifies documentation by incorporating the plan of care into the progress notes. Documentation is entered for each nursing diagnosis during every shift, using the acronym "PIE" to structure information according to *problem* (P), *intervention* (I), and *evaluation* (E). Patient assessments are not part of the PIE note because this information is recorded on flow sheets for each shift. Figure 16-4 provides

an example of a PIE nursing note. At the end of a 24-hour period, the nurse reviews patient documentation to ascertain the patient's response to therapeutic intervention and progress. In this way, he or she can eliminate outdated problems and add new problems to the documentation record. This daily review of patient progress helps promote continuity of care.

Variations for the PIE system can be used when appropriate. To designate new problems or abnormal assessments, "A" can be added to the numbered problem (i.e., APIE), allowing the nurse also to provide pertinent assessment data in the documentation. When appropriate, an intervention or an evaluation can be documented without writing the entire PIE statement.

Advantages of the PIE system of documentation include increased efficiency and flexibility; care planning focus; better tracking of patient problems, nursing interventions, and patient outcomes; and less redundancy. This system easily adapts to automated charting, and patient care can easily be audited. A disadvantage of the PIE system is that it is not multidisciplinary; it provides a documentation system only for nursing. Although the PIE system uses a nursing plan of care format, there is no written plan of care, which necessitates review of previous documentation to become knowledgeable about current nursing diagnoses.

Focus DAR Notes

The **FOCUS system** of documentation organizes entries by *data* (D), *action* (A), and *response* (R). This system is broader in its view because a focus can be a problem area (e.g., nursing diagnosis) but does not need to be. An entry can be made on a significant event, positive growth, or learning that occurs during a teaching session. In this way, patient documentation can focus on the patient's strengths as well as problem areas.

The data portion of the statement describes subjective and objective data that support the focus of the note. Interventions and treatments are included in the action section of the note, whereas the patient's response to therapy is discussed in the response section. Some notes may include all three sections, but flexibility permits the nurse to chart data, actions, and responses singularly or in combination. An example of a FOCUS nursing note appears in Figure 16-5.

PLAN OF CARE

A **plan of care** should be generated at admission and revised to reflect changes in the patient's condition. The trend is to involve the patient and all team members in the development and revision of the plan of care; however, the nurse often is the point person to promote good communication among all team members. The plan of care contains nursing diagnoses or problems, goals, outcome criteria, interventions, and evaluation. Standardized plans of care designed for patients with specific medical diagnoses may be used, but these plans must be individualized. The plan of care is part of the permanent patient record and is discussed in great detail in Chapter 14.

2/4/16 04:00	Problem #1	Caregiver role strain related to chronically ill spouse, lack of immediate family support, and financial stress.
	Intervention for P(#1)	IP(#1): Acknowledge and talk with caregiver about stress involved with 24-hour care for loved one.
		IP(#1): Allow caregiver to express feelings.
		IP(#1): Help caregiver identify possible supports within the family and community.
	Evaluation for P(#1)	EP(#1): Caregiver discussed the strain of caring for her husband; crying and demonstrating signs of anxiety, e.g., "I just don't think I will be able to do this for long and then what is going to happen to us all? Sometimes it seems so hopeless." Stated she felt her children were supportive but they lived in another state and could not help with the day-to-day problems. —R. Wolfe, RN
		Note: as additional data are charted for the problem of caregiver role strain, Problem #1 is used to identify the problem.

FIGURE 16-4 Example of a PIE nursing note arranging information by problem (P), intervention (I), and evaluation (E).

Date/ Time	FOCUS	NOTE
2/13/16 15:00	Injection Instruction	**Data:** Referred to injection room for teaching re-injection technique as wife will be discharged and needs IM injections of Compazine for nausea control. Husband states willingness to learn, yet states anxiety re-"sticking wife and causing her pain." **Action:** Demonstrate injection technique including drawing up medication in syringe, locating site, injecting medication, keeping record of medication administered. Have husband verbalize steps and then demonstrate technique. **Response:** Husband able to draw up medication correctly in syringe and verbalize steps to injection technique without cuing. Husband injected model, hands shook, and needed verbal cuing to aspirate. —J. Morales, RN
2/14/16 11:00	Injection Instruction	**Response:** Husband demonstrated good technique giving wife injection, without cuing. Wife will be discharged in AM with visiting nurse follow-up. —J. Morales, RN

FIGURE 16-5 Example of a FOCUS nursing note arranging information by data (D), action (A), and response (R).

CLINICAL PATHWAYS

With increasing interest in outcomes of care, many institutions and agencies have moved to the use of **clinical pathways** (sometimes referred to as collaborative pathways or care maps) as a way to guide the care of patients who have specific and generally predictable conditions. Based on scientific knowledge about best practices, clinical pathways serve as models for ensuring quality of care. The pathway may be for patients who require complex care (e.g., after organ transplantation) or for frequently encountered situations (e.g., home care visits for patients who have undergone hip replacement surgery). Pathways may look like flow sheets and may use CBE documentation. (See Chapter 14 for an example of a clinical pathway.)

Clinical pathways serve as multidisciplinary tools, identifying the expected progression of the patient toward discharge. They provide direction about major interventions to be performed: assessments, diagnostic tests, procedures, medications, teaching, activity, diet, and discharge planning. Documentation may occur on the pathway form, and then the nurse is required to sign his or her initials when a specific intervention has occurred or an outcome has been met. A **variance** occurs when the patient does not proceed along the pathway as planned. Any variances are documented in detail, usually with the use of nursing progress notes.

The provider initiates the clinical pathway for a specific patient through standard orders that match those identified in the pathway. Additional orders are written as needed to individualize care. The pathway is then placed in the patient's record, providing orders for care.

The clinical pathway provides a concise means for all members of the healthcare team to view the patient's continuing needs and progress toward discharge. This decreases the length of stay because care is coordinated. Review of variance data can help institutions seek improvements in care and can lead toward changes in pathways themselves.

WRITTEN HANDOFF SUMMARY

Handoff, or transfer of care for a patient from one health provider to another, significantly increases the risk of errors. Receiving staff must have up-to-date assessment data to safely care for the patient. Traditionally, nurses think of handoff occurring during shift change, but handoff also occurs when a patient is transferred from one area of the hospital to another. For example, handoff occurs when a postoperative patient moves from the postanesthesia care unit (PACU) to the surgical floor or back to the medical unit following dialysis or an invasive diagnostic procedure. Transfers also occur when a patient is transferred from one healthcare facility to another (e.g., from a hospital to a skilled nursing unit or a rehabilitation unit).

To minimize potential errors from lack of information, agencies often provide specific assessments on a written transfer summary in addition to a verbal report. Some agencies have created specific forms for this transfer of information, while others require documentation in the progress notes.

NURSING DISCHARGE SUMMARY

A nursing discharge plan is started at the initiation of care, indicating potential discharge needs and patient teaching that will take place. The discharge summary notes the patient's condition at discharge and provides specific information about care after discharge. A copy of the discharge summary may be given to the patient or sent to a home health nurse or extended care facility.

Nursing discharge summary forms are usually standardized and contain space to write specific instructions for the patient. Such information includes medications, diet, activity, follow-up care, and special instructions, such as circumstances that require notification of the physician (e.g., signs of wound infection). Sometimes these forms are completed in multiple copies so that a copy can be given immediately to the patient. More recently, computer-generated discharge forms can be individualized for the patient and obtained from software programs installed on the agency computer. Nursing discharge summary forms also contain space for documentation of vital signs, condition at discharge, method of discharge, time, and to whom and where the patient was discharged.

When a patient is transferred to a different facility (e.g., from the hospital to a skilled nursing facility), a form must be completed to provide necessary information for the patient's continued care. Forms vary, but the basic information includes provider orders, nursing orders, specific patient needs, patient limitations, and other pertinent data for planning care.

Document any pertinent discharge information on the nursing progress notes if it is not on the nursing discharge summary (e.g., assessment of the patient's home environment, support system, and self-care abilities). Record your educational assessment as well as any educational goals and knowledge or skill criteria to be met by discharge. Document the patient's response to patient teaching throughout the hospital stay and any written information or teaching plans given to the patient. A note to the receiving healthcare provider should mention any further health education needs.

MEDICATION ADMINISTRATION RECORD

The medication administration record (MAR), or electronic medication administration record (eMAR), documents medication administration (Fig. 16-6). The nurse should document administration of medications promptly to avoid confusion about missed doses and prevent inadvertent double dosing.

The inpatient medication record distinguishes between routine and "as needed" (prn) medications. Typically, a pharmacist verifies information (allergy, appropriate dosage, incomplete order, drug interactions) that could pose patient safety risks. The eMAR identifies routine times for medication administration (e.g., "08:00, 12:00, and 16:00"). When the nurse logs on to the system, the nurse's signature automatically appears beside the administered dose. It is essential for the nurse to log off the computer after administering the medication so that his or her name is not noted when the next medication is administered by another nurse.

When giving a prn drug, record the time it is given as well as the drug's indication and effectiveness. If the patient refuses or does not receive a medication for any reason, note the reason the patient did not receive the drug. The eMAR will have a space to include comments.

In the home care setting, nurses monitor patient self-administration of medications. Therefore, an important function of the admission visit is to review all prescribed and over-the-counter medications that the patient is using, with current dosing. This information must be compared with the discharge orders or provider referral, with discrepancies clarified. The record must be updated regularly in accord with changes in the patient's medications and patterns of use. If the patient is using a medication dispenser, any copies of the medication

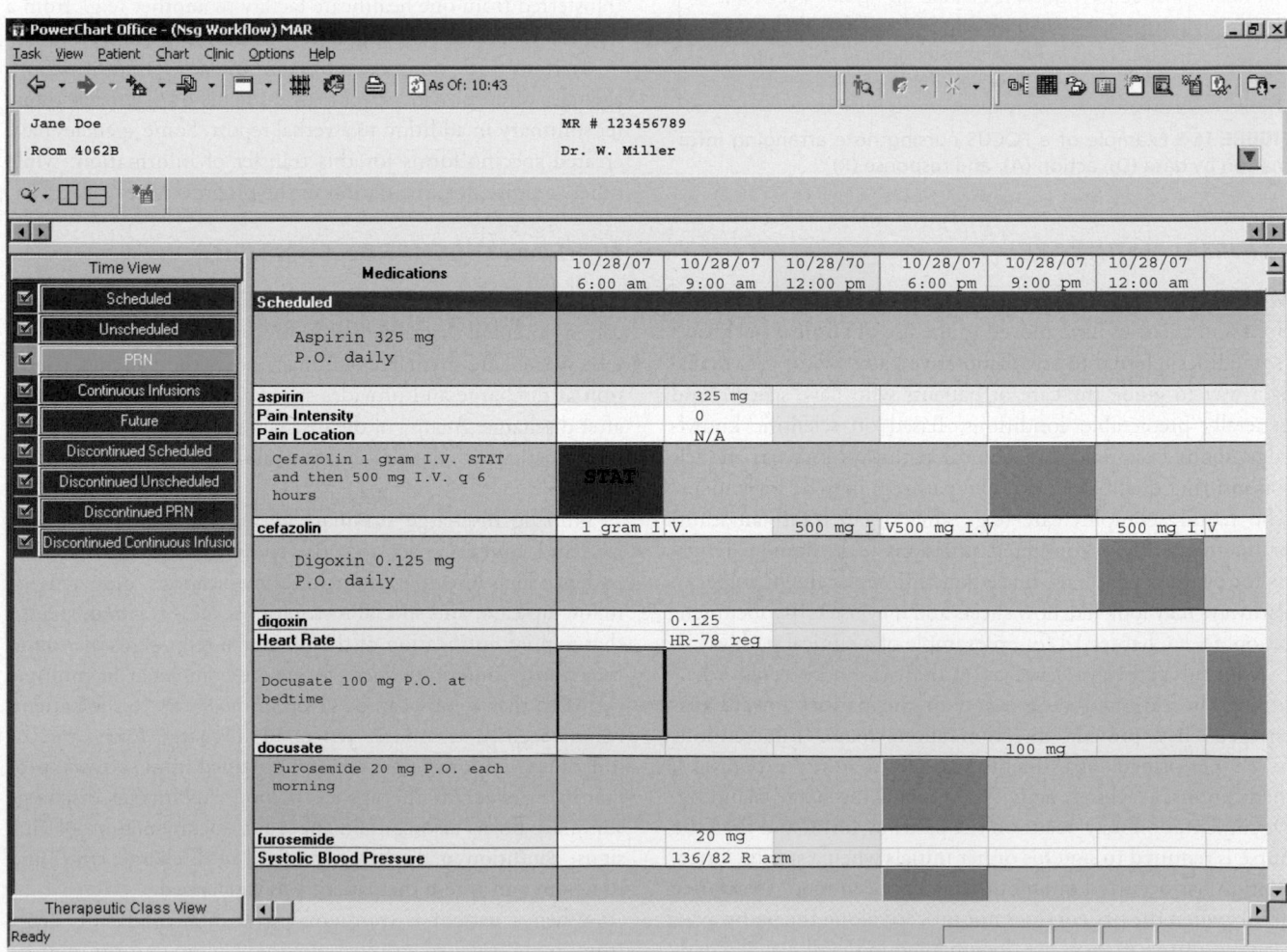

FIGURE 16-6 Example of an electronic medication record.

record left in the home also must be updated. Documentation of medication-related activities during home visits is then completed in the patient record.

DOCUMENTATION OF CARE IN NON–ACUTE CARE SETTINGS

Each work setting has unique requirements with respect to documentation. Many of the specific forms addressed in this chapter had their origins in acute care settings. As more care is provided outside these settings, the structure of documentation is changing. The need for efficient and complete charting in the ambulatory care setting may lead to a single form of one or two pages that encompasses technical, educational, and psychosocial dimensions of care. Documentation in the home care setting takes place during or immediately after each home visit. It includes such information as the reason for the visit, the patient's health status, nursing interventions performed, and evaluations of interventions or outcomes. Plans and recommendations for future home visits are also included. Nurses within each practice area need to become well versed in the ways in which their agency documentation addresses the primary principles of documentation of the nursing process.

Home Care Documentation

In 2000, the federal government mandated that home care agencies must use the **Outcome and Assessment Information Set (OASIS)** in the initial and ongoing assessment of all patients they care for to qualify for Medicare or Medicaid reimbursement. The OASIS tool accurately measures the patient's status at various specified points during an episode of care, thus providing the basis for measuring patient outcomes (CMS, 2013). OASIS data items include sociodemographic data, environmental information, support systems, health status, and functional status of all adult home care patients. Additional education of nurses is necessary because of the complexity of the OASIS system. Assessment is performed initially and to reassess the effectiveness of interventions and measure if the patient is meeting outcomes.

Long-Term Care Documentation

The **Resident Assessment Instrument (RAI)** governs documentation in long-term care settings. The RAI tracks goal achievement among long-term care residents and includes (a) minimum data set, (b) triggers, (c) resident assessment protocols, and (d) utilization guidelines. The goal of RAI is to coordinate the efforts of all members of the healthcare team to optimize the resident's quality of care and quality of life. The care team completes assessment and planning, with participation from social work, physical therapy, and other disciplines. The RAI is a comprehensive assessment tool. Skilled nursing facilities are mandated to collect and report a "minimum data set (MDS)" for Medicare review. The object of this national program is to identify common problems and to seek improvements in care.

INCIDENT REPORT

An **incident** is any unusual happening, such as a fall, medication error, malfunction in equipment, or injury to a patient,

visitor, or employee, that occurs during the performance of healthcare activities. Each agency has a standardized form on which the witnessing or documenting nurse can record patient or visitor incidents. The form includes the date and time of the incident, the events leading up to it, the patient's response, and a full nursing assessment. Nurses must avoid sounding judgmental or accusatory when documenting incidents. There should be a place on the form for provider notification, which usually is required, and an area for additional medical orders and assessment.

Facilities should use incident reports as a way to evaluate the quality of care. These may be called **quality assurance memos** (QAM). These reports are used to assess patterns of errors and the need to change the procedures or processes involved. For example, a monthly review of QAM may reveal three identical errors by three different nurses, with the same medication involved in each instance. Discussion with each nurse may reveal that a simple change in the medication's packaging could prevent further incidents. Although admitting that a mistake was made can be difficult, it is essential to document the error for the patient's sake and to prevent future errors. For legal reasons, do not attach incident reports to the patient's chart. When an error occurs, accurately document what occurred in the patient's chart but do not highlight any mistakes that could result in litigation. For example, if a medication is given at the wrong time, the time that the medication was actually given should be indicated in the chart, but explanation that this was a medication error should not be documented in the patient's record. See Chapter 4 for more information.

VERBAL COMMUNICATION

Verbal communication is essential to maximize patient outcomes and create a safe, supportive environment for care delivery. Between nurses and primary care providers, verbal communication can provide a concise summary of the patient's current status and any recent changes. Between nurses and other departments, it provides critical current information to enhance patient care. Verbal communication occurs face-to-face, on the telephone, by taped messages, or voice mail. It should be organized, complete, and professional. With increasing computer access in many settings, the sending of electronic messages (email) or text messages may be used as a written form of reporting to communicate simple messages. Text messages can be typed into the pagers of physicians or other personnel to relay simple information or emphasize the urgency of a request. In this case, the nurse must become knowledgeable about the institutional policies governing the use and storage of these messages.

Verbal communication needs to be organized, complete, accurate, concise, and respectful. Safe and effective care depends on reliable and standardized communication among all caregivers. When there is a breakdown of communication, the risk of potential harm to a patient increases. This is especially true during patient transfers and nursing handoffs or reports as well as when critical events are taking place.

Reporting, because it involves face-to-face communication, is influenced by nonverbal communication as well as the actual spoken words. It is important for nurses to maintain eye contact and to give their undivided attention during any reporting situation. Negative nonverbal cues such as lack of respect, inattention, or irritation might negatively affect the quality or completeness of the report. Differences in communication style also influence reporting. Nurses are often instructed to be very descriptive and detailed in their communication, whereas physicians tend to be more concise and focus on objective facts (Haig, Sutton, & Whittington, 2006). Providers may become impatient and inattentive with nurses who provide a rambling report. If a nurse, especially a student or a new graduate, experiences a hostile or disrespectful response when giving a report, he or she might hesitate or delay reporting significant information in the future.

Nurses use critical thinking and clinical judgment to determine what information to include in a verbal report, how quickly to report the information, the proper team member to receive the information, and what method of reporting (e.g., face-to-face, telephone, text message) is most appropriate. Some reporting is scheduled at specific times—for example, shift change handoff. In other situations, the nurse decides whether an assessment finding or a change in the patient's status requires immediate or routine notification of the provider. For example, if a stable patient tells the nurse caring for him at 3:00 AM that he has not had a bowel movement in 2 days, the nurse waits until the primary provider's rounds in the morning to report this and get an order for a laxative. Conversely, if a patient's blood pressure is low and she is NPO (nothing by mouth) for surgery, the nurse contacts the provider for an IV order to prevent severe dehydration. If the situation is acute and potentially life threatening, the nurse may activate and report to a rapid response team. In this way, the nurse uses assessment information and clinical judgment to take appropriate steps to ensure patient safety.

Verbal Handoff

A handoff occurs any time one provider transfers the responsibility and accountability for the care of a patient to another. Other industries such as aviation, power plants, and the NASA Space Center have studied and standardized handoffs to prevent errors, but only recently has the healthcare industry started paying attention to handoffs. Effective communication at handoff is critically important to create a shared mental model around the patient's condition, which creates situational awareness or knowing what is going on around you (Haig et al., 2006). The greater the number of handoffs and the more caregivers involved, the greater the risk for errors (Dracup & Morris, 2008).

In 2007, the Joint Commission developed a National Patient Safety Goal that required agencies to develop a standardized approach to handoff communications, including the opportunity to ask and respond to questions. Box 16-2 lists common handoff situations and strategies for effective handoff communication.

BOX 16-2   Handoff Reporting

Handoff Defined

A handoff takes place any time one provider transfers the responsibility and accountability for the care of a patient to another to provide continuity of care.

Common Handoff Situations

- At change of shift, when a new nurse is assigned to care for the patient
- When a nurse leaves for a meal or a break
- When a change in status requires transfer of the patient to another unit, such as the intensive care unit
- When the surgical patient is transferred from the operating room to the PACU or from the PACU to the surgical floor
- When the patient is admitted from the emergency department to a medical–surgical unit or to the intensive care unit
- When the patient moves to or from a procedural care area for a diagnostic procedure or treatment (cath lab, gastrointestinal [GI] lab, dialysis unit)
- When hospitalists or medical staff change coverage

Strategies for Effective Handoff Communication

- Communicate in a respectful, professional manner.
- Use a standardized format such as SBAR for handoffs so that all important information is presented in a predictable, concise, clear manner.
- Communicate with face-to-face verbal update of current status and historical data with interactive questioning.
- Assure limited interruptions.
- Use "read back" policies to ensure that both parties agree and comprehend.
- Use written documentation to supplement the verbal handoff.
- Cross monitor the handoffs of others with written and verbal communication.
- Ask if the person receiving report has any questions.

Things to Avoid

- Don't discuss routine care or normal assessments that are documented in the patient's medical record.
- Don't gossip or socialize.
- Don't be critical of patients or staff.
- Avoid negative nonverbal signs of impatience or irritation (e.g., rolling eyes, sighing).

Source: Clancy, C. (2006). Care transitions: A threat and opportunity for patient safety. *American Journal of Medical Quality, 21*(6), 414–417.

TEMPLATE FOR COMMUNICATION

Situation, Background, Assessment, and Recommendations (**SBAR**) is a shared mental model for improving communication between and among clinicians. Note that situation, background, and assessment are all based on the collection of complete and accurate assessment data. The last piece, recommendations, encompasses the nurse's suggestions for the next interventions.

- *Situations:* What is happening at the present time?
- *Background:* What are the circumstances leading up to this situation?

- *Assessment:* What do I think the problem is?
- *Recommendations:* What should we do to correct the problem?

Prior to giving an SBAR report, it is important to assess the patient and review the patient record for necessary information. Sometimes, it is helpful to write out information to help organize your thoughts. Although this tool was first used for the nurse to provide critical patient information to the physician, it is becoming the standard process for all verbal communication among health team members in some agencies. The SBAR display in this chapter demonstrates a home health nurse using SBAR to communicate with the provider. Additional examples of SBAR communication are provided in the Collaborating With the Healthcare Team display found in many of the clinical chapters in the text.

CHANGE OF SHIFT HANDOFF

In inpatient settings, the handoff that occurs when a new shift starts is sometimes referred to as the change of shift report. This ensures continuity of patient care from one shift to the next, allowing the oncoming nurse to be updated regarding the patient's status or plan of care (Fig. 16-7). Historically, the report occurred in the nurses' station with all nurses listening to the report on all patients. Many agencies are adopting bedside report including the patient in the process and limiting the interchange to the nurses and assistive personnel directly involved with caring for the patient. High-risk interventions, such as neurologic status or infusion rates on high-risk medications infusions, can be double-checked at the bedside to ensure safe and consistent delivery of care. Using understandable language and encouraging the patient to participate can facilitate the patient's involvement and active participation in recovery. Bedside handoff report including the patient has been found to increase patient participation and satisfaction, increase nursing teamwork and accountability, and improve communication among team members (Wakefield, Ragan, Brandt, & Tregnago, 2012).

Variations in shift handoff occur according to the nursing specialty area. For example, the report in a critical care setting may include an in-depth evaluation of each patient's body systems (e.g., respiratory status by assessment and ventilator readings, cardiovascular status by rhythm strips and blood pressure measurements). The report in a long-term care setting might include only significant changes.

REPORTING TO THE PRIMARY HEALTHCARE PROVIDER

Reporting to the primary care provider can occur face-to-face, by telephone, by text messaging, or in some settings (e.g., long-term or home care) by fax. The nurse identifies the appropriate provider to notify by checking the patient record to ascertain the primary provider, surgeon, or nurse practitioner responsible for managing care. Identifying the appropriate provider becomes more complex in a teaching center, where multiple providers are involved in providing care, or during nights or weekends when cross coverage occurs. In these situations, a call schedule helps to determine the appropriate person to contact. Valuable time can be lost if the process and schedule are unclear.

Telephone Communication

If a significant issue or problem occurs, the nurse may need to phone the primary provider to report this information (Fig. 16-8). The nurse may call the provider's office or page the provider to call back. When talking to a provider over the phone, it is important to have the patient's record and important information available for reference. It is important to document the call, including the time, who was called, what information the nurse gave to the provider, and what information the nurse received. Most agencies now limit the use of telephone orders. For agencies that have CPOE, remote

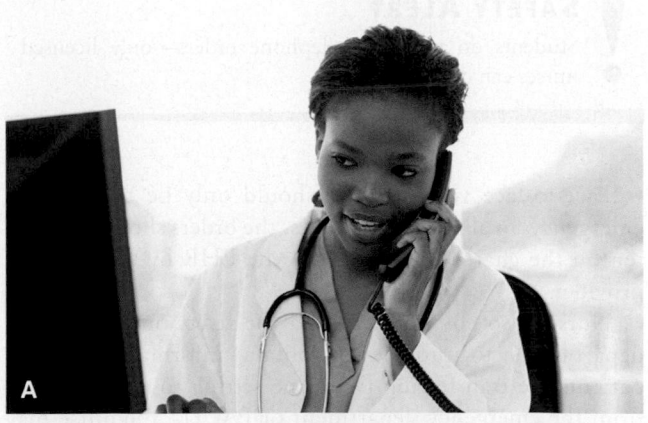

9/1/2016: 2200—Give 1,000 mL NS over 30 minutes STAT, Monitor VS every 15 minutes. Telephone order from Dr. J. Houseman/S. Roberts, RN

B

FIGURE 16-8 A. Nurses may need to communicate with the physician by telephone. **B.** Example of documentation of a telephone order from a physician to a nurse.

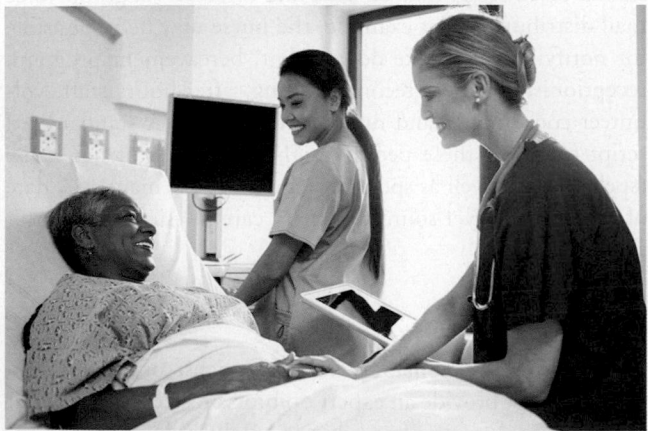

FIGURE 16-7 By reporting to one another, nurses ensure that their patients have continuity of care from one shift to another.

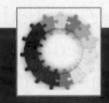

COLLABORATING WITH THE HEALTHCARE TEAM
A Community Health Nurse Contacting a Physician

Nancy Newton, a home health nurse assigned to visit Mr. Jones after his surgery, decides to call his physician using SBAR to report his progress and express her concerns regarding possible postoperative complications.

***S**ITUATION:* This is Nancy Newton, RN, from Community Home Health. I am calling regarding Mr. Jones, because the incision on his left leg is now showing signs of potential infection.

***B**ACKGROUND:* Mr. Jones, a diabetic, is now day 8 post–CABG (coronary artery bypass graft) surgery. He has an area of redness extending 3 inches up from the distal end of the incision and 1.5 inches on either side. The incision itself remains closed, but the skin is swollen and serous drainage can be expressed. Mr. Jones reported he first noticed the redness yesterday when bathing and he has increased pain in the incision. His blood glucose levels have been 180 to 240 mg/dL during the past 12 hours. He states he has had no other signs of infection, and his temperature today is 38°C. He is not taking any medications that would mask a fever at this time.

***A**SSESSMENT:* I am worried about his hyperglycemia and think he may have a surgical site infection.

***R**ECOMMENDATION:* I would like an order to culture his wound and would like you to assess his need for antibiotics and additional insulin.

CRITICAL THINKING CHALLENGE
- The home health nurse is often the eyes and ears of the physician. How might that impact the phone report using SBAR that the nurse gives the physician?
- Consider how the nurse can respond to physician orders in the home setting.
- Discuss how the nurse might document her telephone report to the physician and the importance of doing so.

computer access allows providers to enter orders when they are off-site. If a nurse is taking a telephone order, it is important to write the order and then read it back to the provider to make sure it is correct.

SAFETY ALERT

Students do not take telephone orders—only licensed nurses can do so.

Face-to-face verbal orders should only be taken in an emergency. In all other situations, the orders should be written on the chart or entered into the EHR by the ordering provider.

Nurses also communicate via the telephone with other departments to provide or obtain information. When patients are transferring from one setting to another (e.g., from the emergency department or PACU), the nurse may give the handoff report by phone. Nurses often receive laboratory data, especially critical values, by telephone. For any critical values, all health personnel must read back values obtained over the telephone to ensure accuracy and avoid errors.

When requesting information from another department, be courteous. Identify yourself and the patient. Identify any pertinent identification numbers, the patient diagnosis, and the attending physician to ensure accuracy in patient identification. When you receive a report, read back the information and speak clearly to verify findings.

Likewise, nurses often give reports to other departments. In inpatient settings, the nurse must identify the patient by two separate identifiers such as full name (correctly spelled), medical record number, or date of birth. This is especially important when the patient will undergo procedures or has laboratory analysis of specimens.

The admission of a patient to a service such as hospice may necessitate informing a large group of people. In such cases, a standardized script may be used and directed via group voice mail distribution. For example, the nurse may be responsible for notifying the intake department, bereavement program, receptionist, medical records, billing, after-hours staff, volunteer coordinator, and nursing supervisors. A standardized script for all of these people might note the patient's name (spelled out as well as spoken), names of case managers, date of admission, payer source, primary care physician, and location of care.

CONSULTS

Providers order a **consult** when a specialist or health team member must provide an expert opinion or specialized care for a patient. For example, a physician might order a consult for an infectious disease specialist to see a patient with a significant infection that is not responding to prescribed antibiotics. He or she might request a psychiatrist consult if a patient is having severe problems coping with a new diagnosis or chronic unresolved issues.

Sometimes nurses initiate consults based on their assessments. For example, if the admission assessment reveals significant recent weight loss and anorexia, the nurse might initiate a nutrition consult. When reimbursement is necessary, a provider order may be required.

ROUNDING

In the acute care area, physicians or licensed providers usually visit patients at least once per day to review their progress. Physician rounding is more productive when is includes the nurse assigned to the patient. Some agencies include other key personnel (e.g., case manager, clinical nurse leader), especially for complex patients. The nurse is responsible for communicating nursing issues. Presence during provider rounds helps inform the nurse about key medical problems and the management plan. The nurse can reinforce information with the patient and answer questions that may arise after the provider has left.

Purposeful hourly rounding is a strategy that is being employed in many acute care agencies to increase patient safety and improve patient satisfaction. An RN or assistive partner will check each patient every hour while awake, rather than wait to be summoned to the room by the patient using the call light. The staff is provided with a script where they will question if the patient is comfortable, needs toileting or repositioning, or has any requests. A safety check to make sure the call light is within reach, the alarms are activated, and the bed is in the proper position is done before leaving the room (Kenney, 2011).

CARE PLAN CONFERENCES

Care plan conferences are discussions about patient care, usually involving several disciplines. Interdisciplinary conferences help to coordinate services so that the patient's plan of care can be developed and implemented in the most efficient way. Nurses may initiate these conferences and invite members of the healthcare team from other departments (e.g., physical therapy, social services, dietary). Patients who most benefit from such conferences are those with multiple, complex problems. In some settings, routine conferences are held to review patient progress and services being provided. For example, in the pediatric oncology setting, such conferences may bring together members from inpatient and ambulatory care teams, allowing for each to anticipate services to be provided. In a rehabilitation setting, patient goals and outcome attainment are reviewed since continued reimbursement by third-party payers often depends on appropriate progress toward goals.

VOICE COMMUNICATION BADGES

Small, wearable devices that permit instant two-way voice communication with other team members have been introduced into the clinical setting. The Vocera system allows the nurse to verbally respond to call lights or answer a team member request without breaking sterile technique or interrupting direct patient care. A message can also be transmitted to multiple staff people—for example, "transfer help needed." The system also includes a text message system (Spader, 2009). In some settings, cell phones are given to nurses for communication among coworkers and to receive outside calls—for example, from families or providers.

Changes to Improve Communication

Communication is very complex. Because more than half the medical errors in today's healthcare system can be traced to faulty communication or problems with teamwork, much research and renewed energy is focused on how we can improve this area. TeamSTEPPS™ and the development and use of a checklist are system improvements so that care can be delivered more safely to the patient.

TEAMSTEPPS™

TeamSTEPPS™—Team Strategies and Tools to Enhance Performance and Patient Safety—is a safety curriculum designed to improve patient outcomes by cultivating teamwork among healthcare providers. Developed in 2006 by the U.S. Department of Defense (DOD) Patient Safety Program and the Agency for Healthcare Research and Quality (AHRQ), the TeamSTEPPS™ program is based on the concept of a "just culture" in which everyone, regardless of her or his place in the hierarchy, is relied upon to monitor and speak out in an effort to improve the care being delivered (DOD Patient Safety Program, 2009; Guimond, Sole, & Salas, 2009). This program uses a "train the trainer" model, teaching strategies and standardized tools to promote and evaluate team communication to healthcare workers. It is being adopted by an increasing number of acute care agencies to improve care and keep patients safe. The curriculum contains four teachable–learnable skills: team leadership, situational monitoring, mutual support, and communication, each using various standardized tools that are summarized in Table 16-3.

Checklists

Research conducted on teams using checklists has demonstrated a significant reduction in postoperative complications and resulted in cost savings (Semel et al., 2010). A simple checklist of four to five critical elements could be developed for various clinical situations. Developing standard tools, including simple checklists based on evidence and research, will help us consistently deliver safe and effective care to our patients.

TABLE 16-3 TEAMSTEPPS: STRATEGIES AND TOOLS TO ENHANCE PERFORMANCE AND PATIENT SAFETY

TeamSTEPPS is an evidence-based framework to optimize team performance across the healthcare delivery system. The TeamSTEPPS tools support efficient and respectful exchanges of information to ensure patient safety.

Team leadership	**Brief**: Brief session prior to start to discuss expectations and expected outcomes **Huddle**: Ad hoc planning to reinforce plan in place and assess the need to readjust **Debrief**: Review and informal information exchange designed to improve team performance and effectiveness
Situational monitoring	**Situational awareness**: Knowing what is going on around you **Cross monitoring**: Monitoring the action of all team members, providing a safety net, catching mistakes early **STEP:** 1. Assess *status* of the patient (patient history, vital signs, medications, POC, physical exam, psychosocial status) 2. Assess *team* members (fatigue, workload, skill, stress, task performance) 3. Assess *environment* (equipment, triage acuity, human resources, information) 4. Assess *progress* toward goal (established goals of team status of patients, actions of team, plan still appropriate?)

Mutual support	**Task assistance**: Actively seek and offer assistance to team members to ensure patient safety; protect team members from work overload
	Feedback: Information provided to improve team performance (timely, respectful, specific, considerate, and directed toward improvement)
	Advocacy and assertion
	Two-challenge ruleCUS:
	   I am *concerned*
	   I am *uncomfortable*
	   This is a *safety* issue
	Collaboration

Communication	**SBAR:**
	   Situation
	   Background
	   Assessment
	   Recommendations
	Call out
	Checkback
	Handoff

From: Agency for Healthcare Research and Quality. (2008). *Pocket guide to TeamSTEPPS™: Strategies & tools to enhance performance and patient safety*. [AHRQ Pub. No. 06-0020-2] Washington, DC: U.S. Government Printing.

KEY CONCEPTS

- The purposes of the patient record are communication, assessment, care planning, education, research, auditing, and legal documentation.

- Principles of documentation include confidentiality accuracy, completeness, conciseness, objectivity, organization, timeliness, and legibility.

- The use of computers is increasing in documentation. The entire patient record or just parts of it (e.g., nursing documentation) can be computerized. The universal CPR is designed to bring together all health data on a single patient into a readily accessed form.

- The patient care summary or patient profile contains background information, routine care information, and specific treatments for each patient. It is used when giving care and for handoff reporting.

- The SOAP format organizes information into subjective (S), objective (O), assessment (A), and plan (P) categories. Chronologic narrative nursing progress notes may be

difficult to follow when checking the progress of the patient on a specific problem.

- The PIE format incorporates the plan of care into the progress notes. Information is organized according to problem (P), intervention (I), and evaluation (E).

- FOCUS charting permits documentation on any significant topic, not just patient problems. Information is organized around data (D), action (A), and response (R).

- Flow sheets for vital signs, intake and output, and routine nursing assessment and care make recording quicker and less redundant.

- CBE enables the nurse to check off normal assessments or treatment administered, writing narrative notes only when deviations from standards or norms are found.

- Clinical pathways allow all members of the team to monitor and record patient progress toward discharge based on care-related norms.

- A nursing discharge summary reports the patient's status at discharge and gives instructions for diet, activity, home care, and follow-up.

- Using a standard process and template such as SBAR (Situation, Background, Assessment, Recommendation) helps organize reporting so that essential information can be provided in a concise manner.

- Handoffs should be comprehensive but brief, highlighting changes or significant issues.

- In telephone reporting, the sender of the message should speak clearly and the receiver should read back the message to avoid errors.

- The nurse must maintain the confidentiality of documentation and respect the patient's right to privacy in reporting care.

- TeamSTEPPS™ includes strategies (e.g., SBAR) to improve how communication occurs in the healthcare system.

PRACTICING FOR THE NCLEX

CHECK YOUR ANSWERS IN APPENDIX A.

1. As a patient is admitted to an intensive care unit, the nurse documents that skin is intact. The patient is in the unit for nearly a month, and a chart audit discovers that no wound care was charted and the wound care nurse consult was not done until the patient was transferred to a medical–surgical unit. At this time, the patient's skin is documented as having a stage II pressure ulcer on her coccyx. What does this lack of documentation indicate?
   a. Appropriate admission assessment
   b. Wound care was not done daily
   c. Medicare reimbursement will be possible
   d. The nursing role of care planning is not apparent

2. Which of the following are elements that improve documentation when using an electronic medical record? Select all that apply:
   a. Nurses are "tasked" to perform scheduled assessments
   b. Reassessment of pain medications is scheduled depending on administration route
   c. Computerized order entry to directly communicate orders legibly and timely
   d. Access codes to track patient care and compare to established standards of care

3. A group of nurses are discussing a patient case in the elevator when a group of people enter the elevator. Which aspect of HIPAA is most directly in violation?
   a. Patient education on privacy protection
   b. Patient recourse if privacy protections are violated
   c. Minimal disclosure of protected health information
   d. Limit use of information to accomplish intended purpose

4. A nurse calls a physician regarding a patient's increased output to a surgical Jackson-Pratt (JP) drain. She relays the following information: "The patient has had 600 cc of serosanguineous drainage from his JP drain over the last two hours; the previous 8 hour shift had a total of 160 cc. He is post-op day #1 for a prostatectomy. He has had no increase in pain but is now hypotensive with a BP of 100/64 and a HR of 98. I think he has a urine leak." What is missing from this SBAR communication?
   a. Situation
   b. Background
   c. Assessment
   d. Recommendation

5. Two nurses are performing a change of shift handoff at the bedside of a patient with a recent abdominal surgery who is receiving a constant infusion of opioids via a patient-controlled analgesia (PCA) IV pump. The off-going nurse provides a thorough report including the plan of care and the biggest safety risks. What else should these nurses do as part of their handoff?
   a. In-depth neurologic assessment
   b. List of all medications ordered
   c. In-depth medical history
   d. Double-check of high-risk infusion rates

REFERENCES

Arditi, C.,Rege-Walther, M., Wyatt, J., Durieux, P., & Burnand, B. (2012). Computer generated reminders delivered on paper to healthcare professionals: effects on professional practice and healthcare outcomes. *Cochrane Database of Systematic Reviews*, (12), CD001175. doi:10.1002/14651858. CD001175.pub3

Centers for Medicare and Medicaid Services. (2013). Outcome and assessment information set (OASIS). Retrieved from http://www.cms.gov/Medicare/Quality-Initiatives-Patient-Assessment-Instruments/OASIS/index.html?redirect=oasis/

Department of Defense Patient Safety Program. (2009). *What is TeamSTEPPS*. Uniformed Services University of the Health Sciences. Retrieved from http://dodpatientsafety.usuhs.mil/index.php?name=News&file=article&sid=31

Dracup, K., & Morris, P. (2008). Passing the torch: The challenge of handoffs. *American Journal of Critical Care*, *17*(2), 95–97.

Guimond, M. E., Sole, M. L., & Salas, E. (2009). TeamSTEPPS. *American Journal of Nursing*, *109*(11), 66–68.

Haig, K., Sutton, S., & Whittington, J. (2006). SBAR: A shared mental model for improving communication between clinicians. *Joint Commission Journal on Quality and Patient Safety*, *32*(3), 167–175.

Jones, B. (2013). Developing a vital signs alert system. *American Journal of Nursing*, *113*(8), 36–44.

Health Insurance Portability and Accountability Act of 1996, Public Law, 104–191. Retrieved June 14, 2011, from www.hhs.gov/ocr/hipaa

Joint Commission. (2014). Sentinel event data: Root causes by event type 2004–2014. Retrieved from www.jointcommission.org/assets/1/18/Root_causes_by_Event_Type_2004-2Q2014

Kahn, J., Aulak, V., & Bosworth, A. (2009). What it takes: Characteristics of the ideal personal health record. *Health Affairs*, *28*(2), 369–376.

Kenney, C. (2011). *Transforming health care: Virginia Mason Medical Center's pursuit of the perfect patient experience.* New York, NY: Productive Press.

Rosenthal, M. B. (2007). Nonpayment for performance? Medicare's new reimbursement rule. *New England Journal of Medicine, 35*(7), 1673–1675.

Semel, M. E., Resch, S., Haynes, A. B., Funk, L. M., Bader, A., Berry, W. R., et al. (2010). Adopting a surgical safety checklist could save money and improve the quality of care in U.S. hospitals. *Health Affairs (Project Hope), 29*(9), 1693–1699.

Spader, C. (2009). Cool tools. Cutting-edge gadgets sharpen nurses' efficiency. *Nursing Spectrum, 18*(11), 20–21.

Wakefield, D., Ragan, R., Brandt, J., & Tregnago, M. (2012). Making the shift to bedside shift reports. *Joint Commission Journal on Safety and Quality, 38*(6), 243–253.

Whittington, J., White, R., Haig, K., & Slock, M. (2007). Using an automated risk assessment report to identify patients at risk for clinical deterioration. *Joint Commission Journal on Quality and Patient Safety, 33*(9), 569.

Wilson, M., Murphy, L., & Newhouse, R. (2012). Patients' access their health information: A meaningful use mandate. *The Journal of Nursing Administration, 42*(11), 493–496.

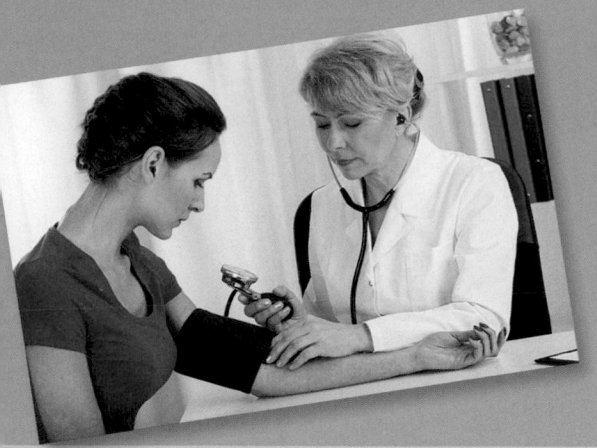

UNIT 3
Clinical Nursing Therapies

CHAPTER 17

Health Assessment

Sharon Jensen

Case Scenario

The history describes your patient as a 38-year-old married woman, the mother of two children in the sixth and eighth grades. She works full time as a paralegal professional. Her past medical history is listed as a tonsillectomy at age 8 years and a urinary tract infection at age 14 years (none since then). She has sought healthcare at this clinic for the last 2 years and had a comprehensive assessment when she entered the system. Her husband says that she has been fatigued for the last 2 weeks and that she gets short of breath on exertion. The patient's reason for seeking care is "stabbing chest pain on my right side when I take a deep breath or cough." Her height is 67 inches (170.2 cm), weight is 160 lb (72.7 kg), and she is alert and oriented. Her vital signs are temperature 102.2°F (39°C), pulse 120 beats per minute and regular, respirations 32 per minute and regular, and blood pressure 152/80 mm Hg. She is coughing up moderate amounts of thick, yellow sputum. A pleural friction rub is present.

Once you have completed this chapter and have incorporated health assessment into your knowledge base, review the above scenario and reflect on the following areas of Critical Thinking:

1. Construct a list of which data presented in the situation are primary data and which are secondary data. Determine which data are subjective and which are objective.
2. Develop the order in which you would collect your assessment information about the patient. Using a functional health, head-to-toe, or body systems framework, cluster the data into meaningful groups.
3. Select which data are of priority and which data are irrelevant at this time.
4. Identify gaps in the priority data. List what further data you will gather. Summarize the procedures you would use to obtain these data.
5. Determine if you are able to make a nursing diagnosis at this time. If yes, identify the diagnosis. If not, explain why.

KEY TERMS

accessory muscles
accommodation
anterior–posterior diameter
ascites
audiometer
auscultation
bronchial breath sounds
bruits
capillary refill time
circulation, motion, sensation (CMS)
clubbing
crepitus
cyanosis
diaphragmatic excursion
edema
erythema
expressive aphasia
focused health assessment
gallops
general survey
Glasgow Coma Scale
health history
inspection
jaundice
kyphosis
lordosis
murmur
nystagmus
objective data
ophthalmoscope
otoscope
pallor
palpation
percussion
point of maximal impulse
primary data
receptive aphasia
resonance
respiratory excursion
retraction
scoliosis
secondary data
skin turgor
stethoscope
subjective data
tactile fremitus
vesicular breath sounds

Upon completion of this chapter, you will be able to do the following:

1. Organize a nursing assessment.
2. Discuss preparation of the patient and the environment to foster data collection.
3. Differentiate between subjective and objective data.
4. Discuss methods to obtain subjective information during the patient interview.
5. Describe the techniques of inspection, palpation, percussion, and auscultation used in the physical assessment.
6. Describe methods to obtain objective data during the physical examination.
7. Individualize the nursing assessment based on lifespan considerations.

INTRODUCTION

A comprehensive health assessment encompasses the physical, psychological, social, and spiritual dimensions of living. Physical health includes basic functions such as breathing, eating, and walking. Psychological health involves intellect, self-concept, emotions, and behavior. Social dimensions of health encompass relationships and interactions among family, friends, and coworkers. Spiritual health refers to belief in a higher being, personal interpretation of the meaning of life, and attitudes toward moral decisions and personal conduct. In performing a comprehensive health assessment, nurses consider all of these dimensions.

A comprehensive health assessment may be performed as a patient makes initial contact within the healthcare system. It should take approximately 45 minutes but can vary in length, depending on the specific patient.

A comprehensive assessment is complete, but it may not always be practical or feasible. Often, nurses must select the most important interviewing questions or assessment techniques to use and perform a **focused health assessment** based on the patient's problems. Components of a focused assessment include performing a **general survey**, taking vital signs, and assessing specific areas that relate to the problem. Nurses need to use critical thinking to determine which assessment skills to use with each patient (Alfaro-LeFevre, 2014).

Assessment includes collecting **subjective data** through interviewing the patient and obtaining **objective data** by physically examining the patient. Subjective data are those symptoms, feelings, perceptions, preferences, values, and information that only the patient can state and validate. Objective data can be directly observed or measured, such as vital signs or appearance (Jensen, 2015).

PURPOSE OF THE HEALTH ASSESSMENT

The purpose of the health assessment is to establish a database for the patient's normal abilities, risk factors that can contribute to dysfunction, and any current alterations in function. A clear description of the patient's health status and health-related problems is the desired outcome of a health assessment. From this information, the nurse and the patient together can plan strategies to encourage continuation of health, prevent potential health problems, and alleviate or manage existing health problems.

The information gathered in health assessment is organized into meaningful groupings to elicit patterns, similarities, and differences. Pieces of information are not used in isolation but rather in combination with other pieces to provide a holistic view of the patient. Unclear data are validated, missing information is collected, and connections between patterns are analyzed.

A complete assessment provides an adequate database to help formulate a conclusion or a problem statement, such as a nursing diagnosis. By comparing the patient's assessment findings with the defining characteristics for the diagnosis, the nurse can determine whether supportive data to meet the diagnosis have been obtained, whether further data should be gathered, or whether another diagnosis is more appropriate. An accurate assessment provides an essential foundation for the care of the patient.

FRAMEWORKS FOR HEALTH ASSESSMENT

The three major frameworks for organizing assessment data are the functional health framework, the head-to-toe framework, and the body systems framework. Each framework helps nurses organize the information they collect and ensure that they do not inadvertently omit important assessment data. Each assessment framework begins with observing the patient's general appearance and obtaining vital signs. Developing a consistent, comprehensive method for assessment is more important than which specific framework a nurse decides to use. Table 17-1 compares data collection using the functional health, head-to-toe, and body systems frameworks.

Functional Health Framework

A functional health assessment evaluates the effects of the mind, body, and environment in relation to a person's ability to perform the tasks of daily living. The functional health

TABLE 17-1 COMPARISON OF FUNCTIONAL HEALTH, HEAD-TO-TOE, AND BODY SYSTEMS FRAMEWORKS

Functional Health Pattern	Head to Toe	Body Systems
Activity–exercise	Upper and lower extremities (pulses and circulation); precordium and anterior thorax, posterior thorax	Respiratory Cardiovascular Musculoskeletal
Nutrition–metabolism	Hair and scalp, head, oral cavity, thyroid, nails, abdomen	Gastrointestinal Integumentary Endocrine
Elimination	Abdomen, pelvis, anus, rectum	Genitourinary Gastrointestinal
Cognition–perception	Eyes, ears, cranial nerves	Sensory Neurologic
Self-perception–self-concept	Roles, coping, and values	Psychosocial
Roles–relationships	Mental health	Psychosocial
Coping–stress tolerance	Mental health	Psychosocial
Sexuality–reproduction	Breasts, testicles, pelvic exam, genitalia	Endocrine Reproductive
Values–beliefs	Mental health	Psychosocial

framework for assessment organizes data collection in terms of Gordon's 11 functional health patterns: health perception–health management, activity–exercise, nutrition–metabolism, elimination, sleep–rest, cognition–perception, self-perception–self-concept, roles–relationships, coping–stress tolerance, sexuality–reproduction, and values–beliefs (Gordon, 2010). Often, nurses collect subjective information using functional health patterns but conduct the physical assessment using a head-to-toe approach. This method is used in this chapter.

Head-to-Toe Framework

The head-to-toe framework is a system for collecting data in an organized manner, starting from the head and proceeding systematically downward to the toes. This framework is used to improve efficiency and to expedite the actual physical examination. Box 17-1 outlines the organization for head-to-toe assessment. The interview is conducted separately, usually before the physical examination, to guide and focus data collection. A typical outline of data collection is skin, head, respiratory, cardiac, abdominal, musculoskeletal, and neurologic.

Body Systems Framework

Body systems is a framework that physicians and advanced nurse practitioners commonly use. It focuses on the pathophysiology involved within specific body systems (e.g., cardiovascular, genitourinary). A body systems approach may be used during the focused assessment of an acutely or critically ill patient to determine function of a particular body system. A focused assessment may be used, for example, after orthopedic surgery, when a musculoskeletal assessment may be important to assess the effects of surgery on mobility and activity. In an

unconscious patient, it is more important to obtain physical assessment data from all body systems because the patient cannot communicate any difficulties.

CONDUCTING A HEALTH ASSESSMENT

The beginning of the interview serves as an introduction to the patient. Demographic information such as name and age are collected. Cultural considerations are included at the beginning to identify the need for an interpreter. The patient and environment are prepared so that comfort is considered.

Demographic Information

Usually, it is possible to obtain some general information about the patient by using **secondary data** sources before introducing yourself. Secondary data sources include sources of data other than the patient, such as the history or other healthcare providers. Such sources help to personalize the interview.

PAST HEALTH HISTORY

If the history is available, note the patient's name, age, primary language, **health history**, and current medications or treatment. Doing so promotes efficient communication with the patient and prevents repetition of the same questions by several different people. If other healthcare providers are available, they may also be able to give information about the patient's symptoms and history. Any information that is shared must be pertinent to the patient's case at this time.

Primary data are gathered directly from the patient. During the initial stage of the assessment, the nurse takes the patient's

BOX 17-1 Physical Assessment Collection Using Head-to-Toe Framework

General
General health state
Vital signs and weight

Cognition
Evaluate cognition
Level of consciousness
Orientation
Mood
Language and memory

Skin, Hair, and Nails
Inspect scalp and hair
Evaluate skin turgor
Observe skin lesions
Assess wounds
Inspect nails

Head and Neck
Cranial nerves
Inspect lymph nodes
Inspect neck veins

Sensory
Sensory function
Inspect and examine eyes
Test vision
Inspect and examine ears
Test hearing

Mouth
Inspect oral cavity and teeth

Respiratory
Inspect and auscultate lungs

Cardiac
Auscultate heart

Breasts
Inspect and palpate breasts

Abdominal
Inspect, auscultate, and palpate four quadrants
Palpate and percuss the liver, stomach, and bladder
Bowel elimination
Urinary elimination

Genitalia
Inspect female patient
Inspect male patient

Peripheral Vascular
Palpate arterial pulses
Observe capillary refill
Evaluate edema

Musculoskeletal
Observe posture
Assess gait and balance
Evaluate mobility
ADLs
Assess joint mobility
Measure strength

Neurologic
Assess sensory function
Assess CMS
Deep tendon reflexes
Inspect skin and nails

vital signs, height, and weight to obtain a general overview of the patient's status. The nurse also interviews the patient to obtain primary data.

Cultural Considerations

At the core of culturally based care is assessment of the patient's health beliefs and practices and, when no safety concerns arise, incorporation of the patient's beliefs and practices into the plan of care. Seeking an understanding of patients' culturally based healthcare practices is essential to nursing because each culture has its own traditional values and beliefs about health and illness that may affect individuals' adherence to treatments. For example, for some individuals, healthcare services may not be affordable or culturally relevant, especially when dietary habits and preferences are not taken into consideration when treatments are ordered. Others, because of the unequal distribution and underrepresentation of ethnic minorities in healthcare, may reluctantly decide to seek conventional care

from a provider who does not represent their own culture after traditional healing remedies prove unsuccessful (Jensen, 2015).

Often, the patient's language, customs, beliefs, and values differ from those of the nurse performing the assessment. A nurse's conscious or unconscious biases can influence his or her interpretation of data. For example, if in the nurse's culture people freely express discomfort and pain, the nurse may misinterpret cues from a stoic patient in whose culture it would be weak or embarrassing to verbalize pain. Be sensitive to communication differences across cultures. For example, in some cultures, it is comfortable to talk close to another's face, whereas in others, additional space is more comfortable. Some cultures find it more comfortable to discuss personal issues (e.g., bowel or bladder elimination) than do others. Additionally, some people regard direct questioning as invasive and are more receptive to a warmer and more casual type of interview. In some cultures, the husband is the family spokesperson and must be present during the health assessment of his wife or children. Knowledge and awareness of these differences among cultures can help prevent inadvertent miscommunication.

USING AN INTERPRETER

When a non–English-speaking patient is being assessed, an interpreter may be needed. Additional time is required when an interpreter is used. Family members are sometimes helpful, but staff or official translators often provide a more objective translation. For example, information that is emotionally difficult for the family, such as that pertaining to a life-threatening illness, could be traumatic and interfere with the translation process. Recognize that even translators who have a good command of English may need explanations for specific medical terms or may use different terms to describe body functions.

When using an interpreter, speak to the patient and use language as if you were speaking directly to the patient. Instead of saying "Ask her if she has pain," say "Do you have pain?" Look and listen to the patient when he or she responds. Observe cues the patient expresses with body language, and listen to the tone of voice. This communication can be very important in understanding what the patient is saying and underlying emotional messages.

Preparing the Patient and Environment

Thoughtful preparation of the patient and the environment is advantageous for both the patient and the nurse. Understanding the process and knowing what to expect helps ensure the patient's physical and emotional comfort. The nurse who is well organized, calm, and efficient reassures the patient.

Most patients undergoing a health examination are anxious. Pain, fear, and embarrassment may all contribute to a patient's distress. Thoughtfully preparing the patient and environment before the assessment can eliminate some controllable sources of anxiety.

ENVIRONMENT

The environment should be comfortable for both nurse and patient. A warm, quiet, well-lit room is ideal. Gather all necessary pieces of equipment in advance, making sure that they are fully functional. Leaving the patient to find equipment is distracting and time consuming.

Privacy and confidentiality are important concerns for the patient who is about to share personal information and submit to a physical examination. The patient should feel confident that others will not view or overhear the interview or physical examination. Providing such privacy can be a challenge if the patient shares a room with another patient. Family members and visitors may leave or stay, depending on the patient's preference. Pull the curtains around the bedside, and position yourself so that you are facing the patient.

Ask the patient if he or she needs to use the bathroom before beginning the assessment, especially if you anticipate an abdominal assessment. When there is an acute or emergent issue (e.g., shortness of breath), interventions may need to occur first (e.g., application of oxygen). Occasionally, you may be unable to provide comfort to the patient who is in

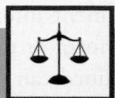

ETHICAL/LEGAL ISSUE

HEALTH ASSESSMENT
Bob Ellis is the student nurse assigned to Mrs. Androni, a 73-year-old widow who was recently admitted for observation after a fall. Bob introduces himself and explains that he needs to ask her some questions and perform a physical examination. Mrs. Androni states, "I just don't feel comfortable having a man examine me. It is against the beliefs and ways of my people. I feel just fine, so you go along and find someone else to practice on."

CRITICAL THINKING CHALLENGE
- How would you feel if you were the nurse in this situation?
- Explain factors that might contribute to Mrs. Androni's feelings.
- Can the healthcare facility provide safe care to Mrs. Androni if Bob avoids performing the physical examination?
- Brainstorm advantages and disadvantages to switching the patient assignment so that Mrs. Androni receives care from a female nurse.

acute pain or distress until you have accomplished a portion of the assessment. When this occurs, acknowledge the distress and promptly begin the assessment, focusing immediately on the patient's primary problem. The assessment and treatment for the problem takes priority when a patient is uncomfortable or acutely ill.

ORGANIZING AND DOCUMENTING DATA

The major portion of the patient interview may be conducted either before the physical examination is performed or during dialogue with the patient throughout the assessment. Document pertinent information (e.g., quotations, abnormal values) during the interview, and complete the remainder of the form after the conclusion. Practice how and what you will document during the conversation to develop skills in documenting without distracting from the conversation.

During most health assessments, use a preprinted form to record information, or enter data into a computer. Health assessment forms vary in title and format, depending on the institution, the patient population, and the purpose of the assessment. Some common titles for health assessment forms are Nursing History, Nursing Admission Form, Patient Database, and Nursing Assessment Form.

The format may be structured, using specific questions and lists of required data, or it may be unstructured, defining broad areas of health. Following a form is useful, particularly when you are learning to perform health assessment, because it provides a structure for moving logically from one health area to another.

It also helps to prevent the omission of any pertinent information. Whenever possible, bring the assessment form or the computer into the patient's room so the data obtained can be documented and validated with the patient.

INTRODUCTION TO THE PATIENT

Introduce yourself to the patient, and explain the nature and purpose of the health assessment. Describe assessment as a series of questions about the patient's past and present state of health, followed by a physical examination. During this introductory phase, tell the patient approximately how long the assessment will take. Reassure the patient that information obtained during the assessment process is confidential and will be shared only with other healthcare professionals participating in provision of care.

OBTAINING SUBJECTIVE DATA: THE INTERVIEW

The health history, or interview, is a goal-directed conversation between nurse and patient. Goals may include the following:

- Obtaining the patient's health history and perceptions of past experiences
- Identifying factors that either positively or negatively influence the patient's health status
- Describing how health status influences the patient's abilities
- Identifying what changes the patient has made to adapt to the health problems

The interview component of a health assessment is often the patient's first encounter with the nurse and therefore the first step toward establishing a trusting and therapeutic nurse–patient relationship. Be professional, concerned, and attentive throughout the interview. When the patient responds to a question, convey interest by maintaining eye contact, occasionally nodding, or verbally responding to his or her remarks (Arnold & Boggs, 2015) (Fig. 17-1). Refer to Chapter 6 for phases of the interview process.

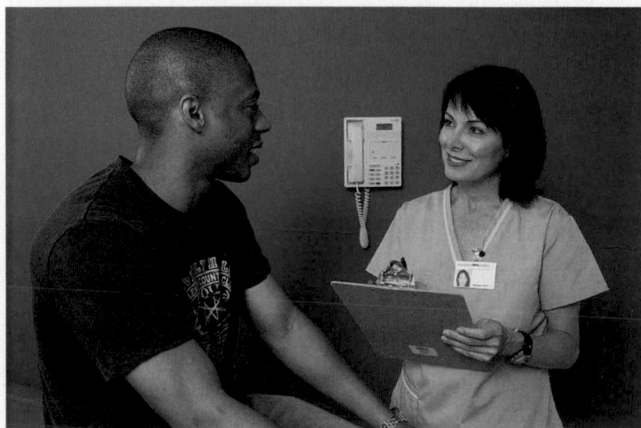

FIGURE 17-1 Maintaining eye contact during the interview demonstrates interest and concern.

Nonverbal behavior, particularly body language, can convey a strong message during an interview. The nurse who sits at eye level with the patient, appears unhurried and alert, and takes notes conveys to the patient that the information being shared is important and deserves attention. In contrast, the nurse who stands over a patient during an interview communicates that the nurse's stay will be brief, and the patient may feel powerless or conclude that the nurse is in a hurry or has more important tasks to do. The nurse who sits on the bed may invade the patient's personal space or appear unprofessional. When the nurse is using a computer, the computer is positioned so that the nurse can face the patient. Throughout the interview, continuously evaluate your verbal and nonverbal messages. These messages can either promote or discourage the patient's trust and confidence.

Questioning patients about their health is a skill that requires study and practice to achieve competence. Before the first assessment and interview, prepare questions in each health area. Some questions, such as those about allergies, can be asked with a closed-ended (yes/no) question. Open-ended questions are preferable in other areas of health concern. For example, the question "Describe what you eat on a normal day" will yield more valuable information than "How is your appetite?" Ask follow-up or probing questions when a problem area is discovered or suggested. Solicit further detail by statements such as "Tell me more about that" or "That seems to concern you."

Special techniques may be necessary to control the interview if a patient is overly talkative, particularly in regard to unrelated information. Many patients have difficulty staying on a topic or limiting their answers to significant points. A sensitive yet effective method for directing the patient might be "Because our time is limited, we won't be able to discuss that in detail now. I would like to hear more about. ..." The ability to skillfully yet sensitively control the interview is essential for obtaining pertinent information in a time-efficient manner.

Reason for Seeking Healthcare

The first subject usually discussed in a patient interview is the patient's specific reason for seeking care (Jensen, 2015). This subject is often called the patient's "chief complaint" or "chief concern." Listen carefully to the patient's description of the primary problem, and document it, when possible, quoting the patient's exact words. In-depth questioning and discussion of this problem should follow. Information obtained during the interview helps to target areas of pain or probable abnormality so that the examination of the affected areas can be especially careful, thoughtful, and thorough.

Health History

During the interview, obtain information about the patient's health history, family health history, and risk factors. Health history information should include known allergies, childhood illnesses, immunization history, previous surgeries, and chronic health conditions. Ascertain what, if any, medications the patient is taking. Some patients may have a written list or be able to show you the bottle with the medication's name. Family history includes a review of major illnesses, listing the family member who is affected (e.g., paternal grandfather, sister). Risk factors can assist with identifying areas of health promotion and teaching.

Pain Assessment

Addressing pain early in the health assessment allows the nurse to individualize the rest of the assessment, avoiding positioning and techniques that are especially uncomfortable for the patient. If the patient is in severe pain, lengthy questioning is best postponed. Acknowledging the patient's pain and verbalizing your efforts to limit discomfort during the assessment are important.

Acute illness, chronic disability, surgical intervention, and treatment modalities can all cause the patient pain. Pain can limit normal function and affect wellness and quality of life. Accurate assessment of pain is necessary to identify and treat the underlying cause of pain. Assessment permits a better understanding of the patient's pain experience.

Because the pain experience is personal and subjective, the patient interview is the best way to collect information to assess pain. Such an assessment should include asking the patient to describe the location, intensity, quality, onset, and chronology of his or her pain experience. Various tools to measure pain are available, and each has its advantages and limitations (D'Arcy, 2011). Also, determine factors that influence the pain experience and methods of effective pain management. Last, explore the impact the pain experience has on daily life and other areas of health.

Questions helpful in soliciting subjective information concerning the patient's pain experience include the following (Jensen, 2015):

- *Location*: "Where does it hurt?"
- *Duration*: "When did it start? How long has it lasted?"
- *Intensity*: "On a scale of 1 to 10, how do you rate your pain?"
- *Quality*: "Tell me what it feels like."
- *Alleviating/aggravating factors*: "What makes it better? Worse?"
- *Pain goal*: "What level of pain is acceptable to you?"
- *Functional goal*: "What would you like to be able to do if you were not in pain?"

Acute pain stimulates the sympathetic nervous system and produces the following objective symptoms: increased blood pressure, increased pulse, increased respiratory rate, dilated pupils, and diaphoresis. This sympathetic response is not present in chronic pain states, and these parameters may be absent if pain has been present for several weeks. Observing the patient's body position and facial features also gives clues to pain. If the patient exhibits any of the following—grimacing, guarded positioning, tense body posture, refusal to move a body part, muscle spasms, or rubbing a body part—these can all indicate pain despite verbal denial.

A "facial mask of pain," in which the patient's facial expression is flat or fixed, the eyes appear dull, and fatigue is evident, commonly occurs in chronic pain. Emotional expression such as crying, moaning, or yelling also can occur during severe pain.

APPLY YOUR CRITICAL THINKING

You are a clinic nurse seeing Mr. Schorr, who has been experiencing back pain for the last 7 months. He is currently out of work and receiving disability. His vital signs are as follows: temperature 37°C, pulse 78 bpm, respirations 18 per minute, and blood pressure 128/78 mm Hg. Mr. Schorr sits very quietly, holding himself in one position during most of the interview. His face is nonexpressive as he describes his pain as incapacitating. "All I can do is lie in bed and watch TV and read. The pain pills I have been taking don't seem to be working anymore." When you ask him to rate his pain, he says 7 on a scale of 1 to 10.

- Classify subjective and objective data in this pain assessment.
- What data have the most validity in this situation? Why?

Check your answer in Appendix B.

Assessment of Health Perception and Health Management

The major focus in health perception–health management is the patient's perception of health status, preventive health practices, compliance with medical treatment, and patient safety (Gordon, 2010). Discuss the patient's health promotion activities, such as exercise, nutrition, routine preventive examinations (e.g., dental, vision, hearing), immunization history, safety precautions (e.g., child safety seats, bicycle helmets), and stress management. Inquire about the use of nicotine (including chewing tobacco; cigarette, pipe, and cigar smoking; and use of nicotine gum or patches), alcohol (amount, frequency, and type), and drugs (recreational and prescription). Assess the patient's overall willingness and ability to follow health-related advice, such as taking medications on schedule or following a prescribed diet. Also, elicit other sources of health advice used by the patient, such as an acupuncturist, herbalist, or naturopath.

Obtain a detailed allergy history, including medication, food, pollen, insect, latex, and any environmental allergens for every patient. Inquire about the specific type of reaction that the patient experienced. Some patients may confuse a medication side effect, such as nausea, with an allergic reaction. Document any allergic reactions, and communicate them to other members of the healthcare team.

Many people live with chronic diseases, such as heart disease, cancer, or stroke. Control of these health problems depends directly on modification of a person's behavior and habits of living. Prevention necessitates eliminating activities that many people enjoy, such as overeating, overindulgence in alcohol, and nicotine use. Prevention also implies doing things that require special effort, such as exercising regularly, eating a healthy diet, seeking regular health examinations, and striving for a harmonious life. Assessment of a person's health perception and health maintenance reveals knowledge, behavior, and attitudes toward preventing disease and living a healthy lifestyle. The following are selected sample interview questions in a health history:

- How would you describe your health?
- When was your last dental, eye, or physical examination?
- Have you ever used tobacco, alcohol, or recreational drugs? What type? How often?
- What safety practices do you follow (e.g., safety belt, bicycle helmet)?

Screening for violence is an important part of the health interview. The term *family violence* is often used interchangeably with the following terms: domestic violence, intimate partner violence (IPV), and violence against women (Khan & Rogers, 2014). Types of family violence include child maltreatment, sibling violence, IPV, and elder abuse. The nurse may encounter all of these types during patient assessments. Nurses can prepare patients for sensitive or difficult questions about violence by prefacing comments with statements such as "Now is the point in the interview where I ask patients about relationships in their family. Who lives in your home with you? How do you feel in that relationship?" It is also common to ask "Because violence is so common for so many people, I routinely ask all patients about violent experiences—those in the past and currently. I wonder if you have experienced or are experiencing violence" (Jensen, 2015).

Assessment of Activity and Exercise

Mobility affects independence and self-care abilities. For patients with no deficits, only a brief discussion of mobility and self-care is necessary. Observing the patient's posture, gait, and movement as he or she enters the room provides much information. If you detect deficits, a detailed evaluation is needed.

POSTURE

Inspect the spine for straight alignment and symmetry. The patient's posture should also be straight, without abnormal curving. In **kyphosis**, the shoulder and upper back tend to curve forward. Many schools screen for **scoliosis**, which is a curvature of a portion of the spine to the side laterally. Scoliosis can be seen better by having the patient bend over and evaluating for symmetry. Also, observe for **lordosis**, commonly known as "swayback," in which the lumbar region curves inward and the sacral region curves outward.

GAIT AND BALANCE

Gait describes a person's manner of walking. Balance refers to stability and equality between both sides of the body. An evaluation of gait and balance contributes to the assessment of a patient's mobility as well as risk for injury due to falling. Gait and balance abnormalities may also indicate dysfunction or disease in other body systems, particularly the brain, spinal cord, muscles, and skeleton. A patient may acquire a slowed, cautious, or unnatural gait as an unconscious means of protection from pain, weakness, or loss of balance.

The nurse may observe gait and balance during many activities that naturally occur in the course of a health assessment. Assess the patient's balance as he or she walks into the room, moves around in bed, rises from the sitting position, or rolls onto his or her side. To assess gait further, ask the patient to walk a distance of about 10 feet (3 m) down a hallway. A normal gait is quick, springy, and rhythmic, with the arms naturally swinging back and forth. Characteristics of abnormal gait include the following: slow, measured steps; limping; leaning to one side; shuffling the feet; shorter steps taken on one side compared to the other; wide outward swinging of one leg; a wide gait or stance; leaning the trunk forward; lifting the knee higher than normal with each step; and short, hurrying steps (Bickley, 2013).

MOBILITY

Foot pain is a common cause of decreased mobility. Inspect the patient's feet for bunions, corns, calluses, ingrown toenails, spurs, and ulcers. If the patient uses any assistive devices for ambulation, such as a cane, crutches, walker, prosthesis, or brace, assess the patient's use of the aid, focusing on coordination, stability, comfort, and safety. For additional information on assessing mobility status, refer to Chapter 25.

Discuss a program of regular physical activity with every patient. Participation in sports and recreational activities contributes to physical and psychological well-being. Determine whether the patient has any pain or discomfort associated with exercise and if he or she can participate in any desired activities. Energy level also affects the desire and ability to be physically active. Fatigue is frequently associated with cardiac or respiratory disease, anemia, or cancer.

When a patient's mobility or self-care functions are compromised, a daily living assessment should be performed. A daily living assessment includes evaluation of the ability to perform self-care skills (bathing, toileting, dressing, grooming, and eating) and simple motor activities (sitting, standing, walking, climbing stairs, and opening doors). Depending on the patient's living situation, an assessment of some home maintenance skills may also be appropriate. These skills include cooking, shopping, housekeeping (making a bed, cleaning, vacuuming, washing dishes), doing the laundry, paying bills, and using the telephone. The architecture of a home, particularly stairs, can complicate independent activity and should be considered.

A scale is used to rate these self-care abilities (Box 17-2). The daily living assessment provides key information about a

BOX 17-2	Self-Care Abilities Scale

0   Full self-care, independent
I   Needs to use equipment or device
II   Needs supervision
III Needs equipment or device and supervision
IV   Unable to perform, dependent

person's ability to live independently or the amount of assistance that he or she requires to do so. If major disabilities are present, an occupational therapist may be consulted for further evaluation.

Mobility assessment is preventive as well as descriptive. Patients with impaired mobility are at risk for accidents and injury. Older people, particularly those who have fallen in the past, are most susceptible. A thorough assessment of risk factors can determine the risk for falling, and appropriate safety precautions may be instituted.

The following are suggested patient interview questions related to mobility:

- Describe your usual activities in a normal day (or week).
- What limitations in ability do you have (eating, toileting, walking, dressing, bathing)?
- Have you recently fallen or consider yourself to be at risk for falling?
- Do you experience fatigue or discomfort during activity?

RESPIRATORY FUNCTION

Assessment of general respiratory status occurs every time you interact with the patient. A survey of skin color, respiratory difficulty, and position the patient takes to breathe is important to determine the acuteness of the patient's problem.

 SAFETY ALERT

For acute respiratory distress, obtain immediate assistance so that appropriate interventions can begin.

Respiratory history should focus on four major areas: risk factors for lung disease (e.g., smoking, occupational exposure to pollutants), signs and symptoms of respiratory dysfunction (e.g., cough, sputum production, dyspnea), impact of respiratory status on activities of daily living (ADLs), and adaptive measures for any respiratory dysfunction. Suggested interview questions that can help to elicit this information include the following:

- Have you been exposed to environmental or occupational materials that have affected your breathing? What are they?
- Have you had allergies, asthma, bronchitis, emphysema, tuberculosis, or other lung problems?
- How often do you cough? Describe the sputum.

- Do any breathing difficulties limit your activity? What are they?
- What position do you assume for sleeping?

CARDIOVASCULAR FUNCTION

Subjective data can be collected concerning adequate peripheral (arm and leg) circulation, evaluating arterial and venous blood flow. Evaluate the patient's use of vasoconstricting agents such as nicotine. The history for cardiovascular assessment includes risk factors for cardiovascular disease (e.g., hypertension, elevated cholesterol level, smoking), signs and symptoms of cardiovascular dysfunction (e.g., pain, dizziness, palpitations), the impact of cardiovascular dysfunction on ADLs, and specific adaptations to cardiac or circulatory impairment. Interview questions to help elicit this information might include the following:

- Describe your normal activity or exercise pattern.
- Do you have a history of heart attack, heart rhythm problems, high blood pressure, or high cholesterol?
- Have you had any chest pain, shortness of breath, cough, swelling in the legs, calf or leg pain, fluttering in the heart, or fatigue?
- How has this problem limited your activities?

Assessment of Nutrition and Metabolism

Assessment of nutrition and metabolism includes dietary habits and metabolic needs. Information reflects how well the patient's body is able to ingest, digest, absorb, metabolize, and use food to maintain tissue integrity, maintain fluid and electrolyte balance, and fight infection.

Assessment of nutrition and metabolism requires specific information about the patient's normal diet and careful observations of the physical features that reflect nutritional state. The nutrition–metabolism assessment should focus on normal food and fluid intake, alterations in normal eating patterns, how dietary changes have affected daily living, and the development of medical problems secondary to altered nutritional status.

Interview questions to focus a nutrition–metabolism assessment might include some of the following:

- Tell me what you've eaten in the last 24 hours.
- What is your usual weight? Has it changed in the past 6 months? How much?
- Do you have any problems with tasting, chewing, or swallowing food?
- Do you have any problems with getting groceries or preparing food?

Weight measurement can provide important information regarding nutritional status. Standardized tables have been developed (e.g., Metropolitan Height and Weight Tables for Men and Women, ages 16 to 59) that recommend ideal body weights for men and women. Standardized tables are also available to evaluate growth in children. Such tables provide a baseline for evaluating the patient's weight. More commonly, the body mass index (BMI) is used as an indication of nutritional status. Deviations from normal body size, ranging from obese to severely underweight, can influence not only the nutritional state but also other areas such as exercise, activity, and self-concept. Obesity in adults is associated with increased mortality and risk for coronary heart disease, hypertension, hyperlipidemia, diabetes, gallbladder disease, certain cancers, and osteoarthritis. Overweight children often become overweight adults, and being overweight in adulthood is a health risk (Centers for Disease Control and Prevention, 2014).

Standardized weight tables are often used to evaluate nutritional status. Determination of the percentage of weight change, which uses the patient's usual weight as the standard, is also helpful. In general, a change in weight of 10% during the last 6 months is considered to be abnormal (Jensen, 2015). A dietitian should be consulted for further evaluation.

Weight measurement can also be used to evaluate fluid status or the response of the patient to medical treatment (e.g., diuretic therapy for congestive heart failure). Rapid weight gain or loss (e.g., 10 lb in 2 weeks) usually results from the gain or loss of body fluid rather than body fat.

Weight measurement can be done on various scales; the choice depends mainly on the patient's status. An upright scale is appropriate for patients with normal mobility who can step onto a platform and maintain balance while weight is determined. A chair scale is used for patients who can transfer to a chair but are unable to support the body in a standing position for accurate weight measurement. A bed scale is used for patients who are too weak or immobile to use other scales safely. Special infant scales are used to determine the height and weight of babies.

Scales can be calibrated in terms of pounds or kilograms, with some scales providing both measures of weight. To convert from pounds to kilograms, divide by 2.2; to convert from kilograms to pounds, multiply by 2.2. For most patients, height and weight measurements are obtained on admission to a healthcare agency. When daily or frequent weights are required to evaluate patient progress, weight is measured at the same time each day (usually before breakfast), using the same scale. **Procedure 17-1** outlines steps in measuring weight.

Height is measured with a measuring stick attached to a standing scale. The patient stands erect without shoes on the scale, and the height is determined by lowering the sliding arm until it rests on the patient's head. Height can be measured in inches or centimeters. To convert inches to centimeters, multiply by 2.54; to convert centimeters to inches, divide by 2.54.

Assessment of Elimination

Elimination assessment focuses on determining the adequacy of bladder and bowel function, identifying risk factors that may contribute to problems in elimination, assessing the impact of bladder or bowel dysfunction on daily living, and understanding the patient's methods of managing and coping with any dysfunction.

Focus on the patient's normal urinary and bowel patterns, noting any recent changes. Questions to elicit such information from the patient include the following:

- What is your normal pattern of urination?
- Have you experienced any changes in your usual urination pattern?
- Have you had any discomfort, pain, frequency, incontinence, or difficulty starting the urinary stream?
- What is your normal bowel pattern?
- When was your last bowel movement?
- Have you had any problems with constipation, diarrhea, or lack of control with bowel movements?

Assessment of Sleep and Rest

The assessment of sleep and rest focuses on the patient's normal sleep patterns, alterations from the normal pattern, and satisfaction with quality of rest and sleep. Sleep habits, problems with obtaining adequate rest or sleep, and any aids that the patient uses to induce sleep are important areas to consider. The following are suggested questions to elicit this information:

- Tell me when you usually go to sleep. Tell me when you usually wake up. Do you awaken during the night?
- Can you easily fall asleep? What do you do to promote sleep?
- Do you feel rested on awakening?
- Do you snore, or have you been diagnosed with sleep apnea?

Most data indicating a dysfunctional sleep pattern are subjective, although a few objective signs may support subjective data. Frequent yawning, decreased attention span, and dark circles or puffiness around the eyes may be related to sleep deprivation. Continual dozing during the day may also occur when the amount or quality of sleep is inadequate. During periods of apparent sleep, note snoring, rapid eye movements, or jerking movements. Observe the patient's pattern of breathing while he or she sleeps.

Neurologic Assessment and Mental Status

Cognitive function refers to a person's ability to think, which is evaluated primarily through written and verbal communication. Factors that contribute to cognition include awareness, thought processes, memory, language, judgment, and attention span. Whereas significant impairment in cognitive abilities is readily noticeable on the first interaction, repeated assessments over time are often required to detect subtle changes or minor deficits in cognitive ability.

Subjective data for appraising mental abilities are gathered throughout the health assessment from the context of a patient's conversation and his or her degree of cooperation during the physical examination. Assess whether the patient has difficulty understanding or answering questions or following directions.

Evaluate the patient's responses to questions in terms of clarity and appropriateness. The patient should be able to express any health concerns in a coherent and clear manner. Assessment can detect early decline or evaluate worsening delirium.

Possible questions to elicit further information concerning a person's cognitive and communication ability include the following:

- Tell me your full name.
- What is today's date?
- Where are you right now?
- Tell me how your memory is. Have you had any recent changes?
- Do you have problems with speaking? Reading? Writing?

The purpose of assessing the patient's sensory status is to determine functioning of the five senses: vision, hearing, touch, taste, and smell. Assessment should also include the impact sensory deficits have on ADLs and any devices the patient uses to cope with sensory impairment.

Sensory losses may be congenital but are often associated with the aging process. Assess older patients carefully for sensory deficits because many adaptive techniques are available to improve the safety, pleasure, and independence of their lives.

Patients are usually aware of sensory loss and can verbalize specific deficits when questioned. During the interview, observe the patient for signs of sensory impairment, such as asking questions to be repeated, watching lips closely during speech, squinting to improve vision, or holding reading material at arm's length. Questions concerning sensory status include the following:

- How is your vision? Do you have glasses, contact lenses, or a prosthesis?
- How is your hearing? Do you use a hearing aid?
- Do you have any numbness or tingling in your hands or feet?
- Have you noticed any changes in your taste or smell?

Assessment of Self-Perception and Self-Concept

The self-perception and self-concept pattern focuses on the content and feelings associated with a person's self-evaluation (Gordon, 2010). The components of self-concept include one's self-knowledge, self-expectation, social self, and self-evaluation. The ways in which others evaluate and interact with a person throughout the lifespan influence self-concept. Body image, the mental picture and feelings about one's body, is an important component of self-concept. Individual beliefs concerning locus of control are also important to explore. Some people believe that life events are self-determined (internal locus of control), whereas others view individual happenings as a matter of fate, luck, or the influence of others (external locus of control).

During a basic health assessment, the goal in assessing self-perception is to describe the patient's general view of self and his or her satisfaction with that image. Patients whose primary health problem directly relates to a disturbance in self-concept (such as psychiatric, chemically dependent, or abused patients) require an extensive evaluation by a mental health specialist. However, many illnesses alter one's self-concept because of changes related to physical strength, appearance, and loss of control. For this reason, consideration of self-concept should be integrated into the health assessment of every patient.

Collect subjective and supporting objective data concerning normal self-concept, recent changes in self-concept, and conditions (e.g., burns, skin disorders, colostomy, mastectomy, obesity) that could threaten or alter body image.

Possible questions that help the patient describe self-perception include the following:

- What are you most concerned about in relation to your health?
- How would you describe yourself?
- How has being sick made you feel differently about yourself?

Eye contact, personal grooming and appearance, posture, body movements, mood, emotions, and voice and speech pattern are nonverbal cues to a patient's self-concept. Poor eye contact, inattention to personal grooming, and body language that conveys embarrassment or shame may reflect low self-concept.

Assessment of Roles and Relationships

Most people fill various roles, such as spouse or partner, parent, worker, student, colleague, friend, coach, and adviser. These roles may be rewarding and stimulating, or they may be overwhelming and stressful.

The goal in a basic health assessment is to identify the patient's major roles in the family, at work, and in their social life and to identify the patient's relative satisfaction or dissatisfaction with each role. The assessment should also indicate how health problems or hospitalization may interfere with a person's ability to fulfill role expectations and maintain relationships. Although the patient normally provides this information, it is often helpful (and sometimes necessary) to consult other members of the family unit to obtain meaningful data. Information you obtain in the assessment should focus on the patient's family configuration and occupation, recent or anticipated changes in the patient's roles or relationships, and the patient's level of satisfaction with current roles and relationships (Gordon, 2010).

Within the family unit, important information includes who shares the household; responsibilities or dependencies of each member; and specific problems, such as issues related to parenting, caring for elderly parents, or marital discord. The illness of a family member may necessitate shifting responsibilities within the family, such as financial support, child care, cooking, and home maintenance. Chronic illnesses often involve the patient in long and sometimes permanent dependence on others. Evaluate the specific circumstances of that dependence, the patient's attitude, and the patient's coping ability.

Roles and relationships related to work are an important area to assess. Factors such as job-related stress, insufficient time for leisure activities, unsafe work environment, job insecurity, inadequate pay, or lack of recognition may negatively affect physical and psychological well-being.

A change in relationships may contribute to the cause or exacerbation of an illness. Explore any areas in which recent change has occurred, such as divorce, death, or illness of a family member, loss of a job, change in job status or pay, increase in job responsibility, or transition from student to worker.

Suggested questions to help obtain this information from the patient include the following:

- Are you employed? Retired? Disabled?
- What do you see as your primary role at work? Home?
- Whom do you live with?
- Whom do you ask for help when you need it?
- Are there any problems at work or home that influence your health?
- Do you have any insurance or financial concerns that you desire help with?

Obtain objective data by watching the interactions of the patient with family members and others. Verbal interactions and nonverbal communication can support what the patient has discussed in the interview. Observing visitors, cards, and flowers can help to validate that the patient has positive relationships with others. Likewise, the absence of visitors and communication from others might suggest a lack of positive relationships.

SAFETY ALERT

Note repeated unexplained injuries, such as bruises, burns, or fractures, as a possible sign of abusive relationships. Frequently, people involved in abusive relationships verbally deny that abuse has occurred.

Assessment of Coping and Stress Tolerance

Stress is an event that disrupts or challenges a person's equilibrium (Gordon, 2010). Although stress is most readily conceptualized as negative, positive life changes also challenge a person and therefore create stress. Examples of positive stressors include marriage, planned pregnancy, job promotion, and a long-awaited vacation. Serious illness, hospitalization, and surgery are universally perceived as stressful events.

Whether something is a stressor depends largely on a person's perception of the event. Each person's response to stress is unique. The way in which a person reacts and, it is hoped, adapts to stress is called a *coping behavior.*

Coping behaviors can be adaptive, producing relief from stress and even growth. For example, a patient who is experiencing work-related stress may cope by exercising more. Coping behaviors can also be maladaptive, leading to further disintegration and disorganization. In assessing coping and stress tolerance, the goal is to identify and acknowledge current stressors the patient is experiencing, determine how the patient has handled stressful events in the past, and identify current methods the patient is using to cope.

Subjective data concerning coping and stress tolerance can be obtained through the interview with the use of open-ended or specific questions. Another technique is to ask the patient to describe a stressful event that occurred in the past and his or her response to it. Such a description can help the nurse identify past stressors and how the patient managed the situation. The manner in which a patient handled past life crises is often a good predictor of how he or she will manage present or future situations. Suggested questions for interviewing the patient regarding coping and stress tolerance include the following:

- Have there been any changes or stress recently in your life? What are they?
- How do you usually handle stress?
- Would you like help to deal with the stress of being sick?

Stress activates the sympathetic nervous system, which produces certain physiologic effects. Sympathetic stimulation may increase the force and rate of the heartbeat; increase respiratory rate and depth; decrease blood flow to the skin, resulting in **pallor** and diaphoresis; and increase blood flow to the muscles. These symptoms may be pronounced in the event of a sudden stressful event. When a person is exposed to chronic stress, the symptoms may be less sudden and less dramatic.

Assessment of Sexuality and Reproduction

Sexuality is the behavioral expression of sexual identity. It may involve, but is not limited to, sexual relationships with a partner. Sexual expression is a complex integration of physiologic, psychological, and social aspects of human nature. Physical illness and its treatment may influence sexual function. For example, impotence is frequently associated with diabetes mellitus, alcoholism, chronic renal disease, and certain drug therapies. Patients may question their own desirability after surgeries such as mastectomy, radical neck dissection, colostomy, and hysterectomy. Diseases that reduce energy, such as heart or lung disease, may limit physical endurance.

Many patients and nurses are hesitant in addressing sexual matters during a health interview. However, sexuality is such an integral aspect of human nature that to ignore it would be neglecting a vital component of health. Including sexuality in the initial patient contact conveys to the patient that sexual health is an appropriate, legitimate concern. The sexual assessment is not meant to illuminate nonexistent problems. Rather, the patient is, in effect, given permission and encouragement to present sexually related questions.

The areas for assessment of sexuality and reproduction include reproductive functioning, sexual role and satisfaction with that role, and potential for alteration in sexual role or function (Gordon, 2010). Discuss the impact of the patient's current health status on sexual role and functioning. Examination of the reproductive organs is not usually performed unless the patient has problems in that area or as part of a preventive health examination.

The best approach to obtaining a sexual history is to introduce subjects of least sensitivity first. Begin by focusing on chronologic events, such as puberty, menstruation, menopause, and reproductive history. Invite the patient to elaborate on any problems or expectations in these areas. Also, determine the patient's knowledge and compliance with preventive health practices, such as breast self-examination, regular Papanicolaou (Pap) smear, and testicular and prostate examination.

A sexual assessment should be adapted to correlate with the patient's developmental level. Many adolescents are concerned about changes in their bodies and early sexual experience. Use this opportunity to educate, support, and guide the adolescent in matters involving sexuality. Married people may have concerns about their own sexuality and concerns related to parenting and sex education for their children. Many elderly patients enjoy sexual relations throughout their lives and may desire acknowledgment and discussion of their concerns.

Selected questions to elicit information concerning the sexual–reproductive pattern should be individualized for each patient and may include the following:

- Are you concerned about pregnancy? What method of contraception do you use? Is this method acceptable to you and your partner?
- Have you ever been diagnosed as having a sexually transmitted infection (gonorrhea, genital herpes, chlamydia, or AIDS)?
- Many men (or women) in your situation have questions about how their illness or surgery will affect the sexual aspects of their lives. What questions do you have?
- Has your illness interfered with you being a mother (or wife, husband, father, partner)?
- *For adolescents*: Many boys (or girls) at your age have questions about dating, becoming intimate, contracting a disease, or getting pregnant. What questions do you have?

When working with a female patient, here are some questions that you may ask:

- At what age did you begin menstruating?
- How long is your typical menstrual cycle?
- What was the date of your last menstrual cycle?
- Do you have any problems related to menstruation?
- How many times have you been pregnant?
- How many children do you have?

Some questions related to breasts include:

- Do you examine your breasts? How often?
- Do you have a family history of breast cancer?

During assessment of the male patient, you may ask the following questions:

- Do you examine your testicles? How often?
- Do you have any concerns about sexual function?

Assessment of Values and Beliefs

Assessment of values and beliefs is also referred to as a spiritual assessment because it focuses on the spiritual dimension of life. Spirituality may be defined as the quality that transcends the physical world; permeates and unifies a person's entire being; and gives life purpose, meaning, and importance (Gordon, 2010). Spirituality usually, but not always, involves a belief and relationship with a higher being. Values and beliefs emerge from one's sense of spirituality and guide one's opinions about what is right, good, proper, and meaningful. Values help determine choices about the conduct of one's life, including health-related decisions concerning personal practices, treatments, and even life or death. The spiritual realm is one aspect of being human that often comes into focus during illness or crisis.

Illness, injury, loss, aging, and disability are spiritual as well as physical and emotional experiences. Serious or life-threatening illness often triggers a person's first encounter with mortality. Crisis often provides the motivation to question one's life, goals, and what is important.

Because body, mind, and spirit are intertwined, distress in any one area affects the health of the whole person. Nurses should include spiritual assessment and care in their daily practice. A nurse who understands a patient's spiritual beliefs is better prepared to support coping strategies and provide resources that are spiritually helpful to the patient.

Assessment of values and beliefs focuses on the significance of religious affiliation and religious practices, the patient's spiritual needs and the resources available to meet those needs, and the relationship between spiritual beliefs and the patient's current state of health (Gordon, 2010).

Mention of spiritual beliefs may arise during discussion of the patient's coping–stress tolerance pattern. If so, smoothly direct the conversation toward the values–beliefs pattern. The following interview questions may be used to discuss the values–beliefs pattern:

- Are any religious or spiritual practices significant to you?
- Has this illness affected any of these practices or beliefs?
- Is there a religious person to contact or a practice to perform that you would like during this illness?

Assessment of the values–beliefs pattern depends primarily on subjective data. However, visible expression of spiritual values is sometimes present. Notice religious articles belonging to patients, such as a Bible, Buddha, Koran, or rosary. You may observe the patient in prayer either alone or with family, friends, or clergy.

OBTAINING OBJECTIVE DATA: THE PHYSICAL EXAMINATION

Physical examination involves the use of one's senses to obtain information about the structure and function of an area being observed or manipulated. The four basic techniques of physical examination are **inspection**, **palpation**, **percussion**, and **auscultation**. It is often suggested that beginning students practice newly learned physical assessment skills on fellow students, friends, or family. Doing so can help students acquire some skill, confidence, and organization before approaching patients. Expertise in the techniques of physical examination can be learned only through practice. Be prepared, however, to follow up if abnormal findings are present.

Positioning and Draping

The patient may need to assume various positions for the physical examination. Patients may need assistance with positioning and, if in pain, should not remain in any uncomfortable position for an extended length of time.

Draping is a method to help ensure privacy. During the examination, cover the patient's body parts that are not included in the specific examination taking place, exposing only the part of the body being examined. As you examine another part of the body, redrape the patient. Draping also keeps the patient warm during examination. Draping materials include paper sheets, linens, or blankets.

Inspection

Inspection is used to make specific observations of physical features and behavior. The nurse's vision is the most valuable tool for this part of the examination. Inspection is the natural beginning to physical examination because it starts immediately on meeting the patient. The initial observations provide an overall impression of the patient's present state of health and whether immediate interventions are indicated. Obtaining vital signs, height, and weight measurements follow these initial observations.

The general survey of the patient begins on your first contact with the patient. It includes apparent state of health, level of consciousness, and signs of distress. The general height, weight, and build can be noted. Also, notice skin color, dress, grooming, and personal hygiene. Facial expression, odors, posture, gait, and motor activity are observed (Jensen, 2015). If the nurse determines that the patient is in acute distress, the comprehensive health assessment is deferred. The nurse may obtain assistance and perform a focused assessment instead. General inspection of a patient focuses on the following areas:

- *Overall appearance of health or illness*: Does the patient appear weak, frail, or older than the stated age?
- *Signs of distress*: Is the patient grimacing as if in pain? Is breathing labored? Is the skin blue or pale?
- *Facial expression and mood*: Does the patient appear anxious, depressed, angry, or uninterested?
- *Body size*: Does the patient appear thin and malnourished or overweight?
- *Grooming and personal hygiene*: Are the patient and his or her clothing clean and neat? Is there an unusual odor?

In addition to the role of inspection in the general survey of a patient, inspection is the first method used in examination of a specific area. The chest and abdomen, for example, are inspected before palpation, percussion, or auscultation is performed.

The optimal conditions for effective inspection are full exposure of the area and adequate lighting. Removal of clothing and bed linen is necessary. Out of respect for the patient's modesty and comfort, expose only the area you are examining. A well-lit room is essential for good visualization. Tangential lighting is provided by indirectly shining light with a lamp or flashlight to create a shadow over the examined area. The shadow brings out subtle differences in contour and movement.

Palpation

Palpation usually follows inspection. Palpation is the use of the hands and fingers to gather information through touch. Palpation is used to discriminate position, texture, size, consistency, masses, and fluid. For patient comfort, the nurse's hands should be warm and the touch should be gentle and respectful.

During palpation, different parts of the hand are more suitable for different tactile sensations. The fingertips are concentrated with nerve endings and can sense fine differences in texture and consistency. They are used to discriminate raised versus flat skin lesions or to evaluate an arterial pulse. The skin over the dorsum of the hand is sensitive to temperature because it is thin and its nerve density is great. Skin temperature over a specific area may be evaluated by comparing its temperature with that of adjacent areas or the opposite side of the body. The palm of the hand is sensitive to vibration and is useful in locating a vibration associated with a heart **murmur**.

In addition to this superficial palpation, nurses use light or deep palpation to examine the abdomen. These two latter types of palpation require the patient to relax because tensed muscles block access to underlying tissue. The nurse will enhance the patient's ability to relax if actions are explained to the patient before touching.

With light palpation, three or four fingers of the dominant hand are used to depress an area of the patient's skin approximately 0.5 to 1 inch (Fig. 17-2A). The fingers evaluate the skin temperature and moistness. Move the hand in a gentle, circular motion to detect abnormal masses and locate areas of discomfort. Using a systematic pattern, lightly palpate and then release. Discomfort is best monitored by observing the patient's facial expression while palpating. A ticklish patient may place his or her hand on top of the nurse's hand to reduce ticklish sensations. This pattern of light palpation always precedes deep palpation. If discomfort is elicited in an area, avoid deep palpation there.

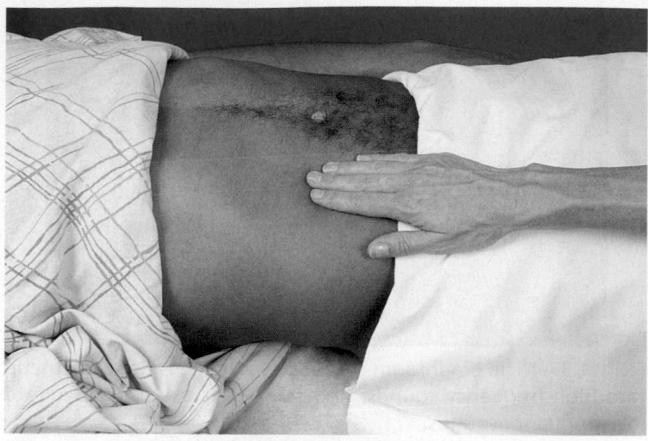

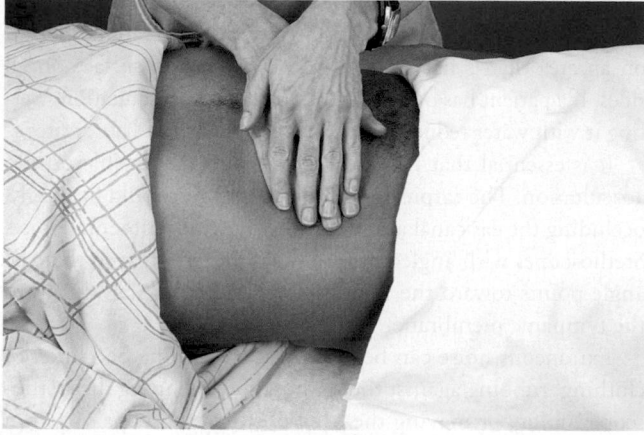

FIGURE 17-2 A. Light palpation. Move the fingertips in a circular motion, depressing the body surface 0.5 to 1 inch. **B.** Deep palpation. Hold the fingers at a greater angle to the body surface than in light palpation, and depress the skin 1.5 to 2 inches.

Deep palpation involves compression of an area to a depth of 1.5 to 2 inches and requires significantly more pressure than light palpation (Fig. 17-2B). In addition, the fingers are placed at a greater angle to the body than in light palpation. One or both hands may be used, depending on the structure being examined. When using both hands, place the fingers of one hand over the fingers of the other hand. The top hand presses and guides the bottom. The purpose of deep palpation is to locate organs, determine their size, and detect abnormal masses.

Percussion

Percussion, which uses the sense of hearing, involves using the fingers and hands to tap an area on the patient to produce sound. The type of percussion tone is determined by the density of the medium through which the sound is traveling. Percussion provides information about the nature of an underlying structure. It is used to outline the size of an organ, such as the bladder or liver. Percussion is also used to determine whether a structure is air filled, fluid filled, or solid. Such findings are important during percussion of the lungs and abdomen.

The degree to which sound propagates is called **resonance**. Sound propagates through air; therefore, air-filled spaces are resonant, whereas solid tissue is not. Percussion produces five characteristic tones: tympanic, hyperresonant, resonant, dull, and flat (Table 17-2).

Characteristically, percussion of the abdomen is tympanic, hyperinflated lung tissue is hyperresonant, normal lung tissue is resonant, the liver is dull, and bone is flat. The sound is also characterized in terms of intensity, or loudness. The more dense the medium, the quieter the percussion sound. Tympanic tones are the loudest, and flat ones are the quietest.

Percussion may be performed directly or indirectly. Direct percussion is accomplished by tapping an area directly with the fingertip of the middle finger or thumb. Indirect percussion interposes a finger between the area to be percussed and the finger creating the vibrations; indirect percussion usually is used (Fig. 17-3). The steps for indirect percussion are outlined in Box 17-3.

Auscultation

Auscultation is listening for sounds of movement within the body. The heart and blood vessels are auscultated for moving blood, the lungs are auscultated for moving air, and the abdomen is auscultated for movement of gastrointestinal contents.

The **stethoscope** collects and transmits sound, selects frequencies, and screens out extraneous sound. Although sound transmitted through the stethoscope seems loud, the stethoscope does not amplify the sound. A Doppler ultrasound device is a machine used to make sound louder if needed.

The head of the stethoscope applied to the skin collects the sound from beneath it. Most stethoscopes have two types of heads,

TABLE 17-2 CHARACTERISTICS OF PERCUSSION TONES

Tone	Quality	Pitch	Intensity	Location
Tympany	Musical, drumlike	High	Loud	Air-filled stomach
Hyperresonance	Booming	Very low	Very loud	Emphysematous lung
Resonance	Hollow	Low	Loud	Normal lung
Dullness	Thudlike	Medium	Medium	Liver, diaphragm
Flatness	Extreme dullness	High	Soft	Sternum, thigh

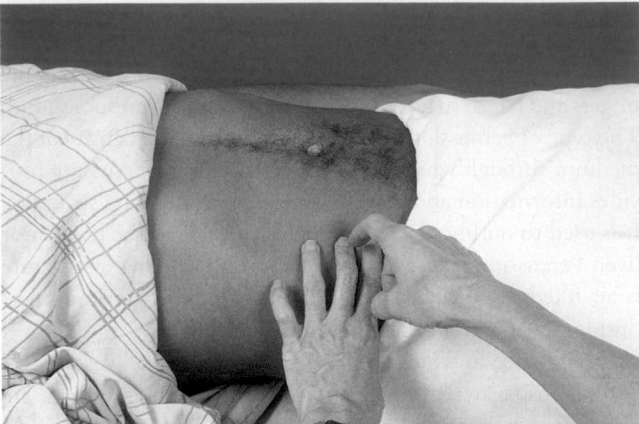

FIGURE 17-3 Perform indirect percussion with two hands, using the finger of one hand to tap on the finger of the other hand.

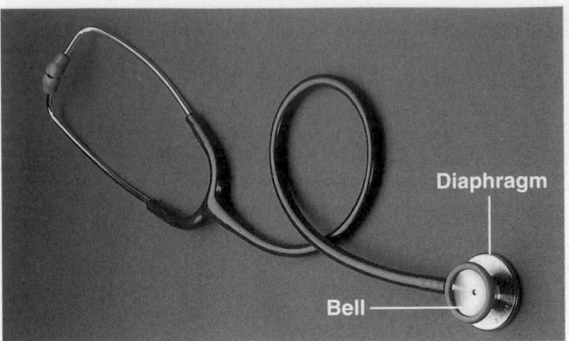

FIGURE 17-4 The diaphragm of the stethoscope is used to auscultate high-frequency sounds, and the bell is used to auscultate low-frequency sounds.

a diaphragm and a bell (Fig. 17-4). The diaphragm is a flat piece that is applied firmly against the skin and responds best to high-frequency sounds. The bell is a funnel- or cup-shaped head that collects low-pitched sounds. The bell should simply be allowed to rest on top of the skin; if too much pressure is applied, the skin is stretched and a diaphragm effect is produced. Some sounds that are very clear with one side may not be audible at all on the other side. Table 17-3 contrasts usage of the diaphragm and bell.

The ability to auscultate clearly also depends on transmission of sound. The tubing should be short (12 to 18 inches) to avoid distortion. The rubber should be thick and heavy to conduct the

sound optimally. The head of the stethoscope must be completely sealed by the patient's skin over the area of auscultation. Place it on an area that is flat enough to touch the skin surface on all sides. If a patient has body hair over the area of auscultation, wetting it with water reduces the crackling sound that hair creates.

It is essential that the room be as quiet as possible during auscultation. The earpieces of the stethoscope should fit snugly, occluding the ear canal and screening out environmental noise. Stethoscopes with angled earpieces should be worn so that the angle points toward the nose, thereby directing sound toward the tympanic membrane.

Extraneous noise can be generated by rustling bed linen or clothing, rubbing against the stethoscope, bumping the stethoscope tubing, or moving the head of the stethoscope. Attempt to hold the stethoscope and other equipment still to avoid these extraneous noises.

Four properties are used to describe sound: frequency, intensity, duration, and quality. *Frequency* is the measure of vibration, expressed in cycles per second, which is heard as pitch. A vibration of many cycles per second (i.e., high frequency) produces a high-pitched sound; one of few cycles per second produces a low-pitched sound. *Intensity* describes the loudness of sound. Breath sounds over the trachea are loud, whereas most heart sounds are soft. *Duration* is the length of the sound. An abnormal heart sound is described according to its duration within the cardiac cycle. Timing of the sound may also be described, such as during inspiration or expiration. *Quality* reflects the musical characteristic of a sound. Blowing, squeaking, and humming are adjectives frequently used when describing the quality of a sound.

BOX 17-3   Steps for Indirect Percussion

The steps for indirect percussion are as follows:
1. Rest the nondominant middle finger flatly against the patient's skin over the area to be percussed. The remainder of this hand should not touch the patient. Identify the interphalangeal joint of this middle finger, because it is the striking area for the opposite hand.
2. Poise the dominant hand about 4 to 5 inches above the striking area, and slightly flex the fingers. Snap this wrist downward, and with the tip of the middle finger, sharply tap the striking area. (The fingernail should be short to facilitate percussing with the tip, not the pad, of the finger.)
3. Deliver several sharp successive blows, rapidly withdrawing.
4. Identify the percussion sound (see Table 17-2).
5. Proceed to the next area, moving from more resonant to less resonant areas.

Perfecting the percussion technique is often difficult; repetition and practice are essential. Additionally, smaller hands generate less sound. Begin by refining the technique over a tympanic area such as the stomach. Once the percussion sound is clearly audible, move to another area and listen for changes in tone and intensity. Try to label the tone and intensity in this second area. Work from areas of tympany to areas of dullness, and repeat the percussion until the tone and intensity are clear.

TABLE 17-3 STETHOSCOPE DIAPHRAGM AND BELL USAGE

	Technique	Purpose	Examples
Diaphragm	Press firmly against the skin	Detects high-pitched sounds	Breath sounds, normal heart sounds, bowel sounds
Bell	Lay lightly on the skin	Detects low-pitched sounds	Abnormal heart sounds, bruits

HEAD-TO-TOE PHYSICAL ASSESSMENT OF FUNCTION

Assessment of Cognition

Objective data concerning the patient's cognitive abilities are obtained through the neurologic examination. This examination also provides information on sensory function. The neurologic examination is a systematic method of assessing the integration of brain function and motor response. Abnormalities often reflect impairment to the brain or spinal cord. If a patient is fully alert and oriented, the nurse may perform a full neurologic assessment to obtain baseline data. In many agencies, comprehensive, detailed neurologic testing is performed by advanced practitioners. See **Procedure 17-2** for a detailed description of how to perform a neurologic assessment.

LEVEL OF CONSCIOUSNESS

Consciousness is awareness of and responsiveness to the surrounding environment. Impairment in consciousness is evaluated on a continuum. At the highest level of consciousness, a person responds to environmental stimuli with appropriate verbal and motor activity. The person is attentive, cooperative, and completely oriented to self, time, and place. A patient may demonstrate impaired consciousness by loss of orientation and inability to follow simple commands. At the lowest level of consciousness—the comatose state—painful stimuli are necessary to induce a verbal or motor response.

The **Glasgow Coma Scale** (Table 17-4) is a standardized assessment tool that is used when serial assessments are done for high-risk patients (e.g., brain tumor, after brain surgery, after a cerebral vascular accident). Nurses are able to detect subtle changes in a patient's consciousness state by reviewing the scale and noticing deviations from baseline. In addition, this tool evaluates the best verbal response and the best motor response so that increased intracranial pressure (ICP) can be detected and treated quickly. The patient's reactions are scored according to the best response that he or she gives, and the results are documented appropriately in the patient's record.

ORIENTATION

Evaluate orientation by asking simple, direct questions about time, place, and person. Orientation × 1 indicates person orientation, such as knowing one's own name, knowing the names of significant others, or knowing the nurse. Orientation × 2 indicates person and place, which includes knowing location, city, or state. Orientation × 3 indicates person, place, and time of day, day of week, or date. It may be necessary to ask the friends or family to verify data the patient provides. A fourth level of orientation is oriented to the situation where the patient should be able to verbalize what is happening—for example, that the patient is in the hospital for tests.

MOOD

Abnormalities of mood may indicate psychological or neurologic problems. Normal mood is described as happy or pleasant. A patient who is unusually overjoyed may be described as elated or euphoric. Depression is being overly sad. Patients who are easily provoked or annoyed are described as irritable. Those with a rapid change of emotions may be described as labile. A patient whose affect is clearly out of context with the situation may be described as having an inappropriate affect. Flat affect describes the patient who expresses few emotions.

LANGUAGE AND MEMORY

Communication and memory are specific aspects of cognitive functioning that are important to achieve effective patient teaching. Speech deficits may take on various appearances. It is important to differentiate between problems in receiving the communication (**receptive aphasia**) and problems in expressing communication (**expressive aphasia**). With receptive aphasia, patients are unable to understand simple directions. With expressive aphasia, the patient understands and follows directions but is unable to verbally communicate effectively with the nurse. Mechanical, muscular, or sensory problems may cause difficulties with articulation of words (dysarthria).

If impaired reading ability is suspected, ask the patient to read aloud a short passage from the newspaper or from a patient education pamphlet and then paraphrase what he or she has read. Some patients are unable to read for reasons other than neurologic deficits, such as illiteracy or understanding a different language. Writing ability involves a complex series of tasks and can simply be evaluated by having the patient write his or her name.

Remote memory is evaluated by asking about birthdays, anniversaries, or social security numbers. Evaluate recent memory by

TABLE 17-4 GLASGOW COMA SCALE	
Best eye-opening response	
Purposeful and spontaneous	4
To voice	3
To pain	2
No response	1
Untestable	U
Best verbal response	
Oriented	5
Disoriented	4
Inappropriate words	3
Incomprehensible sounds	2
No response	1
Untestable	U
Best motor response	
Obeys commands	6
Localizes pain	5
Withdraws to pain	4
Flexion to pain	3
Extension to pain	2
No response	1
Untestable	U

asking the patient to recall events of the day, such as activities, visitors, or meals eaten. Cues to recent memory loss include losing direction easily and inability to remember a discussion that took place earlier in the same conversation. New learning ability includes the ability to remember three or four words and repeat what they were 5 minutes later (Bickley, 2013).

Assessment of Skin, Hair, and Nails

The skin is the largest organ of the body. It protects underlying structures, regulates temperature, and senses stimuli. The epidermis is the outer layer of skin; the dermis below it contains the oil and sweat glands. The subcutaneous tissue is a layer of connective tissue below the epidermis that thins with aging.

Patients may complain of problems with the skin, indicating underlying abnormalities. The skin is a reflection of the body's nutrition and metabolism. Some skin disorders may interfere with the patient's body image, especially if present on the face. Examples of questions used in assessment include the following:

- What is your usual daily care routine for skin, hair, and nails?
- Describe any birthmarks, tattoos, moles, or freckles.
- Have you had any hair loss or change?
- What level of protection do you use against sun exposure?

The skin is examined through inspection and palpation. Assess the skin for color, moisture, temperature, texture, and hygiene. Normal skin color may be pink, tan, brown, black, olive, or yellowish. The color and appearance of the skin and nails may reflect insufficient delivery of oxygenated blood to the tissues because of respiratory or cardiac dysfunction. With a normal supply of oxygen, the nail beds, the tongue, and the lips appear pinkish red in color. Hypoxia (decreased supply of oxygen to the tissues) changes this color to a gray, blue, or purple tone called **cyanosis**. The skin color may also appear pale with hypoxia and anemia; this is known as pallor. **Jaundice** is a yellow tone to the skin and is observed in liver disease. **Erythema** is redness, usually from irritation or inflammation. Abnormal skin colors are more difficult to detect on dark-skinned patients.

The skin is normally dry; either extreme dryness or excessive sweating (diaphoresis) is abnormal. Skin temperature is normally warm; hot may indicate fever, and cool may indicate poor circulation. Skin texture is soft for most of the body but rough over the elbows, knees, and heels of the feet. Observe the skin for past injuries, calluses, stains, scars, needle marks, and insect bites. Note the location of rashes. A diagram is helpful in identifying the location of lesions.

SKIN TURGOR

Assess the amount of fluid in the tissues by checking **skin turgor**. Check for skin turgor by pinching a small area of skin on the medial arm or anterior chest and noting how quickly it returns to the original position when you release it. If skin turgor is poor, the skin remains elevated (tenting) or slowly resumes position. Poor skin turgor may indicate dehydration, but it may also occur with normal aging or with weight loss.

SKIN LESIONS

A skin lesion is an abnormality in the structure of the skin that results from injury or disease. Describe every lesion in terms of size, color, type, and location. Lesions may be measured with a metric ruler to ensure accurate size determination. Take note of the appearance of the border of the lesion and surrounding skin. It is also important to palpate the lesion to distinguish between flat and raised lesions. Lightly press the lesion to determine whether it blanches with pressure. These steps will assist in labeling the lesion and identifying the cause. A lesion that exhibits asymmetry, irregular borders, uneven color, a raised surface, or a recent change in size may indicate malignancy, and the patient should be referred for evaluation.

Wounds

Accidents, pressure, or surgeries may cause wounds. It is especially important to note a wound's color. Yellow or green coloring may indicate infection. A black, brown, or gray color may indicate necrotic (dead) tissue. In a wound, bright pink or red is the color of new granulation tissue, which indicates wound healing. Note the color, character, and amount of any drainage (exudate) from the wound. Creamy, colored drainage indicates infection. Bright red drainage indicates blood. A watery, clear drainage is serum.

SCALP AND HAIR

Inspect the scalp and hair for color, quantity, distribution, texture, hygiene, nodules, and lesions. Hair color may range from pale blonde to deep black; graying begins normally in the third decade of life. Texture may be straight, curly, kinky, fine, or coarse. Examine the base of the hair follicle for pest infestation and dandruff. Loss of hair is known as alopecia.

NAILS

Inspect the nails for shape, color, and texture. **Clubbing** of the nails is a sign of chronic hypoxia. To determine whether clubbing is present, examine the contour of the nail and its adherence to the nail bed. When viewed in profile, normal fingernails present an angle of 160 degrees between the nail bed and the finger. With clubbing, swelling flattens the angle to 180 degrees or less (Fig. 17-5). With advanced clubbing, the nail becomes less adherent to the base of the nail and feels spongy. The nails and fingertips appear large and swollen, sometimes described as "drumstick-like."

Assessment of the Head and Neck

Have the patient open and close the jaw while the joint is palpated. Problems with the temporal mandibular joint (TMJ) include pain or a grating feeling called **crepitus**. Test for nasal obstruction by first occluding one side of the nares and then the other. Inspect the inside of the nose with an **otoscope**. Note any drainage. Palpate the nasal sinuses for tenderness.

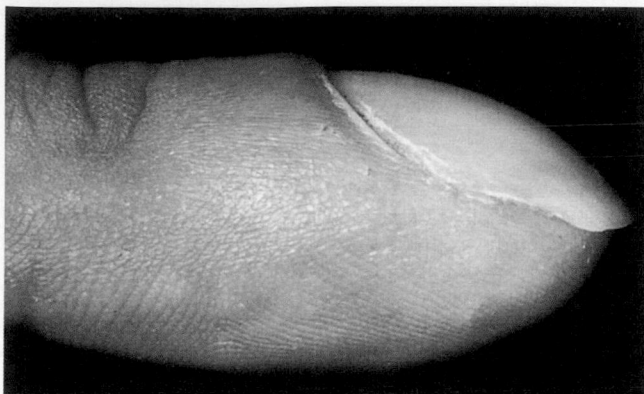

FIGURE 17-5 Clubbing of the nail and fingers.

Auscultation of the neck is used to detect **bruits**, which are abnormal arterial sounds, similar to murmurs, caused by increased turbulence of blood flow. Bruits can be detected by placing the stethoscope over major blood vessels, such as the carotid artery. Bruits occur when an artery is partially obstructed or distended, which prevents blood flow from moving straight through the vessel. Palpate the lymph nodes for enlargement, mobility, and tenderness. The lymph nodes may become enlarged or tender with inflammation or infection. Evaluate the veins in the neck for distention, which often occurs with fluid volume excess. Figure 17-6 identifies the technique for inspection of jugular venous distention.

The trachea is normally in a straight, vertical position. Some lung disorders, such as large masses and pneumothorax, can cause a shift in the trachea from its normal midline position. Stand behind the patient and reach across the patient's shoulders, placing the index finger on each side of the trachea in the suprasternal notch. The space on either side of the trachea and the ends of the suprasternal notch should be equal. To palpate the thyroid, place the fingers on either side of the trachea below the cricoid cartilage. Using the fingers on the left, push the trachea to the right and ask the patient to swallow as you palpate the gland. Do the opposite to palpate the left side of the thyroid (Fig. 17-7).

Evaluate cranial nerve XI by having the patient shrug the shoulders and turn the head. Evaluate strength by having the patient perform these movements against resistance. Movements should be of equal strength on both sides.

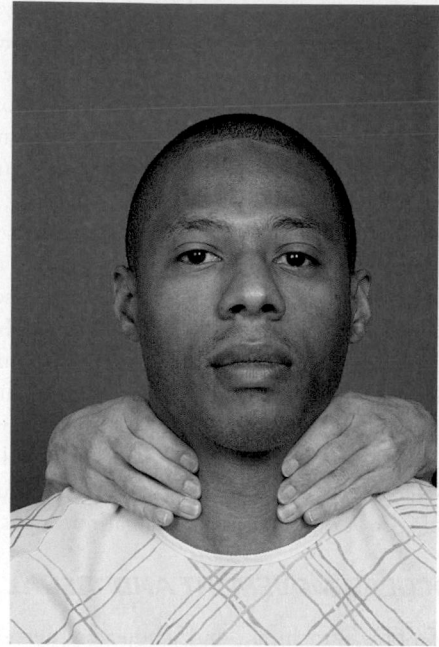

FIGURE 17-7 Palpation of the thyroid.

Assessment of Sensory Function

Physical examination of the senses usually is not performed in a basic health assessment unless evidence of impaired function is uncovered during the patient interview. Physical examination of the senses is a routine part of a health screening examination, such as hearing or vision screening in elementary schools.

SENSORY AIDS

Document the use of glasses, contact lenses, hearing aids, and other assistive devices in the patient's health assessment. The proper care of such devices should also be solicited and written in the patient's record. Doing so helps to ensure proper use and care of expensive devices during the patient's stay in a healthcare agency.

VISUAL ACUITY

To test the patient's near vision, hold newsprint 14 inches from the patient's face. If the patient is unable to focus well enough to read, experiment with the distance to determine whether improvement

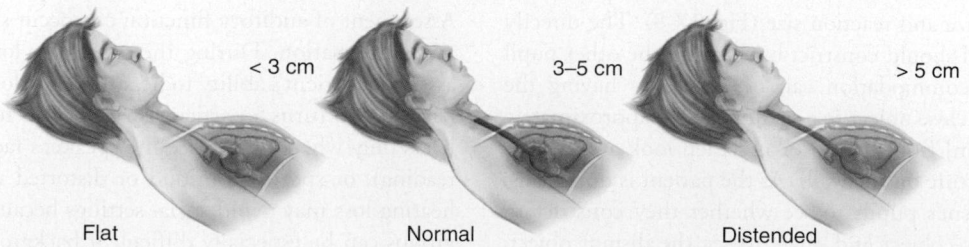

Flat   < 3 cm   Normal   3–5 cm   Distended   > 5 cm

FIGURE 17-6 Height of jugular venous pressure is measured in relation to the sternal angle at the second intercostal space. Normal height is less than 3 cm at 45 degrees.

occurs when the print is moved closer or farther away. Visual problems with close objects occur more frequently after the age of 40 years. To test far vision, ask the patient to read the time on a clock across the room or to read a sign across the hall or room. If problems are detected, refer the patient for further testing.

The Snellen "E" is used for assessing distant visual acuity. Position the patient 20 feet from a Snellen chart (6.1 m) that has been placed at eye level. Test each eye separately and then both eyes together. As the patient covers one eye, direct the patient to read the smallest line that he or she can see. Young children who do not yet know the letters of the alphabet may be tested with another chart that has pictures. Compare the patient's distance from the chart (20 feet) to the number by the smallest line that the patient can read. For example, if the patient can read the 100-foot line, report visual acuity as 20/100. Refer any person with less than 20/20 acuity to an ophthalmologist or optometrist for evaluation.

EXTRAOCULAR MOVEMENT AND VISUAL FIELDS

The oculomotor, trochlear, and abducens nerves control the horizontal, vertical, and diagonal movement of the eyes. Assessment of peripheral visual fields and the six ocular movements is important in a comprehensive visual assessment. To evaluate extraocular movements, ask the patient to visually follow an object (such as a pencil) through various positions (horizontal, vertical, and diagonal). The patient's head remains still as the eyes move to follow the object. At each position, pause to evaluate for **nystagmus** (involuntary, rhythmic oscillations of the eyes) as well as evaluate whether the patient's eyes can follow the object smoothly.

Peripheral vision can be tested in a similar manner. Have the patient look straight ahead, and cover one of the patient's eyes as you bring your finger or another object from far away to within the field of vision. Repeat for each eye from different fields (temporal, upward, downward, and nasal).

PUPILS AND PUPILLARY REFLEXES

As a beam of light is directed through the pupil and onto the retina, stimulation of cranial nerve III causes the muscles of the iris to constrict. Evaluate pupils bilaterally for size, shape, **accommodation**, and reaction to light. Normally, pupils are black and round, and they constrict briskly when exposed to a bright light source. To test pupils, first dim the light in the room. As the patient gazes straight ahead, shine a penlight into the pupil from the side of the head. Observe both pupils and estimate initial size and reaction size (Fig. 17-8). The directly illuminated pupil should constrict briskly and the other pupil consensually. Accommodation can be tested by having the patient look at a close object (e.g., a finger held approximately 4 inches [10.2 cm] from the nose) and then look at a distant object (e.g., a picture on the wall). As the patient is doing this, observe the patient's pupils to see whether they constrict to focus on the close object and dilate to see the distant object. Normal pupil assessment data are recorded as PERRLA: pupils equal, round, reactive to light and accommodation.

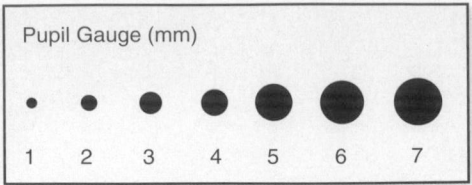

FIGURE 17-8 Pupil size chart. To test the pupil reflex, the nurse shines a penlight from the side into the pupil, observing the rate and amount of pupil constriction. The pupils should constrict briskly and be equal in size after constriction.

Pupils can appear cloudy when cataracts are present. Dilated pupils can occur when glaucoma is treated with drops or neurologic impairment is present. Unilateral changes in pupil reflexes can signify increased ICP caused by tumor, trauma, or cerebral vascular accident. Report changes in pupillary response to the physician.

CRANIAL NERVE ASSESSMENT

Intact cranial nerve function is important for normal sensory functioning. Vision depends on normal functioning of cranial nerves II, III, IV, and VI. Cranial nerve VIII is important for hearing, and cranial nerve I is important for the sense of smell. Cranial nerves V, VII, IX, and XII are important in the coordination of facial movement or reflex activity. During an initial neurologic assessment, or at specific intervals for high-risk patients, evaluate normal functioning of the cranial nerves. Table 17-5 lists the cranial nerves and techniques used to assess their functioning.

EXTERNAL AND INTERNAL EYE STRUCTURES

External eye structures should be free from lesions or inflammation. A blink reflex should be present. An **ophthalmoscope** is the instrument used to assess internal eye structures (Fig. 17-9A). Usually, advanced practitioners with additional training and practice perform such examinations. Ophthalmic examination permits visualization of the retina, optic nerve disc, macula, fovea centralis, and retinal vessels. As the fundus is observed through the ophthalmoscope, a round red glow (the red reflex) is noted (Fig. 17-9B). Normal findings include uniform red reflex; round, white, or pink optic nerve disc; reddish retina; and bright red arterioles and dark red veins (Fig. 17-9C).

AUDITORY ASSESSMENT

Assessment of auditory function can occur simply during normal conversation. During the interview, lower your voice to assess the patient's ability to hear. Hearing loss is suggested in a patient who turns a particular ear or leans toward the speaker, hears only when able to see the speaker's face (evidence of lip reading), or speaks in a loud or distorted voice. People with hearing loss may avoid social settings because conversation in groups can be especially difficult if background noise is present. Other physical symptoms associated with the ear are tinnitus (ringing in the ears) and vertigo (dizziness).

TABLE 17-5 CRANIAL NERVE FUNCTION AND ASSESSMENT

Number	Name	Function	Method of Assessment
I	Olfactory	Sense of smell	Ask patient to identify different mild aromas, such as vanilla, coffee, chocolate, cloves.
II	Optic	Vision	Ask patient to read Snellen chart.
III	Oculomotor	Pupillary reflex Extraocular eye movement	Assess pupil reaction to penlight. Assess directions of gaze by holding your finger 18 inches from patient's face. Ask patient to follow your finger up and down and side to side.
IV	Trochlear	Lateral and downward movement of eyeball	Assess directions of gaze. Test with cranial nerve III.
V	Trigeminal	Sensation to cornea, skin of face, nasal mucosa	Lightly touch cotton swab to the lateral sclera of the eye to elicit blink. Measure sensation of touch and pain on the face using cotton wisp.
VI	Abducens	Lateral movement of eyeball	Assess directions of gaze. Test with cranial nerve III.
VII	Facial	Facial expression Taste—anterior two thirds of tongue	Ask patient to smile, frown, raise eyebrows. Ask patient to identify different tastes on tip and sides of tongue: sugar (sweet), salt, lemon juice (sour).
VIII	Auditory	Hearing	Assess ability to hear spoken word.
IX	Glossopharyngeal	Taste—posterior tongue Swallowing Movement of tongue	Ask patient to identify different tastes on the back of the tongue as above. Place a tongue blade on posterior tongue while patient says "ah" to elicit a gag response. Ask patient to move tongue up and down and side to side.
X	Vagus	Swallowing Movement of vocal cords Sensation of pharynx	Assess with cranial nerve IX by observing palate and pharynx move as patient says "ah."
XI	Spinal accessory	Head and shoulder movement	Ask patient to turn head side to side and shrug shoulders against resistance from examiner's hands.
XII	Hypoglossal	Tongue position	Ask patient to stick out tongue to midline, then move it side to side.

If hearing loss is suspected, inspect the patient's external ear canal for inflammation or cerumen (ear wax). Using an otoscope (the instrument for examining the ear), visualize the canal after pulling the pinna up, out, and back to straighten the ear canal. In an infant, pull the pinna down and back. A buildup of cerumen may prevent visualization of the tympanic membrane. Insects or other foreign objects may be present in the ear canal. Because these objects can temporarily impede normal hearing, remove them before performing further assessment related to hearing.

An advanced practitioner usually performs visualization of the inner ear structures. To do this, insert the otoscope into the external ear canal as far as is comfortable to the patient. Support the otoscope by resting a finger against the patient's head or cheek, and wiggle the auricle until the tympanic membrane is visualized (Fig. 17-10A). The normal tympanic membrane is pearly, gray, shiny, translucent, and intact. A cone-shaped reflection of the light from the otoscope is usually seen between the 5 and 7 o'clock positions. The small bones of the ear may also be visualized (Fig. 17-10B).

Health screening may include hearing tests using an **audiometer**. For this test, the patient wears headphones that are capable of transmitting sounds of different frequencies. The patient indicates when he or she hears a sound by raising the hand. Such tests may also be administered to high-risk patients who are receiving medications (e.g., aminoglycoside antibiotics) that can cause hearing impairment.

The Weber test and the Rinne test, which require a tuning fork, can be used to evaluate hearing loss further. The *Weber test* can evaluate lateralization of sound (Fig. 17-11A). Activate the tuning fork, and place it at the top of the patient's head. Normally, the patient will hear vibrations equally in both ears. Patients with conduction deafness will best hear vibrations in the affected ear, whereas in those with sensorineural loss, the sound lateralizes to the unaffected ear.

The *Rinne test* discriminates between bone conduction and air conduction of sound. Strike the tuning fork, and place its stem firmly against the mastoid process (Fig. 17-11B). When the patient can no longer hear the tuning fork, remove it from the bone and allow sound to conduct through the air near the ear. Normally, the patient should hear the sound of the tuning fork when it is placed near the ear, indicating that air conduction of sound is greater than bone conduction. When the patient does not detect sound until the tuning fork is placed on the mastoid process, bone conduction of sound is greater than air conduction because of a conductive hearing loss.

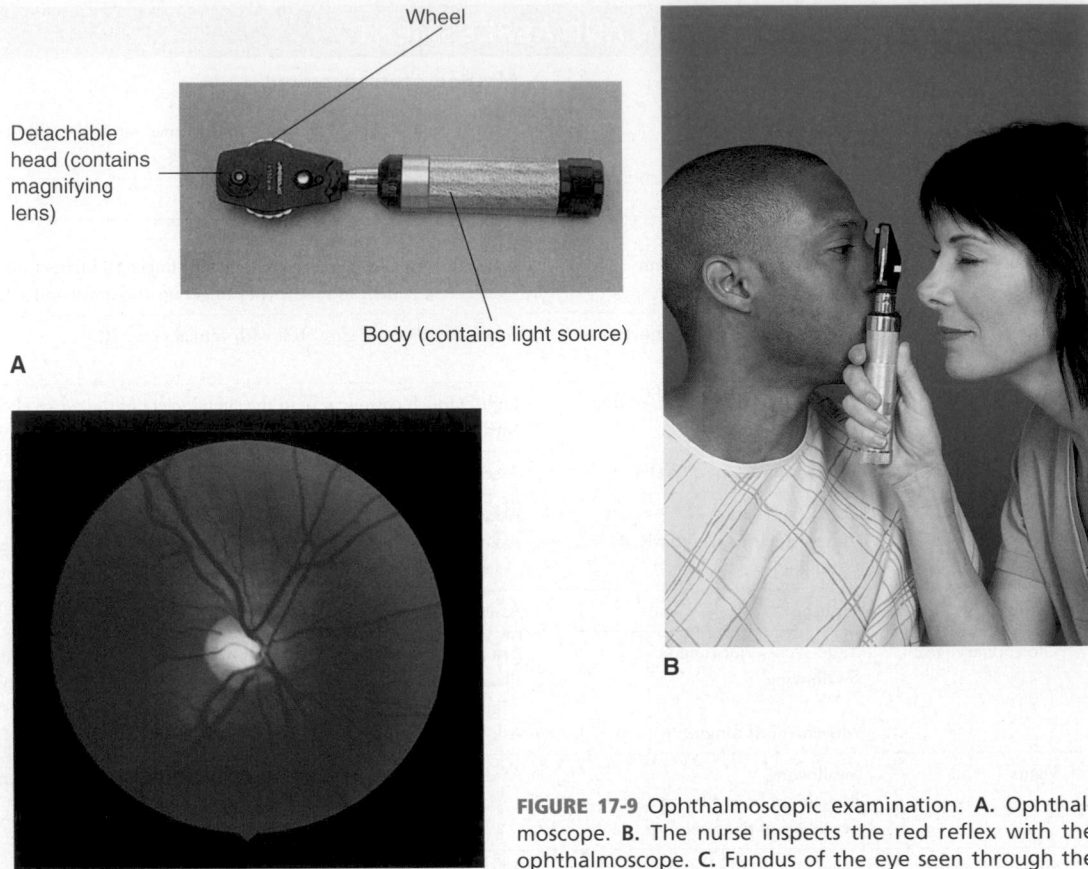

Wheel

Detachable head (contains magnifying lens)

Body (contains light source)

A

B

C

FIGURE 17-9 Ophthalmoscopic examination. **A.** Ophthalmoscope. **B.** The nurse inspects the red reflex with the ophthalmoscope. **C.** Fundus of the eye seen through the ophthalmoscope.

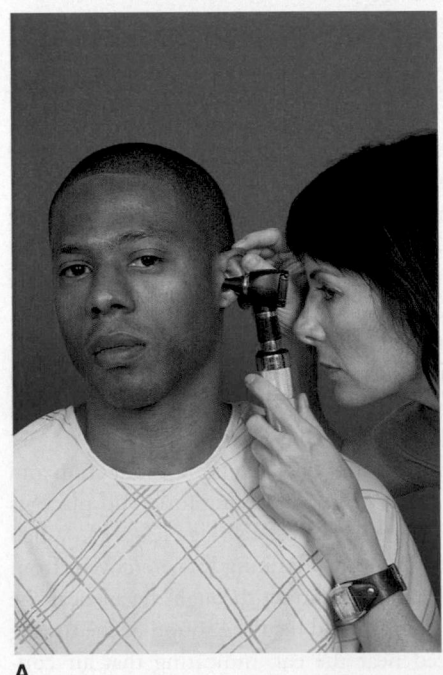

A

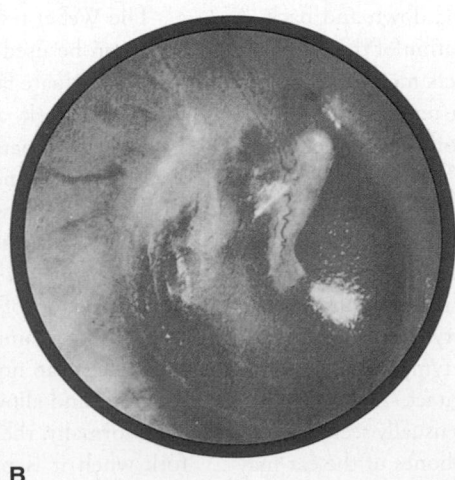

B

FIGURE 17-10 Internal ear examination. **A.** Inserting the otoscope into the ear. **B.** Normal eardrum with cone of light, malleus, and incus visible.

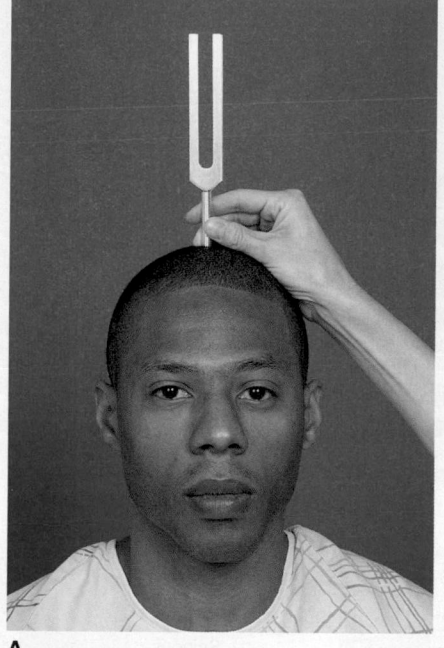
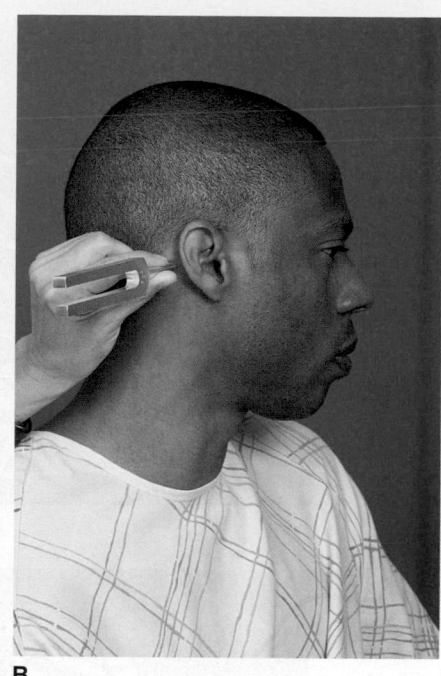

A   B

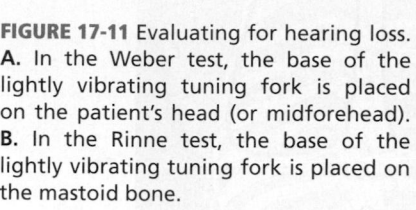

FIGURE 17-11 Evaluating for hearing loss. **A.** In the Weber test, the base of the lightly vibrating tuning fork is placed on the patient's head (or midforehead). **B.** In the Rinne test, the base of the lightly vibrating tuning fork is placed on the mastoid bone.

Assessment of the Mouth

Examination of the mouth includes the buccal mucosa (cheek), teeth, lips, gums, tongue, tonsils, and uvula (Fig. 17-12). Evaluate the lips for color, moisture, cracks, and lesions. Use a bright light and a tongue blade to inspect the mucous membranes, teeth, and gums. Remove and inspect dental appliances, especially if the patient complains of pain or has ill-fitting dentures. Mucous membranes should appear pink and moist. Observe for lesions in the mouth, gums, or tongue. Candidiasis, an oral fungal infection, appears as cheesy white plaque on the tongue and frequently occurs in patients on antibiotic therapy or chemotherapy. Ask the patient to say "Ahh" while the uvula is observed; it should rise symmetrically. The tonsils should be pink, symmetric, and slightly visible. Inspect the teeth for stability and overall hygiene. Evaluate the bite. A major concern when examining the mouth is to detect any abnormalities that might impede the patient's ability to taste, chew, swallow, or enjoy food.

Respiratory Assessment

Physical assessment of the respiratory system includes inspection, palpation, percussion, and auscultation. Discussing findings with an experienced nurse or respiratory care practitioner helps refine assessment skills and verify results.

ANATOMIC LANDMARKS OF THE CHEST AND LUNGS

Nurses use anatomic landmarks and imaginary reference lines during the assessment of structures that lie within the thorax (chest). During lung auscultation and percussion, these lines

FIGURE 17-12 Structures of the mouth.

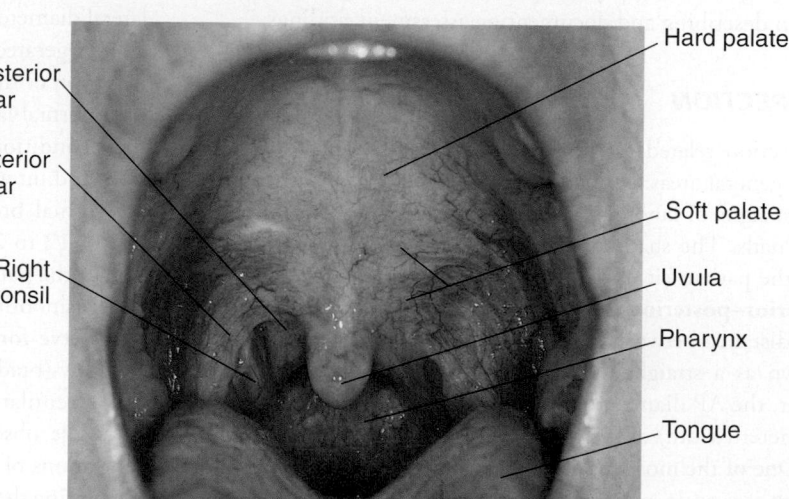

Posterior pillar

Anterior pillar

Right tonsil

Hard palate

Soft palate

Uvula

Pharynx

Tongue

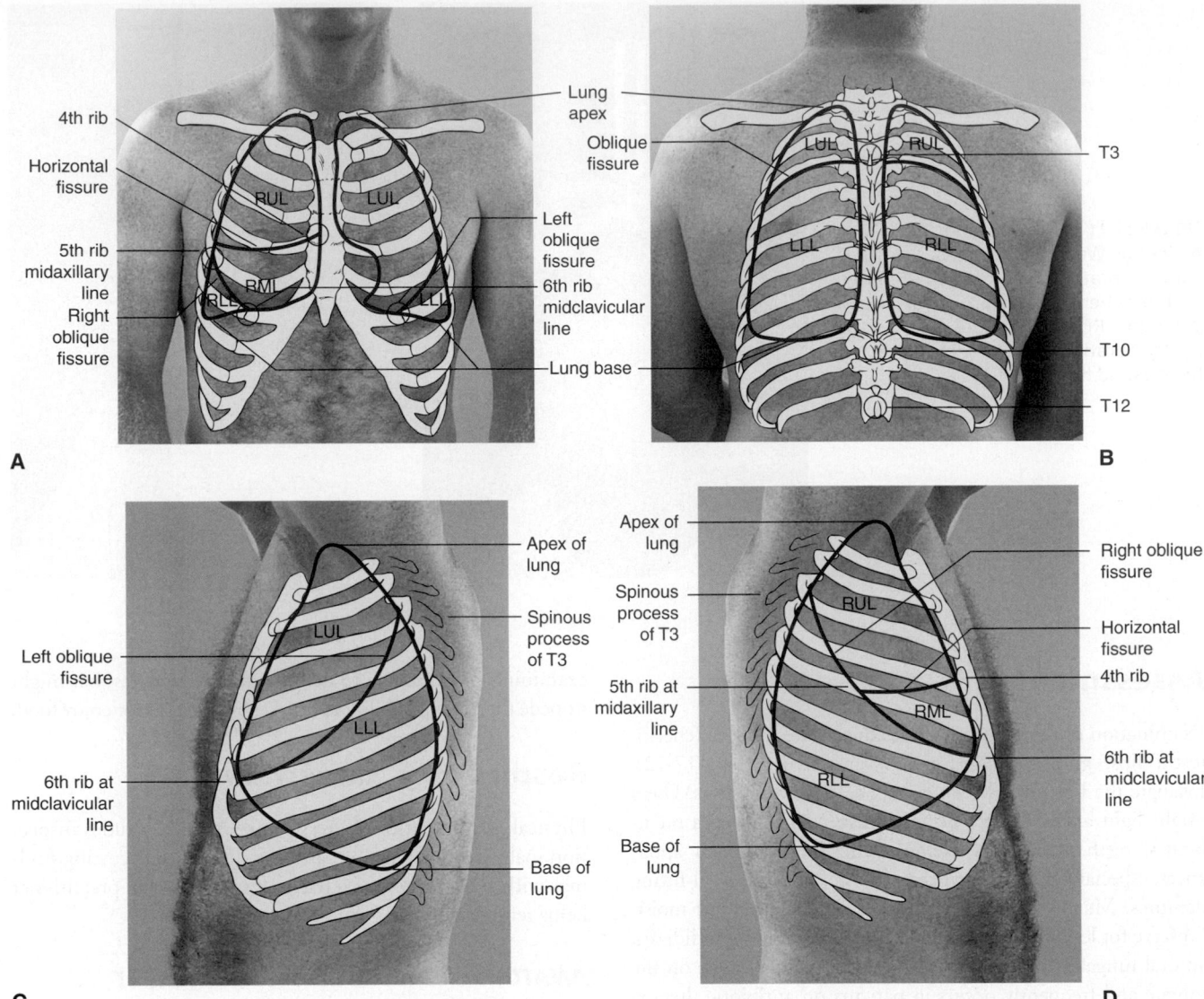

FIGURE 17-13 Landmarks of the anterior and posterior chest wall. **A.** Anterior. **B.** Posterior. **C.** Left lateral. **D.** Right lateral.

and landmarks define the specific area of the lung being examined (Fig. 17-13). They also provide a standard vocabulary for use in describing and documenting assessment findings.

INSPECTION

Inspection related to the respiratory examination focuses on four general areas: configuration of the thorax, breathing patterns, signs of labored breathing, and observation of the skin and nails. The shape of the thorax is best examined by having the patient sit upright with the chest area unclothed. The **anterior–posterior (AP) diameter** is a term used to describe the distance between the sternum and the vertebral column, drawn as a straight line through the thorax. In the normal adult, the AP diameter is approximately one half of the lateral diameter (width) of the chest.

One of the most common abnormalities of thorax configuration is seen in patients with chronic obstructive pulmonary disease. These patients exhibit a "barrel-shaped" chest in which the AP diameter is enlarged and approximately equal to the lateral diameter. Other thoracic abnormalities include *kyphosis*, an exaggerated convex curve of the spine; *scoliosis*, a lateral deviation of the spinal curve; and *kyphoscoliosis*, a combination of abnormal lateral and convex curvature of the spine. Any of these conditions may deform the rib cage, impede lung expansion, and interfere with breathing.

Normal breathing is silent and effortless and occurs at a rate of 12 to 20 times per minute in adults. Careful observation of the patient's breathing should normally reveal a pattern that is smooth, regular, symmetric, and rhythmic. Conditions to observe for include breathing that is too fast (tachypnea), too slow (bradypnea), too shallow (hypoventilation), too deep (hyperventilation), or irregular (Cheyne–Stokes breathing).

While observing the patient's breathing pattern, look for indications of respiratory distress or increased effort in breathing, noting the position that the patient has assumed to breathe.

Patients experiencing respiratory distress will be sitting upright and may be leaning forward or need a pillow for support. Symptoms such as nasal flaring, facial straining, and pursed-lip breathing indicate abnormal respiratory effort. Abnormal effort during inspiration is evidenced by active, visible use of the scalene and sternomastoid muscles of the neck and shoulders. These muscles are called **accessory muscles**. Contraction of the abdominal muscles, which assists upward movement of the diaphragm, may also be observed. During inspection of the patient's breathing, observe the intercostal spaces. Airway obstruction or decreased lung compliance may result in **retraction** of the intercostal spaces during inspiration, whereas some respiratory diseases (e.g., emphysema) can cause bulging of the intercostal spaces during expiration.

PALPATION

Palpation is used in respiratory assessment to evaluate painful or abnormal areas on the chest wall, to test for symmetry of chest expansion, and to detect tracheal deviation. To examine any areas on the chest where the patient has complained of discomfort, or where visible abnormalities are present, lightly palpate the area and surrounding area. Note any tenderness, masses or bulges, or a crackling feeling (crepitus), which may indicate air leaking into the subcutaneous tissue. **Tactile fremitus** is a vibration of the patient's chest wall produced by vocalization. It is assessed while the patient says "1, 2, 3," or "99." Normal fremitus is symmetric; it may be increased in pneumonia and decreased with a pneumothorax.

Normal chest expansion during inspiration is symmetric, indicating equal expansion of both lungs. To evaluate **respiratory excursion**, stand behind the patient, place your thumbs at the level of the 10th rib, and wrap your hands around the lateral rib cage (Fig. 17-14). Ask the patient to inhale deeply, and observe your thumbs for equal, outward movement.

PERCUSSION

Percussion of the lung normally reveals a hollow, loud, low-pitched, resonant sound because the lung is filled with air. Percussion that reveals dullness or reduced resonance may indicate masses, fluid, or tissue-filled lung space. Percussion that is hyperresonant indicates hyperinflation of the lung such as with the air trapping that occurs with emphysema. Diagnostically, examination of the chest radiograph has largely replaced chest percussion. **Diaphragmatic excursion** can be assessed by percussing the posterior diaphragm and measuring the difference between complete exhalation and full inhalation. The patient takes a deep breath in, and the nurse percusses until the sound turns dull. The patient then exhales and the nurse percusses to find the resonant sounds again, usually one rib space away.

AUSCULTATION

Lung auscultation involves listening with a stethoscope over the anterior and posterior chest wall for variations in breath sounds. The movement of air in and out of the airways

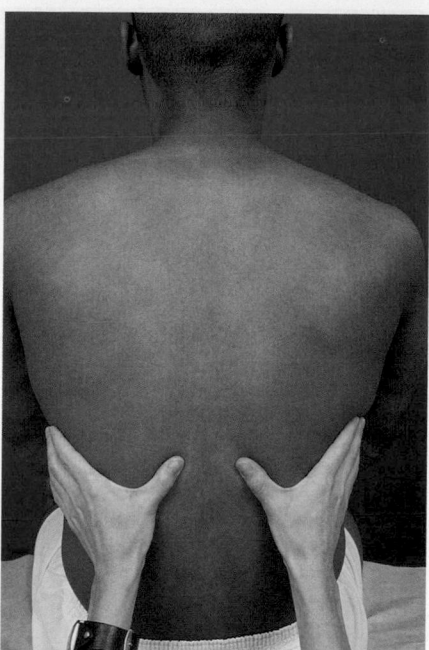

FIGURE 17-14 Palpation of thoracic excursion. In the posterior approach, the nurse's hands are placed at the level of the 10th rib and observed for equal outward movement as the patient inhales.

with each inspiration and expiration creates breath sounds. Auscultation of the lungs reveals direct, objective data about the patient's ventilatory status. Data gathered through auscultation provide important clues to underlying pathophysiology. Refer to **Procedure 17-3** for the steps in pulmonary auscultation.

Normal Breath Sounds

Normal breath sounds are classified as bronchial, bronchovesicular, and vesicular. They are described according to location, ratio of inspiration to expiration, intensity, and pitch, as summarized and illustrated in Table 17-6.

Bronchial breath sounds are loud and high pitched, with a hollow quality often compared to the sound of air blowing through a pipe. Expiration is longer and louder than inspiration with bronchial breath sounds. They are normal when heard over the trachea but indicate a lung abnormality when heard elsewhere. Abnormal bronchial sounds may be associated with pneumonia, pleural effusion, tumor, or atelectasis.

Vesicular breath sounds are normally heard over all areas of the lung except over or near the major airways. Vesicular sounds are described as soft and breezy, with inspiration markedly longer than expiration.

Bronchovesicular breath sounds are intermediate in character between bronchial and vesicular sounds. They are described as breezy but softer and lower pitched than bronchial sounds. Inspiratory and expiratory times are approximately equal. Bronchovesicular sounds are normally heard in two areas only: on the anterior chest over the bifurcation of the main bronchi in the first or second intercostal spaces and posteriorly between

TABLE 17-6 NORMAL BREATH SOUNDS FROM ANTERIOR LOCATION

Location	Description	Ratio of Inspiration to Expiration	Intensity	Pitch
Bronchial	Blowing, hollow sounds over the trachea	Inspiration / Expiration	Expiration is markedly longer and louder.	Expiration is higher.
Bronchovesicular	Intermediate sounds over first and second anterior intercostal spaces and posteriorly between scapula	Inspiration / Expiration	Medium and similar	Medium and similar
Vesicular	Soft and breezy sounds over all lung area except airways	Inspiration / Expiration	Inspiration markedly longer and louder	Inspiration is higher.

the scapulae. Like bronchial sounds, bronchovesicular sounds should not be detected elsewhere over the chest.

Adventitious Breath Sounds

Adventitious breath sounds are abnormal sounds that occur from air passing through fluid, narrowed airways, or from an inflammation of lung pleura. The major adventitious breath sounds are crackles, wheezes, and friction rubs (Fig. 17-15). These sounds are often superimposed over normal breath sounds and take much practiced listening to discern. Chapter 26 describes adventitious breath sounds in detail.

When you detect abnormal breath sounds in a patient, continue to listen, requesting the patient to say words or sounds. If consolidation or atelectasis is present, the words (such as "ninety-nine") will sound louder and clearer than they usually do. This is known as bronchophony. Also, if the patient says "ee," the sound will transmit as "ay"; this is known as egophony.

Cardiac Assessment

Activity and exercise are impeded when the heart cannot work effectively to pump blood or when the vasculature is unable to supply the perfusion of blood that body tissues need. Assessment of cardiac and peripheral vascular status provides clues about circulation and oxygenation to every part of the body.

Inspection, palpation, and auscultation are the three basic techniques used to assess the precordium and vasculature. Percussion may be used to estimate the size of the heart, but radiographic examination has generally replaced this method.

Obtain objective data about the patient's cardiovascular status by assessing vital signs, the heart, and arteries and veins. Significant deviation from normal heart rate and blood pressure may be the first indicator of a serious problem in circulatory function.

Crackles

Wheezes

Pleural friction rubs

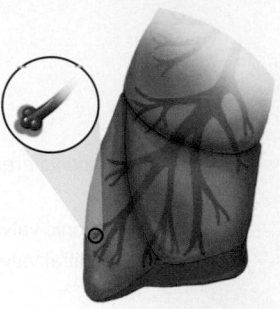

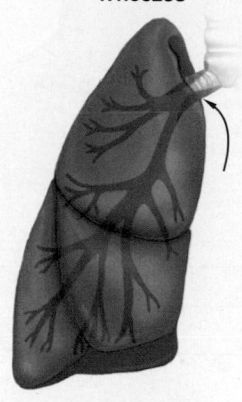

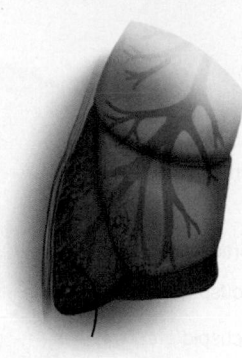

FIGURE 17-15 Adventitious breath sounds.

Crackles: high-pitched, discrete, noncontinuous cracking sounds heard during the end of inspiration

Coarse crackles: loud, bubbly noise heard during inspiration, not cleared by a cough

Fine wheeze: musical noise sounding like a squeak; may be heard during inspiration or expiration

Coarse wheeze (rhonchi): loud, low coarse sounds like a snore heard at any point of inspiration or expiration; coughing may clear sound (usually means mucus accumulation in large trachea or large bronchi)

Pleural friction rub: dry rubbing, or grating sound, usually caused by inflammation of pleural surfaces; heard during inspiration or expiration; loudest over low lateral anterior surface

> ! **SAFETY ALERT**
> Treat any chest pain, if present, as heart pain. Stop the assessment and notify the physician. Treatment should begin immediately.

LANDMARKS FOR CARDIAC ASSESSMENT

The precordium is the area on the anterior chest that overlies the heart and its great vessels. Knowledge of the location of structures within the precordium is necessary to perform effective cardiac assessment.

There are four major areas on the precordium for examining the heart (Fig. 17-16). Each area corresponds to one of the heart's four valves' sounds:

- Aortic area—second intercostal space, right sternal border
- Pulmonic area—second intercostal space, left sternal border
- Tricuspid area—fifth intercostal space, left sternal border
- Mitral (or apical) area—fifth intercostal space, just medial to the midclavicular line

INSPECTION

Inspect the entire precordium for movement. Using tangential light across the chest and observing the heart at eye level can enhance inspection. Normally, movement is seen only in the mitral valve area. A visible pulsation occurs with ventricular contraction as the left side of the heart strikes the anterior chest wall. This pulsation is called the **point of maximal impulse** (PMI). Often, the PMI is not visible, especially in patients with thick chest walls or large breasts. Abnormal movements over the precordium include

forceful movement around the area of the PMI, called a *heave*; anterior movement of the sternum, called a *lift*; and small areas of pulsation in the intercostal spaces or around the sternum.

PALPATION

Palpation follows and complements inspection. Palpate in each of the four precordial areas, noting any vibrations (termed *thrills*) or pulsations. The fingertips are the most sensitive to pulsation, whereas the heel and ulnar surfaces of the hand are most sensitive to vibration. Feel for the PMI in the mitral area, and note its exact location and size. The normal PMI is a light tap, located at the fifth intercostal space at the midclavicular line, confined to the area of one intercostal space. A PMI lateral position to this may indicate an enlarged heart. Pulsations or vibrations over the aortic, pulmonic, or tricuspid areas may indicate problems with those heart valves.

AUSCULTATION

Valuable information can be obtained from listening to heart sounds. Learning the basic techniques of cardiac auscultation is enhanced by using a consistent pattern to auscultate the precordium and concentrate on one heart sound or phase in the cardiac cycle at a time. Positioning the patient in the left lateral position or sitting forward will help to move the heart closer to the chest wall and make the heart sounds easier to hear. **Procedure 17-4** details steps in auscultation of heart sounds.

Normal Heart Sounds

Normal heart sounds include the first and second heart sounds (S_1 and S_2, respectively). Systole (ventricular contraction) is the period from the beginning of S_1 to the beginning of S_2.

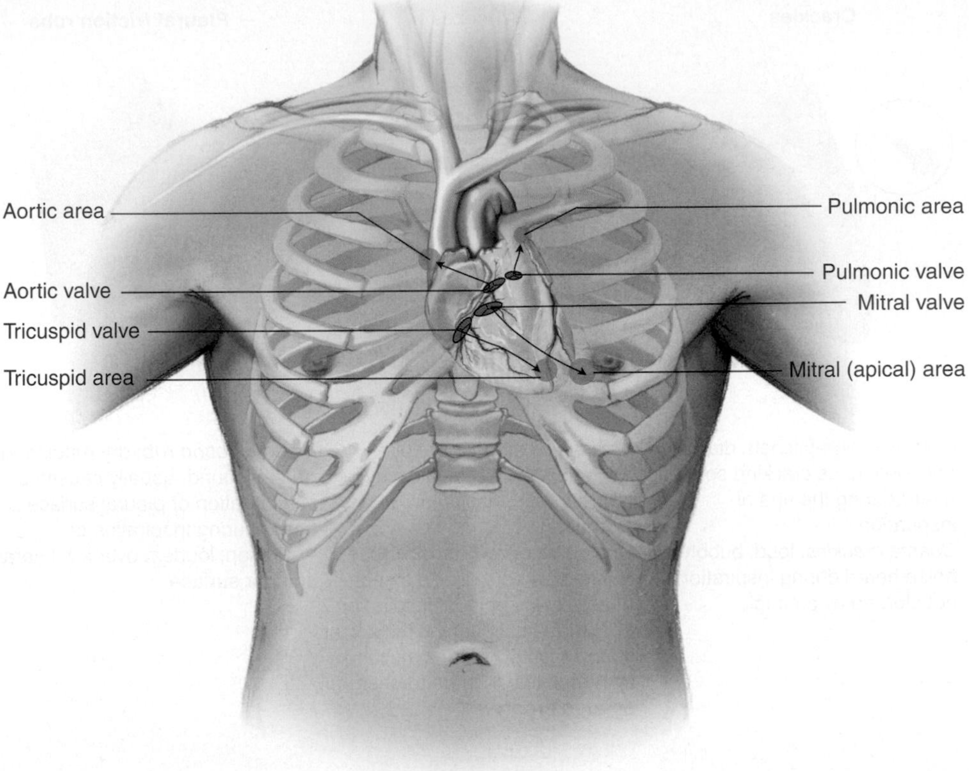

Aortic area

Aortic valve

Tricuspid valve

Tricuspid area

Pulmonic area

Pulmonic valve

Mitral valve

Mitral (apical) area

FIGURE 17-16 Heart sounds are referred from valvular points of origin to the auscultatory or precordial landmarks. Sound travels in the direction of blood flow and may be heard some distance from the valve.

Diastole (ventricular relaxation) is the period from the beginning of S_2 to the beginning of the next ventricular contraction.

S_1 coincides with the beginning of systole, when the mitral and tricuspid valves close. S_1 is louder at the mitral and tricuspid areas. When an audible difference in closure of the two valves is detected, S_1 is said to be *split*. Because the force generated in the left ventricle is much greater than that in the right ventricle, S_1 is dominated by the mitral valve and is best heard in the mitral (apical) area. S_2 coincides with the beginning of diastole, when the aortic and pulmonic valves close. S_2 is heard more loudly in the aortic and pulmonic areas.

S_1 and S_2 are high-pitched sounds that are best heard with the diaphragm of the stethoscope. When the heart rate is slow, it is easy to differentiate the two sounds. Systole is shorter than diastole, so two "paired" sounds (S_1 then S_2) sound like "lub-dub" and are followed by a pause. When the heart rate is faster, the pause is less distinctive or even absent. To distinguish S_1 from S_2 in this situation, feel the patient's carotid pulse when listening to the heart. The carotid pulse and S_1 occur almost simultaneously.

Extra or Abnormal Heart Sounds

The third heart sound (S_3) is an extra heart sound that occurs early in diastole as the ventricle rapidly fills. It can be normal in healthy children or young adults, but in older people, it often signifies heart failure. An S_3 is an important clinical finding to look for in a patient who is at risk for heart failure. The fourth heart sound (S_4) is an extra sound that occurs late in diastole, just before S_1. It coincides with atrial contraction, when blood is actively propelled into the ventricle. S_4 is thought to result from a stiffened left ventricle and is frequently associated with

hypertension and coronary artery disease. The development of an S_4 is not as serious as an S_3 and does not necessarily indicate heart failure. Auscultation of S_3 and S_4 is clearest at the apex when the patient is positioned on the left side. These sounds are commonly called **gallops**. Figure 17-17 illustrates where S_3 and S_4 occur in the cardiac cycle.

A murmur is vibrating sound that results from turbulent blood flow through the heart, especially across the valves. The more common causes for a murmur include partially obstructed flow through a valve opening (stenosis), increased blood flow across a normal valve, backward blood flow (regurgitation) caused by a leaky (incompetent) valve, blood flow into a dilated chamber, and blood flow through an abnormal opening between heart chambers. Murmurs resemble blowing or swishing noises and may occur during systole or diastole. They may be low pitched or high pitched, so both the bell and the diaphragm of the stethoscope are appropriate for detecting murmurs. When a murmur is heard, note whether it occurs during systole (between S_1 and S_2) or during diastole (after S_2) and where it is heard on the precordium. Figure 17-18 illustrates where systolic and diastolic murmurs fall in the cardiac cycle. Heart disease

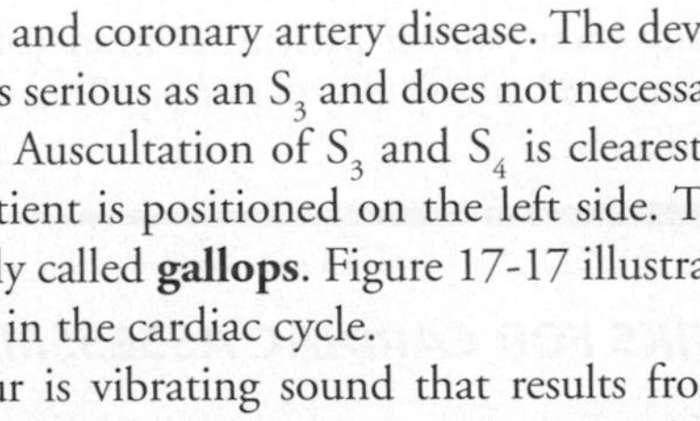

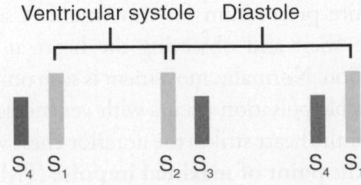

Ventricular systole   Diastole

S_4 S_1 S_2 S_3 S_4 S_1

FIGURE 17-17 Occurrence of the third and fourth heart sounds (S_3 and S_4, respectively) in the cardiac cycle.

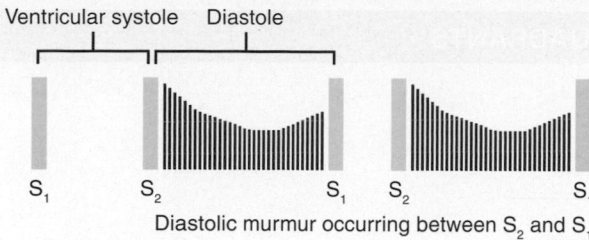

Diastolic murmur occurring between S₂ and S₁

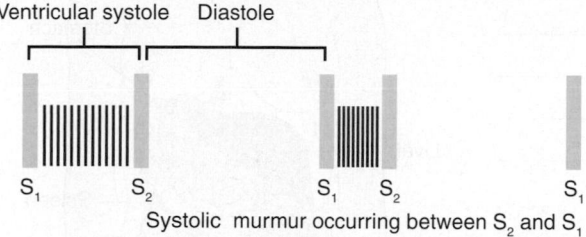

Systolic murmur occurring between S₂ and S₁

FIGURE 17-18 Location of heart murmurs in the cardiac cycle.

almost always causes diastolic murmurs; systolic murmurs may be related to heart disease but frequently are benign.

Assessment of Breasts

Breast examination is important in early detection of breast cancer (American Cancer Society, 2013). This procedure should be conducted as a joint activity of the patient and the nurse, with the nurse's primary role as educator. Although breast cancer is rare in men, a brief examination of the male breast is also appropriate.

INSPECTION

Teach the patient to do a breast self-examination while you are performing the breast examination. Normal breasts appear rounded and essentially symmetric, although one breast is often slightly larger than the other. The skin should be smooth and intact, with the areola darker in color, round, and symmetric. The nipple should be everted and without discharge or lesions. Abnormal findings include flattening, bulges or changes in breast size, marked asymmetry, redness, dimpling, and **edema.**

PALPATION

Palpation is done to determine whether masses or lumps are present in the breast. Palpate the breast with the patient in the supine position with his or her hands behind the head. Palpate each breast for tenderness, nodules, or masses. Use three or four fingers, pressing the flat part of the fingers in small circles and moving the circles slowly around the breast. Follow a sequential pattern of palpation so that all breast areas are included. Begin at the outer edge of the breast, gradually working toward the nipple. The tail of the breast extends into the axillary area. Because most breast cancers occur in the upper outer quadrant of the breast, it is especially important to palpate this area carefully. The final step in breast examination

is gentle squeezing of the nipple to check for discharge. Again, during the palpation, teach the woman how to perform breast self-examination.

Abdominal Assessment

The abdomen contains organs for digestion of food, organs for elimination of waste, major arteries and veins, and organs of reproduction in the female. Problems arising from this area may be difficult to diagnose. Elimination is the excretion of waste products from the body through the gastrointestinal and urinary systems. Elimination assessment focuses on determining the adequacy of bowel and bladder function, observing characteristics of feces or urine, identifying risk factors that may contribute to problems in elimination, assessing the impact of bowel or bladder dysfunction on daily living, and understanding the patient's methods of management and coping for any bowel or bladder problems.

BOWEL ELIMINATION

Some patients may consider bowel function to be a private matter, but it is important for nurses to develop ease in asking patients questions regarding their bowel status. Basic abdominal assessment consists of inspection, auscultation, and palpation. Abdominal assessment provides clues to general gastrointestinal function and any related problems.

Landmarks for Abdominal Assessment

For descriptive purposes, the abdomen is divided into four quadrants. An imaginary horizontal line through the umbilicus separates the upper and lower quadrants. An imaginary vertical line between the xiphoid and symphysis pubis separates the right and left quadrants. Table 17-7 lists and illustrates the structures underlying each of the four quadrants.

Inspection

During inspection, note the contour, skin, and movement of the abdomen. Observe the patient at eye level from the side, from the foot of the bed, and from directly over the abdomen. Use tangential lighting across the abdomen to accentuate subtle changes. Evaluate the contour of the abdomen by placing the patient supine and viewing at eye level from the side. Possible descriptions are *flat, rounded, protuberant,* or *scaphoid* (boat shaped or hollowed). **Ascites** is the accumulation of serous fluid in the peritoneum. This fluid may cause the shape to become protuberant, or distended and firm. A distended abdomen may also be measured to provide more specific data.

In relation to elimination, observe the abdomen for distention, which can signify decreased peristalsis in the intestines. When *distention* is present, the abdomen appears larger than usual; in severe distention, the skin appears stretched and taut. The patient may be able to verify that the abdomen appears larger than usual or that clothes are tighter.

The abdominal skin is similar in color and texture to skin on other areas of the body. Note the presence and location

TABLE 17-7 ORGANS IN THE FOUR ABDOMINAL QUADRANTS

1—Upper Right Quadrant	3—Upper Left Quadrant
Liver	Left lobe of liver
Gallbladder	Stomach
Duodenum	Spleen
Head of pancreas	Upper lobe of left kidney
Right adrenal gland	Pancreas
Upper lobe of right kidney	Left adrenal gland
Hepatic flexure of colon	Splenic flexure of colon
Section of ascending colon	Section of transverse colon
Section of transverse colon	Section of descending colon
2—Lower Right Quadrant	**4—Lower Left Quadrant**
Lower lobe of right kidney	Lower lobe of left kidney
Cecum	Sigmoid colon
Appendix	Section of descending colon
Section of ascending colon	Left ovary
Right ovary	Left fallopian tube
Right fallopian tube	Left ureter
Right ureter	Left spermatic cord
Right spermatic cord	Part of uterus (if enlarged)
Part of uterus (if enlarged)	

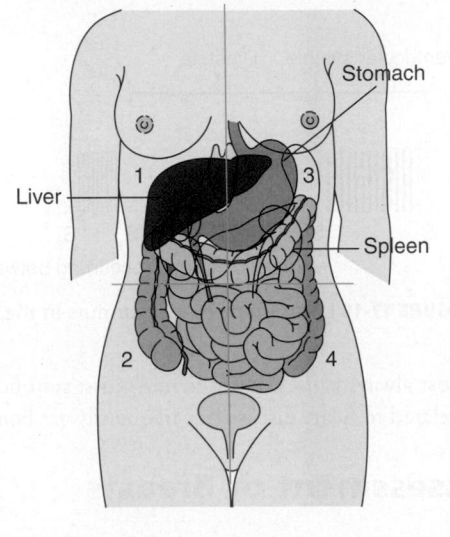

Note: The uterus and urinary bladder fall in the lower midline.

of scars, rashes, lesions, petechiae (small, red, hemorrhagic spots), or striae. *Striae* are streaks caused by rapid or prolonged stretching of the skin. Recent striae are pink or blue; they turn silvery white with age. Pregnancy, ascites, and weight gain or loss are common causes of striae. Fine veins may normally be visible on the abdomen, especially in the inguinal area. Distended, prominent veins are abnormal and are frequently associated with liver disease. Scars provide clues about previous surgeries.

Visible movement over the abdomen is not uncommon. Wavelike movements of intestinal peristalsis may be seen in thin patients. A normal aortic pulsation is frequently visible in the epigastrium. A rise and fall of the abdomen synchronized with respiration is frequently seen, especially in men.

Auscultation

Always auscultate the abdomen before palpating or percussing because touching can alter motility of the bowel and increase the sounds. Bowel sounds are created as air and fluid mix in the intestine. **Procedure 17-5** outlines the method of abdominal auscultation.

Normal bowel sounds are tinkling, gurgling noises that occur every 5 to 20 seconds. Bowel sounds of increased frequency and loudness are called *borborygmi*, or hyperactive bowel sounds. Borborygmus reflects increased intestinal peristalsis, which may be related to diarrhea, laxatives, emotional

upset, or intestinal obstruction. Borborygmus heard before a meal is better known as "stomach growling."

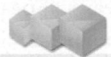 **Concept Mastery Alert**

Nurses must be careful when distinguishing between hypoactive bowel sounds and an absence of bowel sounds. A complete lack of audible bowel sounds during a period of 3 to 5 minutes constitutes an absence of bowel sounds. Bowel sounds that are audible, but infrequent, are documented as being hypoactive.

Percussion

Percussion is used to detect the location of organs that are not normally palpable and to give clues about the characteristics of the masses underlying the skin. Generalized tympany is present over the intestines, although varying degrees of tympany will be audible depending on the location of food and stool masses. The liver is percussed at the right midclavicular and midsternal lines, and the sound elicited is dull. The gastric bubble in the left lower rib cage is normally very tympanic. The spleen is found at the left 9th to 10th rib posterior to the midaxillary line and is dull (see Table 17-7).

Palpation

Light palpation is performed to obtain information about pain or discomfort. Palpate all four quadrants, reserving the area of suspected pain or abnormality until last. Relaxation of the abdominal wall is necessary for an accurate assessment. Promote relaxation by positioning the patient with knees slightly flexed and arms at the sides or across the chest. During deep palpation, avoid areas of pain found through light palpation. With deep palpation, masses of stool may normally be palpable in the abdomen. The liver border may be assessed during palpation, although it normally is not palpable at the midclavicular line in adults. Note the location and approximate size of any abnormal masses or enlarged organs.

> **! SAFETY ALERT**
>
> Do not palpate the abdomen of a patient complaining of sudden, severe abdominal pain, because doing so could rupture an inflamed appendix, causing peritonitis.

Perirectal Area

Palpation and inspection of the perirectal area should reveal smooth, intact skin without stretching or shininess. To palpate the rectum, insert a gloved, lubricated index finger in the rectum and direct it toward the umbilicus (Fig. 17-19). Document internal or external hemorrhoids, polyps, or abnormal masses. Frequently, a rectal examination is performed to detect the presence and consistency of stool in the rectum. Hard, dry stool may indicate a fecal impaction, which may require manual removal.

URINARY ELIMINATION

Inspection

Assessment of the bladder for distention due to urinary retention is warranted if a patient complains of lower abdominal (or bladder) discomfort or reports a history of difficulty urinating, or if a prolonged time has elapsed since the last

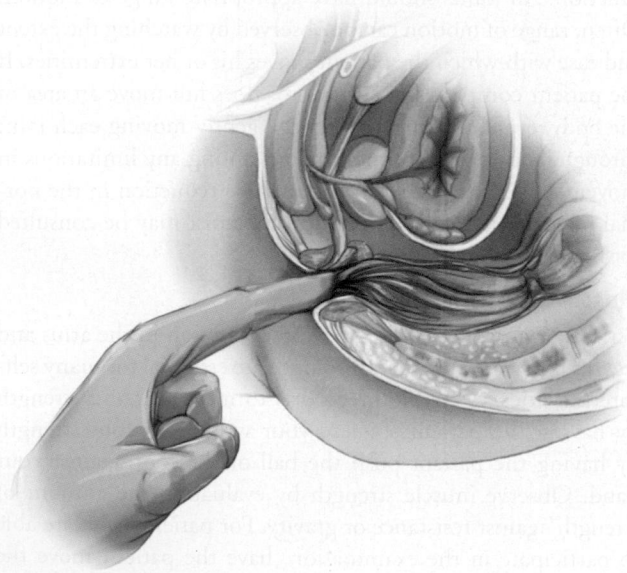

FIGURE 17-19 The nurse inserts a gloved, lubricated index finger into the rectum to detect stool or abnormalities.

voiding occurred. Inspect the bladder for signs of distention, which appears as a swelling of the lower abdomen, just above the symphysis pubis. Observation of urinary distention may be difficult in the obese person. If the bladder contains less than 500 mL of urine, no bulge is present on inspection.

Percussion

Percussion of the lower abdomen follows inspection to identify a distended bladder. Percussion begins at the umbilicus and proceeds toward the symphysis pubis. If the bladder is empty or contains only a small amount of urine, a tympanic note is heard when the bladder is percussed; percussion over a full bladder produces a duller sound. Bladder ultrasound has replaced the need for percussion to determine urinary retention in many instances.

Palpation

Often, the patient exhibits signs of sensitivity or discomfort when the full bladder is being palpated. In this case, palpation may be deferred. Light palpation can provide additional data if the patient can tolerate it. Palpate from the umbilicus to the symphysis pubis, using the fingertips. With light palpation, you will feel a firm ridge or mass as you locate the bladder. Be aware that palpation can stimulate voiding. If the bladder is full, a more complete assessment includes scanning the bladder with an ultrasound device.

Assessment of the Genitalia

ASSESSMENT OF A FEMALE PATIENT

Examination of female internal reproductive organs is not commonly part of the basic health assessment unless the nurse is working in a specialized area such as a gynecology clinic or labor and delivery. Frequently, the nurse is present with the patient during a pelvic examination. The following measures can assist relaxation and comfort:

- Assist the patient to assume the lithotomy position, and drape the patient to maintain privacy and warmth.
- Warm the speculum.
- Have a mobile or pictures on the ceiling to focus the patient's attention.
- Encourage rhythmic breathing (breathing deeply and slowly through the mouth).
- Ask the patient to concentrate on relaxing body muscles with each exhalation.
- Remind the patient not to hold her breath.

Inspection of the female external reproductive organs includes examining the labia minora, labia majora, clitoris, and vaginal opening. The color of these organs should be pink, with some blue or brown pigments occasionally seen. Bright red color or obvious areas of excoriation are abnormal and often occur with infection or irritation. Normal vaginal secretions are white, colorless, and odorless. Foul-smelling, purulent drainage is abnormal.

ASSESSMENT OF A MALE PATIENT

Examination of the testicles in men is important for early detection of testicular cancer. The examination should be undertaken as a joint activity, with the nurse as educator.

Inspection of the external male reproductive organs includes the glans, foreskin, and shaft of the penis as well as the scrotum. The man may be circumcised or uncircumcised. If the patient is uncircumcised, gently retract the foreskin during the examination to inspect the glans and the urethral opening. Replace the foreskin to the previous position after the inspection. Inspection of the penis should reveal no lesions or abnormal discharge. *Smegma* is a normal white discharge that may collect around the glans, especially in the uncircumcised man. The scrotal sac is wrinkled in appearance, with the left scrotal sac usually hanging lower than the right.

Perform palpation of the male genitalia to detect the testicle in each scrotal sac and the absence of pain, swelling, or growths. Palpate one scrotal compartment at a time by grasping the scrotum gently between the thumb and forefinger. Roll the testicle gently to palpate. The testicles should feel round, smooth, and freely movable within the scrotum.

Assessment of Extremities

INSPECTION

Inspection can be used to assess peripheral circulation. Examine the skin for color and temperature. Poor peripheral circulation may be associated with hair loss and skin discoloration or scaling. Observed varicosities (swollen, twisted veins) can indicate venous problems. Edema, or fluid, may also be detected through inspection. Arterial problems are associated with pallor; dependent rubor; shiny, cool, hairless skin; weak or absent pulses; decreased capillary refill; and sharp calf pain with increased activity. Venous problems are associated with edema; warmth; brown pigmentation; flaky dermatitis; achy, chronic pain; and ulcers that heal slowly.

PALPATION

Palpation is important in peripheral vascular assessment. Skin temperature is best evaluated using the back of the hand. Symmetric coolness or warmth may be normal; unilateral coolness may indicate decreased blood flow; unilateral warmth may indicate local infection. Generalized cool skin accompanied by pallor and moistness may indicate peripheral vasoconstriction due to circulatory shock.

Arterial Pulses

Palpate arterial pulses, noting rate, rhythm, amplitude, and symmetry. Use the brachial, radial, ulnar, femoral, popliteal, posterior tibial, and dorsalis pedis pulses. Comparing pulses between sides is helpful in evaluating for differences in circulation. Also, it can generally be assumed that if a distal pulse is present, the more medial pulses also are present in the same extremity. A grading scale is used to compare the strength of the pulses (Box 17-4).

> **! SAFETY ALERT**
>
> If the peripheral pulses are newly absent, it may be an emergency situation, and the physician should be immediately notified.

BOX 17-4 Grading Scale for Pulses

0—Absent
1+—Diminished thready easily obliterated
2+—Normal not easily obliterated
3+—Increased full volume
4+—Bounding hyperkinetic

Capillary Refill

Palpation is also used to assess capillary refill. **Capillary refill time** is a simple test of circulatory status that uses the nail beds. Press down on the nail bed until it turns white, and then note how quickly the color returns after you release the pressure. Normal refill time is 3 seconds or less; a prolonged capillary refill time indicates poor circulation.

Veins

Observe the arms and legs for swollen or varicose veins during sitting and standing. Normally, veins will become more swollen when standing and become smaller when lying. Observe for any red, tender, or swollen areas that may indicate phlebitis.

Edema

Edema is evaluated through palpation. Edema is fluid accumulation in the tissues. The degree of edema is estimated by noting how long the tissue remains indented when pressed. Assess edema in dependent areas such as the hands, feet, ankles, and lower legs. Press firmly with the thumb, for at least 5 seconds, behind the medial malleolus, over the dorsum of the foot, and over the shin. If the patient is bedridden, the dependent areas are the back and sacrum. A grading system, ranging from +1 to +4, is often used to record edema. Lower limbs may also be measured for circumference to evaluate for changes in edema and symmetry.

Joint Mobility

Joint movement is also important to activity and exercise function. All joints should have appropriate range of motion. Often, range of motion can be observed by watching the extent and ease with which the patient moves his or her extremities. If the patient complains of stiffness or does not move an area of the body, evaluate joint mobility by gently moving each joint through its full range of motion and noting any limitations in movement. Generally, greater than 10% reduction in the normal range is abnormal. A physical therapist may be consulted for further evaluation.

Muscle Strength

Perform a simple screening of motor function in the arms and legs, as limb movement and strength are essential for many self-care activities. A simple method is to measure hand strength by having the patient squeeze your wrists and foot strength by having the patient push the ball of the foot against your hand. Observe muscle strength by evaluating the amount of strength against resistance or gravity. For patients who are able to participate in the examination, have the patient move the limb against your resistance. Other patients may be asked to

<table>
<tr><td>

BOX 17-5 **Grading Scale for Muscle Strength**

0—No detectable muscle contraction
1—Barely detectable contraction
2—Complete range of motion or active body part movement with gravity eliminated
3—Complete range of motion or active movement against gravity
4—Complete range of motion or active movement against gravity and some resistance
5—Complete range of motion or active movement against gravity and full resistance

</td></tr>
</table>

hold a limb in a position, with gravity acting as the resistance. The response is then graded (Box 17-5). Evaluate symmetry of strength. It is expected that muscle strength is slightly greater in the dominant arm. Notable differences in strength or overall difficulty in performing these tests reveals problems with movement or weakness in the arms. Report any deficits to the physician or to a nurse specialist for a more comprehensive and detailed assessment of muscle function.

Sensory Assessment

Loss of tactile sensation may occur with various conditions, such as diabetes, peripheral vascular disease, spinal cord injury, brain trauma, tumor, or vascular lesion. Patients with decreased tactile sensations are at risk for injury from heat or cold, prolonged pressure, or shearing force. Sensory function is also evaluated in patients who are recovering from surgery with spinal anesthesia, who are receiving epidural pain medication, or who have spinal cord injuries. Dermatomes are sensory fibers from a single spinal nerve that serve a particular skin surface (Fig. 17-20). Evaluate function in dermatomes around and below (distal to) the problem area. Evaluate sensory perception by observing the patient's response to light touch, vibration, and pain. With the patient's eyes closed, touch various body areas with a wisp of cotton to assess light touch, with a tuning fork to test vibration and with a toothpick to test pain. You may use water of different temperatures to assess temperature discrimination. Documentation should include the inability to sense stimuli and the affected location of the body. Report any abnormal sensations such as paresthesias, numbness, or tingling.

Circulation, Movement, and Sensation

When an acute problem with a limb is possible, **circulation, motion, and sensation** (CMS) are evaluated. Assess circulation

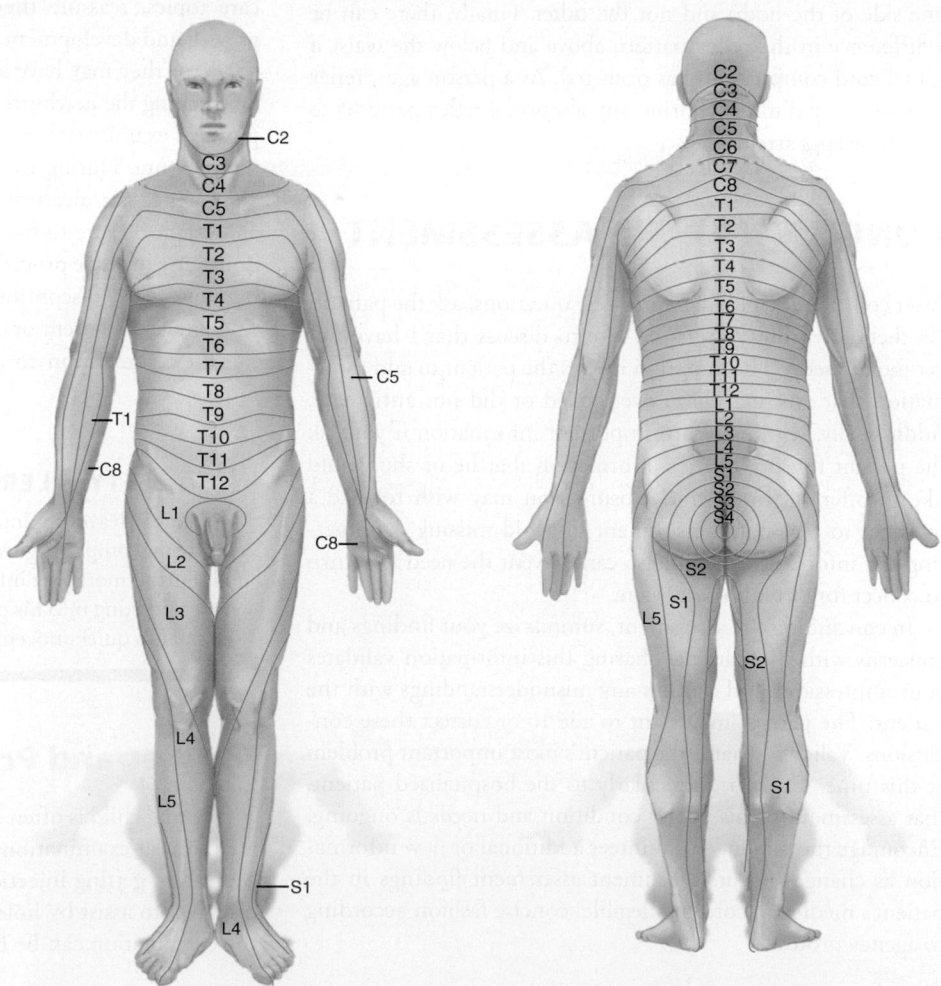

FIGURE 17-20 Dermatomes are sensory fibers from a single spinal nerve that serve a particular skin surface. They are used to evaluate sensory function for high-risk individuals (e.g., after epidural analgesia, spinal anesthesia, spinal cord injury).

by color, temperature, pulses, and capillary refill. Assess movement by asking the patient to voluntarily move the extremity. Assess sensation by asking the patient to say when he or she feels the touch. Also, question the patient about *paresthesias*, or sensations of numbness and tingling. CMS is normal if the skin is warm, pulses are present, and capillary refill takes place within 3 seconds. The patient should be able to wiggle the toes or fingers and to report the nurse's touch. No paresthesias should be present.

Deep Tendon Reflexes

Testing of deep tendon reflexes may be indicated in high-risk patients in specialized practice settings. Use a reflex hammer to tap various tendons in the body to see whether the appropriate reflex arc through the spinal cord is elicited. Normally, a brisk contraction of the muscle occurs. Reflex response can be graded, with 0 indicating no reflex activity; +1, minimal activity; +2, normal response; +3, more activity than normal; and +4, hyperactive response. Common reflexes that may be tested include the biceps, the triceps, the patellar, and the Achilles. Table 17-8 illustrates these reflexes and explains the procedures for testing them.

Three significant variations from the normal reflex pattern may be found. First, reflexes on the same side of the body may be different. Second, cortical damage may affect reflexes on one side of the body and not the other. Finally, there can be a difference in the reflex pattern above and below the waist if spinal cord compression has occurred. As a person ages, reflex response may diminish. Bring any abnormal reflex patterns to the physician's attention.

CONCLUDING THE ASSESSMENT

After covering the planned interview questions, ask the patient, "Is there anything you would like to discuss that I have not yet mentioned?" This question invites the patient to add information that you may have overlooked or did not anticipate. Additionally, you may learn important information if you ask the patient for any further information that he or she would like to offer. Before formal closure, you may wish to take a moment to review the assessment to avoid missing or forgetting any information. Doing so can prevent the need to return to collect forgotten information.

In concluding the assessment, summarize your findings and concerns with the patient. Sharing this information validates your impressions and clarifies any misunderstandings with the patient. The patient may want to add to or correct these conclusions. Validate what is the patient's most important problem at this time. Explain, particularly to the hospitalized patient, that assessment of his or her condition and needs is ongoing. Encourage the patient to volunteer additional or new information as changes occur. Document assessment findings in the patient's medical record in a legible, concise fashion according to agency protocol.

LIFESPAN CONSIDERATIONS

Developmental stage and other age-related factors are important in planning, focusing, and performing a functional health assessment. Nurses should be knowledgeable about common problems of each age group so that they can include appropriate screening measures that permit early detection of potential or actual problems. Awareness of the patient's cognitive development is essential so that questions can be phrased appropriately. Understanding the patient's emotional development helps make the examination less traumatic and anxiety provoking.

Newborn and Infant

Nursing assessment is made shortly after birth and at 24 hours of age. If parents are present during the assessment, explain what the examination includes and why it is being performed. Whenever possible, reassure parents about findings that are normal. Permitting parents to see their newborn and participate can help parent bonding and allay fears.

During the first year of life, nurses frequently assess infants during well-baby examinations. These examinations provide an opportunity to educate family caregivers on various infant care topics, reassure them about the wide range of normal growth and development, and allow time for discussion of any concerns they may have about their child.

Keeping the newborn or infant properly covered during the physical examination is important to prevent a drop in body temperature. During the first year of life, head and chest circumference are measured, the infant is weighed, and reflexes are tested. Be sure to finish inspection and auscultation before doing any invasive procedure. Such techniques can frighten the infant or cause discomfort, which may cause the infant to cry. Encourage the parent or other caregiver to hold the infant during the examination to decrease fear and help the child feel more secure.

> **! SAFETY ALERT**
> Never leave an infant on an examining table without being properly guarded. Infants can move quickly and fall. Furthermore, the infant must be properly restrained when you are looking into his or her ears, eyes, nose, or throat so that the infant's quick movements do not result in injury.

Toddler and Preschooler

The young child is often afraid to be examined and may associate physical examination with the discomfort of invasive procedures or getting injections. Encouraging the parent or other caregiver to assist by holding and comforting the child during the examination can be helpful. Explain in simple terms what

TABLE 17-8 ASSESSMENT OF DEEP TENDON REFLEXES

Reflex	Procedure		Normal Response
Biceps	Flex patient's arm at the elbow with his or her forearm resting on the thigh, palm up. Place your thumb on the base of the biceps tendon in the antecubital fossa. Strike your thumb with the reflex hammer.	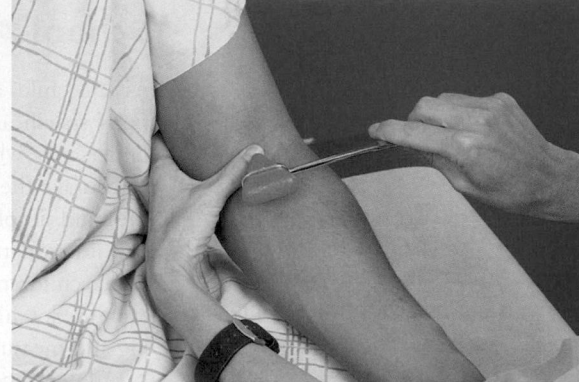	Flexion of forearm at the elbow
Triceps	Hold patient's arm across his or her chest, flexing the elbow at a 90-degree angle. Support wrist as patient allows forearm to become limp. Strike the tendon just above the olecranon process.	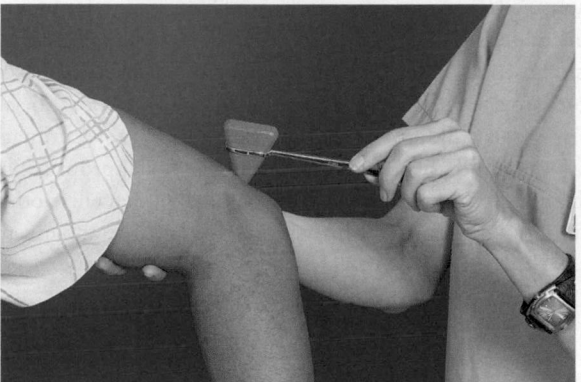	Extension at the elbow
Patellar	Patient sits upright with legs hanging loosely over side of bed. If patient remains supine, support back of knee while leg is flexed at a 45-degree angle. Strike patellar tendon just below the patella.	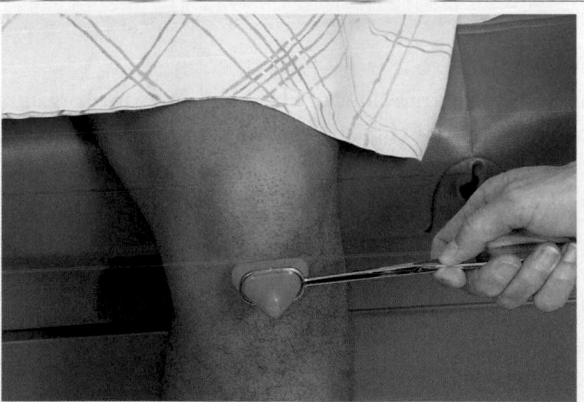	Extension of lower leg at the knee
Achilles	Patient's knee should be slightly flexed while foot is dorsiflexed. Strike Achilles tendon 1 inch above heel. The blunt end of the reflex hammer may also be used.	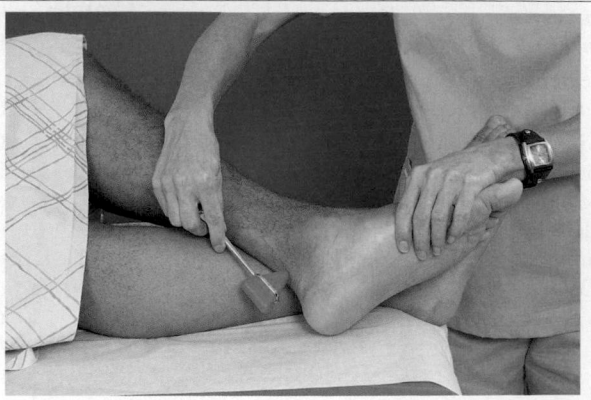	Plantar flexion

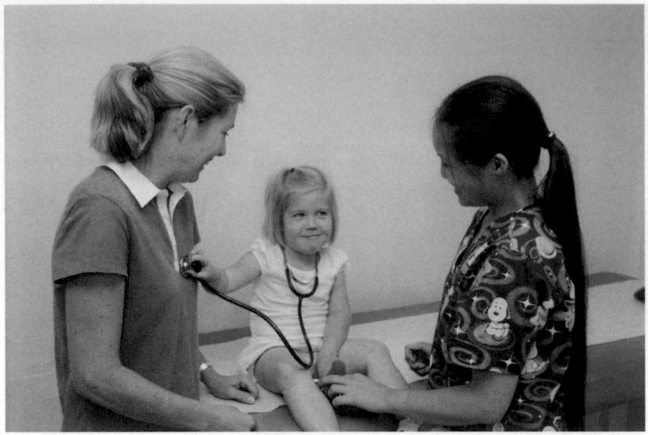

FIGURE 17-21 Allowing the toddler to play with the equipment allays her fears.

you plan to do. Demonstrating how equipment works can help alleviate some anxiety in toddlers and preschoolers. Allowing the child to touch the stethoscope or see the shining light of the otoscope can help prepare the child for examination procedures (Fig. 17-21). For some children, it may be helpful to use a puppet or allow the child to role-play examining a doll or stuffed animal. Be honest with children. If the child is going to experience pain, it is best to say, "This will hurt for a while, but I'll try and make it quick." Plan uncomfortable procedures toward the end of the examination. Then, perform them immediately after the explanation so that anxiety does not escalate.

School-Aged Child and Adolescent

As the child ages, nurses can direct more assessment questions specifically to the child. Use vocabulary the child can understand when asking questions or explaining procedures. Encourage the child to ask questions. Whenever possible, give the child simple choices. The child can be distracted during the examination through conversation or playing simple games. Some children are ticklish, especially when the abdomen is examined. Children at this age can be modest, so proper draping and measures to ensure privacy are important.

Adolescence is a period of rapid physical and emotional development. During this time, the youth is often examined alone, unaccompanied by a parent. Sensitive questioning and honest answers to any questions the teen asks help develop good rapport. Because sexual maturation occurs during this period, the examination includes assessment of the sexual organs and appropriate health teaching. Be aware of the sensitivity of adolescents about the body during this time. Discuss any concerns the adolescent has about the maturation process.

 THERAPEUTIC DIALOGUE: HEALTH ASSESSMENT

SCENE FOR THOUGHT

The nurse practitioner in the pediatrics clinic of a health maintenance organization visits Georgie Stevens, who is 5 years old. Georgie's mother brought him to the clinic because he has a fever of 2 days' duration. He says he is feeling "bad."

LESS EFFECTIVE		MORE EFFECTIVE	
Nurse:	Hi, Ms. Stevens. How's Georgie doing? I see he's had a fever lately. (*Looking at the history.*)	**Nurse:**	Hi, Georgie, remember me from last time?
Mother:	Yes, and coughing all night and sniffles and wheezing. (*She looks weary.*)	**Georgie:**	Yeah, you're Theresa. Can I play with the hearing tube again?
Nurse:	Let's see what we can find out here. (*Examines Georgie while talking to his mother. Keeps all equipment out of his reach. Doesn't explain what she's doing.*)	**Nurse:**	Sure you can. You can warm it up before I use it to listen to your breathing. I'm going to talk to your mom now.
		Georgie:	Okay. (*Plays with stethoscope contentedly.*)
Mother:	Is it pneumonia? (*Looks worried. Georgie looks worried, too, when he sees his mother's face.*)	**Nurse:**	How long has he had this fever?
		Mother:	Two days. And sniffles and coughing all night long and wheezing. I'm worried it might be pneumonia. (*She looks tired.*)
Nurse:	No, it's just a bad cold. I'll recommend some medications you can buy at the pharmacy. And then give him lots of fluids and get him to wash his hands before he eats and after going to the bathroom so the rest of the family doesn't catch it, too. Okay, Georgie?	**Nurse:**	I can see it's been a long 2 days. I'm going to examine him and then see what I can recommend so he and you can get some rest. Georgie, here's what my plan is. (*Tells child how she'll proceed with the examination, explaining each step. Georgie is cooperative and "assists" Theresa by holding the tongue depressor, warming the stethoscope, and so forth.*)

THERAPEUTIC DIALOGUE: HEALTH ASSESSMENT (*Continued*)

Georgie: (*He stopped paying attention when he heard it wasn't pneumonia. He's playing with the paper on the examining table, making little decorative rips in it. He looks up guiltily.*) Uh-huh. Can we go home now, Mommy?

Nurse: Bye, Ms. Stevens. See you next time, Georgie.

Nurse: Okay, Georgie, you've been a great help to me today. You have a cold, my friend, and here's what you need to do. (*Proceeds to tell Georgie and his mother about the importance of fluid intake, getting rest, using cough medicine appropriately, and the like. Includes Georgie in decisions about what kind of fluids he likes and the flavor of the cough syrup they should buy as well as agreeing to wash his hands before he eats or drinks anything and after going to the bathroom.*)

Georgie: I'll do everything you say, Theresa, because I want to get better and go back to school.

Nurse: Georgie, you're a smart person, and I know you'll get better soon. Call me if you have any questions, Ms. Stevens.

CRITICAL THINKING CHALLENGE

- List the subjective data each nurse had at her disposal.
- Based on her behavior toward him, detect what Theresa knew about Georgie that the first nurse did not know.
- Explain the benefits of including Georgie in decisions.
- Judge whether Theresa could treat all of her 5-year-old patients this way, and give your reasons.

Adult and Older Adult

By the time a person has reached adulthood, multiple exposures to physical examinations and assessments have occurred. Some adults feel apprehensive and dislike having private areas examined. It is important to prepare the patient for all procedures and to provide for privacy. Include health teaching regarding desirable screening measures, such as breast self-examination, testicular self-examination, and routine gynecologic examinations, in the health examination for an adult.

During later years of adulthood, a person may have chronic health problems that necessitate adaptation of the physical assessment. Arthritic joints or decreased mobility may make getting onto an examination table more difficult.

Holding various positions required for examination, especially for long periods, may be tiring. Lengthy examinations may be fatiguing and should be planned for when the patient is well rested, if possible. Hearing loss may necessitate speaking more loudly and clearly to facilitate communication. Elderly persons can easily become chilled, so proper draping in a warm examination room is important for patient comfort.

KEY CONCEPTS

- A health assessment consists of the collection of subjective and objective data about the patient's health and health-related problems or concerns.

- Frameworks for organizing the assessment include functional health patterns, head to toe, and body systems.

- Adequate psychological and physical preparation of the patient is important for effective assessment.

- The nurse uses interviewing techniques to obtain subjective (patient perception) data concerning each functional health pattern.

- The nurse collects objective data through the techniques of inspection, palpation, percussion, and auscultation during the physical examination.

- Assessment of health perception and health management should focus on the patient's perception of health status, preventive health practices, compliance with medical treatment, and safety.

- Assessment of activity and exercise includes posture, gait and balance, mobility, and respiratory and cardiovascular function.

- Assessment of nutrition and metabolism should focus on food and fluid intake in relation to metabolic demands, skin integrity, and wound healing.

- Urinary and bowel elimination may be part of the health management and the abdominal assessment.

- Assessment of sleep and rest involves eliciting the patient's perception of sleep, rest, and relaxation.

- Cognition and perception are assessed in the conscious patient through verbal communication, pain level, and sensory–perceptual capabilities such as vision, hearing, and pain.

- Assessment of self-perception and self-concept focuses on the patient's perception of self, such as body image and sense of worth.

- Assessment of roles and relationships describes the quality of a person's family, work, and social roles.

- Assessment of coping and stress tolerance describes current stressors that the patient is experiencing, past coping methods, and the effectiveness of current coping methods.

- Assessment of sexuality and reproduction describes reproductive function, sexual role, and the impact of current health status on sexual role function.

- Assessment of values and beliefs includes the significance of religious affiliation and religious practices, resources available to meet the spiritual health needs of the patient, and the relation between spiritual beliefs and the current state of health.

- Altered cognitive function is assessed through the neurologic examination including level of consciousness and the Glasgow Coma Scale.

- The head and neck, eyes and ears, and mouth are assessed when assessing the head.

- The skin, hair, and nails are assessed throughout the examination as a reflection of processes that occur throughout the body, such as nutrition and oxygenation.

- Respiratory and cardiac function are evaluated through inspection, palpation, percussion, and auscultation using normal landmarks of the thorax and pericardium.

- The patient is evaluated for normal and adventitious breath sounds as well as normal and abnormal heart sounds.

- Assessment of the abdomen should focus on normal excretory function (bowel and bladder) and specific management to assist normal function.

- The breasts and genitalia are examined with an emphasis on health promotion and self-examination.

- The extremities are evaluated for peripheral vascular, musculoskeletal, and neurologic function.

- Lifespan considerations are important in individualizing assessment techniques to obtain important information from the patient.

PRACTICING FOR THE NCLEX

CHECK YOUR ANSWERS IN APPENDIX A.

1. A patient is admitted to the unit following a left total hip repair. The nurse conducts a focused health assessment. Which of the following findings would be most appropriate? Select all that apply:
   a. Sensation, movement, and temperature of left leg
   b. Effects on role as primary household provider
   c. Hip pain rated 8/10
   d. Wife's ability to provide care upon discharge

2. A nurse is conducting a health history on a newly admitted patient. Which of the following should be included? Select all that apply:
   a. Reason for seeking healthcare
   b. Past surgical history
   c. Perception of health status
   d. Significant spiritual practices
   e. Auscultation of lung sounds

3. The four basic techniques of physical examination include:
   a. Interview, inspection, percussion, and auscultation
   b. Inspection, palpation, percussion, and resonance
   c. Interview, subjective data, objective data, and closure
   d. Inspection, palpation, percussion, and auscultation

4. You are assessing a patient with a diagnosis of glioblastoma, a type of malignant brain mass. The patient responds to his name and is unable to follow simple commands, states that he is at home, and presents with a left mouth droop. Which of the following assessment statements are appropriate? Select all that apply:
   a. Expressive aphasia
   b. Receptive aphasia
   c. Orientation × 1
   d. Lack of accommodation
   e. Impairment of cranial nerve VII

5. Which of the following assessment might be seen in a patient with congestive heart failure? Select all that apply:
   a. Clubbing of the nail bed
   b. Crackles in the bases of the lungs
   c. Vesicular breath sounds
   d. Pitting of ankles

6. A nurse is assessing respiratory function on a patient with a pneumothorax by asking him to say "99." This is a technique used to determine which of the following?
   a. Egophony
   b. Fremitus
   c. Excursion
   d. Friction rub

7. A nurse determines that ascites is present in assessing a patient with end-stage liver failure. Which of the following is congruent with this finding? Select all that apply:
   a. Striae
   b. Scaphoid shape
   c. Visible peristalsis
   d. Borborygmi

8. A nurse is assessing a patient receiving epidural pain medication. Which of the following are related to the resultant decrease in sensation and pain relief? Select all that apply:
   a. Prolonged pressure on the heels
   b. Risk for fall or injury
   c. Need for focused dermatome assessment
   d. Documentation of numbness and tingling

9. Assessment of genitalia of a teenager should include which of the following? Select all that apply:
   a. Examination of the teenager unaccompanied by the parent
   b. Utilizing simple games for distraction during the exam
   c. Emphasis on health promotion and self-examination
   d. Examination as a joint activity, with the nurse as educator

10. The nurse is concluding the patient assessment. Which of the following actions would be most appropriate?
    a. Acquire secondary data to verify health problems.
    b. Summarize findings and concerns with the patient,
    c. Discuss patient's history with other providers.
    d. Apply interventions appropriate for patient condition.

REFERENCES

Alfaro-LeFevre, R. (2014). *Applying nursing process: The foundation for clinical reasoning* (8th ed.). Philadelphia, PA: Wolters Kluwer Health/Lippincott Williams & Wilkins.

American Cancer Society. (2013). Can breast cancer be found early? Retrieved on July 5, 2014 from http://www.cancer.org/cancer/breastcancer/detailedguide/breast-cancer-detection

Arnold, E., & Boggs, K. U. (2015). *Interpersonal relationships: Professional communication skills for nurses* (7th ed.). Philadelphia, PA: W. B. Saunders.

Bickley, L. S. (2013). *Bates' guide to physical examination and history taking* (10th ed.). Philadelphia, PA: Lippincott Williams & Wilkins.

Centers for Disease Control and Prevention. (2014). Childhood obesity facts. Retrieved July 1, 2014 from http://www.cdc.gov/healthyyouth/obesity/facts.htm

D'Arcy, Y. (2011). *Compact clinical guide to acute pain management: An evidence-based approach for nurses* (2nd ed.). New York, NY: Springer.

Gordon, M. (2010). *Manual of nursing diagnoses* (12th ed.). St. Louis, MO: Mosby.

Jensen, S. (2015). *Health assessment: A best practice approach* (2nd ed). Philadelphia, PA: Lippincott Williams & Wilkins.

Khan R., & Rogers, P. (2014). The normalization of sibling violence: Does gender and personal experience of violence influence perceptions of physical assault against siblings? *Journal of Interpersonal Violence* 30(3), 437–458.

Procedure 17-1 Measuring Weight

Purpose	1. To provide baseline data from which to assess total fluid balance or nutritional status. 2. To provide baseline data to determine drug dosages or information for diagnostic testing with dye or radioactive injections.

Equipment	• An appropriate scale. *Note*: Use the same scale each time you weigh the patient. • Protector towel or plastic sheet

Assessment	• Assess necessity for baseline, daily, or weekly weight measurements. • Review previous weight measurements, if available. • Identify time of day previous weights were measured. Check your facility's current policy regarding when serial weight is measured. • Assess patient's mental and physical status to determine whether a standing, sitting, or bed scale is appropriate. A scale is built into many hospital beds so weight can easily be obtained especially for the bedridden patient.

Procedure

1. **Perform hand hygiene.**

   Rationale: Reduces microbe transmission.

2. **Identify the patient.**

   Rationale: Ensures correct patient receives proper assessment or treatment and reduces errors.

3. **Close door or bed curtains and explain the procedure to the patient.**

   Rationale: Ensures patient privacy, increases patient compliance, reduces patient anxiety, and promotes learning.

4. **Have patient void before weighing.**

   Rationale: A full bladder, wet gowns, and saturated dressings affect the measurement.

5. **Use the same scale and measure the weight at the same time each day. Patient should wear same clothing for each weight measurement. He or she should remove slippers or shoes before measurement.**

   Rationale: Using the same scale and measuring weight at the same time each day increases the accuracy of measurement because weight can vary significantly during a 24-hour period.

6. **Place protective paper or cloth on scale.**

   Rationale: Helps prevent the transfer of microorganisms.

7. **Check that scale registers zero. Adjust as necessary.**

   Rationale: Ensures accuracy of readings.

Weight with Standing Scale

8. **Assist patient onto scale (Fig. 1). Patient must stand in center of platform and not lean or hold onto supports.**

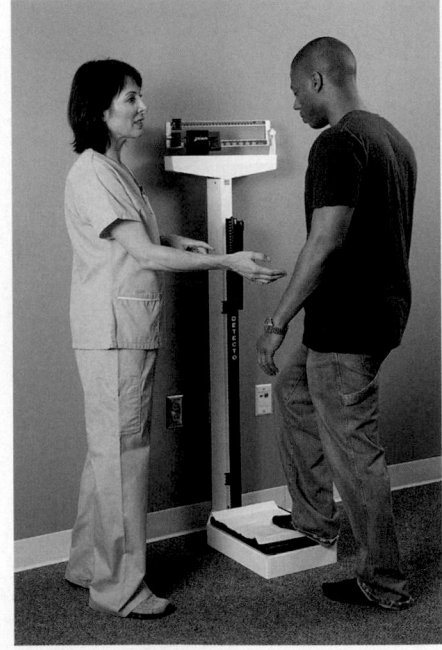

FIG. 1 Assist patient onto scale.

Rationale: Depending on type of equipment, movement may cause inaccurate weight.

Procedure 17-1 *continued*

9. Read digital display or adjust counterweights to determine patient's weight (Fig. 2).

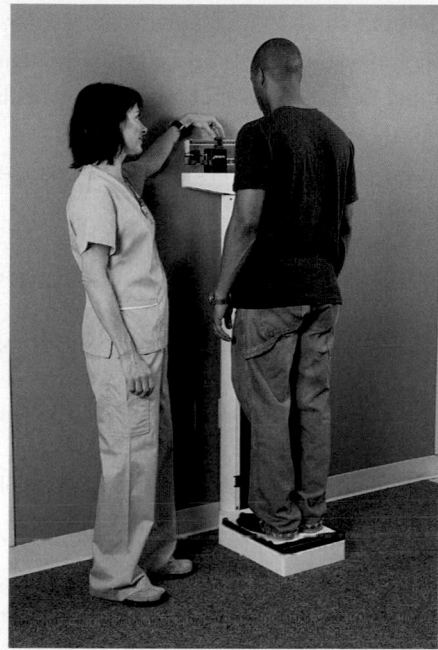

FIG. 2 Adjust counterweights to determine patient's weight.

Rationale: This helps ensure accurate weight measurement.

10. **Assist patient from scale and record weight in the patient's record.**

   Rationale: Prompt, accurate recording of data provides information for other members of the healthcare team.

Weight with Chair Scale

8. **Place scale beside patient and lock wheels.**

   Rationale: Safety measures prevent accidental falls.

9. **Transfer patient onto chair. If arm of chair is removable, unlock and remove before transfer. Lock back into place after transfer.**

   Rationale: Provides security and prevent accidental falls. Some scales allow wheelchairs to be wheeled onto scale.

10. Read digital display or adjust counterweights to determine patient's weight (Fig. 3).

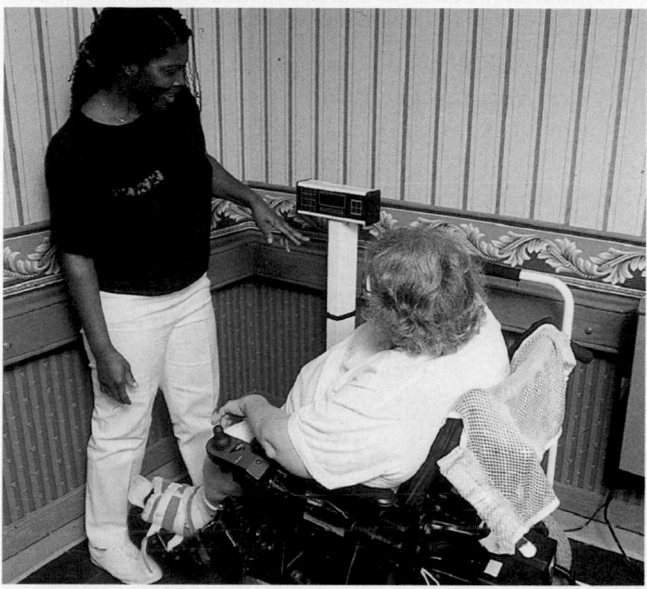

FIG. 3 Read digital display to determine patient's weight.

Rationale: Helps ensure accurate weight measurement.

11. **Transfer patient back to bed or wheelchair.**

   Rationale: Provides for the patient's safety and comfort.

12. **Clean the scale according to agency policy.**

   Rationale: A clean scale helps prevent transfer of microorganisms.

13. **Return scale to proper location and plug in.**

   Rationale: Keeps battery charged for next use.

Weight with Bed Scale

8. **Elevate patient's bed to level of stretcher scale.**

   Rationale: Avoids back injury to nurse.

9. **With one or two assistants, turn patient on the side with back toward the scale.**

   Rationale: Prepares for a smooth transfer to the scale.

10. **Roll scale toward the bed, lock wheels in place, and lower stretcher onto bed.**

   Rationale: Provides for safe transfer.

11. **Position folded stretcher under patient. Roll patient onto stretcher.**

   Rationale: Provides for safe transfer of patient to bed scale.

12. **Attach stretcher arms to stretcher and gradually elevate stretcher about 2 inches above mattress surface. Inform patient before elevating. Reassure the patient that he or she will not fall but the head may feel lower than the body.**

   Rationale: Decreases the patient's anxiety and improves cooperation.

13. **Determine that the stretcher is not touching any equipment. Lift all drains and tubing away from stretcher.**

    Rationale: Equipment alters measurement and affects accuracy.

14. **Read digital display for patient's weight (Fig. 4).** *Note*: **This is a good time to change patient's linen as he or she is elevated off the bed.**

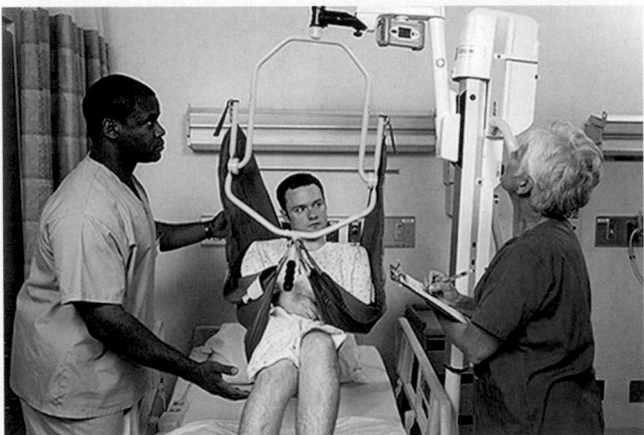

FIG. 4 Determine that the stretcher is not touching any equipment, and read digital display to determine patient's weight.

Rationale: Clusters care for efficiency.

15. **Gradually lower stretcher to the bed. Remove stretcher arms and transfer patient off stretcher. Remove stretcher.**

    Rationale: Ensures the patient's safe transfer.

16. **Unlock bed scale wheels and move away from bed.**

    Rationale: Bed scale will not move with wheels locked.

17. **Assist patient to comfortable position.**

    Rationale: The patient may shift so a change of position may be necessary.

18. **Clean stretcher and scale according to agency policy. Return to proper location and keep plugged in for next use.**

    Rationale: Prevents the transfer of microorganisms and keeps battery charged for next use.

19. **Record weight, and note any extra linen or equipment weighed with the patient.**

    Rationale: Documentation provides communication of trends.

Documentation

4/1/17: 10:30—weight, 73.9 kg on bed scale with patient in gown.

—B. Bond, NA

Lifespan Considerations

- Infants are usually weighed nude. Be careful that room temperature is warm because infants' body temperature can fluctuate severely because of their immature thermoregulatory system.
- Infants often roll and kick. The nurse's hand should always be within 1 to 2 inches of the child's body to prevent accidental falls.

Home Care Modifications

- Encourage patients requiring serial weights to keep a written log of their weights.
- Instruct patients to weigh themselves at the same time each day, usually in the morning before breakfast, and to wear similar-weight clothing for each measurement.
- If visual problems restrict the patient's ability to read the scale, family members may be able to assist.

Collaboration and Delegation

- Unlicensed nursing personnel (UAP) usually assess patients' weights. Inform UAPs of any patient's mobility restrictions and safety precautions that are important. Ask them to notify you of any significant (1 kg/d) change in a patient's daily weight from previous measurement.

Procedure 17-2 Assessing the Neurologic System

Purpose

1. To obtain baseline information about the patient's neurologic status.
2. To assess the patient's orientation to his or her environment.
3. To evaluate the patient's cognitive function and ability to make judgments.
4. To assess the integrity of motor and sensory pathways and the patient's ability to ambulate safely.
5. To detect increased ICP.
6. To detect changes in neurologic status.

Equipment

May need all or part of equipment depending on comprehensiveness of assessment:

- Toothpick
- Cotton applicator or cotton ball
- Vials of hot and cold water
- Tongue blade
- Penlight
- Vials of coffee, vanilla, or clove extracts
- Vials of salt, sugar, and lemon solutions
- Snellen chart
- Tuning fork
- Reflex hammer

Assessment

- Explain to the patient what you plan to do and approximately how long it will take. A complete neurologic assessment can be lengthy. Decide how extensive the assessment should be, based on the patient's diagnosis, level of consciousness, and physical disabilities. An efficient nurse learns how to integrate components of the neurologic assessment with other parts of the patient's functional assessment (e.g., assess cranial nerves during head and neck examination, evaluate mental status during nursing history, and test reflexes during musculoskeletal assessment).
- Determine whether any immediate need (e.g., pain, urge to urinate) is distracting the patient. Attend to that need first.
- Ask significant others whether they have noted memory loss or changes in the behavior of the patient.
- Question the patient about headache, seizures, dizziness, visual changes, or numbness or tingling of any body parts.
- Review medication history for any drugs that can alter level of consciousness or cause behavioral changes (e.g., analgesics, sedatives, antidepressants, antipsychotics, central nervous system stimulants).

Procedure

1. **Perform hand hygiene.**

   Rationale: Reduces microbe transmission.

2. **Identify the patient.**

   Rationale: Ensures correct patient receives proper assessment or treatment and reduces errors.

3. **Close door or bed curtains and explain the procedure to the patient.**

   Rationale: Ensures patient privacy, increases patient compliance, reduces patient anxiety, and promotes learning.

Cognitive–Sensory Assessment

4. **Assess the patient's level of consciousness by asking direct questions that require a verbal response. Note appropriateness of response and emotional state.**

   Rationale: Irritability, decreased attention span, inability or unwillingness to cooperate, and an abnormal perception of the environment may be signs of decreased level of consciousness.

5. **Evaluate patient's speech patterns.**

   Rationale: Normally, speech should be clear, well paced, and coherent. Language should seem appropriate for educational level.

6. **Observe general appearance: hygiene and appropriateness of clothing to setting and weather.**

   Rationale: Unkempt appearance or inappropriate clothing for weather conditions may give clues to patient's altered mental status.

Procedure 17-2   *continued*

7. If patient responses are inappropriate, ask direct questions related to person, place, and time (e.g., "What is your name?" "Where are you right now?" "What city do you live in?" "What day is this?").

   Rationale: Measures the patient's orientation to immediate environment. As consciousness deteriorates, patients become disoriented to person, place, and time. Note: Be sure a communication or language problem is not causing the patient's inappropriate response.

8. If patient doesn't respond or inappropriately responds to orientation questions, give simple commands (e.g., "Squeeze my fingers," "Wiggle your toes"). If the patient gives no response to verbal commands, test response to painful stimuli by applying firm pressure on patient's sternum or fingernail bed with your thumb.

   Rationale: Level of consciousness can vary from fully alert and oriented to unable to follow commands to unresponsiveness to external stimuli. Note: Avoid pinching patient's skin to elicit a pain response.

9. Document cognitive or sensory assessment objectively by stating specific patient responses to verbal or tactile stimulation. Use of Glasgow Coma Scale (see Table 17-4) helps documenting of frequent level-of-consciousness testing.

   Rationale: Assessments are more objective and consistent. Subtle changes can be more apparent when tools such as the Glasgow Coma Scale are used to quantify changes and see trends.

10. Assess function of cranial nerves (see Table 17-5).

    Rationale: An increase in intracranial pressure (ICP) puts direct pressure on the optic nerve (C-II). The oculomotor (C-III), the trochlear (C-IV), and the abducens (C-VI) exit the brain stem at the level of the tentorial notch. When ICP increases and the brain shifts downward, changes in the functions of these nerves are noted.

11. Assess sensory pathways:

    a. Patient's eyes are closed during all sensory tests.

       Rationale: Tests are valid only if patient doesn't see where stimulus strikes skin.

    b. Apply stimuli to skin in a random, unpredictable order while comparing one side of body with the other.

       Rationale: Patient should feel sensations equally on both sides of the body. Random stimuli prevent patient from anticipating and correctly guessing where stimulus is.

    c. Patient should verbally state when he or she feels a particular stimulus. If you detect an area of altered sensation, note which spinal cord segment is affected by referring to a dermatome chart.

       Rationale: Boundaries of sensory dysfunction can be found by testing responses about every 2.5 cm in a localized area.

12. Test pain sensation first by lightly touching the pointed, then the blunt, end of sterile toothpick to proximal and distal aspects of the arm and legs.

    Rationale: Assess intactness of spinothalamic tract. If pain sensation is intact, nurse may omit tests for temperature.

13. Test temperature sensation by touching skin with vials of hot, then cold, water.

    Rationale: Patient should identify hot versus cold sensation.

14. Lightly stroke proximal and distal aspects of patient's arms and legs with a cotton applicator or ball (Fig. 1). Ask patient to tell you when and where each stroke is felt.

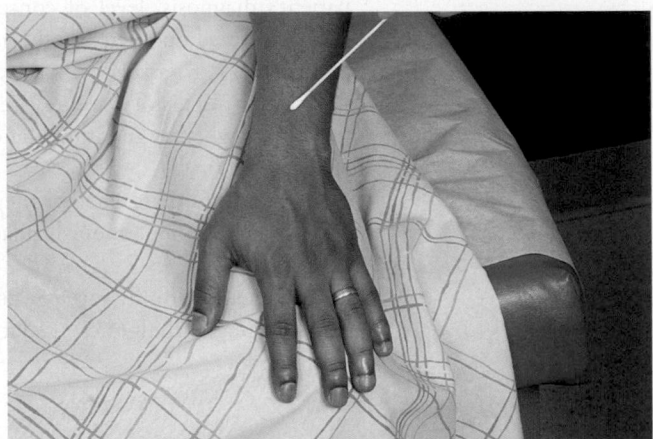

FIG. 1 Assess light touch sensation with cotton applicator.

Rationale: Testing the patient's perception of light touch assesses intactness of the posterior column. Loss of any of these sensations may indicate a lesion of the posterior column on the same side as the loss.

Procedure 17-2   *continued*

15. Apply a vibrating tuning fork to the distal interphalangeal joints of fingers and great toe (Fig. 2). Ask patient to describe what he or she feels and when it stops. *Note*: If patient does not feel vibration, move the tuning fork proximally to the next joint until sensation is felt.

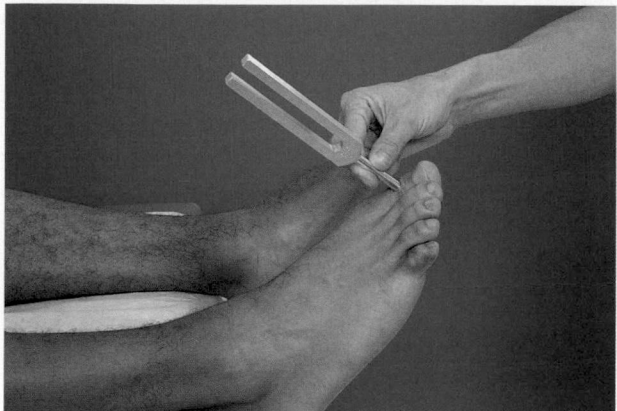

FIG. 2 Assess vibratory sensation with a tuning fork.

Rationale: Testing the patient's response to vibration and position also assesses intactness of the posterior column. Loss of any of these sensations may indicate a lesion of the posterior column on the same side as the loss.

Activity–Mobility Assessment

4. Inspect arm and leg muscles for atrophy, tremors, fasciculations, or other abnormal movements.

   Rationale: Abnormal movements may indicate disease.

5. Assess strength of specific muscle groups by having patient extend or flex individual joints against resistance provided by examiner's hands. Test biceps, triceps, wrist, leg muscles, and ankle (Fig. 3).

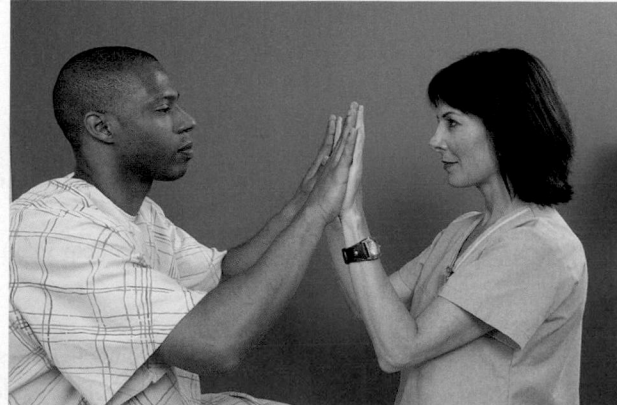

FIG. 3 Test biceps strength by having patient extend arms against resistance.

Rationale: Lack of symmetry of same muscle groups can indicate neurologic impairment.

6. Ask patient to close eyes and hold arms in front of body with palms up. Have patient hold position for 30 seconds and observe for pronation of hands or drifting of arms (pronator drift). *Note*: Notice weaknesses on one or both sides.

   Rationale: This test detects deformities, reduced mobility of joints, or decreased muscle strength. Upper and lower extremities of dominant side are usually stronger than nondominant side.

7. Evaluate coordination and balance.

   a. Perform a series of rapid alternating movements.

   b. Have patient pat upper thigh by rapidly alternating his or her palm and back of the hand (Fig. 4).

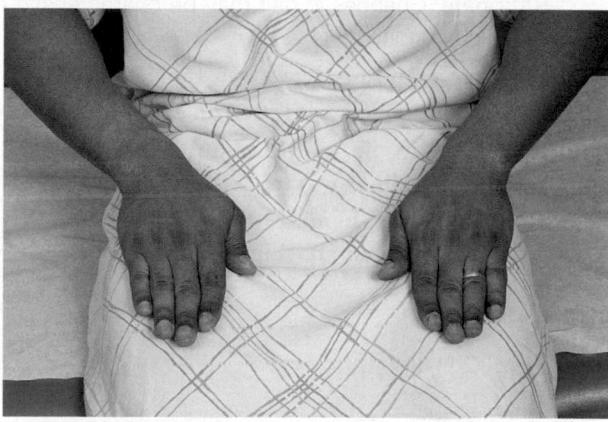

A

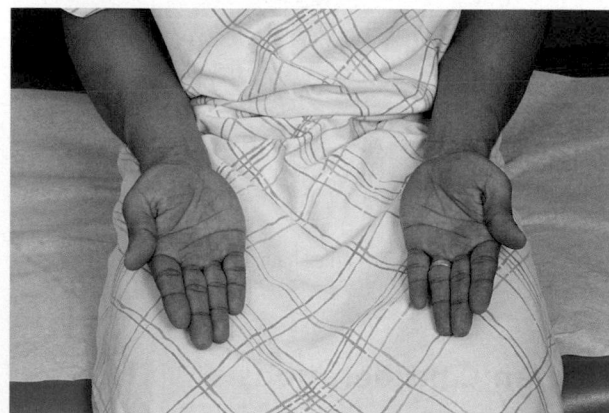

B

FIG. 4 Have patient perform rapid alternating movements by having patient pat the upper thigh with the palm of his hand (**A**) and the back of his hand (**B**).

   c. With dominant hand, have patient touch his or her thumb to each finger on that hand as quickly as possible.

   d. Have patient use his or her dominant forefinger to first touch your forefinger, then his or her nose. Instruct patient to repeat this many times as fast as he or she can.

   Rationale: Difficulty performing any of these tests may suggest that further evaluation for cerebellar disease is indicated.

Procedure 17-2 *continued*

e. Romberg test: Ask patient to stand with feet together, arms at sides. Have patient maintain this position for 30 seconds with eyes open, then 30 seconds with eyes closed. Assess for swaying. Stay close to patient to assist in case he or she begins to fall.

Rationale: Patients with cerebellar disease may not maintain balance with eyes open or shut; problems with proprioception cause difficulty only with eyes shut. Stay close to avoid injury.

f. Ask patient to walk across the room. Observe gait for symmetry, rhythm, limping, shuffling, or other abnormalities.

Rationale: Changes in gait may be characteristic of specific neurologic diseases.

8. Assess deep tendon reflexes (see Table 17-8).

a. Compare symmetry of reflex on each side of body.

b. Extremity to be tested should be completely relaxed and slightly extended.

c. Hold the reflex hammer loosely and allow it to swing freely in an arc (Fig. 5).

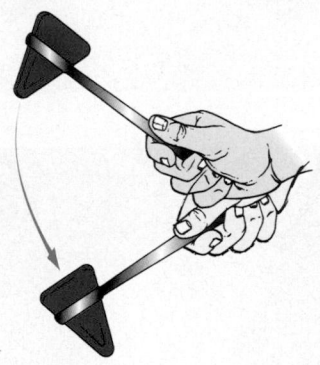

FIG. 5 Swing reflex hammer in an arc.

d. Tap tendon briskly.

e. Document reflexes by grading from 0 to 4+ on stickman, comparing bilaterally (Fig. 6).

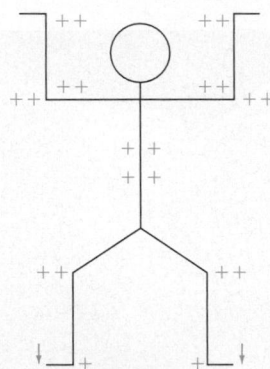

0 —no response
1+—diminished reflex (may be normal)
2+—normal
3+—brisker than normal (may be normal)
4+—hyperactive—upper neuron disorder
       suspected

FIG. 6 Document reflexes by grading from 0 to 4+ on a stickman.

Rationale: The quality of a reflex response varies among individuals and by age.

Documentation

10/1/17: 08:30—Patient not oriented to person, place, or time; responds to nail bed pressure by withdrawal of hand, Glasgow Coma Scale 6/15; no significant change in neurologic state for last 6 hours.

—S. Roberts, RN

Lifespan Considerations

Newborn and Infant

- The infant at birth has little or no voluntary control over muscular movements. Much of the infant's motor activity is seen as mass responses to stimuli, and the infant has built-in reflexes:
  - *Rooting reflex*—Infant turns head toward a warm object placed against his or her cheek; function is to help infant locate the mother's breast when nursing.
  - *Sucking reflex*—Swallowing and gagging reflexes are well developed in healthy infants at birth.
  - *Moro reflex*—In response to loud noise or sudden movement, infant extends arms in tense, quivering embrace and often cries.
  - *Tonic neck reflex*—When relaxed or asleep on back, infant has head turned to one side with arm and leg of that side extended, whereas extremities of opposite side are flexed.
  - These reflexes disappear as the infant's neurologic state matures.

Toddler and Preschooler

Children are often fearful of strangers and of examining equipment. Spend several minutes becoming acquainted with the child. Allow the child to handle the equipment before the examination. Using a "This is a game" approach often helps allay the fear. Several screening tools are available, such as the Denver Development Test, which is designed to evaluate cognitive and psychomotor skills of infants and children of varying ages.

Older Adult

- A lengthy examination may exhaust the older adult. You may need to complete it in phases.
- Arthritic changes in joints may limit range of motion and physical mobility and should be considered when evaluating assessment data.
- Some reflex responses may become less intense as a person ages. The Achilles reflex and the plantar reflex may be difficult to elicit.
- Short-term memory may be decreased in the older adult; long-term memory is usually unaltered.
- Being in an unfamiliar place or situation can be stressful and promotes confusion.

Collaboration and Delegation

- For high-risk patients, the neurologic assessment may be performed at the bedside by the assigned nurse and nurse coming on duty during handoff.
- Report abnormal findings to the physician/neurologist.
- Nurses who do not frequently work with neurologic patients may collaborate with clinical nurse specialists to perform comprehensive neurologic assessment for high-risk patients or compare abnormal findings with a more experienced nurse.

Procedure 17-3 Auscultating Breath Sounds

Purpose

1. To listen for variations in breath sounds that may indicate airway obstruction or disease process.
2. To assess the effectiveness of medications or therapies in opening or clearing airways.
3. To detect fluid volume excess or pulmonary edema.

Equipment   Stethoscope

Assessment

- Explain to the patient what you plan to do and approximately how long it will take.
- Determine if any immediate need is distracting the patient (e.g., pain, need to void). Attend to that need first.
- Provide for privacy so that the patient is not concerned about being viewed or overheard. You may ask visitors and family members to leave the room.
- Ensure that the room is warm and quiet.

Procedure

1. **Perform hand hygiene.**

   Rationale: Reduces microbe transmission.

2. **Identify the patient.**

   Rationale: Ensures correct patient receives proper assessment or treatment and reduces errors.

3. **Close door or bed curtains and explain the procedure to the patient.**

   Rationale: Ensures patient privacy, increases patient compliance, reduces patient anxiety, and promotes learning.

4. **Assist the patient to an upright sitting position. Remove patient's gown to expose chest.**

   Rationale: Upright position improves chest excursion. Assessing breath sounds through clothing would muffle or distort sounds.

5. **Warm the diaphragm of the stethoscope by holding it between your hands for a short time.**

   Rationale: A warm stethoscope is more comfortable for the patient and helps put the patient at ease.

6. **Ask patient to breathe deeply through the mouth. Patient should breathe slowly.**

   Rationale: Mouth breathing enhances volume of breath sounds; nasal breathing decreases volume and can simulate adventitious sounds. A slow breathing rate is necessary to avoid hyperventilation.

Auscultate Anterior Chest

7. **Place diaphragm of stethoscope about 1 inch below the middle of the right clavicle, making sure it lies between the ribs. Listen to one full inspiration and exhalation. Repeat the process at the corresponding site on the left side.**

   Rationale: Placement of stethoscope over intercostal space improves sound quality. Representative sounds of right and left upper lobes are audible here.

8. **Note normal and adventitious breath sounds at each point on the chest as you proceed (Fig. 1).**

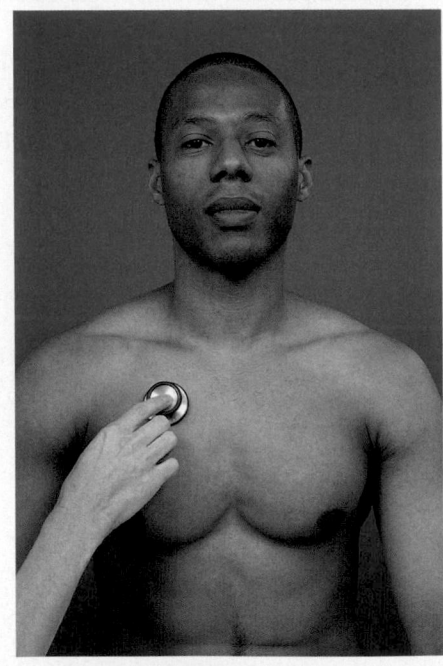

FIG. 1 Auscultate anterior thorax for breath sounds.

   Rationale: Movement of air through airways produces characteristic sounds. Abnormal sounds are indicative of airway disturbances.

9. **Move stethoscope downward about 1.5 to 2 inches along midclavicular line. Note sounds; move stethoscope laterally to opposite side.**

   Rationale: Air movement through other (larger) airways of upper lobes can be heard here. Listening to sounds at corresponding points on opposite sides of sternum allows you to compare similar lung fields.

Procedure 17-3   *continued*

10. Move stethoscope downward another inch or two along midclavicular line to fifth intercostal space. (This space lies just below the nipple line on men, approximately across from the head of the xiphoid process of the sternum.) Note sounds, and then move to same spot on opposite side.

    Rationale: Right middle lobe and corresponding segments on left can be heard here.

Auscultate Posterior Chest

7. Instruct patient to lean forward and cross arms in front.

    Rationale: This position separates scapulae and facilitates listening to posterior breath sounds.

8. Begin by auscultating the area about 2 inches below the shoulders and 2 inches to the right of the spine. Note sounds, and then move to corresponding point on left (Fig. 2).

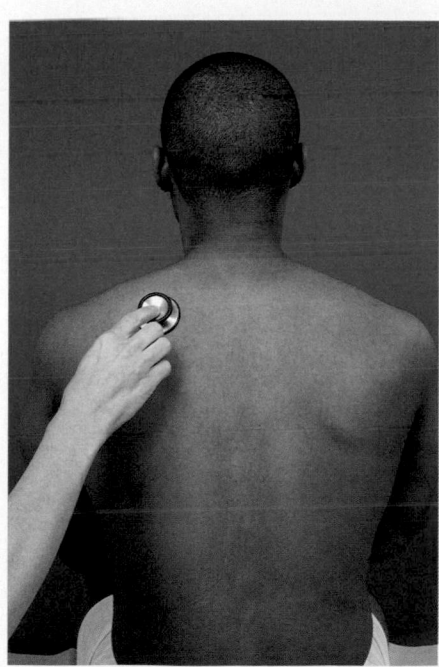

FIG. 2 Auscultate posterior thorax for breath sounds.

Rationale: These positions allow comparison of breath sounds of posterior segments of the upper lobes.

9. Move stethoscope directly downward 2 or 2.5 inches; note sounds, then move stethoscope laterally, and listen on the right.

    Rationale: Superior segments of lower lobes are audible here.

10. Repeat process, moving downward 2 to 2.5 inches; listen to corresponding opposite side.

    Rationale: Each placement of stethoscope allows you to hear sounds of different segments of the lung.

11. Move stethoscope downward to area just below scapula. Listen on right and left. Listen also to areas laterally along lower rib cage.

    Rationale: The lower lobes end at the level of the 10th thoracic vertebra (about 1.5 inches below scapulae) and follow the contour of the lower ribs. Their large size and the fact that many clinical problems can affect the lower lobes make lateral assessment essential.

12. Replace patient's clothes and assist the patient to a comfortable position.

    Rationale: Avoids chilling the patient and provides privacy.

13. Discuss your findings with the patient.

    Rationale: Discussion provides an opportunity for patient feedback on the effectiveness of therapies and provides directions for patient teaching if new therapies are to be initiated (e.g., cough, deep breathing, incentive spirometry).

14. Record assessment findings. Be specific as to description and location of adventitious sounds.

    Rationale: Provides timely information to health care team which can impact treatment decisions.

Documentation

> 8/1/17: 14:30—RR 18 breaths per minute, shallow. Chest movements symmetric, no use of accessory muscles. Crackles noted in RLL.
>
> —S. Roberts, RN

Lifespan Considerations

Newborn and Infant

- Newborns have difficulty maintaining body temperature. Uncover only the body area that you are directly assessing.
- At 8 to 12 months of age, infants become fearful of strangers. Spend several minutes becoming acquainted with the child before proceeding with the examination.

Procedure 17-3   *continued*

Toddler and Preschooler

- Children 2 to 5 years of age are often afraid of examining equipment. Letting them handle the stethoscope and using a "This is a game" approach often help allay the fear.
- Auscultate breath sounds before performing any invasive examination, which may cause the child to cry.

School-Aged Child and Adolescent

- Older children are modest. They may or may not want a parent to be with them during the examination; give the child the choice. Protect modesty through the use of gowns or drapes.

Older Adult

- A lengthy physical examination may be exhausting for the older adult and may need to be completed in phases.
- Older adults can become easily chilled. Provide warmth through adequate draping or gowning.

Collaboration and Delegation

- Review your assessment findings with physicians or respiratory therapists (RTs) to improve and refine your skills.
- Collaborate with RT to develop a plan for patients who have adventitious breath sounds.
- Report any significant abnormal findings or respiratory distress to the physician.

Procedure 17-4 Auscultating Heart Sounds

Purpose
1. To assess normal and abnormal functioning of the heart valves.
2. To detect cardiac problems.

Equipment   Stethoscope with a bell and diaphragm

Assessment
- Determine whether any immediate need is distracting the patient (e.g., pain, urge to urinate). Attend to that problem first.
- Explain to the patient what you plan to do and approximately how long it will take.
- Provide for privacy so that the patient is not concerned about being viewed or overheard. Visitors and family members may be asked to leave the room.
- Ensure that the room is warm and quiet.

Procedure

1. **Perform hand hygiene.**
   Rationale: Reduces microbe transmission.

2. **Identify the patient.**
   Rationale: Ensures correct patient receives proper assessment or treatment and reduces errors.

3. **Close door or bed curtains and explain the procedure to the patient.**
   Rationale: Ensures patient privacy, increases patient compliance, reduces patient anxiety, and promotes learning.

4. **Assist the patient to the supine position for auscultation (Fig. 1). You may want to re-examine the patient in the upright sitting position and a left lateral position. Lift patient's gown to expose the chest.**
   Rationale: Certain positions accentuate some heart sounds.

5. **Warm the diaphragm of the stethoscope by holding it between your hands for a few moments.**
   Rationale: A warm stethoscope is more comfortable and will not startle the patient, which could alter his or her heart rate.

6. **Listen in the mitral area using the diaphragm. Identify the first and second heart sounds (S$_1$ and S$_2$). Count the heart rate, noting whether the rhythm is regular or irregular. If the rhythm is irregular, count the heart rate for a full minute. Also, note whether the irregularity has a pattern or whether it is totally unpredictable.**
   Rationale: Auscultation is best performed systematically, concentrating on one sound at a time in each area.

7. **Listen in the aortic area using the diaphragm. Concentrate first on S$_1$, then S$_2$, noting whether splitting occurs. Shift your concentration to systole and then diastole; listen for extra sounds, such as murmurs.**

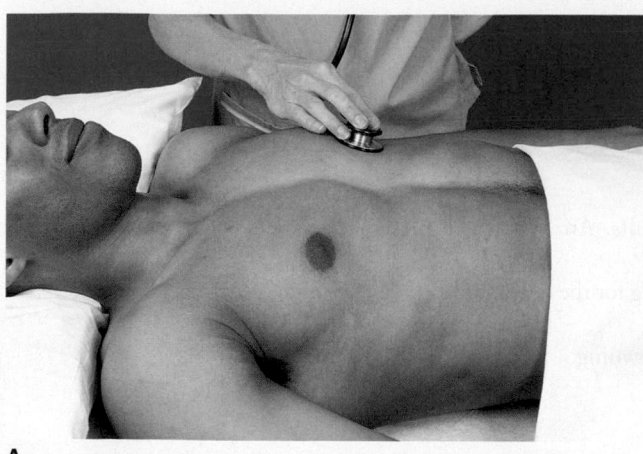

A

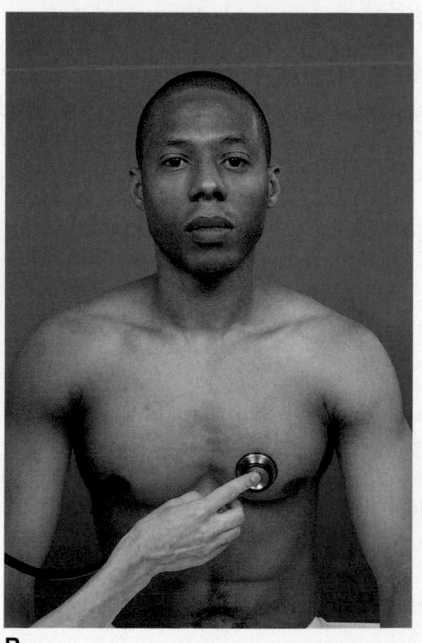

B

FIG. 1 Auscultate the heart in supine position (**A**) and forward sitting position (**B**).

Procedure 17-4   *continued*

Rationale: The diaphragm of the stethoscope transmits the high-pitched sounds of S$_1$ and S$_2$. Murmurs are best heard over the valvular areas in the direction in which the blood is flowing through the heart.

8. **Listen in the pulmonic area, still using only the diaphragm. Repeat the sequence described in step 7, concentrating on S$_1$, S$_2$, systole, and diastole. Compare the loudness of S$_2$ in the aortic and pulmonic areas.**

   Rationale: Loudness of S2 in the aortic area relates to the systemic arterial blood pressure and can be louder than normal in adults with hypertension. Loudness of S2 in the pulmonic area relates to the pulmonary artery pressure and may be louder than normal in patients with chronic obstructive pulmonary disease. It is abnormal for the pulmonic S2 to be louder than the aortic S2 in those older than 40 years of age.

9. **Move the diaphragm and listen to the tricuspid and mitral areas.**

   Rationale: Listen to all areas to hear sounds transmitted from each valve.

10. **Return to the aortic area, this time using the bell of the stethoscope. As before, concentrate individually on S$_1$, S$_2$, systole, and diastole.**

    Rationale: The bell and diaphragm pick up different sounds.

11. **Repeat the same process, using the bell, in the pulmonic, tricuspid, and mitral areas. Especially in the mitral area, concentrate during diastole to detect a third or fourth heart sound (S$_3$ and S$_4$).**

    Rationale: The lower-pitched sounds of the mitral and tricuspid valves, as well as an S3 or S4, are best transmitted through the bell of the stethoscope. Note: To increase your ability to hear an S3 or mitral murmur, have the patient lie on the left side (brings the heart closer to the anterior chest wall) while you auscultate with the bell. An S3 often disappears when the patient sits up.

12. **Replace the patient's clothes. Assist the patient to a comfortable position.**

    Rationale: Provides comfort and warmth before leaving.

13. **Record your assessment findings, describing the intensity, quality, and location of the sounds.**

    Rationale: Communicates findings and establishes baseline.

Documentation

4/2/17: 09:45—Apical pulse 86 regular, PMI palpated at fifth ICS, 2 cm in diameter, no extra heart sounds, murmurs, or rubs.
—S. Roberts, RN

Lifespan Considerations

Newborn and Infant

- Newborns have difficulty maintaining body temperature. Uncover only the body area that you are directly assessing.
- Heart rates are normally very rapid, so S$_1$ and S$_2$ are often difficult to discern.
- At 8 to 12 months of age, infants become fearful of strangers. Spend several minutes becoming acquainted with the child before proceeding with the examination.

Toddler and Preschooler

- Children 2 to 5 years of age are often afraid of examining equipment. Letting them handle the stethoscope and using a "This is a game" approach often help allay the fear.
- Auscultate heart sounds before performing any invasive examination, which may cause the child to cry.

School-Aged Child and Adolescent

- Older children are modest. They may or may not want a parent to be with them during the examination; give the child the choice. Protect modesty through use of gowns or drapes.
- An S$_3$ is normal in children and young adults.

Older Adult

- An S$_3$ may indicate heart failure in older adults. An S$_4$ may be present in patients with coronary artery disease or hypertension.
- A lengthy physical examination may be exhausting for the older adult and may need to be completed in phases.
- Older adults can become easily chilled.
- Provide warmth through adequate draping or gowning.

Collaboration and Delegation

- Assessing heart sounds takes much practice. Consult with cardiac nurses or cardiologists to compare your assessment findings.
- Notify the physician or cardiologist of new abnormal heart sounds.

Procedure 17-5 Auscultating Bowel Sounds

Purpose	1. To determine the presence or absence of intestinal peristalsis.
Equipment	Stethoscope
Assessment/ Planning	• Explain to the patient what you plan to do and how long it will take. • Determine whether any immediate need is distracting the patient (e.g., pain, urge to urinate). Attend to that problem first. • Plan to auscultate the abdomen before palpating or percussing if performing a complete abdominal examination. Rationale: Stimulation of the abdominal wall may alter bowel motility. • Provide for privacy so that the patient is not concerned about being viewed or overheard. • Ensure that the room is warm and quiet. • If the patient has a nasogastric tube with suction, turn off the suction during auscultation.

Procedure

1. **Perform hand hygiene.**

   Rationale: Reduces microbe transmission.

2. **Identify the patient.**

   Rationale: Ensures correct patient receives proper assessment or treatment and reduces errors.

3. **Close door or bed curtains and explain the procedure to the patient.**

   Rationale: Ensures patient privacy, increases patient compliance, reduces patient anxiety, and promotes learning.

4. **Ask the patient when he or she last ate.**

   Rationale: Bowel sounds may be increased shortly after eating or if a meal is long overdue.

5. **Have the patient urinate before the examination.**

   Rationale: An empty bladder enhances validity of observations and promotes patient comfort.

6. **Assist the patient to a supine position with abdomen exposed.**

   Rationale: Supine position prevents tension in the abdominal muscles.

7. **Visually divide the abdomen into four quadrants using the umbilicus as the central crossing landmark (see Table 17-7).**

   Rationale: Consistent landmarks facilitate accurate description of assessment findings.

8. **Place the stethoscope diaphragm in each of the four quadrants. Listen for pitch, frequency, and duration of bowel sounds at each site (Fig. 1).**

Rationale: Active bowel sounds are irregular, gurgling noises that occur every 5 to 20 seconds.

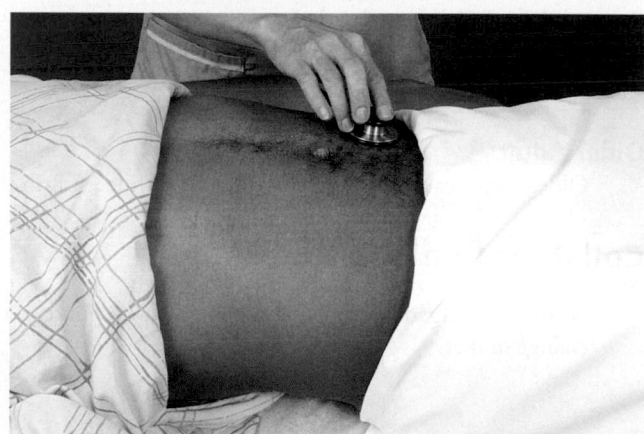

FIG. 1 Auscultate bowel sounds with diaphragm of stethoscope.

9. **If you do not hear bowel sounds, listen for 3 to 5 minutes in all quadrants before concluding that they are absent.**

Rationale: Bowel sounds are very irregular and require longer assessment to confirm that they are absent and not hypoactive. Absent or hypoactive bowel sounds indicate inhibited intestinal motility. It may not be practical for the nurse to listen for an extended period of time in each quadrant; hypoactive bowel tones can be recorded if bowel tones are not detected in an appropriate time period.

Procedure 17-5   *continued*

10. **Proceed with the rest of the physical examination or cover the patient's abdomen and assist him or her to a comfortable position.**

    Rationale: Avoids chilling the patient and provides for privacy.

11. **Document your findings.**

    Rationale: Communicates and establishes baseline.

Documentation

1/16/17: 11:40—Bowel sounds hypoactive in all quadrants, no flatus, no abdominal distention or complaints of nausea.
—S. Roberts, RN

Lifespan Considerations

Newborn and Infant

- Newborns have difficulty maintaining body temperature. Uncover only the body area that you are directly assessing.
- At 8 to 12 months of age, infants become fearful of strangers. Spend several minutes becoming acquainted with the child before proceeding with the examination.

Toddler and Preschooler

- Children 2 to 5 years of age are often afraid of the examining equipment. Letting them handle the stethoscope and using a "This is a game" approach often help allay the fear.
- Auscultate bowel sounds before performing any invasive examination, which may cause the child to cry.

School-Aged Child and Adolescent

Older children are modest. They may or may not want a parent to be with them during the examination; give the child the choice. Protect modesty through use of gowns or drapes.

Older Adult

Older adults can become easily chilled. Provide warmth through adequate draping or gowning.

Collaboration and Delegation

Notify the surgeon when the patient's bowel sounds return postoperatively, because this development usually warrants a change in diet.

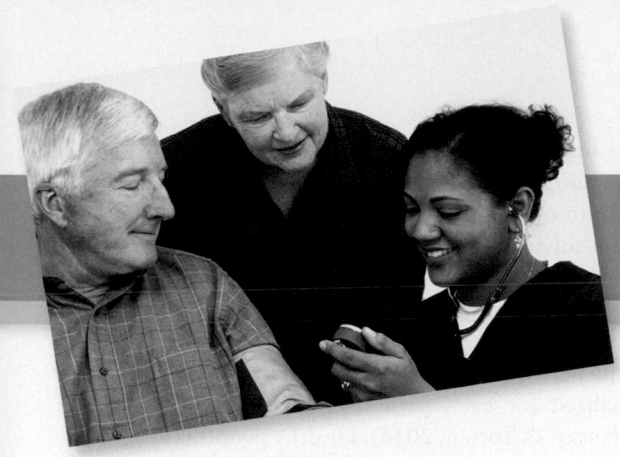

CHAPTER 18

Vital Signs

Christine M. Henshaw

Case Scenario

A couple in their 50s is shopping in a mall where a health fair is set up. You are a nurse participating at a booth offering blood pressure readings. After much coaxing, the woman persuades her husband to have his blood pressure taken. You obtain a reading of 168/94 mm Hg. The wife reacts strongly, saying, "I told you that your lack of exercise and overeating would catch up with you one day. How am I going to manage being a widow at such an early age?" The husband responds by saying, "Don't worry about me. I'm just as healthy as ever, and I plan to live until I'm 99 years old. I'm sure there's something wrong with that machine." Both of them turn to you. The wife says, "Tell him it's not the machine and that he isn't taking care of himself!"

Once you have completed this chapter and have incorporated vital signs into your knowledge base, review the above scenario and reflect on the following areas of Critical Thinking:

1. Identify possible interpretations of an isolated blood pressure reading of 168/94 mm Hg. List factors that may have affected the reading's accuracy.

2. Analyze the man's reaction to this situation. Indicate the teaching points about blood pressure that may be appropriate at this time.

3. Outline potential ways to deal therapeutically with the wife's anxiety, describing possible verbal and nonverbal interactions.

KEY TERMS

afebrile
apnea
auscultatory gap
blood pressure
bradycardia
bradypnea
core temperature
diastolic blood pressure
dyspnea
eupnea
hypertension
hypotension
Korotkoff sounds
paradoxical blood pressure
postural (orthostatic) hypotension
prehypertension
pulse deficit
pulse pressure
stridor
stroke volume
systolic blood pressure
tachycardia
tachypnea
tidal volume
wheezing

LEARNING OBJECTIVES

Upon completion of this chapter, the student will be able to do the following:

1. Describe the procedures used to assess the vital signs: temperature, pulse, respirations, and blood pressure.

2. Describe factors that can influence each vital sign.

3. Identify equipment routinely used to assess vital signs.

4. Identify rationales for each route of temperature assessment.

5. Identify the location of commonly assessed pulse sites.

6. Describe how to assess postural (orthostatic) hypotension.

7. Recognize normal vital sign values among various age groups.

Vital signs—body temperature (T), pulse (P), respirations (R), and blood pressure (BP)—indicate the function of some of the body's homeostatic mechanisms. Measurement and interpretation of the vital signs are important components of assessment that can yield information about underlying health status. Patient teaching concerning the vital signs is a key aspect of health promotion.

Typical or normal ranges of values for vital signs have been established for patients of various age groups (Table 18-1). During initial measurement of a patient's vital signs, the values are compared with these normal ranges to determine any variation that might indicate illness. When several sets of vital signs have been obtained, this information forms a baseline for comparison of subsequent measurements. Single vital sign values are less helpful; a series of values should be taken and evaluated to establish trends for the patient. Vital sign trends that deviate from normal are much more significant than are isolated abnormal values.

The tasks involved in measuring vital signs are simple and easy to learn, but interpreting the measurements and incorporating them into ongoing care and assessment require knowledge, problem-solving skills, critical thinking, and experience. Although measuring vital signs is usually part of routine care, they provide valuable information, and their evaluation should not be taken lightly.

The frequency with which to assess vital signs should be individualized for each patient (Johnson, Winkelman, Burant, Dolansky, & Totten, 2014). Healthy people may have vital signs checked only during annual physical examinations. Patients seen in ambulatory settings, wellness clinics, or psychiatric institutions may require infrequent vital sign checks. Most inpatient settings have a policy regarding the frequency of vital sign assessment, minimally every 8 hours for stable patients. Providers order additional vital sign checks at specific intervals based on the patient's condition (e.g., postoperatively or after an invasive diagnostic procedure). The nurse

THERAPEUTIC DIALOGUE: BLOOD PRESSURE

SCENES FOR THOUGHT

Mr. Richards is sitting up in bed with an IV in his left arm and ECG leads attached to his chest. Being careful to use his right arm, the nurse prepares to take his blood pressure.

LESS EFFECTIVE		MORE EFFECTIVE	
Nurse:	Hi, Mr. Richards. I'm here to take your blood pressure.	**Nurse:**	Hi, Mr. Richards. I'm Cheryl Bianco, and I'll be taking care of you today. How's it going?
Mr. Richards:	Again? They just took it 20 minutes ago. *(Looks irritated.)*	**Mr. Richards:**	Okay, I guess. Are you going to take my blood pressure again? *(Looks irritated.)*
Nurse:	Sure, we have to do that on heart patients. Just let me get this cuff on, and I'll be out of your way in a minute, okay?	**Nurse:**	Yes, I am. You look irritated about that. Are you? *(Exploring her observation.)*
Mr. Richards:	I guess so. Everyone else does. *(Continues to look annoyed.)*	**Mr. Richards:**	Well, yes. I mean, I'm not annoyed at you, but ever since I had the heart attack, people have been taking my pressure every 10 minutes, it seems, and I don't like it. *(Stopping to breathe.)*
Nurse:	There, all done. I'll be back to change your bed and get you up in the chair in a little bit.	**Nurse:**	It feels like the staff is focusing on your pressure. *(Restating.)*
Mr. Richards:	Bye. *(Sinks back onto the pillows.)*	**Mr. Richards:**	Are they worried? Am I going to have another heart attack? Should I be worried? I'm confused. *(Looking upset.)*
		Nurse:	It sounds like you're looking for some information. Let's talk about it. *(Opportunity to provide information and allay his fears.)*

CRITICAL THINKING CHALLENGE

- Analyze the significance of his blood pressure as Mr. Richards sees it.
- Detect his feelings regarding the blood pressure readings.
- Infer what his thinking might do to all of his vital signs if he is upset about frequent blood pressure readings.

TABLE 18-1 NORMAL VITAL SIGN RANGES ACROSS THE LIFE SPAN

	Pulse	Respirations	Temperature (°F)	Blood Pressure (mm Hg) Systolic	Diastolic
Newborn (>96 h)	70–190	30–60	96.0–99.5	60–90	20–60
Infant (>1 mo)	80–160	30–60	99.4–99.7	74–100	50–70
Toddler	80–130	24–40	99.0–99.7	80–112	50–80
Preschooler	80–120	22–34	98.6–99.0	82–110	50–78
School age	75–110	18–30	98.0–98.6	84–120	54–80
Adolescent	60–90	12–20	97–99	94–120	62–80
Adult	60–100	12–20	97–99	90–120	60–80
Older adult (>70 y)	60–100	12–20	95–99	90–120	60–80

caring for the patient may decide to monitor vital signs more frequently if the patient's condition changes.

Provide the patient with values obtained when vital signs are monitored. This is an excellent opportunity to teach patients the significance of the values obtained, the importance of a healthy lifestyle, and how they can optimize their own health. Positive changes in vital signs provide objective data to motivate individuals to continue a healthy lifestyle.

BODY TEMPERATURE

Humans are warm-blooded creatures, meaning that they maintain a consistent internal body temperature independent of the outside environment. The body's surface or skin temperature can vary widely with environmental conditions and physical activity. Despite these fluctuations, the temperature inside the body, the **core temperature**, remains relatively constant, unless the patient develops a febrile illness. The body's cells, tissues, and organs require this constant internal temperature and function optimally within a relatively narrow temperature range.

Normal body temperature when measured orally usually ranges between 36.5°C and 37.5°C (97.6°F and 99.6°F). This state of normal body temperature in a patient is termed **afebrile**. When temperature exceeds 37.5°C, this is termed *hyperthermia, fever,* or *pyrexia.* Body temperature can fluctuate with exercise, changes in hormone levels, changes in metabolic rate, and extremes of external temperature. In general, rectal temperatures may be 0.5°C (1°F) higher than oral

temperatures and axillary temperatures 0.5°C (1°F) lower than oral temperatures, although it is difficult to accurately convert temperatures obtained at different sites (Sund-Levander & Grodzinsky, 2009). Temperatures measured over the temporal artery tend to be close to oral temperatures, while tympanic temperatures fall approximately midway between normal oral and rectal temperature measurements. Refer to Table 18-2, which lists normal adult temperatures at different body sites.

Regulation of Body Temperature

Body temperature regulation requires the coordination of many body systems. For the core temperature to remain steady, heat production must equal heat loss. The thermoregulatory center in the anterior hypothalamus is the body's built-in thermostat. It can sense small changes in body temperature and stimulates the necessary responses in the nervous system, circulatory system, skin, and sweat glands to maintain homeostasis (state of dynamic equilibrium).

Heat Production

The body continually produces heat as a by-product of chemical reactions that occur in body cells. This collective process is known as metabolism. The process of thermoregulation keeps core temperature fairly constant regardless of where the heat is being produced. The basal metabolic rate (BMR) reflects the amount of energy the body uses, and thus the amount of heat produced, during absolute rest in an awake state. Physical exercise, increased production of thyroid hormones, and stimulation of the sympathetic nervous system can increase heat production.

HEAT LOSS

Just as the body is continually producing heat, it is also continuously losing heat through the skin and lungs. Heat is lost through four processes: radiation, conduction, convection, and evaporation.

TABLE 18-2 NORMAL ADULT TEMPERATURE RANGES FROM DIFFERENT BODY SITES

Oral	Axillary	Rectal	Tympanic
97.6°F–99.6°F	96.6°F–98.6°F	98.6°F–100.6°F	98.2°F–100.2°F
36.5°C–37.5°C	35.8°C–37.0°C	37.0°C–38.1°C	36.8°C–37.9°C

Exposure to a cold environment increases radiant heat loss. All objects with temperatures above absolute zero constantly lose heat through infrared heat rays. Covering the body with closely woven dark fabric can reduce radiant heat loss. Conduction is the transfer of heat from one object to another. The body loses a considerable amount of heat to the air through conduction. It can also lose heat to water during swimming or tepid baths. Convection is the loss of heat through air currents such as from a breeze or a fan. Evaporation causes heat loss as water is transformed to a gas. Examples of evaporation include diaphoresis (sweating) during strenuous exercise or when one is febrile.

Factors Affecting Body Temperature

Understanding the factors that can affect body temperature can help nurses accurately assess the significance of body temperature variations.

AGE

Newborns have unstable body temperatures because their thermoregulatory mechanisms are immature. They lack the ability to decrease heat loss in response to environmental temperatures and usually cannot mount a robust fever response to infection. Some older adults may have body temperatures less than 36.4°C (97.6°F) because baseline body temperature may drop as an individual ages. The febrile response may be blunted, leading to a delay in therapy if the nurse waits to report fever based on expectations for younger adults (Sloane et al., 2014). Remember this fact when evaluating low-grade temperatures in the elderly or identifying those at risk for hypothermia.

ENVIRONMENT

Ordinarily, changes in environmental temperatures do not affect core body temperature, but core body temperature can be altered by exposure to hot or cold extremes. The degree of change relates to the temperature, humidity, and length of exposure. The body's thermoregulatory mechanisms are also influential especially in infants and older adults who have diminished control mechanisms. Death may occur if a person's core body temperature drops to 25°C (77°F) or rises to 45°C (113°F).

TIME OF DAY

Body temperature normally fluctuates throughout the day. Temperature is usually lower in the early morning and higher in the late afternoon and early evening, varying by as much as 2°C (3.6°F). Theorists attribute this variation to changes in muscle activity and digestive processes, which are usually lowest in the early morning during sleep. Even greater variation in body temperature at various times of the day is found in infants and children.

EXERCISE

Body temperature increases with exercise because of increased breakdown of carbohydrates and fats to provide energy. Strenuous exercise, such as running a marathon, can temporarily raise the temperature to as high as 40°C (104°F).

STRESS

Emotional or physical stress can elevate body temperature. When stress stimulates the sympathetic nervous system, circulating levels of epinephrine and norepinephrine increase. As a result, the metabolic rate increases, which, in turn, increases heat production. Stressed or anxious patients may have an elevated temperature with no underlying pathology.

HORMONES

Women usually have greater variations in their temperature than do men. Progesterone, a female hormone secreted at ovulation, increases body temperature 0.3°C to 0.6°C (0.5°F to 1°F) above baseline. By measuring her temperature daily, a woman can determine when she ovulates, which is the basis for the rhythm method of birth control (see Chapter 41). After menopause, mean temperature norms are the same for men and women. Thyroxine, epinephrine, and norepinephrine also elevate body temperature by increasing heat production.

Factors Affecting Body Temperature Measurement

External factors can lead to false temperature readings. Small alterations in oral temperature readings can occur after smoking or chewing gum or when oxygen is administered by mask or cannula. Hot or cold drinks may also cause variations in oral temperature readings. Diaphoresis or air blowing over the face may affect temporal artery measurements; stool in the rectum can affect rectal temperatures.

Assessing Body Temperature

Temperature measurement establishes a baseline for comparison as a disease progresses or therapies are instituted. The reliability of a temperature value depends on selecting the most appropriate site, choosing the correct equipment, and using the correct procedure.

SITES

Use judgment when selecting the route to measure temperature. The most commonly used sites are the mouth, rectum, ear (tympanic), forehead (temporal artery), and axilla. In most clinical situations, any of these sites is satisfactory if the nurse uses proper technique and accounts for normal variations for the different sites, although the axilla is the least accurate. Additional sites are the bladder, esophagus, and pulmonary artery, all of which are considered core temperatures and require special probes. Because body temperature can vary with age, sex, and measurement site, a baseline should be obtained and used to evaluate subsequent changes for the individual. Refer to Table 18-2 for normal temperature ranges.

Oral

A common site for temperature measurement is the mouth. Advantages of the oral route include easy access and patient comfort. Drinking hot or cold liquids can affect temperature measurement; wait 15 to 30 minutes to allow the patient's mouth temperature to return to baseline before placing the thermometer (Quatrara et al., 2007). Oral temperature assessment is not prudent or safe for infants, young children, unconscious or delirious patients, or patients with seizure disorders.

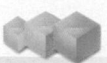

Concept Mastery Alert

Oral temperature assessment should not be used with infants and young children, due to the safety risks and difficulty in obtaining an accurate reading. Tympanic or forehead (temporal artery) methods are appropriate options.

Rectal

Rectal temperature measurement, once thought to be the most accurate and commonly used clinically, is usually replaced by less invasive procedures. Patients often do not tolerate rectal temperatures well because of discomfort and embarrassment. If this route is used, take care to avoid placing the thermometer into fecal material, which may falsely elevate the temperature reading.

The rectal route is contraindicated in patients with diarrhea, those who have undergone rectal surgery, those with rectal diseases, and those with cancer who are neutropenic. In selected patients (e.g., those with tetraplegia), rectal temperature measurements may cause vagal stimulation, which can result in bradycardia and syncope.

SAFETY ALERT

Rectal thermometers are contraindicated in infants because they may cause trauma to the rectal mucosa.

Ear

Since the development of the tympanic membrane thermometer, the ear has been added to the list of sites where temperature can be measured easily and safely. Measuring temperature at this site has many advantages but also has a high degree of variance when compared to the oral route (Lawson et al., 2007). The tympanic membrane receives its blood supply from the same vasculature that supplies the hypothalamus; thus, tympanic temperature readings closely reflect core body temperature. Cerumen in the ear canal, crying, or otitis media

will not significantly alter temperature readings. Smoking, drinking, and eating, which may alter oral temperature measurement, do not affect tympanic temperature measurement. The ear is readily accessible and permits rapid temperature readings in very young, confused, or unconscious patients. Because the ear canal harbors fewer pathogens than do the oral or rectal cavities, infection control is a minor concern with the tympanic site.

Poor measurement technique is often responsible for errors in measurement using the ear. To obtain an accurate reading, hold the pinna and gently pull the ear slightly upward and backward to straighten the ear canal (pull the pinna down and straight back for a child 2 months to 3 years old), fit the probe snugly in the patient's ear canal, and angle it toward the jawline. Home-use tympanic thermometers can be used for fever screening but should be verified by other routes to decide patient follow-up.

Forehead (Temporal Artery)

Recently developed devices allow fast, safe measurement of temperature across the forehead, over the distribution of the temporal artery. The limited research available using these devices indicates that they may be more accurate than tympanic thermometers and comparable to oral thermometers in accuracy. They are easy to use and well tolerated by infants and young children. Measurements are consistent when taken on either the right or left side of the forehead but may be affected by perspiration or air blowing over the face (Carr et al., 2011; Lawson et al., 2007).

Axillary

The axillary route is considered the least accurate and least reliable site because several factors can influence the measurement obtained. For example, if the patient has bathed recently, the reading may reflect the temperature of the water used. Sweat and ambient air temperature may influence the reading. The axillary route may be recommended for infants but is of limited value in assessing fever in adults.

EQUIPMENT

Equipment used for temperature measurement includes electronic thermometers, tympanic membrane thermometers, temporal artery thermometers, disposable paper thermometers, and noncontact infrared thermometers. Mercury thermometers, no longer used due to the dangers of exposure to mercury, may be found in homes and should be replaced with other equipment with the mercury thermometers properly disposed of.

Tympanic Membrane Thermometers

The tympanic membrane thermometer is a portable, handheld device resembling an otoscope that recharges using a battery pack (Fig. 18-1). It records temperature through a sensor probe placed in the ear canal to detect infrared radiation from the eardrum. It is noninvasive and fast to use, but studies show discrepancies between tympanic membrane and oral measurements, resulting in both false-positive and false-negative readings.

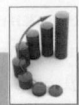

OUTCOME-BASED TEACHING PLAN

Sylvia Yantes, 16 years old, has just given birth to her first child, a boy weighing 5 lb, 10 oz. Her son had three elevated temperature readings during the first 24 hours of life. Before Sylvia and her son can go home, she needs to be able to monitor his temperature.

OUTCOME

Before discharge, Sylvia (the mother) will be able to demonstrate accurate assessment of axillary temperature.

STRATEGIES

- Assess the mother's experience in monitoring temperature and her ability to read a digital thermometer.
- Encourage the mother to wash her hands first, explaining its importance before handling the baby.
- Have the mother turn on the thermometer.
- Demonstrate placement of the thermometer in the axilla, explaining the importance of leaving it in place until a final reading is obtained (it will beep).
- Stress the importance of holding the thermometer in place and never leaving the infant unattended while taking the temperature.
- Have the mother demonstrate the procedure until she feels comfortable. Give positive feedback.
- Instruct the mother to check the temperature once every evening unless the baby becomes febrile.

EVALUATION

> 8/12/17: 09:00—Mom was able to demonstrate obtaining accurate axillary temperature on her baby without cueing.
> —S. Roberts, RN.

OUTCOME

During the first postpartum week, the mother will keep a record of daily temperature and bring log to first physician's visit.

STRATEGIES

- Provide the mother with a log indicating date and times and a place to fill in the temperatures obtained.
- Provide the mother with written appointment card requesting that she bring the temperature log to that baby visit.
- When you review the log at the first baby visit, give the mother positive feedback.
- Stress that the mother reports any temperature elevation above 98.6°F, which could indicate infection.

EVALUATION

> 8/12/17: 09:00—Mom verbalized willingness to keep temperature log and report any temperature readings above 98.6°F.
> —S. Roberts, RN.

These discrepancies can be minimized by using the same ear and device for measurement each time and by ensuring that the user is well trained. Because discrepancies are usually small, the convenience, safety, and efficiency of tympanic temperature measurement outweigh its disadvantages.

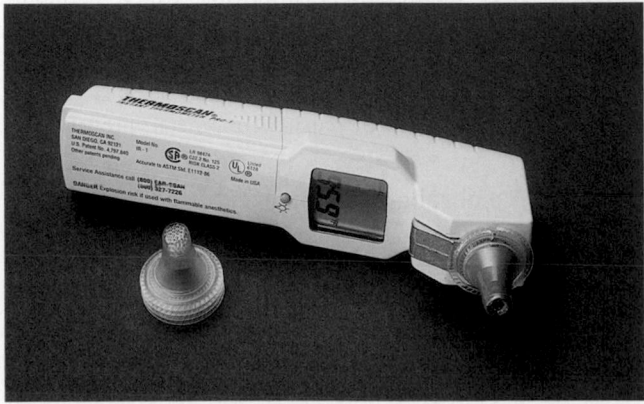

FIGURE 18-1 Tympanic membrane thermometer.

The tympanic membrane thermometer is appropriate for infants older than 2 months or very young children who may have difficulty remaining still for extended periods. Because recordings are obtained within 2 seconds, the tympanic membrane thermometer often is preferred for fever screening in emergency departments or other areas where assessments must be made quickly. Tympanic thermometers should not be used on people with ear drainage or scarred tympanic membranes.

Temporal Artery Thermometers

The temporal artery thermometer is a handheld device that scans the forehead and measures temperature over the temporal artery (Fig. 18-2). The temporal artery thermometer corrects for radiant heat loss from the forehead by measuring the ambient temperature at the same time the skin temperature over the temporal artery is measured. The thermometer then adjusts the temperature measurement to discount radiant heat loss. Measurement of temperature over the temporal artery does not require contact with mucous membranes, but the head must be uncovered since bandages or clothing will trap heat.

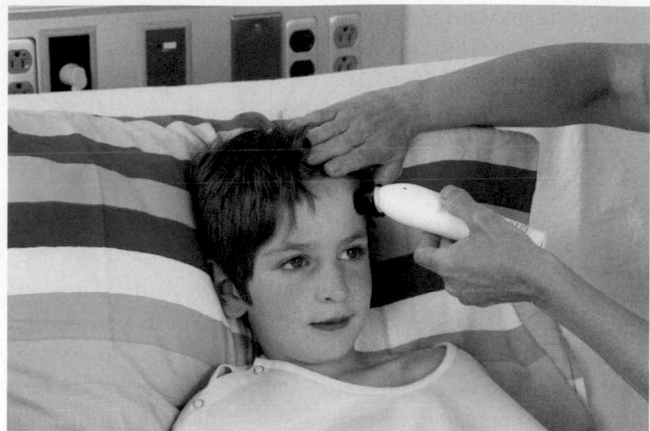

FIGURE 18-2 Temporal artery thermometers are noninvasive and well tolerated by young children. For an accurate reading, move hair to expose forehead and hairline.

Disposable Paper (Chemical) Thermometers

Single-use paper thermometers (Fig. 18-3) are thin strips of chemically treated paper with raised dots that change color to reflect the temperature. Disposable thermometers are convenient when infection control is a concern since they are discarded following a single use; however, they may not be accurate if stored incorrectly. For oral temperature measurement, they are placed deeply in the posterior sublingual pocket and left in place for 60 seconds. If used for axillary temperatures, the strips are placed vertically against the trunk of the body and held in place by the upper arm for 3 minutes.

Electronic Thermometers

Healthcare facilities use electronic thermometers extensively. Many types are on the market, but all have similar characteristics. The thermometer consists of a battery-powered display unit and a temperature-sensitive probe connected to the display unit by a thin cord. A disposable plastic sheath covers the probe to prevent the transmission of infection. Electronic thermometers provide readings in less than 60 seconds. When used orally, they are most accurate if placed in the posterior sublingual pocket. The thermometer displays results based on the Celsius or Fahrenheit scale; some thermometers can display readings from both scales.

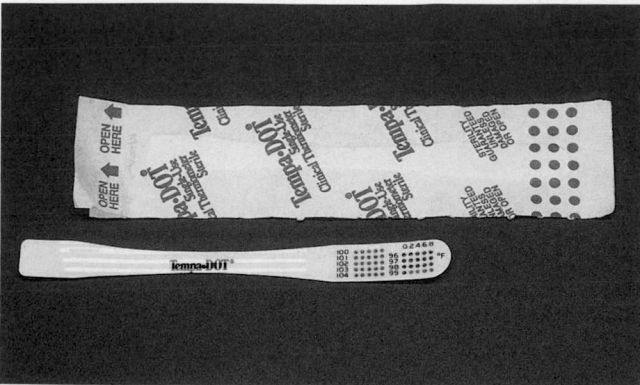

FIGURE 18-3 Disposable paper thermometer. The dots change color to indicate temperature.

The electronic thermometer is ideally suited for use with children because the sheath is unbreakable and the time necessary for accurate measurement is relatively short. A separate probe (often red) must be used for rectal temperature measurement.

Noncontact Infrared Thermometers

Infrared technology allows measurement of body temperature without contact with skin or mucous membranes. This allows rapid temperature measurement without cross-contamination between patients. Holding the thermometer close to the forehead detects heat being emitted from the body. Although accuracy is variable, ease of use is an advantage. The primary use is in determining that the patient does not have a fever, rather than in assessing exact temperature (Wang et al., 2014).

Glass Mercury Thermometers

Mercury thermometers are no longer sold in retail stores; however, some homes still have glass thermometers. They are not used in healthcare environments because of the risks of mercury exposure to people and the environment if the thermometer breaks. Patients should be instructed to safely dispose of mercury thermometers and purchase new, safe equipment. Pharmacies may accept mercury thermometers for disposal, or patients should check with their waste disposal company.

SCALES

Temperature can be measured on the Celsius or Fahrenheit scale (Fig. 18-4). The scale used varies among agencies. Nurses do not routinely have to convert from one scale to the other;

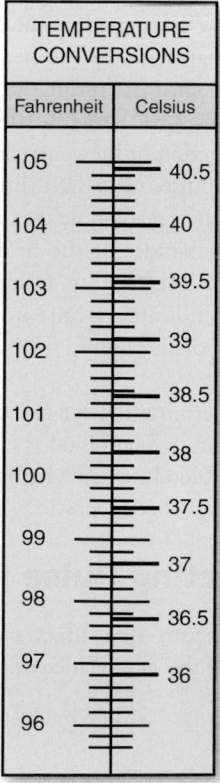

TEMPERATURE CONVERSIONS	
Fahrenheit	Celsius
105	40.5
104	40
103	39.5
102	39
101	38.5
100	38
99	37.5
98	37
97	36.5
96	36

FIGURE 18-4 Temperature conversion chart.

however, if conversion is necessary, use the simple conversion guide provided in Figure 18-4.

METHODS

Nurses often delegate temperature taking to unlicensed assistive personnel (UAP). Nurses use critical thinking to interpret temperature measurements, document the results, and report abnormal values. Whenever possible, measure and record temperature measurements at the same site, using the same device, so that fluctuations may be interpreted accurately. See **Procedure 18-1** for specific details on how to obtain a temperature measurement using different routes and equipment.

PULSE

Contraction of the ventricles of the heart ejects blood into the arteries. The force of the blood entering the aorta from the left ventricle causes stretching or distention of the elastic aortic wall. As the aorta first expands and then contracts, a pulse wave is created that travels along the blood vessels. The pulse wave or pulsation can be felt as a throb or tap where the arteries lie close to the skin surface.

Characteristics

Characteristics of the pulse include rate or frequency, rhythm, and quality. Rate or frequency refers to the number of pulsations per minute. Rhythm refers to the regularity with which pulsation occurs. Quality refers to the strength of the palpated pulsation.

Specialized cells that make up the heart's conduction system establish the rate and rhythm of the pulse. An electrical impulse in the sinoatrial (SA) node of the right atrium initially simulates contraction of the ventricles. In adults, the SA node initiates the impulse 60 to 100 times per minute. The electrical impulse then spreads quickly through the conduction system to the remainder of the heart so that the heart muscle contracts in a synchronous fashion. Irregularities of heart rhythm usually indicate a failure in the conduction system or the generation of an impulse from a site other than the SA node.

Several factors determine the quality of the arterial pulse, including the force with which blood is ejected from the ventricles, the amount of blood ejected with each heartbeat (stroke volume), and the compliance or elasticity of the arteries.

Factors Affecting Pulse Rate

Understanding the factors that affect pulse rate helps with accurate assessment of the significance of pulse rate variations.

AGE

The average pulse rate of an infant ranges from 100 to 160 beats per minute. The heart rhythm in infants and children often

varies markedly with respiration, increasing during inspiration and decreasing with expiration. The normal range of the pulse in an adult is 60 to 100 beats per minute. Table 18-1 shows the normal pulse ranges for various age groups.

AUTONOMIC NERVOUS SYSTEM

Stimulation of the vagus nerve in the parasympathetic nervous system (dominant activation during resting states) results in a decrease in the pulse rate. Normally, parasympathetic nervous system input slows the pulse rate below 100 beats per minute. Conversely, stimulation of the sympathetic nervous system results in an increased pulse rate. Sympathetic nervous system activation occurs in response to various stimuli, including pain, anxiety, exercise, fever, ingestion of caffeinated beverages, and changes in intravascular volume.

MEDICATIONS

Various categories of medications affect heart rate. Medications that decrease intravascular volume, such as diuretics, may cause a reflex increase in pulse rate. Other medications mimic or block the effects of the autonomic nervous system. For example, atropine inhibits parasympathetic input, causing an increased pulse rate. Other medications such as metoprolol, a beta-blocker, block the action of the sympathetic nervous system on beta receptors, resulting in a decreased heart rate.

Assessing the Pulse

Baseline pulse, rhythm, and quality are established during the initial nursing assessment and are used for comparison with future measurements.

SITES

The pulse can be assessed in any location where an artery lies close to the skin surface and can be compressed against a firm underlying structure such as muscle or bone. The most commonly assessed pulses are the temporal, carotid, apical, brachial, radial, femoral, popliteal, pedal, and posterior tibial (Fig. 18-5).

Temporal

The temporal artery courses across the temporal bone of the skull. The pulsation of the temporal artery is most easily palpated just in front of the upper part of the ear.

Carotid

The sternomastoid muscles, which stand out when the jaw is clenched forcefully, run from below the ear to the clavicle and sternum. Beneath the sternomastoid muscles lie the carotid arteries. The carotid artery is most easily palpated at the lower half of the neck, along the medial border of the sternomastoid muscle. Palpating the carotid artery in the upper part of the neck may result in stimulation of the carotid sinus, which causes a reflex drop in pulse rate. The carotid pulse best

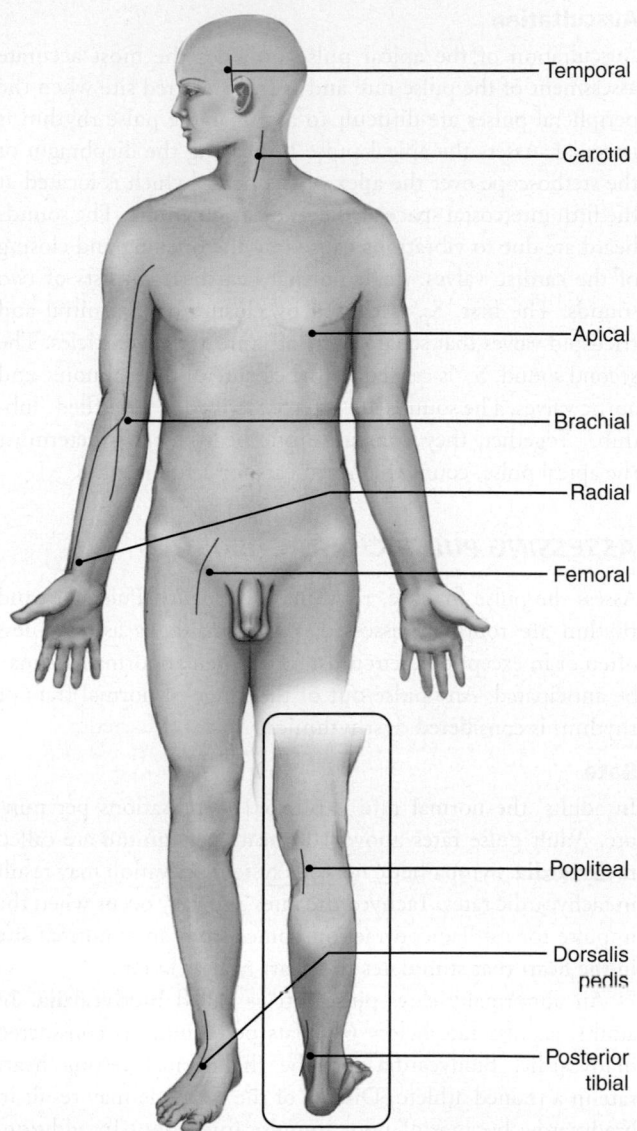

Temporal

Carotid

Apical

Brachial

Radial

Femoral

Popliteal

Dorsalis pedis

Posterior tibial

FIGURE 18-5 Pulse sites. The insert shows the right leg. The posterior tibial pulse is on the medial aspect of the ankle.

represents the quality of pulsation in the aorta because of its proximity to the central circulation.

SAFETY ALERT

Always palpate the carotid artery in the lower half of the neck to avoid stimulating the carotid sinus. Never palpate bilateral carotid pulses simultaneously because this can seriously impair cerebral blood flow.

Apical

The contraction or beating of the heart ventricles also can be palpated with the hand or auscultated with a stethoscope placed over the area of the left ventricle. Normally, this area is at the level of the fifth intercostal space at about the midclavicular line.

Brachial

The brachial artery lies between the groove of the biceps and triceps muscles in the inner aspect of the upper arm. The brachial pulse is palpated most easily with the patient's arm extended at the elbow and supported by the examiner to prevent muscle contraction, which may obscure the pulse.

Radial

The radial artery is the site most commonly assessed in the clinical setting. The radial pulse is palpated on the thumb side of the inner aspect of the wrist.

Femoral

The femoral pulse is palpated in the anterior, medial aspect of the thigh, just below the inguinal ligament, about halfway between the anterior superior iliac spine and the symphysis pubis. Deep palpation may be required to detect the femoral pulse beneath the subcutaneous tissue.

Popliteal

The popliteal pulse is palpable behind the knee in the lateral aspect of the popliteal fossa (the hollow area at the back of the knee joint). The pulse is best assessed with the knee flexed and the leg relaxed. The patient may be supine or prone.

Pedal

The pedal pulse or dorsalis pedis pulse can be felt on the dorsal aspect of the foot (the area of the foot that is on top in a standing position). The pulse is palpated lateral to the tendon that runs from the great toe toward the ankle. The dorsalis pedis pulse may be congenitally absent in some patients.

Posterior Tibial

The posterior tibial pulse is located behind the malleolus (the rounded protuberance of bone) of the inner ankle. The pulse is palpated by curving the fingertips over the bone.

EQUIPMENT

A stethoscope and a Doppler ultrasound device may be used to measure pulse rate.

Stethoscope

Auscultation of the apical pulse requires a stethoscope. The stethoscope should have snugly fitting earpieces and thick-walled tubing about 12 inches (30 cm) long for optimal sound transmission. The stethoscope should be equipped with a bell and a diaphragm.

Doppler Ultrasound Device

Peripheral pulses that cannot be detected by palpation may be assessed with an ultrasonic Doppler device. A conductive gel is first applied to the skin to reduce resistance to sound transmission. The transmitter of the device is then placed over the artery to be assessed (Fig. 18-6). High-frequency waves directed at the artery from the transmitter are disturbed by the pulsating flow of blood and are reflected back to the ultrasound device. The sound disturbances (Doppler shifts) are amplified and heard through earpieces or a speaker attached to the device.

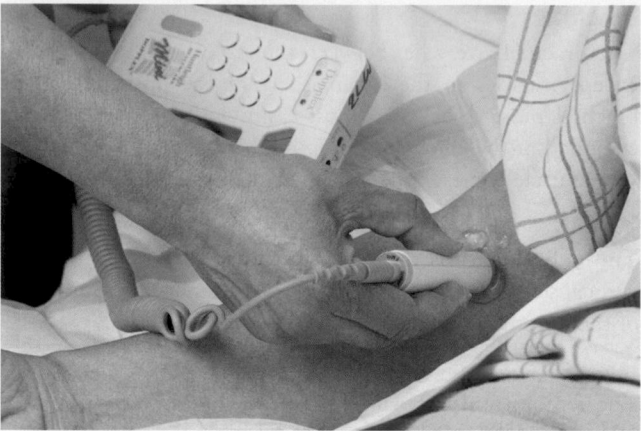

FIGURE 18-6 An ultrasonic Doppler device can be used to assess a peripheral pulse.

Doppler assessment of the pulse is generally used to determine the adequacy of blood flow to an area for which occlusive vascular disease threatens the blood supply or for postoperative assessment where peripheral circulation can be occluded. Doppler also may be useful when obesity or edema obscures the pulse, in situations of cardiopulmonary collapse where peripheral vasoconstriction makes pulses difficult to palpate, or to assist in placement of vascular access devices. When a Doppler is used to assess a pulse, be sure to document that the pulse was found by Doppler.

METHODS

Palpation and auscultation are methods used to assess pulse rate.

Palpation

The pulse is palpated using the first and second or second and third fingers of one hand. The fingers should be placed parallel to the course of the artery. Use light pressure initially to locate the area of strongest pulsation. More forceful palpation may be applied to count the rate, determine the rhythm, and assess the quality of pulsation. Count the number of pulses for 30 or 60 seconds and multiply as necessary to yield pulses per minute. The time interval used to assess the pulse depends on the patient's condition and the agency's norms. Patients with irregular or abnormally slow or fast pulse rates are best assessed for 1 full minute. Patients with regular rhythms and normal rates may be assessed for a shorter time. Intervals of 15 seconds may be used for patients with regular rhythms when reassessing the pulse frequently, as during recovery from anesthesia.

Regardless of the time interval selected, count the initial pulsation as zero. Do not count pulses at or after completion of the time interval. Counting the first pulse as one or counting pulses after the period of assessment results in overestimation of the pulse. The error is multiplied when intervals of less than 60 seconds are used to assess the rate. Counting even one extra pulsation in a 15-second pulse assessment results in overestimation of the pulse rate by four. **Procedure 18-2** provides detailed instructions on taking a pulse.

Auscultation

Auscultation of the apical pulse provides the most accurate assessment of the pulse rate and is the preferred site when the peripheral pulses are difficult to assess or the pulse rhythm is irregular. Assess the apical pulse by placing the diaphragm of the stethoscope over the apex of the heart, which is located at the fifth intercostal space at the midclavicular line. The sounds heard are due to vibrations caused by the opening and closing of the cardiac valves. Each normal heartbeat consists of two sounds. The first, S_1, is caused by closure of the mitral and tricuspid valves that separate the atria from the ventricles. The second sound, S_2, is caused by the closure of the pulmonic and aortic valves. The sounds are often described as a muffled "lub-dub." Together, they constitute one heartbeat. To determine the apical pulse, count the heartbeats for 1 full minute.

ASSESSING PULSE CHARACTERISTICS

Assess the pulse for rate, rhythm, and quality. Pulse rate and rhythm are routinely assessed; pulse quality is assessed less often or in exceptional circumstances when abnormalities may be anticipated. Any pulse out of the range of normal (rate or rhythm) is considered dysrhythmic.

Rate

In adults, the normal rate is 60 to 100 pulsations per minute. Adult pulse rates above 100 beats per minute are called **tachycardia**. Sympathetic nervous system activation may result in tachycardic rates. Tachycardic rates also may occur when the impulse for cardiac contraction comes from an abnormal site in the heart that stimulates the heart to beat faster.

An abnormally slow pulse rate is called **bradycardia**. In adults, a pulse rate below 60 beats per minute is considered bradycardic. Bradycardia may be the normal resting heart rate in a trained athlete. Disease of the SA node may result in bradycardia because of poor impulse formation. In addition, enhanced parasympathetic nervous system activity (e.g., stimulation of the carotid sinus) may cause bradycardia.

Rhythm

Normally, cardiac contractions occur at evenly spaced intervals, resulting in a regular rhythm. Infants and children often have increased pulse rates during inspiration and decreased rates during expiration.

Heart disease, medications, or electrolyte imbalances may alter the heart's normal rhythmic beating, causing an irregular pulse. An irregular pulse rhythm that still displays a consistent pattern is called *regularly irregular*. An example is pulsus bigeminus, in which a normal heartbeat initiated in the SA node is followed by a heartbeat initiated in a different part of the heart. The second beat is early and often weaker than the first, resulting in a regularly irregular pulse.

If the pulse has no pattern, it is called *irregularly irregular*. Irregularly irregular pulses may be a component of many conditions, including atrial fibrillation. In atrial fibrillation, the atria do not contract in a synchronous fashion, and the primary impulse for the heartbeat does not come from the SA node. Consequently, the time interval between successive ventricular contractions varies, and an irregularly irregular pulse is detected.

When you note an abnormal pulse rhythm, consider using the auscultatory method to obtain an apical pulse rate. Also, determine if irregularity of the pulse is a new finding for the patient.

> ### ❗ SAFETY ALERT
> Many people have chronically irregular pulse rhythms, but a new finding of pulse irregularity requires immediate investigation to determine the causes and to assess the need for treatment.

Quality

Pulse quality generally refers to the strength of pulsation and may be rated on a numeric scale (Table 18-3). Because there are multiple scales for grading pulses, it is best to describe what you feel. The normal quality of the pulse is described as full or strong and can be palpated easily. Weak pulses are obliterated easily by the examiner's fingers and may be described as thready. A bounding pulse is stronger than normal and difficult to obliterate. Pulse quality reflects the stroke volume, the compliance or elasticity of the arteries, and the adequacy of blood delivery. When stroke volume is decreased, as in severe hemorrhage, the pulse is often thready and may be difficult to palpate in the peripheral arteries. The pulse is usually palpated more easily in the central areas, such as the carotid or femoral arteries. With aging, the arteries lose elasticity, and the pulse becomes bounding. The combination of rapid pulse rate and increased stroke volume with exercise results in a pulse that the patient can feel and is sometimes called a pounding heart.

Palpate pulses bilaterally (except for carotids) to compare quality. Equality of pulsation provides information about local blood flow. For example, partial occlusion of a right femoral artery would result in weaker femoral, popliteal, pedal, and posterior tibial pulses on the right compared to the left. Bilateral pulse comparison is used to monitor for complications after procedures that are invasive to the arteries, such as arteriography. After an arteriogram, during which a large artery is punctured and injected with radiographic dye, the normal clotting to seal the artery may cause total arterial occlusion. Weakened or absent pulses distal to the puncture site would signal an occlusion.

Pulse Deficits

In some situations, stroke volume may vary from beat to beat during cardiac contraction, resulting in a pulse wave so weak that it cannot be perceived by palpation at a peripheral site. It is important to recognize this situation because it provides information about the heart's ability to perfuse the body adequately. When some of the ventricular contractions do not perfuse, a difference exists between the apical and peripheral pulses—a **pulse deficit**. When a pulse deficit is present, the radial pulse rate is always lower than the apical pulse rate. Document and report to the provider any new finding of a pulse deficit so that evaluation and follow-up can occur.

RESPIRATIONS

Respiration is a term used to summarize two different but related processes: external respiration and internal respiration. External respiration is the process of taking oxygen into and eliminating carbon dioxide from the body. Internal respiration refers to the use of oxygen, the production of carbon dioxide, and the exchange of these gases between the cells and the blood.

The process of inspiration is active. Inspiratory muscles contract, resulting in increased intrathoracic volume as the lungs expand. The pressure in the airway becomes negative and air flows inward. At the end of inspiration, natural lung recoil occurs, the airway pressure becomes slightly positive, and the air flows out as the muscles relax. Expiration is basically a passive process.

Normal breathing is automatic and involuntary. At rest, the normal adult respiratory rate is 12 to 20 breaths per minute. Normal **tidal volume** (the amount of air moving in and out with each breath) is 500 mL or 6 to 8 L per minute. In people with healthy respiratory systems, the normal stimulus to breathe is hypercarbia, an increased carbon dioxide level. Chemoreceptors throughout the body sense changes in carbon dioxide levels and stimulate the respiratory center, which increases or decreases respiratory rate and depth accordingly. Chapter 26 provides an in-depth explanation of respiratory control.

Factors Affecting Respirations

Several factors can affect respiratory rate, rhythm, and depth. Familiarity with these factors allows the nurse to determine the significance of alterations.

AGE

Normal growth from infancy to adulthood results in an increased lung capacity. As lung capacity increases, lower respiratory rates are sufficient to exchange air. As the adult ages, lung elasticity decreases. With this decrease in elasticity, respiratory rate increases to allow for adequate air exchange.

TABLE 18-3	SCALE TO RATE PULSE QUALITY
0	No pulse detected
1⁺	Thready, weak pulse; easily obliterated with pressure; pulse may come and go
2⁺	Pulse difficult to palpate; may be obliterated with pressure
3⁺	Normal pulse
4⁺	Bounding, hyperactive pulse; easily palpated and cannot be obliterated

MEDICATIONS

Sympathomimetic drugs (e.g., albuterol) can be used to dilate bronchioles, increasing the person's ability to move air into and out of the lungs. Inhaled corticosteroids decrease airway inflammation. Opioids may decrease respiratory rate and depth.

STRESS

Stress or strong emotions can change a person's respiratory pattern because such conditions stimulate the sympathetic nervous system. Stressors, including pain, anxiety, infection, and fever, increase the rate and depth of respirations.

EXERCISE

When people exercise, their tissues consume and process more oxygen. Also, exercise produces extra carbon dioxide and heat that the body must eliminate. The body responds to these needs by increasing the rate and depth of respirations.

ALTITUDE

Because of a decrease in atmospheric pressure with altitude, the oxygen content of the air decreases. The percentage of oxygen in the air (about 21%) does not change with altitude. To compensate for the decreased oxygen content, the rate and depth of respirations increase to improve the oxygen supply available to body tissues.

GENDER

Because men normally have a larger lung capacity than do women, men may have a lower respiratory rate.

Assessing Respirations

Assess respirations during every vital sign evaluation. Establish a set of normal baseline measurements of rate, rhythm, depth, and quality for each patient so comparisons can be made.

The respiratory assessment can provide valuable information and insight into a patient's condition. When assessing a patient's respiratory status, keep in mind the patient's normal pattern, the influence of any disease conditions, and the influence of any medication or therapies that could affect the patient's respiratory status.

RATE

Respiratory rate changes with age (Table 18-1). At rest, the normal respiratory rate for an infant is 30 to 60 breaths per minute, decreasing to 12 to 20 breaths per minute for an adult. **Tachypnea** is an abnormally fast respiratory rate (usually above 20 breaths per minute in the adult). **Bradypnea** is an abnormally slow respiratory rate (usually less than 12 breaths per minute in the adult). **Apnea**, the absence of respirations, is often described by the length of time in which no respirations occur (e.g., a 10-second period of apnea). Continuous apnea is synonymous with respiratory arrest and is not compatible with life.

RHYTHM AND DEPTH

Eupnea refers to normal respiratory rhythm and depth. Regularity refers to the pattern of inspiration and expiration. Expiration is normally twice as long as inspiration. Assess depth by observing the movement of the chest wall. Also, note the use of accessory muscles. Table 18-4 describes abnormal patterns, such as Biot respirations, Cheyne–Stokes respirations, and Kussmaul respirations.

QUALITY

Respirations are usually automatic, quiet, and effortless. When assessing respirations, be attentive to changes from the normal quality. Abnormalities in quality are usually characterized by effort or noise.

TABLE 18-4 ABNORMAL BREATHING PATTERNS

Abnormal Breathing Pattern	Description	Conditions
Bradypnea	Respiratory rate below 12 beats/min	Neurologic disturbances, electrolyte disturbances, opioid or barbiturate overdose, postanesthesia
Tachypnea	Persistent respiratory rate above 20 beats/min	Trauma, injury, stress, pain; respiratory, cardiac, liver disease
Biot's	Cyclic breathing pattern characterized by shallow breathing alternating with periods of apnea	Neurologic problems (meningitis, encephalitis), head trauma, brain, abscess, heatstroke
Cheyne–Stokes Apnea	Cyclic breathing pattern characterized by periods of respirations of increased rate and depth alternating with periods of apnea	Congestive heart failure, drug overdose, increased intracranial pressure, impending death
Kussmaul Duration 1 Minute	Increased rate (above 20 beats/min) and depth of respirations	Metabolic acidosis, diabetic ketoacidosis, renal failure

Dyspnea describes respirations that require excessive effort. Respirations can be painful or labored. Patients may report being unable to catch their breath. Dyspnea can occur at rest or with activity; dyspnea that occurs with activity is called exertional dyspnea. Healthy people who are not in good physical condition may experience exertional dyspnea.

Breathing also can be noisy. Several terms are used to describe the different types of noisy respirations that can be heard without a stethoscope. **Stridor** is a harsh inspiratory sound that may be compared to crowing. It may indicate an upper airway obstruction. Stridor is commonly heard in children with croup or after aspiration of a foreign object. **Wheezing** is a high-pitched musical sound. It is usually heard on expiration but may be heard on inspiration. It is associated with partial obstruction of the bronchi or bronchioles, as in asthma. Sighs are breaths of deep inspiration and prolonged expiration. Everyone sighs, and sighing aids in the expansion of alveoli. However, frequent sighing may indicate stress or tension.

METHODS

Perform the respiratory assessment without patients being aware that you are doing so. If patients are conscious of the procedure, they may alter their breathing patterns or rate. Assess the respiratory rate after or before taking the radial pulse, while holding the patient's wrist. If respirations are very shallow and difficult to visually detect, count them while observing the sternal notch, where respiration is more apparent. If the patient is sleeping, rest a hand gently on the patient's chest to detect its rise and fall. With an infant or young child, assess respirations before taking the temperature so the child is not crying, which alters the respiratory status. See **Procedure 18-3** for details on assessing respirations.

BLOOD PRESSURE

Blood pressure is the force that blood exerts against the walls of the blood vessels. The pressure in the systemic arteries is most commonly measured in the clinical setting. Blood pressure is stated in millimeters of mercury (mm Hg).

Physiologic Factors Determining Blood Pressure

The contractions of the heart result in a pulsating flow of blood into the arteries. The pressure is highest when the ventricles of the heart contract and eject blood into the aorta and pulmonary arteries. The blood pressure measured during ventricular contraction (cardiac systole) is the **systolic blood pressure**. During ventricular relaxation (cardiac diastole), blood pressure is due to elastic recoil of the vessels, and the measured pressure is the **diastolic blood pressure**. The mathematical difference between the measured systolic and diastolic blood pressures is the **pulse pressure**. For example, a systolic pressure of 120 mm Hg and a diastolic pressure of 80 mm Hg result in a pulse pressure of 40 mm Hg.

Blood pressure is a function of the flow of blood produced by contraction of the heart and the resistance to blood flow through the vessels. The pressure, flow, and resistance relationship is described mathematically as pressure equals flow multiplied by resistance ($P = F \times R$).

BLOOD FLOW

Blood flow is essentially equal to cardiac output. Cardiac output is the product of **stroke volume** (the amount of blood each ventricle pumps with each heartbeat) and heart rate. A stroke volume of 70 mL and a heart rate of 72 beats per minute result in a cardiac output of 5,040 mL per minute, or about 5 L per minute. Average cardiac output in a resting man is 5.5 L per minute.

Poor cardiac pumping (as occurs with a failing heart) or reduced blood volume (as in severe hemorrhage) may reduce stroke volume, which in turn decreases cardiac output. Bradycardia also may cause decreased cardiac output. Conversely, a rapid heart rate and larger stroke volumes would be expected to increase cardiac output.

The magnitude of output change created by increases or decreases in one factor (either heart rate or stroke volume) is influenced by the other factor's concurrent response. An increase in heart rate in response to a decrease in stroke volume to maintain a normal cardiac output is an example of a compensatory response. If compensation does not occur or is incomplete, cardiac output will decrease, and the blood pressure will be lower.

RESISTANCE

Friction among the cells and other blood components and between the blood and the vessel walls causes blood flow resistance. The friction within the blood components reflects the blood's viscosity and is largely due to the number and shape of the blood cells. Normally, the number and type of blood constituents do not vary greatly, and viscosity is a constant factor.

Friction between the blood and the vessel walls varies with the dimensions of the vessel lumen. Contraction and relaxation of the smooth muscle in the vessel walls control the diameter of the blood vessel. The autonomic nervous system regulates this vascular tone. Constricted vessels offer greater resistance, thus increasing blood pressure; dilated vessels offer less resistance, thus decreasing blood pressure.

Factors Affecting Blood Pressure

Major factors affecting blood pressure include age, the autonomic nervous system, circulating volume, medications, and normal fluctuations.

AGE

Blood pressure gradually increases throughout childhood and correlates with height, weight, and age. These normal changes make it difficult to identify abnormal blood pressure levels for children at various developmental stages. The National Institutes of Health (NIH) states that children and adolescents with blood pressure levels of 120/80 mm Hg or above but less than the 95th percentile are considered to have **prehypertension**. Blood pressure consistently above the 95th percentile for age indicates a need for diagnostic evaluation (NIH, 2005).

In adults, systolic and diastolic blood pressure increase gradually as age advances. In part, this trend is due to increased systemic vascular resistance, reflecting arterial narrowing and decreased vessel elasticity due to atherosclerotic vessel disease. The increase in systolic blood pressure is proportionally greater than the increase in diastolic blood pressure; therefore, pulse pressure widens. Table 18-1 shows normal blood pressures for various age groups.

AUTONOMIC NERVOUS SYSTEM

The autonomic nervous system influences heart rate, cardiac contractility, systemic vascular resistance, and blood volume. Increased sympathetic nervous system activity results in increased heart rate, stronger contraction of heart muscle, changes in vascular smooth muscle tone, and increased blood volume due to retention of water and sodium. The cumulative effect is increased blood pressure. Therefore, factors that enhance sympathetic nervous system activity (such as pain, anxiety, fear, smoking, and exercise) result in elevated blood pressure readings.

Exceptions occur when sympathetic nervous activity cannot keep up with a stressor. An example is a patient with severely diminished blood volume resulting from hemorrhage. The sympathetic nervous system is activated to maintain adequate blood pressure, but it may not be enough to compensate for the volume loss. Measured blood pressure may be quite low, although sympathetic nervous system activity is increased markedly.

CIRCULATING VOLUME

A decrease in circulating volume, either from blood or fluid loss, results in lower blood pressure. Fluid volume deficit can occur with abnormal, unreplaced losses such as diarrhea or diaphoresis. Insufficient oral intake also can cause fluid volume deficit. Excess fluid, such as in congestive heart failure or renal failure, can cause elevated blood pressure readings.

MEDICATIONS

Any medication that alters one or more of the previously described determining factors may cause a change in blood pressure. Examples are diuretics, which decrease blood volume; cardiac medications, which affect the heart's rate or contractile force; opioid analgesics, which reduce pain and sympathetic nervous system activity; and specific antihypertensive agents.

NORMAL FLUCTUATIONS

Blood pressure fluctuates from minute to minute in response to various stimuli. Increased ambient temperature causes blood vessels near the skin surface to dilate, decreasing resistance and blood pressure. Blood pressure also fluctuates with the respiratory cycle, increasing during expiration and decreasing during inspiration.

In addition to these fluctuations, there is a discernible circadian pattern to blood pressure. Investigators have documented a consistent variation in blood pressure throughout the day, with blood pressures at their highest in the morning.

Assessing Blood Pressure

Blood pressure may be measured directly with a catheter placed into an artery. Direct measurement provides a continuous reading of blood pressure and is used in critical care settings. More commonly, blood pressure is measured by indirect methods, using an inflatable cuff to temporarily occlude arterial blood flow through one of the limbs. As the cuff is deflated and flow returns, the blood pressure is determined by palpation, auscultation, or oscillations. Table 18-5 summarizes potential sources of error in blood pressure measurement. **Procedure 18-4** provides detailed instructions for measuring blood pressure.

SITES

Blood pressure can be measured in either the upper or lower extremity. For accurate data interpretation, note the site of blood pressure measurement.

Upper Extremity

The blood pressure is usually measured in the upper arm. Wrap a cuff around the upper part of the limb and auscultate or palpate blood flow at the brachial artery. Blood pressure also may

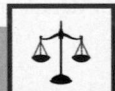

ETHICAL/LEGAL ISSUE

DELEGATING VITAL SIGNS

You are working on a busy day surgery center. You delegate to a nursing assistant every-5-minute vital sign assessments for a postoperative patient. The nursing assistant is using an automated monitor to obtain blood pressure and pulse readings every 5 minutes. The vital signs she records on the patient's record appear stable.

When the patient has been back from the operating room about 30 minutes, you notice that her hand (distal to the automated cuff) is purple. You quickly release the cuff, but color does not return to the patient's hand.

CRITICAL THINKING CHALLENGE

- If the patient sustains permanent injury due to the malfunction of the automated monitoring system, who might be considered negligent (the hospital, nursing assistant, the registered nurse [RN], the doctor, the manufacturing company)?
- What factors make this patient especially vulnerable?
- What could be done to prevent similar situations from occurring?

be determined by auscultation or palpation of the radial artery in the wrist with an appropriately sized cuff applied to the forearm. Blood pressure readings will differ when measured in the upper and lower arm, so it is important to note the site of blood pressure measurement.

⚠ SAFETY ALERT

Do not measure blood pressure in any arm with a venous access device, especially an internal arteriovenous fistula, a peripheral vascular access for hemodialysis, or a PICC line. Also, if the patient has had a mastectomy, blood pressure monitoring on the same side can further impede circulation, contributing to lymphedema, and so should be avoided.

Lower Extremity

The blood pressure can be measured in the lower extremity if the patient has arteries in the upper extremity that cannot be palpated, if the upper extremity is covered by dressings or splints, if the patient has a vascular access device, or if the patient has had a mastectomy. Wrap the cuff around the thigh or above the ankle.

Thigh pressure measurement requires a larger, appropriately sized cuff. Place the patient in a flat, supine position with the

cuff centered midthigh over the popliteal artery. Auscultate or palpate blood flow at the popliteal fossa. When an appropriately sized cuff is used, blood pressure measurements should vary only slightly from readings measured in the upper extremity (unless the patient has peripheral vascular disease). Using a cuff that is too small will result in falsely high readings.

Sometimes, ankle blood pressure measurements are taken to calculate an ankle-brachial index (ABI) to determine if it is safe to use compression therapy for venous ulcers. To measure blood pressure in the ankle, place the patient in a flat, supine position, and place a standard arm cuff just above the malleolus. Auscultate or palpate the posterior tibialis or dorsalis pedis pulse as you deflate the cuff. A lower blood pressure in the lower extremity than in the upper arm may indicate poor arterial circulation to the leg.

EQUIPMENT

There are several different pieces of equipment that can be used to measure blood pressure: the sphygmomanometer, stethoscope, Doppler ultrasound, and automated devices.

Sphygmomanometer

A sphygmomanometer consists of an inflatable bladder enclosed in a nondistensible cuff. The bladder is connected to an inflating mechanism such as a bulb or pump, a valve for

TABLE 18-5 POTENTIAL ERRORS IN BLOOD PRESSURE MEASUREMENT

Error	Cause	Recommendation
Falsely low readings	Environmental noise	Turn down television or radio; stop talking; avoid moving stethoscope or tubing; position earpieces snugly in ear canal.
	Hearing deficit	Use hearing-amplified stethoscope or hearing aid.
	Earpieces fitting poorly	Angle ear pieces forward to fit snugly into ear canal.
	Stethoscope tubing too long	Shorten tubing to 30–38 cm (12–15 in).
	Failing to pump cuff up high enough	Palpate systolic pressure to avoid missing auscultatory gap.
	Cuff too large	Measure arm circumference: Bladder width should be 40% to 50% and length should be 80% to 100% of arm circumference.
	Arm above heart level	Reposition arm at level of heart, generally the fourth intercostal space.
	Releasing valve too rapidly	Practice slow release of 2–3 mm Hg/s.
	Reading taken at inspiration (in selected high-risk patients, COPD, pulmonary embolism, hypovolemic shock)	Consistently try to record BP at end expiration.
Falsely high readings	Measuring BP when a patient has just eaten, is in pain, is anxious, or has a full bladder	Try to assess BP during basal state, or adjust interpretation accordingly.
	Cold hands or stethoscope	Warm hands and stethoscope before measuring BP.
	Viewing meniscus from below eye level	View meniscus from eye level.
	Cuff too small	Bladder width should be 40% to 50% and length should be 80% to 100% of arm circumference.
	Wrapping cuff unevenly or loosely	Rewrap cuff snugly.
	Deflating cuff too slowly	Practice steady deflation of cuff at 2–3 mm Hg/s.
	Venous congestion	Wait 2 min before reinflating cuff to retake BP; elevate arm to promote redistribution of blood.
	Unsupported arm	Support arm on table to prevent muscle contraction.
	Back unsupported, legs dangling	Provide support for legs and back.
	Arm below heart level	Reposition arm at heart level, usually at the fourth intercostal space.
Inaccurate readings	Needle not at zero	Recalibrate or service equipment.
	Faulty valves or leaky tubing	Replace equipment.
	Examiner digit preference	Do not round up or down.
	Forgetting measurement	Record immediately in the room.

COPD, chronic obstructive pulmonary disease; BP, blood pressure.

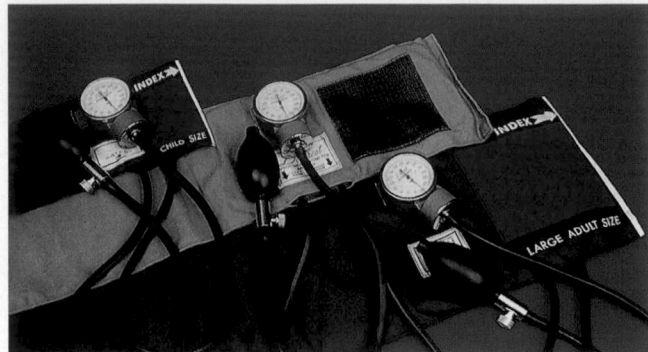

FIGURE 18-7 Three cuff sizes: a small cuff for a child or a small or frail adult; a normal-sized cuff; and a large cuff, called a leg cuff, for measuring blood pressure on a leg, or for use on an obese adult.

deflation, and a manometer (Fig. 18-7). The manometer may be an aneroid or gravity mercury type. The gravity mercury type has been the standard for clinical blood pressure measurement but has been phased out in most healthcare settings because of environmental concerns.

Aneroid manometers have a circular gauge marked in 2-mm increments. The pressure transmitted from the cuff causes movement of a metal bellows within the manometer, a movement indicated by a needle on the gauge. Aneroid manometers require at least yearly calibration with a properly functioning mercury manometer or other pressure standard. These routine checks of manometer function should be made throughout the range of pressure measurement to ensure the device's accuracy. Aneroid manometers with a stop peg at the zero point or an external reset are not recommended because verifying the accuracy of the manometer is impossible.

The tubing and hand bulb in all sphygmomanometers must be free from cracks or holes, and connections must be airtight to prevent leaks that cause poor transmission of pressure and consequently inaccurate readings. To allow the operator to control the rate of deflation, the deflation valve must function smoothly.

Stethoscope

A stethoscope is necessary for the auscultatory method of blood pressure measurement. The stethoscope should have snugly fitting earpieces and thick-walled tubing about 12 inches (30 cm) long for optimal sound transmission. The stethoscope should be equipped with a bell and a diaphragm.

Doppler Ultrasound

The Doppler method is useful during low-flow states or when the blood pressure is difficult to auscultate by stethoscope. A standard cuff is used to occlude an artery while the ultrasound transducer is placed over the artery distal to the site of occlusion. Systolic blood pressure is the point at which continuous pulsatile flow is heard. Diastolic blood pressure is not identified with a Doppler, and the blood pressure may be recorded as the systolic number over "D" for Doppler, for example, 120/D.

Automated Devices

Automated oscillometric blood pressure devices are frequently used to monitor blood pressure in hospital and ambulatory settings and for home monitoring. The electronic units determine blood pressure by analyzing the sounds of blood flow or measuring oscillations. Although automated blood pressure measurement is easier than manual measurement, allows for frequent reassessment, and can provide printouts or a digital record, it is more likely to provide false readings. Very irregular heart rates or excessive movement from shivering, transporting the patient, or the use of a rapid-cycling ventilator can interfere with blood pressure readings. Treatment should not be based on an isolated automated blood pressure reading, and if there is any question about the accuracy of the reading, the blood pressure should be taken manually.

Systolic, diastolic, and mean arterial blood pressure and heart rate are displayed on the monitor (Fig. 18-8). The machine can be set to record these values automatically at a preset interval (e.g., every 15 minutes). The data obtained are stored in the machine and can be retrieved easily as needed. Although electronic devices are appropriate for monitoring blood pressure, diagnosis of hypertension requires measurement of blood pressure using auscultation with a sphygmomanometer.

! SAFETY ALERT

When using automatic blood pressure devices for serial blood pressure recording, check the cuffed limb frequently to ensure adequate arterial perfusion and venous drainage between measurements.

METHODS

Ideally, measure baseline blood pressure with the patient in a resting state, after he or she has been sitting quietly for 5 minutes or more. The patient should be in a warm, quiet environment

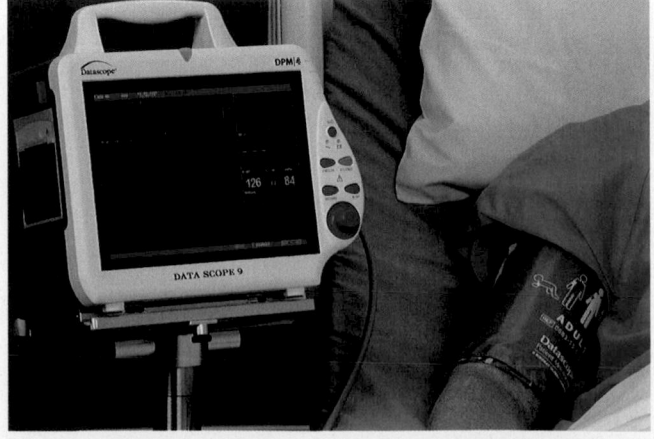

FIGURE 18-8 The automatic blood pressure monitor reports systolic, diastolic, mean blood pressure, heart rate. (Photo by B. Proud.)

with the back supported and feet flat on the floor, if sitting. Blood pressure increases when legs are crossed at the knee. At least 30 minutes should elapse between smoking, exercising, or eating and measuring blood pressure. Sometimes, blood pressure must be measured when the patient is anxious or in pain, but these readings may differ from those made if the patient were in a basal state.

Proper Cuff Size

The American Heart Association has made specific recommendations about cuff size and application (Table 18-6). Using an inappropriately sized cuff or incorrect cuff placement may lead to an erroneous reading. Base cuff size on the circumference of the limb that you are using. The width of the cuff bladder should be at least 40% of the circumference of the midpoint of the limb. An average adult arm requires a bladder with a 12- to 14-cm width, although mean arm circumferences (including those for children and adolescents) are increasing in the US population as the incidence of obesity increases. The bladder length should be 80% to 100% of the limb circumference, or approximately twice the bladder width.

Apply the cuff snugly around the limb, and center the bladder over the artery. Using a cuff that is too small or loosely applied results in falsely high readings. Using a cuff that is too large results in falsely low readings (Fig. 18-9).

Proper Positioning

Measure blood pressure with the arm at heart level. Elevating the arm above heart level results in a falsely low measurement; positioning the arm below heart level results in a falsely high

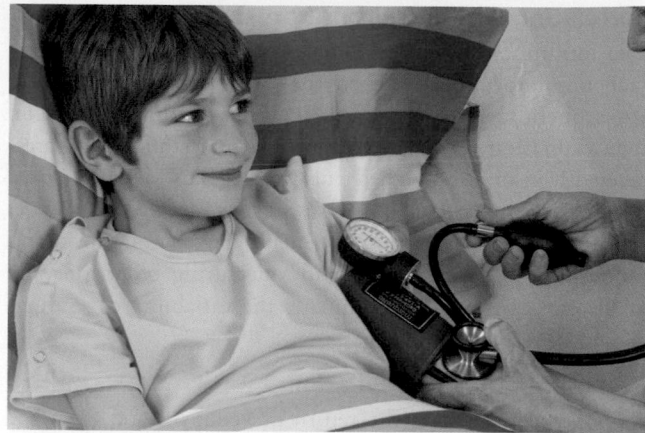

FIGURE 18-9 It is especially important to use a proper-sized cuff and bladder when measuring blood pressure in a child.

reading. If the patient is sitting or standing, support the forearm horizontally at the level of the heart (generally considered the level of the fourth intercostal space, where the ribs join the sternum). Failure to support the arm causes the patient to contract the arm muscles, elevating the blood pressure. When the patient is supine, the arm may need to be elevated to heart level on a pillow.

APPLY YOUR CRITICAL THINKING

Ms. George arrives at the clinic for a blood pressure check and an infusion of intravenous medications. She appears red in the face and states she hurried over during her lunch hour. Observe the medical assistant taking Ms. George's blood pressure in the accompanying photograph. Identify factors that might result in an inaccurate reading if the assistant uses this technique. It might be helpful to refer to Table 18-5.

Check your answer in Appendix B.

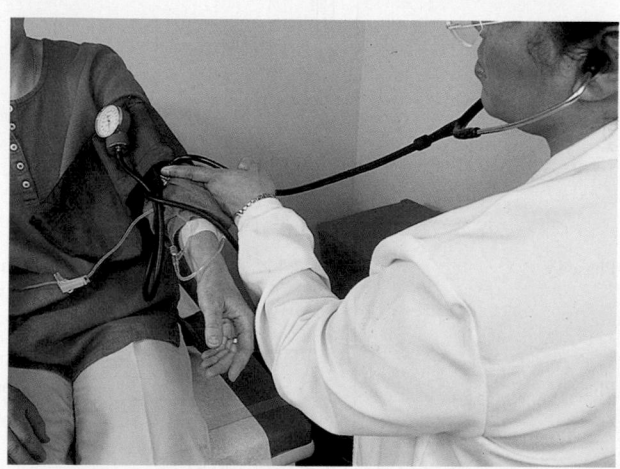

Cuff	Bladder Width (cm)	Bladder Length (cm)	Arm Circumference Range at Midpoint (cm)
Newborn	3	6	≤6
Infant	5	15	6–15[†]
Child	8	21	16–21[†]
Small adult	10	24	22–26
Adult	13	30	27–34
Large adult	16	38	35–44
Adult thigh	20	42	45–52

TABLE 18-6 ACCEPTABLE BLADDER DIMENSIONS (IN CENTIMETERS) FOR ARMS OF DIFFERENT SIZES*

*Here is some overlapping of the recommended range for arm circumferences in order to limit the number of cuffs; it is recommended that the larger cuff be used when available.
†To approximate the bladder width to arm circumference ratio of 0.40 more closely in infants and children, additional cuffs are available.
Source: Pickering T, et al. (2005). Blood pressure measurement in humans: A statement for professionals from the Subcommittee of Professional and Public Education of the American Heart Association Council on High Blood Pressure Research. *Hypertension*, 45, 142–161.

Correlation With the Respiratory Cycle

The intrathoracic pressure changes that occur during a normal respiratory cycle affect the heart and great vessels. Consequently, blood pressure is lower during inspiration than expiration. Exaggerated decreases in systolic blood pressure with inspiration (called pulsus paradoxus or **paradoxical blood pressure**) occur in diseases such as cardiac tamponade, constrictive pericarditis, emphysema, hypovolemic shock, and pulmonary embolus. Consistently measuring blood pressure at the end of expiration eliminates the variability of readings caused by respiratory changes.

Proper Inflation and Deflation

An inflated cuff slows the return of venous blood from the extremity back to the heart. Increased venous pressures are transmitted back to the arterial side of the circuit, which leads to a corresponding rise in arterial pressures. Slow, prolonged, or frequent cuff inflation promotes venous congestion. Inflate the cuff rapidly when taking a reading and deflate it completely after measurement. At least 1 to 2 minutes should elapse before sequential cuff inflation on any one limb. Elevating the arm above the head between cuff measurements speeds venous return to the heart.

Auscultation

When determining the blood pressure by the auscultatory method, use an inflatable cuff to temporarily occlude blood flow through a limb. As you deflate the cuff and blood flow returns, the **Korotkoff sounds** can be heard with a stethoscope placed over the artery. Five distinct phases are identifiable, as shown in Table 18-7. The onset of phase I Korotkoff sounds is the recorded systolic pressure. Diastolic pressure is indicated by the onset of phase V sounds in adults. In children, the definition of diastolic pressure is controversial, with some using phase IV Korotkoff sounds as the indicator and some using phase V (absence of sound). Documentation of all three phases may be used—for example, 120/72/66.

Because the Korotkoff sounds are low in frequency, the bell of the stethoscope is best used for auscultation, although most practitioners use the diaphragm because of its larger shape and ease of placement. If the sounds are inaudible with the diaphragm, try the stethoscope bell. Do not press the head of the stethoscope too firmly against the skin; doing so may partially occlude blood flow and alter the reading.

An **auscultatory gap** is the absence of Korotkoff sounds between phases I and II. Failure to identify an auscultatory gap may result in underestimation of the systolic blood pressure or overestimation of the diastolic pressure. Find the auscultatory gap by palpating the brachial or radial pulse while inflating the cuff. Inflate the cuff about 30 mm Hg above the number where palpable pulsation disappears. In addition to detecting an auscultatory gap, palpation gives an initial estimate of systolic blood pressure and eliminates the need to inflate the cuff to extremely high pressures in people with normal or low blood pressure. When you detect an auscultatory gap, record

TABLE 18-7 KOROTKOFF SOUNDS

Phase	Interpretation	Description	Recording
Phase I	← 120 Systolic	Initiated by the onset of faint, clear tapping sounds of gradually increasing intensity	Recorded as systolic pressure
Phase II	← 110	Sound has a swishing quality.	
Phase III	← 100	Marked by crisper, more intense sounds; clear intense tapping	
Phase IV	← 90 First diastolic	Characterized by muffled, blowing sounds	Often recorded as diastolic pressure in children
Phase V	← 80 Second diastolic	Absence of sound	Recorded as diastolic pressure in adults; may be recorded as diastolic in children

BP=120/90/80

the systolic and diastolic pressures as usual, and note the magnitude and range of the auscultatory gap (e.g., 196/90; auscultatory gap from 184 to 150).

Palpation

When Korotkoff sounds are inaudible, blood pressure may be estimated by palpation. Apply the cuff, inflate as previously described, and palpate the brachial or radial artery during cuff deflation. Systolic blood pressure is the point at which pulsation returns. Diastolic blood pressure is difficult to determine reliably with palpation but is indicated by a snap or whipping palpable vibrations. Palpated blood pressure is usually recorded as a systolic reading over "P" (for *palpated*, e.g., 110/P).

ABNORMALITIES

Hypertension, hypotension, and orthostatic hypotension are three abnormalities of blood pressure.

Hypertension

Hypertension is the condition in which blood pressure is chronically elevated. Although in industrialized societies there is a trend toward increased blood pressure with advancing age, hypertension is a dangerous disease associated with an increased risk of morbidity and mortality due to cardiovascular complications, such as stroke or heart failure. Therefore, chronically elevated blood pressure is treated aggressively in adults of any age. Adults with blood pressure above 140/90 mm Hg should be evaluated for hypertension. Those 60 and older should be treated to a goal blood pressure of less than 150/90. Individuals aged 30 to 59 should be treated to a goal diastolic blood pressure of less than 90 (James et al., 2014). Hypertension is diagnosed on the basis of serial elevated values rather than a single measurement. Studies have shown that some patients demonstrate higher recorded blood pressure in the physician's office than in the home setting. This is referred to as the "white coat effect." Ambulatory blood pressure measurements refer to blood pressure values obtained away from the clinical setting while the person is engaged in normal activity. Ambulatory blood pressure measurements are helpful in diagnosing hypertension accurately and in planning treatment. Chapter 27 covers hypertension in greater detail.

Hypotension

Hypotension is blood pressure below 100/60 mm Hg. Low blood pressure readings can be normal for some healthy, young adults and are no cause for concern. Even in older individuals, a low reading without symptoms may not be significant. A sudden drop in blood pressure, significantly below the normal range for a person, causes hypotension. For example, a hypertensive patient who usually has blood pressure readings of 180/94 mm Hg would be considered hypotensive if his or her blood pressure fell to 120/80 mm Hg. Once again, a significant change from baseline values is more important than any one specific measurement.

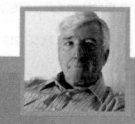

Vital Signs PICO

The woman from the opening scenario comes back to you. She tells you that her husband hates going to see doctors. She's heard about supplements that help prevent heart disease. She pulls out a small piece of paper from her bag and shows it to you. It reads, "CoQ10." The woman asks you, "Do you think this will help prevent heart problems for my husband?" You open up the Cochrane Library on your smartphone to look for evidence. The PICO statement you use is, *"In adults, how does Coenzyme Q10 supplements compare to no therapy to prevent heart disease?"*

P = Adults
I = Coenzyme Q10 supplements (CoQ10)
C = no therapy
O = prevent heart disease

You find a systematic review that analyzed six randomized controlled trials with 218 participants. Two of the studies reviewed patients who were taking only the supplements. The other four studies compared the CoQ10 with patients who were on statin drugs. The review did not show strong evidence that CoQ10 supplements alone were beneficial for blood pressure, high-density lipoprotein, or triglycerides. The participants using statin meds and CoQ10 also did not show statistical evidence of improvement of their blood pressure or lipid levels. The reviewer concluded that there are more studies in progress that might shed light on the beneficial use of CoQ10. The current information was based on only a few short-term studies.

You share the findings with the woman and encourage her to talk to her husband about visiting his primary care provider.

REFERENCE:

Flowers, N., Hartley, L., Todkill, D., Stranges, S., & Rees K. (2014). Co-enzyme Q10 supplementation for the primary prevention of cardiovascular disease. *Cochrane Database of Systematic Reviews*, (12), CD010405. doi: 10.1002/14651858.CD010405.pub2

Orthostatic Hypotension

In adults, moving from a flat, horizontal position to a vertical position results in pooling of blood in the lower extremities. People with healthy, intact autonomic nervous systems reflexively compensate for the volume shift by increasing the rate and force of myocardial contraction and by vasoconstriction, thus maintaining adequate blood pressure. Even with normal compensation, however, a position change usually results in a drop in systolic blood pressure and an increase in heart rate, but these changes are temporary.

Inadequate reflex compensation upon position change results in **orthostatic or postural hypotension**. Symptoms of orthostatic hypotension are those related to decreased cerebral perfusion, such as dizziness, weakness, blurred vision, syncope, and marked changes in blood pressure and heart rate. Orthostatic blood pressure changes may indicate hypovolemia or a failure of the autonomic nervous system protective reflexes. Hypovolemia or impaired vasoconstriction is signaled by decreased blood pressure and increased heart rate. Autonomic nervous system dysfunction is indicated by decreased blood pressure without marked increases in heart rate. Orthostatic hypotension is a drop in systolic pressure of at least 20 mm Hg or a drop in diastolic pressure of at least 10 mm Hg, accompanied by an increase in heart rate of at least 10 beats per minute when moving from lying to sitting or standing.

> ! **SAFETY ALERT**
> The person experiencing orthostatic hypotension is at risk for falling. Therefore, checking postural vital signs is one way of screening to ensure patient safety.

Instruct patients with chronic orthostatic hypotension to change positions slowly, allowing several minutes to elapse between positions when moving from lying to sitting to standing.

Measure orthostatic blood pressure in patients exhibiting symptoms of dizziness, blurred vision, or weakness when changing position; patients taking diuretic medications; and patients with a history of volume loss. The best data for determining and monitoring therapy will come from systematic, consistent technique in assessing blood pressure and heart rate response to position change. **Procedure 18-5** gives a step-by-step description for assessing orthostatic hypotension.

Patients experiencing severe orthostatic hypotension may be unable to tolerate a standing position long enough for you to obtain the blood pressure and heart rate.

> ! **SAFETY ALERT**
> If the patient becomes severely symptomatic while standing, he or she should be assisted back to bed without completing the measurements.

Record the blood pressure and heart rate values and the position of the patient when the values were obtained. Document any symptoms of diminished cerebral perfusion.

DOCUMENTING VITAL SIGNS

Nurses are responsible for ensuring accurate assessment and documentation of vital signs. Frequently, they delegate vital sign monitoring to UAPs. It is essential to provide health team members with clear guidelines so that abnormal readings can be reported promptly. Some vital sign measuring equipment may link directly to the electronic health record (EHR) for automatic documentation when vital signs are taken. After assessing trends, report abnormal findings to the provider. Data entered into an EHR may be viewed in a graph format that allows trends to be seen easily. Trends may reflect normal variations or a change in response to disease or therapy. For example, the normal trend is toward a decreased body temperature in the early morning. If the graph shows increasing values during the night and early morning, this trend may indicate fever and would require further investigation. Increasing pulse rate, with or without a drop in blood pressure or rise in temperature, may indicate infection.

LIFE SPAN CONSIDERATIONS

Knowledge of developmental considerations is important for accurate measurement and interpretation of vital signs. Table 18-1 summarizes normal ranges for the vital signs across the life span.

Newborn and Infant

Temperature, pulse, and respirations fluctuate widely in newborns. Their thermoregulatory mechanisms are immature, and ambient temperature may affect body temperature of the newborn markedly. Pulse and respiration increase rapidly above resting values when a newborn is active, crying, or startled. The apical pulse is the most reliable method of assessing heart rate because peripheral pulses are faint and difficult to palpate and accurately count. Healthy newborns may exhibit periodic apnea. Blood pressure is not assessed routinely in the healthy newborn or infant because the information obtained is unreliable. Conditions in which children younger than 3 years should have blood pressure measured include prematurity, very low birth weight, congenital heart disease, recurrent bladder infections, and kidney disease.

Safety considerations are important when monitoring the vital signs of newborns and infants. Temporal artery, tympanic, or axillary temperature monitoring is preferred because rectal temperature monitoring can cause mucosal tearing or perforation, and infants cannot safely hold oral thermometers in their mouths. Regular-sized tympanic probes may be too large for the ear canals of premature infants or infants younger than 2 months. Infants move quickly, so protecting them from falling or injury during vital sign monitoring is essential.

Toddler and Preschooler

As a child enters the 2nd year of life, vital signs fluctuate less. The pulse rate decreases to a normal range of 80 to 120 beats per minute, and respirations fall to 22 to 40 breaths per minute. Normal blood pressure ranges from a systolic

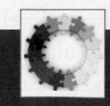

COLLABORATING WITH THE HEALTHCARE TEAM
Calling the Physician Concerning Change in Vital Signs

You are working evenings on a surgical unit and caring for Mrs. Cho, a 70-year-old widow who had a colon resection this morning. You call the physician to report a change in vital signs.

SITUATION: I am calling about Mrs. Cho in room 257, who had a colon resection this morning, to report a change in her condition. Are you covering for Dr. Moran?

BACKGROUND: Her current vital signs are temp 37.4, B/P 100/60, p 98, and r 20. Preoperatively, her vital signs were temp 37, B/P 128/80, p 80, and r 16. She has not voided since surgery. Her dressing is dry, and her pain is well controlled. We have no labs since surgery.

ASSESSMENT: I am concerned about Mrs. Cho's hypotension, increased heart rate, and inability to void since surgery.

RECOMMENDATION: Could you provide an order to catheterize Mrs. Cho so that we can see if she is producing adequate amounts of urine? Would you also like to get a Hct to rule out postoperative bleeding? There were no parameters for vital signs, so it would be helpful if you would provide guidelines for when nursing should call you. I would feel most comfortable if you would come to assess this patient.

CRITICAL THINKING CHALLENGE

- Reflect on data to collect prior to calling a physician to report a change in vital signs. What additional data could this nurse have presented to the physician?
- How do you decide when it is important to notify a physician concerning a change in a patient's vital signs? Are the criteria you use different for different patients?
- How can you work with nursing assistants to ensure that vital signs are monitored and documented appropriately and you are kept informed?
- Would the information you provide be different if you are reporting to the attending surgeon or a physician who is covering for the primary doctor?

---

pressure of 80 to 112 mm Hg over a diastolic pressure of 50 to 80 mm Hg. Blood pressure is monitored routinely after the age of 3 years, using an appropriately sized cuff.

Toddlers and preschoolers may become fearful of procedures involving vital sign measurement. At this age, verbal explanations do little to allay fears. Permitting children to play with stethoscopes or push the buttons on electronic thermometers may help calm their fears. Having parents or other caregivers hold and talk to frightened children can be comforting.

Safety concerns continue to be important. Monitor temperature using the tympanic, temporal artery, or axillary route until the child is 4 or 5 years old and can follow directions about holding the thermometer in the sublingual pocket.

School-Age Child and Adolescent

The broad range of normal values for children reflects the wide variability in their vital signs. In general, temperature, pulse, and respirations gradually decrease through childhood, but blood pressure increases and correlates with height and weight.

Children in this age group are familiar with vital sign assessment and seldom exhibit fear during monitoring. Health teaching about normal values and the reason for taking vital

signs helps to educate them. A child may try to experiment by putting the thermometer under hot water or near a light source, so validate any unlikely temperature readings.

Adult and Older Adult

Vital signs are usually stable during young adulthood. As adults age, the effects of lifestyle and chronic diseases become evident in the vital signs. Chronic respiratory disease and exposure to pollutants, such as cigarette smoke, can influence respiratory rate and pattern. Cardiovascular diseases may cause changes in the heart rate and rhythm. The incidence of hypertension is increasing in the United States. The American Heart Association estimates that about one in three adult Americans has high blood pressure. By 2030, that number will rise to an estimated 44% (American Heart Association, 2014). Conversely, orthostatic hypotension is common in older adults, although the actual incidence is unclear. It is uncertain whether orthostatic hypotension is a result of normal aging or related to existing disease states. Older adults also have lower normal ranges for body temperature.

Adults often ask nurses about the values obtained during monitoring. This discussion is an excellent opportunity for patient education.

KEY CONCEPTS

■ Temperature, pulse, respirations, and blood pressure are considered the vital signs because significant deviations from normal ranges are not compatible with life.

■ Vital sign assessment is an important nursing function that permits the nurse to detect alterations from normal and evaluate the patient's progress.

■ Body temperature can be monitored in five sites: the mouth, rectum, ear, forehead, and axilla.

■ Factors that can affect body temperature include age, environmental conditions, time of day, exercise, stress, and hormone levels.

■ Equipment to monitor body temperature includes electronic thermometers, tympanic membrane thermometers, temporal artery thermometers, noncontact infrared thermometers, and chemically treated paper thermometers. Glass mercury thermometers are no longer used.

■ As the heart contracts and ejects blood into the circulation, pulsations can be palpated at various arterial sites in the body.

■ Evaluation of the pulse should include rate, rhythm, and quality.

■ Factors such as age, autonomic nervous system stimulation, and medications can affect the pulse.

■ An irregular pulse should be counted for 1 full minute, preferably at the apical site.

■ A pulse deficit occurs when a cardiac contraction creates a pulse wave that is weak and not palpable at peripheral sites.

■ Age, medications, stress, exercise, altitude, gender, body position, and fever can influence respiratory rate, rhythm, and depth.

■ Abnormal breathing rates include tachypnea (more than 20 breaths per minute), bradypnea (less than 12 breaths per minute), and apnea (interval of absent respirations).

■ Abnormal breathing patterns include Biot respirations, Kussmaul respirations, and Cheyne–Stokes respirations.

■ Blood pressure is a function of the flow of blood produced by the heart and the resistance to blood flow through the vessels.

■ Systolic pressure occurs during ventricular contraction, and diastolic pressure occurs during ventricular relaxation. Pulse pressure is the difference between systolic and diastolic pressure.

■ Factors that can affect blood pressure include age, autonomic nervous system input, circulating volume, medications, and circadian rhythms.

■ Blood pressure is usually measured indirectly using a sphygmomanometer and a stethoscope.

■ Auscultation of blood pressure reveals five different phases known as Korotkoff sounds. The first Korotkoff sound corresponds to systolic pressure and the fifth (fourth in children) to diastolic pressure.

■ Selecting proper cuff size, keeping the arm at heart level, avoiding venous congestion, and detecting an auscultatory gap are important steps in obtaining accurate blood pressure readings.

■ Orthostatic hypotension occurs when a person experiences a decrease in blood pressure when changing from a supine to an upright position.

■ Normal variations in vital signs occur throughout the life span.

PRACTICING FOR THE NCLEX

CHECK YOUR ANSWERS IN APPENDIX A.

1. A nurse obtains an oral temperature of 35.9°C on a 70-year-old woman before morning change of shift (05:00). Which is/are possible explanations for this reading? Select all that apply:
   a. Elderly adults may have a lower baseline temperature reading related to age
   b. Stress of hospitalization
   c. Postmenopausal state
   d. Time of day

2. A nurse needs to check an ill infant's temperature at the pediatrician's office. Which site would be most appropriate for this age?
   a. Ear
   b. Rectum
   c. Temporal artery/forehead
   d. Mouth

3. A nursing student is checking an apical pulse on a patient who has just returned from surgery. Which of the following is an important element of this procedure?
   a. Place the diaphragm of the stethoscope at the third intercostal space at the midclavicular line.
   b. Count the pulse for 60 seconds.
   c. Count the first audible pulsation as "one."
   d. Count S_1 and S_2 sounds separately.

4. A patient has just returned from surgery, and upon taking his vital signs, the nurse assesses a respiratory rate of 10 breaths per minute. Which factor is most likely the cause of this patient's decreased respiratory rate?
   a. Male gender
   b. Opioid medication use
   c. Stress
   d. Pain

5. A child is exhibiting marked trouble breathing and complains of feeling short of breath. A high-pitched musical sound is heard on inspiration and expiration. How would the nurse best classify this dyspnea?
   a. Stridor
   b. Unlabored
   c. Exertional dyspnea
   d. Wheezing

6. A nurse needs to take the blood pressure of a new patient admitted to the unit. The patient has an arteriovenous fistula in her left lower arm and a right-sided mastectomy. Which is the best site and proper technique to measure blood pressure on this patient?
   a. Left upper arm, standard cuff size, auscultate brachial artery
   b. Left thigh, appropriate-sized cuff, supine patient position
   c. Left ankle, standard cuff size, auscultate dorsalis pedis
   d. Right lower arm, appropriate-sized cuff, auscultate radial artery

7. A patient is postoperative day 1 following prostatectomy surgery. He complains of dizziness on standing and when checked is found to have a lying blood pressure of 116/84 with a heart rate of 88 and a standing blood pressure of 98/76 with a heart rate of 110. Which advice would be appropriate for this patient with orthostatic hypotension? Select all that apply:
   a. "You are at risk for falling related to your low fluid volume and low blood pressure."
   b. "You should change positions slowly to prevent dizziness and falls."
   c. "Please call for assistance when you are ready to get out of bed."
   d. "Ambulate more frequently to help you feel steadier on your feet."

8. A nurse is about to assess a patient's blood pressure while the patient is out of bed in the chair. Which of the following should be considered in relation to patient position?
   a. The patient's arm should rest on the arm of the chair.
   b. The patient should hold the arm even with the fourth intercostal space.
   c. Blood pressure should not be taken while the patient is upright.
   d. The nurse should support the arm even with the fourth intercostal space.

9. A nurse is checking the radial pulse rate of a patient with renal disease. Which of the following should he do first?
   a. Position the patient with the forearm at the side with the wrist extended.
   b. Apply gel to the end of the Doppler probe or radial site, if not easily palpable.
   c. Count for 30 seconds and multiply by two if the pulse is regular.
   d. Place the fingertips of your first two fingers in the groove at the base of the thumb.

10. A nurse is checking the respiratory rate of a toddler, previously admitted with asthma. The child is crying and upset by the hospital and the process of taking her vital signs. What should the nurse do?
   a. Note respiratory pattern and rate, including a comment that the child is crying.
   b. Call the provider since the respiratory rate is 60 and extremely labored.
   c. Wait to assess respirations until the child is not crying.
   d. Measure the respiratory rate before the temperature.

REFERENCES

American Heart Association. (2014). *High Blood Pressure: Statistical Fact Sheet, 2014 Update.* Retrieved from http://www.heart.org/idc/groups/heart-public/@wcm/@sop/@smd/documents/downloadable/ucm_462020.pdf

Carr, E., et al. (2011). Comparison of temporal artery to rectal temperature measurements in children up to 24 months. *Journal of Pediatric Nursing, 26*(3), 179–185.

James, P., Poaril, S., Carter, B., Cushman, W., Dennison-Himmelfarb, C., Handler, J., et al. (2014). 2014 evidence-based guidelines for the management of high blood pressure in adults: Report from the panel members appointed to the Eighth Joint National Committee (JNC 8). *JAMA, 311*(5), 507–520. doi: 10.1001/jama2013.284427

Johnson, K. D., Winkelman, C., Burant, C., Dolansky, M., & Totten, V. (2014). The factors that affect the frequency of vital sign monitoring in the emergency department. *Journal of Emergency Nursing, 40*(1), 27–35. doi: http://dx.doi.org/10.1016/j.jen.2012.07.023

Lawson, L., et al. (2007). Accuracy and precision of noninvasive temperature measurement in adult intensive care patients. *American Journal of Critical Care, 16*(5), 485–496.

National Institutes of Health (NIH). (2005). *The Fourth Report on the Diagnosis, Evaluation, and Treatment of High Blood Pressure in Children and Adolescents (NIH Pub. No. 05–3790).* Retrieved from http://www.nhlbi.nih.gov/health/prof/heart/hbp/hbp_ped.htm

Quatrara, B., et al. (2007). The effect of respiratory rate and ingestion of hot and cold beverages on the accuracy of oral temperatures measured by electronic thermometers. *Medsurg Nursing, 16*(2), 100, 105–108.

Sloane, P. D., Kistler, C., Mitchell, C. M., Beeber, A. S., Bertrand, R. M., Edwards, A. S., et al. (2014). Role of body temperature in diagnosing bacterial infection in nursing home residents. *Journal of the American Geriatrics Society, 62*(1), 135–140. doi: 10.1111/jgs.12596

Sund-Levander, M., & Grodzinsky, E. (2009). Time for a change to assess and evaluate body temperature in clinical practice. *International Journal of Nursing Practice, 15*, 241–249.

Wang, K., Gill, P., Wolstenhholme, J., Price, C., Heneghan, C., Thompson, M., et al. (2014). Non-contact infrared thermometers for measuring temperature in children: Primary care diagnostic technology update. *British Journal of General Practice.* doi: 10.3399/bjgp14X682045

Procedure 18-1 **Assessing Body Temperature**

Purpose
1. Obtain baseline temperature data for comparing future measurements.
2. Screen for alterations in temperature.
3. Evaluate temperature response to therapies.

Equipment
Digital or electronic thermometer
Disposable plastic thermometer sheaths or probe covers
Water-soluble lubricant and disposable gloves (for rectal temperature)
Pen and vital sign documentation record

Assessment
- Identify patient's baseline temperature.
- Assess for clinical signs and symptoms of temperature alteration.
- Assess for factors that influence body temperature measurement:
  - Ingestion of hot or cold foods or liquids in last 30 minutes (oral)
  - Smoking within last 30 minutes
  - Recent exercise
  - Age, hormones, and drugs that cause variations in body temperature
- Determine site most appropriate for temperature measurement.

Procedure

1. **Perform hand hygiene.**
   Rationale: Reduces microbe transmission.
2. **Identify the patient.**
   Rationale: Ensures correct patient receives proper assessment or treatment and reduces errors.
3. **Close door or bed curtains, and explain the procedure to the patient.**
   Rationale: Ensures patient privacy, increases patient compliance, reduces patient anxiety, and promotes learning.

Assessing Oral Temperature With an Electronic Thermometer

4. **Remove electronic thermometer from the battery pack, and remove the temperature probe from the recording unit, noting a digital display of temperature on the screen (usually 34°C [94°F]).**
   Rationale: The electronic thermometer is stored in a battery pack to ensure that it is always charged and ready for use. Extending the temperature probe prepares the machine to measure and record temperature. The digital display of temperature indicates that it is charged.

5. **Place the disposable cover over the temperature probe and attach securely (Fig. 1). Grasp the base of the probe.**

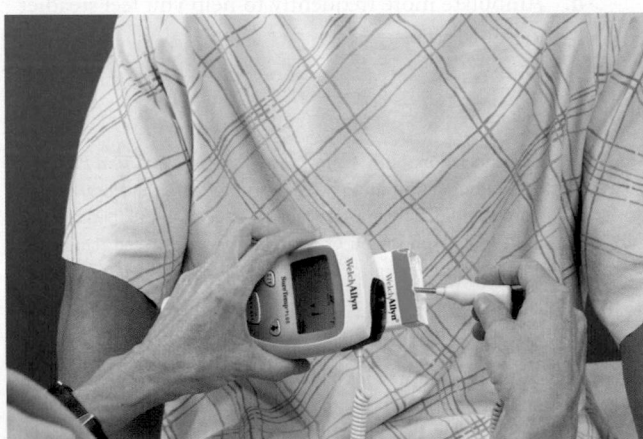

FIG. 1 Cover temperature probe with disposable cover.

Rationale: Ensures snug fit of the probe cover and prevents the transmission of microorganisms.

Procedure 18-1 *continued*

6. **Insert the probe below the patient's tongue and into the posterior sublingual pocket of the mouth. Ask the patient to close his or her lips around the probe. Hold the probe, supporting it in place (Fig. 2).**

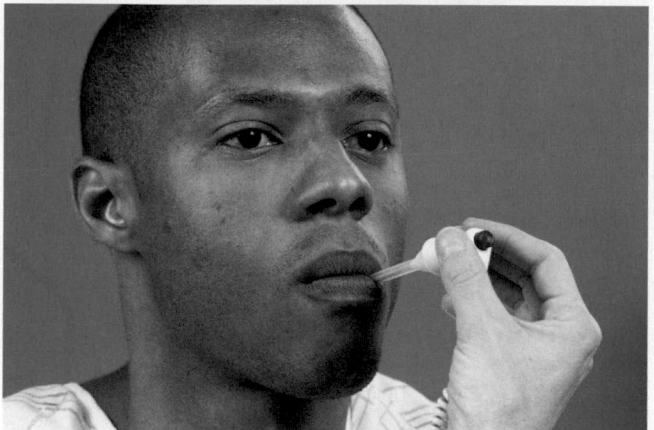

FIG. 2 Hold probe in posterior sublingual pocket.

Rationale: Inserting the probe into the posterior sublingual pocket obtains the most accurate temperature. The weight of the probe will displace it from the sublingual pocket if left unsupported.

7. **Wait for a beep indicating the measurement is complete. Note the temperature displayed on the unit and remove the probe from the patient's mouth (Fig. 3).**

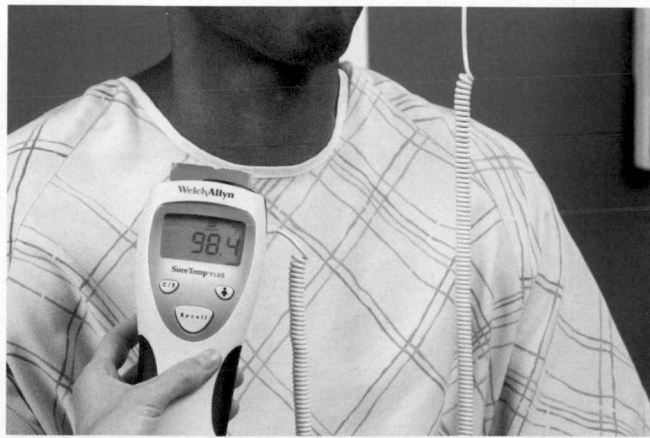

FIG. 3 Note temperature displayed on the unit before removing the probe from the patient's mouth.

Rationale: The beep indicates the reading is complete and the thermometer may be removed.

8. **Hold the probe over a waste container, and displace the probe cover by pressing the probe release button (Fig. 4).**

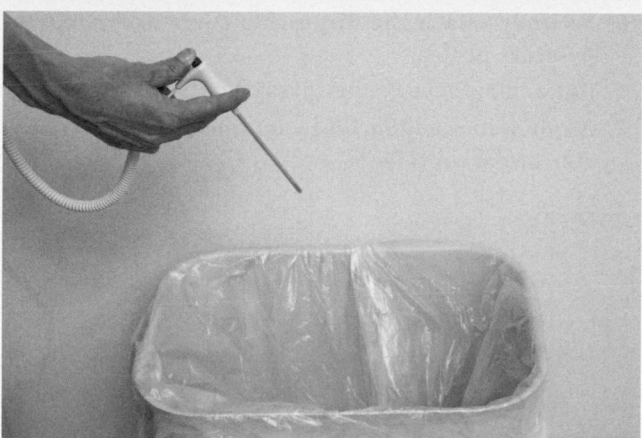

FIG. 4 Release probe cover into waste receptacle.

Rationale: The contaminated probe cover can be removed without touching the nurse's hands, thus preventing the transmission of microorganisms.

9. **Return the probe to the storage place within the unit, and return the thermometer to the battery pack. Cleanse according to agency policy.**

Rationale: Proper storage prevents damage to the sensitive temperature probe and ensures that the unit will be recharged and ready for use. Adequate cleansing prevents transmission of microorganisms when the thermometer is used for another patient.

10. **Record temperature on vital sign documentation record, indicating "O" for oral site. Discuss findings with patient if appropriate.**

Rationale: These actions ensure proper documentation and encourage the patient's participating in and understanding of health status.

Assessing Rectal Temperature With an Electronic Thermometer

4. **Assist patient to Sims' position with upper leg flexed. Expose only anal area.**

Rationale: Lateral position exposes the anal area for thermometer placement.

5. **Remove rectal (red) electronic thermometer from battery pack, and extend the temperature probe from the unit, noting a digital display of temperature on the screen.**

Rationale: Ensuring that the rectal (red) probe only is used for monitoring rectal temperature prevents cross-contamination of the oral probe with rectal bacteria.

Procedure 18-1 *continued*

6. **Securely attach the disposable cover over the temperature probe.**

   Rationale: Prevents transmission of microorganisms.

7. **Apply water-soluble lubricant liberally to thermometer probe tip (Fig. 5).**

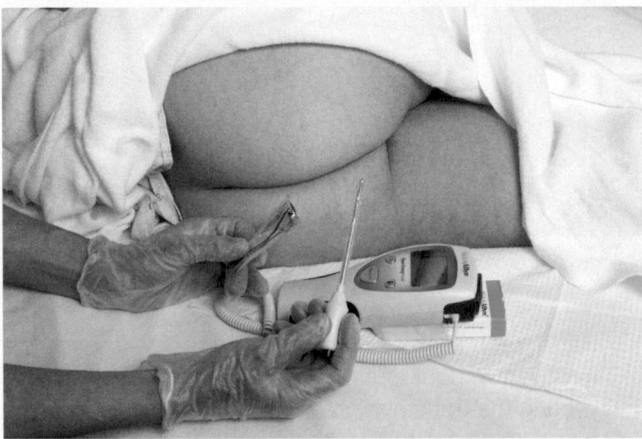

FIG. 5 Lubricate thermometer probe.

   Rationale: Lubricant facilitates insertion of the thermometer without irritating or traumatizing the rectum.

8. **Don nonsterile exam gloves.**

   Rationale: Protects nurse from patient's body fluids.

9. **Separate patient's buttocks with one gloved hand until the anal sphincter is visible.**

   Rationale: Visual exposure of the anus ensures accurate placement of the probe.

10. **Ask patient to take a deep, slow breath. Insert thermometer into anus in direction of umbilicus, 1 inch (2.5 cm) for a child and 1.5 inches (4 cm) for an adult (Fig. 6). Do not force.**

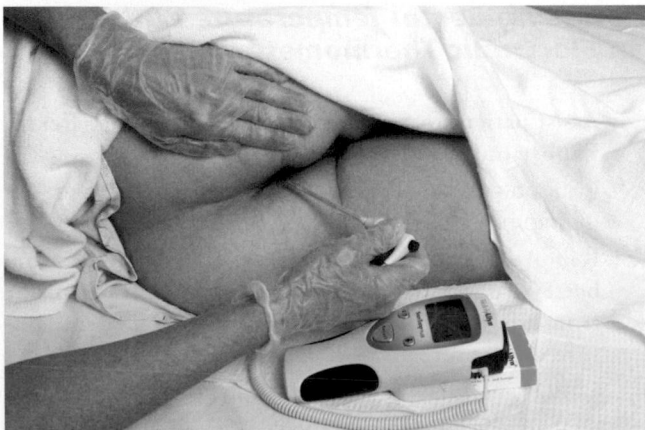

FIG. 6 Gently insert into anus.

   Rationale: A deep, slow breath allows the patient to relax the external sphincter. Insertion depth allows adequate exposure of the probe to blood vessels in the rectal wall.

11. **Hold the probe in place until machine emits a beep (Fig. 7). Obtain reading.**

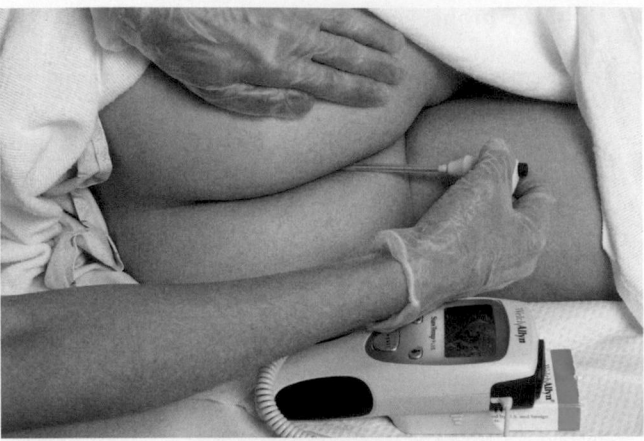

FIG. 7 Hold thermometer in place.

   Rationale: Holding the thermometer prevents rectal damage or perforation caused by the patient moving with the thermometer in place.

12. **Follow steps 7 through 9 in Assessing Oral Temperature With an Electronic Thermometer. Document "R" for rectal site.**

Assessing Temperature Using a Tympanic Membrane Thermometer

4. **Remove tympanic thermometer from recharging base, and check that the lens is clean. Attach tympanic probe cover to sensor unit (Fig. 8).**

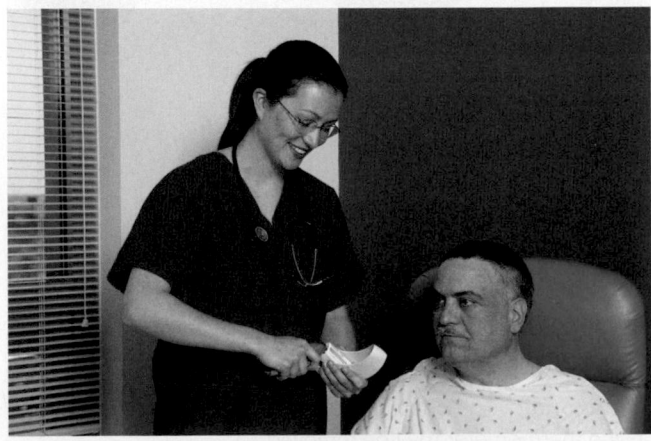

FIG. 8 Attach probe cover to sensor unit.

   Rationale: A clean lens is important to detect infrared radiation from the eardrum. Dirty lenses are a common cause of inaccurate measurements. The probe cover keeps the unit clean and prevents the transfer of microorganisms.

Procedure 18-1 *continued*

5. **Insert probe into ear canal, making sure the probe fits snugly (Fig. 9). Avoid forcing the probe too deeply into the ear. Pulling the pinna back, up, and out in an adult will straighten the ear canal. Some manufacturers recommend moving the thermometer in a figure-of-eight pattern. Rotate the probe handle toward the jawline.**

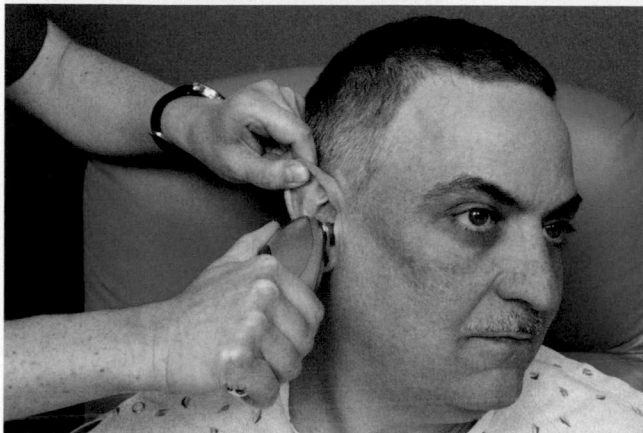

FIG. 9 Insert probe snugly into ear canal.

Rationale: Straightening the ear canal permits better exposure of the tympanic membrane. Snug fit into the ear canal is also necessary for accurate temperature detection. Forceful deep insertion could result in injury to the eardrum. Angling the probe toward the jawline ensures an accurate reading.

6. **Activate the thermometer, and note the temperature readout, which is usually displayed within 2 seconds (Fig. 10).**

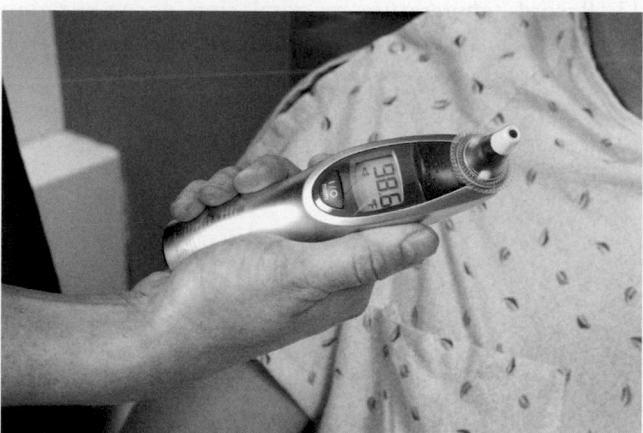

FIG. 10 Note the temperature readout.

Rationale: Temperature assessment occurs very quickly with the tympanic membrane thermometer.

7. **Eject sensor probe cover directly into waste container, cleanse according to agency policy, and return tympanic thermometer to base for storage or recharging. Store away from temperature extremes.**

Rationale: Preventing contamination of equipment by microorganisms is important. Recharging the tympanic thermometer will prepare the thermometer for later use. Proper storage will help ensure accurate functioning of the equipment.

8. **Record temperature on vital sign documentation record. Document "TM" for tympanic membrane site. Discuss findings with patient if appropriate.**

Rationale: These actions ensure proper documentation and encourage the patient's understanding of his or her health status.

Assessing Temperature Using a Temporal Artery Thermometer

4. **Remove thermometer from storage base. If low battery indicator shows, replace battery.**

5. **Inspect the thermometer lens. If not shiny, clean by first wiping with alcohol, then rinsing with water-dampened swabs. Allow to air-dry. Lens should be cleaned daily.**

Rationale: Buildup of skin oils can cause inaccurate readings.

6. **Attach disposable cover.**

Rationale: The probe cover keeps the unit clean and prevents the transfer of microorganisms.

7. **Move hair to expose forehead and hairline. Measure only exposed side of forehead. If patient is lying on side, measure "up" side only. If patient is perspiring heavily (diaphoretic), consider alternate method (e.g., oral).**

Rationale: Anything covering the skin will insulate it and keep heat from dissipating, which may lead to a falsely high reading. Diaphoresis causes skin cooling, which may cause a falsely low reading.

Procedure 18-1 *continued*

8. **Place probe flush against the center of the forehead and depress button (Fig. 11). Slowly slide probe straight across forehead to hairline (Fig. 12). Keeping button depressed, lift the probe from the forehead and touch it briefly against the neck just behind the earlobe (Fig. 13).**

Rationale: Measurement of both the forehead and behind the ear may compensate for skin cooling due to diaphoresis.

9. **Release the button and read the recorded temperature within 15 seconds (Fig. 14). If repeated measurements are necessary, wait at least 30 seconds.**

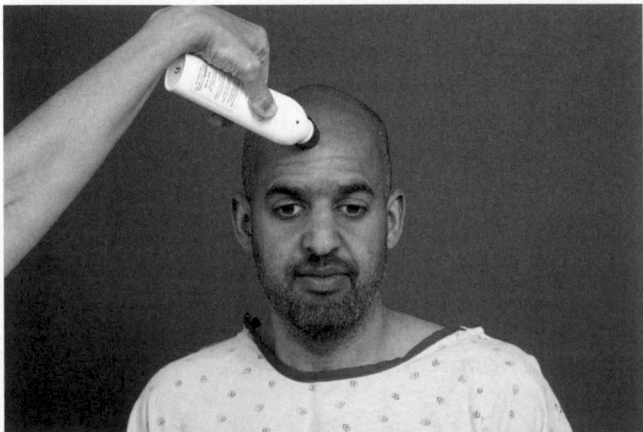

FIG. 11 Place probe against center of forehead.

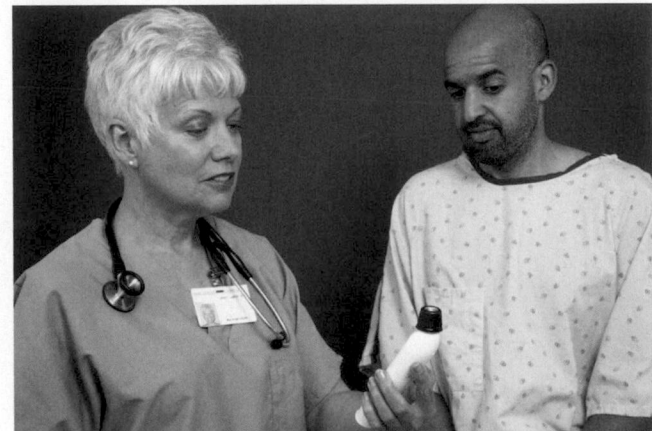

FIG. 14 Read recorded temperature within 15 seconds.

Rationale: Skin cooling may occur with rapidly repeated measurements.

10. **Eject probe cover directly into waste container or keep at bedside to use again on the same patient, cleanse according to agency policy, and return temporal thermometer to storage base. Store away from temperature extremes.**

Rationale: Preventing contamination of microorganisms from equipment is important. Proper storage will help ensure accurate functioning of the equipment.

11. **Record temperature on vital sign documentation record, indicating "TA" for temporal artery site. Discuss findings with patient if appropriate.**

Rationale: These actions ensure proper documentation and encourage the patient's understanding of his or her health status.

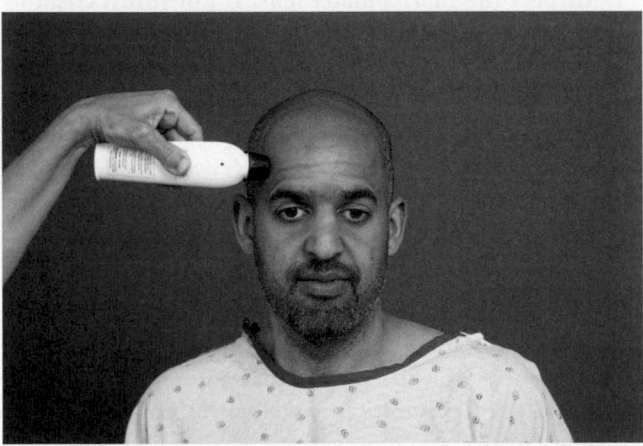

FIG. 12 Slide probe straight across forehead.

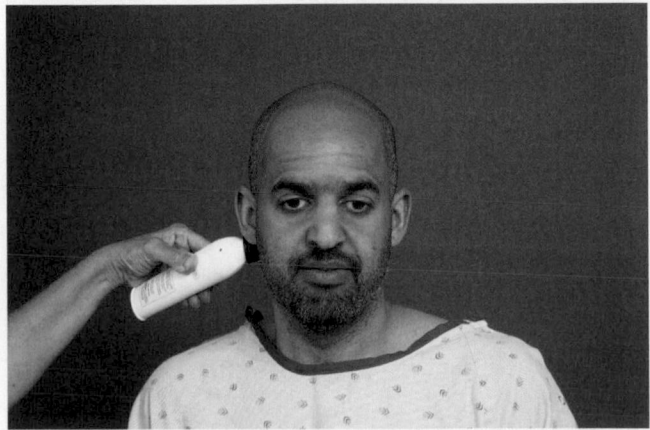

FIG. 13 Touch probe against the neck behind the earlobe.

Procedure 18-1   *continued*

Assessing Axillary Temperature With an Electronic Thermometer

Follow steps 1 to 6 in Assessing Oral Temperature With an Electronic Thermometer.

7. Assist patient to comfortable position, and remove clothing to expose axilla (Fig. 15).

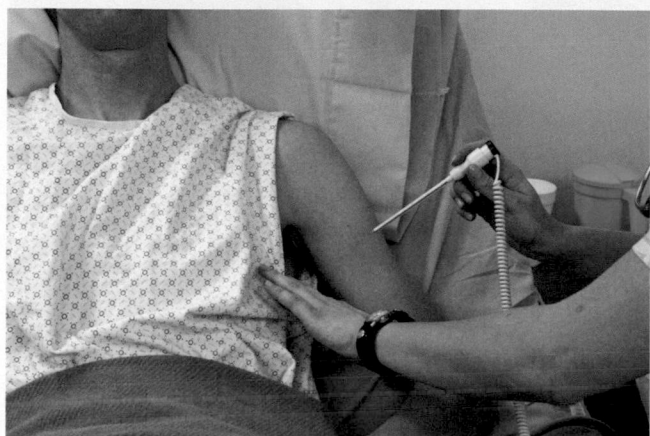

FIG. 15 Exposing axilla to assess temperature.

Rationale: Clothing in the axilla area could interfere with accurate temperature measurement.

8. Place thermometer against middle of axilla; fold patient's arm down and place across chest, enclosing thermometer in axillary area (Fig. 16).

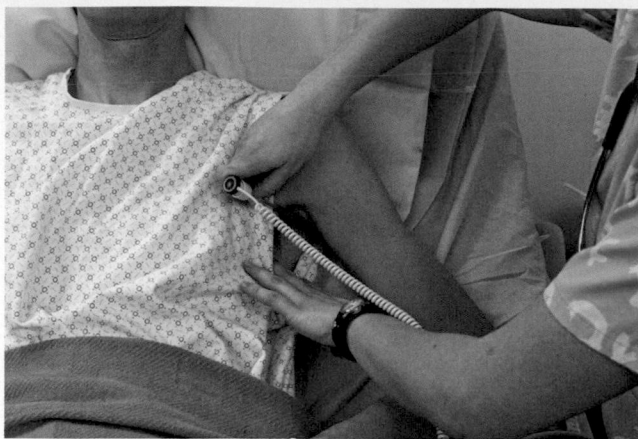

FIG. 16 Place thermometer against middle of axilla.

Rationale: This position maintains correct position of the thermometer against blood vessels in the axilla.

9. Wait for a beep indicating the measurement is complete. Note the temperature displayed on the unit and remove the probe from the patient's axilla.

Rationale: The beep indicates the measurement is complete and the thermometer may be removed.

10. Follow steps 8 and 9 in Assessing Oral Temperature With an Electronic Thermometer. Document "A" for axillary site.

Documentation

7/14/16: 01:30—Axillary temp 37°C at 08:00. No complaints of chills or diaphoresis. Afebrile for last 36 hours.
—S. Roberts, RN

Life Span Considerations

Newborns, Infants, and Children

- Newborn thermoregulation is ineffective and immature. Environmental temperatures greatly affect the body temperatures of infants.
- A child who has a very high temperature reading (>38.5°C) should have the temperature rechecked at a different site.
- Temporal artery, tympanic, or axillary temperature measurement is the preferred method for infants older than 2 months and children younger than 6 years because these areas are easily accessible. Noncontact infrared thermometers may be used. Younger children have limited attention spans and a more difficult time holding their lips closed long enough to obtain an accurate oral temperature reading. Also, with the temporal artery, tympanic, or axillary route, there is no chance of rectal perforation if the infant or child moves suddenly. Remember that tympanic temperature readings can be affected by devices such as incubators, radiant warmers, or fans.
- When taking a tympanic membrane temperature measurement in children under 3 years old, pull the pinna down and straight back (Fig. 17). In children older than 3 years, pull the pinna slightly upward and straight back, as you would with an adult patient (Fig. 18).

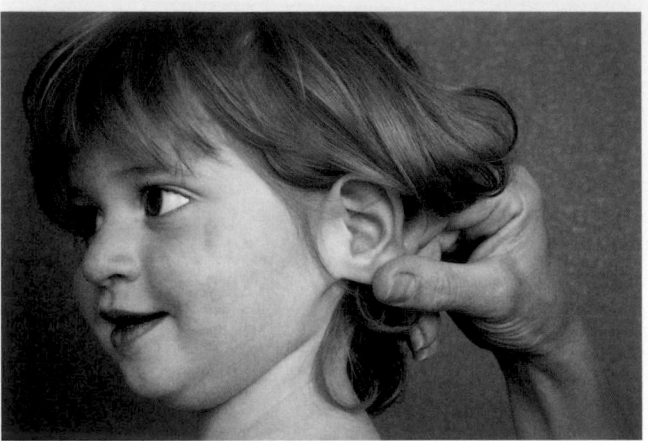

FIG. 17 Pull the pinna down and straight back in children under 3 years old.

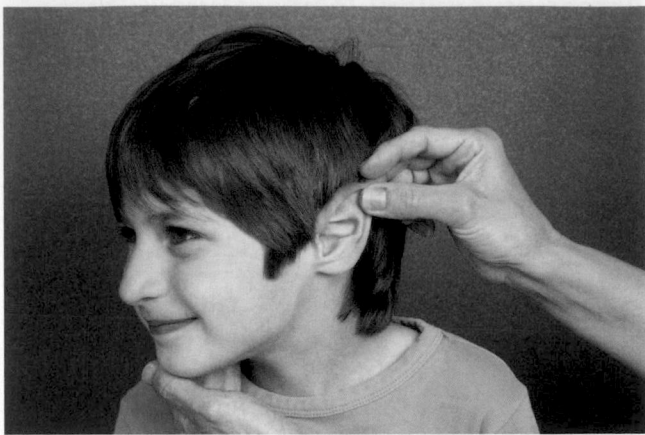

FIG. 18 Pull the pinna slightly upward and straight back in children older than 3 years.

Older Adults

- Older adults may have difficulty flexing their legs and assuming the left lateral position for rectal temperature measurement. Thermometer may be inserted with both legs straight.
- Normal body temperature drops to an average of 36°C in the older adult.

Home Care Modifications

- Advise purchase of a digital or battery-operated thermometer to replace any glass mercury thermometers that are still being used in the home since they pose an environmental hazard. Temporal artery, tympanic, and noncontact infrared thermometers are becoming less expensive and are a good choice for quick, accurate temperature screening in the home.
- Clean thermometer after each use or use disposable probe covers to prevent transmission of infectious organisms between family members.
- If family members need to assess temperature of patients, they may need to know the following:
  - How frequently to monitor temperature
  - When to notify home care nurse or provider
  - Not to measure temperature orally in children younger than 6 years or in any confused or unconscious person

Collaboration and Delegation

- UAPs routinely monitor patients' temperatures. Remind them to promptly report any temperature elevation above 38°C to the RN for follow-up.
- Instruct UAPs that they must report even low-grade fevers in certain patients (e.g., those who are immunocompromised or elderly).
- Providers usually want to be notified of any temperature greater than 38.5°C (101°F).

Procedure 18-2 Obtaining a Pulse

Purpose	1. Obtain a baseline measurement of heart rate, rhythm, and quality.
	2. Evaluate the heart's response to various therapies and medications.
	3. Peripheral pulse may be palpated to assess local blood flow to an extremity or to monitor perfusion to an extremity following surgery or diagnostic procedures (e.g., cardiac catheterization).
Equipment	Wristwatch or wall clock with second hand
	Vital sign flow sheet and pen, or electronic health record
	Doppler and conducting gel (for difficult-to-palpate pulses)
	Stethoscope
Assessment	• Review medical history to determine risk factors for alterations in pulse rate (heart disease, fluid or electrolyte imbalances, pain, hemorrhage).
	• Assess for physical signs and symptoms of alteration in cardiac or vascular status (dyspnea, chest pain, palpitations, syncope, edema, cyanosis).
	• Identify factors that influence pulse (age, medications, fever, and exercise).
	• Identify site most appropriate for pulse assessment.
	• Review previous and baseline pulse assessments, if available.

Procedure

1. **Perform hand hygiene.**
   Rationale: Reduces microbe transmission.
2. **Identify the patient.**
   Rationale: Ensures correct patient receives proper assessment or treatment and reduces errors.
3. **Close door or bed curtains and explain the procedure to the patient.**
   Rationale: Ensures patient privacy, increases patient compliance, reduces patient anxiety, and promotes learning.

Obtaining a Radial Pulse

4. **Position patient comfortably with forearm across chest or at side with wrist extended.**
   Rationale: Relaxed position of lower arm with wrist extended allows easier artery palpation.
5. **Place fingertips of your first two or three fingers along the groove at base of thumb, on patient's wrist, parallel to the artery (Fig. 1).**

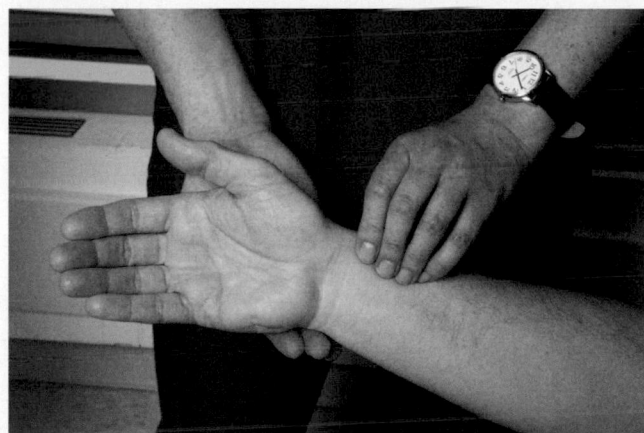

FIG. 1 Use fingertips to palpate radial pulse.

Rationale: Fingertips are the most sensitive part of the hand for palpating pulses. Do not use the thumb to palpate—it has a strong pulse that you may confuse with the patient's pulse.

6. **Press against radial artery to obliterate pulse, then gradually release pressure until you feel pulsations; assess for regularity and strength.**
   Rationale: Moderate pressure is needed to accurately assess the pulse's rate and regularity.

Procedure 18-2   *continued*

7. **If pulse is not easily palpable, use Doppler.**

   a. **Apply conducting gel to end of probe or to radial site.**

      Rationale: Doppler works by ultrasound, which transmits sound better with the airtight seal that gel provides.

   b. **Press "on" button and place probe against skin on pulse site. Reposition slightly, using firm pressure, until you hear a pulsating sound.**

8. **If pulse is regular, count pulse for 30 seconds and then multiply by two. If pulse is irregular, count for 1 full minute. If irregular pulse is a new finding, assess apical and radial rates simultaneously to detect a pulse deficit. Count the initial pulse as zero.**

   Rationale: Prevents overestimation of pulse. If pulse is irregular, a longer counting period ensures a more accurate pulse rate determination. Assessing for pulse is helpful to determine if irregular beats are strong enough to perfuse to peripheral pulse sites.

Obtaining an Apical Pulse

4. **Position patient in supine or sitting position with sternum and left chest exposed (Fig. 2).**

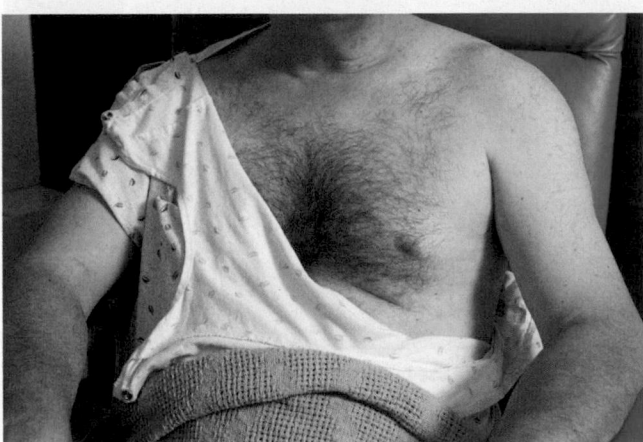

FIG. 2 Expose sternum and left chest.

   Rationale: This position allows easy access for selection of correct site. Rustling from clothing or bed linens will not distract the nurse from hearing the pulse.

5. **Warm diaphragm of stethoscope by holding it in the palm of your hand for 5 to 10 seconds.**

   Rationale: A cold metal or plastic diaphragm can startle the patient when placed directly on the chest. This could alter the pulse rate.

6. **Use an alcohol swab to clean the stethoscope and earpieces before using.**

   Rationale: Maintains asepsis.

7. **Locate apex of the patient's heart by palpating the space between the fifth and sixth rib (fifth intercostal space) and moving to the left midclavicular line (Fig. 3).**

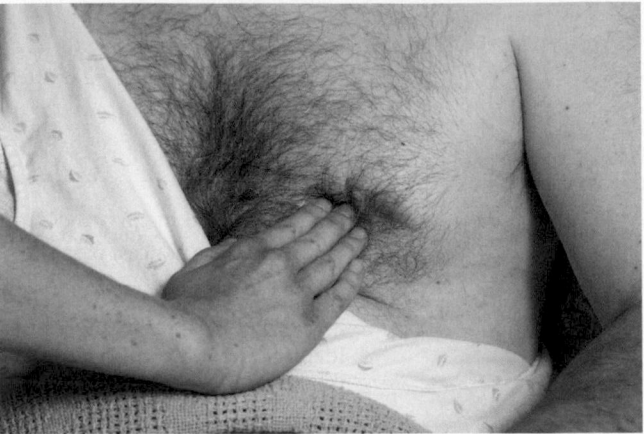

FIG. 3 Locate apex of patient's heart.

8. **Insert the earpieces of stethoscope into your ears, and place diaphragm over apex of patient's heart (Fig. 4).**

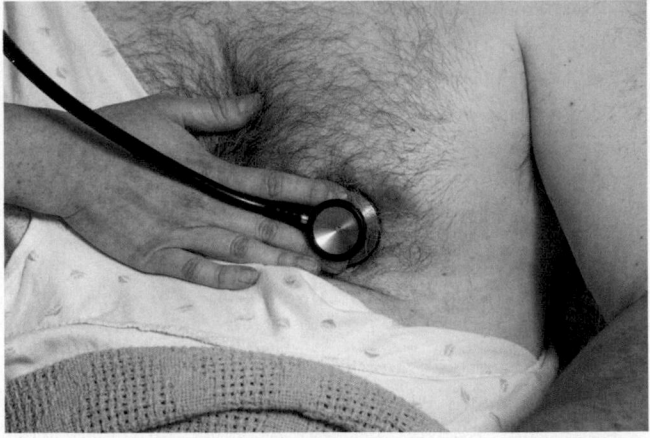

FIG. 4 Place diaphragm over apex of patient's heart.

   Rationale: The heartbeat is usually heard loudest at the fifth intercostal space, near the midclavicular line.

9. **Assess the heartbeat for regularity and dysrhythmias.**

   Rationale: Frequent irregularities within 1 minute may indicate inadequate cardiac perfusion.

Procedure 18-2   *continued*

10. **If rhythm is regular, count the heartbeat for 30 seconds and then multiply by two (Fig. 5). Count for 1 full minute if the rhythm is irregular. Count the initial pulse as zero.**

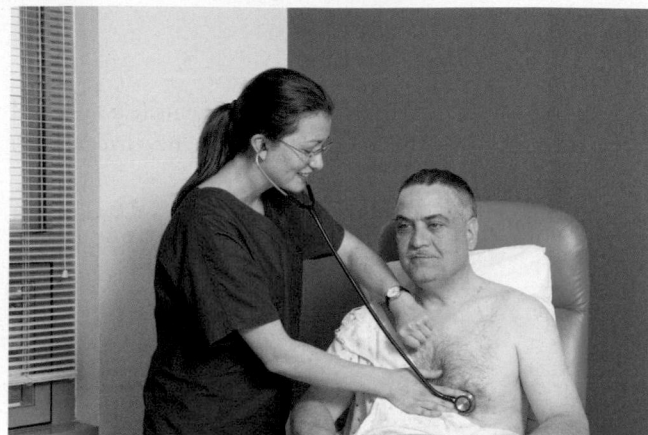

FIG. 5 Count heartbeat for 30 seconds.

Rationale: Prevents overestimation of pulse. Heart rate is more accurate when counted over a longer period if the rate is irregular.

11. **Replace the patient's gown and assist the patient to return to a comfortable position (Fig. 6).**

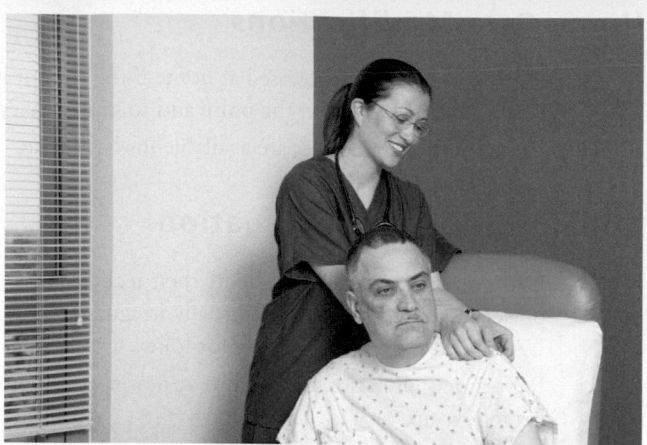

FIG. 6 Replace patient's gown.

Rationale: Provides for patient comfort.

12. **Share results of assessment with patient, if appropriate.**

Rationale: Promote the patient's understanding of health and response to therapies.

13. **Document pulse on vital sign record or EHR. Specify in the documentation that you obtained an apical pulse (e.g., "AP").**

Rationale: Maintains legal record and communicates with health team members.

Documentation

> 7/15/16: 08:00—AP 77 at resting state, regular rhythm and consistent with baseline 70–85.
>
> —S. Roberts, RN

Life Span Considerations

Infants and Children

- Newborns and children younger than 2 years have weak radial pulses. Assess apical pulses for heart rate.
- The apex of the heart on an infant is at the third to fourth intercostal space, to the left of the midclavicular line.
- Crying greatly increases the pulse rate. Minimize the effect of crying by taking the pulse while the child sits in a parent's or caregiver's lap or by distracting the child with toys before disruptive procedures.

Older Adults

- If patient is taking cardiac medications such as digitalis preparations or beta-blockers or has a history of cardiac dysrhythmias, obtain a more accurate assessment of heart rate and rhythm using the apical pulse site for 1 full minute.

Procedure 18-2   *continued*

Home Care Modifications

- Pulse may need to be assessed at home if the patient is taking various cardiac medications. Teach the caregiver or patient how to locate and count the pulse and to keep a diary of daily pulse rate to take to healthcare appointments.
- Digital pulse rate devices are available for home use.

Collaboration and Delegation

- UAPs often assess pulses. Validate their technique for accuracy. Provide specific information about patients (e.g., if apical pulse is required or if pulse is usually irregular). Indicate what assessment data (e.g., pulse <60 or >100; new irregularity) UAPs need to report promptly for follow-up.
- Report new alterations in rhythm or new episodes of unexplained tachycardia or bradycardia to the provider/cardiologist for follow-up.

Procedure 18-3 Assessing Respirations

Purpose	1. Assess respiratory status by evaluating rate and quality.
	2. Evaluate the influence of medications and therapies on respiration.

Equipment	Watch or wall clock with second hand
	Vital signs documentation sheet or computer documentation record

Assessment	• Identify risk factors for altered respiratory status (chest trauma, respiratory disease, smoking history, respiratory depressant medications).
	• Assess for physical signs and symptoms of altered respiratory status (cyanosis, clubbed fingers, reduced level of consciousness, pain during inspiration, dyspnea, coughing, retractions, nasal flaring, grunting, orthopnea, use of accessory muscles).
	• Review pertinent laboratory studies (arterial blood gases, oxygen saturation, complete blood count).
	• Determine baseline respiratory rate.

Procedure

1. **Perform hand hygiene.**

   Rationale: Reduces microbe transmission.

2. **Identify the patient.**

   Rationale: Ensures correct patient receives proper assessment or treatment and reduces errors.

3. **Close door or bed curtains and explain the procedure to the patient.**

   Rationale: Ensures patient privacy, increases patient compliance, reduces patient anxiety, and promotes learning.

4. **After or before assessment of pulse, keep your fingers resting on patient's wrist and observe or feel the rising and falling of chest with respiration (Fig. 1). If patient is asleep, you may gently place your hand on the patient's chest so you can feel chest movement. Do not explain procedure to patient.**

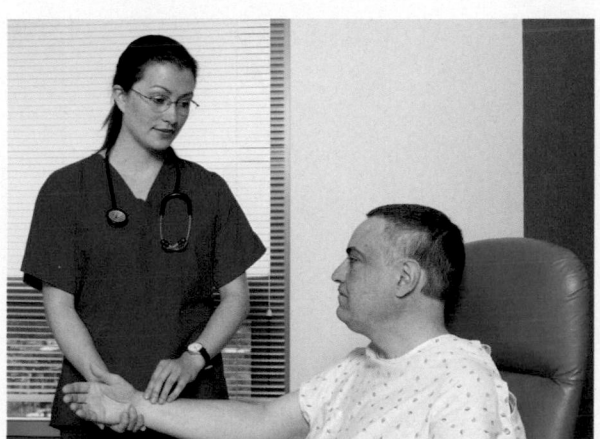

FIG. 1 Palpate the radial pulse. Observe rise and fall of the chest.

Rationale: Explaining the procedure may make the patient self-conscious about respirations and could cause him or her to alter the respiratory pattern.

5. **When you have observed one complete cycle of inspiration and expiration, and if respiration is regular, look at second hand of your watch and count the number of complete cycles in 1 full minute (Fig. 2).**

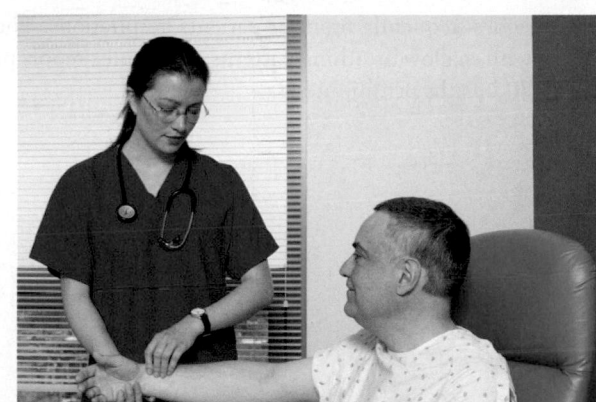

FIG. 2 Look at the second hand of your watch and count the number of complete cycles in 1 full minute.

Rationale: Ensures accuracy of assessment.

6. **If respirations are shallow and difficult to count, observe at the sternal notch.**

   Rationale: Respirations are more visible at the sternal notch.

Procedure 18-3   *continued*

7. Note depth and rhythm of respiratory cycle.

   Rationale: Respiratory characteristics give additional data about alterations in respiratory status.

8. Discuss findings with patient and document respiratory rate, depth, rhythm, and character.

   Rationale: Maintains legal record and communicates with healthcare team.

Documentation

> 7/16/16: 08:00—RR 16, shallow and regular, no use of accessory muscles.
>
>   —S. Roberts, RN

Life Span Considerations

Infants and Children

- A crying child's respiratory rate cannot be accurately assessed. Count respirations when the child is sleeping, if possible. If the child is crying, attempt to quiet him or her before assessing respirations. If the child cannot be soothed, indicate "crying" on the vital signs documentation sheet.

Home Care Modifications

- High-risk infants may be placed on apnea monitors so that parents can be quickly alerted if respirations slow dangerously or stop.

Collaboration and Delegation

- UAPs frequently monitor patients' respirations. They must take care to accurately assess the rate, especially for patients with shallow breathing patterns. They must report promptly any alterations of rhythm or rate fewer than 12 or more than 20 breaths per minute.

Procedure 18-4 Obtaining Blood Pressure

Purpose
1. Evaluate the patient's hemodynamic status by obtaining information about cardiac output, blood volume, peripheral vascular resistance, and arterial wall elasticity.
2. Obtain baseline measurement of blood pressure.
3. Monitor the hemodynamic response to various therapies or disease conditions.
4. Screen for hypertension.

Equipment
Stethoscope
Sphygmomanometer with bladder and cuff of correct size for patient and site
Vital signs flow sheet or computerized record

Assessment
- Assess blood pressure on initial patient examination.
- Identify factors that may alter blood pressure (medications, exercise, age, emotional conditions, smoking, postural changes).
- Assess best site for obtaining blood pressure.
- Review previous blood pressure readings, if available.
- Consider any factors that limit site selection (e.g., mastectomy, dialysis access, vascular access).

Procedure

1. **Perform hand hygiene.**
   Rationale: Reduces microbe transmission.

2. **Identify the patient.**
   Rationale: Ensures correct patient receives proper assessment or treatment and reduces errors.

3. **Close door or bed curtains and explain the procedure to the patient.**
   Rationale: Ensures patient privacy, increases patient compliance, reduces patient anxiety, and promotes learning.

4. **Clean stethoscope head with alcohol or approved cleaning solution.**
   Rationale: Maintains asepsis.

5. **Assist patient to a comfortable position with forearm supported at heart level and palm up (Fig. 1). Verify that you have a correctly sized blood pressure cuff.**

   Rationale: Variations in blood pressure can occur with patient in different positions. Blood pressure increases when the arm is below heart level and decreases when above heart level. Diastolic blood pressure may increase 10% if the arm is unsupported, secondary to isometric muscle contraction used to support the arm. Inappropriate cuff size produces inaccurate readings.

6. **Expose the upper arm completely. Palpate the brachial artery.**

   Rationale: Accurate placement of cuff and stethoscope requires complete exposure of the upper arm. Locating the brachial artery assures correct placement of the cuff.

7. **Wrap deflated cuff snugly around upper arm with center of bladder over brachial artery (Fig. 2). Lower border of cuff should be about 2 cm above the antecubital space (nearer the antecubital space on an infant).**

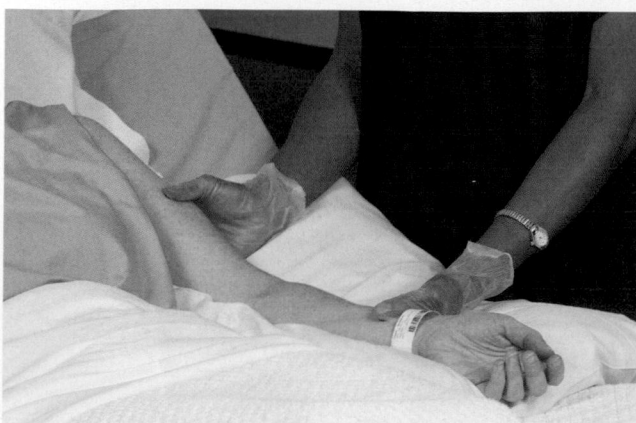

FIG. 1 Proper positioning for blood pressure assessment using the brachial artery. (Photo by B. Proud.)

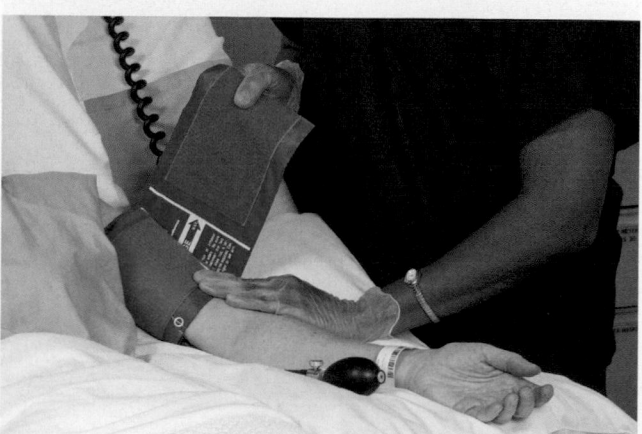

FIG. 2 Palpating the brachial pulse. (Photo by B. Proud.)

Procedure 18-4   *continued*

Rationale: Placing the bladder directly over the brachial artery ensures proper compression of the artery during cuff inflation. Loose or uneven application can result in falsely high readings.

8. **Palpate brachial or radial artery with fingertips (Fig. 3). Close valve on pressure bulb and inflate cuff until pulse disappears. Slowly release valve and note reading when pulse reappears.**

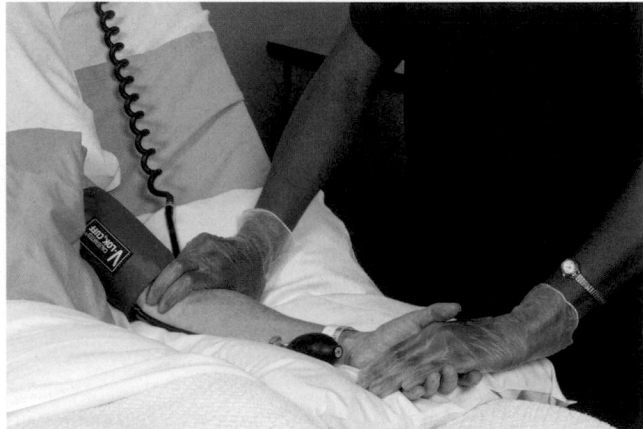

FIG. 3 Placing the blood pressure cuff. (Photo by B. Proud.)

Rationale: Identifies the approximate systolic blood pressure reading to prevent underestimating systolic blood pressure in the event the patient has an auscultatory gap. It is most important to use the two-step method during the initial screening to detect an auscultatory gap.

9. **Fully deflate cuff and wait 1 to 2 minutes.**

Rationale: A waiting period prevents falsely high readings by allowing blood trapped in the vein to be recirculated.

10. **Place stethoscope earpiece in ears. Repalpate the brachial artery, and place stethoscope bell or diaphragm over site (Fig. 4).**

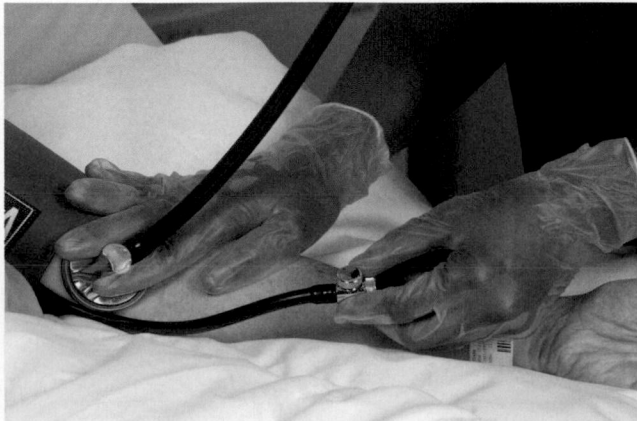

FIG. 4 Pump bulb to inflate cuff. Inflate cuff to 30 mm Hg above reading where brachial pulse disappeared.

Rationale: Blood pressure is a low-frequency sound that is best heard with the stethoscope bell, but the diaphragm is widely used because it is easily placed and more generally available.

11. **Close bulb valve by turning clockwise. Ensure gauge starts at zero. Pump bulb to inflate cuff. Inflate cuff to 30 mm Hg above reading where brachial pulse disappeared.**

Rationale: Ensures accurate assessment of systolic blood pressure.

12. **Open valve on manometer, and then slowly release valve so pressure drops about 2 to 3 mm Hg per second.**

Rationale: Inaccurate measurements may occur if deflation rate is too fast or too slow.

13. **Identify manometer reading when first clear Korotkoff sound is heard (Fig. 5).**

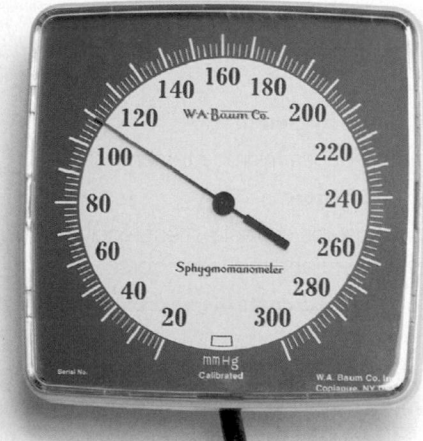

FIG. 5 Measuring systolic blood pressure.

Rationale: Indicates systolic pressure reading.

14. **Continue to deflate, and note reading when sound muffles or dampens (fourth Korotkoff) and when it disappears (fifth Korotkoff) (Fig. 6).**

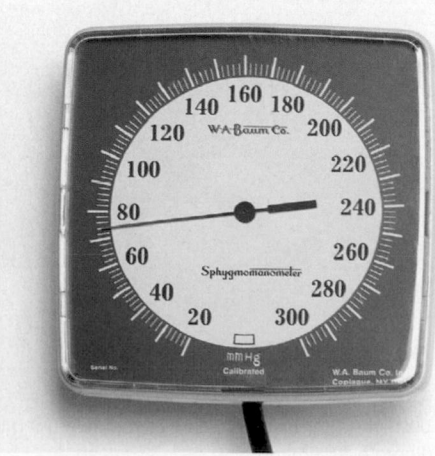

FIG. 6 Measuring diastolic blood pressure.

Procedure 18-4 *continued*

Rationale: The American Heart Association recommends using the fifth Korotkoff sound as diastolic pressure in adults and the fourth Korotkoff in children; however, some use the fifth Korotkoff phase in children. In all patients, if the fourth and fifth Korotkoff are 10 mm Hg or greater apart, note all three readings.

15. **Deflate cuff completely and remove from patient's arm.**

    Rationale: Removes all air from the cuff so it will be ready for the next use.

16. **If cuff will be used on another patient, clean cuff according to agency requirements and allow to air-dry.**

    Rationale: Prevents transfer of microorganisms to another patient.

17. **Record blood pressure. Record systolic (e.g., 130) and diastolic (e.g., 80) in the form "130/80." If three pressures are to be recorded, use the form "130/80/40" (40 is the fifth Korotkoff). Abbreviate as "RA" or "LA" to indicate right or left arm measurement.**

    Rationale: Maintains legal record and communicates with health team members.

18. **Assist patient to comfortable position and discuss findings with patient, if appropriate.**

    Rationale: Encourages the patient's understanding of his or her health status and promotes compliance with therapies.

Documentation

7/16/16: 08:00 B/P: 110/74 mm Hg— in RA in sitting position at end expiration.

—S. Roberts, RN

Life Span Considerations

Infants and Children

- Selection of a proper-sized cuff and bladder is critical for obtaining accurate blood pressure measurements in children and adults. The bladder width should be at 40% to 50% of the circumference of the limb.
- In infants, Korotkoff sounds may be too faint for accurate measurement. Accurate assessment of systolic pressure can be obtained using a Doppler ultrasonic device.
- When monitoring blood pressure in children, take respirations and pulse rate first since they are less invasive and less likely to cause anxiety and pain.

Older Adults

- Adults with hypertension or peripheral artery disease are prone to auscultatory gaps in blood pressure. Estimation of systolic pressure using the brachial artery palpation technique will prevent inaccurate readings secondary to auscultatory gap.
- Diastolic pressure often increases with age as a result of decreased compliance of the arteries.

Home Care Modifications

- Teach patients with hypertension to monitor their blood pressure at home. Various monitors for home use are available, including devices able to store measurements and transmit via telephone or computer for review by the healthcare provider. Verify that the patient uses a correctly sized cuff. Teach the patient the following:
  - To avoid caffeinated beverages, smoking, and exercise for 30 minutes before measurement
  - To use the same arm and correct body position for each measurement
  - At what measurements the patient should alert the nurse or provider
  - To bring their home monitor to appointments yearly to compare to measurements taken in the clinical setting and to verify correct cuff size, which may change over time with weight gain or loss

Collaboration and Delegation

- Frequently, UAPs monitor patients' blood pressures. Validate their techniques for accuracy and provide specific patient information (e.g., how frequently to monitor, appropriate size of cuff, site limitations). If the patient has been experiencing hypertension or hypotension, verbalize what readings he or she needs to promptly report for follow-up.
- Report any cases of significant hypertension or hypotension to the provider. Providers frequently establish parameters of notification.

Procedure 18-5 Assessing for Orthostatic Hypotension

Purpose

1. Assess the compensatory status of the cardiovascular and autonomic nervous systems to changes in body position.
2. Assess for fluid volume deficit.
3. Assess patient's safety in getting up and ambulating.

Equipment

Stethoscope
Sphygmomanometer
Watch or clock with second hand
Vital sign documentation form or EHR

Assessment

- Identify patients at risk for postural drops in blood pressure:
  - Volume depletion
  - Inadequate vasoconstrictor mechanisms secondary to prolonged bed rest
  - Autonomic insufficiency secondary to spinal cord injury or drugs (beta-adrenergic blockers, calcium channel blockers)
- Assess patient for complaint of dizziness or light-headedness during position changes.
- Review baseline blood pressure measurements, if available.

Procedure

1. **Perform hand hygiene.**
   Rationale: Reduces microbe transmission.
2. **Identify the patient.**
   Rationale: Ensures correct patient receives proper assessment or treatment and reduces errors.
3. **Close door or bed curtains and explain the procedure to the patient.**
   Rationale: Ensures patient privacy, increases patient compliance, reduces patient anxiety, and promotes learning.
4. **Position patient supine with head of bed flat for 10 minutes.**
   Rationale: Allows blood pooled in lower extremities to re-enter circulation.
5. **Check and record supine blood pressure and pulse (Fig. 1). Keep blood pressure cuff attached.**

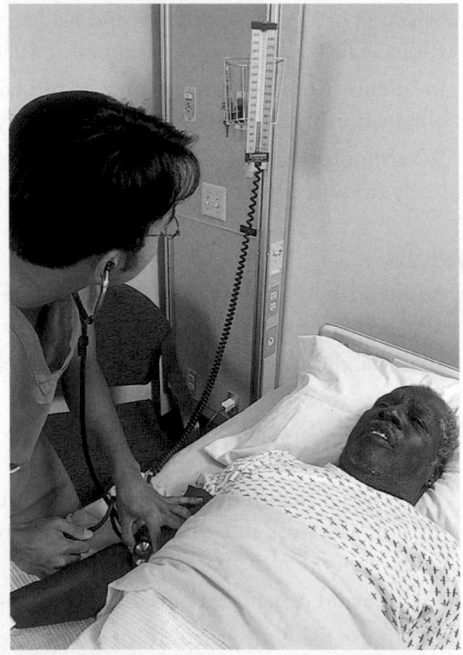

FIG. 1 Obtain blood pressure and pulse with the patient in supine position.

Rationale: Provides baseline information with which to compare measurements after position changes. Assess pulse rate to help differentiate the cause of postural hypotension. During position changes, if pulse rate rises as blood pressure falls, secondary to sympathetic stimulation, the cause may be volume depletion. If the pulse does not increase when the blood pressure falls, the cause may be related to the lack of sympathetic response.

Procedure 18-5   *continued*

6. **Assist patient to a sitting position at edge of bed with feet flat on the floor (Fig. 2). Wait 2 minutes and check blood pressure and pulse rate.**

   Note: **The waiting period is a convenient time to auscultate the patient's lung fields.**

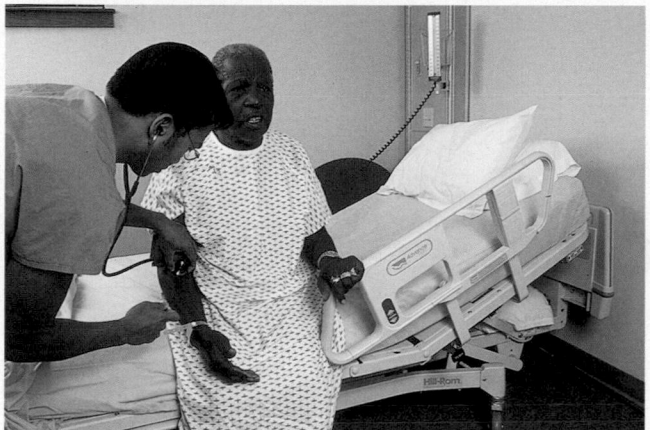

FIG. 2 Obtain blood pressure and pulse with the patient sitting at edge of bed with feet flat on floor.

   Rationale: Two minutes provides adequate time for the autonomic nervous system to reflexively compensate for volume shifts due to position change in the normal person.

7. **Assist patient to standing position, then wait 2 minutes and check blood pressure and pulse rate (Fig. 3). Be alert to signs and symptoms of dizziness.**

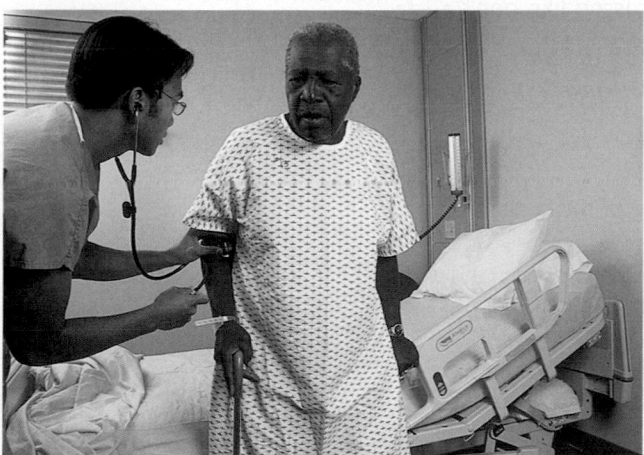

FIG. 3 Obtain blood pressure and pulse with patient in standing position.

   Rationale: If blood pressure drops significantly, the patient may become light-headed and may need to be returned to bed before test completion.

8. **Assist the patient back to a comfortable position.**

9. **Record measurements and any symptoms that accompanied the postural change. Report a drop of 20 mm Hg in systolic pressure or a drop of 10 mm Hg in diastolic pressure, and note pulse change.**

   Rationale: Maintains legal record and communicates with healthcare team.

10. **Discuss findings with patient, if appropriate.**

   Rationale: If there is a significant postural blood pressure drop, advise the patient to sit on the edge of the bed for several minutes before walking to avoid dizziness and possible falls. The patient should have assistance when ambulating.

Documentation

9/13/16: 08:00
- Lying: 142/80, p 72
- Sitting: 110/60, p 96
- c/o of dizziness, returned to bed and MD notified.

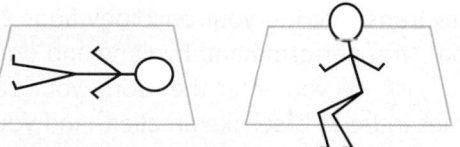

Stick man drawing.

—S. Roberts, RN

Collaboration and Delegation

- Nurses frequently delegate postural blood pressure monitoring to UAPs. Reinforce the order for taking blood pressures: supine first, then sitting, and then standing. Caution that safety is always the most important consideration. If the patient becomes dizzy, the assessment must stop and the patient should return to bed.
- If other health professionals report that the patient complains of dizziness upon rising, validate by obtaining postural vital signs.

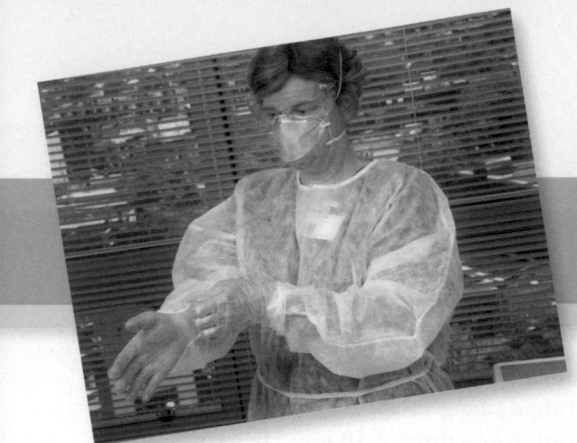

CHAPTER 19

Asepsis and Infection Control

Penny Gilliatt

Case Scenario

Your patient has been undergoing outpatient treatment for leukemia and was hospitalized in the critical care unit last week with pneumonia and respiratory failure. His pneumonia was diagnosed as community-acquired MRSA. He was transferred to your oncology floor 2 days ago. Before you enter the room, you perform hand hygiene and don an isolation gown, gloves, and a mask. As you enter the room, your patient says, "Finally, someone comes in here. I feel like an alien, and you are dressed like one."

Once you have completed this chapter and have incorporated asepsis into your knowledge base, review the above scenario and reflect on the following areas of Critical Thinking:

1. How do contact precautions differ from standard precautions?
2. Identify reasons staff members may want to avoid taking care of this patient or entering his room.
3. Reflect on possible ways to respond to this patient. What are his concerns? What might he be feeling? How might you communicate with him considering these things?
4. Decide how you will talk with other members of the healthcare team about the patient's observation and concerns. Explore possible ways to approach the subject with other staff members.

KEY TERMS

antiseptic
asepsis
bactericidal
bacteriostatic
carriers
disinfectant
extended-spectrum beta-lactamases (ESBLs)
hand hygiene
healthcare-associated infection (HAI)
infectious disease
isolation
medical asepsis
multidrug-resistant organisms (MDROs)
nosocomial infection
opportunistic infections
pathogenicity
pathogens
personal protective equipment (PPE)
prions
sepsis
specificity
standard precautions
sterilization
surgical asepsis
virulence

LEARNING OBJECTIVES

Upon completion of this chapter, you will be able to do the following:

1. Identify the six components of the chain of infection.
2. Identify ways that infection may occur.
3. Describe factors that increase the risk of infection in various settings.
4. Discuss the role of healthcare personnel and health agencies in infection control.

5. Identify ways that caregivers can increase their protection against infectious exposure.
6. Explain ways that caregivers can decrease the transmission of infection to patients.
7. Differentiate between medical and surgical asepsis.
8. Demonstrate good hand hygiene technique and identify key occasions and reasons for incorporating it as an integral part of practice.
9. Describe appropriate situations for using cleaning, disinfection, and sterilization.
10. Describe proper use of barriers also known as personal protective equipment (PPE).
11. Discuss the two-tier system of isolation.
12. Identify age-related and cultural considerations in preventing the transmission of infectious diseases.

Regardless of where they practice, preventing the transmission of microorganisms is a concern of all nurses. One way that nurses accomplish this goal is by **asepsis**.

Asepsis means to make free from disease-producing organisms. A large number of microorganisms live and multiply on every surface. They are in the air, grow on the skin, and flourish in the digestive tract. Certain microorganisms are necessary for normal body function. Some microorganisms help produce food and maintain the planet's ecology. Most of the time, humans and microorganisms live in harmony. When this balance is upset, however, microorganisms are capable of causing infection.

Infectious disease is one of the most common reasons people contact healthcare providers and accounts for multiple clinic and physician office visits in the United States. Preventable infectious diseases are common worldwide, resulting in great suffering and the unnecessary loss of many lives. The economic costs of preventing and treating infection are great. Recent years have shown an alarming increase in **multidrug-resistant organisms (MDROs)**, such as *Clostridium difficile*, carbapenem-resistant Enterobacteriaceae (CRE), *Neisseria gonorrhoeae*, tuberculosis, Enterococci, *Staphylococcus aureus*, and certain bacteria (e.g., *Escherichia coli*, *Klebsiella pneumoniae*, *Acinetobacter baumannii*, and *Stenotrophomonas maltophilia*) that produce **extended-spectrum beta-lactamases (ESBLs).** ESBLs are enzymes that gives bacteria immunity to both penicillin and cephalosporin antibiotics. Eradicating these bacteria is becoming increasingly difficult (Centers for Disease Control and Prevention [CDC], 2013). Additional emerging infectious diseases that underscore the need for precise infection control practices include viral hemorrhagic fevers (Ebola & Marburg viruses and the recently identified South African Lujo virus, first described in 2009), Enterovirus D68, Hantavirus, human influenza A H5N1 (avian flu), human influenza A H1N1 (2009) and H3N2 (2014), and Middle East respiratory syndrome (MERS). The 2014 Ebola outbreak, which affected multiple countries in West Africa, was the largest and most widespread in history and was the first to bring cases to the United States. Across the globe, this outbreak brought renewed focus to infection prevention practices and practices related to donning and doffing **personal protective equipment** (PPE) (CDC, 2014a). Nursing practice focuses on providing a safe and therapeutic environment to protect patients, family members, and healthcare providers from acquiring infections. The chapters on skin integrity and wound healing (see Chapter 30) and infection (see Chapter 31) provide additional information on specific infectious diseases and diagnostic and treatment procedures.

ROLE OF MICROORGANISMS IN INFECTION

Microorganisms that are capable of harming people are called **pathogens** or pathogenic. When pathogens enter and multiply within body tissues, they disrupt normal physiologic processes and produce an infection. The organisms and/or their toxins disrupt normal cell function or kill the cells entirely. **Sepsis**, a term that means poisoning of tissues, is often used to describe serious infection. Transport of an infection or the products of infection throughout the body by the blood is known as *septicemia* or *bacteremia*.

In common usage, "infected" and "septic" are often used interchangeably, but they are not the same. In most instances when a patient is said to be infected, it means that he or she has a disease caused by microorganisms. When the patient is referred to as septic, it means that he or she is displaying the manifestations of a systemic inflammatory state triggered by two things: widespread immune response chemicals released into the blood to fight the infection and microbial destruction of tissues. This systemic condition refers to the pathologic events that result from the invasion and multiplication of microorganisms in a host. Toxins and enzymes produced by the microorganisms cause tissue injury. This injury produces manifestations of infection: fever; rashes; malaise; nausea and vomiting; diarrhea; purulent discharge from wounds; a hot, red, tender area around wounds or puncture sites; aches and pains; or total body collapse.

Healthcare practitioners devote a major portion of their time, energy, and talent to developing and maintaining practices to control the spread of microorganisms. These practices, known as aseptic techniques, are used in the broader context of infection control. Aseptic techniques, which start and end with handwashing, include the processes of cleaning, disinfection, and **sterilization**. The use of barriers to prevent the spread of microorganisms, such as gloves, masks, hair coverings, gowns, and patient **isolation**, is part of aseptic practice.

Agents Causing Infection

Agents causing infection include bacteria, viruses, fungi, parasites, **prions**, and MDROs.

BACTERIA

Bacteria are single-celled, independently living microorganisms, some of which are capable of causing disease in humans. Bacteria may be transmitted through air, food, water, soil, vectors, or sexual activity. They differ in size and shape, growth and replication requirements, and the method by which they inflict harm to the host. All bacteria are capable of diminishing organ function by invading tissues and initiating inflammation. Some are capable of producing metabolic toxins, which they secrete into the host (exotoxin producers). Examples of exotoxin producers are diphtheria, botulism, and tetanus. Others can produce poisons that are contained in their cell walls and released after the death of the microorganism (e.g., gram-negative endotoxin producers). Gonorrhea and meningococcal meningitis are examples of gram-negative endotoxins.

VIRUSES

Viruses are living microorganisms composed of particles of nucleic acid and protein that are often membrane bound. They reproduce inside living cells and cause various diseases. Some viral infections are acute and controlled by the host's defense mechanisms; others spread throughout the body and cause severe tissue damage or result in chronic illness, such as hepatitis and HIV. One virus in particular, Norovirus, causes an estimated 21 million gastroenteritis illnesses annually in the United States and 50% of the worldwide outbreaks of gastroenteritis (CDC, 2011).

FUNGI

Fungi are single-celled organisms that include molds and yeasts. *Candida albicans*, present as part of the normal human flora on mucous membranes and skin and in the gastrointestinal tract and vagina, can cause yeast infections of the mouth, skin, vagina, and intestinal tract in immunocompromised adults. *Candida* infections are known as **opportunistic infections** because they do not result in disease in individuals with properly functioning immune systems. Because *Candida* is an element of normal human flora and has the ability to live on many environmental surfaces, hospital-acquired (nosocomial) *Candida* fungal infections are becoming increasingly common and potentially fatal. Fungal infections of the hair, skin, and nails also frequently occur in humans. Fungi also infest and destroy plant life and cause fermentation in food and milk.

PARASITES

Parasites are multicellular organisms that live on other organisms without contributing anything to their hosts. Examples of parasites include protozoa, helminth, and arthropod species. Sexual contact, insects, and domestic animals frequently carry parasites to humans.

Protozoa are free-living microorganisms that commonly thrive in water. Humans often contract diseases related to protozoa through unsanitary conditions surrounding food preparation or handling. Malaria and sleeping sickness are examples of diseases caused by protozoa. Helminths are worms that infect the gastrointestinal tract or other body tissues of humans. Examples of helminths include tapeworms, hookworms, and trichinae (or pork worm). Arthropods, including mites, fleas, and ticks, are often responsible for skin and systemic diseases.

PRIONS

Prion diseases, also called transmissible spongiform encephalopathies (TSEs), are rapidly progressing neurodegenerative diseases affecting both animals and humans that are untreatable and always fatal. Prions are infectious agents composed primarily of proteins that cause an abnormal folding of proteins in the brain and neural tissue, leading to brain damage. The most common prion diseases are bovine spongiform encephalopathy (BSE; also known as "mad cow" disease) and Creutzfeldt-Jakob disease (CJD) in humans.

MULTIDRUG-RESISTANT ORGANISMS

Microbes, just like humans, adapt to an ever-changing environment to compete for survival. In the 1940s, strains of staphylococcus emerged that were immune to the antimicrobial activity of penicillin. Scientists developed new penicillins to treat these drug-resistant strains effectively. With time, increasing numbers of microbial organisms have developed drug-resistant strains and have caused problems for patients and healthcare workers in the hospital and the community. Each year in the United States, at least 2 million people become infected with bacteria that are resistant to antibiotics, and at least 23,000 people die each year as a direct result of these infections. Many more people die from other conditions that were complicated by an antibiotic-resistant infection. In 2013, the CDC published a report titled "Antibiotic resistance threats in the United States, 2013" outlining three levels of concern regarding MDROs—urgent threats, serious threats, and concerning threats (see Box 19-1).

BOX 19-1 Threatening Multidrug-Resistant Organism (CDC, 2013)

Urgent Threats
- *Clostridium difficile*
- CRE
- Drug-resistant *N. gonorrhoeae*

Serious Threats
- Acinetobacter
- Drug-resistant *Campylobacter*
- Fluconazole-resistant *Candida*
- ESBL-producing Enterobacteriaceae
- Vancomycin-resistant *Enterococcus* (VRE)
- Multidrug-resistant *Pseudomonas aeruginosa*
- Drug-resistant nontyphoidal *Salmonella*
- Drug-resistant *Salmonella typhi*
- Drug-resistant Shigella
- Methicillin-resistant *Staphylococcus aureus* (MRSA)
- Drug-resistant *Streptococcus pneumoniae*
- Drug-resistant tuberculosis

Concerning Threats
- Vancomycin-resistant *Staphylococcus aureus* (VRSA)
- Erythromycin-resistant group A *Streptococcus*
- Clindamycin-resistant group B *Streptococcus*

Factors that have contributed to the evolution of resistant microbial organisms include the following:

- Overprescription of antibiotics
- Use of inappropriate antibiotics for the infecting organism
- Incomplete use of antibiotic prescriptions as symptoms subside
- Harboring and spreading of resistant organisms by **carriers** who remain symptom free, usually unaware that they have been infected
- Increased use of antibiotics in farming, thus contaminating milk and meat

Resistance to the drugs used to treat these organisms is emerging rather quickly, limiting treatment options and increasing mortality and healthcare costs. Therefore, prevention and control of infections are crucial. The CDC has outlined four prevention strategies and seven control strategies to lessen the risk of infection. Prevention strategies include the following:

1. Infection prevention that includes the use of bundles to provide diligent care for vascular and urinary catheters and ventilators (see Chapters 21 and 32)
2. Swift and precise diagnosis and treatment for the infectious organism
3. Accurate use of antimicrobials
4. Meticulous adherence to evidence-based transmission prevention strategies

Control strategies include administrative support, judicious use of antimicrobials, surveillance, standard and contact precautions, environmental measures, education, and decolonization. It is well documented that healthcare workers' hands serve as vehicles, transmitting MDROs from one patient to another; this is why handwashing remains the most effective method of transmission prevention.

SAFETY ALERT

MDROs pose considerable health risks to the general population and specifically to healthcare workers. The infections they cause are increasingly difficult to treat and, in some cases, cannot be effectively destroyed by any known antibiotic. Using effective infection control practices, especially proper handwashing technique, is critical in these instances.

Chain of Infection

The life cycle of pathogens is frequently described as an uninterrupted chain of events. For organisms to spread disease, they must grow, reproduce, and move from one source to another. Nursing interventions are directed at stopping the transmission from the source to the patient and controlling other links in the chain, thereby controlling infection. The "chain of infection" includes the infectious agent, the source, the portal of exit, the mode of transmission, the portal of entry, and a susceptible host (Fig. 19-1).

INFECTIOUS AGENT

The first link in the chain of infection is the microbial agent, which may be a bacterium, virus, fungus, prion, or parasite. The ability of the infectious agent to cause disease depends on its **pathogenicity**, **virulence**, invasiveness, and **specificity**. Pathogenicity is the organism's ability to harm and to cause disease. Virulence relates to the vigor with which the organism can grow and multiply. *Invasiveness* describes the organism's ability to enter tissues. Specificity refers to the organism's attraction to a specific host. The more pathogenic, virulent, and invasive the organism, the more likely it can overcome normal body defenses, causing an infection. These four characteristics are determined by the structure or chemical composition of the microorganism, which includes the organism's ability to attach to skin and mucous membranes, the production of enzymes that counteract the immune system's response to invasion, and the production of toxins.

SOURCE

The sources of organisms, also called reservoirs, are elements in the environment. Inanimate objects (fomites), human beings, and animals are sources. Inanimate objects include medications, air, food, water, or any other material on which organisms can find nourishment or lie dormant and survive. Human sources include other patients, healthcare personnel, family

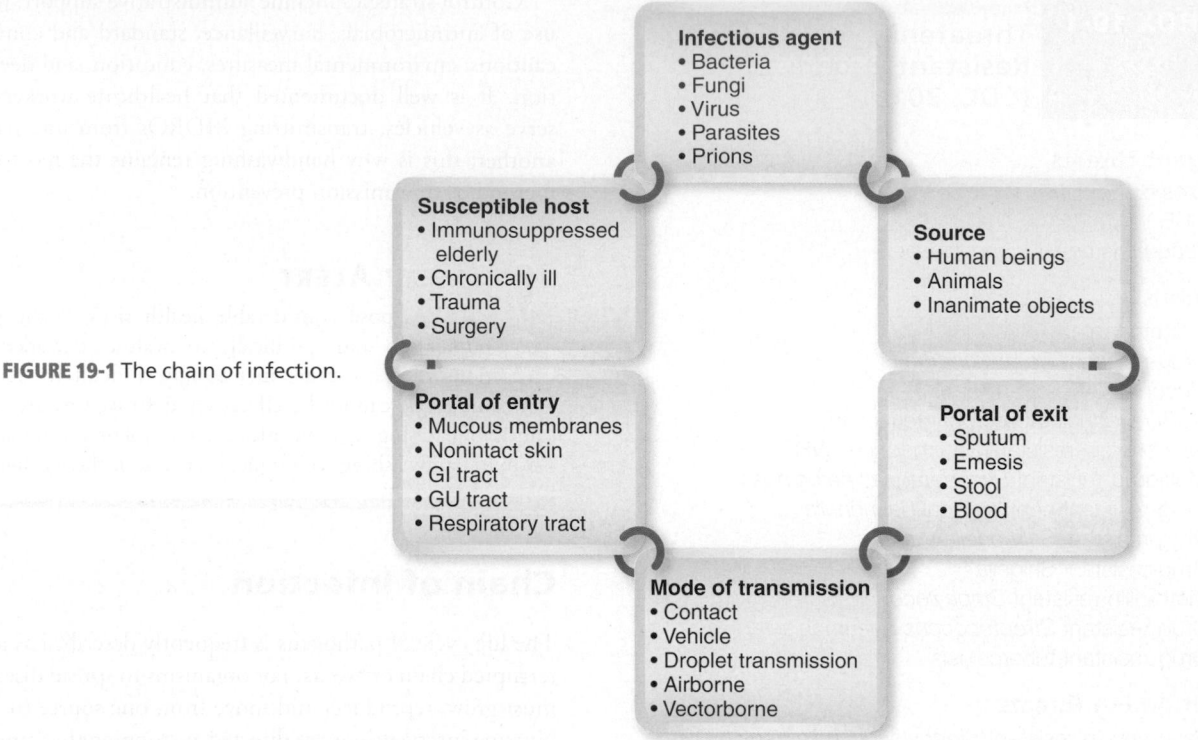

Infectious agent
• Bacteria
• Fungi
• Virus
• Parasites
• Prions

Susceptible host
• Immunosuppressed elderly
• Chronically ill
• Trauma
• Surgery

Source
• Human beings
• Animals
• Inanimate objects

Portal of entry
• Mucous membranes
• Nonintact skin
• GI tract
• GU tract
• Respiratory tract

Portal of exit
• Sputum
• Emesis
• Stool
• Blood

Mode of transmission
• Contact
• Vehicle
• Droplet transmission
• Airborne
• Vectorborne

FIGURE 19-1 The chain of infection.

members, visitors, and patients themselves. Patients may become infected from people who have active disease, people in the incubation portion of their disease, or people who harbor pathogens but have no symptoms of disease (known as carriers). A person's own bacterial flora may cause contamination when it is transferred to another organ or tissue. For example, endogenous microorganisms from the patient's gastrointestinal tract cause disease if they become established in the lungs, urinary tract, or a wound.

Animals are often sources of disease for human beings. Insects and rats have been responsible for historic epidemics in the past and continue to spread disease today. Scientists are particularly concerned with the threat of a pandemic outbreak of influenza, from one of the multiple avian influenza virus strains, including (1) the new H7N9 strain in China, which emerged in 2013; (2) the highly pathologic avian influenza H5N1 strain (HPAI H5N1); (3) the H5N2 and H5N8 strains prevalent in 2014; or (4) the swine influenza (H1N1 strain) (CDC, 2014b; CDC, 2014c). Currently, human risk is low because human-to-human transmission is rare. Unfortunately, the influenza virus continues mutating, and there have been cases in which people have been infected through contact with domestic poultry and swine. There is concern that further mutation may increase human-to-human susceptibility. Because of this continuing mutation, drug resistance is a very real risk.

PORTAL OF EXIT

The portal of exit provides a means for the microorganism to leave the source. Sputum, emesis, stool, urine, blood, wound drainage, or genital secretions all permit microorganisms to exit the source. Animal discharge or blood organisms carried by mosquitoes also can provide a means of escape.

MODE OF TRANSMISSION

Mode of transmission refers to the way in which the organism moves or is carried from the source's portal of exit. The five main routes of transmission are contact, vehicle, droplet, airborne, and vector borne.

Contact Transmission

Contact transmission is the most frequent means of transmitting infections in healthcare facilities. Contact transmission is by direct or indirect contact.

Direct contact involves body surface–to–body surface contact causing the physical transfer of organisms between an infected or colonized person and a susceptible host. Healthcare personnel can transfer organisms to patients during care such as bathing, dressing changes, and inserting invasive devices. Direct transfer also may occur between two patients, with one acting as the source and the other as the host. *Indirect* contact occurs when a susceptible host is exposed to a contaminated object, such as shared patient care devices (e.g., multipatient-use blood pressure cuffs, electronic thermometers, glucose monitoring devices), shared toys in a pediatric setting, needles, or inadequately cleaned surgical instruments.

Vehicle Transmission

Vehicle transmission involves the transfer of microorganisms by way of vehicles or contaminated items that transmit pathogens. For example, food can carry *Salmonella*, water can carry *Legionella*, drugs can carry bacteria from contaminated infusion supplies, and blood can carry hepatitis and HIV.

Droplet Transmission

Droplet transmission occurs when mucous membranes of the nose, mouth, or conjunctiva are exposed to secretions of an infected person who is coughing, sneezing, or talking. Droplets do not remain suspended in the air for very long and seldom travel more than 3 feet; thus, transmission is not via the airborne route. However, investigations of smallpox and the global SARS outbreak of 2003 suggest that droplets from these two infections could reach 6 feet or more from the source (CDC, 2007).

Airborne Transmission

Airborne transmission occurs when fine particles are suspended in the air for a long time or when dust particles contain pathogens. Air currents widely disperse organisms, which can be inhaled by or deposited on the skin of a susceptible host. Special air handling and ventilation systems called airborne infection isolation rooms (AIIRs) are needed to contain and remove the infectious agent (CDC, 2007).

Vector-Borne Transmission

Vectors can be biologic or mechanical. Biologic vectors are living creatures that carry pathogens, such as rats, insects, or birds. Transmission by biologic vectors is of great concern in tropical areas, where mosquitoes transmit diseases such as malaria. Mechanical vectors are inanimate objects that are contaminated with infected body fluids. Central line catheters, which are used for medications, blood draws, and total parenteral nutrition, and ventilators are examples of mechanical vectors. Contaminated needles and syringes shared by intravenous (IV) drug users are also examples of mechanical vectors. CA-MRSA, hepatitis B, and HIV are commonly spread in this manner.

PORTAL OF ENTRY

The portal of entry permits the organism to gain entrance into the host. Pathogens can enter susceptible hosts through body orifices such as the mouth, nose, ears, eyes, vagina, rectum, or urethra. Breaks in the skin or mucous membranes from wounds or abrasions increase opportunities for organisms to enter hosts. The practice in modern medicine of placing central venous catheters (CVCs) for long-term IV therapies or tubes for gastric feedings and drainage of body cavities further increases the number of potential routes of entry into the body, thus increasing the risk of infection. According to a 2011 CDC survey, 25.6% of the estimated 721,800 **healthcare-associated infections** (HAIs) that year were device-related infections (Magill et al., 2014).

SUSCEPTIBLE HOST

A host is a person whose own body defense mechanisms, when exposed, cannot withstand the invasion of pathogens. The body has numerous defense mechanisms that naturally resist entry and multiplication of pathogens. These factors are discussed in detail in Chapter 31. When infectious disease occurs in a human, the agent of infection has overcome the body's ability to resist infection. A primary focus of nursing practice is identifying patients whose defenses may be compromised and working to enhance their defenses.

Healthcare-Associated Infections

HAI is a term that encompasses infections contracted in all healthcare settings and is now used in place of the older term, **nosocomial infection**, which refers only to hospital-acquired infection. The change in terminology is due to the increasing infection rates and risks across all healthcare settings. Shorter hospital stays require increased reliance on outpatient facilities (e.g., clinics, surgery centers, dialysis centers) as well as extended care and rehabilitation facilities. This movement through the healthcare system increases the opportunity for infection transmission and cross-contamination among facilities (CDC, 2007). Infections contracted while the patient is in the healthcare setting may not be apparent at the time due to the infection's incubation period, delaying needed treatment and posing risks to the patient and to others in contact with him or her. The type, prevalence, and severity of pathogenic organisms vary within each setting. Knowledge of the population, the environment, and the pathogens most likely found in that environment permits nurses to focus their efforts on preventing the spread of infection.

RISK FACTORS IN THE DEVELOPMENT OF HEALTHCARE-ASSOCIATED INFECTIONS

The longer a patient is in a healthcare facility, the greater is his or her risk of infection. Exposure to the facility's environment changes the patient's own normal body flora. Risk factors that contribute to the development of HAIs can be grouped into three categories: environment, therapeutic regimen, and patient resistance. They interact in varying patterns of importance, but all must be considered when attempting to decrease the patient's risk.

Environment

Hospitals, outpatient clinics, extended care facilities, the home, and schools are reservoirs of organisms that pose threats to the increasing number of people who have decreased resistance. The sources of these organisms include the air; other patients; families and visitors; and contaminated equipment, food, and personnel. One multicenter sampling study found bacterial growth in 90 of 92 bath basins cultured (98%), indicating a possible source of transmission of HAI (Johnson, Lineweaver, & Maze, 2009). Pneumonia and influenza can spread rapidly among patients and other people in all types of facilities. Equipment that is not thoroughly cleaned, disinfected, or sterilized can spread many pathogens.

Therapeutic Regimen

Multiple factors involved in therapies used to treat patients also can contribute to the risk of infection. Drugs such as steroids, immunosuppressive agents, and cancer therapy, as well as prolonged use of antibiotics, predispose patients to infection. Equipment such as IV catheters, urinary catheters, feeding tubes, and ventilators provide routes for bacterial and fungal invasion. Inadequate dressing techniques for wounds can provide media for bacterial growth. Identifying treatments that pose risk and discontinuing their use as soon as possible decrease the chances of infection.

Patient Resistance

Changes in the physical or psychological status of a patient can affect his or her resistance to infection. Any break in the integrity of the skin or mucous membranes increases the chance of infection. For example, surgical site infections (SSIs) pose a very serious and common threat to postoperative patients. (See the display on SSIs in Chapter 22.) Stress, fatigue, poor nutrition, poor hygiene, and chronic illness also can decrease the patient's ability to ward off infection by impairing normal defenses. The elderly are extremely susceptible to infection because of age-related changes to major body systems. Immunocompromised patients are the most susceptible to infection because they are unable to invoke the immune response necessary to fight off infection-causing pathogens. Nurses play an important role in decreasing these risk factors by providing proper nursing care and education to all patients.

INFECTION RISKS IN VARIOUS HEALTHCARE SETTINGS

Patients can acquire infection in various obvious and not-so-obvious healthcare settings. These settings include acute care settings, long-term care facilities (LTCFs), ambulatory care settings, homes, schools, and the workplace.

Acute Care Settings

In a 2011 study, the CDC estimates that 712,800 hospital-acquired infections occurred in that year in the United States, down from its previous estimate of 1.7 million in 2007. Of those 712,800 infections, two infections tied for most prevalent—both pneumonia and SSIs were just under 22%. The third most prevalent infection was gastrointestinal infections (17.1%), of which 70.9% were *C. difficile*. Urinary tract infections (12.9%) and primary bloodstream infections (9.9%) rounded out the top five infections. *C. difficile* was the most prevalent pathogen, followed by *S. aureus*, *K. pneumonia* or *K. oxytoca*, *E. coli*, and *Enterococcus* species (Magill et al., 2014).

As MDROs continue developing, as people live longer, as more extensive surgeries are performed, and as more technology is used, the focus on HAI prevention must increase in importance. Controlling HAI rates will control healthcare costs and prevent the proliferation of difficult-to-treat, drug-resistant pathogens.

Long-Term Care Facilities

LTCFs, psychiatric care facilities, drug and alcohol treatment centers, and group homes for the mentally or physically impaired are associated with high risks for infection. Frequently, such institutions are understaffed, and available personnel may lack extensive training in infection control measures. Residents, sometimes debilitated from chronic medical or psychiatric conditions, may be incapable of maintaining their own personal hygiene. Communicable diseases are common in these

facilities, with the underlying medical problems of patients often placing them at risk for infections.

Ambulatory Care Settings

Patients come to ambulatory care settings for wellness visits and diagnosis and treatment for health problems. Procedures used by personnel frequently involve invasive techniques that increase the risk of infection. Waiting rooms in such facilities may contain people with active infections, increasing the risk of infection transmission. This is especially true for pediatric clinics, where children who are ill often come in contact with healthy children. Children frequently play with office toys or interact with one another, thus increasing the risk of infection.

Home Care

Shortened lengths of hospital stays and earlier discharges to the home decrease the incidence of hospital-acquired infections. However, patients being discharged to home care can be seriously ill and may require sophisticated invasive treatments to be performed at home, thus increasing the risk of infection in that setting. Treatments such as indwelling urinary catheters, IV infusions for medications or nutrition, and care of extensive open wounds and drainage collection systems are being seen more frequently in homes. Because caregivers in the home are assuming the primary responsibility for these treatments, they need education about how to perform prescribed procedures using aseptic practices to reduce the patient's risk. Caregivers must also learn how to care for family members with communicable illnesses and how to prevent spread of infection. Providing rationales during teaching improves understanding, retention, and compliance among patients and caregivers.

 APPLY YOUR CRITICAL THINKING

You are making a home visit to a single mother with three children younger than 5 years. When you arrive, the mother tells you that the oldest child has had a fever for 2 days, is lethargic, and has little appetite. After assessing the child, you suspect that he has influenza. Based on your knowledge that influenza is an airborne communicable disease, what health teaching regarding infection transmission is appropriate for the mother and family at this time?

Check your answer in Appendix B.

Schools

Classrooms, athletic departments, and school health clinics pose risks of infection to students and their teachers due in part to the proximity of individuals as well as the unknown infection risk during the incubation period. The incidence of communicable illness is high among children grouped together for study and play. Schools often employ nurses to teach health classes, monitor immunization schedules, and develop and monitor infection control practices and outbreaks of communicable diseases.

Their responsibility also includes evaluating children who may be infectious to help ensure proper treatment and prevent spread of infection to others.

Workplace

Employees are exposed to, and can expose their coworkers to, infections. Working conditions and materials that workers use may carry infectious risks. Farmers and other people who work with animals, for example, have a high risk of contracting diseases carried by animals. Sinks, bathrooms, lunchrooms, and food utensils may be sources of infection in the workplace. Many industries employ nurses to screen employees for communicable diseases, to collaborate with building maintenance personnel to maintain hygienic conditions, and to supervise waste disposal.

INFECTION CONTROL

Prevention and control of infections are important concerns for all types of healthcare agencies, and good infection control practices generate cost savings and improved outcomes for patients. Acute care hospitals have organized infection control programs. The infection control practitioner is usually a nurse with advanced training in infection control practices and methods for tracking the source and spread of infections (epidemiologic studies). Each department in the hospital must have written policies and procedures for the control of infection. Caregivers and support personnel (e.g., housekeepers, transport personnel) must have periodic educational updates on infection control, usually mandated annually. Various state and federal regulatory agencies require other healthcare facilities to have infection control policies.

Regulatory Agencies

Several local, state, regional, provincial, and national agencies are involved in overseeing institutional safety practices designed to protect patients, staff, and the community from infectious disease. Physicians' offices, school nurses, health clinics, LTCFs, and various acute care facilities must report episodes of infection to these agencies as required by law. In addition, over half of the states require public reporting of infection rates, with more being added annually. Guidelines as to what is a reportable disease vary according to location and circumstance. Good communication and rapport among clinical and regulatory agencies are necessary to optimize infection control and to prevent severe outbreaks of infectious disease. Agency statistics on the incidence of the disease in the area provide practitioners with information on control and treatment.

Both the CDC and the Joint Commission publish guidelines for monitoring and adhering to several evidence-based infectious disease control strategies. While several strategies focus on improving **hand hygiene**, the guidelines also focus on proper storage, cleaning and disinfection, and use of equipment and supplies. For example, the CDC publishes guidelines on both standard and transmission-based precautions.

Improved training of new hires and more in-service training sessions for employees are also recommended by these agencies to improve patient safety through infection control. The Joint Commission sets requirements that healthcare agencies must meet to obtain accreditation. The CDC does basic research on infectious disease and conducts large multicenter studies on data gathered by local centers. The Occupational Safety and Health Administration (OSHA) of the U.S. Department of Labor develops standards and regulations to protect the safety and health of workers (see Chapter 23).

Employee Health

Healthcare agencies maintain personnel health service programs as part of their infection control efforts. Infection control nurses often are involved in employee education programs. The objectives of such programs include stressing good health practices in diet, exercise, rest, and personal hygiene; monitoring and investigating potentially harmful infectious exposures and outbreaks of infections among personnel; providing care to personnel for work-related illnesses or exposures; identifying the infection risks related to employment; and instituting appropriate measures for preventing exposure and transmission of infectious disease.

MONITORING AND COUNSELING OF PERSONNEL

Almost all institutions require a personal health and safety education lecture as part of the orientation process and on an annual or semiannual basis. Some institutions require laboratory screening for high-risk diseases and offer their employees routine immunization programs. Mechanisms for prompt diagnosis and management of job-related illnesses and provision for prophylaxis of preventable diseases are important to ensure the health of all employees.

Access to health counseling about infections is especially important for women of childbearing age. Pregnant nurses may not be allowed to care for patients who have diseases that pose risks to fetuses. Among the diseases that pose particular risks to fetuses if contracted by pregnant women are rubella, parvovirus, rubeola, syphilis, hepatitis B, hepatitis C, group B streptococci, herpes simplex virus, varicella-zoster virus, cytomegalovirus, and HIV.

> **SAFETY ALERT**
> Personnel who are or who might become pregnant should be informed about potential risks to the fetus due to work assignments and about preventive measures that reduce those risks.

TRANSMISSIBLE DISEASES

Because hospital personnel are at risk for contracting and transmitting vaccine-preventable diseases, maintenance of current immunization status is a good health practice. Employees who

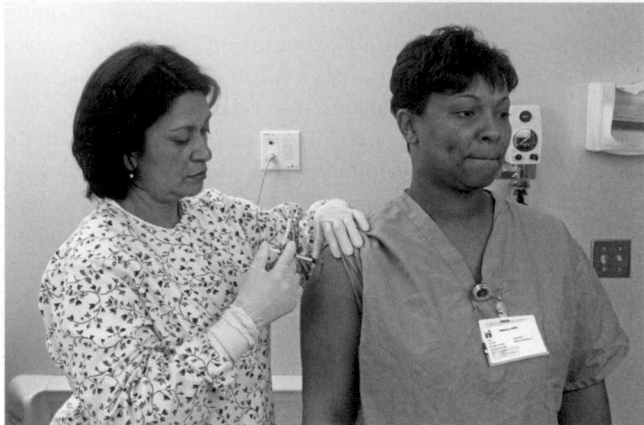

FIGURE 19-2 A flu vaccine is recommended for healthcare workers.

work in high-risk areas such as pediatric, dialysis, burn, or transplantation units are usually required to prove a current immunization status as a condition of employment. Chapter 31 contains a list of available vaccines and their effectiveness. Along with the mandatory purified protein derivative (PPD) test to screen for tuberculosis and vaccine policy for hepatitis B, the CDC also strongly recommends that all healthcare personnel with direct access to patients be vaccinated annually for influenza (Fig. 19-2). Despite these recommendations, for the

2013 to 2014 flu season, only 75.2% of all healthcare workers received the influenza vaccine (CDC, 2014d). Common reasons why healthcare personnel refuse to receive the influenza vaccine include the misconceptions that the vaccine may cause the flu and that their personal risk for contracting the flu is minimal. However, healthcare workers are often the source of influenza outbreaks: Many healthcare workers who are contagious with the flu virus do not exhibit symptoms, leaving the patients in their care at risk. It is also important to remember that with all illnesses, there is a period between the time when the pathogen enters the host and when clinical symptoms appear, known as the *incubation period*. Several states have made influenza vaccination mandatory for healthcare workers or require the individual to sign an informed declination. For those healthcare workers who refuse immunization, a mask may be required when providing care. Many other states have set regulations for personnel in LTCFs. According to the CDC, receiving the influenza vaccine is the responsibility of all healthcare personnel in the name of patient safety.

SIGNIFICANT EXPOSURE

Institutional policies and employee restrictions are designed to prevent exposure to, and contraction of, infectious disease. Any "significant" exposure is investigated to protect employees,

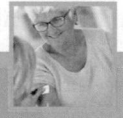

Asepsis and Infection Control PICO

Working on the oncology unit has increased your awareness of how susceptible immunosuppressed patients are to infection. You now support your hospital's decision to make annual flu immunization mandatory for all staff. You worry that many elderly, who are also immunocompromised, do not always get flu immunization. You decide to find a way to reach the senior citizens in your community to encourage influenza shots before the flu season hits. In the past, the public health department has tried sending information out to the seniors, but the responses were poor due to various factors such as cost, access, and knowledge deficits. You decide to use the Cochrane library to get some new ideas and evidence on how best to reach the senior community. The following PICO question guides your search: *In senior communities, how does having access to the flu vaccine compared to no access influence the rate of vaccination?*

P = senior communities
I = access to flu vaccine
C = no access to flu vaccine
O = influence rate of vaccination

You find an article that evaluated several interventions. The meta-analysis examined 57 randomized control trials involving 896,531 participants. The interventions focused on changing societal perception of the flu vaccine, ways to enhance more access, and involving providers to take an active role in encouraging the vaccine during annual exams. The overall results of these interventions showed statistically significant increase in the rate of vaccination. In particular, enhancing vaccination access included such things as group visits to physicians and nurses, home visits, and free influenza vaccinations. The latter two interventions seem to be effective in influencing seniors to get vaccinated.

You take the information from the study to discuss strategies with your manager to help the seniors of your community.

REFERENCE

Thomas, R. E., & Lorenzetti, D. L. (2014). Interventions to increase influenza vaccination rates of those 60 years and older in the community. *Cochrane Database of Systematic Reviews*, Issue 7. Art. No.: CD005188. doi: 10.1002/14651858.CD005188.pub3.

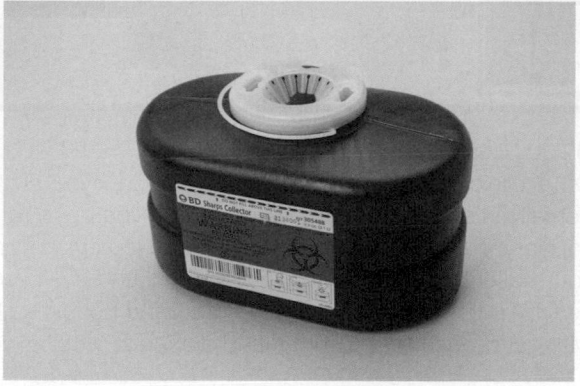

FIGURE 19-4 Disposal container for contaminated sharps.

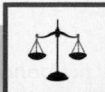

ETHICAL/LEGAL ISSUE

INFLUENZA VACCINE

As a registered nurse on a geriatric ward, you learn that your facility has initiated a new requirement that all personnel receive a flu vaccine or be terminated. The nurse manager presents the rationale for this decision as the responsibility to protect vulnerable patients from inadvertent exposure to the flu that could increase their hospital stay and contribute to increased morbidity and mortality.

CRITICAL THINKING CHALLENGE

- Explore your views about flu vaccine enforcement. How is mandatory flu vaccine different from other mandatory testing or vaccines (e.g., tuberculosis or hepatitis B) required by your employer?
- What reasons would you give your employer if you did not want the vaccine or did not agree with your employer for forcing you to get the vaccine? Are your reasons personal or evidence based?
- What responsibilities, if any, do you feel you have to the patients in your care regarding the flu vaccine?
- How would you respond to a patient you encouraged to get a flu vaccine who asks you If you received the vaccine?

Percutaneous Injuries

One potentially serious exposure for healthcare personnel is percutaneous injuries, which include needlesticks, sharps injuries, cuts, punctures, and percutaneous exposure incidents (PEIs) such as splashes, all of which may transmit bloodborne pathogens such as hepatitis B, hepatitis C, and HIV. The World Health Organization (WHO) reports that 2 million healthcare workers across the world experience percutaneous exposure to infectious diseases each year (Parantainen et al., 2008). The CDC estimates that 385,000 percutaneous injuries occur in U.S. hospitals each year. Prevention of occupational transmission of bloodborne pathogens requires a multifaceted approach to reduce blood contact and percutaneous injuries, which includes safer medical devices (e.g., needleless systems), technique changes to reduce handling of sharps, and the use of PPE (CDC, 2009). In the past, used needles were recapped, bent, or broken. The CDC strongly advises all institutions to educate their employees about the dangers of these practices (Fig. 19-3). Puncture-proof plastic units, often referred to as sharps containers, are provided in all patient areas for safe and immediate needle disposal (Fig. 19-4). Needle-housing systems and needleless systems have been developed and widely used to decrease the incidence of needlestick injuries (Fig. 19-5). Needlestick injuries decrease when needleless systems are used.

patients, and the institution. An exposure's significance is determined by the type and duration of exposure, with consideration of the mode of transmission, whether the host was susceptible, and whether precautions were taken. The infection control nurse commonly investigates exposures to hepatitis, rubella, meningococcal meningitis, tuberculosis, varicella (chickenpox), HIV, Norovirus, and novel influenza A (H5N1, H1N1, H5N2, and H5N8) (CDC, 2014b). Most exposures require timely reporting by staff members to expedite prophylaxis (if any is available) and to qualify for labor and industry insurance coverage should an illness result. If an employee contracts an infectious disease, it must be reported to the local health department.

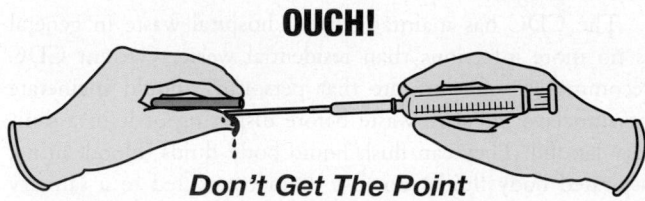

OUCH!

Don't Get The Point

NEVER RECAP NEEDLES

Use your NEEDLE DISPOSAL Container

Protect yourself - follow hospital, state, and national recommendations: NEVER RECAP NEEDLES

FIGURE 19-3 Sample needlestick hazard poster.

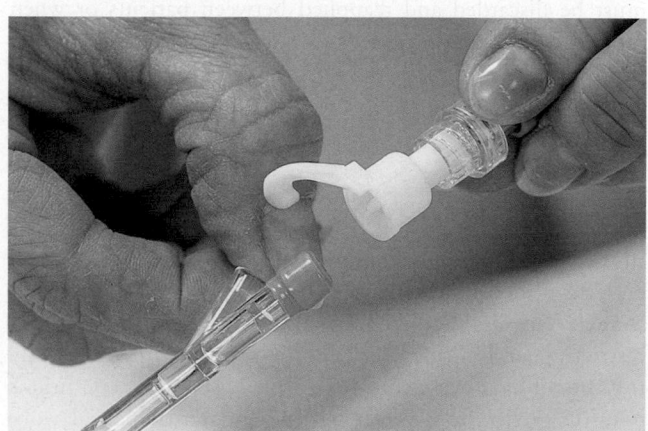

FIGURE 19-5 Needleless equipment prevents needlestick injuries. No needles are used, so stick injuries are avoided.

ETHICAL/LEGAL ISSUE

NEEDLESTICKS

On a clinical rotation as a nursing student, you accidentally stick yourself with a lancet after you perform a capillary fingerstick to obtain a blood glucose level for your patient. Your patient is 86 years old and has been healthy most of his life but now has been hospitalized with cardiovascular problems and diabetes.

CRITICAL THINKING CHALLENGE

- Explore your concerns after the needlestick injury. What risks are there (if any) for you and for the patient?
- When you disclose the incident to your clinical instructor, she explains that you and the patient must have blood drawn so that testing can be done to make certain you have not been exposed to blood-borne pathogens. You are worried about money and realize these tests will cost more than $300. Do you have the right to refuse testing? Weigh the consequences of having the testing versus not having the testing.
- If testing is done, what measures need to be taken to protect your confidentiality and that of the patient?
- Think about measures you or the agency could take to prevent this type of incident from happening in the future.

Gloves

Gloves cannot protect all personnel in every situation, but increased use of gloves during contact with all mucous membranes, nonintact skin, and moist body substances, in combination with good handwashing practices, makes a difference in cross-contamination between patients and staff. Gloves must be discarded and reapplied between patients or when moving from dirty to clean body surfaces. Be sure to *perform hand hygiene after each removal* to avoid spreading microorganisms from one patient to another or from one body surface to another.

WORK RESTRICTION

Ill healthcare employees should not be in contact with patients if their illnesses pose threats to patients or other personnel. Agencies should have well-defined policies directed at restricting or limiting work for personnel with potentially transmissible diseases. Table 19-1 lists the conditions requiring relief from direct patient contact or partial work restriction.

SAFETY ALERT

To avoid transmitting infection, healthcare personnel with diseases characterized by profuse coughing, sneezing, or frequent diarrhea should practice good self-care and stay home until their symptoms resolve.

HEALTHCARE WORKERS WITH AIDS

Personnel considered to have any of the clinical features associated with the AIDS spectrum should be counseled about the risks they pose to patients and to themselves in the work environment. Healthcare workers who perform invasive procedures in which a needlestick or scalpel injury would expose their blood to that of the patient pose the greatest risk. All personnel with AIDS should wear gloves for direct contact with mucous membranes or nonintact skin of all patients. Any healthcare worker with HIV/AIDS and exudative lesions or weeping dermatitis should refrain from all direct care and handling of patient care equipment until the lesions clear. All healthcare workers with AIDS need to be meticulous in adhering to infection control practices.

HIV impairs the immune system, making people with AIDS more likely to acquire infectious diseases or to experience more serious complications. These staff members also should be counseled about risks to themselves from coworkers and patients.

Waste Disposal

Local health agencies and the Joint Commission require hospitals to develop programs for disposal of wastes categorized as infectious, injurious, or hazardous to employees, patients, visitors, the general public, and the environment. Box 19-2 lists common materials within each category of institutional waste for which proper waste disposal protocol must be followed. Most waste that hospitals produce is not infectious, injurious, or hazardous. "Safe" waste includes paper, plastic, metal, and glass products used for a multitude of purposes within the healthcare agency.

The CDC has maintained that hospital waste in general is no more infectious than residential waste. Current CDC recommendations indicate that personnel should incinerate or autoclave infective waste before disposing of it in a sanitary landfill. They can flush liquid body fluids (blood, urine, aspirated body fluids) down a drain connected to a sanitary sewer system, based on local and state sewage requirements. Healthcare agencies use separate waste containers, clearly marked "Biohazard," for infectious waste, such as blood-contaminated items (Fig. 19-6). Because the cost of disposing of contaminated waste is great, it is important not to dispose of all waste in such containers.

TABLE 19-1 INFECTIOUS CONDITIONS REQUIRING WORK RESTRICTION

Infectious Condition	Direct Patient Care Restrictions and Duration
Conjunctivitis	Until discharge ceases
Diarrhea (with other acute symptoms)	Until 3 d symptom free and *Salmonella*, *C. difficile*, and Norovirus infections are ruled out
Group A streptococcal infection	Until 24 h after the start of treatment
Hepatitis A	Until 7 d after the onset of jaundice
Hepatitis B (acute)	Partial patient care restriction with gloves worn for procedures involving tissue trauma and mucous membrane or nonintact skin contact until signs of acute infection resolve (several weeks to 6 mo)
Hepatitis B (chronic)	Until antigenemia resolves
Herpes simplex (hands)	Until lesions resolve
Herpes zoster (acute)	Exclusion from care of patients until all lesions are dry and crusted, or in the absence of vesicular lesions, until no new lesions have appeared for 24 h
Herpes zoster (postexposure)	From days 8 to 21 after exposure or until all lesions are dry and crusted
Measles (active)	Until 7 d after rash appears
Measles (postexposure)	From days 5 to 21 after exposure
Mumps (active)	Until 5 d after onset of parotitis
Mumps (postexposure)	From days 12 to 26 after exposure
Norovirus	Until 3 d after symptoms resolve
Rubella (active)	Until 5 d after rash appears
Rubella (postexposure)	From days 7 to 21 after exposure
Scabies	Until treated
S. aureus skin lesions	Until lesions resolve
Upper respiratory tract infections	Until acute symptoms resolve with exclusion from care of patients at high risk for infection
Varicella (acute)	Until all lesions are dry and crusted
Varicella (postexposure)	From days 10 to 21 after exposure

BOX 19-2   Categories of Institutional Waste

Infectious Waste
Blood and blood products
Pathology laboratory specimens
Laboratory cultures
Body parts from surgery
Contaminated equipment (e.g., dialysis materials, suction receptacles)

Injurious Waste
Needles
Scalpel blades
Lancets
Broken glass
Pipettes
Aerosol cans

Hazardous Waste
Radioactive materials
Chemotherapy solutions
Caustic chemicals

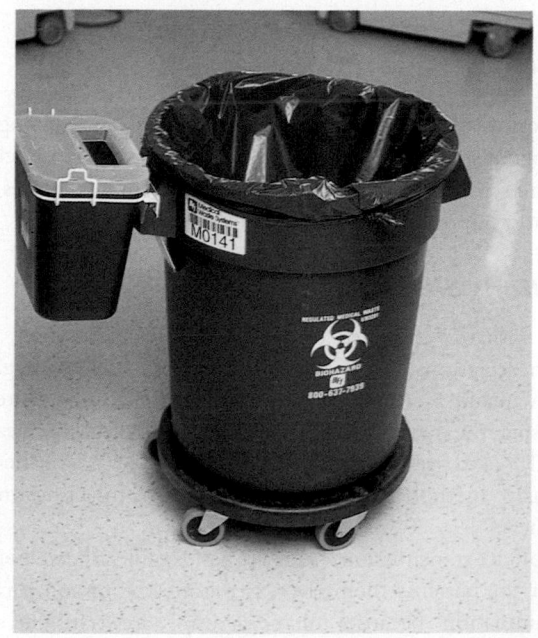

FIGURE 19-6 Waste container used for infectious waste in a dialysis unit.

ASEPTIC PRACTICES

The dramatic reduction in the incidence of infectious disease that occurred during the late 1800s and early 1900s resulted largely from the understanding that microorganisms cause disease and that they can be controlled through aseptic practices. Established control methods include use of physical agents, such as **disinfectants**, on agents outside the body; use of chemical agents, such as **antiseptics**, on inanimate objects and on the body surface; and use of chemotherapeutic agents, such as antibiotics, to combat microorganisms on body surfaces and inside the body.

The two major categories of aseptic practice are **medical asepsis** and **surgical asepsis**. Medical asepsis refers to measures taken to control and reduce the number of pathogens present. It is also known as "clean technique." Measures used to prevent the spread of organisms from place to place include hand hygiene, gloving, gowning, and disinfecting to help contain microbial growth. Surgical asepsis refers to "sterile technique." To be sterile, an object must be free from all microorganisms. Sterile technique is used to prevent the introduction or spread of pathogens from the environment into the patient. Sterile technique is employed when a body cavity is entered with an object that may damage the mucous membranes, when surgical procedures are performed, and when the patient's immune system is already significantly compromised. Procedures requiring sterile technique include insertion of IV catheters, injections, urinary catheterization, some irrigation of drainage tubes that enter sterile parts of the body, and all operative procedures.

For patients whose immune systems are compromised, certain procedures that normally would require clean technique should be performed using sterile technique. Examples of such patients include premature newborns, burn patients, transplant recipients, and patients receiving chemotherapy or radiation.

Medical Asepsis

Medical asepsis includes all measures aimed at reducing the number or spread of microorganisms. Using barriers and cleaning and sterilizing are important medical aseptic measures, but the most important of all is hand hygiene.

HAND HYGIENE

Even with the emphasis on wearing gloves for contact with patient secretions, nothing is more effective than hand hygiene, which includes either handwashing with soap and water or cleansing the hands with a waterless alcohol-based cleanser (Fig. 19-7) to prevent the spread of infection. It is also the least expensive method for decreasing the risk of infecting oneself or others.

Contact transmission, from the hands of healthcare personnel or the patients themselves, is the most common form of contamination because microorganisms are transient flora until the hands are washed. Improved hand hygiene practices

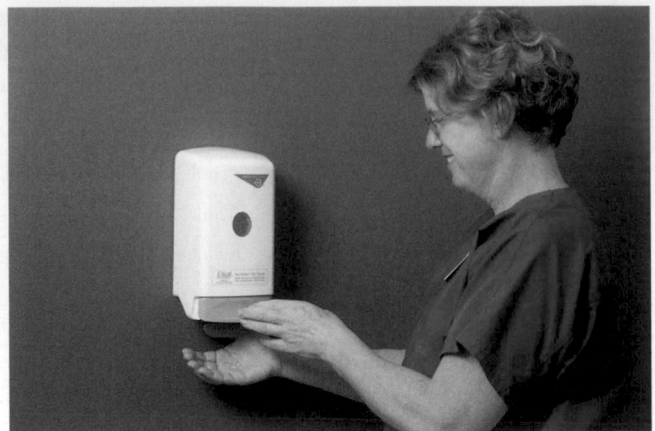

FIGURE 19-7 Alcohol-based hand gel.

can reduce HAIs and the development of antimicrobial resistance, thereby improving patient safety and quality of care.

 SAFETY ALERT
Proper handwashing is the single most effective method to prevent HAIs.

Despite this knowledge, hand hygiene compliance by healthcare workers remains poor. One study indicates that even when optimal conditions are present for hand hygiene to occur, compliance rates are still as low as 50% to 60% (De Wandel, Maes, Labeau, Vereecken, & Blot, 2010). Some factors that contribute to poor compliance with hand hygiene include the following:

- Lack of awareness of patient care activities that require hand hygiene, such as performing routine and "clean" activities, including taking blood pressure or shaking hands with a patient
- Common misperception that wearing gloves and gowns can substitute for hand hygiene
- Understaffing and high workloads leading to perceived time constraints
- Inaccessibility of sinks or dispensers for soap or alcohol-based cleanser
- Skin irritation and dryness

Many lotions counteract the effectiveness of antimicrobial soaps or interact with substances in gloves. Organizations, therefore, purchase appropriate pairs of lotions and soaps. Healthcare providers should not use personal lotions, but rather the lotion provided by the organization, in order to prevent any interaction or diminished effectiveness of soaps or gloves.

The WHO developed and implemented hand hygiene guidelines in 2009. These guidelines include recommendations in nine different areas:

- Indications for handwashing and hand asepsis
- Hand hygiene technique

- Surgical hand preparation
- Selection and handling of hand hygiene agents
- Skin care
- Use of gloves
- Other aspects of hand hygiene
- Healthcare worker educational and motivational programs
- Governmental and institutional responsibilities (WHO, 2009)

Box 19-3 summarizes the major recommendations of these guidelines.

Equipment necessary for hand hygiene (soap, running water, and paper towels or waterless alcohol-based antiseptics) is inexpensive and should be available readily to all healthcare providers.

> **SAFETY ALERT**
>
> Alcohol-based products are *not* effective against *C. difficile* or Norovirus, so handwashing with soap and water is required for any contact with a patient who has diarrhea.

High-risk areas such as newborn nurseries, critical care, transplantation and burn units, and operative suites may also require the use of antiseptic cleansing agents and nail files or sticks. Wash your hands before and after every patient care contact. The use of gloves during patient care does not eliminate the need for hand hygiene. Perform hand hygiene in the following situations:

- At the beginning and end of your shift
- Before contact with a patient

BOX 19-3 Hand Hygiene Guidelines

- Indications for washing hands with soap and water include visibly dirty hands, hands visibly soiled with body fluids, or after using the toilet.
- Handwashing with soap and water is required after exposure to potential spore-forming pathogens, such as *C. difficile* and Norovirus.
- Alcohol-based handrub is preferred in the following situations if hands are not visibly soiled: before and after touching a patient; before handling an invasive device for patient care; after contact with body fluids or excretions, mucous membranes, nonintact skin, or wound dressings; between contact with a contaminated body site to another site on the same patient; after contact with inanimate surfaces and objects; and after removing sterile or nonsterile gloves.
- Handwashing with soap and water is recommended when alcohol-based handrub is unavailable.
- Alcohol-based handrub or soap and water can be used before handling medication or preparing food.
- Concomitant alcohol-based handrub and soap use is not recommended.
- Soap and water handwashing technique includes using a towel to turn off the faucet, thorough drying of hands, and single towel use.
- Acceptable forms of soap are liquid, bar, leaf, or powdered.
- Bar soap racks should allow drainage to ensure that the soap dries.
- Alcohol-based handrub technique includes applying palmful amount of handrub, covering all surfaces, and rubbing hands until dry.
- Surgical hand hygiene recommendations include removal of jewelry, no brushes, and use of either antimicrobial soap or alcohol-based handrub according to the maker's recommendations.
- Selection of hand hygiene agents should consider input from healthcare workers, interaction with other products or gloves, risk for contamination, accessibility and proper

functioning of dispensers, approval of dispensers for flammable materials, and cost comparisons.
- Soap or alcohol-based handrub should not be added to partially empty soap dispensers.
- Skin care irritation in healthcare workers can be avoided by providing educational programs, alternative hand hygiene products for those with allergies or adverse reactions to standard products, and hand moisturizers to reduce irritant contact dermatitis.
- Glove use does not replace the need for handrub or handwashing.
- Gloves should be used if contact with potentially infectious body fluids, mucous membranes, or nonintact skin is anticipated.
- Gloves should be removed or changed after each patient or after contact with a contaminated body site.
- Artificial nails or extenders should not be used, and the length of natural nail tips should be less than 0.5 cm.
- Educational and motivational programs for healthcare workers should focus on behavior, be multimodal, include senior executive support, educate about the advantages and disadvantages of various hand hygiene methods, monitor adherence and provide performance feedback, and encourage partnership between patients, families, and healthcare workers.
- Healthcare administrators should provide and monitor safe, continuous water supply; provide alcohol-based handrub at the point of patient care; prioritize compliance; provide leadership, administrative support, and financial resources; ensure training; implement a multidisciplinary, multifaceted, and multimodal program to improve adherence; and adhere to national safety guidelines and local legal requirements.
- National governments should prioritize adherence; consider funded, coordinated implementation and monitoring; support strengthening of infection control in healthcare settings; promote community hand hygiene; and encourage use of hand hygiene as a quality indicator in healthcare settings.

- Between contacts with different patients
- Before and after contact with wounds, dressings, specimens, or bedclothes
- Before and after performing any invasive procedure
- Before administering medications
- After contact with any patient secretion or excretion
- After body fluid exposure
- After contact with the patient's environment
- Before and after using the bathroom
- After sneezing, coughing, or blowing your nose
- After removing gloves every time
- Before eating

Medical and surgical asepsis vary in the technique for proper handwashing. Hand hygiene performed to ensure medical asepsis is described in **Procedure 19-1**. Handwashing for surgical asepsis usually takes longer, is more methodical, and requires the use of antimicrobial agents. Long-term flora on the hands resides in the nail bed and under the fingernails. Pay special attention to these areas, and use soft sticks or fingernails from the opposite hand to clean them. Ideally, remove all rings before handwashing and place them in pockets or pin them to the uniform during patient care to minimize the places that could harbor bacteria. If you wear a thin wedding band, slide it up on the finger to cleanse the area under the ring properly.

! SAFETY ALERT

Keep fingernails short, and avoid nail polish because cracked or chipped nail polish can harbor bacteria that ordinary handwashing cannot reach. Artificial fingernails present similar reservoirs for infectious agents and are typically not allowed.

If the hands become dry or cracked or develop dermatitis, a person may be less apt to wash them as often as necessary. This problem is a common complication for people with sensitive skin. Switching to another soap or antiseptic solution, thoroughly drying after every washing, and using skin lotion that is appropriately paired to the type of soap used may help. Alcohol-based hand sanitizers are known to be less abrasive and irritating on skin than washing with soap and water.

! SAFETY ALERT

Always wear gloves during patient care when your skin is abraded. Using alcohol-based hand sanitizers decreases skin irritation and drying that leads to skin breakdown.

All patients and their family members should learn proper handwashing techniques. Provide patients with materials that explain the importance of washing their hands before and after toileting. Instruct all visitors to wash their hands before contact with patients and before leaving a patient's room. Instruct

and empower patients to request all healthcare providers and visitors to wash their hands if they forget to do so. If infection is to be controlled, the paramount importance of adequate handwashing cannot be stressed too often, no matter how unsophisticated it may seem.

 **Concept Mastery Alert**

Hand hygiene, whether performed with soap and water or an alcohol-based rub, does not render the nurse's hands sterile. Hand hygiene greatly reduces the load of infectious microorganisms on the nurse's skin, but it does not produce the complete absence of microorganisms that constitutes sterility.

DISINFECTION AND STERILIZATION

Disinfection and sterilization remove potentially pathogenic microorganisms.

Disinfection

Disinfection refers to chemical or physical processes used to reduce the number of pathogens on an object's surface. These processes do not necessarily remove all potential for infection because spores, capable of growing at a later time, may remain. A chemical used on lifeless objects is called a disinfectant. A chemical used on living objects is called an antiseptic. Solutions that are disinfectants at higher concentrations may be diluted to be used as antiseptics on living objects. A chemical is **bactericidal** if it kills microorganisms; an agent that prevents bacterial multiplication but does not kill all forms of the organism is called **bacteriostatic**. To be useful, the method chosen must kill or retard growth of the pathogens without damaging the material or person being treated.

Sterilization

Sterilization refers to the complete destruction of all microorganisms, including spores. Sterilization processes are caustic because they require extremes of heat, potent chemicals, or gas that cannot be used on body tissues. Any process used to sterilize equipment must be effective in killing organisms but not destructive to the equipment.

Most items are purchased as sterile or are sterilized by steam sterilization in an autoclave. If the items might be destroyed by the heat used during autoclaving, ethylene oxide gas or chemical solutions may be used. Two of the most popular methods of sterilization are steam sterilization and gas sterilization with ethylene oxide. Chemical indicators, which change color when the object being sterilized has been exposed to steam penetration for a specific period, are placed outside and inside the object's package. This practice enables the healthcare worker to know when sterilization of an object has been effective (Fig. 19-8). Load stickers are also used to trace the sterilization process back to a specific sterilizer. Contamination can occur at a later time, so packaging should be checked for integrity. The sterility of a package does not change with the passage of time,

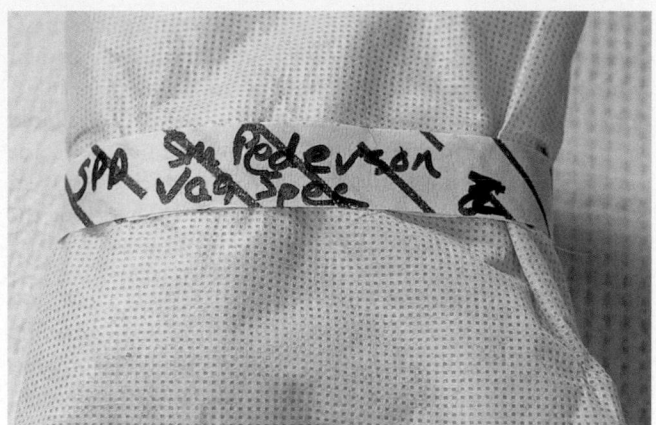

FIGURE 19-8 Color indicator strips change color indicating one or more of the conditions necessary for sterilization have been achieved within the package.

but it may be affected by certain events (e.g., amount of handling) or environmental conditions (e.g., humidity) (Conner, 2014, p. 564).

> ! **SAFETY ALERT**
>
> Any item entering sterile tissues or the vascular system, such as surgical instruments, IV and urinary catheters, implants, IV fluids and medications, and needles, must be sterile.

USE OF PERSONAL PROTECTIVE EQUIPMENT

Techniques or equipment that prevents the transfer of pathogens from one person to another are referred to as "barriers" or PPE. Their aim is to contain pathogens by establishing aseptic barriers around the patient and personnel. Recommendations for specific PPE are outlined later in this chapter in Box 19-4 and Table 19-2. The most commonly used PPE and barriers are masks and respirators, gowns, gloves, private rooms, waterproof disposal bags for linen and trash, labeling and bagging of contaminated equipment and specimens, and control of airflow into sterile areas and out of contaminated areas. With the advent of AIDS and other serious infections, goggles or face shields have been added to the list when splashing is likely to occur, as well as check valves on masks used in mouth-to-mouth resuscitation. Staff awareness about the need to prevent cross-contamination of people, equipment, and supplies is most important. See **Procedure 19-2:** Applying and Removing Personal Protective Equipment.

Masks and Respirators

Masks prevent transmission of infectious agents through the air. They protect the wearer from inhaling both large-particle droplets, which are transmitted by close contact and usually travel only a short distance (up to 3 feet), and small-particle droplets, which remain suspended in the air and may travel farther. Masks lose their effectiveness if they are wet or are worn for long periods. They also are ineffective when they are

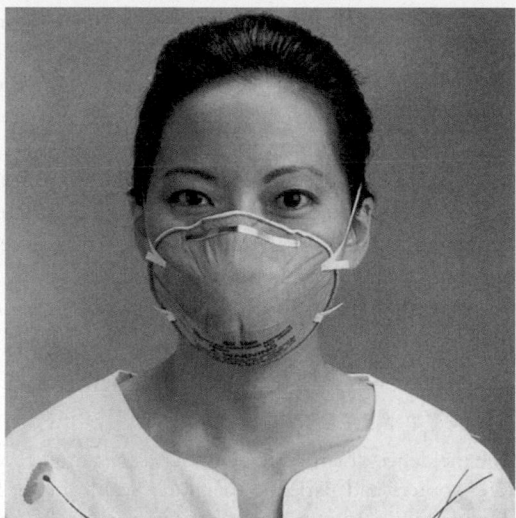

FIGURE 19-9 Particulate respirator fits tightly to the face and filters out organisms as small as 1 μm.

not changed after caring for each patient. Masks should not be worn away from patient care activities.

Disposable particulate respirators (N95 or higher level) are indicated whenever a caregiver is working with a patient who has, or is suspected of having, contagious airborne diseases such as tuberculosis (Fig. 19-9). Respirators look like masks but fit the face more tightly and are able to filter out particles or organisms as small as 1 μm. Individual mask fitting is recommended because a tight seal must be maintained. Nurses working in communities with high-risk populations need to carry respirators and use them whenever indicated.

Gowns

Gowns should be worn when the caregiver's clothing is likely to be soiled by infected material. Many agencies use paper disposable gowns. Use gowns only once, and change gowns when they become moist. Always remove gowns using proper technique and dispose of gowns in a proper laundry or disposal container before exiting the patient's room.

Caps and Shoe Coverings

Caps are used to cover the hair, and special covers are available for shoes. Surgical hats should cover ears and all hair (including the nape of the neck). Hoods should be worn to cover sideburns and beards. Products are available for use in high-risk areas (e.g., labor and delivery, emergency room) to shield body parts from accidental exposure to contaminated body secretions.

Gloves

Gloves protect personnel from acquiring infective organisms on their hands. They also reduce the likelihood that personnel will transmit their own or other patients' microbial flora from their hands to patients. Wear clean, nonsterile gloves when direct contact with moist body substances from any patient is anticipated. Change and discard gloves between patients or when they become torn or grossly soiled. Do not wash and reuse gloves. Perform hand hygiene before gloving, when changing gloves during care due to soiling or tearing, and after glove removal.

Latex and synthetic latex-free gloves, such as vinyl, are two categories of gloves widely used clinically. Latex gloves are made of natural rubber and are more flexible and durable. Although they are more expensive, latex gloves are preferred when lengthy exposure is anticipated or fine motor skills are required. The use of latex gloves for routine care activities is unnecessary, adds to the cost of care, and increases the risk of latex allergy. Many facilities are providing only latex-free clean gloves at point of care. When latex gloves are used, wash hands after removing gloves to help decrease the potential for development of an allergy over time.

> ! **SAFETY ALERT**
> The incidence of latex allergy is increasing among health-care workers and patients; therefore, healthcare facilities must be sure that neither personnel nor patients are allergic to latex when latex gloves and products are used. If a latex allergy is suspected, special latex-free gloves and other equipment are available.

Vinyl gloves made of polyvinyl chloride, a synthetic rubber, fit loosely and offer less protection than do latex gloves but are usually adequate for routine patient care activities, such as emptying bedpans, handling specimens, or providing hygiene.

Gloves can give a false sense of security; therefore, there are important safety measures to keep in mind when using gloves. Hand hygiene must be performed before donning gloves and every time gloves are removed. Working from clean to dirty on body surfaces and work surfaces will decrease the chance of spreading infection. Avoiding unnecessary touching of self or objects in the environment will reduce contamination. Double-gloving is indicated during activities when gloves may tear or puncture, such as during surgical procedures.

Goggles or Face Shields

Goggles and face shields are used as personal protection when splashing is likely, such as during wound irrigation or when contamination from respiratory secretions or blood splatter is possible. Goggles provide protection for the eyes, and face shields provide protection for the eyes, mouth, nose, and facial area. Never substitute personal eyewear for goggles or face shields.

Private Rooms

Separation of patients into private rooms decreases the chance of transmission of infection by all routes. If this is impossible, place a patient with an infection in the same room as another patient who is infected with the same microorganism. Special AIIRs (formerly called negative airflow rooms) are indicated for patients infected with tuberculosis or other organisms transmitted by the airborne route. High risk infected individuals who may require a private room include children younger than 5 years, patients with altered mental status, and patients with large, draining wounds or blood loss that cannot be contained in dressings.

Whenever possible, avoid transporting patients with infections who need a private room. If transport to another department is necessary, change the patient's gown and dressings before leaving the room and make sure that the patient wears appropriate barriers, such as a mask or gown. If the infection is transmitted by the airborne route, the patient should wear a mask and the transporters should be immune to the disease. Be sure to notify the department to which the patient is being transported so that staff members are aware of the patient's status and can take appropriate precautions.

Equipment and Refuse Handling

Special handling of articles and linen soiled by any body fluid is indicated. Place these articles in impervious bags before they are removed from the patient's bedside. Bagging in watertight containers is indicated to prevent exposure of personnel and contamination of the environment. Do not contaminate the outside of the bag when placing articles inside it. Each hospital and community agency has procedures for labeling and decontaminating exposed articles. Rinse items that are visibly soiled with body substances and place them in plastic bags or clearly marked containers, often labeled as "Contaminated," in dirty utility rooms before returning them to the central processing areas. If the outside of the bag becomes contaminated, place that bag in another bag (double-bagging).

ISOLATION SYSTEMS

Isolation refers to techniques used to prevent or limit the spread of infection. Some form of isolation has been used for centuries, whether to protect a high-risk person from exposure to pathogens or to prevent the transmission of pathogens from an infected person to others.

The first two manuals published by the CDC recommended only category-specific isolation. Increased episodes of hospital-associated infections (especially among immunocompromised patients) and the AIDS epidemic in the 1980s fostered the development of two new systems—universal precautions and body substance isolation. Universal precautions relate to blood and certain body fluids and are designed to protect healthcare workers from patients who may be carrying HIV, hepatitis B virus, or other bloodborne pathogens. Body substance isolation involves the use of barriers to provide protection from all moist body secretions. In 1995, the CDC introduced guidelines for a two-tiered system of isolation precautions that includes **standard precautions** and transmission-based precautions:

1. Standard precautions for all patients to protect against blood and body fluid transmission of potential infective organisms
2. Transmission-based precautions to protect against the spread of highly transmissible or epidemiologically significant pathogens in patients with documented or suspected infection

This two-tiered system is an attempt to synthesize different systems and to improve adherence to appropriate infection control practices. Transmission-based precautions are used in addition to standard precautions when organism have been identified and the route of transmission is known.

Isolation systems are costly in terms of equipment, supplies, and the time that they require from caregivers. However, even more expensive are breaks in isolation technique that result in infection. All healthcare personnel and staff, including physicians, nurses, technicians, students, and housekeepers, are responsible for understanding and complying with isolation precautions. Furthermore, all personnel are ethically responsible for tactfully calling observed infractions to the attention of those who do not comply. Compliance is best obtained by using a consistent, simple system; educating staff; and instilling a sense of personal responsibility in all caregivers. The infection control committee usually examines all systems of isolation and decides on guidelines and procedures to use throughout the particular healthcare agency.

Standard Precautions

Standard precautions decrease risk of transmission from bloodborne pathogens and transmission from moist body substances. This system protects against the transmission of both undiagnosed and identified infections. The use of standard precautions protects healthcare providers and patients using healthcare services. Box 19-4 details the guidelines of standard precautions.

Transmission-Based Precautions

When highly transmissible or significant pathogens have been identified, additional isolation may be required to prevent the spread of infection. Depending on the organism identified and its mode of transmission, airborne precautions, droplet precautions, or contact precautions may be instituted. Combined protocols may be used if the organism has more than one mode of transmission. See Table 19-2 for a complete description of transmission-based precautions.

Airborne Precautions. Airborne precautions are used to protect against microorganisms transmitted by small-particle droplets that can remain suspended and become widely dispersed by air currents. The patient should be cared for in an AIIR. Healthcare personnel should wear an N95 respirator mask when performing patient care and make sure that the patient wears a mask when transported out of the room.

Droplet Precautions. Droplet precautions are used for microorganisms transmitted by larger-particle droplets, which disperse into air currents. For droplet precautions, make sure the patient is in a private room or with a person who is infected with the same microorganism. An AIIR is not required. Use masks when working within 3 feet of the patient. The patient should wear a mask when outside the room.

Contact Precautions. Contact precautions are used with organisms that can be transmitted by hand- or skin-to-skin contact, such as during patient care activities or when touching the patient's environmental surfaces or care items. When patients are known to be infected with significant organisms (e.g., MDROs), extra care is required to prevent transmission, and contact precautions are instituted. The patient is cared for in a private room or has a roommate who is infected with the same organism. Use gloves when entering the room, and change the gloves when exposed to potentially infected material during care delivery. Remove gloves before leaving the patient's room. Use gowns and other protective barriers when contamination is likely, either from the patient, the environmental surfaces, or the patient's room.

BOX 19-4   Standard Precautions

A. Wear clean gloves when touching:
   1. Blood, body fluids, secretions, and excretions, and items containing these body substances
   2. Mucous membranes
   3. Nonintact skin
B. Perform handwashing immediately:
   1. When there is direct contact with blood, body fluids, secretions and excretions, or contaminated items
   2. After removing gloves
   3. Between patient contacts
C. Wear a mask, eye protection, and face shield during procedures and patient care activities that are likely to generate splashes or sprays of blood, body fluids, or secretions and excretions.
D. Wear a cover gown during procedures and patient care activities that are likely to generate splashes or sprays of blood, body fluids, secretions, or excretions, or cause soiling of clothing.
E. Remove soiled protective items promptly when the potential for contact with reservoirs of pathogens is no longer present.
F. Clean and reprocess all equipment before reuse with another patient.

G. Discard all single-use items promptly in appropriate containers that prevent contact with blood, body fluids, secretions and excretions, contamination of clothing, and transfer of microorganisms to other patients and the environment.
H. Handle, transport, and process linens soiled with blood, body fluids, and secretions and excretions in such a way as to prevent skin and mucous membrane exposures, contamination of clothing, or transfer to other patients and the environment.
I. Prevent injuries with used needles, scalpels, and other sharp devices by:
   1. Never removing, recapping, bending, or breaking used needles
   2. Never pointing the needle toward a body part
   3. Using a one-handed "scoop" method, special syringes with a retractable protective guard or shield for enclosing a needle, or blunt-point needles
   4. Depositing disposable and reusable syringes and needles in puncture-resistant containers
J. Use a private room or consult with an infection control professional for the care of patients who contaminate the environment or who cannot or do not assist with appropriate hygiene or environmental cleanliness measures.

TABLE 19-2 TRANSMISSION-BASED PRECAUTIONS

	Precautions	Indications
Airborne	Private AIIR with adequate filtration; mask; mask worn by the patient during transport out of room	Transmission via airborne route (small-particle droplets); tuberculosis, measles, varicella
Droplet	Private room or cohabitation with the patient infected with same organism; mask required when working within 3 feet of the patient; mask worn by the patient during transport	Transmission of large droplets through sneezing, coughing, or talking; *Haemophilus influenzae*, multidrug-resistant strains, *Neisseria meningitidis*, diphtheria, rubella, *Mycoplasma pneumoniae*
Contact	Private room or cohabitation with the patient infected with same organism; gloves at all times (don before entering room and remove before leaving) with change after exposure to organism; handwashing immediately after removal of gloves; gown and protective barriers when direct contact with organism occurs; daily cleaning of bedside equipment and patient care items; exclusive use of items such as stethoscope and sphygmomanometer for infected patient with terminal disinfection when precautions are no longer necessary	Serious infections easily transmitted through direct contact; any multidrug-resistant strains, *C. difficile*, *Shigella*, impetigo, and others

Protective Isolation

Protective isolation may still be used in high-risk situations to prevent infection for people whose body defenses are known to be compromised. Patients who are neutropenic (neutrophils less than 500/mm³) as a result of chemotherapy, radiation therapy, or immunosuppressive medications are prime candidates. Patients with extensive burns or dermatitis are also at high risk for infection. Such patients are placed in private rooms. Everyone practices strict and meticulous handwashing, including the patient and his or her family. Visitors are restricted. No fresh fruits or vegetables are allowed, only canned and cooked foods. Flowers, either in water or soil, are not permitted because soil harbors fungus and standing water supports the growth of microorganisms. All of these measures help to ensure that the patient's environment stays as free from pathogens as possible, thereby decreasing the chance of infection.

Psychological effects of being separated from healthcare personnel, family, and friends may occur when isolation precautions are used. Patients spend more time alone. The bodies, hands, and faces of caregivers are covered. Patients may mistakenly feel dirty or untouchable, especially if they have diseases that are considered socially unacceptable. Lack of social interaction can be psychologically injurious, especially to children and their parents. Maintaining the patient's social support before, during, and after care by being present, listening to the patient's concerns, and answering questions while adhering to infection control practices is crucial for the patient's well-being and healing. Answering call lights promptly to alleviate feelings of abandonment is also important.

Surgical Asepsis

The purpose of sterile technique is to prevent the introduction of microorganisms from the environment to the patient. Surgical asepsis is used in the following circumstances:

- Surgical procedures
- All procedures that invade the bloodstream

- Procedures that cause a break in skin or mucous membranes (e.g., intramuscular injections)
- Selected dressing changes and wound care
- Procedures involving insertion of catheters or devices into sterile body cavities (e.g., bladder)
- Care for selected high-risk people or groups (e.g., transplant recipients, burn patients, immunosuppressed patients)

When all organisms and their spores have been destroyed, the item is deemed sterile. These items are clearly labeled as sterile on their packaging. The packaging must not be torn, punctured, wet, or outdated. During any sterile procedure, care must be taken to keep all sterilized equipment sterile. Adhering to proper sterile technique can help eliminate breaks in sterile procedure, but if breaks in technique do occur, replace sterile equipment before resuming the procedure.

PRINCIPLES OF SURGICAL ASEPSIS

Surgical asepsis starts with thorough planning and preparation of the environment, supplies, and personnel. Although surgical asepsis is carried out in many settings, the operating room is the area where surgical asepsis is used most extensively. Staff members in the operating room require special training in maintaining aseptic technique for various operative procedures. Operative suites are specially constructed rooms that provide for no-touch surgical scrub handwashing at sinks controlled by foot pedals, have special airflow patterns, and control traffic into and out of areas.

Good personal hygiene is basic behavior for all personnel. A shower should be taken before beginning the workday. Staff members who are ill with respiratory infections or who have conditions that cause diarrhea, vomiting, or skin lesions should not participate in sterile procedures. All scrub attire must be hospital washed. Street attire is not generally worn in the operating room or in other hospital areas where sterility is important. In certain situations (observers, vendor representatives, etc.), personnel can enter the operating areas in street attire that is completely covered by a "bunny suit." Shoes must be

THERAPEUTIC DIALOGUE: ASEPSIS

SCENE FOR THOUGHT

Arnie McKellan is 43 years old, with acute lymphocytic leukemia, and has been admitted to the oncology unit for treatment for a serious MDRO. The nurse is meeting him for the first time and is wearing a mask, gown, and gloves.

LESS EFFECTIVE

Arnie: Well, well, another astronaut entering the forbidden planet. And who are you, spaceperson?! *(Looks annoyed and depressed but sounds cheerful.)*

Nurse: Well, I'm Sally Ride, the first woman astronaut! How's it going with you today? *(Very cheerful, answers with the same tone of voice.)*

Arnie: Couldn't be better with all the space people coming in here. I get lots of company and nobody's done anything awful to me yet. How can I complain? *(Looks strained, and his eye contact begins to slip.)*

Nurse: Well, I'm not here to change that part yet. I'm really Sheila Evans, your nurse for the evening shift. I need to take a history and do a nursing assessment. It won't take long. I can see you're tired. *(Sits down in the chair next to the bed and begins to write.)*

Arnie: Yes, I really am. I'd appreciate it if you'd make it quick. *(Continues to look strained.)*

Nurse: Sure, no problem. *(Proceeds to ask some assessment questions. Arnie makes jokes and answers questions shortly, usually with sarcasm.)* You know, I can't tell if you're serious or joking sometimes! Makes it hard to fill out this assessment.

Arnie: Well, I'll try my best to be serious all the time from now on! Are you done yet? *(Sounds irritated.)*

Nurse: Yes, I am, for now. I'll let you rest now and I'll be back with your dinner tray. We can talk some more then. *(Leaves thinking, "Just what I need. An angry patient!")*

Arnie: *(Turns to the wall and sighs.)*

MORE EFFECTIVE

Arnie: Well, well, another astronaut entering the forbidden planet. And who are you, spaceperson?! *(Looks annoyed and depressed but sounds cheerful.)*

Nurse: I'm Susan O'Shea, Mr. McKellan, your nurse for the evening shift. You sound cheerful today. Are you? *(Stands next to the bed.)*

Arnie: Of course! Wouldn't you be, getting to spend all this time alone and space people coming to see you every 5 minutes? *(Says this with great sarcasm.)*

Arnie: No, I'd be lonely and annoyed. *(Says this quietly and seriously.)*

Arnie: *(Looks away and stays quiet for awhile. So does Susan.)* I don't want to feel depressed about this admission, Susan. I know it's going to be one of many. So I guess I've been a little loud and sarcastic. I can tell you won't let me get away with it. *(Smiles.)*

Nurse: *(Laughs.)* We can get loud together later, but we have other work to do first. Maybe I could start with the reason for the "spacesuits" and then we could go on to a short history and physical. How does that sound? *(Makes an alliance with Arnie, being sure to laugh rather than smile, which is hidden by the mask.)*

Arnie: Okay, okay. Especially the part about the masks and everything. I'm not used to it. Makes me feel terminal already!

Nurse: Sounds like we have a lot to talk about. Let's get to it. *(Explains about the reason for the isolation, what's involved, how long it will go on, and so forth. Arnie listens carefully, asks questions, and makes a few jokes but appears more relaxed.)*

CRITICAL THINKING CHALLENGE

- List behaviors that indicate Arnie is angry, afraid, apprehensive, and annoyed.
- Compare and contrast how Sheila and Susan responded to these behaviors.
- Identify each nurse's concerns.
- Appraise your emotional reaction when you're confronted by an irritated, sarcastic person, and describe what you do.
- Examine the aspects of communication that are lost with a mask.

covered with shoe covers, and beards and hair must be covered by hoods and caps. Surgical hats/hoods should not be removed while in surgical scrubs, to prevent spreading of hair and microorganisms into the air. Jewelry should not be worn on the hands. Other jewelry must be covered by scrub attire. General principles of surgical asepsis are discussed in Table 19-3.

SKIN PREPARATION

Skin preparation reduces microorganisms present on the skin. Bacteria on the skin include both transient and resident flora. The transient microorganisms are held in place by sweat, oil, and debris. They can be removed easily with soap and water or ETOH-based solution (e.g., chlorhexidine gluconate) and by

TABLE 19-3 PRINCIPLES OF SURGICAL ASEPSIS

Technique/Principle	Rationale
Moisture causes contamination. • Handle liquids carefully near sterile fields to prevent splashing. • Place wet objects in sterile, water-impermeable surfaces, such as sterile basins.	Microorganisms travel more easily through moist environments. When a sterile surface becomes moist, microorganisms may be transmitted from an unsterile surface by capillary action.
Never assume that an object is sterile. • Check to see that it is labeled as sterile. • Always check the integrity of the packaging. • Always check the expiration date on the package. • If there is any doubt about the sterility of an object, it should be considered unsterile.	Commercially prepared products are labeled as sterile on their packaging. Special indicators are used to show that objects have completed their sterilization process, such as tapes on the outside of packages or chemically impregnated paper inside containers. Packages that are torn, punctured, or moist cannot be considered sterile. All packaging materials should have clearly visible dates that indicate when sterility cannot be guaranteed. Items that have passed that date cannot be used.
Always face the sterile field.	The area defined as sterile for the purposes of the procedure is the "field." Objects that are out of the line of vision may be inadvertently contaminated, and their sterility is never guaranteed.
Sterile articles may touch only sterile articles or surfaces if they are to maintain their sterility.	Anything considered unsterile may transfer microorganisms to the sterile object it touches. An object used on an unsterile surface, such as swabs used in cleaning the skin, must be used once and then discarded because skin cannot be sterilized. Keep unsterile objects away from the field.
Sterile equipment or areas must be kept above the waist and on top of the sterile field. • Drapes hanging over the edge of the table are not considered sterile.	Waist level is the limit of good visual field. By defining only the top of the field as sterile, maximum visibility of all sterile objects used in the procedures is ensured. The front of the sterile gown should be considered sterile only from the chest to the level of the sterile field. The neckline, shoulders, axilla, and back of the surgical gown should be considered contaminated. Gown sleeves should be considered sterile from 2 inches above the elbow to the cuff, circumferentially.
Prevent unnecessary traffic and air currents around the sterile area. • Close doors. • Unfold drapes or wrappers slowly. • Do not sneeze, cough, or talk excessively over the sterile field. • Do not reach across sterile fields.	Microorganisms cannot be completely excluded from the air even with the best filtration and airflow designs. Movement creates air currents that circulate organisms in the air. Masks do not contain all organisms expelled from the oral or nasal cavities and become moistened more quickly from talking. Move around a sterile field or turn the field slowly by reaching under the drapes if an object is not convenient to a sterile person.
Open, unused sterile articles are no longer sterile after the procedure.	Once the protective wrappings have been removed, the article is being contaminated by the air. Even if it is untouched and resting on a sterile surface, it must be discarded or resterilized before it is used. Liquids opened during the procedure that remain in their original container are also considered to be contaminated.
A person who is considered sterile who becomes contaminated must re-establish sterility.	If a "scrubbed" person punctures the gloves or is contaminated accidentally by touching an unsterile object, he or she must change the contaminated article. If a scrubbed person leaves the area of the sterile field, he or she must go through the procedure of rescrubbing, gowning, and gloving.
Surgical technique is a team effort. • A collective and individual "sterile conscience" is the best method of enhancing sterile technique.	Staff members must rely on one another to maintain sterile technique. Individuals who are considered sterile must have access to sterile supplies delivered to them by circulators in the operating room or prepared by themselves at the bedside. Team members must be open to critiques by other members about their technique and respond to their suggestions that objects or their clothing have been contaminated or that they have contaminated an object. Periodic review of procedures and infection control surveillance reports enhance everyone's sterile technique.

the friction of scrubbing. Resident flora adheres to epithelial cells and extends into hair follicles and glands in the skin and varies according to location on the body.

Antiseptic agents are used in skin preparation and surgical scrubs to reduce the number of transient microorganisms. They do not penetrate into the dermis, nor are they able to remove all resident floras. The mechanical action of scrubbing and rinsing with water helps remove organisms from deeper layers of the skin, but a portion of these bacteria remains. When surgical gloves are worn, especially for extended periods, resident flora grows and replicates from deeper skin layers.

The following are the objectives of surgical scrubs and patient skin preparation:

• To remove dirt, oil, and microorganisms from the skin
• To reduce bacterial counts to subpathogenic levels
• To avoid abrading the skin
• To leave a layer of antimicrobial material on the skin that inhibits the growth of microbes for an extended period

Typically, a patient's skin preparation consists of several steps. Unless contraindicated, patients should perform two perioperative baths or showers with 4% chlorhexidine gluconate before surgery (Conner, 2014). Hair removal is accomplished by clipping with electric clippers. Shaving, once ordered before surgery, is no longer performed because tiny nicks in the skin may predispose the patient to infection.

SURGICAL HANDWASHING

Surgical hand scrubs differ in both technique and length from general handwashing that the nurse performs during most patient encounters. A disposable scrub sponge is usually impregnated with antimicrobial scrub solutions. The solution is either an iodophor solution or 4% chlorhexidine gluconate. Follow the manufacturer's guidelines for all surgical hand preparations. Sterile nail cleaners made of plastic or metal should also be available. Antiseptic soap containers that dispense solution by knee or foot pressure must be located above or next to a splash-proof sink.

Before starting the scrub, remove all nail polish. Keep fingernails short and without sharp edges that can puncture surgical gloves. Make sure your hands are free from lesions, cuts, or abrasions, because traumatized skin can harbor bacteria. Always hold hands higher than the level of the elbows and away from the body to allow water to run off at the elbows. Water running down the arms to the hands can cause contamination. Thoroughly dry your hands on a sterile towel.

STERILE FIELD

A sterile field is an area free from microorganisms on which sterile items can be placed. This provides a work surface to facilitate maintaining sterility during a sterile procedure. Drapes or sterile wrappers can be used to create a sterile field. Sterile items are transferred to the surface by peeling back packaging and dropping the item onto the field without contact with anything nonsterile. See **Procedure 19-3**: Preparing and Maintaining a Sterile Field.

> **❗ SAFETY ALERT**
>
> Always place sterile objects on a dry surface and avoid splashing liquids when pouring; moisture causes contamination.

STERILE GLOVES

Sterile gloves are mandatory for all procedures that require surgical technique. Gloves are worn to prevent contamination of wounds, equipment, supplies, and the sites of invasive procedures. Sterile gloves are donned after the hands have been thoroughly cleaned. For procedures performed at the bedside, it is common to use the open method of gloving, which is outlined in **Procedure 19-4**.

In the operative suite or during invasive procedures, the preferred method for donning gloves is to be gloved by another team member who is already in surgical attire. The first practitioner uses the closed technique and then assists others.

In the closed method, don the sterile gown and slide your hands into the sleeves until the cuff seam is reached. Keep the hands inside the gown sleeve. Then, using the dominant hand, pick up a cuffed glove for the other hand. Draw the glove over the nondominant hand, and pull the sleeve onto the wrist. Glove the dominant hand in the same manner using the sterile glove on the other hand.

> **❗ SAFETY ALERT**
>
> If your gloves become punctured or torn during a sterile procedure, change them immediately to reduce the chance of contamination. Any puncture or tear of gloves during sterile procedures allows organisms on the hands to contact an open wound.

LIFE SPAN CONSIDERATIONS

Newborns and Infants

Prevention of infection in newborns begins by protecting the fetus from infection exposure during pregnancy. Maternal infections can be transmitted to the fetus during pregnancy, resulting in minor or major congenital anomalies or fetal death, depending on the time of exposure and the organism involved. In general, the earlier in pregnancy the mother is infected, the more severely the fetus is affected. A very mild or asymptomatic infection in the mother can have serious consequences for the fetus. Very early in pregnancy, when exposure is most dangerous, the mother may be unaware that she is pregnant. Adequate prenatal care is important in decreasing the incidence of maternal infection.

> **❗ SAFETY ALERT**
>
> All women of childbearing age should have up-to-date immunizations. Urge pregnant women, or those trying to get pregnant, to avoid exposure to infectious disease whenever possible.

The most frequent mode of transmission of organisms to the infant is from direct contact with the skin and hands of caregivers and, to a lesser extent, through contaminated infant formula. Handwashing is the single most important means for preventing hospital-associated infections in the newborn. Teaching all caregivers the importance of scrupulous handwashing and general good hygiene is an important role for nurses. Another area important to infection prevention is immunizations, which begin during infancy and continue through childhood. Nurses can provide parents and other caregivers with immunization schedules and teach them the important role vaccination plays in preventing many contagious diseases.

Toddlers and Preschoolers

Young children frequently become infected because normal behavior at this age fosters transmission of microorganisms. These children usually are not toilet trained and have poor personal hygiene. Playing on the floor, continually putting objects in the mouth, and even playing with bodily secretions all contribute to exposure to potential pathogens. For both toddlers and preschoolers, increased exposure to groups of children in day care or preschool is another factor affecting the spread of infection. Upper respiratory tract and subsequent ear infections are common among these age groups.

Teaching about hygiene practices that limit infectious exposure is important for toddlers and preschoolers. Proper handwashing after use of the bathroom and before meals is an important habit for young children to develop. If children of this age are exhibiting signs of infection, advise parents and other caregivers to avoid exposing them to other children so that infection transmission can be minimized.

School-Age Children and Adolescents

During the school years, the incidence of many infections decreases because of children's more mature immune systems and completion of routine childhood immunizations. Direct contact and airborne transmission of infections are more common in the winter months because children crowd into schoolrooms and engage in indoor recreational activities. Often, skin eruptions such as impetigo and lice infestations occur because these children may share personal hygiene aids, clothing, and sports equipment. Reinforcement of proper handwashing and hygiene practices is important.

Adolescence brings new elements of exposure. Injuries occur more frequently and may predispose teens to infection. The incidence of sexually transmitted infections (STIs) and mononucleosis starts to rise when adolescents begin sexual activity. Respiratory infections and viral diseases are common because many group activities keep adolescents in close quarters.

School nurses play a significant role in detecting and preventing the spread of infections among older children and adolescents. Health teaching is also important in preventing injury and STIs among these groups.

Adults and Older Adults

By adulthood, most people have acquired immunity to many communicable diseases. However, infection as a complication of injury and STIs continues to be a threat. As adults increase their independence and travel, especially to foreign countries, they may be exposed to new infectious organisms. Elective surgical procedures can also pose infection risks. In addition, monitoring to ensure current immunization status for the adult is important because adults frequently forget to update immunizations as necessary. Also, in working with adult populations, stress the importance of preventive health practices to reduce the risk of developing chronic disease states (e.g., diabetes, cardiovascular disease, drug and alcohol dependence, cancer), thereby decreasing infection risk.

Complications of long-standing chronic diseases in older adults predispose this population to higher incidences of infection. Older adults may be predisposed to serious infections because of decreased nutritional status, waning immunologic responses, decreased activity level, poor circulation, frequent breaks in skin integrity, urinary retention, and impaired mechanical clearance mechanisms. Previous diseases such as tuberculosis and herpes zoster can be reactivated, and older adults may be more vulnerable to the various microorganisms that cause community and HAIs. Severely disabled older adults are at particular risk because they often cannot perform their own personal hygiene. Immobility, incontinence, and dysphagia also greatly increase infection risk, and if invasive devices are needed for these dysfunctions, the infection risk is even higher.

Hospitalized older adults incur hospital-associated infections at two to five times the rate of younger patients. They have higher rates of pneumonia, urinary tract infections, bacteremia, and SSIs during their hospital stays, and they usually require treatment with vigorous courses of antibiotics. If patients are placed in LTCFs while receiving continuing antibiotic regimens, they risk developing antibiotic-resistant infections. When these patients, who are potential reservoirs for transmission to others in their LTCFs, are readmitted to acute care hospitals, they become reservoirs for the new facility. Thus, they may require several acute care admissions and pass on more virulent organisms with each round trip.

Cultural Considerations

The concepts of personal hygiene and infection control develop very early in an individual and are greatly influenced by family, community, and the culture of origin. Hygiene practices can vary widely within the same culture and different groups living in the same country or area.

The WHO created a task force to look at religious and cultural aspects of hand hygiene. Their findings are reported in the *WHO Guidelines on Hand Hygiene in Health Care* (WHO, 2009) and discuss cultural and religious considerations surrounding the issue of hand hygiene. Two purposes for this task force were to create guidelines that could be spread throughout the entire globe, into all regions, cultures, and religious environments, and to consider both behavioral and transcultural issues in the plan to promote hand hygiene to both healthcare workers and patients.

These guidelines discuss such topics as:

- Generic hand hygiene practices that are influenced by religious and cultural factors. For example:
  - Buddhism—washing hands after every meal and washing hands of the deceased
  - Christianity (Catholics)—washing hands after handling holy oil
  - Hinduism—washing hands after prayer, after any unclean act (e.g., toileting), before and after any meal

- Islam—washing hands before prayers five times a day, before and after any meal, after toileting, after touching anything soiled (e.g., a dog, shoes, or a cadaver)
- Judaism—washing hands first thing in the morning, before and after each meal, and after toileting
- Sikhism—washing hands in the early morning, after each meal, and after taking off or putting on shoes
- Hand gestures with different meanings in different cultures
- The concept of "visibly dirty" hands in the context of different cultures, different skin colors, and different perceptions of dirtiness
- The prohibition of alcohol use in the Buddhist, Hindu, Islamic, and Sikh faiths

The WHO recommends taking all cultural and religious beliefs into consideration when both interacting with patients and families and when considering goals and plans for patient education.

KEY CONCEPTS

- Infectious disease is the most common reason people contact healthcare providers and accounts for more clinic and physician office visits than any other cause in the United States.
- Agents that cause infection, such as bacteria, viruses, fungi, prions, and parasites, occur everywhere in the environment—on body surfaces, in food, and in products used in normal activities of daily living.
- The chain of infection includes the infectious agent, the source, the portal of exit, the mode of transmission, the portal of entry, and a susceptible host.
- The three common modes of transmission are contact, droplet, and airborne. Vectors also account for the spread of some diseases.
- Contact transmission of infectious organisms on the hands of caregivers is the most frequent mode of transmission of infection in healthcare facilities.
- Resistance to the drugs used to treat MDROs is emerging rather quickly, limiting treatment options and increasing mortality and healthcare costs.
- The incidence of infections associated with healthcare delivery (HAIs) can be decreased with strict adherence to evidence-based infection control practices.
- Risk factors in the development of HAIs include environment, therapeutic regimen, and patient resistance.
- Effective infection control measures have a favorable cost–benefit ratio.
- Hand hygiene is the *single most important* infection control practice. All caregivers and patients and their family members should learn hand hygiene techniques.
- To aid in the fight against infection and to increase compliance with handwashing, alcohol-based handrubs are recommended for all healthcare delivery sites.
- Intact skin and mucous membranes are major barriers against organisms and transmission of infection. Invasive procedures and surgeries can jeopardize this line of defense.

- Regulatory agencies at local, state, regional, and national levels are involved in the control of infection and institutional waste to protect patients, staff, and the community.
- Employee health programs to monitor and counsel personnel are important components of institutional and community infection control programs.
- Institutional waste disposal methods are important factors in infection control programs.
- Aseptic practices are those techniques used to keep people or objects free from microorganisms. Cleaning, disinfection, and sterilization can be accomplished by various methods and agents.
- The use of barriers, also known as PPE, such as gloves, gowns, caps, and shoe coverings, is important in preventing the spread of infection.
- Gloves should be worn whenever there could be contact with the patient's body secretions.
- Private rooms are used to decrease the chance of transmission of infection by all routes.
- Sterile technique is used to prevent the introduction of microorganisms from the environment to the patient during surgery, invasive procedures, or in selected high-risk situations.
- An item is sterile when all organisms and spores on the object are destroyed.
- Infectious exposures and the risk of contracting infectious disease change during a person's life span.

PRACTICING FOR THE NCLEX

CHECK YOUR ANSWERS IN APPENDIX A.

1. A patient diagnosed with pneumonia is exhibiting an elevated temperature, high white blood count, and low blood pressure with increased heart rate. Which of the following would describe the patient's condition?
   - a. Sepsis
   - b. Infectious disease
   - c. Opportunistic infection
   - d. Nosocomial infection

2. A patient is identified as having MRSA in his sputum. Which of the following transmission routes would be most appropriate?
   - a. Contact
   - b. Vehicle
   - c. Airborne
   - d. Droplet

3. What type of PPE would be appropriate for assisting with respiratory care of a pediatric patient with pertussis (whooping cough)?
   - a. Gown and gloves
   - b. Gown, gloves, and mask
   - c. Gown, gloves, and mask with eye shield
   - d. Gown, gloves, and respirator

4. HAIs are gaining attention as preventable conditions among hospitalized patients. Which of the following include common HAIs? Select all that apply:
   a. Pneumonia
   b. Urinary tract infections
   c. SSIs
   d. Central IV line infections

5. A nurse is finished changing a wound dressing for a patient on contact precautions for *Clostridium difficile*. Which of the following would be appropriate hand hygiene? Select all that apply:
   a. Before and after dressing change
   b. Using soap and water after removing gloves
   c. Before medication administration
   d. Using alcohol-based gel when leaving room

6. Which of the following terms best describes the synthesis of major features of decreasing risk of transmission of bloodborne pathogens and body substance isolation?
   a. Universal precautions
   b. Medical asepsis
   c. Standard precautions
   d. Protective isolation

7. A nurse has completed caring for a patient with MRSA in the sputum. As she exits the room, what is the most appropriate way to remove her PPE and wash hands?
   a. Remove gloves, wash hands, remove gown, face shield, and mask
   b. Remove gloves, wash hands, face shield, gown, mask, and wash hands
   c. Remove gloves, gown, face shield, mask, and wash hands
   d. Remove gown, wash hands, gloves, mask, goggles

8. A nurse is inserting an indwelling catheter into a female patient (a sterile procedure). Which is the most important first step in maintaining a sterile field?
   a. Never turn your back to the sterile field.
   b. Unfold sterile drape away from your body.
   c. When adding sterile supplies, hold 10 to 12 inches above the field and allow them to drop.
   d. Inspect the sterile kit for package integrity, contamination, or moisture.

9. A nurse is assisting a surgeon with the placement of a chest tube at the bedside. She begins to apply sterile gloves by inserting her nondominant hand into the glove. What does she do next?
   a. Unfold the cuff using the inside of the glove.
   b. Adjust the fingers and glove fit, keeping the hands above the waist.
   c. Slip gloved hand inside second gloved cuff.
   d. Insert dominant hand, extending cuff down the arm.

10. A nurse is explaining the transmission of hepatitis A to a new public health nurse. Which of the following explanations of the chain of infection would be most correct?
    a. Infected human → stool → vehicle transmission → gastrointestinal tract
    b. Infected human → vector-borne transmission → blood → nonintact skin
    c. Infected human → gastrointestinal tract → contact transmission → stool
    d. Contact transmission → stool → gastrointestinal tract → infected human

REFERENCES

Centers for Disease Control and Prevention. (2007). *Guideline for isolation precautions: preventing transmission of infectious agents in healthcare settings.* Retrieved January 11, 2015, from www.cdc.gov/hicpac/2007IP/2007isolationPrecautions.html

Centers for Disease Control and Prevention. (2009). *Influenza vaccination and exposure management modules.* Retrieved January 11, 2015, from www.cdc.gov/nhsn/PDFs/HSPmanual/5_HPS_fluVacc.pdf

Centers for Disease Control and Prevention. (2011). Updated Norovirus Outbreak Management and Disease Prevention Guidelines. *Morb Mortal Wkly Rep, 60,* (3). Retrieved January 2, 2015, from http://www.cdc.gov/mmwr/pdf/rr/rr6003.pdf

Centers for Disease Control and Prevention. (2013). *Antibiotic resistance threats in the United States,* 2013. Retrieved September 20, 2014 from http://www.cdc.gov/drugresistance/threat-report-2013/

Centers for Disease Control and Prevention. (2014a). Infection Prevention and Control Recommendations for Hospitalized Patients with Known or Suspected Ebola Virus Disease in U.S. Hospitals. Retrieved January 2, 2015, from http://www.cdc.gov/vhf/ebola/hcp/infection-prevention-and-control-recommendations.html

Centers for Disease Control and Prevention. (2014b). Avian Influenza A Virus Infections in Humans. Retrieved January 2, 2015 from http://www.cdc.gov/flu/avianflu/avian-in-humans.htm

Centers for Disease Control and Prevention. (2014c). Avian Influenza A (H7N9) Virus. Retrieved January 2, 2015 from http://www.cdc.gov/flu/avianflu/h7n9-virus.htm

Centers for Disease Control and Prevention. (2014d). Influenza Vaccination Information for Healthcare Workers. Retrieved January 11, 2015 from http://www.cdc.gov/flu/healthcareworkers.htm

Conner, R. (Ed.). (2014). *Perioperative standards and recommended practices, 2014 edition.* Denver, CO: Association of periOperative Registered Nurses (AORN).

De Wandel, D., Maes, L., Labeau, S., Vereecken, C., & Blot, S. (2010). Behavioral determinants of hand hygiene compliance in intensive care units. *American Journal of Critical Care, 19*(3), 230–239.

Johnson, D., Lineweaver, L., & Maze, L. M. (2009). Patients' bath basins as potential sources of infection: A multicenter sampling study. *American Journal of Critical Care, 19,* 31–40.

Magill, S., Edwards, J., Bamberg, W., Beldavs, Z., Dumyati, G., Kainer, M., et al. (2014). *Multistate Point-Prevalence Survey of HealthCare–Associated Infections. N Engl J Med, 370,* 1198–1208. doi: 10.1056/NEJMoa1306801

Parantainen, A., Anthoni, M., Valdes, A., Lavoie, M. C., Hellgren, U. M., & Verbeek, J. H. (2008). Prevention of percutaneous injuries with risk of hepatitis B, hepatitis C, or other viral infections for health-care workers (Protocol). *Cochrane Database of Systematic Reviews,* Issue 2. Art. No.: CD007197. doi: 10.1002/14651958.CD007197.

World Health Organization. (2009). *WHO guidelines on hand hygiene in health care.* Retrieved January 11, 2015, from http://www.who.int/gpsc/5may/tools/9789241597906/en/

Procedure 19-1 **Hand Hygiene**

Purpose	1. Reduce the numbers of resident and transient bacteria on the hands.
	2. Prevent transfer of microorganisms from healthcare personnel to the patient and others.

Equipment	Warm, running water
	Soap (most agencies supply liquid soaps, containing a germicidal agent, in dispensers at each sink.)
	Paper towels
	or
	Alcohol-based hand gel

Assessment	• Inspect hands for breaks or cuts in skin or cuticles.
	• Identify appropriate times for handwashing before, during, and after patient contact.
	• Identify need to repeat handwashing if hands become contaminated during a procedure.
	• Determine whether waterless alcohol-based product is appropriate or if soap and water are necessary.

Procedure

1. **Remove all rings except a plain wedding band. Push watch 4 to 5 inches above wrist.**

   Rationale: Microorganisms lodge in the irregular surfaces of jewelry.

For Alcohol-Based Product

2. **Apply a generous amount of waterless alcohol-based gel to the palm of your hand (Fig. 1).**

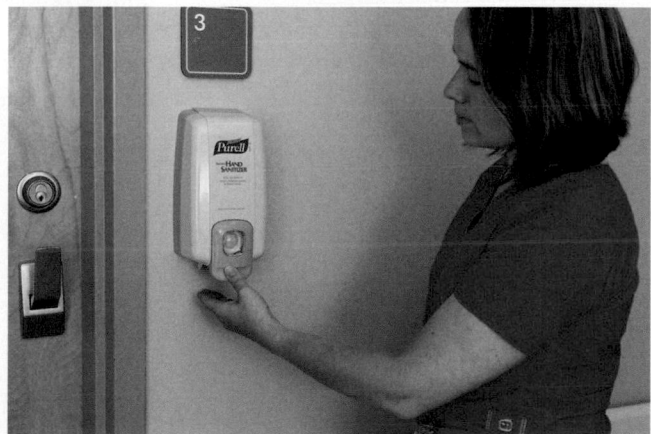

FIG. 1 Apply alcohol-based gel.

   Rationale: Enough gel must be available to moisten all skin surfaces of the hands for adequate cleansing to occur.

3. **Spread gel to all skin surfaces by rubbing palms of hands together (Fig. 2), rubbing each palm over the top of the other hand and then interlacing fingers, alternating so each skin surface comes in contact with gel (Fig. 3).**

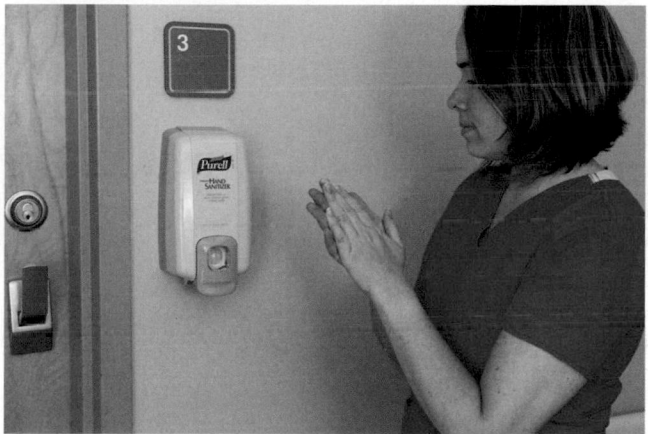

FIG. 2 Spread to all skin surfaces.

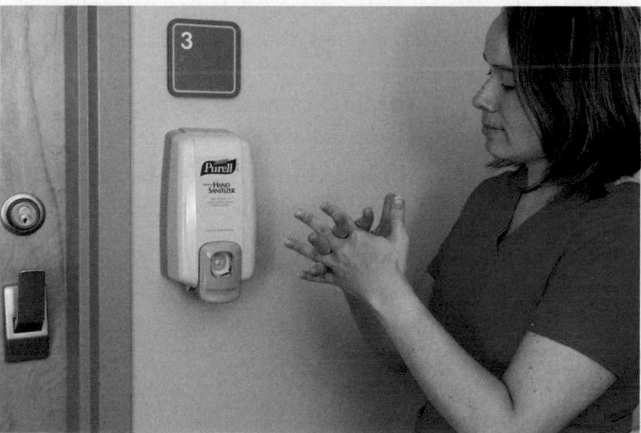

FIG. 3 Interlace fingers.

   Rationale: Covering all skin surfaces and friction removes transient bacteria and promotes antimicrobial action.

Procedure 19-1   *continued*

4. **Rub hands together for several seconds until alcohol product is dry. If applying gloves, allow time for hands to dry completely.**

   Rationale: Provides adequate time for antimicrobial action to work and eases application of gloves.

For Soap and Water

1. **Remove all rings except a plain wedding band. Push watch 4 to 5 inches above wrist.**

   Rationale: Microorganisms lodge in the irregular surfaces of jewelry.

2. **Turn on the water and adjust temperature to warm (Fig. 4). Do not splash water or lean against the wet sink. Faucets may be controlled by your hands or may be operated by knee levers or foot pedals**

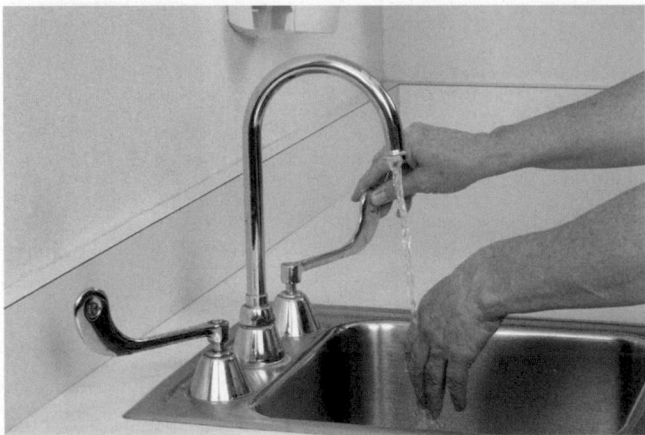

FIG. 4 Turn on water and adjust temperature.

   Rationale: Warm water removes fewer protective oils from the skin than hot water does and reduces chapping of hands from frequent handwashing. Microorganisms need moisture to thrive. Avoid water splashing and sink contact with clothing to prevent contamination.

3. **Hold hands lower than elbows, and thoroughly wet hands and lower arms under running water (Fig. 5).**

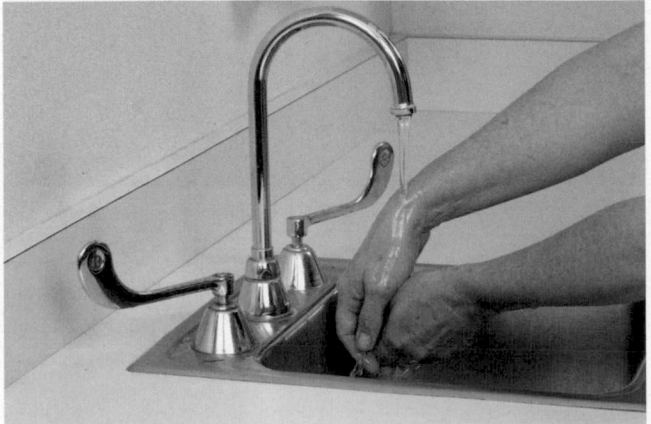

FIG. 5 Wet the hands, holding the wrists below the elbows.

   Rationale: Hands are more contaminated than lower arms; water should flow from least to most contaminated areas.

4. **Apply soap, and rub palms, wrists, and back of hands firmly with circular movements. Interlace fingers and thumbs, moving hands back and forth. Wash at least 1 inch above the area of contamination. If there is no visible soiling, wash to 1 inch above wrists. Continue using plenty of lather and friction for 15 to 30 seconds on each hand (Fig. 6). Timing of scrub may vary depending on purpose of wash and amount of contamination.**

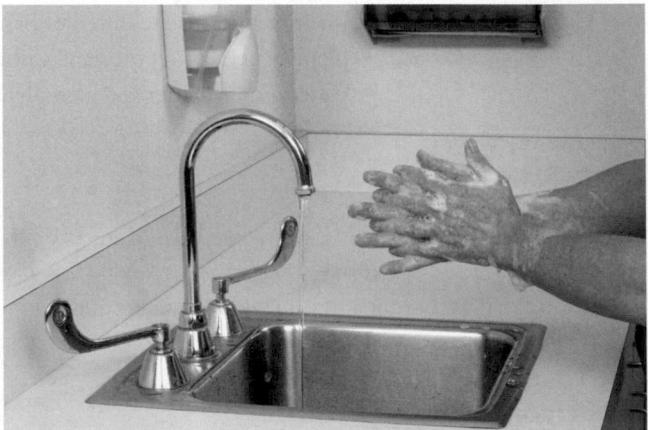

FIG. 6 Lather soap using friction.

   Rationale: Friction mechanically loosens and removes dirt and microorganisms on all hand surfaces.

5. **Clean under fingernails using fingernails of other hand and additional soap. Use orangewood stick if available (Fig. 7).**

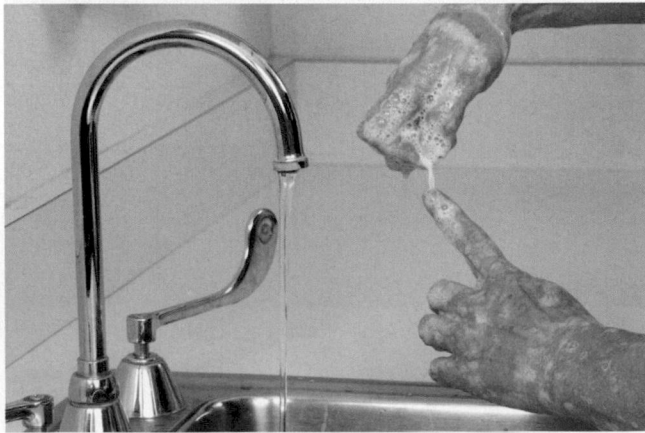

FIG. 7 An orangewood stick can be used to clean under fingernails.

   Rationale: Microorganisms are frequently harbored under nails.

6. **Rinse hands and wrists thoroughly with hands held lower than forearms.**

   Rationale: Rinsing using this technique washes away microorganisms and dirt and prevents recontamination of clean skin surfaces.

Procedure 19-1   *continued*

7. Dry hands and arms thoroughly with paper towel, wiping from fingertips toward forearm (Fig. 8). Discard paper towel in proper receptacle.

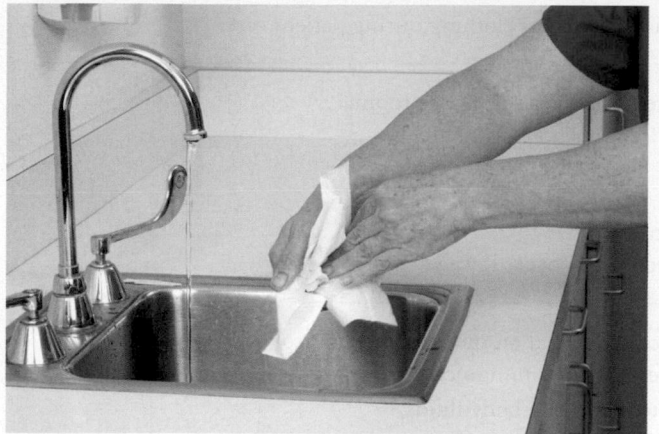

FIG. 8 Dry the hands with paper towel.

Rationale: Drying hands prevents chapping and cracking of skin. Dry from cleanest area (fingertips) toward least clean area to reduce chances of contamination.

8. Turn off water using clean, dry paper towel on faucets (Fig. 9).

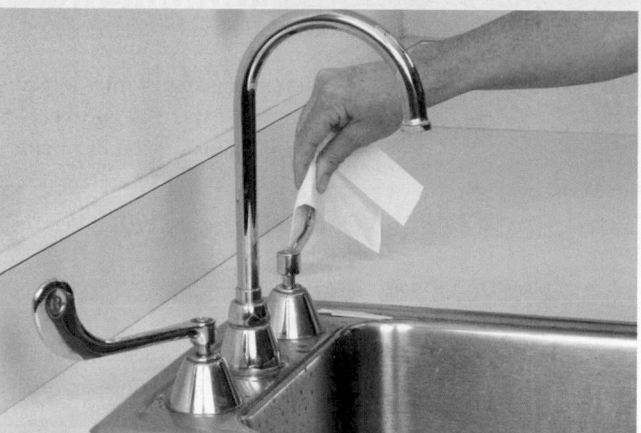

FIG. 9 Turn off faucet with clean paper towel.

Rationale: Paper towel prevents transfer of microorganisms from faucet to the hands.

9. Apply oil-free lotion, especially if skin is dry.

Rationale: Keeps skin soft and prevents chapping that could create cracks in the skin, posing an infection risk.

Documentation

> It is unnecessary to document this procedure.

Home Care Modifications

- Alcohol-based cleaning agents are used frequently in the home setting to effectively cleanse hands that are not visibly contaminated. If you are visiting a patient in the home setting, bring alcohol-based cleansing agents with you. Patients can buy such products for home use and should be encouraged to do so, especially if infection control is an issue or household members are immunocompromised.

Collaboration and Delegation

- All healthcare personnel are responsible for following appropriate handwashing technique during care delivery. Monitoring and reminding one another are important steps to ensure 100% compliance.

Procedure 19-2 Applying and Removing Personal Protective Equipment

Purpose

1. Prevent transfer of microorganisms via the contact, droplet, and airborne modes of transmission from one patient to another.
2. Prevent transmission of microorganisms to self or clothing during patient care.

Equipment

Often, all necessary PPE is kept in a receptacle as you enter the room:
Gloves
Mask
Gown
Goggles or face shield (if splash is expected)
Alcohol-based hand sanitizer or soap, water, and paper towels

Assessment

- Determine the type of equipment necessary based on the infection control practices for the suspected or diagnosed organism, infection, or communicable disease.
- Determine the potential of exposure to blood and body fluids.
- Determine availability of necessary equipment.
- Post a sign at the entrance to the room notifying all staff of necessary precautions.

Procedure

1. **Perform hand hygiene.**
   Rationale: Clean hands reduce the number of microorganisms that could be transferred if gloves accidentally puncture or tear.

Applying PPE

2. **Unfold the gown in front of you.**
   Rationale: Allows you to don clean gown first, then apply mask and gloves.
3. **Place your arms through the sleeves and tie at the neck and back (Fig. 1).**

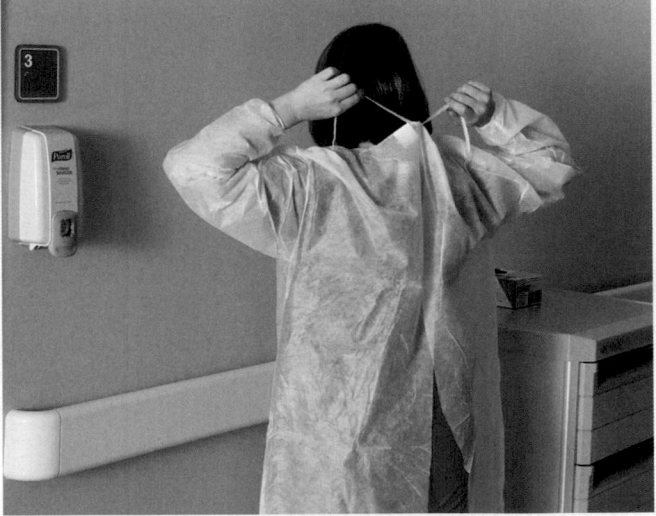

B

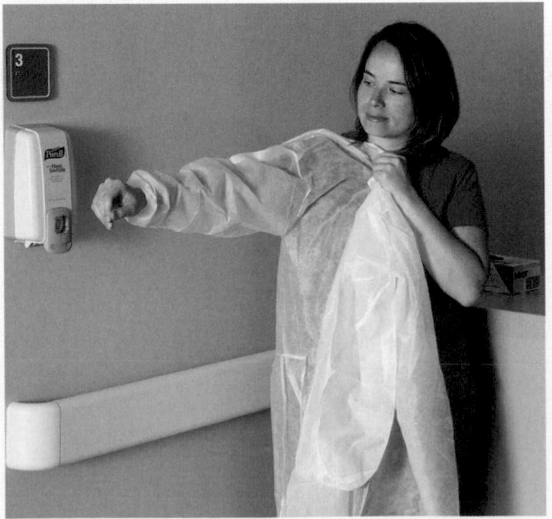

A

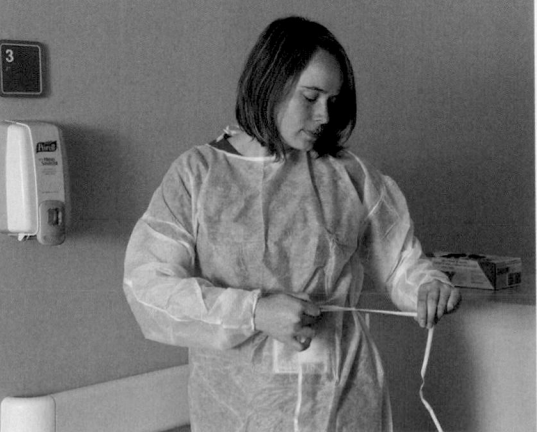

C

FIG. 1 Place the arms through sleeves **(A)** and tie at the neck **(B)** and at the waist **(C)**.

Procedure 19-2   *continued*

Rationale: Loose-fitting gowns may interfere with care and may expose clothing to infectious microorganisms.

4. **Place the mask at your lower face, secure around the ears, and pull down the mask to cover below chin and fit the nose area securely. If the mask has ties, secure the ties above the ears and around the neck (Fig. 2). When wearing glasses, be sure to position the mask edge under the glasses. Make sure the mask fits securely and comfortably.**

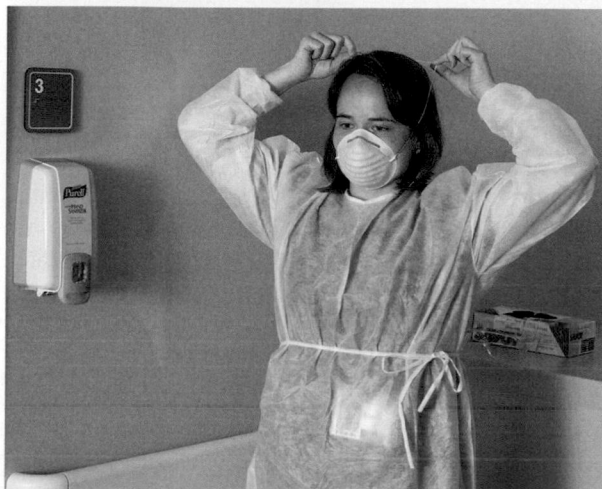

A

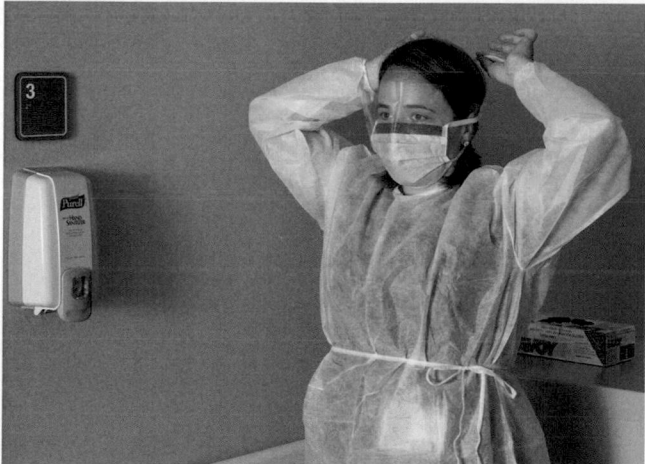

B

FIG. 2 Secure mask on the face **(A)**. If mask has ties, secure ties above the ears first **(B)**.

Rationale: Covering the nose and mouth will prevent exposure to airborne and droplet modes of transmission. Adjusting the fit of the mask after the procedure begins predisposes you to infection risk by touching your face with contaminated hands. If the mask is not tucked under glasses, the glasses may cloud, decreasing vision.

5. **If splash is anticipated, put on goggles, making sure they fit securely (Fig. 3). Alternatively, a face shield with mask can take the place of the mask and goggles.**

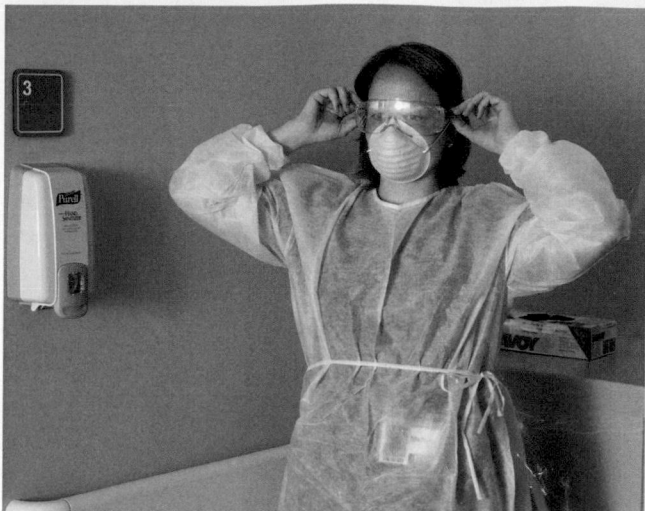

FIG. 3 Apply goggles if splash could occur.

Rationale: Adjusting to fit now will ensure that no adjustments will have to be made during the procedure, such adjustments may expose you to infection risk. Placing the goggles on after the mask allows the mask to fit nicely under the rim of the goggles for better visibility.

6. **Don gloves last so that the cuffs of the gloves fit snugly over the cuffs of the gown (Fig. 4).**

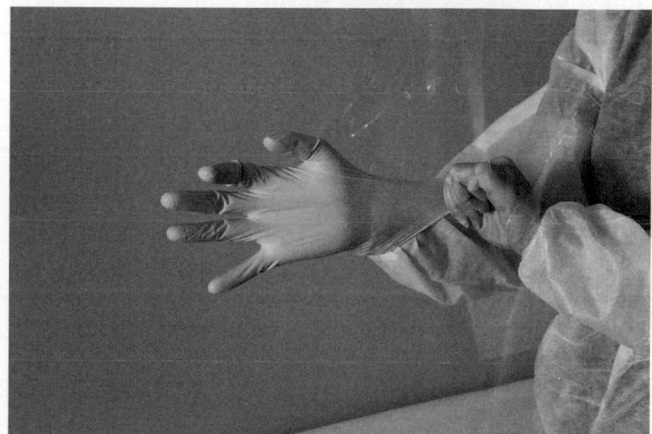

FIG. 4 Fit gloves snugly over cuffs of gown.

Rationale: Placing the glove cuff over the gown cuff provides an impenetrable seal from microorganisms.

Removing PPE

1. **Remain inside the patient's door while removing PPE. PPE must never be reused.**

Rationale: All PPE worn inside the patient's room must be considered contaminated, regardless of the procedure performed. Removing the PPE outside the patient's room risks transmission to others.

Procedure 19-2 *continued*

2. **To remove gloves: First, grasp outside of one glove near the cuff without touching the wrist with your gloved hand. Pull it inside out off your hand. Continue to hold the discarded glove in the other gloved hand. Slide fingers of the ungloved hand under the remaining glove at the wrist. Peel off this glove over the first glove turning the glove inside out over the discarded glove (Fig. 5). Dispose in appropriate waste container. Wash hands.**

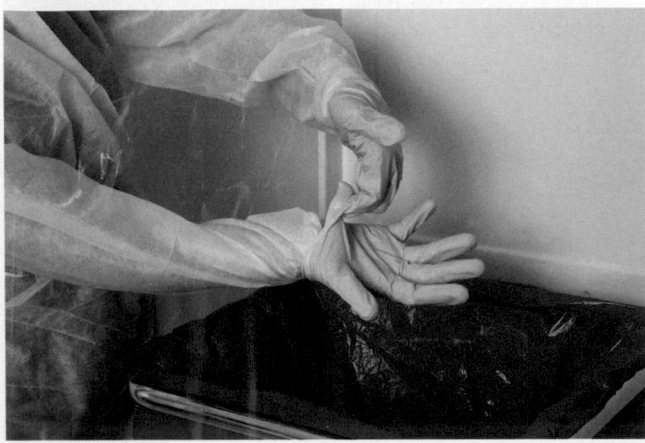

A

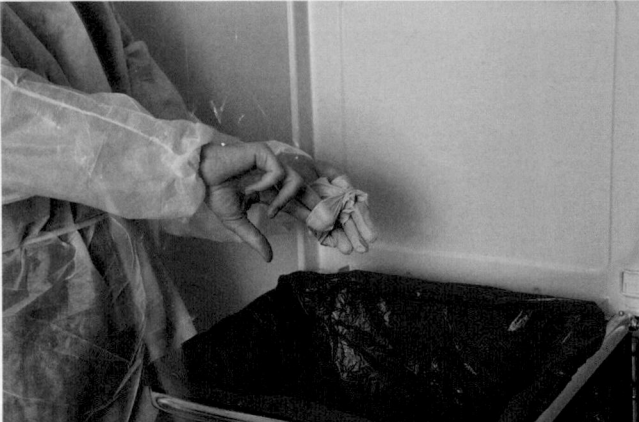

B

FIG. 5 Grasp outside of first glove without touching the wrist to remove **(A)**. Slide bare hand under second glove and peel off to remove **(B)**.

Rationale: Removing the soiled gloves first safeguards against contamination of your face or eyes when removing your mask and goggles or your neck when you are removing the gown. Peeling gloves off inside out and not touching any exposed skin surfaces also prevents contamination.

3. **To remove gown: Untie and pull the gown away from you near the neck, grasping from the inside and avoiding touching the outside. Roll it into a ball, inside out, and keep the sleeves inside the ball. Discard in appropriate waste container (Fig. 6).**

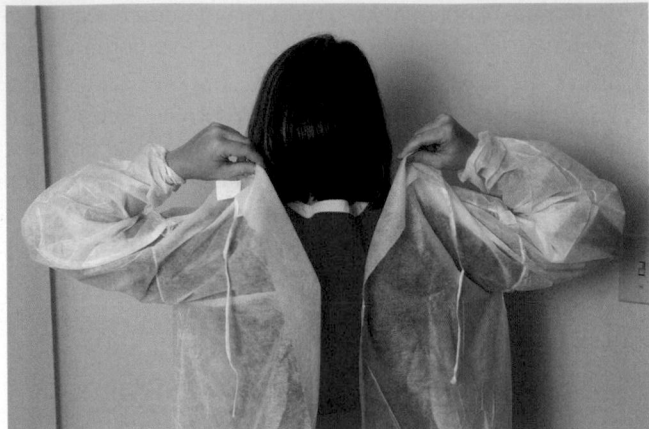

FIG. 6 Untie gown at the neck, grasping inside of gown to pull forward.

Rationale: Ungloved hands can become contaminated if they touch the outside of the gown. Keeping the sleeves in the center of the ball prevents the area that is most likely to be contaminated from contaminating you or objects in the room.

4. **To remove goggles or face shield: Hold only the headband or ear pieces. Lift away from the face. Place in designated receptacle for reprocessing or in an appropriate waste container (Fig. 7).**

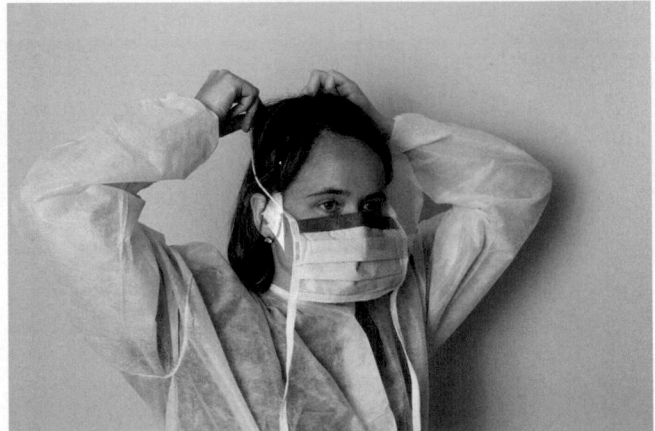

FIG. 7 Holding upper ties bend slightly forward and lift away from the face.

Rationale: The outside of the goggles or face shield is contaminated. Prevents transmission of microorganisms.

5. **To remove mask: Hold only by earbands or ties (bottom tie first, then top) and move the mask away from the face. Discard in appropriate waste container.**

Rationale: According to the CDC, masks should be removed last to prevent respiratory transmission of infection. The front of the mask is considered contaminated whether visibly soiled or not. Removing the bottom tie first prevents the mask from falling forward, possibly contaminating your clothes. When removing a respirator (N95), you may be just outside the room to prevent airborne exposure.

Procedure 19-2   *continued*

6. **Wash hands thoroughly with an alcohol-based hand sanitizer unless hands are visibly soiled; if they are, use soap and warm water. If the patient has diarrhea or the Norovirus, use soap and water.**

Rationale: Wearing PPE does not eliminate the need for thorough handwashing after patient care. Alcohol-based products are ineffective against *Clostridium difficile* and the Norovirus.

Documentation

It is unnecessary to document this procedure.

Procedure 19-3 **Preparing and Maintaining a Sterile Field**

Purpose	1. Create an environment to prevent the transfer of microorganisms during sterile procedures.
	2. Create an environment that helps ensure the sterility of supplies and equipment during a sterile procedure.

Equipment	Flat work surface
	Commercially prepared sterile kit or tray
	Sterile wrapped drape
	Sterile supplies as needed (sterile gauze, sterile basin, liquid solutions, scissors, forceps)

Assessment	• Assess what sterile supplies are necessary for the procedure.
	• Select an area at or above waist height that is free from clutter.
	• Assess the area on which the sterile field will be established for potential sources of contamination (e.g., moisture, soiling) and clean if necessary.
	• Assess for the sterility of all supplies by noting the package integrity, the color strip indicator (see Fig. 19-7), or the expiration date on the package.
	• Assess the order in which supplies will be used during the procedure so that supplies used first can be added to the field last.

Procedure

Preparing a Sterile Field Using a Commercially Prepared Sterile Kit or Tray

1. **Perform hand hygiene.**

   Rationale: Reduces the number of transient bacteria on the hands, helping to prevent microbial contamination.

2. **Inspect the sterile kit for package integrity, contamination, or moisture (Fig. 1).**

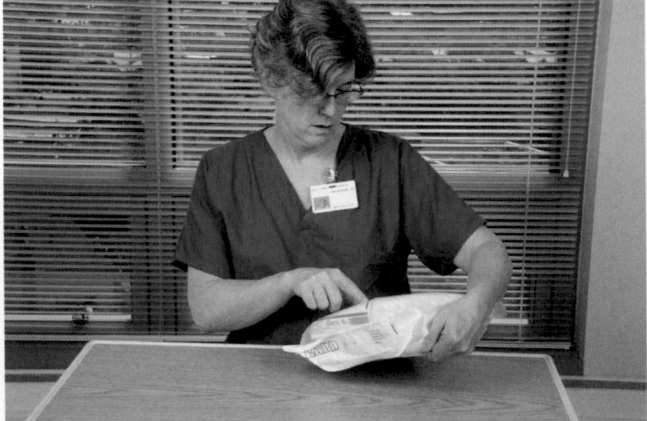

FIG. 1 Inspect the sterile package for package integrity, contamination, or moisture.

   Rationale: Moisture, breaks in package integrity, and visible contamination indicate that the contents are no longer sterile and must be discarded.

3. **During the entire procedure, never turn your back on the sterile field or lower your hands below the level of the field.**

   Rationale: Sterility of the field cannot be certain.

4. **Remove the sterile drape from the outer wrapper and place the inner drape in the center of the work surface, at or above waist level, with the outer flap facing away from you.**

   Rationale: Maintains sterility of the package and allows for opening the drape in a manner that will not contaminate the sterile field.

5. **Touching the outside of the flap only, reach around (rather than over) the sterile field to open the flap away from you (Fig. 2).**

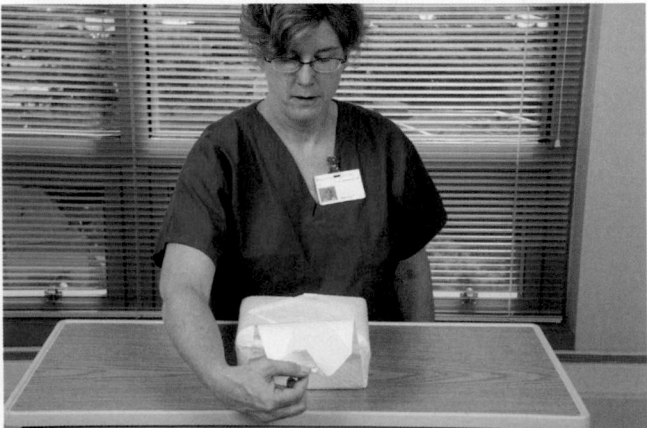

FIG. 2 Reach around the sterile field to open the flap away from you.

   Rationale: Maintains sterility of the field.

Procedure 19-3   *continued*

6. Open the side flaps in the same manner, using the right hand for the right flap and the left hand for the left flap (Fig. 3).

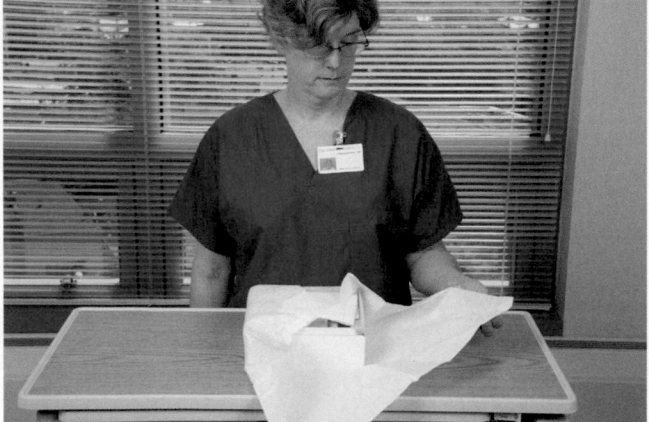

A

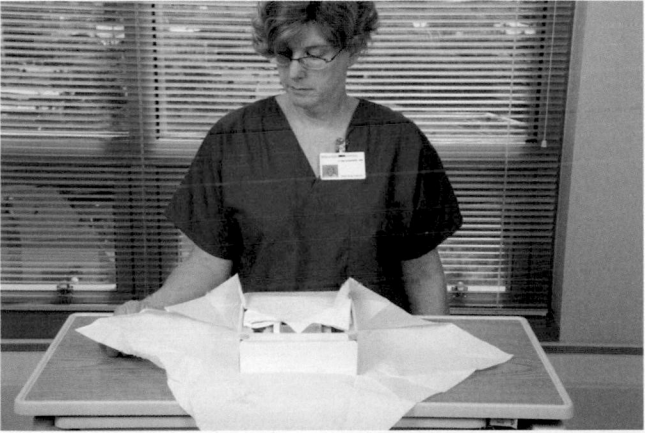

B

FIG. 3 Use your left hand to open the left flap **(A)** and your right hand to open the right flap **(B)**.

Rationale: This maintains sterility by avoiding crossing over the field.

7. Last, open the innermost flap that faces you, being careful that it does not touch your clothing or any object (Fig. 4).

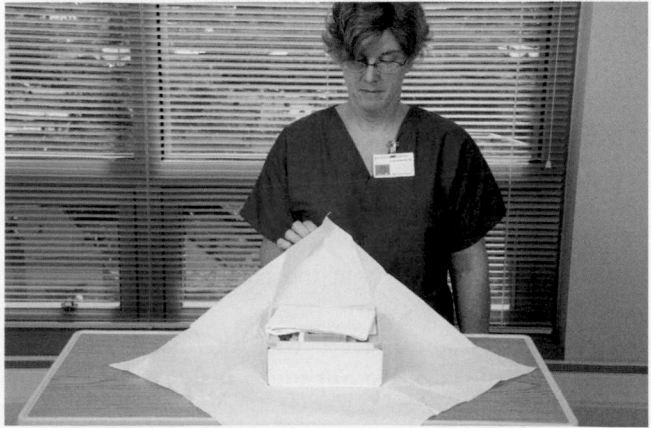

FIG. 4 Open the innermost flap without touching your clothes.

Rationale: Maintains sterility of the field.

Preparing a Sterile Field Using a Packaged Sterile Drape

1. Open the outer covering of the drape (Fig. 5).

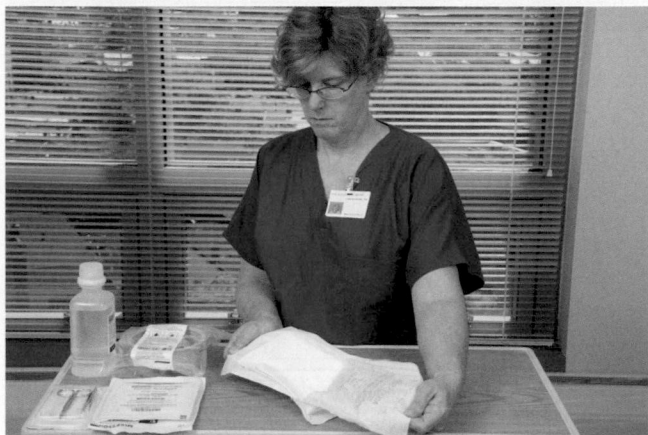

FIG. 5 Open the outer covering of the drape.

Rationale: Removes sterile drape from sealed package.

2. Remove the sterile drape by carefully pinching over the top edge (1 inch) of the two corners so that you are touching only the underneath of the sterile drape (bottom, moisture-proof side). Lift the drape carefully out of the package, holding it away from your body and above your waist and work surface (Fig. 6).

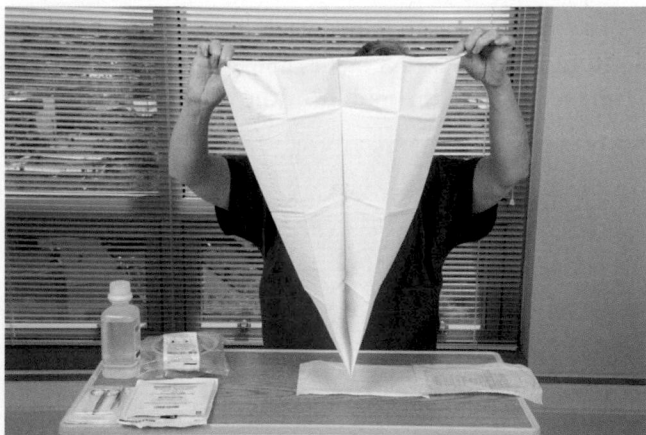

FIG. 6 Carefully pinch over the top edge (1 inch) of the two corners and lift the drape carefully out of the package, holding it away from your body and above your waist and work surface.

Rationale: Pinching over the two top corners maintains the sterile field. Touching the drape in any other location or contact of the drape with any other surface would contaminate the sterile field.

3. Continuing to hold only by the pinched-over corners, allow the drape to unfold away from your body and any other surface.

Rationale: Contact with any surface would contaminate the field.

Procedure 19-3 *continued*

4. **Position the drape on the work surface with the moisture-proof side down (shiny or blue side) (Fig. 7). Avoid touching any other surface or object with the drape.**

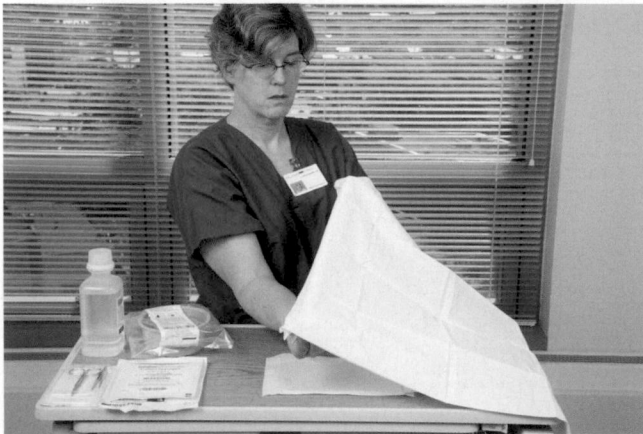

FIG. 7 Position the drape on the work surface with the moisture-proof side down.

   Rationale: The moisture-proof side prevents contamination of the field if it becomes wet.

Adding Sterile Supplies to the Field

5. **Open prepackaged sterile supplies by peeling back the partially sealed edge with both hands or lifting up the unsealed edge, taking care not to touch the supplies with your hands.**
   Rationale: Maintains the sterility of the supplies and object.
6. **Hold supplies 6 to 8 inches above the field and allow them to fall to the middle of the sterile field (Fig. 8).**

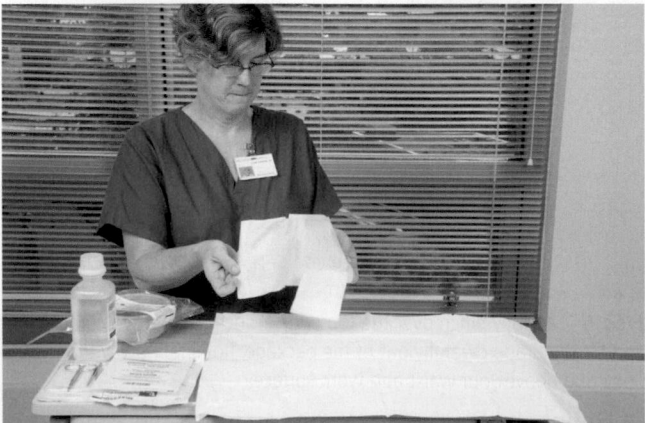

FIG. 8 Hold supplies 6 to 8 inches above the field and allow them to fall to the middle.

   Rationale: Holding supplies too close to the field may cause hand contact that would contaminate the entire field. Holding supplies too high may cause them to land on the edge of the field, also resulting in contamination. The edges of the field are not considered sterile.

7. **Add wrapped sterile supplies by grasping the sterile object with one hand and unwrapping the flaps with the other hand (Fig. 9).**

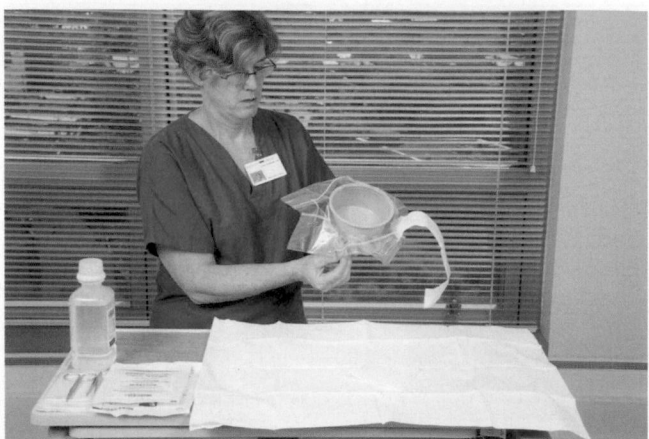

FIG. 9 Grasp the sterile object with one hand and unwrap the flaps with the other hand.

   Rationale: Maintains sterility of the object.
8. **Grasp the corners of the wrapper with the free hand and hold them against the wrist of the other hand while you carefully drop the object onto the middle of the sterile field (Fig. 10).**

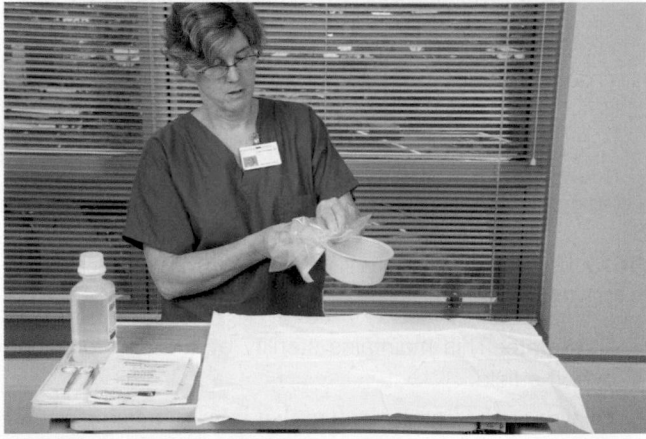

FIG. 10 Grasp the corners of the wrapper with the free hand and hold them against the wrist of the other hand while you carefully drop the object onto the middle of the sterile field.

   Rationale: Maintains sterility of the object and the field.

Adding Solutions to a Sterile Field

9. **Read the solution label and expiration date. Note any signs of contamination.**
   Rationale: Ensures that the correct solution is used and that it is sterile.
10. **Remove cap and place it with the inside facing up on a flat surface. Do not touch inside of cap or rim of bottle.**
    Rationale: Maintains sterility of the solution and bottle.

Procedure 19-3   *continued*

11. **If bottle has been opened previously, "lip" it by pouring a small amount of solution into a waste container (Fig. 11).**

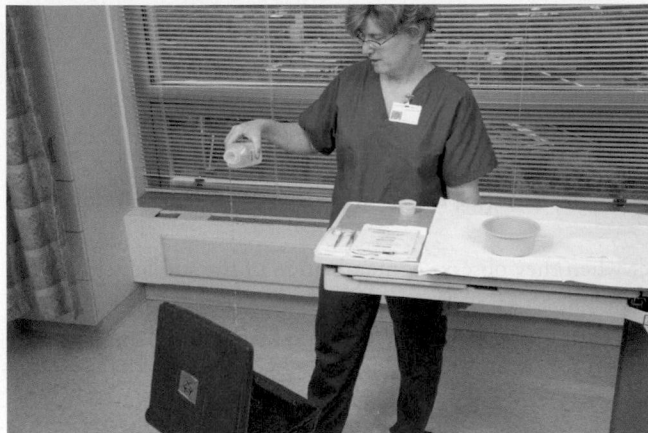

FIG. 11 If bottle has been opened previously, "lip" it by pouring a small amount of solution into a waste container.

Rationale: This cleanses the lip of the bottle.

12. **Hold the bottle 6 inches above container on the sterile field and pour slowly to avoid spills (Fig. 12). Label solution.**

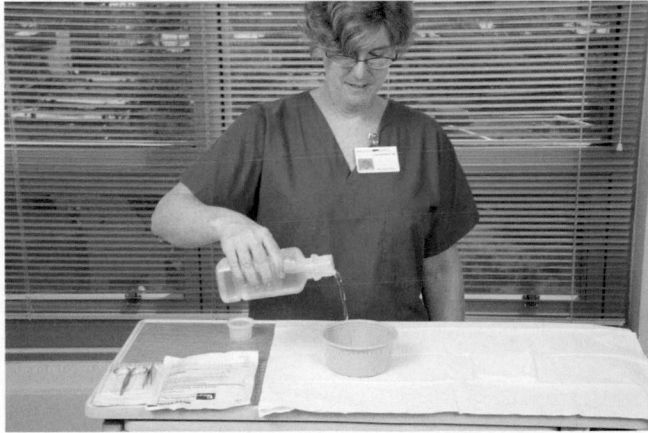

FIG. 12 Hold the bottle 6 inches above the container and pour slowly.

Rationale: Spilling fluid on the sterile field could result in contamination because a wet surface allows microorganisms to wick up from the support surface, which is not sterile.

13. **Recap the solution bottle and label it with date and time of opening if the solution is to be reused.**

Rationale: Keeps solution in the bottle sterile and avoids use of solution that has passed its expiration date.

14. **Add any additional supplies and don sterile gloves before starting the procedure.**

Rationale: Donning sterile gloves just before beginning the procedure helps to ensure sterility.

Documentation

Usually unnecessary unless breaks in sterility occurred that placed the patient at risk.

Procedure 19-3   *continued*

Home Care Modifications

- Select a clean area in the home to set up a sterile field. Avoid areas that pets frequent and areas that are visibly dirty. Alcohol can be used to clean surface areas. Often, clean rather than sterile technique is used in the home setting.
- Self-contained, prepackaged, disposable sterile kits are convenient for use in the home.
- Use waterproof plastic bags to dispose of contaminated waste.

Collaboration and Delegation

- Nonprofessional staff with appropriate training often set up sterile fields, especially in areas such as the operating room or delivery room.
- All coworkers must be responsible for informing each other when they observe contamination of the sterile field so that sterility can be re-established.
- At times, it is more convenient to have one person gloved and sterile with another person opening and handing sterile supplies as they are needed.

Procedure 19-4 Applying and Removing Sterile Gloves

Purpose	1. Prevent transfer of microorganisms from hands to sterile objects or open wounds.

Equipment	Packaged sterile gloves in correct size Flat working surface

Assessment	• Identify the necessity of wearing sterile gloves.
	• Inspect the glove package to determine whether it is dry and intact. Also note expiration date, making sure that the date is still valid.
	• Assess that nails are filed short and all jewelry is removed from hands.
	• Examine ungloved hands for open cuts or lesions, which may harbor microorganisms and prevent the nurse from participating in a sterile procedure.
	• Assess for potential latex allergy.

Procedure

Applying Gloves

1. **Perform hand hygiene.**

   Rationale: Clean hands reduce the number of microorganisms that could be transferred if gloves accidentally puncture or tear.

2. **Remove outside wrapper by peeling apart sides (Fig. 1).**

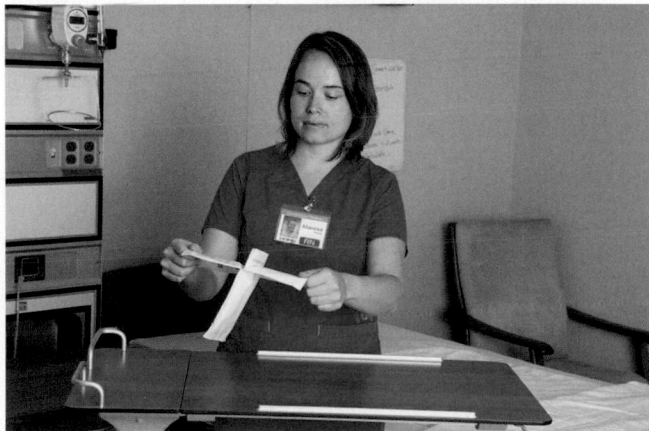

FIG. 1 Peel down to remove outside wrapper.

Rationale: This protects inner package from inadvertently opening and contaminating the gloves.

3. **Lay inner package on clean, flat surface about waist level. Open wrapper from the outside, keeping gloves on inside surface (Fig. 2).**

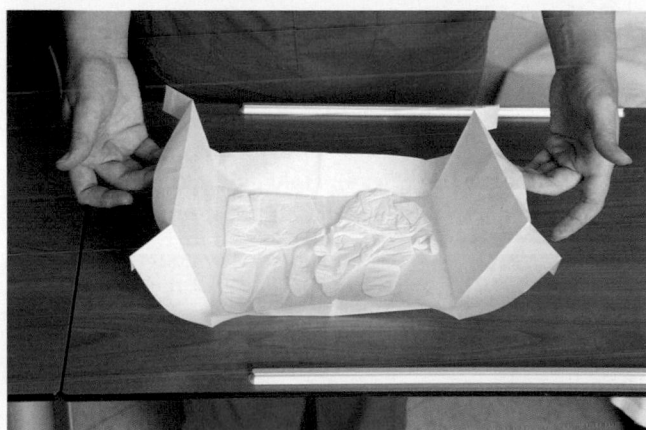

FIG. 2 Open inner wrapper, providing sterile field for glove application.

Rationale: Objects below waist level are considered contaminated. The inner surface of the wrapper is considered sterile.

Procedure 19-4 *continued*

4. Grasp inside edge of the folded cuff of glove with thumb and first two fingers of your dominant hand. Holding hands above waist, insert your nondominant hand into glove. Leave the cuff folded until the opposite hand is gloved (Fig. 3).

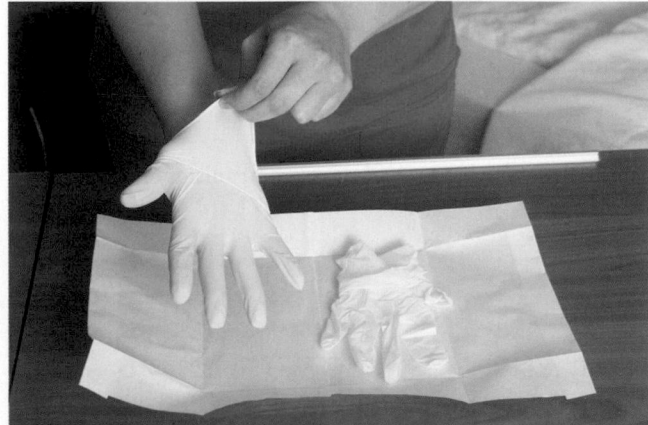

FIG. 3 Grasp first glove by inside cuff and slide on.

Rationale: The inner edge of the cuff unfolds against skin of the hand and is not sterile once applied. Contamination occurs if the ungloved hand contacts the gloved hand.

5. Slip gloved hand inside the second gloved cuff still in package and pull over dominant hand, extending the cuff down the arm (Fig. 4). Hold gloved thumb out of the way so it doesn't come in contact with ungloved hand.

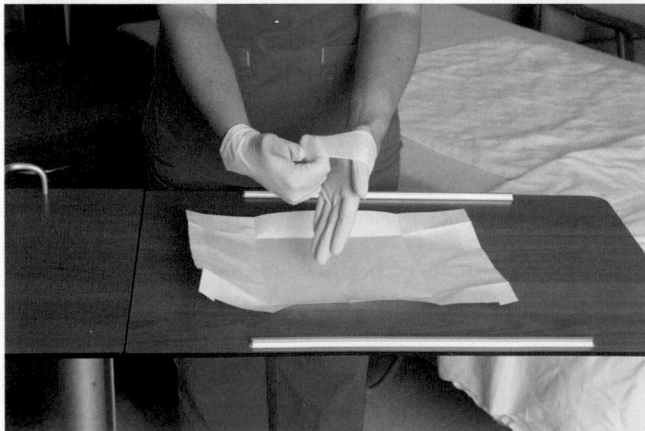

FIG. 4 Slip gloved fingers underneath cuff of second glove and pull over hand.

Rationale: The sterile cuff protects fingers of the gloved hand from being contaminated. The thumb of the gloved hand can easily become contaminated.

6. Keeping hands above waist, adjust fingers inside the glove, touching only sterile areas (Fig. 5).

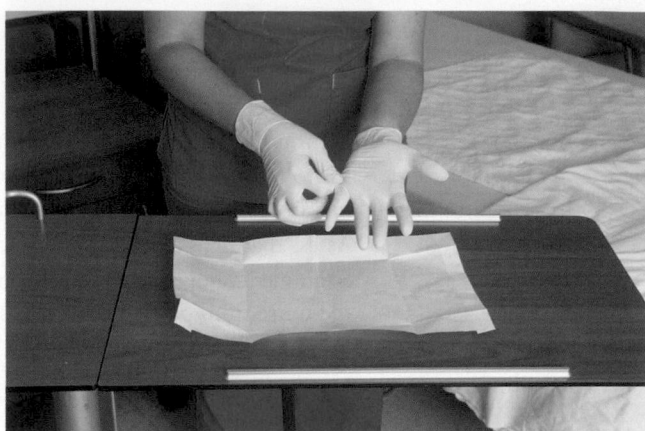

FIG. 5 Adjust gloves as needed, taking care to keep both gloves sterile.

Rationale: These actions prevent contamination while ensuring a smooth fit over fingers.

Removing Gloves

7. With dominant hand, grasp outer surface of nondominant glove just below thumb. Peel off without touching exposed wrist (Fig. 6).

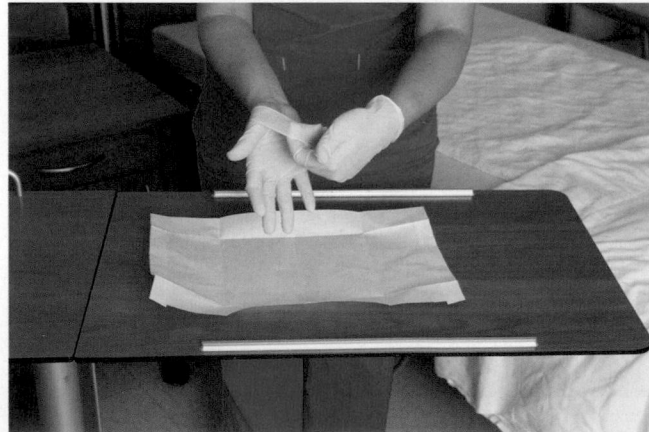

FIG. 6 Grasp outer surface of glove and peel off glove without touching the exposed wrist.

Rationale: After use, the outer surface of the gloves is contaminated and could transfer microorganisms to the nurse's wrist.

Procedure 19-4   *continued*

8. **Place ungloved hand under thumb side of second cuff and peel off toward the fingers, holding first glove inside second glove (Fig. 7). Discard into appropriate receptacle.**

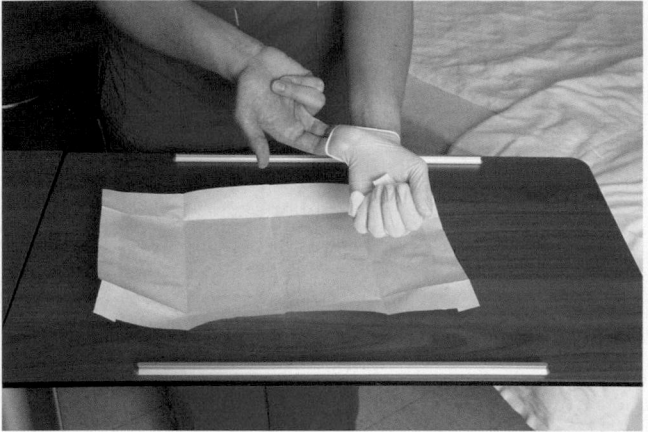

A

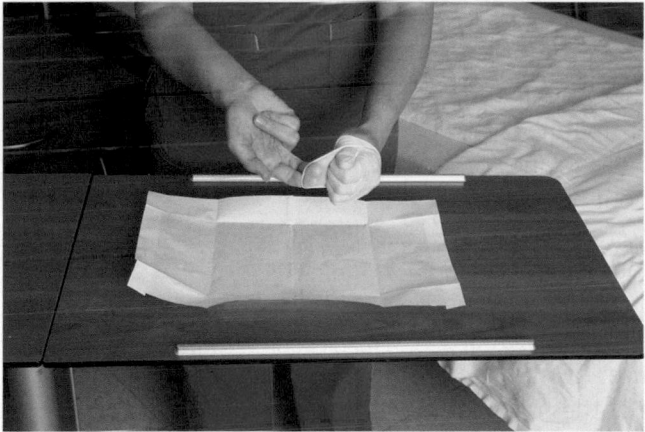

B

FIG. 7 Slide ungloved hand under second glove (**A**). Peel off second glove toward your fingers, holding first glove inside second glove (**B**).

Rationale: Folding contaminated glove surfaces toward the inside minimizes the chance of transfer of microorganisms.

9. **Complete hand hygiene.**

Rationale: Hands can become contaminated even when gloves are worn, especially if not removed correctly.

Documentation

> It is unnecessary to document this procedure.

Home Care Modifications

- For many procedures in the home, clean gloves are used rather than sterile gloves.

Collaboration and Delegation

- Encourage coworkers to notify one another of any observed breaks in sterility, either when gloves are applied or when breaks in technique cause glove contamination. Hand sterile gloves to staff members who are performing sterile procedures.

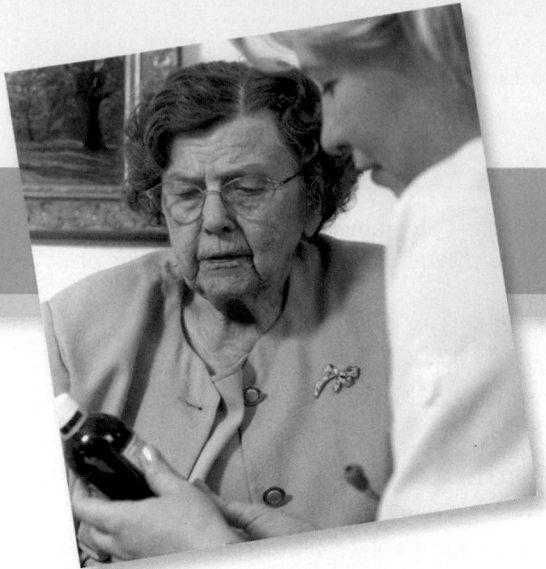

CHAPTER 20

Medication Administration

Niki Kirby

Case Scenario

You are making a nursing visit to a 78-year old woman in her retirement facility. She was recently discharged from the hospital after treatment for a gastric ulcer that resulted from pain medications she was taking for arthritis. During your initial conversation, as you inquire about her health, you notice that the patient appears distracted and seems to have difficulty following questions and giving answers. When you ask about her current medications, her responses indicate that she is unsure about what they are for and how to take them. When you ask her to show you her medications, she produces a large brown paper bag with about 10 bottles: two bottles of a diuretic labeled "Take two tablets twice a day," three bottles of potassium chloride labeled "Take five tablets a day in divided doses," one bottle of a histamine blocker labeled "Take one capsule daily," one bottle of analgesic containing oxycodone to take "as needed arthritis pain," one bottle of extra-strength acetaminophen, one bottle of stool softener capsules to take "as needed," and one bottle of another analgesic containing codeine to take "every 4 hours as needed." As you continue inquiring about which medications she takes and when she takes them, you learn that she has age-related macular degeneration and is legally blind.

Once you have completed this chapter and have incorporated medication administration into your knowledge base, review the above scenario and reflect on the following areas of Critical Thinking:

1. Describe the direction that your assessment might take in this situation.

2. From the information the woman shared with you, identify possible factors that may make it difficult for the patient to adhere to her medication regimen, possibly threatening her health.

3. Propose a course of timely and appropriate nursing actions.

4. What other individuals or healthcare professionals might you want to collaborate with concerning this situation?

KEY TERMS

absorption
adverse drug event
anaphylactic reaction
antagonism
botanicals
buccal
chemical name
controlled substances
distribution
drug incompatibility
excretion
generic name
herbal medications
intradermal
intramuscular
intravenous
medication reconciliation
metabolism
parenteral
pharmacodynamics
pharmacokinetics
prescription
subcutaneous
sublingual
synergism
teratogenic
therapeutic effects
trade or brand name
transdermal
unit dose

Upon completion of this chapter, you will be able to do the following:

1. Describe essential components of a medication order.
2. Discuss pharmacokinetic principles of drug action.
3. List the six rights of proper medication administration.
4. Calculate proper drug dosage, using different systems of drug measurement.
5. Discuss the importance of designing systems within healthcare institutions for medication administration that emphasize patient safety.
6. Discuss important assessment data to obtain from the patient during the initial interview and before and after medication administration.
7. Develop an individualized teaching plan to improve patient knowledge of medications.
8. Incorporate evaluation of medication effectiveness and documentation into safe medication administration practices.
9. Describe recommended guidelines and procedures for medication administration by each route.

Today's nurse plays an important role in medication administration, whether in the acute care, long-term care, or home setting. Not only is the nurse responsible for ensuring that the correct medication is administered to the correct patient in the correct dose via the correct route but also he or she is responsible for knowing the actions and side effects of medications as well as incompatibilities and interactions with other medications and food. Beyond the administration itself, the nurse must be aware of the moral, ethical, and legal aspects of medications. Today's nurse is accountable for his or her practice. No longer is it acceptable to blame providers or pharmacists for medication errors that could have been intercepted and prevented by the nurse. The nurse is the last line of defense for the patients for whom he or she cares.

Nurses play a major role in promoting and maintaining patient health by encouraging patients who need medications to be proactive consumers. By doing so, nurses help patients develop an active understanding of medications, clarify confusing information, insist on being consulted in every aspect of medication prescribing, and responsibly share decision making with other healthcare providers.

In many ways, the success of health promotion depends on patients seeing themselves as healthcare participants with responsibility for choices about treatment and medications—whether alternative, prescribed, or over-the-counter (OTC) medications.

TYPES AND FORMS OF MEDICATIONS

Medications are given at least three different names: a **chemical name** based on its molecular structure, a **generic name** (not owned by a company) that is given by the United States Adopted Names Council and is the drug's official name throughout its lifetime, and the **trade or brand name** used by the pharmaceutical company for a 17-year period in which it has the exclusive rights to make and sell the drug. For example, Tylenol is the trade name for the drug whose chemical name is *N*-acetyl-para-aminophenol. The generic name is acetaminophen. Note that only the trade name is capitalized, and it is usually accompanied by a circled letter "R" for registered trademark. For a single chemical name, there is only one generic name but there may be several different trade names, depending on how many companies manufacture the drug. Medications may be ordered or labeled using either a generic name or a trade name; thus, it is critical for nurses to be aware of both.

Medications may be classified in many ways (e.g., according to their chemical composition, clinical actions, or **therapeutic effect** on body systems). Understanding general medication classifications aids in learning about the actions, side effects, and precautions needed for unfamiliar medications. Table 20-1 lists classes of medications that may be used to promote the patient's health.

Medications are prepared in various forms. Table 20-2 lists different medication preparations. Because of the wide range of available medication forms and dosages, nurses must pay close attention to medication orders and administer the specified form requested.

MEDICATION STANDARDS

Because medications vary, the government establishes and controls standards guiding medication quality. The official list of medications in the United States is contained in two texts, the *United States Pharmacopeia* (USP) and the *National Formulary* (NF). The USP and NF describe medication products according to their source, physical and chemical properties, tests for purity and identity, method of storage, category, and normal dosages. Because medications vary according to their properties of purity, potency, bioavailability, efficacy, and safety and toxicity, medication standards must provide an appropriate range of quality for these properties.

TABLE 20-1 CLASSES OF MEDICATIONS TO PROMOTE NORMAL FUNCTION

Health Pattern	Drug Classes	Actions
Activity and exercise	Antihypertensives	Decrease blood pressure
	Antiarrhythmics	Regulate heart rhythm
	Inotropes	Strengthen cardiac contraction
	Antianginals	Increase coronary blood flow
	Anticoagulants	Decrease clot formation
	Bronchodilators	Open airways
Nutrition and metabolism	Antibiotics	Decrease or prevent infection
	Antiemetics	Decrease nausea
	Antacids	Decrease gastric acidity
	Insulin	Decrease blood glucose levels
	Corticosteroids	Decrease inflammation
	Thyroid	Regulate metabolic rate
	Vitamins and minerals	Supplement inadequate dietary intake
Elimination	Laxatives	Promote stool evacuation
	Antidiarrheals	Decrease diarrhea
	Diuretics	Increase urine production and elimination
Sleep and rest	Sedatives, hypnotics	Induce sleep
Cognition and perception	Analgesics	Decrease pain
	Antipsychotics	Decrease psychotic symptoms (e.g., hallucinations)
Coping and stress tolerance	Antianxiety agents	Decrease anxiety
	Antidepressants	Decrease depression
Sexuality and reproduction	Ovarian hormones	Provide hormone replacement
		Provide birth control

TABLE 20-2 DRUG PREPARATIONS

Type of Preparation	Description
Oral preparations	
Capsule	Gelatinous container to hold powder or liquid medicine
Elixir	Liquid preparation of medication with alcohol base
Emulsion	Suspension within an oil base
Enteric coated	Coating that causes drug absorption in intestines rather than the stomach; prevents stomach irritation
Lozenge (troche)	Tablet held in the mouth to be dissolved
Powder	Finely ground drug; frequently mixed with liquid before administration
Spansule	Time-release drug capsule, which dissolves more slowly to provide an effect over a long period
Suspension	Medication in liquid, which must be shaken before administration because it separates
Syrup	Medicine dissolved in sugar and water
Tablet	Compressed hard disk of powdered medication; may be scored for easy breaking; may be sugar coated or have film coating for cohesion
Tincture	Potent solution with alcohol base made from plants; dosage usually small
Topical preparations	
Cream	Nongreasy, semisolid preparation for topical application
Gel or jelly	Translucent or clear semisolid substance that liquefies when applied to the skin
Liniment	Oily liquid used on the skin
Lotion	Emollient liquid, clear solution or suspension, which is applied to the skin
Ointment	Drug combined with oil base for external application
Paste	Thick ointment used for local application to the skin
Suppository	Medicine contained within a gelatinous base (shaped for easy insertion into the body), which dissolves at body temperature, slowly releasing the drug
Transdermal patch	Medicine in a patch, which, when applied to the skin, permits gradual, controlled absorption

SOURCES OF INFORMATION ABOUT MEDICATIONS

A fundamental rule of safe medication administration is to never administer an unfamiliar medication. Before giving any medication, first understand the condition of the patient for whom the medication is ordered. This knowledge, combined with knowledge of the ordered medication, explains if and why the medication is appropriate for that patient. Be familiar with dosage ranges of the medication being given, the expected therapeutic effects, and possible adverse actions and interactions with other medications. Also, be prepared to teach the patient the medication's purpose and to answer questions about the medication's use.

Making a habit of consulting a standard drug reference is a way to stay up-to-date on medications, dosages, purposes, routes of administration, and side effects. The Institute for Safe Medication Practices (ISMP) publishes *ISMP Medication Safety Alert and Nurse Advise–ERR*, which describes errors and how to make medication administration safer. These can be obtained online (www.ismp.org).

The American Hospital Formulary Service publishes individual monographs on single generic and groups of medications that are kept current by ongoing electronic updates. These monographs organize drug information by pharmacologic properties and index the medications by common brand names, generic name, and therapeutic class. Most hospitals prepare their own formularies, compiling information on all medications available within the individual facility. In addition, drug manufacturers' package inserts provide detailed data on the product contained in a packaged unit. Healthcare agencies frequently have drug information systems on computers for easy access.

The information sources that nurses use most frequently are drug handbooks and computer software reference guides. A nursing drug handbook not only provides information about specific medications but also emphasizes the nursing implications for medication administration. Many drug handbooks, which usually are updated annually, are sold with digital access and resources. Most healthcare facilities have hard copy references and computer programs available. Most nursing students are required to purchase a nursing drug handbook and are expected to know how to access facility drug software programs. Due to the speed with which information is disclosed to the Food and Drug Administration (FDA), information is changing all the time, and hard copy drug references are often out-of-date before they reach the bookstores. Online web-based drug references, such as Lexicomp (www.lexi.com) and Epocrates (www.epocrates.com), are available and are continuously updated as new information is provided. These companies also provide apps for download, enabling healthcare providers to have up-to-date information at their fingertips anywhere and anytime.

The pharmacist is also a resource for information including potential medication interactions or contraindications. A clinical pharmacist may be assigned to specific units or located on the unit so that discussion about patients' medications can frequently occur. A pharmacist may also participate in patient rounds with the healthcare team so that he or she actively participates in developing the plan of care when it involves medications.

SYSTEMS OF MEDICATION DISTRIBUTION

Currently, medication distribution systems vary among healthcare institutions. There is, however, ongoing effort within the healthcare industry to standardize medication distribution systems. The following medication distribution systems will be described below:

- **Unit dose**
- Automated medication-dispensing system
- Self-administered supply
- Bar code medication administration (BCMA)

Regardless of the distribution system, in accordance with opioid control laws, all controlled substance medications are kept in locked drawers in all patient care areas.

Unit-Dose System

A unit-dose system involves the pharmacy or manufacturer prepackaging and prelabeling an individual patient dose. The individual unit dose is a prescribed amount of medication dispensed at a specified time.

This type of system is used widely in large healthcare facilities and is considered the gold standard in hospitals. The pharmacy dispenses medications individually packaged by the manufacturer and labeled with the medication name and dose. If a drug is not available from a manufacturer in unit-dose packaging, pharmacists will prepare patient-specific unit-dose medications labeled not only with medication name and dose but also with the patient's name and medical record number (MRN). The nurse administers the medications directly to the patient from the unit-dose package.

Many extended care facilities use a patient-specific unit-dose system. The pharmacy packages and labels a medication in the specified dose for a specific person in a multi–unit-dose packet sometimes referred to as a "bingo card" (Fig. 20-1). Each "bubble" on the bingo card contains 1 dose; the card as a whole may contain as many as 60 doses. This method is used in healthcare settings where the average length of stay for patients is longer than 2 weeks and no pharmacy is on-site.

Automated Medication-Dispensing System

The automated medication-dispensing system is common in healthcare facilities (Fig. 20-2). The system consists of a machine containing medications such as routine medications, as-needed (prn) medications, controlled drugs, and emergency

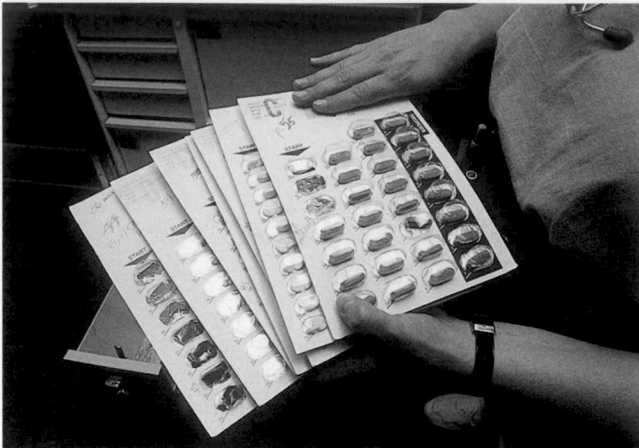

FIGURE 20-1 In long-term care settings, "bingo cards" are a cost-effective method of dispensing medications. Each bubble contains one dose for the patient.

medications. The machine operates similarly to an automated bank machine. Nurses access the system by using a password or by scanning a finger so the machine can identify their fingerprints and then select a function from choices offered by the computerized menus to obtain the desired medication for a patient. The medication is delivered in a unit-dose package. The automated medication-dispensing system keeps an account of all medications used for billing and controlled substance record keeping.

Bar Code Medication Administration

This system uses a lightweight handheld laser scanner, a laptop computer attached to a medication cart, and bar codes. Patients wear bar-coded identification bracelets. The nurse must enter

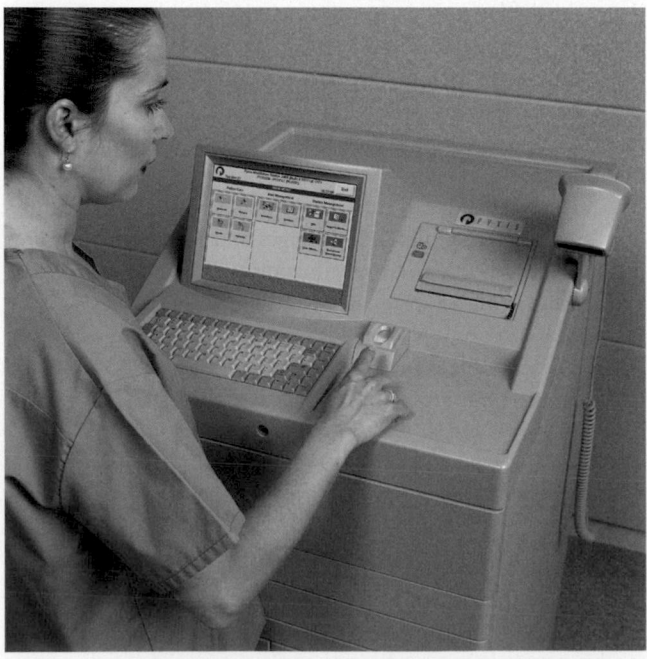

FIGURE 20-2 An automated medication system.

a password to access the computer system. When the nurse passes the scanner over the patient's identification bracelet, the computer screen displays the patient's medication record. The nurse then selects medications from a drawer on the medication cart and scans the bar code on each unit-dose packaged medication. At this time, this system confirms patient identity, medication, dose, and route. It also tracks the actual time of administration and the identity of the nurse administering the medication. The system will warn of a potential error if the action does not meet five of the six rights of medication administration (right patient, right medication, right dose, right route, right time, and right documentation). A legible, real-time medication administration record (MAR) is created and available for review by the nurse, pharmacist, and provider. This system also can display assessment results such as vital signs and laboratory findings. Many organizations recommend the use of bar code systems to improve patient safety, including the Institute of Medicine (IOM), the National Patient Safety Foundation, the American Society of Health-System Pharmacists, and the National Alliance for Health Information Technology. The FDA now requires bar codes on the labels of most prescription drugs and many OTC drugs.

Self-Administered Medication System

The self-administered medication system supplies each patient with his or her prescribed doses and quantities for a given period. Each medication is supplied in a separate container or plastic bottle and is used for one patient only. Medications can be stored at the patient's bedside, allowing the patient to administer his or her own medication doses. This system allows for patient independence and responsibility while simultaneously allowing nursing supervision, teaching, and evaluation for patient adherence and safe medication management before facility discharge.

NONPRESCRIPTION AND PRESCRIPTION MEDICATIONS

Medications can be categorized into those requiring a prescription and those that can be purchased without a provider's order. Nurses administer and provide teaching about prescription and nonprescription medications.

Nonprescription Medications

Many medications can be obtained without a written order from a healthcare provider. They are sold OTC because they generally are regarded as safe enough for use without medical or nursing supervision. Common examples of OTC medications include cold remedies and mild analgesics, such as aspirin and acetaminophen. The FDA maintains control over the safety, effectiveness, and advertising of nonprescription medications. The FDA approves drugs for OTC availability, including the transfer of drugs from prescription to OTC status. At times, additional testing is required prior to OTC approval and additional information must be included on the label to help consumers use the medication safely.

Nonprescription medications are considered safe when used as directed. The dangers of these readily available medications lie in their misuse, which can result in dangerous side effects in the consumer. In addition, people may persist in self-medicating with nonprescription drugs and delay seeking professional help, possibly causing a minor problem to develop into a major one because of early mistreatment. There also is a danger of serious drug interactions.

> ! **SAFETY ALERT**
> Always determine which (if any) nonprescription medications the patient has been taking and ensure that he or she takes no medications without the healthcare provider's knowledge.

Herbs and Other Botanicals

Although the use of medicinal herbs and other **botanicals** or plant products is widespread, botanical medications have not consistently been included in a patient's history until recently. It is important to assess for the use of these products before administering any other OTC or prescription medication. Some of the most commonly used botanicals are *Hypericum perforatum* (St. John's wort), used for mild depression; *Echinacea* (coneflower), used as a mild antibiotic; and *Ginkgo biloba* (maidenhair tree), used to increase blood circulation and to improve cognitive function. Some botanicals can cause toxic effects and drug–drug interactions. For example, *Ginkgo biloba* can cause bleeding when taken with medications such as aspirin or warfarin (Coumadin).

Patients generally think that these products are safe because they are advertised as "all natural," but judging their safety and efficacy can be difficult. Unlike other medications, herbs and botanicals lack quality standards and regulation; their ingredients or quantities may or may not be as stated on the label. Dosages are less exact because the potency of a botanical can vary depending on how it was prepared and the particular plant source used.

The government established the National Center for Complementary and Alternative Medicine (NCCAM) to encourage study of **herbal medications** and botanicals according to rigorous scientific method. Controlled, randomized studies have been done on some botanical preparations; other scientific investigations are beginning to provide clinically relevant information.

Think of botanical products as medications. Any time a person puts a substance into the body, this chemical can cause unknown or unexpected effects. Therefore, assess the patient for use of botanical tablets, teas, extracts, and tinctures, and consult herbal formularies as needed for specific information.

Prescription Medications

A **prescription** is a legal order for the preparation and administration of a medication. Certain medications require medical supervision, often because of a narrow margin of safety between a therapeutic and a toxic dose. Physicians, advanced practice nurses, physician assistants, and dentists are the only healthcare professionals legally responsible for prescribing medications.

MEDICATION ORDER

When discussing medication orders, it is important to consider the components of the order and various types of orders.

Components

The prescriber of a medication conveys an order by specifying the patient's name, the medication's name, the amount and frequency of the dose, and the route of administration. He or she also should include the purpose of the medication. The date and time the prescription was written and the signature of the prescribing healthcare provider must be present. The patient's first and last name must be written with the medication order to avoid confusion between two patients with the same last name. The patient's identification number or MRN can be written with the order as further identification.

Computerized provider order entry (CPOE) allows providers to enter medication orders directly into the patient's electronic medical record, thus ensuring that all entries are legible to avoid potential errors.

MEDICATION NAME

The name of the medication can be the generic or trade name. The name of the medication, if handwritten, should be written clearly because many medications are similar in spelling but different in drug action. Electronic medical records may automatically enter "tall man lettering" on the computer screen when generic drug names are ordered. Tall man letters (e.g., hydrOXYzine and hydrALAZINE) help distinguish look-alike medication names on screens to minimize the risk of selecting the wrong medication name.

> ! **SAFETY ALERT**
> Always clarify with the provider any medication order that is unclear or seems inappropriate.

MEDICATION DOSAGE

The medication dosage can be written using the metric, apothecary (rarely used), or household measurement systems. The strength and frequency of the dose also are indicated (e.g., digoxin 0.125 mg daily). If a medication is dispensed in only one dose, the provider may indicate the number of tablets or pills to take (e.g., multiple vitamin one daily by mouth). A recommended mistake-proofing practice is always to use leading zeros for doses less than one measurement unit (e.g., 0.3 mg, never .3 mg) and never to use trailing zeros (e.g., 5 mg, never 5.0 mg). Another safety practice is the differentiation of the numerals 2 and 7 in handwritten doses by adding a cross on the downstroke of the numeral 7 (e.g., 7) .

ROUTE OF ADMINISTRATION

The route of administration must be included in the medication order. Many medications can be given by several routes, such as orally, intravenously, or intramuscularly. The route of administration is commonly abbreviated as a part of the written order.

> **! SAFETY ALERT**
> If an order specifies a certain route of administration and the patient's condition changes, making the ordered route inappropriate or possibly unsafe, notify the provider so that he or she can change the route of administration.

PURPOSE

All medication orders also should include the purpose or indication for use of the medication (e.g., oxyCODone 5 mg orally every 4 hours as needed for moderate pain). This recent addition to medication ordering assists in evaluating drug effectiveness, since some drugs can be prescribed for more than one purpose. For example, gabapentin (Neurontin) can be used to control seizures or to control chronic pain.

SIGNATURE

Because the written order is a legal request, the provider's signature must follow the written order. An unsigned order is invalid and should not be carried out until the provider signs the order. Electronic signatures are valid.

Types of Orders

There are several different types of medication orders, including routine or standing orders, prn orders, standing protocols, one-time orders, stat orders, telephone and fax orders, and verbal orders.

ROUTINE OR STANDING ORDERS

The routine medication order is one that should be carried out for a specified number of days (e.g., antibiotic) or until another order cancels it. In some healthcare agencies, the standing orders must be reviewed and rewritten within a specified time frame or they are canceled automatically.

PRN ORDERS

A prn order (from the Latin *pro re nata*) does not indicate a specific time period for administration of a medication. Rather, it states guidelines so that the medication can be administered

as needed. Analgesic medications, antiemetic medications, and laxatives are often ordered on a prn basis. Good judgment is essential to determine when a medication is needed and when it is safe to administer the medication. Once administered, evaluation of the effectiveness of the medication is necessary and must be documented.

STANDING PROTOCOLS

Standing protocols are written for medications to be administered in specific situations with criteria for administration outlined clearly for patients on a specific unit or service. For example, a standing protocol might be written for a nurse working on a cardiac unit to administer a certain heart medication if the patient develops an irregular rhythm.

ONE-TIME ORDERS

The one-time or single order is written for a medication that will be given only once. An order for a preoperative medication to help calm the patient before surgery is an example of a one-time order.

STAT ORDERS

A stat order (from the Latin *statim*) is a single order for a medication that must be given *immediately*. An example of this order is "furosemide 20 mg IV stat" for fluid volume excess.

VERBAL ORDERS

A verbal order is a situation when the provider and the nurse are physically present in the same room. A verbal order is accepted only in emergencies (e.g., cardiopulmonary resuscitation or other lifesaving interventions). The provider gives the order verbally, and the nurse then reads back the order in its entirety to the provider for verification. At all other times, when the provider is present, he or she enters the order into the medical record.

TELEPHONE AND FAX ORDERS

At times, the nurse and provider may discuss a patient's condition over the telephone and decide to change the patient's medication regimen. Because the provider is not available to write and sign the order, the nurse may accept the telephone order and write the order on an order sheet or enter it into the electronic medical record. The accepted practice is for the nurse to write the order on a medication order sheet while the provider and nurse are on the telephone; the nurse then reads back the order in its entirety to the provider for verification. The order must include the date and time, correct name of the patient, medication name, and dose, frequency, route, and purpose of the medication. The nurse indicates telephone order (e.g., "T.O. by Dr. Phillips" or "Susan Brown, ARNP"), signs his or her own name, and verifies that the provider cosigns the new order at a later time, usually mandated within 24 hours by facility policy. The nurse must read back the order to verify it.

Sometimes, nurses, especially when working in skilled nursing facilities or the community, communicate with a provider about a patient's condition by fax or e-mail. In writing, the nurse may briefly describe a change in the patient's condition and request a new medication order or change in a current medication order. The nurse sends this request to the provider's office. The provider sends a return message indicating any necessary changes. The nurse then writes the order in the patient's chart. Because the fax machine uses telephone lines, the fax order is considered a telephone order, and the provider must cosign it at a later time, pursuant to facility policy. Some providers using CPOE have remote computer access to the patient's medical record, enabling them to directly enter the new order. When the computerized medical record and CPOE become the standard in the healthcare industry, handwritten, telephone, and fax orders will become unnecessary ensuring greater patient safety.

> **SAFETY ALERT**
>
> To ensure accuracy when taking telephone orders, always repeat the order to the provider after writing it down. The provider must cosign the order within a specified time, usually 24 hours. Do not take verbal orders except in an emergency situation (code), because the risk for error is very great. Direct the provider to write the order.

LEGAL ASPECTS OF MEDICATION ADMINISTRATION

To ensure safe administration of medications, a nurse must be knowledgeable concerning the law, the Nurse Practice Act, best policies, and patients' rights. The FDA is the chief governmental agency that oversees drug safety.

Food and Drug Administration

The FDA, a division of the U.S. Department of Health and Human Services, regulates the manufacture, sale, and effectiveness of medications. It also requires drug testing in laboratory animals and in humans (through controlled, three-phase clinical trials) before a drug is approved for use. The FDA also is charged with keeping ineffective or unsafe drugs off the market and recalling inadequately tested or dangerous drugs. Additional functions include identifying which medications can be obtained with or without a prescription, setting and enforcing standards of purity and potency, overseeing all drugs, and controlling drug advertising to the medical profession.

Nurse Practice Acts

Nursing legislation controls the administration of medications by nurses. Nurse practice acts, established to describe legitimate nursing functions, vary among states and provinces.

Be informed about how your region's nurse practice act defines the boundaries of your functions. Also, recognize your own individual limits of knowledge and skill.

Under current nurse practice laws, nurses are responsible for their own actions regardless of the provider's written order. If an order is ambiguous or inappropriate, the nurse must clarify the medication order with the prescribing healthcare provider. If the nurse is dissatisfied with the provider's response and still believes that the order is incorrect or unsafe, he or she must notify a supervisor.

> **SAFETY ALERT**
>
> You have the right and responsibility to decline to administer a medication if you believe it jeopardizes patient safety.

Prescribing and dispensing medications (i.e., ordering and preparing a medication that someone else will deliver) are not legal practices for registered nurses (RNs) in most states, with the exception of nurses in advance practice roles. Whereas providers prescribe and pharmacists dispense therapeutic agents, it *is* within the nurse's legal domain to administer medications in a safe and timely manner.

> **SAFETY ALERT**
>
> Do not give any medication prepared by another nurse unless the unit-dose label identifies the drug and the seals are intact.

Institutional Medication Policies

Nurses work in various settings, including schools, hospitals, skilled nursing facilities, home healthcare agencies, and private industries. RNs, licensed practical (or vocational) nurses, and nursing students supervised by an RN can administer medications. Institutions may place restrictions on the types of medications that nurses can give or on the degree of supervision or experience that they require. Every institution is governed by its own medication administration policies and procedures. Be aware of the practice within your institution.

Patients' Rights

Patients have the right to expect safe and appropriate drug administration by the nurse (see Chapter 7). To accomplish this, the nurse must observe "six rights": the right patient, the right medication, in the right dose, by the right route, at the right time, followed by the right documentation.

In addition to these six rights, the patient has the right to refuse to take medications. The nurse has the duty to explain to the patient as fully and clearly as possible the purpose of taking the medication. If a patient refuses the prescribed medication, attempt to clarify the patient's concern about the medication and notify the provider of the patient's refusal while explaining the patient's concerns. Many times, these are valid reasons, and the nurse serves as the patient advocate.

Controlled Substances

As a result of rising drug abuse and increasing public concern in the late 1960s, the U.S. Congress enacted the Comprehensive Drug Abuse Prevention and Control Act of 1970, which includes the Controlled Substances Act. **Controlled substances** are drugs that are considered to have either limited medical use or high potential for abuse or addiction. The Controlled Substances Act categorizes controlled substances into five groups (I, II, III, IV, and V) based on their potential for abuse and their medical usefulness. Table 20-3 describes the five groups. Under this law, possession of a controlled substance without a valid prescription is illegal, and the number of times a prescription can be filled is limited. The primary reasons for the Controlled Substances Act were to prevent drug abuse and dependence, provide treatment and

rehabilitation for people who are dependent on drugs, and strengthen drug abuse laws.

Hospitals and other healthcare settings keep controlled substances in a locked drawer or automated medication-dispensing unit as an additional safety measure. Only providers or other healthcare providers registered with the Department of Justice Bureau of Opioids and Dangerous Drugs can order controlled substances. The facility must keep a record for each controlled substance administered. Individual pharmacies provide various types of controlled substance records. Information generally required includes the name of the patient receiving the controlled substance, the date and hour the medication was given, the amount of the controlled medication used, the name of the healthcare provider prescribing the controlled substance, and the name of the nurse administering the controlled substance.

Healthcare facility personnel perform a count of controlled medications at specified times (e.g., at each change of shift or when removed from an automated dispensing machine). Before administering a controlled medication, the count in the drawer must be verified, and the control sheet must be signed (handwritten or electronic) to indicate that the medication has been removed. If all or part of a dose is discarded,

TABLE 20-3 SCHEDULES OF CONTROLLED SUBSTANCES CATEGORIZED BY THE CONTROLLED SUBSTANCES ACT

Schedule	Characteristics	Dispensing Restrictions	Examples*
I	High abuse potential No accepted medical use—for research, analysis, or instruction only	Approved protocol necessary; not dispensed with Rx	Heroin, LSD, marijuana, mescaline, methaqualone, peyote tetrahydrocannabinols
II	May lead to severe physical or psychological dependence High abuse potential Accepted medical uses	Written Rx necessary; fax OK for hospice and long-term care Only required amount may be prescribed No Rx refills allowed Container must have warning label	Amphetamines, cocaine, codeine, meperidine, morphine, opium, oxycodone (OxyContin), oxycodone with aspirin or acetaminophen (Percodan, Percocet), pentobarbital, secobarbital, Ritalin
III	Less abuse potential than drugs in schedules I and II Accepted medical uses May lead to moderate or low physical dependence or high psychological dependence	34-d supply limit Written or oral Rx required Rx expires in 6 mo No more than five Rx refills allowed within a 6-mo period Container must have warning label†	Preparations containing limited quantities of opioids or combined with one or more active ingredients that are noncontrolled substances Codeine combinations (Tylenol with codeine), hydrocodone combinations (Vicodin, Lortab)
IV	Low abuse potential compared with drugs in schedule III Accepted medical uses May lead to limited physical or psychological dependence	Written or oral Rx required Rx expires in 6 mo No more than five Rx refills allowed Container must have warning label	Alprazolam, barbital, clorazepate, chlordiazepoxide, chloral hydrate, diazepam, fenfluramine, flurazepam, lorazepam meprobamate, oxazepam, phenobarbital, propoxyphene, temazepam, zolpidem
V	Low abuse potential compared with drugs in schedule IV Accepted medical uses May lead to limited physical or psychological dependence	May require written Rx No limit on refills Rx expires in 12 mo	Medications, generally for relief of coughs (Robitussin A-C) or diarrhea, containing limited quantities of certain opioid controlled substances

*The examples cited constitute a partial listing. Individual hospital council should be consulted for a complete list for a particular state.
†*Caution*: Federal law prohibits the transfer of this drug to any person other than the patient for whom it was prescribed. From Uniform Controlled Substances Act; see www.justice.gov/dea/

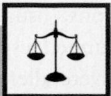

PATIENT'S REFUSAL OF MEDICATIONS

You are a nursing student assigned to care for George Saunders, a 47-year-old homeless man who was admitted last evening for pneumonia. He has a history of alcohol abuse and mental illness. When you approach his room with his scheduled antibiotic and antipsychotic medications, he starts yelling, telling you to "get that poison away from me." You talk with staff members about his reaction, asking them what to do. One staff person tells you to mix the medications in the patient's food when he is not looking. Another tells you to chart that the patient refused the medications.

CRITICAL THINKING CHALLENGE

- Explore whether Mr. Saunders has the right to refuse his medication.
- Evaluate possible factors that might have affected Mr. Saunders' ability to make an informed decision regarding whether to take his medication.
- Determine whether you have the right to trick him into taking his medications. Discuss why or why not and any possible ramifications in doing so.
- Outline possible positive and negative consequences of allowing Mr. Saunders to refuse medication.
- Would you respond any differently if Mr. Saunders were a middle-class business executive?

a second nurse must witness the discarding and countersign the control record. Automated medication-dispensing systems automatically count and track controlled substances as they are taken from the system, eliminating the need for two nurses to count controlled drugs at shift change.

Substance Abuse

The illegal use of drugs by any health professional jeopardizes patient welfare and professional credibility. Stringent rules and procedures help prevent diversion of patient medications to healthcare personnel. Each nurse has the ethical and legal obligation to maintain accurate medication records and to report any discrepancies. The law further requires nurses to report any known diversion of controlled substances by colleagues.

! SAFETY ALERT

The chemically impaired nurse cannot be trusted to exercise optimal clinical judgment. Such individuals must be identified in order to protect patient safety and so that the nurse can obtain treatment.

PRINCIPLES OF DRUG ACTION

An understanding of the ways by which drugs exert their effects is an important component of medication administration. **Pharmacokinetics** is the process by which a drug moves through the body and is eventually eliminated. **Pharmacodynamics** refers to the physiologic and biochemical effects of a drug on the body. Understanding these processes assists the nurse in evaluating therapeutic and adverse effects of medications.

Pharmacokinetics

Pharmacokinetics involves the absorption, distribution, metabolism, and excretion of a medication. Each medication has its own characteristic rate and manner by which it is absorbed by body tissues, delivered to reactive cells, transformed to harmless substances, and removed from the body.

Absorption is the process by which a medication enters the bloodstream. The route of administration affects how quickly and completely a medication is absorbed. Intravenous (IV) administration offers the quickest rate of absorption, followed in descending order by intramuscular (IM), subcutaneous, and oral (PO) routes. **Distribution** is the process by which the medication is delivered to the target cells and tissues. The effectiveness of the circulatory system, the amount of medication bound to protein, and the tissue specificity of the drug affect distribution.

Metabolism is the process of chemically changing the drug in the body. Metabolism takes place mainly in the liver. Alterations in liver function, including decreased function that occurs with aging or disease, affect the rate at which drugs are metabolized.

Excretion is the process of removing the drug or its metabolites from the body. The kidneys excrete most drug metabolites. Some excretion also occurs in the lungs and the intestines. Decreased kidney function adversely affects drug excretion.

Pharmacodynamics

Drug activity is the result of chemical interactions between a medication and the body's cells to produce a biologic response. Most drugs interact with a cellular component to initiate a series of biochemical and physical changes, resulting in the drug's effects. These biochemical and physiologic effects can be local or systemic. For example, local effects are seen when moisturizing lotion is applied to chapped skin. Systemic effects can affect one or more body systems. For example, when analgesics (pain medications) are administered, effects on sedation (nervous system), respiratory rate and depth (lungs), and constipation (gastrointestinal tract) are seen.

Medication effects are monitored by changes in the patient's clinical condition. Generally, improvement in physical or psychological symptoms occurs when medications are effective. In addition to clinical observations, laboratory measurements of the concentration of medication in the blood can be obtained.

THERAPEUTIC EFFECTS

A medication's desired and intentional effects are called its therapeutic effects. These effects vary with the nature of the medication, the length of time the patient has been receiving it, and the patient's physical condition. Interactions with other medications also can affect a drug's therapeutic action. The onset of action of medications varies widely depending on the medication, the route of administration, and the half-life of the drug.

ADVERSE EFFECTS

An **adverse drug event** is any effect other than the therapeutic effect. Adverse effects can result from excessive therapeutic effects (e.g., severe hypotension when an antihypertensive agent is administered). Some adverse effects are minor (e.g., constipation) and can be treated easily. Others may pose serious health risks for the patient (e.g., respiratory depression). Adverse effects increase in patients who are very ill and receiving many medications.

The FDA has developed the MedWatch program to encourage voluntary reporting of any serious adverse drug effects. Any healthcare professional can report, without proof of direct causation, any unexpected response to drug therapy or medical devices. The FDA correlates data collected to update drug information that it gives to the public.

Side Effects

Minor adverse effects are called side effects. Many side effects are essentially harmless and can be ignored. Some, however, are undesirable and potentially harmful. Especially when a new medication is started or added or when a dose is increased, nurses must be alert for adverse drug reactions or side effects in patients.

Tolerance

Tolerance to a medication occurs when a patient develops a decreased response to it, requiring an increased dosage to achieve the therapeutic effects. Some agents that produce tolerance include nicotine, alcohol, opiates, and barbiturates.

Allergic Reactions

Allergic reactions result from an immunologic response to a medication to which the patient has been sensitized. A foreign substance or antigen has been introduced into the body, and the body responds by producing antibodies. Patients respond to certain medications as they would to this foreign substance and develop symptoms of an allergic reaction. These symptoms range from mild to severe. Mild allergic reactions, commonly manifested by hives (urticaria), pruritus, or rhinitis, can occur within minutes to 2 weeks after medication administration.

Skin reactions, including hives, rashes, and lesions, usually improve soon after use of the medication is discontinued, especially with concomitant use of antihistamines. Severe allergic reactions producing symptoms such as wheezing, dyspnea, angioedema of the tongue and oropharynx, hypotension, and tachycardia occur immediately after the medication is given.

> **! SAFETY ALERT**
>
> A severe allergic reaction, called an **anaphylactic reaction**, requires immediate medical intervention because it can be fatal. Treatment includes discontinuing use of the medication and administering epinephrine, IV fluids, steroids, and antihistamines.

Toxicity

Medication toxicity results from overdose or buildup of medication in the blood due to impaired metabolism and excretion. Careful attention must be given specifically to the dosage and to toxicity monitoring, such as assessing laboratory values of liver and kidney function. Drug levels can be assessed for drugs that have a narrow therapeutic range. Some medications can produce toxic effects almost immediately; others do not produce toxic effects for days or weeks.

Toxicity can affect, and permanently damage, organ function. Common drug toxicities include nephrotoxicity (kidney), neurotoxicity (brain), hepatotoxicity (liver), immunotoxicity (immune system), ototoxicity (hearing), and cardiotoxicity (heart). Knowledge about potential drug toxicity permits focused nursing assessments for early detection, thus preventing permanent damage.

INTERACTIONS

A medication interaction occurs when a medication's effects are altered by the concurrent presence of other medications or food. This interaction may result in potentiation or **synergism**, which increases a drug's effects. Interaction also can result in **antagonism**, by which drug effects decrease. Sometimes, foods influence a drug. An example of a food–drug interaction is the deactivation of the antibiotic tetracycline by dairy products.

COMPATIBILITY

In some cases, a drug will precipitate from solutions, or chemically inactivate, if mixed with other medications. This is known as a **drug incompatibility**. When giving two medications in a syringe or when mixing IV medications in tubing, it is important to assess whether the drugs are compatible and can safely be mixed during administration. Almost all drugs interact adversely with at least one other drug. Therefore, it is not always possible to avoid prescribing drugs that interact adversely. However, drugs that are incompatible need to be administered separately. It is the nurse's role to evaluate incompatibility. This is different from a drug interaction and needs to be looked up using an IV drug book or online medical resource.

SAFETY ALERT

Always be aware of the possibility of drug incompatibilities and interactions in order to protect patients from harmful effects. Refer to incompatibility charts and check with the pharmacist for valuable information.

MEDICATION ASSESSMENT

To administer medications safely to any patient, information must be collected during the initial assessment. In addition to these baseline data, a medication-specific assessment is part of the ongoing nursing assessment to determine medication effectiveness and promptly identify adverse effects. Assessment is also necessary in planning appropriate patient teaching to promote adherence with therapy.

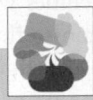

THERAPEUTIC DIALOGUE: MEDICATION ADMINISTRATION

SCENE FOR THOUGHT

As the nurse brings Mr. Abramson, age 58, his heart medication, he turns his attention from the television on the wall to her.

LESS EFFECTIVE

Mr. Abramson: Kirsten, I don't want those pills. I told the doctor I don't need them. They give me headaches, and I don't want them.

Nurse: *(Stops in surprise just inside the room. Sits in chair next to Mr. Abramson.)* You sure seem upset about this. Tell me what happened.

Mr. Abramson: I just get headaches from them, that's all. And she said I'd have to take them for the rest of my life! I can't live with headaches for the rest of my life. *(Looks angry and powerless.)*

Nurse: I can tell this bothers you a lot. Do you have a headache now?

Mr. Abramson: No, but after I take that little white pill, I always do.

Nurse: Which pill is it? I don't seem to have one to give you right now. *(Shows him the three capsules in the cup, two blue and one white with a yellow stripe.)*

Mr. Abramson: *(Looks in confusion.)* It isn't there. Maybe she changed it already.

Nurse: I think that's what happened. There was a medication order change this morning after she made rounds, and the pharmacy just sent these new blue capsules for you. Do you feel better about it now? *(Pours fresh water into a glass so he can take the medication.)*

Mr. Abramson: Sure, sure. At least I won't have those headaches. *(Looks somewhat relieved but still skeptical.)*

Nurse: Yes. I'm glad we got that straightened out! Call me if you need me. *(Goes out to finish giving meds.)*

MORE EFFECTIVE

Mr. Abramson: Christine, I don't want those pills. I told the doctor I don't need them. They give me headaches, and I don't want them.

Nurse: *(Stops in surprise just inside the room. Sits in chair next to Mr. Abramson.)* You seem upset about this. Tell me what happened.

Mr. Abramson: I just get headaches from them, that's all. And she said I'd have to take them for the rest of my life! I can't live with headaches for the rest of my life. *(Looks angry and powerless.)*

Nurse: I can tell this bothers you a lot. Did you mention the reason you don't want this medication to your provider?

Mr. Abramson: Yes. She said she'd change it. *(Sounds irritated.)*

Nurse: Let me check for you. *(Checks the med order the provider wrote that morning. The medication has been changed.)* Well, she did change it, Mr. Abramson. This is the new medication she ordered. *(Shows him the capsule.)*

Mr. Abramson: *(Takes it reluctantly.)* How do I know this won't affect me the same way?

Nurse: I would like to come back and give you some information about it after I've given out the other medications on the unit. Would that help?

Mr. Abramson: Yes, indeed. *(Looks relieved but still a little skeptical.)*

Nurse: And maybe we can talk about your concerns that you'll have to take it for the rest of your life. That sounds like a separate issue but still important. Have I read that right?

Mr. Abramson: I think so, Christine. I'll think about that while you're gone. *(Gives a small smile, almost sheepish.)*

CRITICAL THINKING CHALLENGE

- In both dialogues, Mr. Abramson received the correct medication. Detect what he didn't receive in the first dialogue.

- Explain what concerned Christine about Mr. Abramson's remark about having to take the medication for the rest of his life.

Information Collected During Initial Assessment

During the initial assessment, it is important to perform a medication history, assess for a history of any allergies and medication intolerances, evaluate the patient's medical history, and determine the patient's pregnancy and lactation status.

MEDICATION HISTORY AND MEDICATION RECONCILIATION

During the initial interview, determine the names, dosages, schedules, and patient understanding of the purposes of any medications he or she takes routinely. When available, use the electronic medical record from the patient's primary care clinic or provider as a point of reference to reconcile the names and doses of all patient medications. Historical paper records or "old charts" also can be used. **Medication reconciliation** (or medication verification) is an important safety procedure during patient handoffs between healthcare providers or agencies. Examples of patient handoffs include new and intermittent clinic visits, emergency department visits, hospital admissions, transfers between hospital units, and discharge from one healthcare facility to another or to home. Medication reconciliation prevents medication errors such as omitting a medication, failing to restart administration of a medication that was temporarily withheld, or double-dosing medication. Additional information may be obtained from family members, who may provide information that the patient does not volunteer. An example is, "Mom doesn't take her water pill in the evening because she doesn't like to go to the bathroom at night."

While hospitalized, the patient usually is required to send all medications home or the medications are stored in a secure location until discharge. Alert the physician or other prescribing provider to all medications the patient has been taking so that necessary medications can be ordered. This is especially important if the patient is taking antidiabetic agents, anticonvulsant medications, or cardiovascular medications.

Also, discuss the patient's use of any OTC medications. A question such as "What medications do you buy without a prescription?" may help elicit this information. A patient may overlook common medications, such as aspirin, acetaminophen, herbal remedies, supplements, or laxatives, when asked to list medications. In particular, patients may not consider eyedrops, nasal sprays, skin lotions, food supplements, and herbal remedies to be medications.

If patients are taking multiple medications, cannot remember the names of all of them, or if their medication profile differs from their clinical status, ask the patient or family to collect all medications and bring them in for you to look at. Access to the patient's medications allows the nurse to make a complete list of prescribed medications and to identify actual or potential medication problems. Note whether prescriptions have expired, whether all medications are stored separately in correctly marked containers, whether the prescriptions are actually this patient's or those of another person, and whether the number of pills in a bottle is correct.

ALLERGIES AND INTOLERANCES

During the initial interview, ask the patient about allergies to any medications. If the patient indicates any medication allergies, ask follow-up questions about the allergic symptoms noted with each drug. This information allows differentiation between a medication that caused a true allergic response and a medication that caused side effects. True allergic reactions that are dangerous include hives, kidney pain, difficulty breathing, and lowered pulse with shock (anaphylaxis).

Patients in the hospital or in long-term care facilities will have all allergies listed in one standard location, most effectively in a computerized record, so that any changes in allergies can be clearly communicated. MedicAlert bracelets or pendants might also be worn to identify drug allergies (Fig. 20-3).

 SAFETY ALERT

To avoid potentially fatal anaphylaxis, always check a patient's allergy history before giving any medication.

MEDICAL HISTORY

Before administering any medication to a patient, be aware of the patient's medical diagnosis and general medical history. Any renal, hepatic, cardiac, respiratory, endocrine, or neurologic dysfunction is important to ascertain before administering any medication. This information can be used to identify patients who are at greater risk for drug toxicity or who may require extra care in drug administration.

Drug or alcohol abuse also is important to determine before medication administration. The patient who has used opiates or alcohol frequently may require higher doses of sedatives or opiates to obtain the desired effect. Patients who have not previously or do not routinely use opiates for chronic conditions will require lower doses and close monitoring during therapy to avoid respiratory depression.

PREGNANCY AND LACTATION STATUS

Drugs known to cause birth defects are called **teratogenic**. Drug references categorize drugs (A, B, C, D, and X) in terms of their risk of causing harm during pregnancy. Studies have

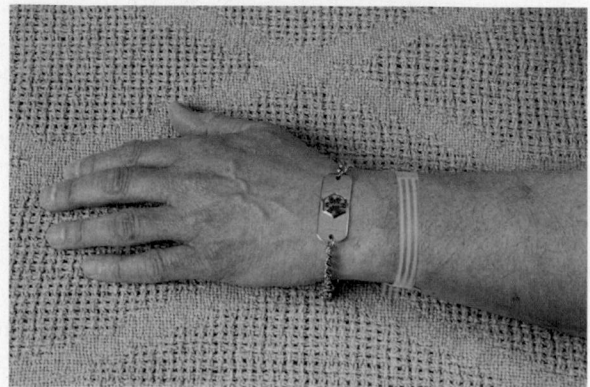

FIGURE 20-3 Patients with medication allergies might wear a MedicAlert bracelet.

demonstrated no risk for drugs in category A, whereas significant risk has been demonstrated for category X. Pregnant women should avoid taking any known teratogenic drug and any drug that has not been thoroughly evaluated. Rarely (e.g., in a pregnant patient with difficult-to-control epilepsy), the use of a potentially harmful drug during pregnancy is indicated. The provider discusses the risks and benefits of such treatment with the patient before prescribing the drug. This discussion is documented in the medical record. Late in pregnancy, women avoid the use of hepatotoxic medications because of increased risk of liver damage to the woman.

A medication may be excreted through breast milk and ingested by a nursing baby. Many medications are excreted in low dosages that do not affect breast-feeding babies, but some (e.g., opiates, antibiotics, anticoagulants, anticonvulsants, histamine antagonists, tranquilizers) can be excreted in amounts great enough to affect babies. If a woman must receive a medication that is excreted in large concentrations in breast milk, bottle feeding may be recommended.

Assessment Before Medication Administration

Before administering any medication, it is important to check the patient's medication record, evaluate the current diet and fluid orders, assess the patient's laboratory values, and perform a quick physical assessment. Medications may affect blood pressure, heart rate, and respiratory rate. Before giving a medication that can affect vital signs, measure and record the value. Measure blood pressure before administering antihypertensive medications or coronary vasodilators. If the patient's systolic blood pressure is low (usually less than 90 or 100 mm Hg systolic), the drug may be held. Often, the parameters are written on the electronic medication administration record (eMAR) for cardiac medications. If no parameters are written, ask the provider to do so to ensure safety. The apical heart rate is counted for 1 minute before giving medications that slow the heart rate. If the heart rate is slow (usually less than 60 beats per minute), withhold the medication and contact the provider. Count the respiratory rate before giving a medication, such as an opiate, that may depress the respiratory rate.

MEDICATION RECORD

Before giving a patient any medication, check the patient's eMAR. The patient may have several medications ordered to treat the same problem. Checking the patient's eMAR allows the nurse to see which medication has been used most recently and whether it is time for the medication to be administered. Knowing a patient's current medications also allows the nurse to avoid giving a medication that may interfere with, or add to the effects of, another medication the patient has received.

DIET AND FLUID ORDERS

A patient may have fluids and food withheld in preparation for surgery or for a diagnostic test. When a patient is ordered to have nothing by mouth (NPO), remind the patient that only the most important medications are given. When the patient is receiving medications that should not be discontinued abruptly (e.g., blood pressure medication, digoxin, anticonvulsants), contact the provider concerning alternative orders for medication administration. In some situations, providers order that oral medications be administered with a small sip of water even though a patient is NPO. When a patient with diabetes is NPO, contact the provider regarding specific orders for holding oral hypoglycemic medications or adjusting the insulin dose.

LABORATORY VALUES

Laboratory tests may be used to monitor serum drug levels, medication effects, and medication side effects. Dosages of certain drugs (e.g., digoxin, vancomycin, phenytoin) are evaluated by monitoring serum drug levels to determine the proper dosage for the patient. Assess these serum drug levels, and notify the provider if values are outside the therapeutic range. Doing so permits the provider to change the medication dosage to ensure therapeutic effects without causing toxicity.

Laboratory tests also may be used to monitor a medication's direct effects. Serum levels can be used to determine proper dosing of medications such as iron, potassium, and thyroid preparations. Anticoagulants also are monitored for therapeutic effects by drawing venous blood to assess coagulation status. Make sure to assess these before administering them.

Side effects are also monitored with the use of laboratory tests. Many diuretics are potassium wasting; thus, serum potassium levels are measured to detect hypokalemia. Many types of chemotherapy cause decreased numbers of white blood cells (increasing risk of infection) or platelets (increasing risk of bleeding). Therefore, blood counts are monitored before and after chemotherapy. If medications are known to cause kidney dysfunction, kidney function tests (e.g., serum creatinine, blood urea nitrogen) are done at regular intervals. If medications can potentially cause liver damage, liver function tests (e.g., alanine aminotransferase [ALT], aspartate aminotransferase [AST]) may be ordered and evaluated.

PHYSICAL ASSESSMENT

Before giving a medication, quickly assess the patient's physical ability to take the medication. The ability to swallow and normal gastrointestinal motility are important considerations for oral medications. Adequate muscle mass and venous access are important for parenteral medications. If the medication is likely to affect vital signs or the function of a body system, appropriate assessments are made before medication administration.

Ability to Swallow

Before administering an oral medication, be sure the patient has an adequate swallowing reflex. Adhere to any swallowing precautions as ordered. If you suspect that a patient cannot safely swallow, position the patient sitting fully upright, give the patient a few sips of water. If the patient coughs or chokes on the water, do not give the medication and inform the provider. A few sips of water prior to the pill help to moisten the mouth and assist with swallowing if the mouth is dry.

Gastrointestinal Motility

If a patient's gastrointestinal function is abnormal (e.g., recent surgery, nausea, or vomiting), perform a quick abdominal assessment. If the patient's abdomen is distended and firm and bowel sounds are hypoactive or absent, gastrointestinal dysfunction is present. Contact the provider to check whether oral medications can be given by another route.

Adequate Muscle Mass

Premature babies and debilitated patients may have limited amounts of lean muscle mass. If an irritating medication is given into subcutaneous tissue or into a very small muscle, pain, inadequate absorption of medication, or tissue damage could occur. Contact the provider to determine whether another route of administration could be used.

Adequate Venous Access

Before giving an IV medication, be sure the IV catheter is located in an adequate vein and is patent. Assess the catheter insertion site for temperature, redness, swelling, and pain. If the needle is out of the vein, or there is infection or inflammation, do not administer medication into the site.

Body System Assessment

To assess the effect of a medication, the appropriate body system must be assessed before it is given. For example, drugs that open the lungs may be inhaled by a patient with chronic obstructive lung disease to treat wheezing. Before beginning the treatment, assess the patient's respiratory system. This quick assessment includes counting the respiratory rate, asking the patient to rate his or her ease of breathing, noting the use of accessory respiratory muscles, and listening to the patient's breath sounds. After the treatment, this assessment is repeated. Judge the effect of the treatment by noting a reduction in wheezing and improved ease of breathing.

SAFE MEDICATION ADMINISTRATION

To administer medications safely, the following actions are necessary:

- Accurately interpret the provider's order.
- Accurately calculate the amount of drug to give for the prescribed dose.
- Develop a systematic and safe procedure, using the six rights for drug administration, including accurate identification using two separate identifiers.
- Document medication administration according to best practice principles.
- Explain the purpose of the medication to the patient.
- Recognize and prevent potential medication errors.
- Promote clear communication with the patient and members of the healthcare team.
- Promote healthcare planning and home- or community-based care.
- Evaluate the patient's response to medications.

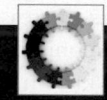

COLLABORATING WITH THE HEALTHCARE TEAM:
Calling the Provider Concerning Holding a Medication

You decide to hold Mr. Brady's morning dose of digoxin because his pulse rate is 62 and irregular and his serum potassium level is 2.9 mEq. You report Mr. Brady's status and your actions and request orders for follow-up using the SBAR communication tool.

S*ITUATION:* I held Mr. Brady's morning digoxin because his pulse is 62 and irregular and his serum potassium is 2.9 mEq.

B*ACKGROUND:* Mr. Brady, 86, was admitted for a fractured hip repair 2 days ago. His pulse usually runs in the 80s, and this is the first time his pulse has been irregular. Since surgery, his potassium has been dropping, but this is the lowest it has been. He also has a history of some renal insufficiency.

A*SSESSMENT:* I held Mr. Brady's digoxin because I think he may be dig toxic, especially with low serum potassium and renal impairment.

R*ECOMMENDATION:* Could we get a dig level to see if he is dig toxic? Do you want to order some potassium or get another serum potassium level? We would also like parameters when you want the digoxin held (e.g., pulse below 60 or irregular).

CRITICAL THINKING CHALLENGE

- Reflect on how a tool like SBAR helps you organize your thoughts before discussing important information with other health team members.
- Consider the advantages and disadvantages of providing this information to the provider over the phone or via a text message.
- Discuss the rationale of holding the digoxin when Mr. Brady's pulse was 62. Many references state to hold digoxin if the pulse is below 60.
- Are there other data you could collect to support your assessment that Mr. Brady is digoxin toxic?

Interpreting the Order

The nurse is responsible for safe interpretation of the medication order. If the order is illegible, he or she can easily misinterpret the intended medication request. If the written order is not completely clear or contains unusual or unacceptable abbreviations, always consult the provider for clarification. Clarification also may be necessary if important information, such as the route or frequency of administration, is omitted.

Evaluate whether the amount and route ordered are safe for the patient. Know or research the dosage range, route of administration, contraindications, and side effects before giving any medication. If you question the safe use of any prescribed medication, you have the legal responsibility to consult with the provider rather than administer a medication that could cause harm.

Computerized provider order entry (CPOE) systems are now common, especially in large healthcare institutions. Errors related to illegibility of written medication orders are virtually eliminated. In addition, these computerized information systems alert providers, pharmacists, and nurses to potential errors related to drug–drug interactions, inappropriate dosing, or critical patient allergies. However, computers cannot prevent an order from being entered into the wrong patient's electronic record.

Calculating Adult Medication Dosages

Medication orders are usually written in metric units of measure and supplied the same way. Occasionally, liquid medications or commonly used oral medications may be ordered in household units of measure. If a medication is ordered in one unit of measure and supplied by the pharmacy in another unit of measure, calculate the amount of medication needed in the measurement system ordered. Expertise in medication calculation and administration is essential for safe medication administration. Regular self-testing of medication calculation skills is recommended.

! SAFETY ALERT

If the calculated dosage of a medication seems unusual (e.g., consists of more than two tablets, less than a half tablet, more than one unit dose of a liquid medication) or if you have any doubts about the accuracy of your calculation, ask another nurse or a pharmacist to check the dosage calculation.

If the medication is ordered and supplied in the same measurement system, use the following formula to calculate the amount of medication needed:

$$\frac{\text{Dose on hand}}{\text{Quantity on hand}} = \frac{\text{Dose desired}}{X}$$

where X is the quantity desired.

Example: 400 mg of an antibiotic is ordered, and you have 200-mg tablets on hand.

$$\frac{200\ \text{mg}}{1\ \text{tablet}} = \frac{400\ \text{mg}}{X}$$
$$200X = 400$$
$$X = 2\ \text{tablets}$$

Example: You have 0.25 mg of digoxin ordered IV. The vial the pharmacy sent says 0.125 mg = 1 mL.

$$\frac{0.125\ \text{mg}}{1\ \text{mL}} = \frac{0.25\ \text{mg}}{X}$$
$$0.125X = 0.25$$
$$X = 2\ \text{mL}$$

Conversions within the metric system can be calculated using this formula or by remembering that the metric system is based on units of 10. Equivalents are computed by multiplying or dividing—moving the decimal point to the right or left, respectively. Only three basic units in the metric system are used to calculate medication dosages: gram (g), milligram (mg), and microgram (μg). The equivalents among these three units are 1 g = 1,000 mg = 1,000,000 μg.

To change grams to milligrams, multiply the grams by 1,000 (because there are 1,000 mg in 1 g) or move the decimal point three places to the left. An example of this conversion in an equation is 0.8 g = 800 mg.

Calculating Children's Medication Dosages

Children's dosages are most often calculated using the child's weight or body surface area. Most drugs are ordered specifically for a child and are not computed from an adult dose. Take into account the many differences in sizes of children and the individual metabolic rate, which influences the therapeutic dose. Observing the child's response to the medication may determine whether the dosage needs to be adjusted for the benefit of the individual child.

Administering Medications According to the Six Rights

Validating the order, calculating the proper drug dose, and following the six rights of medication administration can ensure accurate administration of a medication. The six rights are summarized in Box 20-1.

! SAFETY ALERT

Each time you administer a medication, be sure that you give the right patient the right medication, in the right dose, by the right route, at the right time, followed by the right documentation.

- Identify the *right patient* using two identifiers (e.g., name, birth date, MRN).
- Select the *right medication*.
- Give the *right dose*.
- Give the medication by the *right route*.
- Give the medication at the *right time*.
- Ensure the *right documentation* of medication administration.

THE RIGHT PATIENT

The first "right" of administering medications, the right patient, means that the medication is given to the patient for whom it is intended (Fig. 20-4). Always use two separate identifiers when administering medications. Examples of identifiers include the patient's name (first and last names), MRN, or birth date. Match the two identifiers listed on the patient's MAR with the patient's identification bracelet or the patient's verbal report of the identifiers before administering all medications. Examples of high-risk situations that could lead to medication being administered to the wrong patient include the following:

- Patients with similar names are located in the same areas of an agency.
- Healthcare personnel fail to perform standard patient identification procedures.
- The nurse omits standard identification and relies on memory from previous interactions with a patient.

THE RIGHT MEDICATION

The second "right" of administering medications, the right medication, means that the medication given is the medication that was ordered and that is appropriate for the patient. Medication errors involving this right may occur when:

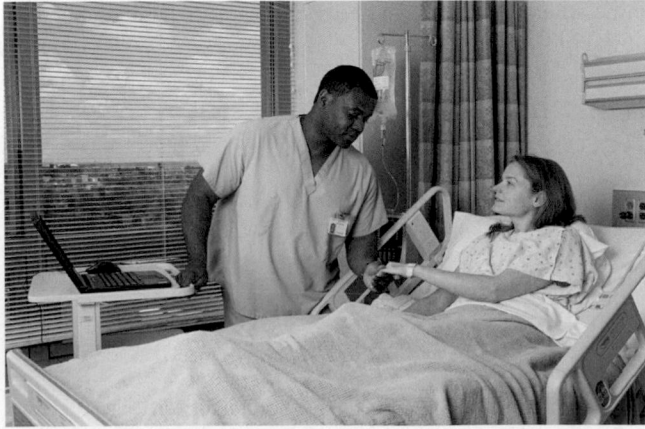

FIGURE 20-4 Always check the patient's identification bracelet for two identifiers. If the patient is conscious, ask the patient to state his or her name and a second identifier.

- The pharmacy incorrectly dispenses a medication that looks similar to the ordered medication.
- A pharmacist or nurse incorrectly dispenses or administers a medication that has a name similar to the medication ordered.
- The prescribing provider orders a medication that is not appropriate for the patient.
- The nurse administers a medication that he or she has not prepared.
- The nurse incorrectly identifies a medication.

Be alert for clues from the patient such as "This doesn't look like the same pill I took before." If you hear a comment like this, recheck the medication order immediately.

THE RIGHT DOSE

The third "right" of administering medications, the right dose, means that the medication is given in the dose ordered and that the dose ordered is appropriate for the patient. Incorrect dosages may be given if the provider orders a dose that is inappropriate for a patient, if the pharmacist dispenses or if the nurse administers an incorrect amount of medication, or if a pharmacist, nurse, or support staff transcribes an order incorrectly onto the patient's medication record.

These errors may be avoided if the nurse and pharmacist are aware of the usual dosage ranges of medications, the nurse double-checks with the provider whenever questions concerning the accuracy of a dosage arise, and the nurse and pharmacist correctly calculate the amount of medication required. Many errors may be eliminated if a computerized order entry system is used.

Triple-check medication dosages whenever you encounter the following situations, which are suggestive of an incorrect medication dosage:

- A patient suggests that the dose he or she is used to taking is different from the dose the nurse is administering.
- Multiple tablets are needed to supply a single medication dose.
- Large or abrupt changes in medication dosages are ordered.
- The amount of medication supplied by the pharmacist does not match the amount needed for the ordered doses.

THE RIGHT ROUTE

The fourth "right" of administering medications, the right route, means that the medication is given by the ordered route and that the ordered route is safe and appropriate for the patient. The provider's medication orders always specify the route of administration. If a route is not specified or seems inappropriate, check with the provider to clarify which route to use.

To ensure that a medication is given by the proper route, know the medication's usual route or routes of administration and the safety of administering the medication by the ordered route.

THE RIGHT TIME

The fifth "right" of administering medications, the right time, means that the medication is given with the correct frequency and at the time ordered according to best policy. Routine medication administration schedules vary among institutions. For example, one agency may specify 9 AM (0900), 1 PM, 5 PM, and 9 PM (2100) as times for medications ordered four times a day. Another agency may specify these times as 8 AM (0800), 12 PM, 4 PM, and 8 PM (2000). Policies defining the meaning of "on time" also vary. Many institutions consider a medication to be given "on time" if it is administered within 30 minutes to 1 hour before or after the scheduled dose time.

Many factors influence the schedules a facility uses to administer medications:

- A medication may be more effective if it is given on an "around-the-clock" schedule.
- A medication that interacts with food may need to be given before meals.
- A medication that causes gastric irritation may need to be given with meals.

Be aware of the scheduling requirements of the medication being given and the routine scheduling times the agency uses.

> **SAFETY ALERT**
>
> Before giving any medication, always check the patient's MAR or eMAR to note when the medication was last administered and if a change has occurred in medication orders. Another advantage of computerized charting is that the computer will alert the nurse of overdue medications.

THE RIGHT DOCUMENTATION

The sixth "right" of administering medications, the right documentation, means that the administration of the medication is appropriately documented according to best practice. An agency's medication policies define the time and type of medication documentation that is required. Medication documentation includes the time, route, dosage, site of administration (for intradermal [ID], subcutaneous, or IM injections), and the nurse's initials and signature (Fig. 20-5). The click of a mouse may meet all of these requirements with computerized charting.

Specific documentation is required if a nurse does not give a scheduled medication. The eMAR allows you to right-click to add a note why the medication was not given or was given late. For paper charting, nurses circle the time of administration when they have withheld a medication. Nurses must indicate why they did not give the medication. At times, this can simply be a matter of indicating NPO next to the designated time for administration. At other times, the reason is more complex and an explanation needs to be written in other appropriate places on the MAR or patient record.

Nurses also are responsible for documenting the therapeutic effects and side effects of any medication administered. For example, if an opiate is administered for pain, document

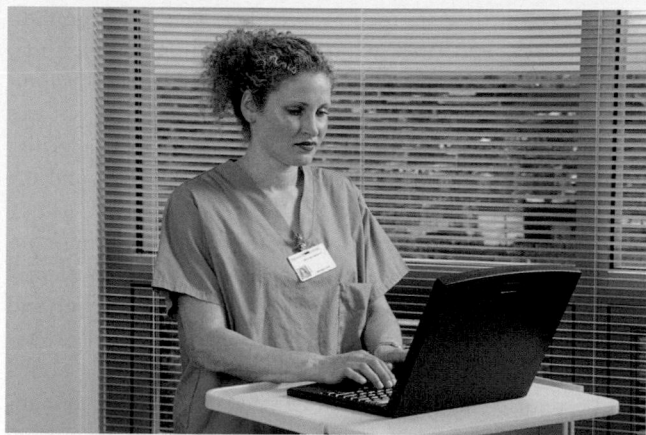

FIGURE 20-5 Documentation of medication administration is an important nursing activity.

the amount of pain relief the patient obtains within the specified time frame (e.g., 30 minutes for IV administration, 60 minutes for PO administration). If a patient develops a rash after the administration of an antibiotic, describe the onset and type of rash in detail in the patient's record. Notify the provider.

> **SAFETY ALERT**
>
> To avoid medication errors, always document immediately after giving a medication.

Preventing Medication Errors

Medication errors are one of the most common types of medical errors. Adverse drug events are the most common source of healthcare mishaps, placing patients at risk every day. Medication errors harm 1.5 million people and account for several thousand deaths per year (Kim & Bates, 2013).

Examples of medication errors include the following:

- A medication is not administered as ordered.
- A medication is administered according to the order, but the order is unsafe or inappropriate for the patient.
- Documentation is inaccurate (the medication was given but not charted, or the medication was not given but was charted as given).
- IV medication is given at the wrong rate.
- Medication is given in the wrong dose.
- Medication is given at the wrong time.
- The wrong medication is given because it was not properly labeled.

Errors of medication substitution may occur with increased use of generic medications. Nurses must be sure that the name of the medication supplied is the same as, not just similar to, the name of the medication ordered. Less common errors include giving a medication by the wrong route or to a patient with a known allergy to that medication.

High-risk medications, such as anticoagulants, opioids, insulin, and sedatives, are more likely to cause harm to a patient even if they are used as intended. The most common types of harm associated with these medications are bleeding, hypoglycemia, delirium, and hypotension. When a medication error occurs, document it by charting the medication as it was given in the patient's MAR or eMAR and completing a facility incident report. Inform your supervisor, the provider, and the patient as appropriate.

The prevention of serious injuries to patients resulting from medical errors is a high priority for healthcare professionals and institutions. According to the IOM (2006), by identifying and preventing medication errors, an estimated 1.5 million adverse drug events can be prevented each year. Adverse drug events can be reduced by implementing safety measures, redesigning delivery systems, creating safety cultures, and maximizing communication. One method is the "it takes two" standard implemented in many institutions. This is a double-check with two RNs independently using the six rights when administering high-risk medications. Both nurses check the patient (with two indicators, name, MRN, birth date, etc.), medication, route, dose, and time and document the administration in an attempt to eliminate medication errors (Institute for Safe Medication Practices, 2014).

Medication errors are generally divided into those caused by systems issues and those caused by individual professional practice issues (see Chapter 4). Systems factors include lack of adequate staffing, increased patient acuity levels, lack of access to medication information, organizational routines, and issues with organizational communication channels (Institute for Safe Medication Practices, 2014; Kim & Bates, 2013). Systems issues may be addressed by healthcare organizations in several ways, including purchase of automated medication carts to dispense medications, utilization of a single type of medication pump for IV medications hospital wide, and implementation of a bar code system for medication administration (Seibert, Maddox, Flynn, & Williams, 2014). Some hospitals have integrated electronic medical records with links to online resources for medication information.

Individual healthcare professional issues that contribute to medication administration errors include failure to comply with policies and procedures, distractions, improper dosage calculation, increased workload, inadequate knowledge about medications, and care delivery models that increase risk of error (Kim & Bates, 2013).

PROMOTING STANDARDIZED COMMUNICATION

Safe and effective medication administration depends on reliable and standardized communication between all caregivers. When there is a breakdown of communication, the risk of harm to a patient increases. This is especially true during patient transfers, during nursing handoffs or report, and when critical events are taking place. The Joint Commission has recognized this and has issued a requirement as part of the 2015 National Safety Goals (NPSG.03.06.01) that reads:

> Record and pass along correct information about a patient's medicines. Find out what medicines the patient is taking. Compare those medicines to new medicines given to the patient. Make sure

the patient knows which medicines to take when they are at home. Tell the patient it is important to bring their up-to-date list of medicines every time they visit a doctor.

When transferring care of a patient from one provider to another, mention any medications that were not given or any unusual reactions to medications that were administered.

Home and Community Care

Assessment and risk identification for factors influencing a patient's ability to adhere to the medication regimen and appropriate patient teaching are the keys to successful community-based care. In the home, most individuals are responsible for their own medication regimens, but in some instances, this responsibility falls to a caregiver.

ASSESSMENT OF KNOWLEDGE AND ADHERENCE

Patient knowledge about a prescribed medication varies with the person and depends on many factors. Some patients desire to receive detailed information about the medications they are taking, whereas other patients want only minimal information. Determine what the patient already knows and what he or she needs to know to take the medication safely. Then, ask questions to elicit this information. Clearly document inadequate knowledge or gaps in important areas so that an individualized teaching plan can be formulated.

Assessing the patient's cognitive ability is important for individualizing the teaching plan and determining whether the patient can independently manage self-medication. Cognitive impairment, confusion, and psychiatric disorders may increase the potential for difficulty with the medication regimen. Learning disabilities may necessitate creative teaching to ensure understanding and adherence to therapy. Include family members or the caregiver in the teaching sessions. Physical and sensory disabilities may also impact the patient's ability to comply with medication regimens. Especially with older adults, visual and hearing impairments may make it difficult for the patient to understand written or verbal instructions. They may have trouble identifying the correct medication container if they are unable to read the labels.

Adherence to a medication routine means that the patient takes the medication exactly as prescribed. Lack of adherence can occur in many ways—for example, when the patient:

- Does not take any of the prescribed drug
- Does not take the proper number of doses of the drug
- Takes extra doses of the drug
- Does not follow the dosage schedule as prescribed
- Discontinues the medication prematurely
- Excessively uses a prn order
- Takes medications that were ordered previously for another condition
- Takes a medication that was prescribed for someone else

Adherence to a medication routine is more likely to occur when the patient understands and agrees with the rationale for using the medication, the routine for taking the medication, and the desired effect of the medication. Patients are more likely to follow simple medication routines that suit their lifestyles.

A patient's attitude about medical care and about specific medications can influence his or her adherence with drug therapy. Begin by asking general questions such as, "Do you believe that these medications will help you get better?" Be alert to comments that indicate a patient's lack of confidence in prescribed drug treatment. Cultural and religious groups may follow certain healing traditions and may favor the use of herbs or alternative forms of treatment. Patients who believe in folk medicine may have strong opinions about certain home remedies and values concerning health and healing.

Lifestyle and financial considerations also affect compliance with drug therapy. The patient with a regular income, health insurance, and a stable home is more likely to obtain medications and to organize routines to remember to take them. But when a patient does not have a home, income, or health insurance, buying, storing, and remembering to take medications regularly can be difficult.

PATIENT TEACHING

Set your priorities for teaching by determining what the patient needs to know to take medications safely. Present the information in everyday, nontechnical language, both verbally and in writing. Provide brief but practical information about the following topics:

- Name of the medication
- Reason for taking the medication
- How and when to take the medication
- How long to take the medication
- Foods, drinks, and prescription or OTC medications that may affect the medication's action
- Any activities that may be affected when taking this medication
- Usual adverse effects of the medication and their treatment

A proven instructional method that can be used to assess a patient's understanding of his or her medication regime is a method call teach-back. When using teach-back, the nurse should use simple language and phrases and speak slowly and clearly. Only two or three concepts should be introduced to the patient at a time, and the nurse should assess for understanding by asking questions such as, "Please tell me the words that I said to you about your medication" (Tamura-Lis, 2013). Depending on the patient's learning style, verbal instruction can be augmented with written instruction and illustrations. The nurse can reiterate any information that the patient cannot recall and ask the patient to teach the information back again to assess comprehension. This cycle should be repeated until the patient is able to provide the correct information to the provider.

If a medication is being given to improve a bothersome symptom (e.g., a metered-dose inhaler [MDI] to treat shortness of breath), warn against using more than the ordered dosage. Without this warning, a patient who thinks "if a little is good, more is better" may take excessive amounts.

Safe disposal of unused medications is discussed, and patients are encouraged to discard unused medications promptly and never share them with others. Some pharmacies are now providing secure locked bins where unused medications can be discarded; flushing them down the toilet may harm the environment because the ingredients will eventually enter the water system. Controlled substances cannot be disposed of in this manner.

Begin teaching about medications as soon as possible. Teaching about administration techniques that require learning new psychomotor skills, such as those used for injecting insulin, start at least 24 hours before discharge from a hospital or extended care facility. The patient is unlikely to learn a complex psychomotor skill without frequent demonstrations and practice. Learning complex psychomotor skills typically requires several clinic or home visits for reinforcement and refinement.

Document any patient teaching. Indicate topics discussed, to whom the teaching was given (patient only or patient and family members), use of any audiovisual aids or written materials given, and any learning barriers (e.g., limited language, visual or hearing impairment) and what was done to address them. Matching medication routines and teaching materials to individual patients; ensuring frequent, ongoing follow-up; encouraging involvement of family or friends in assisting the person with medication adherence; and discussing adherence issues with the patient may help improve patient adherence to medication routines.

MEDICATION ADMINISTRATION IN THE HOME

Medication administration in the home is becoming increasingly common. Home health nurses will either administer medications or teach the patient and family members how to safely and accurately administer different types of medications in a home setting. When supervising or administering medications in the home, nurses must be sure that this nursing intervention is within the scope of the state's nurse practice act. Many states allow delegation of medication administration in the home setting to unlicensed assistive personnel (UAP) with adequate training and supervision (Reinhard, Young, Kane, & Quinn, 2006). If controlled substances are administered in the home, nurses must carefully comply with the law regarding appropriate drug storage, documentation, and disposal. Doing so protects against suggestions of improper diversion of the controlled substances and accounts accurately for controlled substances administered in the home.

TYPES OF MEDICATIONS

Oral medications, such as antibiotics and pain relievers, have always been prescribed for patients to take at home, and this practice continues to be common. Long-term IV antibiotic or chemotherapeutic medications are also being administered with various portable IV drug infusion devices. Sometimes, home health nurses administer these medications at regular intervals. More often, however, family caregivers must learn to administer the medications.

In such situations, patient education becomes a major nursing focus for maintaining accuracy and minimizing risks. Of equal concern is having help quickly available in case of emergency.

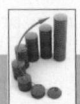

OUTCOME-BASED TEACHING PLANS

Laura Calley, 12 years old, was diagnosed with type 1 diabetes mellitus. You will provide diabetic teaching for her. Her parents are with her. It is clear that the entire family is upset over Laura's newly diagnosed diabetes.

OUTCOME

Before discharge, Laura and her parents will be able to demonstrate the ability to accurately assess Laura's blood glucose level.

STRATEGIES

- Assess Laura's and her parents' readiness to learn by their interest and comfort while watching you perform blood glucose monitoring.
- As you test Laura's blood glucose, verbally explain the procedure.
- At first, encourage Laura to participate by holding equipment and cleansing her own finger.
- Give Laura and her parents written information detailing blood glucose monitoring.
- Verbally cue Laura and/or the parents through blood glucose monitoring.
- Observe a return demonstration by Laura and by her parents.
- Allow Laura to express fears and feelings regarding how frequent glucose monitoring might affect her life.

OUTCOME

After a teaching session, Laura and her parents can verbalize type, dosage, and time of administration for prescribed insulin and list signs and symptoms of hyperglycemia and hypoglycemia.

STRATEGIES

- Provide Laura and her parents with the insulin order in writing.
- Explain the difference between basal and nutritional insulin, providing in writing approximate times for onset, peak, and duration for each type.
- Relate signs of hyperglycemia to Laura's symptoms before diagnosis.
- Compare and contrast the signs of hyperglycemia and hypoglycemia, providing a written list.
- Based on the type of insulin Laura is taking, explain when she may experience hypoglycemia.

- Have Laura and her parents verbalize signs of hypoglycemia and hyperglycemia.

OUTCOME

Before discharge, Laura and her parents will demonstrate the ability to accurately draw up and administer insulin.

STRATEGIES

- Provide Laura and her parents with written information, including illustrations, for drawing up insulin, selecting appropriate site, and performing the injection.
- Periodically review written material with Laura and her parents, allowing time for questions.
- To help Laura overcome any fear of self-injection, avoid long explanations and teaching before giving injection.
- Provide Laura with the dose drawn up and supportively guide her insulin injection.
  - Point to appropriate site.
  - Explain the angle to insert the needle.
  - Stretch or pinch to firm skin.
  - Dart needle through skin and inject insulin dose.
- With successive doses, allow Laura to choose appropriate site, assisting as necessary until Laura is confident with site selection.
- After fear of injecting has passed, verbally cue and observe Laura while she draws up the correct insulin dose, including:
  - Gently rotate insulin to mix suspension.
  - Inject an equal amount of air into vial.
  - Accurately withdraw the ordered amount of insulin.
- Observe a return demonstration of insulin injection into the correct site by Laura and by her parents without cuing and prompting. If they demonstrate that they are unable to complete the steps properly, assess how you can correct the problems to ensure proper insulin administration. Make referrals if needed.

EVALUATION

9/12/17: 03:00—Laura demonstrated her ability to perform blood glucose testing accurately. She was less efficient but stated that she would keep practicing. Both her and her family stated the dose, time, and type of insulin. They listed the signs and symptoms of both high and low blood glucose and the intervention for each. Continue reinforcing knowledge acquisition.

—S. Roberts, RN

In some areas, pharmacies may contract with patients to administer and manage medication administration within the home.

ORGANIZING MEDICATION REGIMENS IN THE HOME

An important aspect of accurate home medication administration is ensuring a schedule that is easy to remember and suits the patient's lifestyle. Arranging administration of medications by linking it with normal events in the patient's life (e.g., meals, bedtime) promotes adherence and accuracy. Be sure to assess the hours when these events occur so that medication administration is staggered appropriately.

For some patients, especially older ones, remembering to take medications and knowing which ones to take can present problems, as illustrated in this chapter's Critical Thinking Challenge. A sectioned medication-dispensing device may be helpful. Such a device may be as simple as an egg carton, divided dish, or envelopes or a commercially available medication pill pack with compartments for a 1-day supply or a weekly supply (Fig. 20-6). These devices may require someone to set up the medications in the appropriate compartments, usually once a week for the entire week. The patient then follows instructions to take medications from the appropriate compartment at the appropriate time. The use of such a device may not prevent all errors, but medication administration with the device may be considerably safer and can help the caregiver evaluate whether medications have been taken.

ADMINISTRATION OF MEDICATIONS BY ROUTE

There are several different routes of administration for medications, including oral, sublingual or buccal, topical, inhaled, and parenteral. It is essential to know how to correctly administer medications by each specific route.

Oral Medications

Medications that are given by mouth (oral), often referred to as PO (per os), are designed to be swallowed. Refer to Procedure 20-1, Administering Oral Medications. Many oral medications

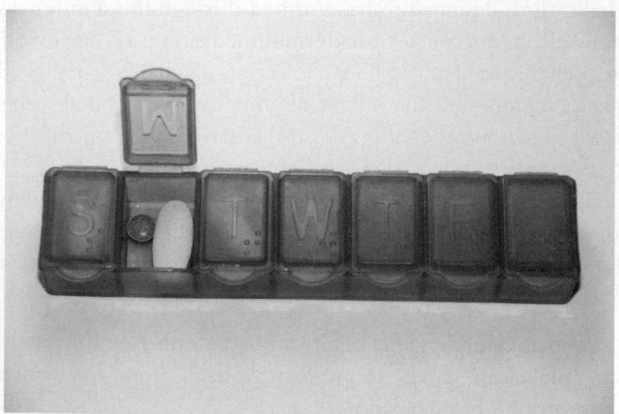

FIGURE 20-6 A sectioned medication-dispensing device.

can also be administered into feeding tubes placed into the stomach, duodenum, or jejunum.

Giving medications by mouth is usually the simplest and easiest way. It minimizes patient discomfort and is associated with the fewest side effects of any route. Oral medications tend to be less expensive and more widely available than medications given by other routes.

If the patient cannot swallow water or fluids or is nauseated or vomiting, oral medications are usually discontinued or given by another route. If a patient is NPO before a test or surgery, the provider may continue selected oral medications, given with sips of water. If the patient is NPO after major surgery, oral medications are usually withheld or administered by another route until intestinal function resumes. If the patient is being treated with gastric suction, oral medications usually are withheld or given by another route. Occasionally, a provider may order a specific medication to be administered through a nasogastric tube, ordering that the gastric suction be discontinued for a specified time (usually 30 minutes) after medication administration to allow absorption of the drug.

ORAL ADMINISTRATION

Position the patient sitting with the head of the bed elevated. Have the patient drink liquid to ensure that the medication moves into the stomach and does not lodge in the esophagus. Even patients with normal swallowing reflexes may have problems swallowing and moving large tablets or capsules down the esophagus. Drug-induced esophagitis, an inflammation of the esophagus, may occur if a tablet or capsule lodges in the esophagus and begins to dissolve there. Whenever possible, encourage the patient to drink about 100 mL of fluid after swallowing a capsule or tablet. If the patient senses that a medication is stuck in the throat, offer a small portion of a soft food, such as a piece of bread or banana, to help move the medication.

Several techniques may be used to administer medications to a patient who can swallow soft foods but not whole capsules or tablets. A capsule may be opened and the contents added to a small amount of the patient's food, such as pudding or applesauce. Some medications have an unpleasant taste when crushed and are mixed with a soft food to minimize the unpleasantness. Many tablets can be crushed and added to soft foods. Be alert to medications that cannot be crushed, including enteric-coated and sustained-release tablets.

! SAFETY ALERT

Never crush enteric-coated or sustained-release tablets. Crushing enteric-coated tablets allows the irritating medication to come in contact with the oral or gastric mucosa, resulting in mucositis or gastric irritation. Crushing a sustained-release medication allows all of the medication to be absorbed at the same time, resulting in a higher-than-expected initial level of the medication and a shorter-than-expected duration of action.

Antifungal liquid medications, such as nystatin, that work through contact with the mucous membranes in the mouth are given by the "swish and swallow" technique. The patient puts the liquid in his or her mouth, moves the liquid back and forth in the mouth several times, and then swallows it. When giving multiple medications at one time, administer any swish and swallow medications last to ensure prolonged contact with the oral mucous membranes. The same is true if it is ordered "swish and spit."

Often, liquid medications come premeasured in unit-dose packages or syringes from the pharmacy. If not, facilities provide calibrated medicine cups and syringes for accurate measurement of prescribed doses of liquid medications. When measuring liquids in a cup, keep the measuring container at eye level on a table and pour the medication to the indicated level. An elliptical curve, called the meniscus, is produced because the solution clings to the side of the measuring container. The lower part of the meniscus should rest on the calibration line of the dose being measured (see **Procedure 20-1**).

Administration of Medications Through Tubes

Oral medications may be administered through nasogastric, gastric (percutaneous endoscopic gastrostomy [PEG]), nasointestinal, or jejunal tubes. When giving oral medications through small-bore feeding tubes, take special care to decrease clogging of the feeding tube. The risk of aspiration (movement of matter into the lungs rather than into the stomach) decreases if the patient is properly positioned with the head up whenever he or she is receiving food or medications. Additionally, the head of the patient's bed remains elevated for at least 30 minutes after medication administration or whenever feedings are administered.

Most liquid medications can be given through feeding tubes. Tablets may be given through a feeding tube if they can be crushed into fine particles and dissolved in water. Enteric-coated, sustained-release, sublingual, and buccal medications may not be crushed. Before and after administering a medication, flush the feeding tube with a minimum of 20 to 45 mL of warm water. If it becomes difficult to instill fluid into the tube, try obtaining an order for pancreatic enzymes to unclog the occluded tube. This may help to dissolve food or medication particles within the tube, possibly restoring tube patency. Research has not demonstrated cranberry juice's effectiveness in unclogging tubes (Knox & Davie, 2009). Do not give water-attracting gels such as Metamucil through feeding tubes, because these agents tend to attract water and solidify within the feeding tube.

Administration by the Sublingual and Buccal Routes

Both the sublingual and buccal routes of administration permit very rapid absorption of medication and avoid first-pass metabolism that causes rapid inactivation of many drugs. Examples of oral drugs given via these routes include nitroglycerin for chest pain and morphine sulfate for breakthrough pain. When administering a **sublingual** medication, a tablet is placed under the tongue and allowed to dissolve. If the patient's mucous membranes are dry, use 1 mL of normal saline solution or water to wet the membranes underneath the tongue so that absorption can occur. Patients should not swallow sublingual tablets. When a medication in a capsule is ordered to be given sublingually, the fluid must be aspirated from the capsule and placed under the tongue. A capsule will not absorb sublingually and may be completely inactivated. Some patients are able to bite into the capsule to free the liquid for absorption under the tongue.

The **buccal** route involves placing medications in the side of the mouth. Transmucosal buccal is given between the teeth and the cheek, and buccal tablets are placed between the cheek and the second molar. The patient should receive oral medications first and should be instructed not to chew, drink, eat, or smoke. Various medications for buccal administration are available, including opiates, antiemetics (for nausea), tranquilizers, and sedatives.

Topical Medications

Topical medications are placed on the skin surface or mucous membranes. They may also be placed in body cavities.

LOTIONS, CREAMS, AND OINTMENTS

Lotions, creams, and ointments may be used to treat a skin or wound infection or skin disease, or they may be used to decrease symptoms of skin disorders. Whenever applying topical medications, protect your hands from inadvertent absorption through your skin by wearing clean gloves. Lotions such as hand and body moisturizers prevent complications associated with excessively dry skin. Sunscreens form a protective covering against ultraviolet light. Lotions are rubbed into the skin until no longer visible.

Creams, such as the antifungal agent miconazole, the corticosteroid hydrocortisone, or the antibiotic silver sulfadiazine, may be applied to skin surfaces with a sterile swab, a sterile tongue depressor, or gloved fingers. Clean and dry the skin surface before applying most creams. Ointments, such as zinc oxide, are applied to protect skin against chafing or moisture associated with bowel and bladder incontinence. Clean the skin and completely pat it dry before applying ointments.

TRANSDERMAL MEDICATIONS

Medications designed to be absorbed through the skin for systemic effects are called **transdermal** medications. They usually are prepared as patches. The medication patches are made with special membranes that allow the medication to be absorbed slowly. These patches allow controlled amounts of medication to be supplied over a 24- to 72-hour period.

Nitroglycerin, scopolamine, estradiol, nicotine, and fentanyl are examples of commonly used transdermal patches. Although the manufacturers' guidelines for application of specific transdermal patches vary, these are general guidelines (Fig. 20-7):

1. Perform hand hygiene before and after applying the patch.
2. Apply clean gloves to protect yourself from inadvertent absorption of medication.

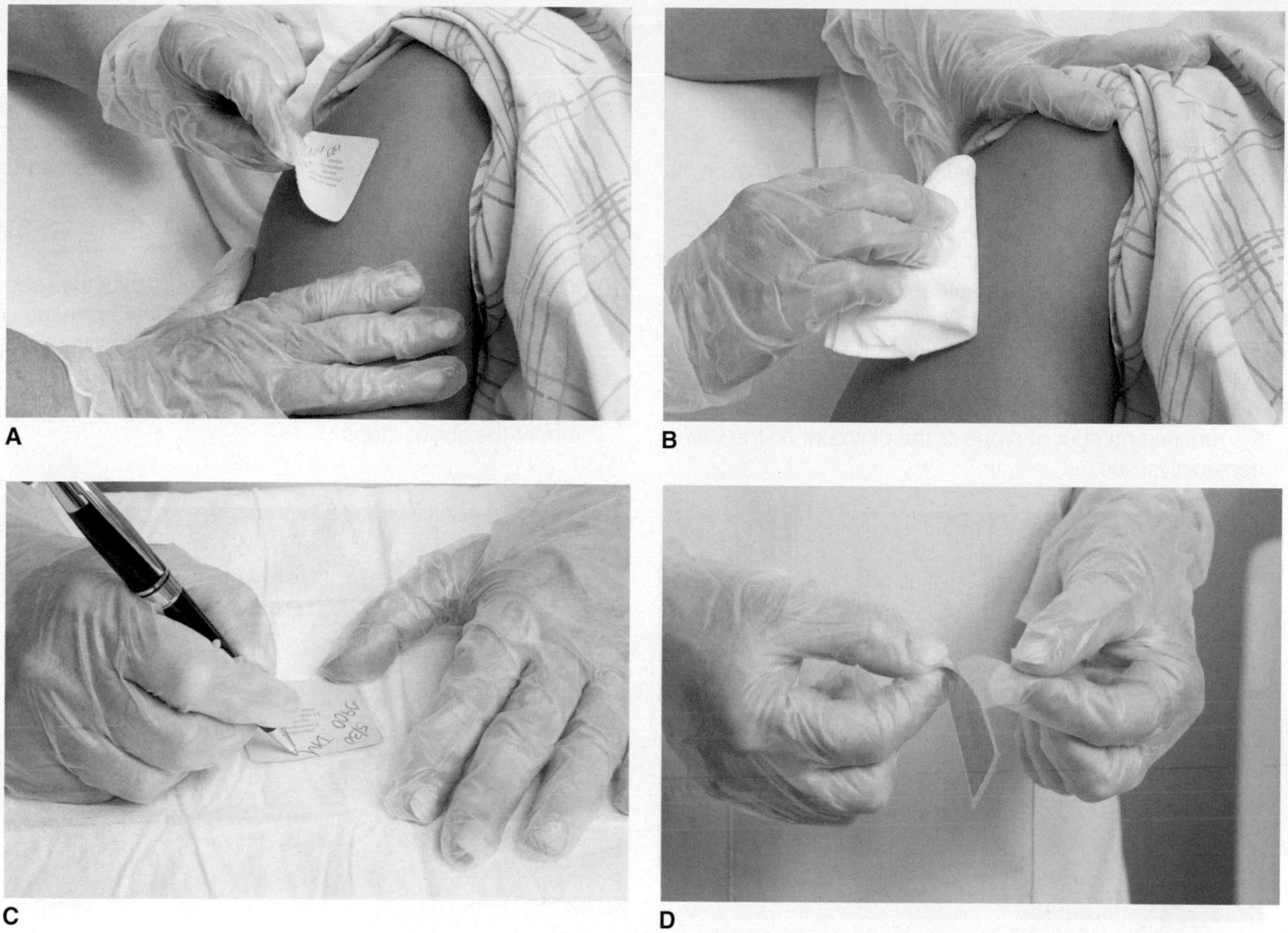

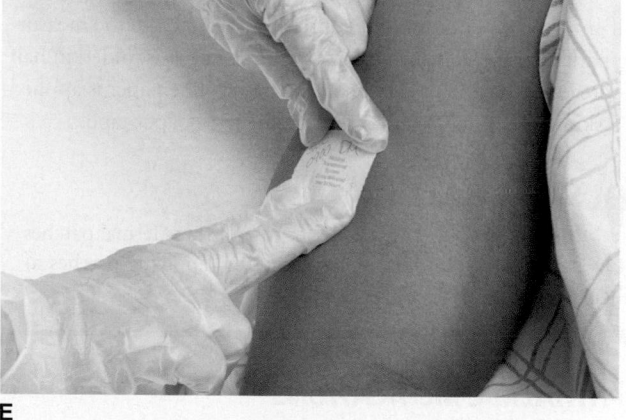

FIGURE 20-7 Transdermal medications are absorbed through the skin. **A.** Remove a previously placed patch. **B.** Clean application site. **C.** Date, time, and initial new patch. **D.** Remove protective covering. **E.** Apply new patch to the skin.

3. Remove a previously placed patch and any remaining traces of medication.
4. Dispose of used transdermal patches carefully.
5. Fold the patch in half and avoid touching the inner surface containing the medication.
6. Apply the new patch to a clean, dry, hairless, intact area of skin, rotating sites.
7. Note the date, time, and your initials on the new patch.
8. Apply the patch immediately after removing the protective liner.

Transdermal patches containing opiate medications should be disposed of in facility-approved containers. Some agencies require two nurses to witness and document disposal of opiate patches. Because heat increases the absorption rate of most transdermal medications, a fever greater than 102°F or the use of heating pads, sun lamps, or other sources of direct heat is usually a contraindication for continued use of the transdermal patch.

Nitroglycerin, sometimes used to control hypertension in acute care settings, also comes in an ointment form that is applied to nitroglycerin paper. The paper is marked with

BOX 20-2   Instilling Eye Medications

1. Assist the patient to sit in an upright position with the head hyperextended.
2. Provide the patient with tissues to blot any medication or tears that spill from the eye during the instillation.
3. Cleanse the eyelid and eyelashes of any drainage. Use each area of the cleaning surface only once, moving from the inner toward the outer canthus.
4. Ask the patient to look toward ceiling.
5. Place the finger or thumb on lower bony orbit, and gently pull the lower lid down.
6. With other hand resting on the patient's forehead, instill the required number of drops or the ointment on the lower conjunctival sac.

7. Avoid touching the eyelids, lashes, or eyeball with either hand or with the applicator.
8. Avoid dropping a solution onto the cornea directly; this causes discomfort.
9. Release the lower lid, and allow the patient to close the eye.
10. Instruct the patient to apply finger pressure over the naso-lacrimal duct for 30 seconds. This prevents drainage of the medication into the nasopharynx, which sometimes causes a tickling sensation or an unpleasant taste.
11. If the patient blinks and the medication is not instilled, repeat the above steps.

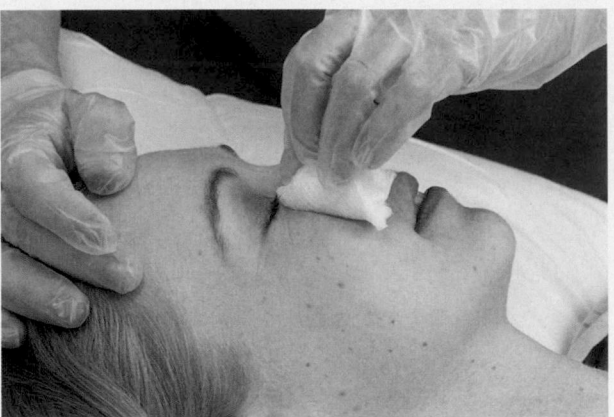
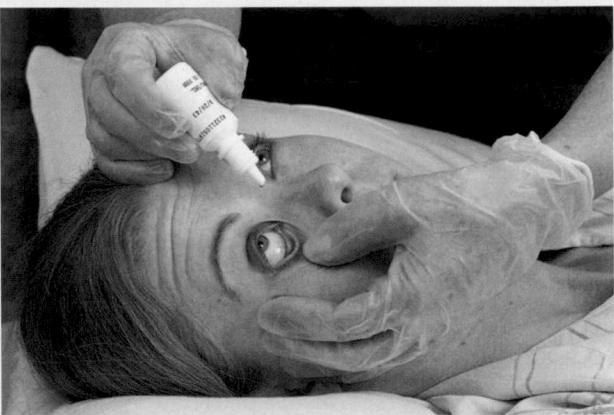

half-inch increments, and the ointment is applied to the measuring paper using a continuous motion. The paper is folded in half to spread the ointment evenly on the paper. The paper is applied to a skin surface and secured to the skin with paper tape.

! SAFETY ALERT

Instruct patients at home to dispose of transdermal patches carefully due to the danger of children applying patches to themselves.

OPHTHALMIC MEDICATIONS

Ophthalmic solutions and ointments may be used to treat eye irritation, infections, or glaucoma. Gently retract the lower eyelid, and place the solution or ointment in the conjunctival sac (lower eye) (Box 20-2). Avoid touching the patient's eye or eyelid with the tip of the ointment tube or dropper. Instruct the patient not to rub the eye after the medication is applied.

OTIC MEDICATIONS

Solutions may be dropped into the ear to treat external ear infections or to soften and remove ear wax. Always use solutions at body temperature because using hot or cold solutions in the ear can cause vertigo, nausea, and pain (Box 20-3).

NASAL MEDICATIONS

Solutions are usually sprayed into the nose to treat nasal congestion. OTC nasal sprays may contain decongestant and adrenergic medications (which stimulate the sympathetic nervous system to constrict vessels). Frequent use can cause systemic effects, such as increased heart rate and increased blood pressure. Rebound nasal congestion, or nasal congestion that is as bad as or worse than the original symptoms, commonly occurs if a patient uses decongestant nasal sprays too frequently or for several days. Corticosteroid nasal sprays are commonly used to treat nasal congestion associated with seasonal or perennial allergies. When consistently used, these nasal sprays are effective as local anti-inflammatory agents to relieve nasal congestion without systemic effects. The nasal route is increasingly used to deliver medications to prevent osteoporosis (calcitonin). When used on a daily basis, alternate nares to avoid irritation.

When administering a nasal spray, have the patient sit up and lean his or her head back or raise the head of the bed and allow the patient to rest his or her head back against the pillow. While holding the medication bottle in one hand, place the top of the bottle just inside the nostril, aiming the spray applicator top toward the midline of the nose (Fig. 20-8). While the patient inhales, squeeze the bottle.

BOX 20-3   Instilling Eardrops

1. Have the patient sit or lie with head turned to unaffected side.
2. Warm solution to body temperature to prevent discomfort during instillation.
3. Prepare appropriate amount of medication in dropper.
4. Straighten the auditory canal by gently pulling the pinna (cartilaginous portion of outer ear) up and back in older children and adults (as shown) and down and back for infants and children younger than 3 years.
5. Instill eardrops on side of the auditory canal to allow the drops to flow in and to continue to adjust to body temperature.
6. Release the pinna, and gently massage tragus of the ear.
7. If permitted, place a cotton ball or wick in the outer ear to keep medication in the canal.
8. If drops are required in the opposite ear, wait a few minutes, and repeat the procedure in that ear.

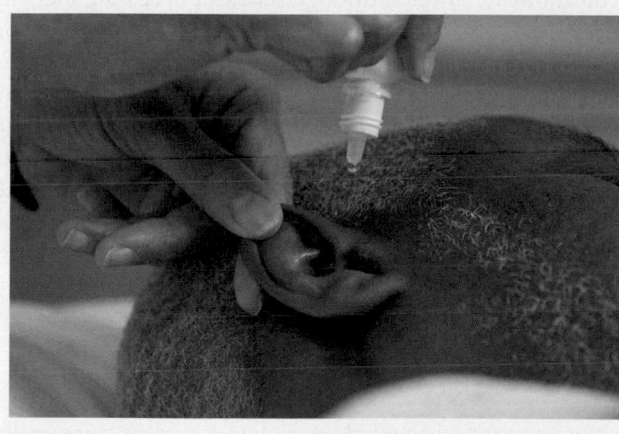

RECTAL MEDICATIONS

Medication in suppository form (a small, cylindrical, waxy base) may be placed in the rectum to treat systemic complaints or as a laxative to encourage bowel movements. Antiemetic suppositories may be used to treat nausea if the patient is at risk for vomiting. The nurse puts on gloves, places the patient in a side-lying position exposing the rectal area, lubricates the end of the suppository, and instructs the patient to exhale as the suppository is gently inserted past the internal anal sphincter (about 1 inch). Suppositories are absorbed through the rectal mucosa, so insert the medication against the mucosa and away from stool. The technique for inserting suppositories is shown in Figure 20-9.

Liquid medications may be instilled into the rectum using an enema to encourage bowel movements or to treat patients with elevated potassium levels. Small-volume enemas are usually given in volumes of about 100 mL and are usually meant to be retained by the patient for 5 to 10 minutes. Large-volume enemas may be up to 1,000 mL. An enema of resin-containing fluid may be used to remove potassium from the bowel of a patient with an elevated potassium level. The procedure for administering large- and small-volume enemas is discussed in Chapter 33.

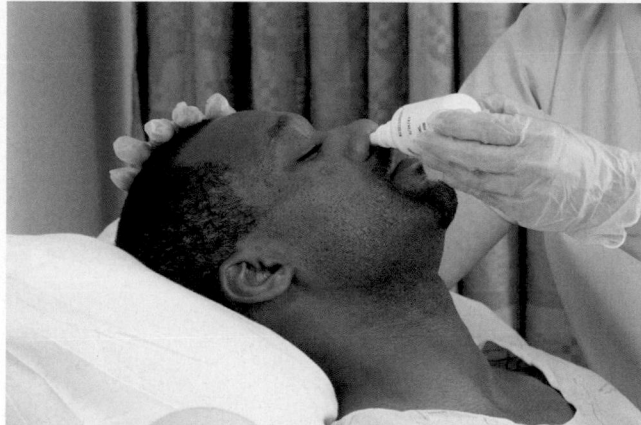

FIGURE 20-8 Nasal medications. Place the top of the bottle just inside the nostril, and aim the spray applicator top toward the midline of the nose.

VAGINAL MEDICATIONS

Medications given vaginally come in various forms: foams, jellies, liquids (douches), creams, tablets, or suppositories. These medications may be used for contraception, to help kill bacteria in the vaginal area before gynecologic surgery, to treat vaginal itching or infection, or to induce labor. Prostaglandin vaginal suppositories cause uterine contractions and induce labor in

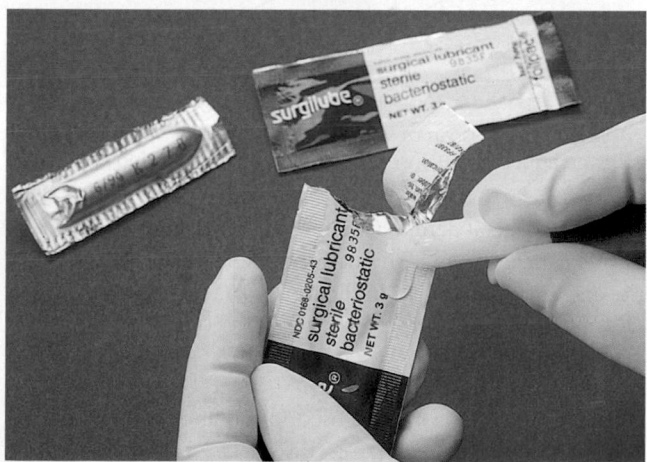

A

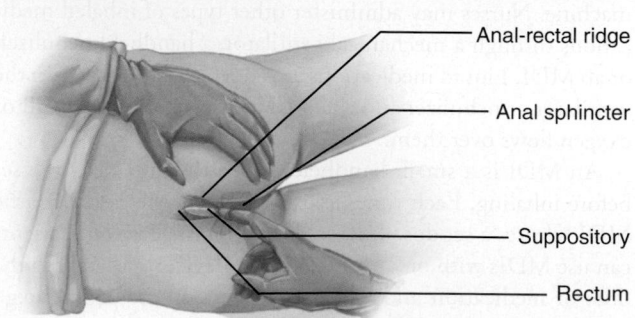

B

FIGURE 20-9 Insertion of rectal suppositories. A. Prepackaged suppositories. B. Insert the suppository past the internal anal sphincter against the rectal wall.

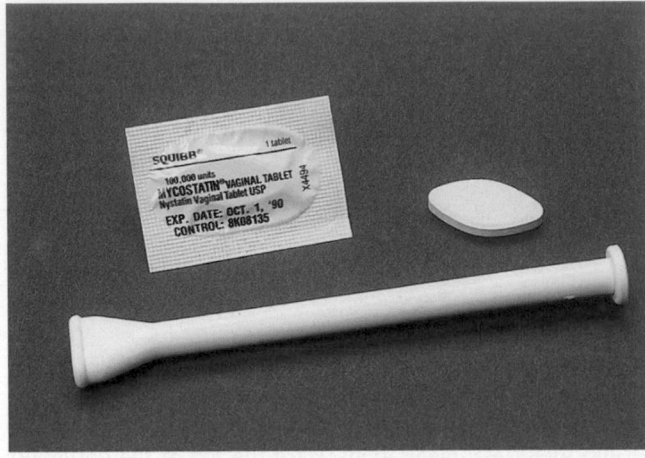

A

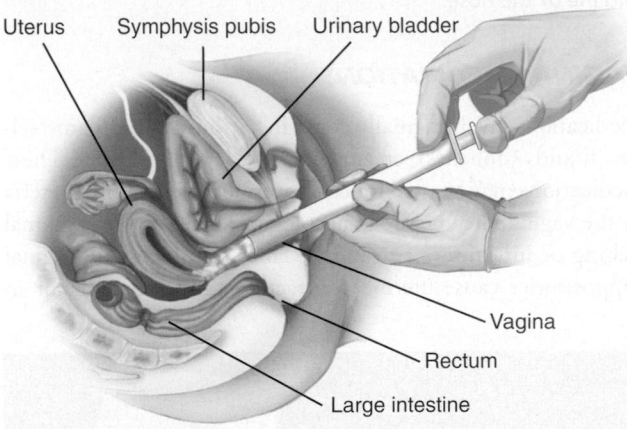

Uterus   Symphysis pubis   Urinary bladder

Vagina

Rectum

Large intestine

B

FIGURE 20-10 Insertion of vaginal medication. **A.** Vaginal suppository and applicator. **B.** Insertion of vaginal cream using applicator.

women after fetal demise (when death of the fetus occurs early in pregnancy). The technique for instilling vaginal suppositories and creams is shown in Figure 20-10.

Inhaled Medications

Inhaled medications may be used to induce anesthesia during surgery and to treat respiratory disorders. Anesthesiologists or nurse anesthetists administer anesthetic medications through a machine. Nurses may administer other types of inhaled medications through a mechanical ventilator, a handheld nebulizer, or an MDI. Liquid medications are added to a receptacle in the ventilator or nebulizer and changed into a gas form when air or oxygen flows over them.

An MDI is a small, handheld device that a patient presses before inhaling. Each time he or she presses the cartridge, the MDI releases a set dose (metered dose) of medication. Patients can use MDIs with or without a spacer device. Spacers trap the dose of medication and are especially useful for people (e.g., children, older adults) who cannot inhale slowly or cannot coordinate pressing the canister while inhaling. Inhaled medications have rapid effects on the lungs and are rapidly absorbed by the systemic circulation.

Bronchodilator medications, used to open lung airways and to promote easier breathing, are frequently administered through MDIs or nebulizers. Assess the patient's respiratory status (reported ease of breathing, breath sounds, respiratory rate, and use of accessory respiratory muscles) before and after administering an inhaled medication (**Procedure 20-2**).

Parenteral Medications

The **parenteral** route refers to medications that are given by injection or infusion. Parenteral medications may be injected into ID, subcutaneous, or IM tissue, into IV or intra-arterial circulation, or into intraspinal or intra-articular spaces. The ID, subcutaneous, and IM routes are discussed in this chapter. IV bolus, IV intermittent infusions, and continuous IV infusions are discussed in Chapter 21.

Medications given by a parenteral route usually are absorbed more completely and begin acting more quickly than do medications given by oral or topical routes. Parenteral medications are injected through the skin; bypassing the skin barrier makes infection more likely if aseptic technique is not used when preparing and administering parenteral medications. Complications may occur if parenteral medications are not given into the intended tissue site or space. Tissue damage may occur if the pH, osmotic pressure, or solubility of the medication is not appropriate to the tissue where the medication is given. Specialized equipment required for parenteral administration usually makes medications given by these routes more expensive than medications given by other routes.

EQUIPMENT

Equipment used when administering medications parenterally may include syringes and needles, vials, and ampules.

Syringes and Needles

Syringes, usually made of plastic, consist of a barrel, plunger, and syringe tip (Fig. 20-11). The plunger fits snugly within the syringe barrel. Moving the plunger out of the barrel allows

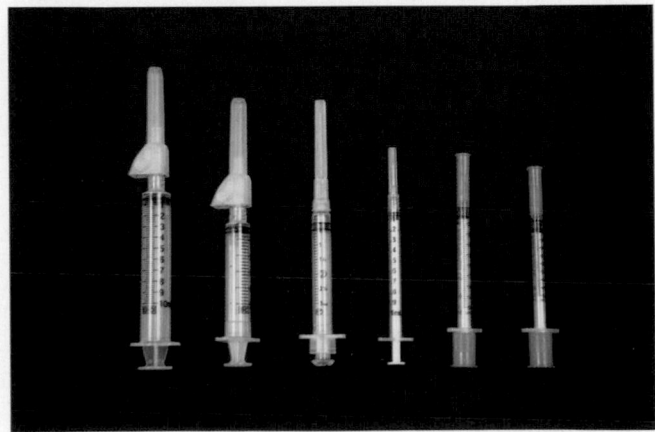

FIGURE 20-11 Syringes (*left to right*): 10 mL, 5 mL, 3 mL, tuberculin, insulin, and low-dose insulin.

fluid or air to move into the syringe, and pushing the plunger into the barrel allows fluid or air to move out of the syringe. A safety needle is attached to the syringe tip (the narrow end of the syringe).

Safety needles have either an active or passive safety design feature. Active design safety needles require the nurse to activate the safety mechanism after use to protect against accidental needlestick injury (Shelton & Rosenthal, 2004). Passive design safety needles use a safety mechanism that deploys automatically during use. Although the passive safety needle is preferred, some facilities may use active design safety needles. Syringes may be packaged with or without attached safety needles.

Needle gauge (diameter size) varies from 14 to 29. Needles with the smallest gauges are labeled with the largest number. For example, an 18-gauge needle has a larger diameter than does a 25-gauge needle. Needle length varies from 0.4 to 3 inches (Fig. 20-12).

The three common types of syringes are tuberculin, insulin, and standard syringes. Tuberculin syringes are 1-mL syringes that are calibrated with 0.1-mL markings and supplied with a small-gauge (26- to 28-gauge), short (0.5- to 0.625-inch) needle. Tuberculin syringes are used to administer tuberculin or sensitivity (allergy) tests. They may also be used for subcutaneous injections of less than 1 mL of medication.

Insulin syringes, calibrated in units of insulin (100 U per 1 mL), are used to administer insulin. Insulin syringes are made in 0.5- and 1-mL sizes, with very small–gauge needles (26- to 30-gauge) attached. Insulin syringes are never used to administer anything other than insulin.

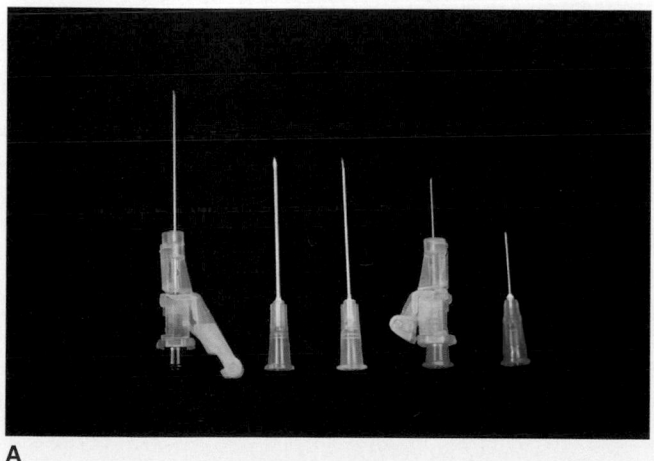

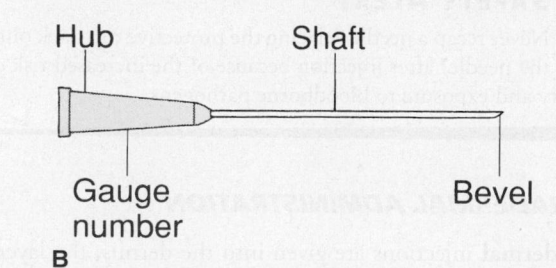

FIGURE 20-12 Needles. **A.** Safety needles of different gauges and lengths (some have safety glide attached). **B.** Parts of a needle.

Hub   Shaft

Gauge   Bevel
number

B

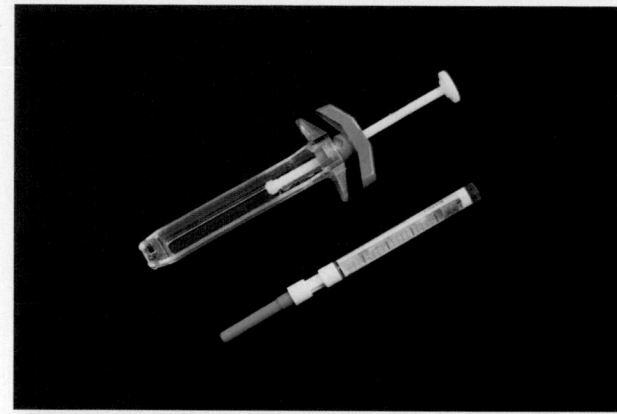

FIGURE 20-13 Prefilled medication cartridges and injector devices.

Standard syringes are supplied in 3-, 5-, or 10-mL sizes. Standard syringes may be supplied without needles or with 18-, 21-, 22-, 23-, or 25-gauge needles that are 0.5 to 3 inches long. IM injections are usually administered to adults via a 3-mL syringe with a long (1- to 1½-inch), medium-gauge (21-, 22-, or 23-gauge) needle. Larger-gauge needles are used to administer viscous medications or to mix IV medications.

Prefilled syringes, prepared by a medication manufacturer or pharmacy, may be used to supply medications. Systems of prefilled syringes that require a specially designed outer injector device are in widespread use. Medications such as opiate analgesics and heparin are supplied in a syringe by the manufacturer with an attached needle. The needle and syringe fit into a metal or plastic injector device with attached plunger (Fig. 20-13). Air and any extra medication are expelled from the syringe, and the medication is injected. Because the needle is fused to the medication syringe, needle gauge and length cannot be changed. The nurse must use the needle supplied or transfer the medication into a standard syringe if a different needle size is required.

Filter Needles

A filter needle is used to trap any rubber or glass fragments that may be drawn up with the medication in a vial or ampule. The nurse must replace the filter needle with a regular needle before injecting the medication into the patient.

Vials

Vials are plastic or glass containers that hold one or more doses of medication. The vial is opened by removing a plastic cap that covers a rubber diaphragm at the top of the container. A needle is used to pierce the center of the diaphragm, and the correct amount of medication is withdrawn into a syringe. Vials can also be fitted with adaptors that permit access through a valve system without a needle (Fig. 20-14). Blunt tip needles are also used to access vials while avoiding the risk of needlesticks.

Medications that are not stable for long periods may be supplied in a vial in powdered form. A diluent (sterile liquid specified by the drug manufacturer—usually sterile water or saline) is mixed with the powder to reconstitute it. Most hospitals with on-site pharmacies prepare medications from vials in the pharmacy and then dispense the labeled syringe into the automated

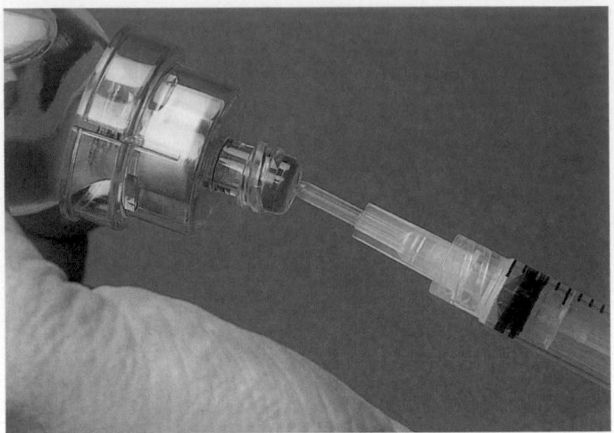

FIGURE 20-14 Use syringe (without needle) to withdraw medication.

dispensing machine. Nurses working in extended care facilities or in home care may need to prepare medications from vials.

Ampules

Ampules are thin-walled glass containers that hold a single dose of a liquid medication. An ampule is shaped like a bowling pin; it has a wide base, narrow neck, and pointed top. Using a gauze pad, the neck of the ampule is snapped off and the medication is withdrawn with a filter needle and syringe.

MEDICATION PREPARATION TECHNIQUES

Techniques for preparing parenteral medications include drawing up the medication, reconstituting the medication, mixing the medication, and disposing of equipment.

Drawing Up Medications

Drawing up medications is the process of moving medications from a vial or ampule into a syringe (**Procedures 20-3** and **20-4**). When withdrawing medication from a vial, first withdraw and inject an equal amount of air into the vial; then, turn the vial over and withdraw the proper dose of medication. When withdrawing medication from an ampule, first open the ampule and then remove the needle cap from the syringe. Place the filter needle directly into the open ampule, and pull the syringe plunger back until all medication enters the syringe.

When drawing up medication from a vial or ampule, air may also be drawn into the syringe along with the liquid medication. To dispel the air, take the syringe out and hold the syringe with the needle pointed upward. If any medication has adhered to the top of the syringe in the air bubble, tap the barrel of the syringe until the liquid moves down the barrel to the rest of the medication. Expel the air and any volume of unneeded medication slowly.

> **! SAFETY ALERT**
> To avoid medication errors, always label syringes with the name of the patient, the medication, and the dose after you draw up the dose. Deaths have occurred when unlabeled medication has been injected into the wrong patient.

Reconstituting Medications

Medications are reconstituted by adding the proper amount and type of diluent to a powdered medication. Vials of powdered medications may be packaged along with vials of the proper type and volume of diluent. The manufacturer's directions printed on the medication box or vial indicate the amount and type of diluent to add. To reconstitute the medication, remove the caps from both the medication and diluent vials, and clean the tops of both vials with an alcohol wipe. Draw up the diluent into the syringe, and inject it into the medication vial. Hold the medication vial and mix the medication and diluent until the medication has dissolved. Draw the reconstituted medication into a syringe, and remove air and unneeded medication from the syringe. Administer the medication as directed.

Mixing Medications

Mixing medications, such as two types of insulin, in the same syringe may allow a patient to receive fewer injections at a lower cost. Medications may be mixed only if they are compatible. Pharmaceutical companies study the compatibility of medications (the ability to mix medications without affecting their constituents or actions). Medication references usually present compatibility information. Medications are mixed in a syringe by first injecting appropriate amounts of air into each vial, then drawing up one medication into the syringe, and expelling any air and unneeded volume of medication. The ordered volume of the second medication is then slowly added to the syringe containing the first medication. If the medication is added rapidly, too much of the second medication may be drawn up. If this occurs, the syringe and medications must be discarded. Refer to **Procedure 20-5** for more information.

Equipment Disposal

Discarding equipment carefully decreases the risk of needlestick injuries and exposure to a patient's blood. Needlestick injuries expose healthcare providers and ancillary workers to dangerous bloodborne pathogens, including HIV and hepatitis B and C viruses. After administering an injection, activate an active design safety needle, if used, and then immediately place the syringe and needle in a needle disposal box or sharps container (see Chapter 19). A sharps container is the only acceptable receptacle for used needles.

> **! SAFETY ALERT**
> Never recap a needle (placing the protective cap back onto the needle) after injection because of the increased risk of injury and exposure to bloodborne pathogens.

INTRADERMAL ADMINISTRATION

Intradermal injections are given into the dermis, the layer of tissue located beneath the skin surface. ID injections are commonly used for allergy testing and the tuberculosis skin test

(TST). They are administered into the inner forearm area, the upper arm, and across the scapula (**Procedure 20-6**).

The TST, also referred to as the purified protein derivative (PPD) test or the Mantoux test, is the most commonly administered ID injection. The TST is the standard screening method for identifying persons infected with *Mycobacterium tuberculosis*. The inner forearm is the site for the test. The test is administered with a tuberculin syringe—a 1-mL syringe with a short, half-inch, small-gauge (26- to 28-gauge) needle. After the skin is cleansed with an alcohol wipe, allow the site to dry. While holding the syringe with the bevel of the needle up, almost parallel to the skin, insert the needle until the entire bevel lies under the skin. Slowly inject a small volume of medication (usually 0.1 mL). A wheal (or bleb) will rise under the epidermis.

Do not apply pressure or massage the injection site; the dermal tissue will quickly absorb the medication. Because the medication is administered into dermal tissue and the injection site is not touched after the injection, the use of gloves is considered optional. Document the location of the injection and time of the test. Forty-eight to seventy-two hours after the injection is given, the test area is inspected and palpated for evidence of induration (palpable swelling). When reading a test, palpate the site and measure the induration. Measure the diameter of the indurated area in millimeters across the width of the forearm. Do not measure erythema (redness). Interpretation of the TST results (positive or negative) is based on the millimeters of induration and the risk category of the person being tested. An induration of more than 5 mm is classified as positive in high-risk people (e.g., those who have had recent close contact with persons with active tuberculosis, those infected with HIV). An induration of more than 10 mm is considered a positive reaction in people with moderate risk (e.g., injection drug users, immunocompromised people, healthcare workers employed in high-risk settings). An induration of more than 15 mm is considered a positive reaction in people in low-risk groups.

SUBCUTANEOUS ADMINISTRATION

Subcutaneous injections are given into the subcutaneous tissue, the layer of fat located below the dermis and above the muscle tissue (Fig. 20-15). When a medication is injected into

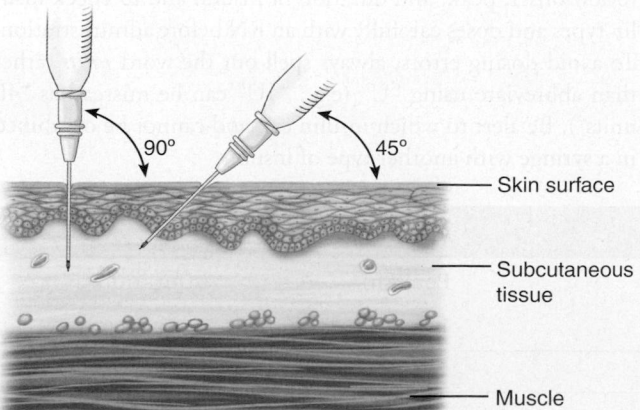

FIGURE 20-15 Subcutaneous injection deposits medication in subcutaneous tissue at a 45- or 90-degree angle.

subcutaneous tissue, absorption is usually slow, sustained, and complete. Small amounts (0.5 to 1 mL) of medication may be injected subcutaneously using a syringe with a short (½- to ⅝-inch), small-gauge (26- to 30-gauge) needle. Subcutaneous injections may be given in the upper arm, upper back, abdomen, upper buttocks, or thigh (Fig. 20-16).

APPLY YOUR CRITICAL THINKING

You are giving heparin subcutaneously for the first time. Your patient has heparin 7,500 U ordered, and the available heparin vial contains 10,000 U/mL.

Calculate how much (in milliliters) you need to administer to give 7,500 U.

What type of syringe would you select to give the heparin?

Discuss specific administration guidelines to safely give this heparin.

Check your answer in Appendix B.

Aspiration (pulling back on the plunger of the syringe to assess the presence of blood, indicating you are in a blood vessel) is not required for subcutaneous injections since the area is less vascular and injection into the bloodstream is rare (American Diabetes Association [ADA], 2011; Centers for Disease Control and Prevention [CDC], 2011).

The speed of absorption varies with the site selected. Medications injected into the abdomen are absorbed most rapidly, those injected into the arms are absorbed intermediately, and those injected into the thigh and upper buttocks are absorbed most slowly. Avoid sites of abnormal subcutaneous tissue, such as areas underneath burns, birthmarks, inflamed tissue, or scars, because of unpredictable medication absorption. Absorption also may be slow or incomplete if subcutaneous medication is administered to a patient with generalized edema or severe peripheral vascular disease or to a patient in cardiac shock. Medications may be absorbed faster than expected if subcutaneous injections are administered to patients with little subcutaneous tissue, such as premature babies or malnourished adults.

Heparin, low-molecular-weight heparin, and insulin are the most commonly administered subcutaneous medications. Nonirritating, water-soluble medications, such as opiates, also may be administered by subcutaneous injection. See **Procedure 20-7** for guidelines for administering subcutaneous injections.

SAFETY ALERT

If a patient has little or abnormal subcutaneous tissue or abnormal blood flow to subcutaneous tissue, check with the provider to see whether you can use an alternative route of administration.

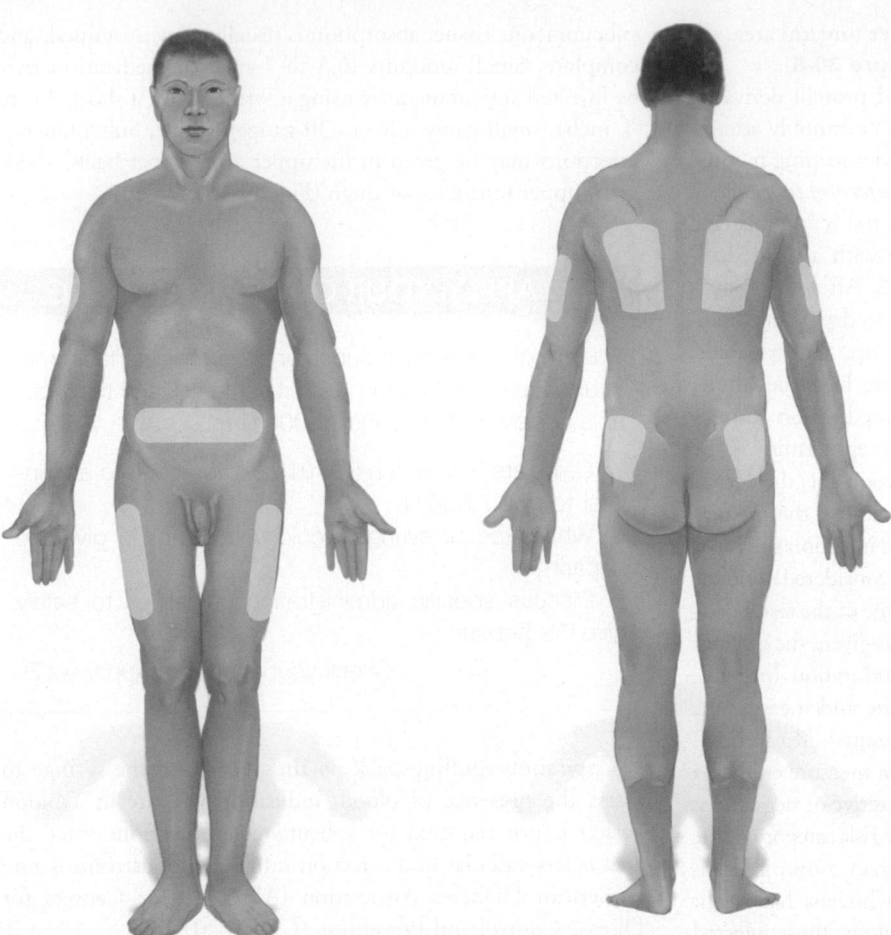

FIGURE 20-16 Sites used for subcutaneous injections.

Insulin Administration

Insulin is administered subcutaneously using an insulin syringe (1-mL syringe with 26- to 30-gauge nondetachable needle) to regulate a patient's blood glucose levels. The syringe is calibrated in units. Insulin vials typically contain 100 U/mL and should be given using syringes designed for that concentration (referred to as U-100 syringes). Although U-500 insulin (500 U/mL) is also available, it is used with extreme caution because miscalculations could result in a patient receiving five times the prescribed dose. When insulin is administered, the number of units, rather than the number of milliliters, is prescribed and measured in the syringe. Low-dose insulin syringes (0.3 mL, 30 U or 0.5 mL, 50 U) permit better visualization when small insulin doses (e.g., less than 30 U) are given.

Insulin pens are also available for the administration of insulin. Pens are advantageous for patients who wish to self-administer insulin but who are visually impaired or lack the manual dexterity required for a regular syringe (e.g., someone with arthritis). Twisting the barrel of the pen sets the dose; an audible click assists with dose identification. Nurses educate patients in the proper use of insulin pens. Insulin is available in rapid-, short-, intermediate-, long-acting, and around-the-clock formulations (see Table 20-4).

The complexity of insulin therapy has risen sharply in the past decade. Insulin is considered a high-alert medication. The patient is most likely to experience hypoglycemia when the insulin administered is at its peak action. Nurses are advised to review onset, peak, and duration of insulin and to check insulin types and doses carefully with an RN before administration. To avoid dosing errors, always spell out the word *units* rather than abbreviate using "U" (e.g., "4U" can be misread as "40 units"). Be alert to which insulin can and cannot be combined in a syringe with another type of insulin.

TABLE 20-4 INSULIN PREPARATIONS

Insulin Type	Insulin	Onset	Peak (h)	Duration (h)
Rapid	Lispro, aspart, glulisine	<15 min	1–2	2–4
Short	Regular	0.5–1 h	2–3	3–6
Intermediate	NPH	2–4 h	4–12	12–18
Long	Detemir, glargine	2–4 h	Peakless	20–24

From: American Diabetes Association. (2014). Retrieved July 23, 2014, from http://www.diabetes.org

Insulin may be administered subcutaneously in the upper arm, anterior or lateral aspects of the thigh, buttocks, or abdomen (avoiding a 2-inch radius around the umbilicus). Rotate the site for each injection systematically about 1 inch from the previous injection site. Rotation within one area is preferred to rotation to a new body area with each injection in order to minimize daily variability in absorption associated with different sites (ADA, 2011). Plan and document site rotation well to prevent repeated use of the same site. Insulin need not be refrigerated for short-term use. A 10-mL vial of insulin will maintain its potency for 1 month without refrigeration if the vial is kept cool and away from heat and sunlight. For teaching, observe patients injecting their insulin because technique problems can affect dose administration and absorption.

In addition to being classified by time of onset, peak, and duration of action, insulin is also identified by its purpose. Those types of insulin that mimic the natural action of the pancreas (long-acting insulin) are called *basal* insulin. Intermediate-acting insulins are sometimes used as a basal insulin. Insulin given routinely with meals to manage the carbohydrates in the food is called *nutritional* insulin. This is most commonly a rapid- or short-acting insulin. Insulin given on an as-needed basis to manage elevations in blood glucose level is called *correctional* insulin. The goal is to manage the insulin needs of diabetic patients with basal and nutritional doses of insulin; ideally, this would mean correctional insulin is not needed. However, hospitalization usually changes the diet and activity of patients, and the illness itself changes the body's glucose management, so correctional insulin is often needed in hospitalized patients. Some nondiabetic patients may also need insulin, for example, those receiving glucocorticoid medications such as prednisone. Typically, those patients will not need insulin after being discharged, but some may continue on insulin after returning home.

Heparin or Enoxaparin Administration

Subcutaneous heparin or enoxaparin (low-molecular-weight heparin) is used to help prevent deep vein thrombosis (blood clots in the legs) and subsequent pulmonary embolism (blood clots in the lungs). Because subcutaneous injections of heparin frequently cause bruising, precautions are necessary. Heparin is considered a high-alert drug, and student nurses are advised to check the dose with an RN before administering it to the patient. Recommendations for administering heparin are included in the modifications for heparin administration in **Procedure 20-7**.

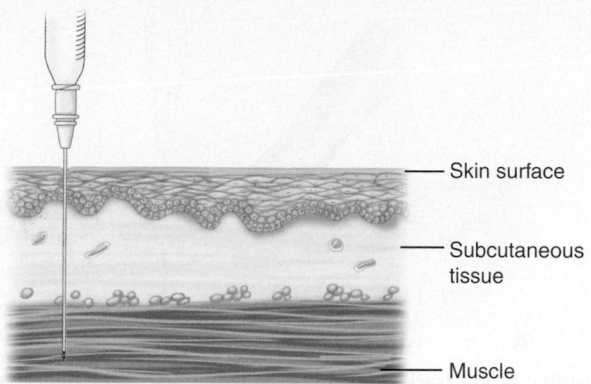

FIGURE 20-17 The IM injection deposits medication into the muscle at a 90-degree angle.

INTRAMUSCULAR ADMINISTRATION

Intramuscular injections are given into the muscle layer beneath the dermis and subcutaneous tissue (Fig. 20-17). According to the CDC (2011) and Crawford & Johnson (2012), needle aspiration is not required for IM injections since no large blood vessels exist at the recommended injection sites. Medications administered by IM injection are usually absorbed more slowly than IV administration but more rapidly than subcutaneous injections. A larger volume of medication per injection and a wider variety of medications may be administered into IM sites than into subcutaneous sites. Refer to Table 20-5 for appropriate sites and volumes of medication to inject for patients of different ages.

Medications in solution or suspension (including antibiotics, antiemetics, opiates, and vaccines) may be injected into IM sites. IM injections are administered with a 3-mL syringe and a 20- to 25-gauge, 1- to 3-inch needle. The larger-gauge needles are used when the medication solution is very thick. Longer needles are used for larger adults. A 23-gauge, 1.25-inch needle is commonly used for IM injections for average-sized adult patients. **Procedure 20-8** discusses administration of IM injections.

Most medications that are appropriate for IM injection can be given using the technique described in **Procedure 20-8**. Depot IM preparations (i.e., Depo-Provera) allow for very slow absorption from the muscle, providing prolonged action over days or weeks. Medications that irritate SC tissue (e.g., hydrOXYzine) or that discolor subcutaneous tissue (e.g., iron) should be given by the Z-track method (Fig. 20-18), which also is described in **Procedure 20-8**. Although the

TABLE 20-5	INTRAMUSCULAR SITES: SAFE VOLUMES TO ADMINISTER (ML)				
Site	Infants (<18 mo)	Toddlers (<3 y)	Preschoolers (<6 y)	School Age (<13 y)	Adolescents and Adults
Deltoid	N.R.	0.5	0.5	0.5–1.0	1.0
Rectus femoris	0.5	1.0	1.5	1.5	2.0
Vastus lateralis	0.5	1.0	1.5	2.0	2.0
Ventrogluteal	0.5	1.0	1.5	2.0	2.5–3.0

N.R., not recommended.

Note: Individual assessment of muscle mass is necessary before giving injection. For small or wasted muscles, the volumes listed may be inappropriate.

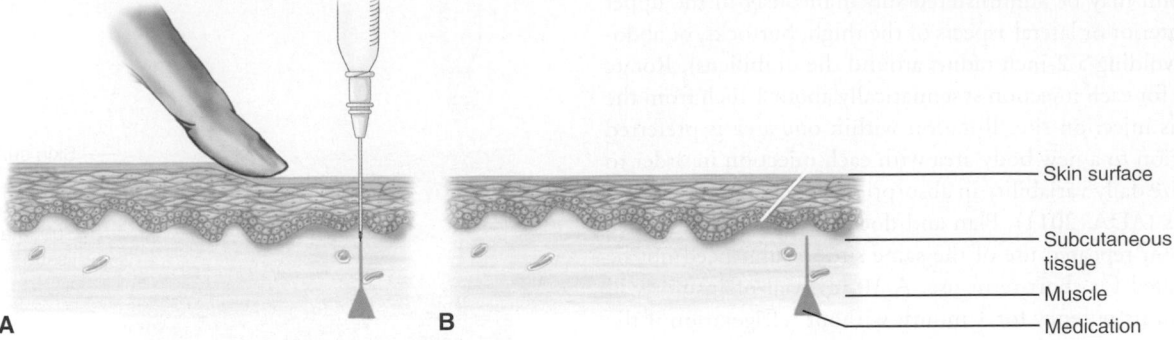

FIGURE 20-18 Z-track method. **A.** Pull skin and subcutaneous tissue 1 to 1.5 inches to one side of the injection site while injecting medication. **B.** Release traction to allow skin to fall back, sealing medication in site.

Z-track technique is generally used with medications that are irritating to the tissues, it can be used routinely for all IM injections, provided that the overlying tissue at the chosen site can be displaced by at least 1 inch (Encyclopedia of Nursing Practice, 2011). The Z-track technique allows medication to be administered into the muscle tissue with no tracking of medication in the subcutaneous tissues as the needle is removed. If these techniques are not followed or if site selection is not accurate, complications can occur (see Table 20-6).

TABLE 20–6 COMPLICATIONS ASSOCIATED WITH INTRAMUSCULAR MEDICATION ADMINISTRATION

Complication (Signs/Symptoms)	Causes	Nursing Measures
Pain with injection (the patient reports discomfort)	Muscle tensing during injection Medication irritating to IM tissue Inadvertent tracking of medication or alcohol through subcutaneous tissue	Encourage the patient to relax muscles during injection. Use Z-track technique when administering medications that are irritating to subcutaneous tissue. Change needle after drawing up medication. Use an air lock when giving irritating medications. Let alcohol skin prep dry before giving injection.
Damage to subcutaneous or IM tissue, including sterile abscesses (collection of undissolved medication), subcutaneous tissue discoloration, hematomas, and muscle contractions (tissue nodules or indurations [indentations], bruising, brown discoloration, or pain in IM injection site; muscle contracture [in infants] characterized by difficulty crawling 4 wk to 1 y after receiving IM injections)	Multiple injections given into same area Injection given into abnormal tissue Injection of drug that is not water soluble (e.g., Dilantin, Valium) IM administration of heparin IM route used for patient with a low platelet count Subcutaneous deposition of iron supplements (e.g., Imferon)	Give an injection at least 1 inch away from recently administered injections or from scars, burns, or areas of abnormal subcutaneous or IM tissue. Rotate injection sites (give injections at least 1 inch away from recent injection). Record sites used for all injections. As soon as possible, change from IM route to another route. Be sure that medication is recommended for IM administration. Check with provider before administering IM injection to a patient whose platelet count is under 30,000/mL. Do not administer IM injections into atrophied muscle. Decrease risk of knee contractures for infants with passive range-of-motion exercises and applying warm soaks and massage to the thighs. Give iron supplements (e.g., Imferon) using the Z-track technique.
Nerve injury (shooting pain down limb, temporary or permanent paralysis)	Nerve struck during injection Medication injected close to nerve	Use careful visual inspection and palpation of landmarks to locate injection site. Avoid use of deltoid site whenever possible.
Bone injury (pain or bone damage)	Bone struck during IM injection	Use a short needle (1.25 inch) when giving injections into the deltoid or ventrogluteal sites. Use visual inspection and palpation to locate injection sites.
Speed shock or rapid absorption of medication (unexpectedly rapid onset of action of medication; may lead to increased heart rate and respiratory rate, decreased level of consciousness, and cardiovascular collapse)	Medication administered directly into a vein or artery	Use proper administration techniques. Administer IM injection at the correct angle and appropriate injection site to avoid injection into an artery or vein.
Infection of muscle or bone (muscle or bone pain in injection site, skin redness or warmth, localized swelling)	Organism introduced into tissue or bone during injection	Follow strict aseptic technique when administering IM injections.

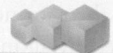

Concept Mastery Alert

The Z-track method is solely used when administering IM injections. It is never used to administer subcutaneous injections.

IM injections may be administered into sites in the upper arm (deltoid muscle), hip (ventrogluteal), or thigh (vastus lateralis or rectus femoris). Factors that influence the site choice include the age of the patient, the medication to be injected, the amount of medication, and the patient's general condition. The CDC recommends deltoid and vastus lateralis sites for vaccines (CDC, 2011). Injections are not given into abnormal muscle tissue, such as tissue underneath burns or scars.

Deltoid Site

The deltoid site has a small amount of muscle mass with little overlying subcutaneous fat. Medication injected into this site is absorbed rapidly. Because the muscle is small and lies close to the radial nerve and the brachial artery, the deltoid site is usually only used for vaccines that are small in volume.

The deltoid site is located by drawing an imaginary line two to three fingerbreadths (2.5 to 5 cm) below the lower edge of the acromion (shoulder) process. The injection is given into the thickest area of muscle that lies in the center of an imaginary triangle whose base is the central half of this horizontal line and whose apex is formed inverted on the midpoint of the lateral aspect of the arm in line with the axilla (Fig. 20-19).

To give the injection, slightly angle the needle toward the acromion process or insert it at a 90-degree angle. This site may be higher than you have had with previous injections but is evidence based.

 SAFETY ALERT

If you must use the deltoid site, locate the site carefully, using anatomic landmarks to decrease the risk of injury to the radial nerve and brachial artery.

Rectus Femoris and Vastus Lateralis Sites

Injection sites in the thigh, the vastus lateralis and rectus femoris sites, offer rapid rates of medication absorption. Because these muscles contain no large blood vessels or nerves, they are safe to use for IM injections for most patients.

The rectus femoris is located midway between the patella and the superior iliac crest, in the center of the anterior thigh (Fig. 20-20). An injection is administered into this site by lifting the muscle away from the bone and inserting the needle at a right angle to the muscle. This site is convenient for patients who self-inject medication.

The vastus lateralis site is used for IM injections for infants, children, and adults. In adults, the vastus lateralis site is the area between one handbreadth above the knee and one handbreadth below the greater trochanter on the medial outer portion of the thigh. An injection is administered into this site by lifting the muscle away from the bone and inserting the needle at a right angle to the muscle.

In infants and children, the vastus lateralis site is located in the middle third of the area between the greater trochanter and the knee on the medial outer aspect of the thigh (Fig. 20-21). Use short needles (not exceeding 1 inch) to administer injections into the vastus lateralis site in children.

Ventrogluteal Site

The ventrogluteal site on the lateral hip is free of major blood vessels, nerves, and fat. It is considered the safest and least painful site for delivering IM injections. To locate the ventrogluteal

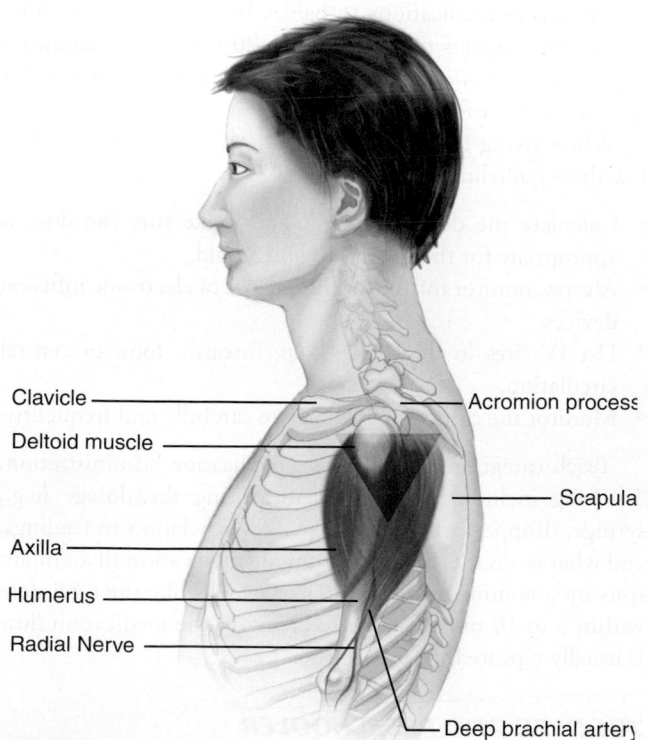

Clavicle

Deltoid muscle

Axilla

Humerus

Radial Nerve

Acromion process

Scapula

Deep brachial artery

FIGURE 20-19 Deltoid muscle injection site. The site is located by imagining a line extending one to two fingerbreadths (or 2.5 to 5 cm) from the acromion process. A triangle is formed that indicates the injection site.

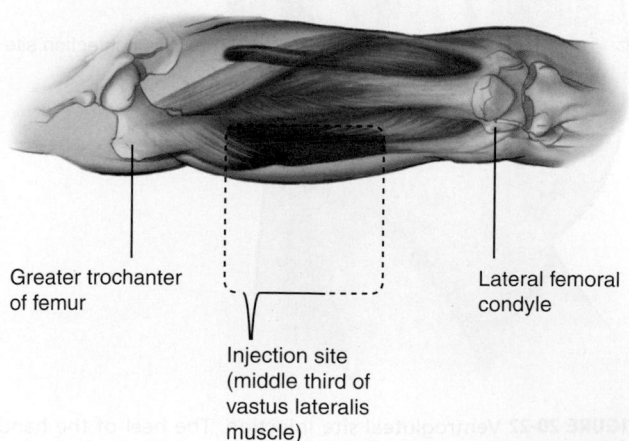

Greater trochanter of femur

Lateral femoral condyle

Injection site (middle third of vastus lateralis muscle)

FIGURE 20-20 Location of rectus femoris and vastus lateralis sites for injection.

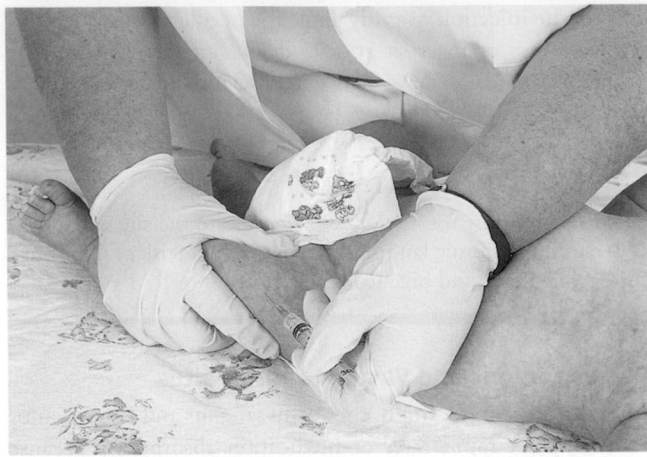

FIGURE 20-21 Administration of an injection to an infant in the vastus lateralis site. Note the right angle of short needle.

site, place the heel of the opposite hand (for right hip, use left hand; for left hip, use right hand) over the greater trochanter, with the index finger pointing toward the anterior superior iliac spine and the middle finger stretched dorsally toward but below the iliac crest. Give the injection in the center of the triangular area thus formed, with the needle directed at a 90-degree angle to the skin or angled slightly toward the iliac crest (Fig. 20-22).

Dorsogluteal Site

The dorsogluteal site of the buttocks has been used commonly for IM injections in the past. However, because of its proximity to the sciatic nerve and superior gluteal artery and the possibility of administering the injection subcutaneously into

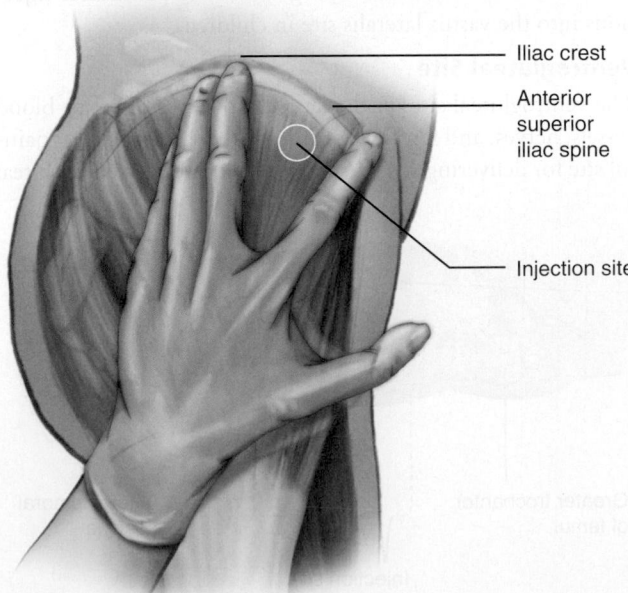

— Iliac crest

— Anterior superior iliac spine

— Injection site

FIGURE 20-22 Ventrogluteal site injection. The heel of the hand is placed over the greater trochanter, and the middle finger reaches toward the iliac crest while the index finger is angled toward the anterior superior iliac spine.

the thick layer of fat over the dorsal gluteal muscle, the routine use of this site for IM injections is not recommended (Malkin, 2008). Patients may describe numbness, tingling, or weakness if the sciatic nerve has been injected.

INTRAVENOUS ADMINISTRATION

Intravenous medications may be given by IV push (bolus), intermittent infusion (IV drip), or continuous infusion. Intravenous techniques via these routes will be discussed in-depth in Chapter 21. IV pain medication may be delivered via epidural or self-delivered with equipment known as a patient-controlled analgesia (PCA) device (see Chapter 35).

Life Span Considerations

NEWBORN AND INFANT

Special considerations are important when giving oral, subcutaneous, IM, and IV medications to newborns and infants. Liquid oral medications are preferred for newborns and infants. If such medications are unavailable, crush the solid medication and dissolve it in water. Using a syringe to draw up and give oral medications also may be helpful. Babies receive oral medications on an empty stomach unless otherwise noted. Infant formulas may alter medication absorption, and infants are less likely to spit up medications they receive before feedings.

Administer parenteral medications to newborns and infants with special care. The subcutaneous route is rarely used for administering medications to babies because they have little or no subcutaneous tissue. See Table 20-6 for information on appropriate IM injection sites and amounts of medication that are safe to inject for various IM sites.

When giving IV medications to newborns and infants, follow these guidelines:

- Calculate the dose accurately, and make sure the dose is appropriate for the infant or young child.
- Always monitor infusions with the use of electronic infusion devices.
- Use IV sites in the hand, scalp, forearm, foot, or central circulation.
- Monitor the catheter insertion site carefully and frequently.

Teach caregivers about correct medication administration. Teaching includes methods of measuring the dosage (e.g., syringe, dropper), the dosage schedule in relation to feedings, and what to do if the child spits up the medication (if an infant spits up a volume of medication that looks like the total dose within 5 to 10 minutes after receiving it, the medication dose is usually repeated).

TODDLER AND PRESCHOOLER

Physical changes during the toddler and preschool years have implications for medication administration. Oral medications are still given in liquid form, or, if necessary, tablets are crushed and mixed with food. Children younger than 3 years of age have straighter, stiffer external auditory canals than do older children and adults. Therefore, when administering eardrops to this age group, pull the pinna of the ear down and back before dropping the medication into the ear canal (Hockenberry & Wilson, 2011).

Many young children fear injections, so give them as promptly as possible to avoid escalating anxiety and fear. Often, children must be carefully immobilized, usually by another person who is not their parent, to ensure safety during the procedure. EMLA cream, a cream containing a mixture of local anesthetics, can be applied to the skin 1 hour before painful procedures such as IV insertions. The area of application is covered with clear plastic. EMLA cream is helpful only when painful procedures can be anticipated.

Children in these age groups are beginning to explore their world and learn about themselves and their environment. Accidental poisoning is a particular risk. Urge parents, grandparents, and caregivers to store all medications in a protected area out of children's reach and to make sure that medications are packaged in containers with childproof caps. Make sure that children are aware that medications are not candy. Also, instruct caregivers to have the telephone number of a poison control center readily available in case of accidental ingestion of medications.

Explain procedures in simple terms, appropriate to a child's experiences and level of understanding. Reassure children that the medication is not a punishment. Whenever possible, allow children to make choices about therapy (e.g., which arm to use for the IV, which fluid to drink with the oral medication).

Effective teaching materials for toddlers and preschoolers might include coloring books, dolls, or puppets. Dolls and puppets can be used to demonstrate a procedure, and, if necessary, children can return the demonstration on the doll.

SCHOOL-AGE CHILD AND ADOLESCENT

As children mature and develop, nurses can direct more teaching and responsibility for medication administration toward them. Most school age children can swallow tablets and capsules. To increase adherence, the dosage schedule avoids school hours whenever possible. When medication administration is necessary during school hours, most schools require that medications be deposited with the school nurse in the original prescription container.

Many school-age children still fear injections and worry about crying or losing control when injections are administered. Although these children understand the importance of remaining still during injections, sudden movement may occur as the needle pierces the skin. Support of the extremity and judicious positioning help ensure safety during the injection. By the time children have reached school age, all injection sites may be used because all muscles have adequately developed.

Teaching school-age children and their caregivers about medication administration is a key component of patient education. Many medications are given in the home, making the child and caregiver responsible for administration. If medication is being given by injection, the child and caregiver need to learn how to administer the injection properly (Fig. 20-23).

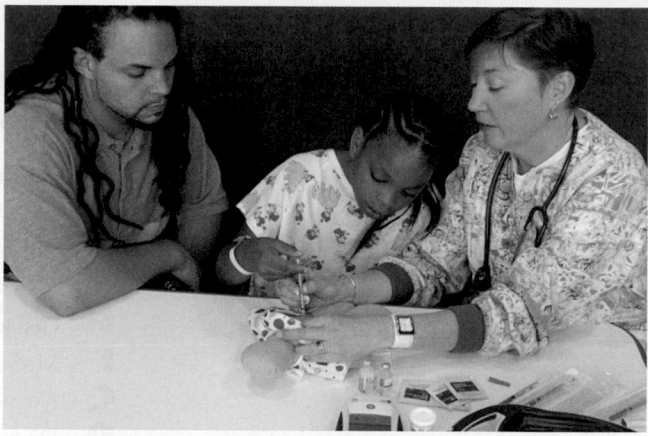

FIGURE 20-23 The nurse supervises instruction with medical equipment to help the child and caregiver learn how to administer an injection.

Teaching during the adolescent years emphasizes the importance of not taking any prescription medication that has not been ordered specifically for the person. Nurses need to explore possible use of illegal drugs or alcohol with adolescents.

ADULT AND OLDER ADULT

As adults age, they may need more medications to treat chronic health problems. Adhering to complex medication schedules can be difficult, especially for older adults who have cognitive deficits. Most adults can swallow tablets, but neurologic problems may interfere with swallowing.

Physical conditions (e.g., weight loss, obesity) may influence which IM sites are chosen for adults. Thin adults may retain muscle mass in the ventrogluteal site longer than in other IM sites.

Visual deficits may make reading drug information and prescription labels difficult. Decreased fine motor skill and tactile sensation may increase the difficulty of administering eyedrops or injections such as insulin.

Older adults are at increased risk for drug toxicity because of their altered renal excretion and hepatic metabolism of drugs. Decreased circulation can affect the absorption of ingested drugs. Observe older adults very carefully for drug toxicity, especially if renal or hepatic disease is present.

Drug misuse can occur when adults save medications for future use or share their prescription drugs with friends who report similar symptoms. Older adults on a fixed income may find that the expense of many medications stresses an already limited budget. Although these problems can occur among all age groups, they are more common among older adults because of their increasing dependence on medications to improve health and functioning.

The Hartford Institute for Geriatric Nursing (2011); www. hartfordign.org, has a list of medications that may cause side effects on its website, located in the "Try This" series. Some of the medications may cause delirium, lethargy, hypotension, confusion, vertigo, and agitation when given to an older adult. These side effects can contribute to falls and potential injury. Nurses and providers should be familiar with the items on this list.

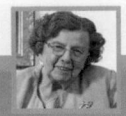

Medication Administration PICO

The nurse in the chapter-opening scenario refers the patient in that scenario to the local Senior Health Clinic to perform a medication review due to concerns about polypharmacy. A student nurse that is following this case wonders if medication reviews such as this are helpful in reducing prescribing errors. He uses the Cochrane library and the following PICO question for his search: *In geriatrics, how does medication review compared to no review help decrease medication errors?*

P = Geriatric

I = Medication review

C = No medication review

O = Decrease medication errors

He finds a systematic review that evaluated twelve studies. The review looked at various interventions including educational programs, medication review by pharmacists, and computerized programs that assisted providers to select the correct treatment for patients. Although the evidence is limited due to multiple factors impacting geriatric care, there is affirmation that some of these interventions may decrease medication errors and prevent inappropriate prescribing—especially with multidisciplinary care. More rigorous studies are recommended to fully assess if these interventions are helpful in improving clinical outcomes.

After reading the study and reflecting on the case, the student feels that utilizing the given resource would be beneficial for the patient's plan of care.

REFERENCE:

Patterson, S. M., Cadogan, C. A., Kerse, N., Cardwell, C. R., Bradley, M. C., Ryan, C., et al. (2014). Interventions to improve the appropriate use of polypharmacy for older people. *Cochrane Database of Systematic Reviews*. Issue 10:Art. No.: CD008165. doi: 10.1002/14651858.CD008165.pub3

Cultural Considerations

With the increase in diverse cultures and ethnicity in the United States, it is important to consider the cultural perspectives of your patients with respect to medication. Research has been done on immigrant populations to look at medication and treatment compliance. Some cultures believe strongly in herbal preparations and may not adhere to prescribed medication regimens. Some immigrants come from countries where antibiotics and other medications are available without prescriptions, but these drugs require prescriptions in the United States. Some cultures may support sharing of medications.

Religious and cultural beliefs impact how patients think of their health. For example, patients of Hispanic or Asian origin may believe that their illness is based on hot/cold concepts (Avery, 2007). They may not adhere to their prescribed medication regimen because they believe the medication is too "hot" for what they consider a "hot" illness (e.g., fever). Some religious groups do not believe in treating illness with medication because they believe that prayer will heal them. Trust in Western healthcare providers and the healthcare system may be an issue for some cultures. The patient may not be truthful about taking the medication or following treatment protocols.

Non–English-speaking patients have been found to have a higher incidence of nonadherence to prescribed medication regimens. Often, the older adult immigrant may rely on the younger generation to interpret in the healthcare setting but becomes upset when the age-based power structure is reversed and ultimately refuses to comply with suggested medication treatments.

Because cultural and religious beliefs have a significant impact on adherence to prescribed medication regimens, it is critical that nurses address these factors in patient interviews and assessments.

KEY CONCEPTS

- Medication administration is a significant nursing responsibility that requires solid understanding of pharmacologic principles, assessment skills, and ability to individualize patient teaching.

- Medications can be identified by three different names: chemical name, generic name, and brand name.

- Written and computer drug references provide healthcare professionals with specific information on each medication. Nurses are responsible for using drug reference resources to obtain knowledge about each drug they administer.

- Medication distribution systems include the automated medication-dispensing system, unit-dose system, self-administered medication, and bar-coding system.

- A medication order must include the patient's name, the date of the order, the medication's name, the dose, the frequency, the route of administration, and the provider's signature.

- Types of medication orders include routine, prn, one-time, stat, telephone, and verbal. It is the nurse's responsibility to interpret accurately and carry out safely the provider's orders.

- Federal legislation controls the way medications are manufactured, marketed, and controlled. The nurse must practice within the state's nurse practice act and the agency's policies and procedures concerning medication administration.

- To ensure patient safety, the nurse must follow the "six rights" (the right patient, the right medication, in the right dose, by the right route, at the right time, followed by the right documentation) whenever a medication is administered.

- A medication's activity is the result of chemical interactions between the medication and the cells of the body, which produce a biologic or physiologic response. This response can be altered by drug absorption, distribution, metabolism, or excretion.

- Therapeutic effects are the desired effects obtained from medication administration. Adverse effects are any effects other than therapeutic effects and may include side effects, toxicity, tolerance, and allergic reaction. Interactions with other drugs or food also can occur.

- Nursing assessments are done to obtain baseline information concerning a patient's medication use, to evaluate the effectiveness of medications, to identify adverse effects, and to individualize patient teaching concerning medications.

- Many forms of medications, such as tablets, capsules, syrups, and elixirs, are appropriate for oral administration. Oral medications may be swallowed or administered through gastric or intestinal tubes. Sublingual or buccal administration allows for very rapid absorption from the oral mucosa.

- Topical medications include those that are applied to the skin or inserted in a body cavity. Solutions, creams, lotions, ointments, and transdermal patches are applied to the skin. Topical medications can be administered into the eye, ear, nose, rectum, or vagina.

- Parenteral medications are given by injection or infusion into ID tissue, subcutaneous tissue, IM tissue, or the venous (IV) circulation.

- Sites commonly used for IM injections include the deltoid, ventrogluteal, vastus lateralis, and rectus femoris muscles. Anatomic landmarks must be used to identify each site properly.

- IV medications enter the venous circulation by IV push, intermittent infusion, or continuous drip.

- Changes occurring during the life span are important to consider when administering medications and may necessitate adjustments in the techniques for administration.

- Cultural and religious beliefs may impact adherence to prescribed medication regimens.

PRACTICING FOR THE NCLEX
CHECK YOUR ANSWERS IN APPENDIX A.

1. A nurse is covering for a colleague at lunch when the patient requests a prescribed medication, unfamiliar to the nurse. What is the most appropriate action?
   a. Delay the administration until the primary nurse returns.
   b. Refuse to treat the patient because the patient's condition is not fully known by this nurse.
   c. Look up the prescribed medication to see if it is appropriate at this time.
   d. Call the doctor to ask if it is appropriate to administer.

2. A patient requests pain medication for pain at a surgical site of 8/10. There is a prn, or "as-needed," order for 10 mg PO of oxycodone for pain greater than 6/10 on the pain scale. What is the first thing the nurse should do?
   a. Administer the oxycodone.
   b. Assess the effects of the medication.
   c. Document the administration of the medication.
   d. Determine if the order is appropriate.

3. A nurse is reviewing medication orders when she realizes that a patient with renal failure has been prescribed Bactrim (an antibiotic contraindicated in patients with severe renal impairment). What action would be most appropriate according to nursing practice laws?
   a. Administer the medication as ordered and then discuss with the physician.
   b. Refuse to administer the medication since it is contraindicated for this patient.
   c. Call the physician who ordered the medication to discuss this inappropriate order.
   d. Administer the medication and perform frequent assessments for drug effects.

4. At shift handoff, a nurse receives a confused patient who has been refusing antihypertensive medications because she believes it is poison. Which nursing action would be most appropriate?
   a. Crush the medication and mix it with applesauce.
   b. Chart the medication as not given and attend to the other patient's medications.
   c. Discuss what the medication is for and why it is important to take it.
   d. Ask the patient why she has been refusing her medications.

5. A nurse administers a prescribed dose of IV morphine for pain. The next day, the patient reports constipation. Which of the following best describes this adverse reaction?
   a. Tolerance
   b. Side effect
   c. Allergic reaction
   d. Anaphylactic reaction

6. A nurse administers a medication to a patient at the end of her shift. She brings in a blue pill in a medication cup, places it on the dinner tray, and states "Remember to take that, Betty" before leaving to document and give shift report. Which of the following "rights" were not done? Select all that apply:
    a. Right patient
    b. Right medication
    c. Right route
    d. Right documentation

7. A new nurse is hanging a bag of continuous infusion IV fluids. The medication-dispensing cart releases the wrong bag, and the nurse infuses the wrong type of fluids. Another nurse notes the error, the correct fluids are infused, and there is no harm done to the patient. Which nursing action would be most appropriate in acknowledging this error?
    a. Call the physician to report the error.
    b. File an incident report per organizational protocol.
    c. Discuss the error with the patient.
    d. Not tell anyone as no harm was done.

8. A nurse is about to administer a dose of supplementary potassium (40 mEq) PO. Which information should be checked prior to administration? Select all that apply:
    a. MAR to confirm dose, time, route, medication
    b. Adequate venous access
    c. Ability to swallow and diet order
    d. Serum potassium lab value

9. A nurse is administering a 5,000 U/0.5 mL dose of subcutaneous heparin. The medication is stocked in single-dose glass vials. What should the nurse select as an appropriate needle for subcutaneous injections? Select all that apply:
    a. ½ to ⅝ inches
    b. 1 to 3 inches
    c. 20 to 23 gauge
    d. 26 to 30 gauge

10. A 2-year-old is seen in a well-child checkup and needs a flu vaccine (1 mL). How should this be administered?
    a. As an IM injection in the deltoid
    b. Z-track method must be used
    c. As an IM injection in the vastus lateralis
    d. Using a long needle (more than 1 inch)

REFERENCES

American Diabetes Association. (2011). *Insulin administration*. Retrieved March 16, 2011, from http://care.diabetesjournals.org/content/27/suppl_1/s106.full

Avery, K. (2007). *Medication non-adherence issues with refugee and immigrant patients*. Retrieved March 26, 2010, from http://ethnomed.org/clinical/pharmacy/medication-non-adherence-issues-with-refugee-and-immigrant-patients/

Centers for Disease Control and Prevention. (2011). *Epidemiology and prevention of vaccine-preventable diseases. The pink book: Course textbook* (12th ed.).

Crawford, C., & Johnson, J. (2012). Research corner. To aspirate or not: An integrative review of the evidence. *Nursing, 42*(3), 20–25. doi: 10.1097/01Nurse.0000411417.91161.87

Encyclopedia of Nursing Practice. (2011). Z-track method. Retrieved August 9, 2011, from www.enotes.com/nursing-encyclopedia/z-track-injection

Hartford Institute for Geriatric Nursing. (2011). *Nursing standards of practice protocol: reducing adverse drug events*. Retrieved August 9, 2011, from http://consultgerirn.org/topics/medication/want_to_know_more

Hockenberry, M., & Wilson, D. (2011). *Wong's nursing of infants and children* (9th ed.). St. Louis, MO: Mosby Elsevier.

Institute for Safe Medication Practices. (2011). *ISMP Newsletters*. Retrieved March 17, 2011, from http://ismp.org/default.asp

Institute for Safe Medication Practices. (2014). *Independent Double Checks: Undervalued and Misused: Selective Use of This Strategy Can Play an Important Role in Medication Safety*. Retrieved July 23, 2014 from http://www.ismp.org/Newsletters/Acutecare/showarticle.aspx?id=51

Joint Commission. (2015). *2015 National Safety Goals*. Retrieved July 28, 2015 from www.jointcommission.org/assets/1/6/2015_OBS_NPSG_ER.pdf

Kim, J., & Bates, D. (2013). Medication administration errors by nurses: adherence to guidelines. *Journal of Clinical Nursing, 22*(3/4), 590–598. doi:10.1111/j.1365-2702.2012.04344.x

Knox, T., & Davie, J. (2009). Nasogastric tube feeding—which syringe size produces lower pressure and is safest to use? *Nursing Times, 105*(27), 24–26.

Malkin, B. (2008). Are techniques used for intramuscular injection based on research evidence? *Nursing Times, 104*(50/51), 48–51.

Reinhard, S., Young, H., Kane, R., & Quinn, W. (2006). Nurse delegation of medication administration for older adults in assisted living. *Nursing Outlook, 54*(2), 74–78.

Seibert, H., Maddox, R., Flynn, E., & Williams, C. (2014). Effect of barcode technology with electronic medication administration record on medication accuracy rates. *American Journal of Health-System Pharmacy, 71*(3), 209–218. doi: 10.2146/ajhp130332

Shelton, P., & Rosenthal, K. (2004). Select a safer needle. *Nursing Management, 35*(6), 25–32.

Tamura-Lis, W. (2013). Teach-back for quality education and patient safety. *Urologic Nursing, 33*(6), 267–298. doi:10.7257/1053-816X.2013.33.6.297

Tarnow, K., & King, N. (2004). Intradermal injections: Traditional bevel up versus bevel down. *Applied Nursing Research, 17*(4), 275–282.

Procedure 20-1 Administering Oral Medications

Purpose
1. Provide a safe, effective, economical route for administering medications
2. Provide sustained drug action with minimal discomfort

Equipment
MAR or electronic medication administration record (eMAR)
Medication supply
Disposable medication cups or oral syringe
Water, juice, or milk with straw if not contraindicated
Pill-crushing or pill-cutting device (when necessary)

Assessment
- Consult a nursing drug handbook, computer resource, or other standard references about unfamiliar drugs.
- Assess the patient's allergy history.
- Assess the patient's ability to take oral medications:
  - Level of consciousness and cooperativeness
  - Active swallow reflex
  - Complaints of nausea and vomiting
  - Recent gastrointestinal surgery or bowel obstruction
  - Nasogastric tube connected to suction
  - Current diet order
  - Ability to sit upright
- Identify and perform individual preadministration assessments of pulse, blood pressure, laboratory data, and other factors as indicated by the medication being administered.
- Ensure that the correct medication and dosage are available at the time scheduled.

Procedure

1. **Review provider's orders for accuracy and completeness, including patient's name, drug name, dosage, route, and time and indications.**
   Rationale: Prevents errors.

2. **Perform hand hygiene.**
   Rationale: Reduces transfer of microorganisms from hands to medication.

3. **Arrange eMAR or MAR next to medication supply.**
   Rationale: Organizes work space to save time and reduce the chance of error.

4. **Prepare medications for only one patient at a time. Check patient allergies before removing any medications.**
   Rationale: Prevents errors during preparation.

5. **Remove ordered medications from supply. Compare label on medication with the MAR or eMAR (Fig. 1), and check the six rights of medication administration. Scan bar code if using BCMA. If a discrepancy exists, recheck the patient's chart and medication orders.**

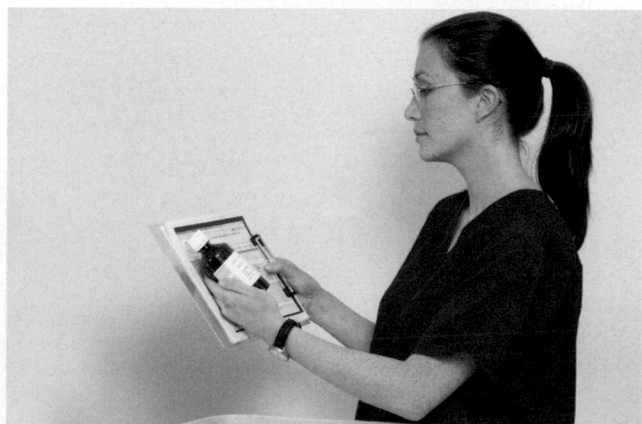

FIG. 1 Compare medication, container label, and medication record.

Rationale: Check the six rights of medication administration twice. The first check occurs when removing the medication from the storage area.

6. **Calculate correct drug dosage if necessary.**
   Rationale: Prevents dosage errors.

Procedure 20-1 *continued*

7. **Prepare selected medications.**

   a. **Unit dosage:** Place packaged medications directly into medicine cup or lay them on tray without unwrapping them (Fig. 2A).

   b. **Medications from a multidose bottle:** Pour tablets or capsules into the container lid, and transfer them into medicine cup. Return any extra tablets to the bottle. Label all unlabeled medications. Break only scored tablets, if necessary, using a pill cutter to obtain proper dosage (Fig. 2B).

   c. **Medications from a bingo card:** Snap the bubble containing the correct medication directly over the medication cup. Do not touch the medication.

   d. **Swallowing difficulty:** If the patient has trouble swallowing tablets, grind with mortar and pestle or other drug-crushing device until smooth (Fig. 3). Mix powder in small amount of pudding or applesauce. Do not crush enteric-coated tablets or extended-release tablets.

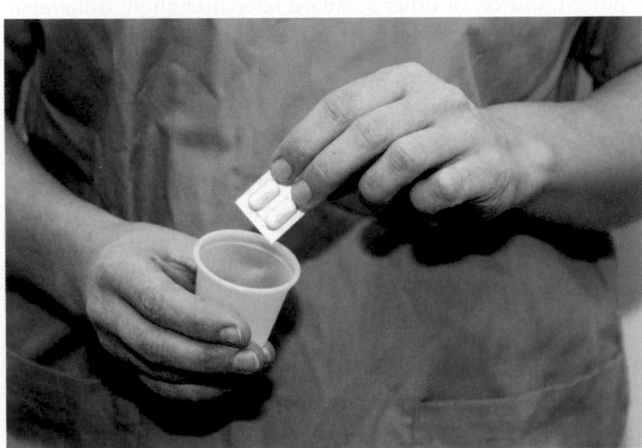

A

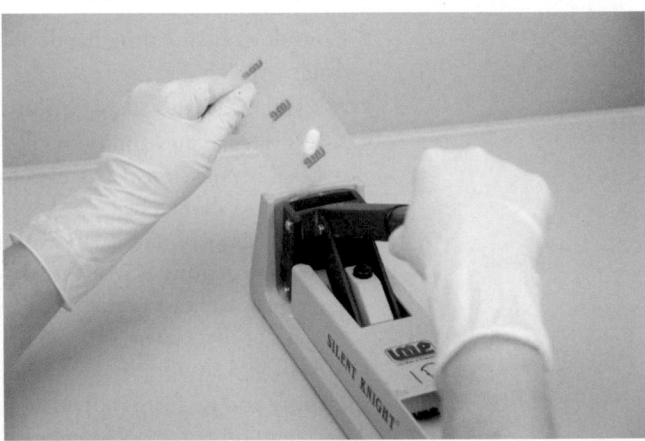

A

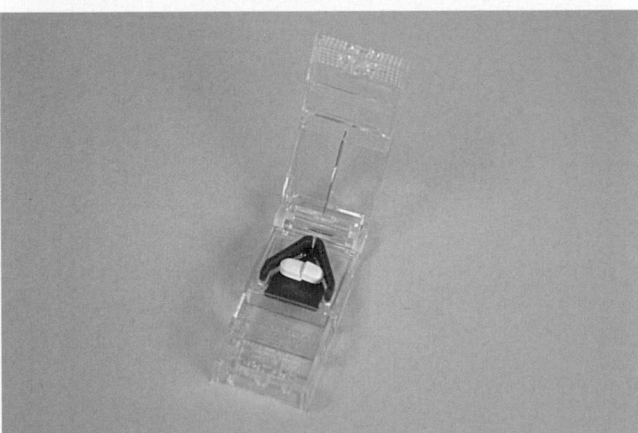

B

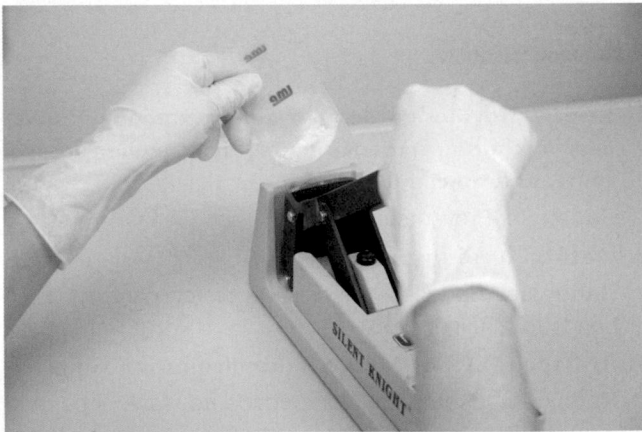

B

FIG. 2 **A.** Place tablet in a medicine cup. **B.** Use a pill cutter to break scored tablets.

Rationale: Maintains cleanliness of drugs. All medications taken from the supply should be labeled so that the final check of the six rights can occur at the bedside.

FIG. 3 **A.** Place packaged tablet in pill crusher. **B.** Pill crusher grinds the tablet into a powder.

Rationale: Crushed enteric-coated tablets irritate gastric mucosa, and crushed extended-release tablets alter drug absorption and duration of drug effects.

Procedure 20-1   *continued*

e. **Liquid medications: Remove cap and place on countertop with the inside up. Hold bottle so label is against palm of hand. Fill until bottom of meniscus (the surface of the fluid that appears curved) is at desired dosage (Fig. 4). Discard excess poured liquid from cup into sink; do not pour it back into the bottle. Label medication.**

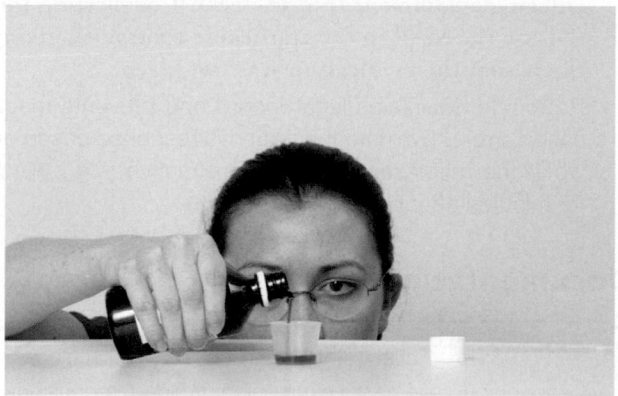

FIG. 4 Pour liquid medication into a medicine cup.

Rationale: Prevents soiling of label when pouring medication and contamination of the medication in the bottle. All medications taken from the supply should be labeled so that the final check of the six rights can occur at the bedside.

8. **Take medications directly to the patient's room. Keep medications in sight at all times.**

Rationale: Prevents medication errors.

9. **Compare name on MAR with name on patient's identification band using two separate identifiers (e.g., name, MRN, Social Security number, or birth date). Do not administer medications if the patient is not wearing an identification band. Scan patient's identification bracelet if using BCMA (Fig. 5).**

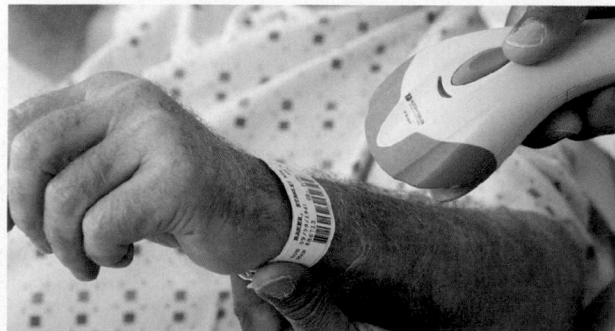

FIG. 5 Scan patient's identification bracelet when using BCMA.

Rationale: Careful checking ensures administration of drugs to the proper patient.

10. **Complete any preadministration assessment (e.g., blood pressure, pulse) required for the specific medication to be given.**

Rationale: Medications that have a direct action, such as decreasing pulse rate or blood pressure, require assessment to determine if the medication can be given safely at that time.

11. **Compare medication to eMAR or MAR, and recheck the six rights of medication administration (Fig. 6). If using unit-dose medication, unwrap the medication and place it in the cup before checking the six rights of the next medication.**

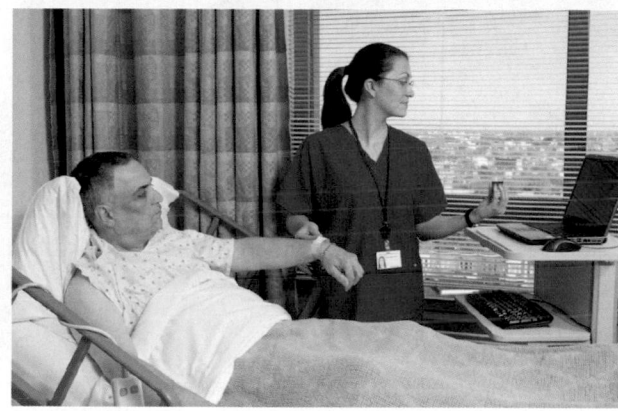

FIG. 6 Compare medication to MAR and recheck the six rights of medication administration.

Rationale: The second check of the six rights occurs before administration to the patient.

12. **Explain the medication's purpose to the patient.**

Rationale: Protects the patient's rights and encourages the patient's participation in care and begins teaching about medications. The patient may detect discrepancies from the usual medication regimen.

13. **Assist the patient to sitting position if necessary. Give the medication cup and glass of water to the patient (Fig. 7).**

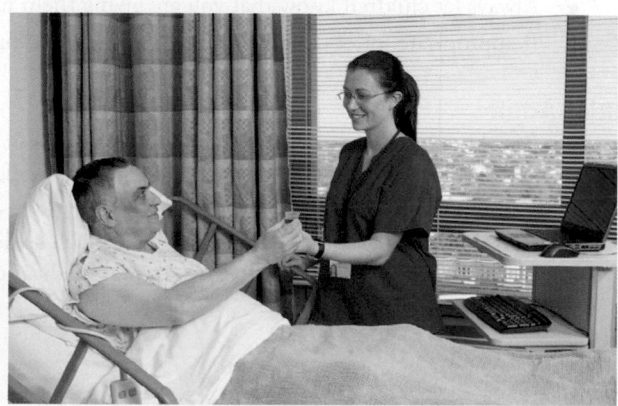

FIG. 7 Give the medication to the patient.

Rationale: The sitting position facilitates swallowing and prevents aspiration.

Procedure 20-1   *continued*

14. **If the patient cannot hold the medication cup, place it to the patient's lips and introduce the medication into his or her mouth. If a tablet or capsule falls on the floor, discard and repeat preparation.**

    Rationale: Medication that has fallen on the floor is contaminated.

15. **Stay with the patient until he or she swallows all medications (Fig. 8). Look inside the patient's mouth if the patient is cognitively impaired or has difficulty swallowing.**

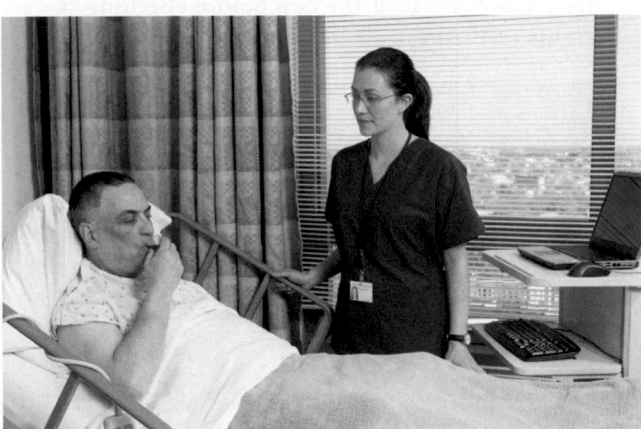

FIG. 8 Stay with the patient while medications are swallowed.

Rationale: The nurse is responsible for ensuring that the patient receives the ordered medications.

16. **Dispose of soiled supplies, and wash hands.**

    Rationale: Maintains asepsis.

17. **Document time at which medication was administered and any preadministration assessments. Note the time that postadministration assessments to assess effectiveness are due for prn medications. If a medication has been held, note this (usually by entering a comment into the eMAR or circling initials on the MAR in the applicable time slot), giving the reason the medication was not given.**

    Rationale: Maintains legal record and prevents medication errors. Evaluate the patient's response based on when the medication should be effective (e.g., 30 to 45 minutes after oral administration).

Documentation

> 7/15/17: 08:00—Patient states pain 7 on a 0–10 scale. Appears diaphoretic, facial expression strained, repositioning and guarding left abdomen. Given oxycodone 5 mg orally. Patient stated pain 2 on a 0–10 scale in 30 minutes. Patient with relaxed facial expression, resting comfortably with head of bed at 30-degree angle. Will reassess in 30 minutes.
>
> —S. Zoe, RN

Life Span Considerations

Infant and Child

- Tablets and capsules are not recommended forms of oral medication in children younger than 5 years. Young children may not swallow them safely. Use liquid preparations (available for most oral medications), and measure the preparation appropriately. Some come with calibrated droppers for measuring small amounts of medication for infants. Do not interchange droppers among medications. Different companies use different-sized droppers, and medications may be inaccurately measured.

- Always let children know that you are giving them medicine, not "candy."

- If appropriate, offer children a choice about what fluid to take with the medication.

Older Adult

- Be aware that the normal physiologic changes that occur with aging, such as decreased salivation, resulting in a dry mouth and delayed esophageal clearance, may impair swallowing, and the patient may have difficulty taking oral medications. Use a liquid form of medication as necessary.

- Additional changes that occur with aging, such as decreased stomach peristalsis, gastric acidity, and colon motility, may also affect the patient's ability to take oral medications. Refer to Table 10-2 for a list of medications that are especially problematic for the elderly.

Procedure 20-1   *continued*

Home Care Modifications

- Assess the patient or caregiver's knowledge of medication therapy.
- Assess the patient's sensory function (sight, hearing, touch) to determine whether he or she needs special teaching or administration strategies. Be sure the patient wears eyeglasses or hearing aid during teaching sessions.
- Patients with arthritis may have difficulty opening childproof caps and can request special packaging from the pharmacist.
- Assess the patient's ability to read. The patient may be unable to read prepared booklets or medication labels.
- Instruct the patient or caregiver in purpose of medications, dosage schedule, common side effects, whom to call with problems, and what to do about missed doses.
- Give guidelines for drug safety as appropriate: discarding outdated drugs, keeping drugs out of children's reach, and refrigerating medications.
- Devise learning aids if needed. Examples include calendars for each week that contain separate zip-top bags with medications to take at specific times, egg cartons with color-coded sections for medications to take at specific times, and commercially available divided containers to provide 1 week of medication at a time.
- Document patient teaching, including the use of learning aids.

Collaboration and Delegation

- Clarify with provider any unclear orders. Do not accept orders that are unclear or include unapproved abbreviations.
- Notify provider of any changes in a patient's status that necessitate a change in medication orders. See the Collaborating With the Healthcare Team display.
- Do not ask UAP to administer medications to patients in the hospital. Instruct them in how to observe for and report therapeutic effects and side effects when caring for patients. Also, urge them to notify the nurse caring for the patient about any patient complaints or changes.

Procedure 20-2 Administering Medication by Metered-Dose Inhaler

Purpose
- Deliver a premeasured dose of medication to the bronchial airways and lungs

Equipment

MAR or eMAR
Medication canister
Inhaler mouthpiece
Spacer device (optional)

Assessment
- Review the patient's medical history, medication history, and allergy status.
- Assess the patient's respiratory status, including ease of breathing, respiratory rate, accessory muscle use, and breath sounds (Fig. 1).

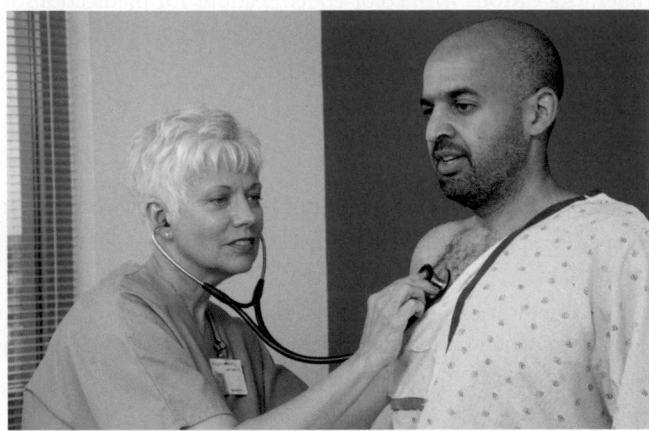

FIG. 1 Assess the patient's respiratory status.

Procedure

1. **Review physician's order for type of medication, dosage, and route, and assess patient allergies (see Procedure 20-1, steps 1 through 6).**

2. **Close door or bed curtains and explain the procedure to the patient.**
   Rationale: Ensures patient privacy, increases patient compliance, reduces patient anxiety, and promotes learning.

3. **Assist the patient to sitting or standing position.**
   Rationale: Sitting or standing enhances full chest expansion, allowing deeper inhalation of the medication.

4. **Perform the second medication check of six rights. Compare name on MAR with name on patient's identification band using two separate identifiers (e.g., name, MRN, Social Security number, or birth date). Do not administer medications if the patient is not wearing an identification band. Scan the patient's identification bracelet if using BCMA.**
   Rationale: The second check occurs before administration of the medication to the patient. Checking the six rights minimizes the risk of medication errors.

5. **Instruct the patient on assembly of medication canister, inhalation mouthpiece, and spacer device if needed.**

Instruct the patient to attach the medication canister to the inhaler mouthpiece by inserting the metal stem into the long end of the mouthpiece. Teach the patient to shake the canister and spacer several times.
Rationale: Shaking the canister mixes the medication and ensures uniform dosage delivery.

6. **Steps 6 through 8 need to occur smoothly, one right after the other. Ask the patient to breathe out through his or her mouth (Fig. 2).**

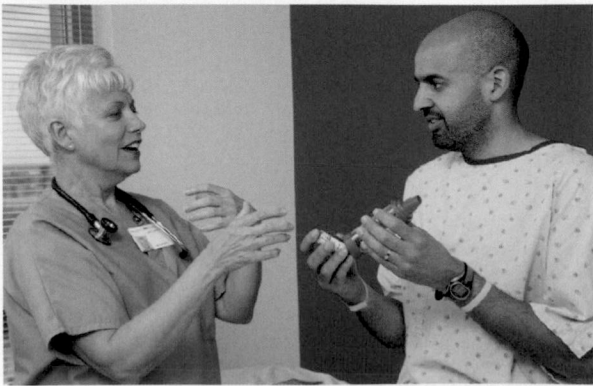

FIG. 2 Instruct the patient to breathe through the mouth.

Rationale: Empty lungs facilitate deeper inhalation of medication.

Procedure 20-2   *continued*

7. **Assist the patient to position the mouthpiece 1 to 2 inches from his or her open mouth. If using a spacer, have the patient place spacer's mouthpiece into the mouth, forming a secure seal (Fig. 3). Instruct the patient to breathe in slowly through the mouth. As the patient starts inhaling, instruct the patient to press the canister down to release one dose of the medication.**

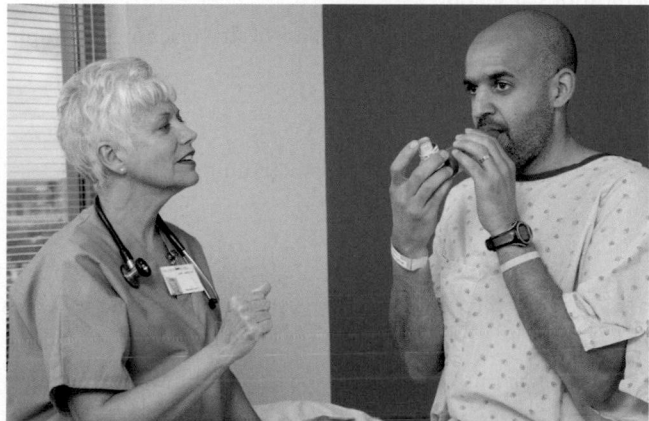

FIG. 3 The patient places the mouthpiece of the spacer in the mouth, closes the lips around it, and inhales.

Rationale: When a spacer is not used, releasing the medication 1 to 2 inches away from the mouth allows medication to form a mist and to be delivered more accurately by inhalation to the bronchial airways rather than being trapped in the oropharynx and then swallowed.

8. **Instruct the patient to hold his or her breath for 10 seconds (if possible) and then to exhale slowly through pursed lips (Fig. 4 illustrates a spacer).**

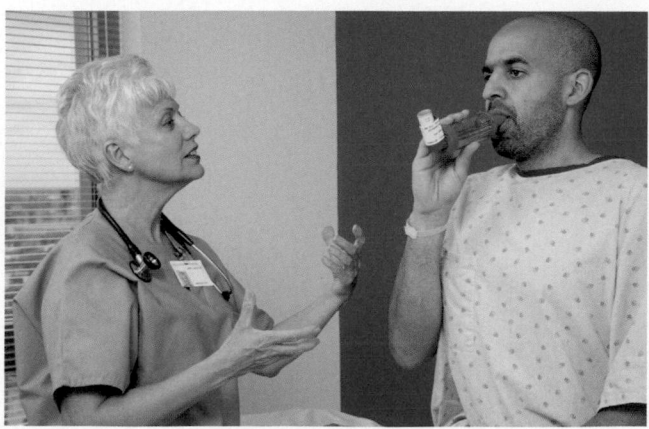

FIG. 4 With a spacer, the patient breathes in and out.

Rationale: Enhances absorption of the medication.

9. **Wait at least 1 minute before administration of a second puff by MDI.**

Rationale: Waiting allows medication from the first dose to be distributed and absorbed often opening up airways so additional puffs can absorb better. Usual orders prescribe two puffs.

10. **Wash hands and clean mouthpiece. If steroid medication was administered, have the patient rinse mouth.**

Rationale: Washing hands and equipment minimizes spread of infection and maximizes inhaler efficiency. Oral fungal infections can occur if inhaled steroid medication remains in the oral cavity.

11. **Reassess ease of breathing, respiratory rate, accessory muscle use, and breath sounds.**

Rationale: Follow-up assessment provides data to evaluate the effectiveness of inhaled medications.

12. **Document medication administration and patient status before and after administration.**

Rationale: Documentation helps maintain accurate patient records, including effectiveness of the medications, and prevents medication errors.

Modification for Using a Spacer With a Metered-Dose Inhaler

13. **Attach the spacer to the inhaler mouthpiece. Instruct the patient to exhale and then place the mouthpiece in the mouth, closing his or her lips around the mouthpiece. Depress the medication canister and have the patient inhale until the medication from the chamber is gone. Advise the patient to take two or three short breaths to get all the medication from the spacer.**

Documentation

6/14/17: 08:00—PRN Rescue MDI with albuterol administered due to complaints of dyspnea, RR 24, O₂ sat 88%, expiratory wheezes, and coarse crackles noted on auscultation. Spacer used. Posttreatment assessment RR 20, O₂ sat 90, and patient verbalizes less distress. Crackles and expiratory wheezes still present. Will continue to monitor every 30 minutes.

—S. Zoe, RN

Procedure 20-2 *continued*

Life Span Considerations

Infant and Toddler

- Use a spacer or nebulizer with a face mask to deliver medications by inhalation for an infant or toddler.
- Teach caregivers about symptoms that require prn bronchodilator treatment.

Child and Adolescent

- School-age children often require treatment during school hours or in emergencies. Inform the school nurse of the need for the MDI, and check school policies regarding use of medications at school.
- Children may be embarrassed to use MDIs at school. Provide encouragement, support, and health teaching regarding respiratory function.

Adult and Older Adult

- Use spacers for older adults, especially if they have difficulty with manual dexterity or deep breathing.

Home Care Considerations

- Teach the patient which MDI to use in an emergency (β_2 agonist) and when to seek medical treatment.
- Caution against overuse of the MDI.
- Review infection control measures, including daily rinsing of the inhaler in warm, running water and biweekly washing of the mouthpiece with soap and water.
- Teach the patient to always have a spare canister on hand to avoid running out of medication. The patient can determine how much medication remains in the canister by placing it in a container of water. A full canister will sink to the bottom; an almost-empty canister will float.

Collaboration and Delegation

- Respiratory therapists may provide initial instruction on how to use an MDI. Consult them as needed when problems occur with MDI use.
- Report worsening respiratory symptoms to the provider or pulmonary specialist as soon as possible.

Procedure 20-3 **Withdrawing Medication From a Vial**

Purpose	• Withdraw a precise amount of medication from a vial while maintaining asepsis.
Equipment	MAR or eMAR Vial with medication Alcohol wipes or antiseptic swabs for cleaning vial Sterile syringe and needle Sterile water or normal saline solution for reconstituting medication if it is in powder form (optional; usually, reconstitution is done in the pharmacy) Needle with filter if needed to prevent drawing solid matter into the needle and syringe (optional)
Assessment	• Review the order and assess the intended medication administration route (e.g., subcutaneous, IM, IV) before selecting the needle and syringe. • Inspect the ordered medication for clarity, crystals, and expiration date.

Procedure

1. **Check medication order and compare the name of the ordered medication with the label on the medication vial. Complete steps 1 through 6 in Procedure 20-1.**

2. **Assemble needle and syringe.**
   Rationale: Prevents infection.

3. **Pick up vial. If medication has been reconstituted or is in suspension, place the vial between your palms, rotating or rolling the vial back and forth (Fig. 1). Do not shake the vial.**

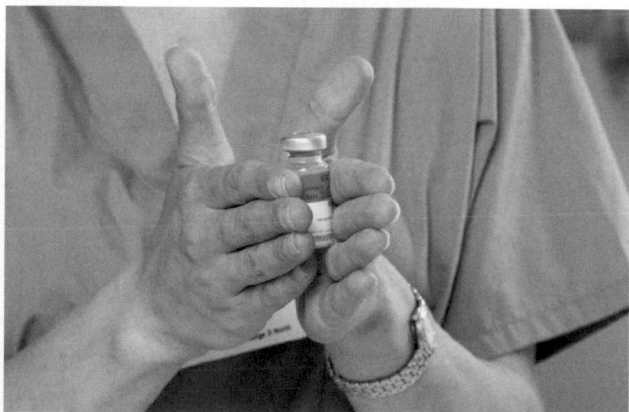

FIG. 1 Place the vial between your palms, rotating or rolling the vial back and forth.

Rationale: The rolling motion mixes and disperses the medication. Shaking can cause bubbles that interfere with accurate measurement.

4. **Remove metal cap from vial and remove guard from needle. If multidose vial is being used (e.g., withdrawing insulin), date the vial when opened and discard on expiration date. Cleanse the vial top with alcohol prior to withdrawal (Fig. 2).**

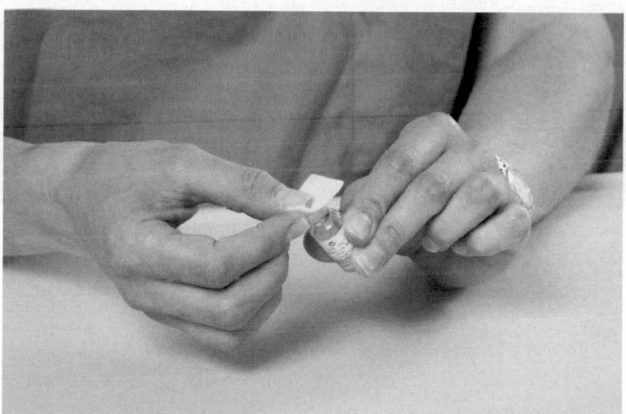

FIG. 2 Cleanse top of vial with alcohol wipe.

Rationale: Maintain asepsis.

5. **Pull back on barrel of syringe to draw in a volume of air equal to the volume of the ordered medication dose. Holding the vial between the thumb and fingers of the nondominant hand, insert needle through the rubber stopper into the air space—not the solution—in the vial and inject air (Fig. 3).**

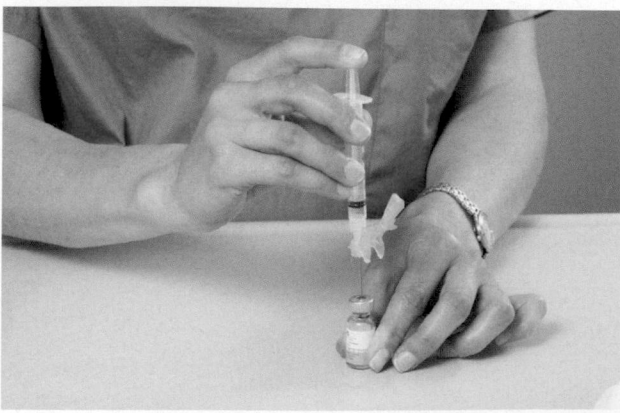

FIG. 3 Add air to the vial.

Procedure 20-3   *continued*

Rationale: Injecting air into the air space in the vial prevents creation of negative pressure within the vial, allowing easy withdrawal of medication. Injecting air into the solution would create bubbles and could interfere with withdrawing an accurate dose of medication.

6. **Invert the vial and withdraw the ordered dose of medication by pulling back on the plunger (Fig. 4). Make sure that the needle is in the solution to be withdrawn and observe if fluid is moving into the syringe.**

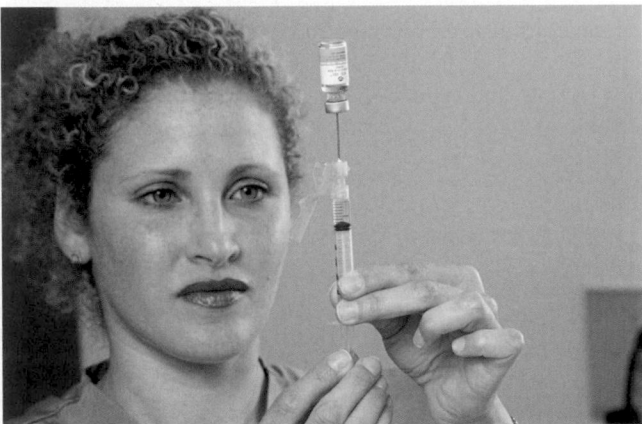

FIG. 4 Withdraw medication from the vial.

Rationale: Inverting the vial brings the needle in contact with the solution so that medication can be withdrawn.

7. **Expel air bubbles and adjust dose if necessary.**

Rationale: Air bubbles inadvertently drawn into the medication solution take up space, which impacts accurate dosage measurement.

8. **Remove needle from vial and cover the needle with guard. Perform hand hygiene.**

Rationale: Maintains asepsis and reduces the risk of needlesticks.

Procedure 20-4 Withdrawing Medication From an Ampule

Purpose
- Withdraw the full dose of medication from an ampule safely while maintaining asepsis

Equipment

MAR or eMAR
Ampule with medication
Sterile syringe and filter needle
Sterile gauze pad or alcohol wipe

Assessment
- Same as in Procedure 20-3

Procedure

1. Check medication order and make sure the solution in the ampule matches the ordered solution. Complete steps 1 through 6 in Procedure 20-1.
2. Assemble filter needle and syringe.
3. Pick up ampule and flick its upper stem several times with a fingernail (Fig. 1).

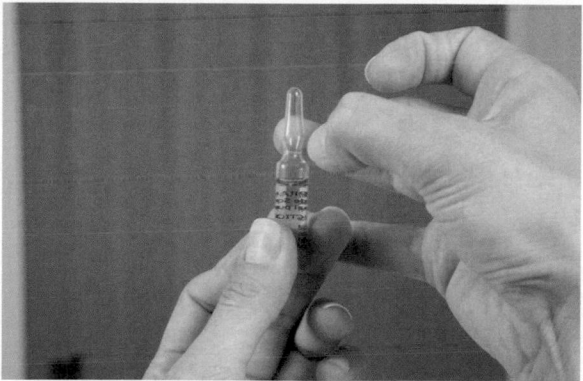

FIG. 1 Flick upper stem to release medication.

Rationale: The sharp, flicking motion releases medication trapped in the ampule's upper chamber.

4. Wrap a sterile gauze pad or alcohol wipe around the ampule's neck before breaking the neck along the scored line with an outward snapping motion (Fig. 2). Always break away from your body.

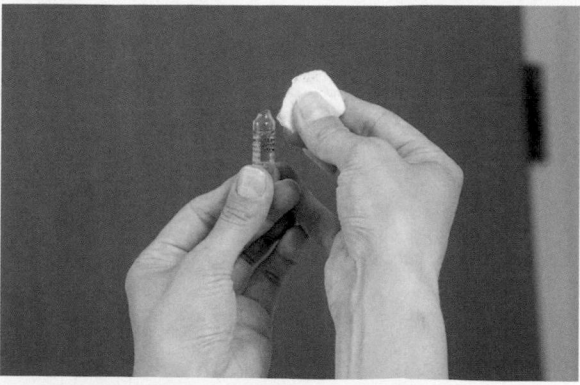

FIG. 2 Break neck of ampule.

Rationale: The sterile gauze barrier protects the fingers from broken glass, possibly trapping sharp fragments and preventing accidental injury to the hand.

5. Discard the broken neck appropriately, and prepare to withdraw medication from the ampule using one of the following methods:

   a. Place the ampule upright on a flat surface, insert the needle in the solution, and withdraw the correct amount of medication by pulling up on the plunger (Fig. 3). Do not touch the needle to the glass rim.

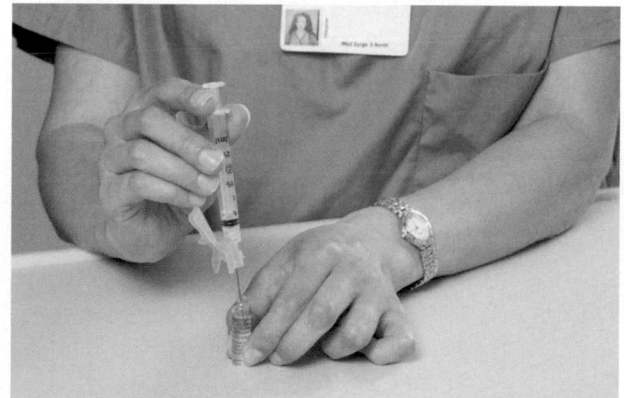

FIG. 3 Withdraw medication from upright ampule.

   Rationale: Contact between needle and ampule contaminates the needle. There is no need to inject air.

   b. Tilt the ampule sideways. Withdraw the proper dose of medication.

   Rationale: Keeping the needle in the solution keeps air out of the dose of medication.

6. Remove the needle from the solution. Hold the needle upright, inspect the syringe, and dispel any air that may have been drawn into the syringe. Make sure that the syringe contains the right amount of medication. Expel any extra medication. Label syringe.

Procedure 20-4   *continued*

Rationale: Ensures accurate measurement of dose. Labeling the syringe will allow proper identification in the patient's room.

7. **Cover the filter needle with a safety guard and change the needle. Discard filter needle and ampule in sharps container.**

Rationale: Proper disposal protects healthcare personnel from injury. A filter needle is used to trap glass particles and should not be used for injection.

8. **Perform hand hygiene.**

Rationale: Reduces microbe transmission.

Procedure 20-5 Drawing Up Two Medications in a Syringe

Purpose
1. Minimize the number of injections a patient receives
2. Prevent contaminating one vial of medication with medication from the other vial

Equipment
MAR or eMAR
Two vials of ordered medication
Sterile 1- to 3-mL syringe with appropriate gauge and length needle
Antiseptic swabs

Assessment
- Review medication order.
- Review drug literature to ensure compatibility of the two medications.

Procedure

1. **Check medication order and compare the name of the ordered medication with the label on the medication vial. Complete steps 1 through 6 in Procedure 20-1.**
2. **Cleanse tops of both vials with antiseptic (Fig. 1).**

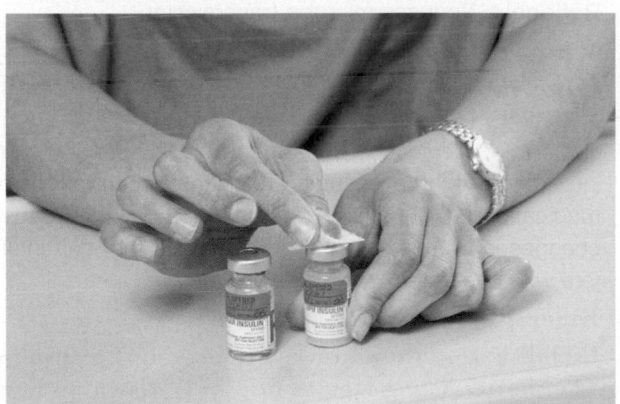

FIG. 1 Cleanse tops of both vials with antiseptic.

Rationale: Maintains asepsis and prevents introduction of organisms into vials.

3. **With syringe, aspirate a volume of air equal to the medication dose from first medication (Vial A).**
4. **Inject air into Vial A, being careful that the needle does not touch the solution (Fig. 2).**

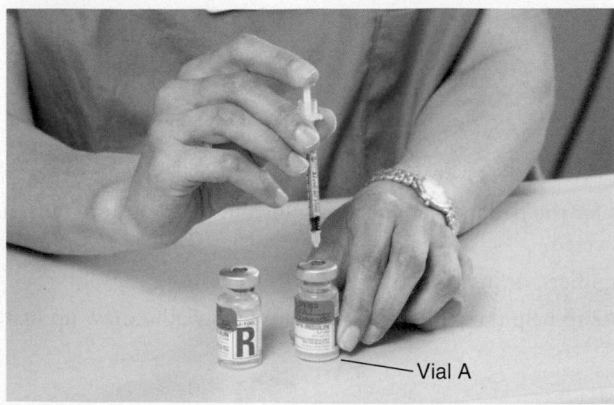

FIG. 2 Inject air into Vial A.

Rationale: Air in vial creates positive pressure to facilitate solution withdrawal. The same needle will be used to withdraw medication from second vial, so it must not have medication from Vial A on it.

5. **Remove syringe from Vial A without withdrawing medication.**
   a. **Aspirate volume of air equal to the medication dose from second medication (Vial B) (Fig. 3).**

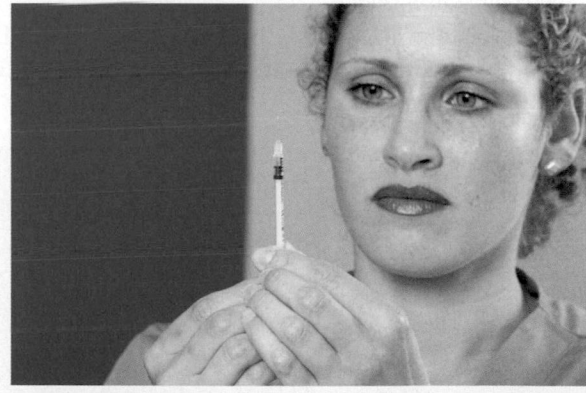

FIG. 3 Aspirate volume of air equal to the medication dose from Vial B.

   b. **Inject air into Vial B (Fig. 4).**

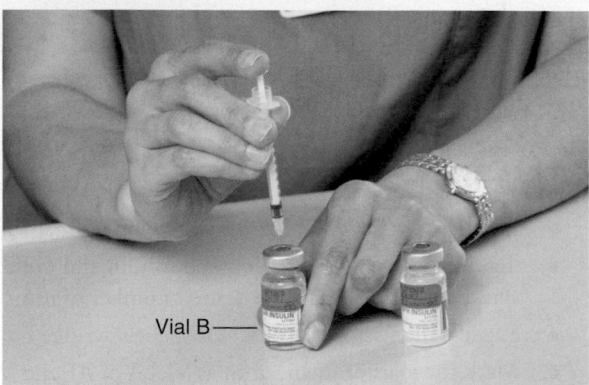

Vial B

FIG. 4 Inject air into Vial B.

Rationale: Same as for step 4.

Procedure 20-5　*continued*

6. **Invert Vial B, and withdraw the required volume of medication into syringe (Fig. 5). Expel all air bubbles, and withdraw needle from Vial B.**

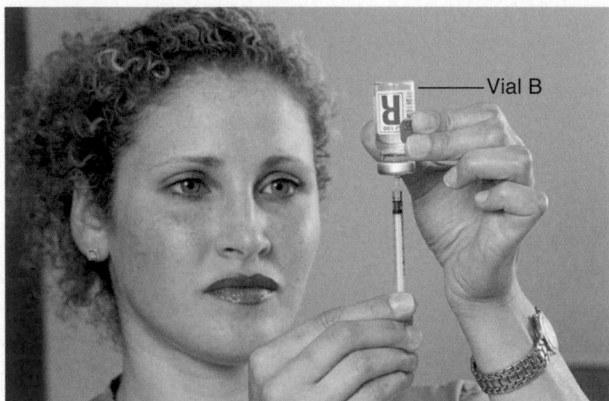

FIG. 5 Withdraw medication from Vial B.

Rationale: Expelling air permits accurate dosage measurement.

7. **Determine what the total combined volume of the two medications would measure on the syringe scale.**

Rationale: Prevents accidental withdrawal of excess medication from Vial A.

8. **Insert needle into Vial A, invert vial, and carefully withdraw required volume of medication (as in step 6) (Fig. 6).**

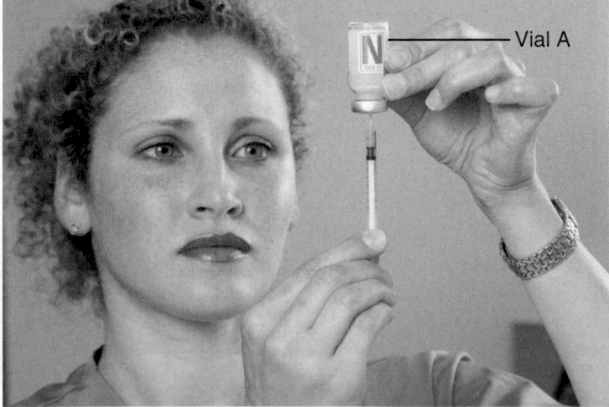

FIG. 6 Insert needle into Vial A and withdraw medication.

Rationale: If required volume is exceeded, the procedure must be started over with step 1.

9. **Withdraw needle from Vial A and replace needle guard.**

Rationale: Prevents injury to healthcare workers.

10. **Check medication and dosage before returning or discarding vials. Label syringe with medication.**

Rationale: Rechecking dosage reduces the risk for medication errors. Labeling syringe allows final medication check at bedside.

Modification for Insulin

Equipment

U-100 insulin syringe
Vials of prescribed U-100 insulin

1. **Perform hand hygiene**

Rationale: Reduces microbe transmission.

2. **When preparing insulin in suspension, gently rotate vials between palms of hands to mix the suspension.**

Rationale: Medication separates from suspension during storage. Mixing ensures accurate concentrations of medications throughout. Shaking vigorously can cause changes in potency of insulin or bubbles that can interfere with accurate measurement.

3. **Follow steps 2 through 10 as above.**

4. **Establish a routine order for drawing up insulin. The shorter-acting regular insulin is drawn up first, followed by the cloudy intermediate-acting insulin. Glargine (Lantus), detemir (Levemir), and glulisine (Apidra) insulins cannot be mixed with other types of insulin.**

Rationale: Use of a standard sequence while mixing insulins prevents errors (CDC, 2011).

Home Care Considerations

- If patients are having difficulty drawing up medications from two vials, assist with drawing up a week's supply.
- Teach caregivers how to draw up insulin and prefill syringes for the patient. Patients using insulin pens can program the syringe by clicking on the desired number of units to be delivered.
- Suggest the use of adaptive aids such as syringe holders, magnifiers, or insulin pens.
- Mark the vials of medication as Vial A or #1 and Vial B or #2 to help the patient remember which vial to draw up first.

Procedure 20-6 **Administering Intradermal Injections**

Purpose
- Administer medication into the dermal tissue to screen for an allergic (antigen–antibody) dermal reaction, to screen for tuberculosis, or to administer local anesthesia

Equipment
MAR or eMAR
Antiseptic swab
Vial of medication
Sterile syringe and needle (1-mL syringe with 26- to 28-gauge 0.5-inch needle)
Gloves

Assessment
- Review medication order for type of medication, dosage, and route.
- Assess the patient for anxiety related to fear of injections.
- Inspect site for lesions, rash, or ecchymosis.
- Review patient history for possible allergies.

Procedure

1. **Check medication order. See Procedure 20-1, steps 1 through 6.**
2. **Assemble needle and syringe.**
3. **Remove needle guard and withdraw medication from vial (see Procedure 20-3).**
4. **Identify the patient by two identifiers (name, MRN, Social Security number, or birth date), checking identification bracelet. Scan bracelet if using BCMA. Repeat check of six rights.**

   Rationale: Repeated checking prevents errors before medication is administered to the patient.

5. **Close door or bed curtains and explain the procedure to the patient, and then educate the patient about medication.**

   Rationale: Ensures patient privacy, increases patient compliance, reduces patient anxiety, and promotes learning.

6. **Don gloves. Select injection site that is relatively hairless and free from tenderness, swelling, scarring, and inflammation (Fig. 1).**

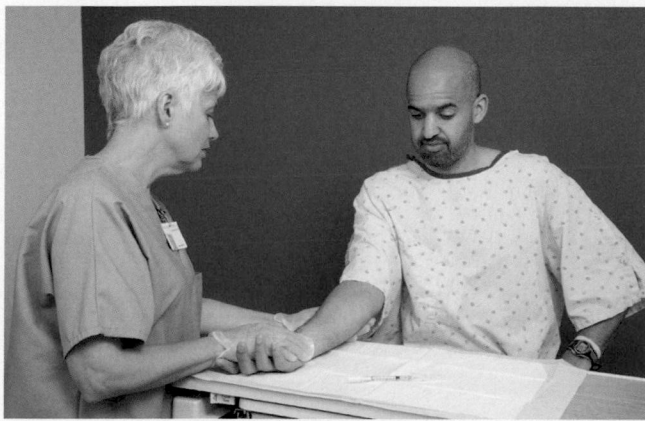

FIG. 1 Select injection site.

Rationale: Injection into skin areas with abnormal characteristics could impair drug absorption or interfere with subsequent interpretation of skin reaction.

7. **Cleanse the site with an antimicrobial swab and then allow the skin to dry (Fig. 2).**

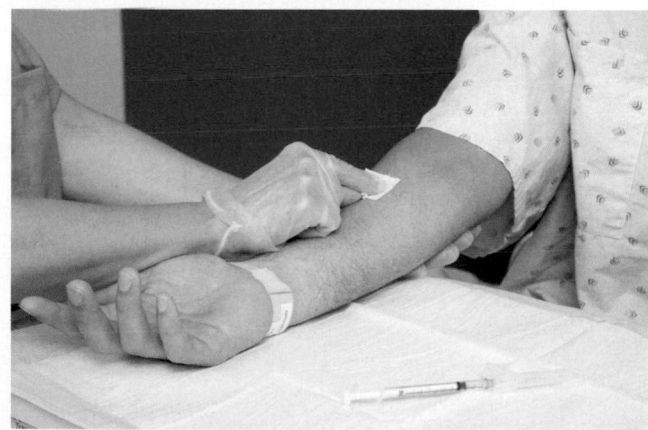

FIG. 2 Cleanse the site with an antimicrobial swab.

Rationale: Pathogens on the skin can be forced into the tissues by the needle. Allowing the skin to dry prevents introducing alcohol into the tissues, which can be irritating and uncomfortable.

8. **Remove needle guard. Hold syringe in dominant hand. Gently pull skin distal to intended injection site taut with nondominant hand.**

   Rationale: Pulling skin taut helps to stabilize the injection site and ensures administration into dermal tissue.

9. **Holding syringe from above, at a 10- to 15-degree angle (almost parallel to skin), gently insert needle, bevel up, about 1/8 inch until dermis barely covers bevel (Fig. 3).**

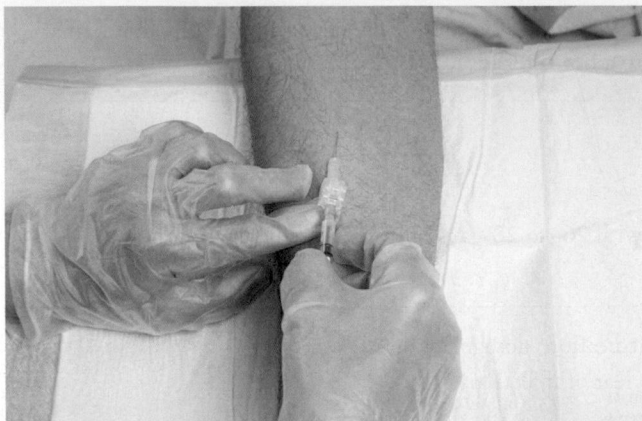

FIG. 3 Gently insert the needle, with the bevel up, until the dermis barely covers the bevel.

Rationale: Accurate delivery of medication into dermal tissue is very important. An angle more than 15 degrees will deliver medication into subcutaneous tissue. Visualization of wheal will occur with the needle bevel up and barely covered by dermis. Patients report that bevel up is more comfortable (Tarnow & King, 2004).

10. **Stabilize needle; inject medication slowly over 3 to 5 seconds while watching for a small wheal or blister to appear (Fig. 4).**

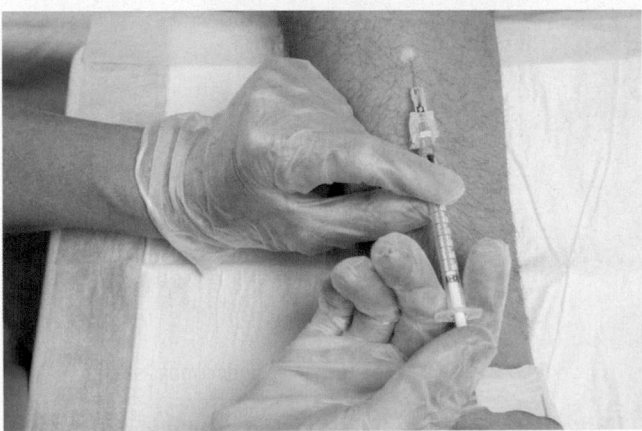

FIG. 4 Inject medication slowly; wheal will gradually form at site.

Rationale: Slow medication injection prevents discomfort from injection and ensures that medication is being delivered correctly as wheal gradually forms at injection site.

11. **Withdraw needle at the same angle at which it was inserted. Do not wipe or massage site.**

Rationale: Wiping or massaging may remove or promote absorption into subcutaneous tissue.

12. **Do not recap needle. Dispose of syringe and needle in sharps container.**

Rationale: Proper disposal protects the nurse and other healthcare workers from accidental needle injury.

13. **Record time and site of injection according to best protocol.**

Rationale: Maintains legal record and communicates to the healthcare team.

14. **Instruct the patient when to return for reading of response—15 to 60 minutes after injection for allergy testing and usually 48 to 72 hours after injection for PPD.**

Rationale: Appropriate timing of site assessment is necessary to accurately interpret antibody response.

Documentation

7/15/17: 13:00—Administered tuberculin PPD 5 US units subcutaneous on underside of right forearm. Good wheal present. Will check results in 48 to 72 hours.

—B. Tsang, RN

Procedure 20-7 Administering Subcutaneous Injections

Purpose
1. Ensure more rapid absorption and action of a drug than can be achieved orally
2. Administer drugs to patients who are unable to take oral medications (e.g., unconscious, nausea/vomiting, NPO status)
3. Administer medications that are not active by the oral route or are inactivated by digestive enzymes (e.g., heparin, insulin)

Equipment
MAR or eMAR
Antiseptic swabs
Vial or ampule of ordered medication
Sterile gauze squares for opening an ampule and for applying pressure to the injection site
Sterile syringe and needle (0.5-, 1-, or 2-mL syringe with 25- to 29-gauge, ½- to ⅝-inch needle)
Gloves

Assessment
- Review patient's medical history, medication history, and allergy status.
- Assess for any contraindications to receiving subcutaneous injections, such as circulatory shock or localized body areas of reduced tissue perfusion that would interfere with drug absorption.
- Assess for anxiety related to fear of injections.
- Review chart for documentation of previous injection sites. Note rotation schedule when administering insulin or heparin.
- Inspect administration site for lesions, rash, ecchymosis, lipid dystrophy, and other abnormalities.
- Refer to drug literature to determine appropriateness of medication and dosage, common side effects, and nursing implications.

Procedure

1. **Check medication order. Assess allergies. See Procedure 20-1, steps 1 through 6.**
2. **Assemble needle and syringe.**
3. **Remove needle guard and withdraw medication from container (see Procedures 20-3 and 20-4).**
4. **Identify the patient by two identifiers. Scan bracelet if using BCMA. Recheck six rights.**
   Rationale: Checking allergies and the six rights before medication is administered to the patient prevents errors.
5. **Close door or bed curtains and explain the procedure to the patient, and then educate the patient about medication.**
   Rationale: Ensures patient privacy, increases patient compliance, reduces patient anxiety, and promotes learning.
6. **Don gloves.**
   Rationale: Gloving maintains Standard Precautions in case blood leaks from the injection site.
7. **Select an injection site that is free from tenderness, swelling, scarring, and inflammation.**
   Rationale: Injection into skin areas with abnormal characteristics could impair drug absorption or increase the chance of abscess or infection.

8. **Cleanse site with antiseptic swab, using a circular motion from center toward outside (Fig. 1). Allow area to dry thoroughly.**

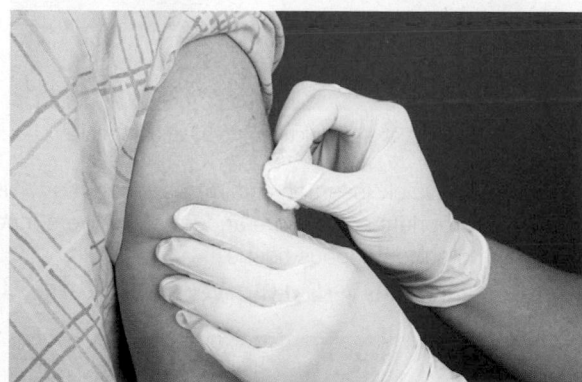

FIG. 1 Cleanse site with a circular motion.

Rationale: Cleanse the site from the cleanest toward more contaminated areas, pulling any contamination away from the intended injection site.

9. **Remove needle guard. Hold syringe in dominant hand. Place nondominant hand on either side of injection site. Spread or bunch skin to stabilize site and identify subcutaneous tissue (Fig. 2).**

Procedure 20-7   *continued*

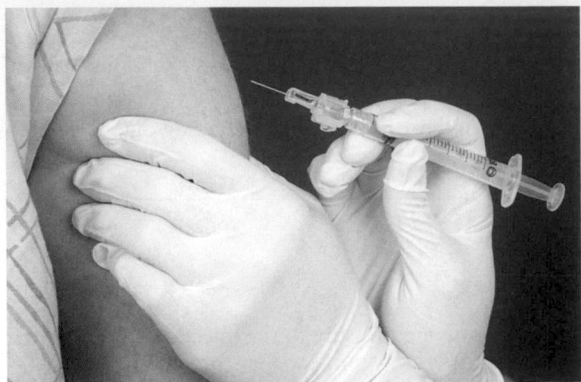

FIG. 2 Bunch skin to stabilize site.

Rationale: The amount of subcutaneous tissue varies among sites and individuals. Nursing judgment is necessary to decide if spreading or bunching the skin will more accurately deliver the medication into subcutaneous tissue.

10. **Hold syringe between thumb and forefinger of dominant hand (like a dart). Inject needle quickly at a 45- to 90-degree angle depending on the amount of subcutaneous tissue (Fig. 3). Release bunched skin.**

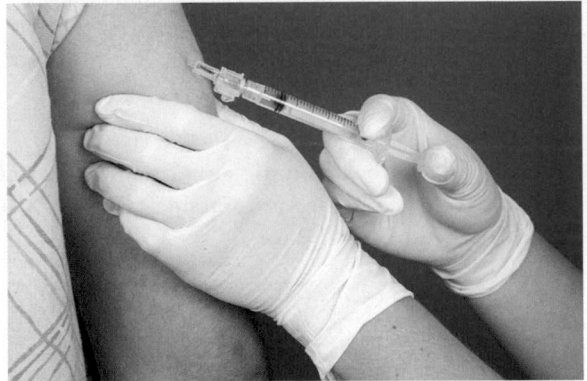

FIG. 3 Inject at a 45- (pictured) to 90-degree angle.

Rationale: Quick insertion minimizes discomfort. Use of the appropriate angle more accurately delivers medication into subcutaneous tissue.

11. **Inject medication with slow, even pressure (Fig. 4).**

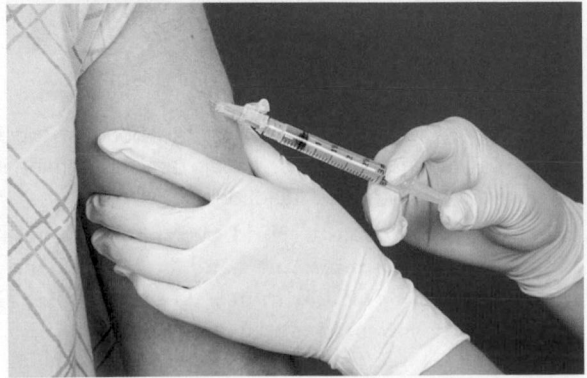

FIG. 4 Inject medication slowly.

Rationale: Slow, even pressure promotes patient comfort and prevents tissue damage.

12. **Remove needle quickly at the same angle at which it was inserted while supporting the surrounding tissue with your nondominant hand. Apply gentle pressure to the site with a gauze square after the needle is withdrawn. Do not massage the site.**

Rationale: Patient discomfort is minimized by supporting the tissues while withdrawing the needle.

13. **Assist the patient to a position of comfort.**

14. **Do not recap needle. Activate the needle guard. Dispose of syringe and needle in sharps container.**

Rationale: Protects healthcare workers from accidental needle injury.

15. **Perform hand hygiene.**

Rationale: Reduces microbe transmission.

16. **Document according to best protocol.**

Rationale: Documentation maintains accurate patient records and prevents medication errors.

Modifications for Insulin Administration

- Routine aspiration is not necessary (ADA, 2011).
- Systematically rotate injection sites to prevent lipodystrophy and variable insulin absorption.
- Explain to the patient that absorption differs depending on the site. The abdomen allows the fastest absorption, followed by arms, thighs, and buttocks (ADA, 2011). Exercise of a muscle group increases absorption.
- Instruct patients who self-administer insulin to always check the bottle label and draw up insulin in the same order each time.
- Insulin pens are increasingly used by diabetic patients for insulin administration. To use an insulin pen:
  1. Load cartridge with prescribed insulin.
  2. Screw on pen needle.
  3. Dial in desired dose (Fig. 5).

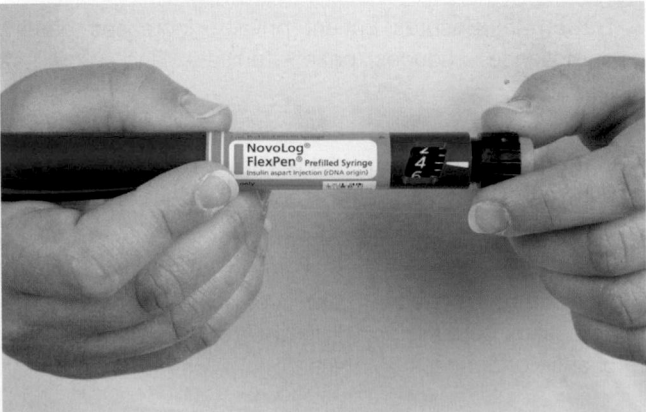

FIG. 5 Dial in desired dose.

Procedure 20-7 *continued*

4. Inject needle into appropriate site and press button to deliver insulin (Fig. 6).

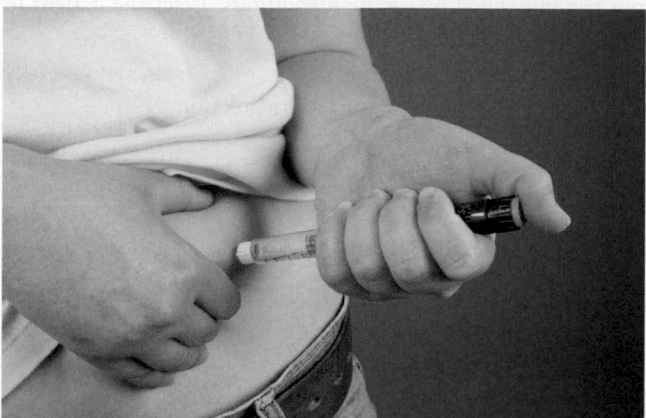

FIG. 6 Inject needle into appropriate site and press button to deliver insulin.

5. Remove and properly dispose of needle.

- For premixed insulins, prior to dosing, shake pen to mix insulins well.

Modifications for Heparin Administration

- The abdomen (avoiding the area 1 to 2 inches on either side of the umbilicus) is the most frequently used site because the lack of major muscle groups or muscle activity in the abdomen is thought to reduce the chance of hematoma formation.
- Roll or gently bunch the tissue between thumb and forefinger to ensure that heparin is administered into subcutaneous tissue. Do not tightly pinch the skin.
- Because heparin is an anticoagulant, do not aspirate for a blood return or massage the site after injection.
- After injection, slowly and smoothly withdraw the needle to prevent leakage into subcutaneous tissue.

Documentation

7/15/17: 21:30—Administered enoxaparin 75 mg subcutaneously in right abdomen. Stated slight discomfort but no bruising noted.

—C. Garcia, RN

Life Span Considerations

Infant and Child

- Securely restrain infants and children up to about 5 years of age for injections. Quick movement by the child once the needle is injected could cause trauma and loss of medication.
- Enlist the help of an assistant to restrain the child. To convey that you are asking for cooperation, tell the child, "I will help you to hold still."
- Do not perform painful procedures in the child's bed, which is a "safe zone." Remember that parents also are regarded as "safe protectors" and should not help restrain the child during a painful procedure. Let the parent comfort the child after the injection.
- Offer praise, bandages, and "good job" stickers as rewards for children for a job well done.
- Do not tell a child that the injection will not hurt. Instead, honestly describe the sensations to be expected to increase future cooperation.

Obese Adult

- Obese patients have a layer of fatty tissue above the subcutaneous layer, so select an appropriate needle length to deliver medication to the subcutaneous skin layer.
- Bunch the skin at the site and inject the needle below the tissue fold to deliver medication to the subcutaneous layer.

Home Care Modifications

- If a visually impaired patient must self-administer injections, teach family members how to preload several syringes to help increase the patient's independence.
- Assist a patient who requires multiple or daily injections to develop a pattern of site rotation to minimize trauma and scarring of body tissues. Provide the patient with a sheet to record each site.
- Review proper insulin storage. Insulin vials not being used should be refrigerated, but insulin used for injection should be at room temperature.

● The patient may be taught not to cleanse the skin with alcohol when giving self-injections to simplify the procedure. However, always stress the need for proper handwashing.

● Some patients reuse syringes to decrease cost, but this is not recommended by the manufacturers. Refer the patient to programs that might help decrease the cost of equipment.

● Stress proper disposal of syringes in a plastic container that will prevent needlestick injuries. In most areas, syringes may not be discarded in normal waste, so check with area waste management companies for local regulations.

Procedure 20-8 Administering Intramuscular Injections

Purpose

1. Administer medication deeply into muscle tissue, without injury to the patient
2. Administer a medication that requires absorption and onset of action quicker than the oral route without irritating the subcutaneous tissues

Equipment

MAR or eMAR
Antiseptic swabs
Vial, ampule, or prefilled cartridge syringe of medication
Syringe or tubex: 2 to 3 mL for adult
Sterile syringe and needle (21 to 23 gauge for adult, 1.5- to 3-inch needle for adult)
Gloves

Assessment

- Review patient's medical history, medication history, and allergy status.
- Assess for contraindications to receiving IM injections, such as circulatory shock, reduced blood flow, or muscle atrophy.
- Assess injection site; avoid injecting into sites that may be bruised, tender, hard, swollen, inflamed, or scarred.
- Assess for anxiety related to fear of injection.
- Review chart for documentation of previous injection sites if the patient is receiving multiple injections.
- Refer to drug literature to determine appropriateness of medication and dosage, common side effects, and nursing implications.
- Assess adipose tissue and muscle mass of the patient to determine correct needle size.

Procedure

1. **Check medication order. See Procedure 20-1, steps 1 through 6. Assemble needle and syringe.**

2. **Prepare needle, syringe, and medication by following the appropriate steps in Procedure 20-3 or 20-4. If medication is known to be irritating to subcutaneous tissues, replace needle after withdrawing medication.**

   Rationale: Prevents medication that adheres to outside of needle from irritating and burning subcutaneous tissues as the needle passes into muscle.

3. **Assess for allergies. Perform the second medication check of six rights. Compare name on MAR with name on patient's identification band using two separate identifiers (e.g., name, MRN, Social Security number, or birth date). Do not administer medications if the patient is not wearing an identification band. Scan patient's identification bracelet if using BCMA.**

   Rationale: The second check occurs before administration of the medication to the patient. Checking the six rights minimizes the risk of medication errors.

4. **Close door or bed curtains and explain the procedure to the patient, and then educate the patient about medication.**

   Rationale: Ensures patient privacy, increases patient compliance, reduces patient anxiety, and promotes learning.

5. **Don gloves. Assist the patient to a comfortable position, and expose only the area to be injected.**

   Rationale: Maintains Standard Precautions should blood leak from the injection site. Exposing as little area as possible promotes comfort and privacy.

6. **Select appropriate injection site by inspecting muscle size and integrity. Consider volume of medication to be injected.**

   Rationale: Larger muscles can absorb larger volumes of medication.

7. **Use anatomic landmarks to locate the exact injection site (Fig. 1; also see Figs. 20-18 through 20-22).**

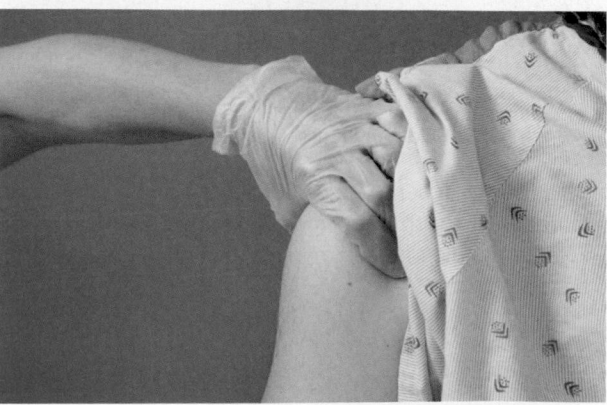

FIG. 1 Locate the exact injection site.

Rationale: Injection into the proper site prevents trauma to bones, nerves, or blood vessels.

8. **Cleanse the site with antiseptic swab, wiping from center of site and rotating outward (Fig. 2).**

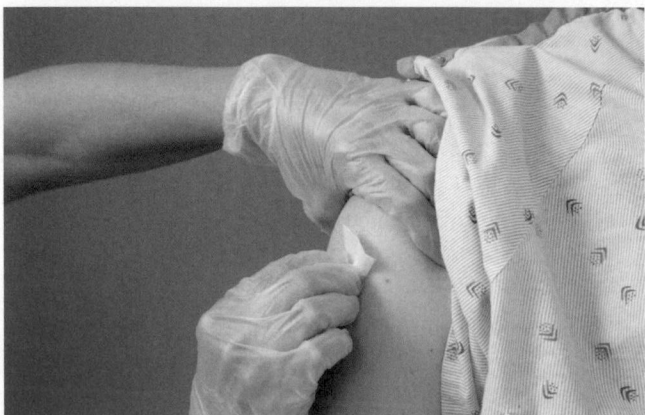

FIG. 2 Cleanse the site with an antimicrobial swab.

Rationale: Cleanse the site from the cleanest to most contaminated areas, pulling any contamination away from the intended injection site.

9. **Remove needle guard. Hold syringe between thumb and forefinger of dominant hand, like a dart. Spread skin at the site with nondominant hand. Encourage the patient to relax the muscle or use distraction techniques.**

10. **Insert needle quickly at a 90-degree angle to the patient's skin surface (Fig. 3).**

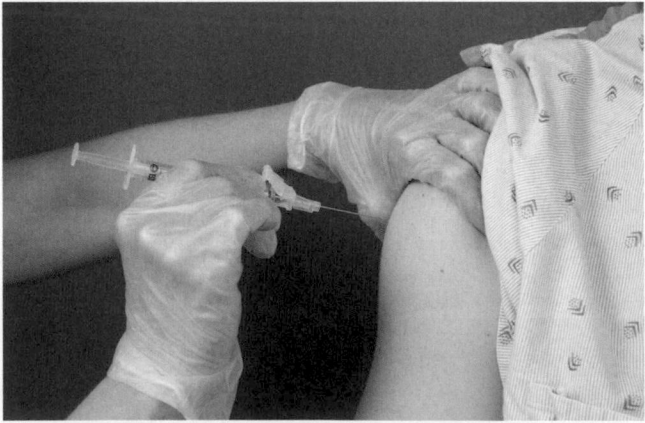

FIG. 3 Quickly insert needle at a 90-degree angle.

Rationale: Insertion at a 90-degree angle enables the needle to reach deep muscle layers (see Fig. 20-16). Rapid needle insertion minimizes patient discomfort.

11. **Stabilize syringe barrel by grasping with nondominant hand (Fig. 4). Slowly inject medication (Fig. 5).**

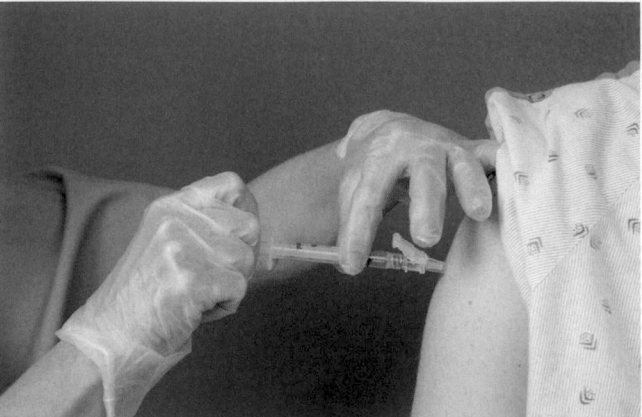

FIG. 4 Optional: Aspirate slowly for blood return.

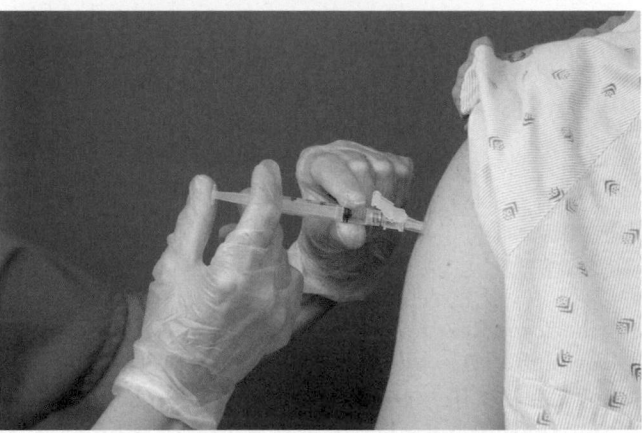

FIG. 5 Slowly inject medication.

12. **Withdraw needle while pressing antiseptic swab above site.**

Rationale: Minimizes discomfort by supporting tissues during needle withdrawal.

13. **Apply gentle pressure at the site with swab or dry gauze.**

Rationale: Stops possible bleeding and decreases discomfort.

14. **Do not recap needle. Activate needle guard. Dispose of equipment in sharps container.**

Rationale: Proper disposal protects nurse and other healthcare workers from accidental needle injury.

Procedure 20-8 *continued*

15. **Perform hand hygiene.**
    Rationale: Maintains asepsis and minimizes the risk for infection transmission.
16. **Document medication administration and patient response according to best protocol.**
    Rationale: Proper documentation provides information about the patient's status, maintains accurate patient records, and reduces the risk for medication errors.

Variations for Z-Track Injection

Manufacturers' guidelines for certain medications advise "for deep IM use only" or "given deeply into the body of a relatively large muscle." Z-track method is then the recommended technique.

1. **When preparing the injection site, pull the skin and subcutaneous tissues about 1 to 1.5 inches to one side of the selected site.**
   Rationale: Creates a zigzag track through the tissues, which prevents back-leaking of medication when needle is withdrawn.
2. **Insert the syringe at a 90-degree angle. Do not release your nondominant hand that is stretching the skin to stabilize the syringe.**

Rationale: Releasing tension of the skin to stabilize the syringe will reverse the zigzag track that is needed to administer medications using the Z-track technique.

3. **Administer medication while continuing traction on skin.**
   Rationale: If traction on the skin is released, the medication can exit the muscle and irritate tissue.
4. **Leave needle inserted an additional 10 seconds.**
   Rationale: Allows medication to disperse and muscle to begin absorption.
5. **Simultaneously remove needle along the line of insertion and release traction on skin.**
   Rationale: Zigzag pathway seals medication into the muscle tissue.

Documentation

7/15/17: 09:30—Administered pneumococcal vaccine PPV 23 0.5 mL intramuscular in right deltoid. No swelling or bruising at injection site.

—L. Brown, RN

Life Span Consideration

Infant and Child
- See Procedure 20-7.
- Use a 1- to 2-mL syringe and 0.5- to 1-inch, 25- to 27-gauge needle for a child.
- Vastus lateralis is the preferred site for infants, and the deltoid can be added for toddlers and children with adequate muscle mass.
- EMLA (a mixture of lidocaine and prilocaine) can be applied topically over the injection site 60 minutes before the injection to decrease pain (Hockenberry & Wilson, 2011).

Home Care Considerations

- Teaching injection technique to caregivers requires time to decrease anxiety and master psychomotor skills.
- Use a hard plastic jug (e.g., liquid detergent or fabric softener container) for safe collection of used needles and syringes. Check with local waste management companies about how to dispose of contaminated and sharps waste because they cannot be disposed of in normal garbage.

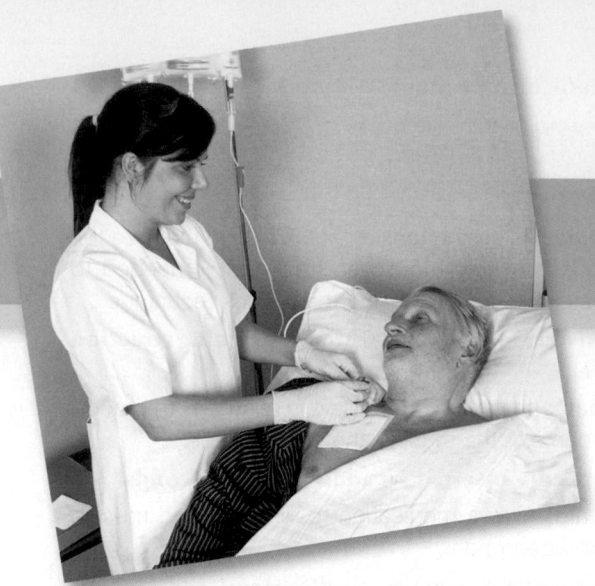

CHAPTER 21

Intravenous Therapy

Terry F. Cicero

Case Scenario

Sue is assigned to care for a 59-year-old man who is having nothing by mouth (NPO) and receiving intravenous (IV) therapy following a bowel resection. He is receiving D5½NS with 20 mEq KCl at 110 mL per hour, administered through an electronic infusion device (EID). The device begins alarming, and Sue assesses and troubleshoots the problem.

Once you have completed this chapter and have incorporated IV therapy into your knowledge base, review the above scenario and reflect on the following areas of Critical Thinking:

1. Describe further assessment data that you will collect.
2. List the factors to check in the infusion system, giving rationales.
3. Identify additional data you would want to know about this patient's IV therapy.
4. Prioritize possible problems that may exist in this situation.
5. Plan how you will correct the problem.

LEARNING OBJECTIVES

Upon completion of this chapter, you will be able to do the following:

1. Explain the purpose of intravenous infusion therapy.
2. Identify the two major types of solutions administered intravenously.
3. List equipment necessary to administer peripheral and central intravenous therapy.
4. State guidelines for site selection in peripherally inserted venipuncture.
5. Outline the nurse's role in initiating, monitoring, maintaining, and discontinuing intravenous therapy.
6. Describe differences in the nursing care and maintenance of central venous catheters and peripheral catheters.
7. Discuss the purpose of total parenteral nutrition (TPN) and monitoring considerations.
8. Discuss indications for blood component therapy and safe transfusion practices.
9. Describe potential complications of intravenous therapy, TPN, and blood transfusions.
10. Identify principles of patient and family education associated with intravenous therapy.

Patients in various healthcare settings receive IV therapies. **Intravenous (IV) therapy** is the infusion of a fluid into a vein to prevent or to treat fluid or electrolyte imbalance or to deliver medications, nutrition, or blood products. The therapeutic goal of IV therapy may be maintenance, replacement, treatment, diagnosis, monitoring, palliation, or a combination. IV therapy may be prescribed for many reasons, including provision of the following:

- Maintenance or replacement fluids for daily fluid requirements
- Electrolytes to maintain normal electrolyte balance
- Glucose and nutrients for patient use as an energy source
- An access route to administer medications intravenously
- Venous access to administer blood products
- Venous access for emergencies

IV therapy may be administered in outpatient settings, in acute and long-term care facilities, and in a patient's home.

PRINCIPLES OF INTRAVENOUS THERAPY

Principles of IV therapy include the types of IV solutions used, the equipment used for vein access and infusion, catheter site selection, determination of flow rates, and prevention of complications.

Types of Intravenous Solutions

IV solutions are classified as **crystalloid** (fluids that are clear) or **colloid** (fluids that contain proteins or starch molecules).

Crystalloids can be further classified as isotonic, hypotonic, or hypertonic, according to how closely the solution's osmolarity matches that of plasma, which is between 275 and 295 mOsm per liter. **Osmolarity** refers to the number of particles or solutes that are in a liter of solution. Therefore, osmolarity is measured in milliosmoles per liter (or mOsm/L). Specific patient fluid and electrolyte needs determine which solution is prescribed.

CRYSTALLOID SOLUTIONS

Because of the permeability of cellular membranes, water will move across membranes based on the osmolarity within the body's three fluid compartments. Figure 21-1 presents the relationship of osmotic pressure to isotonic, hypotonic, and hypertonic solutions. Table 21-1 presents nursing considerations relative to the osmolarity of IV solutions.

Isotonic Fluids

Isotonic fluids have an osmolarity of 250 to 375 mOsm per liter, which is the same osmotic pressure as that found within the cell. Isotonic fluids are used to expand the intravascular compartment and thus increase circulating volume. Because these solutions do not alter serum osmolarity, interstitial and intracellular compartments remain unchanged (Smeltzer, Bare, Hinkle, & Cheever, 2010). An isotonic solution is helpful for hypotension caused by hypovolemia in dehydration. Examples of an isotonic solution include normal saline (0.9% NaCl) and lactated Ringer's.

Hypotonic Fluids

Hypotonic fluids have an osmolarity below 250 mOsm per liter or a lower osmotic pressure than does the cell. When a hypotonic solution is infused, it lowers serum osmolarity,

ISOTONIC

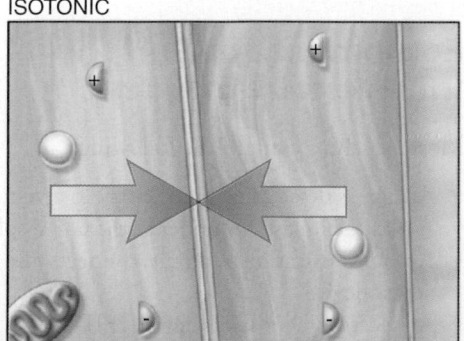

HYPERTONIC

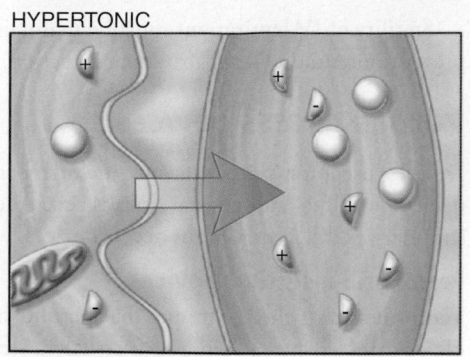

HYPOTONIC

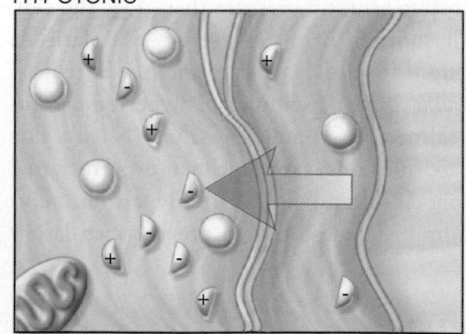

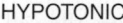 Vascular space

☐ Interstitial space

FIGURE 21-1 Isotonic, hypotonic, and hypertonic solutions. In isotonic fluids, cells maintain normal size because of fluid balance. In hypotonic solutions, the body fluids shift out of the blood vessels and into cells and the interstitial space. In hypertonic solutions, the fluid is pulled from the cells and the interstitial tissues into the vascular space.

TABLE 21-1 NURSING CONSIDERATIONS IN ADMINISTERING INTRAVENOUS SOLUTIONS

Solution Type and Examples	Indications	Nursing Considerations
Isotonic Normal saline Lactated Ringer's	**Isotonic solutions cause no fluid shifts.** Vascular expansion, electrolyte replacement	Monitor closely for signs of fluid overload, especially if the patient has a history of renal or cardiovascular disease. Avoid use of lactated Ringer's in patients with liver disease or those in metabolic acidosis.
Hypotonic 0.45% NaCl	**Hypotonic solutions move fluid into cells and interstitial space.** Cellular dehydration	Monitor regularly because these solutions can cause a sudden shift of fluid into the cells. This can lead to intravascular fluid depletion and cardiovascular collapse. Don't give to patients at risk for increased intracranial pressure (ICP)—(head trauma, neurosurgery, cerebrovascular accident). Increased ICP can result from shift of fluid into brain cells. Don't give to patients at risk for abnormal fluid shifts into the interstitial compartment (third spacing),burn victims, trauma, liver failure, and severe protein malnutrition.
Hypertonic 3% NaCl	**Hypertonic solutions draw fluid from the intracellular to the intravascular.** Intravascular dehydration with interstitial and intracellular fluid overload and sepsis	Closely monitor the patient for fluid overload because these solutions expand the intravascular compartment. Avoid use in patients with renal or cardiac impairment. Avoid use in patients with intracellular dehydration such as diabetic ketoacidosis. Rarely used clinically outside the intensive care unit.

causing body fluids to shift out of the blood vessels and into the cells and interstitial space. For this reason, hypotonic fluids are administered when a patient needs cellular hydration. One-half normal saline (0.45 NaCl) is an example of a hypotonic solution. A solution, such as D5½NaCl, though an isotonic solution before administration, quickly becomes a hypotonic solution once in the body because this small amount of dextrose is quickly metabolized.

Hypertonic Fluids

Hypertonic fluids have an osmolarity of 375 mOsm per liter or higher and a greater osmotic pressure than does the cell. When a hypertonic solution is infused, serum osmolarity is increased, pulling fluid from the cells and the interstitial tissues into the vascular space. Examples of hypertonic solutions include 3% saline (NaCl) and 5% saline (NaCl). The primary use for these solutions is management of intracranial hypertension and shock (Strandvik, 2009). Hypertonic solutions should be administered slowly to prevent circulatory overload.

COLLOID SOLUTIONS

Infusion of a colloid solution increases intravascular osmotic pressure (pressure of plasma protein) within the intravascular space, and the pressure gradient pulls fluids into the vascular space.

Blood Products

Whole blood or specific components of blood may be infused directly into a person's circulatory system. Commonly infused blood components include packed red blood cells (RBCs, for anemia), white blood cells (WBCs, to prevent infection), platelets (to help clotting), plasma, albumin (as a volume expander), and cryoprecipitate (a clotting factor). Nursing responsibilities associated with transfusion therapy are discussed in greater detail later in this chapter.

Parenteral Nutrition

Parenteral nutrition refers to nutritional elements supplied through an IV route, usually a central vein. **Total parenteral nutrition (TPN)** is a hypertonic solution containing 20% to 50% dextrose, proteins, vitamins, and minerals that is administered into the venous system. TPN is indicated when there is interference with nutrient absorption from the gastrointestinal tract or when complete bowel rest is necessary for healing. Parenteral nutrition is discussed later in this chapter.

Equipment for Peripheral Intravenous Infusion

Most IV setups contain the following:

- An access device that gains entry to a vein
- A plastic or glass container with the IV solution
- An administration set that connects the IV bag with the access device
- An electronic infusion device (EID)
- Various needleless connectors

Sterility of IV equipment must be maintained during use to prevent potentially life-threatening infection.

VENOUS ACCESS DEVICES

Devices used for venous access include peripheral insertion devices, midline, and central venous access devices. Table 21-2 summarizes different venous access devices.

Peripheral Insertion Devices

Venipuncture is the technique that permits insertion of a needle or catheter into a vein and is strictly a sterile procedure. In some facilities, nurses are responsible for starting IV therapy.

TABLE 21-2 TYPES OF COMMON INTRAVENOUS CATHETERS

Catheter Type	Advantages	Disadvantages
Peripheral catheters	Choice of many sites Easy to insert and remove Lower infection rates	Short-term use Infiltration and phlebitis more common Inability to infuse hyperosmolar solutions Inability to use for blood draws
Midline catheters	Easy to insert and remove Intermediate use Lower infection rates May be used to infuse TPN and for blood draws	Thrombosis, phlebitis, air embolism more common than with peripheral lines
PICC	Easy to insert and remove Long-term and home care use May be used for blood draws May infuse all solutions	Higher thrombosis rates than tunneled or implanted catheters Small diameter limits flow rates. Catheter longevity less than tunneled or implanted catheters Greater incidence of malposition
Nontunneled CVC	Choice of sites Easy to insert and remove Multiple lumens available	Short term—in-hospital use Higher risk of complications
Tunneled CVC	Lower infection rate than nontunneled CVC Long-term use Multiple lumens available	More complex insertion and removal
Implanted port	Long-term use No external catheter: • Cosmetically attractive • Low maintenance • May swim, shower, bathe Lower infection rate than tunneled catheters	Surgical insertion and removal More difficult for frequent, repeated access

CVC, central venous catheter.

Competency should be validated by the facility at time of employment and on an ongoing periodic basis (INS, 2011). In other agencies, a team of specialized infusion nurses are responsible for all IV starts; in some instances, this team also oversees general IV maintenance. The use of specialized, dedicated IV therapy teams to provide staff education, to review and revise IV policies, and to assist with obtaining vascular access has been demonstrated to decrease complications and improve patient outcomes, specifically in relation to a reduction in hospital-acquired bloodstream infections (O'Grady et al., 2011). The most common method of accessing the venous system is through insertion of a needle or flexible catheter into a peripheral vein (vein in the extremities). The peripheral veins usually provide the quickest and easiest approach to establishing IV access for administration of solutions and medications.

Over-the-needle IV catheters are the access devices most commonly used for peripheral IV therapy (Fig. 21-2). These are plastic catheters that are placed over metal stylets or introducer needles. The metal stylet is used to pierce the skin and enter the vein, and then the plastic catheter is threaded into the vein and the metal stylet is removed. Many of these devices have springback, rigid housing to protect against inadvertent sharp exposure following insertion. Winged infusion or small vein needles may be used for short-term or one-time infusion therapies or may be used with infants and small children. These are short, beveled needles with plastic flaps or wings.

IV catheters are available in various sizes. The lumen size is measured in gauges; odd numbers designate winged infusion needles (19, 21, 23), whereas even numbers designate catheter sizes. The most common adult catheter sizes are 22, 20, and 18. As the numbers increase, the lumen size decreases; thus, a 22-gauge needle is smaller in diameter than is an 18-gauge needle. Various catheter lengths are also available. Usually, the shortest length possible is used. Most catheters are 1 or 1¼ inches long. The small, winged needles are approximately ¾ inch long and range in diameter from 19 to 27-gauge bore.

Midline Infusion Device

A midline catheter is a catheter that is 4 to 6 inches in length and inserted near the antecubital fossa and terminates in the vasculature, just before the axilla (Fig. 21-3). These catheters are suitable for patients who need moderate-term parenteral therapy (1 to 4 weeks) or who have limited peripheral access (Hadaway et al., 2010; Perucca, 2010). They are more durable than are standard peripheral catheters but may not be suitable for TPN, hyperosmolar infusions, or vesicant therapy (INH Standards, 2011).

Central Venous Access Devices

Central venous therapy involves placement of a flexible catheter into one of the patient's large veins, with the tip of the catheter placed in either the superior vena cava or the right atrium. Central venous therapy may be required when infusing hypertonic solutions or when the patient's peripheral venous access is inadequate for the duration or type of IV therapy required. When patients require long-term or home IV therapy, specially trained nurses may insert peripherally inserted central venous catheters (PICCs) or the patient may have a

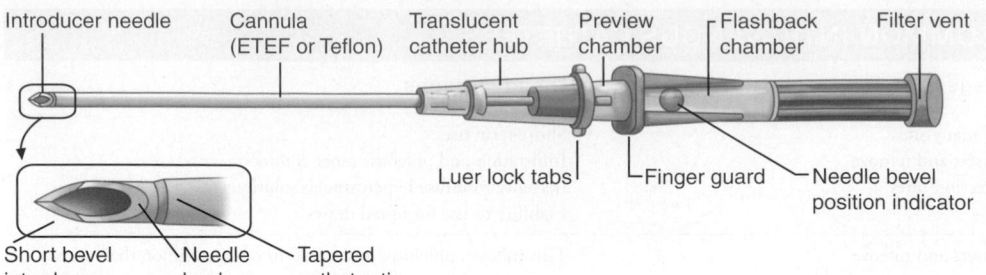

Introducer needle — Cannula (ETEF or Teflon) — Translucent catheter hub — Preview chamber — Flashback chamber — Filter vent

Luer lock tabs — Finger guard — Needle bevel position indicator

Short bevel introducer — Needle heel — Tapered catheter tip

FIGURE 21-2 Parts of the over-the-needle catheter.

tunneled or implanted catheter placed by a physician. Access to central veins is often necessary for infusion of irritating medications and TPN, when peripheral vein access is not available, or when long-term venous therapy is anticipated. When central access is necessary, a wide assortment of products may be used to facilitate cannulation of the central vein. There are four main categories of central venous catheters:

- *Single- or multilumen catheters*: These catheters are placed into the superior vena cava or the right atrium. They can have one, two, or three lumens that permit simultaneous infusion of fluids, medications, and blood products. They are used in the hospital for short-term therapy.
- *PICC*: A long-line catheter inserted in the antecubital area and advanced into a central vessel. An advantage of a PICC is that surgical insertion is not required and it is appropriate for long-term therapy in the hospital or home.
- *Tunneled catheters*: A tunneled catheter is used when long-term therapy is required. The catheter contains a Dacron

cuff that causes adhesions to form in the chest, stabilizing the catheter and decreasing the incidence of infection.

- *Implanted access port*: A surgically implanted central access port is placed within the chest and into a central vein that can be accessed when needed. An implanted access device is often used for oncology patients so that they can be free from external tubing between treatments.

Physicians usually insert central venous catheters, but nurses with advanced training may insert some types. Central venous access devices are associated with a risk of complications such as pneumothorax and air embolism because the tip lies in the superior vena cava or right atrium. The risk of central **catheter-related bloodstream infection (CRBSI)** is prominent in the healthcare literature. There are four recognized routes for catheter contamination. The most common route of infection is colonization of the catheter tip due to migration of skin organisms from insertion site. Direct contamination of the catheter or catheter hub is also a contributing factor (O'Grady et al., 2011). Less common, the catheters may be contaminated by organisms that migrate from infections in other areas of the patient, and rarely, the infusion itself may be contaminated. Additionally, the material the catheter is made from may contribute to CRBSI. Silastic catheters are associated with higher risk of catheter infections due to surface irregularities that allow development of a biofilm formation along the catheter's inner lumen (O'Grady et al., 2011). The use of catheters coated or impregnated with chlorhexidine and silver sulfadiazine, minocycline and rifampin, and silver ion have been associated with a reduced risk of catheter-related infections (INS, 2011; Mermel et al., 2009). National estimates of CRBSI are available on the Center for Disease Control (CDC) website: http://www.cdc.gov/nhsn/dataStat.html. In response to the growing concern of central CRBSI, the Institute for Healthcare Improvement (IHI) has identified the Central Catheter Care Bundle, incorporating evidence-based science into recommendations for best practice to reduce rates of infections (The Joint Commission, 2014). See the "Evidence-Based Bundles to Improve Patient Care" box regarding the prevention of catheter-related bloodstream infections.

Multilumen Central Catheters. The most commonly used **central venous catheters** are the basic single-lumen catheter and the multilumen catheter, which has either two or three lumens and is made of nonthrombogenic material such as Teflon or polyurethane, making it more resistant to adherence

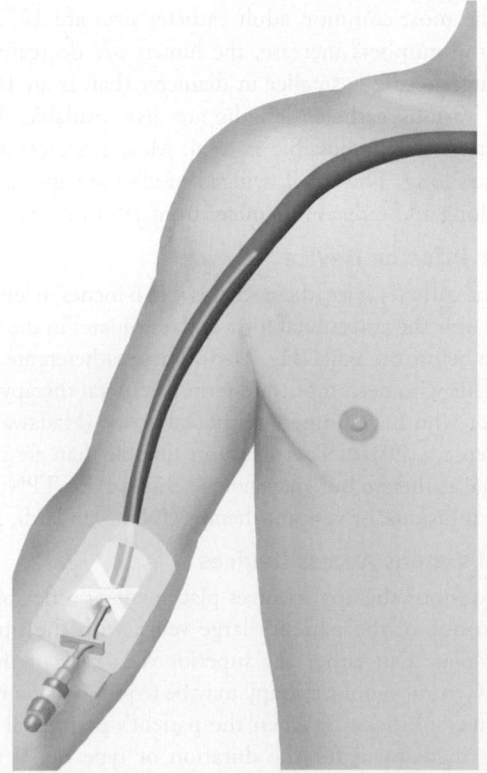

FIGURE 21-3 A midline catheter is 4 to 6 inches long and inserted in the antecubital fossa, terminating in the vasculature.

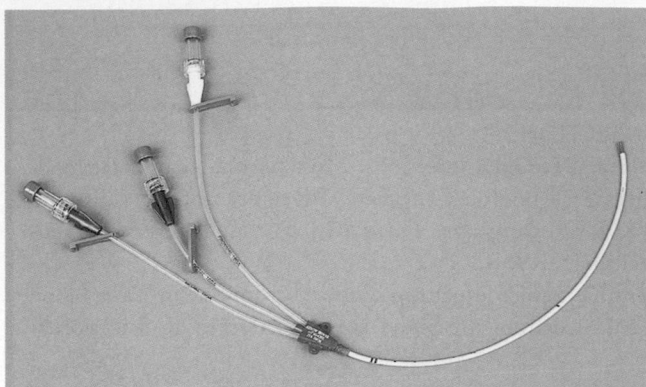

FIGURE 21-4 Multilumen catheter with three distinct catheters in one sheath.

to microorganisms (O'Grady et al., 2011). The central vein catheterization is a sterile procedure that is often performed at the bedside. Following informed consent, the insertion site is prepared and the vein is accessed with an introducer. The catheter is then inserted through the introducer and secured in place with an adhesive securing device. Ultrasound guidance, if available, may be used to reduce the number of cannulation attempts and associated mechanical complications. Placement is confirmed by x-ray. Because the catheter tip is placed in the superior vena cava or at the entrance of the right atrium, central venous catheters also allow the nurse to monitor central venous pressure in specialized patient populations. The multilumen catheter's obvious advantage is that as many as three separate catheters can be housed in one sheath, allowing multiple drugs to be administered simultaneously

without the risk of incompatibility of solutions (Fig. 21-4). Because of the risk of complications, multilumen, nontunneled catheters are used only in hospitalized patients. If a patient's condition necessitates long-term IV therapy, numerous additional options are available.

Peripherally Inserted Central Catheters. The **peripherally inserted central catheter (PICC)** is a long-line catheter made of soft silicone or Silastic material; it is placed peripherally but delivers medications and solutions centrally (Fig. 21-5). The basilic vein is usually used, but the median cubital and cephalic veins in the antecubital area also can be used. PICC lines are threaded so the catheter tip terminates in either the axillary or subclavian vein or the superior vena cava (Infusion Nurses Society [INS], 2011). A nurse specially trained in PICC insertion inserts the catheter and usually anchors the line with sutures. A radiograph confirms correct placement of the catheter tip, and then the catheter can be used for infusion therapy. PICC lines are used for patients who require intermediate- to long-term venous access. Because PICC lines can be left in place for several months, they are very useful for home as well as acute care. PICC lines have a small diameter, which makes them ideal for use in the very young and the elderly. The catheter flexibility does not restrict arm movement. These lines have been shown to be associated with fewer severe complications, such as pneumothorax, air embolism, and sepsis, than other central lines. Patients and their caregivers require instructions on the care and maintenance of the PICC as well as information about potential complications and appropriate interventions should complications occur.

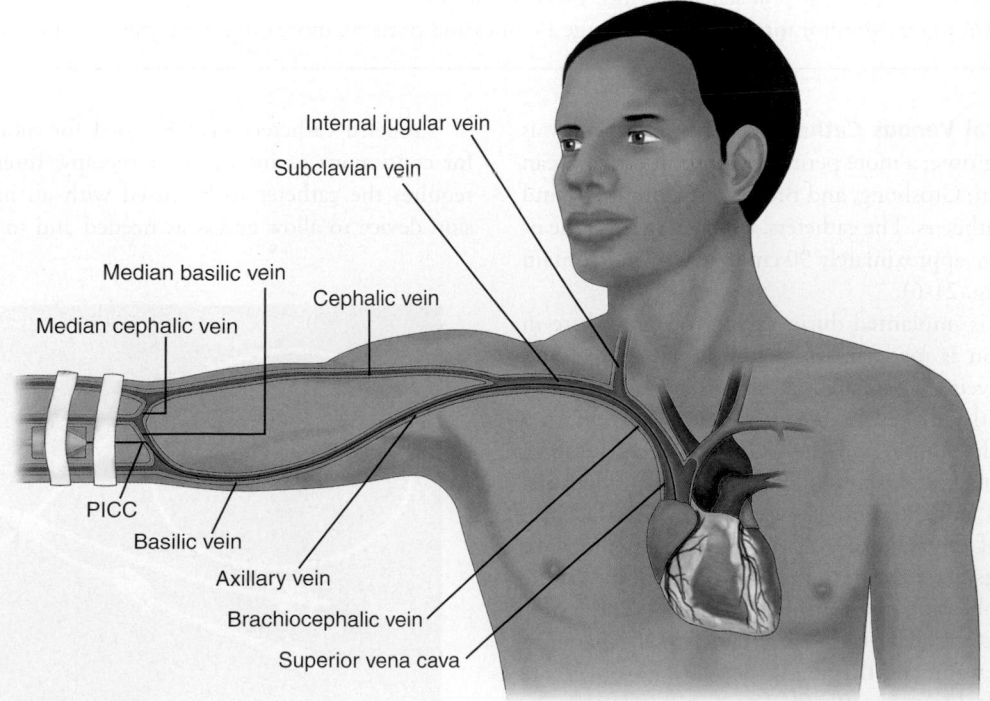

FIGURE 21-5 PICC access device is a peripherally inserted catheter that terminates in the subclavian vein or the superior vena cava.

EVIDENCE-BASED BUNDLES TO IMPROVE PATIENT CARE

PREVENTION OF CATHETER-RELATED BLOODSTREAM INFECTIONS

From 1970 to 2002, the CDC collected data on incidence of hospital-acquired infections. Most hospital-acquired bloodstream infections are associated with the use of central venous catheters. CRBSIs are associated with significant morbidity and mortality. Prevention is a key intervention in the IHI's "1,000,000 Lives" campaign. There are five evidence-based components of care identified by the CDC endorsed by the IHI for preventing CRBSIs.

  Definition of catheter-related bloodstream infection: The patient has a microorganism cultured from one or more blood cultures less than 48 hours after admission, and the organism cultured from the blood is not related to an infection at another site (Meyer, 2009).

EVIDENCE-BASED RECOMMENDATIONS

1. *Hand hygiene:* Wash hands with antiseptic soap, water, and/or gels before and after all patient contact.
   Nursing implications: Specialized IV teams, staff education and training, and adequate nursing staff levels.
2. *Site of catheter insertion:* Skin flora at the site of catheter insertion is a major risk factor:
   * Central venous catheters should be placed in the subclavian site whenever possible.
   * Femoral site should be avoided.
3. *Maximal sterile barrier precautions during insertion:*
   * Cap, mask, sterile gown, sterile gloves, and large sterile drape
   Nursing implications: Patient advocacy
4. *Skin asepsis:*
   * 2% chlorhexidine (CHG)-based products for skin prep prior to insertion
   Nursing implications: Dressing changes:
   * 2% CHG to disinfect skin
   * Use of either sterile transparent semipermeable dressing or sterile gauze to cover site
   * CHG-impregnated patch with semipermeable dressings
   * Change of dressing 24 hours after insertion
   * Change of dressing every 7 days or if visible bloody or soiled
5. *Daily review of line necessity:*
   * Prompt removal of unnecessary line
   * Routine catheter replacement at scheduled intervals discouraged
   Nursing implications: Monitor for adherence. Change IV lines and ports no more often than every 72 hours.

Tunneled Central Venous Catheters. When IV therapy is needed for a long time, a more permanent type of catheter can be used. Hickman, Groshong, and Broviac are common brand names of these catheters. The catheters, which may have one or several lumens, are approximately 90 cm in length and contain a Dacron cuff (Fig. 21-6).

The catheter is implanted during a surgical procedure in which an incision is made in the deltopectoral groove and the subclavian vein is isolated. A subcutaneous pathway or tunnel is gently formed with a pair of long forceps to a point between the nipple and the sternum—thus the term *tunneled catheter*. The Dacron cuff is positioned between the skin incision and the vein. The catheter is threaded into the lower part of the vena cava at the entrance to the right atrium. Dressings placed at both incision sites require simple cleaning and application of an antimicrobial agent and a sterile occlusive dressing. The catheter is taped to the patient's chest to lessen tension and tugging. Eventually, fibrous tissue grows around the Dacron cuff, which stabilizes the catheter in place, decreases infection rates, and permits use as a long-term venous access route (Fig. 21-7).

Tunneled catheters may be used for months, even years, for continuous or intermittent therapy. Intermittent therapy requires the catheter to be fitted with an intermittent infusion device to allow access as needed and to keep the system

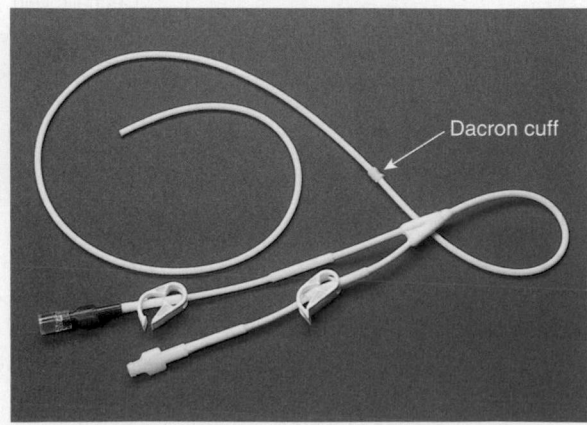

FIGURE 21-6 Double-lumen Hickman catheter showing the two ports and clamps.

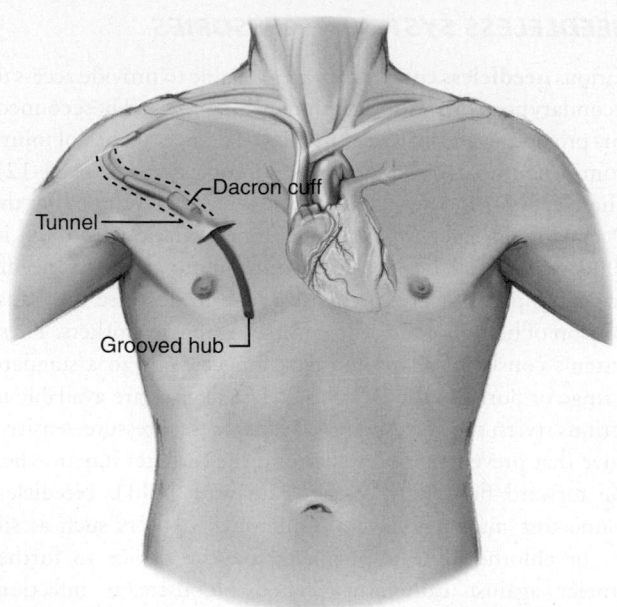

FIGURE 21-7 Insertion technique of indwelling tunneled catheter. A tunnel is formed from the vein to an area between the sternum and the nipple. The catheter tip is placed in the superior vena cava.

otherwise closed and intact. Catheter patency is maintained with periodic diluted heparin flushing. Because of its unique design, the Groshong catheter requires irrigation with normal saline rather than heparin.

Implanted Vascular Access Devices. Totally implantable access devices have been developed to allow long-term access without having a catheter protrude from the skin (Fig. 21-8). The system includes the subcutaneous injection port and a Silastic catheter, which is usually inserted into the superior vena cava. The device has a self-sealing septum or port, which allows repeated use without the risk of air entering the system.

With the patient under local anesthesia, the system is surgically implanted and sutured into a subcutaneous pocket (see Fig. 21-8A). When venous access is desired, the location of the injection port must be palpated. The system is then accessed with a noncoring needle, such as a Huber-point needle

(see Fig. 21-8B). As with other central venous systems, patency is maintained by periodic flushing. The implanted port systems require flushing with a diluted heparin solution.

Intraosseous Devices

Intraosseous (IO) devices provide a temporary, emergency vascular access device that may be inserted in emergency situations for fluid and medication administration when intravenous cannulation is not available (Neuman et al., 2010). IO access is widely accepted for emergency care in the pediatric population (Kleinman et al., 2010). The proximal tibia is the most acceptable insertion site for the IO needle. Additional information on IO access and maintenance is beyond the scope of this text.

SOLUTION CONTAINERS

Containers for IV fluid include glass bottles and plastic bags (Fig. 21-9). Plastic bags have become the industry standard unless a particular infusate is unstable in plastic. Plastic bags collapse as they empty and therefore require no vent to equalize pressure. However, the plastic bag's semirigid nature makes it difficult for healthcare personnel to accurately measure the amount of remaining fluid. Another disadvantage of plastic bags is that certain drugs (e.g., insulin) bind with the plastic; this makes IV administration of these drugs in plastic bags difficult.

Bottles and bags come in various sizes. Usually, 1,000-mL containers are used for routine hydration purposes. Smaller bags (e.g., 250 to 500 mL) may be used for children or when fluid is infusing at a very slow rate. Smaller containers (50, 100, or 250 mL) also are used to dilute and dispense medications.

ADMINISTRATION SETS

An IV administration set is tubing that connects the IV bag or bottle to the access device. Parts of the administration set are shown in Figure 21-10. Normally, an IV administration set includes the following features:

- A piercing pin or spike to permit the tubing to access the IV container.
- A slide clamp to stop fluid flow and a roller clamp to manually regulate the flow rate.

FIGURE 21-8 Implantable access system. **A.** Placement of the implantable system beneath the skin. **B.** Access to the system with a noncoring needle.

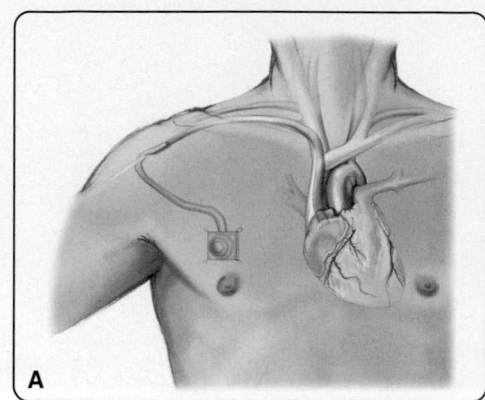

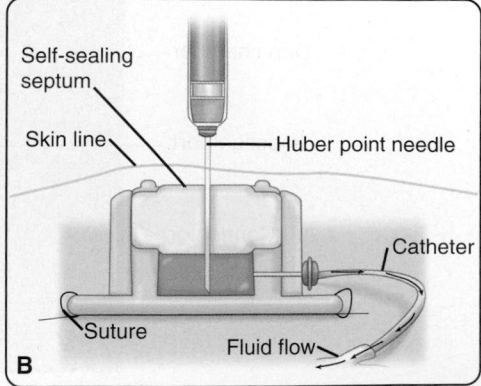

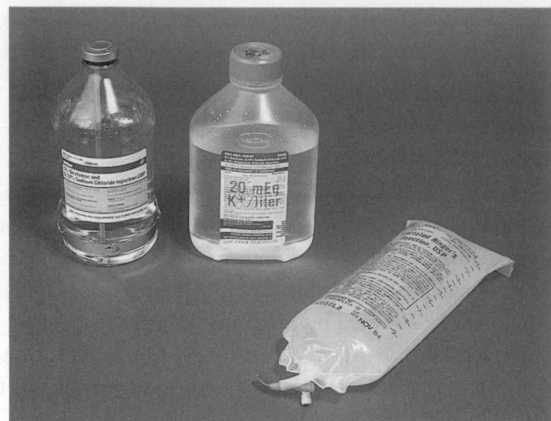

FIGURE 21-9 Examples of solution containers.

- An in-line filter to trap any particles and prevent them from entering the patient's bloodstream.
- A cassette that fits into an EID or a drip chamber to allow the nurse to visualize and count the drops of IV fluid if an EID is not being used.
- Needleless connector ports to permit the administration of medications, blood products, flushing, or other IV therapies.
- A connector at the end of the tubing for connecting the tubing to the needle or cannula. Although the connectors have various designs (slip tip or Luer lock), the dimensions are standard and fit all needle and cannula hubs.

Although specialized volume-controlled administration sets also are available, such as Buretrol or Soluset (Fig. 21-11), there is no substitute for the use of EIDs to provide accuracy and safety in controlling the infusion of IV fluid. For an unvented bottle system, there is tubing available that provides an air vent in the drip chamber to equalize pressure and provide easy fluid flow from the bottle to the patient.

The IV tubing should have a label applied to identify the date and time the tubing was initiated. Refer to the agency policy and procedures for frequency of changing tubing. The IV solution container should also be labeled with the patient's name as well as the date and time the infusion was initiated.

NEEDLELESS SYSTEM ACCESSORIES

Various **needleless connectors** are available to provide access to secondary ports on IV tubing or for flushing access. These connectors provide an alternative to needles to reduce the risk of injury from contaminated sharps during IV procedures (Fig. 21-12). The Needlestick Safety and Prevention Act developed by the Occupational Safety and Health Administration (OSHA) in 2000 requires all healthcare institutions to use safer needle devices as part of a comprehensive plan to decrease the transmission of bloodborne pathogens to healthcare workers. These systems consist of adaptors that connect easily to a standard syringe or ports on the IV tubing. The devices are available in various styles; the newest device available is a pressure-sensitive valve that prevents blood reflux into the catheter lumen when the forward fluid flow ceases (Hadaway, 2011). Needleless connectors may also have antimicrobial barriers such as silver or chlorhexidine impregnated on the device to further protect against catheter-associated bloodstream infection. The needleless connector should be consistently disinfected using alcohol, tincture of iodine, or chlorhexidine gluconate/alcohol combination prior to each access. The needleless connector should be changed whenever the needleless connector is removed, if there is blood within the needleless connector, and prior to drawing a blood culture sample from the catheter (INS, 2011).

! SAFETY ALERT

Any add-on device should be of a Luer lock–type configuration; add-on devices also require the healthcare staff to use aseptic technique.

Intermittent Infusion Devices

Intermittent infusion devices are used when the patient is to receive solutions or medications intermittently. Adaptors with a needleless connector can convert any IV catheter to an

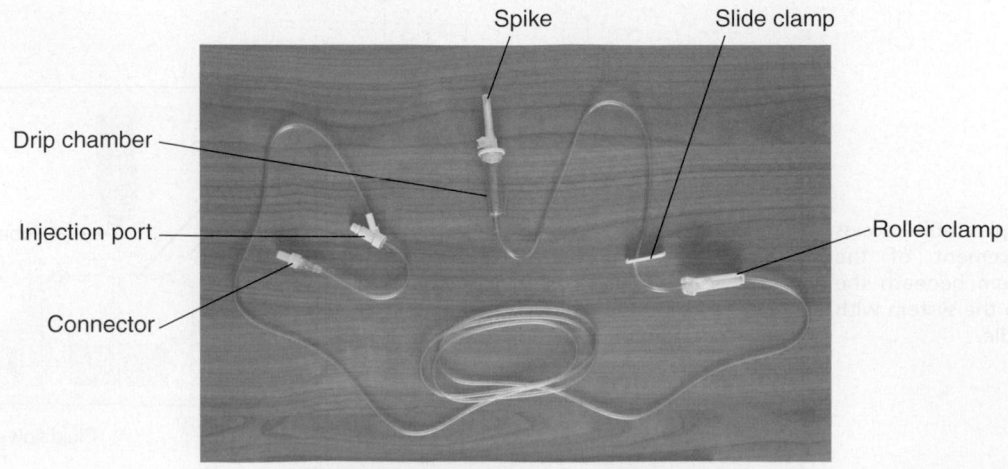

FIGURE 21-10 Administration set.

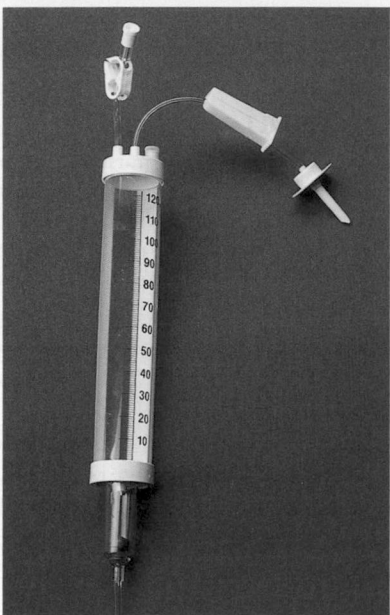

FIGURE 21-11 Volume-controlled set.

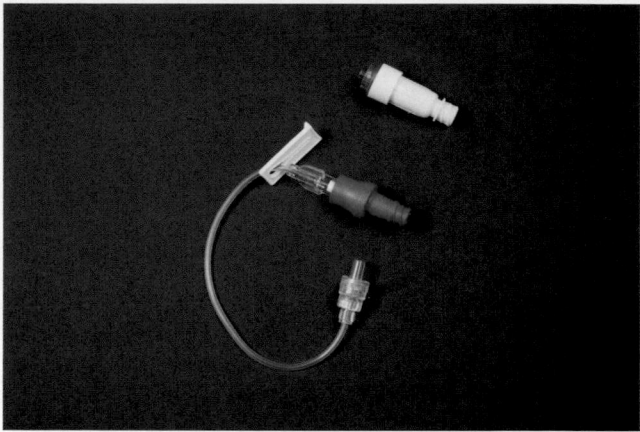

FIGURE 21-13 Adaptors used to convert indwelling IV catheters or infusion sets to intermittent infusion devices.

intermittent infusion device (Fig. 21-13). Intermittent infusion devices maintain venous access without requiring the patient to receive a continuous infusion, thus allowing increased mobility and minimizing the risk of fluid overload. Attaching an extension set (tubing with a clamp, sometimes referred to as a Y-connector) between the IV catheter and the IV tubing simplifies conversion to an intermittent infusion device, because the adaptor is already in place. To prevent blood clot formation, the devices are irrigated with a small quantity (3 mL) of sterile, preservative-free sodium chloride (NaCl) from a large-barrel (10 mL) syringe. The large-barrel syringe is used to decrease pressure during irrigation and hence decrease the risk of catheter damage (Gorski, 2009c). Prefilled NaCl syringes have been shown to have less risk of transmitting bloodborne pathogens (Delahanty & Myers, 2009). Flushing with positive, pulsing

pressure prevents reflux of blood into the cannula lumen and maintains patency (INS, 2011).

Intravenous Flow Rates

There are two important concepts to keep in mind when setting and maintaining IV flow rates: regulation of flow rates and factors that affect flow rates.

REGULATING FLOW RATE

Regulation of the flow rate can be done by either electronic or manual regulation. Use of EIDs, however, is highly recommended and is by far the safest and most widespread practice.

Electronic Regulation

An IV **electronic infusion device (EID)** accurately regulates the infusion rate, especially if fluid administration must be watched very carefully, such as when infusing fluid to an infant or administering certain medications. The INS standards state that EIDs should be used when warranted by the patient's age, condition, setting, and prescribed therapy (INS, 2011). Various types of EIDs are available commercially. In general, the EID pump uses positive pressure to deliver the prescribed fluid volume, whereas the controller senses the drops infusing to maintain a precise flow rate (Fig. 21-14). They are powered by electricity or battery pack and are programmed electronically.

> **SAFETY ALERT**
>
> Because many different types and models of EIDs are used, be knowledgeable about the specific operating guidelines for the machine you are using. Never turn off the alarm until the underlying problem has been discovered and resolved.

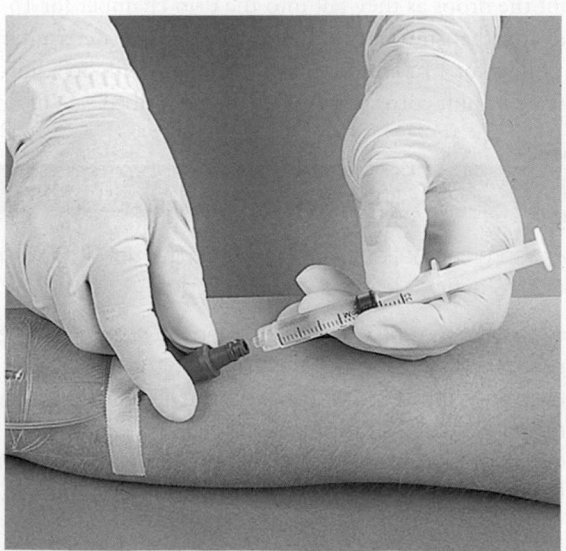

FIGURE 21-12 A needleless port allows the nurse to administer IV medication without risk of needlestick injury.

The healthcare provider enters the amount of fluid in milliliters and the rate of infusion in milliliters per hour. The instrument displays how many milliliters have infused and how much fluid remains in the IV container at any given time. In addition, programmable syringe pumps are useful for precise

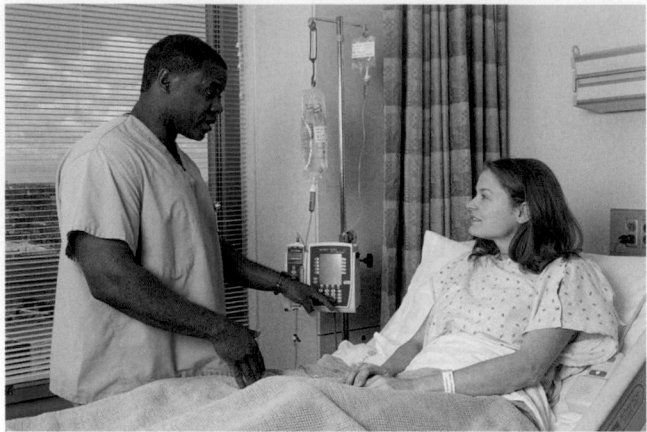

FIGURE 21-14 The nurse teaches the patient about the EID.

administration of small-dose, high-potency medications at rates of 0.01 to 99.9 mL per hour. These pumps are useful alone or piggybacked to a continuous infusion.

Electronic regulating devices also have sensors that can trigger an alarm when fluid cannot be delivered at the prescribed rate for any reason (e.g., the container is empty, the tubing is kinked, air is in the line, the vein is occluded). Because many EIDs are on the market, refer to the manufacturer's guidelines for setting up and troubleshooting each device.

Smart Pumps

In 1999, the Institute of Medicine published the classic article *To Err Is Human: Building a Safer Health System* (Institute of Medicine, 1999), which reported that up to 98,000 patient deaths every year in the United States were caused by medical errors. In response, government agencies, healthcare professionals, and healthcare organizations have looked to evidence-based practices to reduce medication errors (Hertzel & Sousa, 2009). The Joint Commission (2009) and the National Coordinating Council for Medication Error Reporting and Prevention (2008) have both set goals to prevent medication errors. Additionally, the Institute for Safe Medication Practices (2008) reported that the most serious medication errors involved IV administration, especially high-alert medications, such as insulin, heparin, and morphine. Technology responded and rapidly developed smart pumps to help prevent medication errors. **Smart pumps** are an enhanced EID that has an embedded computer safety software program, also known as a "dose error reduction system" (Hertzel & Sousa, 2009). Healthcare teams from individual agencies, including pharmacy, nursing, medicine, and information technology, work collaboratively to determine which drug libraries will be downloaded to the smart pump computer system (Longshore, Smith, & Weist, 2010). The software is also configured to match specialty patient populations within the organization, such as critical care, acute care, oncology, neonatal, and pediatrics. When the pump is turned on, the nurse identifies a clinical practice area and then programs the pump with the patient's name, weight, and so on. Features built into the pump include safety features such as concentrations, predetermined dose limits, and administration guidelines. Limits can be set to allow for overrides that the user will first be prompted to confirm

(soft limits). Additional limits can be programmed that will not allow the user to override (hard limits), due to safety limitations.

❗ SAFETY ALERT
EIDs do not replace diligent nursing assessment of the IV system; the nurse is still responsible for identifying the cause of any problems and making corrections to ensure proper infusion. However, the use of smart pump technology in combination with critical thinking by the nurse has great potential to promote medication safety.

Manual Regulation

In instances when an EIC is not used, the flow rate can be calculated and manipulated manually to ensure proper infusion. Tubing is available as macrodrip and microdrip (minidrip). The choice of tubing depends on the nurse's judgment and which rate is easiest to count. Macrodrip tubing delivers 10, 15, or 20 drops per milliliter, depending on the manufacturer (usually 10 drops per milliliter). Macrodrip tubing generally is used for adult patients, especially when large-volume replacement may be required.

Microdrip tubing delivers 60 drops per milliliter and is used for small-volume administration. After the administration set is selected, the infusion drip rate can be calculated from the physician's order using the following formula:

$$\text{Drops per minute} = \text{total volume identified} \times \text{drop factor (drops per milliliter)}$$

The drop factor, which can be found on the administration set packaging, represents the size of the drop that the administration set creates. To calculate the drip rate of an IV that is to infuse 125 mL per hour using tubing that has a drop factor of 10, the nurse would use the previous formula, obtaining a rate of 21 drops per minute. Once the IV drip rate has been calculated, the infusion can be regulated manually after it is connected to the patient. A roller clamp adjusts the flow rate according to drops per minute counted in the drip chamber. Count the drops as they fall into the drip chamber for 15 seconds, and then multiply this number by 4 to determine the rate of flow for 1 full minute. Use the roller clamp to adjust the flow rate until it corresponds with the prescribed rate of flow.

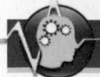 APPLY YOUR CRITICAL THINKING

Your surgical patient has an IV order for 1,000 mL 5%D/NS every 8 hours.

- Calculate the infusion rate for an IV controller to be programmed using milliliters per hour.
- Calculate the drip rate using a gravity infusion with a drop factor of 20 drops per milliliter.
- Calculate the drip rate for a gravity infusion with a microdrip (60 drops per milliliter) tubing using a simplified formula.

Check your answers in Appendix B.

FACTORS AFFECTING FLOW

Factors that affect the flow rate include the height of the solution container, position of the extremity, a tubing obstruction, position of the IV access, IV patency, vein integrity, and air vents on the tubing.

Height of the Solution Container

If an EID is not used, the height of the IV bag or bottle can affect the rate of infusion. As the height of the container from the infusion site increases, gravitational force will be greater and the fluid will flow faster. Conversely, as the distance between the bottle and IV site decrease, the fluid will infuse more slowly. This may occur when the patient gets up and walks in the hall, pushing his or her IV pole with the hand into which the IV is flowing.

Position of the Extremity

When the extremity is elevated, the fluid will infuse more slowly. Bending the extremity at a point of flexion, such as the wrist or the elbow, or leaning on the arm can slow the rate of infusion and cause the EID alarm to sound.

> **SAFETY ALERT**
>
> Take extra care to monitor an IV that appears to be positional. As the infusion slows down, the EID will alarm. If this happens repeatedly, the interruptions of the infusion could potentially decrease the amount of fluid that is infused to the patient. Stabilizing the joint with an arm board or splint may facilitate accurate IV infusion.

Tubing Obstruction

Constriction or kinking of IV tubing also can contribute to altered flow rates. Tubing can become kinked if inadvertently placed under the patient. Tubing also can be obstructed if tape is applied too tightly or if edema develops when the tape interferes with venous blood return in the extremity. If the tubing becomes obstructed, the EID will alarm to alert the nurse.

Position of the IV Access

The position of the needle or catheter within the vein can affect the rate of flow. Position changes can cause the needle bevel or catheter to rest against a vein wall. This is known as a **positional IV**. If the flow is interrupted, the EID will alarm. Careful selection of the IV site prior to insertion can help eliminate this problem.

IV Patency

Catheter patency is important to ensure proper infusion of fluids. Whenever fluid flow is interrupted for any reason (e.g., bending at a joint, kinking of tubing), a blood clot can form at the end of the catheter, stopping the infusion. If the clot does not completely obstruct the lumen of the catheter, the flow rate may slow and become sluggish. If the flow decreases below the set rate on the EID, the pump will alarm. This is often a prob-

lem when IVs are infusing very slowly to keep the vein open (to keep open [TKO] or keep vein open [KVO]). When a KVO rate is ordered, intermittently flush the catheter with saline to prevent clot formation.

> **SAFETY ALERT**
>
> Never irrigate the catheter if you meet pressure when attempting to flush; irrigation may push the clot into the circulatory system.

ROLE OF THE NURSE IN INTRAVENOUS THERAPY

Nurses are responsible for initiating, monitoring, maintaining, and discontinuing the IV infusion and for patient teaching related to the infusion. Although many patients who receive IV fluids are admitted to healthcare facilities, it is increasingly common for patients to receive IV fluids at home or in special ambulatory or short-stay settings. The physician orders the type and amount of IV fluid and electrolyte replacement. Components of an IV order include the following:

- Type and amount of solution
- Other medications or electrolytes to be added to the solution
- Length of time for infusion to be given or infusion rate

Initiating Intravenous Therapy

IV therapy requires an order from a licensed provider. The nurse is responsible for checking the order to determine the volume of solution to be infused, the rate of flow per hour, and any additives to the solution. Once the order has been verified and the solution is available, the nurse gathers needed equipment and prepares the patient for venipuncture. Step-by-step guidelines for initiating IV therapy are provided in **Procedure 21-1**.

PREPARING THE PATIENT

Educating the patient or caregiver about the prescribed infusion therapy and plan of care as well as obtaining informed consent, if necessary, is a major component of patient preparation. Teaching should include the purpose, goals of treatment, infusion-related care, and potential complications (INS, 2011). Continuous nursing supervision and assessment is available in the hospital or long-term care settings, but the patient at home requires in-depth instruction and support from a home health nurse.

SELECTING THE SITE

The patient's history, diagnosis, allergies, activity level, vein condition, therapy type, and anticipated duration of therapy are all important to consider when determining the IV

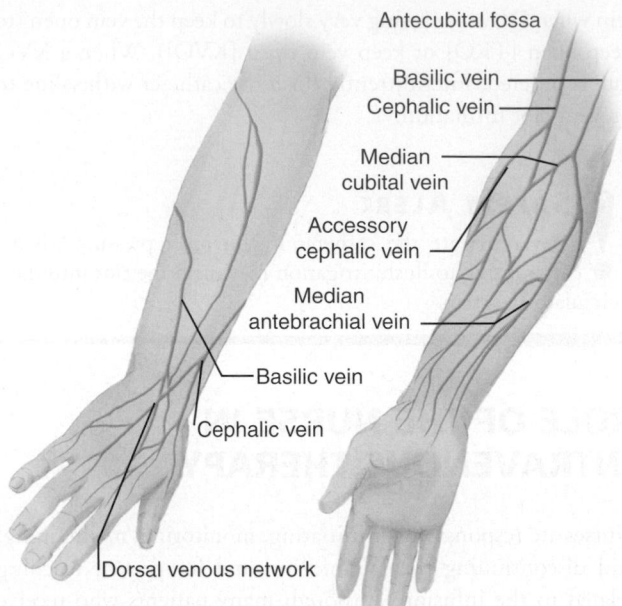

Antecubital fossa

Basilic vein

Cephalic vein

Median
cubital vein

Accessory
cephalic vein

Median
antebrachial vein

Basilic vein

Cephalic vein

Dorsal venous network

FIGURE 21-15 Adult IV insertion sites.

placement site. In the adult, the veins of the hand and forearm are commonly used for IV infusion (Fig. 21-15). When the basilic or cephalic vein is used, the ulna and radius act as natural splints, allowing the patient greater freedom of movement. Whenever possible, larger veins are used and the distal portion of the vein is punctured first, leaving the more proximal sites for later venipunctures (Gorski, 2009b). Avoid veins located directly over movable joints, because at these sites, the IV is more likely to dislodge and infiltrate or the patient is more likely to develop phlebitis. Use a site where the bone acts as a natural splint. Avoid veins of the lower extremities whenever possible; using these sites limits mobility and increases the incidence of thrombophlebitis.

Various techniques are helpful to locate and visualize veins before venipuncture. Visually inspect the patient's veins, avoiding any areas that appear bruised or sclerosed. Place a tourniquet on the extremity 4 to 6 inches above the intended venipuncture site to distend the vein with blood. Other techniques include lowering the extremity below the level of the heart, asking the patient to open and close the fist several times, tapping lightly over the selected vein, or using warm soaks for 5 minutes before venipuncture to vasodilate the selected vessel. In some agencies, ultrasound devices are available to identify vein location.

PREPARING THE SITE

Adequate site preparation is necessary to avoid infection. Clip any hair around the site as necessary. Shaving is avoided because microscopic nicks or abrasions can provide entry sites for microorganisms. Prepare the site with a single application of 2% chlorhexidine in 70% isopropyl alcohol, using gentle pressure in a side to side, back and forth motion (McGoldrick, 2010; O'Grady, 2011). For patients with chlorhexidine allergies, use povidone–iodine swabs, using an expanding circular motion, allowing one minute

contact time. Remove povidone–iodine with an alcohol pad. Allow the solutions to air-dry. Institutional policy dictates the use of local anesthetics before venipuncture. The most common agents used are intradermal lidocaine and EMLA cream (INS, 2011).

PERFORMING THE VENIPUNCTURE

Assemble all equipment before attempting venipuncture. Cut tape and have all equipment within reach. Wear gloves, as in any invasive procedure. Identify the patient with two separate identifiers. Stretch the skin taut over the intended venipuncture site with the thumb and index finger. Stabilize the vein, using a backward pull. Keep the vein stabilized until the needle is withdrawn from the skin. With the bevel up, hold the needle to enter the skin at a 21- to 30-degree angle. As the skin is pierced, decrease the angle of the needle to 15 degrees. This will permit entry into the vein at an angle and decrease the risk of puncturing through a vein. Watch for blood return, which indicates placement in the vein. When using an IV catheter, thread the plastic catheter into the vein, after inserting the needle and cannula, until the catheter hub is situated against the skin. Then remove the stylet while the catheter is fully inserted within the lumen of the vessel. When placement of the needle or catheter in the vein is ensured, attach the tubing and release the tourniquet. If cannulation is unsuccessful, repeat the entire procedure with a new catheter at another site. The same nurse should not attempt cannulation more than two times because of undue stress on patient and nurse (INS).

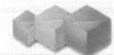 **Concept Mastery Alert**

When inserting a patient's peripheral IV, it is unnecessary to wear sterile gloves. Clean gloves are sufficient to protect yourself and to ensure asepsis is maintained during the procedure.

❗ SAFETY ALERT

When performing venipuncture, observe standard precautions to limit provider exposure to bloodborne pathogens, especially hepatitis B and HIV. Be sure your hepatitis B vaccinations are current. To avoid needlestick injuries, dispose of needles in appropriate biohazard containers, do not attempt to recap needles, and utilize self-retracting safety needles when performing venipuncture. Use needleless adaptors whenever possible for all other IV maintenance and medication administration.

SECURING THE VENIPUNCTURE DEVICE

Tape the cannula flush with the skin using ½-inch-wide tape. Place another strip of tape under the hub, adhesive side up. Secure one end tightly and diagonally over the cannula and repeat with the other end. Repeat this with the other end of the tape crossing the

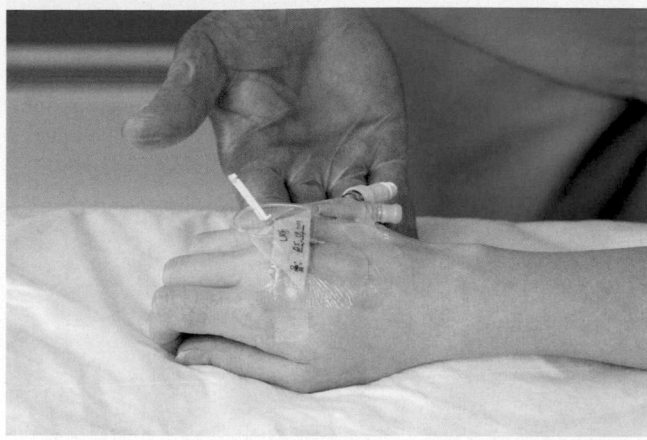

FIGURE 21-16 Venipuncture device properly secured.

first. This secures the cannula and prevents sideways movement. Then loop the tubing and anchor it with tape. Apply a transparent dressing over the infusion site (Fig. 21-16). Alternatively, manufactured stabilizing devices may be used to secure the IV site in some healthcare agencies. Documentation includes the time, date, IV site location, and IV catheter length and gauge.

Maintaining Intravenous Infusions

The nurse is responsible for maintaining and monitoring IV infusions to ensure that the fluid infuses at the proper rate and that complications of IV therapy are detected promptly. The steps in monitoring the IV infusion are outlined in **Procedure 21-2**.

MONITORING AND DOCUMENTATION

The patient's condition, type of access device, practice setting, and agency protocols all determine the frequency of monitoring an IV device. Document pertinent assessment data, including condition of the IV site, infusion rate, vital signs, intake/output data, and the patient's response to therapy at a minimum of every 4 hours (INS, 2011). In the home setting, instruct patients and their caregivers to monitor the IV site for redness, swelling, and patency. If problems are noted, a home healthcare nurse should be notified.

> ❗ **SAFETY ALERT**
>
> In an acute or long-term care facility, evaluate the patient's IV at least once each hour. If the patient is a child, perform this assessment more frequently.

DRESSING CHANGES

Institutional and agency policies specify expectations for site care, in accordance with the Nursing Standards of Practice defined by the INS and the recommendations from the Centers for Disease Control and Prevention (CDC). Visually inspect and palpate the site for tenderness often. If tenderness, fever without obvious source, or symptoms of local or bloodstream infection are present, remove the dressing and inspect the site directly. There is no evidence to support use of transparent, semipermeable dressing over gauze dressings, and the dressing should not be removed if the patient has no clinical sign of infection (Gilles et al., 2003; O'Grady et al., 2011). When performing site care, take extra care not to dislodge the catheter. The steps in performing site care are outlined in **Procedures 21-3** and **21-4**.

CHANGING INTRAVENOUS SOLUTIONS AND TUBING

The nurse is responsible for changing the IV bag as needed and changing IV tubing according to institutional or agency policy. The IV bag is changed when the previous container is empty, when there is a change in IV orders, or when the IV bag has been hanging for more than 24 hours.

All IV bag and tubing changes must be done under strict aseptic technique to prevent infection. Intravenous administration sets, including secondary sets and add-on devices, should be changed no more frequently than every 96 hours (Gilles et al., 2005; O'Grady, 2011). Tubings used for blood administration, intralipids and TPN require more frequent changes. Most facilities have policies that indicate the frequency and protocol for these procedures. **Procedure 21-5** outlines the steps involved in changing IV solution and tubing. See PICO display for evidence-based practice recommendations.

INTERMITTENT FLUSHING OF AN INFUSION LOCK

An existing IV catheter may be converted to an intermittent infusion device by using a needleless adaptor (**Procedure 21-6**). Peripheral intermittent lines are usually flushed with preservative-free 0.9% NaCl before and after each medication administration and every 8 hours when medications are not being given. Flushing protocols for central venous catheters remain controversial. Many studies report equivalent outcomes when central venous catheters are flushed with diluted heparin solutions compared to saline locking (Mitchell et al., 2009; INS, 2011). However, flushing with diluted heparin can affect the coagulation status of a patient or cause heparin-induced thrombocytopenia (HIT). If agency protocols recommend flushing the central catheter with diluted heparin solution, the nurse should monitor for signs and symptoms of HIT and discontinue all sources of heparin, if suspected. The frequency, quantity, and type of flush solution depend on the manufacturer's recommendation and the organization's policy.

Assessing for Complications

Monitoring the patient for possible complications of IV therapy is an important nursing responsibility. The most significant complications of IV therapy include infiltration, phlebitis, infection, and fluid overload. Air embolism and pneumothorax are potentially life-threatening complications associated more commonly with central venous therapy. Catheter breakage is another complication occasionally seen with long-term therapy and central venous access devices. For more information, see Table 21-3.

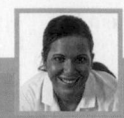
Sue, the nurse from the chapter-opening scenario, is on the intravenous (IV) committee, and she is in the process of updating one of the policies. The current standard in her hospital is to change IV tubings every 3 days to reduce the risk of infection. The policy she is reviewing was written 4 years ago. She doesn't think that this policy is based on the current evidence. She decides to search the Cochrane library for the latest research using the following PICO statement: *In patients with intravenous catheter, how does replacing administration sets (or tubing) every 72 hours (h) compare to other frequent intervals (24h, 48h, or 96h) decrease infection rates?*

> **P** = patients with intravenous catheter
> **I** = replacing administration set every 72 hours
> **C** = replacing it at other frequencies (24, 48, 96 hours)
> **O** = decrease infection rate

Sue finds a current systematic review that evaluated 16 randomized control trials with 5,001 participants (both neonates and adults). The review included studies that analyzed infection rates in central, peripheral, venous, and arterial catheter tubings/administration sets over a range of days. Overall, the review concluded that IV tubing that did not contain blood, blood products, or lipid could be used up for 96 hours without risk for infection. However, in neonates the risk for infection was higher and led to mortality if tubing was not changed frequently. The authors noted that the quality of evidence was considered low to moderate due to poorly described methods in some of the studies. Sue decides to bring the article to the next committee meeting to open it up for discussion with the team before revising the policy.

REFERENCE

Ullman, A. J., Cooke, M. L., Gillies, D., Marsh, N. M., Daud, A., McGrail, M. R., et al. (2013). Optimal timing for intravascular administration set replacement. *Cochrane Database of Systematic Reviews*, (9): CD003588. Doi: 10.1002/14651858.CD003588.pub3.

TABLE 21-3 COMPLICATIONS OF INTRAVENOUS THERAPY

Complication	Signs/Symptoms	Action	Prevention
Infiltration	Swelling, coolness, and discomfort at site Slowed infusion rate Absence of blood return	Discontinue IV and restart in another location. Apply warm soaks to decrease swelling.	Select a site that is over long bones that act as splint. Avoid sites over joints. Consider using manufactured stabilization devices.
Phlebitis	Pain, warmth, and redness at site Vein may feel hard and cordlike Slowed infusion rate	Discontinue IV and restart in another location. Apply warm soaks to decrease discomfort. Do not irrigate.	Change IV sites every 72 h. Use large veins and large-gauge needles rather than catheters. Dilute medications well and infuse slowly. Use central line for very irritating solutions.
Infection	*Local*: Redness, warmth, and purulent drainage at the IV site *Systemic*: Fever, chills, malaise, and elevated WBCs	Discontinue IV and restart in another location. Culture catheter tip and draw blood cultures. Treat with appropriate antibiotics.	Maintain strict asepsis when dealing with IVs. Use good handwashing. Change tubing and dressings every 96 h according to agency protocol.
Fluid overload	Elevated blood pressure, increased pulse and respirations, dyspnea, crackles, neck vein distention, weight gain	Slow IV to "keep open" rate and notify physician. Place patient in high or semi-Fowler position. Administer oxygen as needed.	Monitor rates carefully, especially for high-risk patients (elderly, infants, congestive heart failure, or renal disease). Use EID. Don't catch up when IV gets behind for high-risk patients.
Air embolism (central venous catheters	Pain in chest, shoulder, or back; dyspnea; hypotension; thready pulse; cyanosis; loss of consciousness	Place on left side in Trendelenburg position. Notify the physician. Monitor vital signs closely.	Tape all connectors or use Luer lock connectors. Use air-eliminating filters. Use EID for all central venous catheters. Instruct the patient to use Valsalva's maneuver when changing tubing or discontinuing a central line.

INFILTRATION

When IV solutions inadvertently leak into the subcutaneous tissues, it is called **infiltration**. This is referred to as **extravasation** if the solution or medication is a vesicant. **Vesicants** are highly irritating and can cause extensive tissue damage when they leak into the subcutaneous tissues (Doellman et al., 2009). Chemotherapy and solutions with high or low pH are examples of vesicants. Infiltration can occur if the needle or catheter slips out of the vein or if IV fluid leaks from the vein into subcutaneous tissue. When infiltration occurs, the patient may complain of pain and may have swelling around the infusion site, which usually becomes cool to the touch. The IV usually infuses more slowly because of increased pressure within the subcutaneous tissues, causing the EID to alarm. Ask the patient to promptly notify staff of pain, burning, or swelling at the site so that prompt corrective action can be taken.

PHLEBITIS

Phlebitis refers to inflammation of the vascular endothelial wall. If a blood clot accompanies the inflammation, it is referred to as **thrombophlebitis**. Factors that contribute to the development of phlebitis include catheter gauge, size, and material; length of time the catheter is in a vein; type and pH of solution administered; and use of small veins or veins of the lower extremities, where blood flow is relatively sluggish. Clinical manifestations of phlebitis include complaints of discomfort and a vein that appears red and feels warm and hard (almost cordlike) when palpated (Dos Reis, Silveira, Vasques, & de Carvalho, 2009; Webster, Osborn, Rickard, & Hall, 2010). The IV will be sluggish, especially if a clot is present. The catheter should be removed if phlebitis develops.

CHANGING THE CATHETER

Recent guidelines on caring for peripheral intravenous catheters have emphasized routine changing of the catheter to prevent complications such as phlebitis and catheter-related infections. A systematic review by Webster et al. in (2010) revealed no conclusive evidence that routine replacement of peripheral intravenous catheters was more beneficial than was clinically indicated replacement. Current recommendations are to replace the peripheral catheter if clinically indicated, rather than routine replacement (Ken & Daphne, 2012).

THERAPEUTIC DIALOGUE: INTRAVENOUS THERAPY

SCENE FOR THOUGHT

The evening nurse enters the room of Delores Davis, a 65-year-old social worker with a wide smile who has an IV in her left arm. She greets the nurse warmly as she assesses the IV site, infusion rate, and EID.

LESS EFFECTIVE		MORE EFFECTIVE	
Delores:	Hi there. How are you this evening? *(Big smile.)*	**Delores:**	Hi there. How are you this evening? *(Big smile.)*
Nurse:	Just fine, Ms. Davis. How are you this evening? *(Gently palpates the area around the IV site.)*	**Nurse:**	Just fine, Ms. Davis. How are you this evening? *(Gently palpates the area around the IV site.)*
Delores:	Don't touch that, please. *(Winces and pulls back.)*	**Delores:**	Don't touch that, please. *(Winces and pulls back.)*
Nurse:	*(Stands still; moves hand to gently rest on Delores's hand.)* Is the IV bothering you?	**Nurse:**	*(Stands still; moves hand to gently rest on Delores's hand.)* Is the IV bothering you?
Delores:	Well, yes, it is, actually. *(Her face now looks worried, her eyes searching those of the nurse.)*	**Delores:**	Well, yes, it is, actually. *(Her face now looks worried, her eyes searching those of the nurse.)*
Nurse:	Let me check everything out now. *(Thoroughly examines the site, EID, drip rate, tubing.)* I can untangle this tubing a bit for you, but I don't see anything else wrong. Tell you what, I'll be back later on this evening to check on it again, and, if something is wrong, we'll fix it. Okay? *(Pats her hand reassuringly and smiles as she leaves.)*	**Nurse:**	Tell me a little more.
		Delores:	It started this evening after supper. I'm afraid I pulled on it when I was reaching for my tea. The other nurse put the tray where I couldn't reach it, and I didn't want to bother her, so I just reached for it and then the skin felt a little sore there. Did I do something wrong? *(Face is still worried.)*
Delores:	Okay, I guess. *(Face has no expression except for two frown lines between her eyes.)*	**Nurse:**	Well, let's see what the area is like. *(Talks to Delores while examining.)* I don't see any redness or swelling where the needle enters your skin, the pump seems to be functioning fine, and the fluid is dripping at just the right rate. I think everything is working properly. One thing I can do is untangle the tubing a little so you'll have more room to move. How's that?

(Continued)

THERAPEUTIC DIALOGUE: INTRAVENOUS THERAPY *(Continued)*

Delores:	*(Looks relieved.)* Better. I'm pleased to hear that I didn't do any damage. I've never had one of these **before. (Smiles but not as widely as before.)**
Nurse:	Sounds like you're still a little worried about it. Anything I can help with?
Delores:	No, I'm fine. But could you come back and check again later? It would put my mind at ease.
Nurse:	I'd be delighted. I was going to suggest that myself. By the way, it isn't a bother to set your tray up more comfortably for you. Please ask next time. We're here to make you feel better, not to make you struggle!
Delores:	Thank you so much. I appreciate it. *(Big smile.)*

CRITICAL THINKING CHALLENGE
- Analyze how the second nurse reassured Delores.
- Explain how you can tell from behavior that a person is reassured.
- Determine when reassurance becomes patronizing.
- Assess what was missing between the nurse and patient in the first dialogue.

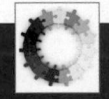

COLLABORATING WITH THE HEALTH CARE TEAM
Requesting Consultation for a Problem With an Intravenous Site

You have been assigned to care for Mr. Raymond, who was admitted yesterday with a potassium level of 3.0 mEq per liter. He is currently NPO and has maintenance fluid of D51/2NS with 40 mEq KCl infusing at 125 mL per hour. It is infusing through an EID, but the alarm indicating an occlusion has been activated a few times this morning. However, this time when you look at the insertion site, you see it is swollen, and Mr. Raymond says it is more painful than earlier in the day. You place an order for an IV team consult for a site assessment and a possible restart. The IV RN approaches you for more information prior to entering Mr. Raymond's room.

SITUATION: Mr. Raymond's IV site is swollen, and he tells me it is painful.

BACKGROUND: The IV site was placed yesterday when he was admitted. He is currently NPO and has a 25-gauge IV site in his right wrist with D51/2NS with 40 mEq Kcl infusing at 125 mL per hour. I've been having trouble with the site today, with it alarming a lot saying it was occluded; however, it seems to be a positional site since he's right handed. The site is now swollen and red and the infusion has been stopped. I also placed a warmed cloth on the swollen site.

ASSESSMENT: Mr. Raymond's IV site is infiltrated, and he needs a new IV site placed.

RECOMMENDATION: I would recommend a larger-gauge IV site be placed in a larger vein of his left upper extremity.

CRITICAL THINKING QUESTIONS
- What gauge IV would you recommend?
- Consider the impact of 40 mEq KCl infusing in the IV. Would this impact your assessment of the IV status?
- What is the danger of infiltration in this situation, and what can be done to prevent injury?
- List interventions that can decrease the risk of infiltration.

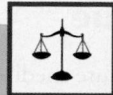

CLINICAL JUDGMENT IN INTRAVENOUS MANAGEMENT

Mr. Brown, an elderly patient with end-stage prostate cancer, is admitted to an acute care facility with sepsis secondary to a urinary tract infection (UTI). Mr. Brown has an advance directive requesting no artificial nutrition or life-sustaining treatments. The provider has ordered IV ciprofloxacin and a 1 L bolus of lactated Ringer's. The family has been notified of Mr. Brown's admission and are said to be on their way to the hospital. Mr. Brown is not fully conscious, opens his eyes intermittently, and moans.

CRITICAL THINKING CHALLENGE

- Do you have enough information in this situation to determine a course of action?
- Would your plan of care include starting the IV line and begin the fluids and antibiotics as ordered?
- How does Mr. Brown's advance directive influence your decision?

INFECTION

Infection can occur at the IV infusion site or systemically. The longer an IV is in one site, the greater the chance for infection. Infection can occur with central venous catheters, especially when the patient is at risk. Meticulous hand hygiene, site preparation, and use of sterile technique during insertion and maintenance are essential to minimize the risk of infection. Signs and symptoms of infection can be local or systemic. If infection is suspected, notify the physician. Consistent use of the IHI Central Line Bundle is aimed at decreasing central line infection rates.

FLUID OVERLOAD

Fluid overload may occur if the patient receives IV fluid too rapidly. The very young, the elderly, and patients with cardiac or renal impairment are particularly vulnerable. Fluid overload can occur if the nurse tries to "catch up" when the IV infusion gets behind. Assessments such as increased weight, decreased urine output compared to intake, and crackles (rales) upon lung auscultation often indicate fluid overload.

AIR EMBOLISM

The entry of air into the patient's circulatory system is called an **air embolism**. Air embolism is more common when central venous catheters are used; air entry is due to the change in intra-

SAFETY ALERT

Preventing fluid overload is crucial by carefully monitoring all IVs and using EIDs.

thoracic pressures during respiration. Luer lock connections on all IV devices and ports are a vital step in prevention. A significant amount of air must enter the peripheral venous circulation before it poses a significant health risk for the patient. Smaller amounts of air are significant when a central venous catheter is used for IV therapy. Symptoms of air embolism include complaints of chest, shoulder, or back pain; dyspnea; hypotension; cyanosis; tachyarrhythmias; and loss of consciousness. At the first sign of air embolism, clamp the existing catheter and/or occlude the puncture site if the catheter has been removed to prevent additional air from entering the bloodstream. Immediately position the patient on her or his left side in the Trendelenburg position to allow the air to rise into the right ventricle and allow blood to pass into the lungs (Gorski, 2010; INS, 2011; Smeltzer & Bare, 2010). This can be a life-threatening situation, so get help promptly. Refer to Table 21-3 for recommendations from the INS to prevent air embolism.

PNEUMOTHORAX

Pneumothorax may occur during insertion of a central venous catheter if the catheter inadvertently punctures the lung or pleural membrane since it closely underlies the access point. Symptoms of pneumothorax include chest or shoulder pain, sudden shortness of breath, tachycardia, and absence of breath sounds on the affected side. After all central venous catheter insertions, a chest x-ray verifies the position of the catheter before infusion of any solutions or medications. The chest x-ray also will detect pneumothorax.

CATHETER BREAKAGE OR DAMAGE

Catheter breakage or damage, although rare, may occur at any point along the IV catheter. This damage can be in the form of tiny pinholes or a complete fracture of the catheter. The most serious risk to the patient is if the catheter breaks and the fractured fragment embolizes to the heart or pulmonary artery. All IV devices are made of radiopaque materials, so radiographic evaluation will assist in locating the catheter fragments. To avoid catheter damage, use needleless systems and syringes 10 mL or greater to flush the catheter. Additionally, avoid inserting catheters near or over joints. Upon removal of a catheter, assess the catheter's integrity before disposal and document this.

Discontinuing an Intravenous Infusion

An infusion is discontinued when all ordered fluids have infused or when complications develop. Before discontinuing an infusion, don disposable gloves. Position the roller clamp to the "off" position and turn the EID off. Carefully remove the tape from the outside to the insertion point while supporting the catheter. Once the tape is loose, withdraw the catheter with one steady motion. Then apply pressure over the site and a bandage once bleeding has stopped. Assess the integrity of the catheter and insertion site. Document the amount of fluid infused, the time the infusion was discontinued, the condition of the site, any complications of therapy that occurred, the integrity of the catheter, and any nursing measures taken (such as application of a warm compress).

When removing a central venous catheter or a PICC, special precautions are taken to prevent complications related to air embolism and catheter breakage. To prevent air embolism, place the patient in the Trendelenburg position and remove the catheter while the patient performs Valsalva's maneuver. If resistance is felt while attempting to remove the catheter, stop the procedure and notify the physician. Immediately after catheter removal, cover the site with an occlusive dressing, which should remain in place for 24 to 72 hours. Inspect the integrity of the catheter after removal. The catheter tip should be sent to the laboratory for culture if infection is suspected. Document the procedure.

ADMINISTERING INTRAVENOUS MEDICATIONS

IV medications may be administered by IV push (bolus), intermittent infusion, and continuous infusion.

Intermittent Infusion Technique

The intermittent infusion technique is used to administer IV medications that need to be infused for an intermediate length of time (usually 20 to 60 minutes). Medications administered by intermittent infusion are supplied either in bags that contain 50 to 250 mL of IV fluid (0.9 normal saline or 5% dextrose in water) or in 20- to 60-mL syringes to be used with an infusion pump. The pharmacist prepares the medication and labels the bag or syringe with the patient's name and medical record number, medication name, type of IV fluid or diluent, and suggested infusion rate (**Procedure 21-7**). When administering IV medication, be sure of the following:

- The medication supplied is the medication ordered.
- The medication, as ordered, is safe for the patient.
- The IV catheter is patent (i.e., the catheter is still in the vein, the catheter is not clogged, and the catheter site is not reddened or swollen).
- The medication is infused at the proper rate and time.

Intravenous Push (Bolus) Technique

The IV push (bolus) technique is used to administer medications that are given over one minute for rapid therapeutic effect. IV push medications can be given into a continuous infusing IV or into a capped IV port. See **Procedure 21-8**.

 SAFETY ALERT
Research the infusion rate recommended by the manufacturer prior to administration as too rapid infusion can cause serious, even lethal complications. Because of the potential risks associated with IV push medications, they are generally not performed independently by students.

Continuous Infusion Technique

The continuous infusion technique is used to infuse medications that must be given continuously to achieve the desired effect (e.g., vasopressors, dobutamine, dopamine) and medications that are toxic if given over short periods (e.g., cisplatin, potassium). Medications ordered by continuous infusion are supplied in IV bags containing 250 to 1,000 mL of IV fluid. Generally, students will not be administering these medications independently because of the high risks associated with them.

SAFETY ALERT
Agency protocols require the use of smart pumps or at least an EID for administration of continuous IV medications.

The machines can be programmed to deliver a set volume of IV fluid over a specific time frame, usually a certain number of milliliters per hour. Smart pumps have preset limits that increase safety by preventing too rapid infusion of medication. Controlled delivery is important to prevent overdose of IV medication. The machines also have audible alarms that temporarily stop the infusion while simultaneously alerting the nurse to check the system. The alarm will be set off if there is air in the tubing or an occlusion (kinked tubing, clot formation at the catheter tip, bent catheter), if the infusion is complete, and if the bag is empty.

Patient-Controlled Analgesia

PCA devices permit patients to administer opiates intravenously as needed for pain control. A PCA device is programmed electronically to deliver a set amount of pain medication through a prefilled syringe connected to an IV tubing. Specific dosages and time intervals can be programmed into the machine to prevent overdose; medication is delivered when the patient pushes a control button. Refer to Chapter 35 for more information on PCA.

Epidural Analgesia

Pain medication also can be administered through a catheter that has been placed in the epidural space that surrounds the spinal cord. Opiates and local anesthetic agents can be administered to manage pain during labor and delivery or during the postoperative period. The infusion can be set on a continuous rate (basal mode) or an intermittent mode controlled by the patient (patient-controlled epidural analgesia [PCEA]). Refer to Chapter 35 for more information on epidural analgesia.

LIFE SPAN CONSIDERATIONS

Newborn and Infant

Newborns and infants present the nurse with unique challenges regarding IV therapy. Their veins are tiny and are difficult to locate and cannulate. Umbilical veins may be used

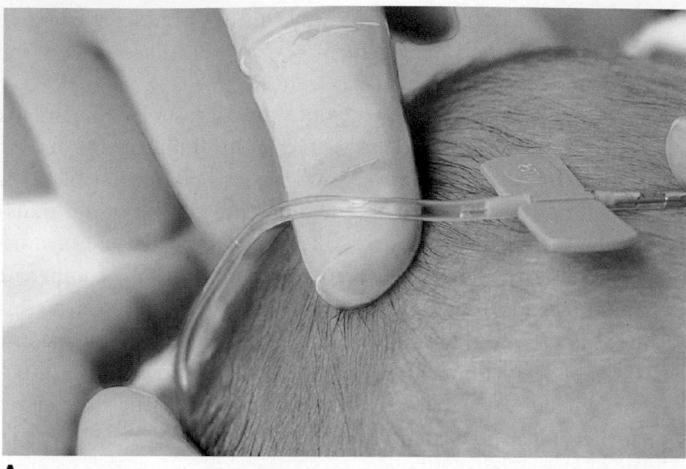
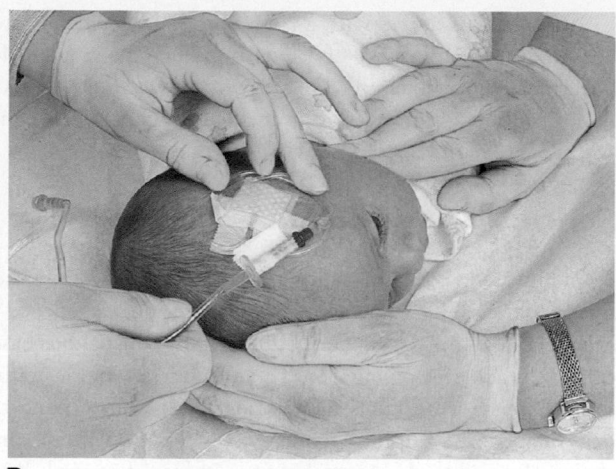

FIGURE 21-17 Site of IV therapy in infants. **A.** Butterfly scalp vein needles are used in infants. **B.** The nurse monitors the patency of the infant's scalp vein infusion site.

for neonates and can be used for up to 14 days (O'Grady, 2011). For infants younger than 9 months, scalp veins in the temporal region are often used (Fig. 21-17). IV therapy delivered into a scalp vein can prove very upsetting for parents, so provide teaching, support, and comfort. Never ask parents to restrain a baby but allow them to comfort the child during or after the procedure. Secure the IV site well so that the parents can hold and comfort the infant without fear of dislodging the IV.

Administering IV medications can pose challenges not encountered with adults. Small-volume catheters are essential to ensure that all of the medication is infused and not retained in the catheter or tubing. In addition, flushing of the catheters, if multiple medications are given, can contribute to volume overload. The amount of fluid used for flushing must be included when calculating the infant's total fluid requirements. To minimize risk of fluid overload, the volume of the solution container is based on the age and size of the child as well as the child's 24-hour fluid needs. IV solutions in 250- and 500-mL containers may be used instead of the 1-L containers used for adults. Additionally, small-volume buretrols may be used in addition to EID to protect against inadvertent volume infusion. Due to the small lumen size of catheters used in pediatrics, occlusion is a potential complication, especially for central venous catheters that are used intermittently. These catheters are usually flushed twice a day with saline, followed by a flush with 10 units per milliliter of heparin (Kramer, Doellman, Curley, & Wall, 2013). Refer to agency and manufacturer policies for further detail.

> **SAFETY ALERT**
>
> For very young patients, always use an EID for continuous IV infusions because too rapid an infusion of fluid could be lethal.

Toddler and Preschooler

After explaining the IV insertion procedure to parents, ask them if they would like to stay. The parent's presence is for the child's comfort; their role is not to restrain the child. Be honest in explanations to the young child, and provide information in terms that she or he can understand (Breiner, 2009).

The child's room, whether at home or in the hospital, should be a place where the child can feel safe and comfortable. For this reason, perform painful or unpleasant procedures in a different room.

Selecting appropriate IV sites for children can be a challenge. Avoiding the areas over joints is important because of children's increased activity level. Since infants and young children have very small veins, IV sites may include the metacarpal and cephalic veins in the upper extremities and the dorsalis pedis and great saphenous veins in the lower extremities. Use small-gauge catheters and monitor IV infusions with an EID. Smiley faces or stickers can be placed close to the IV site. A security device, such as an IV house, can help protect the site from bumping and tugging (Fig. 21-18).

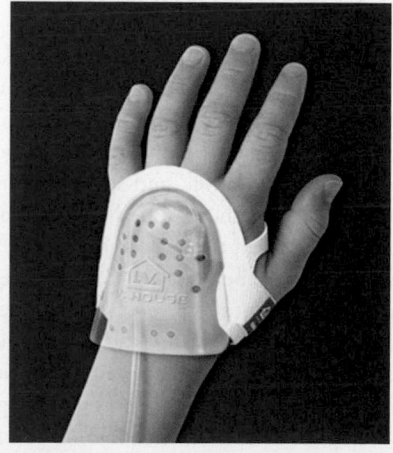

FIGURE 21-18 IV house over the IV site on a child's hand.

Intraosseous access with a large-bore rigid needle inserted into the medullary cavity of a long bone may be required for the critically injured child who needs emergency fluid, medication, or blood administration if adequate venous access is not accessible (Kleinman et al., 2010).

School-Age Child or Adolescent

Fear of invasive procedures, such as injections or IVs, is common for the older child, who may have had previous experience or heard about it from classmates. Individualize explanations based on the child's developmental level and readiness. Demonstrating the procedure using dolls or coloring books that outline the treatment can be helpful. Giving the child or adolescent some choice, if possible, decreases the sense of loss of control. Body image is very important for the adolescent, and IV treatment, especially with long-term catheters, can be stressful.

Adult and Older Adult

The older adult patient receiving IV therapy requires special care because of the normal age-related changes in the skin and vessels. As people age, subcutaneous fat and elasticity decrease, the dermis thins, and the collagen tissue diminishes. The veins become more fragile, appear tortuous, and are likely to roll. These changes require the nurse to alter the insertion technique.

Using a tourniquet may cause blood to leak around the puncture site into surrounding tissue. The older adult patient's veins might fill sufficiently for the IV start simply by placing the patient's arm in a dependent position without using a tourniquet. To stabilize the large, tortuous veins during IV insertion, apply tension or downward pressure on the vein below the insertion site. Avoid using veins in the feet and lower extremities; impaired circulation at those sites increases the potential for complications. To prevent tearing fragile skin, take special care with the site dressing and tape. Older people, especially those with poor cardiac or renal function, are prone to fluid overload. Frequent cardiovascular assessment during infusions and the use of EIDs are essential.

Cultural Considerations

Culturally sensitive care is an expected competency for all healthcare professionals. Many factors influence how closely an individual identifies with his or her cultural or ethnic group. Some of these include gender, age, generation, primary language spoken at home, degree of acculturation, and socioeconomic status. It is particularly helpful to gather cultural information at admission. If language is a barrier, the use of well-trained interpreters is imperative. Family members should not interpret because of their own biases. The patient should always be addressed directly, and the interpreter will then transmit the patient's response.

There may be cultural differences in expression of pain. This may be an important consideration during venipuncture for IV therapies. People from different cultures may be stoic and silent during painful procedures, or they may be very expressive. The culturally sensitive nurse would be attentive to prevention and management of pain regardless of how the patient manifests the pain experience.

Individual cultural and religious practice, such as in patients who are Jehovah's Witnesses, may contraindicate the use of blood components. Jehovah's Witnesses believe that blood is sacred and represents life. Their religion prohibits the transfusion of blood or blood products. However, the use of nonblood alternatives may be acceptable. The culturally competent nurse recognizes that adult patients have the right to make this choice. However, for minors, the physician may obtain a court order to allow administration of blood or blood products, especially for lifesaving situations. Bloodless treatment alternatives are available and a suitable option.

TPN AND PPN

Parenteral nutrition is a form of nutritional support that supplies protein, carbohydrate, fat, electrolytes, vitamins, minerals, and fluids to patients who are unable to assimilate nutrients from the gastrointestinal tract.

TPN constitutes a hyperosmolar solution exceeding 10% dextrose and/or 5% protein. TPN must be administered through a central venous catheter. Peripheral parenteral nutrition (PPN) contains the same components as TPN except the final concentrations are dextrose 10% or lower and/or protein 5% or lower. This provides a formula that is less than 900 mOsm per liter to prevent thrombosis of the peripheral vein. Because PPN contains a lower concentration of dextrose and protein, it provides fewer calories than does TPN and is used more commonly for supplemental nutrition.

The indications for parenteral nutrition have greatly expanded since the 1960s when Dudrick first demonstrated the efficacy of parenteral nutrition in pediatric populations with short gut and failure to thrive conditions (Dudrick, Wilmore, Vars, & Rhoads, 1968). Malnutrition is a serious problem for hospitalized patients (Butterworth, 1994). Currently, parenteral nutrition is indicated when enteral nutrition is contraindicated or when enteral nutrition is not meeting the patient's nutrition requirements. Enteral nutrition is always preferred to parenteral nutrition whenever possible (Cahill, Dhaliwal, Day, Jiang, & Heyland, 2010). A comprehensive nutritional assessment of all patients is recommended as a means to screen for patients who are malnourished or are nutritionally at risk. Early identification of patients at risk for malnutrition is especially important because compromised nutritional status decreases the patient's ability to respond to metabolic stress and impairs the immune system (Sriram & Mizock, 2010). The laboratory evaluation of serum albumin, prealbumin, or transferrin and total lymphocyte count and assessment of body mass index (BMI), height, and weight are indicators of the patient's current nutritional status (Jensen, 2015). The four key steps before starting parenteral nutrition are as follows:

- Assessing the patient's nutritional status
- Determining the patient's energy needs

- Evaluating gastrointestinal function
- Estimating the duration of required therapy

Chapter 29 further discusses nutritional assessment.

TPN solutions contain essential nutrients, including protein, carbohydrates, electrolytes, vitamins, water, and trace elements. The proportion of each ingredient is individualized based on the patient's clinical condition. The carbohydrate source is often a 50% dextrose solution. Protein is provided as synthetic crystalline amino acids. The patient's caloric need is assessed carefully to provide the number of calories required to maintain an anabolic state. Electrolytes, vitamins, and trace elements are added based on laboratory assays. Additionally, some common medications, such as histamine blockers and insulin, can be added to the parenteral nutrition solutions. Compatibility data should be evaluated carefully before adding any medications to parenteral nutrition solutions.

To supply all necessary nutrients, a 10% to 20% lipid emulsion, derived from egg yolks and soy or safflower oil, is often given with TPN. Intralipids are milky in appearance, are compatible with TPN, and can be infused simultaneously. Single-solution containers with admixtures of dextrose, amino acids, and lipid emulsions are also available.

Administration

TPN must be administered through central venous access because it is a hyperosmolar solution. Irritation and sclerosing of the vein and sudden fluid shifts are less likely to occur when the hypertonic solutions are infused into large vessels with rapid blood flow and dilution. When TPN is a short-term intervention (less than 4 weeks), the subclavian and jugular veins are commonly used. When TPN is anticipated for an extended period (greater than 4 weeks), a long-term catheter (PICC line, tunneled catheter, or an implanted vascular access device) may be placed.

TPN and PPN must be administered through tubing with an in-line filter and monitored with an EID (INS, 2011). A 0.2-μm filter is sufficient for administering solutions without lipid additives. The lipids then are administered through separate tubing attached below the filter of the main IV administration set to prevent separation of the emulsified fats in solution. If placed above the filter, the large particles of fat will clog the TPN filter.

When TPN therapy is initiated, the solution is administered to provide nutrition at a consistent rate over 24 hours. The use of an EID ensures an accurate rate of administration. The parenteral solution and tubing are changed every 24 hours to decrease the risk of microbial growth (INS, 2011). See **Procedure 21-9** for more information.

Parenteral nutrition is discontinued gradually. If the infusion is terminated abruptly, hypoglycemia may develop due to the continued release of insulin from the pancreas (INS, 2011). Dextrose 10% may be administered to prevent rebound hypoglycemia, which includes symptoms of weakness, diaphoresis, shakiness, faintness, or confusion (Smeltzer et al., 2014).

Cycling Parenteral Infusions

After the patient has stabilized in tolerance of the TPN therapy, the physician may prescribe a cyclic infusion. **Cycling**, or the interruption of infusion for a period of time, may be used for patients to permit increased freedom for activities of daily living, because nutrition is delivered during sleeping hours (Stout & Cober, 2011). Orders and regimens for cycling vary but usually mean that the patient receives a 24-hour volume of TPN during a 10- to 14-hour period. Some providers may order a ramping schedule for cycling TPN. A ramping schedule allows the administration rate to begin slowly over 2 hours, reach and sustain the peak hourly rate over a period of time, and then decrease slowly over the last 2 hours of the infusion. Tapering the TPN rate allows the body's endogenous insulin production to increase or decrease as the body's biofeedback system dictates. Abrupt discontinuation of TPN in adults has been shown to produce a decrease in blood glucose; however, symptoms of hypoglycemia have not been report in the studies (Stout & Cober, 2011). In contrast, abrupt discontinuation of TPN in children less than 2 to 3 years old has been associated with increased incidence of hypoglycemia compared to tapering the infusion over 1 hour (Stout & Cober, 2011).

Complications of Total Parenteral Nutrition

Patients receiving parenteral nutrition are at risk for various complications. Many potentially serious complications, such as pneumothorax and air embolism, are associated with central line placement and have been discussed previously. Other complications include infection, fluid overload, and metabolic alterations.

INFECTION

Infection is a potentially serious complication of parenteral nutrition due to the high dextrose concentration, which readily supports microbial growth. Prevention of infection at the site and in the solution is accomplished by using strict aseptic technique during catheter manipulations, dressing changes, and tubing and bottle changes. TPN solutions are prepared under laminar flow hoods in the pharmacy to further decrease microbial contamination. Before hanging a new container, observe the solution for any changes in color or cloudiness. Assess the insertion site frequently. Document any inflammation at the site, and culture any drainage.

> **SAFETY ALERT**
>
> When using a multilumen central venous catheter, keep one lumen dedicated strictly for administering parenteral nutrition. Never draw blood, administer other medications, or take central venous pressure measurements through the TPN lumen. The infusate bag and tubing should be changed every 24 hours (INS, 2012).

Patients receiving TPN are often immune compromised as a result of malnutrition; these patients are highly susceptible to infections. The infection's origin may be catheter-related sepsis. If the patient spikes a temperature during TPN therapy, blood cultures are usually drawn to evaluate for sepsis. If the fever source cannot be identified, the catheter may be removed and cultured. There is also increasing opinion that the use of parenteral nutrition may predispose patients to an increased risk of noncatheter-related infection because they are not being fed enterally. This predisposition is thought to be related to changes in intestinal morphology and increased permeability of the intestinal mucosa due to lack of nutrients passing through the gut. The increased permeability allows translocation of endotoxins and bacteria from the gut to cross into the vascular system. To prevent sepsis from this cause, nutritional support administered by way of the enteral route is recommended whenever possible (De Aguilar-Nascimento, Dock-Nascimento, & Bragagnolo, 2010).

FLUID OVERLOAD

Fluid overload can occur if the hyperosmolar solution is infused too quickly, which may draw fluid into the circulatory system. Risk is increased for patients who have a history of congestive heart failure or renal insufficiency. Always use an EID to regulate TPN infusions, and avoid sudden shifts in fluid rate. Monitor fluid balance through serum electrolytes, daily weights, lung auscultation, and intake and output measurements.

METABOLIC COMPLICATIONS

Metabolic complications also may present a problem for the patient receiving TPN. Most commonly, patients experience hyperglycemia if they are unable to tolerate the high glucose content of the TPN solution. When therapy is initiated, the infusion rate is usually tapered up over a period of a day or two. Blood glucose is monitored every 6 hours or before meals, if eating, and insulin is administered as needed. Hypoglycemia may occur when the TPN is discontinued, especially if the infusion rate is not tapered gradually. Assess electrolytes daily to detect and treat imbalances of potassium, sodium, calcium, magnesium, phosphate, and trace minerals. Lipid emulsions may cause reactions, especially in patients who are allergic to eggs. If the patient experiences fever, chills, vomiting, chest pain, or rash, alert the physician and nutrition support team to evaluate if discontinuation is needed.

BLOOD TRANSFUSION

Blood **transfusion** refers to the introduction of whole blood or blood components (packed red cells, plasma, platelets) directly into a patient's circulatory system. Transfusions are given primarily to improve the oxygen-carrying capacity of the blood, restore coagulation factor deficiencies, increase the number of circulating platelets, and increase WBCs to decrease the chance of infection.

Blood Components

The components of blood include whole blood, packed RBCs, WBCs, platelets, fresh frozen plasma (FFP), and albumin. Each component has unique requirements for storage and processing to maximize the longevity of the cells and factors.

WHOLE BLOOD

Whole blood contains all blood components and is rarely transfused since patients can be successfully treated with component therapy. However, it may be transfused to patients who need both RBCs and volume replacement to reverse the effects of hypothermia, acidosis, and coagulopathy or after significant blood loss related to disasters or wartime injury (Cassella, Appenzeller, & Stich, 2009).

RED BLOOD CELLS

RBC component contain a concentration of RBCs with most plasma removed. A unit of RBCs provides the same oxygen-carrying capacity as whole blood but without the volume. RBCs do not provide viable platelets or provide significant amounts of coagulation factors (Gernsheimer, 2010). Problems of fluid overload and electrolyte imbalances can be avoided because packed cells contain less volume and also less sodium and potassium. Current guidelines recommend adhering to a restrictive transfusion practice, with the goal of minimizing exposure to allogenic blood and minimizing potential reactions (Carson, 2012). These guidelines from the AABB, formerly American Association of Blood Banks are based on the patient's hemoglobin levels, clinical symptoms and comorbidities (Carson et al., 2012). The recommendations are summarized in Table 21-4. To prevent an allergic response, RBCs can be washed to remove most antibodies from the cells. Decisions to transfusion RBC in infants and children is based on indications similar to adults,

TABLE 21-4 RED BLOOD CELL—CLINICAL PRACTICE TRANSFUSION GUIDELINES FROM THE AABB	
Patients	Recommendations
Hospitalized, stable patients	The AABB recommends adhering to a restrictive transfusion policy based on hemoglobin 7–9 g/dL.
Hospitalized, patients with preexisting cardiovascular disease	Consider transfusion for patients who are clinically symptomatic or have hemoglobin 8 g/dL or less.
Hospitalized, hemodynamically stable patients with acute coronary syndrome	The AABB cannot recommend for or against either liberal or restrictive transfusion policy, due to in conclusive evidence.
All patients	Transfusion decisions should be influenced by clinical symptoms as well as hemoglobin levels.

Source: Carson et al. (2012).

such as blood volume, hemoglobin levels appropriate for the age group, and the ability to tolerate blood (AABB, 2010).

WHITE BLOOD CELLS

WBCs, also called granulocytes, can be administered to patients with a low or abnormal WBC count. Infusion of white cells may be indicated for infections that are unresponsive to antibiotic therapy (AABB, 2010). They are given to patients with cancer who have low white cell counts due to chemotherapy or the effects of the cancer.

PLATELETS

Platelet transfusions consist of platelet concentrates and platelet-rich plasma. The major function of platelets is to participate in blood clotting and hemostasis. One common indication for platelet transfusion is thrombocytopenia following chemotherapy. Platelets must be maintained at room temperature and agitated during storage (Gernsheimer, 2010).

FRESH FROZEN PLASMA

FFP is administered to provide clotting factors to patients with coagulation deficiencies who are bleeding or about to undergo an invasive procedure. One unit of FFP is approximately 250 mL and must be ABO compatible.

FACTOR CONCENTRATES (CRYOPRECIPITATE)

Cryoprecipitate is a plasma protein rich in fibrinogen and blood clotting factor VIII. Cryoprecipitate may be pooled from several units of blood and administered to patients with fibrinogen deficiencies who are predisposed to bleeding problems because genetically they lack factor VIII. Commercially prepared factor VIII concentrates are also available in a powder purified from human plasma. The concentrate is treated with heat or detergent solvent to reduce the risk of virus transmission. Alternatively, a synthetic protein purified from genetically engineered nonhuman cells is available for transfusion. Cryoprecipitate is indicated for patients with low platelets who are either bleeding or immediately prior to an invasive procedure (Gernsheimer, 2010).

ALBUMIN

Albumin is a plasma protein contained within the plasma. It is used to restore intravascular volume and to maintain cardiac output in patients with hypoproteinemia. Another advantage of albumin is that, unlike whole plasma, it carries no risk of hepatitis transmission and may be given without regard to the patient's ABO group or Rh factor. It is available in 5% or 25% concentrations (Smeltzer et al., 2014).

Blood Compatibility

Blood typing refers to identifying the patient's blood group. Cross-matching (or compatibility testing) is the process of ensuring that the patient's blood group is compatible with the donor blood. Before administration, blood components are tested for infectious diseases and ABO typing (Smeltzer et al., 2014).

 SAFETY ALERT

Except in life-threatening circumstances, compatibility or cross-match testing is required on all RBC transfusions to ensure that donor blood is compatible with the patient's blood.

BLOOD GROUPS

Testing for antigens on the erythrocyte can determine ABO blood groups. The population can be divided into four blood groups: types A, B, AB, and O. The erythrocytes of a person in group A have the A antigen; group B, the B antigen; group AB, both A and B antigens; and group O, neither A nor B antigens. In addition to containing antigens, each blood group also houses naturally occurring antibodies (agglutinins) in the serum. Group A has anti-B antibodies, group B has anti-A antibodies, group AB has no A or B antibodies, and group O has anti-A and anti-B antibodies in the serum. Anti-A antibodies destroy A antigens, and anti-B antibodies destroy B antigens (AABB, 2010). This results in red cell destruction known as **hemolysis**. People with group O negative blood are often referred to as universal donors for packed cells because type O blood has neither A nor B antigens, and people with other blood types can safely receive it. Likewise, patients with AB positive blood are often referred to as universal recipients because the lack of antibodies enables transfusions from other blood groups to be accepted. The ABO blood groups are summarized in Table 21-5.

RH FACTOR

It is important to determine Rh factor before transfusion to prevent blood incompatibility. Five antigens in the Rh system, the most important of which is D, are located on the surface of the erythrocyte. The recognition of the D antigen means that the person is Rh positive (85% of Caucasian people), whereas the lack of this antigen means that the person is Rh negative

TABLE 21-5	ABO BLOOD GROUPS: ANTIGENS AND ANTIBODIES	
Blood Group	Antigens on Red Cells	Antibodies in Plasma
A	A	Anti-B
B	B	Anti-A
AB	A and B	No anti-A or anti-B thus universal recipient
O	No A or B	Anti-A and anti-B thus universal donor

(15% of Caucasian people). Antibodies against Rh factor do not occur naturally; those antibodies form only when Rh-negative blood is exposed to Rh-positive cells. After antibodies form, only on subsequent exposure to Rh-positive blood does a reaction (agglutination) occur where there is hemolysis of cells.

Rh factor is especially important in obstetrics. If an Rh-negative mother carries an Rh-positive fetus, antibodies can form in the mother's blood. If the mother should become pregnant again with an Rh-positive fetus, Rh antibodies can enter the circulation of the fetus and cause a hemolytic reaction. The mother receives RhoGAM, a commercial name for antibodies directed against Rh factor, after the first miscarriage, abortion, or pregnancy to prevent future problems.

Selection of Blood Donors

Nurses may be responsible for screening prospective blood donors and overseeing the blood collection process. The nurse is responsible for ensuring the safety of the blood donor and the blood recipient. To do this, the nurse interviews the prospective donor to rule out any history of hepatitis or recent hepatitis exposure, recent infectious exposure, syphilis or malaria, and recent immunizations and any recent blood component transfusions. The nurse also ascertains the donor's possible exposure to HIV through high-risk behaviors such as IV drug abuse or homosexual or bisexual activities. Screening ensures the safety of the blood supply by identifying high-risk people and preventing them from donating blood. To protect the blood donor, people cannot donate if they are pregnant or anemic, do not meet minimum weight restrictions, have abnormal blood pressure, or have given whole blood within the past 56 days.

Extensive testing procedures are used to screen the blood supply for viruses. Blood is tested for antibodies to HIV 1 and 2, hepatitis B and C, syphilis, cytomegalovirus, and the West Nile virus. The chance of the patient contracting AIDS through a blood transfusion has been reduced significantly because all blood is now screened for antibodies to HIV. Nevertheless, the viral screening may be unreliable if the donor is undergoing seroconversion. New, more sensitive nucleic acid amplification testing has reduced the risk of transfusion-transmitted HIV infection still further. The risk of transmission of HIV and hepatitis C is less than 1 in 1,900,000 and less than 1 in 1,000,000 units of blood, respectfully (Gernsheimer, 2010). The blood donor is not at risk for acquiring any infectious disease, including AIDS, because all blood is collected under strict aseptic conditions.

Transfusion Technique

Before administering any blood component, the nurse must understand correct administration technique and be aware of complications. **Procedure 21-10** lists steps for administering a blood transfusion.

Important considerations when administering blood components include obtaining informed consent, properly identifying

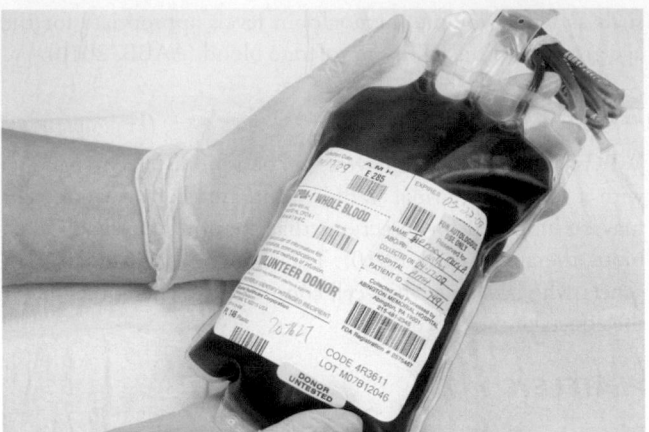

FIGURE 21-19 Example of a labeled blood component bag.

the intended recipient of the blood component unit, using a 150- to 260-μm standard blood filter, using only compatible IV solutions of normal saline to prevent cell hemolysis, and using a 20-gauge or larger IV catheter (INS, 2011). IV infusion pumps must be documented as safe for use with blood products. Proper identification of the patient using two identifiers with information on the labeled blood component bag is essential to prevent serious errors (Fig. 21-19). Two licensed providers are required; students are not allowed to perform these checks, but they may assist with assessment of vital signs and symptoms. Frequently assess the patient for signs of a transfusion reaction, which can range from mild to life threatening.

Complications of Blood Transfusion

Complications of blood transfusion include febrile reactions, allergic reactions, hemolytic reactions, transfusion-related acute lung injury, circulatory overload, and septic reactions.

FEBRILE REACTIONS

Febrile reactions to blood components can occur if the recipient is hypersensitive to antigens on cell components, particularly the leukocytes. The patient develops a fever and chills and may complain of headache and malaise. Sometimes, patients are given antipyretics before the transfusion to prevent shaking and chills. If symptoms occur after the infusion has started, stop the transfusion immediately and keep the IV open with normal saline. Notify the physician and the blood bank, and monitor vital signs. Leukocyte-reduced blood components can be ordered for patients with a history of febrile reactions.

ALLERGIC REACTIONS

Allergic reactions may occur if the patient is sensitive to donor plasma proteins. Symptoms include flushing, urticaria (hives), wheezing, and a rash with itching. Once again, stop the transfusion, keep open the IV with normal saline, and notify the physician. An antihistamine may be ordered to decrease the severity of the reaction and to make the patient more comfortable. If hives are the only manifestation, the physician may elect to continue the infusion at a slower rate. Monitor the patient carefully for manifestations of a more severe reaction, which could cause respiratory difficulty. Washed RBCs or platelets should be ordered for all patients with a history of severe (anaphylactic) allergic reactions. Premedication with antihistamines may also be prescribed.

HEMOLYTIC REACTIONS

Acute hemolytic transfusion reactions, the most serious of the acute complications, although rare, can be life threatening. A **hemolytic transfusion reaction** occurs if the donor's blood is incompatible with the recipient's blood. This may occur if even a small amount of incompatible blood is mistakenly administered to a patient. Hemolysis, or destruction of RBCs, occurs when the antibodies in the recipient's blood quickly react to the donor's blood cells. The resultant clumping or agglutination of RBCs obstructs the capillaries, disrupting the flow of blood and oxygen to vital organs. Free hemoglobin from the ruptured RBCs may block renal tubules, resulting in renal failure. Symptoms, which are immediate, include facial flushing, fever, chills, headache, low back pain, tachycardia, dyspnea, hypotension, and blood in the urine. Prompt intervention is essential to prevent death.

The physician will order drugs to treat the hypotension and will have the patient monitored closely. Blood from the donor and recipient will be tested to assess whether a hemolytic reaction has occurred. A urine specimen may also be collected to determine if renal involvement is present.

> ### ! SAFETY ALERT
> Always monitor and record vital signs before starting the infusion and during the first 5 minutes, when the blood is infusing slowly. A transfusion should be stopped immediately whenever a transfusion reaction is suspected and the IV site kept open for venous access if needed (Gernsheimer, 2010; INS, 2011).

TRANSFUSION-RELATED ACUTE LUNG INJURY (TRALI)

Transfusion-related acute lung injury (TRALI) is the number one cause of patient death related to blood transfusion in the United States (Clark, 2009). The term *TRALI* was identified in 1983 following a landmark study that reviewed reports of severe respiratory symptoms following blood transfusions (Popovski, Abel, & Moore, 1983). TRALI is thought to occur when the donor plasma contains an antibody against the patient's leukocyte-specific antigen (Gernsheimer, 2010). It occurs most frequently following transfusion with blood products containing plasma, particularly FFP (Casey, 2011). TRALI is suspected when symptoms of dyspnea, hypotension, and fever develop within 30 minutes to 6 hours following a blood transfusion and the chest radiograph shows diffuse infiltrates (Gernsheimer, 2010). Additionally, the patient has

new-onset symptoms of noncardiac pulmonary edema, tachycardia, tachypnea, and severe hypoxia (Casey, 2011; Clark, 2009). Aggressive therapy with ventilatory support, oxygen, and fluids is often required.

TRANSFUSION-ASSOCIATED CIRCULATORY OVERLOAD

Transfusion-associated circulatory overload (TACO) can occur if blood components are infused too quickly or too voluminously. Transfusion-associated circulatory overload is more likely in the very young patient or the older adult with poor cardiac or renal function. Symptoms include increased venous pressure, distended neck veins, dyspnea, coughing, and abnormal breath sounds. Circulatory overload can be minimized by infusing packed RBCs (rather than whole blood) and volume-reduced platelets for high-risk patients and carefully monitoring the infusion rate of blood components. If circulatory overload is suspected, stop the infusion of blood, position the patient in an upright position with feet dependent, and notify the physician.

SEPTIC REACTIONS

Septic reactions can occur if bacteria have contaminated the blood components. These reactions are most often seen in patients receiving contaminated single-donor apheresis platelet transfusions because all platelets are stored at room temperature (20°C to 24°C) for as long as 5 days. The patient will likely have a rapid onset of fever and chills and perhaps vomiting, diarrhea, and hypotension. If this occurs, stop the transfusion, keep the IV open, and notify the physician. To minimize the risk of bacterial growth within the blood component, refrigerate RBCs and thawed FFP until used and then infuse them within 4 hours (AABB 2010; INS, 2011). The longer blood components remain at room temperature, the more likely bacteria will grow and multiply.

HOME AND COMMUNITY CARE

Home IV therapy and nutritional support have become a thriving part of the home care industry during recent decades. Long-term antibiotic therapies, once given only in the acute care facility, are administered frequently in the home setting, thus allowing patients to avoid long hospital stays. The ability to provide home IV and nutritional support has increased because of advances in IV catheter materials, placement techniques, and the simplicity and portability of EIDs.

Planning for home IV or nutritional support requires a careful assessment of the patient, family/caregiver, and home environment. Patients receive their medications or TPN solutions at home with the support of an interdisciplinary team, including the physician, nurse, dietitian, and pharmacist. Successful home therapy depends on the following: medical stability, emotional stability, the patient's lifestyle, intellectual ability, the patient or primary caregiver's visual acuity and manual dexterity, and evaluation of the home environment.

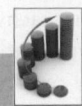

OUTCOME-BASED TEACHING PLANS

Mr. Tambuli is being discharged home after treatment for a serious bone infection. He requires IV antibiotic therapy for 4 more weeks. Mr. Tambuli has a PICC line in place. He and his wife will be caring for the PICC line and administering the antibiotics through it at home.

OUTCOME

Before discharge, Mr. Tambuli and his wife can demonstrate safe care and flushing of the PICC line.

STRATEGIES

- Assess Mr. and Mrs. Tambuli's readiness to learn, cognitive ability, and psychomotor dexterity.
- Provide the Tambulis with a pamphlet about PICC line care, using the illustrations to explain where the catheter is placed and why it is important to use strict asepsis and prevent any air from entering the system.
- Ask them to read the pamphlet together, and then review it with them.
- Arrange for a time with the Tambulis to demonstrate how to flush the catheter using aseptic technique.
- Verbally list the steps as they are completed. Provide them with a written list of steps to review. Allow them time to practice with additional equipment.
- Have both Mr. and Mrs. Tambuli demonstrate the flushing procedure repeatedly until they voice comfort and confidence with the procedure.
- Positively reinforce behaviors; answer questions and provide feedback as necessary.

OUTCOME

Before discharge, Mr. Tambuli and his wife will demonstrate safe administration of antibiotics through the PICC catheter.

STRATEGIES

- Review their knowledge of the PICC catheter.
- Discuss the antibiotic ordered, how it is to be prepared, and frequency of IV administration.
- Develop a schedule for administration based on their usual daily routine.
- When you administer Mr. Tambuli's IV antibiotic, verbally list the steps as you complete them.

- Provide a written list of information about the medication and the procedure of administering it IV through a PICC line. Allow them time to practice with equipment.
- Ask Mr. and Mrs. Tambuli to describe the procedure with administration of next dose.
- Have both Mr. and Mrs. Tambuli demonstrate administration of the IV antibiotic until they can voice comfort and confidence with the procedure.
- Give positive feedback and repeat instructions as necessary.

OUTCOME

Mr. and Mrs. Tambuli can verbalize when to call for help and how to contact the IV home management company should the need arise.

STRATEGIES

- Provide Mr. and Mrs. Tambuli with the phone number of the IV home management agency that will be working with them after discharge and with the name of the nurse who will manage their care. (*Note:* Often, this nurse does the IV teaching while the patient is still in the hospital.)
- Review the signs and symptoms of possible complications that may occur.
- Provide written guidelines for complications that require notification of this nurse (inability to flush the line, redness or pain at the site, signs of infection).
- Provide the Tambulis with some hypothetical problems that might occur, and ask them to discuss what they would do.
- Ask if the Tambulis have any questions, and encourage them to call if they have any questions or concerns.

EVALUATION

8/12/17: 04:00—Following the teaching session, Mrs. Tambuli flushed the catheter while Mr. Tambuli read the directions for flushing aloud. She washed her hands before the flushing and maintained asepsis. She administered the 10 AM antibiotic with cuing from the nurse. Plan to have her repeat once or twice before discharge. A home care nurse will visit on day of discharge.

—S. Roberts, RN

Patient Teaching

Patient education is a vital component of effective home infusion therapy and reduces the risk of infusion-related complications. Although the patient will be monitored at home by the home care nurse, the patient is responsible for living day to day

with the infusion device and is likely to be participating in self-infusion and dressing changes. Training should include written instructions and demonstration/return demonstration in aseptic technique, preparation and storage of solutions, operation of the infusion device, self-monitoring, detection of complications, and troubleshooting. The patient and family's readiness to learn and limitations must be assessed. Encourage the patient or caregiver to have a plan in place about handling equipment malfunctions or problems with IV therapy. Telephone numbers for the supplier and nurse should be provided. Developing hypothetical problems and asking the patient to think of solutions is a good method of evaluating problem-solving abilities and skills.

Monitoring

The patient receiving home IV or nutritional support is monitored by both a home care nurse and the physician. It is best if the home care nurse is present to start the initial nutritional support at home, set up all equipment, and make sure that all supplies, including glucose monitoring equipment, are present. This is an opportunity to teach the patient to watch for symptoms that she or he needs to report to the physician. The patient and/or caregiver must learn to detect and report fever, catheter redness, or any unusual symptoms. Catheter-related bloodstream infection is the most common major complication for patients receiving home TPN (Santarpia et al., 2010), although the overall risk of infection in patients receiving home infusion therapy is lower than inpatient settings (Gorski, Hankins, & Perucca, 2010).

The frequency of monitoring varies widely. Stable long-term patients need infrequent laboratory studies and monthly measurement of weight, whereas other patients may require weekly intake and output measurements and more frequent laboratory studies. Outcomes of nutritional support therapy are an important focus of monitoring. Often, a patient is taught to keep a record that can be evaluated by the healthcare team. The regimen's nutritional adequacy and the patient's weight gain are included as objective outcome measures.

KEY CONCEPTS

- Homeostasis of body fluids, electrolytes, and nutrition may need to be supported through the use of IV therapy, parenteral nutrition, or transfusions.
- Venous access devices include peripheral access devices, central access devices (single- or multilumen devices, PICC, tunneled catheters), and implanted ports.
- Strict asepsis must be used to avoid serious infection and possible sepsis when initiating or handling IVs.
- Important nursing interventions include teaching patients and initiating, regulating, monitoring, and discontinuing an IV infusion.
- Potential complications of IV therapy include infiltration, phlebitis, infection, air embolism, and fluid overload.
- TPN is a hypertonic solution administered through a central catheter that provides protein, carbohydrates, electrolytes, vitamins, and minerals. Lipids can also be given.
- Blood transfusions are administered to restore circulating volume, to improve the blood's oxygen-carrying capacity, to restore coagulation factors, and to increase WBC count to decrease the risk of infection.
- To prevent serious adverse reactions from blood administration, careful screening and matching of donor and recipient blood are necessary.

PRACTICING FOR THE NCLEX
CHECK YOUR ANSWERS IN APPENDIX A.

1. Which of the following are advantages to having a dedicated IV insertion team? Select all that apply:
   a. Assist unit staff
   b. Decrease complication rates
   c. Update IV policies and procedures
   d. Improve patient outcomes

2. A patient is hypotensive related to extensive bleeding in surgery. Which type of fluid would be most appropriate to administer to this patient?
   a. Hypertonic 3% saline (NaCl)
   b. Hypotonic D5W + ½ NaCl
   c. Isotonic lactated Ringer's (LR)
   d. Colloid total parenteral solution

3. A nurse is connecting an intermittent infusion of cefazolin antibiotic to a peripheral IV site. What should the nurse do first?
   a. Flush using pulsing, positive pressure
   b. Irrigate the line with 3 mL of sterile, preservative-free sodium chloride
   c. Wipe the needleless connector for 15 seconds with mechanical friction
   d. Flush with diluted heparin to prevent clotting in the line

4. A patient is receiving frequent blood draws and has poor venous access. Which type of line would be most appropriate to use for routine blood draws?
   a. Peripheral
   b. Midline
   c. Dialysis access
   d. PICC

5. A patient is receiving a chemotherapy drug that is a known vesicant. Which type of line is most appropriate? Select all that apply:
   a. Peripheral
   b. Midline
   c. Hickman catheter
   d. PICC

6. A nurse is discontinuing a peripherally inserted venous (PIV) line. She removes the tape and withdraws the catheter, noting that the catheter is jagged at the end. Which of the following complications has occurred?
   a. Infiltration
   b. Toxicity caused by a vesicant
   c. Air embolism
   d. Catheter breakage

7. A toddler is receiving continuous IV fluids. Which of the following precautions are recommended for this age group? Select all that apply:
   a. IV house
   b. No tourniquet
   c. EID
   d. Metacarpal or great saphenous veins

8. A patient is receiving cyclic infusions of TPN at night only. The nurse knows that the rationale behind this schedule is a result of which of the following facts?
   a. TPN must only be given in 12-hour shifts to prevent hyperglycemia.
   b. Night scheduling promotes independence of activities of daily living independent of the infusion pump.
   c. Metabolism of TPN is improved when the patient is sleeping.
   d. Fluid overload can occur if the patient has oral intake and TPN concurrently.

9. A patient is receiving a unit of RBCs for transfusion and begins to experience an itchy rash on her chest. Which of the following should the nurse do first?
   a. Notify the physician of a transfusion reaction
   b. Provide the patient with education on how to prevent future transfusion reactions
   c. Place a nonrebreather mask on the patient and start supplementary oxygen
   d. Stop blood administration infusion

10. A mother is pregnant with her second child and needs blood during the delivery. She is Rh negative, group O, and her first child was Rh positive, group A. Which nursing intervention is appropriate for blood administration to this patient?
    a. Administration of blood at a reduced rate to prevent fluid overload
    b. Administration of antihistamine drugs to prevent reaction
    c. Administration of RhoGAM to prevent hemolytic reaction
    d. Blood administration is not appropriate in this patient

REFERENCES

American Association of Blood Banks (AABB). (2010). *Primer of Blood Administration*. Bethesda, MD: American Association of Blood Banks.

Alexander, M., Corrigan, A., Gorski, L., Hankins, J., & Perucca, R. (2010). *Infusion Nurses Society infusion nursing an evidence-based approach* (3rd Ed.) St. Louis, MO: Saunders.

Breiner, S. M. (2009). Preparation of the pediatric patient for invasive procedures. *Journal of Infusion Nursing*, 32(5), 252–256.

Butterworth, C. E. (1994). The skeleton in the hospital closet. *Nutrition*, 10(5), 435–441.

Cahill, N. E., Dhaliwal, R., Day, A. G., Jiang, X., & Heyland, D. K. (2010). Nutrition therapy in the critical care setting: what is "best achievable" practice? An international multicenter observational study. *Critical Care Medicine*, 38(2), 395–401.

Carson, J. L., Grossman, B. J., Kleinman, S, Tinmouth, A. T., Marques, M. B., Fung, M. K., et al. (2012). Red blood cell transfusion: a clinical practice guideline from the AABB. *Annals of Internal Medicine*, 157(1), 49–58.

Casey, G. (2011). Blood transfusion: the high-risk life-saving therapy. *Kai Tiaki Nursing New Zealand*, 17(4), 21–25.

Cassella, D., Appenzeller, G., & Stich, J. (2009). From donor to patient in 21 minutes: emergency resuscitation with whole blood during operation Iraqi Freedom. *Critical Care Nurse*, 29(2), 27–32.

Clark, C. R. (2009). Transfusion-related acute lung injury clinical features and diagnostic dilemmas. *Journal of Infusion Nursing*, 32(3), 132–136.

De Aguilar-Nascimento, J. E., Dock-Nascimento, D. B., & Bragagnolo, R. (2010). Role of enteral nutrition and pharmaconutrients in conditions of splanchnic hypoperfusion. *Nutrition*, 26(4), 354–358.

Delahanty, K. M., & Myers, F. E. III. (2009). Nursing 2009 I.V. infection control survey report. *Nursing*, 29(12), 24–30.

US Food and Drug Administration. (2010). Infusion pump risk reduction strategies for home health nurses. http://www.fda.gov/Medical Devices/ProductsandMedicalProcedures/GeneralHospitalDevices andSupplies/InfusionPumps/ucm205411.htm. Accessed June 1, 2010.

Doellman, D., et al. (2009). Infiltration and extravasation: update of prevention and management. *Journal of Infusion Nursing*, 32(4), 203–211.

Dos Reis, P. E., Silveira, R. C., Vasques, C. I., & de Carvalho, E. C. (2009). Pharmacological interventions to treat phlebitis: systematic review. *Journal of Infusion Nursing*, 32(2), 74–79.

Dudrick, S. J., Wilmore, D. W., Vars, H. M., & Rhoads, J. E. (1968). Long-term total parenteral nutrition with growth, development, and positive nitrogen balance. *Surgery*, 64(1), 134–142.

Gernsheimer, T. (2010). *Blood component therapy 2010*. Seattle, WA: Puget Sound Blood Center.

Gilles, E., O'Riodan, E., Carr D., O'Brien, I., Frost, J., & Gunning, R. (2003). Central venous catheter dressings: a systematic review. *Journal of Advanced Nursing*, 44, 623–632.

Gilles, D., Wallen, M. M., Morrison, A. L., Rankin, K., Nagy, S. A., & O'Riordan, E. (2005). Optimal timing for intravenous administration set replacement. *Cochrane Database of Systematic Reviews*, (4):CD003588: Doi: 10.1002/14651858.CD003588.pub2.

Gorski, L. A. (2009a). Reducing the risk of air embolism. *Journal of Infusion Nursing*, 32(2), 71–72.

Gorski, L. A. (2009b). Standard 37: site selection. *Journal of Infusion Nursing*, 32(3), 125–126.

Gorski, L. A. (2009c). Standard 60: catheter clearance. *Journal of Infusion Nursing*, 32(5), 245–246.

Gorski, L., Perucca, R., Hunter, M. (2010). Central venous access devices: care, maintenance, and potential complications. In M. Alexander, A. Corrigan, L. Gorski, J. Hankins, R. Perucca, (Eds.). *Infusion nursing: An evidence-based approach* (3rd ed., pp. 495–515). St. Louis, MO: Saunders/Elsevier.

Hadaway, L. (2010). Infusion therapy equipment. In M. Alexander, A. Corrigan, L. Gorski, J. Hankins, R. Perucca, (Eds.). *Infusion nursing: An evidence-based approach* (3rd ed., pp. 391–436). St. Louis, MO: Saunders/Elsevier.

Hadaway, L. (2011). Needleless connectors: improving practice, reducing risks. *Journal of the Association for Vascular Access*, 16(1), 20–33.

Hertzel, C., & Sousa, V. D. (2009). The use of smart pumps for preventing medication errors. *Journal of Infusion Nursing*, 32(5), 257–267.

Hind, D., Calvert, N., McWilliams, R., et al. (2003). Ultrasonic locating devices for central venous cannulation: meta-analysis. *BMJ*, 327(7411), 361–375.

Infusion Nurses Society. (2011). Infusion nursing standards of practice. *Journal of Infusion Nursing*, 29(Supp1. 1), s1–s110.

Infusion Nurses Society (2011). Standards of practice. *Journal of Infusion Nursing*, 34(Suppl. 1):21–110.

INH Position Paper. (2010). The role of the registered nurse in determining distal tip placement of peripherally inserted central catheters by chest radiograph. *Journal of Infusion Nursing*, 33(1), 19–20.

INH Position Paper. (2012). Recommendations for frequency of assessment of the so I have no more current additions Peripheral Catheter Site. Retrieved June 29, 2014, from http://www.ins1.org/files/public/07_05_12_Assessment_Position_Paper_BOD_FINAL.pdf

Institute for Healthcare Improvement. (2014). *Implement the central line bundle.* Retrieved June 29, 2014, from www.ihi.org/resources/Pages/Changes/ImplementtheCentralLineBundle.aspx

Institute for Safe Medication Practices. (2007). Actions needed to prevent serious tissue injury with IV promethazine. *ISMP Newsletter*, 5(1), 1.

Institute for Safe Medication Practices. (2008). *ISMP's list of high-alert medications.* Retrieved April 4, 2010, from www.ismp.org/Tools/highalertmedications.pdf

Institute of Medicine. (1999). *To err is human: Building a safer health system.* Washington, DC: National Academies Press.

Jensen, S. K. (2015). *Nursing health assessment: A best practice approach* (2nd ed.). Philadelphia, PA: Lippincott Williams & Wilkins.

The Joint Commission. (2009). *National patient safety goals.* Retrieved April 3, 2010, from www.jointcommission.org/PatientSafety/NationalPatientSafetyGoals

The Joint Commission. (2014). Preventing Central Line–Associated Bloodstream Infections: Useful Tools, An International Perspective. Nov 21, 2013. Accessed 06/29/14, Care Medicine, 38(2), 690–691. Staun, M. http://www.jointcommission.org/CLABSIToolkit

Kaler, W., & Chinn, R. (2007). Successful disinfection of needleless access ports; A matter of time and friction. *Journal of the Association for Vascular Access*, 12(3), 140–142.

Ken, H. H., & Daphne, C. S. (2012). Guidelines on timing in replacing peripheral intravenous catheters. *Journal of Clinical Nursing*, 21, 1499–1506.

Kleinman, M. E., Chameides, L., Schexnayder, S. M., Samson, R. A., Hazinski, M. F., Atkins, D. L., et al. (2010). Part 14. Pediatric advanced life support 2010 American Heart Association Guidelines for Cardiopulmonary Resuscitation and Emergency Cardiovascular Care. *Circulation*, 122, 876.

Kramer, N., Doellman, D., Curley, M., & Wall, J. L. (2013). Central vascular access device guidelines for pediatric home-based patients: driving best practices. *JAVA*, 18(2), 103–113.

Longshore, L., Smith, T., & Weist, M. (2010). Successful implementation of intelligent infusion technology in a multihospital setting. *Journal of Infusion Nursing*, 33(1), 38–47.

Ludeman, K. (2007). Choosing the right vascular access device. *Nursing*, 37(9), 38–41.

McGoldrick, M. (2010). Infection prevention and control. In: M. Alexander, A. Corrigan, L. Gorski, et al. (Eds.) *Infusion Nurses' Society Infusion Nursing: An Evidence-Based Approach* (3rd ed., pp. 204–218). St. Louis, MO: Elsevier.

Mermel, L., Allon, M., Bourza, E., Craven, D. E., Flynn, P., O'Grady, N. P., et al. (2009). Clinical practice guidelines for the diagnosis and management of intravascular catheter related infection: 2009 update by the Infectious Diseases Society of America. *Clinical Infectious Diseases*, 49, 1–45.

Meyer, J. (2009). A broad-spectrum look at catheter-related blood stream infections. *Journal of Infusion Nursing*, 32(2), 80–86.

Mitchell, M., Anderson, B., Williams, K., & Umscheid, C. (2009). Heparin flush- ing and other interventions to maintain patency of central venous catheters: a systematic review. *Journal of Advanced Nursing*, 65(10), 2007–2021.

National Coordinating Council for Medication Error Reporting and Prevention. (2008). *What is a medication error?* Retrieved April 3, 2010, from www.nccmerp.org/aboutMedErrors.html

Neuman, R. W., Otto, E. W., Link, M. S., Kronick, S. L., Shuster, M., Callaway, C. W., et al. (2010). Part 8. Adult advanced life support 2010 American Heart Association Guidelines for Cardiopulmonary Resuscitation and Emergency Cardiovascular Care. *Circulation*, 122, 729.

O'Grady, N. P., Alexander, M., Burns, L. Q., Dellinger, E. P., Garland, J., Heard, S. T. et al. (2002). Guidelines for the prevention of intravascular catheter-related infections. *MMWR. Recommendations and Reports: Morbidity and Mortality Weekly Report*, 51(RR-10), 1–29.

O'Grady, N. P., Alexander, M., Burns, L. Q., Dellinger, E. P., Garland, J., Heard, S. T. et al. (2011). *Guidelines for the prevention of intravascular catheter-related infections.* The Healthcare Infection Control Practices Advisory Committee (HICPAC). http://www.cdc.gov/hicpac/pdf/guidelines/bsi-guidelines-2011.pdf accessed August 2015.

Popovski, M. A., Abel, M. D., & Moore, S. B. (1983). Transfusion-related acute lung injury associated with passive transfer of anti-leukocyte antibodies. *American Review of Respiratory Disease*, 128(1), 185–189.

Perucca, R. (2010). Peripheral vascular access devices. In M. Alexander, A. Corrigan, L. Gorski, J. Hankins, R. Perucca, (Eds.) *Infusion nursing: An evidence-based approach* (3rd ed., 456–479). St. Louis, MO: Saunders/Elsevier.

Phillips, L. D. (2010). *Manual of IV therapeutics: Evidence-based practice for infusion therapy* (5th ed., pp. 303–401). Philadelphia, PA: FA Davis.

Rosenthal, K. (2006). Guarding against vascular site infection. *Nursing Management*, 37(4), 54–67.

Ryder, M. A. (2005). Catheter-related infections: It's all about the biofilm. *Topics in Advanced Practice Nursing Journal*, 5(3).

Santarpia, L., Alfonsi, L., Tiseo, D., Creti, R., Baldassarri, L., Pasanisi, F., et al. (2010). Central venous catheter infections and antibiotic therapy during long-term home parenteral nutrition: an 11 year follow-up study. *JPEN, Journal of Parenteral & Enteral Nutrition*, 34(3), 364–362.

Smeltzer, S., Bare, B., Hinkle, J. L., & Cheever, K. H. (2014). *Brunner & Suddarth's textbook of medical-surgical nursing* (4th ed.). Philadelphia, PA: Lippincott Williams & Wilkins.

Sriram, K., & Mizock, B. A. (2010). Critical care nutrition: are the skeletons still in the closet? *Critical Care Medicine*, 38(2), 690–691.

Staun, M., Pironi, L., Bozzetti, F., Baxter, J., Forbes, A., Joly, F., et al. (2009). ESPEN guidelines on parenteral nutrition (HPN) in adult patients. *Clinical Nutrition*, 28(4), 467–479.

Stout, S. M., & Cober, M. P., (2011) Cyclic Parenteral Nutrition Infusion: Considerations for the Clinician. *Practical Gastroenterology*, 11–24.

Strandvik, G. F. (2009). Hypertonic saline in critical care: a review of the literature and guidelines for use in hypotensive states and raised intracranial pressure. *Anaesthesia*, 64, 990–1003.

Webster, J., Osborn, S., Rickard, C., & Hall, J. (2010). Clinically-indicated replacement versus routine replacement of peripheral venous catheters. *Cochrane Database of Systematic Reviews*, (3): CD007798. Doi: 10.1002/14651858.cd007798. PUB2.

Procedure 21-1 Initiating Intravenous Therapy

Purpose
1. To maintain or replace fluids for daily body fluid requirements
2. To provide electrolytes to maintain or restore electrolyte balance
3. To deliver glucose and nutrients for use as an energy source
4. To deliver medication or blood products

Equipment
Clean gloves
Tourniquet
IV access device
IV labels
IV start kit with chlorhexidine applicator or povidone–iodine swabs (if allergic to chlorhexidine)
IV solution
IV administration set and EID
Transparent semipermeable dressing
Tape (nonallergenic)
Towel or disposable pad
Topical or local anesthetic (according to agency policy)
Extension set tubing, if necessary

Assessment
- Review the patient's medical record for allergies and disease history; note vital signs, intake and output record, and any pertinent laboratory tests that may affect therapy.
- Review physician's order for type and amount of IV solution, infusion rate, and any additives that may be ordered, and compare with the solution on hand.
- Determine whether EID is needed to carefully regulate infusion rate.
- Inspect the container and solution for intactness and clarity.
- Assess the patient's understanding about the need for IV therapy. Ask the patient about previous IV therapy administration and previous history of IV device insertions. Ascertain the patient's dominant extremity. Inspect the patient's nondominant extremity for an appropriate insertion site.

Procedure

1. **Verify the physician's order for IV therapy including solution type, amount, additives, and infusion rate.**
   Rationale: Confirms that the patient will receive the correct solution and prevents medication errors
2. **Gather all equipment and bring it to the patient's bedside.**
   Rationale: Enhances efficiency
3. **Perform hand hygiene.**
   Rationale: Reduces microbe transmission

4. **Identify the patient using two separate identifiers (Fig. 1).**

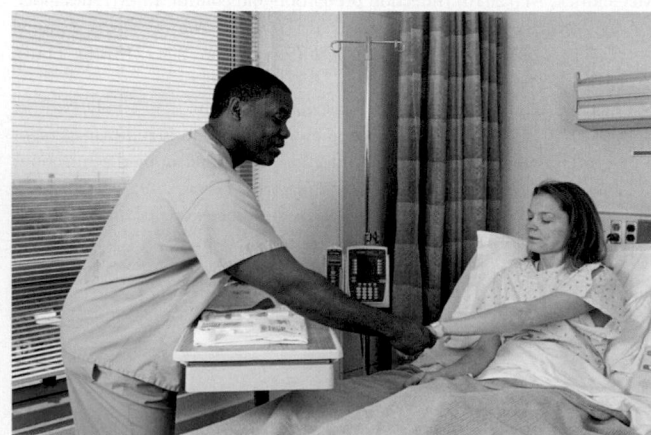

FIG. 1 Identify the patient.

Rationale: Ensures that the correct patient receives proper assessment or treatment and reduces errors

Procedure 21-1 *continued*

5. Close door or bed curtains and explain the procedure to the patient (Fig. 2).

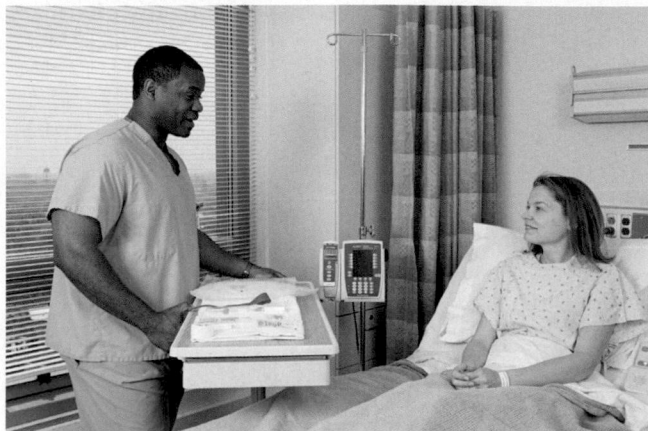

FIG. 2 Explain the rationale for IV therapy and the procedure.

Rationale: Ensures patient privacy, increases patient compliance, reduces patient anxiety, and promotes learning

Preparing the Solution

6. Remove the IV solution bag from the outer plastic covering (Fig. 3). Open all other equipment packages, maintaining sterility of the equipment.

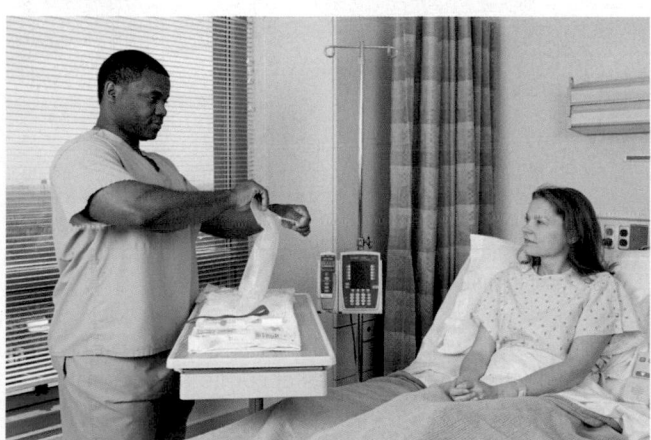

FIG. 3 Open and set up equipment.

Rationale: Removing the outer plastic covering allows access to the solution container and its ports. Maintaining equipment sterility is essential to prevent infection.

7. Grasp the IV administration set and close the flow clamp on the tubing (Fig. 4). Attach an extension set tubing to the administration set if necessary.

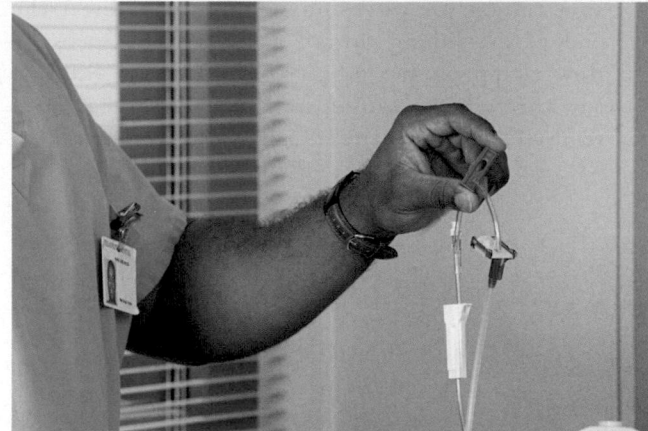

FIG. 4 Clamp the tubing.

Rationale: Closing the flow clamp prevents fluid flow through the tubing once the solution container is accessed. Use of extension set tubing may be necessary to reduce the risk of device manipulation and exposure to blood, depending on the type of IV access device being used. Some new devices do not require the use of a separate extension set.

8. Remove the protective cap or tear the tab from the tubing insertion port on the solution container; remove the protective covering from the spike on the administration tubing, maintaining sterility of the system. Hold the port carefully and firmly with one hand, and then quickly insert the spike into the port with the other hand (Fig. 5).

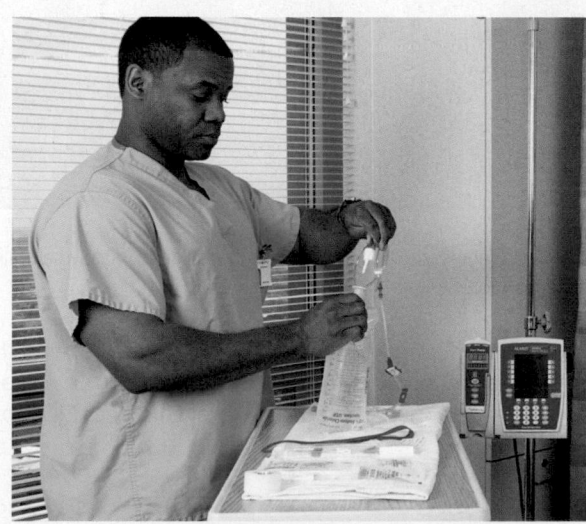

FIG. 5 Insert the spike into the port.

Rationale: Inserting the tubing into the solution container accesses the solution and creates a closed system.

Procedure 21-1   *continued*

9. **Invert the solution container and hang it on the IV pole with the infusion pump. Compress the drip chamber until it is approximately half full (Fig. 6A). Remove the protective cap from the end of the infusion tubing (or extension set, if used); direct the end of the tubing toward a receptacle. Open the flow clamp on the tubing and allow the fluid to run through the tubing until all the air has been removed and the entire length of the tubing is filled with solution; then close the flow clamp (Fig. 6B).**

10. **Attach the solution and tubing to the infusion control device according to the manufacturer's instructions (Fig. 7A). Apply label to the solution container if one has not already been applied by the pharmacy (Fig. 7B).**

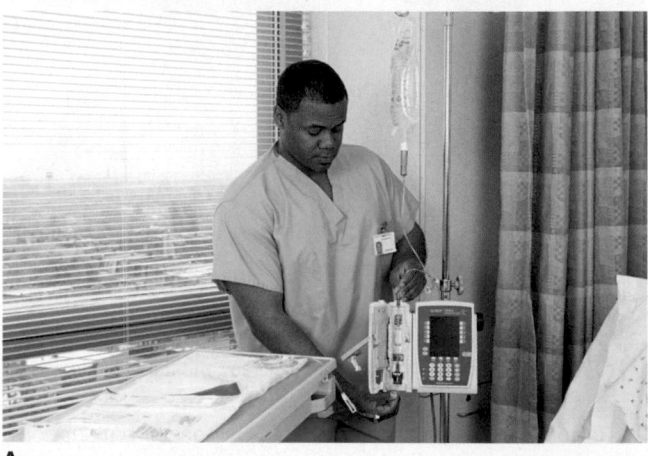

A

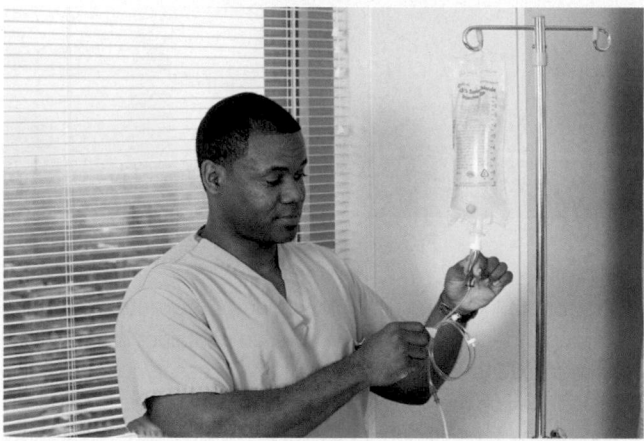

A

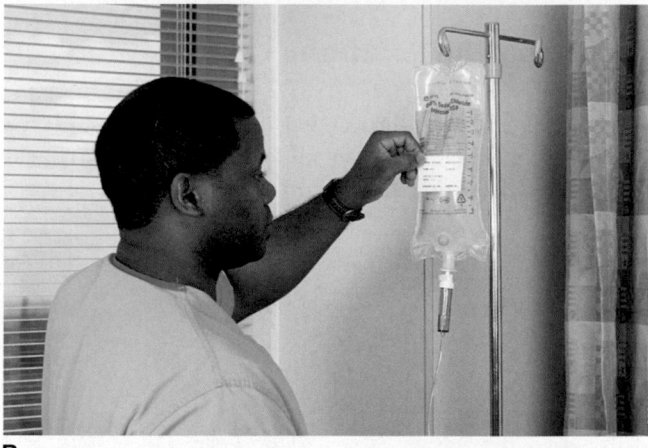

B

FIG. 7 A. Attach the solution and tubing to the infusion control device. **B.** Apply label to the solution container.

Rationale: Correctly attaching the solution to the infusion control device ensures accurate administration of the solution.

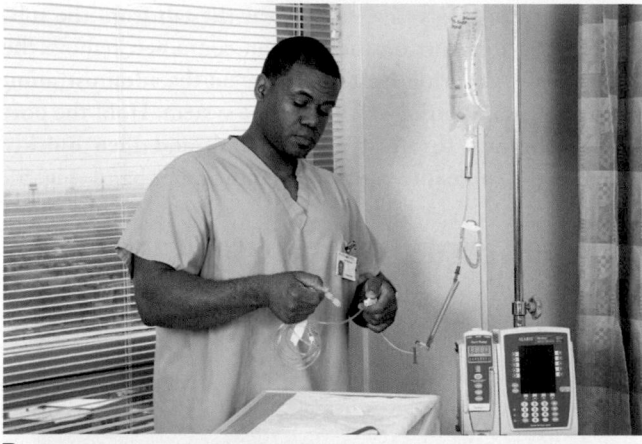

B

FIG. 6 A. Compress the drip chamber until it is approximately half full. **B.** Prime the tubing.

Rationale: Filling the tubing with solution prevents the introduction of air into the patient's vascular system once therapy is initiated and prevents the EID from alarming.

Procedure 21-1 *continued*

Selecting the Insertion Site

11. Place the patient in a comfortable, reclining position, leaving the arm in a dependent position. Place a towel or protective pad under the extremity to be used. Inspect and palpate the patient's extremity to identify an appropriate vein (Fig. 8). Select the puncture site. If long-term therapy is anticipated, start with a vein at the most distal site so that you can move proximally as needed for subsequent IV insertion sites.

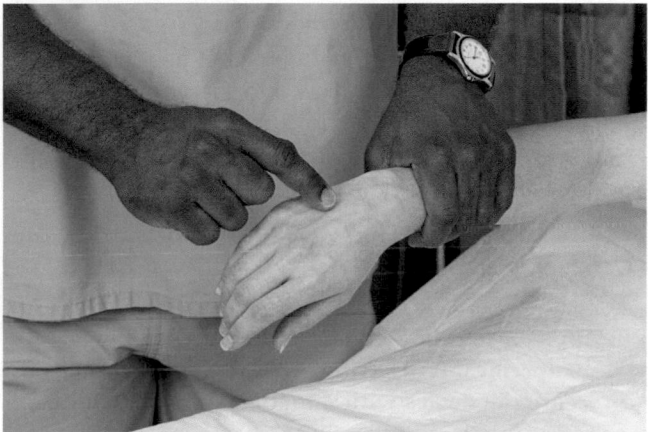

FIG. 8 Inspect and palpate the patient's extremity to identify an appropriate vein.

Rationale: Selecting an appropriate vein reduces the risk of trauma and discomfort to the patient.

12. Put on clean gloves and apply a tourniquet about 6 inches (15 cm) above the intended puncture site (Fig. 9). Ensure that the ends of the tourniquet are positioned away from the intended insertion site. Check for a radial pulse. If it isn't present, release the tourniquet and reapply it with less tension.

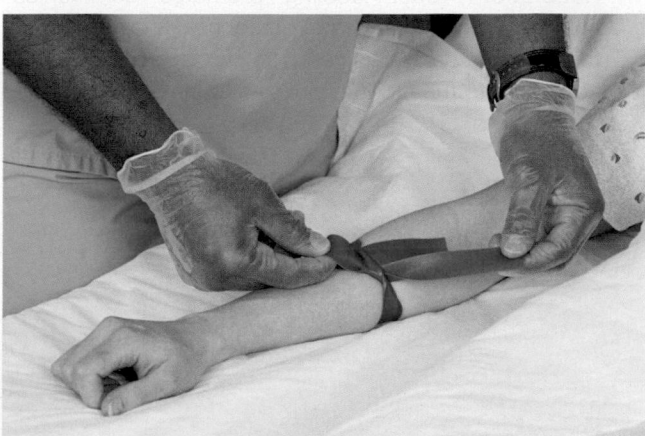

FIG. 9 Apply a tourniquet about 6 inches (15 cm) above the intended puncture site.

Rationale: Applying the tourniquet dilates the vein without compromising arterial blood flow. Arterial occlusion can occur if the tourniquet is applied too tightly. Keeping the ends of the tourniquet away from the insertion site prevents contamination of the site.

13. Lightly palpate the vein with the index and middle fingers of your nondominant hand. Stretch the skin to anchor the vein. If the vein feels hard or ropelike, select another site.

Rationale: The vein must be distended to insert the IV device.

Inserting the Device and Initiating Therapy

14. Administer a local anesthetic according to agency policy (e.g., 0.1 to 0.2 mL lidocaine 1% without epinephrine injected intradermally). If a transdermal analgesic cream (EMLA) is ordered, ensure adequate time from the application of the topical agent to insertion.

Rationale: Use of a local anesthetic reduces the pain associated with insertion. Topical anesthetics require approximately 1 hour to become effective.

15. If facility policy permits, clip hair around the intended insertion site for a distance of up to 2 inches. Do not shave or use depilatory creams, which may injure the skin and increase risk of infection. Clean the site using the approved antimicrobial agent (chlorhexidine gluconate or povidone–iodine) according to facility policy (Fig. 10). Using gentle pressure, cleanse area in a side to side, back and forth motion. Allow agent to dry.

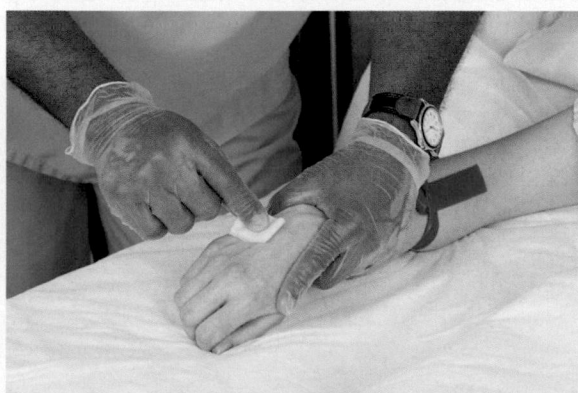

FIG. 10 Clean the site.

Rationale: Cleaning the site reduces the risk of infection transmission. Clipping the hair if necessary reduces the risk of nicking the skin (allowing a portal of entry for microorganisms) and removes microorganisms that can attach to the hair.

Procedure 21-1 *continued*

16. **Grasp the device. Using the thumb of your nondominant hand, stretch the skin taut below the puncture site. If using a vein in the hand, position the hand in a slightly flexed position to keep the skin taut (Fig. 11). Tell the patient that you are about to insert the device and that you need him or her to remain still.**

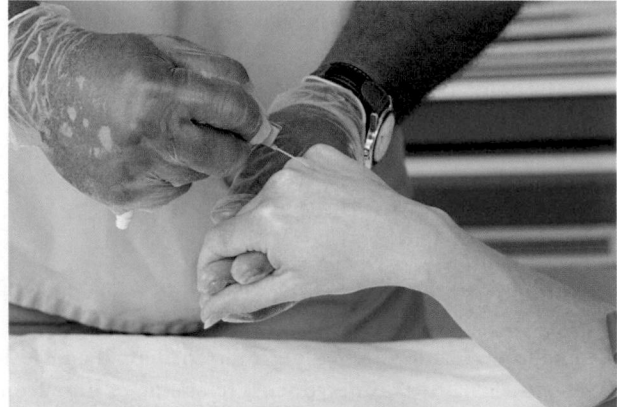

FIG. 11 Stretch the skin taut below the puncture site.

Rationale: Keeping the skin taut helps to stabilize the vein. Informing the patient about what will happen helps to reduce anxiety and facilitates cooperation.

17. **Hold the needle bevel up at a 20- to 30-degree angle, depending on estimated depth of the vein, and enter the skin parallel to the vein. Decrease the angle of the needle to 15 degrees until almost parallel with the skin, and advance the device into the vein in one motion either from directly over the vein or from the side (Fig. 12). You will feel a sense of release or a pop as you enter the vein. Check for blood return and then advance the device, maintaining the device parallel to the skin until the hub is at the insertion site.**

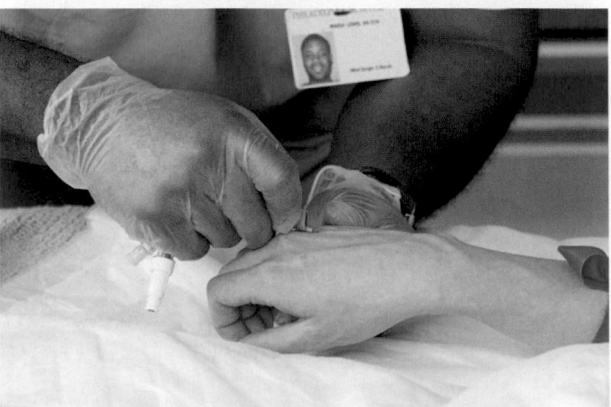

FIG. 12 Advance the device, maintaining the device parallel to the skin until the hub is at the insertion site.

Rationale: The device must be inserted completely to prevent it from becoming dislodged. A blood return indicates that you are in the vein.

18. **Hold finger pressure over end of catheter while removing needle stylet.**

Rationale: Slight pressure prevents bleeding from catheter before attaching the IV tubing. Many styles of IV catheters are available with safety features to prevent against an inadvertent stick with a contaminated needle.

19. **Remove the tourniquet quickly. While holding the hub with your nondominant hand, attach the end of the infusion tubing to the device.**

Rationale: Removing the tourniquet and initiating the infusion allows fluid to flow into the vein, maintaining patency. Holding the hub stabilizes the device and prevents dislodgement. Infiltration indicates that the device is no longer in the vein.

Applying a Dressing

20. **Apply a dressing (most commonly a transparent, semipermeable dressing) to the site. Alternatively, secure the device with nonallergenic tape and cover with a 2 × 2 gauze.**

Rationale: Dressing helps to secure the device in position. A transparent dressing allows air to pass through but is impervious to microorganisms. It also facilitates assessment of the insertion site.

21. **Loop any IV tubing on the patient's extremity and secure with tape.**

Rationale: The loop allows some slack to prevent dislodgement of the IV device.

22. **Label the dressing with the date and time of insertion; device type, gauge, and size; and your initials.**

Rationale: Proper labeling promotes communication with other healthcare personnel. It also ensures that tubing, dressings, and solutions are maintained according to the facility's policy and standards of care.

Procedure 21-1   *continued*

23. **Begin the infusion, setting the infusion pump to the prescribed rate of flow (Fig. 13A). Assess the flow of the solution and infusion control device function. Inspect the site for signs of infiltration (Fig. 13B).**

24. **Dispose of all equipment and remove gloves. Perform hand hygiene.**

    Rationale: Reduces the risk of infection

25. **Apply site protection device and secure as necessary.**

    Rationale: Helps to stabilize the device position and prevents unnecessary motion that could lead to dislodgement and subsequent infiltration or inflammation

26. **Assist the patient to a comfortable position. Assess the patient's tolerance of the procedure.**

    Rationale: Promotes patient comfort and provides information for documentation

27. **Document the procedure, including the date and time of the venipuncture; device type, gauge, and length; location of insertion site and appearance; type and flow rate of the IV solution; patient's response (including adverse reactions); patient teaching performed; and patient's understanding of the teaching.**

    Rationale: Documentation provides communication among healthcare team members to ensure continuity of care.

28. **Monitor infusion rate, condition of IV site, and patient complaints, initially approximately 30 minutes after beginning the infusion and then according to facility policy. Change dressing, tubing, and solutions according to facility policy.**

    Rationale: Ongoing monitoring provides information related to the effectiveness of IV therapy and aids in early detection of complications.

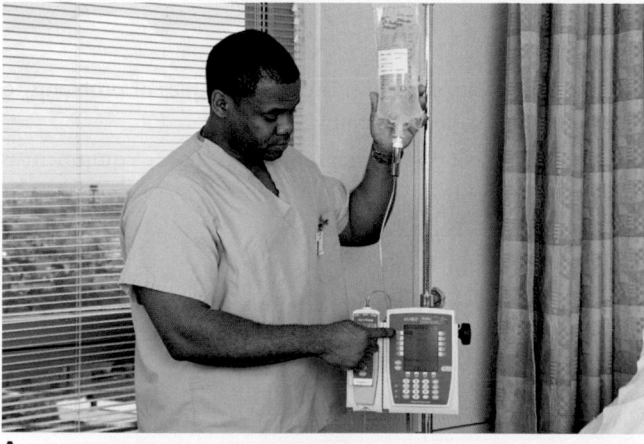

A

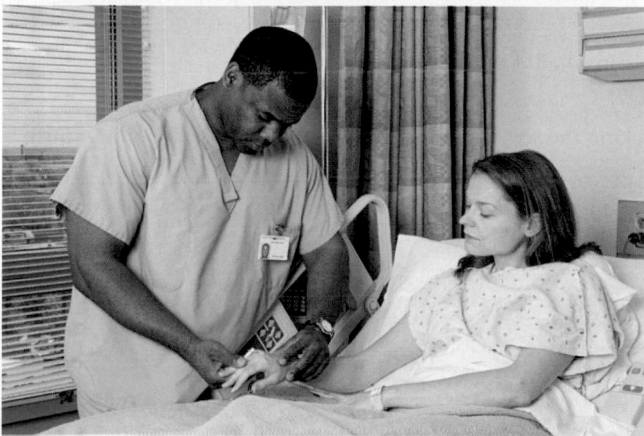

B

FIG. 13 **A.** Set the infusion pump to the prescribed rate of flow.
B. Inspect the site for signs of infiltration.

Documentation

7/1/17: 13:15—IV inserted in right hand with 20-gauge, 1¼-inch catheter following intradermal injection of 0.1 mL 1% lidocaine. Patient tolerated procedure well. IV patent, infusing well, no complications at this time.

—S. Roberts, RN

Life Span Considerations

Infant and Child

- Consider the use of topical anesthetics prior to insertion to minimize the child's pain.
- Use scalp veins for IV insertion only in infants less than 6 months of age; use dorsal veins in the foot for toddlers.
- Use the smallest IV gauge possible to reduce the risk of trauma to the child.
- Do not use chlorhexidine in neonates less than 7 days of age or if gestational age is less than 26 weeks.

Older Adult

- If the vein is easily palpable but not sufficiently dilated, one or more of the following techniques may help raise the vein. Place the extremity in a dependent position for several seconds, gently tap your finger over the vein, rub or stroke the skin upward toward the tourniquet, or have the patient open and close his fist several times. If the patient's skin is cold, warm it by rubbing and stroking the arm, or cover the entire arm with warm compresses for 5 to 10 minutes to help distend the veins.

Procedure 21-1 *continued*

- Perform venipuncture quickly and efficiently and remove the tourniquet promptly in older patients to prevent bruising due to the fragility of their veins.
- An older adult's veins appear tortuous because of the skin's increased transparency and decreased elasticity.
- To help stabilize the vein for insertion, stretch the skin proximal to the insertion site and anchor it firmly with your nondominant hand.

Home Care Modifications

- Teach the patient and caregivers how to care for the IV site and identify complications. Include examples of problems to report, such as "the solution stops infusing" or "the IV site becomes red, swollen, or painful."
- When teaching, use the equipment and supplies that the patient will be using at home; sometimes, home equipment is different from that used in the facility.
- Ensure that the patient has the necessary supplies available at home for use before discharge.
- Arrange for a referral to home healthcare to provide continued support in the home.
- Provide patient and caregiver with written instructions, troubleshooting guides, and phone numbers for home care nurse.
- Provide patient and caregiver with clear instructions on intravenous care during bathing.

Collaboration and Delegation

- All IV orders must be written by the patient's healthcare provider. The nurse is responsible for properly administering them.
- IV teams often start and maintain IVs in hospitals and are consulted if problems arise with the IV.
- PICCs are inserted by providers certified in their insertion.
- Verify IV solutions just as you would any medication, checking the six rights. Additionally, verify the rate of administration and compatibility.
- Instruct unlicensed assistive personnel to promptly notify you if the patient complains about the IV or if the IV alarm is sounding. They should not turn off the alarm.

Procedure 21-2 Monitoring an Intravenous Infusion

Purpose	1. Provide a safe, patent route for infusion of IV therapy.
	2. Ensure correct infusion of IV fluids.
	3. Detect IV complications promptly.

Equipment	Prefilled 10-mL syringe with sterile NaCl
	Alcohol or Betadine wipe
	Clean, disposable gloves
	Dressing supplies

Assessment	• Review the patient's chart for diagnosis and medical plan for IV therapy.
	• Assess the patient for clinical signs of fluid or electrolyte imbalances.
	• Check the physician's order for type of IV solution, additives, and infusion rate.
	• Calculate hourly infusion rate in milliliters (mL) per hour when an EID is used or in drops per minute if IV is gravity controlled. The INS strongly recommends that an EID be used for intravenous infusions.

Procedure

1. **Perform hand hygiene.**

   Rationale: Reduces microbe transmission

2. **Identify the patient using two separate identifiers.**

   Rationale: Ensures that the correct patient receives proper assessment or treatment and reduces errors

3. **Close door or bed curtains and explain the procedure to the patient.**

   Rationale: Ensures patient privacy, increases patient compliance, reduces patient anxiety, and promotes learning

4. **Compare IV fluid currently infusing with the ordered solution.**

   Rationale: Comparison ensures prompt recognition and correction of errors.

5. **Inspect the rate of flow at least every hour (Fig. 1). For gravity-regulated IVs, check actual flow rate for 15 seconds and multiply by 4 for the minute rate. Compare the assessed rate with prescribed flow rate. If the infusion** is ahead of schedule, slow it so the infusion will complete at the planned time. If infusion is behind schedule, review hospital policy and complete patient assessment before increasing flow rate; some agencies require a physician's order to increase the rate of flow. If EID is used, the hourly infusion rate in milliliters per hour is programmed into the machine.

   Rationale: Fluids that are infused too rapidly may cause circulatory overload with resultant pulmonary edema and cardiac failure. Fluids that are behind schedule deliver insufficient fluids and nutrients.

6. **Inspect the system for leakage; if present, locate the source (Fig. 2). Tighten all connections within the system. If leak persists, slow the IV flow rate to keep the vein open and replace tubing with sterile set.**

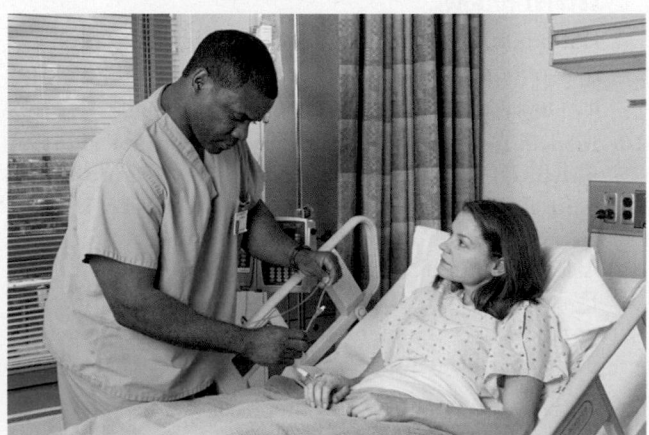

FIG. 2 Inspect the tubing.

Rationale: IV therapy is a sterile procedure. A break or leak in the tubing allows microorganisms to enter and contaminate the entire system.

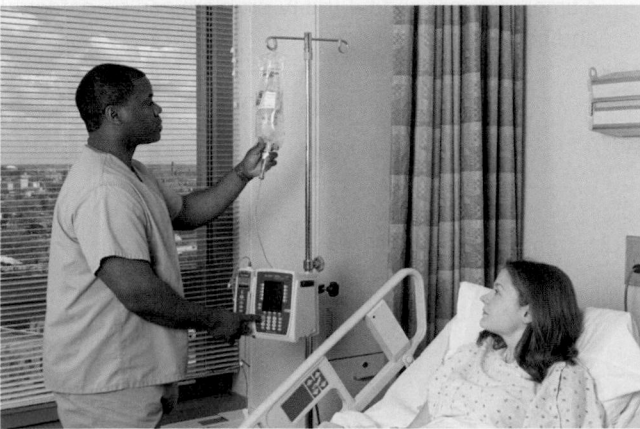

FIG. 1 Inspect the rate of flow at least every hour.

Procedure 21-2 *continued*

7. **Inspect the tubing for kinks or blockages. Loosely coil tubing and place it on the bed.**

   Rationale: Blockages in the tubing impede the solution flow, and the patient may not receive the necessary fluids and nutrients or the EID will alarm.

8. **Inspect the insertion site and dressing for leakage of IV solution (Fig. 3).**

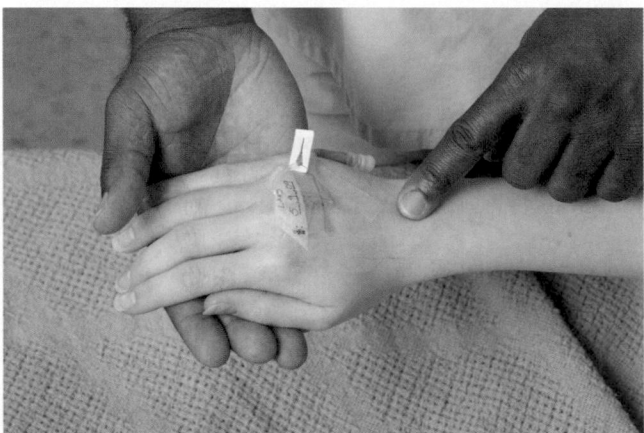

FIG. 3 Inspect the insertion site.

   Rationale: Leakage may occur at the connection of the tubing with the hub of needle or catheter and cause loss of IV solution.

9. **Inspect the infusion site for infiltration. Infiltration occurs when the needle becomes dislodged from the vein and IV fluid flows into the interstitial tissue. Look for signs of infiltration, including decreased flow rate, swelling, pallor, coolness, and discomfort at or above needle insertion site. If signs are present, change the IV site. If a large amount of fluid has infiltrated, elevate the arm above the heart on several pillows.**

   Rationale: Prompt detection is important to promote patient comfort and permit early treatment. Site elevation facilitates venous and lymphatic drainage.

10. **Inspect arm above the insertion point for signs of phlebitis, including redness, swelling, warmth, and pain along the vein above IV insertion site. If present, discontinue the IV and restart in another area. Ask the patient to report burning or pain at the IV site (Fig. 4). If you suspect phlebitis is present, notify the IV team or physician and check agency policy for treating phlebitis.**

   Rationale: Phlebitis may occur as a result of trauma or chemical irritation secondary to IV additives or solution pH. Often, patients experience pain before signs of phlebitis can be observed.

11. **Inspect the insertion site for bleeding.**

   Rationale: Bleeding can be caused by trauma at the insertion site.

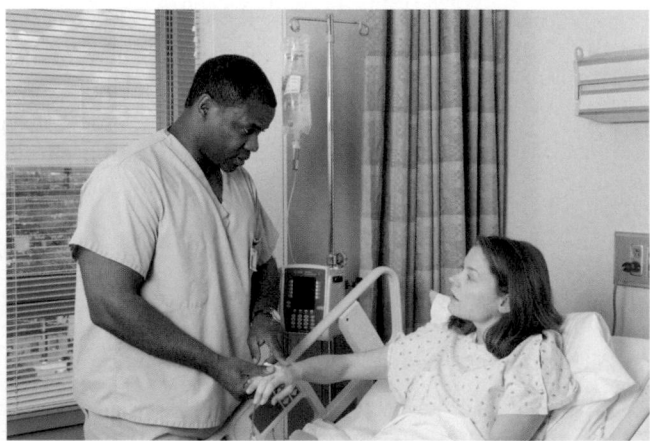

FIG. 4 Ask the patient to report burning or pain at the insertion site.

12. **Inspect the site for local manifestations of infection including redness, pus, warmth, induration, and pain. Inspect the patient for systemic manifestations of infection, including chills, fever, tachycardia, and hypotension, that may accompany local infection. Inspect the patient for additional complications of IV therapy (e.g., fluid overload).**

   Rationale: Prompt detection of complications is important to promote patient comfort and permit early treatment.

13. **Check EID alarm settings. Attend to all alarms in a timely manner.**

   Rationale: Alarms on the EID must always be audible and are usually set at the highest setting. Alarms should never be turned off. All alarms should be attended to in a timely manner so that the IV problem can be detected and corrected.

Procedure 21-2 *continued*

14. Although monitoring IV therapy is a nursing responsibility, if the patient is able to comply, teach him or her to contact the nurse if the following occur:

    a. **The flow rate changes suddenly.**

    b. **The fluid container is almost empty.**

    c. **Blood is in the tubing.**

    d. **The site becomes uncomfortable.**

    Rationale: Allowing the patient to participate in care helps to detect and prevent complications and enhances the patient's feelings of control.

15. Chart any findings indicating complications of IV therapy (e.g., infiltration).

    Rationale: Charting maintains a legal record and communicates with all healthcare team members.

Documentation

7/6/17: 08:30—IV infusing into the right hand @ 125 mL/h on EID. IV patent, no redness, no swelling. Transparent dressing intact. No patient complaints of discomfort.

—S. Roberts, RN

Life Span Considerations

Infant and Child

- Children change position frequently, so their tubing can easily become kinked or disconnected. Tape all connections, and protect the insertion site with a manufactured stabilizing device and rigid arm board to help prolong the patency of the IV.
- Offer emotional support. IV therapy can be stressful for the child and the parents.

Home Care Modifications

- Collaborate with the home care agency that will provide home follow-up. Give the patient the agency's name and phone number and the name of the nurse who will coordinate care.
- Teach the patient or caregiver to do the following:
  - Inspect the insertion site at least four times daily through the transparent dressing.
  - Assess for infiltration, phlebitis, or an obvious dislodged catheter. If any of these occur, the caregiver should clamp the IV tubing and call the nurse.
  - Observe flow rate for sluggishness or lack of dripping. Should this occur, the caregiver should open the roller clamp and look for kinks in the tubing. If the problem continues, contact the healthcare provider.

Collaboration and Delegation

- In acute care agencies, work closely with members of the IV team to ensure safe, efficient IV management.
- If an agency does not have an IV team, consult the anesthesia department if there are problems with IVs or difficult IV starts.
- Teach unlicensed personnel how to safely provide hygiene care and ambulation for patients receiving IV therapy. Instruct them to notify the nurse if the alarm is ringing or the IV bag needs to be changed.

Procedure 21-3 Peripheral IV Site Care

Purpose	1. Protect the IV site from infection. 2. Permit visual inspection of the IV site to promptly detect complications of therapy.
Equipment	2% chlorhexidine solution Antimicrobial swabs Adhesive remover (optional) 1-inch adhesive tape Sterile semipermeable transparent dressing (or sterile gauze dressing) Clean gloves Waterproof pad
Assessment	• Assess the integrity of the dressing to determine if it needs to be changed. **Peripheral IV dressings are not routinely changed unless they are loose, bloody, or wet because changing dressings increases the risk of site contamination or dislodging the catheter.**

Procedure

1. **Perform hand hygiene**
   Rationale: Reduces microbe transmission

2. **Identify the patient.**
   Rationale: Ensures that the correct patient receives proper assessment or treatment and reduces errors

3. **Close door or bed curtains and explain the procedure to the patient.**
   Rationale: Ensures patient privacy, increases patient compliance, reduces patient anxiety, and promotes learning

4. **Put on clean gloves. Place waterproof pad under IV site.**
   Rationale: Maintains asepsis

5. **Inspect site for signs of infection, infiltration, and thrombophlebitis.**
   Rationale: A complication would require changing the IV catheter rather than just changing the dressing.

6. **Hold catheter in place with your nondominant hand and gently remove dressing and tape (Fig. 1). For transparent dressing, gently stretch the film horizontal to the skin.**

Rationale: Stabilization prevents movement or dislodgement of the catheter, which could lead to infiltration.

7. **Clean the entry site with a chlorhexidine solution, using a circular motion and moving from the center outward (Fig. 2). Allow the area to dry completely; do not blow or blot dry.**

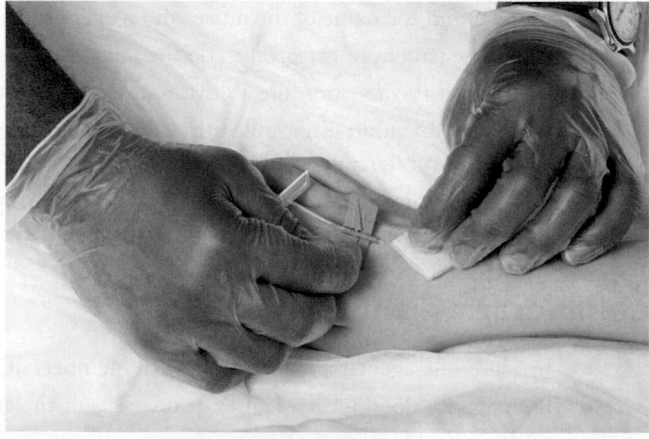

FIG. 2 Clean site.

Rationale: Cleansing from site outward removes microorganisms from the skin and minimizes contamination of the IV site. Allowing the area to dry increases antimicrobial effectiveness.

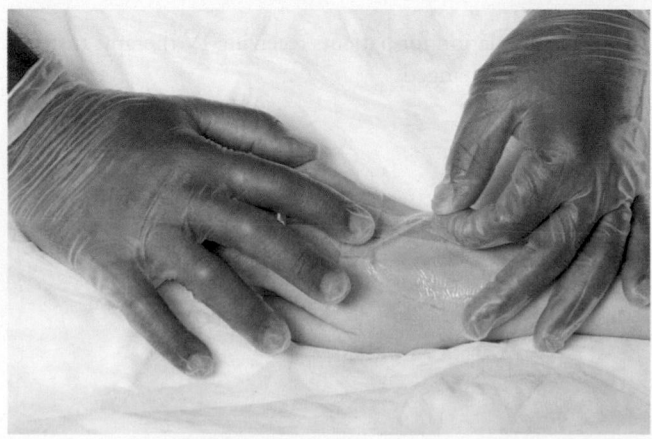

FIG. 1 Remove old dressing.

Procedure 21-3   *continued*

8. **Attach new nonsutured securing device, using extreme care to not dislodge catheter. Apply transparent semi-permeable dressing to the IV site. Take care not to tape over the IV connection or IV tubing (Figs. 3 and 4).**

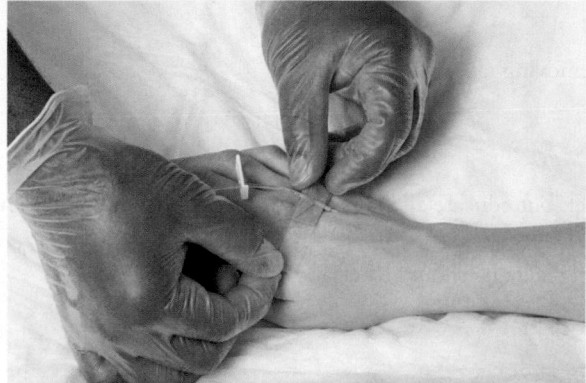

FIG. 3 Reapply tape strip.

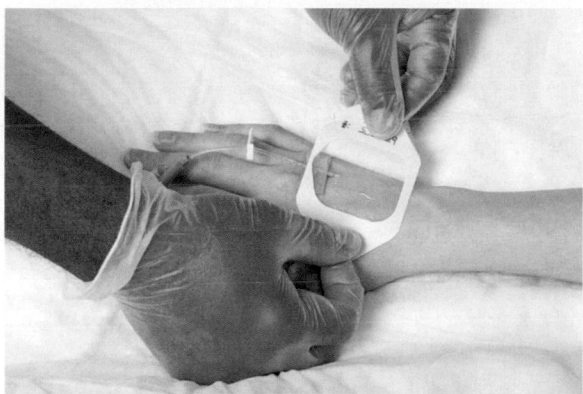

FIG. 4 Apply new dressing.

Rationale: Taping over the IV connection would make it difficult to change the IV tubing without destroying the integrity of the dressing.

9. **Label dressing with date, time, and initials (Fig. 5). Secure IV tubing with additional tape if necessary (Fig. 6).**

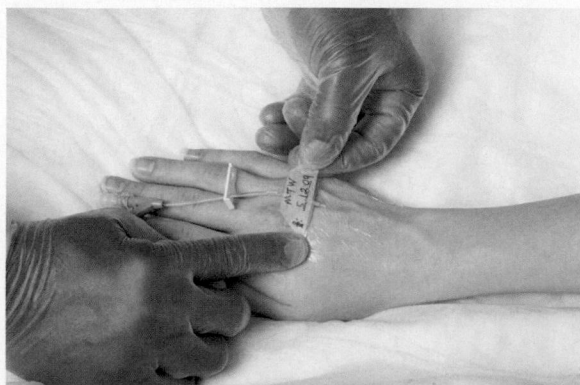

FIG. 5 Label dressing.

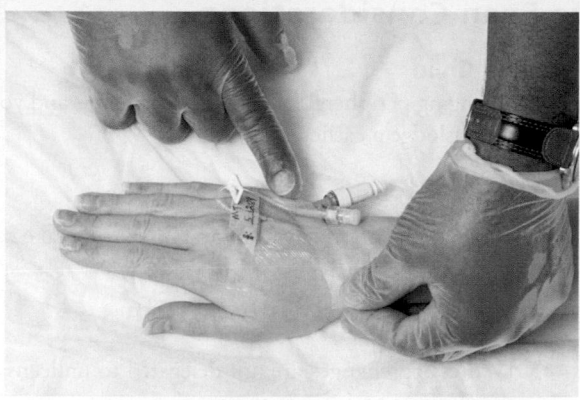

FIG. 6 Secure tubing with additional tape.

Rationale: Labeling communicates information to the healthcare team so that dressing changes can occur on schedule according to agency protocol.

10. **Assess IV flow is accurate and system is patent.**

Rationale: Manipulation of the catheter during the dressing change could have caused dislodgement from vein or changed flow rate.

11. **Remove gloves and perform hand hygiene. Document dressing change and observations.**

Rationale: Documentation maintains a legal record and communicates with the healthcare team.

Documentation

7/6/17: 14:00—Peripheral IV site dressing changed. No signs of infiltration or phlebitis.

—S. Roberts, RN

(*Note:* This would usually be documented on an IV flow sheet.)

Procedure 21-3   *continued*

Life Span Considerations

Infant and Child
- Changing peripheral IV dressings on infants and young children can be especially challenging since their quick movements can dislodge a catheter.

Older Adult
- Older adults often have very fragile skin, so take care when removing tape.

Collaboration and Delegation

- IV dressing changes are not delegated to unlicensed personnel, but educate all team members to notify the nurse when the IV dressing is loose or wet.
- Call the IV team for questions or concerns. Policies on dressing changes should be clear.

Procedure 21-4 Peripherally Inserted Central Venous Access Device (PICC) Site Care

Purpose
1. Protect the PICC site from infection.
2. Permit visual inspection of the PICC site to promptly detect complications of therapy.

Equipment

2% chlorhexidine solution
Antimicrobial swabs
Sterile tape
Sterile semipermeable transparent dressing (or gauze dressing). Agency policy may use chlorhexidine sponge dressing.
Clean gloves
Sterile gloves and two masks
Sterile drape
Sterile skin protectant
Nonsutured catheter securing device
PICC injection caps
Normal saline solution (NSS) vial and 10-mL syringe or prefilled NSS syringe (preferred)
(*Note*: Most IV devices are currently flushed with sterile NaCl. However, a few central IV devices may require diluted heparin flush to ensure patency instead of the NaCl that is described in the following procedures. Please refer to agency policies and manufacturer recommendations.)

Assessment

- Assess agency policy for PICC site care.
- Assess when dressing was last changed to determine need for dressing change.
- Assess type of central catheter to note manufacturer recommendations.

Procedure

1. **Perform hand hygiene.**
   Rationale: Reduces microbe transmission

2. **Identify the patient.**
   Rationale: Ensures that the correct patient receives proper assessment or treatment and reduces errors

3. **Close door or bed curtains and explain the procedure to the patient.**
   Rationale: Ensures patient privacy, increases patient compliance, reduces patient anxiety, and promotes learning

4. **Place patient in a comfortable position.**
   Rationale: Maintains asepsis and increases patient comfort

5. **Apply mask. Have patient put on mask and turn head away from site. Prepare sterile field and place sterile drape around site. Put on clean gloves.**
   Rationale: Strict asepsis is necessary to prevent infection and sepsis.

6. **Assess insertion site for infection and phlebitis (Fig. 1).**

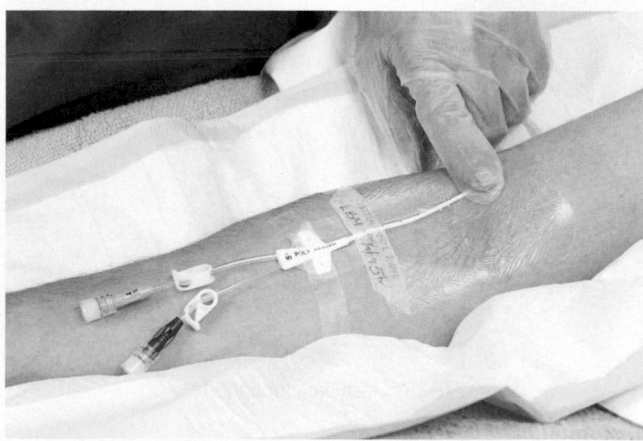

FIG. 1 Assess PICC insertion site.

Rationale: Prompt detection of complications decreases morbidity and mortality and ensures central venous access.

Procedure 21-4   *continued*

7. **Stabilize catheter with thumb. Remove old dressing, stretching horizontally and then working proximally (Fig. 2). Carefully remove securing device. Remove gloves.**

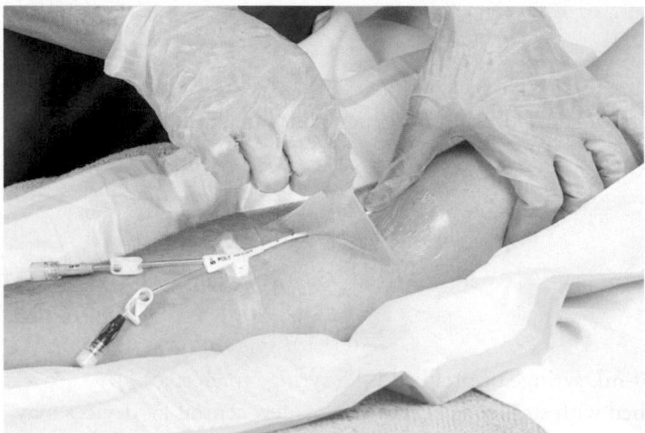

FIG. 2 Stabilize catheter and remove old dressing.

Rationale: Maintains asepsis and prevents dislodgement of catheter

8. **Don sterile gloves and clean the area around the site with a chlorhexidine solution. Move in a circular fashion, cleaning from the insertion site outward 2 to 3 inches (Fig. 3). Allow to dry; do not blow or blot.**

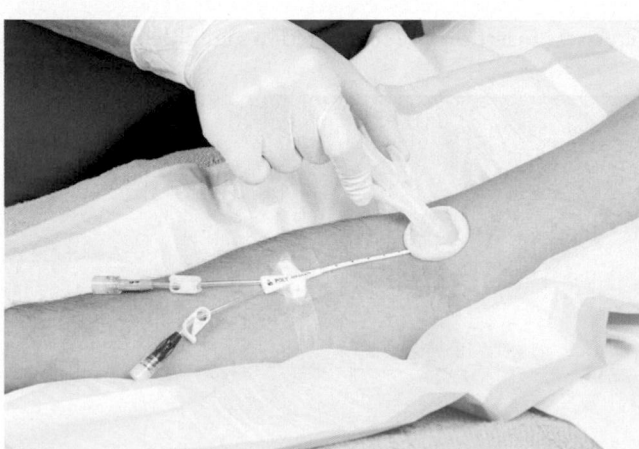

FIG. 3 Clean area around site.

Rationale: Cleansing site moving from clean to dirty removes microorganisms from the skin and minimizes contamination of the IV site. Allowing site to dry increases antimicrobial effectiveness.

9. **Re-dress the site with a transparent semipermeable dressing, according to agency policy (Fig. 4). Secure tubing and all Luer lock connections.**

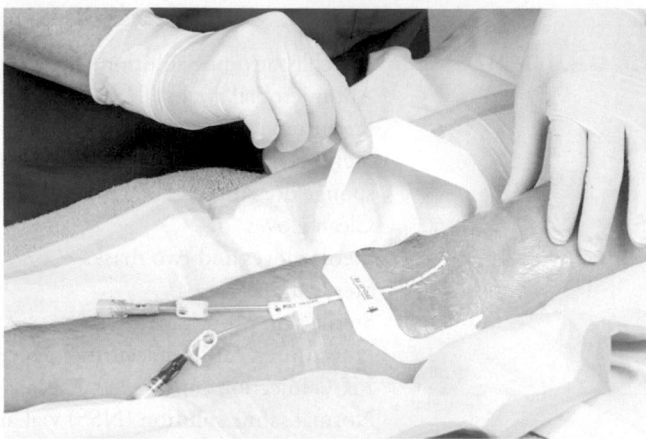

FIG. 4 Apply new dressing.

Rationale: Transparent dressing allows for site inspection. Securing connections and tubing prevents stress and tugging on site.

10. **Label the dressing with date, time, and initials (Fig. 5).**

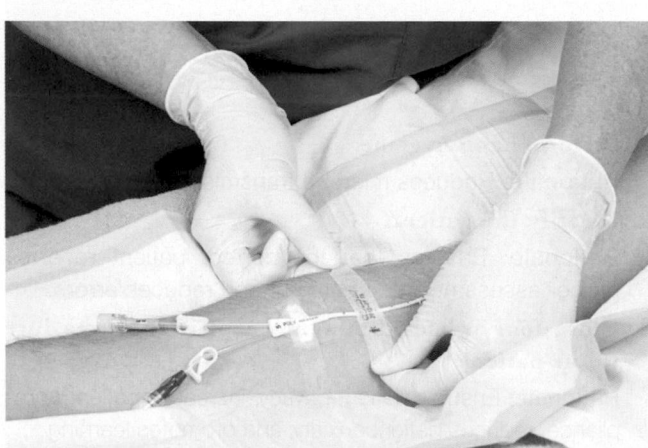

FIG. 5 Label dressing.

Rationale: Labeling communicates information to the healthcare team so that dressing changes can occur on schedule according to agency protocol.

Procedure 21-4   *continued*

11. **Clamp all lines of device and remove injection caps (Fig. 6). Cleanse catheter ends with antimicrobial swab and reapply new injection caps (Figs. 7 and 8).**

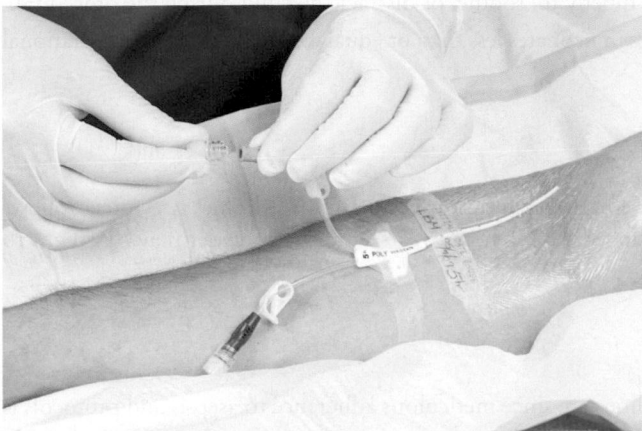

FIG. 6 Remove injection caps.

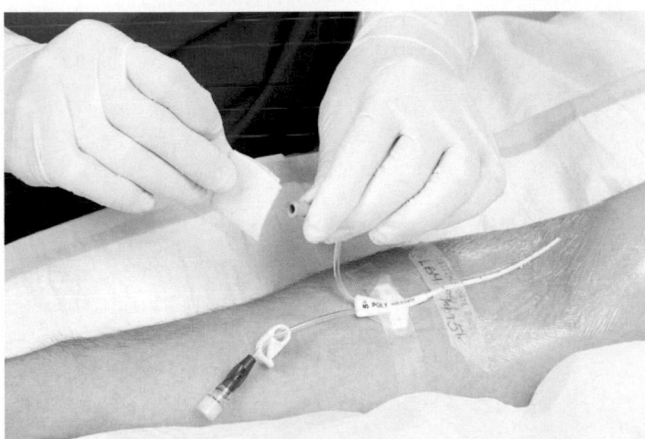

FIG. 7 Swab catheter ends with antimicrobial swab.

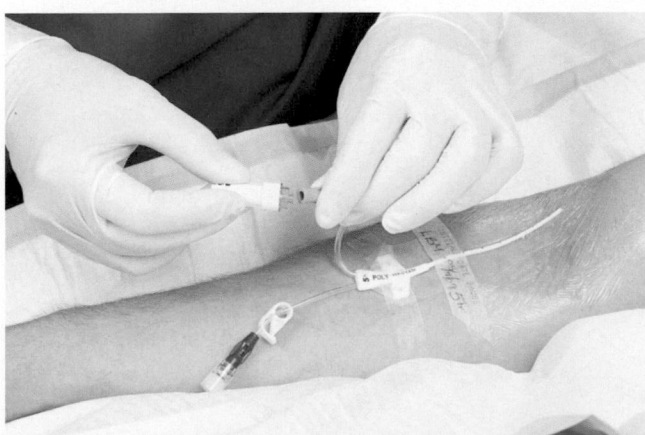

FIG. 8 Reapply new injection cap.

Rationale: Injection caps provide a location for microorganisms that could cause infection.

12. **Flush the catheter according to agency policy using a 10-mL syringe (Fig. 9). Use the "pulse-pause" technique, always ending with positive pressure by clamping prior to ending the flush.**

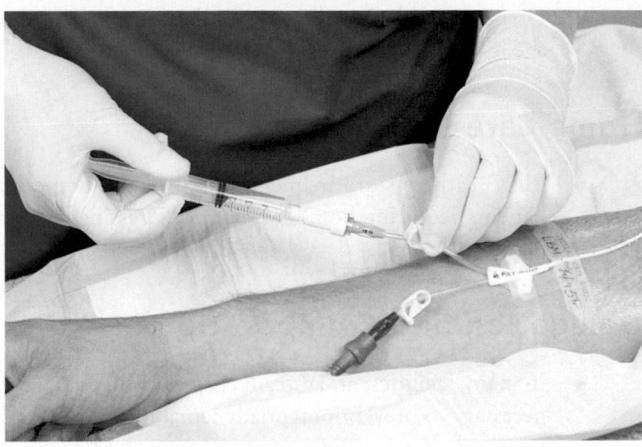

FIG. 9 Flush the line.

Rationale: The pulse-pause technique increases friction during the flush, ensuring the device remains patent. Ending with positive pressure prevents backflow of blood into the catheter, which could contribute to occlusion. A large 10-mL syringe is used to avoid very high pressures that could cause catheter rupture.

13. **Discard all used items properly. Reposition the patient comfortably. Document dressing change and observations.**

Rationale: Documentation maintains a legal record and communicates with the healthcare team.

Documentation

8/23/17: 14:00—CVAD changed, no signs of complications.

—S. Roberts, RN

(*Note:* This is usually documented on an IV flow sheet unless there are complications.)

Procedure 21-4 *continued*

Life Span Considerations

Infant and Child

- Have another care provider stabilize and restrain the infant or child during the dressing change to prevent dislodgement from sudden movement. The parent or caregiver may talk quietly to, soothe, or distract the child during the procedure.
- Do not use chlorhexidine or chlorhexidine sponge dressings in neonates less than or equal to 7 days of age or if gestational age is less than 26 weeks.

Home Care Considerations

- PICC catheters are frequently used in the home setting. Often, an infusion company or a home care nurse follows patients requiring home IV therapy. Dressings may be changed during home visits or a care provider may be taught to perform the skill.

Delegation and Collaboration

- In many facilities, an IV team is responsible for all central line care since meticulous adherence to asepsis and protocols is necessary to prevent potentially lethal infection.
- Notify the IV team about any concerns with a central line. If the agency does not have an IV team, the anesthesiology department is often available for consultation.

Procedure 21-5 Changing Intravenous Solution and Tubing

| **Purpose** | 1. Deliver IV therapy as ordered. |
| | 2. Decrease risk of patient infection. |

Equipment

Sterile container of ordered amount and type of IV solution
Appropriate sterile tubing administration set
Extension tubing with Luer lock connections and injection ports
Premarked strips for labeling container and tubing
Tape for securing tubing
Clean, disposable gloves (for tubing change)
Dressing material and antiseptic solution if IV site dressing is to be changed

Assessment

- Determine what time the next solution container is due. Prepare next solution 1 hour before it is due. Plan to change container when less than 50 mL remains.
- Review physician's orders for IV fluid orders.
- Check label on currently infusing solution and tubing for the date and time they were hung. (IV solutions are not considered sterile if they are open longer than 24 hours.)
- Determine date and time of last tubing change. IV administration sets, including secondary sets and add-on devices, should be changed no more frequently than 72 hours to help ensure the sterility of system.
- Inspect IV system to determine type of tubing required. Many different administration sets are available. Most infusion pumps use specially designed cassette tubing.
- Review the policy of your agency and the manufacturer's recommendations.

Procedure

1. **Perform hand hygiene.**
   Rationale: Reduces microbe transmission

2. **Identify the patient.**
   Rationale: Ensures that the correct patient receives proper assessment or treatment and reduces errors

3. **Close door or bed curtains and explain the procedure to the patient.**
   Rationale: Ensures patient privacy, increases patient compliance, reduces patient anxiety, and promotes learning

Changing Solution Container

4. **Compare the solution with the physician's order (Fig. 1). Assess patient allergies. Adhere to six rights of medication administration, including identifying the patient with two separate identifiers (Fig. 2).**

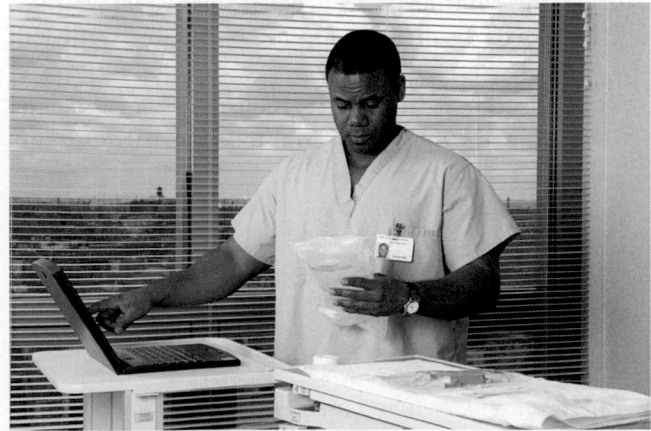

FIG. 1 Compare the solution with the physician's order.

Procedure 21-5   *continued*

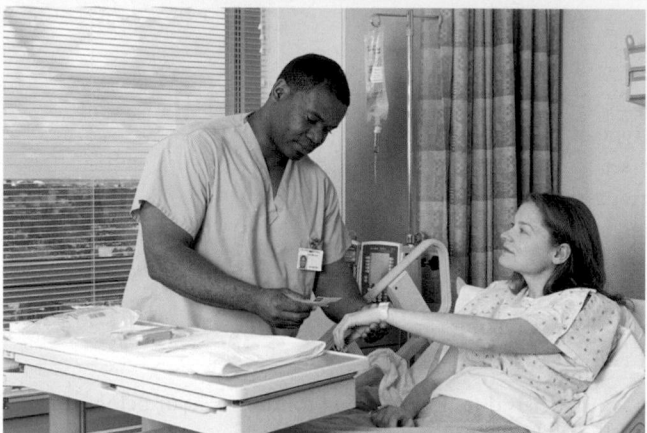

FIG. 2 Identify the patient.

Rationale: IV solutions are considered medications. Errors in administration could have serious negative consequences for the patient.

5. **Remove IV bag from outer wrapper. Look for leaks or impurities in the bag and check the IV fluid bag for expiration date.**

Rationale: Some dampness may occur as plastic on plastic sweats, but distinct leaks would destroy IV bag sterility. Expired bags of IV fluid should not be used.

6. **Label the solution container with the patient's name, solution type, additives, date, and time hung. If labeled by the pharmacy, check prelabeled container with physician's order. Record the solution change in the patient's record.**

Rationale: Proper labeling and documentation helps prevent errors in administration.

7. **Prepare container for spiking:**

   a. **If the solution is in a plastic bag, remove plastic cover from entry nipple. Maintain sterility of nipple end.**

   b. **If solution is in a bottle, remove metal cap, metal disk, and rubber disk. Maintain sterility of bottle top.**

   Rationale: Sterility prevents transmission of microorganisms into container when spike is inserted.

8. **Close the clamp on the existing tubing. If using an electronic device, turn the device to the "hold" position.**

   Rationale: Clamping prevents fluid in drip chamber from emptying and air from entering tubing during changing procedure.

9. **Take the old solution container from the pole and invert it. Quickly remove spike from used container, maintaining spike sterility (Fig. 3).**

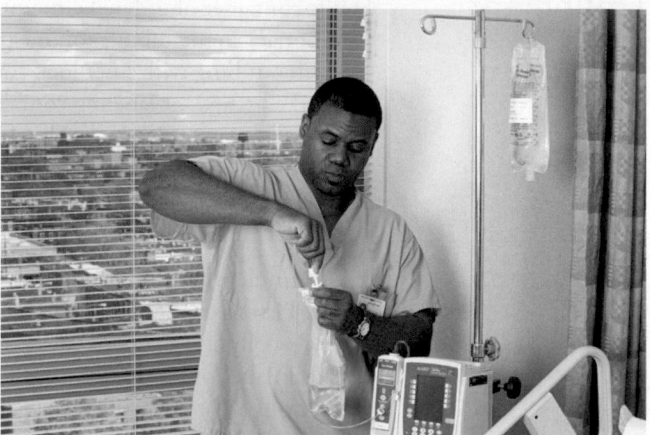

FIG. 3 Remove spike from old container.

Rationale: This position prevents fluid remaining in container from emptying onto the floor when tubing is removed.

10. **Spike new IV container with firm push/twist motion and hang new container on IV pole. Alternatively, you can hang the IV bag and then spike the new container (Fig. 4).**

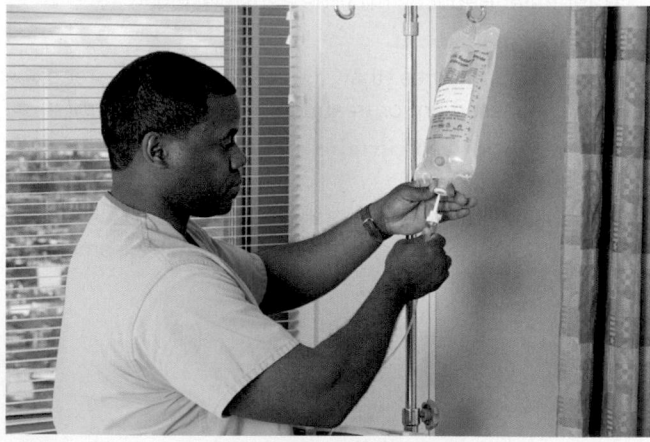

FIG. 4 Spike new IV container.

Rationale: Maintains sterility and allows gravity to augment fluid filling the drip chamber

11. **Inspect tubing for air bubbles, and assess that drip chamber is half full of solution.**

    Rationale: Decreases the risk of air entering the tubing, which would cause the EID alarm to sound

12. **Reopen and adjust clamp to regulate flow rate or program EID, according to orders.**

    Rationale: IV fluids are delivered as ordered to restore fluid balance.

Procedure 21-5 *continued*

Changing Intravenous Tubing Connected Directly into the Hub of the Intravenous Access Catheter

1. Follow introductory steps 1 through 3, above, and steps 4 through 6 of the Changing Solution Container section.
2. Open new tubing package. Keep protective covers on spike and catheter adaptor.

   Rationale: Maintains sterility of new tubing set
3. Adjust roller clamp on new tubing to fully closed position.

   Rationale: Prevents air from entering the tubing
4. Prepare new solution container as directed in step 5 of the Changing Solution Container section.
5. Maintaining sterility, remove protective cover from spike and insert spike into new solution container (Fig. 5).

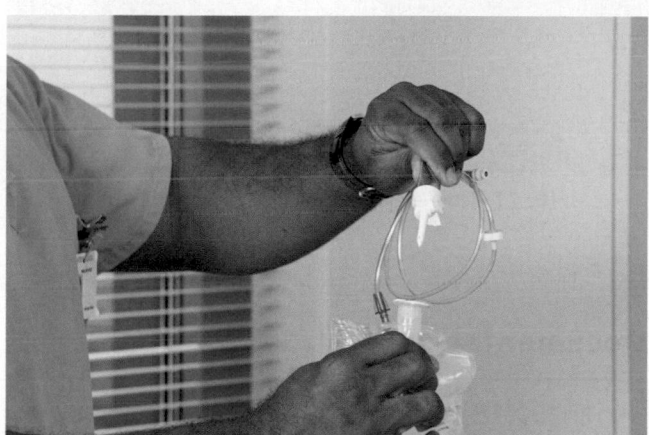

FIG. 5 Insert spike of new tubing into new solution container.

6. Hang container and "prime" drip chamber by squeezing gently, allowing to fill half full (Fig. 6).

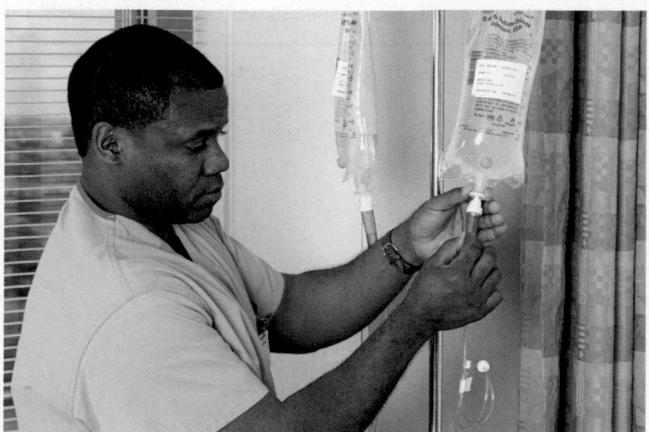

FIG. 6 Prime drip chamber.

Rationale: Prevents air bubbles from entering tubing with the solution

7. Remove protective cap from end of IV tubing (Fig. 7), and adjust roller clamp to flush tubing with fluid. Replace protective cap.

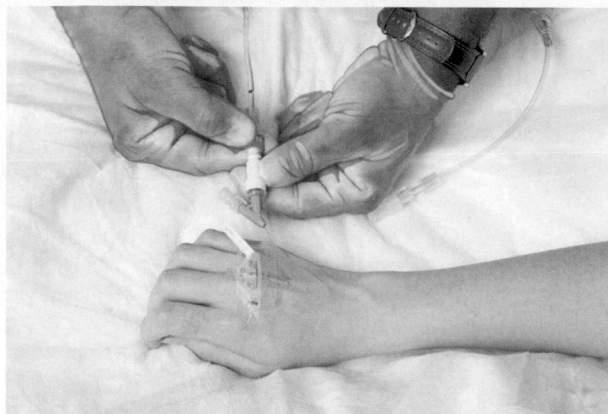

FIG. 7 Remove current infusion tubing from the resealable cap on the short extension IV tubing.

Rationale: Removing air prevents air embolus. Protective cap maintains sterility of system.

8. Adjust roller clamp on old tubing to close fully.

   Rationale: Fluid leakage should be prevented when tubing is disconnected.
9. Place towel or disposable pad under extremity. Don clean, disposable gloves.

   Rationale: Nurse is protected from transfer of microorganisms if blood inadvertently gets on hands.
10. Hold catheter hub with fingers of one hand (may use hemostat). With other hand, loosen old tubing using gentle twisting motion. (*Note*: The dressing may have to be removed.)

    Rationale: Holding the catheter hub firmly maintains needle position in the vein.
11. Cleanse cap with antiseptic swab using friction (Fig. 8). Grasp new tubing, remove protective catheter cap, disconnect IV tubing, and Luer lock new tubing tightly into needle hub while continuing to stabilize catheter hub with other hand (Fig. 9).

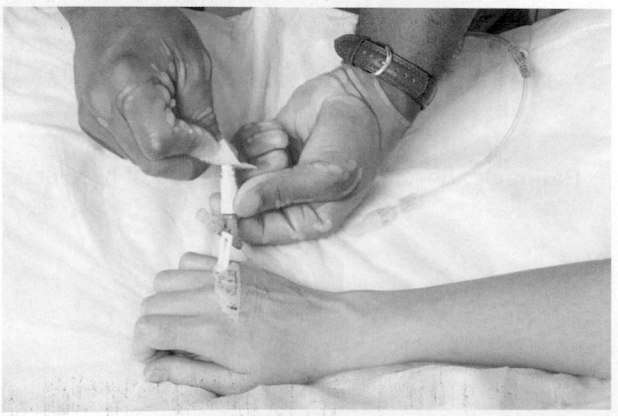

FIG. 8 Cleanse the cap.

Procedure 21-5 *continued*

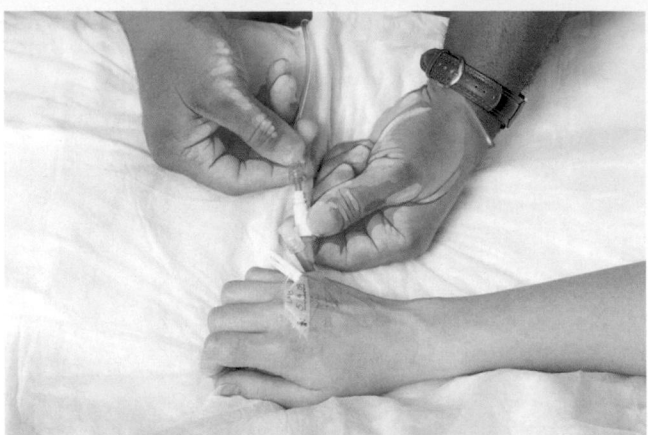

FIG. 9 Insert the new IV tubing into the cap.

Rationale: Stabilizing the catheter hub prevents accidental dislodgement from the vein.

12. **Discard gloves.**

Rationale: Tape will stick to gloves.

13. **Secure tubing with tape.**

Rationale: Securing tubing prevents catheter from becoming dislodged.

14. **If dressing was removed, apply new dressing to IV site according to agency policy.**

15. **Insert cassette into EID (Fig. 10). Program the EID or adjust roller clamp to start solution flowing according to physician's order.**

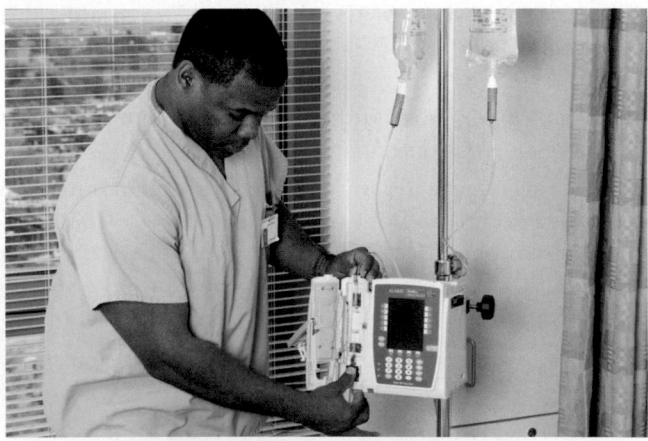

FIG. 10 Insert tubing into EID.

Rationale: Ensures the correct infusion of IV solution

16. **Label new tubing with date, time, and your initials.**

Rationale: The nurses following will know when the next change is needed.

17. **Label solution container with patient's name, solution type, additives, and date and time hung (if not already done). Record solution and tubing change.**

Rationale: Facilitates monitoring by other staff members

18. **Remove old IV solution container and tubing (Fig. 11).**

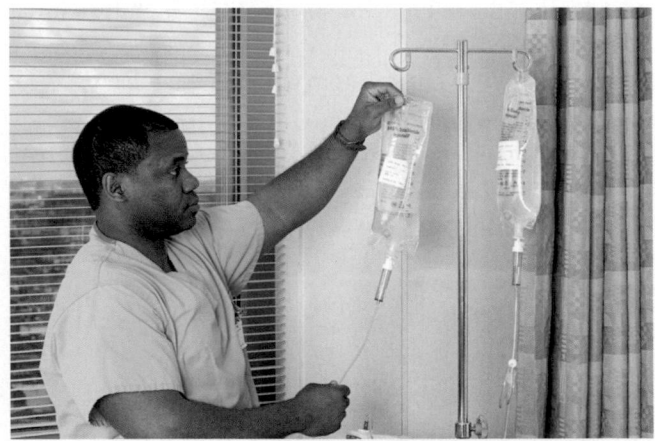

FIG. 11 Remove old IV solution container and tubing.

Rationale:

Documentation

8/12/17: 09:00—1,000 mL D5½NS with 20 mEq KCl @ 125 mL/h on EID. Tubing changed. Alarms on. IV patient. No signs of complications.

— S. Roberts, RN

(*Note:* IV solution and rate is usually documented in the medication administration record [MAR]. IV tubing changes are documented with the IV assessment on the flow sheet.)

Procedure 21-5   *continued*

Life Span Considerations

Infant and Child

- Because infants and children are at risk for circulatory overload, if IV fluids are accidentally infused too rapidly, use IV solutions available in 250- and 500-mL containers. Consider using small-volume buretrols.
- Always use an EID to ensure proper IV infusion in children because fluid overload can be lethal.

Home Care Modifications

- Have the patient/caregiver practice changing IV containers using aseptic technique. Allow time for practice and return demonstration.
- Make sure the patient and caregiver have the name and phone number of their home care company should problems arise.

Collaboration and Delegation

- IV teams may be responsible for routine tubing and dressing changes, especially for central lines.
- Have all unlicensed assistive personnel listen for EID alarms and promptly notify the registered nurse (RN) so that troubleshooting can occur.

Procedure 21-6 Converting to an Intermittent Infusion Device and Flushing

Purpose

1. Maintain patency of IVs used intermittently for medication and emergency IV access.
2. Permit patient increased mobility and freedom if continuous IV infusion is not required.

Equipment

Gloves
Antiseptic swab
Extension tubing set with appropriate intermittent infusion port adaptor (if converting to intermittent infusion device with extension tubing)
Sterile, prefilled NaCl 10-mL syringe
Sterile end protectors
Depending on manufacturer recommendations and agency policy, heparin flush solution; concentration depends on agency policy. Diluted heparin flush (heparin 10 units/1 mL) may be used for some central lines.

Assessment

- Check for order for converting IV line to an intermittent infusion port.
- Identify all pertinent allergies.
- Assess site for signs of erythema, pain, tenderness, and edema.
- Assess label and documentation for date and time of IV device placement.
- Review procedure manual for specific policies regarding flushing locks with saline or heparin.

Procedure

1. **Perform hand hygiene.**

   Rationale: Reduces microbe transmission

2. **Identify the patient.**

   Rationale: Ensures that the correct patient receives proper assessment or treatment and reduces errors

3. **Close door or bed curtains and explain the procedure to the patient.**

   Rationale: Ensures patient privacy, increases patient compliance, reduces patient anxiety, and promotes learning

4. **Assess IV site for signs of phlebitis, infiltration, or infection.**

   Rationale: If complications are detected the IV will need to be discontinued and restarted.

5. **Prepare 10-mL syringe with 3 mL of NaCl (or heparin flush solution according to agency policy or manufacturer recommendations for specific intravascular device). Prefilled 10-mL NaCl syringes are preferred to decrease risk of contamination. Label syringes if not using prelabeled syringe.**

   Rationale: Normal saline has been shown to be as effective as heparin in maintaining patency of peripherally inserted IV locks. Some central lines (Hickman and implanted port) may require intermittent heparin flushes to maintain patency. Label all syringes to prevent medication errors.

Converting to an IID When Extension Tubing Is in Place

6. **Clamp off primary IV tubing.**

   Rationale: Prevents blood loss when IV and tubing are disconnected

7. **Put on clean gloves. Clamp the extension tubing (Fig. 1). Disconnect IV tubing from extension tubing (Fig. 2).**

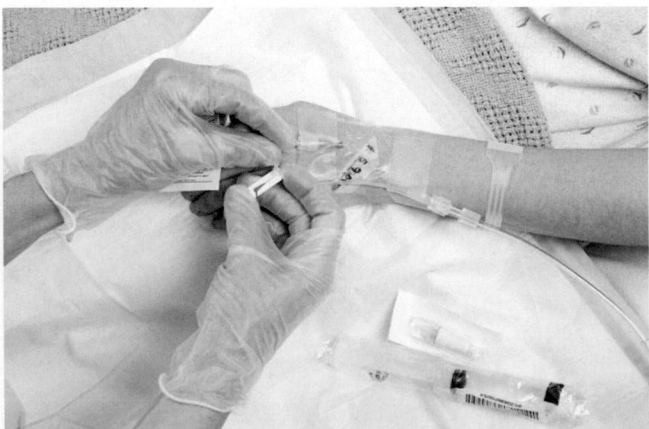

FIG. 1 Clamp the extension tubing.

Procedure 21-6 *continued*

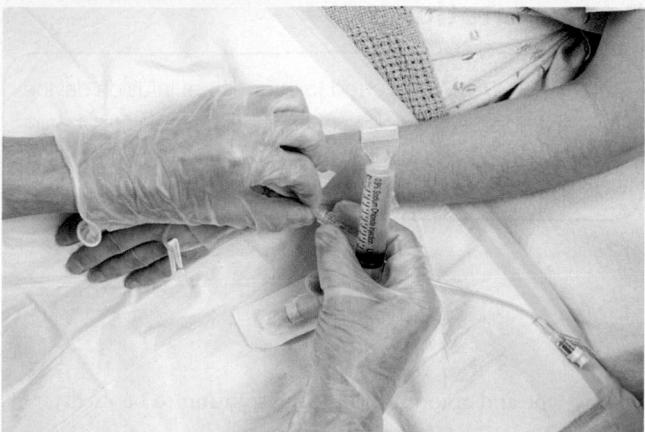

FIG. 2 Disconnect IV tubing from the extension tubing.

Rationale: Clamping prevents air from entering the line.

8. **Cleanse port on extension tubing with antiseptic swab using friction for 15 seconds (Fig. 3).**

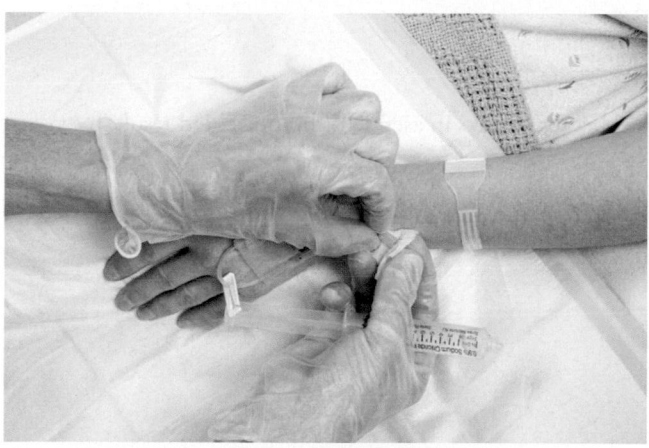

FIG. 3 Cleanse the port on the extension tubing.

Rationale: Reduces risk for contamination

9. **Unclamp the extension set and insert a normal saline or heparin flush syringe into the cap. Flush according to agency policy (Fig. 4). Inject the recommended amount of solution using pulsating technique, ending with 0.5 mL of solution remaining in syringe. Do not force if resistance is met. Reclamp the extension tubing and remove the syringe (Fig. 5).**

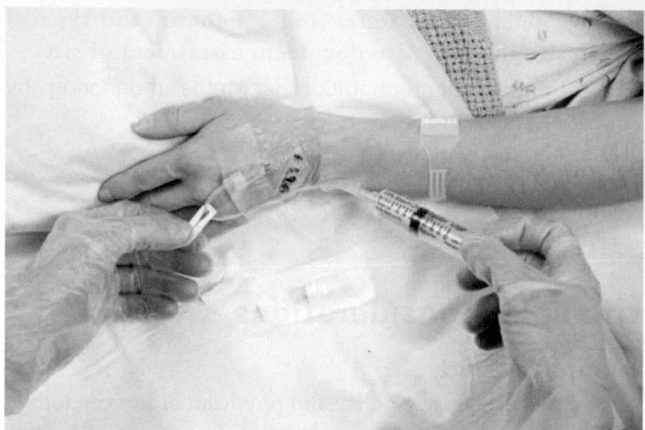

FIG. 4 Flush with normal saline.

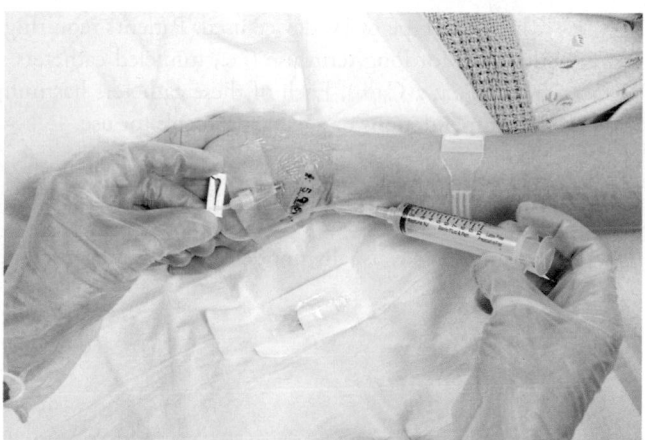

FIG. 5 Reclamp the extension tubing.

(*Note*: **This procedure must be done at least every 8 hours or after each use of the catheter for IV medications to ensure catheter patency. Most agencies recommend changing IV locks every 72 hours to ensure patency and to prevent common complications of IV therapy.**)

Rationale: Positive pressure is maintained, preventing backflow of blood into the catheter, which would increase the chance of occlusion. Forceful flushing can dislodge a clot at the end of the catheter, increasing the risk of complications.

10. **Dispose of syringes in proper container. Remove gloves and dispose of them properly.**

Rationale: Tape will stick to gloves.

11. **Tape adaptor device and extension tubing.**

Rationale: Tape secures the device in the proper position.

12. **Perform hand hygiene.**

Rationale: Deters the spread of microorganisms

Procedure 21-6   *continued*

13. **Document date, time, route, amount, and type of flush solution. Also document assessment of site.**
    Rationale: Documentation facilitates monitoring by other staff members.

Documentation

> 8/4/17: 13:00—IV converted to intermittent infusion device (IID). No redness or swelling at IV site or complaints of pain.
> —S. Roberts, RN

Life Span Considerations

Infant and Child
- Check agency policy and physician orders carefully to determine type and amount of flushing solution to be used.

Home Care Modifications

- Check the type of IV device used. Patients requiring long-term IV access usually have devices placed that are especially designed for long-term use (i.e., tunneled catheters such as the Hickman or Groshong and implantable catheters such as the Port-a-Cath). Each of these catheters has unique flushing requirements and procedures. Refer to manufacturer's recommendations or agency protocols for use.

Collaboration and Delegation

- Flushing IVs is usually not delegated to unlicensed personnel because breaks in aseptic technique could result in sepsis.

Procedure 21-7 Administering Intermittent Intravenous Medications by Syringe Pump

Purpose
1. Maintain therapeutic levels of medication in patient's blood
2. Dilute irritating IV medications.
3. Prevent complications associated with bolus administration by delivering medications over a longer period.
4. Prevent combining incompatible medications.

Equipment
MAR or electronic medication administration record (EMAR)
Medication prepared and labeled in a 20- to 60-mL syringe
IV syringe pump
Microbore extension tubing
Two sterile syringes containing 1 to 3 mL NaCl each
IV lock adaptor or cap
Smart pump (if available), especially for high-risk medications

Assessment
- Review medication order and appropriate rate of infusion.
- Assess the patency of existing IV line.
- Inspect the insertion site for infiltration or phlebitis.
- Determine the patient's drug allergy status.
- Check for possible drug incompatibilities. **Do not administer IV medication through tubing that is infusing blood products or TPN**.

Procedure

1. Check medication order. See Procedure 20-1, steps 1 through 6.

Administering IV Medications When Using Syringe Pump and Intermittent Infusion Device

2. Prepare the medication syringe and IV tubing. Examine the syringe for any air bubbles and expel any that are present. Attach the syringe to the extension tubing, and gently push the syringe plunger to prime the tubing. Cover adaptor.

Rationale: Primed IV tubing prevents air bubbles from entering the patient's vein. The cover on the adaptor maintains the sterility of the system before connection to the primary IV line.

3. Secure the medication syringe into the pump with the flange of the syringe in the clamp's groove (Fig. 1).

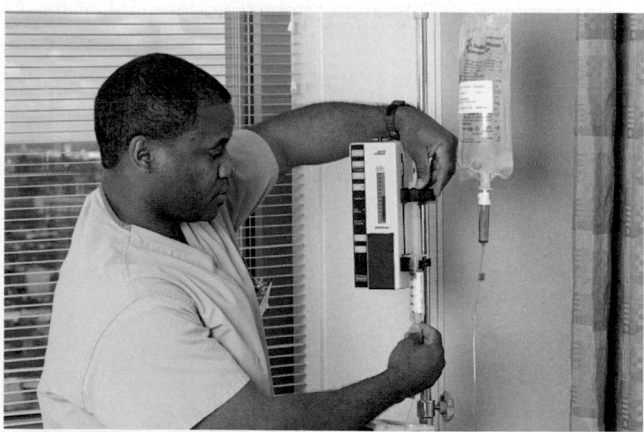

FIG. 1 Insert medication syringe into the pump.

Rationale: The syringe must fit snugly in the pump according to manufacturer's guidelines to function properly.

4. Assess patient allergies. Identify the patient with two identifiers and recheck the six rights. Scan the patient's identification bracelet if using BCMA.

Rationale: Rechecking before administering the medication to the patient prevents errors. With IV medications, mistakes may be lethal because the medication is rapidly absorbed and cannot be retrieved.

Procedure 21-7 *continued*

5. **Assess the IV site for inflammation or infiltration.**

   Rationale: If assessment reveals infiltration or phlebitis, do not administer the IV medication.

6. **Don gloves.**

   Rationale: Prevents spread of microorganisms and adheres to standard precautions

7. **Attach syringe with normal saline into the lock device. Flush lock with normal saline.**

   Rationale: Confirms patency of the IV catheter; assesses for signs of infiltration or phlebitis at IV site

8. **Attach tubing to lock device (Fig. 2). Secure IV tubing to IV site with tape.**

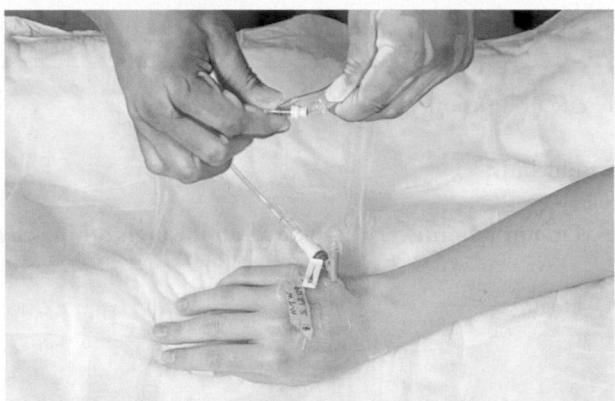

FIG. 2 Attach tubing to lock device.

   Rationale: Prevents inadvertent dislodgement of the IV catheter

9. **Program the pump for the appropriate infusion speed and press the start key (Fig. 3). The medication syringe label often indicates the suggested infusion speed, typically 30 to 60 minutes. If uncertain, consult a drug reference handbook or pharmacist.**

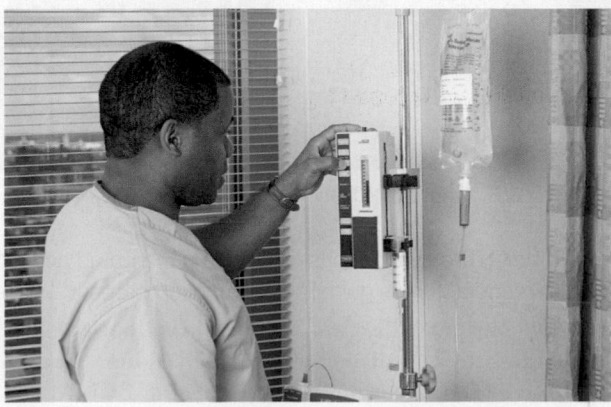

FIG. 3 Program pump to the appropriate rate.

   Rationale: Careful timing ensures safe medication infusion. Too rapid injection of some IV medication causes serious side effects.

10. **Document medication administration.**

    Rationale: Proper documentation reduces the risk of medication errors and serves as communication with the healthcare team.

11. **Assess the patient and infusion device 5 to 10 minutes after infusion has begun.**

    Rationale: Assessment provides information about any adverse reactions to the medication and proper functioning of the infusion pump.

12. **When the completion alarm sounds, return to the patient's room and press the pump's stop key.**

13. **Don gloves. Remove tubing from lock device. Attach syringe with 1 to 3 mL of normal saline and flush lock using push pulse technique ending with positive pressure.**

    Rationale: Flushing the lock immediately after the IV infusion is complete ensures infusion of the entire dose of medication and ensures catheter patency.

14. **Replace lock with new sterile cap.**

    Rationale: Using a new cap maintains sterile system.

15. **Dispose of syringes in proper container. Perform hand hygiene.**

Administering Intermittent IV Medication by Piggyback

Equipment

MAR or EMAR

Medication prepared and labeled in a secondary IV bag (usually 50 to 250 mL)

Secondary IV tubing

20-mL syringe of sterile normal saline flush solution (*optional*— used only if medication is incompatible with primary infusing IV solution to flush IV line of incompatible primary solution both before and after medication is infused)

EID or smart pump

1. **Check medication order. See Procedure 20-1, steps 1 through 6. Prepare medication, tubing, and EID according to procedures described earlier.**

2. **Assess patient allergies. Identify the patient with two identifiers and recheck the six rights. Scan patient's identification bracelet if using BCMA.**

   Rationale: Rechecking before administering the medication to the patient prevents errors. With IV medications, mistakes may be lethal because the medication is rapidly absorbed and cannot be retrieved.

Procedure 21-7 *continued*

3. **Assess the IV site for inflammation or infiltration (Fig. 4).**

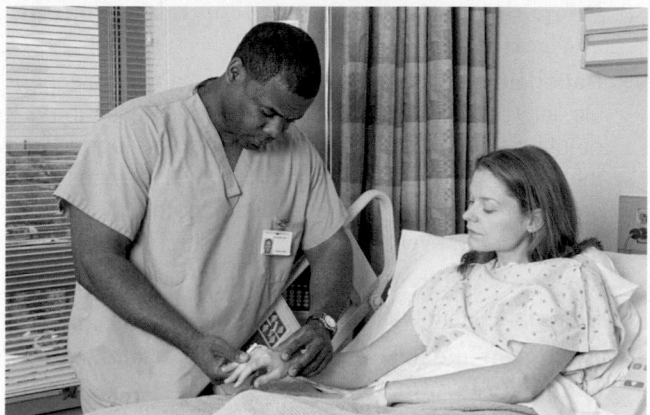

FIG. 4 Assess the IV site.

Rationale: If assessment reveals infiltration or phlebitis, do not administer the IV medication.

4. **Position infusion bags so that the medication (secondary) bag is at or above the level of the primary IV solution (Fig. 5). Insert secondary line into the adaptor port.**

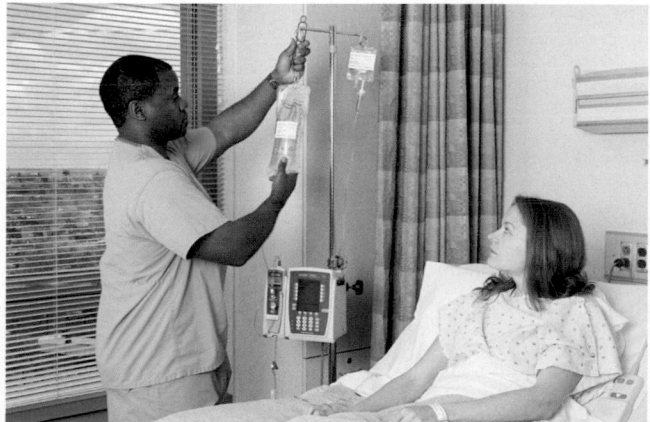

FIG. 5 Position the infusion bags so that medication (secondary) infusion bag is higher than the primary bag during IV piggyback administration.

Rationale: Most infusion sets include back-check valves that stop primary IV solution flow while medication infuses and then automatically open when medication infusion stops. When using these devices, the secondary bag is hung higher than the primary bag, as illustrated here.

5. **Check compatibility of medications to be administered with the IV solution being infused and any other infusing medications. If medication is not compatible with primary IV solution, clamp primary IV tubing above injection port, attach syringe with 20 mL of normal saline flush solution, and flush IV line. Do not administer IV medication through tubing that is infusing blood products or TPN.**

Rationale: Flushing prevents reactions and precipitation of incompatible solutions. Designated line is required for blood products and TPN to avoid incompatibility and reduce infection risk.

6. **Clean the access port on the primary IV infusion tubing using an antimicrobial swab (Fig. 6).**

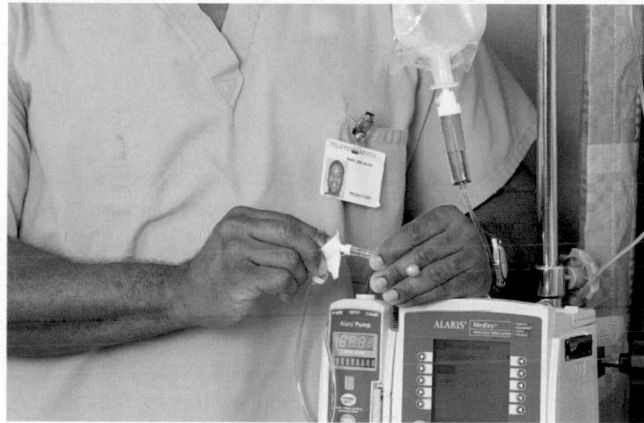

FIG. 6 Cleanse the access port using an antimicrobial swab.

Rationale: Deters entry of microorganisms when piggyback setup is connected to the port

7. **Connect secondary (piggyback) line to injection port or Y-site on IV tubing closest to IV insertion site (Fig. 7).**

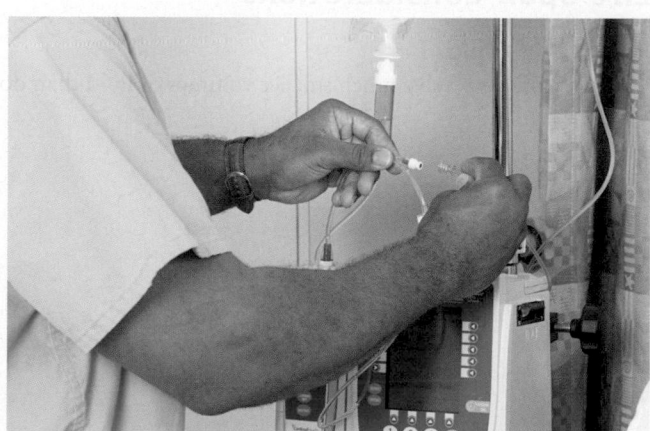

FIG. 7 Connect the piggyback setup to the access port.

Rationale: Increases transit into the vascular system and minimizes amount of drug that will be left in the tubing

Procedure 21-7   *continued*

8. **Program the EID or smart pump with the correct volume and infusion rate for secondary infusion (Fig. 8). Release clamps and press start button.**

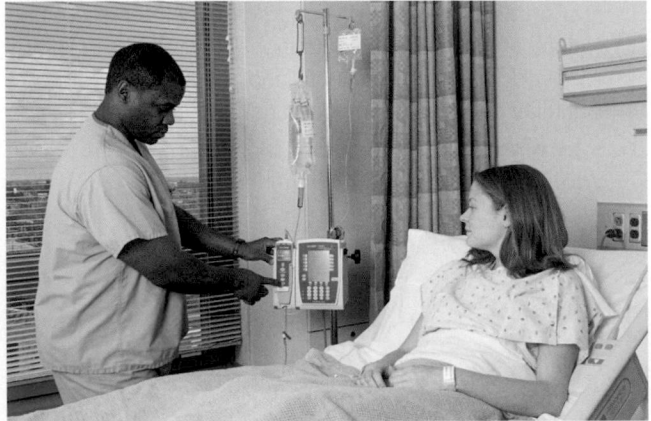

FIG. 8 Program the EID with the correct volume and infusion rate for secondary infusion.

Rationale: Ensures medication infuses at correct rate. Most EIDs allow separate programming of secondary infusions. The EID will infuse the secondary infusion at the programmed rate and then switch to the primary infusion rate when the secondary volume has infused. Smart pumps will indicate whether the rate entered for the medication exceeds limits that have been set in the pump. Soft limit (can override) and hard limits (cannot override) will ensure safe rate of infusion.

9. **When medication has infused, clamp tubing and leave attached. Discard medication bag and tubing if last dose or if tubing will need to be changed before the next dose. Do not loop tubing together at Y-port.**

Rationale: If medications are given on a routine schedule, leaving the equipment attached decreases the risk of infection. When tubing is detached and looped into the Y-port, infection risk significantly increases. The secondary tubing is then changed according to agency protocol (e.g., every 72 hours).

10. **Perform hand hygiene.**

Rationale: Handwashing maintains asepsis.

11. **Document medication administration and add IV volume to IV intake.**

Rationale: Proper documentation maintains accurate patient records and reduces the risk of medication errors.

Documentation

- Document medication administration on the MAR or EMAR. Include the rate of administration.

Life Span Considerations

Infant and Child

- Infants receive much smaller volumes of fluid than do adults.

Procedure 21-8 Administering Medications by Intravenous Bolus (less than 5 minutes)

Purpose
1. Achieve high blood levels of a medication in a short period.
2. Achieve immediate and maximal effects of a medication.

Equipment
MAR or EMAR
Antiseptic swab
Medication vial or ampule
Watch with second hand or digital display
Syringe; two 5- to 10-mL syringes of NACl (if medication is not compatible with IV solution)
Syringe of appropriate size for medication volume
Sterile needle (if nurse is preparing medication from vial or ampule)
Gloves
Label for each syringe

Assessment
- Check medication orders for type of medication, dosage, route, indications, and time scheduled for administration.
- Assess for compatibilities of medications and solutions to be administered.
- Identify all pertinent allergies.
- Assess IV site for patency, erythema, pain, tenderness, or edema.
- Research all information needed to administer medication safely, including action, purpose, side effects, normal dosage, time of peak onset, and nursing implications. High-risk medication may be administered only when the patient is monitored continuously.
- Obtain pertinent physical assessments (e.g., pulse rate, blood pressure) and laboratory data (e.g., potassium level).

Procedure

1. Check medication order. See Procedure 20-1, steps 1 through 6.
2. If medication has not been prepared and labeled by the pharmacy, the nurse prepares the medication. Draw up ordered medication from vial or ampule. Read package insert for proper amount and solution for dilution. Note rate of administration as well as compatibility with infusing IV solutions. Label syringe with the patient's name, name of medication, and dose. Remove needle and dispose of it properly.

   Rationale: Needleless equipment is used for IV procedures to prevent accidental needlesticks and decrease the risk of infection. Labeling the syringe prevents medication errors.
3. Assess patient allergies. Identify the patient with two identifiers and recheck the six rights. Scan patient's identification bracelet if using BCMA.

   Rationale: Rechecking before administering the medication to the patient prevents errors. With IV medications, mistakes may be lethal because the medication is rapidly absorbed and cannot be retrieved.
4. Close the door or bed curtains and explain the procedure to the patient, and then educate the patient about medication.

   Rationale: Ensures patient privacy, increases patient compliance, reduces patient anxiety, and promotes learning
5. Assess IV site for signs of infiltration or phlebitis.

   Rationale: If assessment reveals infiltration or phlebitis, do not administer the IV medication. Restart the IV in another site.
6. Don clean gloves.

   Rationale: To comply with standard precautions

Procedure 21-8 *continued*

Administering Medication into an Existing Intravenous Line

7. **Select injection port or "Y"-site in IV tubing closest to the IV insertion site. Clean port with antimicrobial swab (Fig. 1).**

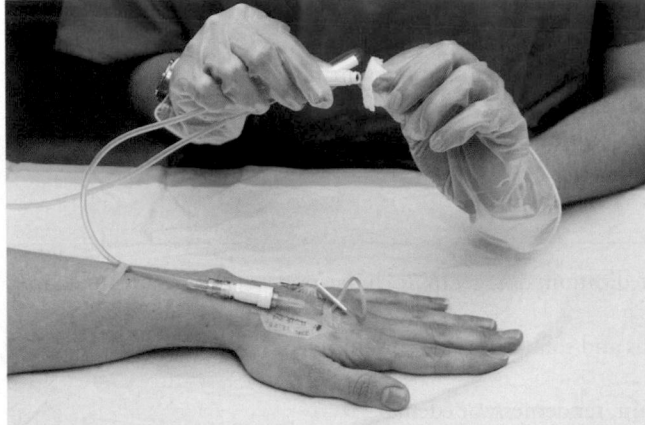

FIG. 1 Cleaning the injection port.

Rationale: Minimizes dilution of the medication and increases transit of medication into patient's vascular system. Close proximity to the insertion site also makes it easier to assess catheter placement by blood return. Cleaning deters entry of microorganisms when the port is punctured.

8. **Uncap the syringe. Steady the port with your non-dominant hand while inserting the needleless device into center of injection port (Fig. 2).**

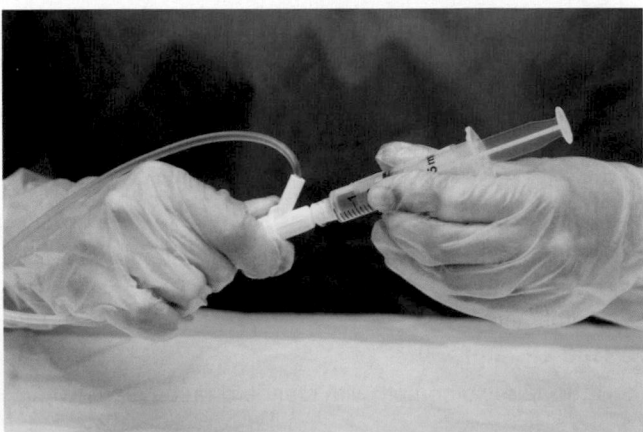

FIG. 2 Inserting the syringe into the injection port.

Rationale: Supports the injection port, lessens the risk for accidental dislodgment of the IV, and helps with entering the port correctly

9. **Pull back on plunger to assess for blood return.**

Rationale: Blood return helps determine if the catheter is still in the vein, ensuring injection of medication into the bloodstream. In some cases, especially with small-gauge catheters, no blood return is observed even when the catheter is in the vein. If no signs of infiltration are present, proceed with IV administration.

10. **Inject the medication slowly into the IV port at the prescribed rate (Fig. 3). It is helpful to use a watch to time the administration rate.**

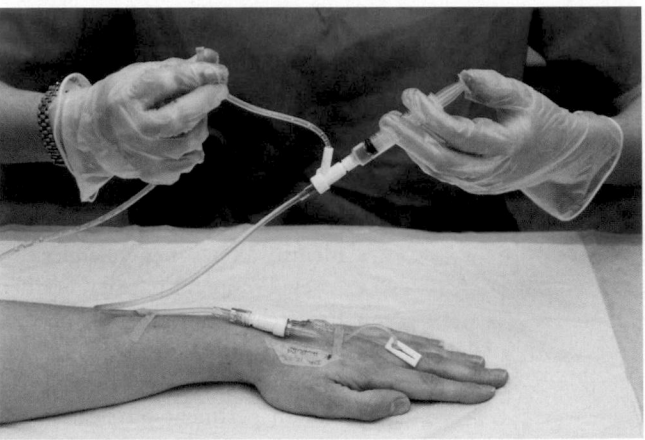

FIG. 3 Injecting medication while interrupting IV flow.

Rationale: Delivers correct amount of medication at the proper interval according to manufacturer's directions. Too rapid injection of some IV medications can be fatal.

11. **If IV medication and IV solution in tubing are incompatible, flush line with normal saline solution while occluding catheter above port. Administer medication at prescribed rate; reflush with 10 mL of sterile normal saline solution and release occlusion.**

Rationale: Flushing before and after with normal saline keeps incompatible solutions from mixing.

Procedure 21-8 *continued*

Administering the Drug into an Intermittent Infusion Device

7. Clean port with antimicrobial swab using friction (Fig. 4).

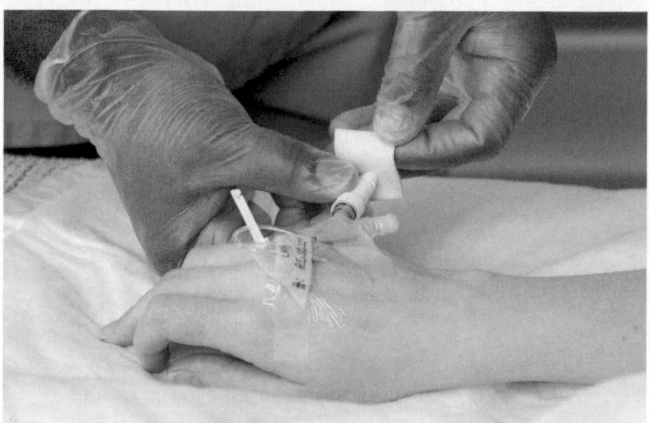

FIG. 4 Clean with antimicrobial swab.

Rationale: Maintains asepsis

8. **Stabilize port with your nondominant hand and insert syringe with 1 mL normal saline solution into injection port.**

   Rationale: Allows for careful insertion into the center circle of the lock

9. **Release the clamp on the extension tubing of the medication lock. Optional: Aspirate gently and check for blood return (Fig. 5).**

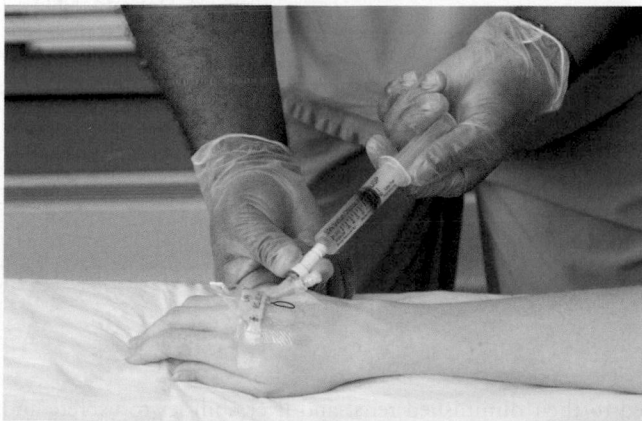

FIG. 5 Optional: Aspirate gently to inspect for blood return.

Rationale: Ensures the catheter is in a vein. In some cases, especially with small-gauge catheters, no blood return is observed even when the catheter is in the vein. If no signs of infiltration are present, proceed with IV administration.

10. **Gently flush with normal saline by pushing slowly on the syringe plunger (Fig. 6) Observe the insertion site while inserting the saline. Remove the syringe.**

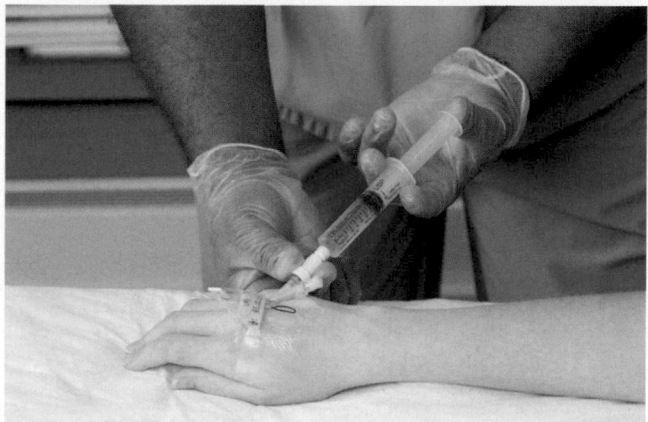

FIG. 6 Flush with normal saline.

Rationale: Flushing confirms patency of catheter; observe for signs of infiltration at the site.

11. **Insert syringe with medication into injection port (Fig. 7). Inject medication slowly at the prescribed rate. Use watch to time administration rate. Remove syringe. Do not force the injection if resistance is felt.**

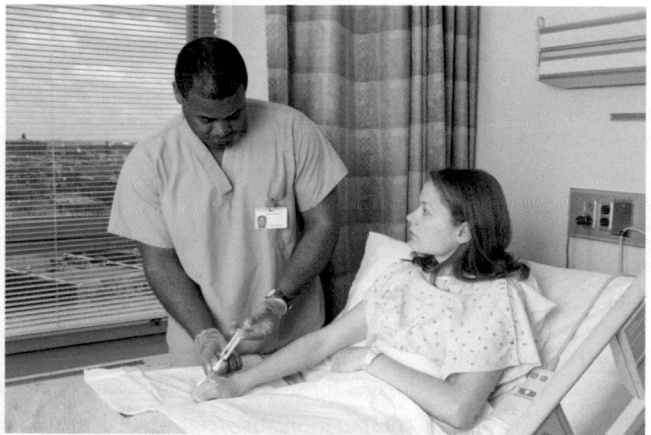

FIG. 7 Insert medication syringe into injection port.

Rationale: Careful timing ensures safe medication infusion. Too rapid injection of some IV medications can be fatal.

Procedure 21-8 *continued*

12. **Insert syringe with 1 to 3 mL of normal saline into injection port and gently flush the port with saline. To gain positive pressue, clamp the IV tubing as you are still flushing with saline using the push pulse technique into the medication lock (Fig. 8). Remove the syringe from the injection port.**

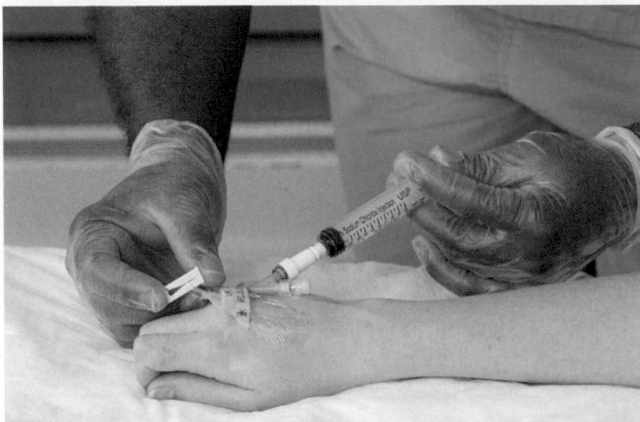

FIG. 8 Clamp the IV tubing as you flush with normal saline.

Rationale: Maintains patency of the IV site

13. **Dispose of used syringes properly, remove gloves, and wash hands**

Rationale: Maintains asepsis

14. **Document medication administration (Fig. 9). Evaluate and chart the patient's response to medication therapy and document according to agency policy.**

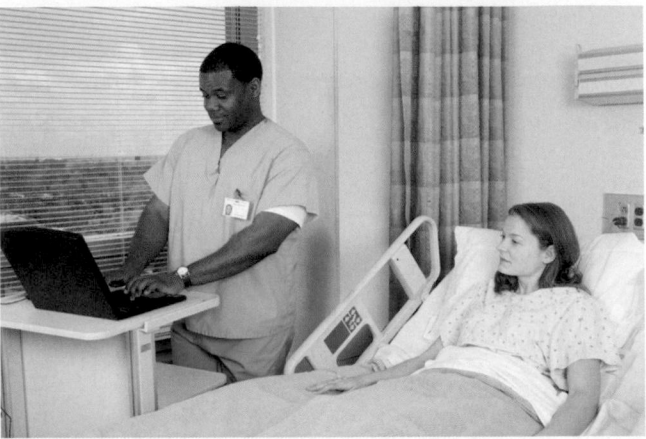

FIG. 9 Document medication administration on EMAR.

Rationale: Accurate documentation is mandatory to prevent medication errors.

Careful and timely assessment is necessary because medications given by IV bolus can have a rapid action.

Documentation

> 6/14/17: 13:00—Administered Ativan 2 mg IV over two minutes for CIWA of 10. No redness or swelling at IV site or complaints of pain. Patient reported feeling more comfortable.
>
> —S. Roberts, RN

Life Span Considerations

Infant and Child

- Medication dosages for infants and children are greatly reduced and are based on their body weight.
- Cross-check computations of weight-based medications with another nurse to verify accuracy and decrease the risk of errors in administration.

Older Adult

- Medication doses for older adults may be decreased related to their diminished renal and liver abilities to excrete and metabolize drugs.

Procedure 21-9 **Monitoring Total Parenteral Nutrition and Administering Intralipids**

Purpose
1. Provide parenteral nutritional support to malnourished patients.
2. Provide parenteral nutritional support to patients who are NPO for extended periods of time.
3. Provide parenteral nutritional support to patients requiring bypass of the gastrointestinal tract for prolonged periods.
4. Provide parenteral nutritional support to patients who have excessive metabolic needs due to trauma, cancer, or hypermetabolic states.

Equipment
TPN solution (prepared by the pharmacy)
Appropriate IV tubing with filter
EID
TPN dressing kit as per hospital protocol (usually contains transparent dressing, acetone swabs, Betadine swabs)
Sterile gloves and mask
Blood glucose monitoring equipment

Assessment
- Assess the patient's nutritional needs.
- Check pattern of weight loss or gain, and intake and output balance.
- Check appropriate lab values (e.g., blood glucose, albumin, electrolytes).
- Check physician's order for TPN, noting additives and rate of infusion.
- Compare the container of TPN with physician's order to ensure that it is correct.
- Assess the patient's knowledge of TPN and need for patient teaching.

Procedure

1. **Perform hand hygiene.**
   Rationale: Reduces microbe transmission
2. **Identify the patient using two separate identifiers.**
   Rationale: Ensures that the correct patient receives proper assessment or treatment and reduces errors
3. **Close door or bed curtains and explain the procedure to the patient.**
   Rationale: Ensures patient privacy, increases patient compliance, reduces patient anxiety, and promotes learning

Monitoring Total Parenteral Nutrition Therapy

4. **Schedule and assist patient with chest x-ray after central catheter insertion.**
   Rationale: X-ray documents that the catheter is in the correct position and determines whether pneumothorax occurred during insertion which is necessary prior to infusing any TPN.

5. **Confirm correct solution against physician's order. Check solution's expiration date. Assess patient allergies. Set the EID for the proper infusion rate (Fig. 1).** (*Note*: Solutions with more than 10% dextrose must be infused directly into a central catheter to rapidly dilute the solution and prevent phlebitis. Constant flow rate helps prevent hyperglycemia and electrolyte imbalances.)

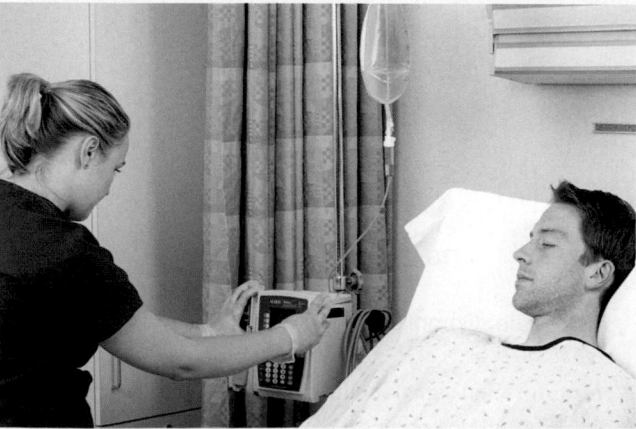

FIG. 1 Set the EID for the proper infusion rate.

Rationale: Careful checking helps prevent medication errors.

Procedure 21-9   *continued*

6. **Inspect tubing and catheter connection for leaks or kinks (Fig. 2). Tape all connections. Change tubing every 24 hours according to agency policy.**

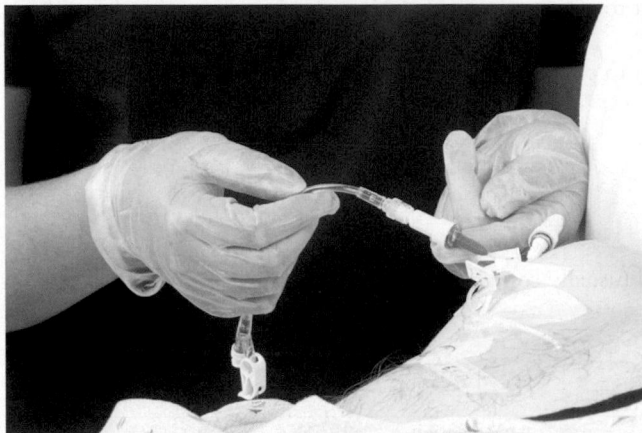

FIG. 2 Inspect tubing and catheter connection for leaks or kinks.

Rationale: Leaks prevent the patient from receiving the prescribed volume of solution and are a potential entry site for bacteria. Kinks in tubing can obstruct flow of solution and result in clotting of the catheter. Taping connections prevents accidental disconnection.

7. **Inspect insertion site for infiltration, phlebitis, or drainage (Fig. 3). If present, notify physician. The physician may order removal of the catheter and culture of the catheter tip if infection is suspected.**

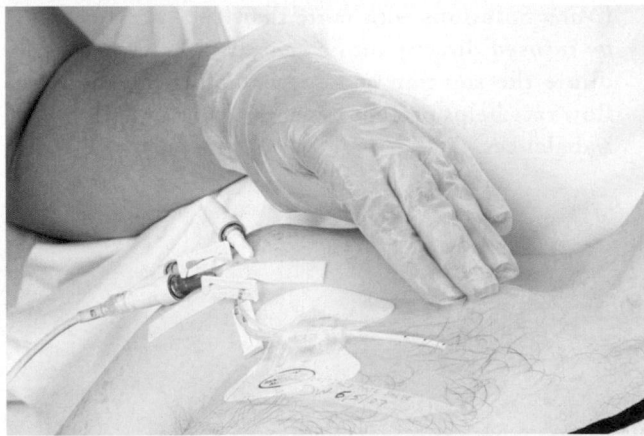

FIG. 3 Inspect the insertion site.

Rationale: Complications are best detected and treated early.

8. **Monitor vital signs, including temperature, every 4 hours.**

Rationale: Unexplained elevated temperature may indicate catheter-related sepsis.

9. **Use the TPN line only for administration of TPN and lipids. Do not use the line for any other reason.**

Rationale: Dedicating the IV line minimizes breaks in integrity of the line to decrease risk of infection.

10. **Monitor patient's blood glucose as ordered (usually every 6 to 12 hours). Notify physician if abnormal.**

Rationale: Hyperglycemia may indicate that the patient needs insulin to help metabolize glucose or may be an early indication of sepsis.

11. **Monitor laboratory tests of electrolytes, blood urea nitrogen (BUN), and glucose, as ordered, and report abnormal findings.**

Rationale: Allows complications to be detected and treated immediately

12. **Maintain accurate record of intake and output to monitor fluid balance.**

Rationale: Allows complications to be detected and treated early

13. **Weigh patient daily and record.**

Rationale: Allows complications to be detected and treated early

14. **Inspect dressing once a shift for drainage and intactness. Change dressing whenever loose or moist, and perform site care at least every 48 hours (Fig. 4).**

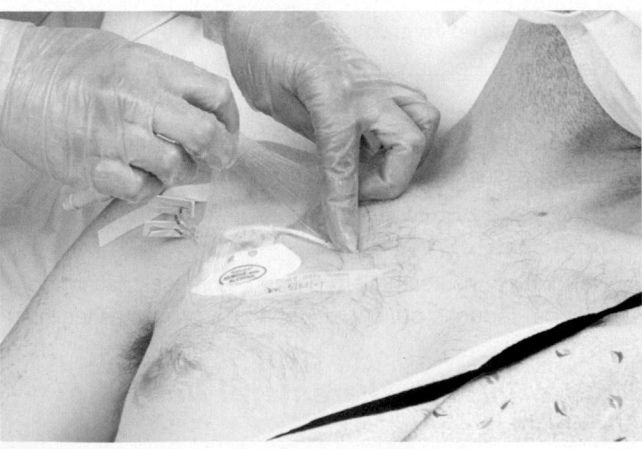

A

FIG. 4 **A.** Position the patient with the head turned away from the site. Apply mask if necessary. Stabilize catheter and remove dressings.

Procedure 21-9   *continued*

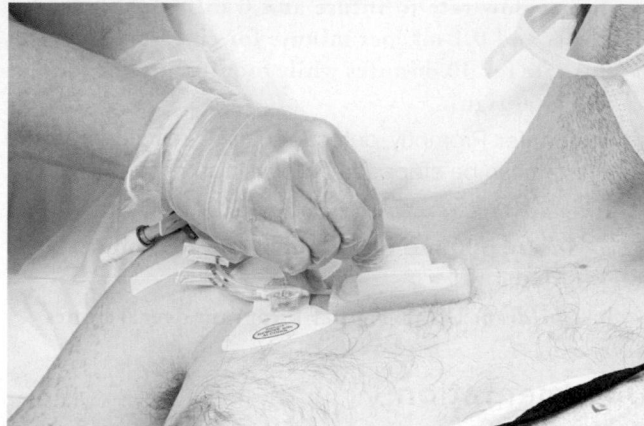

B

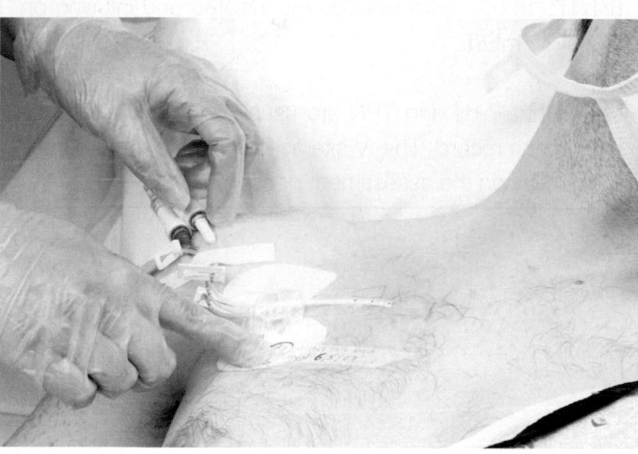

C

FIG. 4 (*Continued*) **B.** Don sterile gloves and clean site area with chlorhexidine solution, moving in a circular fashion from insertion site outward. **C.** Redress the site with a semipermeable dressing, according to agency policy. Label the dressing with date, time, and initials.

Rationale: Intact and dry dressings help prevent infection and keep patient comfortable.

Administering Intralipids

1. **Check lipid solution against physician's order. Inspect solution for separation of emulsion into layers or for froth. Do not use if present.**

   Rationale: Solution may become contaminated or spoiled.

2. **Assess patient allergies to egg yolks or soy products.**

   Rationale: Intralipids are derived from fats from egg yolks, soy, or safflower oil.

3. **Attach fat emulsion tubing to bottle (Fig. 5). Prime tubing as for a conventional IV (Fig. 6).**

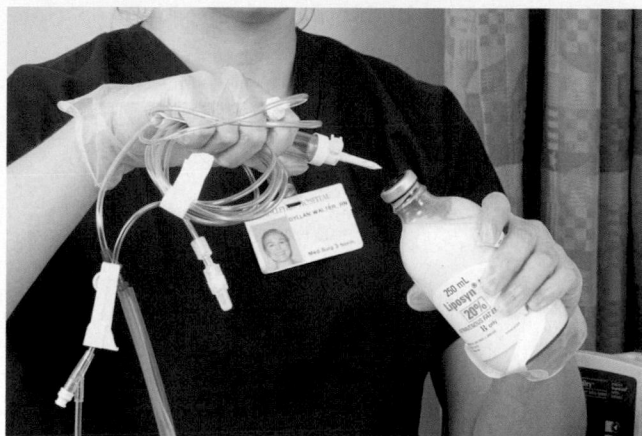

FIG. 5 Attach fat emulsion tubing to bottle.

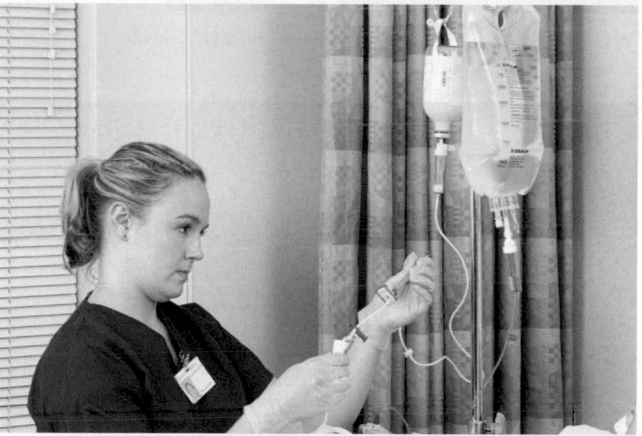

FIG. 6 Prime tubing as for a conventional IV.

Rationale: Tubing has no in-line filter to cause separation of the emulsion.

4. **Identify patient using two separate identifiers. Adhere to the six rights of medication administration.**

   Rationale: Prevents medication errors

Procedure 21-9   *continued*

5. Identify Y-port on tubing (below in-line filter). Cleanse Y-port with antiseptic swab (Fig. 7). Allow to dry. Insert connector into port (Fig. 8). Secure with tape. (*Note*: Lipids can be infused into a peripheral IV.)

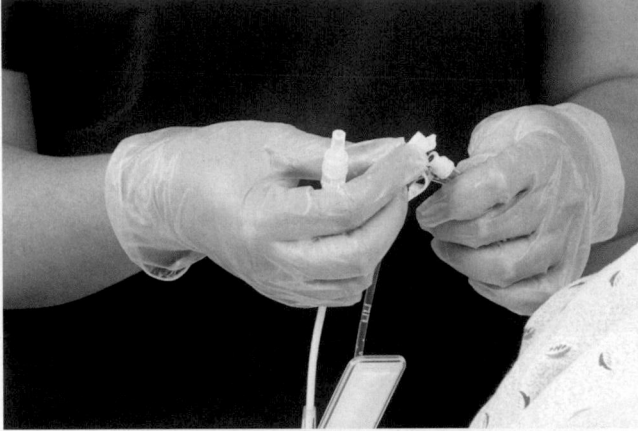

FIG. 7 Cleanse Y-port with antiseptic swab.

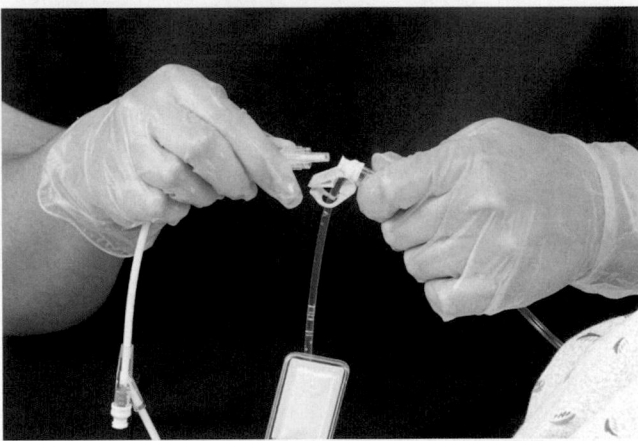

FIG. 8 Insert connector into port.

6. Adjust flow rate to infuse at 1.0 mL per minute for adults and 0.1 mL per minute for children. Infuse at this rate for 30 minutes while monitoring the patient and vital signs.

   Rationale: Promptly detects adverse reactions so the infusion can be stopped and physician notified

7. If no adverse reactions occur, adjust flow rate:
   a. *Adults*: 500 mL intralipid over 4 to 6 hours, or as ordered
   b. *Children*: Up to 1 g per kilogram over 4 hours

Documentation

8/1/17: 16:00—Intralipid 500 mL initiated and infusing on EID @ 83 mL/h.

—S. Roberts, RN

(*Note:* Intralipids and TPN are usually documented in the medication record. The IV site assessment is documented separately on the assessment documents.)

Life Span Considerations

Infant and Child

- TPN solutions for children generally start with a 10% dextrose solution, increased to 25% dextrose. Exogenous insulin is usually not needed because a child's pancreas adapts easily to higher glucose levels. TPN solutions also usually contain higher concentrations of calcium, phosphorus, magnesium, and vitamins.
- Children are usually more active than are adults and require frequent assessment of the tubing to prevent disconnections or obstruction during ambulation or play.
- Instruct parents about preventing accidental disconnection or obstruction of tubing.
- Soft restraints may be necessary to prevent the child from pulling out the catheter. Provide play therapy, books, and stimulation to distract the child.

Procedure 21-9 *continued*

Home Care Modifications

- The healthcare team must determine that the patient or a guardian is responsible and able to safely monitor therapy.
- Identify and consult with a home health nurse who can be available 24 hours a day to troubleshoot complications.
- A long-term infusion device, such as a Hickman or Groshong catheter, should be in place before the patient's discharge.
- Teach the patient or caregiver how to initiate, monitor, and maintain an IV catheter and infusion according to the above protocol.
- Weigh the patient daily. Record intake and output. Monitor blood values at least every other week. Have the patient keep a log.

Collaboration and Delegation

- Nutritionists and pharmacists may be consulted, may write TPN orders, or may complete teaching before the patient is discharged for home management.
- IV teams or home IV companies may be involved in teaching and monitoring patients receiving TPN.

Procedure 21-10 Administering a Blood Transfusion

Purpose
1. Replace blood volume or blood components lost through trauma, surgery, or a disease process.
2. Prevent complications from transfusing incompatible blood products.

Equipment

Packaged blood component from blood bank according to agency protocol
500- to 1,000-mL IV container of sterile 0.9% normal saline
Blood administration set with filter
Blood warmer and pressure bag (*optional*—may be used if infusing large volumes of blood rapidly)
EID (certified to be used to administer blood components)
Alcohol swabs and tape

Assessment

- Review physician's order for transfusion.
- Review informed consent for transfusion that documents the conversation with the patient, family, or guardian by a physician, nurse practitioner, or physician's assistant (*not* a staff nurse) regarding the risks and benefits of and alternatives to blood component transfusion.
- Review chart for pertinent, baseline laboratory values (i.e., complete blood count [CBC], platelets).
- Review chart for previous transfusion history, noting if patient has ever had a transfusion reaction.
- Inspect patient's current IV for catheter gauge (gauge should be 18 or larger), patency, and intactness. Restart if necessary.

Procedure

1. **Perform hand hygiene.**

   Rationale: Reduces microbe transmission

2. **Identify the patient using two separate identifiers.**

   Rationale: Ensures that the correct patient receives proper assessment or treatment and reduces errors

3. **Close door or bed curtains and explain the procedure to the patient.**

   Rationale: Ensures patient privacy, increases patient compliance, reduces patient anxiety, and promotes learning

4. **Ensure informed consent has been signed by provider and patient. Teach patient what to report in the event of an adverse reaction, such as chills, back pain, headache, nausea or vomiting, rapid heart rate, rapid breathing, or skin rash.**

   Rationale: Keeping the patient informed increases participation in care. Teaching the patient to self-monitor for adverse reactions helps to detect any potential problem quickly. Informed consent is required for routine, planned transfusion of blood products. Emergency transfusion should *not* be delayed if informed consent has not been obtained.

5. **Administer premedications, such as diphenhydramine (Benadryl), if ordered.**

   Rationale: May be given to lessen the allergic response in high-risk patients who have developed antibodies from previous blood transfusion.

6. **Obtain patient's vital signs, including temperature.**

   Rationale: Baseline vital signs can be compared against vital signs taken during and after transfusion to detect reactions.

7. **With another RN, a physician, or other licensed staff member at the patient's bedside, verify the blood component and the patient's identity by comparing the laboratory blood record with the following:**

   a. **The patient's name and identification number, both verbally and against patient's identification band**

   b. **The blood unit number on the blood bag label**

   c. **The blood ABO group and Rh factor on the blood bag label**

   d. **The type of blood component and the expiration date on the blood label.**

   Document verification by both RN signatures on transfusion record.

   Rationale: Strict adherence to verification before blood administration greatly reduces the risk of infusing the wrong blood type. Students and other unlicensed personnel are not allowed to verify blood products.

8. **Inspect blood product for integrity of bag and appearance of component (clots, cloudiness, abnormal color). Note expiration date and time on the transfusion report.**

   Rationale: Prevents infusion of contaminated blood and decreases risk of complications

Procedure 21-10   *continued*

9. **Wash your hands. Put on clean gloves.**

   Rationale: Prevents transmission of microorganisms

10. **Open Y-type blood administration set, and clamp both rollers completely.**

    Rationale: Clamping prevents spilling and wasting blood.

11. **Spike blood component unit bag port. Prime drip chamber and tubing with blood component (Fig. 1).**

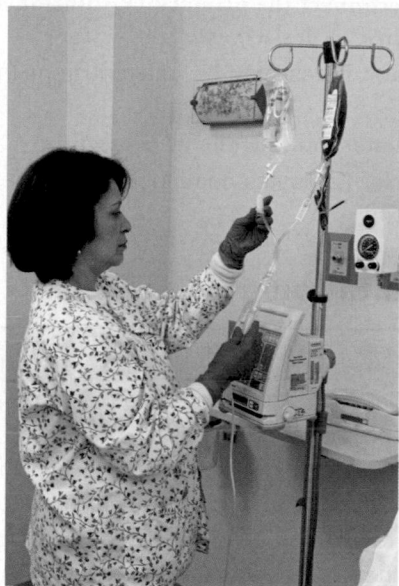

FIG. 1 Prime drip chamber and tubing with blood component.

12. **Spike 0.9% NaCl container with second spike. Keep roller clamp shut.**

    Rationale: Normal saline is compatible with blood. Dextrose solutions will cause hemolysis. Lactated Ringer's should not be used.

13. **Remove primary IV tubing from catheter hub, and cover end with sterile protector.**

    Rationale: If sterility of IV is ensured, it can be reconnected after transfusion.

14. **Attach blood administration tubing to catheter hub, and secure with tape. The IV should be started into an 18- or 19-gauge catheter**

    Rationale: A small-gauge catheter could damage cells that are being transfused.

15. **Open clamp to blood component. Open roller clamp below drip chamber and begin transfusion. Program EID to infuse blood slowly for first 15 minutes (Fig. 2).**

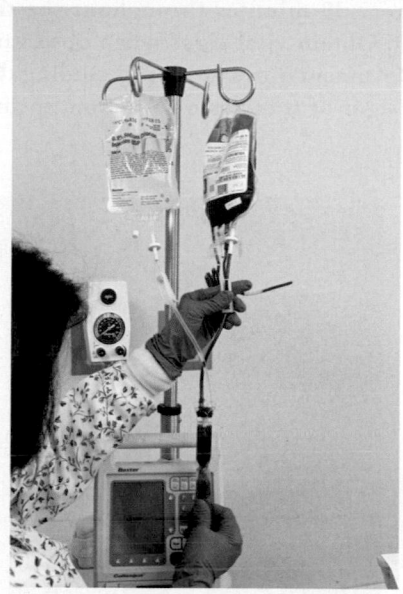

FIG. 2 Infuse the blood product slowly for the first 15 minutes.

Rationale: Most blood reactions occur within first 15 to 20 minutes of transfusion.

16. **Observe and document patient's condition during first 15 minutes, assessing for chilling, back pain, headache, nausea or vomiting, tachycardia, hypotension, tachypnea, fluid overload, or skin rash. (*Note*: If any adverse reactions occur, close clamp to blood, open clamp to 0.9% NaCl, and notify physician immediately. Follow agency policy for laboratory notification and obtaining blood and urine specimens.)**

Rationale: Altered vital signs or other adverse reactions are early indications of a transfusion reaction. Infusing blood slowly during this period limits the amount of blood the patient receives if there is a reaction.

17. **If no adverse reactions occur after 15 minutes, reprogram EID to increase infusion rate according to physician's orders. A unit of RBCs is usually administered over 2 to 4 hours. Observe the patient for signs and symptoms of transfusion reaction at least every 30 minutes throughout the transfusion (Fig. 3). Obtain vital signs when observations warrant. Document observations, including the absence of any signs of transfusion reaction, in the medical record.**

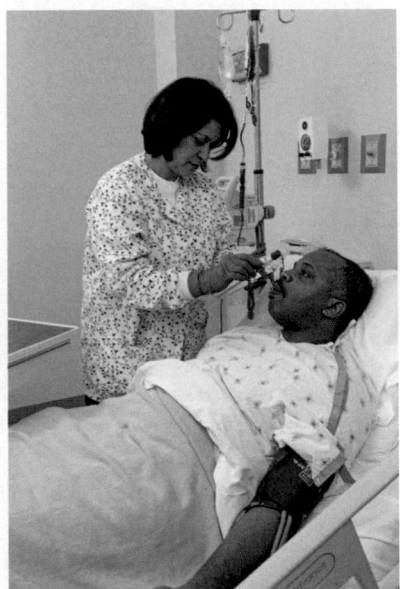

FIG. 3 Monitor the patient every 30 minutes for signs of a transfusion reaction.

Rationale: Patient's appearance or voiced concerns may indicate transfusion reactions or fluid volume overload.

18. **When blood transfusion is complete, clamp roller to blood and open roller to 0.9% NaCl. Infuse until tubing is clear (usually no more than 50 mL of normal saline).**

Rationale: Prevents wasting blood component remaining in tubing and prevents hemolysis of cells from incompatible IV solutions

19. **Obtain and document vital signs.**

Rationale: The finals vital signs need to be identified in case there are changes.

20. **If second blood component unit is to be transfused, slow 0.9% NaCl to keep vein open until next unit is available. Follow verification procedure and vital sign monitoring for each unit.**

21. **If transfusion orders are complete, disconnect the blood administration tubing from the IV catheter hub. Reconnect the primary IV solution and tubing and adjust to desired rate.**

Rationale: Rates may be different from the previous order.

22. **Wash hands and document procedure.**

Rationale: Facilitates communication with the healthcare team

Documentation

8/1/17 13:30—1 unit packed RBC (250 mL) infused over 3 hours. Vital signs stable, no adverse reactions.
CBC redrawn and results pending.
—S. Roberts, RN
(*Note:* The unit number, type, and volume of blood product should be recorded in the I&O record. Blood products are recorded under "colloids" in the fluid record. Vital signs will be recorded in the vital sign record. Some agencies have separate transfusion records for recording specific assessments surrounding administration of blood products. The agency and regional blood bank also require the time, date, and *two* verifier signatures to be recorded on the transfusion record that is provided with the blood product.)

Life Span Considerations

Infant and Child

- Many blood banks have "pedipacks" of RBCs available in 50- and 100-mL volumes for transfusion to children.
- Follow agency protocol for administering blood and blood components to children.

Procedure 21-10 *continued*

Older Adult

- If the patient has heart failure, carefully assess to promptly detect signs of fluid overload. Packed RBCs are often infused to limit the volume being given. The infusion of 0.9% NaCl may be limited to the minimum needed to irrigate the tubing. The infusion time may be increased up to 4 hours from the time RBCs or FFP were removed from refrigeration to decrease the load on the heart. Diuretics may be ordered.

Home Care Modifications

- Blood products are administered in the home only to stable patients. The home care nurse can transport the blood in a special cooler. The caregiver can help verify the identification of the patient and check the unit number. Home care patients can also receive transfusions in short-stay or special procedure units; they leave after the transfusion.

Collaboration and Delegation

- Do not allow unlicensed personnel to verify patient or blood component identification before transfusion; however, they may monitor and record the patient's vital signs during transfusion.

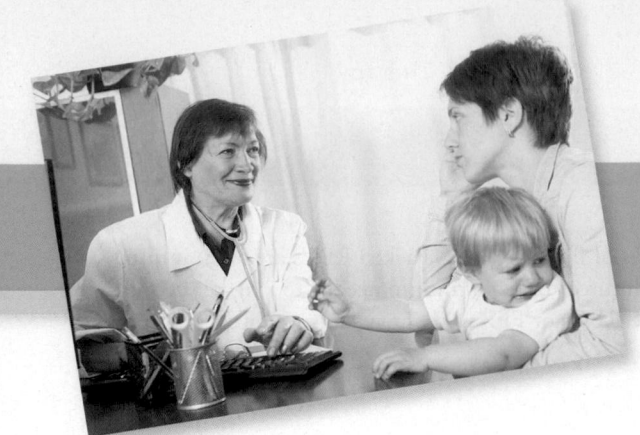

CHAPTER 22

Perioperative Nursing

Kim Leppert

Case Scenario

You are a nurse working in the preadmission surgical unit where preoperative assessment and teaching are performed. A young mother brings in her 2-year-old son, who is scheduled for a bilateral myringotomy (an incision of the tympanic membrane) with tube placement. You talk with the mother about the surgery and then proceed to collect the following information:

- A 12-month history of repeated ear infections, averaging usually between one and two per month
- No known drug allergies
- Currently on no medications
- Vital signs: temperature 37.9°C, pulse 108, respirations 22
- Tenacious, dark tan nasal drainage for last 48 hours
- Lungs clear on auscultation
- Remainder of physical assessment within normal limits

You observe that the mother–child interaction appears appropriate, noting that the mother comforts the child when he begins to cry and actively interacts with him.

Once you have completed this chapter and have incorporated perioperative nursing into your knowledge base, review the above scenario and reflect on the following areas of Critical Thinking:

1. Review age-related considerations for a 2-year-old child having surgery. How will you individualize care for this toddler and his family?
2. Prioritize the most significant assessment data, explaining why you think they are most significant.
3. Plan what teaching is important at this time, and role-play how you will individualize teaching for this family.
4. Demonstrate how you will document or report this information to other team members by preparing a written or oral report to be shared, focusing on the most significant assessment data.

KEY TERMS

anesthesiologist
certified registered nurse anesthetist (CRNA)
circulating nurse
general anesthetic
informed consent
intraoperative phase
local anesthetic
malignant hyperthermia
moderate sedation
paralytic ileus
postanesthesia care unit (PACU)
postoperative phase
preoperative phase
regional anesthetic
scrub person
skin staples
surgical verification
suture

Upon completion of this chapter, the student will be able to do the following:

1. Describe the three phases of perioperative patient management.
2. Discuss the effects of surgery on health and function.
3. Identify life span considerations for the patient undergoing a surgical procedure.
4. Describe appropriate perioperative patient teaching.
5. Discuss emotional support, safety, and asepsis during the intraoperative phase.
6. Identify appropriate nursing assessments in the recovery facility and during the postoperative period.
7. List common postoperative complications and appropriate nursing interventions to prevent or treat each postoperative complication.
8. Develop an appropriate discharge plan for the surgical patient.

In modern culture, surgery has become a common method of treating disease and promoting health. In the last few decades, the complexities of surgery have increased greatly, and entire organ systems can be transplanted to replace nonfunctioning body parts. All surgical procedures can potentially affect a person's functional abilities. The impact can be great and permanent or brief and temporary.

The goal of perioperative nursing practice is to assist patients and their families and significant others to achieve a level of wellness equal to or greater than that which they had before the procedure (Association of periOperative Registered Nurses [AORN], 2014). Perioperative nurses provide specialized care to surgical patients, promoting their return to optimal function. As appropriate, nurses include family members and significant others in this specialized care.

SURGICAL INTERVENTION

Phases of Perioperative Nursing

Perioperative nursing includes three distinct phases: preoperative, intraoperative, and postoperative. The **preoperative phase** includes all activities that prepare the patient for surgery. It begins when the decision for surgery is made and ends when the patient is transferred to the operating room. The **intraoperative phase** includes all those activities that occur from the time the patient is transferred to the operating room until he or she is transferred to the recovery facility. The **postoperative phase** involves the period after the patient is discharged from the recovery facility and ends with the resolution of all surgical consequences. The postoperative phase may be short (less than 1 day) or lengthy (several months or longer), depending on the nature and extent of the surgical procedure and the patient's ability to recover from it. Immediate postoperative care usually is given in a designated area of the hospital or ambulatory care facility. This area is referred to as the **postanesthesia care unit (PACU)**. In each phase, the nurse plays an integral role, using the nursing process to individualize care and meet the surgical patient's specific needs.

Classification of Surgery

Surgery may be performed for many specific reasons: to investigate a problem or set of symptoms, alleviate pain, prolong life, improve mobility, provide vascular access for medications or nutrition, improve function, or improve appearance. Table 22-1 provides general classifications of surgery according to purpose and urgency.

Surgical Facilities

CLINICS AND PHYSICIANS' OFFICES

In the past, surgery performed in a clinic or physician's office was usually limited to minor procedures, such as diagnostic, oral, or gynecologic procedures or removal of skin lesions, and required little in the way of anesthesia. As technology advances and procedures become less invasive, the number of surgeries performed in clinics and physicians' offices continues to grow. Surgery done here is less expensive because less complex equipment is used. Shorter-acting anesthetic agents or nurse-monitored sedation may be used, both of which often result in less need for extensive postanesthesia recovery time and monitoring.

AMBULATORY SURGICAL CENTERS

Ambulatory surgical centers, also known as day surgery units or surgicenters, have proliferated in an attempt to keep down rising surgical costs. These facilities may be affiliated with and located in or near hospitals. Patients typically are admitted on the day of surgery and discharged that same day.

Because ambulatory surgical centers can save time and money, many hospitals are increasing the number of surgeries performed in these centers. This trend is likely to continue in the next decade until most surgeries are performed on an ambulatory basis. The anesthetic and surgical risks and the patient's ability to safely care for himself or herself after discharge from the short-stay facility are important determinants. Increasingly, surgeries once performed only in the hospital, such as cholecystectomies (gallbladder removal), appendectomies, and hernia

TABLE 22-1 TYPES OF SURGERY BASED ON PURPOSE AND URGENCY

Classification	Purpose	Examples
Purpose		
Diagnostic	Confirms suspected diagnosis	Biopsy, culture, endoscopy, fluid tap
Explorative	Confirms the type and extent of a disease process	Laparotomy, joint exploration
Reconstructive	Repairs physical deformities or improves appearance	Rhinoplasty, mammoplasty, skin grafting
Curative	Removes or repairs diseased or damaged body organs or structures and cures the patient	Appendectomy, hysterectomy, fixation of fractures
Transplant	Replaces diseased or damaged body organs and structures with donated or artificial organs	Heart, kidney, cornea, bone, liver, lung, pancreas, or skin transplants
Palliative	Alleviates pain or other disease symptoms, slows progression of diseases but does not cure	Tumor debulking, nerve blocks, placement of feeding tubes
Urgency		
Emergent	Preserves function of body parts or life of patient	Repair of major vessel to stop severe bleeding
Urgent	Requires prompt attention within 24–48 h	Repair of fracture, incision and drainage of wound infection
Required	Indicated for health problem but immediacy not necessary to preserve function or life	Gallbladder removal, excision of cancerous growth
Elective	Satisfies patient's desire but not needed to preserve life or function	Cosmetic surgery

repairs, are being performed with the use of a laparoscope (a tubular optical and surgical instrument) in ambulatory surgical centers. Patients who have procedures using this minimally invasive technology are usually able to avoid the complications often associated with more extensive "open" procedures and are able to return to previous activity levels much sooner. However, ambulatory surgery provides a special challenge to perioperative and postanesthesia nurses, who must provide optimal patient care and teaching within limited time frames.

HOSPITALS

Hospitals are comprehensive facilities for all types of surgery and postsurgical recovery. They have the necessary equipment and personnel available for surgeries requiring intensive monitoring, complex technology, and prolonged recovery periods. Hospitals provide a wide range of services and have extensive emergency backup systems, should they be necessary. Hospital surgeries are generally more expensive than surgeries at either ambulatory surgery centers or clinics. Emphasis on cost containment may prevent admission to a hospital for minor surgical procedures because insurance companies may be unwilling to reimburse for the cost of inpatient hospital care.

Effects of Surgery on Health and Function

HEALTH PERCEPTION AND HEALTH MAINTENANCE

The decision to have surgery is made jointly by the patient and healthcare provider to promote health or improve function. This individual decision is based on a person's perception of health and what actions are appropriate to manage current problems.

Surgery involves many aspects of safety, both psychological and physical. Psychological safety is a feeling of comfort, security, and well-being, which are feelings of trust and confidence in the patient's healthcare that providers and caregivers can enhance. Nurses can do much to promote these feelings. Providing emotional support and promoting an understanding of procedures greatly facilitate this process. When possible, nurses should include family members and significant others in the explanation of surgical procedures. Physical safety considerations include safety with anesthesia, medications, chemicals, electricity, procedures, special equipment (e.g., lasers, radiation units), surgical positioning, and patient transport.

ACTIVITY AND EXERCISE

Depending on the nature of the surgery, the impact on exercise and activity levels can be significant. Such alterations in activity levels may be either temporary or permanent. The woman who is to have a breast biopsy in an ambulatory surgery center will probably need to curtail her regular activities for only a few hours, whereas the patient who is to have surgery on a fractured leg will need to alter activity for several weeks to months, depending on the extent of rehabilitation needed to return to a previous level of functioning. Both patients will experience relatively temporary changes in their activity levels.

Permanent changes in a patient's activity level may also occur as a result of surgery. A person who has a leg amputated secondary to trauma or peripheral vascular disease will need to make permanent changes in activity. Regardless of the specific nature of the changes that surgery brings, all patients will benefit from well-planned and well-implemented nursing interventions directed at returning them to their highest possible level of activity.

During the immediate postoperative period, respiratory and cardiovascular complications may result from inactivity and immobility. Deep breathing and incentive spirometry are beneficial in maximizing air exchange and in preventing atelectasis (alveoli collapse) and pneumonia. Leg exercises, antiembolic hose, and sequential compression devices (SCDs) help maintain peripheral circulation, promote venous return to the heart, and prevent deep vein thrombosis and subsequent pulmonary emboli.

NUTRITION

An optimal nutritional state is essential for safe and successful surgery. It promotes wound healing, increases resistance to infection, promotes physical and psychological well-being, and maintains an adequate energy level and optimal fluid and electrolyte balance. After surgery, a diet with sufficient amounts of protein and vitamins A and C helps rebuild tissues and promotes wound healing. Adequate amounts of carbohydrates and fat are also important to avoid depleting protein stores. Metabolic disorders, such as diabetes mellitus, need to be assessed before surgery and managed well to avoid intraoperative and postoperative complications. Obesity poses a risk for the surgical patient because surgery is often longer, positioning on the operating table is more challenging, and postoperative complications (e.g., wound dehiscence) are more frequent.

After surgery, nutrition may be affected. For example, nausea and vomiting can occur after surgery from the effects of anesthetic agents, pain medications, or manipulation of intestinal organs. In addition, oral fluid and food may be withheld until intestinal motility resumes. Once active bowel sounds are present, the diet is usually advanced as tolerated.

INFECTION

The skin is the primary defense against infection. Surgical site infections (SSIs) are the most common healthcare-associated infection (HAI; CDC, 2014), and the most effective treatment of SSIs is prevention (Rothrock, 2015). Before surgery, detection and treatment for any infection are necessary to promote healing and lessen the chance that the infection will spread or become systemic. During surgical procedures, the risk of infection increases because the skin barrier is broken and trauma occurs. Meticulous intraoperative aseptic practices are necessary to prevent infection. Evidence indicates that additional factors such as close glucose monitoring for diabetic patients and maintenance of intraoperative normothermia also significantly reduce the likelihood that a patient may develop a SSI.

Preoperative skin scrubs can decrease endogenous flora (microorganisms that normally live on the skin), which might otherwise increase the infection risk. Antibiotic prophylaxis is an important prevention strategy. A cephalosporin antibiotic is usually the antibiotic of choice; however, antibiotic prophylaxis depends on the type of surgery, cost, safety, and effectiveness of the prophylaxis (Rothrock, 2015). The antibiotic should be administered within 1 hour of the surgical incision so that the level of medication circulating in the patient's blood will be at a therapeutic range during surgery.

During the postoperative period, key nursing responsibilities focus on monitoring the wound for signs of infection and instituting measures to prevent other infectious complications, such as respiratory or urinary tract infections.

THERMOREGULATION

Normally, body temperature is maintained without difficulty. During surgery, several factors—including decreased ambient temperature in the operating room, vasodilation secondary to the use of certain anesthetic agents, blood loss, intravenous (IV) fluid administration, exposure of body surface area, cool skin preparation solutions, and decreased consciousness—can lead to hypothermia, which has been shown to increase risk for bleeding, impaired wound healing, and SSI (Rothrock, 2015).

In addition, the patient's age can affect thermoregulation. The risk of hypothermia increases in the very young and the very old. Interventions to promote normothermia, such as providing warm blankets and the use of forced-air warming devices, should be initiated in the preoperative area and continued during the intraoperative and postoperative phases. Additional measures such as warming skin preparations and IV solutions and minimizing body surface exposure once the patient is in the operating room will help to alleviate body heat loss. See Figure 22-1 for a photo of a forced-air warmer.

Another potential surgical problem of body temperature regulation is **malignant hyperthermia**, a hypermetabolic disorder of skeletal muscle that can be induced by some anesthetic agents, including certain inhalants and muscle relaxants. Because malignant hyperthermia has been identified as an inherited disease, patients who have a positive family history are particularly susceptible. This complication is manifested by masseter (jaw) muscle rigidity and ventricular dysrhythmias, which are associated with tachypnea (rapid respirations), cyanosis, skin mottling, and unstable blood pressure. These symptoms are followed by an increase in body temperature (possibly 1°C every 5 minutes if untreated), although fever may be a late sign of malignant hyperthermia.

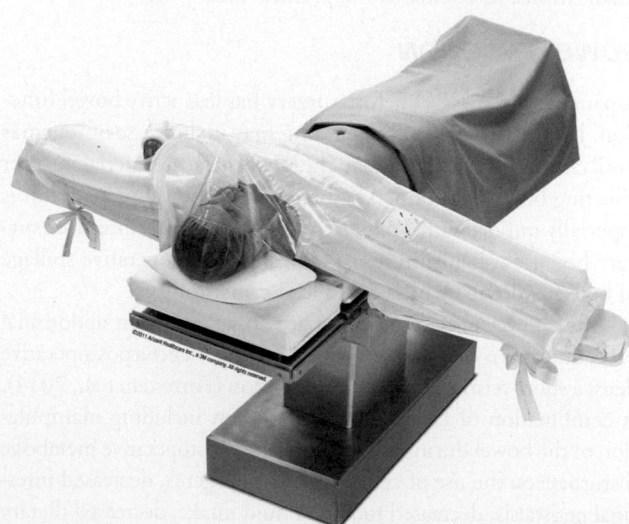

FIGURE 22-1 The Bair Hugger patient warming system. (Reprinted with permission from 3M.)

SAFETY ALERT

If not detected early and treated effectively, malignant hyperthermia can result in cardiac arrest and death. Consequently, in addition to identifying susceptible people, muscle rigidity, vital signs, and body temperature must be monitored closely during and after surgery for all patients, and emergency medications and equipment need to be immediately available.

URINARY FUNCTION

Before surgery, the patient usually receives no food or fluid orally (known as NPO status) to decrease the risk of aspiration during the surgical procedure. NPO status decreases urine production.

Urine output of 30 to 60 mL/hour usually indicates adequate intravascular volume and blood pressure (Phillips, 2013). The patient may have an indwelling urinary catheter placed in the bladder before surgery. If a urinary catheter is not in place, the patient should void immediately before going to the operating room to help prevent bladder distention during or after the procedure. Emptying the bladder also helps make the abdominal organs more accessible during abdominal surgery and prevents accidental injury to the bladder.

During surgery, urine output is monitored closely for all patients with indwelling catheters. Patients who are undergoing shorter procedures (less than 2 to 4 hours) may not have a urinary catheter. For patients with urinary catheters and those without, blood pressure and fluid and electrolyte balance are carefully monitored intraoperatively because these measurements provide information that helps evaluate the adequacy of renal function and circulation.

After surgery, urine output is closely monitored. In this stage, inadequate output may indicate hypovolemia, hemorrhage, electrolyte imbalance, inadequate circulation, hypoxia, or impending shock. Patients without a urinary catheter in place should void within 8 hours after the surgical procedure. Patients without a urinary catheter can have difficulty voiding after surgery because of decreased level of consciousness, pain, medications, or edema in the perineal area.

BOWEL FUNCTION

A patient who is NPO before surgery has less active bowel function. In addition, bowel preparation may include use of "enemas until clear" or laxatives to clean the bowel of fecal material, further affecting bowel function. The preoperative bowel preparation is especially important for patients undergoing gastrointestinal surgery because it helps prevent the possible intraoperative spillage of bowel contents, which could lead to peritonitis.

After bowel surgery (both laparoscopic and open abdominal procedures), it is common for patients to experience a postoperative ileus, a short-term cease of bowel function (Forrester et al., 2014). A combination of factors causes this delay, including manipulation of the bowel during surgery, pre- and postoperative metabolic disturbances, the use of certain anesthetic agents, decreased intestinal peristalsis, decreased food and fluid intake, decreased dietary bulk, pain medications, decreased physical activity, stress, lack of a normal routine, and decreased privacy. Frequently, stool softeners are prescribed after surgery once bowel sounds are present, especially if the patient is receiving large doses of opioid analgesics. Sometimes, laxatives and enemas are necessary.

Postoperative ileus may resolve spontaneously within 2 to 3 days; however, if the lack of bowel function persists 3 days or longer, the condition is known as a **paralytic ileus** (Forrester, Doyle-Munoz, McTigue, D'Andrea, & Natale-Ryan, 2014).

The delay in the return of GI motility can lead to the development of other postoperative complications and extend the length of stay postoperatively; therefore, it is important to treat the symptoms of paralytic ileus (abdominal pain, emesis, abdominal distention, inability to pass flatus or tolerate food) (van Bree et al., 2014). Treatment may include the insertion of a nasogastric tube, analgesics, gum chewing, and IV therapy.

PAIN

Pain has both physical and psychological components. Pain may occur before surgery secondary to a disease process or to a traumatic injury and also after surgery secondary to the surgical incision or procedure. Nursing interventions vital in helping patients cope with pain include obtaining a thorough pain assessment, administering medications, positioning, relaxation techniques, psychological support, distraction techniques, and appropriate referrals to other health professionals. Many hospitals now have a pain service or clinic that may be consulted. Maintaining a restful and comfortable environment is also helpful.

Analgesics often are administered by the IV route, either IV push or via patient-controlled analgesia (PCA), or by epidural administration. These forms of administration are more successful in controlling pain than the use of intramuscular or subcutaneous injections. Nonsteroidal analgesic and adjuvant pain medications are often used in combination with opioid medications to effectively manage pain during the postoperative period. Refer to Chapter 35 for information on pain management.

SLEEP AND REST

The surgical patient may experience disrupted sleep because of preoperative preparation activities, changes in schedule, stress or anxiety related to the impending procedure, medication therapy, physical or emotional pain, separation from family and others, money worries and job uncertainties, and changes in normal diet and activity level. Nursing interventions that can help promote rest include providing a calm environment, clustering care activities, relieving anxiety through patient teaching and emotional support, making referrals to other professionals as appropriate (e.g., mental health professionals, financial counselors, chaplains), and administering medications and treatments as appropriate. Sedatives or antianxiety agents may be administered the evening before surgery and during the postoperative period.

After surgery, adequate sleep and rest are important for wound healing and emotional well-being. The patient who can rest sufficiently and maintain adequate amounts of rapid eye movement (REM) or dream sleep can better handle the stress associated with surgery and recovery. Planning for adequate periods of rest and sleep and maintaining a quiet, restful environment are essential.

DELIRIUM

The surgical patient may experience delirium secondary to medication therapy, unfamiliar surroundings and people, sensory overload, electrolyte imbalances, pain, anxiety, or sleep deprivation. Delirium is an acute abnormal state of cognition that includes inattention, disorganized thinking, and altered level of consciousness. Symptoms fluctuate over time and can manifest as a hyperactive state (agitation, pulling out tubes) or a hypoactive state (lethargy, difficulty focusing). It is important to identify and treat the underlying cause of the delirium. Nursing interventions to assist confused patients include orienting patients to unfamiliar surroundings and people, maintaining a safe and comfortable environment, promoting increased visual and auditory input (e.g., pictures of family and friends, calendars, radio, television) during waking hours, promoting a quiet and restful environment during the hours set aside for sleep and rest, and monitoring medication therapy. Refer to Chapter 37 for detailed information on delirium.

SELF-CONCEPT

For many people, self-concept is closely related to physical appearance, which surgical procedures may alter. The impact of surgery on self-concept depends on the patient's perception of his or her value or image rather than a specific objective measure. The alteration may be minor, such as a small scar, or it may be major, such as a limb amputation or breast removal. Surgical alterations may also involve removal of certain organs (e.g., uterus, portions of the colon), which may result in significant emotional and psychological changes. Such alterations may affect a person's self-concept, which may necessitate intensive, long-term rehabilitation, both physical and emotional.

In addition to providing the patient with the necessary technical care, teaching, extensive rehabilitation, and emotional support, nursing interventions may also include referral to agencies and support groups that can benefit the patient after surgery and discharge from the acute care facility. Such groups include the American Cancer Society (and its numerous affiliates) and the American Heart Association. These organizations sponsor support groups that can assist the patient and family to cope with changes in self-concept.

ROLES AND RELATIONSHIPS

Surgery and the separation that it may entail can affect personal, family, and business relationships. Changes may be temporary or permanent. Usually, procedures from which one recovers quickly allow a person to resume previous roles and relationships without any long-term changes or conflicts. Chronic illnesses and major procedures, however, may lead to long-lasting changes that require much adaptation. Surgery may directly affect energy level, so fulfilling the role of provider, sexual partner, or parent may be more difficult. Moreover, a prolonged recovery period may create problems in a person's work relationships, which can have an impact on financial security.

Appropriate nursing interventions depend on the specific role or relationship and the values or beliefs that are creating conflict. Providing the patient and family members with emotional support and appropriate patient teaching can positively affect role relationships. Referring the patient to another healthcare team professional, such as a social worker, mental health counselor, or a chaplain, may be necessary.

COPING AND STRESS TOLERANCE

Surgery, even a minor procedure, entails significant stress. Coping behaviors and stress tolerance are closely related to how a person defines stress and how that person has managed stress in the past. Nursing interventions should include attempts to identify stress management strategies that were effective for the patient in the past because these strategies may be effective again during the perioperative period. Keep in mind that stress tolerance and coping behaviors are individual matters. What is effective for one person may not be effective for another.

Other interventions to assist a person in coping and managing stress include identifying and promoting effective stress management strategies and coping behaviors, providing emotional support and instruction for the patient and family, and making referrals to other health professionals as necessary.

SEXUALITY

Surgery may temporarily or permanently affect a patient's sexuality and reproduction. Separation, prolonged convalescence, and actual surgical alterations all may significantly affect a person's sexuality and sexual identity. The impact may be physical, psychological, or both. Physical changes that may affect a person's sexuality can result from surgeries that alter appearance, limit mobility, alter reproductive capacity, and limit physiologic functioning.

Box 22-1 lists surgeries that may affect a person's physical appearance, mobility, and functioning, either temporarily or

---

BOX 22-1 Surgical Procedures Affecting Appearance, Mobility, and Functioning

Physical Appearance
Radical neck surgery
Mastectomy
Amputations
Facial surgeries
Oral surgery

Mobility
Bone fusions
Dislocations
Spinal surgeries
Amputations
Joint replacement

Functioning
Vaginectomy
Hysterectomy
Prostatectomy
Ostomies (colostomy, ileostomy)
Oral surgeries

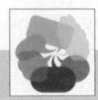

THERAPEUTIC DIALOGUE: POSTOPERATIVE PAIN

SCENE FOR THOUGHT

Alicia Martin, a 52-year-old woman, returned from the operating room last evening. A right leg fracture was repaired and her spleen was removed after a skiing injury yesterday. She has been awake and sitting up in a chair for the last few hours.

LESS EFFECTIVE

Nurse: Hello, Ms. Martin, I'm Robert Henderson, your nurse for the day shift. How are you? *(Good eye contact to indicate that the question is a real one.)*

Alicia: Hello, Robert. Call me Alicia. I'm okay, I guess. *(Looks tired, leaning against the back of the chair.)*

Nurse: You look tired. Do you want to get back into bed?

Alicia: Yes, please. Amazing how just sitting can tire you out. *(Gets back into bed slowly, with help.)*

Nurse: *(Gets Alicia settled and comfortably positioned.)* How does that feel? *(She smiles and nods okay.)* Good. I was wondering if I could talk with you to see if you have any particular questions about the operation or your injuries.

Alicia: I don't have any questions. I just want to go home. *(Looks like she's going to cry.)*

Nurse: I can understand that. No one likes to be in the hospital, especially in the middle of a vacation. *(Puts hand on Alicia's arm in sympathy.)* But I thought you might have some questions that I could help you with. You had quite a difficult accident, and I know it must be hard on you.

Alicia: *(Starts to cry.)* That's true, it is hard on me. And all I want to do is rest right now; I'm not feeling very well at all.

Nurse: Can I get you anything before I go?

Alicia: No, I'll be okay if I just rest a little. *(Closes her eyes.)*

Nurse: Okay, I'll check back with you in a little while.

MORE EFFECTIVE

Nurse: Hello, Ms. Martin, I'm Richard Hines, your nurse for the day shift. How are you? *(Good eye contact to indicate that the question is a real one.)*

Alicia: Hello, Richard. Call me Alicia. I'm okay, I guess. *(Looks tired, leaning against the back of the chair.)*

Nurse: You look tired. Do you want to get back into bed?

Alicia: Yes, please. Amazing how just sitting can tire you out. *(Gets back into bed slowly, with help.)*

Nurse: *(Gets Alicia settled and comfortably positioned.)* How does that feel? *(She smiles and nods okay.)* Good. I was wondering if I could talk with you for a while to see if you have any particular questions about the operation or your injuries.

Alicia: I don't have any questions. I just want to go home. *(Looks like she's going to cry.)*

Nurse: *(Pulls up a chair.)* Tell me a little more about that. *(Leans forward.)*

Alicia: I don't live here; I was just visiting with my husband and children, and I had the accident. And I hurt, a lot. *(Crying while splinting the incision.)* I'm not used to being sick.

Nurse: How about if I get you some pain medication first; then we can talk about the rest after you're a bit more comfortable?

Alicia: That's a good idea. It's hard for me to think clearly with the pain. *(Wipes her eyes.)*

Nurse: I'll be right back. *(Returns with pain medication, which he administers. Alicia reports relief after a few minutes, and they begin to discuss her questions, worries, and fears.)*

Alicia: Thank you, Richard. I think I'll be able to rest now.

Nurse: I'll check back with you in an hour or so to see how you are.

CRITICAL THINKING CHALLENGE

- Both nurses showed caring and sensitivity, but determine what the second nurse did that the first nurse did not do.
- Detect what information the second nurse gathered that the first nurse did not.
- Using Ms. Martin's behavior, analyze the ways pain affects a person psychologically.

permanently. Although any of the surgeries listed may affect a person's psychological and physical functioning, some in particular affect sexual functioning. In addition, some procedures, such as certain types of prostatectomies, orchiectomies (removal of the testes), and certain urinary diversion procedures, may

lead to impotence. Surgically corrective procedures may be available to restore sexual functioning.

Patients need to be fully informed of options regarding surgery or alternative treatments. Nursing interventions focus on performing a thorough assessment of the potential sexual or psychological impact and providing patient teaching, technical skills, emotional support, and referrals as appropriate. The patient also needs to understand clearly the depth and scope of any limitations that the surgical procedure imposes. Some patients may feel uncomfortable discussing sexual matters with healthcare professionals. When working with patients, create as open and comfortable an environment as possible and initiate discussion when appropriate.

VALUES AND BELIEFS

The patient's value–belief system is significant because it guides personal choices and life decisions. A person's cultural background, philosophy, and religious beliefs typically affect choices made with regard to surgery and treatment options.

Choices a person is required to make should be made only when the person is fully informed of the alternatives and the expected consequences of any decisions. After the patient arrives at a decision, expert care, knowledgeable instruction, and emotional support are important nursing interventions. A chaplain or other religious or cultural leader may be useful at this time. Even if healthcare professionals oppose or do not understand the patient's decision, they must maintain a non-judgmental and supportive approach.

Cultural Considerations

Decisions regarding surgery are affected by a person's beliefs and values, which are often influenced greatly by their culture. It is important to consider and respect a patient's religious and cultural beliefs to individualize care for the surgical patient.

Some cultures embrace surgery as a method to treat medical conditions and restore health. Other cultures employ conservative medical treatments, using surgery as a later option. In some cultures, the community leader or the head of the household actively participates in the decision to have a surgical procedure and is consulted by the patient prior to making a decision.

Religions may prohibit certain surgical procedures (e.g., abortion) or include some surgical procedures as part of a religious ceremony performed by religious leaders (e.g., body piercing or circumcision). Some religions (e.g., Jehovah's Witnesses) prohibit their members from receiving blood products. This factor is significant for a person who has experienced major trauma, blood loss, or surgery.

Life Span Considerations

NEWBORN AND INFANT

For newborns and infants, separation from their primary caregivers during a surgical experience is traumatic. Their ability to understand what is happening is limited, and they may perceive the experience as strange, frightening, and lonely. Promote a calm, comfortable environment by holding babies; keeping background noises to a minimum; and providing a stuffed animal, toy, or other diversion as appropriate. Provide

careful explanations to the parents and other caregivers, and include them in their child's care as much as possible. Doing so helps to foster a sense of control over the situation.

An infant's ability to tolerate blood loss and alterations in temperature is significantly less than that of an adult (Phillips, 2013). Therefore, make every attempt to minimize both blood loss and heat loss from the body throughout the perioperative experience. In addition, infant skin is sensitive and easily traumatized. Items such as skin preparation solutions, tape, and dressings can impair skin integrity. Use items that are gentle to the skin, and use extra care when applying and removing dressings. In addition, because of the infant's physical size, instruments, equipment, and medications need to be appropriate to size and physiologic status.

SAFETY ALERT

Always ensure that the medication dosages are calculated correctly for the child's size and weight.

TODDLER AND PRESCHOOLER

Many of the same factors that apply to infants apply to toddlers and preschoolers. At these ages, separation anxiety may be more pronounced because children are more aware of their surroundings. Although these children have an expanded capacity to understand what is going on, they may still perceive the situation as frightening and lonely. Provide careful explanations to children and their families, and elicit their cooperation as needed. Having all instruments and equipment ready in the operating room before a child arrives helps shorten the waiting time before induction of anesthesia. It also helps to maintain a calm, quiet environment. In some situations, allowing the parents to hold the child while medications are being administered is helpful. For example, a suppository may be prescribed to promote relaxation and anesthesia before the child is taken into the operating room. This causes sufficient relaxation so that the child does not perceive other procedures as quite so frightening. Removing the child's clothing, applying the grounding pad, and applying monitoring devices after the child is anesthetized also are helpful. As with the infant, use of appropriately sized instruments and equipment, correct medication dosages, and measures to minimize blood loss and ensure temperature control are essential in promoting a safe and efficient surgical experience.

Planning for a safe recovery phase is another important consideration for toddlers as well as infants. A crib with side rails provides a safe environment. As with all patients, monitor the airway and vital signs carefully and keep children warm after surgery. Family visitation in induction is a commonly accepted practice, though the effectiveness of the intervention is not clear (American Society of PeriAnesthesia Nurses [ASPAN], 2012). Family presence in phase I PACU can reduce the patient's pain, cardiovascular issues, and negative behavior; however, family presence during this critical phase is contingent on assessment of the therapeutic benefits the visit may offer and institutional policy (ASPAN, 2012). In many situations, allowing the parents in the PACU as a child regains awareness of his or her surroundings can help relieve anxiety for both the child and the family (Landriscina, 2009). This also may help ensure children's cooperation with necessary procedures and promote inclusion of parents in care.

SCHOOL-AGE CHILD AND ADOLESCENT

School-age children and adolescents may have an increased understanding of surgery and many of the activities that a surgical procedure will entail. These children usually benefit from a more detailed preoperative teaching program. Many hospitals include a tour of the operating room for school-age children and adolescents and their parents during the preoperative teaching period. A child who has seen the operating room, the operating room bed, the anesthesia machine, and the mask used to administer an anesthetic is usually less frightened than a child who has not had this experience. In addition, because older children are better able to understand the surgery, they are likely to cope better with separation from parents.

Allow school-age children and adolescents to participate in the administration of anesthesia by holding the mask or counting as the anesthetic is administered. Simple choices (e.g., selecting the arm for the IV line) may help give children a sense of control.

Adolescents requiring surgery have special needs. Teenagers usually are concerned with body image and possible disfigurement. They are often self-conscious and embarrassed when private body areas are exposed. Adolescents vary markedly in their ability to cope with the stress of the surgical experience. In striving for identity and independence, they may attempt to hide their feelings. In addition to providing extensive teaching to both adolescents and their families, demonstrate support and acceptance of such feelings and behaviors.

ADULT AND OLDER ADULT

Although surgical intervention is becoming more common for older adults, the risks of surgery and anesthesia are increased for older people with chronic illness (Phillips, 2013). In addition, certain adults may require special considerations when having surgery because of alterations in vision, hearing, or mobility or chronic disease.

If an adult patient is visually impaired, leave the patient's glasses on until just before an anesthetic is administered. Doing so maintains visual orientation and helps to decrease fear and increase confidence. If a patient is having a regional or local anesthetic, operating room personnel may allow the patient to wear glasses or contact lenses during the procedure. Note any visual impairment on the chart so that operating room personnel are aware of this significant deficit.

Older patients may also have hearing impairments. The operating room staff should speak clearly and directly or allow the patient to wear a hearing aid until the anesthetic is delivered. Being able to hear members of the healthcare team fosters

teaching and helps alleviate fear, keeping the patient oriented to the environment. After removal, care for the hearing aid according to the agency's policy.

Document the disposition of glasses or hearing aids in the operative record brought to the operating room. If the patient's glasses are kept in the operating room so that the patient can use them in the recovery unit, label them with the patient's name and medical record number and take special care to avoid losing or misplacing them since the agency may be held liable for their replacement.

Patients with altered mobility, such as those with limited joint mobility, obesity, extreme thinness or fragility, or back problems, may require individualized planning for positioning during the surgical experience. Specific positions necessary for surgical procedures (e.g., the lithotomy, prone, and lateral positions) may need modification or require special padding, positioning devices, or restraints to assist in maintaining required positions.

Alterations imposed by chronic illness, a common consideration in older adults, require specific planning and special monitoring during surgery. Respiratory and cardiovascular problems may affect a person's ability to tolerate certain anatomic positions (e.g., head-down positions may impede breathing for a person with respiratory problems). Kidney or liver dysfunction can affect excretion and metabolism of anesthetic agents. Therefore, the elderly person with severe chronic organ dysfunction is at greater surgical risk. Prior to any surgical procedure, the surgeon will evaluate and review the benefits and risks involved and, together with the patient, will decide whether to proceed with surgery.

PREOPERATIVE NURSING

Nursing Assessment

HISTORY AND PHYSICAL EXAMINATION

Preoperative assessment provides valuable information directly affecting the patient's safety and well-being throughout the perioperative experience. Some of the most significant assessment information in the patient's medical record includes the allergy history, chronic disease history, current cardiovascular and respiratory status, history of surgeries and anesthesia, height and weight, hematology report, and the results of diagnostic studies. Table 22-2 lists rationales for obtaining these data before surgery. Current medication use, especially use of medications that can affect coagulation status (e.g., warfarin, nonsteroidal anti-inflammatory drugs, aspirin), is important and should be reported to the surgeon. In addition, any herbal preparations or nutritional supplements that the patient is taking should be reported. Some of these may interact with other medications or anesthetic agents and need to be discontinued as early as several weeks before surgery.

The collection of physical data is an integral part of the preoperative assessment for many healthcare providers. The physician completes an in-depth patient medical history and

TABLE 22-2 PREOPERATIVE ASSESSMENT DATA AND RATIONALE

Data	Rationale
Interview and Physical Assessment	
Proposed surgery	Individualize patient teaching and preoperative preparation
History of previous surgery	Recognize and avoid problems previously encountered
History of allergies	Avoid patient exposure to allergens eliciting allergic response
Chronic disease history	Provide competent care and necessary medications; alert to possible complications
Smoking history	Identify increased risk for postoperative respiratory complications
Current respiratory and cardiac status	Assess safety of anesthetic and medication administration; minimize risk for postoperative complications
Current height and weight	Determine body surface area for drug dosage calculations
Vital signs	Detect abnormalities; provide baseline data
Mobility restriction	Plan for surgical positioning needs and safe transport
Laboratory and Diagnostic Tests	
Blood studies (complete blood count [CBC], electrolytes, coagulation studies)	Evaluate for actual or potential problems with anemia, infection, fluid and electrolyte imbalances, cardiac dysrhythmias, or bleeding disorders
Urinalysis	Evaluate renal function and absence of urinary tract infection
ECG	Evaluate cardiac function and absence of dysrhythmias
Chest radiograph	Evaluate respiratory status
Blood type and cross-match	Identify blood type; match with potential donor should transfusion be needed

physical examination. The anesthesia provider completes a preanesthetic assessment form. Data collected on this form are particularly important in selecting and preparing safe administration of anesthetic agents.

The nurse also completes an in-depth interview and physical assessment of the patient during the preoperative period. This may be completed days or weeks before surgery during a preoperative visit, by telephone, or in the preoperative care unit just before surgery. With the increasing number of ambulatory surgeries resulting in decreased access to the patient, completion of the preoperative assessment may be a challenge. However, the information obtained is critical; it provides data needed to identify potential and actual nursing diagnoses and to individualize the perioperative plan of care.

ALLERGIES

Assess patient allergies to medications, food, and latex before the surgical procedure, and clearly note them on the patient record. Allergies to latex, tape, and iodine-based solutions (e.g., radiopaque dyes, skin prep solutions) are especially important to note because exposure to these substances is common during surgery.

A recent increase in the number of patients (and staff) sensitized to natural rubber latex products is of concern throughout surgery. The sensitivity may be manifested by a mild type IV allergic reaction (local inflammation, redness, and pruritus), or it may cause a full-blown type I anaphylactic response. Patients at risk include those with many allergies, those who have had multiple surgeries, those with neural tube defects (e.g., spina

bifida, myelomeningocele), healthcare workers, and people with a stated intolerance to objects containing natural rubber latex (e.g., latex balloons, condoms, gloves, underwear).

SAFETY ALERT

A Latex Risk Tool may be used to screen surgical patients. Once a patient is known to be at risk, members of the operating room team should be notified and a latex-safe environment provided for the patient (AORN, 2014).

LEARNING AND DISCHARGE NEEDS

The preoperative assessment also helps to identify learning and discharge needs of the patient and the family. Patient teaching begins during the preoperative period and continues throughout all perioperative phases of care. In the preoperative phase, assess the patient's and family's readiness to learn and their knowledge base so that teaching can be individualized. If the patient will be discharged on the day of surgery, be sure to identify someone who can take the patient home and assist during the postoperative recovery period.

Nursing Diagnoses and Outcome Identification

With the use of the preoperative nursing assessment, actual and potential problems can be identified for the surgical patient. Knowledge deficit, anxiety, pain, disturbed body image, and

TABLE 22-3 SELECTED PREOPERATIVE NURSING DIAGNOSES AND PATIENT GOALS

Nursing Diagnosis	Patient Goals
Deficient Knowledge regarding perioperative procedures related to verbalization of lack of knowledge	Patient will verbalize understanding of perioperative care.
Anxiety related to insufficient knowledge, separation from family, fear of death, or disfigurement	Patient will report decreased anxiety level regarding surgery.
Disturbed Sleep Pattern related to preoperative activities and anxiety	Patient will demonstrate signs of sufficient rest before surgery.

sleep pattern disturbance are common. These problems, stated as nursing diagnoses, are listed in Table 22-3, along with appropriate outcomes.

Nursing Interventions

PATIENT TEACHING

Preoperative teaching helps patients understand what will occur during each phase of the surgical experience and how they can participate in their own recovery. Preoperative teaching includes a general orientation and explanation of the surgical experience, discussion of preoperative activities to prepare the patient for surgery, and description of postoperative care to promote optimal function and recovery. Whenever possible, include family members or significant others in the preoperative teaching sessions.

Preoperative teaching can occur after the patient has been admitted to the surgical unit. However, the patient who is having ambulatory surgery may be instructed before admission. Usually, when the patient is admitted the morning of surgery, little time is available for patient teaching. Moreover, the patient may be anxious and unable to process the information given. Some surgical centers "preadmit" patients a few days or a week before the scheduled surgery. At this time, the nurse can begin preoperative teaching while obtaining a nursing assessment and compiling necessary laboratory test results. Audiovisual materials may be available for the patient to view. Frequently, the patient is sent home with written material explaining what will happen before, during, and after surgery and what the patient can do to participate in his or her own surgical recovery. When the patient is admitted for surgery, any new questions can be answered and a review (reinforcement) of previous teaching can occur.

General Information

A general orientation to the surgical experience should include the following:

- The expected time at which the procedure will begin
- How long the procedure will take
- When the patient will probably return to his or her room (or to the waiting area for same-day surgery)

- Where the patient's family and friends can wait during the surgery
- How the patient will be transported to the operating room
- What type of medications and anesthesia will be administered
- Other factors specific to the surgical procedure

If the patient will be transferred to an intensive care unit after surgery, some facilities offer a tour of the unit for the patient and family.

Preoperative Protocols

Review all preoperative activities and their importance for a successful surgical outcome. Address any specific procedures that must be performed before surgery, such as bowel preparation, skin preparation, and the insertion of urinary or IV catheters or nasogastric tubes. Discuss possible dietary or fluid restrictions, including NPO status.

Postoperative Protocols

Preoperative teaching also provides the patient with information concerning what conditions will be like after surgery. Frequently, patients have specific questions such as "How much pain will I have?" or "What will my scar look like?" Begin by asking patients what questions or concerns they have about their upcoming surgery, and deal with these issues before proceeding with the information that should be presented to each surgical patient.

Before surgery, explain what tubes (IV lines, catheters, nasogastric tubes) will be in place during the postoperative period, the size and location of the incision, and which medications will be ordered to control pain and nausea. Review activities that the patient will participate in, such as turning, deep breathing, using incentive spirometry, coughing, getting out of bed, performing leg exercises, or using a PCA device, to promote recovery and prevent complications.

Because these therapeutic procedures are used for various patients, specific guidelines are included in appropriate clinical chapters in this text and in Table 22-4.

TABLE 22-4 PREOPERATIVE PATIENT TEACHING OF POSTOPERATIVE PROTOCOLS

Procedure	Rationale	Related Chapter
Turning, getting out of bed	Improve postoperative mobility to minimize impact of immobility	Chapter 25: Mobility
Deep breathing, coughing, use of incentive spirometer	Improve postoperative gas exchange and prevent respiratory complications	Chapter 26: Respiratory Function
Leg exercises, SCDs	Improve venous return and prevent deep venous thrombosis postoperatively	Chapter 27: Cardiac Function
Using PCA	Provide optimal pain control postoperatively	Chapter 35: Pain Management

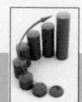

OUTCOME-BASED TEACHING PLAN

Susan Stone is a 15-year-old girl who is preadmitted for a tonsillectomy that will take place in 2 weeks. She has never had surgery before and voices some apprehension. You have 15 minutes to complete preoperative teaching for Susan and her parents.

OUTCOME

At the end of the teaching session, Susan can describe preoperative protocols (informed consent, NPO status, and when to arrive at the surgical center) necessary before her surgery.

STRATEGIES

- Question Susan about what she knows or understands about her upcoming surgery.
- Ask Susan whether she has any questions about her upcoming surgery and address her concerns before any teaching.
- Provide Susan with a preoperative booklet outlining general preoperative and postoperative routines for a tonsillectomy.
- Focus on and discuss the preoperative procedures that will be ordered before Susan's surgery. Highlight the information in the booklet for her to review.
- Answer any questions.
- Ask her to verbalize important preoperative procedures.

EVALUATION

4/12/17: 06:30—Susan accurately verbalized when to arrive for surgery and described NPO status. She said she would read the booklet and write down her questions so they could be answered quickly.

—J. Johnson, RN

OUTCOME

Before surgery, Susan can verbalize discharge care important during the postoperative recovery period (e.g., pain management, diet, when to notify her physician).

STRATEGIES

- Review postoperative care in the booklet, including what will happen after surgery; why vital signs are monitored;

medications that will be ordered for pain and nausea; what to expect when she wakes up in the recovery facility; and expectation of some pain, throat soreness, and drainage.
- Reinforce actions that could irritate surgical site and delay healing.
- Have Susan and her parents verbalize the plan for after-discharge care including pain management, and food and fluids to be included in the diet for the first week after surgery.
- Ask Susan to state actions to avoid that could irritate surgical site and delay healing (e.g., citrus juices, gargling with mouthwash, coughing, and clearing of throat).

EVALUATION

4/12/17: 06:45—Susan and her parents accurately describe postoperative diet and pain management strategies.

—J. Johnson, RN

OUTCOME

Before discharge, Susan and her parents can verbalize appropriate follow-up care and indications that require physician notification during postoperative period.

STRATEGIES

- Review symptoms (bright red bleeding, signs of infection such as temperature above 38°C [100.5°F]); provide them with a written list of danger signs to report.
- Give Susan and her parents telephone numbers to call in case of questions or concerns.
- Provide Susan and her parents with written information regarding a follow-up appointment with the surgeon.

EVALUATION

4/12/17: 14:30—Susan and her parents could verbalize two postoperative situations that would require calling the clinic or doctor. Plan to follow up with a phone call 1 day after discharge.

—J. Johnson, RN

INFORMED CONSENT

The **informed consent** obtained before any surgical procedure is an important legal document. The surgeon is legally responsible for obtaining the patient's informed consent. He

or she fully explains the proposed surgical procedure by providing the patient with all of the information needed to make the decision, discussed in language the patient can understand, and obtains the patient's signature on the consent form. If the patient does not speak or understand the physician's language, an interpreter should be used.

The information usually discussed includes a description of the proposed surgery, the possible risks and benefits of the procedure, the reason the surgery is indicated, the probability of success, the consequences of nonsurgical treatment or no treatment, and any other information that will help the patient reach an informed decision. The surgeon documents this discussion in the patient's record. The patient has the right to ask any questions and to withdraw consent at any point before the surgery begins. In addition to the proposed procedure, the consent form also lists the name of the surgeon and assisting surgeons and the surgical site (e.g., left or right eye, knee, kidney, ear). The surgeon, the patient, and a witness must sign and date the consent form. If the patient is a minor or is not mentally or physically competent to give consent, the consent should be obtained from the patient's parents, spouse, legal guardian, or next of kin. Do not administer any medications that might alter judgment or perception before the patient signs the consent form. Many drugs commonly administered as preoperative medications, such as opioids or barbiturates, can alter cognitive abilities and invalidate informed consent.

The nurse may be involved in obtaining consent, usually by witnessing the patient's signature on the consent document. Be knowledgeable about the healthcare agency's policy regarding informed consent, and ensure that the policy is strictly followed. If the patient seems unsure or indicates lack of understanding, notify the surgeon so that more information can be provided. The nurse is responsible for making sure that the consent form contains all correct and necessary information, is properly signed and witnessed, and is part of the patient's medical record before the surgical procedure begins.

PATIENT PREPARATION

Nurses are responsible for preparing patients physically and emotionally to ensure optimal conditions for surgery. Specific patient preparation is prescribed by the surgeon or indicated by healthcare facility policy, but usually it includes placing the patient on NPO status, starting an IV line, preparing the intestinal tract and skin, and administering preoperative medications.

NPO Status

For any patient receiving general anesthesia, foods and fluids are restricted, and the patient is instructed not to eat or drink anything (NPO) before surgery to prevent possible aspiration during surgery or the immediate postoperative period. To help ensure safe anesthetic administration and prevent vomiting and aspiration, the patient should not have a full stomach. If the surgical patient is receiving necessary medications (e.g., antihypertensive, anticonvulsant, or antiarrhythmic agents) that should not be suddenly discontinued, clarify with the physician how and whether these medications should be administered. Some medications may be taken with a sip of water in certain situations; others may need to be administered parenterally. If the patient is diabetic, insulin and oral hypoglycemic orders should also be clarified. Dosages may be reduced, or the

ETHICAL/LEGAL ISSUE

INFORMED CONSENT

Mr. Willis, a 46-year-old man, is brought to your trauma center after a severe accident. He needs surgery to evaluate abdominal trauma and repair multiple fractures. His vital signs have been unstable, and shock is suspected. His wife is notified and enters the emergency room very distraught. The physician is trying to explain the surgery that needs to be performed and get her consent. Mrs. Willis agrees to the surgery but explains that they are Jehovah's Witnesses and she will not agree to any blood transfusions.

CRITICAL THINKING CHALLENGE

- Discuss factors that are significant for Mrs. Willis at this time in making a decision on her husband's behalf.
- Explore how making a decision for next of kin is different and more complex than making a decision for yourself.
- Role-play how Mrs. Willis can receive the information she needs to make an informed decision about her husband's surgery, yet support her in the decision-making process.
- Try to verbalize your own feelings when dealing with patients who have cultural or religious beliefs that differ significantly from your own.

insulin may be given intravenously immediately before or during the surgery.

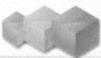 *Concept Mastery Alert*

Until quite recently, it was nearly universal practice for patients to be ordered to fast from the night before surgery. However, the most current recommendations for preoperative fasting allow for the consumption of liquids up to 2 hours prior to surgery.

IV Access

IV access in any surgical patient is important for providing fluid and electrolyte replacement, administering IV medications, providing a route for emergency medication, and administering blood products. Vascular access may be obtained through a peripheral line or a central line. In certain situations, both are indicated. In other situations (e.g., surgery requiring only local anesthesia), an intermittent access device (saline lock) may be adequate. The IV line may be started in the preoperative period to ensure adequate hydration status. For patients who are well hydrated, IV insertion may be delayed until the patient is in the operating room. For any surgical patient, a large-gauge (e.g., 18-gauge) IV device should be used in case a blood transfusion is necessary during the surgical or postoperative period.

Nasogastric Decompression

For selected surgical patients, a nasogastric tube may be inserted to decompress the stomach and allow removal of its contents. Nasogastric decompression may be necessary for patients who have not been NPO before surgery, such as those undergoing emergency surgery. Nasogastric decompression may be indicated when surgery is performed on the stomach or the intestines.

Bowel Preparation

Enemas, suppositories, laxatives, and oral antibiotics (e.g., neomycin) may be given preoperatively to help clear the colon and reduce the level of endogenous bacteria. This decreases the possibility of intraoperative bowel content spillage, which could lead to peritonitis and other complications. Bowel preparation is most important when surgery is performed on the intestines, but it can be indicated for general abdominal surgery.

Skin Preparation

Preoperative skin preparation removes soil and transient microorganisms from the skin, decreasing the number of resident microbes and the chance of infection. Depending on the type of surgery, the agency policy, and the surgeon's preference, the patient may need clipping of body hair, scrubbing of the surgical area, or showering with antimicrobial soap. Usually, the skin preparation focuses on the area that will be involved in the surgery itself and surrounding wide margins. A surgical "prep," or shaving of the hair in the affected area, was a common preoperative procedure a few decades ago. Depending on the length and amount of hair at the site and type of procedure being performed, hair may be removed with clippers, braided away from the surgical site, held away from the surgical site using a nonflammable gel, or left in place. Use of chemical depilatories may cause skin reactions in sensitive individuals, resulting in possible cancelation of surgery. Such agents should only be used if previous skin testing has been done with no resulting skin irritation (AORN, 2014).

Preoperative Medications

Medications, such as those to promote relaxation, decrease nasal and salivary secretions, assist delivery of the anesthetic, relieve pain, and promote sedation, are given just before surgery. The trend in recent years has been to give fewer preoperative medications, except for antibiotics. However, it is important to administer any prescribed preoperative medication on time so that maximum effect can be coordinated with the time of surgery.

! SAFETY ALERT

Make sure that all activities requiring the patient to be out of bed (e.g., showering and voiding before surgery) are accomplished before administering any medications that can alter the level of consciousness. After such medications are given, instruct the patient to stay in bed and keep the side rails up to prevent falling and possible injury.

PREOPERATIVE CHECKLIST

Many hospitals use a preoperative assessment checklist on the day of surgery to summarize the patient's preoperative preparation. These checklists provide such preoperative baseline measurements as level of consciousness, vital signs, and skin integrity and ensure that all required information is in the patient's record before transport to the operating room. Completing the preoperative checklist is a quick way to show that all patient preparation activities have been accomplished and safety measures have been taken. The nurse usually checks off each item as it is completed and then signs the form in the appropriate place.

After all preparation for surgery is completed, the preoperative checklist is filled out, and documentation is completed according to protocol, the patient is ready for transport to the preoperative care unit.

If the patient is transported to a separate preoperative care area, final presurgical assessments are completed. The preoperative care unit nurse and the operating room nurse check the following:

- Patient's name band
- Site and type of surgery
- Location of valuables
- Allergies
- Appropriate dress of the patient
- Surgical consent obtained
- NPO status
- Appropriate records and paperwork
- Laboratory and diagnostic study results entered on the chart
- Blood availability
- Preoperative medication administration
- Status of any additional physician's orders

At this time, IV access and, if necessary, an arterial line may be established. The arterial line provides continual monitoring of blood pressure during the procedure and allows ready access for laboratory studies such as arterial blood gases, hematocrit, and electrolytes. Because arrival to the surgical facility on the day of surgery is now commonplace, the patient may be admitted directly to the preoperative care unit, where these and other final preparations are completed prior to the patient being transported directly to the operating room. If not already in place, SCDs may be placed in the preoperative care area, and prewarming is begun to ensure that normothermia is maintained throughout the perioperative period.

The anesthesia provider may administer the regional block (spinal or epidural), if appropriate. In the operating room, the scrub person and the circulating nurse prepare the instruments, the supplies, and the operating suite environment for the individualized needs of the patient.

In the preoperative care unit, provide a warm, caring environment and offer appropriate emotional support. In some facilities, a limited number of family members may stay in the preoperative care unit with the patient until the patient is transferred to the operating room.

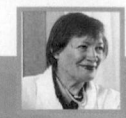

Perioperative Nursing PICO

Nancy, the nurse from the chapter-opening scenario, is making a post-op phone call to a patient that had an abdominal procedure. In the post-op interview, she discovers the patient had "the worst experience" in the holding area because he was "so nervous" waiting for the surgery team. Although the nurse did give him "something in the IV" to calm his nerves, he explained that "it still didn't work." After the phone call, Nancy wondered if alternative interventions such as meditation tapes or music therapy could help patients calm down before surgery. She looks for evidence in the Cochrane Library. Nancy uses the following PICO question for her search: *In preoperative patients, how does meditation or music therapy versus no therapy affect anxiety?*

P = preoperative patients
I = meditation or music therapy
C = no therapy
O = affect anxiety

Nancy does not find current meta-analysis or systematic review about meditation and its effects on preoperative patients. However, she does find a systematic review on how music therapy was used for patients having heart surgery. The study reviewed 26 randomized control trials involving 1,369 patients that listened to music prior to their heart surgery. Several study results indicated consistently that music had a positive effect on reducing psychological stress related to surgery. It decreased heart rate, respiratory rate, and systolic blood pressure. Interestingly, if patients were given the option to choose the type of music they wanted to hear, their anxieties seemed to decrease even more.

   After reading the article, Nancy decides to share her findings with her department to see if they would consider suggesting music therapy as a part of preoperative teaching.

REFERENCE

Bradt, J., Dileo, C., & Potvin, N. (2013). Music for stress and anxiety reduction in coronary heart disease patients. *Cochrane Database of Systematic Reviews*, (12), Art. No.: CD006577. DOI: 10.1002/14651858.CD006577.pub3

Evaluation

While performing interventions in the preoperative phase, continually evaluate the patient's response and document it in the patient's medical record. This information is essential for formulating an individualized plan of care in succeeding phases of the surgical experience.

GOAL

The patient will verbalize understanding of perioperative care.

Possible Outcome Criteria

- During preoperative preparation, the patient asks questions about the impending surgical procedure.
- During preoperative preparation, the patient describes what will happen during the surgical experience.
- After receiving instruction, the patient demonstrates effective turning, coughing, deep breathing, and leg exercises and states why they are important in postoperative recovery.

GOAL

The patient will report a decreased anxiety level regarding surgery.

Possible Outcome Criteria

- During preoperative teaching, the patient discusses fears and concerns regarding the surgical procedure.

- After patient teaching, the patient verbalizes decreased anxiety.
- The patient identifies a support system and strategies to use to reduce stress and anxiety imposed by the surgical experience.

GOAL

The patient will demonstrate signs of sufficient rest before surgery.

Possible Outcome Criteria

- The patient verbalizes feeling adequately rested on the morning of surgery.
- The patient sleeps restfully the night before surgery, as observed by the nurse during the night.

INTRAOPERATIVE NURSING

Nursing Assessment

Assessment continues in the intraoperative period. In addition to planning for the patient's intraoperative needs, assessment allows initial planning for the recovery phase. The operating room nurse is responsible for communicating specific assessment data to the PACU so that recovery personnel can anticipate the patient's individualized needs.

During surgery, assessment is continuous because of the patient's dynamic condition and the potential for serious complications. Monitor all patients appropriately based on the procedure and the patient's condition. Essential assessment parameters include vital signs (blood pressure, heart rate, respiratory rate, temperature), oxygen saturation, electrocardiogram (ECG), and estimated blood loss. Other parameters that may be monitored, depending on the procedure and the patient's condition, include arterial and central line pressures, laboratory values (e.g., hematocrit, blood glucose level, sodium and potassium levels, arterial blood gases, blood pH, clotting factors), and urinary output. Continuous monitoring is necessary to detect and treat any abnormalities immediately. These values and any interventions are recorded in the patient's medical record.

Nursing Diagnoses and Outcome Identification

Although nursing diagnoses and outcomes vary depending on the patient and the surgical procedure, some common problems are Risk for Injury, Risk for Imbalanced Body Temperature, Risk for Infection, Risk for Latex Allergy Response, and Risk for Perioperative Positioning Injury. Table 22-5 lists possible nursing diagnoses and patient outcomes for the intraoperative period.

Nursing Interventions

Nursing interventions during the intraoperative period focus on providing emotional support, ensuring a safe environment and preventing injury, monitoring the patient during anesthetic administration, maintaining asepsis, and promoting wound healing. Both the scrub person and the circulating nurse are responsible for these interventions.

TABLE 22-5 SELECTED INTRAOPERATIVE NURSING DIAGNOSES AND PATIENT GOALS

Nursing Diagnosis	Patient Goals
Risk for Perioperative Positioning Injury related to length of surgery and obesity	Patient will remain free from positioning-related injury.
Risk for Injury related to equipment, electrical, or physical hazards during surgery	Patient will maintain injury free during the surgical procedure.
Risk for Infection related to breaches in asepsis or individual risk factors	Patient will maintain an infection-free wound site postoperatively.
Risk for Latex Allergy Response	Patient will not experience an allergic response from exposure to latex.
Risk for Imbalanced Body Temperature	Patient's temperature will remain within 2°F of baseline.

ROLE OF THE SCRUB PERSON AND CIRCULATING NURSE

The **scrub person** wears a sterile gown, mask, headgear, gloves, and eye protection and provides the surgeon with required instruments, sponges, drains, and other equipment, anticipating what will be needed throughout surgery (Fig. 22-2). Anticipation helps to minimize the time the patient is anesthetized and the wound is open, decreasing potential complications. Other responsibilities of the scrub person include preparing the sterile tables before surgery. A thorough understanding of the principles of asepsis, anatomy, and tissue care, as well as the surgical objectives, is necessary. The scrub person also must have the knowledge and skills to anticipate needs of other members of the surgical team and the ability to make decisions and perform interventions in an emergency situation.

The **circulating nurse** manages patient care in the operating room environment and protects the patient's safety and health needs. Protection involves controlling the environment for cleanliness, temperature, humidity, and lighting. The circulating nurse ensures that the patient's rights are protected and coordinates patient care in the operating room. Coordinating activities of related personnel (e.g., laboratory, x-ray) and monitoring aseptic practices are also the circulating nurse's responsibilities. The circulating nurse and the scrub person are responsible for accounting for all sponges and instruments at the close of surgery.

EMOTIONAL SUPPORT

Providing emotional support for the patient in the operating room can be vital to the success of the procedure. Although some patients may be awake only a short time (half an hour or less) before induction of anesthesia, others are awake during the entire procedure. Attempt to elicit the patient's cooperation and make the patient as comfortable as possible. Doing so helps the patient tolerate the procedure in a calmer, more relaxed manner, which should result in a better outcome. Providing appropriate information and explanations for each phase of the procedure helps prevent unexpected, stressful surprises and promotes a more relaxed, cooperative environment.

Providing emotional support for the patient's family is equally important. Answer the family's questions, provide them with information on the progress of the procedure, and give more detailed information if indicated and if time permits. Also, let the family know when the procedure is completed, how long the patient will be in the recovery facility, and where the patient will go after discharge from the PACU. For ambulatory patients who are to be discharged home after their surgical procedure, the intraoperative nurse may also be involved in planning for discharge and in discharge teaching.

PATIENT AND STAFF SAFETY

Although safety is important in all phases of the surgical experience, equipment safety, electrical safety, chemical safety, radiation safety, **surgical verification**, patient transport and

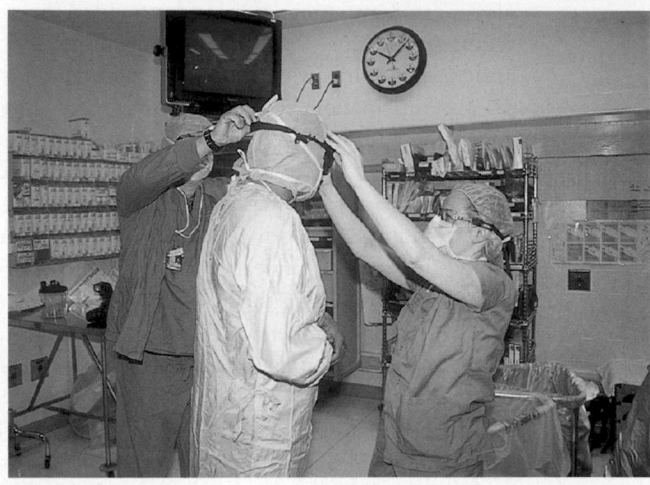
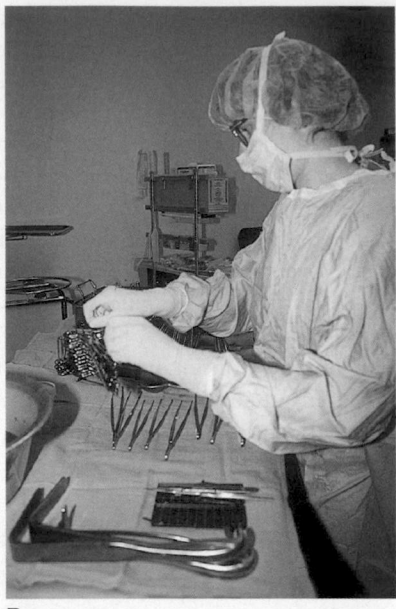

A   B

FIGURE 22-2 Safety is maintained for both the patient and the operating room personnel. **A.** U.S. Occupational Safety and Health Administration (OSHA) requirements mandate protective eyewear in addition to masks to protect personnel from splash exposure to blood. **B.** The scrub person prepares needed surgical instruments.

positioning, and continuous asepsis are particularly important in the intraoperative phase.

Equipment Safety

The operating room nurse routinely checks and maintains equipment used during surgical procedures. Safety policies for patient care equipment should include the following principles and activities:

- Written procedures for the use of equipment
- Special classes and education for the people required to operate and care for equipment
- Routine, periodic maintenance programs for equipment to meet or exceed the manufacturers' recommendations
- Inspection and testing of equipment (e.g., connectors, grounding pads, and settings as required) before each use
- Easily accessed, current, written instructional materials for all people required to use the equipment
- Rapidly available professional assistance if equipment problems arise
- Written documentation for the use, settings, and care of special equipment

Electrical Safety

One of the most significant potential hazards to the patient in the operating room is electricity. Electrical equipment is used in all surgical procedures. Common devices that rely on electricity include lasers, x-ray machines, electrosurgical units (electrocautery), video equipment, physiologic monitors, microscopes, heart bypass machines, cell savers, blood warmers, heating–cooling blankets, ultrasonic devices, cryosurgery units, and surgical spotlights.

SAFETY ALERT

The most common potential threats to patient safety related to electrical devices are electric shock and burns. Appropriate operating room personnel should know how to use the equipment safely, check the equipment for proper functioning, and report and handle problems, especially emergency problems such as fire or explosion. In addition, personnel using electrical equipment should be familiar with the safe use of backup systems should a power failure occur.

Chemical Safety

Chemical safety is another important area of patient and staff safety in the operating room. Common hazardous chemicals found in the operating room include disinfectants and sterilants like glutaraldehyde and hydrogen peroxide; antiseptic agents like alcohol (flammable) and skin prep solutions; methyl methacrylate monomer (the liquid used when mixing bone cement) that is an eye and respiratory tract irritant and is potentially flammable and explosive; housekeeping products used for cleaning and disinfecting (potential eye, skin, and respiratory tract irritants); and waste anesthesia gases like halothane, nitrous oxide, and sevoflurane (AORN, 2014). Personnel working with these chemicals must understand their potential hazards, how to read and follow warning labels, how to use the chemicals safely, how to dispose of them safely, and what to do should an accident occur.

Because of the increase in the number of people who are sensitive to natural rubber latex proteins, perioperative nurses should routinely assess patients for potential risk factors.

Perioperative nurses should continually assess the operating room environment for products that may contain latex so that they can be removed when a potentially sensitive patient is undergoing surgery.

Radiation Safety

Radiation hazards in the operating room may come from the portable x-ray machine, fluoroscopic equipment, diagnostic radiologic devices, radiation implants, and other instruments and compounds used in radiation therapy. Radiation is potentially hazardous because it changes or modifies cells and can lead to genetic defects, thyroid disorders, and cancer.

All personnel who work with radiation sources must strictly adhere to the policies and procedures set forth by the healthcare facility's radiation safety officer. Such practices include wearing monitoring badges, lead aprons, and other shielding devices. Always maintain a safe distance from the radioactive source because the amount of radiation exposure decreases inversely with the square of the distance from the source.

Surgical Verification

The Universal Protocol for Preventing Wrong Site, Wrong Procedure, and Wrong Person Surgery™ has been required by the Joint Commission since 2004 (Joint Commission, 2014). Surgeries performed on the wrong site or wrong patient, or performing the wrong procedure, are sentinel events and are preventable. The protocol was developed to prevent these sentinel events from occurring. The three components of the Universal Protocol are:

1. Preprocedure verification:
   - Verify correct patient, procedure, and site.
   - Involve the patient when possible.
   - Use a standardized list to verify that necessary items are available for the procedure (e.g., x-rays, history, and physical).

2. Mark the procedure site:
   - Mark the site before the procedure and involve the patient if possible.
   - The mark should be at or near the surgical site, visible after surgical draping, and used consistently throughout the institution.
   - Institutions should designate who can perform the site marking.

3. Perform a time-out:
   - This *standardized* process should be completed prior to incision.
   - A designated team member initiates the time-out.
   - All team members should participate in the process (Joint Commission, 2014).

Procedural pauses and protocols for verification should be used when any invasive procedure (e.g., central line placement) is performed in any area of a healthcare facility. See Figure 22-3 for the World Health Organization Surgical Safety Checklist.

Positioning

Proper positioning of the patient is another important safety consideration in the operating room. The ideal position can be defined as the position that provides the best possible exposure for the surgeon, for airway management and monitoring for the anesthetist, and for the patient's physiologic safety. The responsibility for positioning is shared by the anesthesia provider, the surgeon, and the circulating nurse.

Proper positioning helps prevent skin, nerve, and muscle damage, which can be temporary or lead to permanent dysfunction. Circulation is altered during surgery because anesthetic agents disrupt normal vasodilation and constriction, which compromises a patient's ability to make needed hemodynamic adjustments to maintain circulation (Rothrock, 2015).

Use appropriate padding for all body prominences and joints to avoid excessive pressure on the skin and to ensure optimal functioning of the respiratory, nervous, and circulatory systems.

Common surgical positions include the supine, Trendelenburg, reverse Trendelenburg, lithotomy, sitting, prone, and lateral or sidelying positions. Chapter 25 provides illustrations of selected surgical positions. Patients in each of these positions require special padding or support devices to ensure physiologic safety.

ANESTHESIA MONITORING

Monitoring the patient's status during and after the administration of anesthesia is an important responsibility for the nurse in the operating room and in the recovery facility. Knowledge concerning specific anesthetic agents is essential to focus assessment parameters.

Anesthesia may be classified as general, regional, or local. A **general anesthetic** effectively produces analgesia, relaxes muscles, and results in a sleeplike state. A **regional anesthetic** produces decreased sensation and pain in selected body parts by way of nerve blocks, intrathecal blocks, or epidural blocks. A **local anesthetic** depresses superficial peripheral nerves and blocks conduction of pain impulses from their site of origin.

The administration of general or regional anesthesia may be performed by an **anesthesiologist** or a **certified registered nurse anesthetist (CRNA)**. Both of these professionals have specialized education and skills in the administration of anesthetic agents and in monitoring patients during surgical and other procedures. An anesthesiologist is a physician who has specialized education in the administration of anesthesia. Similarly, a CRNA is a registered nurse who has specialized

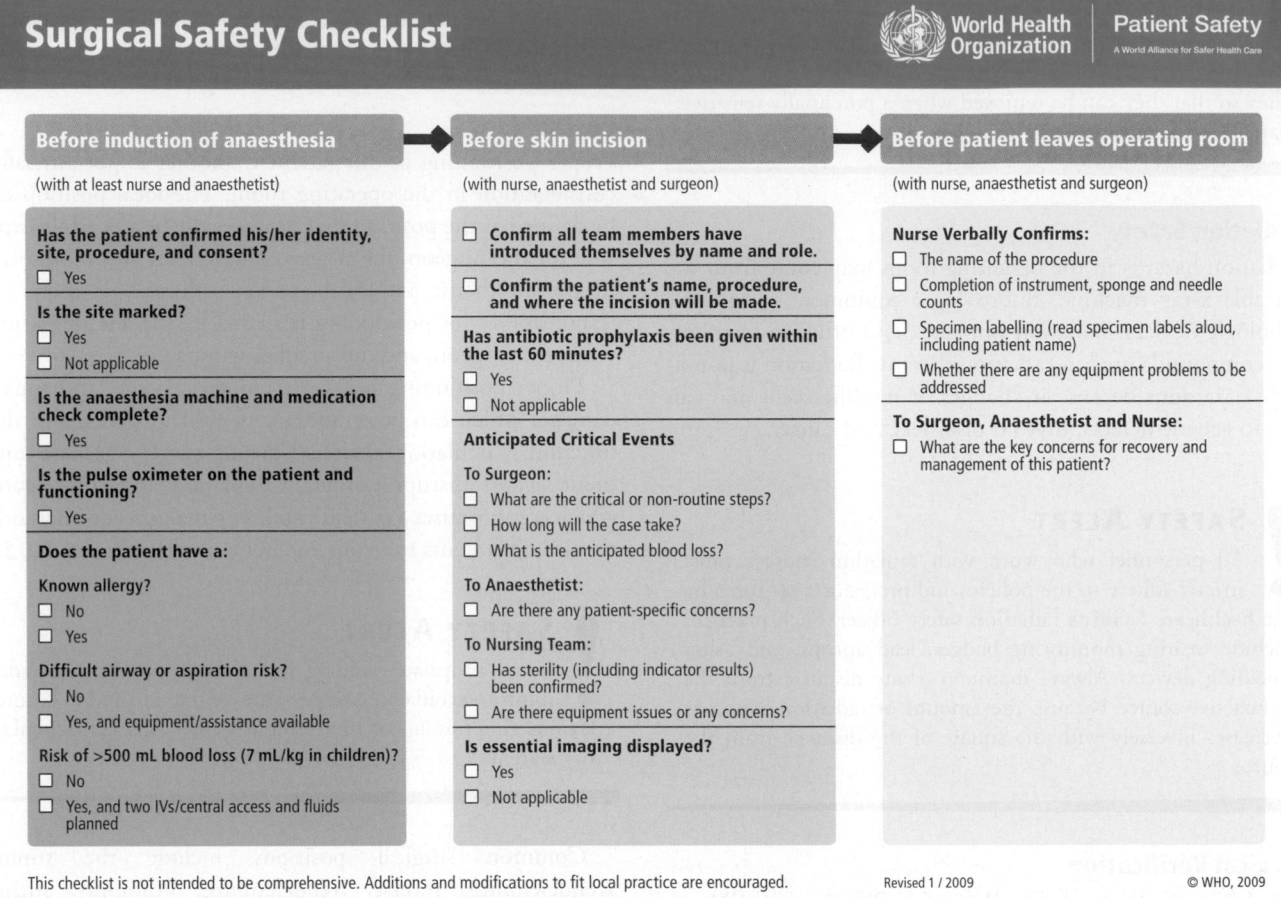

FIGURE 22-3 World Health Organization surgical safety checklist. (Reprinted with permission from the World Health Organization.)

education and certification in the administration of anesthesia. Both professionals are also skilled in managing pain and in placing vascular access lines. The surgeon usually administers local anesthesia at the surgical site.

General Anesthesia

General anesthesia may be administered either intravenously or by inhalation. Inhalation agents (gases) are delivered from the anesthesia machine and tubing by a face mask, endotracheal tube, laryngeal mask airway, or endonasal tube. Some commonly used inhalation agents include nitrous oxide, oxygen, sevoflurane, and isoflurane. IV agents can also be delivered through an established vascular access. These agents include barbiturates (e.g., thiopental), opioids analgesics (e.g., morphine, fentanyl, hydromorphone), and IV anesthetics (e.g., diazepam propofol, ketamine, and midazolam) (Rothrock, 2015).

Muscle relaxants are also commonly administered during surgical procedures and are especially beneficial during wound closure. When an abdominal incision is to be closed with sutures or staples, relaxed abdominal muscles allow the wound edges to be approximated (brought together) more easily than when muscles are tense.

Close monitoring of the patient is necessary during induction of, maintenance of, and emergence from general anesthesia.

Table 22-6 describes the four stages of anesthesia, beginning with induction of anesthesia or analgesia and ending with the toxic stage. As the patient emerges from anesthesia the sequence of stages is reversed. The type of anesthesia administered may vary the transition. Patients who are receiving general anesthesia normally go through the first three stages, which are observed by the anesthetist. The circulating nurse should be present at the patient's bedside to assist the anesthetist as needed to maintain the patient's airway during induction and emergence of anesthesia.

Regional Anesthesia

Regional anesthesia can be a useful alternative to general anesthesia. Instead of placing the entire body in a sleeplike condition, regional anesthesia affects only selected body parts. This type of anesthesia can be used for surgeries of the lower extremities (feet, ankle, knees, hips) and other localized sites, such as the hands and arms. Regional anesthetics are advantageous because they minimize the pulmonary and gastrointestinal complications (e.g., pneumonia, atelectasis, nausea and vomiting) that sometimes occur with general anesthetics. A patient receiving a regional anesthetic usually recovers more quickly from the anesthetic than a patient receiving a general anesthetic. Remember that the patient having a regional anesthesia may be awake during the surgery. Therefore, keep any

TABLE 22-6 PATIENT RESPONSES IN THE STAGES OF ANESTHESIA

Stage	Reflexes	Heart Rate	Respiration	Blood Pressure	Eyes
I. Analgesia amnesia	Present	Normal	Slow rate Increased depth	Normal	Some dilation Reacts to light
II. Dreams and excitement Frequently bypassed with IV induction agents	Active	Increased	Irregular breathing Breath holding	Increased	Pupils widely dilated and divergent
III. Surgical Involves four planes: plane 2 and plane 3 best for surgery	In progression of loss: 1. Lid reflex 2. Pharyngeal (swallowing) 3. Laryngeal (can tolerate oral airway, suctioning, and then intubation) 4. Gag and corneal reflexes lost	Decreased	Progressively depressed until apneic	Normal to decreased	Early plane: constricted pupils, then slightly dilated and centrally fixed
IV. Toxic Extreme depression	No reflexes	Weak and thready	Completely flaccid	Decreased	Widely dilated pupils

conversation appropriate to the situation. Regional anesthesia may also be used for postoperative pain control. Table 22-7 provides examples of regional anesthesia.

Local Anesthesia

Local anesthesia is actually a type of regional anesthesia. It is differentiated here by the people responsible for administering the agent and monitoring the patient. Instead of the anesthetist, the surgeon is usually responsible for administering local anesthetics, and a perioperative nurse is responsible for monitoring the physiologic and psychological status of the patient.

Methods used to provide local anesthesia include topical or direct application of an anesthetic agent to the skin or mucosal surfaces and injection of a local anesthetic agent into the areas surrounding the operative site. This type of anesthesia can be used for localized operations, such as breast biopsies; central line insertions; and surgery of the fingers, hands, nose, eyes, or ears. Patients who are candidates for local anesthetics usually are calm, able to cooperate with the surgical procedure, and have no major systemic medical problems. Local anesthesia has the advantages of regional anesthesia, enhanced by decreased cost to the patient because some healthcare facilities do not charge for local anesthesia services.

The choice of local anesthesia for a patient has many implications for the perioperative nurse. In the absence of an anesthetist, the nurse is totally responsible for monitoring the patient (AORN, 2014). Monitoring includes blood pressure, level of consciousness, respiratory rate, oxygen saturation, skin condition, cardiac rate and rhythm, and maintaining a patent IV access line. Additionally, holistic interventions can be offered to the patient to promote an atmosphere of comfort throughout the procedural experience.

Moderate Sedation and Analgesia

Moderate sedation, sometimes referred to as procedural sedation or conscious sedation, involves the use of IV sedation administered during a surgical or diagnostic procedure to alter the patient's conscious state, thereby allaying fear and anxiety. Combinations of IV opioids and sedatives are employed to decrease consciousness, but to a degree where the patient still can respond to verbal commands and maintain a patent airway. Commonly used drugs include morphine, fentanyl, diazepam (Valium), and midazolam (Versed). Frequently, the nurse is responsible for administering these agents and monitoring the patient. Nurses responsible for administering or monitoring moderate sedation receive special training and validation of their knowledge and skill. Assess each patient receiving IV

TABLE 22-7 REGIONAL ANESTHESIA

Type	Definition and Uses	Examples of Use
Topical	The direct application of an anesthetic agent to skin or mucosal surfaces (mouth, throat, nose, cornea)	Often used before injections (nerve blocks, epidurals) or endotracheal tube placement
Nerve or nerve bundle block (local)	The injection of a local anesthetic agent into a nerve bundle or the nerve supply of the operative site	Breast biopsy, lymph node biopsy, ear procedure, cataract extraction, or cornea transplantation
Epidural or peridural	The injection of a local anesthetic agent into the potential space outside the dura	Lower extremity surgery (foot, ankle, knee), lower abdominal procedures, or for postoperative pain relief
Spinal	The injection of a local anesthetic agent into the subarachnoid space	Useful for surgeries below the xiphoid process or abdominal surgery

moderate sedation physiologically and psychologically, monitoring for reaction to the drugs. A working knowledge of resuscitation and monitoring equipment and the ability to interpret the data obtained are crucial (AORN, 2014).

 SAFETY ALERT

Have drug antagonists naloxone (Narcan) and flumazenil (Romazicon) readily available in the event of overdose.

ASEPTIC PRACTICE

Maintaining asepsis to avoid contamination of the surgical site by microorganisms is the responsibility of all members of the surgical team. AORN, the professional organization for perioperative nurses, has established guidelines for maintaining asepsis (AORN, 2014). Box 22-2 highlights the basic principles of aseptic practice.

Additional policies and procedures have been established in the operating room to ensure asepsis. Every operating room nurse should be familiar with policies concerning the surgical hand scrub, using either an acceptable brushless antimicrobial hand scrub agent or the traditional counted-stroke/timed scrub, cleaning and preparation of the patient's skin before surgery, special considerations for cleaning the operating room environment and disposing of waste products, procedures for sterilizing instruments and supplies, and methods for draping the surgical patient and establishing the sterile field.

WOUND CLOSURE

Nurses often assist surgeons in accomplishing wound closure, and nurses may be directed to remove wound closure devices during the postoperative period. The type of material used for wound closure affects wound healing. In some situations, sutures or staples (or both) are used. For example, a patient may have absorbable sutures closing the viscera and staples approximating the wound edges.

Sutures

A **suture** is the material used to sew an incision together. Sutures can be absorbable (e.g., chromic gut, Vicryl, Monocryl) or nonabsorbable (e.g., nylon, silk). Absorbable sutures used in skin closure absorb into the skin so that removal is not necessary. Nonabsorbable sutures used for closing the skin must be removed after the incision has healed. When used internally, nonabsorbable sutures remain in place.

The type of suture used depends on the size and location of the wound being closed, how strong the suture material needs to be for the type of wound being repaired, the desired cosmetic result, and the surgeon's preference. In general, the less suture material used and the smaller the suture size, the better the wound closure. Sutures represent a foreign body that can potentially lead to infections, such as stitch abscesses.

Staples

The use of skin staples is also an effective wound closure method. **Skin staples** (see Fig. 30-7 in Chapter 30) are made of stainless steel, look like paper staples flat against the skin, and are inserted close to the incision with a staple gun. Skin staples are minimally reactive to the body as a foreign substance and therefore minimize the risk of infection. The use of staples reduces tissue handling and accomplishes wound closure faster than suturing does. Skin staples usually are removed with a staple remover within the first week after surgery, when the incision has healed (Fig. 30-7).

TRANSPORT TO THE PACU

After the intraoperative phase of the surgical procedure has been completed, the circulating nurse, the anesthesia provider, and the surgeon safely transport the patient to the PACU, taking care

---

BOX 22-2   **Basic Principles of Aseptic Practice (AORN, 2014)**

- **Attire:** Operating room attire includes wearing freshly laundered scrubs daily (NO home laundering!): soiled scrubs should be changed when soiled; a scrub jacket for personnel that are not scrubbed in at the sterile field; a head covering and a mask; and clean shoes that are dedicated to the operating room (any outside shoes should be covered with shoe covers). Jewelry that cannot be contained inside the scrubs should be removed.
- **Hand Hygiene:** All OR personnel should complete hand hygiene before starting their shift. Scrubbed personnel should perform a surgical hand scrub prior to donning a sterile gown and gloves. All rings, bracelets, and watches should be removed prior to hand hygiene and the surgical hand scrub. All chipped nail polish should be removed, and artificial nails should never be worn.
- **Sterile Field:** Items in the sterile field should be sterile. All packaged items and containerized instrument sets should be inspected for integrity of the package and container prior to opening to ensure that the sterility of the contents

has not been compromised. Items should be opened using sterile technique. Once a sterile field is created, it should be monitored at all times to ensure that any point of contamination is recognized and corrected. Scrubbed personnel should remain close to the sterile field. Unscrubbed personnel should always face the sterile field and maintain a distance of 12 inches to prevent contamination of the sterile field.
- **Sterile Attire:** The sterile gown and gloves should be applied using sterile technique. The front of the gown should be considered sterile from chest level to the level of the sterile field. The sleeves of the gown are considered sterile circumferentially from the cuff to 2 inches above the elbow. It is recommend that scrubbed personnel wear two pairs of gloves (this is known as double gloving).
- **Drapes:** Sterile drapes are used to establish the sterile field. The top surface of a draped sterile area is considered sterile. Portions of the drape that fall over the sides of a sterile field are not considered sterile.

to maintain the patient's airway during this critical time. Each completes required documentation and provides the recovery facility with reports of the surgical experience. The nurses in the PACU will have been notified of the patient's impending arrival and will have prepared for the patient accordingly.

Evaluation

During the intraoperative period, the results are evaluated and revised as needed. Selected outcome criteria are provided here.

GOAL

The patient will maintain injury-free status during the surgical procedure.

Possible Outcome Criteria

- The patient exhibits no skin injury due to electrical devices or chemicals used during surgery.
- The patient evidences no injury from defective or improper use of surgical equipment.

GOAL

The patient will remain free from signs of positioning-related injury.

Possible Outcome Criteria

- The patient maintains full range of motion and adequate sensation postoperatively.
- The patient exhibits no signs of nerve or muscle damage from inadequate or improper padding or positioning during surgery.

GOAL

The patient will experience an infection-free wound site postoperatively.

POSSIBLE OUTCOME CRITERIA

- The patient's wound site is clean and dry without signs of inflammation or purulent drainage within 24 hours after surgery.
- The patient's wound site appears well approximated and shows signs of normal wound healing 24 hours after surgery.

POSTOPERATIVE NURSING

Nursing Assessment

Systematic assessment is essential during the postoperative period to detect quickly any complications and to individualize nursing care that promotes optimal recovery from the surgery.

ASSESSMENT IN THE PACU

The nurse in the PACU obtains a report from the operating room staff and reads the written documentation of the surgery and the physician's postoperative orders. To plan care effectively, the following information is needed:

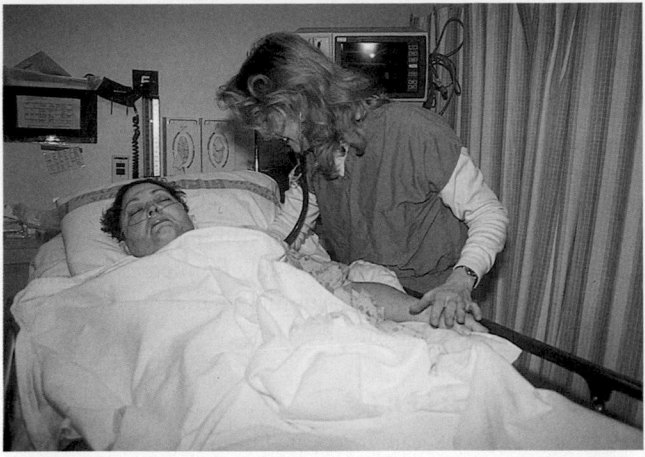

FIGURE 22-4 Close monitoring is needed in the recovery facility.

- Type and extent of the surgical procedure performed
- Type of anesthesia used
- Medication dosages and times medications were given
- Amount of blood lost
- Whether the patient is still intubated
- If any surgical or anesthetic complications occurred

Additional information such as patient allergies, assessment of postprocedure skin integrity, and information relevant to notification of family is also important. Knowing whether the patient will be an inpatient or will return home after recovery from anesthesia is also important. During the immediate postoperative period, assessments are made frequently (Fig. 22-4). Table 22-8 lists important assessments during the immediate

TABLE 22-8 ASSESSMENTS IN THE IMMEDIATE POSTOPERATIVE PERIOD (PACU)

Focus Area	Assessments
Respiratory	Check airway patency and monitor respiratory rate and depth. Auscultate breath sounds. Inspect skin color. Observe chest expansion. Oxygen saturation.
Cardiac	Monitor blood pressure and heart rate and rhythm at least every 15 min.
Neurologic	Check pupillary response. Monitor muscle strength to determine muscle relaxant reversal, if used.
Dressings and drains	Monitor for drainage on dressing and output from drains. Observe for hemorrhage or hematoma formation.
Pain	Assess for both subjective and objective manifestations of pain. Administer analgesics as appropriate.
Renal function	Monitor amounts of urinary output for patients with indwelling catheter (at least 30 mL/h). For patients without a urinary catheter, palpate and percuss for bladder distention or scan with portable bladder ultrasound.

postoperative period. Use airway, breathing, circulation (ABC) to prioritize your assessment.

Assess rate and depth of respirations to detect promptly any signs of hypoxia or airway obstruction. Also evaluate pulse oximetry values, which denote arterial oxygen levels, and compare with baseline data. Assess that oxygen flow is at the prescribed rate. Hypoxia may be first detected as apprehension, anxiety, or restlessness. Loud, irregular respirations may indicate obstruction of the airway, possibly from emesis, accumulated secretions, or patient positioning that allows the tongue to fall to the back of the throat.

❗ SAFETY ALERT

Assessment of cardiovascular function is necessary to detect bleeding promptly. Monitor vital signs every 15 minutes, or more frequently if the patient's condition warrants.

Assess the ECG for cardiac rhythm and rate. Evaluate both the blood pressure and the pulse for trends rather than absolute values. Decreasing blood pressure and an increased pulse rate in the postoperative patient are significant because they may signify hemorrhage or shock. Certain anesthetic agents and muscle relaxants can also cause hypotension. Also, inspect the patient's skin for color (e.g., pale, cyanotic), temperature, and diaphoresis (perspiration). Pale, cyanotic, cool, or clammy skin can indicate impaired tissue perfusion, possibly from shock.

Inspect the dressing for drainage. When present, circle the area of drainage on the dressing with a marking pen and note the time. This provides a baseline from which to track the amount of bleeding. When evaluating incisional bleeding, check for drainage under the patient, where bleeding may not be readily apparent. Catheters, drains, and chest tubes are also assessed for the amount and type of drainage present. Laboratory values (e.g., hematocrit) may also be requested during this period to help evaluate circulatory status.

Perform neurologic assessments to evaluate recovery from the anesthetic agent. Return of reflexes, indicated by swallowing and gagging, occurs when the effects of a general anesthetic are ending. Level of consciousness also changes as the anesthetic agent wears off. Initially, the patient may be unconscious and will not respond to verbal or tactile stimuli. As the anesthetic agent begins to wear off, the patient will respond to loud noises or to his or her name. Finally, the patient becomes oriented to person and place. During this period, the patient may still appear sleepy and will fall into a sleep when not stimulated.

After regional anesthesia, assess the patient for the return of sensory and motor ability. Sensation can be plotted on a dermatome chart (see Chapter 17).

❗ SAFETY ALERT

Autonomic blockade may persist after regional anesthesia, causing severe postural hypotension.

Also, assess the patient's fluid balance, urine output, and pain level during the immediate postoperative period. When administering pain medication, it is important to document whether pain was relieved and what further measures, if any, were needed. Ensure that the IV and all tubes and drains are patent and that all equipment works properly.

ASSESSMENT DURING THE POSTOPERATIVE PERIOD

During the remainder of the postoperative recovery period, systematically assess the patient's status. Table 22-9 lists possible postoperative complications and appropriate nursing assessments for each area.

Each assessment is individualized based on the patient, the surgery that was performed, and the length of time since the surgery occurred. During the first few days after a major surgery, assessments may focus on pain, tissue perfusion, and respiratory function; later in the postoperative course, the patient's ability to perform self-care and to manage at home after discharge may be more important. For an ambulatory surgical patient, self-care capability is a priority in the immediate postoperative period.

Nursing Diagnoses and Outcome Identification

The overall goal for any postoperative patient is to prevent or minimize complications and return the patient to optimal functioning. Although the specific nursing diagnoses vary from patient to patient, Table 22-10 lists some of the more common diagnoses for the postoperative recovery period.

Nursing Interventions in the PACU

The primary responsibilities of the nurse in the recovery facility are assessment and continual monitoring of the patient's condition until the effects of anesthesia subside and the patient's physiologic status stabilizes. A safe patient environment is essential to prevent injury. In the past, family members have not usually been permitted in the PACU, but this practice is changing, especially for young children recovering from surgery.

The PACU nurse maintains a patent airway for the patient through positioning, suctioning, and care of the endotracheal tube, if one is still in place. Fluid replacement and blood administration may be necessary to maintain adequate circulating volume. Pain medications are frequently administered to control postoperative discomfort. As the patient regains consciousness, encourage deep breathing and moving to improve ventilation and circulation.

For the patient to be discharged from the PACU to the postsurgical nursing unit, certain criteria must be met. These criteria usually include the following (ASPAN, 2012):

- Stable vital signs
- Patent airway and adequate respiratory function

TABLE 22-9 POSTOPERATIVE ASSESSMENTS

Function	Potential Complication	Assessments
Health perception–health maintenance	Injury secondary to equipment or body positioning or inadequate recovery from anesthesia	Skin, CMS (color, movement, sensation), patent airway, safe environment (side rails up)
Activity–exercise	Hemorrhage/shock	Vital signs, skin color, bleeding from wound, hematocrit, urine output
	Atelectasis	Respiratory rate and depth, breath sounds, color, arterial blood gases, pulse oximetry, temperature
		Postural blood pressure and pulse
	Deep vein thrombosis	Circulation, movement, sensation (CMS); calf pain or swelling
	Pulmonary emboli	Respiratory rate and depth, other vital signs, oxygen saturation, breath sounds
Nutrition–metabolism	Wound infection	Temperature and other vital signs, wound observation for redness, warmth, swelling, and purulent drainage
	Poor wound healing	
	Dehiscence; evisceration	Wound appearance
	Fluid volume deficit	Intake and output, weight, skin turgor
	Nausea/vomiting	Bowel sounds, abdominal distention
	Malignant hyperthermia	Temperature and other vital signs
	Hypothermia	Temperature
Elimination	Urinary retention	Urine output (especially first 8 h after surgery), bladder distention or discomfort
	Paralytic ileus	Absent bowel sounds, abdominal distention
	Constipation	Lack of stool, abdominal distention, hypoactive bowel sounds
Sleep–rest	Sleep deficit	Sleep duration and quality
Cognition–perception	Pain	Pain level and pain relief after medication, nonverbal indicators
	Delirium	Orientation to person, place, time; level of consciousness, CAM assessment
Self-concept	Altered self-concept	Reaction to wound, drains, tubes
Roles–relationships	Altered role relationship	Perception of alteration in roles or relationships
Coping	Ineffective coping	Anxiety, stress, and lack of coping
Sexuality	Altered sexual function	Impact on sexuality and sexual function
Values–beliefs	Spiritual distress	Surgery or recovery period effects on spiritual beliefs or values

- Satisfactory pain management
- Control of postoperative nausea and vomiting
- Control of bleeding and wound drainage
- Normal thermal state
- Adequate urine output
- Return of sensory/motor function
- Progressive return to baseline level of consciousness and orientation

 APPLY YOUR CRITICAL THINKING

Mr. Johnson is admitted to the PACU immediately after surgery for a bowel resection. He is unresponsive to verbal commands but is breathing on his own. Preoperative vital signs are 134/86, 76, 16. Postoperative vital signs for the last 30 minutes are 128/78, 74, 14 and 142/82, 88, 18. What, if any, conclusions can you draw from these assessment data? What additional assessment data would be important for you to collect?

Check your answers in Appendix B.

After the patient meets the PACU discharge criteria, transfer to the postsurgical nursing unit may occur. The postanesthesia nurse gives a report to the nurse responsible for the surgical patient. This report includes the following information (ASPAN, 2012):

- Patient name and age
- Surgeon and type of surgery performed
- The patient's tolerance of the procedure and any complications
- Type of anesthesia/sedation
- Vital signs
- Patient history
- IV lines
- Blood loss
- Blood and fluid replacement
- Dressings, tubes, and drains
- Urinary and drainage output
- Medications administered
- Level of pain and method of pain control
- Disposition of valuables
- Social support (family, friends)

TABLE 22-10 POSTOPERATIVE NURSING DIAGNOSES AND POSSIBLE PATIENT GOALS

Nursing Diagnosis	Patient Goals
Risk for Aspiration related to anesthesia, decreased level of consciousness	Patient will maintain a patent airway and remain free from aspiration.
Impaired Gas Exchange related to anesthesia, decreased mobility, pain, pain medications	Patient will demonstrate adequate oxygenation of body tissues.
Ineffective Tissue Perfusion related to loss of blood, postoperative edema, anesthetic agents, immobility	Patient will maintain adequate circulation of blood to all body tissues.
Deficient Fluid Volume related to loss of fluids during surgery, decreased oral intake, and abnormal postoperative drainage	Patient will maintain adequate fluid volume.
Risk for Infection related to surgical wounds, invasive lines, decreased nutritional status	Patient will remain free from any postoperative infection.
Urinary Retention related to anesthesia, pain medications, immobility, and edema	Patient will void within 8 h of surgery and without difficulty thereafter.
Constipation related to anesthesia, pain medication, decreased mobility	Patient will resume normal bowel function when normal diet resumes.
Acute Pain related to surgical trauma, inflammation, edema, and invasive procedures	Patient will report that postoperative pain is well controlled.
Impaired Physical Mobility related to pain, fatigue, and tubes, catheters, and drains	Patient will maintain optimal state of mobility, progressively increasing activity daily.
Anxiety related to pain and separation from family, job, and normal activities	Patient will demonstrate adequate coping during the postoperative period.
Deficient Knowledge related to lack of instruction in postoperative activities to prevent complications and promote return to normal function	Patient will verbalize and participate in postoperative activities to prevent complications.
Impaired Home Maintenance related to decreased mobility and decreased energy	Patient will manage normal daily activities at home with necessary assistance from family and friends.
Delayed Surgical Recovery related to length of surgery, age, chronic health problems	Patient will not develop postoperative complications that will delay return to normal activities and increase length of hospital stay.
Nausea related to pain medication, anesthetic agents, decreased gut motility	Patient will not experience nausea or vomiting during postoperative period.

If family members or friends are waiting in the surgery waiting area, they should be informed that the patient is being transferred to another unit.

DISCHARGE FROM THE AMBULATORY SURGICAL CENTER

Most ambulatory surgical centers have two postanesthesia recovery areas for surgical patients: (i) a traditional recovery area where patients are kept recumbent on stretchers and monitored closely until significant effects of anesthesia have subsided and (ii) an area with recliner chairs where patients are encouraged to ambulate, drink fluids, and eat some solids until they meet all the criteria for discharge.

Recovery from anesthesia is usually much quicker when shorter-acting IV anesthetic agents, such as propofol (Diprivan), are administered. Before discharge from an ambulatory surgical unit, the patient should:

- Void (after a spinal or epidural anesthetic or after pelvic surgery)
- Be able to ambulate
- Be alert and oriented
- Have minimal nausea and vomiting
- Have adequate pain/comfort control
- Exhibit no excess bleeding or drainage

Discharge teaching for the patient also must be completed, and a responsible person should be available to accompany the patient home (Fig. 22-5).

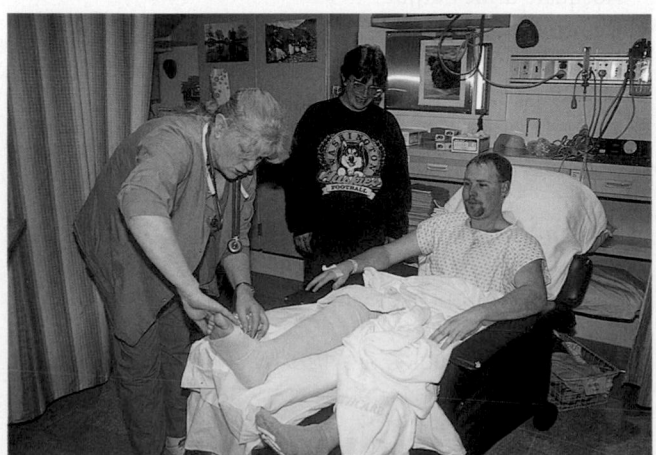

FIGURE 22-5 The patient is assessed in ambulatory day surgery to determine whether criteria for discharge have been met. Patient and family teaching is an important part of care before discharge in the ambulatory surgery facility.

Nursing Interventions on the Surgical Unit

Nursing interventions after the patient arrives on the surgical unit build on patient teaching during the preoperative period. A brief overview of nursing interventions is provided here; in-depth information is provided in selected clinical chapters throughout this text.

RESPIRATORY MAINTENANCE

Aggressive treatment, especially in the immediate postoperative period, is needed to minimize the risk of atelectasis and prevent possible respiratory complications. Deep breathing and coughing, turning and positioning, early and aggressive ambulation, and the use of incentive spirometry are all helpful in preventing postoperative respiratory complications. Refer to Chapter 26 for detailed descriptions of these interventions.

CIRCULATORY MAINTENANCE

Venous stasis resulting from immobility increases the incidence of blood clot formation in the lower extremities. If blood clots lodge in the pulmonary artery (a pulmonary embolus), gas exchange can be severely curtailed and death may occur. Leg exercises, frequent turning and positioning, the use of SCDs and antiembolic stockings, adequate hydration, early ambulation, and anticoagulant prophylaxis all decrease the risk of deep vein thrombosis.

HYDRATION AND NUTRITION

IV fluids are provided during the postoperative period to ensure adequate hydration until the patient can take fluids orally. Fluid volume deficit may occur because of excessive loss of fluids and inadequate fluid replacement. Monitor postural blood pressure on all postoperative patients to detect fluid volume deficits. How long IV fluids will be required depends on the surgery and the patient. Before IV fluids are discontinued, normal bowel sounds are often present, indicating that normal intestinal peristalsis has resumed after the surgery. Peristalsis may resume more slowly if surgery was performed on the gastrointestinal tract.

Progressive dietary intake is ordered after surgery depending on the patient's recovery. Frequently, the physician orders "diet as tolerated" (DAT), and the nurse orders the appropriate diet based on patient assessment. After nausea has subsided and the patient desires food, a clear liquid diet is ordered, progressively followed by full liquids, a soft diet, and a regular diet. As the diet is advanced, continually assess the patient for nausea, vomiting, abnormal bowel sounds, and abdominal distention. Abnormal findings may necessitate a change in diet orders.

ELIMINATION

During the postoperative period, the patient is expected to void within 8 hours after surgery. If the postoperative patient is unable to void because of edema, trauma, medications, or the inability to ambulate to the bathroom, an order for intermittent catheterization may be necessary to relieve urinary retention. An indwelling catheter may be indicated for patients undergoing urologic or gynecologic surgery. Normal urine output is in the range of 0.5 to 1 mL/kg/hour for the average adult (Rothrock, 2015). Urine volumes less than this amount should be reported to the surgeon. When low urine output occurs, challenging the patient with increased IV fluid or administering diuretics may be necessary to ensure adequate urine output.

Surgery may also affect bowel elimination. Normal bowel movements are not expected until normal intestinal motility resumes and the patient has begun eating. Rectal tubes and return-flow enemas may be ordered to help relieve intestinal gas and promote the passage of flatus. Postoperative constipation may occur because of decreased activity, side effects of medications (especially pain medications), fluid volume deficit, or fear of painful evacuation. When the patient has started eating, stool softeners are commonly ordered. Encourage activity, adequate fluid intake, and a diet that promotes normal bowel evacuation. If a bowel movement has not occurred within 3 days after resuming normal dietary intake, laxatives, suppositories, and enemas may be necessary.

WOUND CARE

Wound assessment, aseptic care of the wound, and monitoring of wound drainage systems are all important nursing interventions. Inspect dressings regularly, and note the amount and type of wound drainage. Some surgeons prefer to change the first postoperative dressing, but if the nurse makes the first change, remove it carefully to avoid inadvertent removal of drains. Increasingly, surgeons leave wounds undressed and open to the air to heal. Report symptoms of wound infection (e.g., redness, warmth, purulent drainage, elevated body temperature) to the physician. Finally, removal of sutures and staples is often the responsibility of nursing personnel.

MOBILITY AND SELF-CARE

During the early postoperative period, the patient may require assistance with mobility and self-care. Encourage the patient to increase mobility and independence in self-care progressively to prepare the way for discharge. Early ambulation is indicated for most surgical patients to minimize potential complications. The patient usually sits in a chair or may even ambulate for a brief period on the evening of surgery. Administering pain medication before activity and providing instructions on how best to get out of bed will increase patient comfort. Encourage the patient to ambulate progressively longer distances each postoperative day.

> **❗ SAFETY ALERT**
>
> Medications, postural hypotension, and equipment such as catheters, drains, and IV poles can make ambulation hazardous. Assess the patient's need for assistance prior to ambulation. Safety measures such as gait belts, appropriate footwear, and removal of tripping hazards will help to prevent injury. Always provide standby assistance if the patient is weak or unsteady when ambulating. If the patient complains of dizziness or feels diaphoretic when ambulating, he or she should return to bed.

Adequate hygiene after surgery is important to ensure patient comfort. If the patient has many tubes and has had major surgery, a bed bath may be given on the first postoperative day. Wash off any solutions used to prepare the skin before surgery (e.g., povidone–iodine). Remove compression devices and antiembolic stockings at bath time, and inspect the skin. Always encourage the patient to perform as much self-care as possible. Usually, the surgical patient may shower if surgical dressings and IV sites are covered with a protective, waterproof barrier. Care should be taken when the patient is showering, however, because the warm water can promote vasodilation and hypotension and increase the risk of falls.

COMFORT AND REST

Pain management is an important nursing intervention during the postoperative period. Nonpharmacologic interventions such as positioning, back massage, distraction, and emotional support help the postoperative patient feel more comfortable. Pain medications are administered as needed to control postoperative discomfort. Teaching the patient to recognize and report pain is an important part of pain management. PCA and patient-controlled epidural analgesia (PCEA) are often used postoperatively to allow the patient more control in obtaining effective pain relief. If the dose, frequency, or type of medication ordered by the physician for pain control is ineffective, notify the physician. Many facilities have a pain service whose staff members routinely see postoperative patients and assist physicians in determining appropriate pain management regimens.

Rest is important to promote healing. Hypnotics and barbiturates may be ordered to help ensure rest. Providing a quiet, comfortable environment encourages sleep and rest. Whenever possible, nursing activities, especially during the night, should be grouped together to allow for uninterrupted periods of rest.

Home and Community Care

During the last decade, in-hospital recovery from surgical procedures has been significantly shortened, and an increasing number of surgeries are performed on an ambulatory basis. Much surgical recovery occurs in the patient's home, with family or friends assisting in postsurgical care. Discharge needs vary depending on the surgical procedure and the individual patient. Whereas many patients are discharged and recuperate in the home, others may need to be transferred to a rehabilitation or long-term care facility. Some patients who have sufficiently recovered from their surgical procedure to be discharged home may need the assistance of home care nurses.

Many hospitals and surgical centers have developed special discharge procedures and forms for use when preparing the patient for discharge. Discharge concerns for the surgical patient include pain management, wound care and dressing changes, monitoring for infection, dietary needs, bowel and bladder function, activity restriction, recommended sexual activity, and ability to perform self-care activities. The patient or a responsible caregiver learns to manage any special equipment that is required at home and to perform necessary procedures (e.g., dressing changes) independently. The patient needs to know where to buy needed supplies and how to obtain specialized equipment. A limited number of supplies may be given to the patient to ensure continuing care until the patient can obtain these necessary items.

Include the patient's family or caregiver in the patient teaching session, as appropriate, and give written guidelines. Such guidelines usually include limitations on activity and diet, treatments, and medications necessary during postoperative recovery as well as symptoms necessitating notification of the healthcare provider. Use verbal and written instructions for any prescribed medications, and allow time to answer any questions. Provide the patient, family, or caregiver with instructions concerning a follow-up appointment with the surgeon, along with a phone number.

Explore with the patient what assistance he or she will have after discharge and how he or she plans to manage once home. Asking questions such as "How do you envision your first few days at home?" may help to identify how the patient will cope after discharge. When the identified plan does not seem realistic, help the patient explore alternative approaches or encourage the recruitment of family, friends, or community resources for help.

Evaluation

During postoperative evaluation, determine whether goals have been met. Goals and outcome criteria relate to preventing postoperative complications and returning the patient to optimal functioning. Table 22-10 lists the more common postoperative nursing diagnoses and patient goals. Outcome criteria for four goals are presented here.

GOAL

The patient will state that postoperative pain is well controlled.

Possible Outcome Criteria

- During the postoperative period, the patient reports that pain does not interfere with turning, positioning, ambulating, or self-care activities.
- The patient verbalizes good pain control (less than 3 on a 0 to 10 scale) on oral medications by the time of discharge from acute care facility.

GOAL

The patient will experience normal bowel function when normal diet is resumed.

Possible Outcome Criteria

- The patient passes flatus and verbalizes decrease in abdominal (gas) pain.
- The patient reports passage of usual bowel movement 24 hours after regular diet resumes.

GOAL

The patient will maintain optimal mobility, progressively increasing activity daily.

Possible Outcome Criteria

- The patient sits up in a chair, with the nurse's help, on the evening of surgery.
- The patient walks to the bathroom, with the nurse's help, by 24 hours after surgery.
- The patient walks 200 feet in the hallway on the day after surgery.

GOAL

The patient will manage postoperative treatments and normal daily activities in the home with assistance from family and friends.

Possible Outcome Criteria

- The patient can state discharge instructions before discharge from the hospital.
- The patient or responsible caregiver can demonstrate dressing change and wound drain management before discharge.
- The patient can satisfactorily complete activities of daily living with necessary assistance from a responsible caregiver during the first week after discharge per patient's verbal report.

KEY CONCEPTS

- Perioperative nursing provides individualized care for the surgical patient during the preoperative, intraoperative, and postoperative phases of the surgical experience.

- Surgery may be performed in various clinical facilities, including a physician's office, a clinic, an ambulatory surgical center, or a hospital.

- Surgical procedures can affect all areas of function.

- Life span considerations are important when individualizing care for the surgical patient.

- Preoperative teaching is important to minimize postoperative complications, increase patient compliance, and decrease patient anxiety.

- Informed consent must be obtained by the surgeon before any surgical procedure is performed.

- Preoperative preparation of the patient includes ensuring NPO status, starting IV access, initiating bowel preparation and skin preparation, administering preoperative medications, and, at times, inserting a nasogastric tube.

- Nursing personnel in the operating room provide emotional support, ensure a safe patient environment, and maintain asepsis.

- Anesthesia may be administered by an anesthesiologist or by a CRNA.

- General anesthesia produces a sleeplike state, whereas regional anesthesia decreases pain and sensation in certain areas.

- Sutures or staples may be used to approximate wound edges and promote healing.

- Continual nursing assessment is important in the recovery facility to detect complications promptly and monitor recovery from anesthesia.

- Nursing care during the postoperative period focuses on preventing surgical complications and promoting optimal return of normal function.

- Potential complications during the postoperative period include hemorrhage, shock, atelectasis, deep vein thrombosis, pulmonary emboli, wound infection, fluid volume deficit, nausea, vomiting, malignant hyperthermia, hypothermia, urinary retention, paralytic ileus, sleep deficit, pain, confusion, altered self-concept, altered role relationships, ineffective coping, and altered sexual function.

- To prepare for discharge, instructions regarding activity restrictions, incisional care, and symptoms to be reported to a physician should be addressed.

PRACTICING FOR THE NCLEX

CHECK YOUR ANSWERS IN APPENDIX A.

1. A patient was admitted when a suspicious mass was found in her right breast following mammography. The patient is scheduled for a breast biopsy. What type of surgery would this describe?
   a. Explorative
   b. Diagnostic
   c. Curative
   d. Palliative

2. A postoperative day 1 patient is found to have hypoactive bowel tones. The nurse knows this is an expected (though abnormal) finding because of which of the following reasons? Select all that apply:
   a. The patient was NPO prior to surgery.
   b. The patient is diabetic.
   c. The patient received general anesthetic and opioid pain medications.
   d. The patient has decreased physical mobility.

3. A nurse is caring for a patient following a Whipple procedure (removal of the head of the pancreas, duodenum, part of the stomach, and common bile duct). The patient has nausea and vomiting and absent bowel tones. The nurse inserts a nasogastric tube per physician order to treat which surgical complication?
   a. Pain
   b. Constipation
   c. Fluid volume deficit
   d. Paralytic ileus

4. A patient with reconstructive head and neck skin grafts following mouth cancer is crying when the nurse enters the room and states that she doesn't want to see any

visitors. The surgery's impact on which of the following best explains this behavior?

a. Cognition
b. Self-concept
c. Coping
d. Relationships

5. A surgeon phones the nursing unit and asks the nurse to send the patient to surgery and sign the informed consent. Which of the following is most appropriate?

a. Review surgical complications and procedure with the patient and sign the consent as a witness.
b. Explain procedure and risks/benefits and ask the patient to sign.
c. Ask if the surgeon has explained the surgery and risks, and if so have the patient sign consent if comfortable, and you sign as the witness.
d. Include unsigned consent in the chart and send the patient to the preoperative induction area.

6. Which of the following is the final step before making the first surgical incision?

a. Preoperative teaching
b. Anesthesia induction
c. Procedural pause
d. Skin preparation for infection control

7. Asepsis is paramount during surgery. Which of the following are used to preserve this environment? Select all that apply:

a. Correct donning of sterile gowns/gloves
b. Inspection of sterile equipment packages prior to unwrapping and dispensing

c. Consider a table draped with a sterile drape to be sterile only at table level
d. Keep unscrubbed personnel more than 1 foot away from the sterile field

8. A nurse is receiving a patient from surgery to the post-anesthesia care unit (PACU). She is most interested in which of the following assessment data? Select all that apply:

a. Bowel function
b. Pain
c. Urinary output
d. Pupillary response

9. A postoperative shoulder repair patient (post-op day 3) reports left calf pain. The nurse finds redness and swelling on assessment. What complication best explains these findings?

a. Positioning injury during surgery
b. Wound infection
c. Atelectasis
d. Deep vein thrombosis

10. Hand hygiene is a critical component of aseptic practice. Which of the following demonstrates knowledge of hand hygiene in the intraoperative environment? Select all that apply:

a. Rings and watches removed prior to the surgical hand scrub
b. Presence of newly applied artificial nail tips
c. Performing hand hygiene at the beginning of your shift
d. Presence of intact nail polish

REFERENCES

American Society of PeriAnesthesia Nurses. (2012). *2012–2014 Perianesthesia nursing standards, practice recommendations and interpretive statements.* Cherry Hill, NJ: Author.

Association of Perioperative Registered Nurses. (2014). *AORN standards and recommended practices.* Denver, CO: Author.

Center for Disease Control. (2014). National and state healthcare associated infections progress report. Retrieved from http://www.cdc.gov/hai/progress-report/

Forrester, D. A., Doyle-Munoz, J., McTigue, T., D'Andrea, S., & Natale-Ryan, A. (2014). The efficacy of gum chewing in reducing postoperative ileus: A multisite randomized controlled trial. *Journal of Wound, Ostomy, and Continence Nursing, 41*(3), 227–232.

Landriscina, D. (2009). Care of the pediatric patient. In C. B. Drain (Ed.), *Perianesthesia nursing: A critical care approach* (5th ed., pp. 697–716). St. Louis, MO: Saunders.

Phillips, N. (2013). *Berry & Kohn's operating room technique* (12th ed.). St. Louis, MO: C.V. Mosby.

Rothrock, J. (2015). *Alexander's care of the patient in surgery* (15th ed.). St. Louis, MO: C.V. Mosby.

The Joint Commission. (2014). Facts about the universal protocol. Retrieved from http://www.jointcommission.org/

van Bree, S. H. J., Bemelman, W. A., Hollmann, M. W., Zwinderman, A. H., Matteoli, G., El Temna, S., et al. (2014). Identification of clinical outcomes measures for recovery of gastrointestinal motility in postoperative ileus. *Annals of Surgery, 259*(4), 708–714.

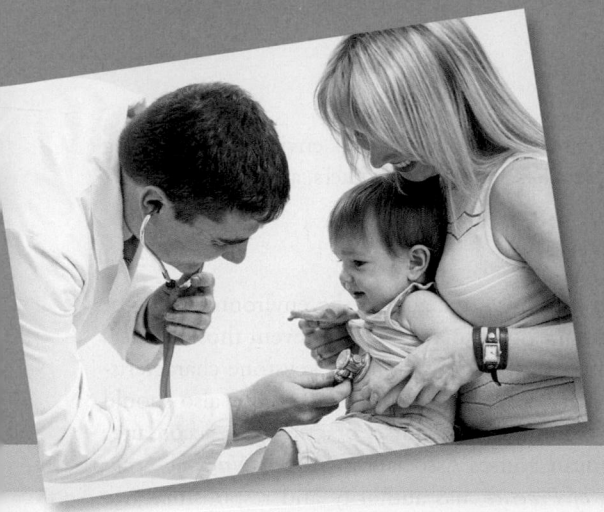

UNIT 4
Clinical Nursing Care

CHAPTER 23

Safety

Christine M. Henshaw

Case Scenario

You are a nurse in a pediatric primary care clinic conducting a well-child assessment for an active toddler and his young mother. As you discuss the home environment, the mother tells you that they live in a two-story house with bedrooms on the second floor and the other rooms on the main floor. The mother tells you that the toddler climbs up and down the stairs and on chairs, gets up on counters and tabletops, and is very curious about boxes and bottles of all types. The mother appears tired and irritated as she tries to hold the toddler still on her lap. He is crying and struggling to get off of her lap.

Once you have completed this chapter and have added safety to your knowledge base, review the above scenario and reflect on the following areas of Critical Thinking:

1. List and analyze your immediate impressions of this family.
2. Describe how you think the mother feels at this time.
3. Propose how you will proceed with your assessment of the mother, toddler, and home environment.
4. Summarize additional information you need to provide further anticipatory guidance to this family.
5. Plan methods for improving the toddler's safety.
6. Reflect on how you can follow up with the mother and her coping strategies.

KEY TERMS

asphyxiation
bioterrorism
burns
electrical shock
falls
ground
poisoning
pollution
RACE
restraint
safety
safety zones
side rails
suffocation

LEARNING OBJECTIVES

Upon completion of this chapter, you will be able to:

1. Recognize the importance of safety in the home and healthcare environments.
2. Relate special safety considerations to specific developmental stages.
3. Identify factors that affect safety and common manifestations of altered safety.
4. Identify safety risks through assessment.
5. Discuss nursing interventions to promote safe homes and healthcare environments.
6. Individualize a teaching plan for individuals with identified safety risks.

Safety is an individual, community, national, and worldwide concern. Society's focus on safety intensifies as awareness increases about the types of dangers that threaten people and places where these dangers exist. A fast-paced society with increased stress and advanced technologies can lead to distracting situations, compromising a person's judgment and resulting in unintentional injury. In healthcare, the scope of safety in hospitals and healthcare agencies has shifted from the context of a single nurse concerned with the physical safety of the patient assigned to his or her care to a realization that safety is a far greater concept with responsibilities distributed among many professionals.

A truly danger-free environment is rare. Consequently, safety promotion involves knowledge about, awareness of, and adherence to safety principles and standards. Teaching the patient and family about safety precautions at home, in the workplace, and in the community is also important.

Nurses work in many different environments, some of which are hazardous, and must minimize their own potential for injury. Safety habits for both patients and nurses ensure an optimal therapeutic environment and promote health. Safety is important on every level of human interaction. Teaching and applying the concepts of safety are part of a seamless approach to injury prevention, regardless of setting.

SAFETY

Safety and security are basic human needs, second in priority in Maslow's hierarchy only to physiologic needs. Safety not only prevents harm and injury but also allows people to feel secure in their actions. The sense of safety reduces stress, which promotes general health. Safety allows a person to meet other basic human needs, such as love, belonging, and self-esteem, and to accomplish personal goals. A positive outlook on life, in turn, results in better mental health and more effective functioning.

Safety can be defined as the state of being free from harm or danger. An injury is a particular form or instance of harm. The term *accident* is no longer used in discussing injury prevention because "accident" implies an event that occurred randomly, was unforeseeable, and therefore was unpreventable. Unlike accidents, injuries have recognizable patterns of occurrence with corresponding controls. Unintentional injury incidents can result in permanent disability, pain, emotional distress, and financial hardship.

The nurse will provide healthcare in a safe manner in all situations. Using critical thinking skills and the nursing process, the nurse is responsible for assessing the patient and the environment, formulating a nursing diagnosis to provide appropriate safe care that includes injury control, and maintaining a safe environment.

The principles of injury control have interventions centered at three primary levels: the individual level, providing education about safety hazards and prevention strategies; the design phase, using engineering and environmental controls (active or passive safety features that can prevent injury from product or equipment use); and the regulatory level, creating, monitoring, and enforcing regulations to ensure safe products and environments among manufacturers, retailers, employers, workers, and product users.

Management

Once a person recognizes dangers in the environment, he or she usually takes measures to avoid or to prevent those dangers and thus practices safety. Prevention is a keystone characteristic of safety. Safety practices involve self-care but also should provide safety for others. The nurse, practicing in accordance with the American Nurses Association (ANA) *Nursing: Scope and Standards of Practice*, has authority and responsibility to protect patients and provide for their safety.

Some people are at greater risk for safety problems because of lifestyle and behavior patterns. A person's lifestyle can involve risky or impulsive behaviors, such as walking alone at night or high-speed driving. Some people enjoy potentially dangerous sports, such as skydiving or mountain climbing, and may not follow prudent safety precautions. The inclination toward risk taking varies widely among people. The use of tobacco, alcohol, and other drugs, unsafe sexual practices, and poor diets also impair safety. These practices can result from lack of awareness of risks, addiction, or neglect of health and safety.

Life Span Considerations

The diverse physiologic and psychological capabilities of people and encounters with various safety hazards across the life span put various age groups at risk for different safety concerns and associated potential injuries. The nurse will encounter people across the life span with differences in ability to perceive danger, to assess and respond to danger, or to perform safety measures. The nurse assesses each person and provides anticipatory guidance and selects interventions geared toward specific age-related concerns.

NEWBORN AND INFANT

Because they lack musculoskeletal and neurologic maturity, newborns and infants are susceptible to falls, choking, burns, and other traumatic injuries. They depend on inarticulate cries and nonverbal communication to signal their needs. With limited ability to adjust to bodily needs (e.g., temperature regulation) or to respond to environmental challenges and no clear method of communication, newborns and infants depend on their caregivers to provide for them and to create safe environments for normal, injury-free growth and development. Providing such safety is a major task of parenting and caregiving. As babies gain function, they learn and explore by pulling objects to themselves and placing things in their mouths.

> **SAFETY ALERT**
> Cords, tablecloths, plastic bags, bottles, and cans are tempting, potentially dangerous objects that caregivers must strive to keep out of reach of infants.

A safe hospital environment for newborns and infants includes a comfortable temperature range, a bulb syringe or suction device to maintain a patent airway, identification bracelets, and equipping each infant with a security tag associated with an alarm system to prevent infant abduction. A safe home environment for newborns and infants also includes a comfortable temperature range, along with nonrestrictive, nonflammable, adequate clothing; warm bathwater; clean air; safe toys; guardrails at staircases and steps; protection with locked, padded rungs or rails for cribs or changing tables; covered electrical outlets; and appropriate car seats for automobile travel. The American Academy of Pediatrics (AAP, 2011a) provides input into the design of child car seats and makes recommendations for use of child seats according to child age, weight, and model of vehicle housing the child. Table 23-1 presents this information.

! SAFETY ALERT

In both environments, parents should be taught to place their infants on their backs when sleeping to prevent sudden infant death syndrome (SIDS; AAP, 2011b).

TODDLER AND PRESCHOOLER

Falls, bumps, and bruises are common during these ages of curiosity and exuberance. Increasing mobility, lack of life experience and judgment, and immature musculoskeletal and neurologic systems lead to potentially hazardous encounters for toddlers and preschoolers.

Improving eye–hand coordination and increasing strength and speed characterize these developmental stages. Caregivers must anticipate the wide-ranging interests of their young explorers. Once upright, toddlers can reach up to new sources of interesting items, although they have not achieved posture stability and are frequently off balance. Life experiences begin to accumulate, however, and learning safe and dangerous behaviors begins. Setting a safe example is an important first step for caregivers of toddlers and preschoolers.

Toddlers and preschoolers delight in opening and closing doors, turning knobs, climbing furniture, and engaging in all sorts of active play. Curiosity still is present. Pets and other animals are new, moveable objects of exploration and fascination. Although these young children usually can communicate their basic needs in words or actions, caregivers must still ensure a comfortable environmental temperature; adequate, nonflammable, nonrestrictive clothing; and warm bathwater. Bathtubs should have nonskid mats or decals to prevent slipping when the child stands erect. Because toddlers and preschoolers lack mature judgment and do not perceive danger near stairs, staircases and steps need guardrails. Open screened windows pose a fall risk for children pushing against the screen to look out the window.

TABLE 23-1 GENERAL CAR SEAT USE INFORMATION

Buckle Everyone. Children Age 12 and Under in Back Seat!

	Age/Weight	Seat Type/Seat Position	Usage Tips
Infants/Toddlers	Birth to at least 2 years *and* until they reach the highest weight or height allowed by their car safety seat's manufacturer	Infant-only seat rear facing or convertible seat used rear facing. *Seats should be secured to the vehicle by the seat belts or by the LATCH system.*	• Never use in a front seat where an air bag is present. • Tightly install child seat in rear seat, facing the rear. • Child seat should recline at approximately a 45-degree angle. • Harness straps/slots at or below shoulder level (lower set of slots for most convertible child safety seats). • Harness straps snug on child; harness clip at armpit level.
	Less than 2 years/20–35 lb	Convertible seat used rear facing (select one recommended for heavier infants) *Seats should be secured to the vehicle by the seat belts or by the LATCH system.*	• Never use in a front seat where an air bag is present. • Tightly install child seat in rear seat, facing the rear. • Child seat should recline at approximately a 45-degree angle. • Harness straps/slots at or below shoulder level (lower set of slots for most convertible child safety seats). • Harness straps snug on child; harness clip at armpit level.
Toddlers/Preschoolers	2–4 years/at least 20 lb to approximately 40 lb	Convertible seat forward facing *or* forward-facing seats with harnesses *Seats should be secured to the vehicle by the seat belts or by the LATCH system.*	• Tightly install child seat in rear seat, forward facing. • Harness straps/slots at or above child's shoulders (usually top set of slots for convertible child safety seats). • Harness straps snug on child; harness clip at armpit level.
Young children	4 to at least 8 years, unless they are 4′9″ (57″) tall or 60 lb.	Belt-positioning booster (no back, base only) or high-back belt-positioning booster *Never use with lap-only belts— belt-positioning boosters are always used with lap and shoulder belts.*	• Booster base used with adult lap and shoulder belt in rear seat. • Shoulder belt should rest snugly across chest, resting on shoulder, and should *never* be placed under the arm or behind the back. • Lap belt should rest low, across the lap/upper thigh area—not across.

From Parents Central. (2015). *Car seat recommendations for children.* Retrieved from http://www.safercar.gov/parents/Right-Seat-Age-And-Size-Recommendations.htm

Toddler toys must be sturdy, free of sharp or rough edges, and without small, removable, or breakable parts that the child could swallow or have lodge in his or her respiratory tract or that could damage an eye. Toddlers and preschoolers usually enjoy tricycles, push cycles, rocking horses, and other active toys that use large muscle groups. Children should use such toys under adult supervision until they understand safety limits. The U.S. government's website, Consumer Product Safety Commission (www.cpsc.gov) and the Toy Industry Association's website (www.toyinfo.org) provide updated information on appropriate, safe toys and games for children at each age level and list the standards on toy product safety.

With the transition to preschool, children begin to learn safety rules and gain better motor control. Preschoolers usually can avoid bumps and learn to climb safely up and down stairs. They also benefit from learning about **safety zones**, which are safe places to stand or sit when a potentially dangerous activity is under way. For example, a kitchen should have a safety zone where children can watch activity but are out of reach of the stove, oven, and knives.

❗ SAFETY ALERT

Outside the home, toddlers and preschoolers need supervision. With caregiver guidance, they will learn about playing away from automobile traffic and avoiding strange animals. In addition, car seats are necessary for travel in motor vehicles.

Preschoolers learn the rules of safe social interaction by trial and error. Striking out and demonstrating aggression usually results from the natural exuberance of this stage rather than from any malicious intent. Caregivers, however, can help their preschoolers by teaching cooperating and sharing. During these stages, caregivers should encourage caution toward strangers. Some law enforcement agencies recommend identification bracelets for children, the fingerprinting of children, and frequently taking photographs of children to ensure that up-to-date photos are available.

Fire safety is a family concern. The United States Fire Administration (USFA, 2014, 2015a) provides educational opportunities for professional and public groups and offers recommendations for parents to protect their families from fire. The USFA website has a page with information and educational materials directed toward children (USFA, 2014). Learning about matches, electrical cords, stoves, and ovens is important for curious preschoolers, who might be tempted to experiment. The whole family should regularly practice crawling on the floor, using escape routes, and having a meeting place outside the home in the event of fire. Local fire departments often have useful information about planning alternative escape routes and other safety procedures.

SCHOOL-AGE CHILD AND ADOLESCENT

Physiologic maturity is almost complete for school-age children. Motor control of large muscles and rapidly developing fine motor control enable school-age children to accomplish

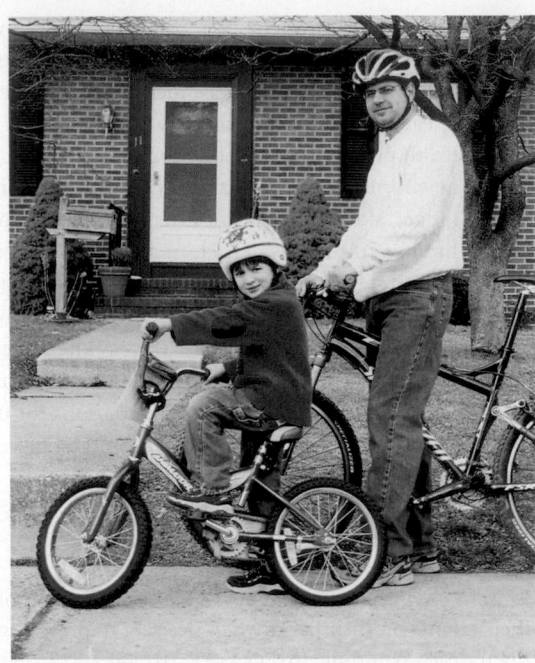

FIGURE 23-1 Helmets are an important part of bike safety. Parents can be role models for children by also wearing bike helmets.

complex tasks. Learning occurs at an astounding rate. Life experiences accumulate, and children use them to make judgments about the appropriateness of behaviors. Their expanding world demands flexible responses and presents opportunities for independent action.

School-age children can make their needs known verbally. Their usually quick reflexes help protect them from burns, falls, and other unintentional traumatic injuries. New activities require new skills, and children of this age group can learn to ski, ride horses, swim, bicycle, sail, or participate in team sports. Safety precautions are important (Fig. 23-1). All children should learn to swim or at least float and tread water. The buddy system, a prearranged agreement between two or more people to provide mutual companionship and to monitor each other's whereabouts and well-being during certain high-risk activities, is an important outdoor and water safety strategy. Many occupational settings use the buddy system for safety.

❗ SAFETY ALERT

Children should wear properly fitted helmets when cycling, riding, or playing contact sports and life jackets when sailing or boating (National Safety Council [NSC], 2015).

Safe examples from adult caregivers continue to influence school-age children. Caregivers should use alcohol in moderation. Guns are locked and ammunition is stored separately. Discussion, rather than force, is used to resolve conflicts.

During adolescence, growth and development occur. Physical maturity of the musculoskeletal system nears completion, and the nervous and cardiovascular systems are fully mature. Adolescents have a physiologic need for 8.5 to 9.5 hours of sleep during this time of accelerated growth and development (American Academy of Pediatrics, 2014). Sleep deprivation as a result of trying to balance many activities can compromise safety. While life experience is accumulating rapidly, so are new responsibilities. Autonomy develops in response to social and societal pressures. Activities that require judgment and independent action include maintaining academic responsibilities, learning to drive a car, coping with pressures from peers or drug dealers to use illicit drugs, beginning to explore sexuality, babysitting, working after school, and developing other life management skills. As they explore opportunities, adolescents may know that certain behaviors are unsafe, but social pressure can persuade them to act against their better judgment. Experimentation is also a common trait of adolescents to explore their limits and capabilities. Increasingly, schools are developing programs on violence prevention to teach teens constructive methods for solving problems and disputes without violence (Centers for Disease Control and Prevention [CDC], 2014).

ADULT AND OLDER ADULT

With physical maturity completed and the attainment of the legal status of adulthood, adults move at will in a world full of potential dangers. Unintentional injuries at home, in the workplace, and during sports are common. Safety habits, no longer reinforced by watchful adults, can become rusty; disregard of judgment, overconfidence, or ignorance can place adults in danger's path. In addition, adults may consume alcohol, which interferes with judgment to interpret the environment and with physical capabilities to operate machinery, thus contributing to injuries.

Motor vehicles continue to be a major cause of death related to unintentional injuries for all age groups to 80 years (CDC, 2013). The use of safety belts with shoulder harnesses and the use of helmets when a person rides motorcycles are mandatory in most states and provinces. Most cars are equipped with air bags for increased safety.

Advancing age entails loss in physical function and usually in acuity of sensory–perceptual function and cognitive judgment. Older adults may have impaired eyesight and hearing and decreased sensing ability to maintain balance and sensitivity to touch. The ability to regulate temperature may become impaired; older adults are at higher risk than are younger adults for hypothermia and heat stroke. Reflex responses slow, and the musculoskeletal system can lose flexibility and strength. Various conditions such as arthritis, osteoporosis, or heart failure can limit the ability to endure sustained physical activity. Medications taken to control conditions such as high blood pressure or Parkinson disease may result in orthostatic hypotension and increase the potential for falling. The principles of a safe environment for older adults follow the same general guidelines as those for all ages: comfortable temperature range; adequate clothing; bathwater of the right temperature (the setting on the hot water heater may need to be reduced); adequate ventilation; lighting that allows for safe navigation throughout the house at all times of day; nonskid surfaces on stairs, in the kitchen, and in the bathroom (throw rugs should be removed); and stable supports for climbing (firm stair rails, grab bars if needed).

Cultural Considerations

Safety practices are individual and often learned as an important value in the family or community. Some families are cautious and very safety conscious, while others are more comfortable with a higher level of risk. Individuals raised in a family that develops and reviews disaster plans, creates a safe home environment, and discusses the dangers in high-risk behaviors will be more likely to value safety and follow safety practices when they become adults. Habits such as smoking and alcohol use are more acceptable and common in certain cultures and geographic areas. Poor neighborhoods and inadequate housing often pose safety risks for immigrants or the poor.

FACTORS AFFECTING SAFETY

Physiologic Factors

The body works to allow a person to recognize unsafe situations and avoid or minimize injury. For example, reflexes withdraw the hand from the flame before conscious thought can do so. A loud noise causes a startle reaction and an immediate increase in level of alertness. The sensation of pain provides important feedback that an activity or situation is dangerous. Immaturity of the systems in early life and aging in later life affect the body; impairments caused by altered conditions or diseases to various systems can affect the body's overall capacity to help maintain safety.

The primary systems that integrate for protection and safety are as follows:

- Musculoskeletal
- Neurologic and sensory
- Cardiovascular and respiratory
- Immune
- Integumentary

Environmental Factors

Humans exist in environments: the home, workplace, community, nature and the outdoors, or healthcare setting. The features of each environment must meet the safety requirements of the human body. These include oxygen, clean air devoid of pollutants and toxic substances, temperature, protection from extreme weather elements, availability of clean safe water and food, and adequate safe sanitation.

POLLUTION

Pollution is harmful or unnatural substances in the air, water, or land. Such toxic substances, which are frequently by-products of manufacturing, increase risks of cancer. Air pollution increases the risk for and severity of respiratory problems, such as asthma and chronic bronchitis. Poor air quality because of pollution often increases allergic symptoms. Polluted water can lead to the spread of disease and infection, either from the direct effects of drinking contaminated water or from contamination of the food supply. Noise pollution from airplanes, trains, heavy automobile traffic, loud music, or public stadiums can harm people by increasing stress and blood pressure levels and by contributing to hearing loss (Environmental Protection Agency, 2012).

RADIATION

Ionizing radiation consists of high-frequency electromagnetic radiation of short wavelength (e.g., x-rays, gamma rays). Such radiation can occur naturally or in devices such as nuclear reactors. The many adverse health effects related to excess exposure to radiation include birth defects, tissue cell destruction, and cancer.

Many healthcare facilities use radiation in diagnosis and treatment. X-ray machines and pharmaceuticals for injection or implantation emit small doses of radiation into the environment. While patients receive the intended dose of radiation, nurses and x-ray technicians are exposed to small doses repeatedly. Procedures for preventing unanticipated exposures are discussed later in this chapter. Increasing concerns about the radiation exposure with CT scans, particularly in children and small adults, have led to research about lowering the dose of radiation and limiting scans to those situations with proven benefit (Food and Drug Administration [FDA], 2015).

TERRORISM

Healthcare facilities need to have a plan to prepare for any type of disaster, including terrorism. During disasters or terrorism attacks, there is both an increase in the numbers of critically ill or injured patients seeking care and a decrease in the full range of usual structures and supports. **Bioterrorism**, or the use of biologic agents to compromise our safety and to cause fear, is one form of attack that could occur.

A facility's emergency disaster plan needs to state specifically how to respond to these kinds of attacks and how to accommodate for lack of the usual administrative support structures. The disaster plan should take into account the type of attack or disaster so that nurses are ready for the potential types of organisms, poisons, and expected injuries so that healthcare personnel know where to turn rapidly for protocols and advice. Nurses need to be prepared to respond according to the agency's emergency plan. This can be accomplished through education, training, and disaster preparedness drills as are practiced in many communities. The resources and needs will be community specific; hence, the healthcare response also needs to be planned for the individual community.

HOME

A safe home environment creates a secure and protective living area that features adequate ventilation; a reliable heating system; smoke alarm and carbon monoxide alarm systems; non-skid bathtub surfaces; well-maintained electrical appliances and electrical cords; sturdy step stools and ladders; and careful labeling, handling, and storing of all potentially toxic substances. Parents should safely lock guns out of children's reach, discard foods and medications on their expiration date, and practice fire escape routes. In addition, parents should locate smoke and carbon monoxide alarms strategically and ensure that the alarms function. Overloading outlets, using appliances with frayed cords, and allowing infants or children to play with plugs or near electrical outlets may result in electrical shock or burns.

Hazards in the home include poorly lighted stairways, throw rugs, slippery floors, cluttered areas, and unstable ladders, all of which can cause falls. The risk of falls increases when a person of advanced age, impaired mobility, or both encounters these hazards. Box 23-1 summarizes possible home hazards.

WORKPLACE

Health and safety hazards and risk of injury are inherent in many jobs. Examples of occupational hazards include noise, hazardous dusts (e.g., asbestos, lead, coal), chemicals, heights, dangerous machines, biologically infectious agents, and violence. Ergonomic hazards, such as heavy lifting and repetitive motion, also contribute to many disabling injuries. Other dangers result when employers or workers do not follow safety precautions, such as wearing protective gear and following safe work practices.

Since 1970, The Occupational Safety and Health Administration (OSHA) has required employers to provide their workers with a safe and healthful work environment. An employer must identify hazardous conditions and exposures present in the workplace, inform workers of their presence, and educate them about the preventive strategies necessary to avoid injury. OSHA also investigates workers' complaints about health and safety issues.

COMMUNITY

The community in which one lives, works, shops, and plays may present safety concerns. Noise (e.g., from trains or planes), air pollution, crime, poor lighting, hazardous waste sites or landfills, busy intersections, dilapidated houses, cliffs, and unprotected creeks are hazards. The community should be free from most of these hazards to lend a feeling of safety and security. Community public health officials and activists work to monitor, report, and remedy unsafe situations.

The level of sanitation affects a community's safety. Sanitation includes clean water supply, adequate sewage system, no insects and rodents, and refrigeration of food supplies. Lack of sanitation can result in increased spread of disease and infection. Impoverished or poorly developed areas may lack sanitation.

BOX 23-1 | Possible Home Hazards

- Poor lighting inside or outside
- Uneven walking areas
- Steps with broken concrete
- Steps without handrails
- Loose mats on steps
- Cluttered steps or clutter near head of stairs
- Slippery tub or shower
- Extension cords across open spaces where people may trip
- Throw rugs on slippery floors
- Folding chairs and cribs that are not properly balanced or secured in place
- Insecure stools or stepladders
- Standing on chairs rather than stools or stepladders
- Items placed precariously on closet shelves
- Bookcases or heavy pieces of furniture that might topple
- Defective smoke detectors
- Oily or dirty rags near heat source
- Stacks of old newspapers or boxes in basement or garage
- Flammable liquids in illegal containers
- Items placed too close to the heat source of the kitchen stove
- Loose-fitting clothes worn while cooking
- Water temperatures that are too hot

- Defective wiring
- Overloaded outlets or frayed cords
- Smoking in bed or alone at night in living room
- Electrical appliances in the bathroom, where they may fall into the bathtub or sink
- Obstructed doorways or pathways in case of fire
- Many medications, or unlabeled medications, in medicine cabinet
- Unlocked cupboards or cabinets with potential poisons
- Improper use of pesticides or other chemicals
- Presence of cracked or peeling lead-based paint
- Poisonous plants where children can reach them
- Unsafe sexual practices
- Pets that may harm children, older adults, or visitors
- Cigarette smoking in a closed area around nonsmokers
- Plastic bags where children may find them
- Cribs near windows or near Venetian blind cords
- Unsupervised children in the bathtub
- Poor hygiene, especially in the bathroom and kitchen
- Improper food preparation
- Rodents or insect infestation
- Guns improperly stored and locked

ALTERED SAFETY

Altered safety is manifested in various harmful and preventable injuries and illnesses. Unintentional injuries include motor vehicle incidents, falls, poisonings, drownings and suffocations, fires and burns, electrical shocks, radiation exposures, infections, stress-related illnesses, respiratory problems, allergies, firearm mishaps, and the effects of hazardous chemicals or pollution.

Manifestations of Altered Safety

MOTOR VEHICLE INCIDENTS

Motor vehicle incidents frequently result from hazardous driving. They can involve one or more drivers or passengers, bicycle riders, skateboarders, and pedestrians.

Motor vehicle incidents are a leading cause of unintentional injury death in the United States and can cause permanent disability, pain, and suffering. Contributing factors include speeding, lack of defensive driving techniques, failure of bicycle riders and skateboarders to use helmets, fatigue, and the use of alcohol and other substances that cause impairment while driving.

> ! **SAFETY ALERT**
> It is important for healthcare providers to educate patients to refrain from driving while under the influence of substances that alter the ability to drive or when sleep deprived.

FALLS

Falls are common inside and outside the healthcare environment, especially among older adults and ill or disoriented people. Falls can cause pain, permanent disability, and even death. Sometimes, falls in older adults result in hip fractures; conversely, spontaneous hip fractures can lead to falls. Variables that increase a patient's risk for falls include gait and balance disorders, weakness, dizziness, environmental hazards, decreased mobility of the lower extremities, sleeplessness, incontinence, confusion, visual impairment, sedating medications, depression, and substance abuse. A cardiovascular problem that causes syncope or hypotension can also lead to a fall. A common scenario involves the older or impaired patient who falls on the way to the bathroom at night. The patient may be disoriented and not see obstacles cluttering the path from the bed to the bathroom. Falls at home commonly involve stairways. Poor lighting, obstacles on the stairs, and slippery or poorly repaired steps are common culprits. In the workplace, risk factors for falls include cluttered or slippery floors and working at heights in construction, such as on a ladder, roof, or scaffold.

POISONING

Poisoning occurs by ingesting, inhaling, or absorbing potentially hazardous substances (Fig. 23-2). The poisons compromise the cardiovascular, respiratory, central nervous, hepatic, gastrointestinal, and renal systems through chemical reactions. Young children are at high risk for poisoning, as are adults who have sensory impairment and communication barriers.

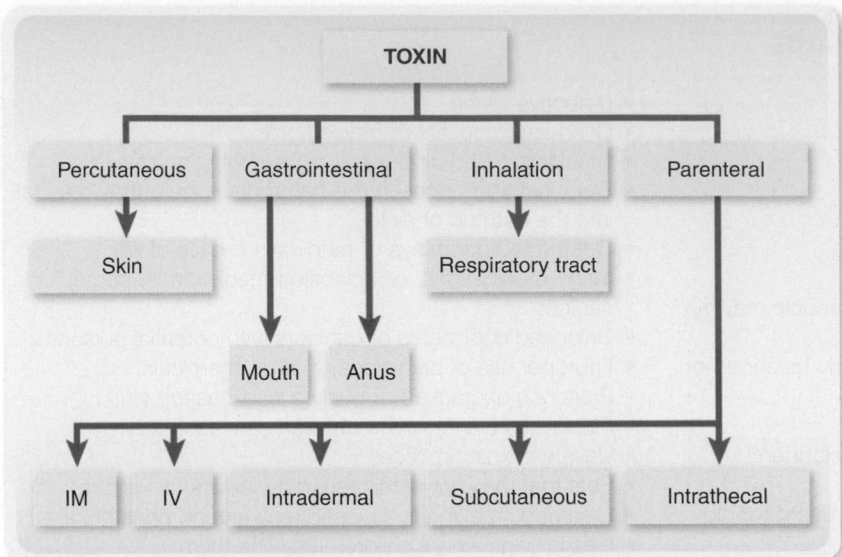

FIGURE 23-2 Routes by which toxins may enter the body.

In the home, children may ingest household cleansers, lawn and garden chemicals, paints and solvents, or medicines that are improperly stored or labeled. Plants are examples of potential household poisons usually not considered hazardous. In older homes, lead-based paint that is chipping or peeling is a hazard to young children, who are prone to placing things into their mouths. Lead dust in the air from paint that is pulverized is inhaled and is a frequent source of lead poisoning. Adolescents and young adults frequently experiment with alcohol and drugs and can overdose inadvertently. Older adults can ingest an overdose of medication because of cognitive impairment or difficulty reading the label as a result of low vision ability, illiteracy, or language barrier. Box 23-2 lists common toxins in the home.

Poisoning can occur in the healthcare environment when pharmaceutical products are administered improperly. Medications can be given to the wrong patient, in excessive dosage, or by the wrong route. Some medications augment the action of concurrently administered medications. In other situations, because of severe illness, the patient cannot eliminate the medications from the body, and these medications become toxic to the patient. Cardiac medications, opioids, insulin, cancer chemotherapy agents, and IV medications are all potentially lethal.

SUFFOCATION AND DROWNING

Suffocation or **asphyxiation** can occur as a result of drowning, smothering, strangling, airway obstruction, or entrapment in a confined space when an individual's airway no longer allows the free flow of oxygenated air. In the home, examples of these kinds of deaths include infants (face down) suffocating in a pillow or blanket; toddlers suffocating from a plastic bag placed over the face or strangling by a shoulder harness, clothesline, or window shade cord; children suffocating as a result of entrapment in an abandoned refrigerator; and older adults choking on poorly chewed food.

Suffocation in the healthcare environment occurs frequently because of airway obstruction caused by choking on foreign objects or aspirating (inhaling) fluid into the small airways of the lungs. Impairment of chewing and a diminished gag reflex, which usually occur in older or neurologically impaired patients, can cause airway obstruction. Improperly fitting dentures and overfeeding of older or neurologically impaired patients can lead to choking and aspiration.

With children, drowning can occur in natural bodies of water, pools, bathtubs, and even large pails or toilets. Lack of supervision, hazardous swimming conditions, careless boating and water sports, and impairment by drugs and alcohol contribute to the risk of drowning.

BOX 23-2   Common Home Toxins

Living Room/Den
Air freshener
Glass cleaner
Rug and upholstery
   shampoo
Houseplant insecticides
Flea collar, bomb
Furniture polish
Permanent ink markers
Typewriter correction fluid
Carbonless copy paper

Bathroom
Toilet bowl cleaner
Disinfectant
Mildew remover
Medicines
Hairspray
Hair color
Home permanent
Nail polish/remover
Lice/flea shampoo

Kitchen/Laundry
Scouring powder, ammonia
Oven cleaner, drain cleaner
Dishwashing detergent
Moth balls
Bleach
Metal polish
Insect spray, rodent killer
Laundry detergent
Spot remover

Garage/Basement
Latex, oil-base paints
Paint stripper
Wood preservative
Adhesives, glues, epoxys
Herbicides, insecticides
Insect repellents, poisons
Fertilizers
Gasoline, fuels
Other chemicals

FIRES

Smoking, faulty electrical equipment, unattended cooking, unsafe sources of heat, and playing with lighters or matches are common causes of fire in the home. Grease fires, originating from faulty equipment or poor work practices, are also common in the home and in some workplaces. Stoves in use may be left unattended; a high flame can easily ignite, splattering grease. These fires can spread to curtains, kitchen cabinets, and clothing. Children left unsupervised near stoves contribute to risks.

Patients in healthcare environments are especially at risk for fire-related injuries because they may be incapacitated or unable to flee without assistance. Flammable gases, such as oxygen and anesthetic agents, contribute to the risk of fires in healthcare environments. Commonly used electrical equipment, such as monitors, heating or cooling units, and respiratory therapy equipment, can malfunction or be used improperly, causing sparks that ignite linens easily in the presence of oxygen. Regular servicing of and education about electrical equipment and strict smoking policies can help reduce the risk of fires.

Four classes of fires exist, based on the type of material burning (USFA, 2015b):

- Class A: Paper, wood, cloth
- Class B: Flammable liquids, such as fuel oil, cooking oil or grease, paint or solvents, and gases (e.g., anesthesia gases)
- Class C: Electrical fires
- Class D: Combustible metals

Firefighting measures, discussed later in this chapter, vary according to fire classification.

BURNS

Burns involve tissue injury from thermal, chemical, or electrical agents and are a major cause of injury and death for infants and children in the home. Children can sustain burns in the home by playing with matches or candles, pulling a teakettle off the stove, being fed formula that is too hot, or playing outdoors without sunscreen protection. Adolescents working in fast-food restaurants are at risk for burn injuries from hot grease or food. Burns also occur in the healthcare environment because of scalds and fires. The person with sensory impairment is at risk for scalds from hot water or steam. A person with diabetic peripheral neuropathy, which damages nerves, may place hands under or step into very hot water and not feel the excessive temperature. Burns also can be sustained from the high electrical pulse needed during resuscitation efforts in the medical procedure of cardioversion.

FIREARMS

Firearms are involved in a significant number of unintentional injuries and deaths as well as homicide and suicide deaths. Gun control typically is handled as a state and local concern. Estimates are that 20,000 separate firearm laws exist in the United States, more than in any other country in the world. Although debate exists over the effectiveness of gun control laws, several studies have shown a decrease in assaults and deaths involving the use of a firearm with more restrictive gun controls (Chapman, 2011).

ELECTRICAL SHOCK

Electrical equipment and outlets present common hazards in the home and healthcare environments. Lighting and electric power lines in the community also create a threat. **Electrical shock** occurs when a current travels to the ground through the body, rather than through electrical wiring, or from static electricity that accumulates on the body's surface. A macroshock can cause superficial and deep burns, muscle contractions, and cardiac and respiratory arrest.

In the home, the use of frayed cords or overloaded outlets, use of electrical appliances near the sink or bathtub, and lack of supervision of children near uncovered electrical outlets or electrical appliances present hazards.

In the healthcare environment, electrical shock is a danger because of the abundant electrical equipment in proximity to the patient. Water from a spilled container, diaphoretic skin, or a leaking IV line increases electricity conduction. Three-pronged plugs that ground electrical equipment help prevent electrical shocks. A **ground** is an electrical connection with a large conducting body (e.g., the earth) that allows dissipation of the electrical charge.

RADIATION INJURY

Radiation injury can result from leakage of ionizing radiation from power plants and industrial sources into the community or from excessive exposure to radiation used to diagnose or treat illness in the healthcare environment. Radiation can injure the skin, reproductive organs, bone marrow, gastrointestinal tract, and other parts of the body. Three factors affect a radiation injury: time, distance, and radiation intensity; therefore, closer proximity to the radiation source and longer exposure to a strong radiation source increase the risk of injury.

Nuclear releases and exposures in communities place large groups at risk for injury. Even if people avoid physical injury, they can incur psychological stress. Federal agencies, such as the Department of Energy and the Nuclear Regulatory Commission, are primarily responsible for establishing and enforcing guidelines for radiation safety.

In healthcare environments, the potential for radiation injury exists when nurses must care for patients with radioactive implants and when technicians or nurses must accompany patients during radiography. Failure to use lead shielding for staff and patients or failure to follow radiation safety procedures when caring for patients with implants contributes to the risk of injury.

RESPIRATORY DISEASES

Respiratory problems can result from air pollution levels in the community or occupational exposure to chemicals, wood dust, asbestos, or other airborne substances. Passive smoke inhalation from living or working with persons who smoke cigarettes can potentially cause respiratory disease. Cigarette smoking and exposure to asbestos have been linked to lung cancer, and smog and dust worsen respiratory allergy symptoms and cause chronic bronchitis. Coal dust from mining causes fibrosis of the lungs, known as "black lung." OSHA has established guidelines to prevent injury to workers from chemical exposures and other hazardous conditions.

ASSESSMENT

Assessment of a person's ability to function safely involves careful investigation of individual and environmental aspects. Questions about safety reveal the manner in which a patient acts at home, at work, and in public. Building trust by being nonjudgmental and supportive will elicit the most accurate information.

Safety assessment begins with a thorough investigation of the patient's perceptions of safety, concerns about safety hazards, and a history of previous injuries. The person at risk for altered safety may report a history of falls, bruises, broken bones, burns, cuts, scratches, and restricted activities. The pattern of past injuries is important; such incidents often relate to periods of emotional stress, fatigue, diminished health, disregard, or lack of awareness about hazards associated with various activities. Individuals can share their fears about unsafe conditions or activities and their concerns about the potential for injury. Many are aware of their risk factors for injury and will share this information if offered nonjudgmental assistance.

Normal Pattern Identification

Current safety practices or plans for management of hazards are part of the assessment; consider these:

- Does the patient use appropriate restraints when in a car?
- Can the patient read traffic signs and anticipate danger warnings?
- Does the pediatric patient have a home that has been made safe and free from dangers?
- Does the patient have up-to-date immunizations?
- Does the patient have knowledge of health and safety practices for the settings in which he or she interacts?
- Does the patient understand the health and safety hazards in the workplace?

Keep in mind the special concerns for each age group to direct questions appropriately. Explore recent changes in the environment (home, school, workplace), in the support system (divorce, change in caregivers, death of family member), or in the developmental stage (transition from infant to toddler). Gather data not only from the patient but also from family members, caregivers, referring health professionals, and others. Be sure to have the patient's permission to solicit data from other sources, unless he or she is underage or declared incompetent. This approach ensures patient confidentiality and promotes trust.

Recall the mother and her active toddler in the case scenario. Use the concept map (Fig. 23-3) to help the mother identify safety habits that need to be followed in the home environment.

Risk Identification

When assessing current safety concerns, consider the patient's reason for seeking healthcare. A recent change in health status related to cognition, perception, sensation, or activity and exercise may have placed the patient at risk for injury. Explore these areas fully, and question the patient about occupation, home environment, lifestyle, habits, and level of knowledge of safety practices. Some questions to ask include the following:

- What medication do you take? What is the dose? When do you take it?
- Do you have any sleepiness or dizziness?
- What medical conditions might increase risk of injury?

State nurse practice laws and other regulations in the United States mandate that nurses are responsible for assessing injuries related to abuse or neglect. This skill requires sensitivity and the ability to evaluate the explanations given by patients. Often, conferring with other health professionals is essential, and a diagnostic workup may be ordered (see the Physical Assessment section). Injuries that seem in excess of the reported cause or occur with unexpected frequency deserve further investigation. No age group is immune to abuse or neglect, and people with higher dependency needs are at higher risk. The groups at highest risk include children, adolescents, older adults, the developmentally disabled, and the debilitated.

Dysfunction Identification

Nurses can determine problems with safety when the patient reports a serious, preventable injury or a recent change in ability to participate safely in activities of daily living (ADLs). A problem also can be evident with unsafe behaviors that the nurse observes or the patient describes. Using specialized knowledge, the healthcare team can determine that the patient is at risk for injury, illness, or infection because of unsafe behaviors or physiologic dysfunction. Unless the patient shares a concern for preventing such developments, there may be no agreement on the existence of a potential problem.

As part of the nursing health history, ask about previous injuries and hospitalizations. Find out the cause of these injuries and whether any unsafe behaviors or hazards were identified and if these have been rectified. For example, a patient may report a history of burns from a fire. Ask the patient what caused the fire. If smoking in bed contributed to the injury, has the patient altered careless smoking practices? If not, does the patient realize the potential for further problems?

Physical Assessment

Physical assessment techniques can help nurses detect injuries and risk factors for injury. Physical assessment should focus on the neurologic and sensory systems, cardiovascular and respiratory systems, skin integrity, and musculoskeletal mobility.

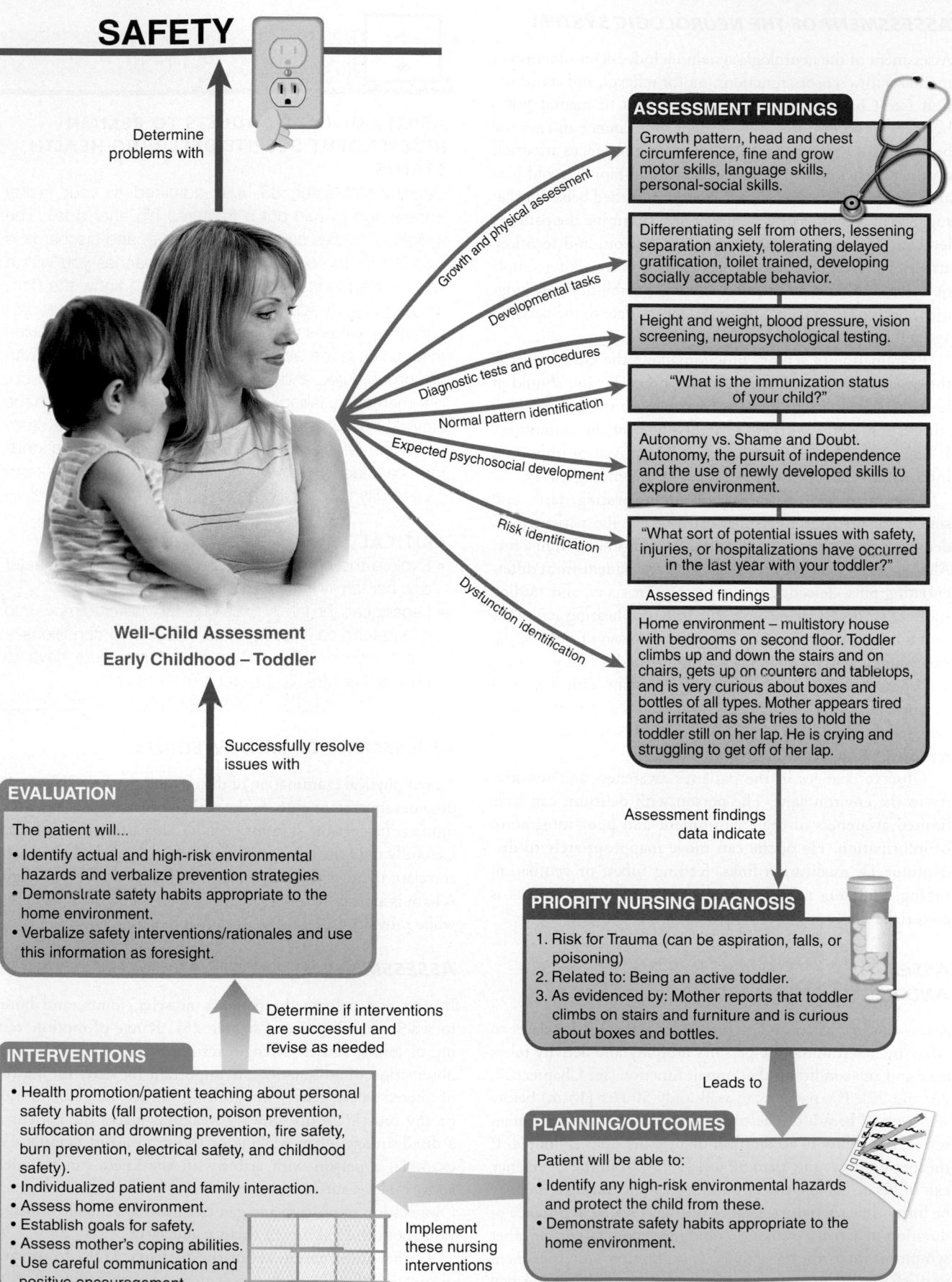

SAFETY

Determine problems with

Well-Child Assessment
Early Childhood – Toddler

Growth and physical assessment

Developmental tasks

Diagnostic tests and procedures

Normal pattern identification

Expected psychosocial development

Risk identification

Dysfunction identification

ASSESSMENT FINDINGS

Growth pattern, head and chest circumference, fine and grow motor skills, language skills, personal-social skills.

Differentiating self from others, lessening separation anxiety, tolerating delayed gratification, toilet trained, developing socially acceptable behavior.

Height and weight, blood pressure, vision screening, neuropsychological testing.

"What is the immunization status of your child?"

Autonomy vs. Shame and Doubt. Autonomy, the pursuit of independence and the use of newly developed skills to explore environment.

"What sort of potential issues with safety, injuries, or hospitalizations have occurred in the last year with your toddler?"

Assessed findings

Home environment – multistory house with bedrooms on second floor. Toddler climbs up and down the stairs and on chairs, gets up on counters and tabletops, and is very curious about boxes and bottles of all types. Mother appears tired and irritated as she tries to hold the toddler still on her lap. He is crying and struggling to get off of her lap.

Assessment findings
data indicate

PRIORITY NURSING DIAGNOSIS

1. Risk for Trauma (can be aspiration, falls, or poisoning)
2. Related to: Being an active toddler.
3. As evidenced by: Mother reports that toddler climbs on stairs and furniture and is curious about boxes and bottles.

Leads to

PLANNING/OUTCOMES

Patient will be able to:

• Identify any high-risk environmental hazards and protect the child from these.
• Demonstrate safety habits appropriate to the home environment.

Implement these nursing interventions

INTERVENTIONS

• Health promotion/patient teaching about personal safety habits (fall protection, poison prevention, suffocation and drowning prevention, fire safety, burn prevention, electrical safety, and childhood safety).
• Individualized patient and family interaction.
• Assess home environment.
• Establish goals for safety.
• Assess mother's coping abilities.
• Use careful communication and positive encouragement.

Determine if interventions are successful and revise as needed

EVALUATION

The patient will...

• Identify actual and high-risk environmental hazards and verbalize prevention strategies
• Demonstrate safety habits appropriate to the home environment.
• Verbalize safety interventions/rationales and use this information as foresight.

Successfully resolve issues with

FIGURE 23-3 Concept map for safety.

ASSESSMENT OF THE NEUROLOGIC SYSTEM

Assessment of the neurologic system includes determination of mental status, sensory functions, motor reflexes, and coordination (see Chapters 36 and 37). Assessment of mental status begins with observation of the patient's appearance and general behavior. For the purposes of safety promotion, focus attention on the patient's ability to detect danger and rapidly avoid hazards. Note any impulsive behavior or diminished behavior that suggests impaired or unsafe judgment. Determine the patient's level of alertness; orientation to time, person, and location; attention span; and basic cognitive function by asking simple questions. Determine decision-making capabilities and judgment by asking "what if" questions appropriate to the patient's age and life experiences.

Examination of sensory function allows the nurse to verify the accuracy and quality of sensory input. Testing should at least include ability to balance, sensitivity to sharp versus dull stimulation, and sensitivity to light touch of the extremities. If sensation is impaired, the patient is deprived of important information that can warn of danger or impending injury.

Assessment includes testing of vision, hearing, taste, and smell. Impaired taste or smell can prevent the patient from detecting spoiled food, a natural gas leak, or smoke from a fire. Alterations in visual acuity can prevent the patient from differentiating pills, detecting uneven terrain or stairs, and reading traffic signs or telephone numbers. Impaired hearing acuity has profound implications when it prevents a person from hearing cars, smoke alarms, or other warning sounds. The gag reflex also should be tested before feeding a patient with decreased alertness or muscle strength. Coordination is important to prevent falls. Observing the patient's gait, muscle strength, and repetitive motions can test coordination.

Observe changes in the patient's awareness and sensitivity to the environment. The person with delirium can have limited awareness of the environment and poor integration of information. He or she can move inappropriately to discontinue IV medication lines, feeding tubes, or ventilation tubing. Ongoing neurologic assessment of some patients is essential.

ASSESSMENT OF CARDIOVASCULAR AND RESPIRATORY SYSTEMS

Assess cardiovascular and respiratory capacity as it relates to safety by determining the person's mobility and activity tolerance and any conditions that impair function (see Chapters 25, 26, and 27). If a patient can walk only 50 feet (15 m) before shortness of breath or chest pain (exertional angina) becomes severe, the ability to accomplish many daily tasks is limited. If this person lives more than 50 feet (15 m) from the emergency exit of his or her apartment building, escape during a fire may be impossible. Activity tolerance is usually stated as distance or duration of activity (walking, standing) before fatigue or other symptoms interrupt the activity; it is an important assessment in discharge planning for a patient's safety outside the hospital environment.

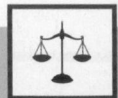

ETHICAL/LEGAL ISSUE

ABILITY OF OLDER ADULTS TO REMAIN INDEPENDENT DESPITE DECLINING HEALTH STATUS

Georgia McMaster, 83, was admitted to your facility 2 days ago to rule out a fractured hip after a fall. The radiology studies came back negative, and discharge is planned for tomorrow. Her son approaches you with a very worried look on his face, saying, "I know the doctor is going to send my mother home tomorrow, but our family worries about her all the time. She has fallen three times in the last month. Her house is cluttered with all sorts of junk, and she is no longer able to keep up. Her memory is failing, and she often leaves pans on the stove, forgetting to turn off the burner. She's so stubborn, she refuses to even talk about going into a long-term care facility. Can we force her to go into a long-term care facility for her own good?"

CRITICAL THINKING CHALLENGE
- Explore the concerns and feelings of Mrs. McMaster and her family in this situation.
- Legally, can the family force Mrs. McMaster to move into a long-term care facility? If so, under what conditions?
- What responsibility do healthcare providers have to ensure that Mrs. McMaster remains safe?

ASSESSMENT OF SKIN INTEGRITY

A brief physical examination of the integument (see Chapter 30) provides important clues to the patient's history of accidents or injuries. Inspect the skin for bruises, cuts, scratches, and scars. Carefully note the location and distribution of the lesions, and correlate them with the patient's explanation of their origin. A bath is an excellent opportunity for assessing the integument while providing a refreshing comfort measure.

ASSESSMENT OF MUSCULOSKELETAL MOBILITY

Inspect and palpate the patient's muscles, joints, and bones to assess mobility (see Chapter 25). Range-of-motion testing of joints, muscle strength testing of the extremities, and observation of ambulation are important for determining risk of altered safety. Any joint showing limited range of motion or any muscle group showing weakness places the patient at a disadvantage when walking or trying to avoid hazards. For example, a person with arthritis in the knees can be safely active on level surfaces but unable to use stairs in an emergency. Observation of posture and gait can provide valuable information about the stability of balance and sway.

Gather information about the patient's ADLs from caregivers and family, but supplement this information with direct observation when possible. Observe the patient moving from bed to chair or commode (and back) when appropriate; for more mobile people, observe them walking from bedroom to bathroom, front door, kitchen, and telephone locations.

Diagnostic Tests and Procedures

Diagnostic tests and procedures are used to determine a person's health status by assessing for medical conditions that can place the person at risk for injury.

Neuropsychological testing can be used to determine the type and source of a cognitive abnormality. Blood pressure assessment, electrocardiogram (ECG) testing, and pulmonary function tests can be used to detect cardiopulmonary capacity and abnormalities. Specific blood tests can identify certain

conditions, such as a complete blood count (CBC) and renal and hepatic function tests to detect an infection, kidney and liver disease, or the ability to eliminate toxins from the body. Laboratory tests can also measure the amount of alcohol, drugs, or lead in a person's blood.

NURSING DIAGNOSES

Nursing diagnoses in the area of safety include Risk for Injury, Risk for Aspiration, Risk for Falls, Risk for Suffocation, and Risk for Trauma. Selected nursing diagnoses are listed in Table 23-2 with associated outcomes (Nursing Outcomes Classification [NOC]) and interventions (Nursing Interventions Classification [NIC]).

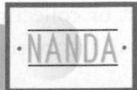 **Table 23-2 SELECTED NANDA-I NURSING DIAGNOSES INVOLVING SAFETY**

Nursing Dx	Related Factors	Dx Statement	NOC*	NIC†
Contamination—exposure to environmental contaminants in doses sufficient to cause adverse harmful effects	Chemical contamination of food or water, exposure to man-made or natural disaster, inadequate sewer, unprotected contact with chemicals, heavy metals, pesticides, smoke, or radiation	Contamination R/T to unhealthy living conditions, exposure to pesticides, lead paint, and animal droppings AEB frequent illness, high serum lead levels, and presence of contaminants found during home visit	Risk Control—L Exposure, Safe Home Environment, Improved Respiratory Status, Community Disaster readiness, Community Disaster Response	Monitor Environment for Safety Status, Collaborate with Community Agencies to Improve Environmental Safety, Educate Regarding Environmental Risks, Assist in Relocation to Safer Environment, Bioterrorism Preparedness
Risk for Suffocation—accentuated risk of accidental suffocation (inadequate air available for inhalation)	Children unattended in water, household gas leaks, playing with plastic bags, objects in airway, vehicles warming in closed garage, lack of education and safety precautions	Risk for Suffocation R/T lack of parent safety precautions in the house and near water for young children	Knowledge: Child Physical Safety, Respiratory Status: Airway Patency, Parenting: Infant/Toddler Physical Safety	Risk Identification, Environmental Management: Safety, Anticipatory Guidance, Teaching: Toddler Safety, Respiratory Monitoring, Airway Management
Risk for Trauma—accentuated risk of accidental tissue injury (e.g., wound, burn, fracture)	Driving when intoxicated, at excessive speeds, or in a mechanically unsafe vehicle; defective equipment; overloaded electrical outlets, plugs, or fuse boxes; nonuse of headgear or seat restraints; emotional difficulties	Risk for Trauma R/T alcohol and drug use, unsafe driving, and risk-taking behaviors	Risk Detection, Risk Control: Alcohol and Drug Use, Personal Safety Behavior, Parenting: Adolescent Physical Safety	Risk Identification, Substance Use: Prevention and Treatment, Vehicle Safety Promotion, Parent Education: Adolescent, Fall Prevention
Risk for Injury (Poisoning)—accentuated risk of accidental exposure to, or ingestion of, drugs or dangerous products in doses sufficient to cause poisoning	Availability of illicit drugs, dangerous product within the reach of children or confused individuals, large supplies of drug in the house stored in unlocked cabinets, emotional difficulties, lack of safety or drug education	Risk for Poisoning R/T medication and toxic substances kept unlocked and within reach of young children	Risk Control, Safe Home Environment, Parenting: Infant/Toddler Physical Safety, Community Risk Control: Lead Exposure	Environmental Risk Protection, Anticipatory Guidance, Environmental Management: Safety, Medication Reconciliation

Dx, diagnosis; R/T, related to; AEB, as evidenced by.
*From Moorhead, S., Johnson, M., Maas, M., & Swanson, E. (2013). *Nursing outcomes classification (NOC): Measurement of health outcomes* (5th ed.). St. Louis, MO: Elsevier.
†From Bulechek, G., Butcher, H., Dochterman, J., Wagner, C. (2013). *Nursing interventions classification (NIC)* (6th ed.). St. Louis, MO: Elsevier.
From Herdman, T. H., & Kamitsuru, S. (Eds.). (2014). *Nursing diagnoses: Definitions and classification, 2015–2017*. West Sussex, England: Wiley-Blackwell.

OUTCOME IDENTIFICATION AND PLANNING

After the nursing diagnosis and related factors have been formulated, patient goals and nursing interventions are identified. Common goals for the patient who is at risk for injury include the following:

- The patient will identify actual and high-risk environmental hazards and avoid the hazards.
- The patient will demonstrate safety habits appropriate to selected environments (home, healthcare setting, workplace, community).
- The patient will experience a decrease in the frequency and severity of injury events.
- The nurse (and nursing staff) will identify safety issues in the work environment and decrease injury events.

These goals must be individualized to reflect the unique needs of the person at risk. Once they are individualized, specific nursing interventions support the goals.

Planning for nursing interventions to promote safety is based on assessment data and resulting nursing diagnoses and patient goals wherever they practice.

IMPLEMENTATION

Nursing interventions related to safety fall into two broad categories: (1) providing safety education for the home, workplace, and community and (2) providing a safe environment in the healthcare setting. Nurses promote these safety interventions.

Health Promotion

HEALTHCARE ENVIRONMENT

Nurses help patients develop personal safety habits. The CDC and OSHA provide guidelines for promotion of health and safety in healthcare settings; the ANA provides strategies for nurses to accomplish these guidelines. The Institute of Medicine (Page, 2004) has added direction and recommendations to creating a safe environment. Each accredited healthcare setting has an ongoing health and safety program.

The patient is at risk for injury in the healthcare environment because of its unfamiliarity and the procedures the patient undergoes. Nurses are responsible for protecting the patient from environmental hazards wherever they provide services. Some of these environmental hazards may be in the equipment being used at the bedside. Nurses are also responsible for anticipating and minimizing the adverse consequences of procedures and treatments. Many nursing policies and procedures are intended to protect the patient and assist the nurse in maintaining a safe healthcare environment.

Initial nursing actions to promote safety and security in a healthcare setting are to introduce staff to the patient and to orient the patient to the immediate environment. If the patient remains overnight, orientation includes instruction on the use of the call-light system and bed controls, location of personal care supplies in the bedside stand, location of the bathroom, operation of lights, and schedule of unit activities. Ensure that the room is uncluttered and free of obstacles between the bed and the bathroom. Use of a night-light and bedside rails is standard protocol. Instruct each patient and his or her significant others about activity limitations, and assist with ambulation as needed. Talk to the patient and answer questions calmly and confidently to increase the patient's sense of security.

Proper identification of the patient prior to providing care and carrying out treatments helps prevent medical errors and ensure patient safety. Proper patient identification is one of the Joint Commission's National Patient Safety Goals (see Chapter 4). Two separate identifiers (e.g., full name, birth date, medical record number, Social Security number) are required prior to administering any medication or blood product or collecting any specimen. Patient room number is not an appropriate identifier because patients may change rooms.

MOTOR VEHICLE SAFETY

Nursing intervention for motor vehicle safety involves patient education about potential hazards and safety measures. The use of seat belts has greatly decreased morbidity and mortality on the highways. Seat belts can reduce the risk of fatal injury in passenger cars by and in light trucks. All 50 states require by law car safety seats or restraint devices for young children. Despite such laws in the United States, hundreds of children die each year because of improper use or lack of restraints.

Approved car seats should properly restrain infants and children when they travel in automobiles. Infants should be in rear-facing car seats as long as possible, up to 3 years of age depending on the child's size, or according to the car seat manufacturer's guidelines. When children are too large for rear-facing seats, they should be in forward-facing car seats. After they have outgrown forward-facing seats, they should be secured in booster seats, still in the back seat of the vehicle. When a child has reached 4 feet 9 inches in height, usually between 8 and 12 years of age, the child may use a properly applied lap and shoulder harnesses (Parents Central, 2015).

 SAFETY ALERT
Never place rear-facing car seats in the front seats of cars with passenger-side airbags.

Motor vehicle safety also includes maintaining a well-functioning vehicle that has met state safety standards and operating the vehicle at a safe driving speed for road and weather conditions. Each driver should avoid substances that impair alertness and reaction time (e.g., antihistamines) while driving motor vehicles. Educate patients about the effects of alcohol and lack of sleep on driving. Teach adolescents to obey state driving restrictions for teen drivers, and advise and reinforce about the danger in riding with friends who are impaired by alcohol or drugs.

THERAPEUTIC DIALOGUE: SAFETY ASSESSMENT

SCENE FOR THOUGHT

Mrs. Jennie Adobo, 45 years old, has been receiving home healthcare for 6 months. During that time, Martha Davis, a community health nurse, has noticed that Jennie's small house has become increasingly cluttered with newspapers, saved paper bags, plastic bags, clean rags, and so forth. Everything is clean and orderly, but the piles seem to be growing at an alarming rate, especially since Jennie's husband left her and her two adolescent children. Jennie has controlled hypertension and is working on controlling her diabetes through diet.

LESS EFFECTIVE

Nurse: Hi, Jennie, how are you this week? *(Acknowledges patient by name.)*

Jennie: Not too good, Martha. I can't seem to get enough sleep or enough to eat lately. *(Fidgets with string she's winding into a ball.)*

Nurse: Let me just get your blood pressure and do a glucose test on you for a minute. *(Does the procedures concentrating on getting the readings correctly. Jennie watches fearfully.)*

Nurse: Everything seems to be okay with your pressure and blood sugar, especially since you seem to have lost some weight. How much would you say you've lost? *(Puts away the equipment and smiles at Jennie.)*

Jennie: About 10 lb, I think. That's good, isn't it? My husband will be so glad when he comes back. He's always saying I should lose some weight. *(Starts to cry and wring her hands.)*

Nurse: Now, don't you worry. Everything will be fine. Your pressure and sugar are down, you look much better than you did with the weight you lost, and I know your kids are helping out with jobs. You'll see. Anything else you'd like to talk about? *(Packs equipment bag.)*

Jennie: No, I'll be fine. I just need to look on the bright side. *(Smiles with her lips.)*

Nurse: That's the ticket. I'll see you in a couple of weeks. Stay well!

MORE EFFECTIVE

Nurse: Hi, Jennie. How are you this week? *(Acknowledges patient by name.)*

Jennie: Not too good, Martha. I can't seem to get enough sleep or enough to eat lately. *(Fidgets with string she's winding into a ball.)*

Nurse: Tell me more about that, Jennie. *(Takes blood pressure, keeping an eye on Jennie's face.)*

Jennie: It's just so hard for me to go to sleep at night. I hear noises and the sirens go off, and I just can't sleep. *(Sounds annoyed.)*

Nurse: Sounds difficult for you. How long has this been going on? *(Puts away the cuff and sits down facing her.)*

Jennie: Since he went away. *(Starts to cry.)*

Nurse: That's been 2 months now, hasn't it? *(Jennie nods.)* Anything else you've noticed besides the sleeping problem? *(Quietly watches Jennie.)*

Jennie: I can't eat. I have no appetite. *(Still fiddling with the string.)*

Nurse: I noticed that you're looking a little thinner. How much weight have you lost?

Jennie: About 10 lb. Actually, I needed to lose the weight, but not this way. *(Crying.)*

Nurse: Something else I've noticed, you've collected a lot more bags and stuff since the last time I was here. Can you tell me about that?

Jennie: I just can't throw them away. We may need them. He's not sending any money. We could sell them and get money to eat! *(Sounds a little panicky.)*

Nurse: You really do seem worried about a lot of things, Jennie. Would it help if we talked about them one at a time? I think we can work together on some resources to help you with the problems you're having.

Jennie: Okay. *(Wipes her eyes.)* I need some help; I can see that. I'm not used to having all these problems all at once.

CRITICAL THINKING CHALLENGE

- Analyze intrinsic and extrinsic factors that are affecting Jennie's behavior with respect to the accumulation of bags, string, and so forth.
- Detect the safety hazards associated with these items.
- Determine what the nurse attended to in the second scenario that was not focused on in the first scenario.
- Identify with what common human emotion insomnia, anorexia, weeping, and sadness are associated.
- Predict what the nurse in the first scenario might discover when she returns in 2 weeks.

FALL PREVENTION

In the home, teach adults, especially older adults, the following measures to prevent falls:

- Remove throw rugs.
- Ensure stairways are well lighted and repaired.
- Remove clutter from stairways and walkways.
- Install handrails wherever needed.
- Avoid use of unstable ladders and step stools.
- Never attempt to do anything beyond reach or physical ability.
- Clean damp areas promptly.

In all healthcare environments, ensure the patient's safety from falls. The room needs to be free from clutter and well lighted during transfers and ambulation. Maintain only necessary equipment in the room, and organize the room well to allow clear access to the bathroom and chair. Anchor side rails and grab bars firmly (Fig. 23-4A). Keep floors nonskid, either carpeted or free from liquid. Wheelchairs, beds, commode chairs, and shower chairs must have working brakes (Fig. 23-4B). These devices must be free from any sharp edges and have a support surface that is comfortable.

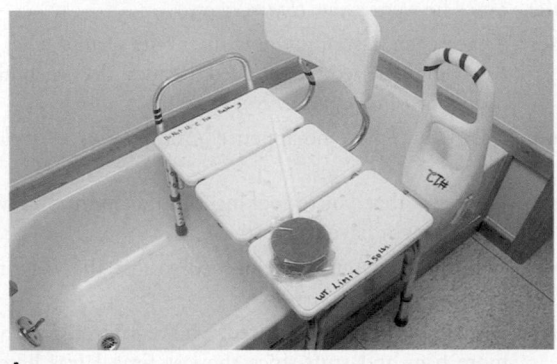

A

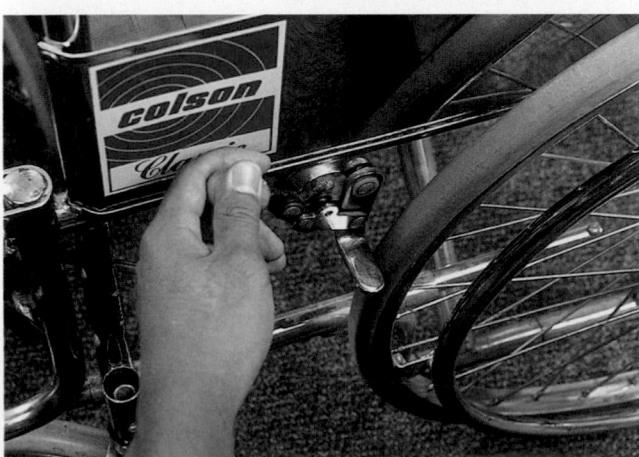

B

FIGURE 23-4 The healthcare facility must provide safety for the patient. **A.** This shower protects the patient with grab bars, safety rails, shower seat, and transfer seat. **B.** The nurse checks wheelchair brakes for safe use.

Teach patients with orthostatic hypotension to change position slowly to allow for blood pressure stabilization. Use nightlights and respond promptly to call lights. During daytime, encourage family members to help weak patients to the bathroom, unless doing so would be unsafe. In some cases, very weak patients need two or more professionals to support them.

Nurses and other healthcare workers are at high risk for back injuries as a result of frequent lifting and transfer of patients, often in awkward positions. Many agencies have developed lift teams to specialize in proper use of devices and in assisting in moving patients. In many instances, a mechanical lifting device assists nursing staff to lift or transfer a patient. New technology and availability of equipment decrease the work effort for the healthcare staff members; attendance at in-service education classes demonstrating how to operate the transfer equipment safely and properly is an important nursing responsibility.

On admission, complete an assessment of the transfer needs required for safe handling and moving of the patient; document and communicate this to the healthcare team. As the patient's condition changes, update this assessment and documentation. An evidence-based fall risk assessment tool should be used to assess the patient's risk.

Prevention of Childhood Falls

Educate parents and other caregivers about children's potential for falling. Prevention includes not leaving infants unattended in the bath, in the bed, or on a table where they can roll or fall off; keeping side rails raised on cribs; using guardrails or gates at the top and bottom of stairs when infants crawl; and supervising children in jumpers, swings, and high chairs. Walkers are particularly dangerous for toddlers, and many have been withdrawn from the market.

RESTRAINTS

A **restraint** is any physical or chemical means of stopping a patient from being free to move. Restraints may be intended to prevent injury to patients but are not risk-free devices. In December 2006, the Centers for Medicare and Medicaid Services (CMS) revised several aspects of their standards regarding restraints and seclusion. Instead of having two separate standards, the final CMS ruling combines the former standards ("Restraint for acute medical and surgical care" and "Restraint and seclusion for behavior management") into one standard, applicable to all instances of restraint and seclusion. The new standard is called "Restraint or Seclusion" (CMS, 2006).

The single consistent definition of restraint is "any manual method, physical, or mechanical device, material, or equipment that immobilizes or reduces the ability of a patient to move his or her arms, legs, body, or head freely; or a drug or medication when it is used as a restriction to manage the patient's behavior or restrict the patient's freedom of movement is not a standard treatment or dosage for the patient's condition" (CMS, 2006, p. 71383). Additionally, "a restraint does not include devices, such as orthopedically prescribed devices, surgical dressings or bandages, protective helmets, or other methods that involve the physical holding of a patient for the purpose of conducting

TABLE 23-3 CATEGORIES OF RESTRAINTS

Restraint	Definition	Example
Physical restraint	Any manual method or physical device, or equipment, that restricts movement or normal access to one's body	Vest, mitt, wrist, or ankle restraints, four side rails up
Chemical restraint	A medication used to control behavior or to restrict a person's freedom of movement that is not a standard of treatment for the person's medical or psychiatric condition	Sedation medication to keep patients safe from harming self or others
Nonviolent/non-self-destructive restraint	Use of a restraint when a patient's behavior interferes with treatment	Physical or chemical restraints used to prevent pulling out tubes or lines that could cause harm to the patient or negatively impact treatment
Violent/self-destructive restraint	Use of restraint when patient is demonstrating aggressive or violent behavior that presents an immediate serious danger to self or others	Four point restraints (each limb) restrained to prevent potentially life-threatening injury
Seclusion	Involuntary confinement of an individual in a room alone for any period of time from which the person is prevented from leaving	Patient wants to leave hospital without provider's order and is prevented from doing so

From The Joint Commission. (2015). *Comprehensive accreditation and certification manual (Edition). Provision of care, treatment, and services: Standard PC.03.05.09*. Retrieved from https://e-dition.jcrinc.com/MainContent.aspx

routine physical examinations or tests, or to protect the patient from falling out of bed, or to permit the patient to participate in activities without the risk of physical harm" (CMS, 2006, p. 71383). Table 23-3 describes different types and categories of restraints.

Citations and fines can ensue when restraints are not used within the guidelines similar to those proposed by the Omnibus Budget Reconciliation Act (OBRA) of 1990 and the revision effective January 1, 2007. These newer guidelines require that restraints be part of the medical treatment after all less restrictive interventions have been considered or tried first, other appropriate disciplines have been consulted, and supporting documentation for their use has been provided. There is little evidence that restraints prevent injury, particularly from falls, and they have many unintended negative consequences.

Restraints may be necessary, however, to limit a patient's physical activity, such as pulling out an IV line or mechanical ventilator tubing, or to prevent movement that would disrupt therapy. Restraints often increase agitation and may not preserve dignity, but they may be clinically justified in selected instances to prevent irreparable harm associated with pulling out therapeutic devices. Box 23-3 lists guidelines for the use of restraints.

The Joint Commission has set standards for use of restraints for nonpsychiatric patients that limit restraint use to clinically appropriate and adequately justified situations. The American Geriatrics Society (AGS) has a policy that limits restraint use to rare, unusual situations (Pellfolk, Gustafson, Bucht, & Karlsson, 2010). Follow healthcare institution guidelines regarding the use of restraints. Be sure to describe the reason for their application in the patient's care record. Nurses can apply restraints in an emergency, without a primary healthcare provider's order; however, nurses should obtain such an order as soon as possible. Use

direct supervision and communication to reassure and reorient the patient. The use of restraints is not a substitute for vigilant nursing care. Types of restraints include a jacket or vest restraint worn on the chest and attached to the bed frame or legs of a chair, a belt restraint on stretchers or wheelchairs used in transporting, mitt or hand restraints that prevent confused patients from using their hands, wrist or ankle restraints that immobilize one or more limbs, and mummy restraints that wrap around a child's body to prevent movement during a procedure.

 **Concept Mastery Alert**

In an emergency, it is appropriate for the nurse to ensure safety by restraining the patient and then promptly inform the physician, obtaining the order. In an emergency situation such as this, the nurse is justified in prioritizing safety. In all other circumstances, it is necessary to obtain an order before applying restraints.

A common form of restraint is **side rails**, which are used on beds, stretchers, and similar equipment. Side rails remind patients not to roll too far to the side, and they provide bars that assist patients when they turn to the side. When side rails are used on beds, the bed must be in the lowest position with the wheels locked. Having side rails raised does not replace careful and frequent observation because patients may still attempt to get out of bed by climbing over the side rails or over the foot of the bed. Having all four side rails raised is considered physical restraint and requires prescriber order and monitoring, the same as other restraints. Deaths have occurred as the result of entrapment of the face or neck between the mattress and rails or within the rails. The need to go to the bathroom is the most frequent reason for patients

BOX 23-3 Recommendations for Restraint Use

Indications and Ordering

- Assess the cause for which the restraint is being considered, develop alternatives to restraint use, and implement these alternatives before applying restraints.
- Restraint use should be considered a temporary solution to a situation.
- Allow the use of restraints only under the supervision of a licensed healthcare provider and for a strictly defined period of time. The patient must be evaluated face-to-face within 1 hour after restraint or seclusion is initiated to manage violent or self-destructive behavior.
- Licensed providers conduct a face-to-face assessment in a predetermined schedule (e.g., 24 hours for nonviolent/non-self-destructive restraints; 4 hours for violent/self-destructive restraints) to determine if restraints are still indicated. If so a new order must be written.
- Obtain informed consent from patient/resident or guardian before use. Patients have the right to be free from restraints. However, if it is determined that a restraint is necessary, explain the reason for the device to the patient/resident and guardian to prevent misinterpretation and to ensure cooperation.

Policies and Training

- Follow local and state laws regarding the use of protective restraint devices.
- Define and communicate a clear institutional policy and staff training on the use of restraints (e.g., alternatives to restraint use, appropriate conditions for restraint use, length of wear time). This written policy also should be available for any patient/resident or any family member.
- Provide in-depth training for staff as regularly as possible, which should include a return demonstration of proper application of restraints.

Nursing Considerations

- Before use, read and follow the manufacturer's directions for use.
- Select the type of restraint that is appropriate to the patient's condition.
- Use the correct size of restraint.
- Note the "front" and "back" of vest restraints, and apply correctly.
- Carefully apply the device and adjust properly, so it maintains body alignment and ensures patient comfort.
- Secure restraints designed for use in bed to the bed springs or frame, never to the mattress or the bed rails, using a quick-release mechanism.
- Emphasize good nursing, rehabilitative, and patient care practices.
- Observe patients in restraints frequently, describing the patient's behavior, the intervention used, and the patient's response to the intervention.
- Continually monitor and assess all patients in restraints. Assess circulation, movement, and sensation (CMS) in limbs, and offer food or fluids. Offer toileting.
- Remove the restraints (one at a time) at least every 2 hours and more often if necessary. Allow for ADLs.
- Continue assessment even after a restraint is used, and discontinue use as soon as feasible.

Documentation

- Clearly document in the patient's record the medical reason for use of the restraint and the type selected.
- Check to make sure there is a current valid order by an appropriate provider. Restraints need to be reordered at least every 24 hours.
- Document according to policies (minimum every 2 hours):
  - Presence and type of restraint
  - Continued need for restraint
  - Assessment data (CMS, cognitive state)
  - Patient needs cared for

---

to try to get out of bed, no matter what kind of restraint may be in place. Anticipating the patient's need to urinate and routinely toileting patients is the primary safety measure that nurses can use.

Many restraints require fastening to an object: the bed, a chair, or a wheelchair. This is usually a buckle that can be undone by the nurse with one hand. Care must be taken that when fastened to a bed, the restraint moves with the patient—for example, as the height of the bed is raised or lowered—to prevent injury to the patient by the restraint.

! SAFETY ALERT

Knots should not be used; rather, restraints should have quick-release connectors so that healthcare providers can release quickly in an emergency.

 APPLY YOUR CRITICAL THINKING

At change-of-shift report, you are told that Mr. Rau was acutely confused during the night shift and that wrist restraints were applied to prevent him from pulling out his IV. When you make rounds, you find Mr. Rau very agitated, pulling hard against the restraints. His fingers are slightly blue and appear swollen. What is the best way to maintain safety for this patient?

Check your answer in Appendix B.

NONRESTRAINT SAFETY DEVICES

Increasingly, nonrestraint safety environments and devices are being developed and used to increase patient safety without the use of typical restraints. Such devices include alarm systems and

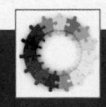

COLLABORATING WITH THE HEALTHCARE TEAM
Requesting a Reorder for Restraints

You call the hospitalist to renew the restraint order for Mrs. Black.

SITUATION: Mrs. Black, in room 345, post-op day 3, restraint order has expired.

BACKGROUND: Wrist restraints were applied yesterday when she became acutely confused 1 day after a total hip replacement. Her family is with her, but she continues to pull at her IV and tries to get out of bed. She is oriented to person but not to place or time. Her serum sodium was 118 mEq/L yesterday, and she is receiving an IV of NS at 75 mL/hour.

ASSESSMENT: She is still confused and needs to be reevaluated.

RECOMMENDATION: Since restraints need to be reordered every 24 hours, please evaluate Mrs. Black this morning so that we are in compliance. Also, could we get another sodium level since this may be causing her acute confusion?

CRITICAL THINKING CHALLENGE
- Nurses must often make sure that restraints are reordered according to policy. What system can be set up to make sure this happens?
- Why did the nurse mention the sodium level to the hospitalist at the same time she requested a restraint reorder?
- Are there any other factors that could cause this patient's acute delirium?
- What other options are available other than restraints to help keep this patient safe?

---

pressure devices. Pressure devices are placed on the bed under the patient's back. When the person sits up, he or she triggers an alarm that alerts the staff that the patient is attempting to get out of bed. Other alarm devices allow the person free movement in bed but trigger an alarm if he or she is about to transfer from the bed. Special cushions can be placed on chairs; these cushions are comfortable to sit on, but because of the angle of the cushion and the material inside, it is extremely difficult for the patient to rise without assistance. Both of these devices permit safety without the use of restraints and involve the nurse or caregiver when the patient ambulates, thereby improving the safety of the patient.

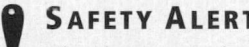

❗ SAFETY ALERT
The alarms must be loud enough to be heard and never turned off so that they can alert staff when a patient is getting out of bed and at risk of falling.

With a comprehensive assessment of the patient and careful and imaginative attention to the environment, nurses can reduce environmental risks and improve safety. Anticipating patient needs for assistance with transfers and responding to the patient's need to go to the bathroom or to change position or location are ways the nurse can help the patient prevent falls and reduce the need for restraints.

POISON PREVENTION

Remind adult caregivers to store medications, including over-the-counter products, in childproof containers out of children's reach. Caregivers should not treat medications as candy.

They should store household cleansers and other potentially toxic products in childproofed or locked cupboards or on shelves out of children's reach. Remind them to keep household chemical products in their original containers with warning labels and emergency information intact.

Caregivers should keep poisonous houseplants out of young children's reach and should supervise children outdoors. Some poisonous plants include azaleas, buttercups, daffodils, mistletoe berries, philodendrons, poinsettias, potato sprouts, tomato greens, and tulip bulbs. Teach children never to eat berries, mushrooms, seeds, or plants found in the wild. Plants can also be poisonous to pets.

Teach patients to keep poison control center telephone numbers posted near telephones. An integrated system of local centers across the United States can provide emergency information when a substance is ingested, inhaled, or splashed in the eyes or on the skin. The American Association of Poison Control Centers (AAPCC, 2011) offers resources and patient management guidelines. The AAPCC no longer recommends using ipecac syrup to induce vomiting in suspected ingestion of poisons; instead, the adult should call the poison control center for instructions.

Poison prevention in the healthcare environment can be accomplished primarily through safe medication preparation and administration practices. Nurses are responsible for checking that the healthcare provider's orders for medications are signed and updated appropriately. Identify the patient with two separate identifiers before administering any medication. High-risk medications are often checked by two nurses or a nurse and a pharmacist prior to administration. Document any significant side effects, and report them to the healthcare provider.

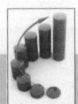

OUTCOME-BASED TEACHING PLANS

When Julie Michaels, the mother of a 1½-year-old toddler named Paula, comes to the clinic for a routine well-child visit, you learn that Paula is becoming increasingly inquisitive. Her mother reports that she has found her getting into the cabinet under the sink and pulling open drawers in the bathroom. She states, "I'm really concerned that she might put something into her mouth before I get to her."

OUTCOME

Julie will verbalize a realistic plan to decrease potential danger of accidental injury from ingestion and to prevent childhood poisoning.

STRATEGIES

- Discuss with Julie common safety measures to prevent Paula's access to potential poisons.
- Review the appropriate handling of medications:
  - Maintain childproof caps on all medications and toxic products.
  - Keep medications and toxic products in their original containers and out of Paula's reach.
  - Measure and give medications in well-lit areas to avoid errors in amount and type of medication.
  - Read labels of medications carefully before administering.
  - Dispose of all medications as recommended by healthcare provider (medications should not be flushed into the water system; some healthcare agencies will accept returned medications).

- Encourage Julie to think of other potential poisoning situations:
  - Keep cleaning products and garden chemicals out of the reach of children.
  - Use chemical and cleaning products in well-ventilated areas.
  - Do not mix chemicals or common household cleaning products.
  - Remove or keep out of Paula's reach any houseplants or natural materials that may be poisonous.
- Review with Julie a plan of response in the event of accidental poisoning, giving positive feedback regarding her concerns:
  - Have the phone number of the poison control center available.
  - Call immediately if you suspected poisoning

EVALUATION

10/15/17: 10:15—Julie was able to list areas in the home (under the bathroom and kitchen sinks and the medicine cabinet) that she would evaluate for toxic substances and childproof them within the next 2 weeks. She has the poison control center number by the phone and verbalizes she would call immediately if accidental ingestion occurred.

S. Roberts, RN

SUFFOCATION AND DROWNING PREVENTION

Drowning can occur not only in pools but also in bathtubs and other sources of water around the home. Caregivers must never leave young children unattended in bathtubs or kiddie pools. They should not leave pails or basins of water within children's reach. Pools should be fenced, and children of all ages must be supervised at pools and beaches. Encourage swimming lessons for children of all ages. Children are required to wear life jackets for boating and fishing and need to be warned not to ice skate or play on ice unless ice thickness is proven safe.

FIRE SAFETY

Fire extinguishers are designed to fight specific types of fires and are labeled appropriately. Table 23-4 describes the various classes of fires and the type of fire extinguisher used for each. Review these topics with children and adults, as appropriate. Individuals should be taught to "Stop, Drop, and Roll" if any clothing catches fire.

TABLE 23-4 CORRECT FIRE EXTINGUISHERS TO USE WITH SPECIFIC CLASSES OF FIRES

Class	Type of Material	Type of Fire Extinguishers
A	Paper, wood, cloth	Water (stored pressure, gas cartridge, soda acid, pump) Multipurpose dry chemical (stored pressure, gas cartridge) Loaded stream
B	Flammable liquids, such as fuel oil, cooking oil or grease, paint, solvents; gases (e.g., anesthesia gases)	Carbon dioxide Regular and multipurpose dry chemical (stored pressure, foam, loaded stream, gas cartridge)
C	Electrical fires	Regular and multipurpose dry chemical (stored pressure, gas cartridge) Carbon dioxide Liquefied gas
D	Combustible metals	Special dry powder

Healthcare agency safety programs emphasize reducing fire hazards by strictly limiting smoking, using nonflammable materials whenever possible, and practicing fire drills and firefighting skills. In the patient care area, each nurse needs to become familiar with emergency telephone numbers; the locations of fire alarms, fire extinguishers, and fire hoses; shutoff valves for oxygen and other flammable gases; evacuation equipment; and exits. Posted wall maps must show evacuation routes.

BURN PREVENTION

Teach patients with sensory impairment to monitor water temperature at home. They may need to reduce the temperature of the thermostat on the hot water heater.

> ### ❗ SAFETY ALERT
> Adults should keep pot handles turned away from the front of the stove top, where young children might reach. They should never allow young children to play unsupervised in the kitchen or near burning fireplaces, barbecue grills, or containers of gasoline.

Teach adults never to smoke around highly flammable liquids such as gasoline or lighter fluid. Smoking in bed or late at night in a chair is hazardous. Smoking materials must be properly extinguished.

Individuals should use sunscreen protection (either barrier creams or clothing) and sunglasses in all outdoor recreation and work activities where exposure to ultraviolet sunlight is a potential hazard. Remind parents to apply sunscreen to children playing outdoors to prevent sunburn. In addition to burns to the skin, extensive exposure to sunlight poses risks for cancer and eye damage.

Burns can be prevented in the healthcare environment by testing bathwater for temperature when the patient has sensory impairment; checking heating pads, heat lamps, and other electrical equipment to be sure they are functioning properly; and assisting patients when handling hot beverages, as needed.

FIREARM SAFETY

Prevention of injuries and fatalities from firearms is an important public health responsibility of nurses. Anticipatory guidance about violence in general, and firearms in particular, is an important nursing role.

Healthcare professionals must ask patients (children and adults alike) about their experience with violence and handguns or other firearms in the home. Advise adults to store unloaded guns in a secured (preferably locked) area, with special attention to keeping them away from children's reach. Warn children not to handle guns unless the older child receives instruction and supervision by an adult.

In addition to increasing counseling efforts during patient care activities, nurses and other healthcare professionals should join community efforts to regulate handguns. Promote product designs that modify guns to make them more childproof (e.g., trigger safety locks, designs that increase the force necessary to discharge a weapon). Such a product-oriented approach has been successful in decreasing other types of childhood injuries.

Injury prevention experts recommend a comprehensive approach to reduce firearm injuries. Elements include firearm surveillance and safety regulation, research, enforcement of restrictions limiting access by minors and other unlawful purchasers, local and state prevention programs, and development of public support. More emphasis is also needed on building community coalitions to make youth environments safer.

ELECTRICAL SAFETY

Nurses must protect themselves and patients from dangerous shocks by keeping their hands dry when manipulating machinery, mopping spilled fluid, ensuring that all plugs are grounded (three pronged), and reporting any equipment damage. Electrical equipment should be serviced regularly.

RADIATION SAFETY

Although the risk of radiation injury in most communities is low, nurses should let the community know about the sources and effects of radiation. Greater public awareness and understanding of radioactive waste and nuclear power can lead to stricter regulation of radiation used in industry.

An international symbol (Fig. 23-5) marks areas where radioactive substances are used. Radioactive implants or ingestion of radioactive materials can make a patient a source of radioactive contamination. Nurses routinely wear radiation detection badges to assist the institution's radiation safety officer in monitoring exposure levels. These badges are collected periodically, and the exposure levels are calculated to ensure that staff stays within safety limits of exposure. The three cardinal rules of radiation protection are (1) minimize time of exposure to the source, (2) maximize distance from the source, and (3) use appropriate shielding.

Safety precautions for staff include distancing and shielding from the radiation source and measuring accumulated dose. Regular inspection and servicing of equipment and licensing of x-ray and pharmacy technicians help minimize risks to the patients and staff. Proper training on safe work procedures is essential for nursing personnel.

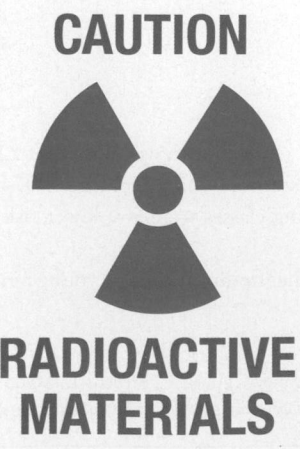

FIGURE 23-5 International radiation symbol.

Nursing care for radiation therapy patients must be well organized so that assistance and support are given efficiently without needless exposure of nurses. Use lead shields or lead aprons if close contact with the patient is required. Wear gloves to prevent skin contact with any body substances (urine, stool, saliva, blood). Encourage patients to do as much of their own care as possible. If the patient is admitted to a healthcare facility, a private room with private bath is essential to prevent exposure of other patients. Keep linens in the room until the radioactive source is removed. Soiled linens, excreta, and other wastes may require special labeling and disposal.

After cessation of therapy, the radiation safety officer will sweep the room with a radiation detector to assess for spills or contamination. After clearance, the room may be cleaned and linens sent to the laundry. If the patient is to go home while receiving radiation therapy through an ingested substance (e.g., iodine-131), the hospital radiation safety manual will list directions for protection of the family, caregivers, and home environment.

CHILDHOOD SAFETY

Make parents and other adult caregivers aware of the need to childproof the home and to supervise children in any potentially hazardous outside area. Teach caregivers to use only cribs and other equipment approved by the U.S. Consumer Products Safety Commission or other regulatory agency.

The use of older equipment that is worn or poorly designed can present a hazard. Toys should be age appropriate.

Teach children safety related to bicycles and sports, such as in-line skating, skiing, soccer, football, and horseback riding. Children should wear helmets to protect against head injury in the event of a fall. Proper signaling and illumination of children and bicycles at night are important measures for injury prevention. Teach adults to check for small children riding low vehicles before driving a car out of a driveway or parking space. Warn children about riding in streets or near driveways.

The care of children in the healthcare environment requires special safety precautions. High staff-to-patient ratios, use of cribs and beds with side rails, carpeting on the floor, play areas with age-appropriate toys and furnishings, locked medications and supply rooms, and protected exits contribute to safety (Fig. 23-6).

OCCUPATIONAL HEALTH AND SAFETY

The work environment brings many rewards and frustrations to both nurses and patients. People spend a large portion of their time on the job—approximately 40% of their waking hours. Workplace hazards take a high toll on employees' lives, causing disability and death. The costs of medical care and lost work time are enormous; however, such estimates do not begin to address the costs associated with pain and suffering or with care provided by family members. The actual number of injuries

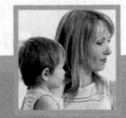

Safety PICO

Mary, a pediatric nurse in the clinic, is performing an assessment on the toddler from the chapter-opening scenario. The mother is a young, single parent who is concerned about the child's safety. She states that her son is extremely active and always getting into things at home. The mother is afraid that her son will hurt himself accidently. She feels exhausted from always trying to protect him. Mary tells the young mother about parenting classes that are offered in the community. The mother questions if attending these classes will prevent accidents from happening to her son. Mary decides to look for evidence in the Cochrane Library. She uses the following PICO statement to guide her search: *Do training programs for parents (compared to no training programs) help promote child safety and prevent injuries?*

Population = parents
Intervention = parent training
Control = no parenting training
Outcome = promote child safety

A meta-analysis research reviewed a total of 22 studies, which included randomized and nonrandomized investigations. Ten randomized controlled studies (which included 5,074 participants) actually showed that children whose families attended *and completed* the parenting training classes were at a lower risk for injuries, compared to the children whose families did not attended any education classes.

Mary shares her findings with the young mother, who agrees that she and her son might benefit from participating in parenting classes.

REFERENCE

Kendrick D., Mulvaney C.A., Ye L., Stevens T., Mytton J.A., & Stewart-Brown S. (2013). Parenting interventions for the prevention of unintentional injuries in childhood. *Cochrane Database of Systematic Reviews*, Issue 3. Art. No.: CD006020. DOI: 10.1002/14651858.CD006020.pub3

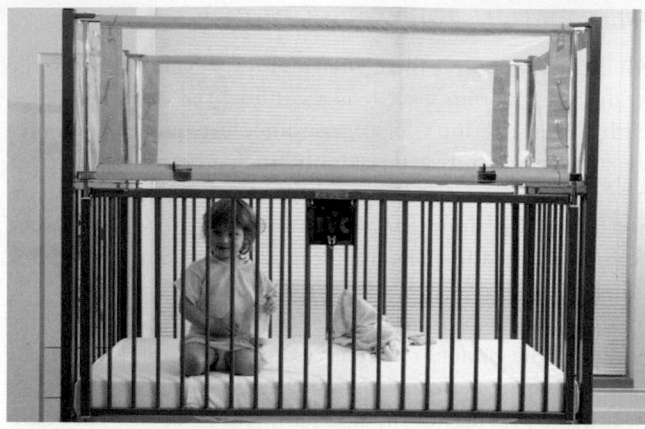

A

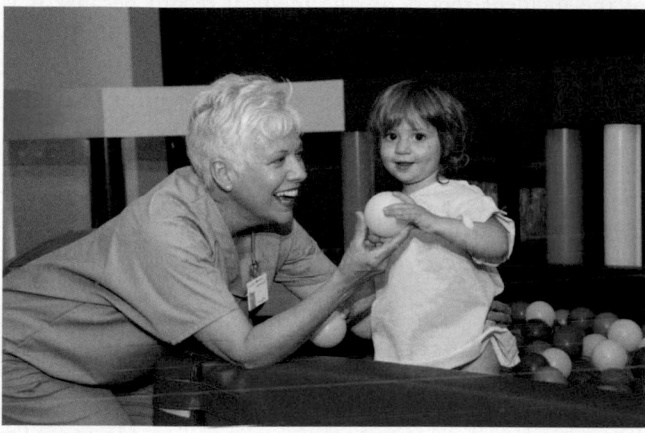

B

FIGURE 23-6 Safety is an essential aspect of pediatric nursing. **A.** A clear plastic cover over the crib prevents the older infant or toddler from climbing out and falling. **B.** A well-organized playroom with age-appropriate toys and activities promotes safety.

and illnesses likely is much higher than reported figures suggest because underreporting of work-related conditions is a significant problem.

The healthcare industry has many occupational hazards, some of which have already been mentioned. Compared with those in other occupations, nursing personnel such as nursing aides, orderlies, and attendants are among those at highest risk for musculoskeletal disorders. Nursing personnel also have the highest back-related workers' compensation claim rates of any occupation or industry (ANA, 2013).

Be aware of the contribution of occupational hazards to the incidence of injuries and illnesses that patients experience. Including an occupational history as part of the basic subjective assessment provides information about the source of certain health conditions as well as the impact that other medical conditions or injuries can have on the patient's ability to resume normal work activities. Patient education should include basic principles about injury prevention, the use of personal protective equipment, and safe work practices when dealing with hazardous exposures.

Nursing Interventions for Altered Safety

Harm to a person or group occurs when safety is not maintained. In the healthcare environment, specific nursing interventions are carried out when preventive measures fail. Nursing interventions for altered safety function include fire evacuation, emergency first aid for poisoning, administration of cardiopulmonary resuscitation, and filing an incident report.

DISASTER PLANS

Some areas are prone to tornadoes, blizzards, earthquakes, floods, and hurricanes. Nurses are responsible for knowing the disaster plans for such emergencies where they work. Understanding and practicing the plan helps nurses remain calm in emergencies. There are two basic types of healthcare agency disasters: internal and external. Internal disasters are those in which the facility itself is in danger. Personnel must take actions to protect employees and patients. In an external disaster, many people are brought to a hospital or clinic for care after a large-scale emergency. Personnel must carry out specific plans when the healthcare agency is notified of any emergency.

FIRE EVACUATION

Annual training for fire evacuation is required of all employees. Often, mnemonics such as RACE or PASS are used to help employees remember what to do should a fire occur (Box 23-4).

In the event of a fire in a patient care area, nurses are responsible for determining which patients are in immediate danger. Direct ambulatory patients toward exits to wait in a safe area. Evacuate bedridden patients using stretchers and wheelchairs if necessary. In severe situations, patients can be carried or dragged

---

BOX 23-4 | **Training to Manage Fire in the Healthcare Setting**

Annual training is required of all healthcare employees so that they will know how to function to protect the safety of patients and all personnel should a fire break out in their agency. The mnemonic *RACE* helps employees remember how to prioritize actions during a fire, and PASS helps employees remember how to use a fire extinguisher.

R Rescue—remove the patient from immediate danger
A Alarm—pull alarm and call "code red," and alert appropriate personnel
C Confine—close all doors and windows
E Evacuate—extinguish fire or evacuate patients if directed by fire department, first horizontally and then vertically
P Pull the pin
A Aim the nozzle
S Squeeze the handle
S Sweep back and forth over fire

on sheets. The local fire department will be notified automatically. If the fire is small, a fire extinguisher can be used, but do not neglect other interventions, because small fires can quickly escalate out of control. Close windows and doors and turn off oxygen in the area to reduce the fire's oxygen supply. Evacuate patients in surrounding areas, if necessary, and give them wet washcloths to breathe through to reduce smoke inhalation.

> **! SAFETY ALERT**
>
> Do not use elevators in the event of a fire. Activate the fire alarm, and notify the healthcare agency's switchboard of the fire's location.

Healthcare facilities are required to have fire evacuation plans with exits clearly marked. Additional staff from the facility and firefighters will respond quickly to help nurses evacuate patients. Never attempt to extinguish fires if the safety of yourself or your patients is in jeopardy. When evacuating patients who require mechanical ventilation, a bag-valve mask can be used for manual respiration. Clamp tubes connected to suction before disconnecting them, and transport IV fluids with the patient.

EMERGENCY CARE IN UNINTENTIONAL POISONING

In the healthcare environment, ingestion of dangerous substances, overdose, or incorrect medication administration can be treated as in the home. Notify the patient's healthcare provider, but if the substance is potentially toxic, notify the local poison control center without delay. The center will require information about the specific poison (the ingredients section on the label may provide this information), quantity ingested, person's age and weight, and apparent symptoms. Nurses may be instructed to induce vomiting if the patient is not unconscious or convulsing or if the substance was not a strong corrosive or petroleum product. Position the patient on his or her side or with the head placed between the legs to prevent aspiration. Gather urine, vomitus, or blood samples as instructed.

If poisonous substances have been instilled into the eye or on the skin, immediate irrigation with lukewarm water for 10 to 15 minutes may reduce harmful effects. Remove contaminated clothing from the skin. Instruct the person to blink as much as possible during eye irrigation. Depending on the type of chemical exposure, be cautious about potential skin contact with the patient or the patient's clothing. Special procedures for handling hazardous materials may be necessary to protect staff and other patients in the area.

CARDIOPULMONARY RESUSCITATION

If a patient chokes, aspirates, or is found cyanotic and apneic, the nurse is responsible for initiating resuscitation efforts (see Chapter 27). Electrical shock also can lead to cardiac arrest requiring cardiopulmonary resuscitation.

FILING AN INCIDENT REPORT

An incident report is filed when an injury event occurs in the healthcare environment. It is a confidential document filed with the institution's legal, insurance, or quality assurance department for internal use only. In it, the nurse describes how an injury occurred, what the effects were on the patient, and what was done for the patient. Incident reports are commonly used for falls, medication errors, and needlestick injuries.

In addition to filing an incident report, the nurse must enter on the patient's medical record a description of the incident and its effects on the patient. Notify the patient's healthcare provider of the incident, and he or she will document the patient's condition. The nurse does not make note of the incident report on the medical record because it is used internally for risk management and quality improvement purposes. The incident report can be reviewed by the institution's attorneys in the event of a lawsuit, and it may be collected by the risk manager to see whether trends in injuries in the workplace are developing. When an injury to the nurse occurs, a workers' compensation claim usually is filed to cover the medical costs of the injury and the costs of any lost work time.

Home and Community Care

Nurses promote safety interventions wherever they practice. For example, school nurses function as safety educators for school-age children. They teach children drug prevention measures and how to tell someone when they do not want to be touched. In most states, school nurses are required to report suspected child abuse. School nurses also may identify children who seem to be at high risk for injury. These children may have a neuromuscular or a sensory–perceptual basis for their injuries and should be evaluated. Screening for problems with vision and hearing is especially important.

The occupational health nurse may be involved in health and safety education and injury prevention at the work site. Adults often need to learn proper body mechanics and may need to use transfer or lifting devices for lifting heavy loads. For the sedentary worker, principles of body alignment and stretching can help prevent muscle strain from prolonged static posture. Proper lighting can improve productivity and prevent eye strain. Occupational health nurses identify ergonomic hazards (e.g., repetitive strain injuries) and hazardous materials in the workplace and encourage appropriate worker protection (adequate ventilation, respiratory protection, ear plugs, protective clothing and eyewear). They also develop instructional health and safety promotion programs to prevent back injury, on-the-job injuries (e.g., falls, needlestick injuries), and illness.

All nurses can act as community activists and advocates for environmental safety in such areas as promoting clean air and water; cleanup of hazardous waste sites; safe, well-lighted pedestrian walkways; and laws supporting seat belt use, air bags, helmet use, and gun control.

HOME CARE MANAGEMENT

Home care nurses identify areas in which the patient is unsafe when performing essential ADLs. They devise a plan that prepares the patient, home caregivers, and the home itself for optimal safety. Box 23-1 lists potential hazards in the home. Other health professionals, such as social workers, occupational therapists, and physical therapists, are involved in the planning process and home care, but the nurse is often considered the most accurate source of information about the patient's function in ADLs. If you work as a home care nurse, observe the patient engaging in transfers and mobility, toileting, hygiene, eating and feeding, and dressing. Observations made during assessments allow the nurse to anticipate the measures that need to be taken to promote safety in these activities at home.

The nurse working with a newly disabled patient in a rehabilitation facility helps the healthcare team anticipate environmental changes that may be needed after discharge. Often, the patient, family, or other caregivers are asked to draw a floor plan of the house, noting especially the width of doorways, configuration of the bathroom and kitchen, stairs approaching the home and within the home, and access to transportation from the home. Special equipment used during the hospitalization may need to be used in the home, and hospital beds, wheelchairs, tub benches, and mechanical lifts may not fit in the home. Early identification of the patient's postdischarge equipment needs will help the family and caregivers to modify the home before the patient is discharged.

Essential to overall safety is the support system. Actively involved family or supportive friends can provide assistance with assessing the availability of additional caregivers, their level of desired participation, and their own capacity for safe judgment. Identify who will be providing care and whether they will be available occasionally, part-time, or 24 hours a day. Determine what training the caregivers need to provide safe care. A home health referral may be needed to allow a home health nurse to visit the patient and caregivers in the home and provide necessary training and supervision.

Community health nurses can help older adults safety proof their homes against falls by removing loose rugs and obstacles in hallways and stairwells. Community health nurses often educate members of the community about safety promotion through health fairs and lectures. Some communities offer a service that telephones the single older adult daily and responds to a help signal activated by a medallion worn around the neck. This system or a buddy system of telephone calls can provide a quick response to injury events for the older adult.

EVALUATION

The effectiveness of nursing interventions to promote safety is determined through nursing observation and feedback from patients, caregivers, and healthcare professionals in the community. Long-term goals include the identification of actual and potential environmental hazards, demonstration of safety habits, reduction in frequency and severity of injuries, and development of safe compensatory strategies for physical deficits. To measure the progress toward these goals, question the patient and caregivers, using "what if" and "what would you do if" questions. Ask for and evaluate the patient's performance of selected safety habits (e.g., transfers in and out of the bathtub). Gather data on the frequency and type of injury incidents. Determine the effectiveness of compensatory strategies: Is the patient using the suggested strategies? What are the potential obstacles to their use? Is the patient satisfied? Does the strategy make the activity easier, safer, or faster to accomplish? Any incident, fall, scrape, bruise, or other trauma requires a nurse's analysis to identify the cause and the best means to prevent recurrence. Nurses have a fundamental responsibility to promote continuous patient safety, and every interaction with the patient is an opportunity to promote and evaluate his or her safety habits.

Goal

The patient will identify actual and high-risk environmental hazards and verbalize prevention strategies.

POSSIBLE OUTCOME CRITERIA

* At home, the patient verbalizes difficulty using stairs to access the bathroom and verbalizes intent to have handrails installed.
* Before discharge, the patient verbalizes a plan for removing obstacles at home to prevent falls.

Goal

The patient will demonstrate safety habits appropriate to selected environments (home, healthcare setting, workplace, community).

POSSIBLE OUTCOME CRITERIA

* Immediately after instructions by the nurse, the patient uses nurse call-light system for assistance each time he or she needs to use the bathroom.
* The patient uses over-the-bed lights, nonskid slippers, and eyeglasses when transferring to chair at first and subsequent times out of bed.
* The patient identifies modifications for home safety (removal of throw rugs, installation of handrails in hallway, better lighting of hallway and stairway) 24 hours after the nurse's instruction about home safety.

Goal

The patient will experience decreased frequency and severity of injury events.

POSSIBLE OUTCOME CRITERIA

* The patient practices safety precautions, as evidenced by absence of falls or other trauma during hospitalization.

Goal

The nurse (and nursing staff) will identify safety issues in the work environment and decrease injury events.

PATIENT PLAN OF CARE
The Patient at Risk for Injury

NURSING DIAGNOSIS
Risk for Injury related to sensory and integrative dysfunction manifested by altered mobility and faulty judgment.

PATIENT GOAL
Patient will demonstrate safety habits to prevent injury when performing ADLs.

PATIENT OUTCOME CRITERIA
- Patient uses nurse call-light system for assistance with any toileting after instruction by the nurse.
- Patient uses over-the-bed lights, nonskid slippers each time when transferring to chair or out of bed.
- Patient identifies modification for home safety (removal of throw rugs, installation of handrails in hallway, better lighting of hallway and stairway) 24 hours after nurse's instruction about home safety.

NURSING INTERVENTION	SCIENTIFIC RATIONALE
1. Position bed in lowest position.	**1.** Low position minimizes the distance to the floor if the patient falls.
2. Place patient call light within reach of hand, and give instructions.	**2.** A call light allows the patient to call for help.
3. Explain all safety modifications of the patient's room: removal of clutter, providing a clear path to bathroom, use of a night-light, installing brakes on bed and chairs, placement of call light.	**3.** The patient and family will feel safer if they are aware of safety promotion strategies.
4. Perform frequent visual checks of the patient.	**4.** The patient may attempt to get out of bed or chair without calling for assistance.
5. Use safety belt in all transfers if the patient is unsteady or has difficulty with balance.	**5.** A safety belt allows for control/monitoring of patient movement without trauma to any body part.
6. Evaluate the patient's ability to use toilet; obtain raised toilet seat or grab bars if indicated.	**6.** Patients with hip muscle weakness may be unable to rise from low toilet seat. Grab bars may assist the weak person to move slowly and safely.
7. Assist the patient to perform hygiene at sink with large mirror; encourage the patient to scan the whole visual field.	**7.** Mirror provides the patient with visual reinforcement of activity.
8. Discuss floor plan of home with the patient and support person. Make suggestions for modifications that will lead to a safer environment.	**8.** Patient and support person need to be involved in planning for patient's safety in the home.
9. Post sign "Do not get up alone. Call for help."	**9.** Reminds the patient and family not to get up without help.

EVALUATION

10/11/17: 13:00—Balance still poor requiring a minimum of one person and gait belt with transfers and ambulation. Attempted to get up by self even after instruction. Teaching reinforced and bed alarm applied. Family instructed of safety plan. Evaluation of home is scheduled before discharge.

S. Roberts, RN

POSSIBLE OUTCOME CRITERIA

- Standards established by the Joint Commission will be enforced daily, and patients will remain safe in the health-care setting.

- The work environment has the proper equipment and staffing levels to allow nursing personnel to care safely for patients and to move patients without injury to the personnel; the environment also allows patients to have safe transport throughout the setting.

KEY CONCEPTS

- Safety is a basic human need that is essential in the healthcare environment, home, workplace, and community.

- Individual and environmental factors affect safety.

- Manifestations of altered safety include falls, fires, burns, lacerations, poisoning, suffocation, electrical shock, radiation injury, and motor vehicle incidents.

- Infants, older adults, and those impaired by illness or medications are at greatest risk for falls.

- Falls in the healthcare environment are frequently associated with walking to the bathroom or early ambulation after illness, injury, or surgery.

- Nursing interventions to promote health and safety involve patient education and providing a safe environment in a healthcare setting, in the workplace, at home, and in the community.

- Nurses must educate parents about the developmental capabilities of infants and children and the special safety precautions needed for their care.

- Nurses must be familiar with emergency interventions for disasters, including fire evacuation and filing an incident report.

- Nurses must be knowledgeable about the health and safety hazards they face in healthcare settings to prevent their own injury and illness.

PRACTICING FOR THE NCLEX

CHECK YOUR ANSWERS IN APPENDIX A.

1. Fall prevention is done on multiple different levels by nurses in the hospital. Which of the following would not be an example of fall prevention done by nursing?
   a. Reminding the patient to use the call light for assistance when getting out of bed
   b. Placing the bed mattress on the floor to prevent injury
   c. Developing an organizational policy for hourly rounding schedules to be performed on each unit to monitor patient needs and comfort level
   d. Applying restraints to patients at risk for falls

2. If a sentinel event occurred in your hospital facility related to a medication error, to which regulatory body/bodies is the hospital required to report the event?
   a. U.S. Department of Labor's OSHA
   b. National Academy of Science's IOM
   c. The Joint Commission Center for Transforming Healthcare
   d. State Department of Health and/or other health agencies
   e. a & d
   f. a & c
   g. c & d

3. Older adults may be at increased risk of injury related to physiologic factors. Which of the following are relevant risk factors unique to this population? Select all that apply:
   a. Decrease in sensory–perceptual function and cognitive judgment
   b. Alcohol impairment
   c. Impaired thermoregulation
   d. Medication side effects

4. Nurses should be aware of various safety hazards in the workplace. Which of the following present safety hazards to nurses? Select all that apply:
   a. Cleaning solution spill
   b. Chemotherapy administration
   c. Needlestick injury
   d. Assisting with patient mobility or transfers

5. An error occurs as the result of the lack of a double-check process on dosing of a high-risk opiate pain medication. The patient becomes oversedated, necessitating reversal of the opioids in order to regain a regular respiratory pattern. Which of the following should the nurse do to document the incident? Select all that apply:
   a. Describe factors that led up to the incident
   b. Document patient assessment findings following the error
   c. Detail contributing factors in patient chart
   d. Include interventions needed to reverse oversedation in incident report

6. A nurse is providing discharge education for a postoperative patient who will be leaving the hospital with a urinary catheter. What statement reflects appropriate environmental safety education for this patient?
   a. "Be aware that you are at risk for falling because the catheter tubing hangs by your feet and is a tripping hazard."
   b. "Your pain medications may cause side effects including drowsiness, so be sure not to drive while you are taking them."
   c. "Because of your incisions, you should be careful to not lift anything heavier than 10 lb."
   d. "Change positions slowly to avoid dizziness."

7. A nurse is assessing a patient for safety upon discharge following a severe cerebrovascular. Which of the following systems would be a priority for this patient's safety? Select all that apply:
   a. Neurologic system
   b. Cardiovascular system
   c. Skin integrity
   d. Musculoskeletal system

8. A nurse is evaluating outcome criteria for a patient following a stroke with Risk for Aspiration assigned as a nursing diagnosis. Which of the following would be appropriate goals for this patient? Select all that apply:

    a. The patient will tuck chin for more effective swallow when drinking thin liquids.

    b. The patient will avoid drinking liquids related to increased risk for aspiration.

    c. The patient will have no signs or symptoms of aspiration (e.g., coughing).

    d. The patient will place food on right side to avoid vision cut.

9. Restraints should be used for patient safety in which of the following situations? Select all that apply:

    a. The patient is attempting to remove mechanical ventilator tubing.

    b. The patient is at risk for falling due to impaired neurologic status.

    c. The patient is confused, impulsive, and wants to leave the hospital unit.

    d. The patient is combative with staff members.

10. In the event of a fire, what is the most important thing that a nurse needs to do?

    a. Give patients wet washcloths to breathe through to reduce smoke inhalation

    b. Close windows and doors and turn off oxygen

    c. Determine which patients are in immediate danger

    d. Evacuate bedridden patients

REFERENCES

American Academy of Pediatrics. (2011a). *Car safety seats: A guide for families in* 2011. Retrieved May 1, 2011, from www.aap.org/healthtopics/carseat-safety.cfm

American Academy of Pediatrics. (2011b). *Technical report: SIDS and other sleep-related infant deaths: Expansion of recommendations for a safe infant sleeping environment.* doi:10.1542/peds.2011-2285

American Academy of Pediatrics. (2014). *Policy statement: School start times for adolescents.* Retrieved from http://pediatrics.aappublications.org/content/134/3/642.full.pdf. doi:10.1542/peds.2014-1697

American Association of Poison Control Centers. (2011). *Out-of-Hospital Patient Management Guidelines.* Available at 1-800-222-1222. Retrieved May 1, 2011, from www.aapcc.org/dnn/default.aspx

American Nurses Association. (2013). *Safe patient handling and mobility: Interprofessional national standards.* Silver Spring, MD: Nursebooks.org.

Centers for Disease Control and Prevention. (2013). *Leading causes of death reports, national and regional, 1999–2013.* Retrieved from http://webappa.cdc.gov/sasweb/ncipc/leadcaus10_us.html

Centers for Disease Control and Prevention. (2014). *About school violence.* Retrieved from http://www.cdc.gov/ViolencePrevention/youthviolence/schoolviolence/index.html

Centers for Medicare and Medicaid Services. (2006). Medicare and Medicaid Programs; hospital conditions of participation: Patients' rights. Final rule. *Federal Register, 71*(236), 71377–71428.

Chapman, S. (2011). Gun control. Australian and US gun deaths compared. *British Medical Journal, 342,* d1005. doi:10.1136/bmj.d1005

Environmental Protection Agency. (2012). *Noise pollution.* Retrieved from http://www.epa.gov/air/noise.html

Food and Drug Administration. (2015). *What are the radiation risks from CT?* Retrieved from http://www.fda.gov/Radiation-EmittingProducts/RadiationEmittingProductsandProcedures/MedicalImaging/MedicalX-Rays/ucm115329.htm

National Safety Council. (2015). *Safe bicycling.* Retrieved from http://www.nsc.org/NSCDocuments_Advocacy/Fact%20Sheets/Bicycling-Fact-Sheet.doc

Page, A. (Ed.). (2004). *Keeping patients safe.* Washington, DC: National Academies Press.

Parents Central. (2015). *Car seat recommendations for children.* Retrieved from http://www.safercar.gov/parents/Right-Seat-Age-And-Size-Recommendations.htm

Pellfolk, T. J., Gustafson, Y., Bucht, G., & Karlsson, S. (2010). Effects of a restraint minimization program on staff knowledge, attitudes, and practice: A cluster randomized trial. *Journal of the American Geriatric Society, 58*(1), 62–69.

Toy Industry Association, Inc. (2015). *Toy safety.* Retrieved from toyinfo.org

United States Fire Administration. (2014). *Keeping kids safe from fire.* Retrieved from http://www.usfa.fema.gov/prevention/outreach/children.html

United States Fire Administration. (2015a). *About the U.S. Fire Administration (USFA).* Retrieved from http://www.usfa.fema.gov/about

United States Fire Administration. (2015b). *Choosing and using fire extinguishers.* Retrieved from http://www.usfa.fema.gov/prevention/outreach/extinguishers.html

Procedure 23-1 Application of Physical Restraints

Purpose	1. Prevent the patient from pulling out tubes or lines that could cause harm to the patient or negatively impact treatment. 2. Manage violent or self-destructive behavior that jeopardizes the immediate physical safety of the patient, staff members, or others.
Equipment	Select appropriate type of restraint: vests, ankle or wrist, mitt, or belt. Select the correct size of restraint for the patient that is appropriate to the patient's condition.
Assessment	• Assess the cause for which the restraint is being considered, develop alternatives to restraint use, and implement these alternatives before applying restraints. • Allow the use of restraints only under the supervision of a licensed healthcare provider and for a strictly defined period of time, seeking an order from a licensed healthcare provider as soon as possible. Obtain informed consent from patient/resident or guardian before use or as soon as possible after the application, if it is an emergent event. Assess for cognitive or physical deficits that could increase the risk for injury. • The need for additional staff to safely apply restraints.

Procedure

1. **Perform hand hygiene.**
   Rationale: Reduces microbe transmission.
2. **Identify the patient.**
   Rationale: Ensures correct patient receives proper assessment or treatment and reduces errors.
3. **Close door or bed curtains and explain the procedure to the patient and patient's family.**
   Rationale: Ensures patient privacy, increases patient compliance, reduces patient anxiety, and promotes learning.
4. **Select the appropriate restraint for the patient.**
   Rationale: Use the least restrictive restraint possible. The correct size is important to maintain safety.

Wrist (or Ankle) Restraint

5. **Wrap the restraint around extremity with soft pad touching skin (Fig. 1).**

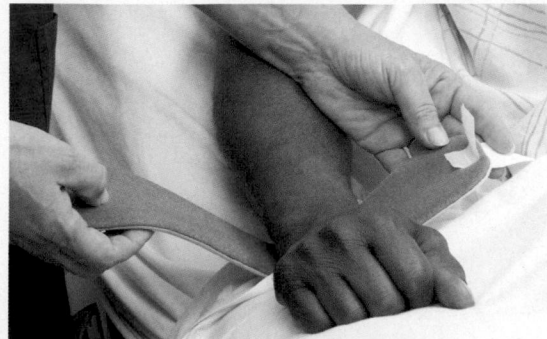

FIG. 1 Apply wrist restraint ensuring that the padded side contacts the patient's skin.
   Rationale: Protects the skin from irritation.

6. **Secure in place by fastening Velcro and/or buckle (Fig. 2). Ensure that two fingers can be inserted between the restraint and the patient's wrist (Fig. 3).**

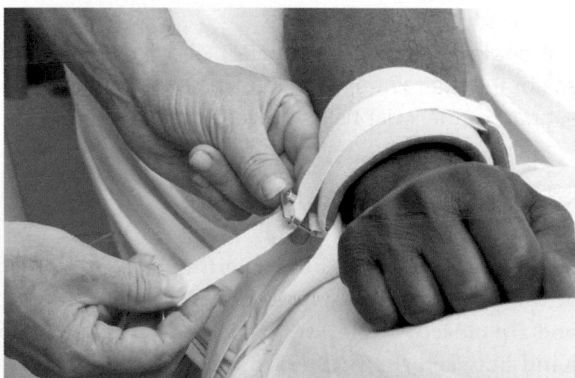

FIG. 2 Secure wrist restraint.

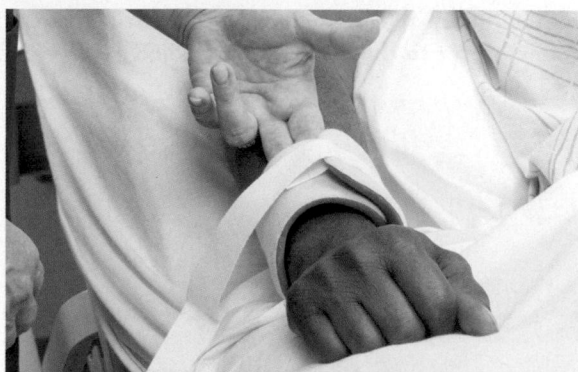

FIG. 3 Ensure that two fingers can be inserted between restraint and wrist.
   Rationale: Maintains adequate blood flow distal to the site of the restraint application.

Procedure 23-1   *continued*

Mitt Restraint

5. Slide patient's hand into mitt restraint. Fingers do not need to go to the tip of the glove. Secure in place by fastening strap and Velcro around the narrowest part of the wrist. Ensure that two fingers can be inserted between the restraint and the patient's wrist. Sometimes a mitt restraint can be secured with a wrist restraint to the bed frame, but often mitts are used independently to prevent use of hands to grab (Fig. 4).

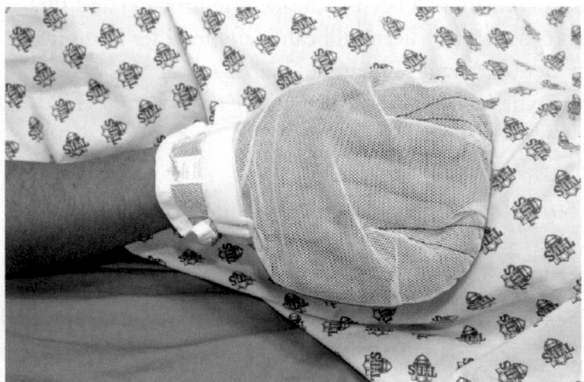

FIG. 4 Using a hand mitt.

Rationale: Maintains adequate blood flow distal to the site of the restraint application. Fastening at the narrowest part of the wrist helps prevent dislodgement.

Vest (Jacket) Restraint

5. Select the correct size of vest noting back versus front of the restraint. Apply front of vest to front of patient and zip closed. Make sure you can slip fingers of your hand between the vest and the patient's abdomen.

Rationale: Ensures proper fit and application, which prevents injury and possible strangulation.

6. Fasten quick-release buckle to the bed springs or frame, never to the mattress or the bed rails (Fig. 5).

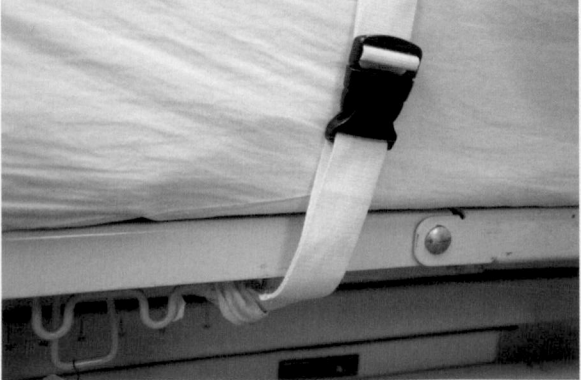

FIG. 5 Attach the restraint to the bed frame, not the mattress.

Rationale: The mattress or bed rails move and may change the pressure and security of the restraints. Quick-release mechanisms allow the patient to be moved quickly in an emergency and are preferred over using knots to attach restraints. Restraints should never be tied with knots that cannot be quickly released.

7. Observe patients in restraints frequently and document according to policy, describing the patient's behavior, the intervention used, and the patient's response to the intervention. The patient must be assessed face-to-face within 1 hour of application and frequently thereafter.

Rationale: Assessing the patient within 1 hour allows the nurse to determine how well the restraint is being tolerated, prevent injury, and assess if it is still needed.

8. Remove the restraints at least every 2 hours and more often if necessary. Allow for ADLs.

Rationale: Check for pressure areas, patient tolerance of restraint, and the need to void.

Documentation

6/15/17: 2:30 PM—Patient confused following return from post-anesthesia care unit (PACU) following total hip replacement. Believes she is at home, and she needs to void. Reassured that she is in the hospital, that a catheter is in place, and that the bed rails are up. However, she continually tries to sit up. After consultation with the physician and family, a vest restraint has been applied as a reminder that she needs to ask for help to get up. Family is present with her and will also remind her. Will reassess the need for the restraint within an hour.

B. Jennings, RN

Procedure 23-1 *continued*

Life Span Considerations

Child

- Children are at increased risk of injury from restraints.
- Use the least restrictive restraint needed to achieve the outcome.
- Swaddling or a mummy restraint may be used for infants.

Older Adult

- Remember that as skin ages, it loses its elasticity and integrity and becomes more sensitive. Avoid tape or restraints that rub because they may tear the skin.
- A skilled nursing facility may not accept a patient who has been in restraints during the last 24 hours.

Home Care Modifications

- When a patient is discharged home, there may no longer be a need for restraints. Caregivers should be cautioned that it is not appropriate or legal to restrain individuals and that they may face criminal charges.

Collaboration and Delegation

- Instruct ancillary staff to observe respiratory, circulatory, and skin status, changes in vital signs, and any other unusual events.
- Instruct staff to observe the face-to-face requirements for assessment as defined by the institution.
- A licensed provider (medical doctor, advanced registered nurse practitioner) must order restraints and reorder at least every 24 hours. Often, nurses remind providers if the order is outdated.

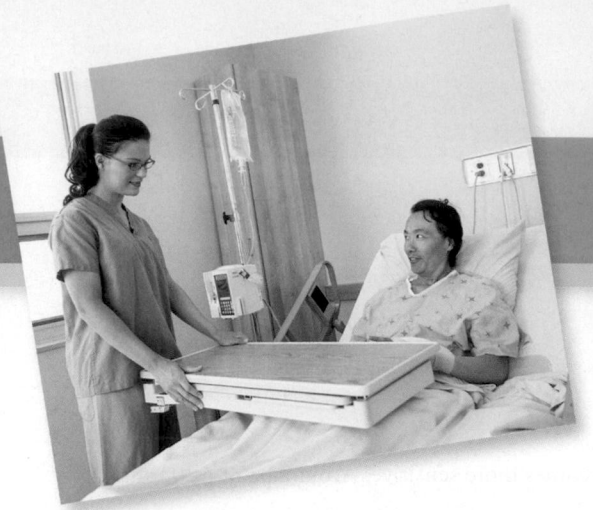

CHAPTER 24

Hygiene and Self-Care

Marisa Gillaspie Aziz

Case Scenario

You are caring for a 37-year-old bachelor who is recovering from urologic surgery. He lived with his mother until her death a few years ago. He works independently as an accountant. This is your patient's first surgery, and although the pathology reports are not back, there is concern that your patient may have bladder cancer. After your morning assessment, you tell your patient that you will help him wash. He states that he does not want to wash and just wants to be left alone. Your assessment reveals dirt under his fingernails, which are untrimmed and jagged; body odor and halitosis, which is easily detected; and dirty tissues all over his bed.

Once you have completed this chapter and have incorporated self-care and hygiene into your knowledge base, review the above scenario and reflect on the following areas of Critical Thinking:

1. Identify factors that might make your patient reluctant to participate in morning care.
2. Discuss the reasons why you as a nurse believe that the patient should participate in morning care.
3. Reflect on your own feelings as you encounter this situation.
4. Identify two or three conclusions that you might draw before obtaining more information from the patient.
5. Predict positive and negative potential consequences of directly approaching this patient and "forcing" him to wash.

KEY TERMS

alopecia
bariatric equipment
caries
cerumen
commode
condom catheter
dysphagia
gingiva
halitosis
hygiene
micturition
pannus
pediculosis
plaque
proprioception
self-care
tartar
urinal
xerostomia

LEARNING OBJECTIVES

Upon completion of this chapter, you will be able to do the following:

1. Discuss the importance of self-care and hygiene in health and illness.
2. Describe the effects of health and illness on the ability to perform self-care.
3. Discuss important subjective and objective areas of assessment when identifying self-care deficits and individualizing a plan for self-care.
4. Demonstrate basic hygiene skills such as bathing, shampooing hair, perineal care, foot care, back massage, toileting, and bed making.
5. Demonstrate proper care of eyes, ears, and teeth, including aids such as dentures, eyeglasses, contact lenses, and hearing aids.
6. List beneficial patient teaching for each of the four areas of self-care.

Self-care refers to a person's ability to perform primary care functions in the following four areas: bathing, feeding, toileting, and dressing without the help of others. **Hygiene** is the observance of health rules relating to these self-care activities. Because these activities are so basic, many people take them for granted. The ability to independently perform appropriate self-care and hygiene practices greatly enhances a person's health status and emotional well-being.

Nurses play a crucial role in helping patients learn or relearn self-care techniques. Because nurses focus on patients' responses to health and illness rather than on disease itself, helping patients gain or regain independence in self-care is one of the most important goals of nursing. When illness or injury interferes with the ability to perform self-care, nurses assist or perform tasks that patients cannot manage, or offer support to family members or other caregivers. The main focus, however, is to help patients achieve as much independence in self-care as possible.

ROUTINE SELF-CARE

Characteristics of Routine Self-Care

Self-care related to hygiene is the ability to bathe and perform normal grooming functions and to dress, feed, and toilet oneself.

BATHING AND HYGIENE

The skin is the first line of defense against microorganisms entering the body. Thus, keeping skin intact and healthy is important in preventing infection. Perspiration interacts with bacteria on the skin to cause body odor, which may be unpleasant, decrease patient comfort, promote bacterial growth, and increase the likelihood of skin breakdown. Regular bathing removes excess oil, perspiration, and bacteria from the surface of the skin. Acute care settings have transitioned from using a bath basin with soap and water for bathing to the use of prepackaged and premoistened, rinse free, disposable washcloths. Research demonstrates that daily bathing with chlorhexidine-impregnated washcloths significantly reduces the risk of acquiring multidrug-resistant organisms and the development of hospital-acquired bloodstream infections (Climo et al., 2013). Other research shows that global infection rates, as well as incidence of specific infections, such as ventilator-associated pneumonia (VAP) and catheter-associated urinary tract infections, were decreased in an intensive care unit when chlorhexidine was used during bathing instead of soap and water (Martínez-Reséndez et al., 2014).

 SAFETY ALERT
To ensure asepsis, always wash from clean areas to dirty areas.

Bathing also increases circulation (from the friction of a washcloth) and helps maintain muscle tone and joint mobility (from the movement of limbs during the bath). In addition, bathing promotes relaxation and comfort as well as gives most people a sense of well-being. A warm bath increases circulation by dilating blood vessels near the skin surface, allowing more blood to flow to the skin.

Bathing allows assessment of the patient's physical condition by noting injured areas, bruises, rashes, overall skin condition, or any other unusual signs, such as skin breakdown. Bathing also can promote psychosocial well-being by allowing conversation and interaction between the patient and nurse, facilitating a trusting, satisfying relationship.

Feet and Nail Care

Healthy feet are crucial in helping people stand and walk. Most people wash their feet along with the rest of the body when showering or bathing. Nails are trimmed as needed. There are many tiny bones, ligaments, and muscles in the foot, and comfortable, properly fitting shoes are essential to healthy feet. Shoes should accommodate the size and shape of the foot and should be large enough so that toenails do not rub on the shoes, causing skin breakdown or ingrown nails. Many people ignore their feet until problems occur. The feet are vulnerable to injury because of their susceptibility to skin breakdown. Seemingly, minor problems, such as ingrown nails, ill-fitting shoes, swollen feet, corns, or abrasions, can jeopardize mobility.

The patient's general condition and health habits affect the nails. Improper diet or fever may cause brittle, broken nails. Water and strong soaps or solutions dry the nails. Torn cuticles around the edges of the nail can be a source of infection. Dirt under the nails can spread infection. Daily care involves cleaning beneath the nails. Nails should be filed rather than cut. Convalescing patients may be able to care for their own nails.

Hair Care

Shampooing removes dirt and oil from the hair and scalp. It also increases scalp circulation. For most people, having their hair shampooed is relaxing. Clean hair makes patients feel good about their appearance and enhances feelings of self-worth. Daily hair brushing and combing help maintain healthy hair by distributing oil across the hair shafts and massaging the scalp. Neatly groomed hair also promotes a good self-image.

Oral Care

Proper care of teeth and gums helps prevent gum deterioration and tooth loss. Cavities in the enamel (**caries**) are caused by deposits of **plaque**, a substance primarily composed of bacteria and saliva that forms on teeth. Bacterial enzymes from plaque combine with carbohydrates from food and organic acids to ferment and break down enamel. Caries form more often when food and plaque remain on the teeth for long periods. When plaque remains on the teeth, it hardens into **tartar**, which cannot be removed by simple brushing; a professional must scrape it off with dental instruments.

Fluoride in small amounts strengthens teeth during their formation and helps prevent caries. Fluoride is added to most water treatment systems at the appropriate concentration—1.0 part per million. Adult caregivers may want to ask their dentist how to give children appropriate supplements of fluoride until the age of 14 years if their water system is not fluoridated. Brushing the teeth with a fluoride toothpaste twice daily, and additional fluoride measures for those at high risk, is recommended to reduce risk of dental caries in all age groups (Centers for Disease Control and Prevention [CDC], 2001).

Healthy gums are important because they provide support for the teeth. The gums are made up of the oral mucosa (**gingiva**), which covers the bone supporting the tooth; the alveolar bone, which forms sockets around the teeth; and the periodontal ligament, which joins the teeth to the bone. Inflammation in these tissues, called gingivitis or periodontitis, can be caused by local irritation from bacteria, plaque, tartar, and food impaction. Mechanical, chemical, or thermal extremes may also contribute to inflammation of the oral mucosa.

Proper oral hygiene includes daily brushing, flossing, and rinsing of the teeth as well as care of dentures or other appliances. Regular dental checkups ensure the health of the teeth and gums. Bacterial colonization of the mouth has been implicated in some nosocomial pneumonias, particularly in those patients requiring mechanical ventilation. The CDC (2004) recommends a comprehensive program of oropharyngeal cleaning and decontamination for patients at risk for developing healthcare-associated pneumonia. The optimal frequency for oral care is unresolved (Coffin et al., 2008).

Eye, Ear, and Nose Care

Under normal conditions, the eyes require little care because the lacrimal fluid bathes them continually, and the lids and lashes prevent foreign material from entering the eye. Special care may be needed for patients who wear glasses, contact lenses, or prostheses; those who have other visual problems; or those who use eye medications.

Ears need little attention, although the external ear should be cleaned while bathing. Patients wearing hearing aids may need special care. Some people may have excess accumulation of earwax (**cerumen**), which requires careful removal. Cotton-tipped applicators should not be used on the inner ear because they can force wax further into the ear canal.

Nostrils can be cleaned by gentle blowing with both nostrils open. Closing one nostril while blowing can force foreign material into the Eustachian tube or cause other damage to the inner canal.

FEEDING

The ability to feed oneself may be the most important self-care skill in terms of independence. Independence or even partial independence in decisions about food choices, and being able to feed oneself can be immensely gratifying and can enhance self-concept for people of all ages. Feeding requires the following activities:

- Desire to make food choices and eat
- Energy and muscular coordination to move food from the plate to the mouth
- Ability to safely chew and swallow

TOILETING

Normal toileting includes feeling the urge to void and defecate; moving to the toilet, commode, or bedpan; rearranging clothing; voiding or defecating; and effectively cleaning the perineal and rectal areas. Although these activities are usually done independently, assistance may be required during periods following injury, acute illness, or chronic debilitating conditions. The hospitalized patient often needs a toileting regimen that provides the use of the restroom or offering of a urinal, commode, or bedpan at set intervals.

Toileting is frequently associated with falls because factors such as altered mental status, cognitive impairment, an inability to rise without assistance, and altered elimination occur in many care settings (Williams, Szekendi, & Thomas, 2014). Tzeng (2010) reported that over 42% of falls in an acute care agency were toileting related, often involving getting out of bed or ambulating to the bathroom, slipping from the toilet or commode, or standing to use the urinal. Another study analyzing falls in an inpatient setting found that 35% of high harm fall events, defined as falls resulting in major injury, occurred when a patient was trying to get to the toilet or toileting. An additional 9% of high harm falls involved use of a commode (Williams et al., 2014).

DRESSING AND GROOMING

Dressing oneself includes being able to get clothes from the closet or drawers, put them on, manage fasteners (such as zippers and buttons), and put on socks and shoes. Routine grooming patterns include the daily brushing and combing of hair. Depending on cultural or personal preferences, some women wear makeup and many shave underarms and legs as a part of grooming. For men, shaving can be extremely important to their physical appearance and self-image. Personal preference and the amount of beard growth may dictate how often shaving is needed. Men with beards or mustaches may need to trim them periodically and remove spilled food particles from them.

Life Span Considerations

NEWBORN AND INFANT

Newborns participate in self-care only by crying and letting others know when they need to be fed or diapered. Parents or other caregivers supply breast milk or formula and perform the necessary bathing, dressing, and grooming. Newborns are born with sucking, rooting, and swallowing reflexes that allow them to ingest milk and liquids. They communicate hunger by crying and indicate satiety by falling asleep. By 3 to 4 months, infants begin to develop eye–hand coordination; by 5 to 6 months, many children have been introduced to solid foods. As gross motor function develops around 7 to 9 months, children can hold a spoon or drink from a cup with help. At 9 to 12 months, children can usually pick up finger food and feed themselves as well as hold and drink from a bottle.

Infants are totally dependent on caregivers for toileting. Urination may occur as frequently as 20 times a day. Stools also are frequent and can be soft or liquid. Frequent diaper changes, skin cleaning, and use of a zinc oxide barrier cream in cases of rash or excoriation will help maintain skin integrity by keeping the skin clean and dry (Oklahoma State Department of Health, 2014). Applied barrier paste should not be completely removed during diaper changes. Instead, wipe off any soiled paste, leaving the paste as intact as possible. Reapply paste as needed to any uncovered areas (Hockenberry & Wilson, 2011).

Changing an infant's diaper is relatively easy in early infancy and becomes more difficult as the child becomes more active.

SAFETY ALERT

During a diaper change, adults should never leave an infant unattended because the child could roll or fall.

TODDLER AND PRESCHOOLER

Self-care abilities increase considerably during this stage, particularly in feeding and toileting. As gross motor development increases, toddlers and preschoolers gain more mastery of their environment. Toddlers' eating patterns are erratic, but most can drink from a cup and use a spoon with some spilling. Small portions of easy-to-handle food are appropriate.

Many children achieve daytime bowel and bladder control between 2 and 3 years. They usually stay dry through the night by 4 years, but some children, especially boys may experience nocturnal enuresis until between 6 and 8 years of age, after which time intervention may be necessary (Hockenberry & Wilson, 2011).

Preschoolers can manage most aspects of bathing and grooming with some support, but children younger than 4 years need support with wiping after toileting, handwashing, dressing, and undressing.

During illness or stress, most children regress in their toileting and feeding habits. Children who are toilet trained may revert to wetting their pants or the bed at night. Children who can feed themselves may want to be fed or drink from a bottle again.

Regression is a common coping mechanism, especially for toddlers and preschoolers. During a stressful period, a child may revert from the most recently learned behavior to an earlier behavior that is more comfortable and satisfying. This "time-out" behavior permits the child to withdraw, conserve energy, and regain control. Regression is a normal reaction, and caregivers should understand and permit it.

CHILD AND ADOLESCENT

Although independent in self-care, some school-age children and adolescents may require reminders to bathe, brush their teeth, and change clothes regularly (Fig. 24-1). They still need direction and encouragement to eat healthy foods and use appropriate table skills. As children approach adolescence,

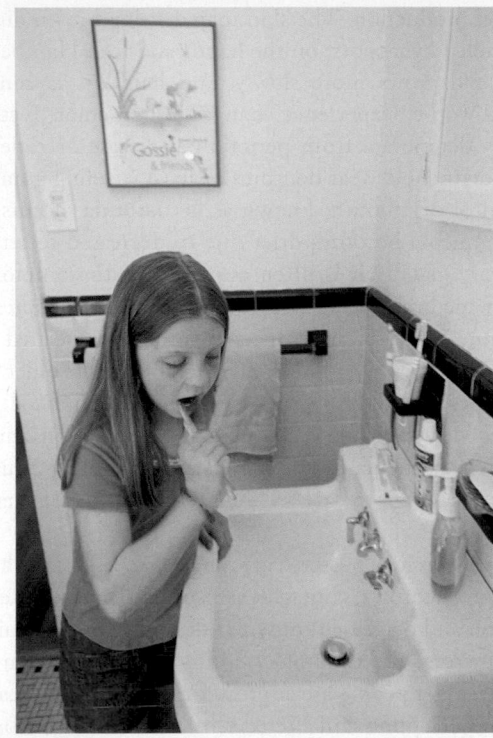

FIGURE 24-1 Using correct technique for brushing teeth helps prevent cavities.

self-care activities become more important as the body begins to mature and physiologic changes start to occur.

Hormonal changes stimulate the growth of axillary (underarm) and pubic hair during adolescence. Boys develop facial hair and may begin shaving. Sebaceous glands become more active and often produce excess oil on the skin. Many adolescents suffer minor skin problems and some experience acne, which can be psychologically devastating to the adolescent's self-image. Sweat glands become fully developed and functional, and adolescents may need to begin using a deodorant or antiperspirant. Daily bathing and shampooing become important to counteract body odor.

Along with these physiologic changes, adolescents undergo extreme psychological and emotional changes. Adolescence is a time of burgeoning independence and self-discovery during which teens begin to develop their own identities. Girls and boys become interested in looking attractive to others. Peer behavior heavily influences dressing and grooming practices because adolescents want others to accept them. Magazine advertisements and media celebrities also influence adolescents, who may copy such hairstyles, makeup, and fashions.

ADULT AND OLDER ADULT

Young and middle-aged adults usually perform self-care independently. By this stage, people have established self-care techniques that enhance their appearance and health. Busy lifestyles that include working and raising families may leave little time for self-care and health maintenance.

Special problems in self-care arise in older adults. Skin becomes drier, less elastic, and less resilient because glands reduce oil production. The skin may develop brown discolorations, called liver spots, on the hands and feet. Hair becomes thinner and grows more slowly, and hair loss is common. Men and women experience changes in hair color. Teeth may gradually deteriorate from periodontal disease or caries, and many older people wear dentures or have receding gums. The sensation of dry mouth, known as **xerostomia**, occurs when the oral mucosa becomes drier due to decreased secretion of the salivary glands. It is often associated with common prescription medications such as diuretics and antidepressants, autoimmune disease, and cancer treatment–associated toxicity (Cotrim, Zheng, & Baun, 2013). The feet of older adults require special attention because reduced peripheral blood flow makes the feet more vulnerable to infection and skin breakdown, particularly after trauma. Some older adults are not mobile enough to care for their feet and may be unable to inspect them easily.

Older adults may need to care for appliances such as hearing aids, glasses, dentures, contact lenses, or artificial eyes. Reduced circulation and decreased muscular flexibility may impair agility and increase the time older adults need to perform tasks. Generally, older people are at greater risk for injury because of decreased perception and altered sensation. This age group has the greatest number of people with physically disabling chronic diseases that affect self-care abilities.

Cultural Considerations

Individuals largely learn self-care routines and practices from the family and community. They form habits around the frequency of bathing, brushing teeth, and changing clothes or eating patterns based on the patterns of family members, friends, and peers within the community. Such preferences may vary widely among individuals and across cultures. For instance, many people in the United States do not feel clean unless they bathe daily and use a deodorant, but people from other countries may consider bathing once a week to be normal and do not feel the need to mask natural body odors. Some people are extremely sensitive regarding privacy during bathing; others are used to communal baths. Selected cultures and religions prohibit personal hygiene being provided by members of the opposite gender, especially males providing such care for females. There is a vast difference in family customs and personal preferences in relation to self-care practices.

FACTORS AFFECTING SELF-CARE

Many people take self-care activities for granted because self-care seems simple and is accomplished routinely throughout life. However, many factors influence how and if a person successfully performs these tasks of daily living.

Self-care requires adequate neuromuscular functioning, muscle strength, mobility, fine motor control, adequate energy, and intact sensory capabilities. Cognitive functioning, psychological factors (motivation, mental status), and sociocultural factors also influence the performance of self-care activities.

Environment

Lack of access to facilities or proper resources for self-care (e.g., poverty or poor living conditions) may affect a person's ability for adequate self-care. Homeless people, migrant workers, and the rural poor may not have access to adequate bathroom facilities or running water, which affects their ability to bathe and wash their clothes. Poverty may limit the resources available to purchase nutritional foods, restrict the quantity of food required to ensure a proper diet, or reduce access to the cooking facilities required to prepare meals.

People in wheelchairs may have problems finding wheelchair-accessible facilities. Bathrooms must be designed so that wheelchairs can move in and out of stalls. Sinks must be at the right height for a wheelchair-bound person. Home alterations may be necessary to allow the person to perform self-care. Legislation has helped to ensure free access to public facilities for disabled persons with mobility restrictions.

Motivation

Motivation can be a powerful factor in achieving independence in self-care. Even though a person is physically capable of self-care, he or she must be motivated to perform self-care and must believe that self-care is important. People with a positive self-image and those who perceive themselves as worthy of attention and care have a greater motivation to attend to self-care.

The nurse or caregiver must value and support the patient becoming as independent in self-care as possible. Efforts must be made to avoid doing "for" the person that which he or she can really do independently. Failing to allow this opportunity decreases patients' perceived control and autonomy and may unnecessarily increase dependency on caregivers. While the caregiver may provide unneeded assistance to save time and effort, allowing a patient to perform tasks independently to the fullest extent possible bolsters self-concept, and enables a person to increase independence and gain self-confidence.

Mental Health

Mental health issues can result in self-care deficits. The inability to perceive reality because of psychosis or schizophrenia may cause inattentiveness to the need for personal care. The patient with these diagnoses may be highly distractible with a short attention span. It can be challenging for these patients to concentrate on basic needs such as eating, grooming, and toileting. Signs of severe dysfunction include wearing inappropriate or no clothing in public or refusing to eat because of a fear of being poisoned.

Depressed people may lack the energy or interest to care for themselves and may be poorly groomed or poorly nourished. In addition, poor grooming may reduce self-esteem and feeling of self-worth, which in turn may further exacerbate feelings of depression. Depression may greatly complicate self-care problems in older people.

Cognitive Abilities

People with unimpaired cognitive and perceptive abilities are usually motivated to perform self-care. Those with limited or altered cognitive abilities may be unaware of the need for self-care, may not know appropriate methods of achieving it, or may be unable to assess what they can perform safely and independently.

Careful assessment of patients with a decreased level of consciousness or confusion due to injury or illness is necessary to determine how much assistance they will need with self-care activities. Although these patients may be physically capable of feeding, dressing, bathing, and toileting, they may not be alert enough to know when they should perform these activities and how to do them safely. Patients with minor deficits need to be reminded to provide self-care, but those with severe disabilities (such as severe head trauma or injuries) are often totally dependent on others and mechanical aids for self-care. Patients with cognitive deficits need careful and individual assessment, often provided by an occupational therapist (OT), to determine what self-care skills they can learn to accomplish independently or with assistance.

Energy

Energy must be available at the cellular level for muscle movement. Acute or chronic illness or injury can jeopardize independence in self-care by decreasing energy levels. Compromised respiratory or cardiac function reduces the body's ability to provide sufficient oxygen to the cells, limiting the patient's ability to participate in self-care without fatigue. Decreased energy and weakness can also result from disrupted diet, infection, disturbed gastrointestinal function, or fluid and electrolyte imbalance or be a response to a medication.

Acute Illness and Surgery

People who have been acutely ill or have undergone surgery often need assistance with self-care. The amount of help needed varies, depending on the course of illness or surgery, the patient's general health, and any sociocultural expectations. Analgesics, fluid and electrolyte imbalance, and hypoxemia can lead to drowsiness and confusion. Nausea and vomiting contribute to general malaise and may lessen motivation to perform self-care. Postoperatively, a temporary decrease in cellular oxygenation from anesthesia, hypovolemia, lowered hematocrit level, and atelectasis can lead to weakness. Weakness combined with postoperative pain also impedes self-care. Casts, splints,

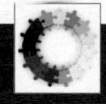

COLLABORATING WITH THE HEALTHCARE TEAM
Consulting With Occupational Therapy

You have just admitted Mr. Shannon, a 76-year-old man who had a right-sided cerebrovascular accident (CVA) 3 days ago, to the rehabilitation unit. The physician has written a referral for occupational therapy to see Mr. Shannon to assess his ability to perform activities of daily living (ADLs).

SITUATION: I see you received the occupational therapy referral for Mr. Shannon. He was transferred to the rehab unit this morning, and it is anticipated that he will be discharged within 5 days.

BACKGROUND: Mr. Shannon suffered an ischemic right CVA on October 4. His vital signs and neuro status have stabilized, but he has weakness on his left side and has been found trying to get out of bed by himself twice. He has a son and daughter, but neither one lives in the area. He is determined to return to his home and live independently.

ASSESSMENT: Mr. Shannon seems impulsive and may overestimate his abilities. His deficits may limit his ability to provide hygiene, grooming, and toileting independently, and he does not have anyone in his family who can provide daily assistance.

RECOMMENDATION: Please let me know the results of your assessment and any recommendations you have to individualize Mr. Shannon's plan so we can add it to his written plan of care. Let me know if occupational therapy will be providing AM care tomorrow so I can alert our nursing assistants.

CRITICAL THINKING CHALLENGE

- On a rehabilitation unit, many disciplines (medicine, nursing, occupational therapy, physical therapy, respiratory therapy, speech, social work) work together to individualize a plan to improve the patient's functional abilities. Reflect on how important interdisciplinary communication is to this process.
- Would a communication tool such as SBAR be helpful in structuring communication during interdisciplinary rounds or care conferences?
- On a rehabilitation unit, what is the primary role of the nurse in communicating with team members and the family? Is this role different from the nurse's role on a medical-surgical unit?

intravenous (IV) lines, incisions, urinary catheters, nasogastric tubes, surgical drains, and anxiety may limit mobility and interfere with the ability to perform activities of self-care.

Pain

Patients experiencing pain may be unable to care for themselves because their ability or willingness to move may be significantly curtailed. Reducing pain through the administration of analgesics prior to self-care may increase patient participation, but these medications also cause drowsiness and light-headedness, placing the patient at risk for falls. Therefore, patients taking such medications should be closely monitored to avoid falls during self-care activities. Bathing and positioning may offer some pain relief. Patients often find bathing or being bathed a relaxing experience and a distraction from pain.

Neuromuscular Function

Self-care activities, such as eating, getting to the toilet, and dressing, require a well-functioning neuromuscular system. To accomplish these tasks, the central nervous system sends messages to the peripheral nervous system and muscle fibers to coordinate the necessary fine and gross motor activities. Normal muscle strength and normal muscle contraction and relaxation are also necessary.

Fine motor control allows the person to have command of small, precise movements (usually of the hands). Fine motor control requires coordination of muscle groups to facilitate activities such as cutting food, opening a milk carton, buttoning a shirt, applying makeup, and wiping after toileting. Gross motor activity involves the coordinated movement of large muscle groups (e.g., climbing in and out of the bathtub, walking or driving to the grocery store, carrying groceries home, getting on and off the toilet). Normal alignment, awareness of the body's spatial position (**proprioception**), and balance are needed to coordinate these large motor movements.

Permanent neuromuscular impairment from conditions such as stroke, spinal cord injury, and some nervous system disorders (parkinsonism, cerebral palsy, myasthenia gravis, and muscular dystrophy) are serious threats to independent self-care. Many of these conditions produce muscle weakness, muscle atrophy, lack of coordination, spasticity, partial or total paralysis, and joint contractures that make walking, talking, eating, and using the extremities difficult or impossible. However, many people with these conditions progress to a high level of independence in self-care with the aid of appliances or other creative adaptations.

Sensory Deficits

People who suffer sensorimotor deficits because of surgery, injury, or infection may need assistance in self-care. Those who have lost some sight may need help with eating or getting to the bathroom. If the visual impairment is prolonged or permanent, the patient may learn to compensate by making adjustments to the environment. For example, placing food and utensils on a tray in a consistent manner makes it easier for a visually impaired person to eat independently. Furniture can be arranged so the person does not bump into objects or fall on the way to the bathroom.

Hearing-impaired people may have difficulty carrying out self-care activities because they cannot hear instructions or verbal cues. Devising alternate methods of cuing and communicating instructions can help them perform self-care independently.

ALTERED SELF-CARE

Nurses often encounter people with self-care deficits in both community and acute care settings. Problems with self-care range from short-term and simple to long-term and complex.

Manifestations of Altered Self-Care

POOR HYGIENE AND GROOMING

Often, the senses provide clues to poor hygiene, inadequate grooming, and problems with self-care. On visual inspection, the skin may be soiled, dry, or flaky or may have rashes and excoriated areas. Hair may be oily, unwashed, and uncombed. Nails may be dirty and broken. Clothes may be soiled, torn, or inappropriate for the weather or setting. Inspection of the mouth may reveal sores, caries, inflamed gums, plaque buildup, and missing or stained teeth. Mouth odor (**halitosis**) is common. Body odor may be present. The smell of urine or feces on soiled clothing may indicate difficulty in toileting.

INABILITY TO DEMONSTRATE SELF-CARE ACTIVITIES

Inability to demonstrate the gross and fine motor coordination needed for self-care activities indicates an impaired ability to perform these functions independently. The ability to get to the bathroom, bathe, dress, and eat is evidence of gross motor skills. The ability to fasten garments, apply makeup, open food containers, and cut food demonstrates fine motor skills. The patient should be able to perform self-care activities without cuing and without excessive fatigue.

VERBALIZATION OF RELUCTANCE TO PERFORM SELF-CARE

Listening to what the patient says provides important clues to self-care. If the patient expresses reluctance or fear to perform self-care activities, a deficit usually is present. Some patients may be reluctant to engage in self-care activities due to depression, altered cognition, or dependent personality. Some may be too fatigued, whereas others may be in too much pain or have fear of not performing the activity successfully. Lack of interest in self-care may be evident because the patient's value system does not attach significance to conventional grooming activities.

Recall the patient in the case scenario at the beginning of the chapter. Use the concept map (Fig. 24-2) to help understand and manage the patient's situation and to plan for his care.

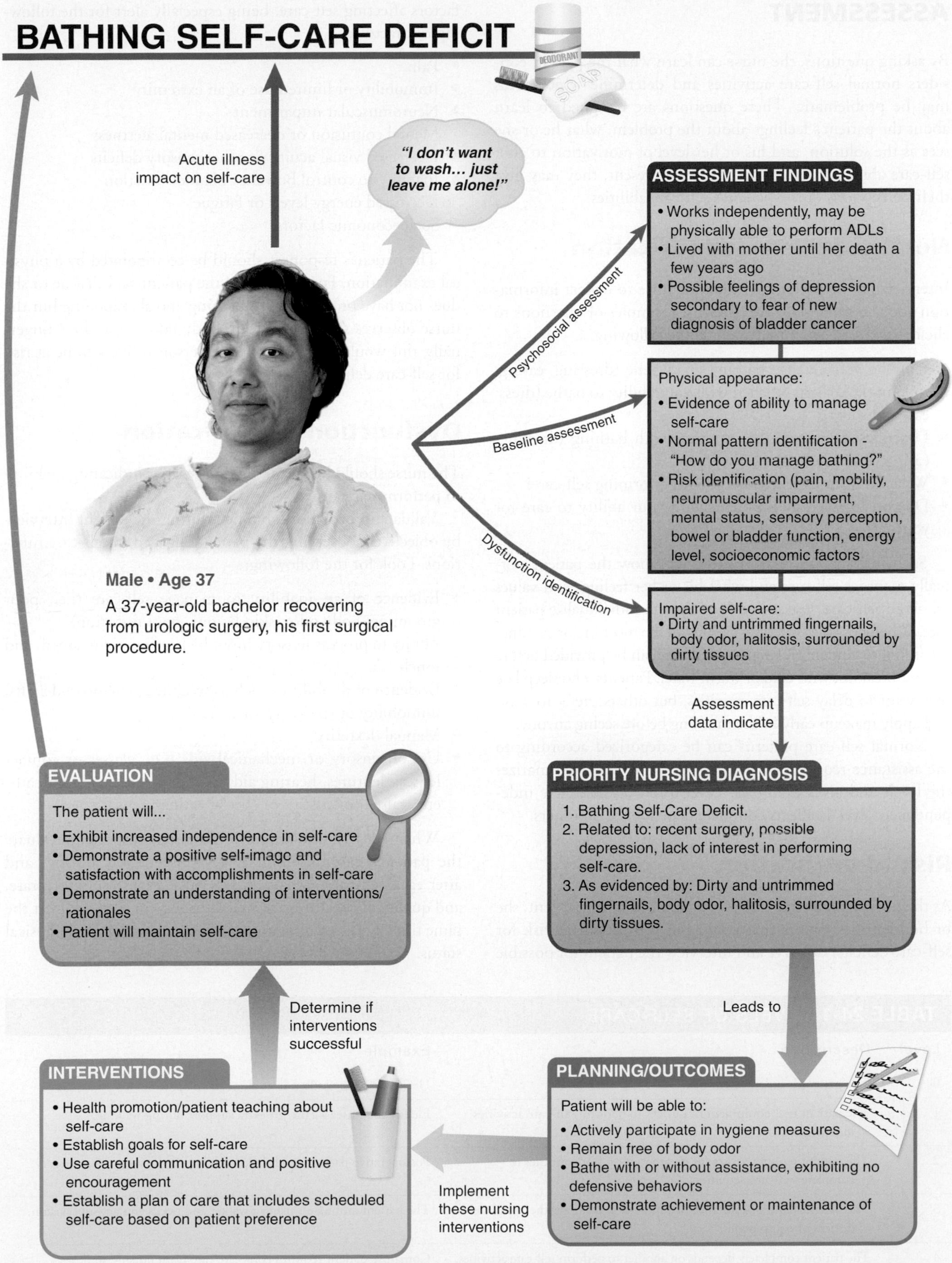

BATHING SELF-CARE DEFICIT

Acute illness
impact on self-care

"I don't want
to wash... just
leave me alone!"

Male • Age 37

A 37-year-old bachelor recovering
from urologic surgery, his first surgical
procedure.

ASSESSMENT FINDINGS

- Works independently, may be
  physically able to perform ADLs
- Lived with mother until her death a
  few years ago
- Possible feelings of depression
  secondary to fear of new
  diagnosis of bladder cancer

Physical appearance:
- Evidence of ability to manage
  self-care
- Normal pattern identification -
  "How do you manage bathing?"
- Risk identification (pain, mobility,
  neuromuscular impairment,
  mental status, sensory perception,
  bowel or bladder function, energy
  level, socioeconomic factors

Impaired self-care:
- Dirty and untrimmed fingernails,
  body odor, halitosis, surrounded by
  dirty tissues

Psychosocial assessment

Baseline assessment

Dysfunction identification

Assessment
data indicate

PRIORITY NURSING DIAGNOSIS

1. Bathing Self-Care Deficit.
2. Related to: recent surgery, possible
   depression, lack of interest in performing
   self-care.
3. As evidenced by: Dirty and untrimmed
   fingernails, body odor, halitosis, surrounded by
   dirty tissues.

Leads to

EVALUATION

The patient will...

- Exhibit increased independence in self-care
- Demonstrate a positive self-image and
  satisfaction with accomplishments in self-care
- Demonstrate an understanding of interventions/
  rationales
- Patient will maintain self-care

Determine if
interventions
successful

INTERVENTIONS

- Health promotion/patient teaching about
  self-care
- Establish goals for self-care
- Use careful communication and positive
  encouragement
- Establish a plan of care that includes scheduled
  self-care based on patient preference

Implement
these nursing
interventions

PLANNING/OUTCOMES

Patient will be able to:

- Actively participate in hygiene measures
- Remain free of body odor
- Bathe with or without assistance, exhibiting no
  defensive behaviors
- Demonstrate achievement or maintenance of
  self-care

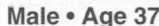

FIGURE 24-2 Concept map for hygiene.

ASSESSMENT

By asking questions, the nurse can learn what the patient considers normal self-care activities and determine which areas may be problematic. These questions are designed to learn about the patient's feelings about the problem, what he or she sees as the solution, and his or her level of motivation to alter self-care ability. If family members are present, they may give their perceptions of the patient's self-care abilities.

Normal Pattern Identification

Interviewing the patient permits the nurse to collect information about normal self-care patterns. Examples of questions to elicit this information may include the following:

- How do you manage bathing or hygiene (dressing, eating, toileting)? Are you satisfied with your ability to bathe (dress, eat, and toilet)?
- Describe any factors that interfere with bathing (dressing, eating, and toileting)?
- What are your expectations about performing self-care?
- Do you foresee any problems with your ability to care for yourself?

Such information helps to determine how the patient normally manages self-care and what his or her feelings and values are about self-care. Use such information to individualize patient care. When possible, schedule bathing in the morning or evening, according to patient preference. Oral care can be provided before or after breakfast with cold or warm water. Patients who sleep late may want to delay self-care activities, but others prefer to wash and apply makeup early in the morning before seeing anyone.

Normal self-care patterns can be categorized according to the assistance required by the patient; Table 24-1 summarizes the levels and gives examples. Level 0 reflects complete independence; level 4 reflects complete dependence on others.

Risk Identification

As the nurse gathers self-care information from the patient, she or he identifies factors that could put the patient at risk for self-care deficits. Observe and interview the patient for possible factors affecting self-care, being especially alert for the following risk factors:

- Pain
- Immobility or limited use of an extremity
- Neuromuscular impairment
- Mental confusion or decreased mental alertness
- Decreased visual acuity or other sensory deficits
- Inability to control bowel or bladder function
- Decreased energy levels or fatigue
- Socioeconomic factors

The patient's responses should be corroborated by a physical examination. For example, if the patient says that he or she does not have problems with bathing and shampooing but the nurse observes skin breakdown, body odors, and dirty fingernails, this would indicate that the person is likely to be at risk for self-care deficits.

Dysfunction Identification

The nurse should be familiar with the signs indicating inability to perform self-care.

Validate information obtained during the patient interview by objectively observing the patient engaged in self-care functions. Look for the following:

- Evidence of an inability to manage self-care (i.e., poor grooming, body odor, skin lesions, poor nutrition)
- Ability to process sensory input by hearing, sight, smell, and touch
- Evidence of disabilities such as weakness, cognitive deficits, immobility or spasticity, or mental lethargy
- Manual dexterity
- Use of sensory or mechanical aids (i.e., glasses or contact lenses, dentures, hearing aid, cane or walker, condom catheter, raised toilet seat, or special eating utensils)

When activity intolerance or fatigue is suspected, evaluate the patient's cardiopulmonary response before, during, and after each self-care activity. Assess pulse rate, respiratory rate, and quality of breathing, as well as change in skin color. At the same time, note any alterations in the patient's normal physical status.

TABLE 24-1 LEVELS OF SELF-CARE

Level	Description	Example
0	The patient is independent in self-care activities.	Healthy college student lives alone in an apartment.
1	The patient uses equipment or devices to perform self-care activities independently.	Elderly man uses a cane for extra support during walking.
2	The patient requires assistance or supervision from another to complete self-care activities.	Postoperative patient needs help with bathing first day after surgery.
3	The patient requires assistance or supervision from another and uses devices or equipment.	The patient ambulates using a walker and needs contact supervision.
4	The patient completely depends on another to perform self-care activities.	Comatose patient requires complete care from nursing staff.

THERAPEUTIC DIALOGUE: SELF-CARE

SCENE FOR THOUGHT

Rick Newfield, 32 years old, was admitted to the rehabilitation unit 2 days ago after being stabilized in the acute unit with a spinal cord injury. He had been in a motorcycle accident, and today is the first day the nurse is meeting him.

LESS EFFECTIVE

Nurse: Hi, Rick. I'm Sarah James, your nurse for the day shift. How's it going today?

Rick: Just great! How do you think, Sarah? I'm a paraplegic, or didn't you know this?! *(Sarcastic tone of voice, swearing, angry face, glaring eye contact.)*

Nurse: I knew. It sounds like you just found out. *(Calm tone and body language.)*

Rick: Yeah, they told me yesterday that all the testing they did showed that paralysis is permanent. I won't be able to walk, go to the bathroom by myself, have sex with my wife, run with my little boy, none of that. *(Turns his head to the wall.)*

Nurse: *(Sits in chair next to the bed.)* Pretty devastated by it all right now, aren't you?

Rick: Wouldn't you be? God, what a waste. *(Lies back in the bed.)*

Nurse: Sure, I'd be devastated, but I wouldn't be so hopeless. There's lots of stuff we can do to help.

Rick: Sure, sure, I know. The doc told me all about the physical therapy and that stuff. Big deal. I'll still be crippled! *(Angry face and voice.)*

Nurse: We don't use that word around here. It means you can't do anything, and there'll be lots you can do. Just hang tight for a bit, and you'll begin to see a big change in yourself. *(Smiles encouragingly.)*

Rick: Yeah, yeah. *(Turns face to the wall again.)*

Nurse: *(Notes his body language.)* I can see you'd rather be alone right now. I'll be back in a bit to check on the incision from the operation and to see if you need anything.

Rick: *(Cries quietly with his face to the wall.)*

MORE EFFECTIVE

Nurse: Hello, Rick. I'm Susan Jacobs, your nurse for the day shift. How's it going today?

Rick: Just great! How do you think, Susan? I'm a paraplegic, or didn't you know this?! *(Sarcastic tone of voice, swearing, angry face, glaring eye contact.)*

Nurse: I knew. It sounds like you just found out. *(Calm tone and body language.)*

Rick: Yeah, they told me yesterday that all the testing they did showed that paralysis is permanent. I won't be able to walk, go to the bathroom by myself, have sex with my wife, run with my little boy, none of that. *(Turns his head to the wall.)*

Nurse: *(Sits in chair next to the bed.)* Pretty devastated by it all right now, aren't you?

Rick: Wouldn't you be? God, what a waste. *(Lies back in the bed.)*

Nurse: *(Sits quietly and says nothing.)*

Rick: Well, what are you in here for? I'm not in pain; I don't need help with anything.

Nurse: You're saying you want to be left alone? *(Continues to sit quietly.)*

Rick: *(Looks up in surprise.)* What do you mean?

Nurse: It seems to me that you're pretty discouraged and angry right now and are having trouble seeing anything but the worst, and so you want to be left alone. Is that right?

Rick: *(Begins to cry quietly and tries to hide it.)* No. I want someone to tell me I'm going to be fine.

Nurse: You will be fine, but you'll be different.

Rick: Don't con me, whoever you are. I don't want to hear any of this.

Nurse: I wouldn't con you. You have lots of work to do on yourself, and some of it won't be easy. We'll be around to help and so will the other guys in the PG.

Rick: What's that?

Nurse: It's a group called the Paraplegia Group. They help each other through the rehab you all have to go through, like the bowel and bladder training, upper body strength exercises, wheelchair races, skin inspection rounds, how to have great sex, and so forth.

Rick: Sounds like fun. *(Said sarcastically but with a spark of interest.)*

(Continued)

THERAPEUTIC DIALOGUE: SELF-CARE (Continued)

Nurse: Jimmy Saguro will be by this afternoon to talk to you about it. Meanwhile, tell me about how your body really feels. You and I have to work together, too, you know. (Smiles.)

Rick: (Smiles back.)

CRITICAL THINKING CHALLENGE
- Name obstacles in the way of Rick's self-care abilities.
- Identify what Susan did that helped him change his perspective that he wouldn't be able to do anything.
- Identify what Sarah did that did not change his perspective.
- Critique timing and how each nurse used or ignored it.

To formulate realistic goals and interventions, the nurse must assess all resources available to the patient. This can mean internal resources (psychological, intellectual, and emotional factors) and external resources (living arrangements, finances). Box 24-1 lists external and internal resources that could be utilized to develop self-care goals and interventions for the patient.

NURSING DIAGNOSES

NANDA-International (NANDA-I, 2014) includes four nursing diagnoses involving self-care deficiencies, namely Bathing Self-Care Deficit, Dressing Self-Care Deficit, Feeding Self-Care Deficit, and Toileting Self-Care Deficit. Table 24-2

BOX 24-1 | Evaluating External and Internal Resources and Influences

External Resources

Housing
- Location, design, access by elevators/stairs, special equipment, kitchen and bathroom facilities, access to telephone, how many people share facilities
- Mobility around home
- Ability to shop for and prepare food
- Access to bathroom for self-care

Water
- Availability of water for drinking
- Hot water for bathing

Neighborhood
- Proximity of shops, hospitals/clinics, available transportation
- Ability to obtain groceries
- Access to healthcare and assistance
- Public transportation

Financial Resources
- Ability to purchase food and self-care products
- Ability to afford healthcare

Support Network and Community Resources
- Family and friends
- Support groups and volunteers such as Meals on Wheels
- Home healthcare

Government and Social Services
- Help with shopping, getting to doctors' appointments, self-care, and meal preparation

- Financial or material assistance for supplies and special equipment
- Assistance with medical bills and the costs of medications

Internal Resources

Inner Strength
Ability to handle physical, mental, and emotional work

Endurance
Stamina or "staying power" to cope with physical, mental, or emotional difficulties

Sensory Input
Ability to attend to and process environmental stimuli to provide a safe environment when attending to self-care needs

Cognitive Abilities
Amount and use of knowledge regarding self-care

Desire
Will or motivation to participate in self-care

Courage
Willingness to take risks and bear hardship to achieve self-care independence

Skills
Abilities regarding psychomotor functions, dexterity, or communication and interpersonal relationships

Communication
Ability to make others understand and make needs known

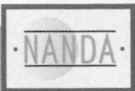

Table 24-2   SELECTED NANDA-I NURSING DIAGNOSES INVOLVING HYGIENE AND SELF-CARE

Nursing Dx	Related Factors	Dx Statement	NOC*	NIC†
Bathing Self-Care Deficit—inability to perform or complete bathing activities for oneself	Decreased strength or endurance, pain, perceptual/ cognitive impairment, neuromuscular problems, depression, lack of motivation	Bathing Self-Care Deficit R/T hemiparesis, right-sided neglect, and depression AEB inability to independently shower and wash parts of the body	Self-Care: Bathing, Adaptation to Physical Disability, Endurance, Coordinated Movement	Self-Care Assistance: Bathing, Perineal Care, Teaching: Foot Care, Energy Management, Environmental Management
Feeding Self-Care Deficit—impaired ability to perform or complete feeding activities for oneself	Decreased strength or endurance, pain, perceptual/ cognitive impairment, neuromuscular problems, depression, lack of motivation	Feeding Self-Care Deficit R/T right hemiparesis, dysphagia, depression, and poor fine motor coordination AEB inability to cut meat and gets food into mouth	Self-Care: Eating, Adaptation to Physical Disability, Nutritional Status: Food & Fluid Intake, Swallowing Status	Self-Care Assistance: Feeding, Swallowing Therapy, Nutrition Management, Fluid Management
Dressing/Self-Care Deficit—the impaired ability to perform or complete dressing activities for self	Weakness, tiredness, pain, lack of motivation, perceptual/ cognitive impairment, neuromuscular problems, environmental barriers	Dressing/ Self-Care Deficit R/T poor fine motor control, cognitive/perceptual problems, depression AEB inability to put clothing on lower body and fasten buttons	Joint Movement: Fingers, Client Satisfaction: Functional Assistance	Self-Care Assistance: Dressing
Toileting Self-Care Deficit—inability to perform or complete toileting activities	Impaired mobility and ability to transfer, neuromuscular impairment, perceptual cognitive impairment	Toileting Self-Care Deficit R/T hemiparesis, weakness, and depression AEB inability to transfer to toilet and manipulate clothing quickly	Self-Care: Toileting, Coordinated Movement, Transfer Performance	Self-Care Assistance: Toileting, Urinary Elimination Management, Dressing, Perineal Care, Bowel Management

Dx, diagnosis; R/T, related to; AEB, as evidenced by.

*From: Moorhead, S., Johnson, M., Maas, M., & Swanson, E. (2013). *Iowa outcomes project: Nursing Outcomes Classification (NOC) (5th ed.).* St. Louis, MO: C. V. Mosby.

†From: Bulecheck, G., Butcher, H., Dochterman, J., & Wagner, C. (2013). *Iowa intervention project: Nursing Interventions Classification (NIC)* (5th ed.). St. Louis, MO: Elsevier.

From: NANDA-International (NANDA-I), (2014). *Nursing diagnoses: Definitions and classification, 2015–2017.* West Sussex, England: Wiley-Blackwell.

provides examples of selected self-care nursing diagnoses with appropriate nursing interventions (Nursing Interventions Classification [NIC]) and nursing outcomes (Nursing Outcomes Classification [NOC]).

OUTCOME IDENTIFICATION AND PLANNING

The following may be included when formulating goals for patients with self-care deficits:

- The patient will actively participate in hygiene measures.
- The patient will safely increase level of independence in eating.
- The patient will actively participate in dressing.
- The patient will manage toileting with standby assistance.

In practice, outcomes are highly personalized and specific. Because of their personal nature, outcomes reflect the patient's wishes and the stage of illness. For example, a chronically ill person who looks at death as a release may have a different response to working toward independence than a person with a favorable prognosis for complete recovery.

IMPLEMENTATION

Health Promotion

Frequently, the nurse is able to stress the relationship between good hygiene, optimal health, and infection prevention. In preschools, nurses can teach young children the importance of proper hygiene after toileting and older children how to detect and prevent the transmission of lice. In prenatal classes, nurses can teach the expectant mother how to bathe a newborn and prevent scalp problems. In a community health center, the nurse can teach proper foot care to an aging population. Providing ongoing education about dental health and regular dental visits is also important.

Nurses can support community and governmental programs that promote self-care for high-risk groups. For example, promoting increased support for shelters and relief agencies so the homeless and mentally ill will have access to showers and bathroom facilities is one way a nurse might support self-care on a community level. Some communities with a large homeless population are encouraging the placement of portable toilets so that toileting can be private and sanitary. Free clinics need to be available and accessible to provide basic healthcare for those in need, such as foot care for patients with diabetes and dental care for low-income families.

Nursing Interventions for Altered Self-Care

The importance of increasing independence in self-care activities needs to be emphasized to all patients. Patient teaching about self-care is a cooperative venture that requires the nurse's knowledge, patience, and effort as well as the patient's motivation to learn and offer information regarding personal preference. Some people have an innate desire to be independent and therefore are very motivated to learn. Others are more inclined to be dependent and may be less willing to relearn how to care for themselves.

People with self-care deficits must often learn new skills. Rehabilitation involves many health team members working together to promote optimal functioning. Table 24-3 lists health team professionals who commonly work with patients to improve self-care abilities. The nurse is often the individual who coordinates care from multiple disciplines and facilitates clear interdisciplinary communication.

Work collaboratively with these healthcare professionals when teaching and reinforcing skills and nurturing the patient's desire for self-care independence. Careful assessment of patient values and interests often reveals motivating factors that might encourage a patient to achieve independence.

Careful patient communication is necessary when teaching or providing assistance with self-care. Explain techniques as simply as possible, avoiding technical or medical terms. Learning or relearning self-care skills takes time and effort. Be patient, supportive, and reassuring. Do not criticize the patient when he or she is unsuccessful. When the patient is successful, regardless of how small or insignificant the task may seem, give reinforcement and encouragement. Do not provide care for patients that they can perform for themselves; receiving unnecessary help fosters a helpless role and dependence upon a caregiver. Focus on patiently teaching toward the ultimate goal of independent self-care within physical or mental limitations.

Nurses can positively influence a patient's progression toward self-care through the use of an individualized,

TABLE 24-3	COLLABORATION TO PROMOTE SELF-CARE
Health Professional	Role
Registered nurse	Assesses abilities and deficits in self-care; coordinates and supports rehabilitation through individualized plan of care and patient teaching
Rehabilitation physician	Directs rehabilitation and medical management of patient enrolled in a rehabilitation program
Physical therapist	Assesses mobility, strengthens muscle groups, and works to improve motor function
Occupational therapist	Assesses ability to perform ADLs; helps patients relearn basic care skills and energy conservation methods
Social worker	Coordinates placement for patients unable to remain in the home; identifies community resources to help patient stay in the home despite deficits
Speech therapist	Evaluates swallowing and retrains safe eating for patients with deficits
Home health nurse	Provides follow-up and coordination for self-care deficits in the home by accessing community resources, teaching, and providing support and direct care

patient-centered plan of care. The core elements of patient-centered care include patient participation and involvement, the relationship between the patient and the healthcare professional, and the context in which care is delivered (Kitson, Marshall, Bassett, & Zeitz, 2013). Ultimately, the patient controls his or her participation in self-care. Positive interventions to encourage self-care include coaxing, rewarding, and educating. Providing assistance with self-care activities gives the nurse an opportunity to develop a trusting, satisfying relationship with the patient. Many of these activities, such as bathing, shampooing, and combing hair, are relaxing and soothing to the patient. Pleasant conversation during these activities can enhance feelings of comfort and self-worth. These activities give hospitalized or long-term care patients a chance to interact with people.

SCHEDULED CARE

Patients with self-care deficits may require assistance in performing hygiene. For the patient's comfort and the nurse's planning, specific types of hygienic care are given at regular intervals. Routine times for providing hygiene care in an inpatient setting may include early morning, morning, afternoon, and evening. Box 24-2 includes common hygiene measures provided.

Hygiene procedures should be individualized according to personal and cultural preferences. Changes in the inpatient setting challenge nurses' ability to provide complete hygiene care to all patients. In general, hospital stays are decreasing in length, patient acuity is increasing, and staffing ratios are

BOX 24-2 Scheduling Hygiene Care

Early Morning Care
Comfort Measures and Preparation for the Day
- Bedpan, urinal, or assistance to bathroom
- Preparation for diagnostic tests or early surgery
- Washing hands and face
- Oral care
- Preparation for breakfast

Morning Care (AM Care)
Hygiene and Grooming
- Bedpan, urinal, or assistance to bathroom
- Bath, shower, or bathing
- Back massage
- Hair care and shaving
- Oral care
- Care for feet and nails
- Dressing
- Bed linen change
- Straightening bedside unit
- Positioning (bed or chair)

Afternoon Care
After Tests, After Lunch, and Before Visitors
- Bedpan, urinal, or assistance to bathroom
- Washing hands and face
- Oral care
- Bed linens and repositioning if needed

Hour-of-Sleep (HS) Care
Comfort Measures and Bedtime
- Bedpan, urinal, or assistance to bathroom
- Washing hands and face
- Oral care
- Back massage
- Bed linens (change soiled linens, fluff pillow, pull out wrinkles)
- Bedclothes
- Straightening unit (place needed night objects within reach)

---

decreasing. Because of staffing and cost constraints, nurses frequently delegate hygiene measures to unlicensed assistive personnel. Specific guidelines for delegating are provided in hospital procedures. Delegating hygiene for a confused or aggressive patient is complex and should be done judiciously, especially if this intervention is to be therapeutic as well as cleansing. Aggression, agitation, and patient discomfort were decreased in individuals with cognitive impairment when bathing was individualized and patient centered (Sloane et al., 2004). Playing a patient's preferred music during personal care is one way to individualize care and to reduce resistance to care behaviors in patients with dementia (Konno, Kang, & Makimoto, 2014).

BATHING AND SKIN CARE

The usual time of day for bathing varies greatly. Some people prefer to bathe in the morning; others find that an evening bath is relaxing and promotes a good night's sleep. It is not always possible to satisfy personal preferences, but patients appreciate the opportunity to wash their face and hands in the morning before breakfast and before going to sleep at night. The frequency of bathing should be determined by the patient's needs rather than by adhering to a rigid bathing schedule that is set for the staff's convenience. Frequent bathing for the older patient can dry skin and contribute to breakdown. The comatose patient or the patient who has excessive body excretions or wound drainage requires bathing every day (sometimes more frequently) to avoid skin irritation, breakdown, and infection.

Some patients are anxious or embarrassed about needing assistance with bathing, grooming, dressing, and toileting.

Be sensitive to the patient's preferences and respect the patient's sense of privacy and modesty. To ensure privacy, curtains should be pulled around beds and doors closed during bathing or dressing. Some patients are sensitive to having these activities performed by someone of the opposite sex. Some healthcare workers may be uncomfortable providing intimate personal care for members of the opposite sex (Inoue, Chapman, & Wynaden, 2006). Agency policies should be clear, and there should be support available for staff. Patient preferences can be indicated on the plan of care so that appropriate assignments can be made whenever possible.

The environment of the long-term care facility should promote self-care independence. Have supplies or equipment available to help patients achieve a higher level of independence. For example, providing a walker to a patient who needs support in getting to the bathroom will help promote more independent self-care.

Methods of Bathing
There are several methods of bathing, depending on the patient's condition and abilities:

- Tub bath
- Stand-up shower
- Sit-down shower with shower chair
- Bed bath (partial or complete)
- Towel or bag bath
- Partial bath at a nearby sink or washbasin

When assessing the type of bath to use, take into account the patient's abilities and adopt the method that allows the most independence in self-care. Consider the patient's

TABLE 24-4 TYPES OF THERAPEUTIC BATHS

Type	Purpose	Nursing Considerations
Sitz bath	To cleanse, soothe, and reduce inflammation of perineal or vaginal area after childbirth, vaginal or rectal surgery, or from local irritation of hemorrhoids and fissures	Water temperature depends on the patient's condition and personal preference but is usually 99°–102°F.
Hot water bath	To relieve muscle spasms and soreness by total immersion	Water temperature should be 113°–114.8°F but may be individualized to patient condition and preference. Remember that older patients, those with sensory deficits, and those with slow or absent reflexes are at risk for burns with hot water. Be alert for vasodilation with resultant orthostatic blood pressure drop and for scalding of the skin.
Warm water bath	To cleanse, promote relaxation, and relieve tension	Adjust water temperature to patient's preference.
Cool water bath	To relieve muscle tension or decrease body temperature in febrile patients	Water should be tepid (98.68°F), not cold. Avoid chilling; shivering may increase body temperature.
Soaks	To soften and loosen secretions during dressing changes or to reduce pain and swelling or itching of inflamed or irritated skin	Medications or topical agents may be added to the water. Apply hot, warm, or cold water to an isolated body part.

energy level and need to conserve energy for other activities, surgical dressings or body parts that may need to be kept dry, the patient's preference, and the need to encourage independent self-care. Table 24-4 lists various types of therapeutic baths.

Some methods are easier for the patient to perform independently or with limited assistance. If the nurse provides the needed equipment, some patients can bathe themselves, although they may need assistance to reach their back and feet. Tub baths or showers are more effective for cleaning and ensuring that the skin is thoroughly rinsed, but they require more mobility and agility. **Procedure 24-1** gives steps in assisting with a bath or shower.

Many institutions provide commercially packaged disposable cloths, which generally remain in a warming unit until needed (Fig. 24-3). Commonly, each package contains six to eight cloths to avoid cross-contamination when washing different body parts. The cleansing solution is a rinse-free formulation. The benefits of these products include convenience for staff and decreased infection risk because research shows that used bath basins are reservoirs for bacteria and may be a source of transmission for hospital-acquired infections (Johnson, Lineweaver, & Maze, 2009).

Washing extremities from distal to proximal stimulates circulation and venous blood return. Preventing excess dryness is important for the skin's health and integrity. Inadequate fluid intake, too frequent bathing with soaps or detergents, use of hot water, and use of defatting solutions on the skin, such as alcohol, exacerbate dry skin. Use practices that reduce skin dryness, such as applying a moisturizer frequently, and teach the patient to do the same.

Some patients are weak or comatose and cannot bathe themselves. Their weakness may necessitate bathing the patient in bed. **Procedure 24-2** outlines steps for this. Often, bathing a patient is delegated to unlicensed assistive personnel.

Perineal Care

If the patient cannot perform adequate perineal and genital care (sometimes referred to as peri care), the nurse must do so. Cleaning the perineum and genitals is usually a part of the bath but may need to be done more frequently if the person is incontinent of urine or feces or has drainage from the perineal area. Nurses also should take the opportunity to teach proper perineal and genital care while bathing the patient.

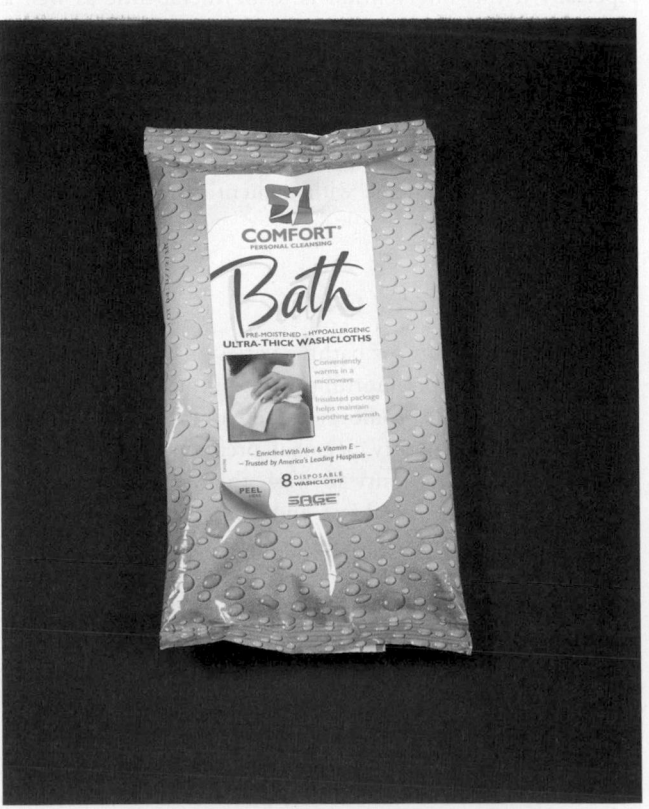

FIGURE 24-3 Disposable bathing cloths.

Perineal care for women involves cleansing the upper inner thighs, the labia majora, and the folds between the labia majora and minora (Fig. 24-4A).

For men, perineal care involves washing the upper inner thighs, penis, and scrotum; in uncircumcised men, the fore-skin is retracted and the glans penis washed (Fig. 24-4B). For both sexes, the buttocks are cleaned after the genitals, from a side-lying position.

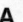

! SAFETY ALERT

Always wipe from front to back to avoid contaminating the vagina or urethra with microorganisms from the anus (Fig. 24-4A).

Perineal tissue is more sensitive than other skin, so avoid temperature extremes. Pouring water over the perineum while the patient sits on the toilet or a bedpan is a comfortable way

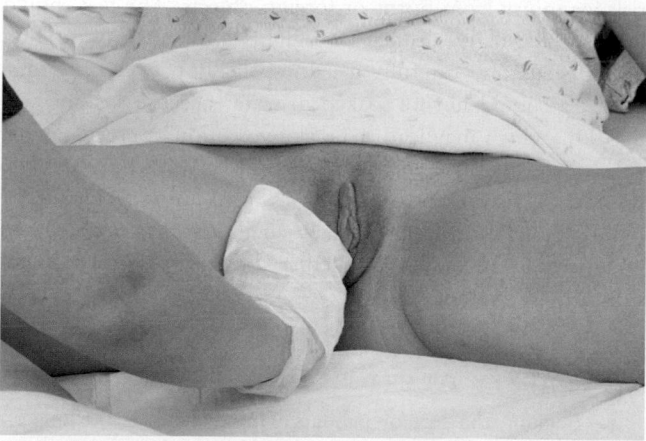

A

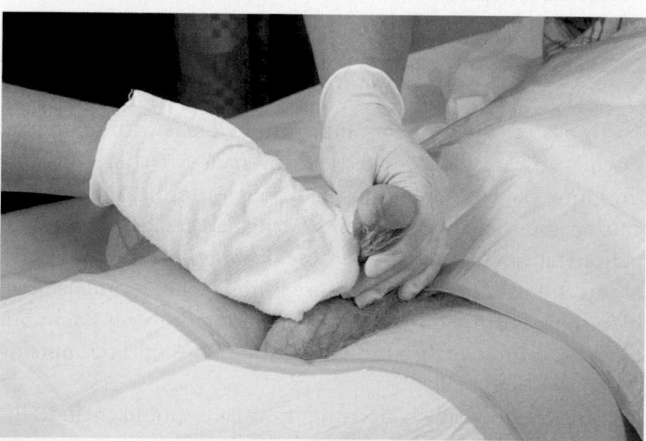

B

FIGURE 24-4 Perineal care. **A.** *Female:* Cleanse the area from the pubic area toward the anus in one stroke. Repeat several times, always using a clean area of the washcloth. **B.** *Male:* Cleanse the tip of the penis from the urethral meatus outward in a circular motion. Cleanse the penile shaft from the tip downward toward the scrotum.

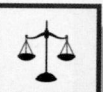

ETHICAL/LEGAL ISSUE

DELEGATION OF CARE TO UNLICENSED PERSONNEL

You are the registered nurse at a long-term care facility, supervising care for over 30 residents. You have one licensed practical nurse (LPN) and three nursing assistants working with you. When you are passing medications, you enter a room where a nursing assistant and the LPN are bathing a comatose patient. They are discussing their boyfriends and their social plans for the upcoming weekend. The patient is completely uncovered and appears cold. At no time do you observe them talking with the patient. They appear rough in the way they move and position him.

CRITICAL THINKING CHALLENGE

- Reflect on your own feelings as you encounter this situation, trying to identify those elements that make you feel uncomfortable.
- Identify underlying assumptions you have concerning what you think is ethically appropriate behavior.
- Refer to the Patient's Bill of Rights in Chapter 7. Do you believe this situation illustrates a breach of this contract?
- Think about three different ways to respond to this situation. Identify a possible approach that might bring about long-term changes in behavior that would improve the quality of care.

of rinsing for the patient who is between baths or cannot use a tub or shower. Certain people are at greater risk for infection and irritation of these areas, including patients with indwelling catheters; those with perineal, rectal, or lower urinary tract surgery; incontinent patients; and women after childbirth. Perineal care is routinely performed frequently by or for these patients.

Many patients can do their own perineal care with minimal assistance. When providing perineal care for a patient of the opposite sex, be direct and professional to help allay embarrassment. Always wear gloves during perineal care and while handling items that may contain exudate from the perineal area.

SITZ BATH

A sitz bath can be helpful in soaking a patient's pelvic area in warm water to decrease inflammation after childbirth or rectal surgery or to decrease the inflammation of hemorrhoids. Immersing only the pelvic region allows for application of local heat without widespread vasodilation that results when the entire body is placed in warm water. A sitz bath can be given in a special chair or tub in which the patient sits. A portable

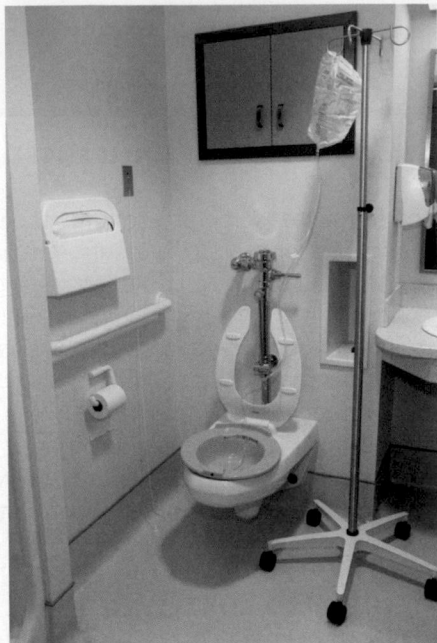

FIGURE 24–5 Disposable sitz bath.

device placed in the toilet also can be used and is illustrated in Figure 24-5. Warm water circulates gradually into the disposable device through tubing attached to a bag of warm water for approximately 20 minutes. Use a bath thermometer to monitor water temperature, and take care not to burn the patient. Start the temperature at 99°F (37°C) and gradually increase to a maximum of 102°F (39°C). If the water feels too warm on the patient's wrist, it is too hot for a sitz bath (Patient and Family Education, 2014).

BACK MASSAGE

Back massage is given to patients to enhance the blood supply to the skin and muscles, to promote comfort, and to promote relaxation. The degree of pressure used varies and should be determined by observing the patient's response or verbal cues. Benefits of massage include increased comfort, relaxation, and improved sleep. Additionally, research demonstrates that the therapeutic effects of massage on patients who have had a stroke include improvements in blood pressure and heart rate. These effects were seen to last up to 3 days after a massage (Mok & Woo, 2004). Similar results, along with a reduction in anxiety, were seen in patients with heart failure (Chen et al., 2013). To prevent pressure ulcers, massage is no longer indicated for high-risk patients because vigorous pressure over bony prominences can damage the underlying tissue (Wound, Ostomy, and Continence Nurses Society, 2010). A lubricant (cream or lotion) permits the hands to glide over the skin. Some young people with oily skin find that alcohol is a cooling and refreshing lubricant, but alcohol is drying to the skin and can cause cracking and skin breakdown in dehydrated patients and older adults.

If possible, have the patient assume a prone position for a backrub. If this is contraindicated or inconvenient, use a side-lying position. With an immobile patient, it may be effective to perform a partial backrub after turning him or her from one side to the other to enhance circulation to the lateral aspect of the hips. **Procedure 24-3** summarizes the back massage.

CARE OF FEET AND NAILS

Assess the appearance of the feet and nails to identify existing problems or patients at risk for foot or nail problems. Table 24-5 lists common foot problems and their causes and treatment.

The skin's color and temperature give clues to the quality of perfusion (blood flow). Cold feet with a dusky skin color may signal poor circulation. People with diabetes mellitus, older people, and patients with poor circulation are at special risk for foot difficulties; therefore, good foot care and education about self-care are essential. Combining teaching with care is a good way to motivate a person with foot problems to improve monitoring and become proficient with care.

Patients with diabetes require special attention to foot care. They have decreased sensation in the feet, placing them at great risk for injury from burns or foreign objects. The feet should be inspected daily, cleaned thoroughly with warm water and a mild soap, and carefully dried, especially between the toes. The feet should not be soaked in water because soaking will dry skin, which may lead to cracking. Lotion or cream can be applied to the tops and bottoms of the feet, but not between the toes. Moisture between the toes from improper drying or lotions can cause infection. The toenails are cut straight across and the edges are filed with an emery board (National Diabetes Education Program, 2012).

> ! **SAFETY ALERT**
> Soaking the feet of patients with diabetes is no longer encouraged because excessive moisture can increase dryness and contribute to skin breakdown (National Diabetes Education Program, 2012).

To protect the feet from injury, individuals with peripheral vascular disease should avoid cutting nails too short and cutting into calluses. Some hospital policies forbid nurses from cutting the toenails of patients with diabetes or people with peripheral vascular disease because healing is slow and the risk of infection after accidental injury is high. These patients often have thick, distorted toenails that are difficult to cut safely, but the nails can be safely filed. **Procedure 24-4** outlines nursing care of feet and nails.

Patient education concerning foot care should include the following:

- Inspect feet daily. You may need a mirror to visualize all areas.
- Never use razors, sharp instruments, or caustic solutions on your feet. Cut nails straight across and file the edges with an emery board, or just use a file.

TABLE 24-5 COMMON FOOT PROBLEMS

Type	Description	Possible Causes	Treatment
Calluses	Flattened thickening of epidermis, often on bottom or side of foot over a bony prominence	Tight shoes or inadequate padding in shoes	Soften by soaking in warm water and abrade with pumice stone.
Corns	Cone-shaped lesion (thickening of the epidermis) usually on the fourth or fifth toe over toe joint	Pressure from tight shoes	The patient should purchase and wear softer, better-fitting shoes or use foam protective pads. Apply keratolytic agents with salicylic acid to keratinous skin.
Plantar warts	Round or irregular, flattened by pressure, surrounded by cornified epithelium; often painful	Virus but may be worsened by inadequate circulation or pressure from tight shoes	Remove by curettage, freezing with solid carbon dioxide, or application of salicylic acid.
Bunions (hallax valgus)	Inflammation and thickening of bursa of the great toe joint; enlargement of joint and displacement of the toe	Heredity, degenerative bone and joint disease, and tight shoes or high heels	Surgical intervention may be needed, or the patient can achieve symptomatic relief by wearing shoes that are wide at the front.
Tinea pedis (athlete's foot)	Redness, scaling, and cracking of the skin especially between toes	Fungus, worsened by moist, unventilated environment	Apply antifungal powder or ointment. Change socks daily; wear 100% cotton socks to absorb moisture.
Ingrown nails	Inflammation, swelling, and tissue pain at edge of the nail	Improper nail trimming, poorly fitting shoes	Prevent by trimming nails straight across and wearing well-fitted shoes. Pain and inflammation are treated with anti-inflammatory agents. Surgical removal of the nail may be required.
Foot odor	Excessive foul odor of the feet	Possibly from fungal foot infections; exacerbated by hot, moist environment	Decrease excess moisture; use deodorant foot powders, 100% cotton socks, well-ventilated shoes.

- Avoid habits that will decrease circulation to your feet (smoking, garters, crossing legs).
- Notify your healthcare provider if you notice abnormal sores or drainage; pain; or changes in temperature, color, or sensation of the foot.
- Select sturdy, well-fitting footwear with a nonskid sole. Shop for shoes in the afternoon or evening when feet are often larger due to swelling. Break shoes in gradually, carefully observing for signs of irritation or skin breakdown.
- Do not walk barefoot.

HAIR CARE

Brushing and Combing

Patients who can brush and comb their hair should be given the equipment and encouraged to do so independently, but patients who cannot comb their own hair need assistance. Brushing hair massages the scalp, stimulates circulation, and facilitates oil distribution along the hair shaft more effectively than does combing. Patients with long hair who must spend an extended time in bed need a hairstyle that minimizes matting; combing the hair daily, braiding it, or tying it back helps. If tangles occur, hair is divided into small sections, brushed, then combed. Tightly curled hair usually requires a wide-toothed comb or a pick and a firm-bristled brush. Combing with the fingers can loosen tangles. A lubricating conditioner may be used to soften hair and avoid breakage.

Shampooing

Shampooing cleans the hair and scalp and helps get rid of excess oil. It promotes circulation to the scalp and provides a relaxing, soothing experience for the patient. Use this opportunity to inspect the hair for dandruff or lice. Shampooing can be done while the patient sits in a shower chair or in bed with a tray to drain the water. Protect the patient from fatigue and chilling during shampooing. **Procedure 24-5** summarizes steps in shampooing the hair of a bedridden patient. Many institutions are using a commercially prepared shampoo in a cap, which is kept in the warmer until needed for use. To use this product, the cap with the cleansing solution is placed on the patient's scalp. Long hair needs to be gathered up under the cap. The nurse or patient massages the cap to work the solution into the hair and scalp. The cap is removed, and the hair is blow dried or allowed to air-dry.

Lice

Infestation with lice is called **pediculosis**. Lice found on the hair of the head, eyebrows, eyelashes, and beard is known as pediculosis capitis. If found in body hair, it is called pediculosis corporis; if found in the hair in the perineal area, it is called pediculosis pubis.

Head and pubic lice attach their eggs, called nits, to hairs with a tenacious substance that makes them hard to remove. Nits, which may be visible with a light and magnifying glass, resemble shiny ovals. To the naked eye, they appear similar to dandruff. Lice live on the skin, and their bites cause itching. Inflamed bites can be seen along the hairline. Body lice suck blood from the skin and tend to live in the clothing, making them hard to detect. Clues to the presence of body lice are scratching and hemorrhagic lesions on the skin.

The usual over-the-counter treatment for pediculosis capitis is permethrin 1% lotion (Frankowski, Bocchini, & Council on School Health, 2010). It is applied to the scalp and hair, left in place for 10 minutes, and then rinsed out. The treatment is repeated 7 days later. The treatment of choice for pediculosis pubis is permethrin 1% or pyrethrins 0.3%/piperonyl butoxide 4% (Workowski & Berman, 2010). Clean clothing must be put on after treatment. Any clothing, towels, or bedding used by the infested person 2 to 3 days prior to treatment must be machine washed and dried using hot water (at least 130°F) and the hot dryer cycle (Global Health—Division of Parasitic Diseases and Malaria, 2013). People with whom the patient has had sexual or intimate contact should also be treated. There are increasing reports of resistance and difficulty successfully treating lice infestations (Gunning, Pippitt, Kiraly, & Sayler, 2013).

Dandruff

Dandruff is a chronic, diffuse scaling of the epidermis of the scalp. It is characterized by itching and flaking of whitish scales that are annoying and embarrassing. Frequent brushing and daily shampooing with a keratolytic shampoo may control the problem, but persistent, severe cases may require medical attention.

Hair Loss

Hair continually grows and renews itself. To promote healthy hair, chemical treatments and excessive heat (drying on the high setting, electric rollers) should be avoided. Cream rinses can be helpful in keeping hair untangled.

Male pattern baldness occurs in middle or older age but can appear much earlier in some men. Premature loss of hair can be stressful, affecting self-image and sexual identity. Treatment includes hairpieces, hair transplants, or drugs that stimulate hair growth.

Acute hair loss can occur due to stress, high fever, certain medications, general anesthesia, or childbirth. Most commonly, hair loss (**alopecia**) is caused by cancer treatment. Warn patients that hair loss may be gradual or sudden and may continue a few weeks after treatment is started. After treatment completion, hair usually regenerates; however, it may grow back a different color or texture. Support the patient during this time, help with selecting a hat, wig, or decorative scarf to wear, or refer the patient to a community agency, such as the American Cancer Society, for support.

Shaving

Shaving may make men feel good about their physical appearance. Most men without beards shave every day; receiving help with shaving can boost the patient's morale. To avoid cuts, soften the beard with warm towels before

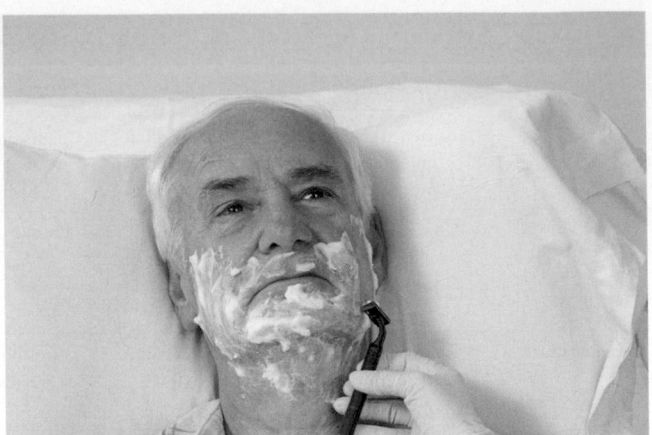

FIGURE 24-6 Shave in the direction of hair growth.

shaving. Use soap lather or shaving cream, pull the skin taut, and shave in the direction in which the hair grows to decrease irritation (Fig. 24-6). Men with decreased energy and impaired fine motor skills find it easier to use electric shavers. Urge patients at risk for excessive bleeding (i.e., those with thrombocytopenia, bleeding disorders, or those taking anticoagulants) to use an electric razor, rather than a safety razor, to avoid cuts. Men with beards or mustaches may need help trimming them and keeping them clean and free from food particles. Facial hair can be washed during a bath or shower. Mustaches or beards are shaved only at the patient's request.

Shaving underarm and leg hair is an important part of grooming for many women. In long-term care settings, nursing staff may perform this function for women who cannot do so independently. This is done using the same shaving technique as for men.

ORAL CARE

Brushing the teeth and cleansing and rinsing the mouth are comfort measures. Rinsing is soothing to the patient with a dry mouth. An unclean mouth can harbor bacteria that can multiply and cause other problems. **Procedure 24-6** gives guidelines for providing oral care.

The nurse or caregiver may need to assist or perform brushing and flossing for patients who are unable to do so. Encourage regular brushing and flossing, which aid in the prevention of caries and periodontal disease and help prevent tooth loss. Providing oral care also permits assessment of the oral cavity.

Brushing and Flossing

Encourage patients who can brush and floss independently to do so. If the patient cannot get out of bed to use the sink, provide the necessary equipment, including a basin for spitting.

For the patient who has difficulty grasping the small handle of an ordinary toothbrush, an electric toothbrush is useful because its larger handle is easier to grasp and requires less manipulation. The handle of a regular toothbrush can be built

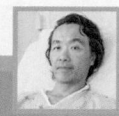

Hygiene and Self-Care PICO

You are the nurse taking care of the patient from the chapter-opening case scenario. He is finally showing some interest in his self-care. As you are setting him up to brush his teeth, he asks you if there is *really* a big difference between using a regular toothbrush and a powered one. In hopes of keeping up his interest in oral hygiene, you tell him that you will look to see if there is any evidence pointing to powered versus manual toothbrushes. You conduct your search by formulating a PICO statement: *Does using a powered toothbrush (compared to regular toothbrush) improve oral hygiene in adults?*

Population = Adults
Intervention = Using powered toothbrush
Comparison = Regular toothbrush
Outcome   = Improve oral hygiene

You discover a meta-analysis study that included 56 studies of randomized controlled trials with 5,068 participants. The evidence looked at both short-term and long-term effects on plaque and gingivitis. The results indicated that in the first 3 months alone, there was an 11% decrease in plaque when using a powered toothbrush. After the 3 months, the results continued to improve with showing a 21% reduction. Gingivitis improved by 6% within the first 3 months and jumped to an 11% after the 3 months.

After you share the results, your patient considers switching to a powered toothbrush when he gets home.

REFERENCE:

Yaacob, M., Worthington, H. V., Deacon, S. A., Deery, C., Walmsley, A. D., Robinson, P. G., & Glenny, A. M. (2014). Powered versus manual toothbrushing for oral health. *Cochrane Database of Systematic Reviews*, (6), CD002281. doi: 10.1002/14651858.CD002281.pub3.

up with tape, a bicycle handlebar grip, or a split rubber ball. Ultrasonic toothbrush systems, which require less manual dexterity, are effective for the older adult.

Flossing finishes the task of removing plaque and debris from between teeth. Waxed dental floss is used to avoid traumatizing the gums. The floss should be long enough so the patient can move easily from a frayed floss section to a new intact section of the floss.

Other oral hygiene measures include cleansing and moisturizing the oral mucosa by rinsing with water, saline, dilute mouthwash, or an antiseptic mouthwash.

Research indicates that bacterial colonization of the oropharyngeal tract plays a significant role in the development of nosocomial pneumonia, particularly in patients receiving mechanical ventilation (Garcia et al., 2009). Ventilator associated pneumonia (VAP) is the leading cause of death among hospital-acquired infections, with an attributable mortality rate of up to 40% and an estimated cost to United States hospitals of $1.03 billion to $1.5 billion per year (American Hospital Association [AHA], 2014). Reducing bacteria has been shown to reduce the potential for VAP development in mechanically ventilated patients (Munro, Grap, Jones, McClish, & Sessler, 2009); therefore, practices that reduce bacteria on the oral mucosa and reduce the potential for bacterial colonization in the upper respiratory tract are considered best practices. Implementing a routine oral care program as part of a ventilator-associated event bundle reduces VAP incidence (AHA, 2014). Evidence-based oral care includes twice daily teeth brushing, swabbing the oral cavity and teeth with an antiseptic

mouthwash at least every 2 to 4 hours, and rinsing with 0.12% chlorhexidine mouth wash at least daily (AHA, 2014).

Patients at risk for altered oral mucous membranes include patients who are NPO (nothing by mouth) or dehydrated, undergoing chemotherapy or radiation therapy for cancer treatment, experiencing trauma or surgery to the oral cavity, malnourished or immunosuppressed, or unable to perform oral care. Feeding tubes, nasogastric tubes, and constant breathing through the mouth can dry mucous membranes. High-risk patients should avoid alcohol-based products, such as commercial mouthwashes or lemon glycerin swabs, because these products are drying to tissues. Patients with drainage or lesions in the oral cavity and those who cannot take fluids by mouth may need rinsing and cleansing as often as every 2 hours. Such patients may have dry lips; a water-based lubricant or petroleum jelly can be applied.

Oral Care in the Unconscious Patient

Special oral care must be provided for patients who are unconscious. External surfaces of the teeth are brushed in the usual way. To protect fingers, place a padded tongue blade between the upper and lower teeth toward the back on one side. Then, using a soft-bristled toothbrush, clean the interior of the teeth and the chewing surfaces. The use of the toothbrush is superior to a foam swab at reducing total plaque. To prevent aspiration, use only small amounts of liquid. Use an oral suction device to remove the fluid safely. See the Variation for the Unconscious Patient section in **Procedure 24-6**.

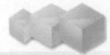

Concept Mastery Alert

When providing oral care for a patient who is unconscious, the patient should be positioned side-lying, with the head of the bed lowered. This position best minimizes the patient's risk of aspiration when providing oral care because it allows fluids to drain easily.

Denture Care

Determine if the patient wears dentures. If so, encouraging the patient to wear them improves eating, talking, and appearance and may boost the patient's self-image.

Dentures collect the same debris, plaque, and tartar as natural teeth. If the patient cannot care for the dentures, the nurse or caregiver needs to do so, using a brushing technique similar to that for natural teeth. Whenever possible, have the patient remove his or her own dentures. If the patient is unable, grasp dentures with a gauze pad to prevent slippage (Fig. 24-7A). Bottom dentures usually remove easily; upper dentures may need to be gently rocked forward or from side to side to break the vacuum seal created with the upper palate. A soft toothbrush is recommended because hard-bristled brushes can produce grooves in dentures. Soap and water is effective, although a mild commercial cleaning agent can be used. To protect dentures from breakage, keep them in a denture cup while carrying them to the sink, and store them in water in a covered container if not worn continuously (Fig. 24-7B). Label them with the patient's name to prevent loss.

The patient should rinse the mouth before reinserting the dentures. The gums and tongue can be cleaned with a soft brush when the dentures are out. Massaging the gums with a brush or thumb and forefinger helps to stimulate circulation and toughen the oral mucosa. Dentures should be removed at night to expose tissues to air.

 APPLY YOUR CRITICAL THINKING

Mrs. Ramirez, an 87-year-old patient, was admitted last evening after a fall in her home. Due to mobility problems and cognitive changes, she has neglected basic hygiene care in recent weeks. Mrs. Ramirez is confused. She has a sore right hip, but all x-rays have been negative for fractures. Develop a plan for providing hygiene care this morning including strategies for encouraging her participation.

Check your answer in Appendix B.

EYE CARE

Some patients need help with eye care, particularly those who have had eye surgery, injury, or infection or who are unconscious and have lost the blink reflex. Assessments include noting if the eyelids are edematous, crusted with secretions, or inflamed with sties and if the lacrimal ducts

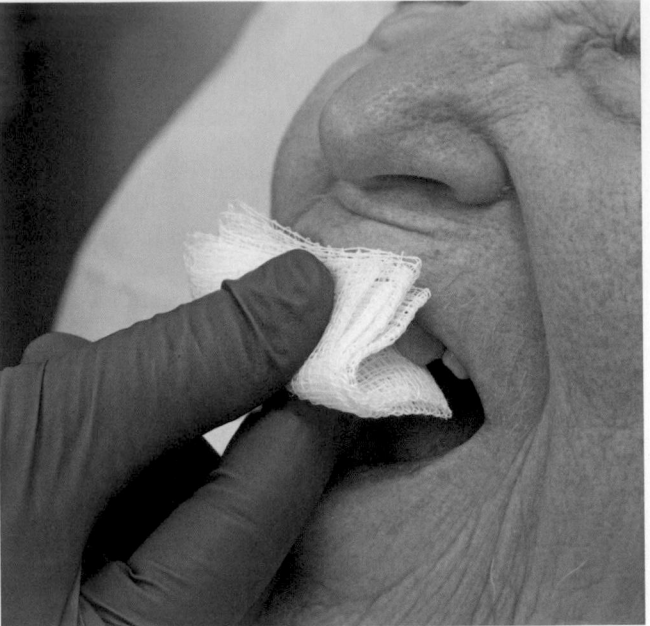

A

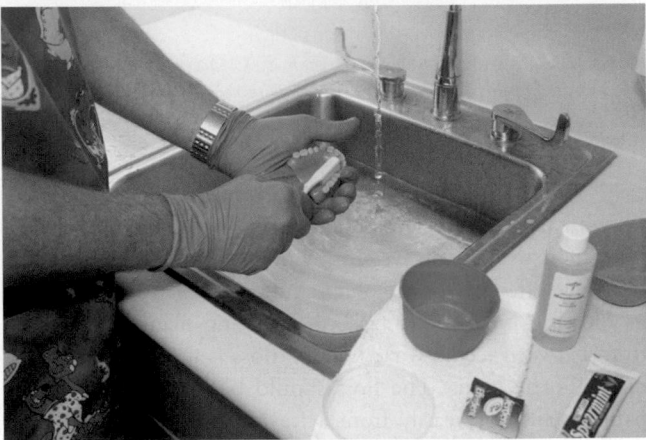

B

FIGURE 24-7 Denture care. **A.** Remove dentures from the mouth by gently rocking to break the seal. **B.** Place a towel in the sink and hold dentures firmly to prevent breakage. Brush as you would do with natural teeth.

are inflamed or tearing excessively. Examine the sclera for discoloration and the conjunctiva for inflammation and degree of redness.

Patients with eye inflammation, draining, or crusting need help cleaning these secretions from the eyes. Eyes should be cleaned with a washcloth or cotton ball soaked with saline or sterile water.

 SAFETY ALERT

Clean from the inside of the eye toward the outside. If infection is not suspected, use a different part of the washcloth for each eye; if infection is present, use a different cloth for each eye. This reduces the potential for spreading infection from one eye to the other.

Eyeglasses and Contact Lenses

Determine if a visual aid is used; locate the aid and encourage its use. Safeguarding these aids contributes to the patient's independence and safety.

Glasses should be cleaned daily, but patients do not often ask for this kind of help. Glass lenses can be washed under warm water, but plastic ones should be washed with a special cleaning solution. Both can be dried with facial tissue or a lens cloth. Store glasses in a secure place where the patient can reach them. Label them with the patient's name to prevent loss. When patients are too ill to manage these activities or have other physical limitations to self-care, the nurse must take responsibility for glasses. Include the glasses' location in the patient's record. This allows the nurse on the next shift, or in the next unit if the patient is transferred, to locate them.

Contact lenses are a common alternative to glasses. These concave plastic disks cover the pupil and float on the tear layer. Contact lenses may be hard, soft, or gas-permeable hard or soft. Hard lenses are made of rigid plastic that does not absorb air or liquid. Because they restrict oxygen supply to the cornea, their use is limited to 14 hours/day. Some kinds of soft lenses are worn during the day and removed at night, but others can be worn for as long as 14 to 30 days. Disposable contact lenses require less care.

Red conjunctiva, excess tearing, and burning pain are symptoms of lens over wear. Secretions and foreign matter (dust, pollen) accumulate under the lenses as they are worn. These substances are irritating to the eye and result in distorted vision and increased risk of infection. Because all contact lenses decrease the flow of oxygen to the cornea to some extent, corneal damage can occur if they are left in place for too long.

Contact lenses must be cleaned and disinfected after removal, using a method that is appropriate for the type of lens. If the patient cannot do so, the nurse must remove and care for the lenses. Refer to **Procedure 36-1**, Removing Contact Lenses. To care for soft lenses, a cleaning solution is used to loosen and remove film and debris. After cleaning, rinsing with a rinsing and disinfecting solution is necessary to remove loosened deposits. Then the lenses are covered with rinsing solution for storage. Before insertion, each lens is rinsed again with the rinsing solution to ensure removal of particulate matter. Recommended care may include a weekly heat or chemical lens cleaning to remove accumulated protein, lipids, and mucin. The patient should bring contact lens supplies from home.

❗ SAFETY ALERT

Do not use sterile saline commonly found in healthcare agencies to clean contact lenses. It may contain additives and may be inappropriate for use in contact lens care.

Artificial Eyes

Artificial eyes are made of glass or plastic. Some are permanent, while others require daily removal for cleaning. Most patients prefer to provide eye care for themselves; the nurse may need to assist by removing the artificial eye if there is evidence of inflammation, if the patient is scheduled for surgery, or if the patient is dependent due to injury or immobility.

To remove an artificial eye, pull down on the lower eyelid and exert slight pressure below the eyelid to overcome the suction holding the eye in place. To ease removal, a small bulb syringe may be used to create suction great enough to counteract the suction holding the eye in the socket. Clean the eye with saline, and store it in saline or water in a covered, labeled container. Clean the edges of the eye socket with saline or tap water and inspect for redness, swelling, or drainage. Because of the proximity of the eye to the sinuses and underlying brain tissue, infection in this area is of great concern. To reinsert the eye, pull down on the lower lid and slip the eye into the socket, lifting the upper lid to permit the eye to slide in.

Eye Care in the Unconscious Patient

Comatose patients are at risk for corneal ulceration, which can cause blindness. When the blink reflex is lost, eyes may remain open and become dry. To prevent these complications, eyes should be kept moist and protected from the air. Liquid tear solution (methylcellulose) or saline can be instilled to prevent drying, or the eyes can be closed and covered with a protective eye patch.

EAR CARE

Healthy ears require little care. Check the external ear for inflamed tissue, drainage, and discomfort. Clean the auricles with a washcloth-covered finger. Excessive cerumen can be removed with the twisted end of a clean washcloth while pulling down the auricle. If this method fails, irrigation may be necessary.

❗ SAFETY ALERT

Emphasize the danger of using bobby pins, cotton-tipped applicators, toothpicks, or other sharp objects to remove cerumen. Bobby pins or toothpicks can rupture the tympanic membrane or traumatize the ear canal; cotton-tipped applicators can push wax into the ear canal, which can cause blockage.

Care of Hearing Aids

A hearing aid is a sound-amplifying device powered by batteries. The aid contains a microphone that picks up sound waves, changes them into electric signals, and transmits them. It also includes an amplifier for magnifying sound, a receiver that transforms the electric signals back to sound energy, and an ear mold that channels the sound to the tympanic membrane. Box 24-3 describes several kinds of hearing aids.

BOX 24-3 Types of Hearing Aids

- **Behind-the-ear aid:** The most common type; fits over the ear. An ear mold fits into the ear, and the case containing the microphone, amplifier, receiver volume control, batteries, and T-coil/microphone (T/M) switch fits behind the ear.
- **In-the-ear aid:** The most compact; has all of the elements located in the ear mold.
- **Eyeglass aid:** Involves a hearing aid in one or both temples of a pair of eyeglasses. It functions similarly to the behind-the-ear aid, but the components are located in the temples of the glasses.
- **Body-type hearing aid:** Used for the most severe hearing losses. The case looks like a pocket-sized transistor radio and can be clipped into a pocket, undergarment, or harness. The case contains the microphone and amplifier and is connected to a receiver that snaps into an ear mold.

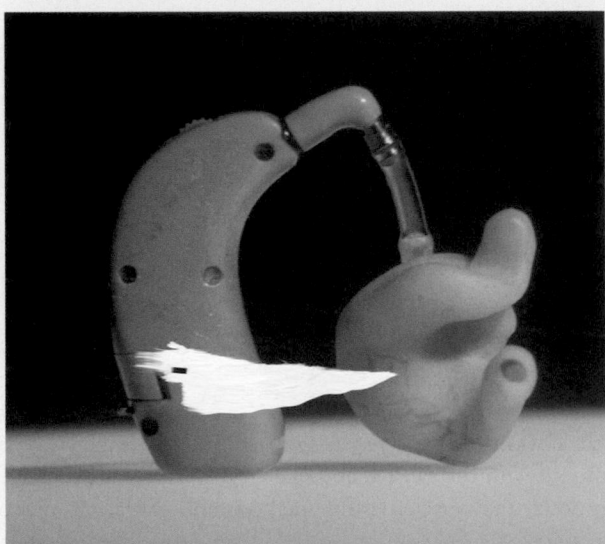

Behind-the-ear

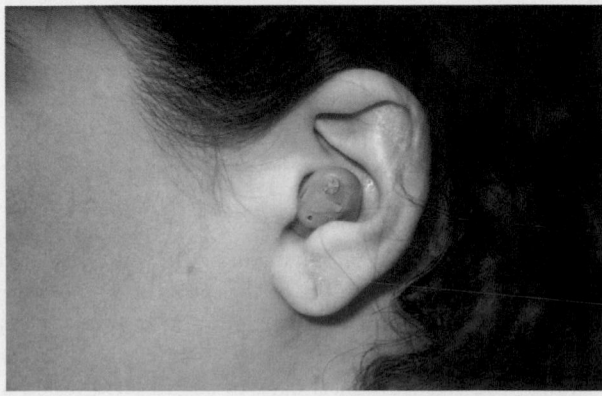

In-the-ear

Hearing aids are expensive and significant to their owners. These devices must be handled and stored safely. When not in use, they should be placed in a container labeled with the patient's name. Note the type of device, how well it functions, how the patient cares for it, and what problems the patient has with it. Care includes careful handling to prevent damage, appropriate use, cleaning of the ear mold, and replacement of dead batteries. To check the batteries, remove the hearing aid from the patient and turn volume slowly to high. A harsh whistling noise is apparent if batteries are in working order. No sound at all indicates that the batteries should be replaced.

When placing the hearing aid in the ear, turn off the device to protect the ear from any sudden loud sound. When the hearing aid is snugly in the ear canal, the volume can be adjusted as needed to promote hearing. See **Procedure 36-2**, Assisting an Adult With Inserting a Hearing Aid.

Although the hearing aid amplifies the sound of voices, it also amplifies background sounds. Patients may continue to have difficulty hearing, especially in a noisy setting. To foster optimal hearing, face the patient, speak slowly and clearly, and rephrase what is said if the patient does not understand. Some hearing-impaired people can lip-read; careful enunciation improves their ability to understand. The telephone company can provide phone amplification for the hearing impaired.

FEEDING

A self-care deficit involving feeding may occur in patients who are weak, fatigued, paralyzed, or have neuromuscular impairments. Assess the patient's feeding ability and the level of support he or she needs for eating. Plan assistance and institute a teaching program if appropriate for the needs of the patient. The nurse should understand that food and eating impact a patient's quality of life.

Often, patients are spoon fed in institutional settings even though they are capable of self-feeding if given adequate time. Verbal prompts and physical guiding can assist the cognitively impaired patient to maintain independent eating, which is preferred over spoon feeding. Quiet, soothing music is thought to be therapeutic during mealtime (Manthorpe & Watson, 2003). Because being fed represents a loss of control, allow the patient some way to participate if possible. This is true for people of all ages. Giving the patient a choice—for instance, the order in which food is eaten—may relieve some helpless feelings. Using bibs and mixing food together decrease the patient's dignity. Because the process of helping with eating is time-consuming, the patient may feel like a burden. The person feeding the patient must avoid reinforcing this belief and should always give the patient ample time to chew and swallow.

Interventions to meet feeding needs vary; Box 24-4 lists examples. Raise the head of the bed if the patient cannot sit on the side of the bed. A high sitting position is necessary to reduce the danger of choking and aspirating food. See **Procedure 29-2** for details on assisting an adult with feeding.

Meeting the Patient's Feeding Needs

- Check chart, computer, or diet list to determine if the patient has limitations on eating (e.g., fasting for laboratory tests or procedures).
- Check each tray for the patient's name and the type of diet. Verify the patient's name by checking the identification band.
- If pain is a factor limiting food intake or self-feeding ability, time analgesia to permit pain relief at mealtime.
- If fatigue is a problem, schedule a rest period before eating to enhance appetite and increase independence.
- Help the patient urinate or defecate before meals as needed.
- Enhance the setting. Turn on the lights if needed. Provide good ventilation. Remove room odors and disturbing sights such as soiled dressings.
- Prepare the patient for mealtime by finding dentures and eyeglasses, brushing teeth, rinsing mouth, and washing hands.
- Help the patient to a comfortable position for eating, usually sitting in high Fowler's position in the bed or a chair.
- Clear the overbed table of extraneous items.
- Determine how much help the patient needs (i.e., uncovering containers, removing food from plastic bags, buttering bread, cutting meat).
- Plan ahead so that you help patients who need assistance while their food is still hot. Have available a microwave oven to heat food that has cooled, provided the temperature is checked for safety to avoid burns.

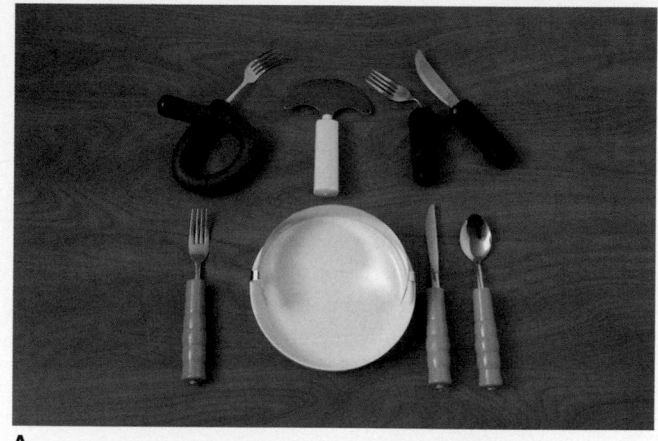

A

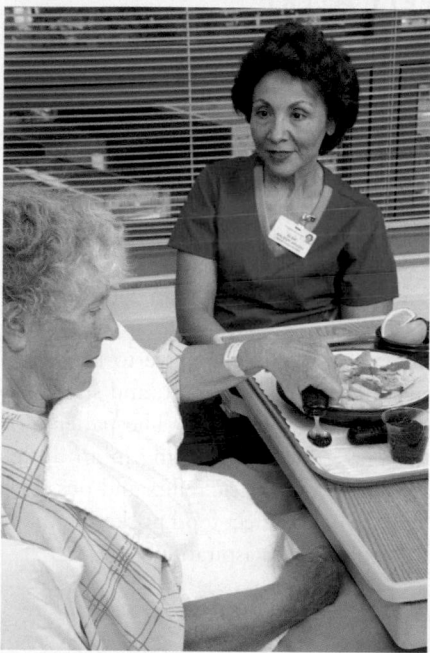

B

FIGURE 24-8 A. Assistive feeding devices. Such devices are made to be easy for patients to grasp and to get food on the utensils. **B.** Assistive feeding devices may be required for patients who are weak, fatigued, paralyzed, or have neuromuscular impairment.

Blind patients can be oriented to the location of food on a plate by referring to the numbers on a clock. The patient may use clockwise references to develop a mental map of the tray by doing a survey with his or her fingertips; then she or he can locate food by gently probing with a fork. Knowing what the foods are helps a blind person plan how best to eat them. For example, knowing that peas and mashed potatoes are on the plate enables a blind person to eat the peas more easily by pushing them against the mashed potatoes.

Many eating aids are available (Fig. 24-8). Plates with guards or lips help the patient get food onto a utensil. Utensil handles can be padded to make them easier to grasp. Cups with spouts help with drinking. Straws may help patients drink without dribbling.

For infant feeding, the atmosphere should be relaxed and free from interruptions. Parents or other relatives should feed children if possible. For feeding solid food, position the infant to face the feeder at eye level. Finger foods allow the older infant to participate in feeding before fine motor skills are developed sufficiently to enable self-feeding with utensils.

When the meal is finished, assess the food and fluid intake and record it if indicated. If a calorie count is ordered, record the precise amount of food eaten. Record any pertinent reaction to the meal. Make necessary adjustments in the diet and the plan of care.

Swallowing Impairment

Adequate swallowing is essential for safe eating. Difficulty swallowing (**dysphagia**) may occur as a result of disease or trauma to cranial nerves. Such damage commonly occurs after a CVA (stroke) or head injury. Diseases such as myasthenia gravis and muscular dystrophy, which cause muscle weakness, may also result in dysphagia. After a stroke or surgical removal of part of the larynx, the patient may need to relearn how to initiate swallowing. Consulting a speech therapist or an OT is important in planning a safe rehabilitation program.

To avoid food aspiration for the patient, carefully assess his or her ability to swallow before feeding. Elicit the gag reflex by stroking the inside of the throat with a tongue depressor. This will cause the pharynx to rise and constrict while the tongue retracts. If the nurse is not certain about the patient's ability to swallow, the patient should not receive any food or fluid by mouth until he or she is properly assessed. This may involve a swallowing evaluation from a speech therapist.

If a patient needs supervision during feeding, this should be indicated on the plan of care. If supervision is delegated to assistive personnel or family members, the nurse must assess that they understand proper feeding technique and emergency care in case of choking.

> ### ❗ SAFETY ALERT
> When there is any doubt as to the patient's ability to swallow, do not try to feed him or her until obtaining a swallowing evaluation.

Keep verbal cues short and simple while feeding. Multiple verbal cues or conversation during feeding may distract and confuse the patient who is cognitively impaired. Use directions like "chew" and "swallow" rather than complete sentences.

Food consistency is important for patients who have difficulty swallowing. Liquids may have to be thickened, while dry food, such as crackers and toast, and sticky food, such as peanut butter, should be avoided. The patient with dysphagia should not use straws. Remaining in an upright position after a meal will prevent gastric reflux and possible aspiration. Check the oral cavity to detect food pocketing that might have occurred and could lead to aspiration.

TOILETING

Patients often require assistance with toileting (i.e., walking to the bathroom or being placed on a bedpan). Needing help with these intimate functions may provoke discomfort for some patients, and nurses will find that a kind approach helps allay embarrassment. Helping patients to be as independent as possible with toileting is an important nursing intervention.

Exercise can affect **micturition** (urination) by strengthening abdominal and perineal muscles, which enhances voiding and helps prevent urinary incontinence. For example, Kegel exercises strengthen the muscles of the perineum. These exercises involve contracting the perineal muscles as if trying to stop micturition or by actually practicing stopping the urine stream while voiding.

Privacy and an opportunity to relax enhance most people's ability to urinate and defecate. If the patient is having difficulty urinating, the following may help:

- Turn on the bathroom water.
- Have the patient visualize his or her bathroom at home.
- Warm the bedpan.

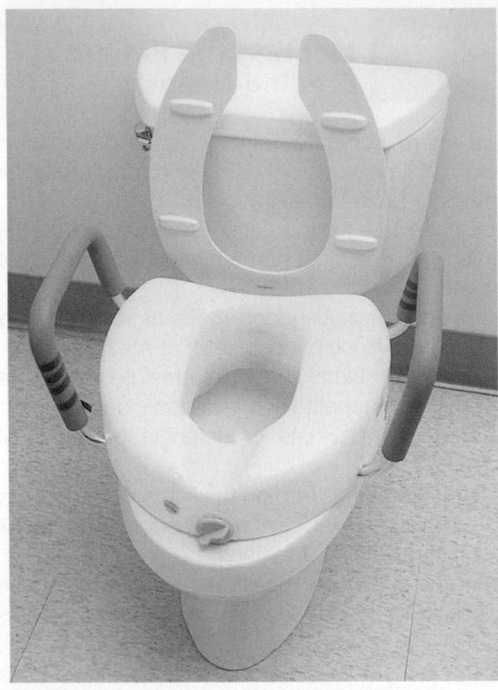

FIGURE 24-9 A raised toilet seat allows a patient who has had hip surgery to safely use the toilet.

- Have the patient assume a comfortable position (standing for men).
- Provide analgesia for pain.
- Pour warm water over the perineum.
- Always provide a call light within easy reach.

(For measures to assist with bowel elimination, see Chapter 33.)

Toilet

Ambulatory patients can walk to and from the bathroom, with assistance if needed, to use the toilet for voiding and defecation. For patients who have difficulty sitting down on and arising from a conventional-height toilet, a raised or elevated toilet seat can be attached so the patient has a decreased distance to lower and raise himself or herself (Fig. 24-9). A raised toilet seat may be required after some types of hip surgery. Based on previous assessment, provide necessary comfort measures for the patient using the bathroom, and give the opportunity for the patient to wash his or her hands when finished.

Bedside Commode

A bedside **commode** is a portable chair with a toilet seat and a waste receptacle beneath that can be emptied. In this way, a patient who cannot walk to the bathroom but can transfer out of bed to a chair can manage toileting. A commode chair can often be wheeled into the bathroom and placed over the toilet after the waste receptacle has been removed (Fig. 24-10). Many commodes have a flat seat that covers the toilet seat so that it can also be used as a chair. Commodes can be rented for use at home if access to the bathroom (e.g., upstairs) or ambulation is difficult during recovery from acute illness or during chronic illness. Before assisting the patient to the commode, assess

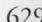

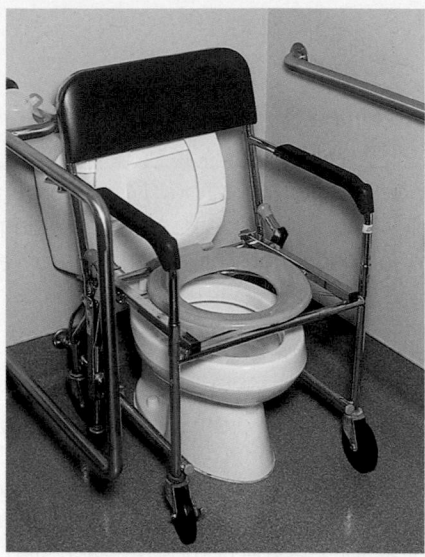

FIGURE 24-10 The commode chair can slide over the toilet when the waste receptacle is removed, allowing patients with mobility problems greater access to the privacy of a bathroom.

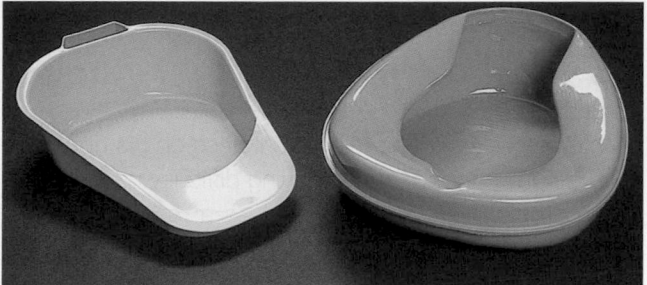

FIGURE 24-11 Two types of bedpans. The fracture bedpan (*left*). Regular bedpan (*right*).

whether or not the patient can safely transfer independently, and if not, determine the support that he or she needs. Always lock wheels on the commode when in use. If the patient is at risk for falling, the nurse or a caregiver should remain with the patient or stand just beyond to give privacy. Provide comfort measures as needed. Give support by providing water, a washcloth, and a towel for self-cleaning, or assist with the cleaning as necessary. Advise patients to notify nursing staff when the commode has been used so that urine measurement can be accurate and prompt cleaning of the receptacle can occur to prevent odor buildup.

Urinal

A male patient who is on strict bed rest or confined to bed due to weakness or disability may use a **urinal**, a plastic receptacle into which the penis can be placed to facilitate urinating without spilling. The urinal needs to be emptied frequently into a toilet to prevent spilling and odors. Assisting the patient to stand at the bedside when using the urinal is physiologically advantageous; however, if standing is contraindicated, the patient must be positioned in bed in as close to an upright position as feasible. In most instances, the patient is able to place and hold the urinal himself. If he is unable to do so, hold the urinal in place while the patient urinates or place the urinal and leave the patient alone for a few moments. When the patient has completed voiding, some patient may place the urinal on an overbed table. However, this should be avoided whenever possible because the patient's tray is placed on the same overbed table and the nurse uses the table for sterile procedures. Be sure to empty the urinal in a timely manner; this eliminates the possibility of anyone spilling its contents and avoids the embarrassment of having the patient's urine clearly visible at the bedside. Men who are incontinent may be more comfortable if the urinal is left in place. If this is done, the scrotum may be padded for protection. Provide

comfort measures as needed and a means of hand hygiene after voiding.

Bedpans

There are two types of bedpans: a regular bedpan has a high rim, and a fracture pan has a lower rim for patients who cannot raise their buttocks or in whom such movement is contraindicated (Fig. 24-11).

Many patients need help to get on a bedpan. Sitting is the most effective position for passing urine or stool. Some patients can use a bedpan alone if it is left on the bed or covered on a nearby chair; encourage such independence. A trapeze on the bed frame also facilitates moving on and off a bedpan. **Procedure 24-7** outlines bedpan use.

Condom Catheter

A **condom catheter** is a rubber sheath that fits over the penis and is connected to a collection tube and bag. A small bag that can be strapped to the leg may promote self-care for the ambulatory man. **Procedure 32-3**, Applying an External Catheter, outlines and illustrates application.

DRESSING

Dressing and undressing may consume a great deal of time and energy, which is why chronically and acutely ill people often become fatigued and discouraged. The following interventions are designed to help patients relearn dressing skills:

- Schedule dressing or undressing at a time when not fatigued, often in conjunction with bathing.
- Encourage the patient to use his or her eyeglasses or hearing aid.
- Provide analgesia if needed.
- Organize carefully and allow ample time.
- Lay clothes out in the order in which they will be needed, and place them within easy reach.
- Choose clothes that are loose and easy to get on and off and have wide sleeves and pant legs and front fasteners. Use Velcro closures when possible. Shoes should be slip-ons or have Velcro closures.
- Encourage the patient to help select clothes. Suggest street clothes, rather than night clothes, when appropriate.
- Assess the patient's ability to maintain balance.
- Ensure privacy (within the limits of safety).

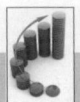

OUTCOME-BASED TEACHING PLANS

Mr. George is experiencing weakness on his right side (he is right-handed) and is having difficulty understanding complex verbal commands as a result of a CVA. He is on the rehabilitation unit and would like to be able to independently dress himself using aids before discharge.

OUTCOME

By the end of the second teaching session, patient can verbalize three energy-saving techniques to use while dressing.

STRATEGIES

- Ask Mr. George to describe his usual dressing routine.
- Evaluate this routine for areas that increase energy expenditure.
- Describe methods that Mr. George can use to reduce energy expenditure.
- Explain the connection between energy expenditure, Mr. George's condition, and success or failure with self-care.
- Develop a written list for Mr. George, identifying measures appropriate for him to use; incorporate use of pictures depicting those measures as necessary:
  - Stress sitting position while dressing.
  - Allow enough time for dressing.
  - Schedule dressing for times when Mr. George is well rested.
  - Use loose-fitting clothes with Velcro fasteners.
- Instruct Mr. George to refer to the list and review it periodically, especially before he dresses each day.
- Provide for assistive devices, such as a long-handled reacher to slip on shoes, as necessary.
- Instruct Mr. George how to use assistive devices.

OUTCOME

By third week of rehabilitation, Mr. George demonstrates ability to put on shoes and loose-fitting clothes with Velcro fasteners without complaints of fatigue or dyspnea.

STRATEGIES

- Tell Mr. George to sit on a chair next to the bed.
- Lay out clothes in the order that Mr. George will put them on.
- Place assistive devices, if used, within easy reach.
- Give simple, concise verbal cues. Provide positive reinforcement as Mr. George completes each step.
- Encourage use of assistive devices as appropriate.
- Assess Mr. George's fatigue level and dyspnea during dressing.
- Provide positive feedback and encouragement even for the smallest accomplishments.

EVALUATION

> 9/15/17: 15:00—Mr. George was able to successfully identify three energy-saving techniques to use while dressing. Mr. George states that he will "allow more time for dressing, sit on the bed to get dressed, and only wear loose clothing that is easy to get on and off." Mr. George has implemented these energy-saving techniques while dressing and has since demonstrated dressing that includes both shoes and clothing without the development of fatigue or dyspnea.
>
> —D. Callum, RN

- If the patient has cognitive deficits, develop a routine to lessen confusion, keep instructions clear and simple, and avoid distractions.
- Teach the use of aids for dressing (e.g., long-handled shoehorn, zipper pull, long-handled reacher [see Fig. 25-10], buttonhook). Help the patient adapt to available equipment to meet specific needs.

CARE OF UNIT ENVIRONMENT

The equipment and supplies that patients use while in the healthcare facility are kept in what is called the patient's unit. It is the responsibility of all nursing staff to make sure that the patient's environment stays tidy and free from clutter. A clean environment is conducive to healing and more pleasant for the patient and family. Before leaving the patient's room, scan to make sure that equipment is within reach. Ask the patient if he or she has everything that is needed. This prevents being called back multiple times and promotes the patient's sense that he or she is receiving attentive care.

Overbed tables, which provide a surface for eating and a work space for nurses, have wheels so that they can be maneuvered to fit over the bed or over a chair. Some overbed tables have a mirror and storage space for toilet articles.

Small stands are placed at the side of the bed to provide storage space for personal belongings, hygiene supplies, a small curved basin (emesis basin), bedpan, urinal, and toilet paper. A towel bar may be attached to the stand. Closet storage for belongings also is provided. A chair, either lightly padded and straight or upholstered, is often provided for the patient or visitors.

In most agencies, oxygen and suction outlets are installed on the wall above the bed, and a sphygmomanometer with a blood pressure cuff is mounted on the wall. The unit lighting usually includes diffuse, less intense lighting for general use; a brighter light for patient reading; and an intense light for use during procedures and when visualization is needed for diagnostic purposes.

A call light, with which the patient can summon the nurse, is attached to the bed. Often, the call light is part of the sound receiver for the television set and the television channel selector. A television and telephone are commonly available. Televisions are usually mounted on the wall to facilitate viewing from a Fowler's or flat position. Explain all equipment to the patient and family at the time of admission.

Beds

Hospital beds can be moved to various positions, providing comfort for the patient, therapy for some conditions, and proper body mechanics for the nurse. Scales are built into most beds so that patients can be weighed. Adjustments in height usually can be made. The high setting permits nurses to perform their tasks without back strain; the low setting permits patients to get in and out of bed easily and safely. Be familiar with prescribed bed positions (Box 24-5) and how to achieve them. Because bed controls are usually accessible to patients, teaching them how to use the bed enhances independence. Controls can be locked if certain positions are contraindicated. Other adjustments that can be made to the beds include the following:

- Elevating the head of the bed to permit eating and other activities
- Simultaneously elevating the head and foot of the bed to prevent sliding toward the feet
- Elevating the foot of the bed when the legs need to be placed above the level of the heart to reduce swelling
- Placing the head of the bed down and the feet up (Trendelenburg position) for certain medical procedures (central line placement)

Several kinds of beds are available for patients who cannot turn themselves and are at risk for skin breakdown; these are

---

BOX 24-5 Bed Positions

Flat position: Mattress is completely flat.
Fowler's position: The lower part of the bed is raised to the following positions:
- *Low Fowler's position:* Head of bed is elevated to semi-sitting position of 15 to 45 degrees. This position also is called semi-Fowler's position.
- *High Fowler's position:* Head and trunk are elevated to 80 to 90 degrees. This position also is called simply the Fowler's position.

Trendelenburg position: The entire bed is tilted with the head downward. This position is not often used because it causes blood pressure to rise and causes hypotension on return to the supine position.
Reverse Trendelenburg position: Entire bed is tilted with feet downward; prevents gastric reflux.

---

discussed in Chapter 30. Mattresses, usually constructed with inner springs to provide good support, are covered with a water- and soil-resistant material to permit cleaning. Most hospital mattresses have some level of pressure redistribution to prevent pressure ulcers, but patients at high risk for pressure ulcers may require specialized mattresses and beds. Side rails, a standard part of beds and stretchers, help prevent accidents caused by patients falling out of bed or getting out of bed by themselves when they are not able to do so safely. They also provide a support for patients to hold while moving in bed and getting up. When all side rails are up, they can be considered a restraint; therefore, it is important to be informed of and follow agency guidelines.

Footboards are boards of wood or plastic placed to form a right angle at the foot of the bed. They remove the weight of bedclothes from feet and legs and support the feet to prevent foot drop. Bed cradles also can remove the pressure of bedclothes from the feet and legs. For patients with injured or swollen legs, feet, or toes, removing the pressure of bedclothes may relieve pain and improve circulation.

Poles used for hanging IV fluid are located near the bedside in most units. A pole can be freestanding or inserted into a hole in the bed frame. IV containers can also be hung from hooks suspended from the ceiling.

Bed Making

A clean, dry, smooth bed enhances the patient's feeling of well-being. Linens are changed on the basis of patient need and cost rather than a fixed routine. Linens that are soiled, wet, or stained need to be changed. When deciding whether or not to change linens, consider the needs and demands of the patient as well. For instance, if the patient is tired and weak, it may be better to pad slightly damp or soiled areas immediately, then wait until the patient has rested to change the linens. Sometimes, straightening and tightening the sheets is adequate. **Procedure 24-8** presents guidelines regarding the making of occupied beds.

To conserve time and energy, pick up all the necessary linens from the linen supply before beginning. Make one side of the bed as completely as possible before moving to the other side. Lowering the head of the bed and raising the bed to a comfortable working height help prevent back strain.

> **SAFETY ALERT**
>
> Asepsis is an important consideration in bed making. Drainage onto used linens may contain microorganisms that can be transmitted through the air when the linens are shaken or through contact with the nurse's hands or clothing. Handle linens carefully without shaking them. Wear gloves during bed making if linen soiling is likely. Avoid touching your clothing, and wash your hands after handling soiled linens.

Put soiled linens immediately into a linen bag. Do not put soiled linens on the floor. If a linen bag is not available, slip a pillowcase over the back of a standard chair to provide a handy receptacle for dirty linens.

Provding Care for the Obese Patient

Special care and equipment is required for obese patients. A person is obese if his or her body mass index (BMI) is greater than 30 kg/m² and is classified as morbidly obese if the increased weight decreases his or her functional ability. Obese patients may be embarrassed and reluctant to ask for assistance with personal care activities. They may also fear hurting a staff person if they should fall or require greater assistance.

Morbidly obese individuals cannot easily get in and out of a standard tub and may have difficulty in a small confined shower. Overweight patients have skin folds that are prone to breakdown and irritation. The **pannus**, a large protuberant abdominal skin fold, provides a dark, moist environment where fungal infection can occur. Other areas that are prone to breakdown include under the breasts and the inner thighs. All skin folds need to be inspected, cleansed, and thoroughly dried at least daily. A hair dryer can be helpful in quickly drying the area. Report any red, raw areas so that they can be evaluated and treated if a fungal infection is present. Extra-large gowns are available but often have to be ordered. Bending over to perform foot care is often impossible for morbidly obese patients, and yet they have a higher incidence of diabetes and foot problems secondary to their increased weight. It is very challenging for the obese individual to clean after toileting, especially after a bowel movement. In the home environment, the obese individual often has figured out how to manage such functions, but independence in the hospital setting is more challenging. Depending on the patient's weight, special **bariatric equipment** may be required to hold the increased weight and provide additional support. Equipment such as bariatric beds, wheelchairs, walkers, commodes, and mechanical lifts may be required to provide safe care for obese individuals.

Home and Community Care

Many people who cannot provide for their own hygiene, feeding, grooming, and toileting live independently in the community. They often need family and community support to ensure adequate functioning. Rehabilitation promotes optimal return of function and ability to cope with limitations while supporting a range of independence.

Before the patient is discharged from the acute care facility, promote as much independence in self-care activities as possible. An OT often helps the patient develop self-care skills. Support this learning daily by incorporating the patient's new skills into the plan of care. Help the patient anticipate self-care problems at home, and develop a plan to successfully manage them.

BATHING

The home environment may need to be altered to enhance self-care. For most patients, getting in and out of the tub poses the greatest problem. In the bathtub or shower, hand grips and nonskid mats can protect against falls. Tub seats can be installed so that patients need not lower themselves down into the tub. Handheld shower appliances can also assist with bathing.

 SAFETY ALERT

The hot water tank thermostat should be set below 48°C (120°F) to avoid burns during bathing.

For the patient who cannot shower or use the bathtub, place a chair in the bathroom so he or she can sit and wash by the sink. This may help to conserve energy. Relatives may be available to visit on a weekly basis to supervise or assist with bathing, but often patients are embarrassed to ask relatives or friends to assist with this private, personal activity. If family support is inadequate, home health aides can visit on a routine basis to provide hygiene care.

SAFETY ALERT

Patients who suffer dizziness, weakness, or mental confusion should not be allowed to take stand-up showers. Obese patients may find it difficult to maneuver into and out of a bathtub and might risk falling. For these patients, using a shower chair (Fig. 24-12) may be more appropriate.

GROOMING AND DRESSING

Assess and promote independent grooming and dressing before discharge. Many patients do not dress in the hospital and are surprised at how draining this activity can be. Before discharge, encourage patients to practice dressing using energy-conserving measures. The patient should sit as much as possible while dressing and should wear clothes that are easy to put on and remove. Because they have no buttons or zippers, sweat suits are often ideal for patients who have difficulty with fine motor skills. Slip-on shoes with nonskid soles are easy to put on, and they

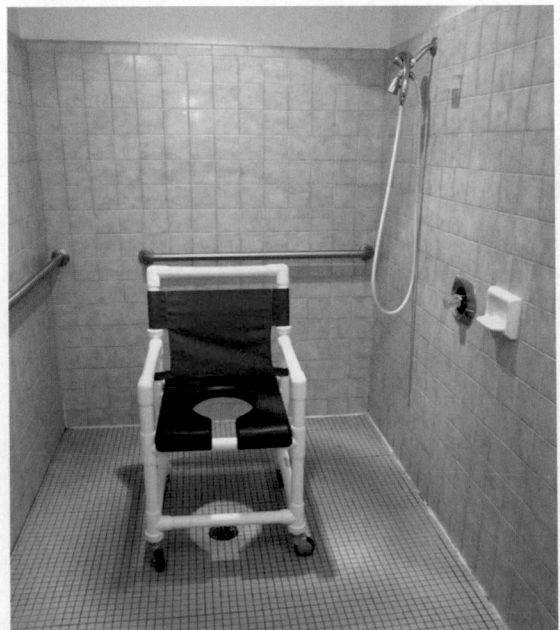

FIGURE 24-12 The use of a shower chair helps reduce the risk of falling.

help prevent falls. Assess the need for assistive devices to help promote independence with dressing. Discuss with the patient the psychological benefits of getting dressed, and work out a plan so that he or she can avoid wearing nightclothes during the day.

Hair care provides a morale boost to homebound patients. Hair should be washed before discharge for patients who might have difficulty with this task. Relatives can take the patient to a local hairdresser for shampoos and hair care, and some beauticians make house calls. Frequently, a family member or friend can be encouraged to provide such a service. Applying makeup is important to some women, and lack of coordination or energy can make this activity difficult.

FOOD PREPARATION AND EATING

Buying and preparing food can be exhausting, so provide instructions for easy, nutritious meals. Frozen foods have improved dramatically in recent years and can be nutritious. Relatives can package single-serving meals to be reheated. Stress safety with regard to food preparation (i.e., burn prevention). Meals on Wheels is a community service that provides hot, well-balanced meals for the homebound person for a nominal fee. Some supermarkets deliver groceries, and friends, relatives, and neighborhood young people can shop for the homebound person.

Eating can consume energy. Encourage rest before and after meals. Patients with fine motor impairment can use special utensils.

TOILETING

Self-care deficit in toileting is an important consideration, so assess home bathroom facilities before the patient is discharged. If the bathroom is on a different floor from the bedroom, the patient may need a bedside commode or a urinal. For the patient who is wheelchair bound, the bathroom doorway must be wide enough for the wheelchair and the bathroom must be large enough to permit the patient to transfer from the wheelchair to the toilet. Some patients find it difficult to lower themselves onto the toilet and get up again. A high-rise toilet seat can be helpful and is indicated for most patients after hip surgery. Hand grips next to the toilet also are helpful. Patients must be able to wipe themselves and wash their hands after toileting. Prepackaged towelettes can be an easy way to wash hands.

COORDINATION OF CARE

Patients with self-care deficits and inadequate support may not be able to manage safely at home and may require transfer to a skilled nursing facility (SNF) or long-term facility. When a patient is transferred to another healthcare agency, communicate his or her level of self-care function to that staff. Transfer forms usually have a place to indicate the patient's abilities in bathing, feeding, grooming, and toileting. Be specific so the patient can maintain optimum independence.

A designated caregiver may have to provide a significant amount of assistance for a patient with severe self-care deficit to remain in the community. The nurse's role expands to include teaching and support for the caregiver. Providing 24-hour care for a patient with severe self-care deficits can be emotionally and physically draining. Providing respite care options (e.g.,

adult day care) or support groups for the caregiver is important to prevent burnout and improve quality of life for all involved.

EVALUATION

Evaluation of self-care deficit is based on the outcome criteria developed from the patient's goals. Collect objective and subjective data from the patient to support successful attainment of patient outcomes. Ideally, the patient should exhibit increased independence in bathing, grooming, feeding, and toileting. The patient should be able to state any limitations regarding these activities and should feel comfortable accepting necessary assistance. The patient should demonstrate a positive self-image and satisfaction with accomplishments in self-care, despite limitations. The patient should be able to use adaptive devices to facilitate self-care, and self-care should occur without injury.

Examples of outcome criteria are listed below. Although some criteria may be important for more than one goal, they should be specific for each patient.

Goal

Patient will safely increase level of independence in eating.

POSSIBLE OUTCOME CRITERIA

- Before discharge, patient verbalizes a plan for managing food preparation at home.
- During next home visit, patient demonstrates using a cup with a built-up handle held with both hands to drink thick liquids.

Goal

Patient will participate in dressing herself.

POSSIBLE OUTCOME CRITERIA

- By the second week of rehabilitation, patient demonstrates the ability to put on a loose-fitting dress with Velcro fasteners.
- By the third week of rehabilitation, patient uses a long-handled reacher to put on slip-on shoes.
- Before discharge from the rehabilitation unit, patient expresses a positive approach to solving problems inherent in relearning to dress self.
- Before discharge, patient demonstrates dressing using energy conservation techniques.

Goal

Patient will manage toileting with standby assistance without cuing.

POSSIBLE OUTCOME CRITERIA

- Within 48 hours, patient is able to recognize and communicate the need to go to the toilet.
- Within 5 days, patient transfers from bed to wheelchair to toilet or from bed to commode with standby assistance.

PATIENT PLAN OF CARE
The Patient With Self-Care Deficit

NURSING DIAGNOSIS
Bathing Self-Care Deficit related to right-sided weakness manifested by impaired ability to wash most body parts.

PATIENT GOAL
Patient will willingly participate in hygiene measures.

PATIENT OUTCOME CRITERIA
- During care, patient states need for assistance to perform hygiene activities that he or she cannot perform alone.
- After teaching session, patient demonstrates bathing face, trunk, and upper extremities, with verbal cuing.
- Before discharge, patient verbalizes a realistic plan for bathing at home.

NURSING INTERVENTION	SCIENTIFIC RATIONALE
1. Assist the patient to identify self-care deficits in hygiene.	**1.** Maximum self-participation can occur with improved self-esteem.
2. Encourage the patient to communicate needs and concerns to nursing staff and significant others.	**2.** Communication reduces energy-consuming stressors such as isolation and worry.
3. Permit and encourage the patient to accept some dependency and verbalize feelings.	**3.** A degree of dependence is a necessary part of recovery and rehabilitation for most people.
4. Ensure safety through monitoring and assistance during bathing and hygiene activities.	**4.** Safety measures reduce the possibility of increased injury due to falls.
5. Schedule hygiene self-care 1 hour after breakfast when the patient feels rested.	**5.** Hygiene self-care is a tiring procedure; fatigue can produce confusion.
6. Lay out objects for hygiene care in the order to be used and place them within the patient's reach and sight. Don't hurry patient.	**6.** Nurse gives support and conserves his or her energy. Placement enables easy access with decreased energy expenditure.
7. Provide for the greatest amount of privacy possible.	**7.** Privacy enhances feeling of dignity and self-worth.
8. Assist the patient to use unaffected hand to wash self, comb hair, and brush teeth within the limits of ability.	**8.** Activities enhance independence while providing help and support as needed. Some programs encourage use of affected side to strengthen and regain function.
9. Evaluate frequently for indications of fatigue by checking pulse and respiratory rate.	**9.** Ability to sustain concentrated effort may be limited until endurance is developed.
10. Coordinate self-care rehabilitation with occupational and physical therapy and any other involved health professionals.	**10.** A team approach is often needed to develop an individualized plan. Represent patient in negotiations and making arrangements for care.

EVALUATION

9/17/17: 08:30—Mr. Shannon achieved his care goals by demonstrating willing participation in hygiene measures. He asked for assistance with some hygiene activities, demonstrating bathing of the upper body, and verbalized his bathing plan at home.

—D. Callum, RN

- Before discharge, patient states plan for managing toileting at home.
- By first home visit, patient demonstrates toileting in own bathroom without experiencing fatigue or activity intolerance.

KEY CONCEPTS

- Self-care and hygiene are important factors in promoting health.

- During stress or illness, children and adults often regress to a lower developmental level that requires more assistance with self-care.

- Factors affecting self-care include culture, values and beliefs, environment, motivation, emotional status, cognitive abilities, energy, acute illness or surgery, pain, and motor deficits.

- Although the primary reason for bathing is to enhance cleanliness, warm water and friction enhance circulation, and movement during bathing provides an opportunity for range of motion. The experience also can be relaxing and promote a positive nurse–patient relationship.

- Care of the eyes, ears, and teeth is important in maintaining optimal health. Care must be taken to avoid damage or loss of glasses, contact lenses, hearing aids, or dentures because they are significant to the patient's functioning and expensive to replace.

- Identification of inability to self-feed is important to promote nutrition and prevent possible aspiration.

- Providing a clean environment and a smooth, wrinkle-free bed helps promote comfort.

PRACTICING FOR THE NCLEX

CHECK YOUR ANSWERS IN APPENDIX A.

1. A nurse is providing oral care to an elderly patient with dentures who has a restricted diet and is receiving nothing by mouth (NPO status). Which of the following is an appropriate action?
   a. Brush dentures and remaining teeth in mouth using toothbrush or swab.
   b. Position the patient in Trendelenburg or side-lying position.
   c. Place your finger in the mouth of the unconscious patient to open the mouth.
   d. Provide oral care daily and as needed to prevent nosocomial pneumonia.

2. The nurse is caring for a patient with hemiplegia following a severe cerebrovascular. In order to promote independence in self-care, which of the following actions would be appropriate? Select all that apply:
   a. Place basin and washcloth on patient's nonaffected side
   b. Assist the patient to bedside commode for toileting
   c. Perform oral care daily
   d. Contact occupational therapy to attain specialized utensils for meals

3. An elderly patient is being seen in relation to her inability to perform self-care. Which of the following should be done first?
   a. Assess feet for poor circulation and signs of infection.
   b. Provide nail care to feet since the patient is unable to perform independently.
   c. Develop plan of care to foster independence in self-care.
   d. Evaluate support system available to assist with self-care upon discharge.

4. Which of the following patients would be most at risk for a self-care deficit?
   a. Toddler who refuses to bathe more than once a week
   b. Patient receiving chemotherapy and experiencing frequent vomiting/diarrhea
   c. Stroke patient who is alert and oriented ×3 and lacks mobility impairment
   d. Surgical patient with pain 5/10

5. In visiting an elderly female patient at home, the nurse notes a smell of urine and that the patient is always in the same chair with her walker parked next to her. Which of the following questions would be appropriate?
   a. "Are you using the bathroom as needed?"
   b. "Do you feel like you are managing okay on your own at home?"
   c. "Are you satisfied with your ability to bathe and toilet yourself?"
   d. "Do you understand that you should be cleaning yourself more thoroughly?"

6. A nurse is developing a plan of care for a patient with failure to thrive following the death of a spouse. Which of the following may be contributing factors? Select all that apply:
   a. Caregiver role strain
   b. Ineffective coping
   c. Powerlessness
   d. Impaired skin integrity

7. The nurse is providing perineal care to an unconscious female patient. Which of the following is the most important step?
   a. Wash front to back to avoid contamination.
   b. Avoid temperature extremes since the perineal tissue is extremely sensitive.
   c. Include cleansing the folds between the legs and labia.
   d. Turn the patient on the side to avoid aspiration.

8. A nurse is interviewing an elderly woman with moderate Alzheimer dementia. What activities of daily living (ADLs) would she most likely be able to do independently?
   a. Dressing
   b. Bathing
   c. Toileting
   d. Feeding

9. The nurse is assessing the influence of external versus internal factors with a patient admitted with failure to thrive and malnutrition. Which of the following would be external factors that may affect this patient's health? Select all that apply:

a. Proximity of grocery stores

b. Ability to prepare food

c. Motivation to perform self-care

d. Support network

10. A nurse is providing skin care for a morbidly obese patient. Which of the following interventions are essential to prevent skin breakdown in bariatric patients? Select all that apply:

a. Elevating heels from bed

b. Drying beneath the pannus

c. Assessing behind ears when using a nasal cannula

d. Cleansing between thighs

REFERENCES

American Hospital Association (AHA), Partnership for Patients, & Health Research and Educational Trust. (2014). *Ventilator Associated Events (VAE) Change Package: Preventing Harm from VTE.* Retrieved from http://www.hret-hen.org/index.php?option=com_content&view=article&id=10&Itemid=134

Bulecheck, G., Butcher, H., Dochterman, J., & Wagner, C. (2013). *Nursing interventions classification (NIC)* (6th ed.). St. Louis, MO: Elsevier Mosby.

Centers for Disease Control and Prevention. (2001). Recommendations for using fluoride to prevent and control dental caries in the United States. *MMWR Recommendations and Reports, 50*(RR-14), 1–42.

Centers for Disease Control and Prevention. (2004). Guidelines for preventing health care associated pneumonia, 2003. *MMWR Recommendations and Reports, 53*(RR-03), 1–36.

Chen, W., Liu, G., Yeh, S., Chiang, M., Fu, M., & Hsieh, Y. (2013). Effect of back massage intervention on anxiety, comfort, and physiologic responses in patients with congestive heart failure. *The Journal of Alternative and Complementary Medicine, 19*(5), 464–470. doi: 10.1089/acm.2011.0873

Climo, M., Yokoe, D., Warren, D., Perl, T., Bolon, M., Herwaldt, L., et al. (2013). Effect of daily chlorhexidine bathing on hospital-acquired infection. *New England Journal of Medicine, 368,* 533–542. doi: 10.1056/NEJMoa1113849

Coffin, S., Klompas, M., Classen, D., Arias, K., Podgorny, K., Anderson, D., et al. (2008). Strategies to prevent ventilator-associated pneumonia in acute care hospitals. *Infection Control and Hospital Epidemiology, 29*(S1), S31–S40. doi: 10.1086/591062

Cotrim, A., Zheng, C., & Baun, B. (2013). Xerostomia. In S. Sonis & D. Keefe (Eds.), *Pathobiology of cancer regimen-related toxicities* (pp. 233–248). New York, NY: Springer Science + Business Media.

Frankowski, B., Bocchini, J. & Council on School Health and Committee on Infectious Diseases. (2010). Head lice. *Pediatrics, 126*(2), 392–403. doi: 10.1542/peds.2010-1308

Garcia, R., Jendresky, L., Colbert, L., Bailey, A., Zaman, A., & Majumder, M. (2009). Reducing ventilator associated pneumonia through advanced oral dental care: A 48 month study. *American Journal of Critical Care, 18*(6), 523–532.

Global Health—Division of Parasitic Diseases and Malaria. (2013). Pubic "Crab" Lice. *Parasites.* Retrieved from http://www.cdc.gov/parasites/lice/pubic/index.html

Gunning, K., Pippitt, K., Kiraly, B., & Sayler, M. (2013). Pediculosis and scabies: A treatment update. *Indian Journal of Clinical Practice, 24*(3), 211–216.

Hockenberry, M., & Wilson, D. (Eds). (2011). *Wong's nursing care of infants and children* (9th ed.). St. Louis, MO: Mosby/Elsevier.

Inoue, M., Chapman, R., & Wynaden, D. (2006). Male nurses' experience providing intimate care for women patients. *Journal of Advanced Nursing, 55*(5), 559–567.

Johnson, D., Lineweaver, L., & Maze, L. (2009). Patients' bath basins as potential sources of infection: A multicenter sampling study. *American Journal of Critical Care, 18,* 31–40. doi: 10.4037/ajcc2009968

Kitson, A., Marshall, A., Bassett, K., & Zeitz, K. (2013). What are the core effects of patient centered care? A narrative review of synthesis of the literature from health policy, medicine, and nursing. *Journal of Advanced Nursing, 69*(1), 4–15. doi: 10.1111/j.1365-2648.2012.06064.x

Konno R., Kang H.S. & Makimoto K. (2014). A best-evidence review of intervention studies for minimizing resistance-to-care behaviours for older adults with dementia in nursing homes. *Journal of Advanced Nursing.* doi: 10.1111/jan.12432

Manthorpe, J., & Watson, R. (2003). Poorly served? Eating and dementia. *Journal of Advanced Nursing, 41*(2), 162.

Martínez-Reséndez, M. F., Garza-González, E., Mendoza-Olazaran, S., Herrera-Guerra, A., Pérez-Rodriguez, E., Mercado-Longoria, R., et al. (2014). Impact of daily chlorhexidine baths and hand hygiene compliance on nosocomial infection rates in critically ill patients. *American Journal of Infection Control, 42*(7), 713–717.

Mok, E., & Woo, C. P. (2004). Effects of slow stroke back massage on anxiety and shoulder pain in elderly stroke patients. *Complementary and Therapeutic Nursing and Midwifery, 10*(4), 209–216.

Munro, C., Grap, M., Jones, D., McClish, D., & Sessler, C. (2009). Chlorhexidine, tooth brushing and preventing ventilator-associated pneumonia in critically ill adults. *American Journal of Critical Care, 18*(5), 428–437.

National Diabetes Education Program. (2012). *Take Care of Your Feet for a Lifetime: A booklet for people with diabetes.* (NIH Publication No. 12–4285, NDEP-4). Retrieved from NDEP4_TakeCareOfFeet_BW_508 (1)

NANDA-International (NANDA-I, 2014). *Nursing diagnoses: Definitions and classification, 2015–2017.* West Sussex, UK: Wiley-Blackwell.

Oklahoma State Department of Health. (2014). *Dermatitis/Diaper.* Retrieved from http://www.ok.gov/health2/documents/Dermatitis%20diaper%20.pdf

Patient and Family Education. (2014). *Having a sitz bath at home.* University Health Network Canada. Retrieved from http://www.uhn.ca/docs/HealthInfo/Shared%20Documents/Having_a_Sitz_Bath_at_Home.pdf

Sloane, P.D., Hoeffer B., Mitchell C.M., McKenzie D.A., Barrick A.L., Rader J., et al. (2004). Effect of person-centered showering and the towel bath on bathing-associated aggression, agitation, and discomfort in nursing home residents with dementia: A randomized, controlled trial. *Journal of the American Geriatrics Society, 52*(11), 1795–1804.

Tzeng, H. (2010). Understanding the prevalence of inpatient falls associated with toileting in acute care settings. *Journal of Nursing Care Quality, 25*(1), 22–30.

Williams, T., Szekendi, M., & Thomas, S. (2014). An analysis of patient falls and fall prevention programs across academic medical centers. *Journal of Nursing Care Quality, 29*(1), 19–29.

Workowski, K., & Berman, S. (2010). Sexually transmitted diseases treatment guidelines. *MMWR Recommendations and Reports, 59* (RR-12), 1–110.

Wound, Ostomy, & Continence Nurses Society. (2010). *Guideline for prevention and management of pressure ulcers.* WOCN clinical practice guideline (No. 2). Mount Laurel, NJ: Wound, Ostomy, and Continence Nurses Society.

Procedure 24-1 Assisting With the Bath or Shower

Purpose
1. Cleanse the skin, control body odors, and promote self-esteem.
2. Stimulate circulation.
3. Provide an opportunity to assess skin and physical mobility.
4. Provide range-of-motion exercises for joints.
5. Promote relaxation and comfort.

Equipment
One or two bath towel(s)
Bathmat
One washcloth
Soap, soap dish, or liquid (nonsoap) cleanser
Personal skin care products (deodorant, powder, lotions, cologne)
Clean gown or pajamas
Laundry bag

Assessment
- Assess the patient's ability to perform self-care and amount of assistance he or she needs. Evaluate activity tolerance, cognitive function, musculoskeletal function, and level of discomfort to determine type of bath. (*Note:* Encourage the patient to be as independent as possible but not to become excessively fatigued. Pain should not be intensified.)
- Assess the patient's preferences for bathing (i.e., frequency, time of day, type of skin care products).
- Review chart to determine other procedures or therapies the patient is receiving to coordinate scheduling and prevent fatigue.
- Identify patients with special considerations for bathing:
  - *Older patients:* Susceptible to dry skin
  - *Immobilized patients:* Pressure areas on dependent and bony parts; need for range-of-motion exercises to joints
  - *Patients with altered sensation:* Risk for burns from hot water
  - *Obese or diaphoretic patients:* Excessive perspiration or moisture on skin surfaces that rub against each other and provide medium for excoriation and fungal growth
- Review history for precautions regarding movement or positioning.
- Assess the patient's knowledge and practice of hygiene to determine learning needs.

Procedure

1. **Perform hand hygiene.**
   Rationale: Reduces microbe transmission.

2. **Identify the patient.**
   Rationale: Ensures correct patient receives proper assessment or treatment and reduces errors.

3. **Close door or bed curtains and explain the procedure to the patient and patient's family.**
   Rationale: Ensures patient privacy, increases patient compliance, reduces patient anxiety, and promotes learning.

4. **Make sure the tub or shower is clean.**
   Rationale: Reduces microbe transmission.

5. **Prepare bathroom by placing towel or disposable bathmat on floor by tub or shower.**
   Rationale: Maintain cleanliness and safety for the patient.

6. **Accompany or transport patient to the bathroom. Some patients may need to use a shower chair for transportation or support.**
   Rationale: Showering or bathing will be tiring. Transportation and/or sitting in a chair will conserve energy.

7. **Place "occupied" sign on door.**
   Rationale: The patient needs privacy while bathing. Doors are not usually locked so that the nurse can come in to assist the patient as necessary.

Procedure 24-1   *continued*

8. **Keep the patient covered with a bath blanket until water is ready (Fig. 1).**

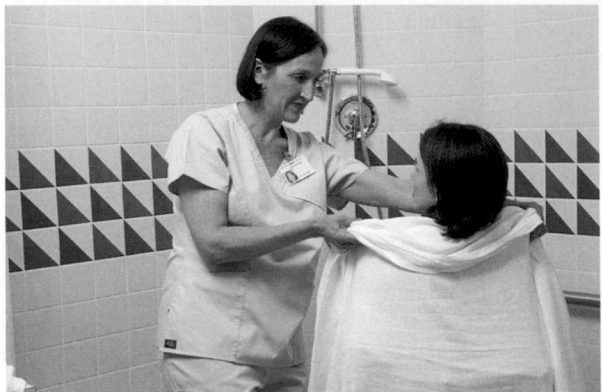

FIG. 1 Wrap the patient in bath blanket.

Rationale: Keeps the patient warm to prevent chills.

9. **Fill bathtub halfway with warm water (105°F [40.6°C]). Test water or have the patient test water (Fig. 2). If the patient is taking a shower, turn on shower and adjust water temperature.**

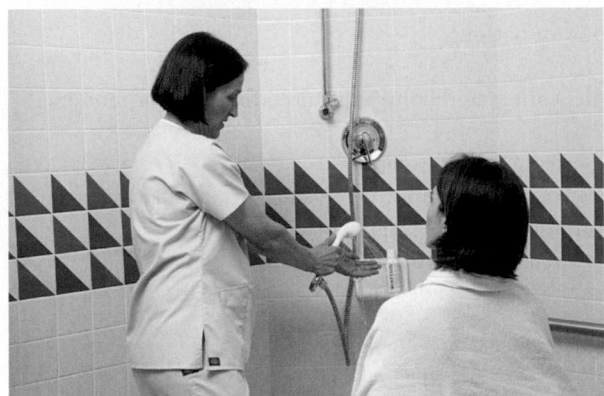

FIG. 2 Test water temperature.

Rationale: Prevents burns.

10. **Help the patient into shower or tub, providing necessary assistance.**

Rationale: Falls can occur in the shower or tub; provide safety for the patient.

11. **Instruct the patient in use of safety bars and call-light signal. The patient may prefer to sit in shower chair to prevent fatigue.**

Rationale: Provide for the patient's safety and comfort.

12. **If the patient is unable to shower independently, stay with the patient at all times. (Two nurses may be necessary for some patients.) Use handheld shower to wet patient. Wash the patient with soap and washcloth using long, firm strokes.**

Rationale: Handheld shower allows the nurse to stay dry.

13. **If the patient is showering or bathing independently, check on patient within 5 to 10 minutes or stay close by. Wash any areas that he or she could not reach.**

Rationale: Prolonged exposure to warm water may cause vasodilation and pooling of blood, which can result in light-headedness and increase fall risk.

14. **Assist with drying (Fig. 3). Help the patient out of tub or shower (Fig. 4). If the patient is unsteady, drain water before helping the patient out of tub.**

Rationale: Prevents falls.

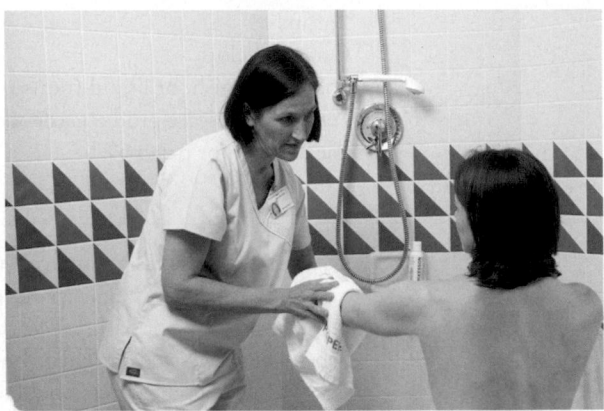

FIG. 3 Dry the patient's arm from hand to axilla.

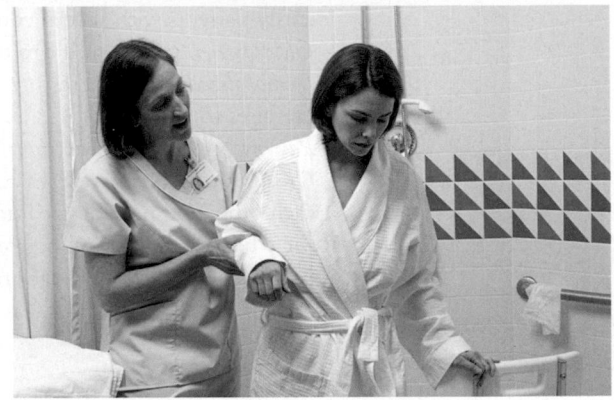

FIG. 4 Assist the patient out of shower.

15. **Assist the patient with dressing and grooming.**

16. **Help the patient to room. Return to bathroom and clean tub or shower according to agency policy. Discard soiled linen. Place "unoccupied" sign on door.**

Rationale: Maintain cleanliness and good infection control practices.

17. **Document procedure.**

Rationale: Maintains legal record and communicates with healthcare team.

Documentation

6/1/17: 16:00— Weekly bath given, tolerated bath without increased pulse rate or dizziness, no areas of skin breakdown observed.

—S. Roberts, RN

Procedure 24-1   *continued*

Life Span Considerations

Newborn and Infant

- To prevent infection, do not submerge an infant in water until the umbilical cord has fallen off (around 7 to 10 days of age).

Child

- To prevent drowning, do not leave children younger than 8 years unattended in a bath.
- Although children often enjoy washing themselves, be sure to supervise so they wash thoroughly.

Adolescent

- Sebaceous glands become active during puberty. Special cleansing agents may be necessary to treat facial acne. Antiperspirants and more frequent baths will help control body odors.

Older Adult

- Older adults are susceptible to dry skin due to reduced sebaceous gland activity, epidermal thinning, and decreased fluid intake. Use lotions, and less soap to reduce the drying effects of aging. Bathing may occur weekly to decrease drying of the skin.
- Check water temperature carefully. Older adults may have decreased sensation and are at risk for burns from hot water.

Home Care Modifications

- Instruct patients at risk for falling to apply lotions and oils after the bath and not put them in bath water. Oils can make the bathtub or shower surfaces more slippery.
- Encourage installation of safety devices, such as tub bars, nonskid tub surfaces, and bathroom carpeting to reduce the chance of falls and promote independence.

Collaboration and Delegation

- Because unlicensed personnel often assist with showers or bathing, be sure to provide assistants with the following information regarding the patient:
    - Any physical limitations or special safety precautions needed
    - Amount of help the patient will require
    - Any drains, casts, or IVs, along with any precautions or limitations that they will impose during the shower/bath
    - Any assessments to report to you (e.g., skin condition under breasts)
- Collaborate with occupational therapy if an OT is seeing the patient. Often, OTs want to assess and work with a patient's ability to perform hygiene, so coordination is important.

Procedure 24-2 Bathing a Patient in Bed

Purpose   1. Same as **Procedure 24-1**.

Equipment   Two bath towels
Two washcloths
Bath blanket
Bag bath packet removed from warmer just before bathing
Personal skin care products (deodorant, powder, lotions, cologne)
Clean gown or pajamas
Laundry bag
Disposable clean gloves for perineal care

Assessment   • Same as **Procedure 24-1**.

Procedure

1. **Identify the patient.**

   Rationale: Ensures correct patient receives proper assessment or treatment and reduces errors.

2. **Close door or bed curtains and explain the procedure to the patient and patient's family.**

   Rationale: Ensures patient privacy, increases patient compliance, and reduces patient anxiety.

3. **Help patient use bedpan, urinal, or commode if needed.**

   Rationale: The patient will be more comfortable and relaxed after elimination.

4. **Close window and door to decrease drafts.**

   Rationale: Provides the patient comfort and minimizes chilling.

5. **Perform hand hygiene.**

   Rationale: Reduces microbe transmission.

6. **Raise bed to high position. Lock up side rail on opposite side of bed from your work.**

   Rationale: Prevents back strain; prevents the patient from falling out of bed.

7. **Remove top sheet and bedspread, then place bath blanket on the patient (Fig. 1). Help the patient move closer to you. If top linen is to be reused, place it on back of chair; otherwise, place it in laundry bag.**

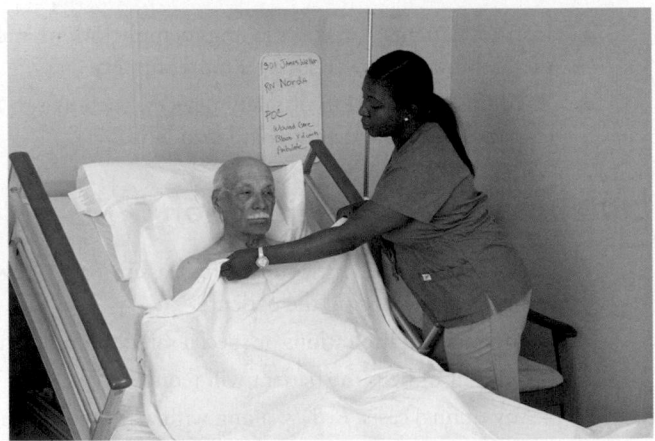

FIG. 1 Place bath blanket on the patient.

Rationale: A bath blanket provides for patient comfort, warmth, and privacy. Bringing the patient closer to you prevents undue muscle strain.

Procedure 24-2   *continued*

8. **Follow package directions to heat the disposable washcloths. Remove first cloth from bag bath packet. Keep the rest of the cloths in the package, selecting new cloths when needed (Fig. 2).**

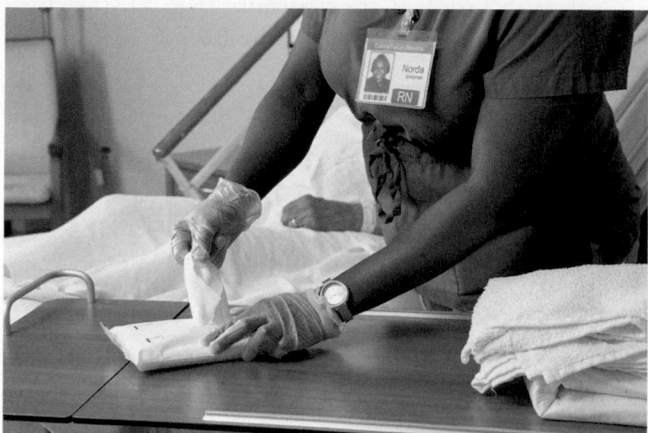

FIG. 2 Remove first cloth from bag bath packet.

Rationale: Following manufacturer's directions will ensure safe use of product. Overheating in a microwave could result in excessive heat, which could burn the patient. Keeping unused cloths in package will keep them warm until use.

9. **Use a cloth to wash face. Cleanse eye, wiping from inner to outer canthus. Use separate corner of cloth for each eye). Offer patient the opportunity to wash face if able (Fig. 3).**

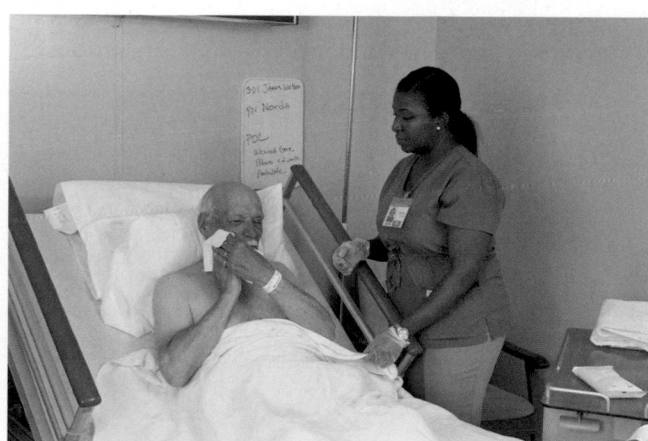

FIG. 3 Offer the patient the opportunity to wash the face if able.

Rationale: Face should be washed first because washing proceeds from clean to dirty areas. Washing the eye from the inner to outer canthus prevents secretions from entering and irritating nasolacrimal ducts. Using separate corners for each eye prevents transfer of microorganisms from one eye to the other. Encouraging patients to wash their face (if able) increases independence.

10. **Fold bath blanket off arm away from you. Place towel lengthwise under arm. Wash the arm using long, firm strokes from the fingers toward the axilla. Wash axilla (Fig.4).**

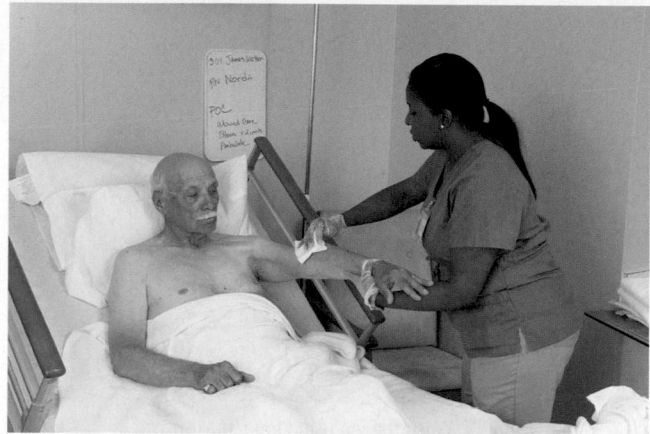

FIG. 4 Wash the arm using long, firm strokes.

Rationale: Stroking from distal to proximal stimulates circulation and facilitates venous blood return.

11. **Repeat for hand and arm nearest you.**

12. **Apply deodorant or powder according to patient's preferences. Avoid excessive use of powder or inhalation of powder.**

Rationale: Hygiene products control excess body moisture and odor. Excessive powder can cause caking, which leads to skin irritation; inhalation can cause respiratory difficulty.

13. **Place bath towel over chest. Fold bath blanket down to below umbilicus.**

Rationale: Keeps the patient warm while preventing unnecessary exposure of body parts.

14. **Lift bath towel off chest, and bathe chest and abdomen with cloth using long, firm strokes. Give special attention to skin under the breasts and any other skin folds if the patient is overweight. Rinse and dry well. Apply a light dusting of bath powder under the breasts or between skin folds.**

Rationale: Bathing provides an opportunity to inspect skin folds to detect any skin problems so that treatment can be initiated promptly.

15. **Help the patient don a clean gown.**

Rationale: Gown prevents exposure of upper body area.

16. **Expose leg away from you by folding over bath blanket. Be careful to keep perineum covered.**

Rationale: Preventing unnecessary exposure of body parts maintains the patient's dignity.

Procedure 24-2 *continued*

17. **Lift leg, and place bath towel lengthwise under leg. Wash leg using long, firm strokes from ankle to thigh (Fig. 5).**

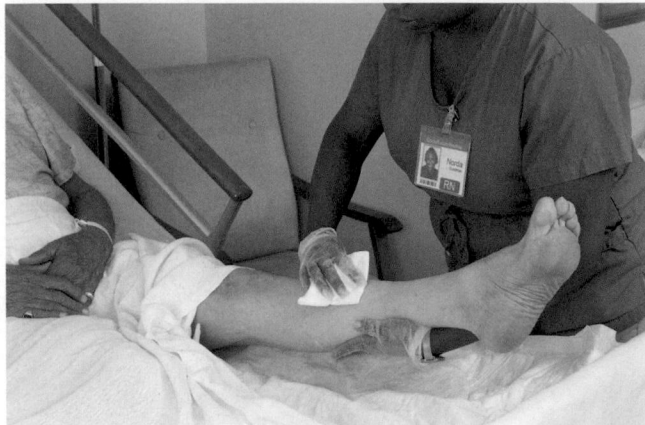

FIG. 5 Wash the leg using long, firm strokes.

Rationale: Washing from distal to proximal stimulates circulation and facilitates venous blood return.

18. **Wash feet. Rinse and dry well. Pay special attention to space between toes (Fig. 6).**

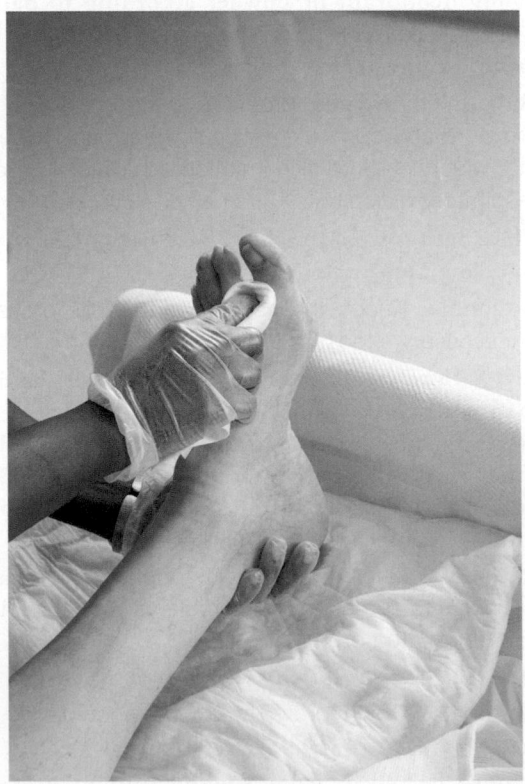

FIG. 6 Wash between the toes.

Rationale: Moisture between toes can foster irritation and fungal growth.

19. **Repeat for other leg and foot.**
20. **Assist the patient to side-lying position. Place bath towel along side of back and buttocks to protect linen. Wash back and then buttocks. Give a backrub with lotion if time permits (Fig. 7). (See also Procedure 24-3, Massaging the Back.)**

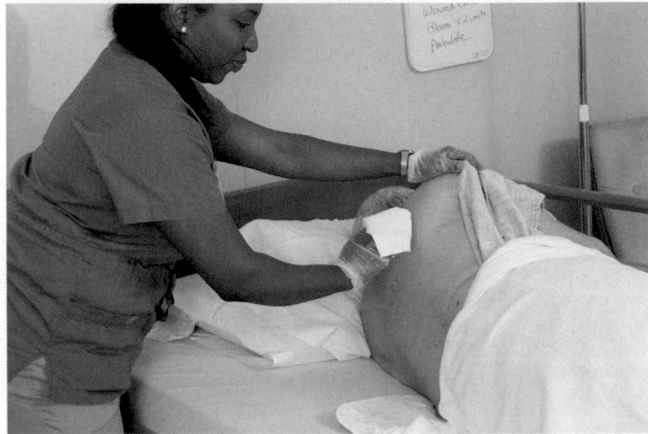

FIG. 7 Wash the back.

Rationale: Always wash from clean areas to more dirty areas. A backrub stimulates circulation and promotes comfort.

21. **Assist the patient to supine position. Assess if the patient can wash genitals and perineal area independently (Fig. 8). If the patient needs help, drape with blanket so that only genitals are exposed. Don disposable, clean gloves. Using a new cloth, wash genitalia and perineum (see text for instructions).**

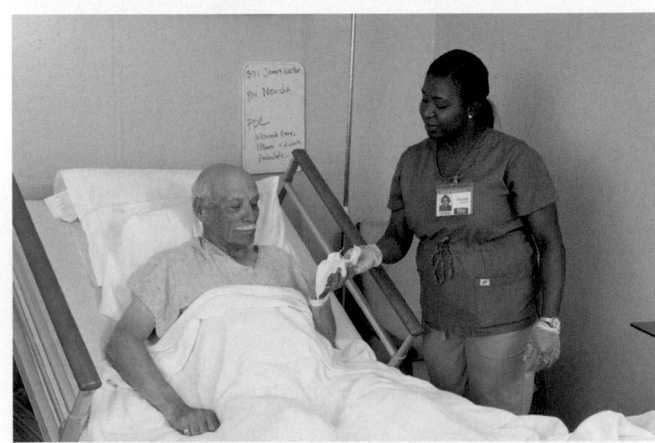

FIG. 8 Ask the patient to wash genitals and perineal area if able.

Rationale: Most patients who are unable to perform perineal care will not ask for assistance with this intimate task, but it is important to keep this area clean to decrease infection risk and prevent odor.

Procedure 24-2   *continued*

22. **Complete care according to patient's preference. Apply powder, lotion, cologne. Assist with hair and mouth care. Make bed with clean linen.**

    Rationale: Involving the patient nurtures self-esteem and self-care efforts.

23. **Clean area, disposing of used cloths and returning hygiene supplies to bedside cabinet. Cloths must never be flushed in the toilet. Perform hand hygiene.**

    Rationale: Maintains cleanliness of the area.

24. **Document procedure.**

    Rationale: Maintains legal record and communicates with healthcare team.

Documentation

- Often noted on a flow sheet, providing information such as complete versus partial bath and the amount of assistance required.

Home Care Modifications

- Arrange for a hospital bed to help prevent caregiver back strain and assist with turning and moving the patient in bed.
- Commercially available disposable cloths can make bathing easier in the home setting.

Collaboration and Delegation

- Same as **Procedure 24-1**.

Procedure 24-3 Massaging the Back

Purpose	1. Stimulate circulation to the skin 2. Relieve muscle tension 3. Promote comfort and relaxation
Equipment	Bath blanket Bath towel (to absorb excess moisture) Lotion or powder (*Note:* Lotion is used to lubricate skin and prevents friction during massage; powder reduces friction and prevents "sticky" feeling on diaphoretic patients. Powder and lotion are not used together.)
Assessment	• Assess the patient for muscle fatigue or stiffness or complaints of back discomfort or tension. • Identify patients with impaired physical mobility who may benefit from back massage. • Assess skin for localized areas of redness on the back, shoulders, or hips. • Assess patient's desire for back massage. • Identify conditions that may contraindicate backrub (rib and vertebral fractures, burns, open wounds, or stage 1 pressure ulcers). • Determine any limitations to positioning.

Procedure

1. **Identify the patient.**

   Rationale: Ensures correct patient receives proper assessment or treatment and reduces errors.

2. **Close door or bed curtains and explain the procedure to the patient and patient's family.**

   Rationale: Ensures patient privacy, increases patient compliance, and reduces patient anxiety.

3. **Help the patient to side-lying or prone position.**

   Rationale: Promotes patient comfort.

4. **Expose back, shoulders, upper arms, and sacral area. Cover remainder of body with bath blanket.**

   Rationale: Covering areas not being massaged prevents unnecessary exposure and chilling while maintaining dignity.

5. **Perform hand hygiene in warm water. Warm lotion by holding container under running warm water.**

   Rationale: Warm hands and lotion prevent a startle response and muscle tension from cold lotion and hands.

6. **Pour small amount of lotion into palms.**

   Rationale: Lubricating palms decreases friction on the skin during massage.

7. **Begin massage in sacral area with circular motion. Move hands upward to shoulders, massaging over scapulae in smooth, firm strokes (Fig. 1). Without removing hands from skin, continue in smooth strokes to upper arms and down sides of back to iliac crest. Continue for 3 to 5 minutes.**

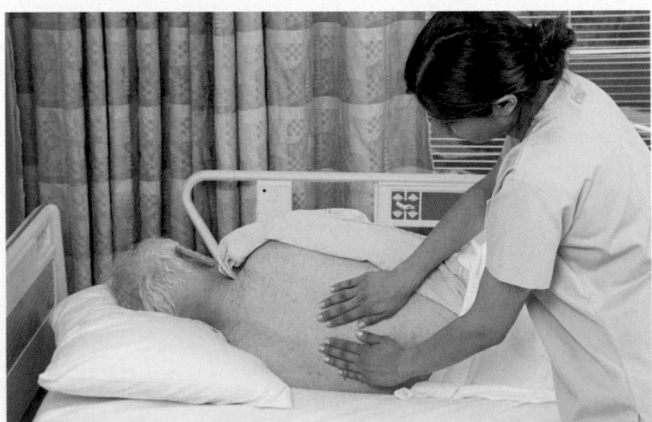

FIG. 1 Move hands upward with firm, circular motion.

   Rationale: Continuous, firm pressure promotes relaxation and stimulates circulation.

8. **While massaging, assess for broken skin areas and whitish or reddened areas that do not disappear. Do not apply pressure over areas of breakdown or redness.**

   Rationale: Pressure from massage can traumatize and damage tissues.

Procedure 24-3 *continued*

9. If additional stimulation is desired, nurse can use pétrissage (kneading) over the shoulders and gluteal area and tapotement (tapping) up and down the spine.

   Rationale: Stroking is the most relaxing of the massage movements.

10. End massage with long, continuous, stroking movements.

11. Pat excess lubricant dry with towel. Retie patient's gown, and assist to comfortable position.

    Rationale: Promotes patient comfort.

12. Perform hand hygiene.

    Rationale: Reduces microbe transmission.

13. Document procedure.

    Rationale: Maintains legal record and communicates with healthcare team.

Documentation

- Document on a flow sheet that massage was given.

Collaboration and Delegation

- Encourage unlicensed personnel to provide back massage, especially at bedtime. In some facilities, volunteers are trained to provide back massages for receptive patients. Communicate any positioning restrictions and assessments that they should report.

Procedure 24-4 Performing Foot and Hand Care

Purpose
1. Maintain skin integrity.
2. Provide for patient's comfort and sense of well-being.
3. Maintain foot function and ability to ambulate.
4. Encourage self-care.

Equipment
Waterproof pad
Washcloth, towels
Washbasin, warm water, soap
Lotion
Disposable gloves
Nail clippers, file
Cuticle stick

Assessment
- Note patient's gait for limping or unusual position. Unnatural gait can be caused by painful feet or bone and muscle disorders.
- Assess footwear worn by patient. Socks should be worn and changed daily to absorb excess perspiration and avoid fungal infections.
- Identify patients at risk for foot or nail problems:
  - Diabetes is associated with changes in microcirculation to peripheral tissues. The patient with diabetes is at high risk for infection from breaks in skin integrity and may have decreased sensation to the feet as a result of neuropathy.
  - Older adult patients' ability to perform foot and nail care may be impeded by poor vision, obesity, or musculoskeletal conditions that limit their ability to bend and maintain balance.
  - CVA may alter the patient's gait due to foot drop, muscle weakness, or paralysis.
  - Conditions associated with foot and ankle edema (renal failure, congestive heart failure) interfere with blood flow to surrounding tissues and impede proper shoe fit.
- Determine patient's ability to perform self-care.
- Inspect nails and skin of fingers, toes, and feet. Assess areas between toes for dryness and cracking.
- Assess patient's knowledge of foot and nail care practices.
- Review agency policy for trimming nails. Some agencies require a physician's order to perform nail trimming on high-risk patients.

Procedure

1. **Perform hand hygiene.**
   Rationale: Reduces microbe transmission.

2. **Identify the patient.**
   Rationale: Ensures correct patient receives proper assessment or treatment and reduces errors.

3. **Close door or bed curtains and explain the procedure to the patient.**
   Rationale: Ensures patient privacy, increases patient compliance, and reduces patient anxiety.

4. **Help the patient to chair if possible. Elevate the head of the bed for bedridden patient.**
   Rationale: Promotes patient comfort.

5. **Fill washbasin with warm water (100°F to 104°F [37.7°C to 40°C]). Place waterproof pad under basin. Soak patient's hands or feet in basin. Do not soak the feet of a patient with diabetes.**
   Rationale: Warm water softens nails, increases local circulation, and reduces inflammation. Soaking increases risk of infection and tissue maceration for patients with diabetes. Peripheral neuropathy puts the patient with diabetes at increased risk for burn.

6. **Place call light within reach. Allow hands or feet to soak for 10 to 20 minutes.**
   Rationale: Softening allows easier removal of dead epithelial cells and reduces possibility of nails cracking during trimming.

Procedure 24-4 *continued*

7. **Dry the hand or foot that has been soaking. Rewarm water, and allow other extremity to soak while you work on the softened nails (Fig. 1).**

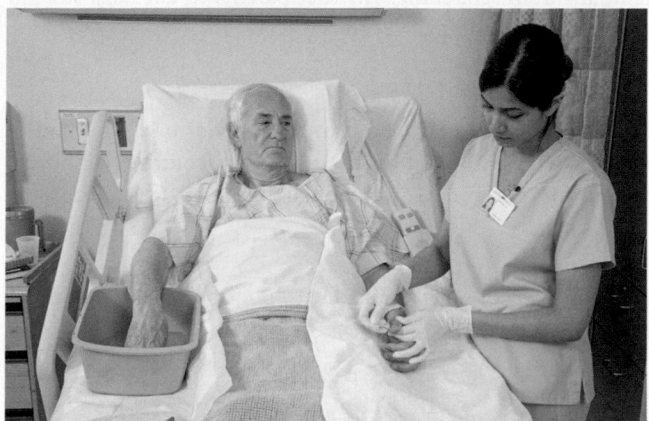

FIG. 1 Continue to soak other extremity while working on softened nails.

Rationale: Soaking the second hand or foot while the nurse works on the first is efficient use of time.

8. **Gently clean under nails with cuticle stick. If nails are thickened and yellow, the patient may have a fungal infection. Wear disposable gloves and eye protection.**

Rationale: Gloves prevent transmission of infection. Eye protection prevents accidental exposure.

9. **Beginning with large toe or thumb, cut nail straight across (Fig. 2). Shape nail with file. File rather than cut nails of patients with diabetes or circulatory problems.**

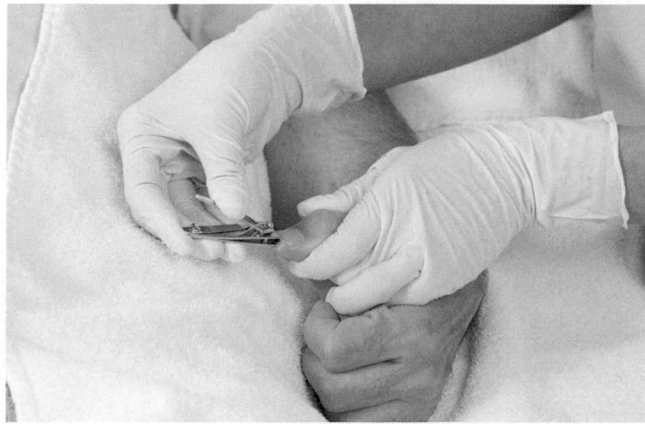

FIG. 2 Cut nails straight across.

Rationale: Trimming straight across prevents nail splitting and tissue injury around nail.

10. **Push back cuticle gently with cuticle stick (Fig. 3).**

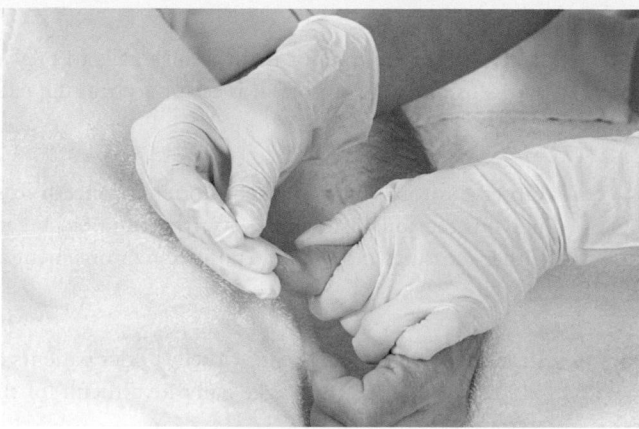

FIG. 3 Use cuticle stick to push back cuticles.

Rationale: Cuticle care reduces inflamed cuticle and hangnail formation.

11. **Repeat procedure with other nails.**
12. **Rinse foot or hand in warm water.**
13. **Dry thoroughly with towel, especially between digits.**

Rationale: Removing excess moisture inhibits bacterial and fungal growth.

14. **Apply lotion to hands or feet. Do not apply lotion between the toes of a patient with diabetes.**

Rationale: Excess moisture between the toes can cause maceration and increase fungal growth.

15. **Help the patient to comfortable position.**
16. **Remove and dispose of equipment.**
17. **Perform hand hygiene.**

Rationale: Reduces microbe transmission.

18. **Document procedure.**

Rationale: Maintains legal record and communicates with healthcare team.

Documentation

6/14/17: 19:00—(*Note:* Routine nail care is often checked off on a flow sheet): Nail care provided at request of patient who has difficulty reaching feet. Toenails thick and very long. CMS+ and no neuropathy noted. Instructed to visit the podiatrist or neighborhood center for nail care after discharge.

—S. Roberts, RN

Procedure 24-4   *continued*

Life Span Considerations

Infant

- Teach parents to care for their infant's nails to prevent the infant from scratching. Instruct parents to cut nails straight across using blunt scissors. It is easiest to trim the nails when the baby is asleep.

Child

- Observe for nail biting, which is often a concern in school-age children. It may be a learned behavior or a symptom of nervous tension. Bad-tasting over-the-counter preparations are available to paint on the nails to discourage nail biting. Other measures may include positive reinforcement and rewards for "good" days with no nail biting.

Older Adult

- Inspect the older adult's nails closely. Older patients often have thickened, horny nails due to poor peripheral perfusion. Mobility problems may make nail care difficult for the elderly.

Collaboration and Delegation

- Refer high-risk patients or those with severely hypertrophied nails to a podiatrist or foot clinic for care. In some institutions the diabetes clinician can provide foot care for high-risk patients.

Procedure 24-5 Shampooing Hair of a Bedridden Patient

Purpose
1. Cleanse hair and scalp.
2. Promote comfort and self-esteem.
3. Apply medication to scalp and hair.

Equipment
Comb and brush
Hair dryer (optional)
Two bath towels, one washcloth
Shampoo (cream rinse is optional)
Water pitcher
Plastic shampoo basin
Washbasin or bucket
Bath blanket
or
Disposable shampoo cap; remove from warmer
Waterproof pads
Cotton balls (optional)
Hydrogen peroxide (optional, to cleanse matted blood from hair)

Assessment
- Assess condition of hair and scalp.
- Determine agency policy about shampooing hair of some patients (e.g., head trauma). Some agencies require a physician's order especially after surgery or trauma involving the head.
- Assess patient's activity level and identify positioning restrictions.
- Assess patient's preference for hair care products. Determine if medicated shampoo has been ordered and is available.

Procedure

1. **Perform hand hygiene.**
   Rationale: Reduces microbe transmission.
2. **Identify the patient.**
   Rationale: Ensures correct patient receives proper assessment or treatment, and reduces errors.
3. **Close door or bed curtains and explain the procedure to the patient.**
   Rationale: Ensures patient privacy and increases patient compliance.
4. **Place waterproof pads under patient's head and shoulders, and remove pillow.**
   Rationale: Keeps bed linen clean and dry.
5. **Raise bed to highest position.**
   Rationale: Reduces strain on the nurse's back.
6. **Remove any pins from hair. Comb and brush hair thoroughly.**

   Rationale: Removing tangles and distributing scalp oils through hair result in thorough cleansing.
7. **Adjust bed to flat position. Place shampooing basin under head. Place bath towel around shoulders and folded washcloth where neck rests on basin.**
   Rationale: Shoulder padding protects the patient from becoming wet. A washcloth protects the neck from strain and discomfort.
8. **Fold bed linens down to waist. Cover upper body with bath blanket.**
   Rationale: The patient should be kept warm and the linen protected from water.
9. **Place wastebasket with plastic bag under spout of shampoo basin on a chair or table at the bedside.**
   Rationale: Water should flow from the face and head into a receptacle.

Procedure 24-5   *continued*

10. Using water pitcher, wet hair thoroughly with warm water (approximately 110°F [43.3°C]) (Fig. 1). Check temperature by placing small amount of water on your wrist.

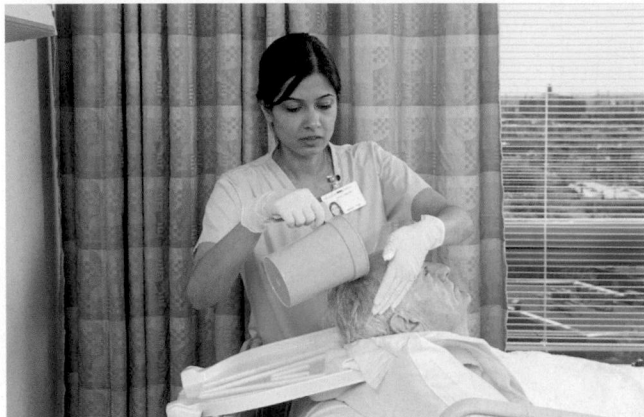

FIG. 1 Run water over the patient's hair.

Rationale: Wetting the hair in this manner protects the face from becoming wet. Checking water temperature prevents burns.

11. Before shampooing, use hydrogen peroxide to dissolve matted blood in hair. Peroxide normally feels bubbly and warm. Reassure the patient that it will not bleach hair.

Rationale: Removing blood before washing will ensure that shampoo will reach and cleanse all hair surfaces.

12. Apply small amount of shampoo. Massage scalp with fingertips while making shampoo lather. Start at hairline and work toward neck (Fig. 2).

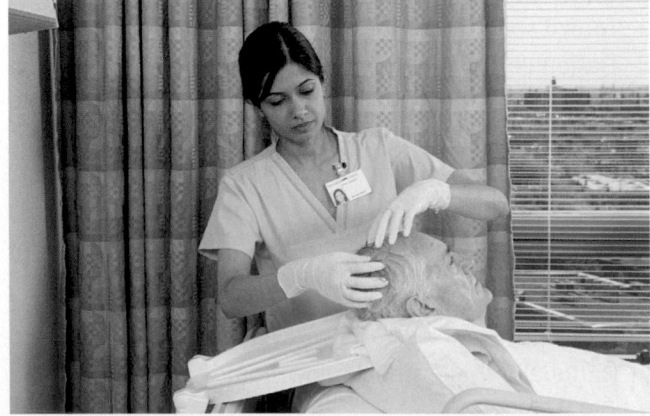

FIG. 2 Massage scalp to lather shampoo.

Rationale: Massage stimulates circulation to the scalp; systematic lathering ensures thorough cleansing.

13. Rinse hair with warm water. Reapply shampoo and repeat massage.

14. Rinse hair thoroughly with warm water. Clean hair "squeaks" when rubbed between fingers.

Rationale: Soap residue in hair may dry and irritate hair and scalp.

15. Apply small amount of conditioner per patient request. Rinse well.

Rationale: Conditioner decreases tangles and makes combing easier.

16. Squeeze excess moisture from hair. Wrap bath towel around hair. Rub to dry hair and scalp (Fig. 3). Use second towel if necessary.

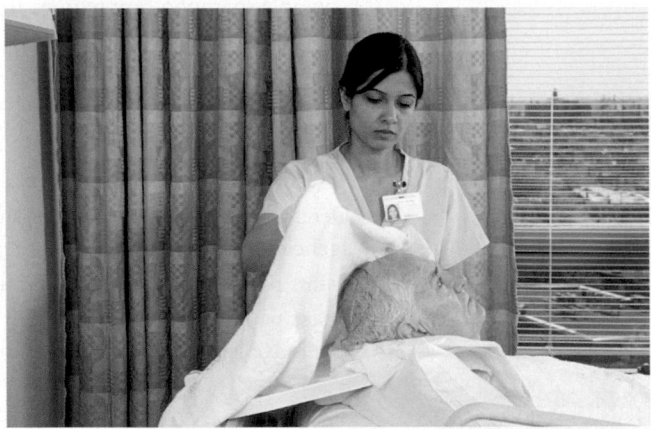

FIG. 3 Pat the patient's hair dry.

17. Remove equipment and wet towels from bed. Place dry towel over the patient's shoulders.

Rationale: Prevents the patient from getting a chill.

18. Dry hair with hair dryer if necessary. Comb and style.

19. Help the patient to comfortable position.

20. Dispose of soiled equipment and linen.

Variation for Using a Dry Shampoo Cap

1. Perform steps 1 through 3 above.

2. Spread towel across patient's chest and place shampoo cap on patient (Fig. 4).

Procedure 24-5   *continued*

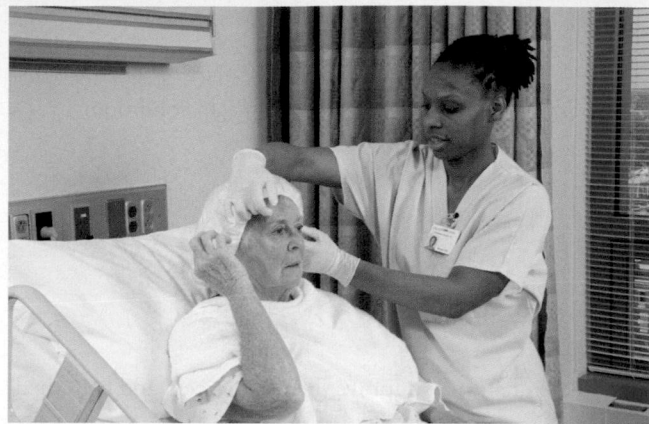

FIG. 4 Apply dry shampoo cap.

Rationale: Provides comfort and prepares the patient for the shampoo.

3. **Massage scalp so that dry shampoo is evenly distributed (Fig. 5).**

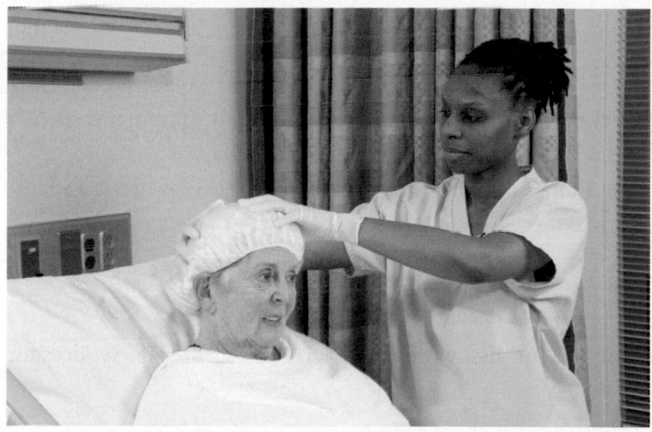

FIG. 5 Massage scalp to lather shampoo.

Rationale: Evenly distributes shampoo to hair shafts to promote cleaning.

4. **Wait 1 to 3 minutes for shampoo to fully saturate hair.**
   Rationale: Allows chemical agent to cleanse hair.
5. **Remove and discard shampoo cap.**
   Rationale: Shampoo caps are used only once.
6. **Use clean towel to dry the patient's hair.**
   Rationale: Promotes comfort and prevents chilling.
7. **Groom and style the patient's hair.**
   Rationale: Promotes the patient's self-esteem.
8. **Document procedure.**
   Rationale: Maintains legal record and communicates with healthcare team.

Documentation

6/14/17: 21:00—Hair shampooed, no dandruff or head lice noted.

—S. Roberts, RN

Procedure 24-5   *continued*

Life Span Considerations

Infant

- Shampooing is usually done during the daily bath to prevent seborrhea (cradle cap), a gray, scaly scalp condition.
- Warm the room and use warmed towels to prevent chilling during the bath.
- Use baby shampoo to decrease eye irritation.

Child

- Assess hair carefully for nits (lice eggs). Pediculosis infestations are common in school-age children.

Adolescent

- Many adolescents shampoo their hair daily. Offering to shampoo their hair may improve their self-esteem and help them foster a therapeutic relationship with the nurse.

Older Adult

- Use warm towels to thoroughly dry hair after a shampoo to prevent chilling. Many older adults have decreased subcutaneous tissue and chill quickly.
- Older adults may have decreased sensation to heat. Use a hair dryer cautiously on a low-heat setting to prevent burning the scalp.

Home Care Modifications

- Ask the family if a relative or friend might provide hair care services. Inform the family about helpful equipment, such as disposable shampoo caps, to purchase if showering or bathing is restricted.
- Assist the family with adapting things in the home (e.g., a dish drainer mat or rolled plastic trash bags) for use as a shampoo tray.

Collaboration and Delegation

- Many long-term care facilities and community-based centers of care contract with a beautician to provide hair services for patients. Encourage and make arrangements for such services.

Procedure 24-6 Providing Oral Care

Purpose	1. Cleanse tooth surfaces to prevent odor and caries.
	2. Maintain hydrated, intact oral mucosa.
	3. Promote self-esteem and comfort.

Equipment

Soft toothbrush (sponge-ended swabs may be used for patients at risk for bleeding)
Toothpaste
Cup with water, straw
Emesis basin
Washcloth, towel
Mouthwash (optional; nonalcohol based is preferable)
Dental floss
Disposable gloves (if the nurse provides oral care)

Assessment

- Inspect lips, buccal membrane, gums, palate, and tongue for lesions or inflammation.
- Assess for caries or halitosis (bad breath).
- Identify patients at risk for oral hygiene complications:
  - Dehydration, NPO status, and nasogastric tubes dry the oral mucosa.
  - Oral airways accumulate secretions and irritate the mucosa.
  - Chemotherapy often results in stomatitis and ulcerations.
  - Anticoagulant therapy or clotting disorders predispose the patient to gum bleeding.
  - Oral surgery or trauma may contraindicate tooth brushing; special rinses may be ordered.
- Determine patient's ability to assist with procedure.
- Assess patient's risk for aspiration.

Procedure

1. **Perform hand hygiene.**
   Rationale: Reduces microbe transmission.

2. **Identify the patient.**
   Rationale: Ensures correct patient receives proper assessment or treatment and reduces errors.

3. **Close door or bed curtains and explain the procedure to the patient.**
   Rationale: Ensures patient privacy and increases patient compliance.

4. **Help the patient to a sitting position. If the patient cannot sit, help to a side-lying position.**
   Rationale: High Fowler's or side-lying position helps prevent choking and aspiration.

5. **Place towel under the patient's chin.**
   Rationale: Protects bed linens and gown from soiling.

6. **Moisten toothbrush with water and apply small amount of toothpaste (Fig. 1). If the patient is anticoagulated or has a clotting disorder, use a very soft toothbrush or a sponge-ended swab to prevent gum bleeding.**

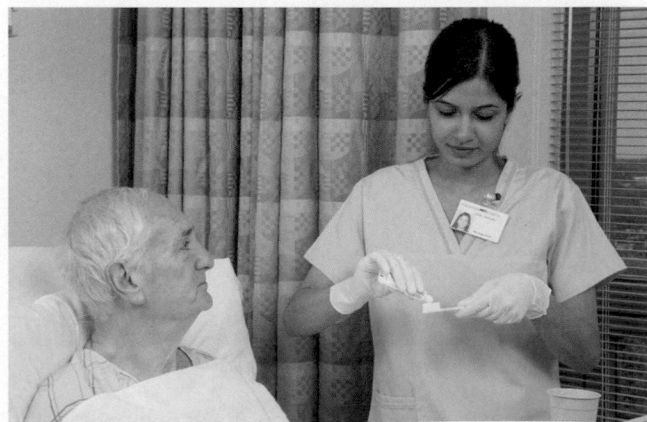

FIG. 1 Moisten toothbrush and apply toothpaste to bristles.

Rationale: Limits trauma to oral mucosa that could cause bleeding.

Procedure 24-6   *continued*

7. Hand toothbrush to patient or don disposable gloves and brush patient's teeth as follows:

   a. **Hold toothbrush at a 45-degree angle to the gum line (Fig. 2).**

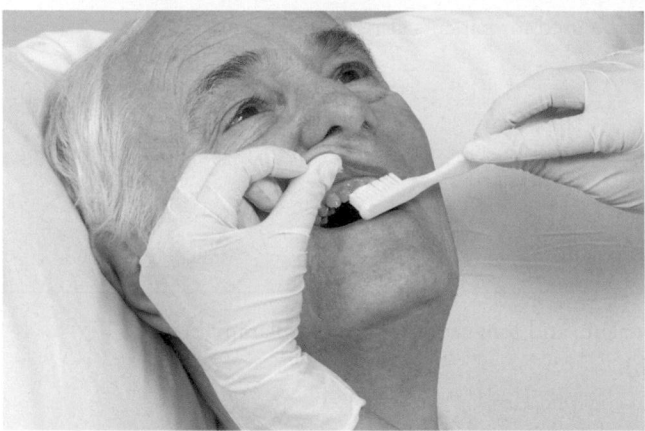

FIG. 2 Place brush at a 45-degree angle to gum line.

   b. **Using short, vibrating motions, brush from the gum line to the crown of each tooth. Repeat until outside and inside of teeth and gums are cleaned.**

   Rationale: Angling the toothbrush allows the brush to reach all tooth surfaces and to penetrate and cleanse under the gum line, where plaque and tartar accumulate.

   c. **Cleanse biting surfaces by brushing with a back-and-forth stroke.**

   d. **Brush the tongue lightly. Avoid stimulating the gag reflex (Fig. 3).**

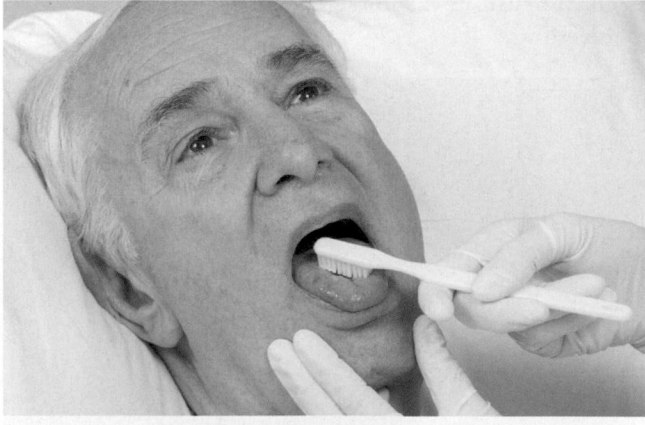

FIG. 3 Brush the tongue.

Rationale: Bacteria accumulate and grow on the tongue surface.

8. **Have the patient rinse the mouth thoroughly with water and spit into emesis basin (Fig. 4).**

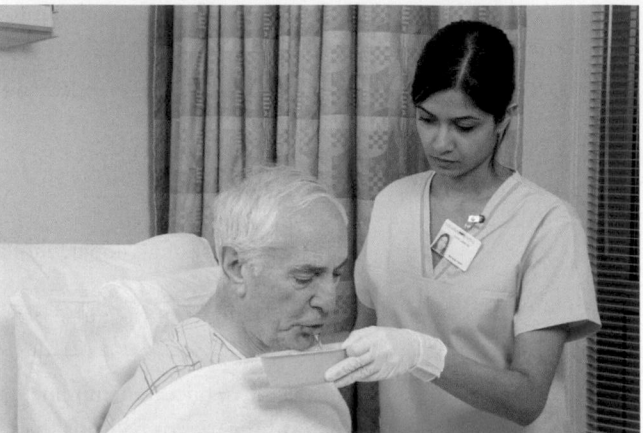

FIG. 4 Offer the patient water and emesis basin to rinse the mouth.

9. **Remove emesis basin, set aside, and dry patient's mouth with washcloth.**

10. **Floss patient's teeth (Fig. 5).**

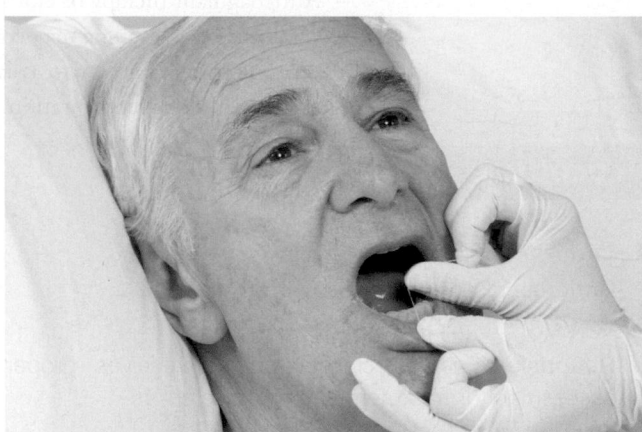

FIG. 5 Floss the teeth.

Rationale: Flossing removes particulate matter trapped between the teeth and below the gum line.

   a. **Cut 10-inch piece of dental floss. Wind ends of floss around middle finger of each hand.**

   b. **Using index fingers to stretch the floss, move the floss up and down around and between lower teeth. Start at the back lower teeth and work around to the other side.**

   c. **Using thumb and index fingers to stretch the floss, repeat procedure on upper teeth.**

   d. **Have the patient rinse the mouth thoroughly and spit into emesis basin.**

Procedure 24-6   *continued*

11. **Remove and dispose of supplies. Help the patient to comfortable position.**

    Rationale: Promotes patient comfort.

12. **Remove gloves and perform hand hygiene.**

    Rationale: The mouth contains many microorganisms, and handwashing prevents the spread of infection.

Variation for the Unconscious Patient

1. **Perform hand hygiene.**

    Rationale: Reduces microbe transmission.

2. **Identify the patient.**

    Rationale: Ensures correct patient receives proper assessment or treatment and reduces errors.

3. **Close door or bed curtains and explain the procedure to the patient's family.**

    Rationale: Ensures patient privacy and increases patient compliance.

4. **Place the patient in a side-lying position.**

    Rationale: Side-lying position prevents aspiration.

5. **Place towel or waterproof pad under the patient's chin.**

6. **Place emesis basin against the patient's mouth or have suction catheter positioned to remove secretions from mouth (Fig. 6).**

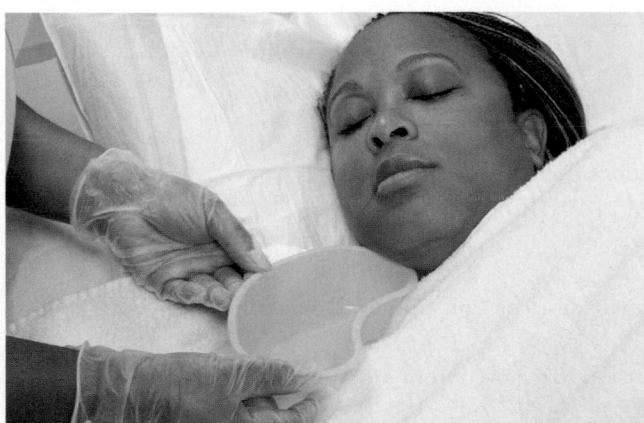

FIG. 6 Place towel across chest and position emesis basin.

7. **Use padded tongue blade to open teeth gently (Fig. 7). Leave in place between the back molars. Never put your fingers in an unconscious patient's mouth.**

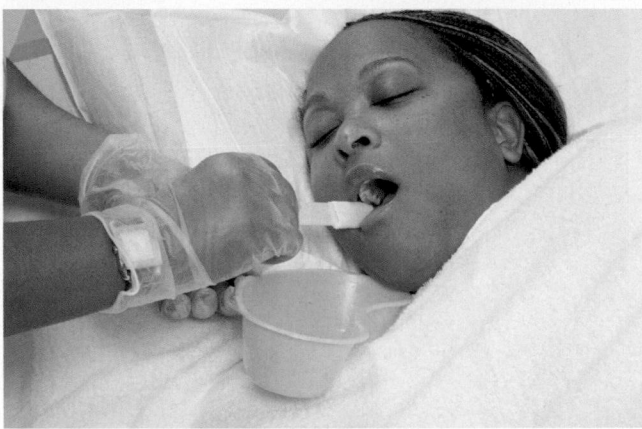

FIG. 7 Using a padded tongue blade, gently open the patient's mouth.

    Rationale: Unconscious patients often respond to oral stimulation by biting down.

8. **Brush teeth and gums as directed previously, using toothbrush or soft sponge-ended swab (Figs. 8 and 9). Cleanse oral cavity using swab.**

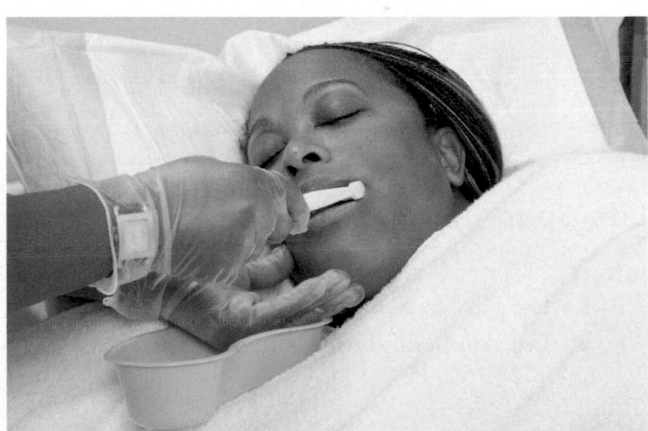

FIG. 8 Carefully brush the patient's teeth.

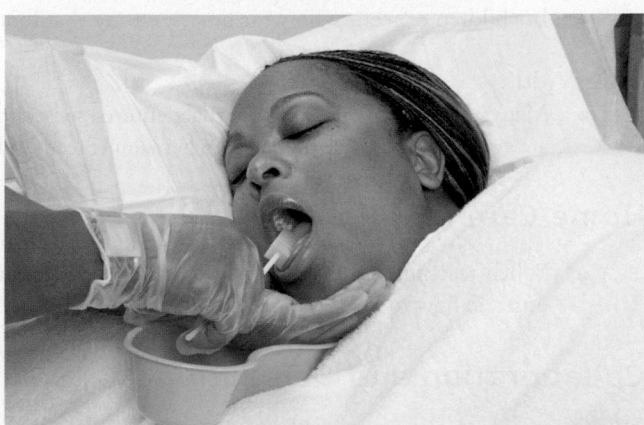

FIG. 9 Using a soft sponge-ended swab, cleanse the teeth and the mouth.

Procedure 24-6 *continued*

9. Use a small bulb syringe or syringe without needle to rinse oral cavity (Fig. 10). Swab or use oral suction to remove pooled secretions (Fig. 11).

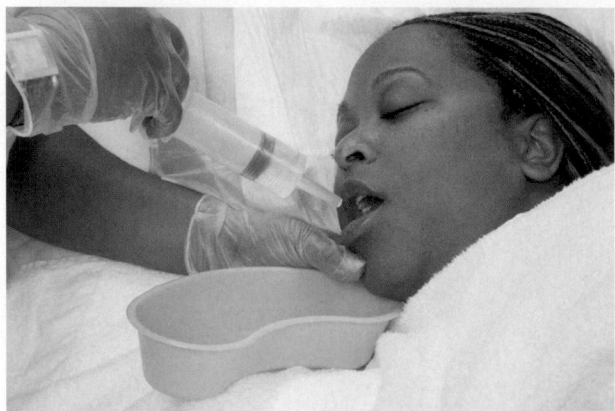

FIG. 10 Use irrigating syringe and a small amount of water to rinse the mouth.

Rationale: Suction is often needed to remove secretions and prevent aspiration in the unconscious patient.

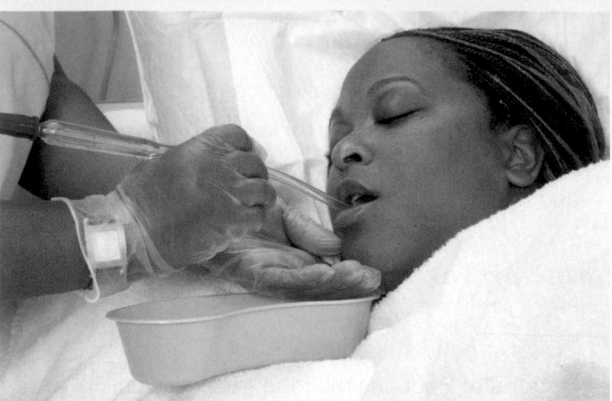

FIG. 11 Use suction to remove excess fluid.

10. Apply thin layer of petroleum jelly to lips to prevent drying or cracking.

Rationale: Prevents lips from drying or cracking.

11. Document procedure.

Rationale: Maintains legal record and communicates with healthcare team.

Documentation

6/13/17: 15:00—Oral care provided every 2 hours. No mouth lesions noted.

S. Roberts, RN

Life Span Considerations

Infant
- Use a dry gauze or washcloth to remove accumulated secretions from an infant's gums.
- Use a small, soft-bristled brush after first teeth have erupted.

Child
- Children younger than 3 or 4 years may not understand what "rinse" or "spit" means. Do not offer them water to rinse with if they are NPO because they will swallow it.
- In children or teens who wear braces, ensure that food particles are removed from the wires.

Older Adult
- Many older adults wear full or partial dentures, so be sure dentures are removed and cleaned regularly. Special denture cleansers are available. Brush the gums or any remaining teeth well. Keep dentures in a labeled denture cup to prevent breakage or loss.

Home Care Modifications

- When teaching family members who are working with a comatose family member, be sure they can verbalize and demonstrate how to avoid aspiration.

Collaboration and Delegation

- Enlist the aid of OTs to work with patients who are relearning oral care procedures.
- Refer the patient to a dentist if you detect gum disease or caries.

Procedure 24-7 Using a Bedpan

Purpose

1. Provide a means for elimination for patients who are confined to bed or unable to get to the bathroom or bedside commode independently or safely.

Equipment

Clean bedpan or fracture pan (see Fig. 24-11 for two types of bedpans)
Toilet tissue
Washcloth, towel, soap
Air freshener (optional)
Specimen container (if needed)
Cover for bedpan (if toilet for discarding is not in patient's room)
Disposable gloves

Assessment

- Assess the patient's normal elimination habits and when he or she last voided or defecated.
- Assess level of mobility, positioning restrictions, and degree of assistance required.
- Review orders to determine if urine or fecal specimens are needed.
- Identify medications the patient is receiving that would alter the color, consistency, or amount of urine or feces obtained.

Procedure

Placing the Bedpan

1. **Perform hand hygiene. Don clean gloves.**
   Rationale: Reduces microbe transmission.

2. **Identify the patient.**
   Rationale: Ensures correct patient receives proper assessment or treatment and reduces errors.

3. **Close door or bed curtains and explain the procedure to the patient and patient's family.**
   Rationale: Ensures patient privacy, increases patient compliance, and reduces patient anxiety.

4. **Position and lock side rail up on opposite side of bed from which you will work.**
   Rationale: Prevents the patient from rolling out of bed when turning on and off the bedpan.

5. **Raise bed to height appropriate for nurse.**
   Rationale: Prevents muscle strain and promotes proper body mechanics.

6. **For the patient who can raise buttocks and assist with procedure:**

   a. **Fold top linen down on your side to expose the patient's hips. (Patient in photographs is exposed for better visualization of procedure.)**
      Rationale: Minimally expose the patient to decrease embarrassment and preserve dignity.

   b. **Have patient flex knees and lift buttocks. Slide waterproof pad under the patient (Fig. 1).**

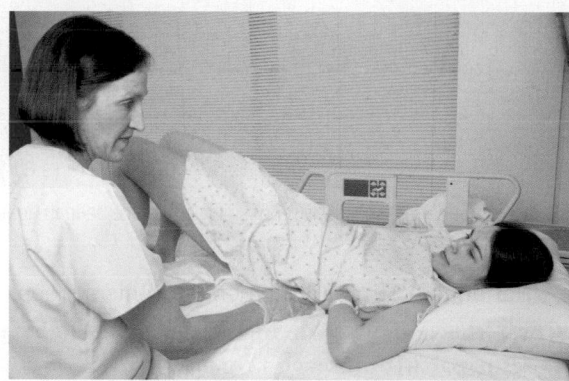

FIG. 1 Place waterproof pad under the patient to protect linens.

Rationale: Lower legs and feet support the patient's body weight. A waterproof pad protects sheets.

   c. **Assist the patient by placing your hand under sacrum, elbow on mattress, and lifting as a lever. Slide rounded, smooth rim of regular bedpan under the patient. If using a fracture pan, slide narrow, flat end under buttocks (Fig. 2).**

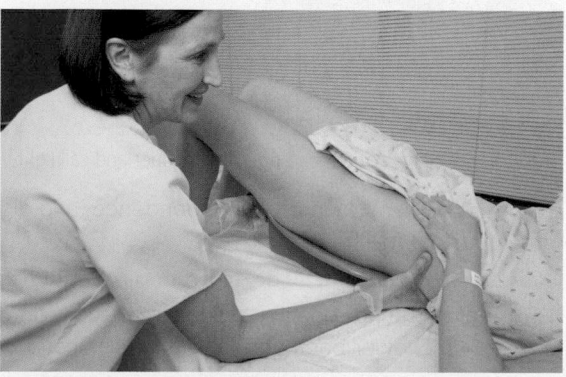

FIG. 2 Correctly place bedpan beneath the patient.

Procedure 24-7   *continued*

Rationale: Proper body mechanics prevent muscle strain. Proper placement prevents spillage and shearing trauma of skin in the sacral area.

7. **For the patient unable to assist by raising buttocks:**

   a. **Lower the head of the bed to flat position.**

   b. **Fold top bed linens down to expose the patient minimally.**

   c. **Help the patient to roll to side-lying position.**

   d. **Place bedpan against buttocks and tucked down against mattress. Hold firmly in place and roll the patient onto back as bedpan is positioned under buttocks (Fig. 3).**

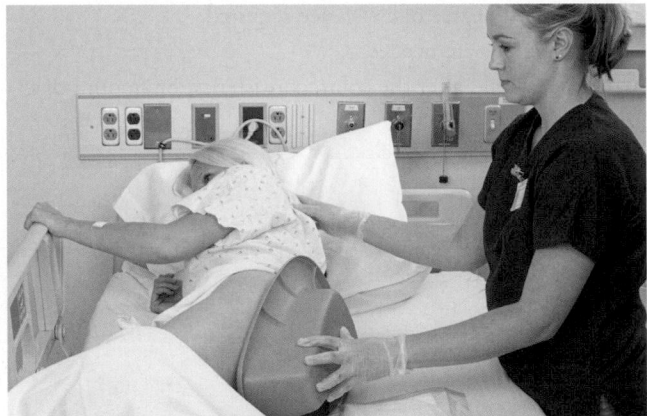

FIG. 3 Assist the patient to side-lying position and place bedpan against buttocks.

Rationale: Correct placement prevents spillage.

8. **Cover the patient with linen. Place call light and toilet paper within reach (Fig. 4).**

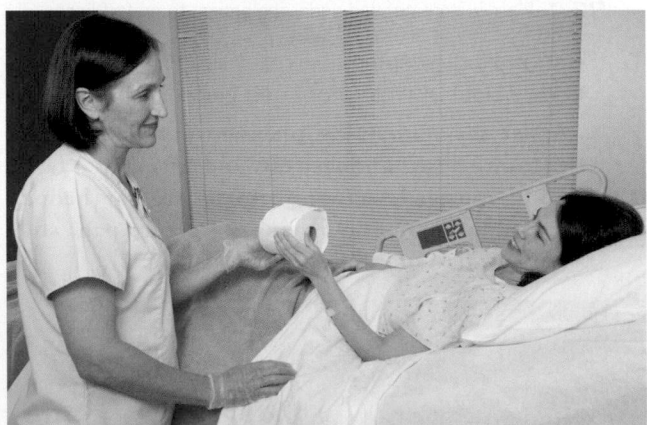

FIG. 4 Cover the patient and offer toilet paper and call light.

Rationale: Privacy, warmth, independence, and dignity are important for the patient.

9. **Raise head of bed 45 to 80 degrees unless contraindicated.**

   Rationale: Sitting position reduces discomfort and strain on the lower back and facilitates elimination.

10. **Lower bed to lowest position. Place side rails up if indicated.**

    Rationale: Ensures patient safety.

11. **Perform hand hygiene. Allow the patient to be alone.**

Removing the Bedpan

12. **Answer call light promptly.**

    Rationale: Sitting on a bedpan for a long period is uncomfortable and can cause pressure on skin.

13. **Place hand hygiene materials at bedside.**

    Rationale: Decreases the transfer of microorganisms and encourages good hygiene practices.

14. **Raise bed to appropriate working height for nurse.**

    Rationale: Prevents muscle strain and promotes proper body mechanics.

15. **Fold back top linens to expose the patient minimally.**

16. **Put on disposable clean gloves.**

    Rationale: Gloves help prevent contamination of hands with body substances.

17. **Assess if the patient can wipe perineal area. If not, wipe area with several layers of toilet tissue. If specimen is to be measured or collected, dispose of soiled toilet tissue in separate receptacle, not bedpan. For female patients, wipe from urethra toward anus.**

    Rationale: Prevents tracking of rectal microorganisms into the urinary meatus. Use as an informal teaching session to reinforce good hygiene practices.

18. **For patient who can raise buttocks and assist with procedure:**

    a. **Lower head of bed.**

    b. **Have the patient flex knees and lift buttocks. Assist the patient by placing one hand under sacrum and supporting bedpan with other hand to prevent spillage. Remove bedpan and place on bedside chair.**

    c. **Offer supplies and encouragement for patient to wash hands and perineal area.**

       Rationale: Washing prevents transfer of microorganisms, promotes good hygiene practices, and prevents skin breakdown.

19. **For the patient unable to assist by raising buttocks:**

    a. **Lower head of bed to flat position.**

    b. **Fold top linen down to expose the patient minimally.**

    c. **Help the patient to roll off bedpan and onto side. Use one hand to stabilize bedpan during turning to prevent spillage.**

    d. **Wipe anal area with tissue. Wash perineum.**

       Rationale: Prevents skin breakdown and excoriation.

Procedure 24-7   *continued*

20. Assist the patient to comfortable position.

21. Cover bedpan and remove from bedside (Fig. 5). Obtain specimen if required. Empty and clean bedpan, and return it to bedside.

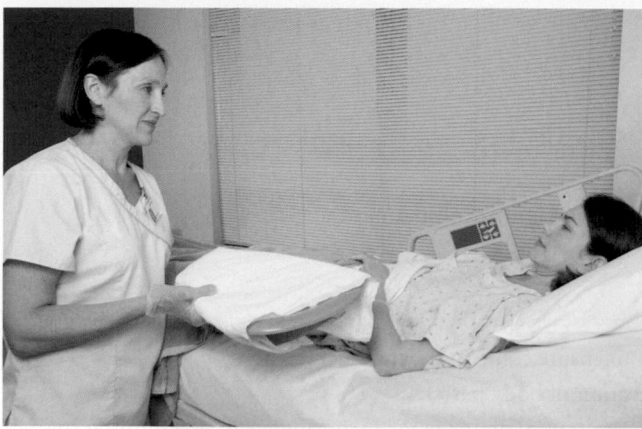

FIG. 5 Cover bedpan and remove from bedside.

Rationale: A clean pan minimizes spread of offensive odor.

22. **Remove and discard gloves. Perform hand hygiene.**

Rationale: Washing reduces spread of microorganisms.

23. **Spray air freshener if necessary to control odor, unless contraindicated (patient with respiratory conditions, allergies).**

Rationale: Odor is embarrassing to patient and visitors. Minimizing embarrassment preserves dignity.

24. **Document procedure.**

Rationale: Maintains legal record and communicates with healthcare team.

Documentation

- Record intake and output or if a stool sample was sent on the appropriate flow sheet.

Life Span Considerations

Child

- If possible, use a potty chair at the bedside for a toddler. A toilet-trained child may be reluctant to use a bedpan because he or she has learned not to urinate or defecate in bed.

Older Adult

- Older adults may find using a regular bedpan difficult because of body movement limitations and arthritis. A fracture pan is less difficult and less painful to use.

Collaboration and Delegation

- Because nurses frequently delegate placing and removing a bedpan to unlicensed personnel, review patient mobility restrictions and the need to measure or collect urine or feces or obtain specimens.

Procedure 24-8 Making an Occupied Bed

Purpose

1. Provide clean linen for patient who is unable to get out of bed.
2. Promote comfort.

Equipment

Bottom sheet
Top sheet
Draw sheet (optional)
Blanket (change only if soiled)
Bedspread (change only if soiled)
Mattress pad, if used by facility (change only if soiled)
Pillowcases
Waterproof pads or bath blanket (optional for incontinent or diaphoretic patients)
Linen bag
Bedside table or chair

Assessment

- Assess pain level and need for analgesia to ensure comfort during linen change.
- Note any position precautions (i.e., elevation of body parts).
- Assess patient's potential for excessive perspiration, drainage, or incontinence in determining special linen requirements.
- Assess agency protocol for linen change. In some long-term care facilities, linen changes occur when the patient gets a bath, weekly or biweekly.

Procedure

1. **Perform hand hygiene.**
   Rationale: Reduces microbe transmission.

2. **Identify the patient.**
   Rationale: Ensures correct patient receives proper treatment and reduces errors.

3. **Close door or bed curtains and explain the procedure to the patient and patient's family.**
   Rationale: Ensures patient privacy, increases patient compliance, and reduces patient anxiety.

4. **Assemble equipment on bedside table or chair. Do not place on another patient's bed.**
   Rationale: Placing linen on a clean surface prevents contamination with microorganisms.

5. **Lock up side rails on side of bed opposite from where you stack the clean linen.**
   Rationale: Side rails prevent the patient from rolling out of bed and give the patient a bar to grasp to assist with turning.

6. **Raise bed to comfortable working position. Lower side rail on your side of bed.**
   Rationale: Promotes good body mechanics and reduces muscle strain on back.

7. **Loosen all top linen from foot of bed. Remove top linen and bedspread or blanket separately. Without shaking, fold each piece and place over back of chair if it is to be reused. If it is soiled, hold it away from your uniform and place in linen bag.**
   Rationale: Folding linen enables the nurse to discard or handle without contaminating the uniform. Shaking linen spreads microorganisms through the air.

8. **Leave top sheet on the patient or cover the patient with a bath blanket; if using bath blanket, remove top sheet from under bath blanket and discard top sheet. (A bath blanket does not appear in photos for better visualization.)**
   Rationale: Provides warmth and prevents unnecessary body exposure during linen change.

9. **Loosen the bottom sheet on your side. Lower head of bed to flat position. If the patient cannot tolerate flat position, lower the head of the bed as far as the patient can tolerate.**
   Rationale: Changing linen is easier when the bed is flat.

10. **Help the patient to roll onto side facing away from you). The patient may grasp side rail to assist. Additional personnel may be needed to assist with patient positioning. Adjust pillow under head.**
    Rationale: Side-lying position provides space for placing clean linen on mattress.

Procedure 24-8 *continued*

11. Tightly fanfold soiled linens (Fig. 1). Tuck under buttocks, back, and shoulders (Fig. 2). Do not fanfold mattress pad unless it is soiled.

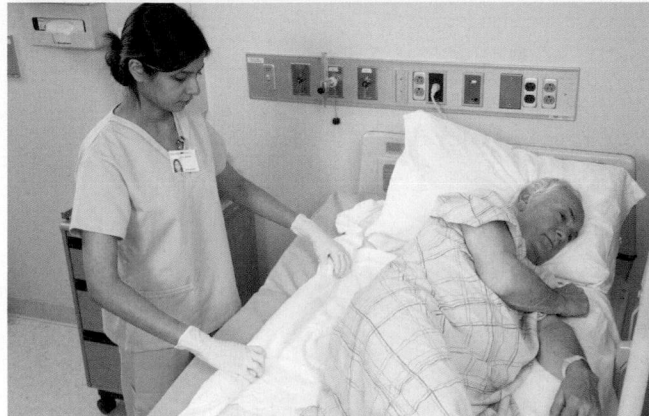

FIG. 1 Fanfold soiled linens.

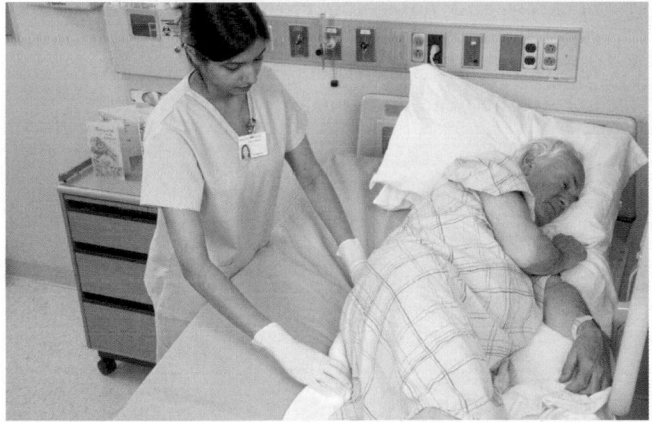

FIG. 2 Tuck soiled linens under the patient.

Rationale: Fanfolds under the patient should be as tight and smooth as possible to provide space for clean linen and enable the patient to eventually roll back over folds.

With Flat Bottom Sheet

12. Unfold lengthwise so bottom edge is even with end of mattress and vertical center crease is at center of bed.

    Rationale: Ensures the sheet will fit properly on the mattress.

13. Bring sheet's bottom edge over mattress sides and fanfold top of sheet toward center of mattress and place next to the patient. Tuck top edge of sheet under mattress. Miter top corner on your side.

    a. Grasp side edge of sheet about 18 inches down from mattress top.

    b. Lay sheet on top of mattress to form a triangular, flat fold.

c. Tuck sheet hanging loose below mattress under mattress without pulling on the triangular fold.

d. Pick up triangular fold, and place it over side of the mattress.

e. Tuck this loose portion of sheet under the mattress.

    Rationale: Mitered corners do not loosen easily when the patient moves in bed.

14. Tuck remaining portion of sheet under mattress. Proceed to step 16.

With Fitted Sheet

15. Secure the top and bottom elastic edges over the side of the mattress nearest you. Fanfold the top of sheet toward center of mattress and place next to the patient (Fig. 3).

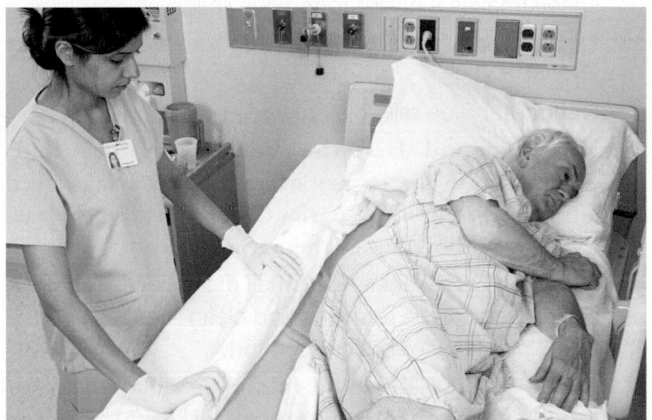

FIG. 3 Fanfold bottom sheet and move toward center of bed.

16. Place draw sheet on bed with center fold at center of bed. Position sheet so it will extend from the patient's back to below the buttocks. Fanfold the top edge and place next to the patient. Tuck excess under mattress. Some agencies use a cloth waterproof pad instead of a draw sheet.

    Rationale: A draw sheet is used to reposition the patient and absorb excess perspiration.

Procedure 24-8 *continued*

17. **Position bottom sheet and draw sheet under soiled sheets (Fig. 4).**

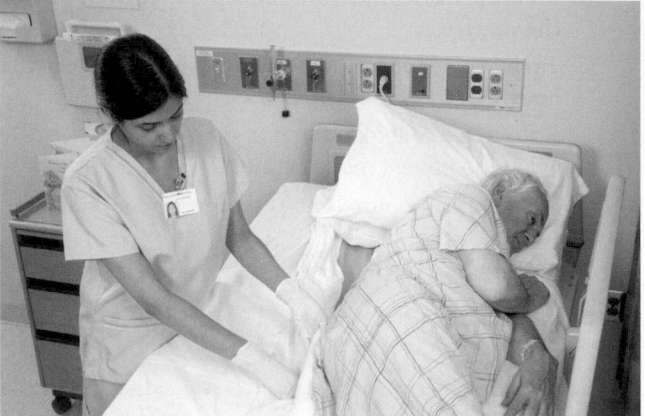

FIG. 4 Position clean linens under soiled linens.

Rationale: Positioning the clean sheet under the soiled sheets makes it easier to remove linens.

18. **Lock up side rails on your side and move to other side of bed.**

Rationale: Side rails maintain the patient's safety.

19. **Lower side rail. Help the patient to roll over folds of linen onto his or her other side. You may need additional help if the patient is unable to move easily. Move pillow under the patient's head.**

Rationale: When the second half of the bed is exposed, soiled linen can be removed and clean linen replaced. A pillow provides for patient comfort.

20. **Remove soiled linen by folding into a square or bundle with soiled side turned in (Fig. 5). Place in linen bag.**

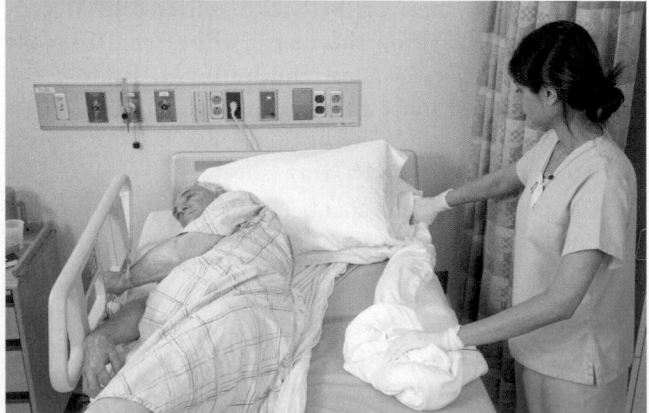

FIG. 5 Loosen and remove soiled bottom linens.

Rationale: Reduces transmission of microorganisms and prevents patient embarrassment at seeing soiled sheets.

21. **Grasp edge of fanfolded bottom sheet and pull from under the patient (Fig. 6).**

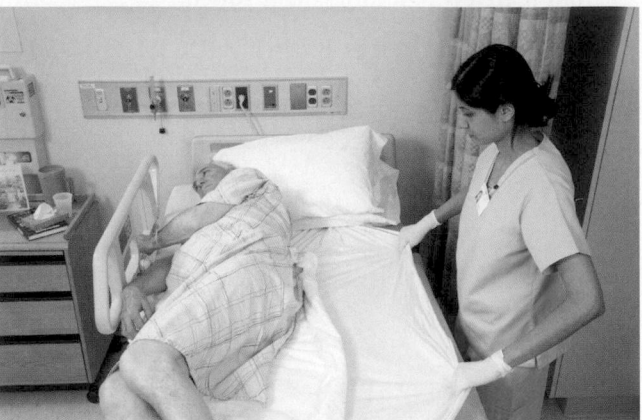

FIG. 6 Pull linen from under the patient.

22. **If using flat sheet, tuck top of sheet under top of mattress and miter top corner. Pull bottom sheet tight and tuck excess linen under mattress from top to bottom. If using fitted sheet, secure elastic corners at the head and foot of mattress (Fig. 7).**

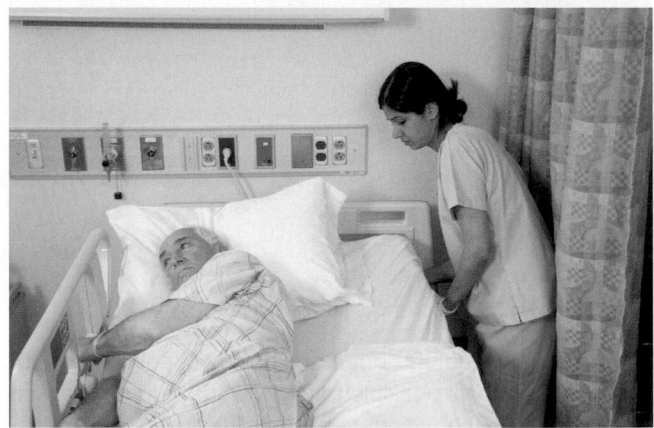

FIG. 7 Secure corner of bottom sheet to mattress.

Rationale: Securing linens under the mattress maintains a sheet's tight fit and eliminates wrinkles.

23. **Unfold draw sheet by grasping at center. Pull draw sheet taut and smooth. Tuck excess tightly under mattress. Tuck the middle first, then the top, and finally the bottom.**

Rationale: Tucking the center first prevents the draw sheet from pulling sideways and causing a poor fit and wrinkles.

24. **Help the patient to center of bed.**

25. **Raise side rail if necessary and move to side of bed where remainder of linen is stored.**

Procedure 24-8   *continued*

26. **Place the top sheet over the patient with center crease lengthwise at center of bed with seam side up. Unfold sheet from head to toe.**

27. **Have the patient grasp the top edge of clean top sheet. Remove bath blanket or soiled top linen by pulling from beneath clean top sheet. Smooth sheet, with excess falling over bottom edge of mattress.**

    Rationale: Limiting exposure of body parts preserves the patient's dignity.

28. **Discard in linen bag.**

29. **Place top sheet on bed with vertical center fold at center of bed. Unfold sheet with seams facing out and top edge even with top of mattress. Smooth sheet, with excess falling over bottom edge of mattress.**

    Rationale: Placing seam side up prevents edges from rubbing and irritating the patient's skin.

30. **Spread blanket or bedspread evenly over bed. Miter the bottom corner, using all layers of linen (sheet, blanket, bedspread). Leave sides untucked. Move to opposite side of bed and repeat (Fig. 8).**

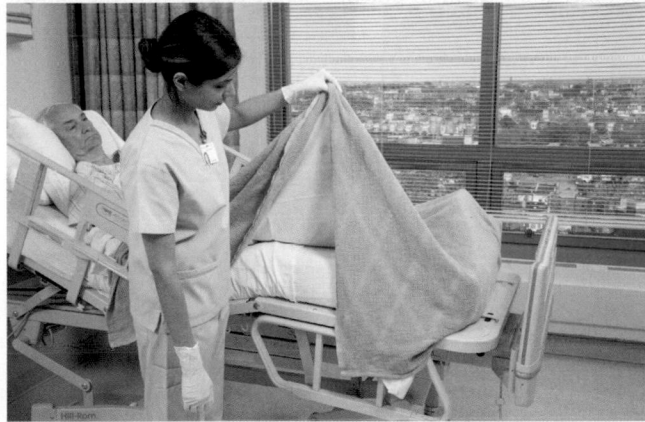

FIG. 8 Miter corner of linens. Grasp side edge of linens; lift up to form a triangle and tuck lower linens under mattress.

    Rationale: Mitering all three layers together saves time and energy. Mitered corners secure top covers but allow easy access in and out of bed by leaving sides free.

31. **Standing at bottom of bed, grasp top covers about 10 inches from bottom of mattress. Loosen linen slightly by pulling on top covers or forming a pleat.**

    Rationale: Additional room for the patient's feet gives comfort and prevents pressure on toes and foot drop.

32. **Put on clean pillowcases:**

    a. **Grasp center of pillowcase with one hand on seamed end.**

    b. **Gather case, turning it inside out over the hand holding it.**

    c. **With same hand, grasp middle of one end of pillow.**

    d. **Pull case over pillow with free hand.**

    e. **Adjust case, so corners fit over pillow.**

    Rationale: Prevents shaking of pillowcase and linen and distributing microorganisms in the room.

33. **Place pillows in center at head of bed.**

34. **Ensure that call light is within the patient's reach and lower bed (Fig. 9).**

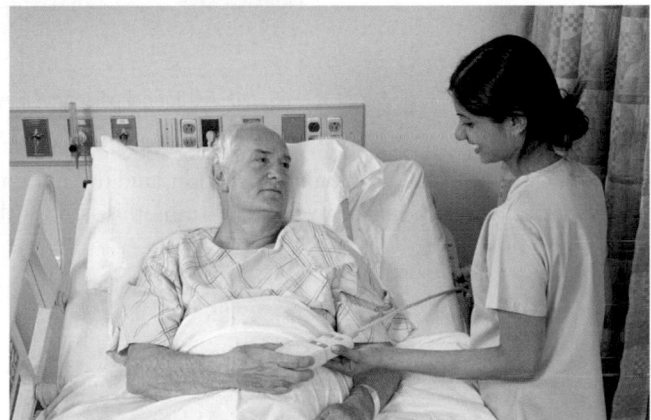

FIG. 9 Place call light within the patient's reach.

    Rationale: A call light within reach helps provide safety for the patient.

35. **Arrange the bedside table, night stand, and personal items within easy reach.**

    Rationale: Provides for patient comfort and prevents falls if the patient attempts to reach for items not close by.

36. **Discard soiled linens and wash your hands.**

    Rationale: Maintains infection control.

37. **Document procedure.**

    Rationale: Maintains legal record and communicates with healthcare team.

Documentation

- It is usually unnecessary to document this procedure.

Procedure 24-8 *continued*

Collaboration and Delegation

- When delegating this task to unlicensed assistive personnel, communicate when help is needed (Fig. 10). This is often done after bathing.

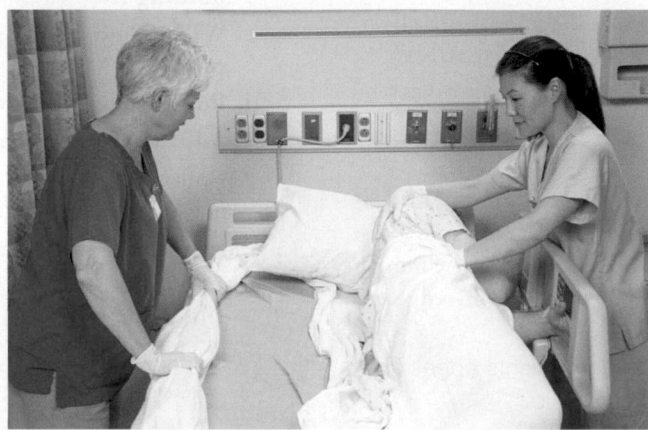

FIG. 10 Additional personnel may be needed to assist with making an occupied bed.

- Communicate positioning restrictions and the amount of assistance that may be required to ensure the patient's safety. If family members/caregivers are learning this skill for the first time, allow them to practice before discharging the patient to home.

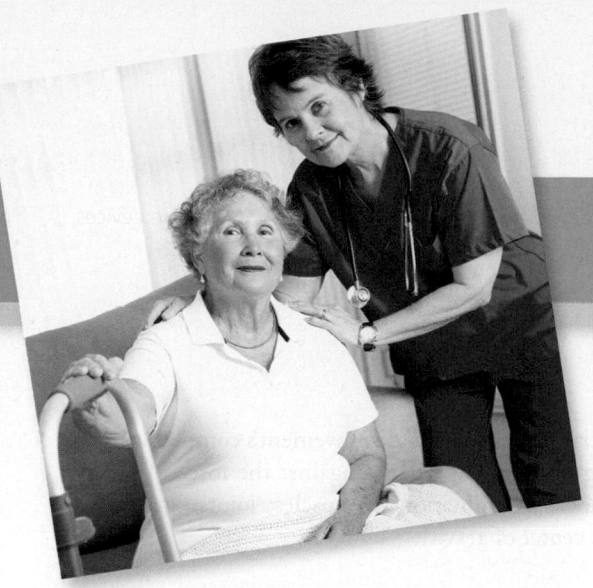

CHAPTER 25

Mobility

Pavla Holman

Case Scenario

You are a home health nurse visiting a new patient, a retired woman recently discharged from the hospital after knee replacement surgery. Her son meets you at the door, looking tired and anxious. He explains that his mother is reluctant to do anything for herself because it still hurts to move. She has been sleeping on the sofa bed in the living room and spends much of the day there. She uses a bedpan rather than walking to a nearby bathroom. Helping her to a recliner has been very difficult for the son, who fears his mother may fall even while using the walker. The son adds that his mother becomes very upset and yells when he encourages her to do more for herself.

Once you have completed this chapter and have incorporated mobility into your knowledge base, review the above scenario and reflect on the following areas of Critical Thinking:

1. Considering the mobility and safety concerns apparent in this scenario, prioritize your assessment.
2. Identify possible causes underlying this patient's reluctance to move. How might this information affect your plan?
3. From the information provided, consider possible nursing diagnoses. Prioritize them, and give rationales for your choices.
4. Propose ways in which collaboration with other healthcare professionals would be beneficial.
5. As you work with this family, discuss ways to ensure their safety.

KEY TERMS

activity intolerance
aerobic exercise
anaerobic exercise
arthroscopy
ataxia
athetosis
atrophy
body mechanics
chorea
contracture
dangling
deep vein thrombosis (DVT)
dystonia
flaccidity
foot drop
gait
isometric exercise
isotonic exercise
lift team
osteoarthritis
paraplegia
range of motion (ROM)
scoliosis
spasticity
tetraplegia
tremor

LEARNING OBJECTIVES

Upon completion of this chapter, you will be able to do the following:

1. Explain normal functions of the musculoskeletal system and characteristics of normal movement.
2. Identify factors, including lifespan considerations that can affect or alter mobility.
3. Describe the impact of immobility on physiologic and psychological functioning.
4. Discuss appropriate subjective and objective data to collect to assess mobility status.

5. Demonstrate nursing interventions such as positioning, ambulating, transferring, providing range of motion, and using assistive devices.

6. Plan strategies to avoid musculoskeletal injury to the nurse and patient during patient care.

7. Develop appropriate community-based nursing interventions for preventing and managing mobility problems.

Mobility, or the ability to move freely within the environment, is fundamental to normal daily functioning. In a highly mobile society, problems affecting mobility are especially significant. Independence is usually defined by a person's ability to perform activities of daily living (ADLs), job-related activities, and role-related activities (e.g., as a parent or spouse). Limitations in a person's ability to move normally and spontaneously can affect all of these areas.

Changes in mobility also create more subtle psychological effects, especially in communication. Facial expressions and gestures are significant in nonverbal communication, and talking with someone at eye level promotes equality between those talking. The person who must look up at someone from a chair or bed may feel that he or she is at a psychological disadvantage. Movement also is significant in diffusing negative feelings and tension. Many people find that jogging and other forms of exercise help to relieve stress and anxiety. Being able to leave uncomfortable or dangerous situations gives most people a feeling of control. Conversely, people confined to bed usually see themselves as sick and may feel less able to participate in the recovery process. Disabilities that affect mobility, such as amputation or a musculoskeletal defect, may alter self-image.

Most people associate mobility with health. Like many aspects of health, mobility can be viewed along a continuum from full mobility to immobility. Full mobility occurs when the person has no physical or psychological factors that limit mobility. Immobility occurs when the person cannot move his or her entire body or a specific body part.

Patients move along this continuum as their abilities change:

*   Therapeutic treatments, such as traction to repair a fracture, may cause temporary changes in mobility.
*   Some conditions lead to progressive disability—examples are muscular dystrophy and severe crippling rheumatoid arthritis.
*   Permanent changes in mobility occur when normal body movement cannot be restored (e.g., spinal cord injuries that result in paralysis or strokes that cause weakness or paralysis on one side of the body).

Rehabilitation is the key to restoring a person with certain disabilities to optimal health. Nurses can play a significant role in this process.

NORMAL MOBILITY

The musculoskeletal system is the supporting framework for the body. The bones and muscles are involved in movement and are responsible for the body's form and shape. Central and peripheral nerves coordinate movement's complex activity. Maintaining posture and balance against the force of gravity requires smooth coordination of muscles, joints, and nerves and a stable center of gravity.

Structures of the Musculoskeletal System

BONES

Bones are a framework on which muscles, tendons, and ligaments are attached. They facilitate movement, protect vital organs (e.g., brain, heart, lungs, liver), store and regulate calcium and phosphate, and form blood cells.

The structure of bones provides for minimum weight and maximum structural strength. Bone tissue is either woven or lamellar. Woven bone is characterized by rapid growth, as occurs in infancy, and is generally found where ligaments and tendons insert into the bones of adults. Lamellar bone is mature with highly organized mineralized plates.

The 206 bones in the body also can be classified by shape: long (arms, legs), short (tarsals, carpals), flat (cranium), and irregular (vertebral). Basic components of the long bones are the diaphysis (shaft) and the epiphyses (ends). Most bone is covered by periosteum, which contains nerves and blood vessels. The outer portion of the long bones is composed of dense, compact bone with a marrow cavity in the center where the blood-forming cells are located.

MUSCLES

Skeletal muscles are connected to the bones at or across joints. Muscles are composed of striated, long muscle fibers usually in parallel alignment. The fibers' formation allows muscles to contract (shorten) or extend (lengthen) as required by movement. Contraction occurs when the overlapping striated fibers slide toward each other, thereby shortening the muscle and increasing its strength.

Muscle contraction requires a complex mechanical, chemical, and electrical interaction. The contraction is initiated when an action potential (electrical charge) moves along a nerve and across the neuromuscular junction to the muscle. Neurotransmitters, which are chemical substances such as acetylcholine, permit neurologic impulses to be transmitted to muscle. The transmitting activity occurs when calcium is released into the sarcoplasmic reticulum (site of storage and release for calcium in the muscle), which initiates a complex series of biochemical events that result in muscle contraction.

Energy for the work of contraction comes from the metabolism of food, especially fats and carbohydrates.

Muscles are covered by a layer of connective tissue that joins with tendon fibers at the end of the muscle fiber where muscle joins bone. Muscle fibers are innervated by motor neurons originating from the anterior horn of the spinal cord. All muscle fibers connected to a single motor nerve are called a motor unit.

During a lifetime, the body has only the number of muscle cells with which it was born; however, the work of the muscle determines the size of the muscle cells. When forceful activity is demanded of the muscle, the muscle hypertrophies (the muscle's diameter increases), increasing the muscle's strength. **Atrophy**, the opposite of hypertrophy, causes the muscle to decrease in strength and size because of disuse. Disuse may be related to lack of exercise, aging, or enforced rest or the use of immobilizing devices.

JOINTS

Joints are the areas where bones meet. The types of joints are fibrous, which do not move (cranial); cartilaginous, which allow minimal movement (costochondral); and synovial, which are moveable (joints of the extremities). Synovial joints are lined with synovial tissue, which has a rich blood supply and produces synovial fluid. Synovial fluid lubricates joints, allowing smooth articulation and easy motion. Terms used to describe joint motion are provided in Box 25-1.

Ligaments and tendons connect and support joints. Ligaments stabilize the bones in the joints and are more

elastic than tendons. Tendons are specialized tissues. They connect muscle to bone and are surrounded by synovial-like tissues.

Normal Physiologic Function

Carrying out coordinated movement is a complex process. Even with a framework of bones held together by ligaments and covered with soft tissue and skin, normal function cannot occur without coordinated muscle activity and neurologic integration.

ALIGNMENT AND POSTURE

Maintaining upright posture requires proper alignment of the bones, muscles, and joints and a stable center of gravity. Alignment is achieved when the joints and muscles are not experiencing extremes in extension or flexion or unusual stress when the person is lying down, sitting, or standing.

Upright posture and movement require a balanced center of gravity: The weight of the body is centered, and the downward forces of gravity are balanced. The usual line of gravity starts at the top of the head and bisects the shoulders, trunk, weight-bearing joints, and base of support; it runs slightly anterior to the sacrum. In older people, the lumbar spine tends to flatten, and the upper spine and head tend to tilt forward, causing the head to fall forward from the usual line of gravity (Fig. 25-1).

BALANCE

Maintaining balance is a complex function of counteracting gravity and reflexes to maintain posture. The reticular formation, a neural network in the brain stem, integrates neural input that is important for maintaining balance. If a person begins to fall to one side, the extensor muscles on that side stiffen while the extensor muscles on the opposite side relax to prevent the fall.

Equilibrium is provided mainly by the vestibular apparatus of the ear. The vestibular apparatus consists of the cochlear duct, the three semicircular canals, and two large chambers known as the utricle and the saccule. The utricle, saccule, and semicircular canals contain tiny hair cells connected to sensory nerve fibers that pass into the vestibular nerve. When the head moves, these hair cells are bent, pulled, or compressed, transmitting signals to the sensory nerves over the appropriate nerve tracts to the area that controls equilibrium and balance.

COORDINATED MOVEMENT

The cerebellum, cerebral cortex, and basal ganglia are responsible for the control of motor functions. The cerebellum coordinates the motor activities of movement, the cerebral cortex initiates voluntary motor activity, and the basal ganglia maintain posture. These systems make up the pyramidal and extrapyramidal tracts. The pyramidal tract (the direct

BOX 25-1	Terms Describing Joint Motion
Adduction	Moving a joint or extremity toward the midline of the body
Abduction	Moving a joint or extremity away from the midline of the body
Rotation, internal	Turning a joint or extremity on its axis toward the body's midline
Rotation, external	Turning a joint or extremity on its axis away from the body's midline
Flexion	Decreasing the angle between two bones
Extension	Straightening a joint
Hyperextension	Moving a joint past normal extension
Supination	Turning the body or a body part to face upward
Pronation	Turning the body or a body part to face downward
Circumduction	Moving a body part in widening circles
Inversion	Turning the feet inward so toes point toward the midline
Eversion	Turning the feet outward so toes point away from the midline
Opposition	Touching the thumb to each finger

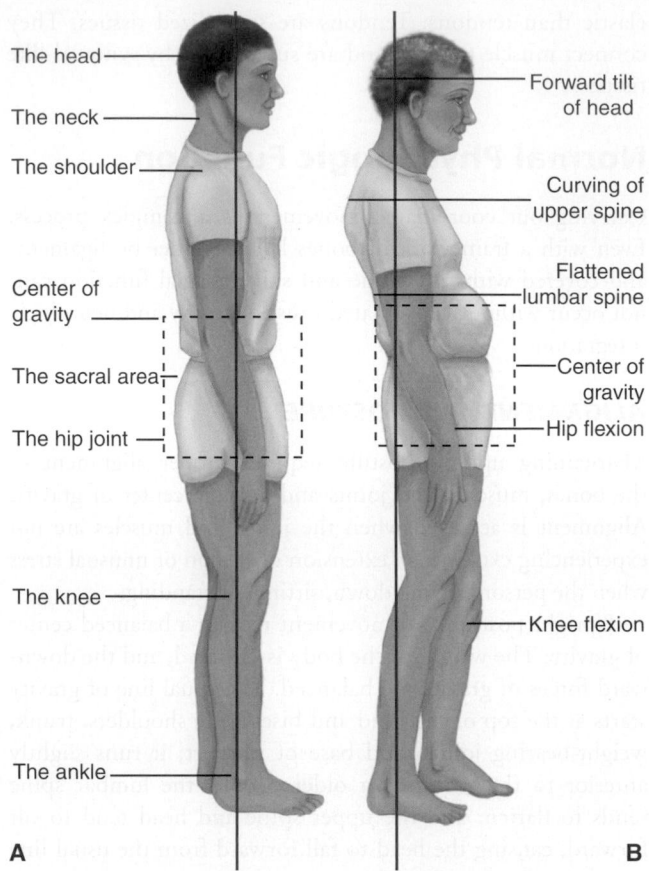

The head

The neck

The shoulder

Center of
gravity

The sacral area

The hip joint

The knee

The ankle

A

Forward tilt
of head

Curving of
upper spine

Flattened
lumbar spine

Center of
gravity

Hip flexion

Knee flexion

B

FIGURE 25-1 Vertical gravity line and posture. **A.** Vertical gravity line and center of gravity. **B.** Postural changes with age.

corticospinal pathway) initiates transmission of impulses to the spinal cord for voluntary movements. The extrapyramidal tract (the indirect corticospinal pathway) dampens and inhibits impulses to promote smooth and coordinated movement.

The cerebellum has a special role in controlling movement. It controls muscles used to maintain steady posture and coordinated, detailed movements. The cerebellum coordinates rapid, automatic adjustments that maintain balance and equilibrium. It refines learned movement patterns. The cerebellum compares the motor commands with proprioceptive information (position sense) and performs any adjustments needed (Martini & Nath, 2014). The result is smooth, coordinated movement and developed fine motor function rather than uncoordinated, arrhythmic movement.

BODY MECHANICS

Body mechanics can be defined as using alignment, posture, and balance in a coordinated effort to perform activities such as lifting, bending, and moving. Proper use of body mechanics promotes safe musculoskeletal function and helps nurses avoid placing undue strain on muscles. When nurses use their bodies to perform therapies, assist patients with movement, or move

equipment, they benefit from effective use of body mechanics to prevent injury to themselves or others. Proper use of body mechanics is explained in **Procedure 25-1**.

Components of Body Mechanics

Using body mechanics effectively means using gravity advantageously in body alignment, posture, balance, and movement. Maintaining a balanced center of gravity, which tends to be in the area of the pelvis slightly anterior to the sacrum, is essential to this process.

Maintaining balance involves keeping the spine in vertical alignment, the feet positioned for a broad base of support, and the body weight close to the center of gravity. When a person lifts or carries a load, that weight becomes part of the body weight; therefore, that additional weight must be balanced over the center of gravity (Fig. 25-2).

The greater the support base, the more stability the person has for changing body position while maintaining alignment, posture, and balance. The weight-bearing joints and skeletal muscles of the legs provide a stable base of support that a person can widen by placing the feet farther apart and flexing the hip and knee joints. These adjustments lower the center of

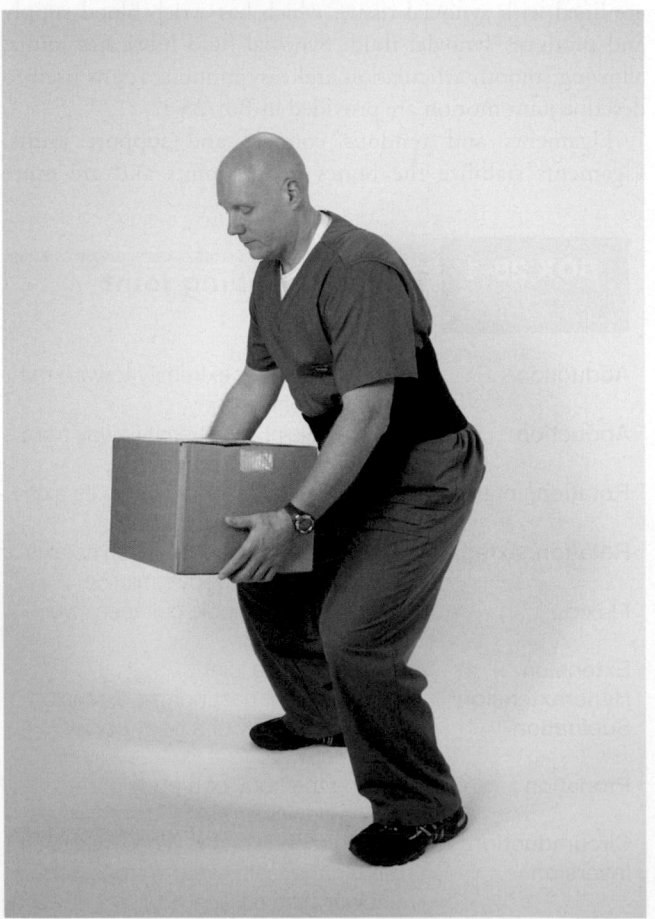

FIGURE 25-2 The nurse demonstrates proper lifting technique to prevent back strain and injury.

BOX 25-2   Principles of Body Mechanics

Scientific Principles Underlying Body Mechanics

- Less energy is used if all body parts are balanced appropriately.
- The greater the base of support, the more stable the body.
- Pelvic tilt (contraction of the abdominal and gluteal muscles to stabilize the pelvis) before activity helps protect the lower back from strain and injury.
- Facing the direction of work reduces the chance of injury.
- Less energy is needed to keep an object moving (momentum) than to initiate movement (inertia).
- Moving an object on a level surface requires less effort.
- Reducing friction between the object moved and the surface on which it is moved requires less energy.
- Holding an object close to the body requires less energy than holding it farther away.
- Muscle strain can be avoided by using the strong leg muscles when lifting, pushing, and pulling.
- Smooth, continuous movements are easier and safer than sudden, sharp, or uncontrolled movements.
- Using rhythmic movements at a normal speed requires less energy.

Applied Principles of Body Mechanics

- Adjust the height of the work area when possible.
- Assume a starting position that will permit freedom of movement in range, direction, and position.
- Keep body balanced over the base of support with knees relaxed and trunk erect (in relation to the pelvis).
- Bend hips and knees to alter position of body, widening the base of support as needed, for effective leverage and use of energy.
- Face the direction of motion, using the muscles of the lower extremities and shifting body weight for lifting, pushing, and pulling actions.
- Hold objects close to the body when lifting.
- Use rhythmic, smooth, and coordinated motions at a reasonable speed.
- Use elbows, hips, and knees as levers when lifting.
- Use mechanical devices when appropriate.
- Holding one's breath during physical activity is an indication of muscle strain and inefficient use of body mechanics.

---

gravity, making a person more stable and allowing flexibility to avoid muscle strain.

Opposing voluntary muscle groups and neuromuscular reflexes coordinate movement. The flexor and extensor muscle groups provide opposing tensions for movement. When the flexors contract to move a joint, the extensors relax; when the flexors relax, the extensors contract. The flexors in the legs are among the largest and strongest muscles in the body and are used for leverage in good body mechanics. The neuromuscular reflexes maintain posture by enabling opposing muscle groups to coordinate movement.

Principles of Body Mechanics

Nurses and patients may fall or incur back injuries as patients are moved from one position or location to another. The more limited the patient's mobility, the more the nurse must rely on good body mechanics. Using assistive devices (e.g., friction reducers) to enhance an ergonomic approach to the necessary lifting can decrease occupational injuries. Box 25-2 lists the principles of body mechanics. Some general rules for body mechanics follow.

The first rule is to assess the situation carefully before acting. Planning is crucial. Unnecessary equipment should be out of the way of the nurse and patient, usually near the head or foot of the bed. Tubing, catheters, intravenous (IV) lines, drains, and wires for cardiac monitoring must be handled by the nurse or positioned to prevent accidental disconnection during a turn or transfer. Using a counting method helps to coordinate the actions of everyone involved in the movement. Counting "one, two, three," with the position change on "three," helps focus everyone's attention and invites the patient's active participation.

❗ SAFETY ALERT

When in doubt, seek assistance before beginning to move a patient. Examine the surroundings for potential obstacles to the desired movement (e.g., equipment, cords, tubing, or other items that could trip the nurse or hamper the patient's free movement).

The second rule is to use the large muscle groups of the legs whenever possible. This is done to provide the force for the movement. The back stays straight, the arms maintain a strong grip with elbows slightly flexed, and the hips and knees are bent. Pushing, pulling, or lifting is then accomplished by orienting the torso in the desired direction of movement and straightening the legs. Back injuries that result from moving patients can usually be traced to asymmetric muscle use. Avoid twisting or moving diagonally.

The third rule is to perform work at the appropriate height. When helping a patient move in bed, raise the bed height to a level close to the nurse's center of gravity, which is usually between the hips and waist. Lowering the side rails allows the nurse to move the patient as close as possible and avoid awkward positioning involved in reaching over side rails to perform tasks. When moving the patient from a bed to a stretcher, the two surfaces should be at the same height so the patient does not need to be lifted.

The fourth rule is to use mechanical lifts or assistance whenever needed to ease a move. Mechanical lifts are recommended when the patient cannot assist or cooperate or when the nurse is uncertain about the safety of the transfer. Stand-up lifts, used when patients can bear some weight and are able to follow simple commands, have been used to decrease injury to staff and patients in long-term care settings and are now being used in acute care settings. Overhead trapezes may provide handholds for patients who wish to assist. In many situations, a lift sheet (also called a turn or drawsheet) is helpful. This sturdy sheet is positioned under the patient in bed so that it extends from the shoulders to just below the hips. Depending on the patient's weight, two or more nurses (equally placed on each side of the bed) can use the lift sheet to move the patient anywhere on the mattress and then to position the patient onto either side. The key to successful use of the lift sheet is coordinated movement by the lifters.

EXERCISE

Exercise that actively requires alignment, posture, balance, and coordinated movement offers many physiologic and psychological benefits. Exercise must be regular and integrated into the person's lifestyle for maximum benefits. A person's family, culture, job, and health may influence his or her participation in and appreciation for exercise. Showing clear evidence of the benefits of an active lifestyle, exercise has become more popular as people have taken responsibility for decreasing risk factors and leading healthier lives.

Types of Exercise

Exercise may be classified by the source of energy (aerobic or anaerobic) and by the type of muscle tension (isotonic or isometric) required:

- **Aerobic exercise** requires oxygen to use the energy provided by the metabolic activities of the skeletal muscles. Aerobic exercise occurs during vigorous, continuous muscle movement (e.g., walking, running, cycling, cross-country skiing, aerobic dancing, playing tennis) when the person's heart rate is high enough to promote cardiovascular conditioning.
- **Anaerobic exercise** occurs when the muscle cannot extract enough oxygen from the blood and anaerobic pathways provide additional energy for a short time. This type of exercise is useful in athletic endurance training. All endurance exercise can become anaerobic when oxygen sources are depleted.
- **Isotonic exercise** is a dynamic form of exercise with constant muscle tension, muscle contraction, and active movement. Most activities (e.g., walking, running, performing ADLs) are isotonic.
- **Isometric exercise** is static exercise by which the patient tenses a muscle, holding it stationary while maintaining the tension. Examples of isometric exercise are quadriceps setting to strengthen the quadriceps muscle and strength training with weights.

Benefits of Exercise

Exercise strengthens muscles, increases endurance, and promotes joint mobility. Cardiovascular health improves as lung capacity increases, resting pulse rate and blood pressure decrease, and the risk of atherosclerosis decreases. Exercise helps to prevent constipation, enhance appetite, and improve sleep quality. Exercise contributes to a feeling of well-being because activity increases circulating endorphins and promotes tension and stress release. Weight loss and improved physical appearance frequently motivate people to continue exercising regularly. The person who does not exercise regularly is at risk for health problems, just as the immobile patient is at risk for problems related to disuse.

Characteristics of Normal Movement

FULL RANGE OF MOTION

Range of motion (ROM) is the ability to move all joints through the full extent of intended function. Each joint must be kept actively moving for the joints to maintain mobility, the muscles to maintain strength, and the cardiovascular system to function adequately.

Active ROM means that the person can initiate and perform exercises in which each joint moves through its complete ROM. The healthy person may complete active ROM as a part of everyday activities and exercise.

Normal joint movement depends on the type of joint. Table 25-1 shows the types of joints and their designated ROMs.

NORMAL GAIT

Walking is the most common form of locomotion. Although most people take the ability to walk for granted, the normal walking **gait**, which is the style and character of a person's walk, is a coordinated process requiring equilibrium and balanced posture. Normal human ambulation requires a complex interactive control between multiple limb and body segments that work congruently to provide the most shock-absorbing and energy-efficient forward movement possible.

The normal walking gait has two phases:

- The stance phase is composed of three events: heel strike, midstance, and push-off.
- The swing phase completes the walking gait with another three events: acceleration, swing through, and deceleration.

Walking is initiated by stepping with a slight forward tilt. The weight of the body is rolled off the ball and toes of one foot and shifted to the heel of the opposite foot and extended leg. In the process, the center of gravity moves from one side of the body to the other and forward at the same time. The body weight is balanced on a narrow base, shifted from one side to the other, and supported alternately on one foot and then the other.

TABLE 25-1 NORMAL MOVEMENT OF BODY JOINTS

Location in Body	Type of Joint	Normal Movement
Neck, cervical spine	Pivotal Spine Cervical	Flexion, extension, lateral flexion, rotation
Shoulder	Ball and socket	Flexion, extension, hyperextension, abduction, adduction, internal rotation, external rotation, circumduction
Elbow	Hinge joints	Supination, pronation, extension, flexion
Forearm	Pivotal	Supination, pronation

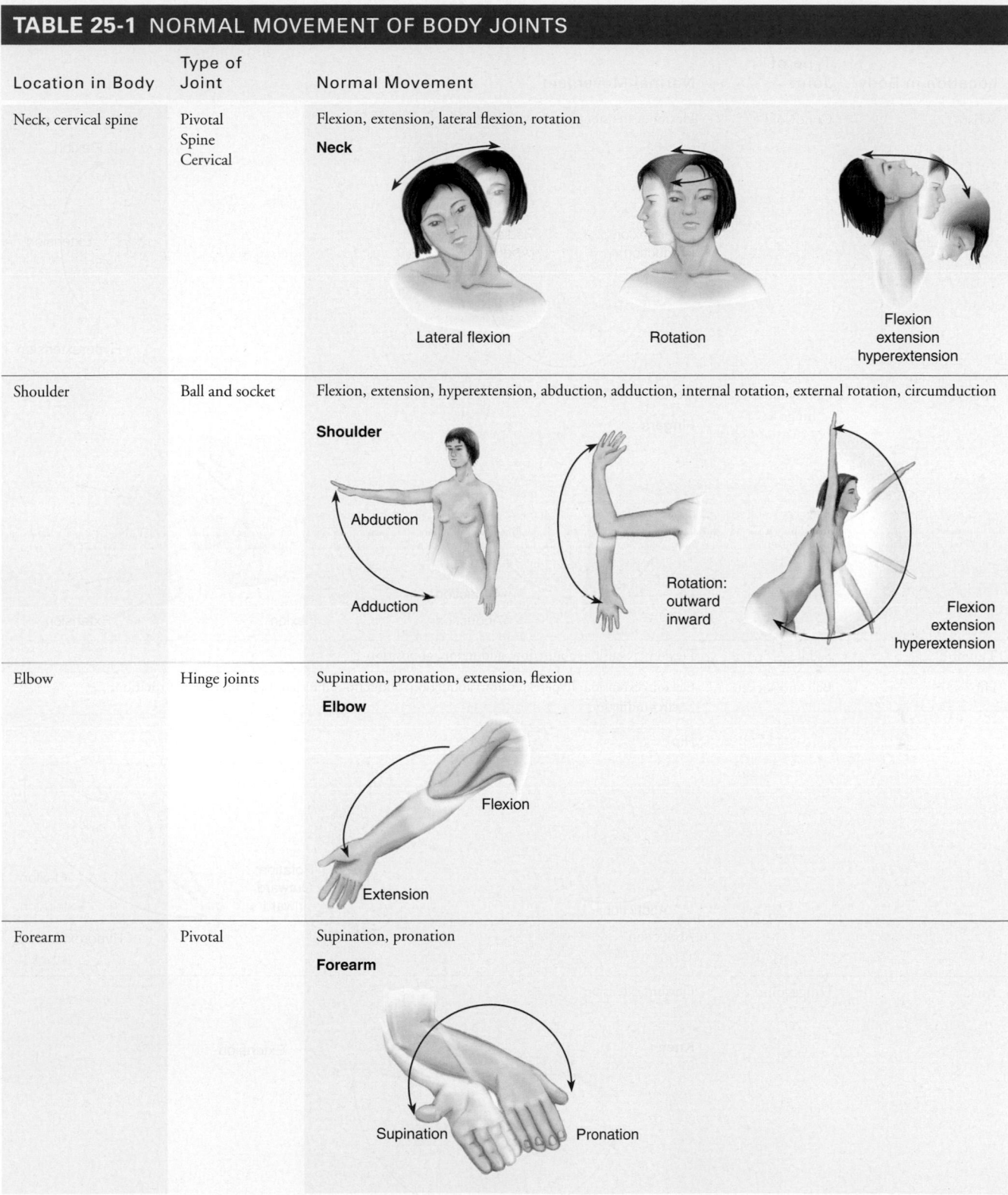

Neck

Lateral flexion   Rotation   Flexion
extension
hyperextension

Shoulder

Abduction

Adduction

Rotation:
outward
inward

Flexion
extension
hyperextension

Elbow

Flexion

Extension

Forearm

Supination   Pronation

(Continued)

TABLE 25-1   NORMAL MOVEMENT OF BODY JOINTS (*Continued*)

Location in Body	Type of Joint	Normal Movement
Wrist	Condyloid	Flexion, extension, hyperextension, adduction, abduction
Fingers	Condyloidal hinge	Flexion, extension, hyperextension, abduction, adduction
Thumb	Saddle	Flexion, extension, abduction, adduction, apposition
Hip	Ball and socket	Flexion, extension, hyperextension, abduction, adduction, internal rotation, external rotation, circumduction
Knee	Hinge joint	Flexion, extension

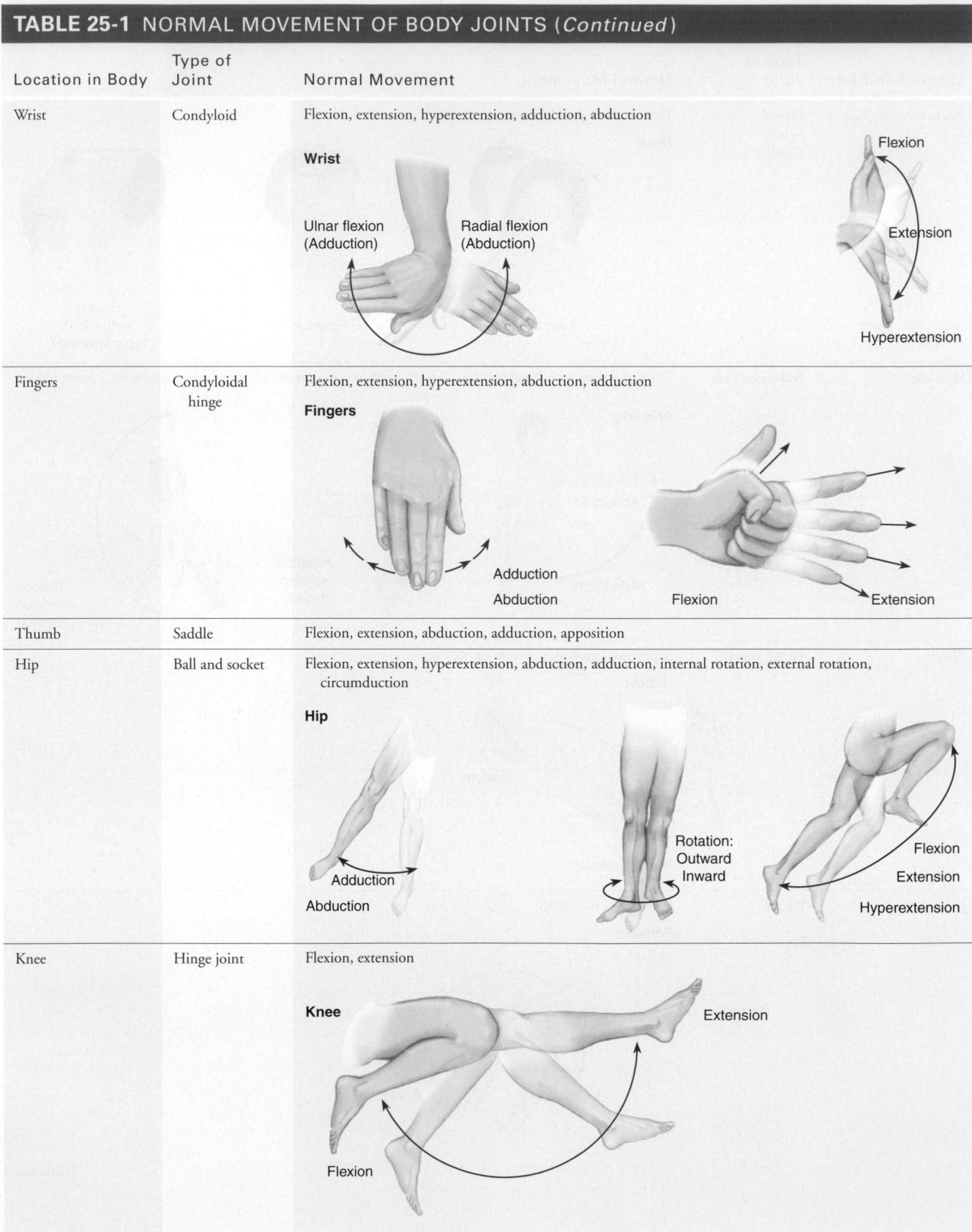

TABLE 25-1 NORMAL MOVEMENT OF BODY JOINTS (*Continued*)

Location in Body	Type of Joint	Normal Movement
Ankle	Hinge joint	Dorsiflexion, plantar flexion
Foot	Gliding	Inversion, eversion
Toes	Condyloid	Flexion, extension, abduction, adduction

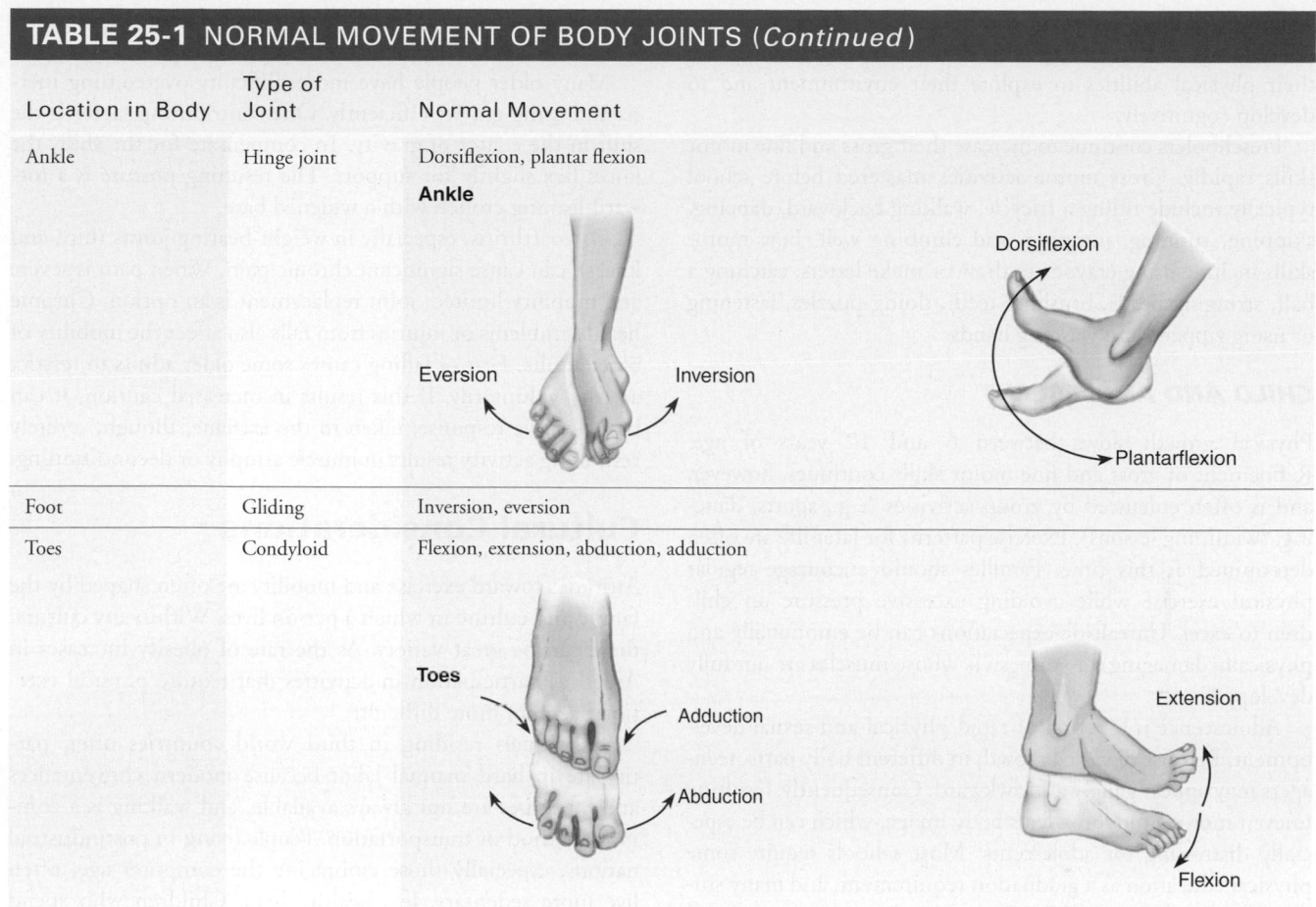

Life Span Considerations

NEWBORN AND INFANT

Movements of newborns are random and reflexive. Survival reflexes include rooting (turning toward the breast when the baby's cheek is stroked) and sucking. Subcortical reflexes (Moro, startle, tonic neck, Babinski) subside as higher brain function matures and exerts an inhibitory influence. Protective reflexes (gag, blink, and withdrawal) persist into adulthood.

The stepping response can be evoked in newborns by holding them on a solid surface and leaning them slightly forward. The shift in the center of gravity and change in equilibrium initiate the stepping reflex. With maturity, infants learn to control and use the same reflex when learning to walk.

Neuromuscular assessment of newborns is important to detect deformities or abnormalities that respond well to early treatment. Some deformities result from the position the baby had in utero and will correct spontaneously as the child grows. Because hip dislocation/subluxation can occur any time during the first year of life, assessing all infants for hip abnormalities during well-baby examinations is crucial.

Control over movement progresses during the infant's first year as the neurologic system matures. Development proceeds from proximal to distal parts and in a head-to-toe fashion; babies progress from being able to control their heads, to rolling over, to crawling, to pulling themselves up to a standing position, to standing, and, finally, to walking (Hockenberry & Wilson, 2011). Each successive task requires increasingly coordinated movement. Refinement of gross motor skills precedes fine motor skills. The ages at which babies accomplish specific tasks vary, but the development always occurs in an orderly progression. Motor activity during the first year characterizes many changes that occur in infants. For this reason, parents and other caregivers frequently rely on motor development as a yardstick to evaluate their infants' progress. Many parents need reassurance that their children are mastering certain physical tasks within the usual age range. Physical milestones provide the order but not the exact time for mastering new physical skills.

TODDLER AND PRESCHOOLER

Refinement of gross and fine motor skills and nearly boundless energy mark the developmental stages of the toddler and preschooler. Most children usually master walking soon after their first birthday. Walking begins with a wide stance and unsteady gait, thus the term *toddler*. In the second and 3rd years of life, common developmental tasks mastered include coordinated walking, running, jumping, climbing stairs, throwing a ball, self-feeding, and scribbling with crayons. Young children use their physical abilities to explore their environment and to develop cognitively.

Preschoolers continue to increase their gross and fine motor skills rapidly. Gross motor activities mastered before school typically include riding a tricycle, walking backward, dancing, skipping, running, jumping, and climbing well. Fine motor skills include using crayons to draw or make letters, catching a ball, stringing beads, brushing teeth, doing puzzles, fastening or using zippers, and washing hands.

CHILD AND ADOLESCENT

Physical growth slows between 6 and 12 years of age. Refinement of gross and fine motor skills continues, however, and is often enhanced by group activities (e.g., sports, dancing, swimming lessons). Exercise patterns for later life are often determined at this time. Families should encourage regular physical exercise while avoiding excessive pressure on children to excel. Unrealistic expectations can be emotionally and physically damaging for youngsters whose muscles are not fully developed.

Adolescence is a period of rapid physical and sexual development. Because of varied growth in different body parts, teenagers may appear gangly and awkward. Consequently, resulting uneven motor function affects body image, which can be especially distressing for adolescents. Most schools require some physical education as a graduation requirement, and many students engage in competitive sports or other school-sponsored physical activities such as dancing.

ADULT AND OLDER ADULT

Between ages 20 and 40 years, relatively few physical changes occur that affect mobility, although late-term pregnancy can limit vigorous physical activity. Young adults may experience altered mobility when trauma (e.g., sprains or fractures) limits normal function. Adults with jobs that require repetitive movement (e.g., assembly line workers, supermarket checkers, computer operators) may develop carpal tunnel syndrome, a nerve compression that causes pain and decreases hand mobility. As adults approach middle age (40 to 60 years), muscle tone and bone density and mass decrease. Joints lose elasticity and flexibility. Bone mass decreases, especially in women with osteoporosis, resulting in an increased incidence of fractures (Tabloski, 2013). In addition, altered coordination affects normal gait, and a slowing reaction time delays the overall body response to stressors.

Aging brings postural changes and chronic joint disorders. Flattening of the lumbar spine and changes in the intervertebral disks and vertebral bodies may cause the head and upper spine to tilt forward, shifting the center of gravity. Joint degeneration and bone demineralization also affect balance and gait. As a result, older adults usually have less extension and swing through and more side-to-side sway; weight is transferred from the ball of one foot to the ball of the other foot, leading to a wide-based, short-stepped, shuffling gait.

Many older people have more difficulty overcoming inertia and using gravity efficiently. One contributing factor is the shift in the center of gravity. To compensate for the shift, the knees flex slightly for support. The resulting posture is a forward-leaning crouch with a widened base.

Osteoarthritis, especially in weight-bearing joints (hips and knees), can cause significant chronic pain. When pain is severe and mobility limited, joint replacement is an option. Chronic health problems or injuries from falls also affect the mobility of older adults. Fear of falling causes some older adults to restrict activity voluntarily. If this results in increased caution, it can be a positive response; taken to the extreme, though, severely restricting activity results in muscle atrophy or deconditioning.

Cultural Considerations

Attitudes toward exercise and mobility are often shaped by the family and culture in which a person lives. Within any culture, there can be great variety. As the rate of obesity increases in America, participation in activities that require physical exertion becomes more difficult.

Individuals residing in third world countries often participate in hard manual labor because modern conveniences and machines are not always available, and walking is a common method of transportation. People living in postindustrial nations, especially those embracing the computer age, often live more sedentary, less healthy lives. Children who spend significant portions of the day watching television or playing computer games are less likely to become physically active adults.

Some cultures may discourage female participation in team sports or vigorous activity as unfeminine. Social norms may include quiet reflective activities. Group exercises such as Qigong or tai chi become a daily spiritual ritual connecting mind and body for some cultures. Folk dancing is unique and practiced by many cultures, especially at times of celebration such as holidays or weddings. Most cultures actively participate in sports and different physical activities, with sports figures often achieving celebrity status. Social norms for male and female participation in sports and physical activities may differ.

FACTORS AFFECTING MOBILITY

Lifestyle and Habits

Regular exercise and optimal nutrition are essential to maintaining mobility and musculoskeletal functioning. If a person has a balanced approach to activity, nutrition, and exercise, he or she should maintain mobility. The maxim "use it or lose it" is particularly true regarding the musculoskeletal system. The person must use it regularly to maintain function. Regular, ongoing exercise is required for optimal conditioning. About 30 minutes of strenuous aerobic exercise three times weekly promotes conditioning. Without this ongoing conditioning, 6 hours of vigorous exercise once a month for a sedentary person may overtax an unconditioned body.

Intact Musculoskeletal System

Anything that interrupts muscle strength, bone resiliency and strength, and full ROM of the joints may impair the musculoskeletal system's ability to facilitate mobility. Fluid and electrolyte levels, exercise, conditioning, nutrition, and condition of tendons, ligaments, or soft tissue influence muscle strength. Exercise increases muscle tone, mass, and strength and enhances the condition of other musculoskeletal tissues and body organs.

The function of the bones and joints depends on the bones' mineral content, which gives them adequate resilience, and the flexibility of joints and their tendons and ligaments. Adequate dietary calcium, phosphorus, and vitamin B are essential to maintaining bone resilience and an intact skeletal system. Joints must be able to move through their entire ROM so the body can move freely and maintain mobility.

Trauma usually results in accidental injury to joints, tendons, ligaments, muscles, or bones. The damage may be minor, affecting mobility for only a short time (e.g., a strain caused by overexerting a muscle or a sprain caused by twisting a joint), or it may be more extensive by involving a dislocated joint, torn tendons, or broken bones. Immobilizing devices are usually used to keep healing body parts in normal alignment.

Demineralization of the bone, as in osteoporosis, increases the risk of fractures. Rheumatoid arthritis, degenerative joint disease (osteoarthritis), and gout also limit mobility because movement causes pain.

Nervous System Control

Normal mobility requires the smooth control of movement provided by the nervous system. Motor ability depends on the integrity of the multisynaptic pathways of the afferent and efferent nerves and the central integration provided by the cerebral cortex. Nerve conduction, in turn, requires adequate circulation and appropriate fluid and electrolyte balance. Balance and stability are the products of equilibrium, which can be affected by some medications, fatigue, or situations that temporarily impair vision or input to the vestibular system in the semicircular canals.

Any disorder that impairs the nervous system's ability to control muscular movement and coordination hinders functional mobility. Usually, these disorders (e.g., muscular dystrophy, Parkinson disease, multiple sclerosis) are progressive; they slowly erode and eventually destroy the ability to move normally, resulting in the person being confined to bed or a wheelchair.

Impairments of the brain or spinal cord can also affect movement. When the spinal cord is severed or severely damaged, paralysis occurs below the level of injury. The term **paraplegia** describes decreased motor and sensory function to the legs. **Tetraplegia**, previously called quadriplegia, describes paralysis of the arms and the legs and all muscle movement below the level of injury.

Infectious processes (e.g., meningitis), tumors, or cerebrovascular accidents (e.g., strokes) can disrupt central nervous system control over movement. Treatment can limit or reverse some damage to the central nervous system, but at times, dysfunction is permanent and severe.

Circulation and Oxygenation

The skeletal muscles need adequate amounts of oxygen to function optimally. The lungs must provide oxygen while removing carbon dioxide, the by-product of aerobic metabolism in the muscles. The heart must adequately pump blood to the muscles and supply other body organs with enough blood to meet the increased demands imposed by exercise. The vasculature must redirect proportionally larger amounts of blood to the muscles, often shunting blood flow away from the gut, during periods of extreme exercise.

Many chronic disorders limit the supply of oxygen and nutrients needed for muscle contraction and movement. Chronic cardiovascular conditions, such as heart failure or peripheral vascular disease, limit effective blood flow, especially during periods of increased need, such as aerobic exercise. Lung disorders decrease the amount of oxygen delivered to all body tissues. Anemia decreases the amount of hemoglobin available for oxygen binding.

Energy

Cancer or other chronic health conditions can strain nutritional stores and thereby deplete energy necessary for movement. Energy for muscle function is derived from using oxygen and the breakdown products of food to produce muscle contraction. There are two primary types of metabolism: aerobic and anaerobic. In aerobic metabolism, the oxidative processes that produce energy occur in the mitochondria of cells; water and carbon dioxide are the by-products. Aerobic metabolism is the most efficient form of energy production for long-term activity.

In anaerobic metabolism, a process known as glycolysis converts stored glycogen to energy. This process provides energy when the oxygen supply is inadequate or delayed; lactic acid is the by-product. The depletion of stored glycogen with lactic acid produces fatigue in a short time, so this type of metabolism is useful only for short bursts of energy.

Congenital Problems

Some conditions, such as spina bifida or cerebral palsy, are present at birth and cannot be cured. Treatment goals are maximal functional mobility and minimal complications. Screening for hip dysplasia should occur at birth and at routine health visits during the first year, since corrective treatment is very effective and can prevent long-term disability. Symptoms include asymmetry of the gluteal and thigh folds, limited hip flexion, or shortening of the femur (Hockenberry & Wilson, 2011).

Affective Disorders

Severe affective disorders can hinder mobility. Depression and catatonic states result in limited mobility not because of physical impairments but because the person lacks the desire to move. Fear, especially of pain on movement, may cause some people to restrict their movements.

Therapeutic Modalities

Sometimes, limiting movement is the treatment for a medical problem. Restrictive devices, such as casts, braces, and splints, can immobilize certain areas of the body to promote healing. Bed rest is another treatment whereby mobility is restricted for therapeutic benefits. A patient may be placed on bed rest for the following reasons:

- To promote healing and tissue repair by decreasing metabolic needs
- To relieve edema (swelling)
- To reduce the body's oxygen requirements
- To decrease pain
- To support a weak, exhausted, or febrile patient
- To avoid dislodging a deep vein thrombosis

The definition of bed rest may vary. Some healthcare providers permit patients on bed rest to use bedside commodes; others insist on strict confinement to bed. Prolonged bed rest can be a significant risk factor, especially for older adults, in adversely affecting mobility.

ALTERED MOBILITY

Manifestations of Altered Mobility

The patient with altered mobility may have various symptoms, including decreased muscle strength and tone, lack of coordination, altered gait, falls, decreased joint flexibility, pain on movement, and decreased ability to tolerate activity.

DECREASED MUSCLE STRENGTH AND TONE

Frequent muscle contraction, which occurs during movement, maintains muscle strength. When movement is limited or abnormal, maximal tension is not applied to muscle groups, which decreases the muscles' ability to contract. Disuse may be accompanied by muscle atrophy, which is a decrease in muscle size.

Decreased strength is apparent when the patient cannot grasp the nurse's hand strongly or can push only weakly with the legs. Weakness may be so severe that the patient's leg muscles cannot support his or her body weight. At other times, decreased strength is less obvious. For example, a patient may be able to extend his or her arms in front of the body, but after a few minutes, the arms begin to drift down as the muscles become too fatigued to provide adequate support.

Muscle tone, or the normal resistance to stretch, also decreases with inactivity. Decreased muscle tone is called hypotonicity or **flaccidity**. Decreased tone can cause the muscles to stretch (if they are held in a lengthened position) or contract (if they are held in a shortened position). Neurologic impairment that results in increased muscle tone, called **spasticity**, also can affect normal movement. Nursing care can be pivotal in caring for the patient with spasticity.

LACK OF COORDINATION

Lack of coordination occurs when neurologic control and movement regulation are impaired. Usually, this is the case when trauma or disease affects the cerebellum. Alcohol and certain drugs, such as barbiturates, also may interfere with normal coordinated movement. Uncoordinated movements appear jerky and uneven and affect the person's ability to move purposefully and efficiently. Many terms are used to describe alterations in coordinated, purposeful movement:

- **Ataxia** is a general term used to describe impaired muscle coordination.
- A **tremor** is a rhythmic, repetitive movement that can occur at rest or when movement is initiated. A tremor usually interferes with fine motor control; however, in Parkinson disease, it also can interfere with coordinated ambulation.
- **Chorea** is spontaneous, brief, involuntary muscle twitching of the limbs or facial muscles; severe chorea hinders mobility.
- **Athetosis** is movement characterized by slow, irregular, twisting motions.
- **Dystonia** is similar to athetosis but usually involves larger areas of the body.

ALTERED GAIT

Abnormal gait can affect the rhythm, steadiness, and speed of walking:

- An *ataxic gait* is characterized by staggering and unsteadiness.
- The gait is called *spastic* when walking appears stiff and toes appear to catch and drag.
- A *waddling gait* is walking with feet wide apart in a ducklike fashion.
- A *hemiplegic gait* occurs when one leg is paralyzed or neurologically damaged, so the leg is dragged or swung around to propel it forward.
- A *festinating gait*, typified by walking on the toes as if being pushed, is common in Parkinson disease.

FALLS

Patients with mobility limitations are likely to fall from gait changes, weakness, postural hypotension, or diminished coordination. Falls can result in musculoskeletal trauma, such as fractures, which can further decrease mobility. Sensory and cognitive changes in older adults, combined with medication usage, further increase the risk of falls for this age group. Fear of repeated falls may cause some patients to limit their mobility. Recognizing risk factors and mobility problems is crucial to preventing falls in all patients. Recent research supports the importance of evaluating patients for previous falls, weakness, gait disturbances, balance impairments, and medications as the strongest predictive risk factors for identifying patients at risk for falling (Tinetti & Kumar, 2010). Research also suggests that geriatric patients are at higher risk for falls (Schwendimann, Buhler, DeGeest, & Milisen, 2008).

Patient falls and falls with injury are the largest category of reportable incidents and a significant problem in hospitals. Falls are devastating to patients, family members, providers, and the healthcare system, especially when they lead to injury. Center for Medicare Services (2008) and many state Medicaid agencies announced that there would be no further reimbursement to hospitals for costs associated with treating injuries incurred by patients who fall during hospitalization (Dykes et al., 2010).

DECREASED JOINT FLEXIBILITY

Decreased joint flexibility typically occurs with altered mobility because decreased movement causes joints to stiffen. Normal ROM decreases because fibrosis and fixation affect the joint structures. Muscles atrophy when they do not regularly shorten and lengthen during normal muscle contraction. Initially, decreased flexibility and altered ROM occur in affected joints, but if the joints remain immobilized, contractures can occur. A **contracture** is the progressive shortening of a muscle and loss of joint mobility resulting from fibrotic changes in tissues surrounding the joint.

PAIN ON MOVEMENT

Impaired mobility is often caused by or accompanied by pain on movement. Pain can result from physical injury, as in sprains, strains, or torn ligaments, or it may result from degenerative and inflammatory processes. **Osteoarthritis** (degeneration of the articular surface of weight-bearing joints) and rheumatoid arthritis (an inflammatory disorder that affects joints) are two common disorders that limit mobility secondary to discomfort/pain on movement.

Incisional pain decreases most patients' willingness to ambulate during the postoperative period. Pain caused by inadequate blood flow to the extremities (intermittent claudication) also can severely decrease mobility. Cancer, low back pain, and other disorders associated with chronic pain also limit movement. Providing nursing interventions

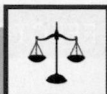

ETHICAL/LEGAL ISSUE

FOLLOWING ORDERS

You are a registered nurse (RN) working at a long-term care facility. When you arrive for duty, the nursing supervisor asks to see you. She tells you that Mrs. Johnson fell yesterday afternoon and was found shortly after you left. She would like you to fill out the Quality Assurance Form (QAF) that outlines the incident. You start to explain that you feel uncomfortable doing this, but the supervisor stops you and states, "I believe I have made myself clear."

CRITICAL THINKING CHALLENGE

- Discuss appropriate ways that a healthcare agency should use a QAF.
- If you were in this situation, identify some of your concerns.
- Explore positive and negative consequences of filling out the QAF.
- Explore positive and negative consequences of not filling out the QAF.
- Did the manner in which the supervisor made the request influence your response to the situation?

to address pain will often have beneficial effects on patient mobility.

ACTIVITY INTOLERANCE

Decreased ability to tolerate activity often accompanies impaired mobility. **Activity intolerance** is when a person has inadequate physiologic or psychological energy to endure or to complete an activity. A balance must occur between the activity and the patient's energy. Symptoms associated with activity intolerance are dyspnea, tachycardia, discomfort, weakness, and fatigue.

Commonly, disorders that affect oxygenation, such as respiratory or cardiac problems, decrease a patient's ability to tolerate increases in activity. Some activity intolerance, however, can be noted in anyone who has been inactive. For example, a 46-year-old man who has been inactive since college will experience activity intolerance if he tries to run 2 miles. Even short periods of immobility can impair activity tolerance.

Impact of Immobility on Physiologic Function

Immobility affects most areas of function (Table 25-2). Recognizing the possible consequences of immobility allows the nurse to intervene to limit or prevent problems. Bed rest can cause many complications that may delay recovery, including

TABLE 25-2 COMPARISON OF THE EFFECTS OF EXERCISE AND IMMOBILITY ON FUNCTION

Functional Area	Effects of Exercise	Effects of Immobility/Inactivity
Health perception–health maintenance	Promotes optimal health and well-being	Increases risk of various chronic health problems (e.g., cardiovascular, diabetes)
Activity–exercise	Strengthens muscles and increases muscle tone Increases endurance Promotes joint mobility Increases cardiac efficiency Decreases resting pulse rate and blood pressure Improves circulation Increases respiratory rate Increases depth of respirations Improves gas exchange	Causes muscle weakness and atrophy, activity intolerance, contractures Decreases ROM Increases cardiac workload Causes orthostatic hypotension Increases risk of thrombus formation Decreases lung expansion Promotes retained secretions Impairs gas exchange
Nutrition–metabolism	Increases metabolic rate, appetite, energy Improves skin tone and turgor	Decreases metabolic rate Causes anorexia, negative nitrogen balance, disuse osteoporosis, impaired immunity, skin breakdown, and pressure ulcer development
Elimination	Increases intestinal tone and motility Increases blood flow to kidneys, promoting optimal excretion of waste products	Decreases intestinal tone and motility Causes constipation, urinary stasis Increases risk of UTI, renal calculi Decreases bladder tone
Sleep–rest	Improves sleep quality	Decreases sleep quality
Cognition–perception	Increases vitality and well-being	Causes sensory deprivation, confusion, hallucinations, pain, and discomfort
Self-perception–self-concept	Improves appearance, body image, self-concept	Impairs appearance, body image, self-concept
Roles–relationships	Fosters relationships if exercise done in groups	Interferes with roles requiring mobility (e.g., going to work, caring for child)
Coping–stress	Reduces stress	Increases stress Produces anxiety, anger, depression, powerlessness
Sexuality	Increases energy available for sexual expression	Can hinder normal sexual expression Immobilizing devices may interfere.

disuse muscle atrophy, joint contractures, and thromboembolic disease (Brower, 2009). Many hospitalized patients spend the bulk of their time in bed, which has been linked to mortality and complications such as developing pressure ulcers, deep vein thrombosis, and falls.

MUSCLE ATROPHY AND WEAKNESS

Reduction in muscle cell size (atrophy) results from the alterations in metabolism that occur during immobility; the body breaks down muscle mass to obtain energy (catabolic metabolism). The resulting changes in muscle strength and mass are substantial and last even after immobility is reversed. Immobility affects the leg muscles more than other muscles. This is thought to be due to the effects of gravity in maintaining muscle tone. The evidence of atrophy can be seen dramatically when a cast is removed and the limbs are compared.

Endurance (the ability to tolerate activity) decreases as the muscle atrophies. In many cases, a vicious cycle ensues. Decreased endurance can discourage the patient from engaging in activity, which contributes to further atrophy.

CONTRACTURES AND JOINT PAIN

In the active, mobile person, movement promotes the formation of new connective tissue deposited around joints and muscles. This tissue is loose and pliable and remains so as long as normal body movement occurs. During immobility, stretching of muscles and movement of joints cease; this results in the deposition of denser, less pliable fibrotic tissue and renders joints more fixed and unable to move normally.

A contracture (progressive shortening of a muscle and loss of joint mobility) results from fibrotic changes that occur when normal mobility is not maintained. Impaired blood flow to the muscle or joint hastens the formation of contractures. Without appropriate intervention, increasing damage occurs and a contracture can become irreversible. An irreversible contracture further decreases the person's mobility because it makes moving the involved muscle difficult or impossible. Contractures also cause disfigurement, which can increase social isolation. Research suggests that splinting joints is not effective in preventing contractures (Lannin, Cusick, McCluskey, & Herbert, 2007).

Flexion contractures are most common in immobilized patients. Patients may assume positions of flexion naturally because these positions require less muscle stress and tension to maintain. Also, flexor muscles (those that allow joints to bend) are usually stronger than their extensor counterparts. Common flexor contractures occur at the joints of the elbow, hip, knee, shoulder, wrist, and ankle. For example, **foot drop** is a contracture in which the foot is fixed in plantar flexion. Boots or high-top sneakers may be used to maintain dorsiflexion and tendon flexibility. Immobility can decrease joint stability as a result of decreased tension exerted by ligaments and muscles secondary to loss of muscle tone. Decreased joint stability is thought to cause the aches and pains that immobilized patients often experience. It also may account for the difficulty ambulating and general stiffness that follow inactivity and bed rest.

INCREASED CARDIAC WORKLOAD

Cardiac workload is increased in the immobilized patient because the heart must work harder when the body is supine than when it is erect. Pooling of blood in the legs usually does not occur in the supine position. With less gravitational pull, blood can be redistributed from the legs to the trunk. This subsequent increase in venous blood returning to the heart means that the heart must work harder to circulate the increased volume. The heart rate also increases in the immobilized patient to accommodate the greater amount of blood that must be pumped.

ORTHOSTATIC HYPOTENSION

Orthostatic hypotension is the decreased ability to maintain systemic blood pressure when changing from a supine to an upright position (see Chapter 18). It is commonly seen after a period of immobility. Position changes do not normally cause systemic blood pressure to drop substantially because arteriolar vasoconstriction prevents large amounts of blood from pooling in the extremities when the person assumes an upright posture. Baroreceptors are stimulated when blood flow decreases in the aortic arch and carotid arteries (i.e., when the person stands). This, in turn, triggers increased sympathetic activity, which causes vasoconstriction.

Immobility decreases the effectiveness of this neurovascular reflex. During inactivity, the body's regulatory adjustments are not used and become inactive. Sympathetic stimulation may still occur in response to standing upright, but peripheral vessels do not respond to this stimulation. Therefore, vasoconstriction does not occur, and a drop in blood pressure results.

Another factor that may contribute to orthostatic hypotension is the ineffectiveness of the muscle pump in promoting venous return. This is especially true of muscles atrophied by immobility. As the calf muscles weaken, they are less effective in compressing the leg veins and less able to promote venous return. Blood pooling in the legs increases, which intensifies postural hypotension.

THROMBUS FORMATION AND EMBOLISM

A thrombus is a blood clot composed of platelets, fibrin, and cellular elements that attaches to the wall of an artery or vein. A thrombus most commonly originates in the large veins of the legs because of the legs' relatively low velocity of blood flow. This condition is called **deep vein thrombosis (DVT)**. Embolus is when the clot breaks away from the vessel wall and enters circulating blood. The clot lodges in the circulatory system as the blood vessel diameter decreases. This most commonly occurs when the thrombus enters the pulmonary vasculature, where it interferes with blood flow to the lung, causing a pulmonary embolus. Large pulmonary emboli can cause immediate death, but small emboli may produce no clinical symptoms.

Immobility promotes venous stasis, which contributes to the development of DVT. When leg muscles are inactive, venous return to the heart decreases. With time, the gravitational effect of the supine position results in the redistribution of body fluids with a net decrease in venous return. The vein's numerous bifurcations and valves are thought to promote further stasis. Poor positioning can cause external pressure on blood vessels, which also contributes to inadequate blood flow and promotes development of thrombi.

Hypercoagulability does not directly result from immobility, but sometimes, immobilized patients become dehydrated, which can increase blood viscosity. Dehydration may partly result from the patient's inability to obtain fluids without assistance. Prophylactic use of heparin or low molecular weight heparin is a common practice to prevent the development of venous thromboembolic problems in high-risk patients.

DECREASED LUNG EXPANSION

The immobilized patient experiences greater-than-normal resistance to breathing, resulting in underinflation of the lungs and increased work of breathing. The healthy person keeps the lungs well inflated with practically no effort. In an upright position, the diaphragm can move up and down freely. An efficient mechanism known as the mucociliary escalator keeps airways cleared of mucous secretions. Periodic sighing and coughing help to keep even the smallest air sacs (alveoli) open and available for gas exchange. Finally, ordinary activity produces enough carbon dioxide to stimulate a smooth, effective breathing pattern.

The immobile patient, however, breathes less deeply and with greater effort. The supine patient must overcome two resistances that do not ordinarily work against breathing. First, the diaphragm is prohibited from free movement by the abdominal organs, which shift against the diaphragm when the patient lies down. To achieve full lung expansion, the patient's diaphragm must push the organs out of the way with each breath. Second, the pressure of the bed against the chest wall limits the patient's chest movement. Together, these factors result in diminished depth of breathing. Because the immobilized patient's activity level is less than normal, less carbon dioxide is produced. This results in a lower level of stimulation for breathing, causing further reduction of tidal volume.

Decreased depth of breathing can result in the collapse of alveoli, which, in turn, hinders the exchange of oxygen and carbon dioxide. This condition of alveolar collapse is known as atelectasis. In addition to limiting the lungs' ability to exchange gases, atelectasis predisposes the patient to pneumonia. The patient's ability to cough deeply is often limited; thus, mucus may become trapped in the lung, which provides a rich medium for microbial growth.

DECREASED METABOLIC RATE

The basal metabolic rate decreases during immobility. Severely restricted activity affects the amount and pattern of thyroid hormone, adrenocorticotropic hormone, aldosterone, and insulin produced by the body. It also alters drug metabolism. Weight loss is thought to result from loss of muscle mass and diuresis.

NEGATIVE NITROGEN BALANCE

In an active person, a balance exists between protein breakdown and protein synthesis. However, immobility raises the rate of protein breakdown, probably because of muscle atrophy. One way to monitor this process is to measure nitrogen, which is excreted in urine as a waste product of protein breakdown. Elevated urine nitrogen levels occur in most immobilized patients. A negative nitrogen balance results when nitrogen excretion exceeds dietary intake. In such cases, the body lacks adequate nitrogen for protein synthesis, which results in nutritional depletion; this, in turn, interferes with wound healing and restoring muscle mass when mobility resumes. More insulin is required during immobility to maintain normal blood glucose levels. Immobilized patients often have concomitant factors that further deplete nitrogen, such as trauma, burns, surgery, coma, cancer, fever, or infection. Patients with chronic illness or poor nutritional balance before immobilization are at increased risk for negative nitrogen balance.

ANOREXIA

Anorexia (loss of appetite) is common in immobilized patients. Decreased metabolic rate is accompanied by decreased caloric need. Moreover, if the patient is confined to a healthcare facility, the institutional food, eating in a supine position, environmental factors, and psychological state can inhibit the appetite.

DISUSE OSTEOPOROSIS

In disuse osteoporosis, bone demineralization occurs secondary to immobility. The bone matrix is always in a dynamic state of formation and destruction. Osteoblastic cells are responsible for the proliferation of bone matrix. In contrast, osteoclastic cells destroy bone matrix by absorbing and removing osseous

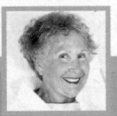

Mobility PICO

Gavin is the home health nurse conducting an initial assessment and plan of care on the patient in the chapter-opening case scenario. The son tells Gavin that his mother has a history of deep vein thrombosis (DVT). He is worried that if his mother does not start moving around more, she might throw a clot. He is inquiring about the continuous passive motion (CPM) machine that was used during his mother's hospital stay and wonders if it can be used to help prevent a DVT during her rehab at home. Gavin is unsure about the answer and decides to look for evidence in the Cochrane Library. She uses the following PICO question to help with her search: *In post-op knee surgery patients with a history of DVT, does using continuous passive motion (compared to not using any external motion machines) prevent venous thromboembolism?*

P = Post-op knee surgery patients with history of deep vein thrombosis
I = Continuous passive motion
C = No external motion machine
O = Prevent venous thromboembolism

Gavin finds a meta-analysis study that used results from eleven randomized control trials. 808 participants were included in the study. According to the meta-analysis, the quality of the studies was variable and showed no clear evidence that using a CPM machine would actually prevent DVTs.

Gavin shares his research findings with the son and reassures him that the DVT concern will be addressed with the surgeon.

REFERENCE

He, M. L., Xiao, Z. M., Lei, M., Li, T. S., Wu, H., & Liao J. (2014). Continuous passive motion for preventing venous thromboembolism after total knee arthroplasty. *Cochrane Database of Systematic Reviews.* (7):CD008207. Doi: 10.1002/14651858.CD008207.pub3.

tissue from the bone. Immobility results in an imbalance between osteoblastic and osteoclastic activity because normal stress and strain imposed on bone through movement are an important parts of osteoblastic processes. In the immobilized patient, osteoblasts continue to lay down bony matrix, but osteoclasts break down bone faster than osteoblasts can build it. The result is a loss of bony matrix. Disuse osteoporosis results in bones that are more porous, brittle, and susceptible to fractures.

IMPAIRED IMMUNITY

The immune system is weakened during immobility. Catabolism of immunoglobulin G doubles, significantly decreasing the normal concentration of circulating antibodies. Leukocytes are less able to engulf and destroy microorganisms. Lymphatic transport may be decreased as well when skeletal muscles are inactive.

PRESSURE ULCERS

Pressure ulcers form when pressure exerted over an area of skin or subcutaneous tissue exceeds the pressure required for adequate blood flow to the area. Cells die because they do not receive oxygen and nutrients and because waste products accumulate. Pressure is usually concentrated on bony prominences but can occur anywhere pressure is great. In the supine position, pressure is greatest over the back of the skull and at the elbows, sacrum, ischial tuberosities, and heels. In the sitting position, the greatest pressure is at the ischial tuberosities and the sacrum.

Reactive hyperemia is a compensatory mechanism that responds to inadequate blood flow. When pressure is removed, blood floods the area in an attempt to prevent tissue necrosis. Reactive hyperemia is effective only if it occurs before cellular damage occurs. The critical time varies from one person to another. Usually, the normal person can sense pressure buildup and can change position to reduce discomfort. The patient with impaired mobility, such as a person with neurologic impairment, may be incapable of movement or unable to sense the need to change positions.

Healing of pressure ulcers is difficult and slow, especially in the immobilized patient. Pressure ulcers can prolong immobility and increase the cost and length of confinement. See Chapter 30 for more information.

URINARY STASIS

Immobilized patients in a hospital or long-term care facility may not want to bother the nurse by asking for a bedpan. Some immobilized patients try to void when they feel the need but have difficulty relaxing the perineal muscles when in the supine position. Delaying voiding causes urine to collect in the bladder. Chronic delay can lead to overstretching the detrusor muscle in the bladder wall, permanent changes in bladder tone, and long-term consequences for normal voiding patterns.

Urinary retention poses significant problems for the immobilized patient. Urinary stasis contributes to urinary tract infections (UTIs) and renal calculi. Bladder distention leads to overflow incontinence, which is embarrassing for the patient and can contribute to skin breakdown.

URINARY TRACT INFECTION

Stagnant urine makes a good medium for bacterial growth. Bladder distention can cause small tears in the delicate bladder mucosa, which contribute to the increased incidence of UTI. When the patient experiences distention, catheterization may be necessary to empty the bladder. With any type of catheterization comes the risk of introducing pathogens and infection into the body.

RENAL CALCULI

Urinary stasis and an increased serum calcium level promote the formation of renal calculi (kidney stones). As serum calcium levels rise (the result of calcium loss from the bones), the kidney excretes more calcium. This increases urinary calcium levels. Because calcium can precipitate from solution to form crystals and because stagnant urine encourages the aggregation of crystals, renal calculi pose a significant problem. Dehydration, common in the immobilized patient, also increases the incidence of calculi formation. Additionally, some urinary infections make the urine more alkaline, which also promotes calculi development.

CONSTIPATION

Even in a healthy person, dietary changes, activity variations, and emotional stress affect normal bowel patterns. The immobilized patient faces additional changes. Abdominal and perineal muscles can be weakened by muscle atrophy, making it more difficult for the patient to bear down and exert pressure to evacuate stool. As stool descends against the rectum, the person feels the stimulus to defecate. In an upright posture, stool descends more quickly into the rectal area, eliciting a strong stimulus. In the supine position, rectal filling is slow, which weakens the stimulus for defecation.

The defecation reflex also can be affected if the person postpones defecation after recognizing the stimulus to defecate. This happens frequently in the immobilized patient, who may feel embarrassed or may need assistance to use a bedpan. When a person delays defecation, the intestine absorbs more water from the feces, making stool passage even more difficult. Dehydration, common in the immobile patient, also can contribute to constipation. The result may be fecal impaction (hard stool in the rectum that cannot be removed naturally by defecation). Often, liquid stool seeps around the obstruction formed by the impaction.

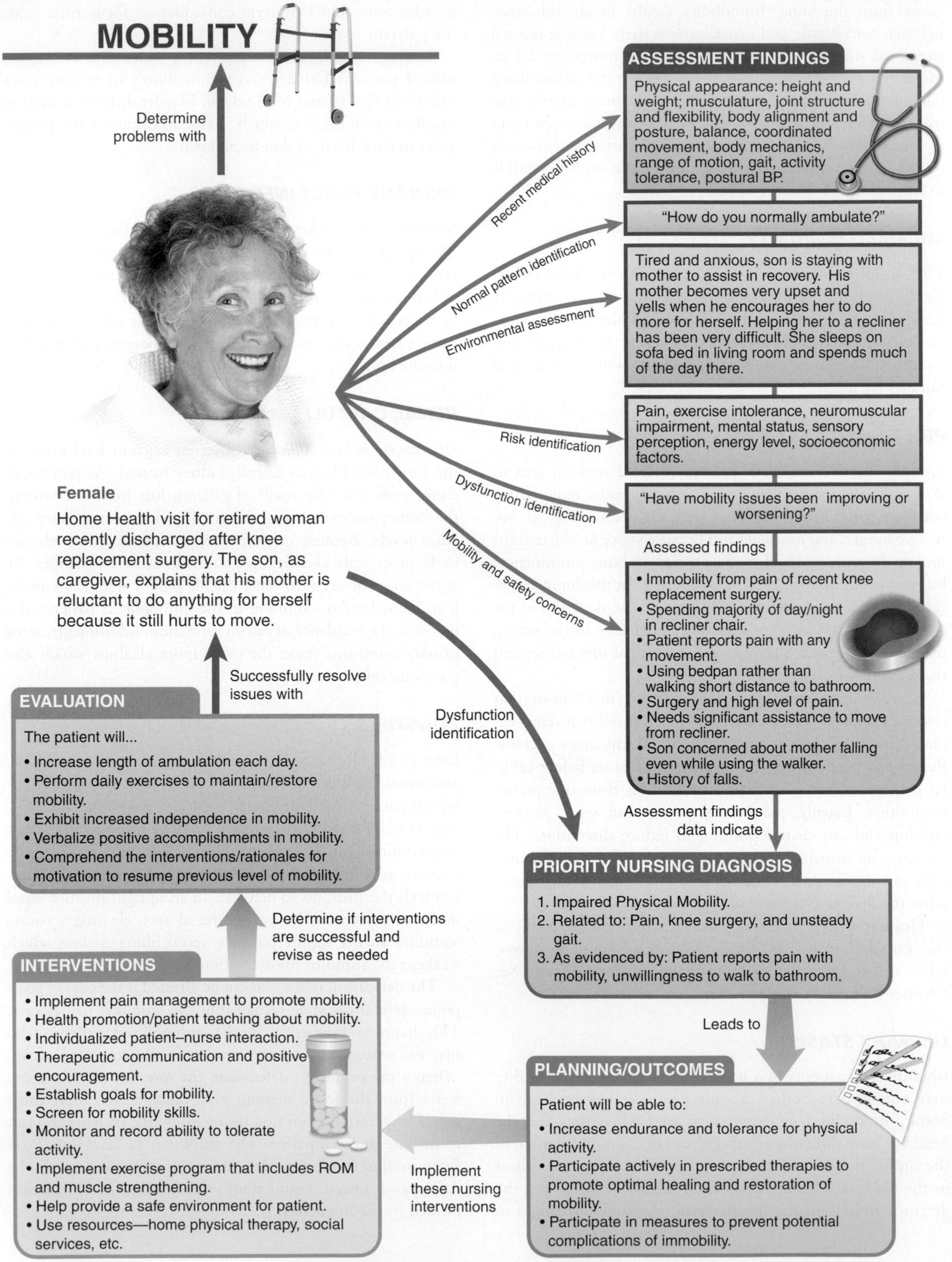

MOBILITY

Determine problems with

Female

Home Health visit for retired woman recently discharged after knee replacement surgery. The son, as caregiver, explains that his mother is reluctant to do anything for herself because it still hurts to move.

Recent medical history

Normal pattern identification

Environmental assessment

Risk identification

Dysfunction identification

Mobility and safety concerns

ASSESSMENT FINDINGS

Physical appearance: height and weight; musculature, joint structure and flexibility, body alignment and posture, balance, coordinated movement, body mechanics, range of motion, gait, activity tolerance, postural BP.

"How do you normally ambulate?"

Tired and anxious, son is staying with mother to assist in recovery. His mother becomes very upset and yells when he encourages her to do more for herself. Helping her to a recliner has been very difficult. She sleeps on sofa bed in living room and spends much of the day there.

Pain, exercise intolerance, neuromuscular impairment, mental status, sensory perception, energy level, socioeconomic factors.

"Have mobility issues been improving or worsening?"

Assessed findings

- Immobility from pain of recent knee replacement surgery.
- Spending majority of day/night in recliner chair.
- Patient reports pain with any movement.
- Using bedpan rather than walking short distance to bathroom.
- Surgery and high level of pain.
- Needs significant assistance to move from recliner.
- Son concerned about mother falling even while using the walker.
- History of falls.

Dysfunction identification

Assessment findings data indicate

EVALUATION

Successfully resolve issues with

The patient will...

- Increase length of ambulation each day.
- Perform daily exercises to maintain/restore mobility.
- Exhibit increased independence in mobility.
- Verbalize positive accomplishments in mobility.
- Comprehend the interventions/rationales for motivation to resume previous level of mobility.

Determine if interventions are successful and revise as needed

INTERVENTIONS

- Implement pain management to promote mobility.
- Health promotion/patient teaching about mobility.
- Individualized patient–nurse interaction.
- Therapeutic communication and positive encouragement.
- Establish goals for mobility.
- Screen for mobility skills.
- Monitor and record ability to tolerate activity.
- Implement exercise program that includes ROM and muscle strengthening.
- Help provide a safe environment for patient.
- Use resources—home physical therapy, social services, etc.

Implement these nursing interventions

PRIORITY NURSING DIAGNOSIS

1. Impaired Physical Mobility.
2. Related to: Pain, knee surgery, and unsteady gait.
3. As evidenced by: Patient reports pain with mobility, unwillingness to walk to bathroom.

Leads to

PLANNING/OUTCOMES

Patient will be able to:

- Increase endurance and tolerance for physical activity.
- Participate actively in prescribed therapies to promote optimal healing and restoration of mobility.
- Participate in measures to prevent potential complications of immobility.

FIGURE 25-3 Concept map for mobility.

SLEEP AND REST

Immobility can interfere with normal sleep patterns. Normal activity, especially physical work, and aerobic exercise produce a sense of fatigue that helps the person fall asleep and obtain restful sleep. The immobilized patient may doze frequently during the day, which disrupts normal nighttime sleep patterns. The immobilized patient may need to be awakened frequently to be turned, monitored, or given treatments and medications. Such wakings, especially when numerous, impair the quality of sleep. In addition, the immobilized patient may sleep in an unfamiliar, noisy environment and may have stressful health concerns that further reduce the amount and quality of sleep.

Impact of Immobility on Psychosocial Function

COGNITION AND PAIN

Because immobility decreases the freedom to interact normally with the environment, the patient receives less sensory information. Preoccupation with somatic complaints, difficulty with time perception, difficulty with understanding and following directions, crying, and other emotional outbursts can occur. Confusion is common but reversible if normal sensory input returns. In severe cases, sensory deprivation can occur, causing the patient to experience visual and auditory hallucinations.

Pain may result from physiologic changes that occur with immobility. Joint stiffness, pneumonia, pressure ulcers, thrombosis, and emboli can contribute to discomfort. The perception of pain also may intensify because focusing on discomfort is more common when diversions are limited.

Think back to the patient in the case scenario who was discharged from the hospital after knee replacement surgery. Recall that she has been reluctant to do anything for herself because she is still in pain. Use the concept map (Fig. 25-3) to help the patient manage her pain and to plan for her care.

SELF-PERCEPTION AND SELF-CONCEPT

Changes in self-perception and self-concept commonly accompany functional motor impairment or immobility. Immobility contributes to a feeling of powerlessness, especially when the patient must depend on others. Motor impairment can alter body image, especially if the impairment results from loss of a body part. Self-concept is altered when the patient must depend on devices such as crutches, wheelchairs, or walkers. Problems with coordination can cause embarrassment (e.g., the patient may worry about appearing awkward or even intoxicated). Altered body image can negatively affect self-esteem and can lead to a feeling of lowered self-worth.

ROLES AND RELATIONSHIPS

Immobility affects role function for many people. For children and adolescents, it disrupts school and social activities

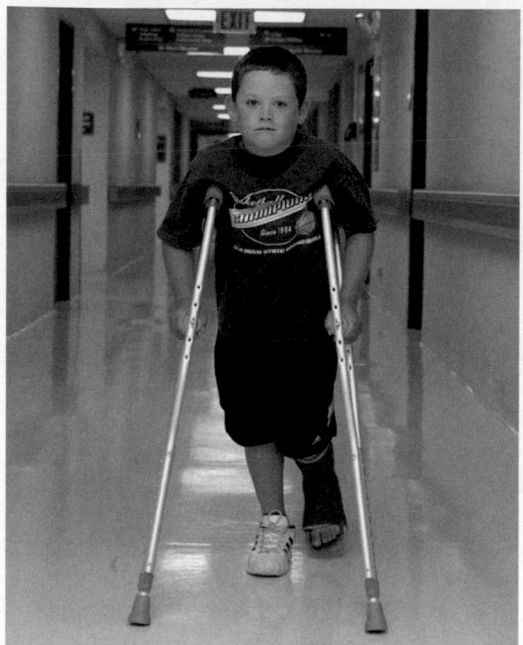

FIGURE 25-4 A broken leg can seem very significant to a child when school and social activities are disrupted.

(Fig. 25-4). For adults, immobility may interfere with the ability to work, resulting in temporary or permanent unemployment with corresponding financial stress. Immobility also disrupts various parental or spousal activities. Child care may be impossible when a parent is hospitalized or immobilized at home.

COPING AND STRESS TOLERANCE

Loss of mobility is not something the patient chooses or desires. With trauma, the loss occurs suddenly. In some cases, the loss is permanent and requires the patient to adapt to different functional abilities. Despite supportive social interactions with family and friends, immobilized patients may spend many hours alone and can be bored or lonely. Depression, anger, and anxiety are common.

Patients who experience stress because of immobility exhibit various behaviors. Some withdraw, limiting social contact even further. Some complain and become demanding. The patient who constantly requests assistance may be responding negatively to the stress of immobility.

SEXUALITY

Mobility limitations may affect sexual feelings and activities. Lack of privacy, depression, fatigue, and physical limitations can contribute to decreased sexual function. Immobility may impede grooming activities that are often important in maintaining sexual identity. For some patients with long-term motor impairments such as paraplegia, sexual function may be permanently altered, so the patient needs to learn new methods of sexual expression.

THERAPEUTIC DIALOGUE: MOBILITY

SCENE FOR THOUGHT

Jeannette Frost is a 73-year-old woman who has suffered shoulder problems during the last year and who had a surgical repair of her right shoulder 6 months ago. She comes to the clinic for assessment of her ROM and pain in the affected shoulder. She drove herself to the clinic.

LESS EFFECTIVE

Nurse: Hello, Mrs. Frost. I'm Nancy Robertson, the nurse practitioner you'll be seeing today. How are you? *(Looks at the chart.)*

Jeannette: Fine. *(She sits quietly and doesn't smile.)*

Nurse: *(Sits down at the desk and pays attention.)* What can I help you with today?

Jeannette: I want to see how much more I can do with my arm. I can only raise it this high. *(Demonstrates, using her left arm to help the right. Looks serious.)*

Nurse: You're concerned about that arm. *(Uses good eye contact.)*

Jeannette: Yes. I live alone.

Nurse: I see that your husband is listed as your emergency contact, but he has a different address. *(Looks through the chart and then at Jeannette questioningly.)*

Jeannette: Yes. I live by myself. *(Looks embarrassed and annoyed.)*

Nurse: *(Realizes this is not a safe subject.)* Well, I can understand you're concerned about doing your housework and cooking and so forth. Let me examine your shoulder and see how much more you might be able to do with your arm. *(Assesses ROM and discusses the swimming and physical therapy that Jeannette is already doing and how they're helping to maintain her current functioning.)* It seems that this is as good as this shoulder's going to get, Mrs. Frost. But it sounds as though you're doing everything you can to keep it in good shape, so I wouldn't worry if I were you. If it gets any worse, feel free to call me, and we'll go over it again. Okay?

Jeannette: *(Gets dressed.)* Fine. *(No eye contact.)*

Nurse: 'Bye now.

MORE EFFECTIVE

Nurse: Hello, Mrs. Frost. I'm Natalie Richmond, the nurse practitioner you'll be seeing today. How are you? *(Looks at the chart.)*

Jeannette: Fine. *(She sits quietly and doesn't smile.)*

Nurse: *(Sits down at the desk and pays attention.)* What can I help you with today?

Jeannette: I want to see how much more I can do with my arm. I can only raise it this high. *(Demonstrates, using her left arm to help the right. Looks serious.)*

Nurse: You're concerned about that arm. *(Uses good eye contact.)*

Jeannette: Yes. I live alone.

Nurse: You live alone, and you're worried you won't be able to manage with your arm the way it is? Am I getting that right? *(Maintains good eye contact.)*

Jeannette: No, I can manage the way it is. I don't want it to get worse. *(Looks more serious.)*

Nurse: I can see how concerned you are. I'd like to examine your shoulder and ask you a few questions, then we can talk about the answers to your questions. Does that sound okay?

Jeannette: Yes, that will be fine. *(After the assessment, Natalie discusses the swimming and physical therapy that Jeannette is doing and how they're helping to maintain the ROM in her shoulder.)*

Nurse: It seems that the exercises you're doing are keeping your shoulder in the shape it is now. If you stop the exercises, you risk losing motion, and it will be harder for you to do your cooking, housework, and entertaining. Otherwise, you're doing a good job. *(Pause.)* Is there something you want to say?

Jeannette: No, I think you answered everything I had on my mind. *(Pause.)* Could I come back and see you again so you can check to see that the shoulder is still okay?

Nurse: Certainly. You can call me, too. Here's my card.

Jeannette: Thank you very much. *(Smiles.)*

CRITICAL THINKING CHALLENGE

- Compare and contrast Nancy's and Natalie's actions and assessment styles.
- Analyze how Nancy talked to Jeannette.
- Recognize the emotions that Jeannette exhibited, and infer emotions from her nonverbal behavior.
- Determine how you might feel working with a patient who is reserved and does not show emotions readily.
- Formulate some helpful skills that could be used when working with Jeannette.

ASSESSMENT

Assessment data help identify the patient's normal mobility, risk factors for potential alterations in mobility, actual mobility impairments, and management techniques or devices the patient uses.

Normal Pattern Identification

First, determine the patient's normal activity pattern. Have the patient describe his or her normal activity and ability to perform ADLs. A rating scale may be useful for documenting the patient's independence, partial independence, and complete dependence in various activities involving mobility such as ambulation, toileting, dressing, bathing, and household chores. Ask the patient to describe any recent change in mobility or activity level. Determine the patient's normal patterns of exercise and leisure. If the patient actively engages in aerobic exercise, determine the frequency and appropriateness of the activity.

Discuss the patient's lifestyle. Some people enjoy sedentary activities and work at sedentary jobs. Others work at jobs that require vigorous physical exertion and take part in sports and physical activities. People who grew up in a family that valued quiet activities commonly carry the pattern of inactivity into adulthood. Assess the patient's satisfaction with his or her current activity level, and note any desire on the patient's part to change the activity pattern.

Risk Identification

Interviewing the patient also can help the nurse identify risk factors that can contribute to impaired mobility. Determine if the patient feels weak or fatigued after routine exercise and activity. Ask the patient to describe any distressing symptoms (e.g., difficulty breathing, pain, or increased heart rate) with activity; document the degree of exercise and the degree of stress. Ask the patient how long the symptoms have occurred and how long they persist after the activity ends.

Evaluate the patient's risk of falls. Assessing for fall risks is particularly important when working with an older adult patient (Schwendimann et al., 2008). Factors that increase this risk include decreased mobility, muscle weakness or atrophy, altered cognition, postural hypotension, and a cluttered environment. Ascertain alcohol or drug use that might impair mobility and contribute to falls. Hypotensive agents and pain medications lower blood pressure and can contribute to falls, anticonvulsants can cause ataxia, antidepressants can contribute to postural hypotension, and corticosteroids can result in muscle weakness and wasting. Research supports that consultation with pharmacists can play an important role in providing information for medication adjustments that may reduce patient fall risk (Cooper & Burfield, 2009).

Document current or chronic health problems that may limit mobility or decrease activity tolerance. Common and notable medical conditions are respiratory disease, cardiac disease, anemia, peripheral vascular disease, arthritis, cerebrovascular accidents, multiple sclerosis, Parkinson disease, brain tumors, head injuries, fractures, spinal cord injuries, and amputations. Evaluate the impact of medical conditions on mobility.

Dysfunction Identification

Document any inability of the patient to move normally and easily upon admission and assess any changes daily. Assessment of the baseline mobility of older adults is especially important. Encourage the patient to explain any problems with mobility or activity tolerance and any adaptations that he or she uses to promote optimal functioning at home. If the patient reports any limitation in mobility, determine the extent of the problem, when it first occurred, and if the patient knows the cause.

Ask the patient if the mobility problem has been improving or worsening and how it affects his or her functional abilities in other areas. Document what the patient can do independently so that independence within his or her capabilities can be encouraged.

Ask the patient if he or she uses devices to assist with ambulation (e.g., prostheses, canes, walkers, crutches). If surgery is planned and if assistive devices will be used afterward, the patient may be asked to demonstrate skills previously learned.

Perform a comprehensive functional health assessment to determine the impact of decreased mobility on all functional health areas. Note any complications resulting from limited mobility (e.g., pressure ulcers or renal calculi). To guide the assessment, review Table 25-2, which describes the effects of immobility on all areas of function.

Discuss how impaired mobility has affected the patient's roles and relationships, self-concept, self-esteem, and body image. Identify family and community support services and evaluate past and present coping strategies.

Physical Assessment

Physical examination findings contribute information about alignment; balance; coordination; gait; joint structure and function; muscle mass, tone, and strength; postural blood pressure; risk of falls; and activity tolerance. For the most part, the nurse uses the technique of inspection to visualize these qualities. When mobility appears normal, more extensive assessment techniques are usually unnecessary; if mobility is impaired, a more detailed assessment may be indicated.

ALIGNMENT

The patient should maintain proper alignment while sitting and standing. When alignment is normal, an imaginary line can be drawn through the earlobe, shoulder, hip, femoral trochanter, knee, and front of the ankle. Note the symmetry of organs and bones. Normal spinal alignment is characterized by concave curvature of the cervical spine, convex curvature of the thoracic spine, and concave curvature of the lumbar spine. Extreme curvature of the spine may be abnormal. **Scoliosis**, a lateral deviation of the thoracic spine, can be detected by watching the patient bend at the waist from a standing position. Lordosis, an abnormal concavity of the lumbar spine, and kyphosis, an exaggerated curvature of the thoracic spine, are less common spinal deviations.

BALANCE

Assess balance by asking the patient to sit or stand with eyes closed. Observe his or her ability to maintain a normal erect posture through postural adjustments. Swaying to one side indicates an inability to maintain balance through normal physiologic mechanisms.

COORDINATION

Watching the patient perform normal activities, including ambulation, allows the nurse to evaluate the coordination of movement. Look for fluid, well-controlled movement. The patient should be able to initiate the desired movement quickly without hesitation. Assess fine motor skills by asking the patient to perform a simple skill such as unbuttoning a shirt or signing papers.

GAIT

To evaluate a patient's gait, watch the patient walk. Normal gait should be rhythmic and even; the stride should be symmetric with full extension. The head should remain erect, and the knees and feet should point forward. Arms should swing alternately with leg movements. The full body weight should be easily supported. For more information about gait, observe the patient's shoes to detect patterns of wear.

JOINT STRUCTURE AND FUNCTION

Observation and palpation can detect redness, swelling, or warmth around the joint. Listen for a crunching or grating sound (crepitus), which can occur when bones rub against one another during movement because of inadequate protection or insufficient joint lubrication. Observe the patient's facial expression and nonverbal signs of discomfort during movement. If observation discloses stiffness or guarding during certain body movements, evaluate joint mobility by moving the involved joint through its full ROM (see Table 25-1). When doing this, note the amount of resistance encountered and whether or not the patient reports discomfort. Compare the right and left sides for symmetry.

MUSCLE MASS, TONE, AND STRENGTH

Normal muscle mass, tone, and strength can vary greatly among individuals. Athletes may have bulging, well-defined muscles and great strength and endurance. Older adults may have weak, small muscles with little tone. Increased strength and tone are usually found on the person's dominant side.

Assess muscle strength by evaluating the patient's ability to perform self-care activities such as feeding, dressing, toileting, and grooming. Estimate strength and coordination by observing the ease with which the patient performs these tasks. Evaluate the strength of specific muscle groups by asking the patient to grip your hand or to use certain muscle groups to push against resistance.

Muscle size in the arms and legs is determined by observation and by comparing measurements. A decrease in circumference in the affected limb usually reflects muscle atrophy from immobility.

POSTURAL BLOOD PRESSURE

To help determine if a patient can safely ambulate, measure postural blood pressure (see Chapter 18 for instructions). A significant drop in blood pressure when the patient changes from a supine to a sitting position suggests a risk for falls. Reports of dizziness, light-headedness, diaphoresis, and tachycardia may accompany orthostatic hypotension and are indications that fainting may occur if ambulation continues.

RISK OF FALLS

Nurses are uniquely positioned to protect patients from falling. Therefore, it is vital for a nurse to determine whether independent ambulation is safe. The incidence of patient falls is a nursing-sensitive indicator that is tracked in acute care. Patient outcomes that are determined to be nursing sensitive are those that improve if there is a greater quantity or quality of nursing care (American Nurses Association, n.d.). Standardized tools such as the Hendrich II Fall Risk Model (Table 25-3) and the Johns Hopkins Fall Risk Assessment Tool allow the nurse to calculate the risk level of a patient and target appropriate interventions for high-risk patients (Hendrich, 2007).

Falls are caused by multiple interacting factors that are different for each patient. They are rarely solely due to environmental hazards but instead are nearly always the result of an interplay between factors related to the individual (Oliver & Healey, 2009).

Risk factors for falls include the following:

- History of previous falls
- Environmental risk factors such as lack of assistive devices/ambulatory aids (e.g., cane, walker), obstacles in the walking path, slippery floors, and low-level lighting
- IVs (particularly an IV with an IV pole), SCDs, or other equipment that is attached
- Altered gait
- Impaired transfer ability
- Urinary frequency, incontinence, and diarrhea
- Confusion/delirium, alcohol induced delirium, and dementia
- Depression
- Poor vision
- History of dizziness, postural hypotension, or syncope
- Use of medications or alcohol that can impair balance, coordination, or cognitive abilities (e.g., anticonvulsants or benzodiazepines) and surgical procedure requiring sedation

ACTIVITY TOLERANCE

In assessing activity tolerance, observe the patient before, during, and after activity to detect abnormal responses. The most common parameters measured are the pulse rate and the respiratory rate. Normally, both increase during activity. Resting vital signs should be within a normal range before activity starts. If activity begins when the patient is experiencing hypotension, tachycardia, or tachypnea (rapid, irregular breathing), he or she has little energy in reserve to meet the body's increased need for oxygen during exercise.

TABLE 25-3 HENDRICH II FALL RISK MODEL

Risk Factor	Risk Points	Score
Confusion/Disorientation/Impulsivity	4	
Symptomatic Depression	2	
Altered Elimination	1	
Dizziness/Vertigo	1	
Gender (Male)	1	
Any Administered Antiepileptics (anticonvulsants): (Carbamazepine, Divalproex Sodium, Ethotoin, Ethosuximide, Felbamate, Fosphenytoin, Gabapentin, Lamotrigine, Mephenytoin, Methsuximide, Phenobarbital, Phenytoin, Primidone, Topiramate, Trimethadione, Valproic Acid)[1]	2	
Any Administered Benzodiazepines:[2] (Alprazolam, Chlordiazepoxide, Clonazepam, Clorazepate Dipotassium, Diazepam, Flurazepam, Halazepam[3], Lorazepam, Midazolam, Oxazepam, Temazepam, Triazolam)	1	
Get-Up-and-Go Test: "Rising from a Chair" If unable to assess, monitor for change in activity level, assess other risk factors, document both on the patient chart with date and time.		
Ability to rise in single movement—No loss of balance with steps	0	
Pushes up, successful in one attempt	1	
Multiple attempts but successful	3	
Unable to rise without assistance during test If unable to assess, document this on the patient chart with the date and time.	4	
(A score of 5 or greater – High Risk)	Total score	

On-going Medication Review Updates:

1. Levetiracetam (Keppra) was not assessed during the original research conducted to create the Hendrich Fall Risk Model. As an antiepileptic, levetiracetam docs have a side effect of somnolence and dizziness which contributes to its fall risk and should be scored (effective June 2010).

2. The study did not include the effect of benzodiazepine-like drugs since they were not on the market at the time. However, due to their similarity in drug structure, mechanism of action and drug effects, they should also be scored (effective January 2010).

3. Halazepam was included in the study but is no longer available in the United States (effective June 2010).

When activity resumes after bed rest or the level of prescribed activity increases, observe the patient carefully for signs of distress, such as dyspnea, diaphoresis, or dizziness. In high-risk patients, such as those with cardiac or respiratory conditions, the nurse may be directed to monitor pulse, respiratory rate, or oxygen saturation during activity and to discontinue the activity if values are outside the prescribed range. After activity, pulse and respiratory rates should return to preactivity baseline values within 3 minutes.

Diagnostic Tests and Procedures

Common diagnostic tests used to evaluate musculoskeletal function are radiographic studies and direct visualization of joints. Laboratory values, such as hemoglobin and hematocrit, may be helpful when assessing activity tolerance because anemia can contribute to generalized weakness and decreased ability to supply muscles with oxygen.

RADIOGRAPHIC STUDIES

X-rays are useful in differentiating traumatic injuries such as sprains, dislocations, and fractures. X-rays also help assess the demineralization of bone that occurs in osteoporosis. Radiographic studies using injected, radiopaque dye can help evaluate problems with the spine or joints. Defects are revealed by an abnormal pattern of dye distribution in the body part. Arthrograms permit visualization of joints and are often used to diagnose tears in ligaments or cartilage. Myelograms rely on radiopaque dye to highlight the spinal column to detect ruptured vertebral disks or other structural defects. Bone mineral density tests detect demineralization of the bone. Results from the proximal femur are helpful in predicting hip fracture risk so that preventive treatment can be started for high-risk individuals (Tabloski, 2013).

ARTHROSCOPY

Arthroscopy is the examination of a joint with a fiberoptic instrument to diagnose abnormalities. Minor corrective surgery also can be performed to remove torn cartilage or repair torn ligaments.

HEMATOLOGIC STUDIES

Hemoglobin and hematocrit values can be used to evaluate the patient's reserve for activity. Patients with low hemoglobin values

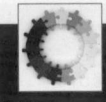

COLLABORATING WITH THE HEALTH CARE TEAM
Consulting with Physical Therapy

You have admitted Mrs. Shannon, a 56-year-old obese woman being treated for heart failure. Moving and ambulating Mrs. Shannon is very challenging, and you decide to consult with physical therapy.

*S*ITUATION: I am Sally, a nurse on the telemetry unit, calling to see if you could help us develop a safe mobility plan for Mrs. Shannon.

*B*ACKGROUND: Mrs. Shannon was admitted last evening for heart failure. She was very short of breath and is receiving diuretics to pull off fluid. Her vitals were 154/92, 94, 24, and oxygen sat 91% on 2 L/min via cannula. She weighs 395 pounds, and it took three staff members to turn and position her in bed. She has orders to get up in a chair this afternoon. She is reluctant to move herself and pleads with us to just leave her alone.

*A*SSESSMENT: I am concerned that Mrs. Shannon will develop complications and have a prolonged hospital stay if she remains immobile. I am not sure how much activity she will be able to tolerate with her heart problems. I am also concerned that a staff member could get injured if we do not work out a better plan.

*R*ECOMMENDATION: Could you please see Mrs. Shannon this afternoon and evaluate her mobility status and make recommendations for how we can safely get her up and progressively assist her with ambulation? She also might need some teaching about energy conservation measures before discharge.

CRITICAL THINKING CHALLENGE
- Is there any additional information that would be helpful to provide before the physical therapist sees Mrs. Shannon?
- Identify why Mrs. Shannon might be reluctant to move.
- Consider how each of the following needs to be considered in individualizing a plan for Mrs. Shannon: her obesity, her heart failure, and her motivation to participate.
- How might staff be proactive in requesting administrative support to prevent staff injuries when moving or lifting patients?

have difficulty transporting adequate oxygen to body tissues. Activity expectations may need to be modified for patients with hemoglobin values less than 10 g per deciliter. Low hematocrit values often reflect blood loss or inadequate volume replacement. When patients have low hematocrit values, they are likely to experience postural hypotension and activity intolerance.

NURSING DIAGNOSES

NANDA-International (NANDA-I, 2014) diagnoses that relate to mobility are Impaired Physical Mobility, Impaired Sitting, Impaired Standing, Impaired Walking, Impaired Wheelchair Mobility, Impaired Transfer Ability, Impaired Bed Mobility, Activity Intolerance, Risk for Falls, and Risk for Disuse Syndrome. Selected nursing diagnoses are included in Table 25-4 with Nursing Outcomes Classification (NOC) and Nursing Interventions Classification (NIC).

OUTCOME IDENTIFICATION AND PLANNING

After nursing diagnoses and related factors have been identified, the nurse, patient, and family plan interventions and expected outcomes.

General goals for patients with impaired mobility might include the following:

- Patient will increase endurance and tolerance for physical activity.
- Patient will participate actively in prescribed therapies to promote optimal healing and restoration of mobility.
- Patient will participate in measures to prevent potential complications of immobility.
- Patient will maintain optimal function despite mobility restrictions.

IMPLEMENTATION

Health Promotion

Health promotion activities in the areas of routine physical exercise, osteoporosis prevention, injury prevention, and fall prevention help keep patients active and safe, improving the quality of life.

PHYSICAL FITNESS PROMOTION

In the United States, machines have reduced the need for physical labor, which has led many people into sedentary lifestyles. This activity decrease has been implicated in the rising incidence of many diseases. Recently, however, the benefits of physical fitness have become more appreciated, spurring many people to walk, jog, and participate in exercise programs. Health clubs are available in most communities, and some employers are incorporating gymnasiums into the workplace for after-hour use. Nonetheless, a relatively small percentage of the population is physically fit. Childhood obesity is on the rise, in part due to the increased number of hours per day spent in front of a television or computer screen. Exercise rates among older adults remain especially low. Research is conclusive that regular exercise improves the quality of life for older adults (Hourigan et al., 2008).

Nurses are frequently in a position to promote physical fitness. By stressing the importance of exercise for physical and emotional health, they help prevent mobility problems.

Physical fitness teaching opportunities occur in many areas of nursing. For example, school nurses can help young people develop good exercise habits. Physical education should be part of the curriculum in all grades, and school nurses should work with physical education teachers and coaches to promote well-balanced programs. Nurses in clinical practice can teach patients about the value of exercise when they make routine visits to healthcare providers and clinics. Nurses are often part of the team for weight reduction programs. Nurses can be role models by remaining physically fit.

People must perform exercise programs regularly for them to be effective. For example, aerobic exercise is most beneficial when performed three to five times a week for at least 30 minutes

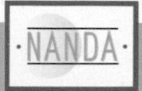

Table 25-4 SELECTED NANDA-I NURSING DIAGNOSES INVOLVING MOBILITY

Nursing Dx	Related Factors	Dx Statement	NOC*	NIC†
Impaired Physical Mobility—Limitation in independent, purposeful physical movement of the body or one or more extremities	Pain; decreased strength, muscle control, or endurance; musculoskeletal, neuromuscular, or cognitive impairment; joint stiffness or contractures; obesity; prescribed movement restriction	Impaired Physical Mobility R/T pain, joint inflammation, obesity AEB inability to ambulate 20 yards without shortness of breath and weakness	Ambulation, Endurance, Physical Fitness, Knowledge: Prescribed Activity, Mobility, Pain Level	Exercise Therapy: Ambulation, Exercise Promotion, Fall Prevention, Pain Management
Impaired Walking—Limitation of independent movement in the environment on foot	Deconditioning, environmental barriers, cognitive impairment, impaired balance, insufficient muscle strength or musculoskeletal impairments, obesity, pain	Impaired Walking R/T left-sided hemiparesis, obesity, cognitive impairment AEB inability to walk more than 50 yards even with a walker	Ambulation, Balance, Coordinated Movement, Endurance, Mobility	Exercise Therapy: Ambulation, Exercise Promotion, Fall Prevention, Pain Management
Impaired Transfer Ability—Limitation of independent movement between two surfaces	Insufficient muscle strength or musculoskeletal impairment, neuromuscular impairment, environmental constraints, cognitive impairment, pain, lack of knowledge, environmental barriers	Impaired Transfer Ability R/T decreased upper arm strength, cognitive decline, and home environment AEB inability to safely transfer from bed to bathroom in home	Body Positioning: Self-Initiated, Transfer Performance, Coordinated Movement	Self-Care Assistance: Transfer, Teaching: Prescribed Activity/Exercise, Fall Prevention, Environmental Management
Risk for Disuse Syndrome—Vulnerable to deterioration of body systems as a result of prescribed or unavoidable musculoskeletal inactivity, which may compromise health	Paralysis, pain, altered levels of consciousness, mechanical or prescribed immobility	Risk for Disuse Syndrome R/T unconscious state	Neurologic Status: Consciousness, Immobility Consequences: Physiologic, Risk Control	Bed Rest Care, Pressure Ulcer Prevention, Exercise Therapy: Joint Mobility, Bowel Management, Embolus Precautions, Cough Enhancement
Activity Intolerance—Insufficient physiologic or psychological energy to endure or complete required or desired daily activities	Generalized weakness, sedentary lifestyle, bed rest or immobility, imbalance between oxygen supply and demand	Activity Intolerance R/T deconditioned state, bed rest for 3 d, and obesity	Oxygen Saturation with Activity; Pulse, B/P, and Respiratory Rate with Activity; Walking Distance and Pace	Energy Management, Exercise Therapy: Ambulation, Teaching: Prescribed Activity/Exercise, Monitoring, Weight Management

*From: Moorhead, S., Johnson, M., Maas, M., & Swanson, E. (2013). *Iowa Outcomes Project: Nursing Outcomes Classification (NOC)* (5th ed.). St. Louis, MO: C. V. Mosby.
†From: Bulecheck, G., Butcher, H., Dochterman, J., & Wagner, C. (2013). *Iowa Intervention Project: Nursing Interventions Classification (NIC)* (5th ed.). St. Louis, MO: Elsevier Mosby.
From: NANDA-International (NANDA-I). (2014). *Nursing diagnoses: Definitions and classification, 2015-2017*. West Sussex, England: Wiley-Blackwell.

of accelerated heart rate. People may drop out of an exercise program because of pain and soreness if they begin too aggressively.

> **! SAFETY ALERT**
>
> Patients should increase exercise tolerance gradually to avoid excessive stress on muscles and joints. Pain during exercise is a signal to stop.

Exercise programs are part of many patients' rehabilitation processes. Extended care facilities often plan group exercise activities. Strength training has been effectively used with older adults in some settings to increase ROM, strength, and balance. Exercise regimens such as tai chi are proving beneficial in enhancing muscle strength and endurance for elderly participants (Li, Xu, & Hong, 2009). A specific exercise program is recommended after a heart attack or cardiac surgery. After a stroke, exercise is useful to improve speed, tolerance, and independence in walking (Saunders, Greig, Mead, & Young, 2010). Many patients with diabetes follow an exercise program to obtain better control over blood glucose levels (Ansari, 2009). The patient who has undergone orthopedic surgery is encouraged to exercise certain muscles and joints. In many healthcare facilities, the physical therapy staff is usually responsible for supervising exercise programs, but nurses can encourage and reinforce the prescribed therapies.

OSTEOPOROSIS PREVENTION

Osteoporosis, the most common bone disease in humans, represents a major public health problem (Cosman et al., 2014). It is characterized by low bone mass, deterioration of bone tissue, and disruption of bone architecture. Osteoporosis is a risk factor for fracture just as hypertension is for stroke. It affects an enormous number of people, of both sexes and all races, and its prevalence will increase as the population ages (Cosman et al., 2014). After age 30 years, bone mass gradually declines for everyone, but this process greatly accelerates for women after menopause because of a decline in estrogen production. Primary risk factors for osteoporosis include the following:

- Postmenopausal status
- Caucasian or Asian race
- Premature or surgical menopause
- Family history of osteoporosis
- History of fragility fractures
- Alcohol abuse or cigarette smoking
- Prolonged immobility or inactivity

Osteoporosis is preventable and treatable. Prevention must begin early to promote adequate mineralization of the bone. Techniques can measure bone density in high-risk individuals. Lifestyle changes recommended for the prevention or management of osteoporosis include smoking cessation, no or limited alcohol and caffeine consumption, a diet rich in calcium and vitamin D, and regular weight-bearing exercise. High sodium intake and low protein intake have also been associated with loss of bone

mass. Increasing research is being done on osteoporosis in men (Shepherd, Cass, & Ray, 2010). Other pharmacologic modalities include calcium supplementation (1,000 to 1,500 mg per day); vitamin D, calcitonin, and bisphosphonates to inhibit bone reabsorption; selective estrogen receptor modulators (SERMs) that cause estrogenlike effects; and new anabolic agents that have the potential to reconstitute destroyed bone (Licata, 2007).

INJURY PREVENTION

Injuries commonly cause impaired mobility, but many injuries can be prevented (see Chapter 23). The nurse can play a significant role in injury prevention:

- Promote automobile safety and instruct patients to wear seat belts and use proper restraint devices for babies and young children.
- Counsel patients about drug and alcohol use.
- Help patients provide a safe environment for themselves and their families.
- Evaluate the ergonomics of workstations to prevent strain on joints and muscles.
- Provide instruction about injury prevention in the workplace.

FALL PREVENTION

Interventions for decreasing fall rates and decreasing the severity of injury if a fall occurs have become a focus to ensure safe patient care. By identifying patients at greatest risk, the nurse can increase and individualize surveillance and preventive interventions. Fall prevention strategies for all patients include the following:

- Orient to the environment, keeping a call light and personal belongings within reach.
- Keep the bed in a low position with brakes locked.
- Clear the environment of clutter, and keep it well lit.
- Encourage nonskid, fitted footwear.
- Monitor patients frequently to proactively take care of requests, especially regular toileting.
- Educate the patient and family regarding fall prevention strategies.

If your assessment determines that your patient is at high risk for falling, individualize the plan based on the specific risk factors. Some things to consider include the following:

- Use of bed or chair alarms for confused patients
- Use of a bowel and bladder program with scheduled toileting
- Physical therapy consult
- Evaluation of medication usage, especially those contributing to postural hypotension or confusion
- Addressing fall risk at handoff and on plan of care
- Keeping nursing staff within visual sight of patient

All staff members need to answer call lights and alarms promptly to prevent falls. Regular purposeful rounding, especially if done hourly, helps attend to patients' needs so that they will not try to get up independently. Regular toileting is especially helpful in fall prevention because most patients fear the embarrassment of not making it to the toilet in time.

> **SAFETY ALERT**
> Never leave a patient who is a high fall risk alone in the bathroom.

Nursing Interventions for Altered Mobility

POSITIONING

Therapeutic positioning is used to prevent complications when mobility is limited. The patient may be placed in specific positions to facilitate diagnostic tests or surgical intervention (Fig. 25-5). Common positioning postures include prone (face down), supine (lying on back), high Fowler's (head of the bed elevated 80 to 90 degrees), semi-Fowler's (head of the bed elevated 30 to 45 degrees), dorsal recumbent (supine with legs flexed in an elevated position), knee–chest position, Trendelenburg (supine with head lower than feet), reverse Trendelenburg (supine with head higher than feet), lateral or side-lying position, and Sims' (semiprone between a prone and side-lying position). Positions most commonly used for the immobile patient include supine, Fowler's, semi-Fowler's, prone, side-lying, and Sims'.

Regardless of the specific position, general principles of body mechanics should be used in any position change. Maintain proper body alignment and support all body parts. Avoid pressure, especially over bony prominences, by adequately padding these areas. Positioning aids such as pillows, splints, footboards, foam rubber, and sheepskin protectors are helpful (Table 25-5). Turning and positioning patients requires various organizational skills. Examples of those skills include the following:

- Think through the task before beginning.
- Ensure that all needed equipment is within easy reach.
- Explain to the patient exactly what will happen before beginning the position change.

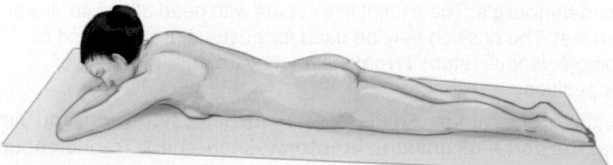

Prone: The patient lies face down. Arms may cushion the head or may be flexed. An alternative position for an immobilized patient, the prone position is contraindicated after abdominal surgery and in patients with respiratory or spinal problems.

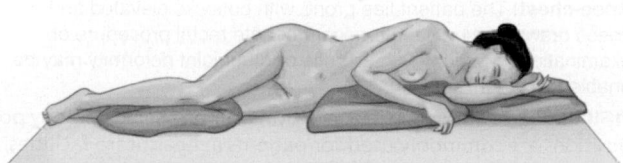

Side-lying: The patient lies on the side with weight on hip and shoulder. Pillows support and stabilize uppermost leg, arm, head, and back. A choice position for patients with pressure on bony prominences of the back and sacral pressure sores, side-lying is not used after hip replacement and other orthopedic surgery.

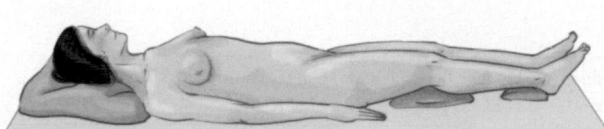

Supine: The patient lies flat on back. Pillows may be used under the head, knees, and calves to raise heels off the mattress. An alternative position for a patient on bed rest, the prone position is used after spine surgery and some spinal anesthesia. It is not used for patients with dyspnea or at risk for aspiration.

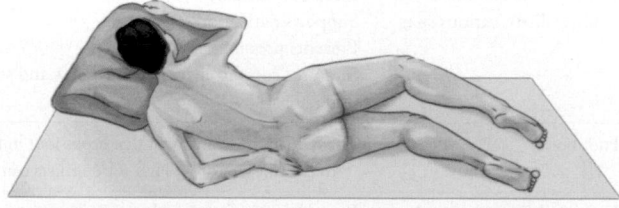

Sims': In this semiprone position the patient lies on the side with weight distributed toward the anterior ilium, humerus, and clavicle. Pillows support the flexed arms and legs. The position is contraindicated in many spine or orthopedic conditions.

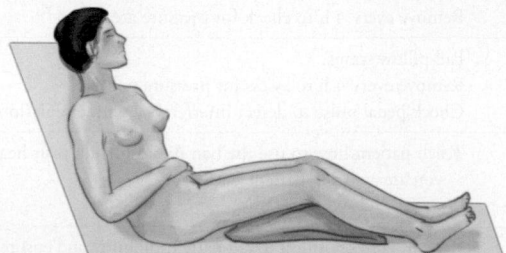

Fowler's: This sitting position raises the patient's head 80° to 90°. Pillows can be used under the head and arms and a footboard may also be used. The position improves cardiac output, promotes ventilation, and eases eating, talking, and watching TV. It is not used after spine or brain surgery.

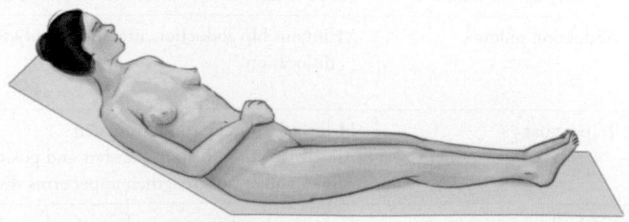

Semi-Fowler's: In this semisitting position the patient's head is elevated 30° to 45°. This position has the same advantages and contraindications as Fowler's position.

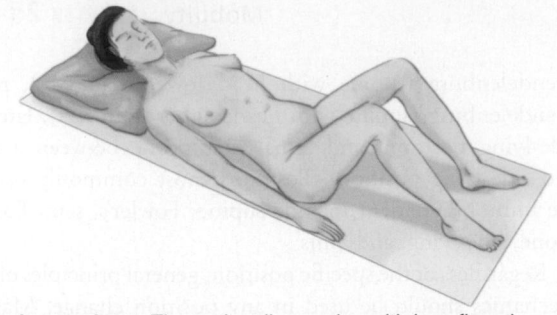

Dorsal recumbent: The patient lies supine with legs flexed and rotated outward. This position is used extensively for vaginal examination but not for abdominal assessment because it promotes contraction of abdominal muscles.

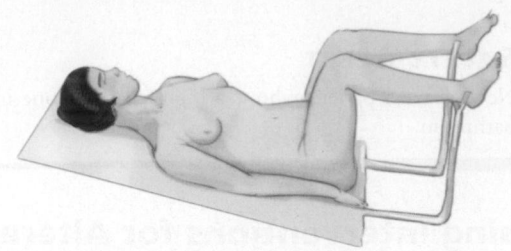

Lithotomy: The patient lies supine with hips flexed and calves and heels parallel to the floor. This uncomfortable and embarrassing position requires draping the patient for privacy. It is used for vaginal and rectal examination and may pose great difficulty for patients with immobilizing arthritis or a joint deformity.

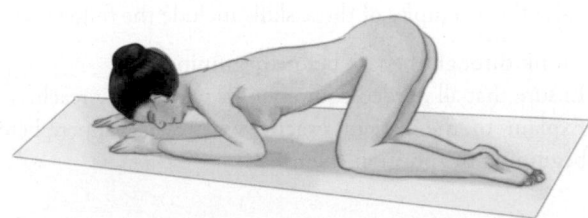

Knee-chest: The patient lies prone with buttocks elevated and knees drawn to the chest to accommodate rectal procedure or examination. A patient with arthritis or other joint deformity may be unable to lie in this position.

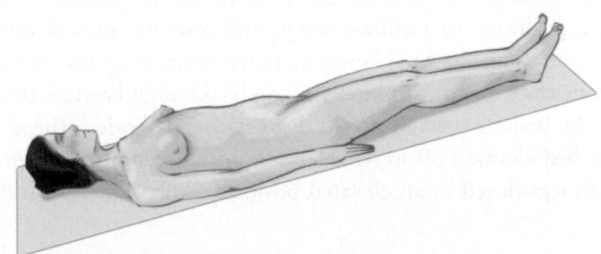

Trendelenburg's: The patient lies supine with head 30° to 40° lower than feet. The position may be used for postural drainage and to promote venous return. Hypotension may be an after-effect of this position.

FIGURE 25-5 Common patient positions. Among selected body positions, the prone, supine, Fowler's, semi-Fowler's, side-lying, and Sims' positions are commonly used for patients in healthcare facilities, whereas the dorsal recumbent, lithotomy, knee–chest, Trendelenburg, and reverse Trendelenburg positions are often used during certain tests and surgical procedures.

TABLE 25-5 POSITIONING AIDS

Aid	Purpose	Nursing Considerations
Pillow (feather, foam, or fiber filled); various sizes	Elevates body part Supports patient on side Prevents pressure on skin Increases comfort by decreasing stress and strain on body parts	Use pillows small enough to maintain proper body alignment. Assess for allergies to feathers before using.
Foot boots	Heavy foam or plastic boot that keeps foot in flexed position to prevent foot drop; high-top sneakers can substitute.	Remove boot a few times a day to inspect skin and provide ROM for the foot.
Hand roll	Keeps hand in functional position Prevents finger contractures	Roll should be large enough to prevent finger flexion and keep thumb in opposition. A rolled washcloth may be used if a manufactured hand roll is unavailable.
Hand–wrist splint	Keeps arm and hand in normal functioning position (slight adduction of thumb and dorsiflexion of wrist)	Individually made for each patient: Pad inside of splint. Remove every 4 h to check for pressure areas.
Heel or elbow protectors (sheepskin or foam)	Reduces mattress pressure on heels or elbows Helps remove elbow friction when patient moves in bed	Launder as necessary. Remove every 4 h to check for pressure areas.
Abduction pillow	Maintains hip abduction after hip surgery to prevent hip dislocation	Pad pillow straps. Remove every 4 h to assess for pressure points. Check pedal pulse to detect interference with circulation.
Trapeze bar	Helps patient raise trunk from bed Allows patient to help in transfers and position changes Allows patient to strengthen upper arms through exercise	Teach patient how to use the bar. Avoid hitting your head when you are assisting patient with care.
Side rail	Helps weak patient turn independently Protects patient from falling out of bed	Keep in raised position to aid patient mobility and ensure patient safety. If all side rails are up, it's considered a restraint.
Turn sheet	Helps reposition patient; can be secured to side rail to support patient in side-lying position	Position from midthorax to below hips. Roll sheet close to patient to obtain better support when moving patient. The turn sheet can be made from bath blankets if manufactured models are unavailable.

- Enlist the patient's assistance whenever possible, giving instructions and encouragement as necessary.
- When the position change has been completed, ask if the patient is comfortable. Reposition as necessary.
- Tell the patient how long he or she will remain in the position. Provide a call device within easy reach.
- Document the position change and indicate to nursing staff when the next position change is due.

 SAFETY ALERT

Decide if you need help from other staff members. If so, ensure that they are in the room before beginning the position change. If there is any possibility that you need help, always request it.

Proper positioning, outlined in **Procedure 25-2**, is important in preventing complications. A patient with partial mobility can usually learn positioning techniques to use with or without the nurse's assistance, but immobile patients rely on the nursing staff or caregiver to reposition them. Helping promote functional mobility is an important independent responsibility of the nurse, who works within mobility restrictions ordered by the healthcare provider or physical therapist. Unless contraindicated, patients should be moved to a chair twice a day (Box 25-3).

Turning Schedules

According to most reports in the nursing literature, immobile patients should be turned and repositioned every 2 hours, but little research shows that this schedule is therapeutic for all patients. More frequent turning may be needed. Significant factors include the amount of adipose tissue, skeletal structure, underlying pathophysiology, adequate blood flow, comfort level, skin condition, and mobility level. Assessing for skin condition and signs of pressure is important in determining

---

BOX 25-3 **Guidelines for Moving Patients**

- Assess the patient's abilities and limitations.
- Medicate the patient to provide optimal pain relief.
- Organize the environment, and request needed help to ensure safety.
- Explain what you are going to do and how you expect the patient to help.
- Permit the patient to do as much as his or her capabilities allow.
- Consider safety precautions (e.g., lock wheels, use transfer belt).
- Follow the principles of body mechanics.
- Keep movements smooth and rhythmic.
- Prevent trauma (e.g., friction against skin, pulling joints, grabbing muscles).
- Check the patient for proper body alignment and comfort, and provide the patient with a call bell before leaving.

---

the turning schedule. Decreased capillary refill and blanched or reddened areas indicate the need for more frequent turning.

Turning schedules should be incorporated in the plan of care and posted at the bedside if the patient is receiving care in the home, a long-term care facility, or a hospital. This helps ensure consistency of care between different shifts and different caregivers. In long-term care facilities, where many patients require frequent position changes, a specific rotation pattern may be developed to ensure that various positions are used in an orderly fashion.

Logrolling

Logrolling (as described in **Procedure 25-2**) is a technique used for turning patients who have had surgery or an injury involving the back or spine. Instruct the patient to keep his or her body as stiff as possible and to avoid any sudden moves during the procedure. A draw or turning sheet can be helpful in logrolling patients smoothly, especially if they are obese. When turning a patient, place pillows between the legs. Leave the pillows in place if the patient remains in the side-lying position.

 SAFETY ALERT

To prevent further trauma and injury, move the body as a unit so that the spinal column does not bend or twist.

Care of Patients With Hip Surgery

Turn patients who have had hip replacement surgery according to the surgeon's orders, taking special care to prevent adduction of the affected hip and leg. For some types of hip surgery, dislocation can result from movement of the leg toward or past the midline of the body (adduction). To avoid this, some orthopedic surgeons order abductor pillows. If an abductor pillow is not ordered, place regular pillows between the patient's legs; an additional staff member should support the affected leg so that it will not fall, even momentarily, during the move. Avoid hip flexion of greater than 90 degrees; keep the operative leg in a neutral position with the toes pointing up.

JOINT MOBILITY MAINTENANCE

Types of Range of Motion

A patient who can perform ROM unassisted is said to have active ROM. A patient who needs the nurse's assistance to perform ROM is said to have passive ROM. Assistive ROM indicates that the patient can participate in ROM exercises with assistance. For example, after a stroke, the patient may have weakness on one side of the body. With direction, the patient may use the strong muscles on the unaffected side to exercise the weaker muscles on the affected side.

SAFETY ALERT

ROM exercises should be done smoothly and gently. Stop movement if the patient complains of pain or if there is resistance.

General Principles of Range-of-Motion Exercises

ROM exercises should be initiated as soon as possible because changes in affected joints can occur after only 3 days of impaired mobility. Allow the patient to participate as fully as he or she can. Perform ROM exercises in a systematic order at a designated time each day (usually during morning care). For high-risk patients, ROM exercises may be indicated more often. In some facilities, physical therapists help immobile patients perform ROM exercises at the bedside.

Support the joint distal to the one being exercised. A healthcare provider's order and specific instructions should be obtained to perform ROM for patients with acute arthritis, fractures, torn ligaments, joint dislocation, or acute myocardial infarction. **Procedure 25-3** details ROM technique.

Automatic Range-of-Motion Equipment

Mechanical devices, such as continuous passive range-of-motion machines (CPM machines), are ordered to provide continuous ROM to a specific joint. Such devices are most commonly used after orthopedic surgery, usually of the knee, when such exercise promotes joint mobility and permits rapid rehabilitation. The equipment extends the joint to a prescribed angle for a prescribed period, continuously cycling according to parameters set by the healthcare provider.

AMBULATION

Early ambulation significantly reduces complications of immobility. Walking exercises almost all body muscles and promotes joint flexibility. Most surgical patients are permitted and encouraged to get out of bed and walk on their first postoperative day. Early ambulation significantly reduces the formation of venous clots and atelectasis, thereby decreasing respiratory and circulatory complications after surgery. Even a short period of immobility decreases a patient's exercise tolerance, so assistance is usually required when the patient resumes walking. Musculoskeletal or neurologic alterations typically require temporary or permanent assistance with ambulation (**Procedure 25-4**).

Muscle Strengthening to Facilitate Ambulation

Certain muscle groups may need strengthening before some patients can walk. Patients on bed rest should learn to contract their quadriceps and gluteal and abdominal muscles regularly because these muscles are important for ambulation. Patients who will use crutches or walkers need to strengthen their arm muscles because increased arm strength will be necessary to support their body weight. *Setting* is a term used to refer to isometric strengthening of muscles. The patient concentrates on one muscle at a time, contracting it for 10 seconds and then permitting it to relax completely. This is repeated a prescribed number of times.

Dangling the Legs

Dangling is a preliminary step to ambulation, especially for patients who may be unable to ambulate initially. The activity involves sitting on the side of the bed with the legs dependent.

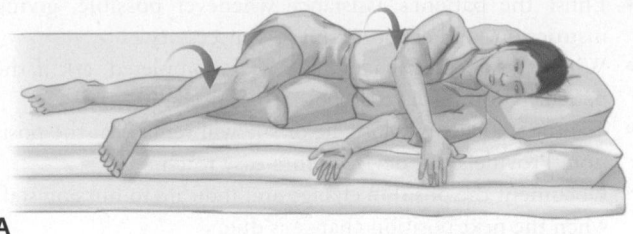

A

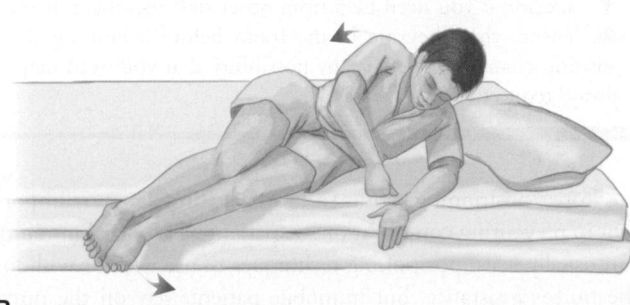

B

FIGURE 25-6 Many patients can reach a sitting position independently when taught the proper method. **A.** The patient rolls over onto his or her side. **B.** The patient grasps the mattress with the lower arm and uses the other hand to push up while swinging the legs over the side of the bed.

Often, dangling is recommended on the evening after surgery or when weight bearing is not permitted. When it precedes the patient's first ambulatory steps, dangling helps to prevent postural hypotension.

When assisting the patient to dangle his or her legs, raise the head of the bed slowly as high as the patient can tolerate. This not only decreases the distance the patient needs to move but also uses the bed to help the patient into a sitting position. To further assist the patient to an upright position, have the patient move as close to the edge of the bed as possible. Face the patient and establish a broad base of support, flexing your hips, knees, and ankles. While supporting the patient under the knees and around the shoulders, move her or him to a sitting position in one smooth movement.

Some patients can independently reach a sitting position. The easiest way to accomplish this is to have the patient roll onto his or her side, grasp the mattress or side rail with the lower arm, and use the other hand to push up while swinging the legs over the side of the mattress (Fig. 25-6). After achieving this position, the patient can maintain it by placing the hands palm down on the mattress for balance.

! SAFETY ALERT

When supporting the patient during dangling, tighten your gluteal and abdominal muscles to avoid back strain or injury.

Assisting the Patient With Ambulation

Assisting the patient to ambulate safely begins by thoroughly assessing his or her muscle strength and coordination. Assist the patient to a sitting position on the side of the bed. If the patient reports dizziness, is diaphoretic, or has orthostatic hypotension (confirmed by blood pressure and pulse measurements), postpone ambulation. If dangling is well tolerated, proceed with ambulation.

> ### ❗ SAFETY ALERT
> Have the patient wear shoes or slippers with nonskid soles, and clear the path of obstacles that might cause the patient to trip. Many hallways have railings that the patient can grip. A weak or unstable patient may prefer to push a chair or wheelchair to provide extra support and balance. Encourage the patient to look straight ahead to promote balance and prevent dizziness.

All equipment (e.g., IV tubing, indwelling catheter, drains) must be secured to a pole. Do not carry equipment while assisting the patient. Keep your hands free to provide support in case the patient falls.

Watch IV lines carefully to promptly detect any problems. Nasogastric suction can usually be discontinued while the patient is ambulating and then reconnected on return to the room. Portable oxygen may be needed to ambulate patients safely who require oxygen. This may require more than one care provider to safely assist ambulating the patient.

🧠 APPLY YOUR CRITICAL THINKING

Mrs. Jones, an 82-year-old retired librarian, had major abdominal surgery yesterday and has not been out of bed. Her vital signs are stable, but her blood pressure is lower than her baseline. She has a hydration IV and patient-controlled analgesia (PCA). Her pain is well controlled with morphine sulfate via the PCA. She complained of some nausea postoperatively and has received an antiemetic. She has a Foley catheter in place and has only had 200 cc of urine during the last 8 hours. Before getting Mrs. Jones out of bed, review factors that may contribute to unsteadiness and difficulty ambulating. How can you promote safety during Mrs. Jones's first time out of bed ambulating?

Check your answer in Appendix B.

Transfer Belts

Transfer belts (sometimes called safety belts, ambulation belts, or gait belts) should be used if the patient is weak or has problems with coordination. The transfer belt is a canvas belt applied around the waist and tightened over clothing (see the example in **Procedure 25-4**).

> ### ❗ SAFETY ALERT
> Grip the transfer belt as the patient walks so that you can provide aid if the patient begins to fall. If the patient becomes dizzy or starts to fall, slowly and gently lower the patient to the floor and call for help. If the patient is at high risk for falls, two nurses may be required to assist with ambulation.

Ambulation Aids

Mechanical devices can help the patient with certain limitations to ambulate safely. During ambulation, walkers, canes, quad canes, and crutches help bear a portion of the patient's weight, promote stability, and maintain balance. The physical therapist is usually responsible for instructing the patient initially with use of these devices; however, the patient often requires additional instruction or supervision from the nurse.

Canes are useful for patients who can bear weight but need support for balance or who have decreased strength in one leg. Canes are made of wood or metal and should be about waist high. Various canes are available, ranging from a simple straight-leg cane to a three- or four-pronged cane (often called a quad cane) (Fig. 25-7).

The cane acts as an additional "leg" by providing the patient with three points of support during ambulation. The patient holds the cane in the hand opposite the weak or injured leg and then moves the affected or weak foot forward with the cane as the weight of the body remains on the stronger extremity. When climbing stairs, the strongest leg advances up the stair first, followed by the cane and the weaker leg. This process is reversed when descending stairs: The cane and the weaker leg are followed by the stronger leg. Instruct the patient to look straight ahead, rather than at the feet, while walking.

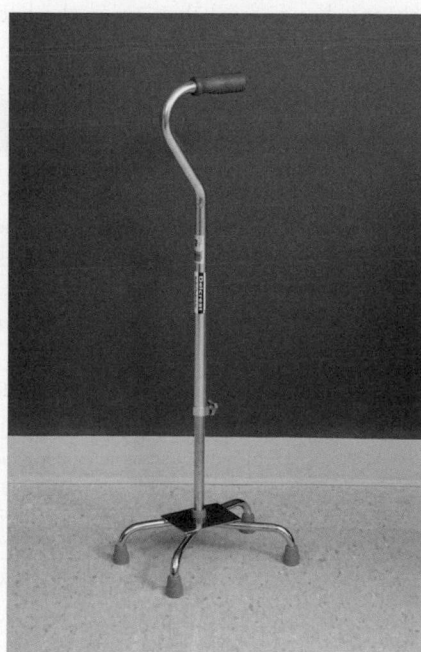

FIGURE 25-7 Quad canes provide greater stability for patients with poor balance or one-sided weakness.

Walkers are lightweight, tubular metal structures that provide more support than canes. Four rubber-tipped legs give walkers a wide base of support. The patient grips the walker, picks it up, and moves it forward (see step 3 in **Procedure 25-4**). The patient may use a two- or three-point gait when ambulating with the walker. Be sure to clear hallways of obstructions before the patient uses the walker. Some walkers have wheels and a seat so that patients who tire can sit and rest or propel themselves by pushing with their feet.

Crutches allow the patient to walk without bearing weight on the legs. Crutches may be indicated when the patient has a sprain, fracture, or nonwalking cast. Underarm crutches usually serve these short-term purposes. The patient must use the arms, not the shoulders, to support the body weight. Using the shoulders can cause skin breakdown at the axilla and nerve damage to the brachial plexus. Underarm crutches must be fitted correctly. About 2 inches should remain between the axilla and the top of the crutch when the crutch is placed 2 inches in front of and 6 inches to the side of the foot.

Crutches also may be used for additional support that weak or paralyzed legs cannot provide for walking. For long-term use, Lofstrand crutches, which have metal bands encircling the forearms, are used. The patient on crutches may use several gaits:

- When the patient can bear partial weight on both feet, the four-point gait may be used. The right crutch is placed forward, followed by the left foot, and then the left crutch is moved forward, followed by the right foot.
- When the patient can bear weight on only one foot, the three-point gait is used. Both crutches and the weaker leg move forward first, followed by the stronger leg.
- The two-point gait requires at least partial weight bearing on each foot, as each crutch moves at the same time as the opposing leg.
- The swing-through gait is often used by paraplegics, who move both crutches forward then swing the body beyond the crutches to propel themselves forward.

To function independently, the patient on crutches must learn how to rise from a sitting position and then climb and descend stairs. This instruction is usually done by a physical therapist. The patient also should be taught to inspect the rubber tips of crutches for wear.

SAFETY ALERT

Prompt replacement of worn tips on crutches can prevent falls.

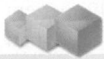 **Concept Mastery Alert**

Some crutches are intended to compensate for a short-term inability to weight bear on one leg. Canes and walkers can be safely and effectively used by many patients who need assistance with balance, but a patient with poor balance would have a high risk for falls if using crutches.

TRANSFERS

Assisted transfers are necessary when the patient is unconscious or extremely weak or has decreased muscle strength or paralysis in the legs. Lateral transfers involve moving the patient from one flat surface to another—for example, from the bed to the stretcher or vice versa (**Procedure 25-5**). Vertical transfers involve moving the patient from the bed to a sitting position either in a chair or wheelchair (**Procedure 25-6**).

Equipment (transfer belts, transfer boards or sleds, roller boards, air-assisted transfer devices, hydraulic lifts, ceiling lifts) can make transfers easier and safer. Table 25-6 describes common transfer aids.

TABLE 25-6 TRANSFER EQUIPMENT

Device	Purpose	Nursing Considerations
Lateral-assist devices	Smooth, flat surface placed under a supine patient to ease the transfer to another flat surface	Use only when transfer surfaces are at the same height. Avoid pinching patient's skin when positioning board.
Roller board	Also assists with transfers from one flat surface to another; consists of metal frame covered with longitudinal rollers encased in a fabric covering	Board is placed in the gap between the bed and the stretcher. A drawsheet may be used to slide patient across.
Transfer belt (also called gait belt, ambulation belt)	Used for support during transfers or ambulation, especially for patients who are weak or dizzy or have poor balance	Fasten belt snugly over clothing. Use whenever ambulation may be unsteady.
Hydraulic lift	Used to transfer immobile patients from bed to chair or bathtub; lift has a canvas sling that fits under patient and hooks into metal frame; patient can then be elevated and transferred using the hydraulic mechanism.	Reassure patients that they will not fall.
Stand-up lift	Assists patients who can bear weight to assume a standing position	When placing the sling, avoid pressure in the axillary area.
Ceiling lift	Sling that can be used to move or reposition patients; attaches to a ceiling tracking device; can be stored when not in use.	The lift is readily accessible whenever needed. There are fewer infection control issues. The ceiling lift is more expensive.
Friction-reducing sheets	Thin, slippery sheets that can be slipped under patient for repositioning in bed	Decreases friction that can increase risk of pressure ulcers

Internationally, there has been a movement recently to address the work-related risks associated with moving patients by limiting manual handling in all patient care situations.

This has been referred to a "no lift" or "zero lift" policy (Nelson & Baptiste, 2006). In the United States, the American Nurses Association has developed a program known as "Handle With Care" to support actions and policies that eliminate manual lifting to promote a safer environment for nurses and patients. Repetitive back strain over the years, especially when staff members consistently use poor body mechanics, contributes significantly to serious back injuries (ANA, 2013).

Lift Teams

Some hospitals have a **lift team** (sometimes referred to as a transfer team) that is called when a patient needs to be transferred. The lift team usually includes two physically fit individuals competent in transfer techniques and well trained on any special equipment who work together to accomplish safe transfers. Implementation of a lift team has led to increased safety for patients and staff, mainly because they eliminate many critical risk factors that contribute to nursing back injuries (Box 25-4) (Nelson & Baptiste, 2006).

Hydraulic Lifts

A hydraulic lift is a mechanical device that permits a patient to be transferred from the bed to a chair (**Procedure 25-7**). It is used when transferring a patient who may pose a safety risk to either him- or herself or to the nurse. Literature supports a stronger emphasis in teaching nurses about the importance of equipment-assisted safe patient lifting, such as regular use of a hydraulic lift, to avoid occupational injuries (ANA, 2013). The hydraulic lift has a canvas or fabric sling that fits under the patient and hooks into a metal frame. Before using any hydraulic device, read the manufacturer's guidelines for proper

BOX 25-4   Factors That Contribute to Back Injuries in Nursing Staff

- Lifts or transfers that are not coordinated
- Lifting pairs with anthropometric disparities
- Fatigue in personnel
- Injured staff who lift
- Lack of available mechanical lifting devices
- Staff who are not trained

From: Nelson, A., & Baptiste, A. (2006). Evidence-based practices for safe patient handling and movement. *Orthopaedic Nursing, 25*(6), 366–379.

operation. Many agencies require instruction and validation of the mechanical lift before staff can use it clinically. The patient may become frightened when lifted away from the bed, so provide verbal support for the patient throughout the lift procedure.

Ceiling Lifts

A ceiling lift allows for vertical movement of a patient and repositioning without lifting manually. The patient is suspended in a sling that is attached to a ceiling-mounted track, allowing the patient to be moved to a different position or location. Since the ceiling lift is available in the room, there are fewer infection control issues and time is not spent looking for the lift. However, installation of the tracking system can be a significant initial expense for a healthcare agency.

Stand-Up Assist Lifts

Stand-up lifts are helpful in assisting patients who can bear weight to assume a standing position. The sling in this lift is placed behind the back and under the arms (without causing pressure in the axillary area), the knees and legs are positioned against a padded support, and the fabric loops are attached to the lift frame (Fig. 25-8). The lift then gently assists the patient to assume an upright position then transfers the patient to a chair or another location. The patient is often unaware of the degree of support the lift provides and thus feels more independent than when moved by a hydraulic lift. The consistent use of stand-up lifts for all high-risk patients can decrease the incidence of back injury to the healthcare provider.

Two- or Three-Person Lifts

Lifts or carries by staff are seldom used in hospitals because they are usually uncomfortable for the patient and pose safety risks for the nurse. Such carries can be used, however, in emergencies. When lifting a patient, place the patient's arms over his or her

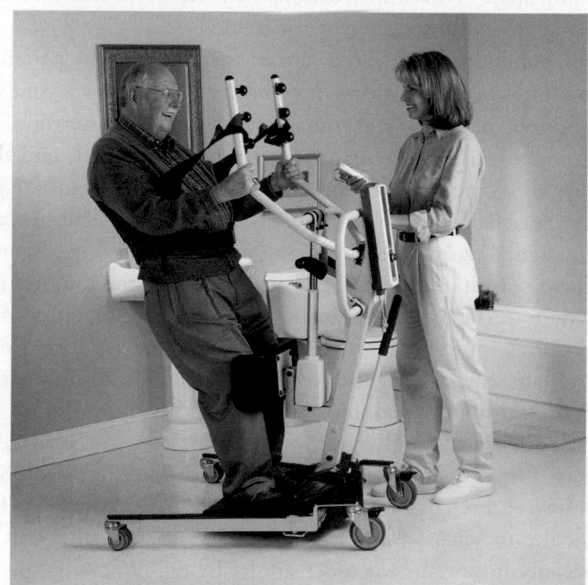

FIGURE 25-8 A stand-up assist lift supports the patient to an upright position when he or she can bear weight.

chest and have colleagues available to lift each body area. When moving the patient to another flat surface, one nurse grasps the patient under the head and shoulders, one under the hips, and a third under the thighs and legs. If the patient is being lifted to a chair, one nurse holds the patient under the arms around the chest while the second supports the hips and legs. Synchronize the lift by counting to three. Using body mechanics is essential to prevent injury to the lifters.

> ! **SAFETY ALERT**
>
> The under-axilla lift techniques, where care providers pull the patient by grasping the arms and under the axilla, should never be employed. This technique is not used because it exerts pressure on the brachial plexus that can affect the nerve function to the neck, shoulder, arm, and hands. It can also subluxate the shoulder. In addition, this technique causes poor body mechanics for the nurse.

Home and Community Care

Many people with mobility problems manage independently in the community and at home. Acute injuries, such as fractures or sprains, are often treated with immobilizing braces until they heal. Many orthopedic surgeries are now performed in same-day surgery centers, allowing the patient to be discharged a few hours after the surgery. With adequate support, even chronic neuromuscular problems (e.g., from stroke, Parkinson disease, or multiple sclerosis) can be managed at home.

Patient teaching aims at helping the patient learn to use special equipment and to live with motor limitations. The patient and family should learn about transfer techniques, ambulation techniques, and special equipment. The physical therapist may provide much of this instruction with reinforcement from the nursing staff. Written instructions help reinforce initial learning and are useful for reference at home.

In some situations, the nurse may assess the patient's home especially for safety. Ask about the physical layout of the house, including the number of stairs, the location of bedrooms and bathrooms in relation to living areas, and the ability to accommodate special equipment in the house (e.g., if a wheelchair can fit through doorways). If disabilities are permanent, reconstruction may be necessary (e.g., ramps built to permit easy wheelchair access). Stress the importance of safety to the patient returning home with impaired motor function. Clutter and area rugs should be removed to prevent falls. Plans should be developed for emergencies. Smoke detectors should be installed, and the person's bedroom should be on the ground floor. The local fire department can provide a special alert sign to place in the handicapped person's bedroom window. A discharge planner or case manager may arrange for someone to telephone or check on the person daily; this is especially important for older adults living alone who are at high risk for falls.

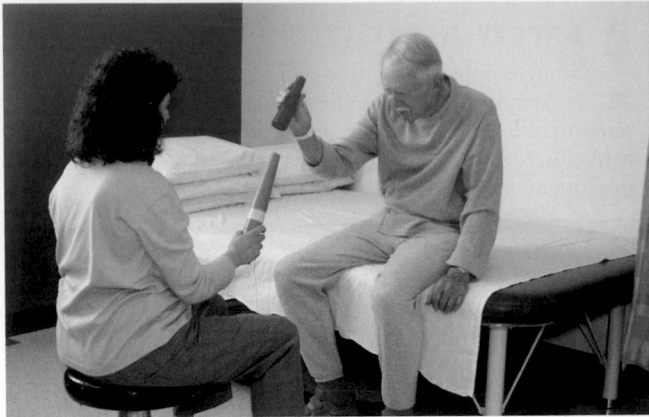

FIGURE 25-9 Outpatient physical therapy sessions can help an older person remain independent as mobility improves after a CVA (stroke).

Arrangements for special equipment and home or community services may be necessary. Sometimes, equipment can be rented, or customized equipment may be made. Written referrals for home nursing care, physical therapy, or other support services may be made as well (Fig. 25-9). Telephoning such personnel to relay preliminary information promotes communication before discharge.

Modifications may be necessary for continued care in the home setting. Ceiling lifts can be installed in the home to aid the caregiver in moving and positioning the patient. When possible, the home situation should be simulated in the hospital before discharge. For example, if a hospital bed will not be available at home, practice transferring the patient in a high-bed position using a transfer sled or board. The patient should discuss how he or she will manage such activities as bathing and cooking. The patient who is place bound due to mobility restriction can use a special reacher to achieve greater independence (Fig. 25-10).

Often, much family support is necessary for the patient to manage at home. Family members should feel knowledgeable and comfortable in assuming this responsibility. They also should

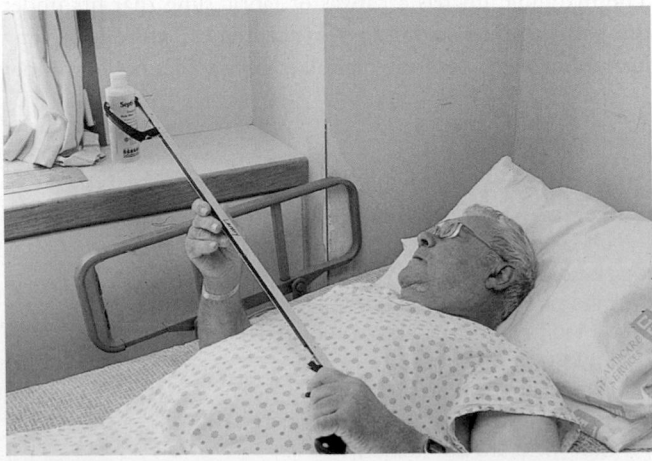

FIGURE 25-10 A reacher is a handy device for the patient with mobility restriction.

You are responsible for discharge teaching for Mr. Block, a 69-year-old retired plumber, who had a total hip replacement 2 days ago. He is an independent man who lives with his wife in a two-story home.

OUTCOME

Mr. and Mrs. Block can verbalize precautions to avoid dislocation of new hip prosthesis.

STRATEGIES

- Assess Mr. and Mrs. Block's readiness to learn and their preferred learning styles.
- Collaborate with the physical therapist to understand the individualized mobility plan that has been developed and how Mr. Block has been doing.
- Review the written sheet outlining hip dislocation precautions with Mr. and Mrs. Block (keep legs abducted or apart, never cross affected leg to midline, never flex hip more than 90 degrees, keep affected leg in neutral position).
- Demonstrate on a model of the hip how crossing legs or flexing at the hip joint causes dislocation.
- Have Mr. and Mrs. Block reverbalize precautions, providing praise when accurately done and gentle correction if needed.

OUTCOME

Mr. Block will demonstrate hip dislocation precautions and verbalize how he will do these after discharge.

STRATEGIES

- When Mr. Block gets out of bed, verbally cue him regarding proper movement of the affected hip.
- Provide a raised toilet seat and demonstrate how to use it.
- Have the Blocks describe their home and plans after discharge. Stress the following measures:
  Take showers rather than baths.
  Avoid using any low, soft chairs or sofas; reclining chairs are good.
  Don't bend over to tie shoes or wash feet.
  Never cross legs.
- Discuss plans for safe transport in the car to the home. (Place the seat in the farthest back position, lead with the unaffected leg when getting into the car, avoid bucket seats, incline the seat back to avoid a 90 degree angle.)

EVALUATION

9/12/17: 09:30—Following instruction, the Blocks could verbalize positions and activities that could cause hip dislocation. They also stated they plan to get a raised toilet seat.

—S. Roberts, RN

PATIENT PLAN OF CARE
The Patient with Impaired Physical Mobility

NURSING DIAGNOSIS

Impaired Physical Mobility related to right-leg above-the-knee amputation, as manifested by inability to move the body purposefully and independently.

PATIENT GOAL

The patient will learn how to move safely after above-the-knee amputation.

PATIENT OUTCOME CRITERIA

- Patient maintains balance and support by standing on left leg (with help of crutches or walker) 1 week after surgery.
- Patient demonstrates safe transfer technique (in and out of bed, commode, wheelchair) by 1 week after surgery.

NURSING INTERVENTION	SCIENTIFIC RATIONALE
1. Keep stump flat and unrotated; do not place pillows under stump.	**1.** Keeping stump flat prevents contracture.
2. Encourage active ROM exercises every 8 hours.	**2.** ROM exercises improve joint flexibility.
3. Provide a program of frequent position changes that includes having patient lie prone for ½-hour intervals every 8 hours.	**3.** Frequent position changes enhance mobility and prevent contractures.

(Continued)

PATIENT PLAN OF CARE (Continued)
The Patient with Impaired Physical Mobility

NURSING INTERVENTION	SCIENTIFIC RATIONALE
4. Avoid long periods of sitting in bed or in a chair.	**4.** Sitting up flexes the stump and can cause contractures.
5. Take postural blood pressure measurements before patient rises.	**5.** This will detect orthostatic hypotension and prevent falls.

6. Encourage patient's active participation in physical therapy.
   a. Discuss value of increasing muscle strength in the remaining leg.
   b. Note time when physical therapy is scheduled, and ensure that patient has eaten and is medicated (if needed) by that time.
	6. Encouraging physical therapy sessions should motivate patient.

7. Remind patient to use abdominal and gluteal muscles to avoid leaning to right side of body when standing.	**7.** Reminding patient which muscles to use while standing promotes better balance.
8. Encourage patient to wear a shoe that provides good support and has a nonskid sole.	**8.** Proper footwear prevents falls and promotes ambulation.
9. Instruct patient to perform good foot care daily.	**9.** Injury to remaining foot will greatly reduce mobility and independence.

10. Show patient how to use trapeze for exercise and in preparation for transfer.
   a. Attach trapeze above bed.
   b. Demonstrate use of trapeze to maneuver in bed and to transfer from bed to sitting position.
   c. Encourage strength in the upper extremities by having patient pull on trapeze to lift body off bed, then lowering himself or herself slowly.
	10. Increase patient compliance with self-transfers. Using trapeze for exercise should strengthen upper extremity muscles.

11. When patient is in wheelchair, encourage him or her to lift body by pushing down on the arms of the wheelchair.	**11.** Muscle strength is increased in upper extremities, preventing prolonged pressure and development of pressure sores.

12. Develop a program of isometric exercises, and have patient perform 10 repetitions three times a day. For example:
   a. Lie on back; squeeze cushion between legs.
   b. Lie on back; spread legs apart against belt buckled around thighs.
   c. Lie on stomach; lift stump toward ceiling.
   d. Lie on back, raise stump, then lower stump and hip, pushing down toward bed.
	12. Isometric exercise should maintain muscle tone in right stump and left leg; spelling out exercises reinforces patient's understanding of them.

13. Teach transfer from bed to chair using stand–pivot technique.
   a. Use transfer belt.
   b. Patient should wear shoe with nonskid sole.
   c. Verbally guide patient through procedure.
   d. Praise successful efforts.
	13. A patient with good strength in remaining leg should be able to transfer safely to chair using this technique.
	   a. Enables you to grip patient better during transfer
	   b. Decreases chance of slipping during transfer
	   c. Provides cueing for movement necessary during transfer
	   d. Psychological support and praise increase patient motivation and reinforce patient's effort.

EVALUATION

10/15/17—During PT session patient demonstrated transfer from bed to chair using good technique. Balance adequate. Required minimal verbal cuing.

—S. Roberts, RN

schedule time for respite from such responsibilities; time off will allow them to recover their strength and enthusiasm. Give relatives telephone numbers of support groups to contact if problems arise. A physical therapist may provide education to caregivers to prevent back and neck injuries, improve general strength and balance, and facilitate the safety and mobility of care recipients.

Great strides have been made in the United States to accommodate people with disabilities. Public buildings have wheelchair access, and special facilities can be found in most public restrooms. Some buses and vans are equipped to handle wheelchairs. Barrier-free, equal accessibility to public buildings is a right guaranteed to all people under the Americans with Disabilities Act of 1990 (Americans with Disabilities Act of 1990).

EVALUATION

Measuring outcome criteria helps determine whether or not the patient has achieved mobility goals. Outcome criteria must be individualized for each patient, but the outcome criteria listed here may be appropriate.

Goal

Patient will exhibit increased endurance and tolerance for physical activity.

POSSIBLE OUTCOME CRITERIA

- Within 24 hours, patient states the importance of gradually increasing activity or exercise.
- Patient increases amount of exercise or degree of activity daily according to preset parameters.
- Patient discontinues exercise or activity if experiencing adverse symptoms (e.g., dyspnea, tachycardia, pain, vertigo).

Goal

Patient will actively participate in prescribed therapies to promote optimal healing and restored mobility.

POSSIBLE OUTCOME CRITERIA

- Patient assists with turning by using trapeze and pushing with legs as instructed during repositioning.
- Patient increases ambulation for a longer period each day.
- Patient demonstrates use of crutches or walker before discharge.
- Patient demonstrates safe transfer technique before discharge.

Goal

Patient will participate in measures to prevent potential complications of immobility.

POSSIBLE OUTCOME CRITERIA

- Patient practices leg exercises every hour to prevent possible thrombus formation during activity restriction.
- Patient practices deep breathing and coughing every hour to minimize pooling of secretions and prevent atelectasis or pneumonia.
- Patient increases fluid intake to eight glasses of water per day for adequate hydration and to prevent UTIs and renal calculi.
- Patient performs ROM exercises daily as instructed to maintain joint flexibility.

KEY CONCEPTS

- The normal functions of the musculoskeletal system are proper body alignment, posture, balance, and coordinated movement.
- Proper body mechanics use alignment, balance, and coordinated movement to perform activities such as lifting, bending, and moving safely and efficiently.
- ROM is the ability to move a joint through the full extent of its normal movement. Active ROM is when a patient can independently move the joint; passive ROM is when another person must do this for the patient.
- Normal walking gait consists of the stance phase and the swing phase. Walking requires coordinated effort, balance, and equilibrium.
- Normal mobility requires an intact musculoskeletal system, nervous system control, adequate circulation and oxygenation, adequate energy, appropriate lifestyle values, and a suitable emotional state.
- Symptoms of altered mobility are decreased muscle strength or tone, lack of coordination, altered gait, decreased joint flexibility, pain on movement, and decreased activity tolerance.
- Immobility affects all areas of function and contributes to many serious complications.
- NANDA-I Nursing Diagnoses in the area of mobility are Impaired Physical Mobility, Impaired Walking, Impaired Sitting, Impaired Standing, Impaired Wheelchair Mobility, Impaired Wheelchair Transfer Ability, Impaired Bed Mobility, Activity Intolerance, Risk for Falls, and Risk for Disuse Syndrome.
- Nursing interventions to assist the patient with mobility problems include turning and positioning, providing ROM exercises, transferring, assisting with ambulation, and teaching how to use ambulation aids.
- Patient goals concerning mobility should focus on promoting optimal mobility, increasing endurance and tolerance to exercise, preventing complications from immobility, and adapting to mobility restrictions.

PRACTICING FOR THE NCLEX

CHECK YOUR ANSWERS IN APPENDIX A.

1. A nurse is planning to help mobilize a patient with lower extremity weakness. Which of the following is/are the priority to ensure patient safety and prevent falls? Select all that apply:
   a. Slide, push, or pull rather than lifting
   b. Lock wheels on bed, stretcher, or wheelchair
   c. Pivot body without twisting back
   d. Use mechanical aids

2. A postoperative patient requests to be repositioned in bed. What should the nurse do first?
   a. Place feet in broad stance and flex knees
   b. Place one arm under the patient's shoulders and one arm under the thighs
   c. Instruct patient to bend legs and put feet flat on the bed
   d. Elevate head of bed and place pillows under head

3. A bilateral below-the-knee amputation (BKA) patient needs assistance moving to his chair using a mechanical lift. Which of the following are appropriate assessments prior to transfer? Select all that apply:
   a. Comfort level
   b. Ability to follow directions
   c. Patient's weight
   d. Limitations of sling/life equipment

4. An elderly patient admitted with malnutrition has positioning aids ordered. Which aids would be most appropriate for this patient?
   a. Trapeze
   b. Bed cradle
   c. Hand roll
   d. Elbow protector

5. A patient is admitted with a cerebrovascular accident (CVA) and right-sided weakness. Which Nursing Diagnosis is most appropriate?
   a. Activity Intolerance
   b. Risk for Disuse Syndrome
   c. Risk for Self-Care Deficits
   d. Impaired Skin Integrity

6. A patient with a diabetic foot ulcer is on bed rest with the affected foot elevated. Which rationale best supports this intervention?
   a. To decrease metabolic needs
   b. To reduce edema
   c. To support a weak patient
   d. To avoid dislodging a DVT

7. A 1-month-old is being examined at a well-child appointment. Which of the following would be normal findings? Select all that apply:
   a. Babinski reflex
   b. Limited hip flexion
   c. Foot drop
   d. Tonic neck

8. A 26-year-old patient is admitted from the recovery room and is identified as at risk for falls. Which of the following best describes the rationale for this nursing diagnosis?
   a. History of dizziness
   b. Depression
   c. Pain medication
   d. Confusion

9. A nursing assistant reports a blood pressure to be 70/49 with a heart rate of 126. What position would be most appropriate for the nurse to use with this patient?
   a. Semi-Fowler's
   b. Sims'
   c. Lithotomy
   d. Trendelenburg

10. A nurse is providing passive ROM to a patient's left lower extremity when he encounters resistance in the ankle. What should the nurse do first?
    a. Assess the ankle for swelling
    b. Continue slow ROM activity to gently increase mobility
    c. Document findings in patient's chart
    d. Stop movement to prevent injury

REFERENCES

American Nurses Association. (2013). Safe patient handling and mobility international standards, Kansas City, MO.

Ansari, R. M. (2009). Effect of physical activity and obesity on type 2 diabetes in a middle-aged population. *Journal of Environmental and Public Health*, *2009*:195285. Retrieved February 25, 2010, from www.hindawi.com/journals/jeph/2009/195285/

Brower, R. G. (2009). Consequences of bed rest. *Critical Care Medicine*, *3*(10 Suppl), S422–S428.

Cooper, J. W., & Burfield, A. H. (2009). Medication interventions for fall prevention in the older adult. *Journal of the American Pharmacists Association*, *49*(3), e70–e82.

Cosman, S., Beur, M., & LeBoff, E. (2014). Clinician's guide to prevention and treatment of osteoporosis. *Osteoporosis International*, *25*(10), 2359–2381.

Dykes, P., Carroll, D., Hurley, A., Lipsitz, S., Benoit, A., Chang, F. et al. (2010). Fall prevention in acute care hospitals: A randomized trial. *JAMA*, *304*(17), 1912–1918.

Hendrich, A. (2007). How to try this: Predicting falls. Using the Hendrich II Fall Risk Model in clinical practice. *American Journal of Nursing*, *107*(11), 50–58.

Hockenberry, M., & Wilson, D. (2011). *Wong's nursing care of infants and children* (9th ed.). St. Louis, MO: Elsevier.

Hourigan, S. R., Nitz, J. C., Brauer, S. G., O'Neill, S., Wong, J., & Richardson, C. A. (2008). Positive effects of exercise on falls and fracture risk in osteopenic women. *Osteoporosis International*, *19*(7), 1077–1086.

Lannin, N. A., Cusick, A., McCluskey, A., & Herbert, R. D. (2007). Effects of splinting on wrist contracture after stroke: A randomized controlled trial. *Stroke*, *38*(1), 111–116.

Li, J. X., Xu, D. Q., & Hong, Y. (2009). Changes in muscle strength, i and reaction of the lower extremities with tai chi intervention. *Journal of Biomechanics, 42*(8), 967–971.

Licata, A. (2007). Update on therapy for osteoporosis. *Orthopaedic Nursing, 26*(3), 162–166.

Martini, F. & Nath, J. (2014). *Fundamentals of anatomy and physiology* (10 ed.). Upper Saddle River, NJ: Prentice Hall.

Nelson, A., & Baptiste, A. (2006). Evidence-based practices for safe patient handling and movement. *Orthopaedic Nursing, 25*(6), 366–379.

NANDA-International (NANDA-I, 2014). *Nursing diagnoses: Definitions and classification, 2015-2017.* West Sussex, England: Wiley-Blackwell.

Oliver, D., & Healy, F. (2009). Falls risk prediction tools for hospital inpatients: Do they work? *Nursing Times, 105*(7), 18-21.

Saunders, D. H., Greig, C. A., Mead, G. E., & Young, A. (2010). Physical fitness training for stroke patients. *Evidence Based Nursing, 13*(1), 18.

Schwendimann, R., Buhler, H., DeGeest, S., & Milisen, K. (2008). Characteristics of hospital inpatient falls across clinical departments. *Gerontology, 54*(6), 252–258.

Shepherd, A. J., Cass, A. R., & Ray, L. (2010). Determining risk of vertebral osteoporosis in men: Validation of the male osteoporosis risk estimation score. *Journal of the American Board of Family Medicine, 23*(2), 186–194.

Tabloski, P. (2013). *Gerontological nursing* (3rd ed.). Upper Saddle River, NJ: Pearson Prentice Hall.

Tinetti, M. E., & Kumar, C. (2010). The patient who falls: "It's always a trade-off." *Journal of the American Medical Association, 303*(3), 258–266.

Procedure 25-1 Using Body Mechanics to Move Patients

Purpose
1. Prevent injury to the nurse's musculoskeletal system.
2. Prevent injury to the patient during transfer.

Equipment
Mechanical aids if necessary.

Assessment
- Evaluate weight of patient to be lifted. Arrange for assistance if necessary.
- Assess position and height of patient to be lifted.
- Assess patient's balance and ability to bear weight.
- Assess patient's knowledge about body alignment and how to maintain it with position changes.

Procedure

1. **Plan movement before doing it.**
   a. **Always lock wheels on bed, stretcher, or wheelchair.**

      Rationale: Unexpected movements may move bed, stretcher, or wheelchair and result in injury to yourself or patient.

   b. **Allow patient to assist during move.**

      Rationale: Patient participation helps overcome forces resisting the move, encourages patient's sense of independence, and provides exercise for patient.

   c. **Use mechanical aids (e.g., transfer belts, mechanical lifts, slide boards, body mobilizers) or additional personnel to move heavy patients (Fig. 1).**

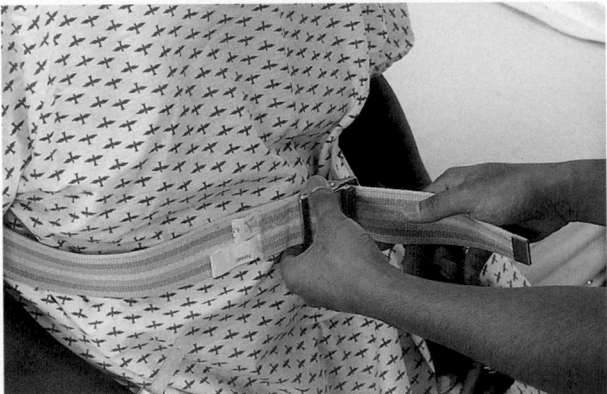

   FIG. 1 Place transfer belt snugly around waist.

      Rationale: Having assistance decreases stress of movement for the patient and nurse, thus reducing risk of injury.

   d. **When possible, slide, push, or pull patient rather than lift or carry.**

      Rationale: Your body weight adds power to muscle work. Rocking your own body weight can balance the patient's weight when assisting to a standing position.

   e. **Tighten abdominal and gluteal muscles before lifting or moving patient.**

      Rationale: Tightening supports the abdomen and stabilizes the pelvis to provide a firm base of support.

   f. **Use smooth, rhythmic, coordinated motions.**

      Rationale: Smooth motions use less energy and lead to less muscle strain than jerky motions.

   g. **If another person is assisting, plan your movements before beginning.**

      Rationale: Planning prevents uncoordinated movements that may result in muscle strain or injury.

2. **Begin all movements with body aligned and balanced.**
   a. **Face patient to be moved, and plan to pivot your entire body without twisting your back.**

      Rationale: Proper positioning avoids back strain and injury.

   b. **Place both feet flat on floor; position your feet and shins alongside the patient's feet and shins; bend knees slightly with one foot slightly in front of the other or one step apart (Fig. 2).**

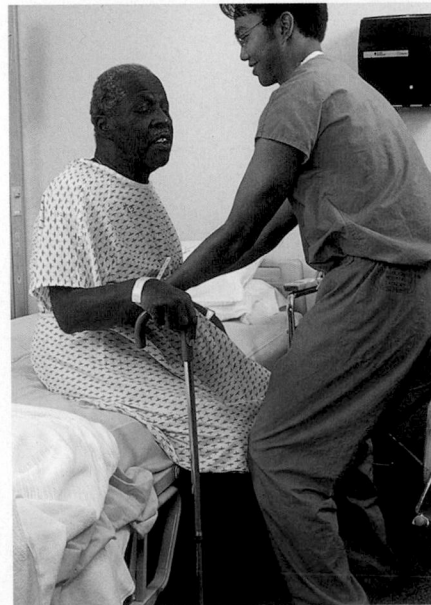

   FIG. 2 With feet flat and slightly apart, lower center of gravity.

      Rationale: Balanced positioning increases base of support and stability. Proper positioning blocks the patient's feet and keeps the patient's knees from buckling as he or she stands up.

Procedure 25-1   *continued*

c. Bend knees to lower center of gravity toward patient to be moved.

Rationale: This maintains body balance, reduces risk of falling, and allows larger muscle groups to work together.

3. **Grasp transfer belt using an underhand grip or pass your arms under the patient's arms, placing your hands on the patient's upper back. Assist patient to stand (Fig. 3).**

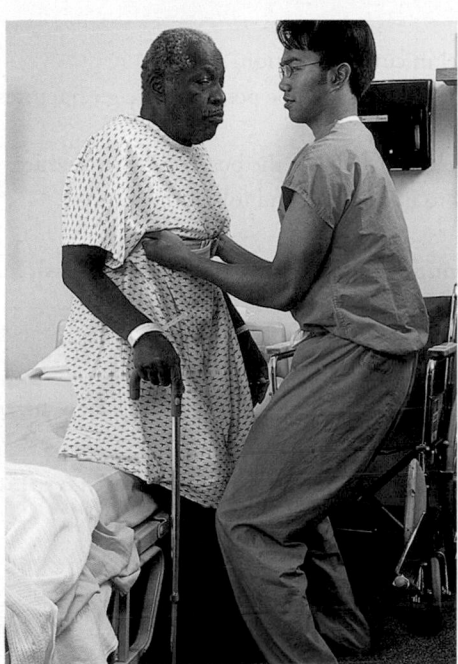

FIG. 3 Assist patient to standing position using a wide base of support and with knees flexed.

Rationale: This provides a firm hold for the nurse and prevents injury to the patient.

4. **When working with a patient in bed, elevate adjustable beds to waist level and lower side rails.**

Rationale: Adjusting the bed and side rails prevents stretching and muscle strain.

5. **Carry objects close to body, and stand as close as possible to work area.**

Rationale: This maintains the workload near the center of gravity to prevent muscle strain and fatigue caused by hyperextension.

Documentation

- It is unnecessary to document.

Home Care Modifications

- Teach caregivers the above guidelines for body movements. Having them demonstrate allows you to evaluate their technique.

Collaboration and Delegation

- Injuries, especially those to the back, are common for healthcare workers who do much lifting. Continually reinforce body mechanics and the use of mechanical aids while expressing concern for the health and well-being of coworkers.
- Physical therapy can provide classes on proper body mechanics for staff review.
- Lift teams to provide transfers for all patients or those at high risk are increasingly being used to prevent injury to staff and patients. Support the formation of a lift team in your agency.

Procedure 25-2 Positioning a Patient in Bed

Purpose	1. Maintain proper body alignment.
	2. Maintain skin integrity and prevent deformities of the musculoskeletal system.
	3. Provide comfort.
	4. Maintain optimal position for ventilation and lung expansion.

Equipment

Pillows
Drawsheet or turning sheet
Side rails

Assessment

- Assess patient's body alignment and comfort level in current position.
- Review chart for conditions that influence ability to move or to be positioned (e.g., fractures, paralysis, head injury, spinal injury).
- Assess for tubes, IV lines, incisions, or equipment that may alter the positioning procedure.
- Assess patient's level of consciousness and ability to understand and follow directions.
- Assess patient's ability to assist with positioning.
- Assess patient's weight and your strength. **Determine if additional assistance is needed.**

Procedure

1. **Perform hand hygiene.**

   Rationale: Reduces microbe transmission.

2. **Identify the patient as well as any positioning or mobility restrictions.**

   Rationale: Ensures correct patient receives proper assessment or treatment and reduces errors.

3. **Close door or bed curtains and explain the procedure to the patient.**

   Rationale: Ensures patient privacy, increases patient compliance, reduces patient anxiety, and promotes learning.

4. **Lower head of bed as flat as patient can tolerate. Raise level of bed to comfortable working height.**

   Rationale: This decreases gravitational pull of upper body and promotes good body mechanics by decreasing back strain.

5. **Remove all pillows from under patient. Leave one at head of bed (Fig. 1).**

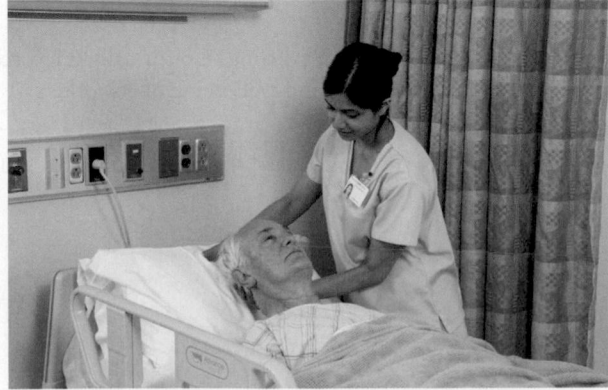

FIG. 1 Remove pillows from under patient's head.

Rationale: Pillows prevent accidental head injury against top of bed frame.

Moving a Patient Up in Bed (One Nurse)

1. **Instruct patient to bend legs and put feet flat on bed (Fig. 2).**

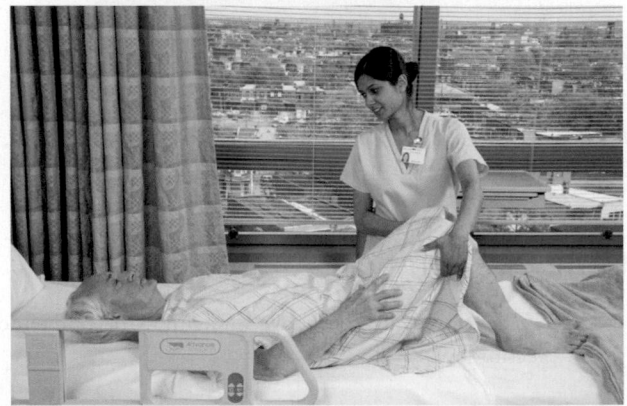

FIG. 2 Assist patient to bend knees.

   Rationale: Patient will be able to assist by pushing legs against bed.

2. **Place your feet in broad stance with one foot in front of the other. Flex your knees and use your thighs.**

   Rationale: Lowering the center of gravity ensures using the legs' large muscle groups.

Procedure 25-2   *continued*

3. Place one arm under patient's shoulders and one arm under thighs. Keep head up and back straight. Ask patient to fold the arms across chest, if able. Have patient lift head and place chin on chest (Fig. 3).

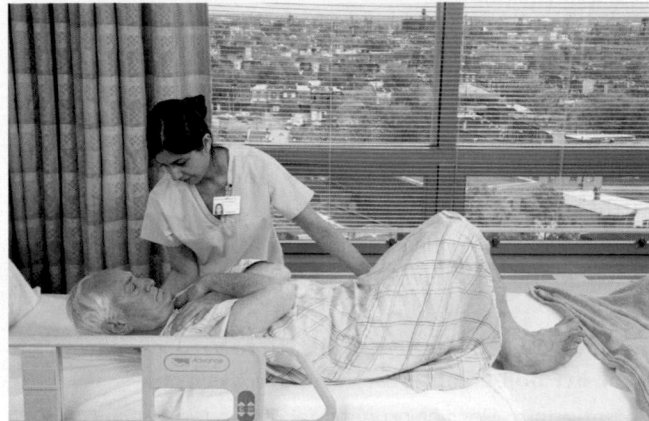

FIG. 3 Properly position hands and head. Assist patient to flex neck with chin on chest.

Rationale: The heaviest parts of patient's body are supported. Avoiding twisting of the back prevents injury.

4. Rock back and forth on front and back legs to count of three. On third count, have patient push with feet as you lift and assist the patient up in bed (Fig. 4).

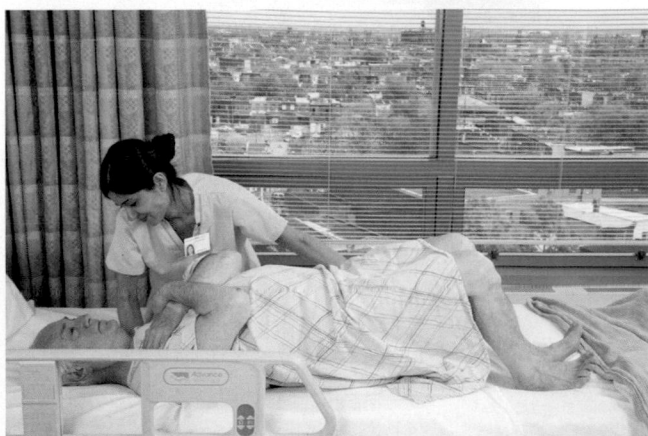

FIG. 4 Assist the patient to move up in bed.

Rationale: Rocking motion develops momentum, which promotes smooth lifting with minimal exertion by the nurse.

5. Elevate head of bed and place pillows under head. Raise side rails and lower bed to lowest level.

Rationale: These actions provide for patient comfort and safety.

Moving Helpless Patient Up in Bed (Two Nurses)

1. One nurse stands on each side of bed with legs positioned for wide base of support and one foot slightly in front of the other.

Rationale: Proper positioning lowers the center of gravity and reduces risk of injury.

2. Each nurse rolls up and grasps edges of turn sheet close to patient's shoulders and buttocks.

Rationale: A turn sheet distributes the patient's weight and prevents shearing injury to the skin by reducing friction during a move.

3. Flex knees and hips. Tighten abdominal and gluteal muscles and keep back straight.

Rationale: Using the legs' large muscle groups and tightening muscles during transfer prevent back injury.

4. Rock back and forth on front and back legs to count of three (Fig. 5). On third count, both nurses shift weight to front leg as they simultaneously lift patient toward head of bed (Fig. 6).

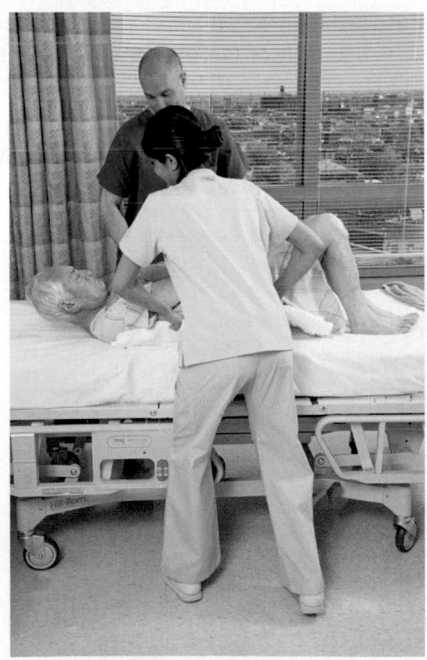

FIG. 5 Moving patient toward head of bed in a coordinated movement.

Procedure 25-2   *continued*

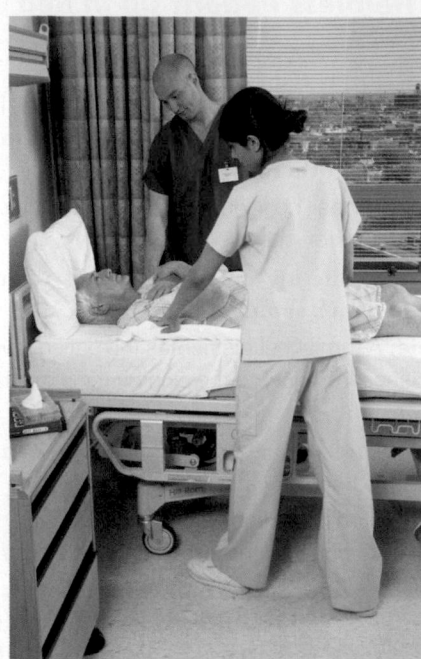

FIG. 6 Patient moved to correct position.

Rationale: Rocking motion develops momentum, which provides a smooth lift of the patient with minimal exertion by the nurses.

5. **Elevate head of bed and place pillows under patient's head. Adjust other positioning pillows as necessary. Put up side rails and lower bed to lowest level (Fig. 7).**

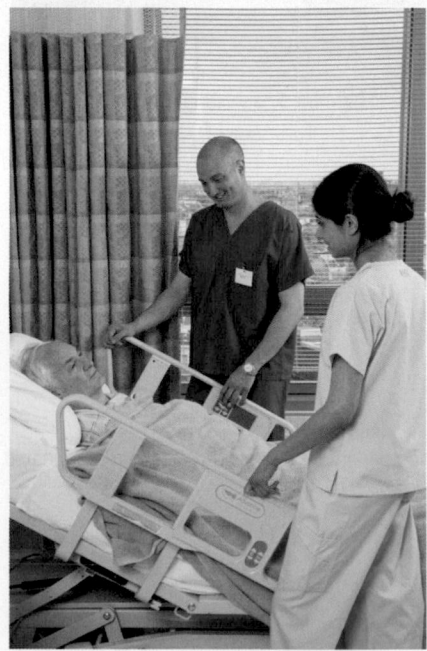

FIG. 7 Adjusting bed to safe and comfortable position.

Rationale: Positioning equipment provides for patient comfort and safety.

Positioning Patient in Side-Lying Position

1. **Elevate and lock side rail on side patient will face when turned.**

   Rationale: Locking the opposing side rail prevents accidental injury from the patient falling out of bed during the turn.

2. **Using drawsheet, move patient to the edge of the bed, opposite the side on which he or she will be turned.**

   Rationale: Provides room so that when the patient is turned, he or she will be positioned in the center of the bed.

3. **Place arm that patient will turn toward away from his or her body. Fold other arm across chest.**

   Rationale: Positioning arms facilitates turning by preventing the patient from rolling onto the bottom arm.

4. **Flex patient's knee that will not be next to mattress after turn. Have patient reach toward side rail with opposite arm (Fig. 8).**

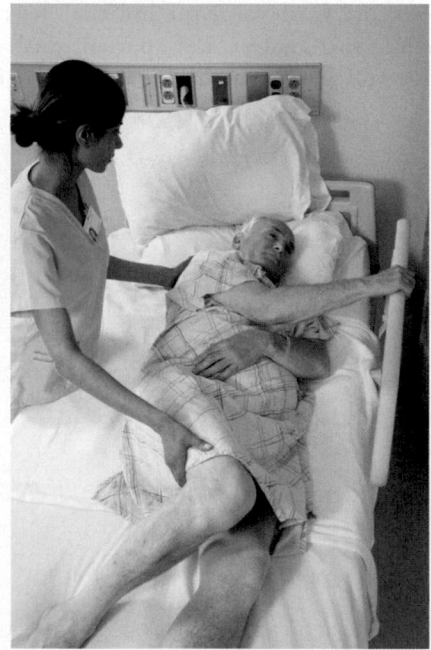

FIG. 8 Have patient reach toward side rail with opposite arm.

Rationale: Encourages the patient to assist with position change.

5. **Assume a broad stance with knees slightly flexed.**

   Rationale: This stance increases balance, lowers the center of gravity, and encourages the use of large muscle groups during movement.

Procedure 25-2 *continued*

6. **Using turn sheet or drawsheet, gently pull patient over on side (Fig. 9).**

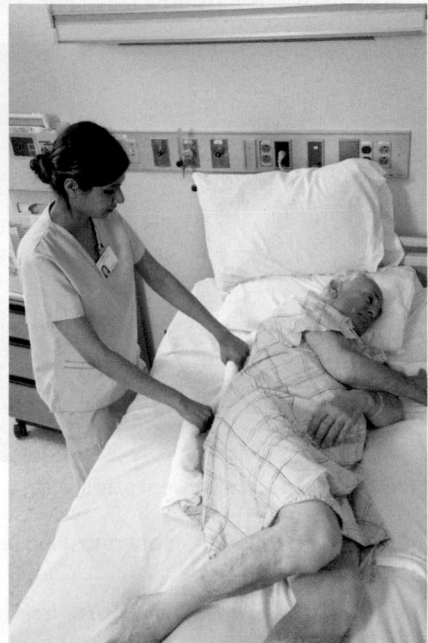

FIG. 9 Using drawsheet to pull patient over on side.

Rationale: You can evenly support the heaviest part of the patient during the turn.

7. **Align patient properly, and then place pillows behind back and under head (Fig. 10).**

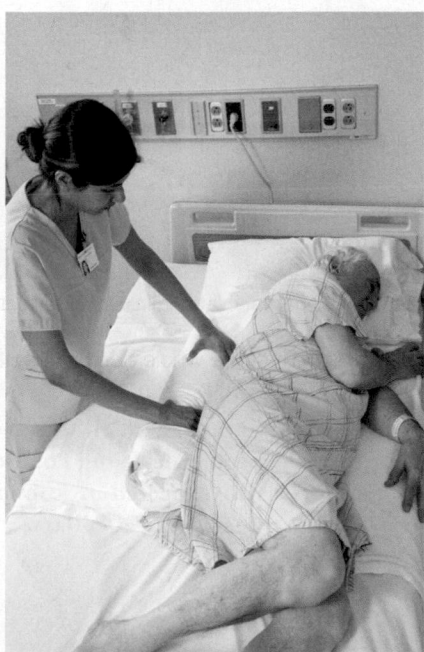

FIG. 10 Placing pillows behind patient's back and under patient's head.

Rationale: Supports the patient in a side-lying position to maintain proper alignment.

8. **Pull shoulder blade forward and out from under patient. Support patient's upper arm with pillow.**

Rationale: Joints are protected from weight and strain. Ventilation also may improve because the chest can expand more fully.

9. **Place pillow lengthwise between patient's legs from thighs to foot.**

Rationale: This keeps leg aligned and prevents pressure on bony prominences.

10. **Cover patient with top linen and blanket (Fig. 11). Elevate head of bed. Put up side rails and lower bed to lower level.**

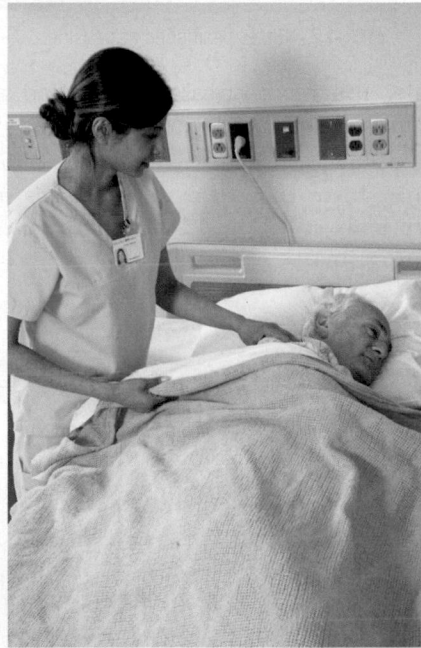

FIG. 11 Ensuring patient comfort.

Rationale: These actions provide for patient comfort and safety.

Logrolling

1. **Obtain assistance. Assess the need for a cervical collar or thoracic braces or jackets to stabilize the spine.**

Rationale: Two or three nurses are usually required. Stabilizing devices must be put on prior to the move.

Procedure 25-2   *continued*

2. Nurses stand with feet apart, one foot slightly ahead of the other (Fig. 12). Flex knees and hips.

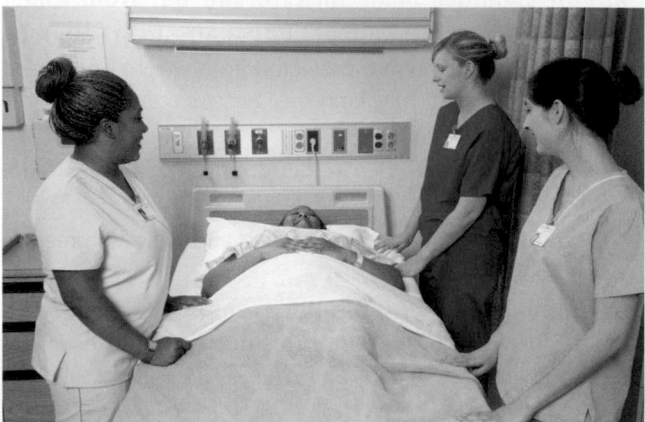

FIG. 12 Nurses positioned at bedside.

Rationale: This stance increases balance and stability and ensures the use of large muscle groups when turning the patient.

3. Use one pillow to support patient's head during and after turn. Instruct patient to fold arms over chest and keep body stiff (Fig. 13). Roll drawsheet toward patient (Fig. 14).

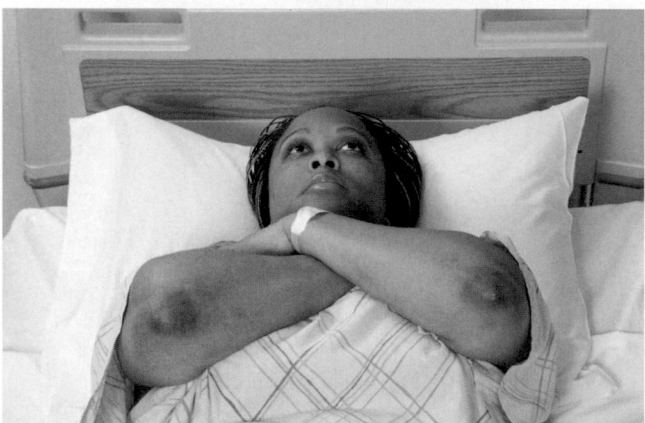

FIG. 13   Patient positioned with head on pillow and arms crossed over chest.

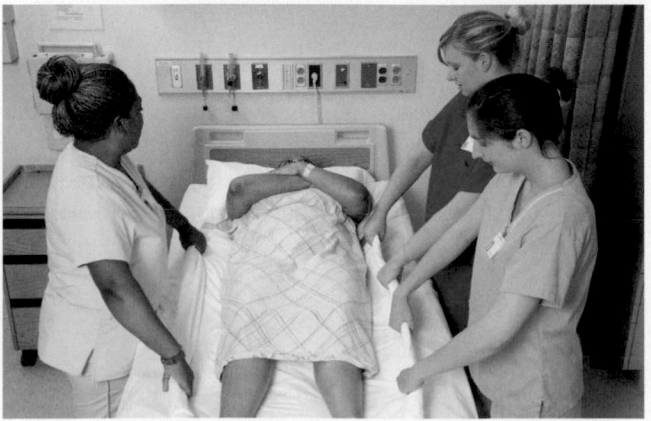

FIG. 14   Prepare to turn patient by rolling drawsheet toward patient.

Rationale: Pillow maintains alignment of the cervical spine during the turn.

4. Place pillows between patient's legs (Fig. 15).

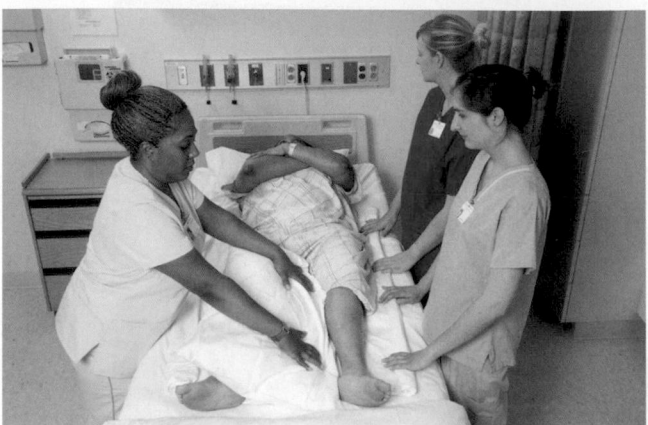

FIG. 15   Place pillow between patient's legs.

Rationale: Pillows support the uppermost leg and prevent adduction during the turn.

5. Reach across patient and support head, thorax, trunk, and legs. On count of three, roll patient in one coordinated movement to lateral position (Fig. 16).

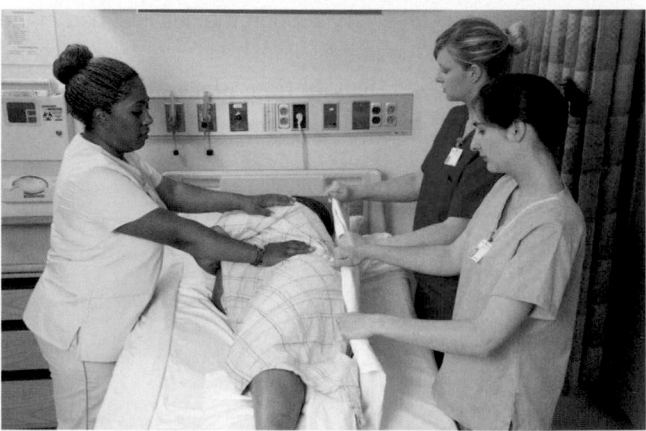

FIG. 16   Roll patient in a coordinated movement.

Rationale: Alignment of the whole body is maintained during the turn.

6. Support patient in alignment with pillows as described in "Positioning Patient in Side-Lying Position" above (Fig. 17). Patients with suspected or known cervical spinal injuries must wear cervical collars.

Procedure 25-2   *continued*

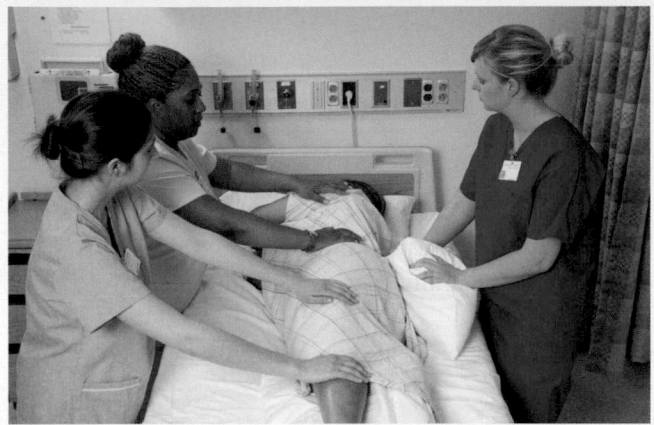

FIG. 17 Support patient's back with a pillow.

Rationale: Support prevents injury to the spinal cord whenever the patient is turned or moved in bed.

Documentation

Position changes should be documented on a flow sheet or turning schedule to ensure that they occur at regular, appropriate intervals.

Home Care Modifications

- Teach caregivers the principles of body alignment.
- Demonstrate how to turn and position a person in bed. Have the caregiver perform a return demonstration of positioning techniques.
- Beds can be placed on blocks to prevent back strain for caregivers if a hospital bed is not available.

Collaboration and Delegation

- Frequently, positioning patients is delegated to unlicensed assistive personnel. Provide clear guidelines regarding limitations and the amount of assistance required.
- Consult with a physical therapist to develop a collaborative plan for any patient with complex positioning problems due to injury or spasticity.

Procedure 25-3 Providing Range-of-Motion Exercises

Purpose	1. Maintain joint mobility. 2. Improve or maintain muscle strength. 3. Prevent muscle atrophy and contractures.
Equipment	No special equipment is required except a bed.
Assessment	• Review medical history to determine specific limitations to joint mobility. • Assess patient's level of consciousness and physical ability to assist or independently perform ROM exercises. • Assess for redness, tenderness, pain, swelling, or deformities around joints.

Procedure

1. **Perform hand hygiene.**
   Rationale: Reduces microbe transmission.

2. **Identify the patient as well as the patient's movement limitations.**
   Rationale: Ensures correct patient receives proper assessment or treatment and reduces errors.

3. **Close door or bed curtains and explain the procedure to the patient.**
   Rationale: Ensures patient privacy, increases patient compliance, reduces patient anxiety, and promotes learning.

4. **Position patient on back with head of bed as flat as possible. Elevate bed to comfortable working height.**
   Rationale: Adjusting the bed promotes proper body mechanics to prevent muscle strain for the nurse.

5. **Stand on side of bed where joints are to be exercised. Uncover only the limb to be exercised.**
   Rationale: This provides warmth and privacy.

6. **Refer to Table 25-1 for illustrations of normal movement for each joint. Perform exercises slowly and gently, providing support by holding areas proximal and distal to the joint. Often, this can be done while providing hygiene.**
   Rationale: This prevents discomfort and muscle spasms from jerky movements.

7. **Repeat each exercise five times. Discontinue or decrease ROM if patient complains of discomfort or muscle spasm.**
   Rationale: Pain may indicate that ROM is causing damage.

8. **Neck:**
   a. Move chin to chest (Fig. 1).

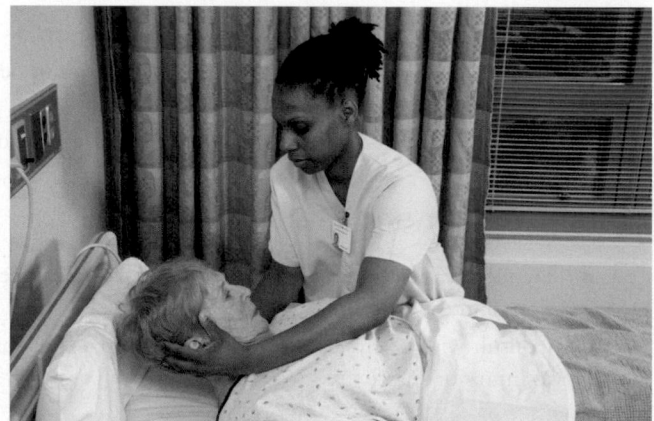

FIG. 1 Move patient's chin to chest.

   b. Return head to upright position (Fig. 2).

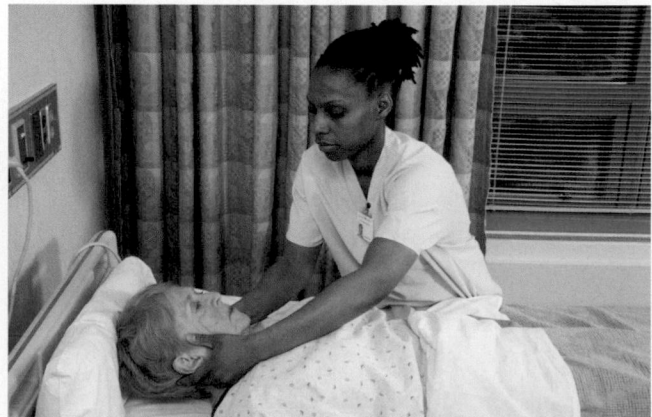

FIG. 2 Hold patient's head upright and neutral.

Procedure 25-3 *continued*

c. Tilt head toward each shoulder (Fig. 3).

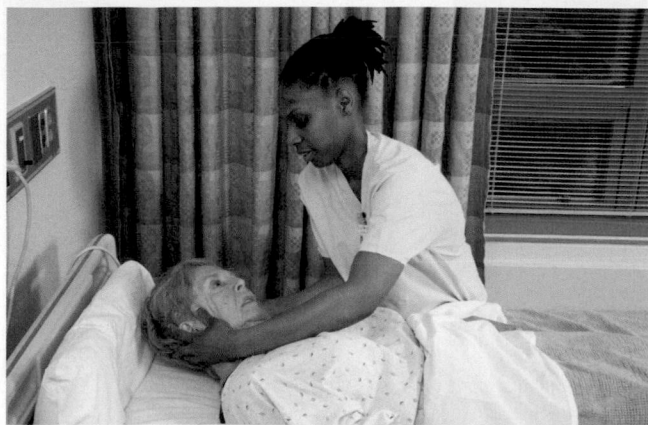

FIG. 3 Tilt head to shoulder.

d. Move chin toward each shoulder (Fig. 4).

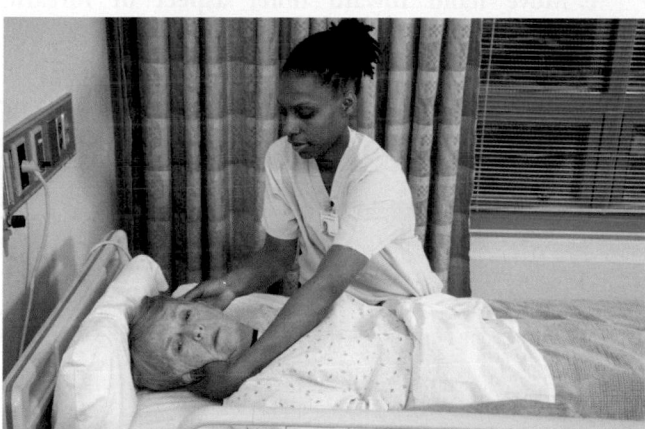

FIG. 4 Move chin toward opposite shoulder.

e. Rotate head in circular motion.

f. Return head to erect position.

9. Shoulder:

a. Raise patient's arm from side to above head (Fig. 5A and B).

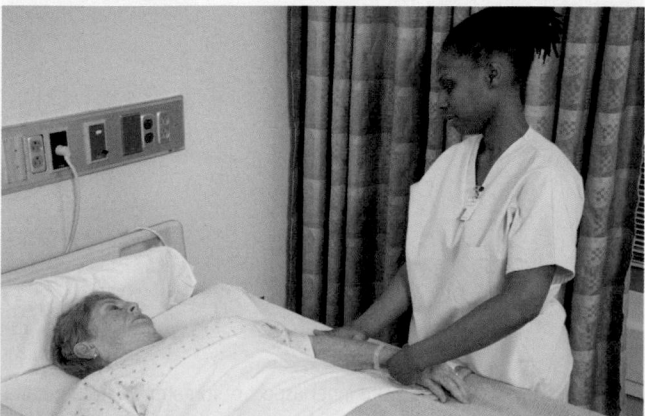

A

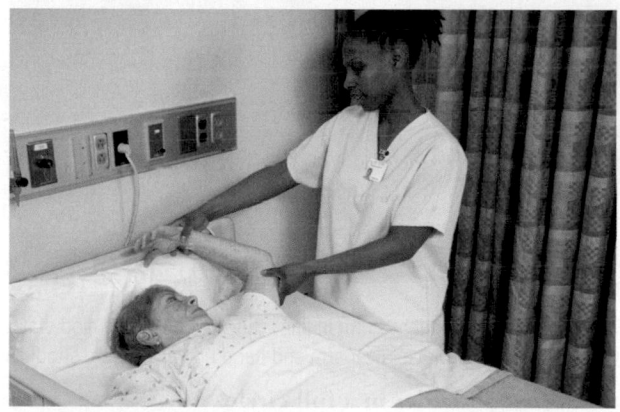

B

FIG. 5 A. Position patient's arm at side. **B.** Raise patient's arm above head.

b. Abduct and rotate shoulder by raising arm above head with palm up (Fig. 6).

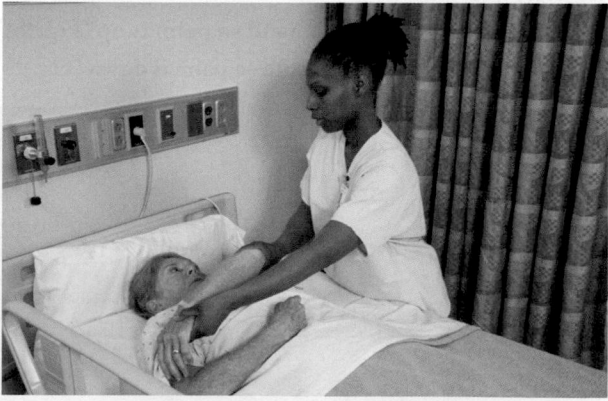

FIG. 6 Move patient's arm laterally to an upright position over head.

c. Adduct shoulder by moving arm across body as far as possible (Fig. 7).

FIG. 7 Move patient's arm across chest.

d. Rotate shoulder internally and externally by flexing elbow and moving forearm so the palm touches mattress; then reverse the motion so that back of patient's hand touches mattress (Fig. 8A and B).

Procedure 25-3 *continued*

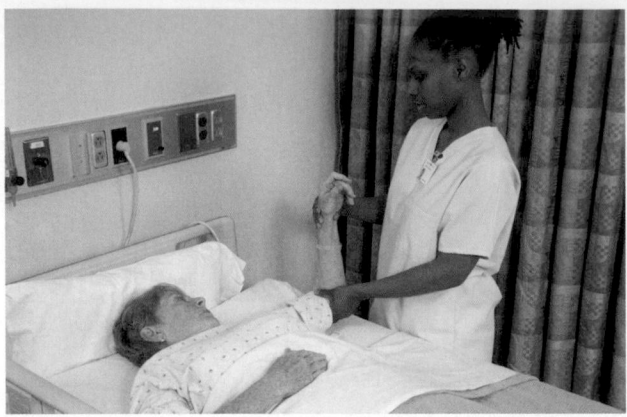

A

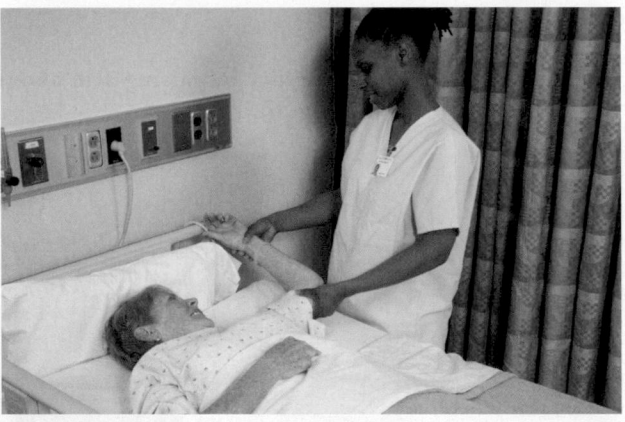

B

FIG. 8 A. Position patient's arm in line with shoulder. Bend elbow at a 90 degree angle. **B.** Move lower arm and hand upward toward shoulder.

    e. Move shoulder in a full circle.

10. Elbow:

    a. Bend elbow so that forearm moves toward shoulder.

    b. Hyperextend elbow as far as possible.

11. Wrist and hand:

    a. Rotate lower arm and hand so palm is up (Fig. 9A).

    b. Rotate lower arm and hand so palm is down (Fig. 9b).

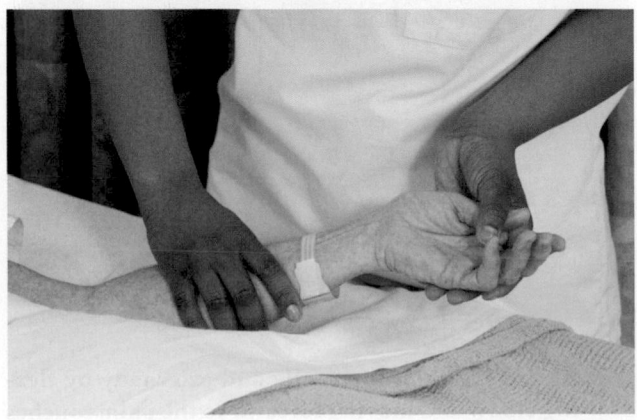

A

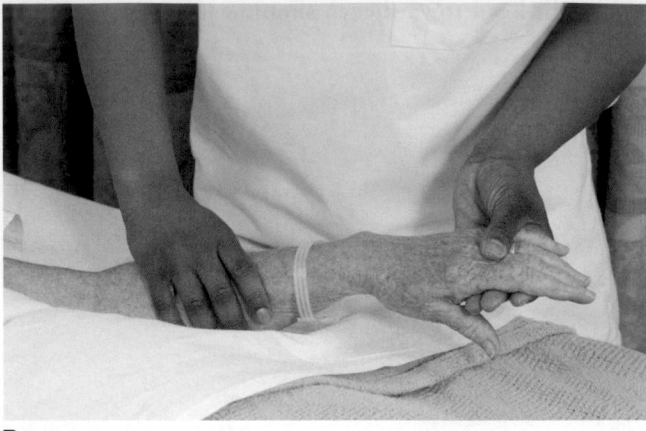

B

FIG. 9 A. Rotate patient's lower arm and hand so palm faces up. **B.** Rotate patient's lower arm and hand so palm faces down.

    c. Move hand toward inner aspect of forearm (Fig. 10A).

    d. Return hand to neutral position (Fig. 10B).

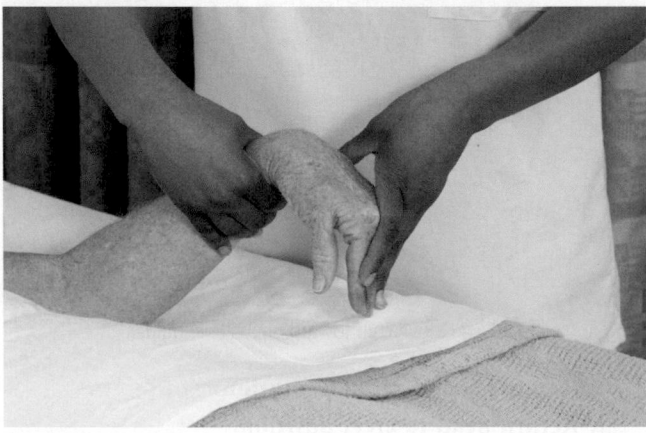

A

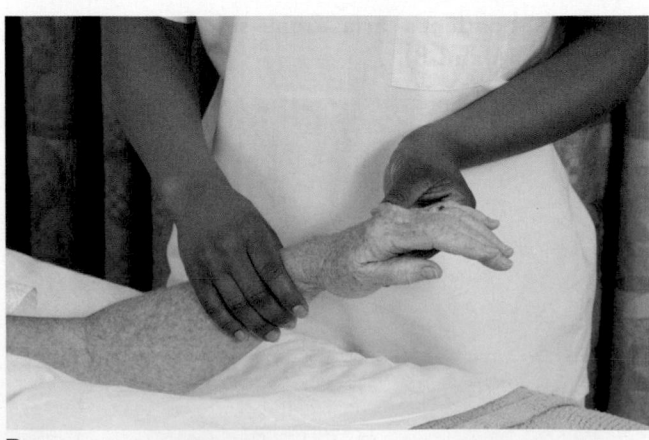

B

FIG. 10 A. Move hand toward inner aspect of forearm. **B.** Return hand to neutral position.

Procedure 25-3 *continued*

e. Bend dorsal surface of hand backward.
f. Abduct wrist by bending toward thumb.
g. Adduct wrist by bending toward fifth finger.
h. Make a fist; extend the fingers (Fig. 11A and B).

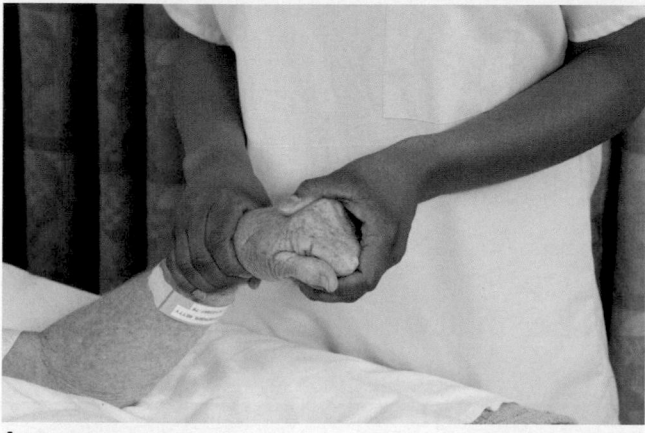

A

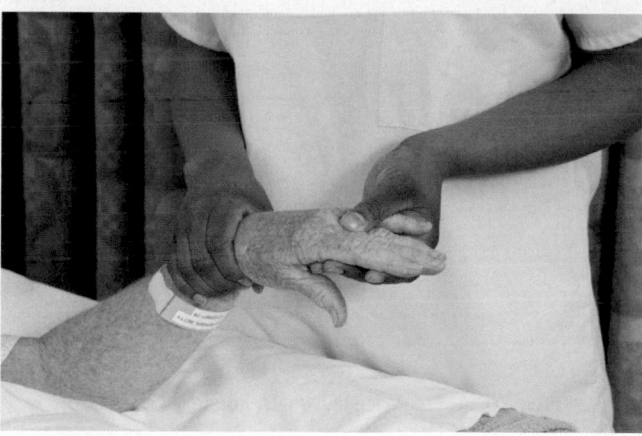

B

FIG. 11 A. Flex fingers to make a fist. **B.** Straighten patient's fingers.

i. Spread fingers apart, then together (Fig. 12).

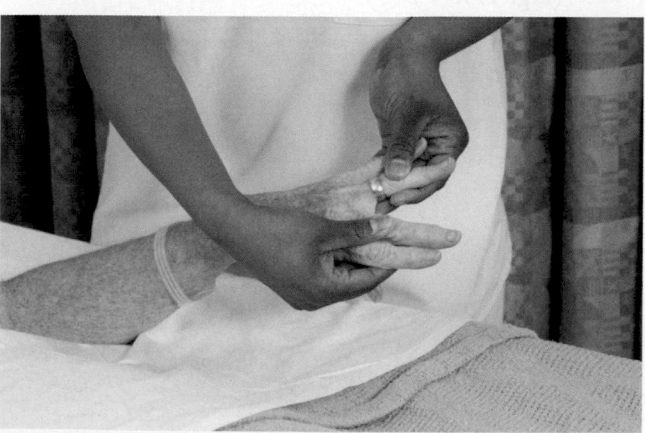

FIG. 12 Spread patient's fingers apart.

j. Move thumb across hand to base of fifth finger (Fig. 13).

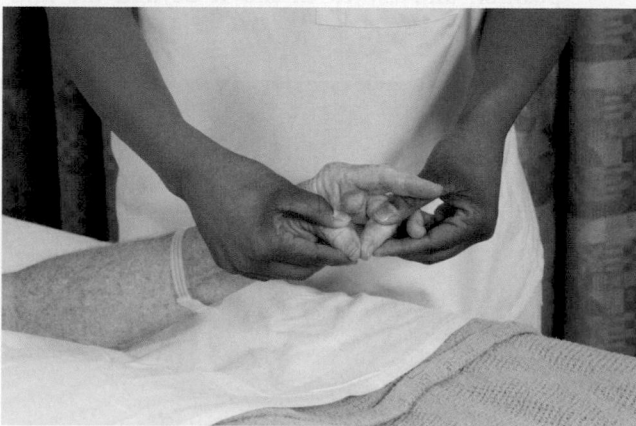

FIG. 13 Touch thumb to each finger.

12. Hip and knee:
a. Lift leg and bend knee toward chest (Fig. 14A). Return leg to straightened position (Fig. 14B).

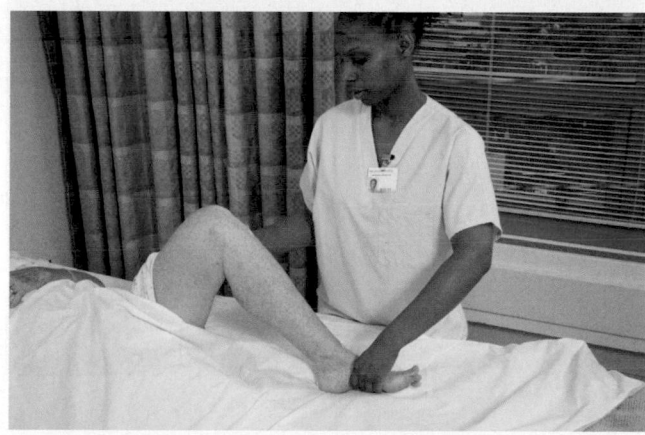

A

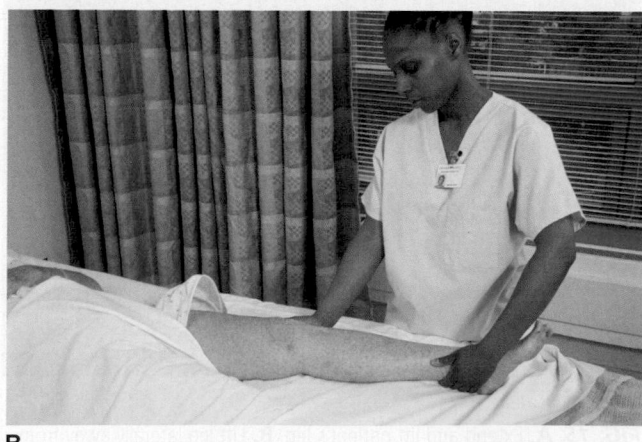

B

FIG. 14 A. Lift leg and bend knee. **B.** Straighten leg.

Procedure 25-3   *continued*

b. Abduct and adduct leg, moving leg laterally away from body (Fig. 15A and B). Return leg to medial position and try to extend it beyond the midpoint (Fig. 15C).

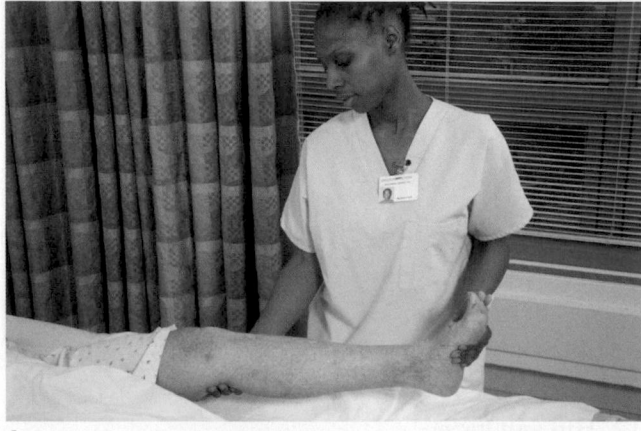

A

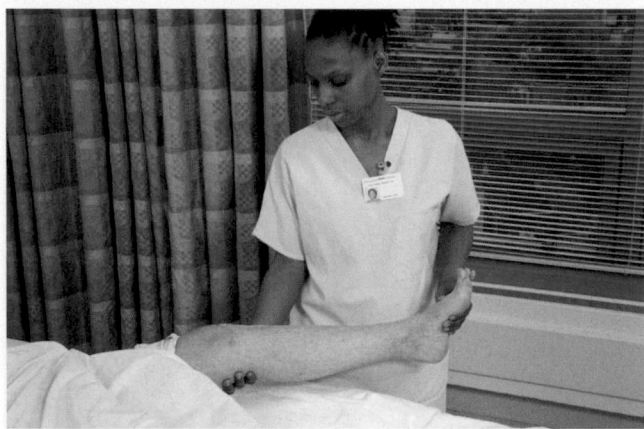

B

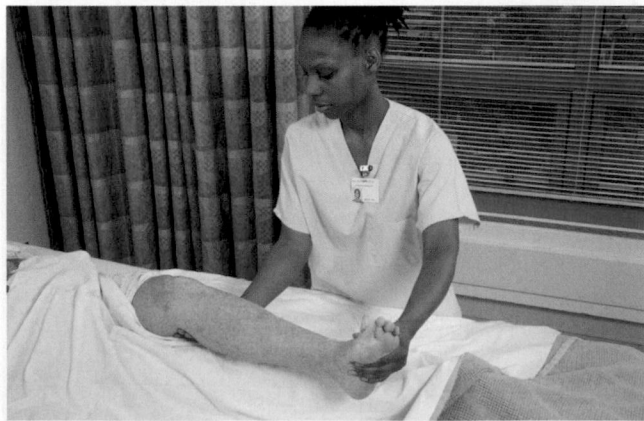

C

FIG. 15 **A.** Extend and lift patient's leg. **B.** Lift leg laterally away from body. **C.** Extend leg beyond midline, if possible.

c. Internally and externally rotate hip by turning leg inward, then outward (Fig. 16A and B).

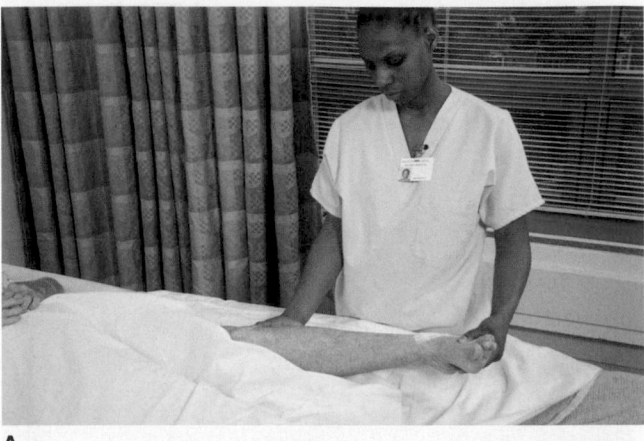

A

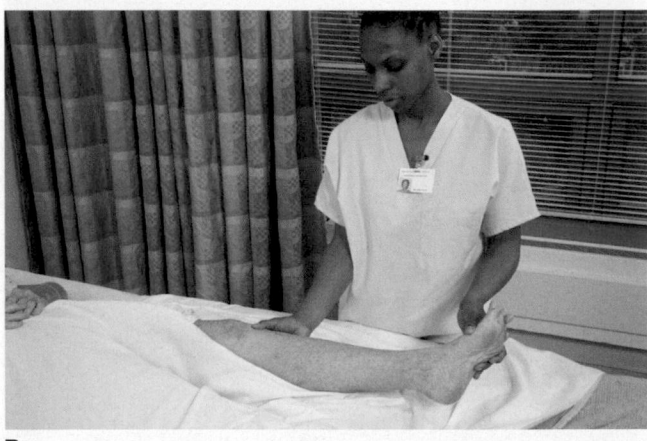

B

FIG. 16 **A.** Rotate leg inward. **B.** Rotate leg outward.

d. Take special care to support joints of larger limbs.

13. Ankle and foot:

a. Dorsiflex foot by moving it so toes point upward (Fig. 17).

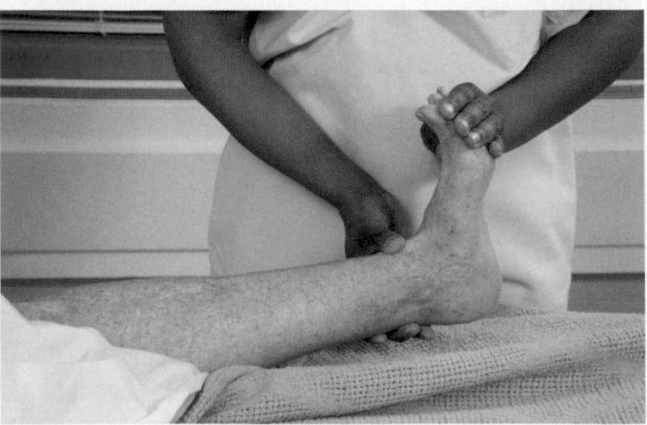

FIG. 17 Dorsiflex foot.

Procedure 25-3 *continued*

b. **Plantarflex by moving foot so toes point down-ward (Fig. 18).**

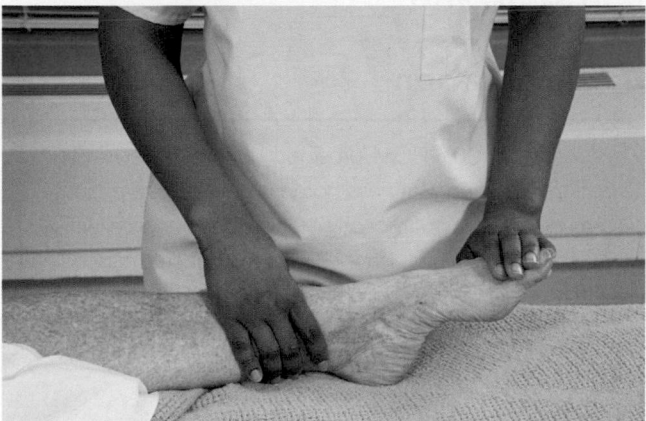

FIG. 18 Plantarflex foot.

c. **Curl toes down, then extend (Fig. 19A and B).**

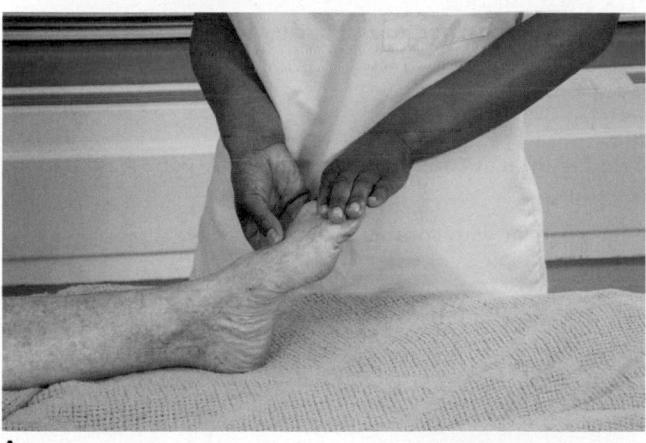

A

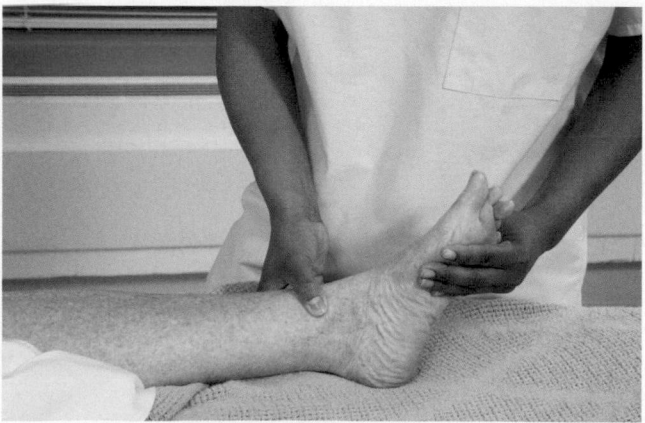

B

FIG. 19 A. Curl toes downward. **B.** Extend toes.

d. **Spread toes apart, then bring together (Fig. 20A and B).**

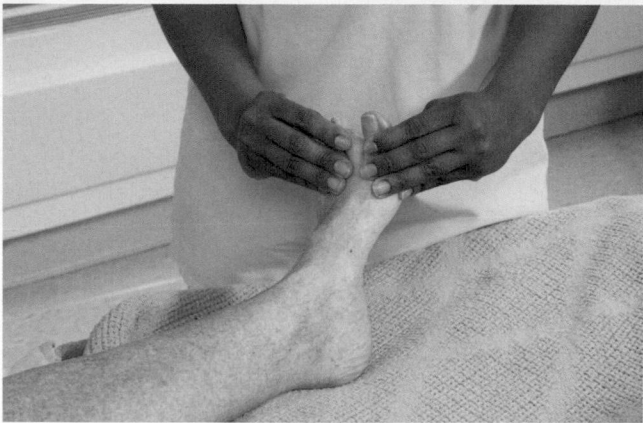

A

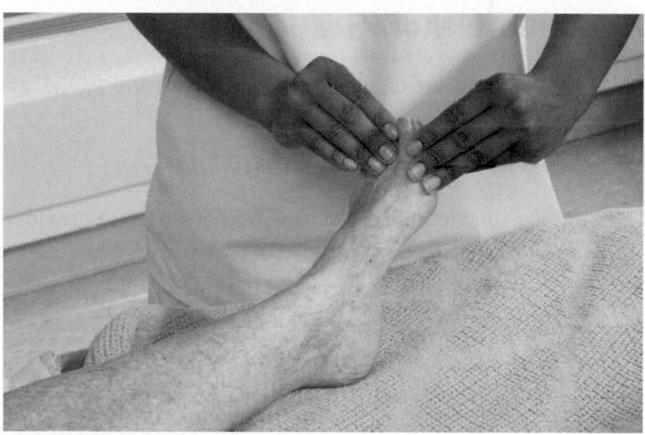

B

FIG. 20 A. Spread toes apart. **B.** Bring toes together.

e. **Invert by turning sole of foot medially (Fig. 21).**

FIG. 21 Turn sole toward midline.

Procedure 25-3   *continued*

f. Evert by turning sole of foot laterally (Fig. 22).

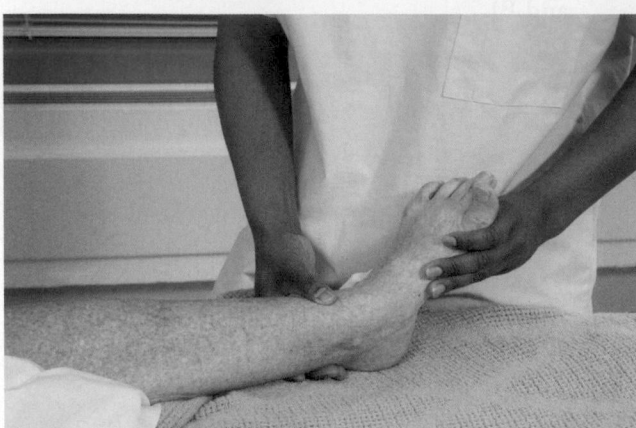

FIG. 22 Turn sole outward.

14. Move to other side of bed and repeat exercises.
15. Reposition patient comfortably.
16. Document ROM.

Documentation

8/14/17: 10:00—ROM provided during AM care with patient assisting. Stiffness noted in right elbow; patient states old injury but recently mobility has become limited and more painful. Physical therapy consult initiated.
—S. Roberts, RN

Home Care Modifications

• Demonstrate to caregivers how to perform ROM, and use return demonstration to evaluate technique.

Collaboration and Delegation

• Encourage unlicensed assistive personnel to provide ROM during hygiene care. Inform them of any patient limitation, and stress that they stop activity whenever a patient experiences pain.

• Consult physical therapy to develop an individualized plan for a patient with contractures or spasticity.

Procedure 25-4 Assisting With Ambulation

Purpose	1. Promote safe ambulation free from falls or injury. 2. Increase muscle strength and joint mobility. 3. Prevent complications of immobility. 4. Promote self-esteem and independence.
Equipment	Ambulation aid (crutches, cane, walker) if required Transfer belt (optional) Robe Well-fitting shoes or slippers with nonskid soles
Assessment	• Review chart for conditions that impair ambulation (e.g., arthritis, fractures, paralysis) and for healthcare provider's orders for ambulation or ambulating aids (e.g., walkers, canes, crutches). • Assess comfort level. Medicate as ordered with analgesics. Plan ambulation for time when analgesics have peak action. • Assess ROM and muscle strength. **Determine if extra assistance is required.** • Obtain baseline vital signs. Obtain postural vital signs if patient has been on prolonged bed rest or is at risk for orthostatic hypotension for other reasons.

Procedure

1. **Perform hand hygiene.**
   Rationale: Reduces microbe transmission.
2. **Identify the patient.**
   Rationale: Ensures correct patient receives proper assessment or treatment and reduces errors.
3. **Close door or bed curtains and explain the procedure and purpose of ambulation to the patient. Decide together how far and where to walk.**
   Rationale: Ensures patient privacy, increases patient compliance, reduces patient anxiety, and promotes learning. Planning helps to ensure safety.
4. **Place bed in lowest position.**
   Rationale: Allows patient to get out of bed safely.
5. **Assist patient to sitting position on side of bed. Assess for dizziness. Obtain orthostatic vital signs if complaints are present. Allow patient to remain in this position until he or she feels secure.**
   Rationale: This minimizes orthostatic hypotension upon standing, which could result in falls or injury.
6. **Help patient with clothing and footwear.**
   Rationale: Being comfortably dressed maintains dignity and safety during ambulation.

One Nurse

7. **Wrap transfer belt around patient's waist (optional according to previous assessment) (Fig. 1).**

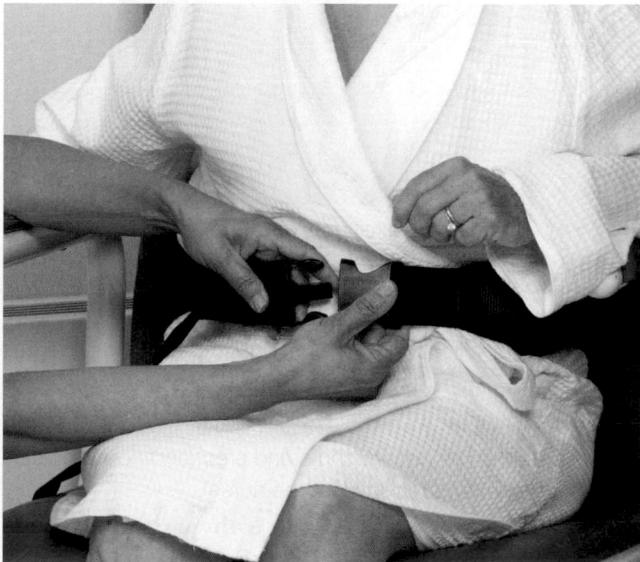

FIG. 1 Place transfer belt snugly around waist.

Rationale: Transfer belt provides a firm hold for the nurse and prevents injury to the patient.

Procedure 25-4   *continued*

8. **Assist patient to standing position and assess patient's balance. Return patient to bed or transfer to chair if he or she is very weak or unsteady. Be sure patient does not grasp your neck for support but places his or her hands around your shoulders or at your waist.**

   Rationale: Keeps both the patient and nurse safe from injury.

9. **Assess patient position when grasping cane (Fig. 2). The handle of the cane should be level with the greater trochanter and should allow approximately 15 degrees of flexion at the elbow.**

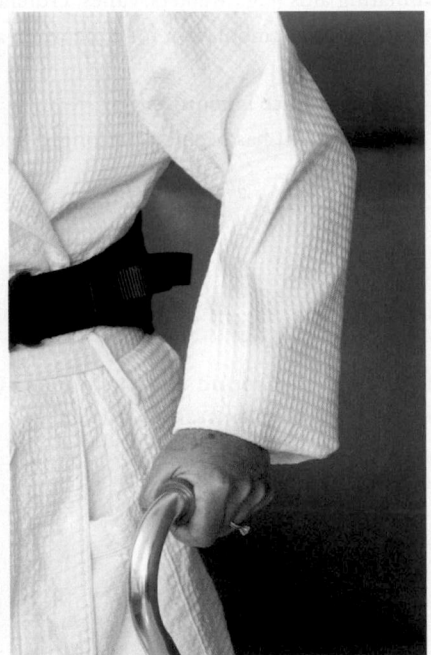

FIG. 2 Ensure proper position of cane.

   Rationale: If the cane is too short, the patient will have to drop the shoulder to lean on it; if the cane is too long, then the patient will have difficulty supporting his or her weight.

10. **Position yourself behind patient while supporting him or her by waist or transfer belt.**

   Rationale: The patient can stand erect and does not lean to one side for support from the nurse.

11. **Take several steps forward with patient (Fig. 3). Assess strength and balance. Encourage patient to use good posture and to look ahead, not down at feet.**

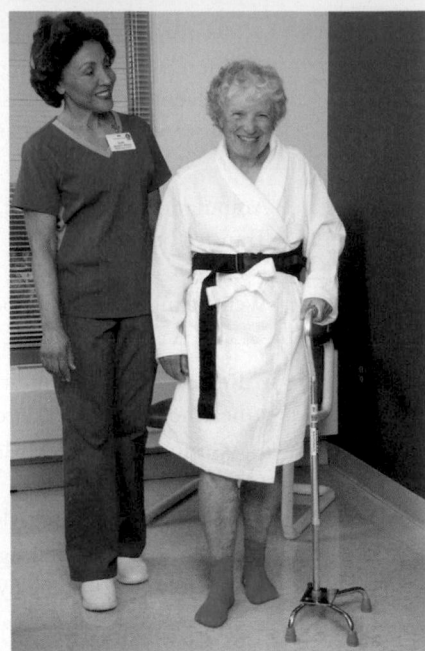

FIG. 3 Walk behind and to the side of patient.

   Rationale: Starting carefully and slowly promotes good balance.

12. **Ambulate for planned distance or time. If patient becomes weak or dizzy, return patient to bed or assist to chair.**

   Rationale: Monitoring the walking encourages exercise tolerance while maintaining patient safety.

13. **If patient begins to fall, place your feet wide apart with one foot in front. Support patient by allowing his or her weight to move backward against your body. Lower gently to floor, protecting head.**

   Rationale: The nurse's foot position widens and stabilizes the base of support and enables the nurse to support the patient's weight with large muscle groups. This protects the nurse from back strain.

Two Nurses

Complete steps 1 through 6.

7. **Assist patient to sitting position as described.**

8. **Assist patient to standing position with one nurse on each side.**

Procedure 25-4 *continued*

9. One nurse grasps the transfer belt to support the patient. The other nurse may carry and manage equipment.

Rationale: Support is provided during ambulation and equipment is managed to prevent falls.

10. Walk with patient using slow, even steps. Assess strength and balance. Encourage patient to look forward rather than down at floor.

Rationale: This promotes the patient's stability.

Using a Walker

Complete steps 1 through 6.

7. Assist patient to standing position. Have patient keep one hand on the arm of the chair or bed while she or he assumes an upright posture.

Rationale: Using the bed or chair for support maintains balance and stability to promote safety.

8. Have patient grasp walker handles. Patient moves walker ahead 6 to 8 inches, placing all four feet of walker on floor. Patient moves forward to walker.

Rationale: Using the walker handles stabilizes the walker and promotes safety.

9. Nurse should walk closely behind and slightly to side of patient (Fig. 4). Use a transfer belt if patient is not steady or is at risk for falling.

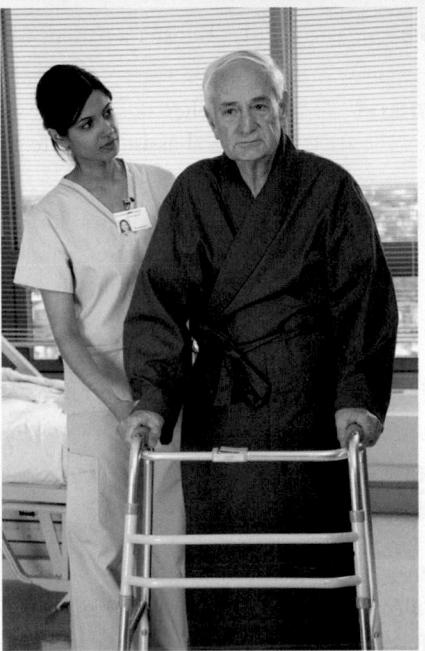

FIG. 4 When assisting the patient using a walker, stand behind and to the side of the patient.

Rationale: If the patient begins to fall, the nurse can support him or her and prevent injury.

10. Repeat above sequence until walk is complete.

Documentation

8/15/17: 15:30—Ambulated length of hall using walker with SBA (standby assist). No significant increase in heart rate or respiratory rate or c/o of dizziness.

—S. Roberts, RN

Home Care Modifications

- To provide safety and prevent falls at home, throw rugs and small pieces of furniture should be removed so the patient will not trip on them.
- The patient should always wear shoes with nonskid soles.
- The bathroom is a common place for falls and injury. Install hand grips and bars to assist with mobility and provide for safety. Place a large rug with a skid-resistant backing on the floor to prevent falls from slipping on wet floors.

Collaboration and Delegation

- Physical therapists often teach and supervise ambulation for high-risk patients (e.g., those who have had orthopedic surgery, amputation, or stroke). Collaborative, individualized plans can be developed and communicated to the rest of the staff.

Procedure 25-5 Transferring a Patient to a Stretcher

Purpose	1. Transfer a patient without injuring nurse or patient.
Equipment	Stretcher Lateral-assist device (e.g., roller boards, transfer boards, slide boards)
Assessment	• Review medical history for conditions that influence or contraindicate ability to move (e.g., fractures, paralysis, spinal injury, generalized muscle weakness, cardiac or respiratory disease that limits exertion). • Assess patient's ROM and muscle strength. • Assess cognitive function or ability to understand and follow directions. • Assess comfort level. Medicate as ordered with analgesics. • Assess patient's weight and your strength. **Determine if assistance is needed.**

Procedure

1. **Perform hand hygiene.**

   Rationale: Reduces microbe transmission.

2. **Identify the patient.**

   Rationale: Ensures correct patient receives proper assessment or treatment and reduces errors.

3. **Close door or bed curtains and explain the procedure to the patient.**

   Rationale: Ensures patient privacy, increases patient compliance, reduces patient anxiety, and promotes learning.

4. **Place stretcher parallel to bed. Raise bed to same level as stretcher. Lower side rails. Lock wheels.**

   Rationale: Positioning equipment makes transfer easier and decreases risk of injury.

5. **One or two nurses stand on side of bed without stretcher. Two nurses stand on side of bed with stretcher (Fig. 1).**

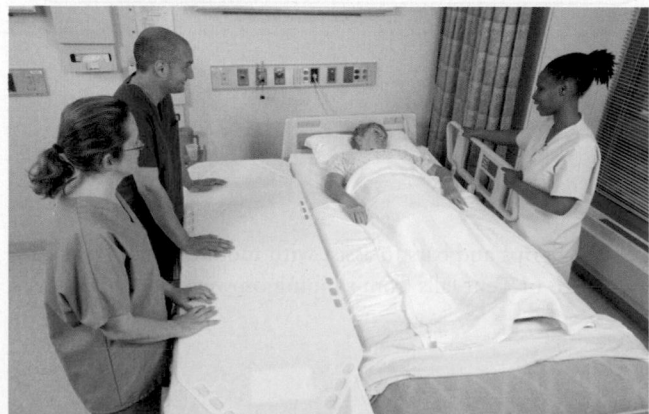

FIG. 1 Move stretcher to side of bed. Position two nurses on side with stretcher and one nurse on side without stretcher.

   Rationale: Team coordination provides for patient safety during transfer.

6. **Loosen drawsheet on both sides of bed or use turn sheet.**

   Rationale: The drawsheet or turn sheet assists in transferring the patient.

7. **Nurse on the side without stretcher helps patient to move toward them onto his or her side. Nurse may use drawsheet to pull patient closer (Fig. 2).**

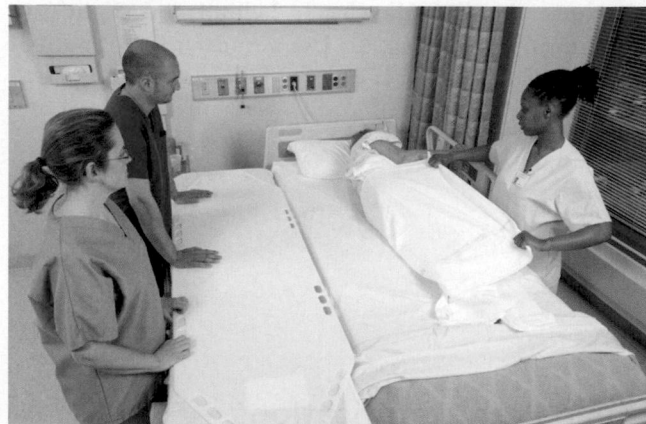

FIG. 2 Move patient to side-lying position using drawsheet.

   Rationale: Side lying position readies patient for transfer board.

Procedure 25-5   *continued*

8. **Nurse(s) on stretcher side of bed slide transfer board under drawsheet and under patient's buttocks and back (Fig. 3).**

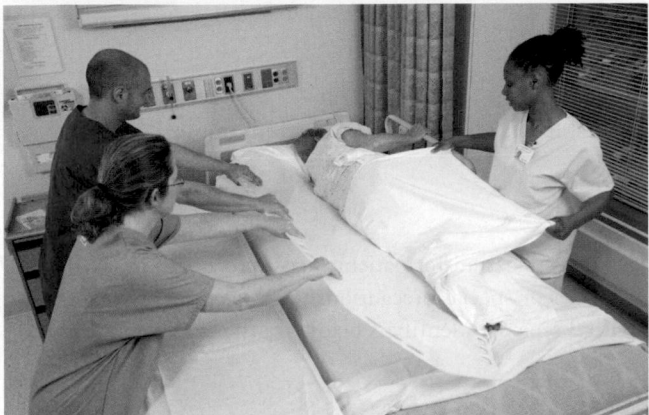

FIG. 3 Position transfer board beneath drawsheet.

Rationale: Transfer board helps slide the patient from bed to stretcher.

9. **Place patient's arms across his or her chest. Using drawsheet, slide patient onto transfer board into supine position (Fig. 4).**

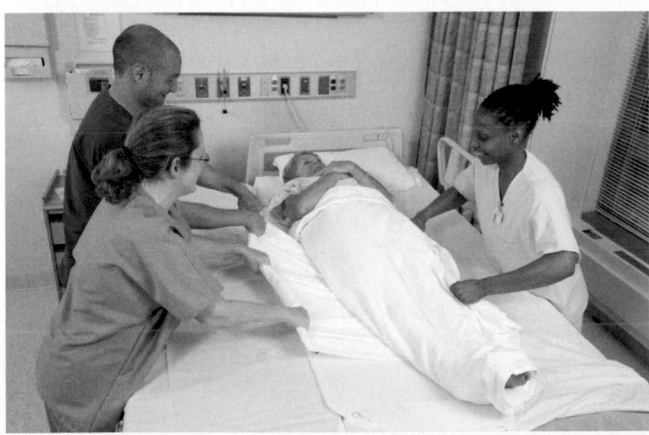

FIG. 4 Slide patient onto transfer board.

Rationale: This prevents injury to arms during transfer.

10. **On the count of three, nurse(s) on stretcher side pulls the drawsheet toward the stretcher. Nurse on side without transfer board lifts the drawsheet, transferring patient's weight to transfer board and pushing patient onto stretcher.**

Rationale: This provides smooth motion for transfer.

11. **Roll patient slightly up onto side, and pull transfer board out from under him or her (Fig. 5). Lock up side rails on bed side of stretcher and move stretcher away from bed.**

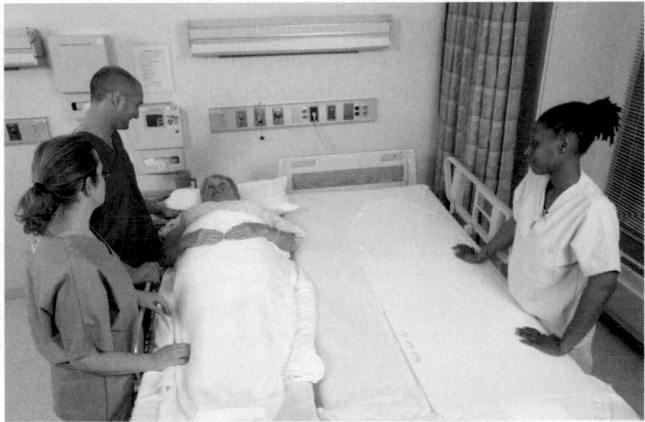

FIG. 5 Remove transfer board. Secure patient on stretcher.

Rationale: This provides for the patient's safety.

12. **Place sheet over patient and lock safety belts across patient's chest and waist. Adjust head of stretcher according to patient limitations.**

Rationale: Comfort, warmth, and safety are provided.

Documentation

> 8/11/16: 14:20—Transferred via stretcher to cath lab.
> —S. Roberts, RN

Procedure 25-5   *continued*

Life Span Considerations

Infant and Child

- Infants can be safely held and moved by one person.
- Children may be moved by one or two people.

Adult

- Depending on level of musculoskeletal function, adults may be able to slide onto a stretcher with minimal assistance.

Collaboration and Delegation

- Acute care facilities and surgical centers often have transport aides that transfer patients via stretcher from one department to another. The nurse communicates any activity restrictions or special precautions (e.g., need for oxygen during transport). The identity of the patient needs to be checked with 2 separate identifiers before transfer to prevent errors.

Procedure 25-6 Transferring a Patient to a Wheelchair

Purpose
1. Increase mobility status using a wheelchair.
2. Decrease complications of immobility.
3. Increase independence and promote self-esteem.

Equipment
Wheelchair
Robe or appropriate clothing
Slippers or shoes with nonskid soles
Transfer belt

Assessment
- Assess musculoskeletal function: joint mobility, paresis or paralysis of extremities, fractures, and amputations.
- Assess cognitive function: ability to understand and follow directions, short-term memory and recognition of physical limitations to movement.
- Assess comfort level. Medicate as ordered with analgesics, and plan transfer when pain is relieved.
- Assess baseline vital signs. Assess for history of orthostatic hypotension.
- Review physician's orders for activity level.
- Ask staff members who had previously transferred patient how much assistance was needed.

Procedure

1. **Perform hand hygiene.**
   Rationale: Reduces microbe transmission.

2. **Identify the patient.**
   Rationale: Ensures correct patient receives proper assessment or treatment and reduces errors.

3. **Close door or bed curtains and explain the procedure to the patient.**
   Rationale: Ensures patient privacy, increases patient compliance, reduces patient anxiety, and promotes learning.

4. **Position wheelchair at 45-degree angle or parallel to bed. Remove footrest and lock brakes.**
   Rationale: This facilitates a smooth, safe transfer.

5. **Lock bed brakes (Fig. 1); lower bed to lowest level, and raise head of bed as far as patient can tolerate.**

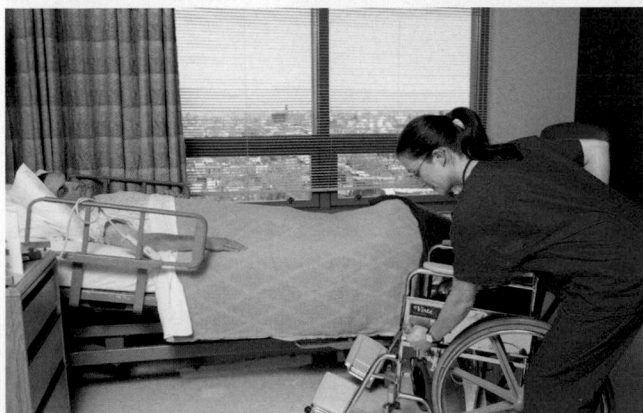

FIG. 1 Position wheelchair at 45 degree angle to bed and lock brakes.

Rationale: Amount of energy needed to move to a sitting position is decreased.

6. **Assist patient to side-lying position, facing the side of bed he or she will sit on. Lower side rail and stand near patient's hips. Nurse positions foot near head of bed in front of and apart from other foot.**
   Rationale: The nurse's center of gravity is placed near the patient's greatest weight to safely assist the patient to a sitting position.

7. **Swing patient's legs over side of bed. At the same time, pivot on your back leg to lift patient's trunk and shoulders. Keep back straight; avoid twisting. Allow patient to independently move to a sitting position if he or she can tolerate it (Fig. 2). Remain close for support.**

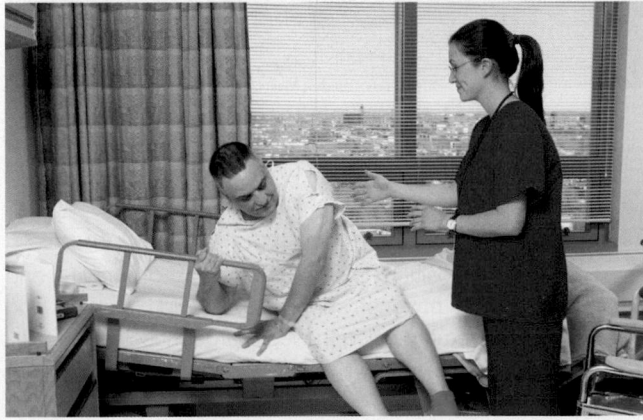

FIG. 2 Have patient independently move to a sitting position if able.

Rationale: Gravity lowers the patient's legs over the bed while the nurse transfers weight in the direction of motion and protects the back from injury.

8. **Stand in front of patient, and assess for balance and dizziness. Allow patient to dangle legs for a few minutes before continuing (Fig. 3).**

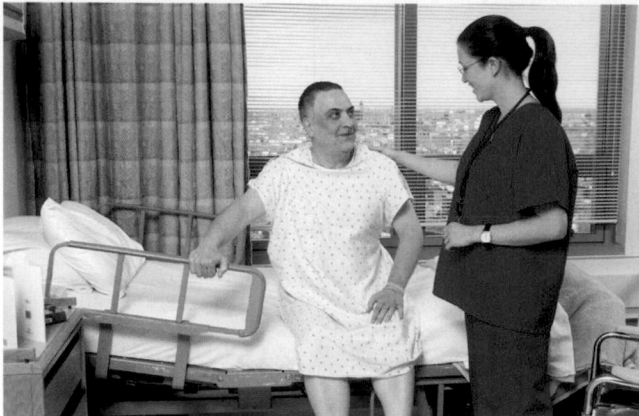

FIG. 3 Allow patient to dangle legs for a few minutes.

Rationale: Assessment prevents falls or injuries from orthostatic hypotension.

9. **Help patient to don robe and nonskid footwear.**
Rationale: Nonskid soles reduce risk of falling.

10. **Apply transfer belt (Fig. 4). Grip belt to assist with transfer.**

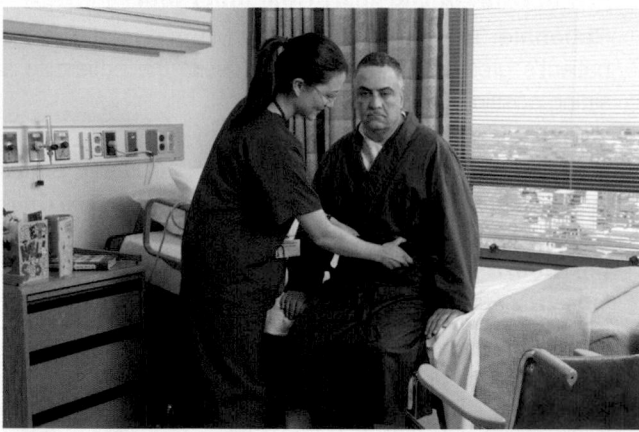

FIG. 4 Secure transfer belt snugly around waist.

Rationale: Transfer belt ensures the patient's safety during transfer.

11. **Spread your feet apart and flex your hips and knees.**
Rationale: Position lowers the center of gravity and broadens the base of support to provide stability and smooth movement using the legs' large muscle groups.

12. **Have patient slide buttocks to edge of bed until feet touch floor.**
Rationale: Position provides balance and support.

13. **Rock back and forth until patient stands on the count of three.**
Rationale: Rocking motion prevents muscle strain by giving the patient's weight momentum and requiring less of the nurse's energy to lift.

14. **Brace your front knee against patient's weak knee as patient stands (Fig. 5).**

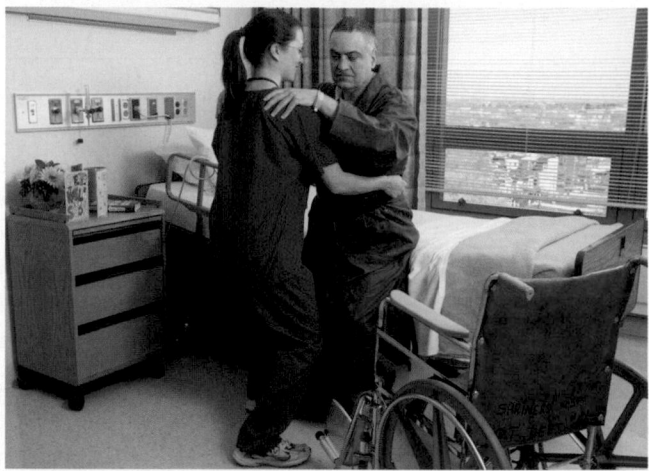

FIG. 5 Brace patient's weak leg and use your legs to help raise patient to standing position.

Rationale: Position prevents the weak knee from buckling and the patient from falling.

15. **Pivot on back foot until patient feels wheelchair against back of legs; keep your knee against the patient's knee (Fig. 6).**

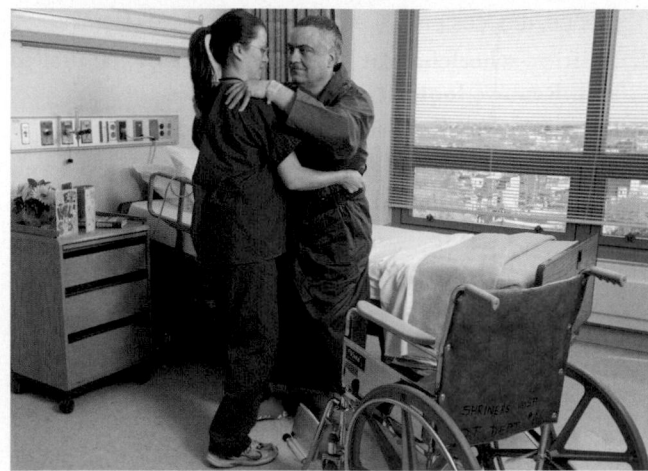

FIG. 6 Pivot on your back foot and patient's strong leg to turn.

Rationale: Ensure proper position before sitting.

Procedure 25-6   *continued*

16. **Instruct patient to place hands on chair armrests for support. Flex your knees and hips while assisting patient into chair (Fig. 7).**

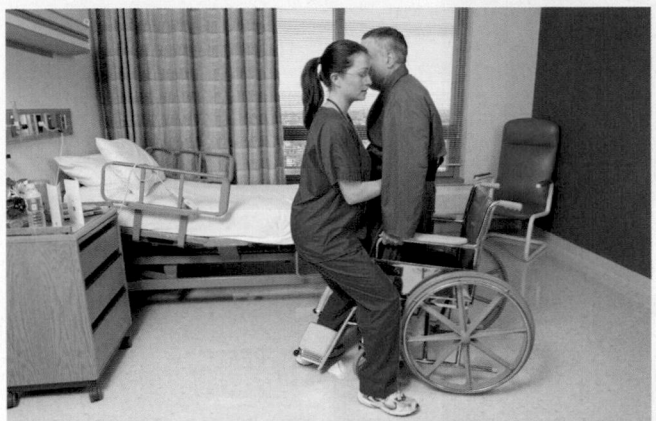

FIG. 7 Assist patient to sitting position.

Rationale: Good body mechanics prevent back injury by supporting weight with large muscle groups.

17. **Adjust foot pedal and leg supports.**

Rationale: Adjustments provide comfort and prevent injury to the leg and foot.

18. **Assess patient's alignment in chair (Fig. 8). Provide call light.**

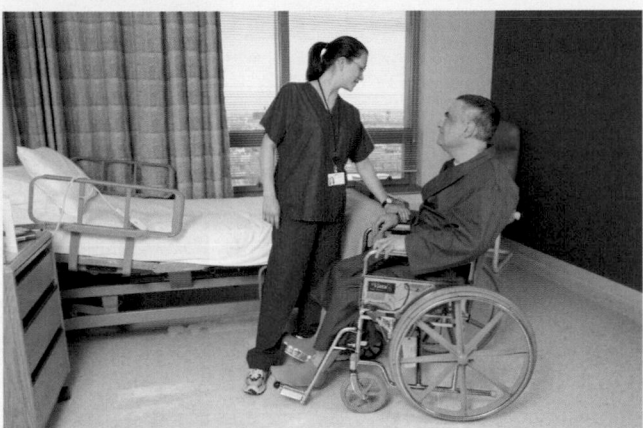

FIG. 8 Assess patient's alignment and comfort in chair.

Rationale: This promotes comfort and provides for safety.

Documentation

9/1/16: 11:30—Transfer to wheelchair with 1 person assist. Good balance and able to pivot with verbal cueing.

—S. Roberts, RN

Home Care Considerations

- Before the patient is discharged, the patient/caregiver should demonstrate safe transfer technique. The patient should master transferring from a wheelchair to a car or van. Motorized wheelchairs, designed for patients who have permanent injuries, permit a greater degree of mobility (Fig. **9**).

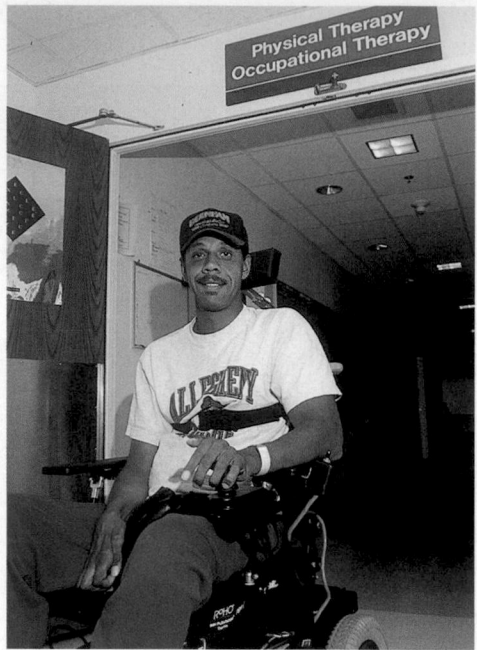

FIG. 9 This patient uses a motorized wheelchair.

Collaboration and Delegation

- Physical therapy may provide assessment and teaching for patients recently experiencing problems that significantly decrease mobility or when increased assistance is required for safe transfers.
- Unlicensed assistive personnel should be required to get assistance when necessary to safely transfer a patient.
- Transfers can be scheduled with a lift team for high-risk patients.

Procedure 25-7 **Procedure for Transferring a Patient From Bed to a Chair Using a Hydraulic Lift**

Purpose

1. To safely transfer a patient from a bed to a chair when safe transfer is not possible without using a hydraulic lift.

Equipment

Hydraulic lift

Assessment

- Assess knowledge of hydraulic lift being used. Most agencies require training and validation of staff before use.
- Assess patient's musculoskeletal function: joint mobility; paresis or paralysis of extremities; fractures, amputations.
- Assess patient's cognitive function or ability to understand and follow directions.
- Assess patient's comfort level. Medicate as ordered with analgesics before transfer.
- Assess patient's weight and your strength. **Determine how much assistance is needed.**
- Determine if patient's weight exceeds sling or lift's recommendation.

Procedure

1. **Perform hand hygiene.**
   Rationale: Reduces microbe transmission.
2. **Identify the patient.**
   Rationale: Ensures correct patient receives proper assessment or treatment and reduces errors.
3. **Close door or bed curtains and explain the procedure to the patient.**
   Rationale: Ensures patient privacy, increases patient compliance, reduces patient anxiety, and promotes learning.
4. **Place the fabric sling evenly under the patient (Fig. 1).**

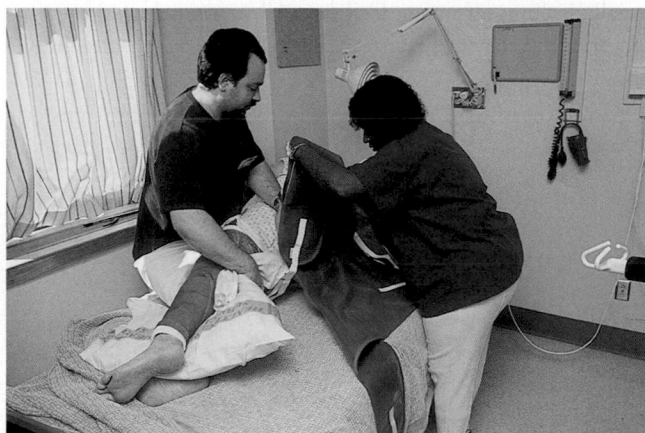

FIG. 1 Place fabric sling evenly under patient.

Rationale: Even distribution of the patient's weight in the fabric sling provides for patient comfort and safety.

5. **Position the lift so the frame can be centered over the patient, then attach the fabric sling to the frame (Fig. 2). Note manufacturer's instructions for the specifics of how the sling should be attached to the frame.**

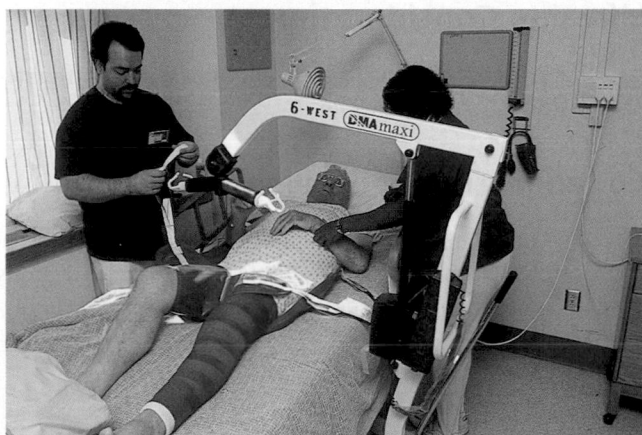

FIG. 2 Position hydraulic lift so that frame is centered over patient. Attach fabric sling to the frame.

Rationale: Improper attachment of the sling to the frame can result in unequal distribution of body weight and possible injury.

6. **Have a nurse on each side of the lift. Warn the patient that he or she will be lifted from the bed. Support head or heavy casts as needed. Engage the hydraulic system to raise the patient from the bed.**
   Rationale: Supporting the patient physically and verbally provides for patient safety and helps reduce fear that often accompanies being lifted from the bed and suspended in midair.

Procedure 25-7   *continued*

7. Carefully wheel the patient in hydraulic lift away from the bed, supporting limbs as needed (Fig. 3). Position patient over chair and gently lower to chair using the hydraulic mechanism.

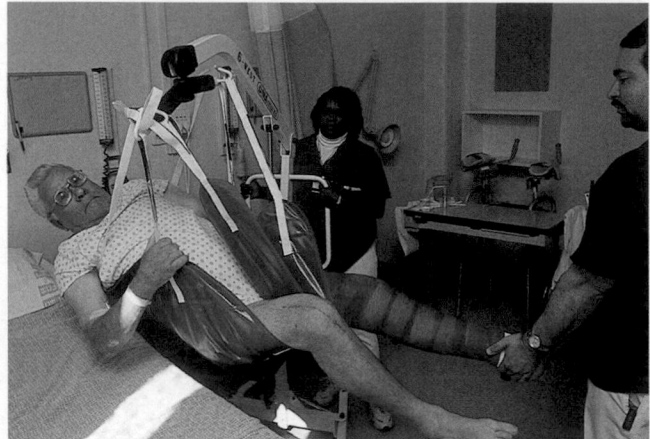

FIG. 3 Wheel patient away from the bed to position him over the chair.

Rationale: Provides for patient safety during transfer.

8. The sling remains in place under the patient and is reattached to the frame when the patient is moved back to bed.

Rationale: Prevents unnecessary removal and replacing of sling under the patient, which is difficult when the patient is sitting in the chair.

Documentation

> 9/12/17: 14:00—Transferred to the chair using hydraulic lift. Patient became very anxious and required reassurance during transfer. Up in chair for 30 minutes, tolerated well.
>
> —S. Roberts, RN

Lifespan Considerations

- Being moved using a hydraulic lift is especially frightening for an older adult who is confused. Physical contact and verbal reassurance are helpful.

Collaboration and Delegation

- Often unlicensed personnel use lifts to move patients, especially in long-term care facilities. All personnel need to complete instruction and be able to provide return demonstration prior to use with patients. Communicate clearly any mobility restrictions or special care in patient transfer using the lift.
- Employ lift teams whenever possible since they have training and expertise on equipment and skill in complex transfers.

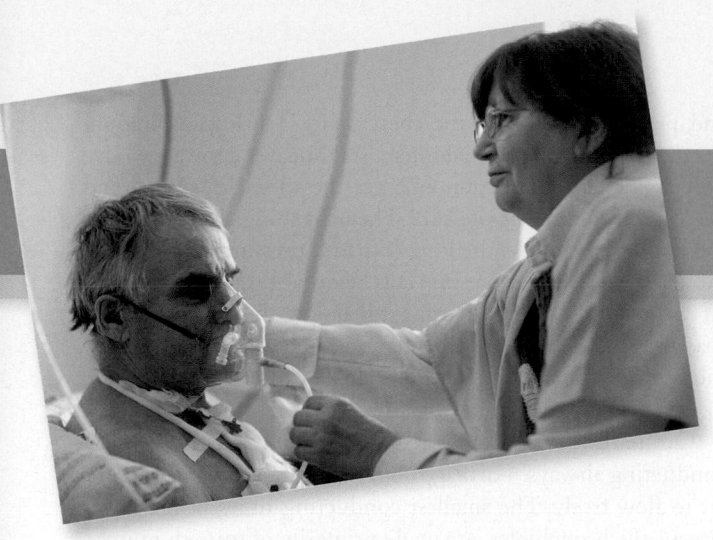

CHAPTER 26

Respiratory Function

Vanessa A. Makareiwicz

Case Scenario

You are a nurse working in a hospital. You have admitted a 55-year-old man, Mr. Garcia, who has a diagnosis of pneumonia. He has a productive cough and decreased lung sounds in the bases of his lungs. His oxygen saturation is 93% on 2 L O_2 with a nasal cannula. He has a history of smoking one pack of cigarettes daily for the past 35 years. Although he tries to eat well, his source of income is public assistance, so he eats primarily starches and very few proteins or fresh vegetables. He is living in a mission with 50 other residents, and he has not yet had his influenza vaccine.

Once you have completed this chapter and have incorporated respiratory function into your knowledge base, review the above scenario and reflect on the following areas of Critical Thinking:

1. What risk factors does Mr. Garcia have for pneumonia?
2. How will you care for Mr. Garcia in relation to his oxygen use?
3. What nursing interventions are indicated because of his diagnosis of pneumonia?
4. What teaching might be indicated for Mr. Garcia in preparation for discharge?

KEY TERMS
alveoli
apnea
arterial blood gas (ABG)
arterial oxygen saturation (SpO$_2$)
atelectasis
bronchioles
bronchospasm
capnography
capnometry
cyanosis
diffusion
dyspnea
EtCO$_2$
fraction of inspired oxygen concentration (FiO$_2$)
hemoptysis
hypercapnia
hyperventilation
hypoventilation
hypoxemia
hypoxia
oxygen saturation
partial pressure of carbon dioxide (PaCO$_2$)
partial pressure of oxygen (PO$_2$)
pulse oximetry
splinting
tracheostomy
ventilation

LEARNING OBJECTIVES

Upon completion of this chapter, you will be able to do the following:

1. Identify factors that can interfere with effective oxygenation of body tissues.
2. Describe common manifestations of altered respiratory function.
3. Discuss life span–related changes and problems in respiratory function.
4. Describe important elements in the respiratory assessment.
5. List three appropriate nursing diagnoses and outcomes for the patient with altered respiratory function.
6. Describe nursing measures to ensure a patent airway.
7. Discuss safe administration of oxygen using different modes of delivery.
8. Identify home care considerations for the respiratory patient.

The respiratory system replenishes the body's oxygen supply and eliminates waste in the form of carbon dioxide. During assessment of respiratory function, nurses gather information from the patients, listen to breath sounds with stethoscopes, interpret laboratory tests, and make important observations to determine the effectiveness of the patient's breathing. Assessment also allows nurses to identify risk factors that cause respiratory impairment.

Nurses are responsible for promoting normal respiratory function regardless of the practice area. School nurses conduct classes about the hazards of smoking. Surgical nurses instruct the patients in deep-breathing techniques. Community nurses screen for and teach tuberculosis prevention. Nurses also help to improve breathing in patients with altered respiratory function. From positioning the debilitated patient in long-term care to managing sophisticated life-supporting ventilator systems, nurses play a vital role in assisting the patient with respiratory disease.

NORMAL RESPIRATORY FUNCTION

Structure of the Respiratory System

Breathing delivers air to the lungs, where gas exchange occurs. Before reaching the lungs, air passes through a series of structures and tubes collectively called the airways (Fig. 26-1). The major components of the upper respiratory tract are the mouth, nose, and pharynx. They are connected by the nasopharynx, which funnels incoming air through the mouth and nose into the lower portions of the pharynx.

The major components of the lower respiratory tract, located in the thoracic cavity, are the trachea, lobar bronchi, segmental bronchi, and the lungs. The bronchi continue to branch in treelike fashion into the **bronchioles**, which connect the larger conducting airways with the lung parenchyma. This gas-exchanging portion of the lung is made up of millions of tiny air sacs called **alveoli**. These thin-walled epithelial structures are in contact with a well-developed capillary network. Oxygen reaching the alveoli crosses the epithelium into the blood for transport to the heart, then to body tissues.

Lung inflation and deflation depend on complex, coordinated neuromuscular activity. The lungs move only passively: They stretch and recoil in response to muscular movement. The diaphragm (which separates the chest from the abdominal cavity) and the intercostal muscles (which lie between the ribs) are the primary muscles of breathing.

Function of the Respiratory System

VENTILATION

Breathing, or **ventilation**, is the physical process of moving air into and out of the lungs so that gas exchange can take place. The mechanical process of ventilation is the result of volume and pressure changes in the chest cavity. During inspiration, the diaphragm and external intercostal muscles contract (active process). Their contraction enlarges the thoracic volume and decreases intrathoracic pressure. The expanding chest wall pulls the lungs outward. As the lungs expand, pressure drops within the airways. As airway pressure falls below atmospheric pressure, air rushes into the lungs. During exhalation, the process reverses (passive process). The diaphragm and intercostal muscles relax, causing the thorax to return to its smaller resting size. Pressure in the chest increases, allowing air to flow out of the lungs.

Ordinarily, little effort is required to draw air through the conducting airways. Cartilage holds open the larger airways for air to flow freely. The smallest conducting tubes of the lower airway, the bronchioles, are made primarily of smooth muscle. Smooth muscle tone helps them remain open and usually provides little resistance to breathing. Because there are millions of bronchioles, they have a collectively large diameter; thus, moving air through these tiny tubes is easy. Inspired air finally reaches the alveoli, which provides an amazingly large surface area for gas exchange.

GAS DIFFUSION

Oxygen and carbon dioxide move between the alveoli and the blood by **diffusion**, the process in which molecules move from an area of greater concentration or pressure to an area of lower concentration or pressure. Breathing continually replenishes the lungs' oxygen supply, so the **partial pressure of oxygen (PAO$_2$)** in the alveoli is relatively high. (The letter after the "p" indicates the location where the gas concentration is being measured. In the alveoli, an uppercase letter is used, "A." When referring to gas in the arteries, a lowercase "a" is used. In veins, a lowercase "v" is used.) Simultaneously, breathing removes carbon dioxide from the lungs, so the **partial pressure of carbon dioxide (PACO$_2$)** in the alveoli is low. Blood flowing to the lungs via the pulmonary arteries is low in oxygen and rich in carbon dioxide. Oxygen diffuses from the alveoli into the blood because PO$_2$ is higher in the alveoli than in the capillary blood. For similar reasons, carbon dioxide diffuses from the blood into the alveolar space. Figure 26-2 illustrates the exchange of gases across the alveolar-capillary membrane. The blood passing through the pulmonary veins returns to the left side of the heart and then enters the systemic circulation as freshly oxygenated arterial blood. When oxygenated blood reaches the tissues, the exchange process occurs again but in the opposite direction.

GAS TRANSPORT

As oxygen crosses the alveolar-capillary membrane into the blood, the blood transports it to the tissues in two forms. Small amounts of oxygen are physically dissolved in plasma (3% of O$_2$), but most oxygen that the blood carries to the tissues is attached to hemoglobin molecules on red blood cells (97% of O$_2$). Hemoglobin has the unique ability to carry oxygen in its molecular form rather than as an ion. This difference is significant because tissues require molecular oxygen for metabolism.

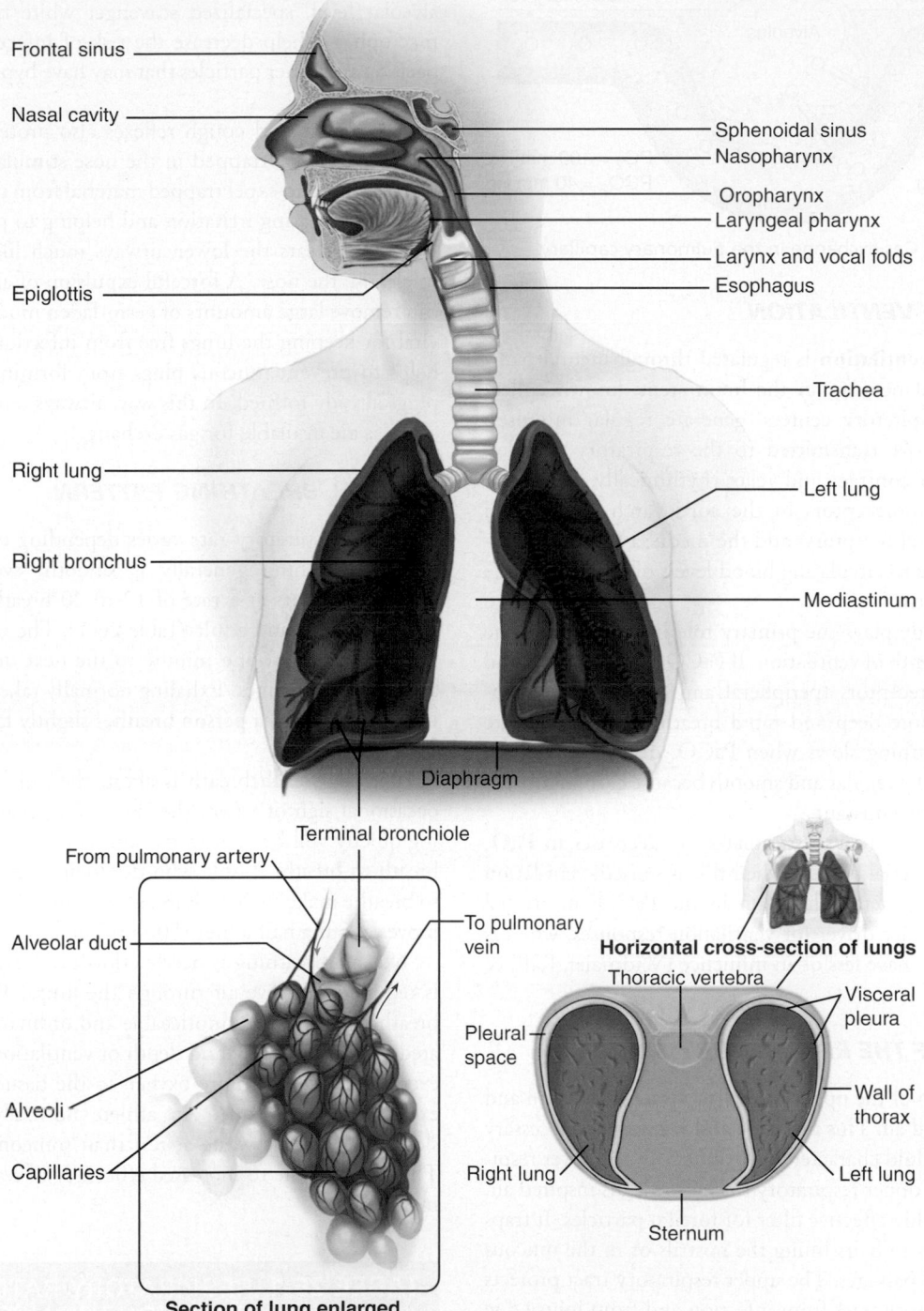

FIGURE 26-1 Respiratory system.

Labels (top figure):
Frontal sinus
Nasal cavity
Epiglottis
Right lung
Right bronchus
Sphenoidal sinus
Nasopharynx
Oropharynx
Laryngeal pharynx
Larynx and vocal folds
Esophagus
Trachea
Left lung
Mediastinum
Diaphragm

Labels (enlarged section):
Terminal bronchiole
From pulmonary artery
Alveolar duct
To pulmonary vein
Alveoli
Capillaries

Section of lung enlarged

Horizontal cross-section of lungs
Thoracic vertebra
Pleural space
Right lung
Visceral pleura
Wall of thorax
Left lung
Sternum

The blood carries carbon dioxide in several forms. Blood transports carbon dioxide in a dissolved state ($PaCO_2$), but carbon dioxide also can combine with some amino acids. The most important transport mechanism for carbon dioxide is in its dissolved form. When combined with water, carbon dioxide dissociates into bicarbonate ions.

$$H^+ + HCO_3^- \rightleftarrows H_2CO_3 \rightleftarrows H_2O + CO_2$$

These ions form the primary component of the bicarbonate buffer system (HCO_3^-), which plays a major role in maintaining the body's acid–base balance. These interactions are discussed later in this chapter.

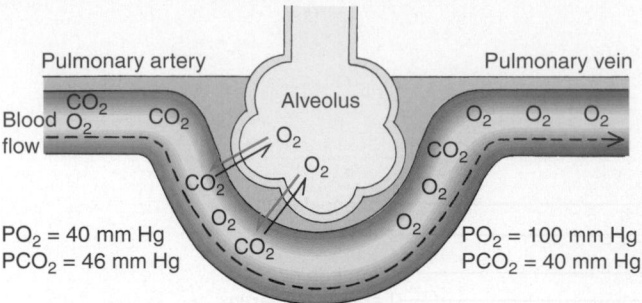

Pulmonary artery
Pulmonary vein
Alveolus
Blood flow
O_2 O_2 O_2
CO_2 CO_2 CO_2
O_2
O_2
CO_2 CO_2 CO_2
O_2 O_2
$PO_2 = 40$ mm Hg
$PCO_2 = 46$ mm Hg
$PO_2 = 100$ mm Hg
$PCO_2 = 40$ mm Hg

FIGURE 26-2 Gas exchange in the pulmonary capillary.

CONTROL OF VENTILATION

The process of **ventilation** is regulated through neural pathways. Specialized neurons in the brain stem, known collectively as the respiratory centers, generate regular impulses. These impulses are transmitted to the respiratory muscles, causing them to contract and relax rhythmically. Peripheral and central chemoreceptors in the aortic arch and carotid arteries (peripheral receptors) and the medulla (central receptors) are sensitive to circulating blood levels of carbon dioxide and hydrogen ions.

Carbon dioxide plays the primary role in determining the frequency and depth of ventilation. If $PaCO_2$ levels in the blood increase, chemoreceptors (peripheral and central) are stimulated, causing more deep and rapid breathing. The opposite is also true: Breathing slows when $PaCO_2$ decreases. Normal breathing is usually regular and smooth because carbon dioxide levels remain fairly constant.

Chemoreceptors are also stimulated by decreases in **PaO_2** and **pH** in the arterial blood. When this is sensed, ventilation will increase. In general, alteration in the $PaCO_2$ in arterial blood is the primary driver for ventilation responses, whereas the PaO_2 and pH have less of an influence (Widmaier, Raff, & Strang, 2013).

DEFENSES OF THE RESPIRATORY SYSTEM

A major function of the upper respiratory tract is to warm and humidify inspired air. This moisture and warmth are necessary to maintain the fluid character of the mucus in the lower respiratory tract. The upper respiratory tract also cleans inspired air. The nose is a highly effective filter for foreign particles. It traps dust and irritants in hairs lining the nostrils or in the mucous layer of the nasal passages. The upper respiratory tract protects the lower respiratory tract from infection and from injury due to aspiration. The epiglottis acts as a trapdoor by preventing large particles of food or foreign matter from being accidentally aspirated.

The lower respiratory tract's conducting tubes further filter and clean incoming air. An epithelial layer containing millions of ciliated cells and mucus-producing glands lines these airways. The mucous membrane produces a "mucus blanket" that efficiently traps bacteria and microscopic foreign particles. The ciliated cells provide motion to the mucus blanket, allowing it to carry trapped matter upward and out of the respiratory tract.

This "mucociliary escalator" protects the airways by constantly sweeping potentially harmful material out of the lungs. At the alveolar level, specialized scavenger white blood cells called macrophages help decrease the risk of infection by engulfing bacteria and other particles that may have bypassed the mucous blanket.

The sneeze and cough reflexes also protect the lungs and airways. Irritants trapped in the nose stimulate sneezing; that reaction helps to expel trapped material from the nasal passages, thereby decreasing irritation and helping to prevent infection. Coughing clears the lower airways much like sneezing helps to cleanse the nose. A forceful expulsion of air from the lungs can remove large amounts of germ-laden mucus. This action is vital for keeping the lungs free from infection. Coughing also helps to prevent mucous plugs from forming and to remove plugs already formed. In this way, airways remain open so that all areas are available for gas exchange.

NORMAL BREATHING PATTERN

Although respiratory rate varies depending on a person's age, normal breathing generally is smooth, even, and regular. Breathing occurs at a rate of 12 to 20 breaths per minute in the older child and adult (Table 26-1). The rate does not vary significantly from one minute to the next unless the person's activity level changes. Exhaling normally takes twice as long as inhaling. Usually, a person breathes slightly faster when awake than when asleep.

Normally, each breath is about the same size. Despite an occasional sigh or yawn, the chest of a person who is breathing quietly will be seen to rise and fall the same amount from breath to breath. People who use their diaphragms effectively to breathe make their abdomens rise and fall. The average adult moves about a half a liter (500 mL) of air per breath.

Normal breathing is nearly effortless. Little muscular work is required to move air through the lungs. That is why quiet breathing is almost unnoticeable and ordinarily has no associated sounds. The rate and depth of ventilation increase during exercise to provide more oxygen to the tissues and to remove excess carbon dioxide. An athlete normally breathes more slowly and deeply while at rest than someone who is less fit. This is likely due to increased efficiency of respiratory muscles in the athlete.

TABLE 26-1	RESPIRATORY RATES THROUGH THE LIFE SPAN
Age Group	Breathing Rate (Breaths per Minute)
Newborn and infant	30–60
1–5 y	20–30
6–10 y	18–26
10 y–adult	12–20
Older adult (60 y and older)	16–25

Life Span Considerations

Like the heart, the lungs perform a lifetime of continual work; however, the structure and function of the respiratory system undergo normal changes that impact respiratory rates across the life span (Table 26-1).

NEWBORN AND INFANT

In the uterus, the fetus's lungs grow rapidly as alveoli continue to develop throughout pregnancy. Until the 24th or 25th week of pregnancy, the fetus's lungs do not have enough properly functioning alveoli to make breathing effective. It takes another 10 weeks or more for fully functional lungs to develop in the fetus. Surfactant, which decreases surface tension and permits alveolar expansion, is not produced in sufficient quantities until late in gestation. For this reason, babies born prematurely may require ventilatory support. Surfactant replacement therapy used in premature newborns has been shown to decrease the severity of respiratory distress syndrome.

Newborns breathe rapidly (30 to 60 breaths per minute), and in general, larger newborns breathe more slowly than do smaller ones. The newborn's breathing pattern is characterized by occasional pauses of several seconds between breaths. This periodic breathing is normal during the first 3 months of life, but frequent or prolonged periods of **apnea** (cessation of breathing of 20 seconds or longer) are abnormal.

TODDLER AND PRESCHOOLER

As children leave infancy, their breathing pattern evens out considerably. The respiratory rate of young children continues to decline. By a child's third year, the rate decreases to around 20 to 30 breaths per minute, and the rhythm is smooth and regular.

During this period, children place things in their mouths, and caregivers must protect them from aspirating foreign objects that can obstruct small air passages. Providing safe toys and avoiding hard candy or small, hard pieces of food are important ways to ensure normal respiratory function for children in this age group.

CHILD AND ADOLESCENT

In growing school-age children, the breathing rate steadily slows to the adult rate of around 12 to 20 breaths per minute. During this period, good respiratory health is the general rule.

During adolescence, 3,200 young men and women begin smoking every day, and most of them will become addicted before age 20 years (Centers for Disease Control and Prevention [CDC], 2014c). One reason for this finding is that adolescents do not believe that they will become addicted to tobacco when they start to smoke. Adolescents' sense of invulnerability leads them to believe that they are not at risk for lung cancer or heart disease because these diseases are commonly associated with older adults.

The use of smokeless tobacco has dramatically increased during the last decade, especially among 16- to 19-year-old males (CDC, 2014a). One study suggested 76% of middle and high schoolers who have used electronic cigarettes within the past 30 days have also used conventional cigarettes. Researchers currently do not know the long-term effects e-cigarettes have on the body but suggest that they can be a "gateway" to conventional tobacco use. Moreover, approximately 51% of calls related to e-cigarette poisoning have involved children under the age of 5, whereas 42% of the calls have involved adults 20 years and older. Poisoning from e-cigarettes is related to the liquid containing the nicotine and occurs by ingestion, inhalation, or absorption through the skin or eyes (CDC, 2014b). One of the nurse's most valuable (and most difficult) functions is to educate adolescents about the health risks of smoking and using tobacco products.

ADULT AND OLDER ADULT

Structural and functional changes occur in the respiratory system in the later decades of life. The thoracic wall becomes more rigid, and the lungs become less able to stretch. There is no significant decrease in total lung capacity, but ventilation of nongas exchange areas of the lungs increases. The lung's protective functions are impaired: There is decreased ciliary activity and stiffening of the chest wall with declining chest muscle strength, and the cough is less propulsive and effective in airway clearance. Finally, gas exchange is affected: Normal PaO_2 decreases, and there is a decreased response to hypercapnia (Tabloski, 2013). These respiratory changes contribute to the activity intolerance and increased incidence of respiratory infections in older adults.

Cultural Considerations

Health literacy, healthcare beliefs, access to healthcare, and confidence in the healthcare system are but a few factors to consider when providing cross-cultural care (Davidson, Lui, & Sheikh, 2010). Furthermore, ineffective cross-cultural communication may hinder determining symptoms to diagnose common respiratory ailments such as asthma. In certain languages, there is not a direct translation for symptom descriptors such as "cough," "wheeze," "whistling," or "hissing," noises that are commonly listed on cross-cultural questionnaire surveys used to obtain information on asthma prevalence (Netuveli, Hurwitz, & Sheikh, 2007). Cultural sensitivity and astute assessment skills are necessary to accurately interpret assessment findings in cross-cultural patients.

FACTORS AFFECTING RESPIRATORY FUNCTION

Respiration is highly complex and depends on many factors, including body position, the environment, level of general health, and lifestyle.

Body Position

An upright posture (standing or sitting erectly) allows for the greatest ease of lung expansion. The diaphragm can move up and down most readily when the abdominal organs are not pressing against it. Breathing requires more effort when lying down because the abdominal contents push against the diaphragm. This is especially evident in people with compromised respiratory function. During the last weeks of pregnancy, breathing may become increasingly difficult in a supine position because the fetus displaces the diaphragm upward.

Environment

The percentage of oxygen humans breathe, referred to as the **fraction of inspired oxygen concentration (FiO$_2$)**, remains stable at around 21% when breathing "room air" (no supplemental oxygen). The atmosphere contains about 21% oxygen. Although the oxygen concentration does not change appreciably, its partial pressure decreases steadily as altitude increases. Lower oxygen pressure at higher elevations means that less oxygen is available to the lungs for gas diffusion. Thus, even healthy people are likely to experience shortness of breath and activity intolerance at higher elevations.

People's reactions to weather conditions are highly personalized. Some tolerate heat and humidity well; others may complain of difficulty breathing under these conditions. People who move to different climates may experience slight changes in breathing patterns until they adjust to their new surroundings. People with chronic respiratory diseases often find breathing more difficult when the weather is hot and humid because humidity makes the air thicker. Some people with asthma breathe more easily in warm, dry climates; others find a damp climate more soothing.

AIR POLLUTION

Industrialized urban areas may have elevated levels of air pollutants. Substances produced by cars and factories interfere with oxygenation by directly damaging the lungs. Carbon monoxide emissions inhibit oxygen attachment to hemoglobin on the red blood cells. Because they are respiratory irritants, pollutants cause increased mucus production and contribute to bronchitis and asthma. Workers in industrial plants or in certain occupations may be exposed to strong concentrations of specific pollutants and harmful dust. These workers may be prone to development of lung problems. The role of secondhand smoke (smoke from someone else's cigarette) continues to attract the attention of researchers for its negative impact on respiratory health. Although e-cigarettes do not appear to produce the same tobacco combustion by-products as regular cigarettes, bystanders are exposed to exhaled nicotine (Czogala et al., 2014). Further research is needed to determine the clinical significance of inhalation of secondhand smoke from e-cigarettes.

POLLENS AND ALLERGENS

Specific substances that cause allergic responses can affect respiration, sometimes severely. The body attempts to rid itself of substances perceived as harmful by releasing chemical mediators that cause an inflammatory response. Substances that trigger an inflammatory response are called allergens. Almost any substance can be an allergen; pollens, dust, and foods are common allergy triggers. The allergic response precipitates a series of events that lead to tissue damage.

Hay fever is the result of allergies confined to the nose and upper airways. Symptoms include dripping nose, itchy eyes, and swollen mucous membranes; they are annoying and uncomfortable but not life threatening. When allergic responses take place in the lungs, breathing difficulties are far more severe. Small airways become edematous, mucus production increases, and inflammatory chemical mediators cause **bronchospasm**. With bronchospasm, the airways narrow and air exchange is limited. These are the hallmarks of common allergic asthma. Severe and uncontrolled allergic asthma can be fatal.

Lifestyle and Habits

SMOKING

Smoking is the most important lifestyle choice affecting respiration. Smokers are far more likely than nonsmokers to experience emphysema, chronic bronchitis, lung cancer, oral cancer, and cardiovascular diseases. By producing more mucus and by slowing the mucociliary escalator, smoking inhibits mucus removal and can cause airway blockage, promoting bacterial colonization and infection. Regardless of whether or not a clinically identifiable lung disease is present, smokers usually breathe more rapidly than do nonsmokers.

DRUGS AND ALCOHOL

Barbiturates, opioids, and some sedatives (legal or illegal) can depress the central nervous system with a resulting decrease in respiration. Alcohol in large doses can achieve the same effect. The intoxicated person is in danger of vomiting and aspirating stomach contents into the lungs. Alcohol depresses the reflexes that protect the airways, so if vomiting occurs, stomach contents can easily slip into the trachea, causing choking and aspiration. If the victim is revived, aspiration is likely to cause pneumonia.

NUTRITION

Without proper diet, the body cannot effectively produce plasma proteins and hemoglobin. In addition, sufficient caloric and protein intake is required for respiratory muscle strength. People with diminished muscle strength work harder at breathing. Adequate nutrition is also essential for maintaining a competent immune system. Malnourished patients (e.g., from poverty or eating disorders) are at greater risk than well-nourished people for contracting pneumonia and other respiratory infections.

In the obese person, chest movement is restricted, especially in the supine position; this restriction causes shallow respirations and increased respiratory rate. The extra work required to carry extra body weight increases oxygen demands. For airways to remain patent, adequate fluid intake is necessary to keep secretions thin and easy to cough up (expectorate).

Increased Work of Breathing

All bodily functions that require muscle movement involve a certain amount of work. For the healthy person, the work of breathing is minimal. Breathing becomes noticeable only during strenuous exercise because normal lung tissue is stretchy and the airways are open to allow air to flow through them.

In altered respiratory function, the amount of work required for breathing becomes significant because the oxygen needs of respiratory muscles increase. Although these muscles ordinarily use less than 5% of the oxygen available in the blood, under extreme conditions (when the work of breathing is very high), muscles may use up to half of all oxygen available to body tissues (Suleman, Riaz, & Heffner, 2013). Because blood oxygen supply is limited, increased work of breathing can deprive other tissues of needed oxygen. The patient who experiences increased work of breathing is at risk for oxygen deprivation and exhaustion. The two general causes of increased work of breathing are restricted lung movement and airway obstruction.

RESTRICTED LUNG MOVEMENT

Certain conditions and diseases may cause the lungs to stiffen or may restrict expansion of the chest. Stiffer lungs (or lungs not allowed to expand fully) tend to collapse, and their alveoli also collapse. This condition is called **atelectasis** and reduces the amount of space available for gas exchange. Some diseases cause lung tissue to swell and thicken. Oxygen has greater difficulty passing through thickened alveolar walls. Because stiff lungs require more work to expand, the respiratory muscles consume an increased amount of oxygen. In any of these situations, less oxygen is available to the blood for the tissues.

Actual stiffening of the lung tissues can result from acute or chronic lung injuries. Smoke inhalation, pulmonary fibrosis, respiratory distress syndrome (in the adult or infant), and infections such as pneumonia are examples of disorders that make lung tissues swell and stiffen. These types of problems are classified as restrictive lung disorders.

Not all restrictive problems are caused by lung injuries or lung diseases. A patient can have perfectly healthy lungs, but other factors may prevent the lungs from expanding completely. Although the reasons for restriction may vary, the same problems with oxygenation can result. Pain from a surgical incision is a common example of this. For the patient with a high abdominal incision, the discomfort of breathing deeply often forces shallow breathing; this is why atelectasis is common in patients after surgery. Other factors that can restrict breathing include severe obesity, chest or abdominal binders, abdominal distention by gas or fluid, medications or anesthesia, rib injuries, musculoskeletal chest deformities, and severe weakness or neuromuscular disorders.

AIRWAY OBSTRUCTION

Any process that reduces the diameter of the conducting airways causes increased airway resistance. Breathing then requires more effort because air must move through a narrower passage.

Airways become obstructed in several ways. They can become plugged by foreign material, mucus, or abnormal growths. Children who aspirate small objects experience airway obstruction. The patient who has chronic bronchitis, cystic fibrosis, or asthma may experience airway obstruction from excessive mucus production. Patients with lung cancer may experience difficulty breathing as tumors obstruct large bronchi.

Inflammation caused by chemical or physical irritants also can increase airway resistance. Inflammation makes airways swollen and edematous. As the walls of the airways thicken, lumen size decreases. Asthma, bronchitis, and bronchiolitis are examples of conditions in which small airways become inflamed and narrowed. Croup and epiglottitis, most common in young children, obstruct upper airways by swelling the throat tissues.

Finally, altered bronchial smooth muscle tone also causes airway obstruction. Normal smooth muscle tone maintains the patency of the smallest airways—the bronchioles. Allergy or injury may cause the smooth muscle to become hyperreactive to stimuli. This greatly increases smooth muscle tone, which narrows airway lumens and makes breathing difficult. Airway hyperreactivity, or bronchospasm, is a common problem for patients with asthma. By contrast, patients with emphysema experience breathing problems because of abnormally low bronchial smooth muscle tone. Years of damage to the bronchiole walls make them floppy and unable to remain open during exhalation. Air becomes trapped in the alveoli, leaving little space for newly inspired air and making full inspiration difficult.

ALTERED RESPIRATORY FUNCTION

Cough

Establish if a cough is ordinarily present and at what times of the day it usually occurs. A cough is usually a reflexive response to irritation in the airways. There is not a "normal" cough. Any cough, regardless of how obvious its origin, is most often an indication that the lungs or airways are being subjected to some form of irritation. Coughs can be triggered by many chemical and physical substances or by physical conditions, such as hot, dry air. Smoke is an irritant, and coughing is the natural response to smoke. A cough's primary function is to help clear substances from the airways. A cough also serves as a warning signal: It should alert the person that possibly harmful stimuli are damaging the airways and that he or she should take measures to prevent further irritation. A cough that accompanies a disease may come from mediators released from inflamed tissues. These mediators, such as histamine, irritate the airways and can trigger a cough.

Not all coughs originate from lung problems. The patient with borderline heart failure, for example, often has a chronic cough. Some people may cough for no apparent reason as a nervous habit. Because coughs are so common, their value as a diagnostic sign is limited. Many people live with a cough, expressing concern only when it changes in severity or frequency. By contrast, some people may have a serious lung disease but a minimal cough.

Sputum Production

Ask the patient how much sputum he or she usually coughs up (a teaspoon, a tablespoon, a half cup?) and about its color. As with a cough, sputum production may be a natural consequence of irritation, but it is never really normal. Respiratory mucus, or sputum, is another protective feature of the airways. Mucus is normally produced in such small amounts that a cough from a healthy person is dry and nonproductive. Raising mucus with a deep cough indicates that the lungs are attempting to clear away irritants. Although the lungs may seem to be the obvious source of expectorated sputum, sometimes coughed-up secretions originate in the nose, mouth, or throat. It is necessary to determine if the patient raises the secretions with a genuine deep cough or if he or she "snorts" and clears them from the nasal passage. It is also necessary to determine if the secretions are cleared from the mouth (appear as frothy oral secretions). When a cough is productive, it is important to establish the source of the sputum and to assess its color, volume, consistency, and other noteworthy characteristics.

Especially frightening can be the coughing up of blood, or **hemoptysis**. Blood-filled secretions that originate in the lungs may indicate a serious condition such as lung cancer or tuberculosis. Often, however, bloody secretions originate in the nose. Drainage from the nose or mouth can drip backward into the throat, mixing with the mucus of the lower airways.

Shortness of Breath

A person who is unable to breathe sufficiently to meet the body's oxygen and metabolic demands experiences the discomfort of breathlessness. This subjective feeling of labored breathing and breathlessness is known as **dyspnea**. Box 26-1 outlines the various levels of dyspnea. The patient may deny usually being short of breath unless you can specify degrees of dyspnea to which he or she can relate. Ask how far the patient can walk before needing to rest (a mile, a city block, a flight of stairs, 20 feet).

The most common cause of dyspnea is the increased work of breathing that occurs with lung disease. Along with increased work of breathing, other causes of dyspnea may need to be assessed. Reduced lung capacity, alterations in oxygen and carbon dioxide levels, or stimulation of receptors on the

BOX 26-1	Levels of Dyspnea
Level I	The patient can walk 1 mile at own pace before experiencing shortness of breath.
Level II	The patient becomes short of breath after walking 100 yards on level ground or climbing a flight of stairs.
Level III	The patient becomes short of breath while talking or performing ADLs.
Level IV	The patient is short of breath during periods of no activity.
Orthopnea	The patient is short of breath lying down.

intercostals or diaphragm can contribute to dyspnea. People with chronic congestive heart failure often experience shortness of breath because of excess fluid in the lungs and low blood oxygen levels. People who become dyspneic during anxiety attacks often have no heart or lung disease.

Shortness of breath is a subjective symptom of lung problems. Some patients with severe lung disease appear to breathe with great difficulty, yet at such times, they may report that their breathing is fine. Others may complain of severe dyspnea even when objective data (e.g., blood gas values or pulmonary function tests) indicate no apparent problem. Family members and people close to the patient are helpful in providing supportive information.

Chest Pain

Ask the patient if he or she has any chest pain and to describe the characteristics of the pain. Chest pain can be associated with various conditions, some of which are respiratory disorders. Diseases characterized by inflammation or infection often cause pain. Inflammatory mediators such as histamine may directly stimulate nerve endings made hypersensitive by the disease process. This occurs in the airways of the patient with bronchitis who complains of a burning sensation with each cough. Acute bronchitis can make the simple act of breathing painful because the flow of cooler air across sensitized nerves can cause them to react. Mediators may also be responsible for edema formation, which can further contribute to pain as swollen tissues exert pressure on nerves. Patients with pneumonia often experience pain with deep breathing because each breath increases pressure on pain receptors that are already compressed and irritated by swollen, inflamed lung tissue.

Various emotions accompany breathing problems. Acute episodes of dyspnea bring anxiety and fear (Fig. 26-3). Panic often accompanies severe dyspnea. Patients with chronic respiratory problems may experience self-consciousness and embarrassment. Because breathlessness may interfere with communication ability, the patient with chronic respiratory problems may feel isolated. This can contribute to frustration, irritability, and eventual depression caused by continued illness and loss of independence.

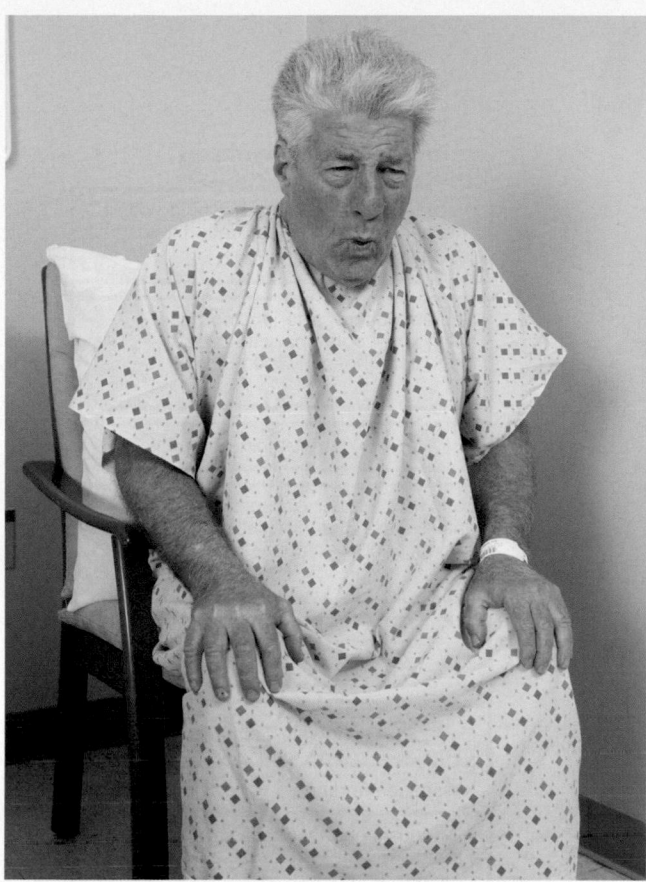

FIGURE 26-3 The patient in acute respiratory distress.

Think about Mr. Garcia, the patient in the case scenario at the beginning of the chapter. Recall that he has been diagnosed with pneumonia and that he has been a chronic smoker for 35 years.

Use the concept map (Fig. 26-4) to help manage the patient's care.

ASSESSMENT

Although it is essential to obtain the patient's history and perform a physical examination, the nurse may find that the patient who is severely short of breath may be unable to respond fully to a series of questions, or the patient with hypoxia may respond with confused answers. Forcing the patient with dyspnea to speak can worsen shortness of breath. Be sensitive to the patient's ability to answer questions; if necessary, wait on less important questions until a better time.

Normal Pattern

Unlike eating, sleeping, or elimination patterns, the patient is likely to have taken no notice of the normal breathing pattern. Few people can provide specific information about how often or how deeply they breathe.

The normal breathing pattern of the person with chronic respiratory problems may differ greatly from that of the healthy person. For example, the patient with chronic asthma ordinarily may breathe with a slight wheeze. Similarly, the patient with

chronic obstructive pulmonary disease (COPD) may grow to accept shortness of breath after walking two city blocks as normal. The patient begins to consider that something is wrong only if exercise tolerance decreases below this standard. These examples show that the nurse must take care in eliciting information about normal breathing patterns. Patients who indicate that their breathing is ordinarily fine or unremarkable may have adjusted to a baseline breathing pattern that is abnormal for most people.

Risk Identification

Causes of the patient's breathing problem may be rooted in long-term habits, occupational exposure, or past illnesses. Assess whether the patient's immunization status is current. Influenza immunization is recommended annually (CDC, 2010), and pneumococcal vaccination is recommended for all adults older than 65 years or anyone with chronic respiratory conditions (CDC, 2014d). Information about smoking habits is most important for providing insight into the patient's condition. The duration and extent of cigarette smoking are sometimes expressed in terms of *pack-years*: 1 pack-year is equal to smoking one pack of cigarettes (20 cigarettes) a day for 1 year. Pack-years are calculated to quickly quantify the risk of chronic disease. A person who has smoked two packs a day for 40 years would be said to have an 80 pack-year smoking history. A person who has smoked 10 cigarettes a day for 6 years would have a pack history of 3 years. To calculate pack-years, multiply the number of cigarettes smoked per day by the number of years smoked and divide by 20 (most packs contain 20 cigarettes). Chronic bronchitis, emphysema, and lung cancer are directly related to smoking and are more likely to occur in patients with a long history of heavy smoking.

Other lifestyle factors can also affect lung health. The patient who has lived in poverty and is malnourished, for example, is more at risk for infections such as tuberculosis. Tuberculosis and other respiratory infections also are more common in people who abuse alcohol. People with substance abuse are likely to have problems fighting infection because of self-neglect and the lowered effectiveness of their immune systems. Work history often provides relevant information. Many occupations involve exposure to fumes or dust, such as silicon and asbestos, which are toxic to lung tissue. Agricultural workers are exposed to organic dusts such as molds that can cause infections and asthma-like symptoms.

Family and personal history are also essential to a thorough evaluation. Cystic fibrosis is genetically transmitted, as is α_1-antitrypsin deficiency, which causes emphysema not related to cigarette smoking that develops in early adulthood. The patient with asthma often recalls a childhood with allergies and eczema. A history of dental problems may explain a patient's bronchiectasis or lung abscess.

Investigate a sleep history by including information about excessive daytime sleepiness, morning headache or sore throat, personality changes, or loud snoring or frequent periods of apnea during sleep reported by the spouse. These symptoms commonly occur in sleep apnea, which is common in obese, middle-aged adults. Sleep apnea causes a significant decrease in oxygenation because of multiple apneic periods during sleep.

RESPIRATORY FUNCTION

Determine problems with

Mr. Garcia • Age 55

Mr. Garcia, a 55-year-old man, has been diagnosed with pneumonia. He has a productive cough and decreased lung sounds in the bases of his lungs.

Physical appearance

Diagnostic tests and procedures

Normal pattern identification

Risk identification

Dysfunction identification

Environmental assessment

ASSESSMENT FINDINGS

Breath rate and pattern, breathing effort, chest shape, oxygen saturation, chest expansion, breath sounds.

Sputum culture, arterial blood gas, chest x-ray, pulmonary function tests, bronchoscopy, skin tests.

"How is your breathing normally?"

Long term habits, occupational exposure, past illnesses, immunization status, socioeconomic status.

"Have your breathing issues been continuous or intermittent?"

Living/social situation

Assessed findings

- Diagnosis of pneumonia.
- History of smoking for past 35 years.
- Altered breath sounds.
- Productive cough.
- Needs supplemental oxygen.
- Poor nutritional intake.
- Low socioeconomic status.
- No influenza vaccine.
- Lives with 50 other people in close quarters.

Assessment findings data indicate

EVALUATION

The patient will...

- Demonstrate knowledge regarding prevention of respiratory dysfunction.
- Demonstrate knowledge regarding optimal management of respiratory dysfunction.
- Mobilize pulmonary secretions.
- Effectively cope with changes in self-concept and lifestyle.
- Demonstrate an understanding of interventions/rationales.

Successfully resolve issues with

Dysfunction identification

Determine if interventions are successful and revise as needed

PRIORITY NURSING DIAGNOSIS

1. Ineffective Breathing Pattern, or Ineffective Airway Clearance, or Impaired Gas Exchange.
2. Related to: Disease process (pneumonia), smoking history, living situation.
3. As evidenced by: A productive cough, altered breath sounds, need for supplemental oxygen.

Leads to

INTERVENTIONS

- Health promotion/patient teaching about smoking cessation, how to prevent further respiratory infections, good hygiene, nutrition.
- Maintain respiratory hygiene precautions.
- Provide influenza and pneumococcal vaccinations.
- Use careful communication and positive encouragement.
- Monitor peak flow.
- Provide adequate hydration.
- Assist with positioning and ambulation.
- Instruct in deep breathing and coughing.
- Instruct in use of incentive spirometer.
- Perform chest physiotherapy.
- Maintain oxygen delivery.
- Assess living environment.
- Utilize resources – social services, etc.

Implement these nursing interventions

PLANNING/OUTCOMES

Patient will be able to:

- Demonstrate knowledge regarding prevention of respiratory dysfunction.
- Have adequate tissue perfusion.
- Mobilize pulmonary secretions.
- Effectively cope with changes in self-concept and lifestyle.

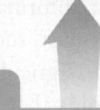
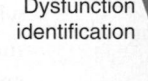
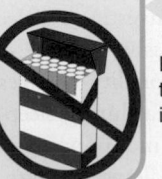

FIGURE 26-4 Concept map for respiratory function.

Dysfunction Identification

When gathering information about the onset and duration of a recent breathing problem, determine if the problem is continuous or intermittent. If the problem seems to be continuous, perhaps, some new exposure, such as new carpeting or a new pet, has triggered an allergic reaction. The patient may have contracted an infection that has progressed or has remained subacute. If the problem is intermittent, ask if the patient can identify the circumstances that bring on the difficulty. Perhaps, the patient's breathing worsens at certain times of the day or when the patient engages in certain activities. Assess cough, sputum production, shortness of breath, and discomfort or pain.

Physical Assessment

The primary techniques used in physical assessment are inspection, palpation, percussion, and auscultation. Sputum is visually examined.

INSPECTION

Observe the rate and pattern of respiration. Very slow breathing can cause **hypoxemia** (low oxygen levels in the blood) and **hypercapnia** (abnormally high carbon dioxide in the blood). Conversely, breathing too fast causes excessive elimination of carbon dioxide, which causes dizziness

THERAPEUTIC DIALOGUE: RESPIRATORY CARE

SCENE FOR THOUGHT

Marvin Ottaway is a 60-year-old man in the hospital for treatment for his pneumonia. He's sitting up in bed with the O_2 nasal prongs lying on his chest and is somewhat short of breath, but smiles when he sees the nurse at the door.

LESS EFFECTIVE

Marvin: Hello, Nancy, it's good to see you again today! I haven't seen you for a week! *(Smiles broadly and breathes rapidly.)*

Nurse: Hello, Mr. Ottaway. *(Speaks slowly and clearly.)* My name is Betsy, actually, and this is the second time I've met you. Who is Nancy?

Marvin: *(Looks confused and somewhat alarmed.)* But … you're Nancy, my sister-in-law!

Nurse: *(Gently replaces the O_2 prongs.)* I'm Betsy, your nurse, Mr. Ottaway. You really need to keep this oxygen on. If you don't have enough oxygen, you're going to get confused. That's why you think I'm Nancy. *(Smiles and speaks in a gentle tone.)*

Marvin: But you are! I know my own kin! Why are you telling me you're not?! *(Becomes agitated and frightened.)*

Nurse: Quiet down, now. The oxygen will start to work soon, then you'll recognize me. *(Still speaks quietly, putting hand on his arm.)*

Marvin: No, I want Nancy! What have you done with her?! *(Becomes more agitated. Finally calms down after nurse administers oxygen and a mild sedative.)*

MORE EFFECTIVE

Marvin: Hello, Nancy, it's good to see you again today! I haven't seen you for a week! *(Smiles broadly and breathes rapidly.)*

Nurse: Hello, Mr. Ottaway. *(Speaks slowly and clearly.)* My name is Barbara, actually, and this is the second time I've met you. Who is Nancy?

Marvin: *(Looks confused and somewhat alarmed.)* But … you're Nancy, my sister-in-law!

Nurse: *(Stands quietly by the bed with hand on his arm. Gently replaces the O_2 prongs.)* I'm Barbara, your nurse, Mr. Ottaway. Tell me a little about Nancy.

Marvin: *(Still breathes somewhat quickly but begins to warm to the subject.)* Oh, she's lovely; been married to my brother for 30 years and always treats me like one of the family. I miss her. She hasn't been to see me lately. *(Looks worried.)*

Nurse: You really like her, don't you? *(Still stands next to the bed.)*

Marvin: *(Looks at Barbara with sudden recognition.)* Oh, now, I remember you. I'm sorry. Sometimes, my mind isn't clear. I can't remember things like I used to. *(Looks embarrassed.)*

Nurse: No need to apologize. Sometimes, lack of oxygen from pneumonia can play tricks with your memory. It's important to keep the oxygen in place so you can get the benefit.

Marvin: Okay, I'll try to remember.

CRITICAL THINKING CHALLENGE

• Explain the relationship between oxygen deprivation, confusion, and anxiety.

• Compare and contrast how the two nurses presented reality.

• Identify dialogue that caused Mr. Ottaway's anxiety level to increase or decrease.

and possibly respiratory alkalosis. Rapid breathing by the severely debilitated patient may lead to exhaustion. Normal respirations should be smooth and regular. Except in the newborn, uneven or irregular breathing can indicate airway obstruction or signal neurologic or muscle problems. Assessment of breathing rate and pattern is described in Chapter 18.

Observe the patient's breathing effort by noting obvious use of shoulder or neck muscles. Healthy people use the muscles of the neck and upper chest to help them breathe deeply during vigorous exercise. The patient with breathing problems may consistently use accessory muscles to ease dyspnea and improve breathing. The patient with COPD often sits in a forward-leaning position, which uses the accessory muscles to help enlarge the chest cavity for more air. This indicates shortness of breath and may be seen as well in patients without COPD who are having other respiratory or cardiac problems. Note other obvious signs of dyspnea, such as gasping, audible wheezing, or panting respirations. In the infant, flaring of the nostrils and retractions of the ribs during inspiration are notable signs of air hunger and extraordinary work of breathing.

In addition to describing the breathing pattern, observe the patient's color. Cyanosis around the lips and under the tongue indicates serious hypoxemia. **Cyanosis** is a bluish skin discoloration caused by a desaturation of oxygen on the hemoglobin in the blood. Hemoglobin, the major carrier of oxygen in the blood, is bright red when saturated with oxygen. When not carrying oxygen, it becomes deep blue. This bluish state should be distinguished from peripheral cyanosis (e.g., blue fingertips on a cold day). Such problems are relatively harmless and indicate only local vasoconstriction, whereas central cyanosis is a late sign of oxygen deprivation and could be life threatening. In people with dark skin tones, cyanosis may be best assessed in the oral cavity and eyelids. See Figure 26-5 for a photo of cyanosis.

SAFETY ALERT

Central cyanosis, seen in the mucous membranes of the eyes and mouth, must never be ignored because it indicates serious oxygenation problems.

Inspect the fingertips and toes. Clubbing is an unusual phenomenon seen in many patients with respiratory or cardiac disease. For reasons that are unclear, the tips of the fingers and toes become rounded and enlarged (see Chapter 17). Long-term tissue **hypoxia** causes the release of platelet-derived growth factor and other mediators that cause dilation of the vessels of the fingertips. Clubbing occurs in lung cancer, cystic fibrosis, and lung diseases such as lung abscess and COPD.

Finally, inspect the chest to detect obvious chest deformities, wounds, or masses. The chest's overall shape is important but less obvious. In COPD, the patient's chest becomes overinflated over time because of an inability to exhale fully. This increases the anterior–posterior chest diameter, resulting in a barrel-shaped appearance (see Figure 26-6).

PALPATION

The nurse's hands are used to assess abnormalities such as swelling or tenderness. Palpation is also used to determine the extent and pattern of thoracic expansion and to note the position of

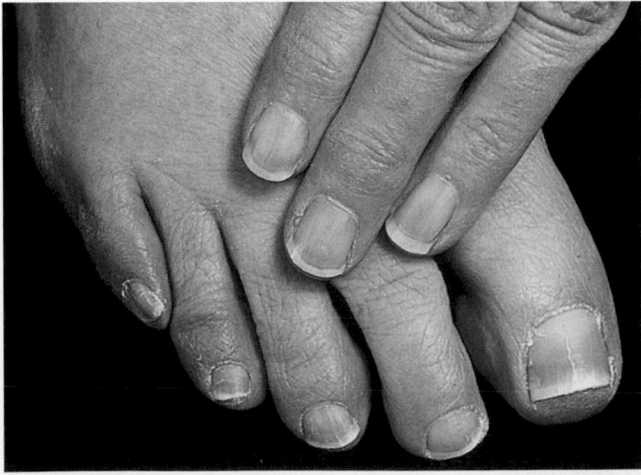

FIGURE 26-5 Cyanosis. (Reprinted with permission from Stedman's Medical Terminology Flash Cards, 2nd Edition. Philadelphia, PA: Lippincott Williams & Wilkins, 2010.)

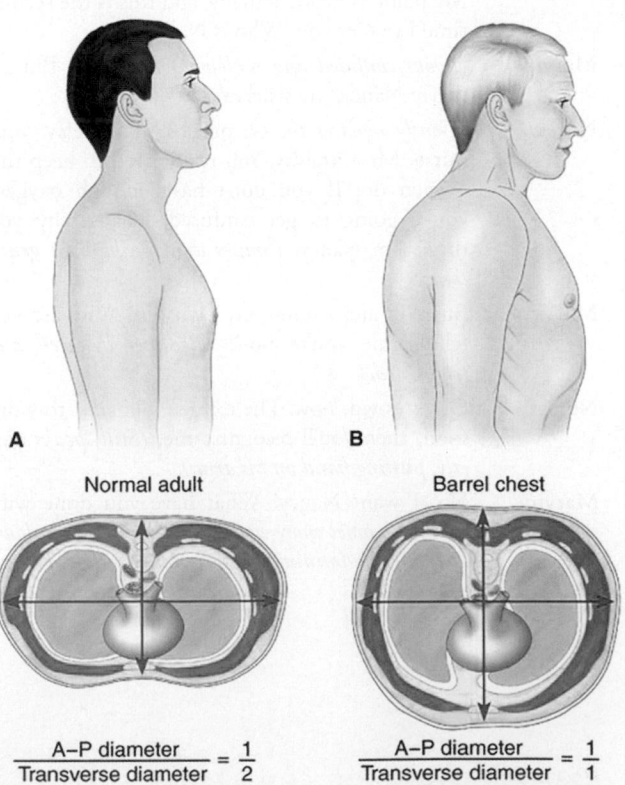

FIGURE 26-6 Barrel chest **(B)**, compared with normal **(A)**. (Reprinted with permission from Hinkle, J. L., & Cheever, K. H. (2014). *Brunner & Suddarth's textbook of medical-surgical nursing* (13th ed.). Philadelphia, PA: Lippincott Williams & Wilkins.)

the trachea. Palpation may detect abnormal chest wall vibrations transmitted through inflamed or fluid-filled lung tissues. Fremitus (the vibration of air movement through the chest wall) is best felt by placing the balls of the palms of the nurse's hand on the patient's back as he or she says "99." The intrascapular space is a good area to feel tactile fremitus because it diminishes as you move out in the lung fields. Increased tactile fremitus can be present in consolidation in the lung, whereas decreased fremitus may occur with pleural effusion, pulmonary edema, emphysema, or bronchial obstruction.

PERCUSSION

Percussion is used to detect fluid-filled or consolidated portions of the lung. A keen ear and experience with pulmonary assessment are needed to interpret correctly the various alterations in pitch, intensity, duration, and quality of percussion notes.

AUSCULTATION

Listening to breath sounds with a stethoscope provides vital information for evaluating the patient's respiratory status. Chapter 17 describes normal breath sounds classified as bronchial, bronchovesicular, and vesicular.

The most important reason for listening to the chest is to determine if air is moving through all areas of the lung. When auscultating with a sensitive stethoscope, you should be able to hear air moving in all lung fields. Breath sounds should be equally loud on both sides of the chest (Fig. 26-7).

Absent or distant-sounding breath sounds in any area of the lung can indicate airway obstruction or can mean that fluid or air has accumulated in the pleural space. A "silent chest" in a patient with asthma who is experiencing severe shortness of breath is a grave sign of poor ventilation and impending respiratory failure (Lewis, Dirksen, Heitkemper, & Bucher, 2014).

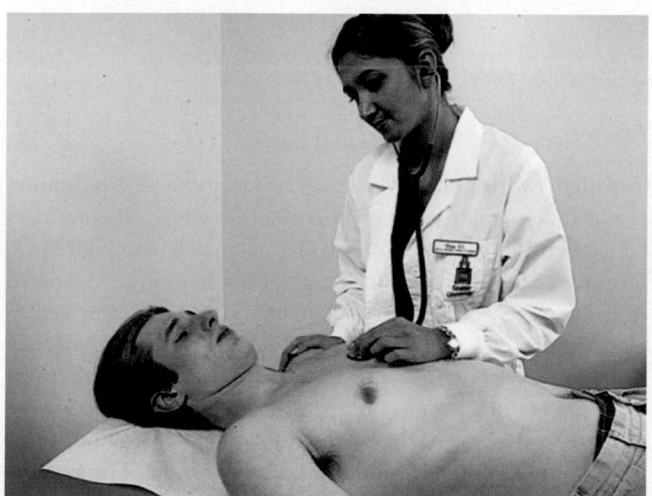

FIGURE 26-7 Auscultation of the chest. (Reprinted with permission from Rosdahl, C. B., & Kowalski, M. T. (2012). *Textbook of basic nursing* (10th ed.) Philadelphia, PA: Lippincott Williams & Wilkins.)

The quality of breath sounds can also be assessed by auscultation. Normal breathing should make soft, rustling sounds, like a breeze blowing gently through leaves on trees. Inspiratory breath sounds are typically louder and longer than expiratory sounds. Nurses must also become familiar with abnormal breath sounds (Table 26-2). Official nomenclature (as developed by the American Thoracic Society) is presented here, but be aware that alternative terminology is commonly used.

Abnormal Breath Sounds

Discontinuous Sounds. *Crackles* (also called rales) are discontinuous sounds heard on inspiration and range from soft, fine sounds to coarse, rattling sounds. Crackles may represent opening of closed airways as in atelectasis, or secretions in the airways. These sounds are often heard in patients with obstructive diseases such as chronic bronchitis, asthma, and emphysema. Late inspiratory crackles may indicate pneumonia, congestive heart failure, or atelectasis.

Coarse crackles (also coarse rales) are low-pitched, rumbling sounds that typically indicate sputum in the airways. These sounds can indicate conditions such as pneumonia, pulmonary edema, and pulmonary fibrosis.

Continuous Sounds. Rhonchi are low-pitched sonorous sounds, typically louder than crackles, representing fluid in the larger airways. Rhonchi often clear with coughing.

Wheezes are typically high-pitched musical sounds associated with narrowed airways. They are commonly heard in patients with emphysema or asthma.

Stridor, the most severe type of inspiratory wheeze, is heard most commonly in children with croup or epiglottitis. If upper airway obstruction becomes too severe, an artificial airway must be used to ensure an open passage for breathing.

A *pleural friction rub* produces a dry rubbing or grating sound caused by inflammation of pleural surfaces rubbing against the chest wall. A pleural friction rub can be heard best on inspiration but also is present during expiration; the rub does not disappear with a cough. This abnormal breath sound is loudest over the lung's lower lateral anterior surface. Unlike a pericardial friction rub, a pleural friction rub disappears when breathing stops.

Diagnostic Tests and Procedures

PULSE OXIMETRY

Pulse oximetry offers a noninvasive and indirect means for approximating oxygenation, whereas arterial blood sampling (an intravenous needle inserted into an artery) provides a precise, direct measure of oxygenation through blood gases. To measure oxygenation through pulse oximetry, a sensor is attached to the patient's finger or earlobe. This allows assessment of heart rate and **oxygen saturation**, either intermittently or continuously. Oximetry is a convenient and painless alternative to needlesticks, is simple to use, and provides immediate data. These advantages make oximetry an invaluable tool for determining the patient's need for oxygen

TABLE 26-2 ADVENTITIOUS BREATH SOUNDS

Abnormal Sound	Characteristics	Location	Source	Conditions
Discontinuous Sounds				
Crackles (fine) Also called fine rales	High-pitched, short, popping sounds heard during inspiration and not cleared with coughing; sounds are discontinuous and can be simulated by rolling a strand of hair between your fingers near your ear.	Alveoli	Inhaled air suddenly opens the small deflated air passages that are coated and sticky with exudate.	Crackles occurring late in inspiration are associated with restrictive diseases such as pneumonia and congestive heart failure. Crackles occurring early in inspiration are associated with obstructive disorders such as bronchitis, asthma, or emphysema.
Crackles (coarse) Also called coarse rales	Low-pitched, bubbling, moist sounds that may persist from early inspiration to early expiration	Peripheral airways	Inhaled air comes into contact with secretions in the large bronchi and trachea.	Can indicate such conditions as pneumonia, pulmonary edema, and pulmonary fibrosis
Continuous Sounds				
Wheeze (sonorous) Also called rhonchi or gurgles	Low-pitched snoring or moaning sounds heard primarily during expiration but may be heard throughout the respiratory cycle. These wheezes may clear with coughing.	Large airways	Same as sibilant wheeze. The pitch of the wheeze cannot be correlated to the size of the passageway that generates it.	Sonorous wheezes are often heard in cases of bronchitis or single-bronchus obstructions.
Wheeze (sibilant)	High-pitched, musical sounds heard primarily during expiration but may also be heard on inspiration	Large or small airways	Air passing through constricted passages caused by swelling, secretions, or tumor	Sibilant wheezes are often heard in cases of acute asthma or chronic emphysema.
Pleural friction rub	Low-pitched, dry grating sound. Sound is much like crackles, only more superficial, and occurs during both inspiration and expiration.	Pleural surfaces	Sound is the result of rubbing of two inflamed pleural surfaces.	Pleuritis

Source: Weber, J., & Kelly, J. (2014). *Health assessment in nursing* (5th ed.). Philadelphia, PA: Lippincott Williams & Wilkins.

therapy and assessing the therapy's effectiveness. The oximeter registers **arterial oxygen saturation (SpO$_2$)**. The pulse oximeter uses infrared light to determine the percentage of hemoglobin that combines with oxygen. An SpO$_2$ greater than 95% is considered normal, whereas values lower than 93% usually indicate the need for oxygen therapy and further assessment.

Several factors affect the accuracy and proper interpretation of oximetry. The patient must have adequate peripheral blood flow for the oximeter to detect a pulse. Conditions such as room lighting, patient motion, cigarette smoking, or dark polish on the patient's fingernails can affect sensor accuracy. Forehead reflectance oximetry is less susceptible to poor tissue perfusion and able to more accurately record oxygen saturation in patients with poor perfusion. Carbon monoxide poisoning results in false high readings; edema at the sensor site produces false low readings. Patients with anemia may have a high SpO$_2$ reading, because most of the hemoglobin has oxygen attached to it. However, because of the anemia, there are fewer hemoglobin molecules in the blood, and therefore, the patient may be hypoxic. Most importantly, interpretation of SpO$_2$ depends on the operator's understanding of hemoglobin and its unique properties. Because of the manner in which hemoglobin combines with oxygen, relatively slight changes in SpO$_2$ may actually reflect large changes in blood oxygenation. Experience and clinical judgment help the skilled practitioner relate oximetry readings to patient condition. Refer to **Procedure 26-1** for guidance using pulse oximetry.

SAFETY ALERT

Pulse oximetry does not measure the adequacy of ventilation. It is not an early indicator of respiratory depression or ventilatory failure. It is one data point that should be combined with other assessment tools to help provide the best information about your patient's oxygenation and ventilation status.

LABORATORY STUDIES

Any sputum the patient coughs up should be inspected. Normal respiratory secretions are clear or white. Normal sputum has no odor and medium consistency. Thick and sticky sputum is usually difficult to expectorate and may indicate that the patient is poorly hydrated. Sputum produced by patients with asthma is stringy, like thickened egg white. Life-threatening pulmonary edema produces frothy, pink secretions.

Sputum that is yellow or green or has a putrid or musty odor may indicate infection. When infection is suspected, collect a sputum sample in a sterile container and send the sample to the laboratory for examination.

Blood-streaked mucus indicates airway inflammation. It commonly occurs during harsh coughing episodes in patients with bronchitis, tuberculosis, or lung cancer. Frankly red, bloody mucus (hemoptysis) is a sign of continual bleeding somewhere in the airways that requires immediate response and thorough investigation.

Sputum Culture

The patient who has a productive cough, is febrile, and shows other signs of infection should have a sputum sample evaluated by the laboratory. A Gram stain can be performed quickly to determine if infection is present and to classify the organism as Gram positive or Gram negative. Sputum is cultured to identify the specific agent causing the infection (this takes 2 to 3 days). A sensitivity test done at the same time will indicate the best antibiotic to use against the causative agent. Once the sputum sample is obtained (see **Procedure 26-2**), the patient may be treated with a broad-spectrum antibiotic until the culture report is back, at which time, the antibiotic may be changed to a drug that is more sensitive to the infectious agent.

Arterial Blood Gas Monitoring

Arterial blood levels of oxygen (PaO_2), carbon dioxide ($PaCO_2$), and pH are the most reliable indicators of gas exchange. PaO_2 is one of the best indicators of how much oxygen is available to tissues. When the PaO_2 is lower than normal, tissues may experience hypoxia. This development is dangerous to all tissues and organs but can be especially damaging to the heart and the brain. Although PaO_2 normally declines with age, an abnormally low PaO_2 always indicates gas exchange problems. PaO_2 decreases in direct proportion to the severity of lung impairment (Box 26-2).

In addition to oxygenation, arterial blood sampling also indicates how effectively the lungs are removing carbon dioxide. The lungs' regulation of this metabolic waste product is essential for the blood's normal acid–base balance. The carbon dioxide level affects many functions, including the drive to breathe, affinity of hemoglobin for oxygen, and cardiac function. The

---

BOX 26-2   Levels of Hypoxemia

Mild:	PaO_2 of 60–80 mm Hg	SpO_2 of 91–95 mm Hg
Moderate:	PaO_2 of 40–60 mm Hg	SpO_2 of 74–91 mm Hg
Severe:	PaO_2 of less than 40 mm Hg	SpO_2 of less than 74 mm Hg

Note: PaO_2 naturally declines with age. For every year over 60, subtract 1 mm Hg from the normal range. For example, a man 70 years of age would be expected to have a PaO_2 of 70 to 90 mm Hg.

Also, the newborn is normally hypoxemic during the first 12 to 24 hours of life. A PaO_2 of 80 to 100 mm Hg is achieved after this time.

$PaCO_2$ stays nearly constant in the person with healthy lungs. A $PaCO_2$ lower than 35 mm Hg indicates **hyperventilation**, or breathing in excess of metabolic needs. Healthy people are able to hyperventilate voluntarily. Hyperventilation is common during an asthma attack and occurs in some patients with head injuries. It may also occur involuntarily during extreme anxiety.

A $PaCO_2$ above 45 mm Hg indicates **hypoventilation**, in which breathing rate and depth are insufficient to clear carbon dioxide adequately from the blood. Severe airway obstruction causes hypoventilation, which is a serious problem for patients with advanced COPD. Respiratory failure is another cause of hypoventilation in patients whose respiratory drive has been diminished by opioids, barbiturates, or trauma.

Arterial blood sampling also indicates the blood's acidity or alkalinity. The pH is a measure of the blood's acid–base balance. Biochemical processes essential to all cellular life require a close balance of acids and bases. Normally, arterial blood pH ranges from 7.35 to 7.45. Arterial pH below 7.35 is described as acidosis, whereas pH above 7.45 indicates alkalosis (Table 26-3). Chapter 28 presents a more detailed discussion of acid–base balance.

End-Tidal CO_2 Monitoring

Exhaled CO_2, measured at the end of exhalation (end tidal), is a sensitive indicator of adequacy of ventilation. Although pulse oximetry may take several minutes to display changes in oxygen saturation of the hemoglobin in the blood, end-tidal CO_2 (**EtCO_2**) changes rapidly in response to changes in the patient's breathing. To monitor $EtCO_2$, the patient wears a nasal sampling device similar in appearance to an oxygen nasal cannula. The sampling device is connected to a monitor that may display the $EtCO_2$ in graphic (**capnography**) or numeric (**capnometry**) form. Normal $EtCO_2$ is 35 to 45 mm Hg. $EtCO_2$

TABLE 26-3   NORMAL ARTERIAL BLOOD GAS VALUES

PaO_2	80–100 mm Hg
$PaCO_2$	35–45 mm Hg
pH	7.35–7.45
HCO_3^-	22–26 mEq/L
Base excess	±2

may be measured in several circumstances. When an endotracheal tube is inserted into a patient, a one-time $EtCO_2$ device may be attached to the end of the tube to assure placement of the tube into the trachea rather than the esophagus. Placement in the trachea would result in a reading of at least 5 mm Hg. Placement of the ET tube in the esophagus would result in a reading less than 5 mm Hg. During CPR, $EtCO_2$ provides an indication of the effectiveness of chest compressions. A reading of 10 to 20 mm Hg indicates good quality compressions. Readings lower than 10 mm Hg suggest inadequate circulation and therefore inadequate compressions.

Continuous $EtCO_2$ readings may be obtained in patients receiving patient-controlled analgesia (PCA). Because medications used in PCA have the potential to suppress respirations, monitoring of respiratory function is essential. Although pulse oximetry may provide information, the readings displayed on the pulse oximeter may lag behind actual oxygenation status by five minutes or more. On the other hand, $EtCO_2$ will drop rapidly when respirations are reduced. This provides an early alert to a potentially dangerous decrease in the patients breathing. See **Procedure 26-3** for instructions on using continuous $EtCO_2$ monitoring.

DIAGNOSTIC PROCEDURES

The most commonly used tests for assessing respiratory status are chest x-ray and pulmonary function tests. More specialized tests include lung scans and pulmonary angiography, bronchoscopy, skin testing for allergies in asthma, and skin tests for tuberculosis.

Chest X-Ray

The chest x-ray is widely used to identify pathologic changes in the lung and chest that may explain the patient's breathing problems. From a chest x-ray, the radiologist can detect abnormal fluid or air in the pleural space or a collapsed lung (pneumothorax). The x-ray can also show if portions of the lungs are consolidated (as in pneumonia) or underinflated (as in atelectasis). Sometimes, routine x-rays initially detect tumors. The chest x-ray is also used to determine the position of catheters and tubes and to monitor a patient's response to therapy. Lung scans and angiography are specialized radiographic techniques used to study blood flow and ventilation in the lung.

Pulmonary Function Tests

Specialized breathing tests measure lung size and airway patency. Spirometry produces graphic representations of lung volumes and flows. These graphs are essential in determining the severity of a patient's restrictive or obstructive lung disease. Common measurements include tidal volume, vital capacity, and forced expiratory volume in 1 second (FEV_1). More highly specialized pulmonary function tests can provide additional information on lung function, characteristics, and capacities.

Bronchoscopy

Bronchoscopy allows the physician to visualize the airways directly. A flexible fiberoptic tube connected to a viewing screen is inserted through the patient's nose. A handheld control directs the scope into the trachea and bronchi. The bronchoscope can be used to collect sterile sputum specimens or tissue samples for laboratory examination or to withdraw large sputum plugs or aspirated objects obstructing the airways. Nursing interventions for a bronchoscopy include ensuring informed consent, teaching before the procedure, and maintaining NPO (nothing by mouth) status until the gag reflex returns after the procedure. Monitoring after the procedure includes frequent assessment for dyspnea, hemoptysis, or cardiac arrhythmias.

Skin Tests

Skin tests can be performed to identify a patient's allergies to specific substances. By determining possible sources of airway hypersensitivity in asthmatic patients, allergists can help them avoid the offending substances. These tests also help the allergist devise serums for desensitizing the patient. Another type of skin test is used to establish whether or not a patient has been exposed to tuberculosis. In the tuberculin skin test (TST), purified protein derivative (PPD) is injected under the skin. A positive reaction helps identify people who may have been exposed to tuberculosis.

NURSING DIAGNOSES

Respiratory nursing diagnoses include Ineffective Breathing Pattern, Ineffective Airway Clearance, and Impaired Gas Exchange (Herdman & Kamitsuru, 2014) (Table 26-4).

OUTCOME IDENTIFICATION AND PLANNING

After nursing diagnoses and related factors have been established, the nurse and patient identify outcomes. The following general areas should be included in the formulation of patient goals and outcomes:

- The patient will demonstrate knowledge regarding prevention of respiratory dysfunction.
- The patient's tissues will have adequate oxygenation.
- The patient will mobilize pulmonary secretions.
- The patient will effectively cope with changes in self-concept and lifestyle.

Patient outcomes differ substantially, depending on the prognosis. For the patient with an acute respiratory problem, the goal is recovery without any residual respiratory complications. Goals for the patient with chronic respiratory problems focus on the patient's ability to live within the limitations the disease imposes and to accept changes in lifestyle and self-concept. For the patient with terminal respiratory problems, goals are to maintain adequate comfort and to accept impending death. Aim interventions at restoring, maintaining, and promoting respiratory health.

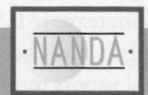 **Table 26-4 SELECTED NANDA-I NURSING DIAGNOSES INVOLVING RESPIRATORY FUNCTION**

Nursing Dx	Related Factors	Dx Statement	NOC*	NIC†
Ineffective Breathing Pattern–state in which a person's inspiration and/or expiration pattern does not provide adequate ventilation	Hyperventilation, hypoventilation, obesity, spinal cord injury, neuromuscular dysfunction, pain, musculoskeletal impairment, perceptual or cognitive impairment, anxiety, decreased energy/fatigue, respiratory muscle fatigue, and neurologic immaturity	Ineffective Breathing Pattern R/T fatigue AEB tachypnea, use of accessory muscles, and poor nutrition	Respiratory Status: Airway Patency, Ventilation; Vital Signs	Cough Enhancement; Oxygen Therapy; Respiratory Monitoring; Nutrition Therapy
Ineffective Airway Clearance–state in which a person is unable to clear secretions or obstructions from the respiratory tract to maintain a clear airway	Smoke, airway spasm, retained secretions, foreign body in the airway, excessive mucus or secretions in the bronchi, neuromuscular dysfunction, COPD, asthma, infection, obstruction, allergic airways	Ineffective Airway Clearance R/T excessive mucus secondary to pneumonia AEB adventitious breath sounds, ineffective cough, and oxygen saturation of 90% on room air	Aspiration Prevention; Respiratory Status: Airway Patency, Ventilation, Gas Exchange	Cough Enhancement; Oxygen Therapy; Fluid Management
Impaired Gas Exchange–state in which a person experiences an excess or deficit in oxygenation and/or carbon dioxide elimination at an alveolar–capillary level	Imbalance of ventilation and perfusion and alveolar-capillary membrane changes contribute to impaired gas exchange.	Impaired Gas Exchange R/T ventilation–perfusion imbalance secondary to asthma AEB hypoxemia, restlessness, and tachycardia	Respiratory status: Gas exchange, Ventilation	Acid–Base Management; Oxygen Therapy; Ventilation Assistance

Dx, diagnosis; R/T, related to; AEB, as evidenced by.
*From: Moorhead, S., Johnson, M., Maas, M., & Swanson, E. (2013). *Nursing outcomes classification (NOC): Measurement of health outcomes* (5th ed.). St. Louis, MO: Elsevier.
†From: Bulecheck, G., Butcher, H., Dochterman, J., Wagner, C. (2013). *Nursing interventions classification (NIC)* (6th ed.). St. Louis, MO: Elsevier.
From: Herdman, T. H., & Kamitsuru, S. (Eds.). (2014). *Nursing diagnoses: Definitions and classification, 2015–2017*. West Sussex, England: Wiley-Blackwell.

IMPLEMENTATION

Health Promotion

Health promotion to prevent respiratory dysfunction has become an increasingly important nursing role. The nurse and other healthcare professionals can work with organizations such as the American Lung Association (ALA) to provide programs to reduce smoking and pollution and to improve working conditions contributing to lung disease. More commonly, the nurse works with people in various settings (e.g., ambulatory clinics, schools, industry, and public health) to teach and promote pulmonary health.

PREVENTING RESPIRATORY INFECTIONS

Health teaching can limit both exposure to and occurrence of acute respiratory infections such as influenza and pneumonia. Promote optimal immune function by encouraging good nutrition. Remind the patient to avoid exposure to known infected people or large crowds during peak flu season. Good hygiene practices, especially hand hygiene, sneezing or coughing into the sleeve rather than hands, and proper used tissue disposal, prevent the spread of communicable respiratory infections.

High-risk patients (e.g., older adults; people with diagnosed diabetes or respiratory disorders such as asthma or COPD; people with immune system dysfunction, such as patients with AIDS, patients undergoing cancer chemotherapy, and transplant recipients; and healthcare workers) should receive annual influenza vaccinations. Influenza vaccines are changed annually based on anticipated new strains; revaccination every fall before flu season is required to produce effective immunity. Pneumococcal vaccination is also recommended for high-risk people. Revaccination is required only for adults older than 65 years or people who are immunocompromised (CDC, 2014d).

ENCOURAGING SMOKING CESSATION

Smoking cessation is a positive step toward health, regardless of the length of time a person has been a smoker. State-of-change theory provides a basis for understanding the process underlying changing an addictive habit. The five stages outlined in the process are as follows:

1. Precontemplation (not thinking about quitting)
2. Contemplation (thinking about quitting in the next 6 months)
3. Preparation (thinking about quitting in the next 30 days)
4. Action (in the process of quitting)
5. Maintenance (abstaining from tobacco use for 6 months or more)

Relapse is common during smoking cessation attempts (Agency for Healthcare Research and Quality, 2008). Provide positive encouragement, and explain that it often takes more than one attempt to successfully stop smoking. Ultimately, it is up to the smoker to be responsible for choosing and carrying out personal change. Often, the diagnosis of lung cancer provides a teachable moment when patients are motivated to stop smoking (Tammemagi, Berg, Riley, Cunningham, & Taylor, 2014).

REDUCING ALLERGENS

Reducing exposure to allergens that can trigger bronchoconstriction and inflammation is an important preventive measure. Although the mortality rate from asthma has declined in the last 20 years, the prevalence of asthma continues to increase (ALA, 2012). More than 400 occupational asthma triggers have been identified; the most common triggers are chemical vapors found in workplaces, such as paper and textile mills, chemical plants, printing plants, and hair salons. Most businesses and workplaces ban smoking, which has significantly reduced exposure to secondhand smoke. Aspirin sensitivity, cold air, or exercise can induce an allergic attack. Seasonal pollens from trees, grasses, and flowering plants frequently exacerbate asthma symptoms in the spring or late summer. Indoor allergens include dust mites, pet dander, cockroach eggs and droppings, and molds. Nurses can be instrumental in working with the patient and family to identify individual asthma triggers and motivate the family to restructure the environment to limit allergen exposure. Allergens can be identified through skin testing, and a program of allergen desensitization (allergy shots) can be instituted.

MONITORING PEAK FLOW

A peak flow meter is a handheld device that measures the highest flow during maximal expiration; the meter indicates how rapidly the patient can breathe out air. Changes in peak flow measurements reflect changes in airway diameter; they occur before symptoms of respiratory distress, such as dyspnea, wheezing, or increased coughing, appear. Peak flow measurement can be used to individualize therapy and prevent the onset of an acute asthma attack. Peak flow measurement may also be useful in patients with chronic bronchitis or emphysema.

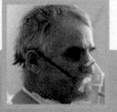

Respiratory PICO

Mr. Garcia from the scenario at the beginning of the chapter is getting ready to be discharged. His doctor added nicotine patches to his discharge medication and wants him to have information about smoking cessation. Jan, a new nurse, is taking care of Mr. Garcia today and has limited knowledge about medications used to help stop smoking. She decides to use the Cochrane Library to find evidence about the effectiveness of smoking cessation meds before talking to Mr. Garcia. Jan started her search by using the following PICO question: *Does use of a nicotine patch (vs. no nicotine patch) help smokers quit smoking?*

P opulation = Smokers
I ntervention = Nicotine patches
C omparison = No patches
O utcome   = Quit smoking

Jan knows that meta-analysis studies reflect the strongest form of evidence. She found an article that compared several smoking cessation drugs (including nicotine replacement therapy [NRT], bupropion [Wellbutrin], and varenicline [Chantix]) with each other and a placebo. The article analyzed 267 studies with 101,804 participants. The results concluded smokers had a better chance of quitting using *any* of these therapies versus no treatment at all. The study showed that NRT is effective alone or it can be paired with bupropion to increase the patient's chances to stop smoking. Jan also learned that for some smokers, treatment options such as varenicline proved to be more successful than nicotine patches, gum, or nasal spray. According to the research, adverse effects with all these drugs were minimal. After reviewing the article, Jan felt like she had a better idea about smoking cessation treatments and their success rates. She felt more confident entering Mr. Garcia's room.

REFERENCE

Cahill, K., Stevens, S., Perera, R., & Lancaster T. (2013). Pharmacological interventions for smoking cessation: an overview and network meta-analysis. *Cochrane Database of Systematic Reviews*, (5), Art. No.: CD009329. doi: 10.1002/14651858.CD009329.pub2.

OUTCOME-BASED TEACHING PLANS

You are a clinic nurse for an allergist. Gina, 8 years old, and her mother are coming in for a follow-up visit. Gina was hospitalized 2 weeks ago for an acute asthma attack. In the hospital, a diagnosis of asthma was made and teaching was begun on asthma management. You are now responsible for continuing this teaching.

OUTCOME

Gina/mother will verbalize preventive measures to decrease exposure to allergens by the next clinic visit.

STRATEGIES

- Assess the patient's and family's knowledge base regarding possible triggers of Gina's asthma attacks.
- Review methods to decrease animal dander (e.g., remove furred or feathered animals from the home or at least prohibit from bedroom, use high-efficiency particulate air [HEPA] filter air cleaners).
- Review methods to decrease dust mite allergens (e.g., encase pillows and mattress in an allergen-proof cover, wash bedding and stuffed animals weekly, remove carpets, vacuum daily using HEPA filter).
- Review methods to decrease environmental pollutants (e.g., no smoking in the home; avoid woodburning fires; avoid exposure to very cold air, perfumes, chemicals, and automobile exhaust).
- Offer to set up home evaluation for allergens.
- Discuss with the family those preventive measures that fit best with their lifestyle and willingness to try.

EVALUATION

- Mother states preventive measures used, including:
  - Methods used to decrease animal dander
  - Methods used to decrease environmental pollutants

OUTCOME

Gina/mother will recognize a worsening of respiratory status and verbalize when they need to consult healthcare professionals by the end of teaching session.

STRATEGIES

- Allow Gina and her mother to express concerns or anxiety they have concerning managing an asthma attack.
- Review peak flow monitoring, asking Gina to demonstrate and verbalize personal "green," "yellow," and "red" zones.
- Review peak flow monitoring log to assess Gina's status, providing positive feedback to her and her parents.
- Review symptoms of respiratory distress that warrant medical attention (e.g., peak flow in red zone, dyspnea that is not relieved with MDI use with a fast-acting bronchodilator, symptoms of respiratory tract infection).
- Demonstrate how to administer epinephrine via an EpiPen should acute symptoms fail to resolve, then call 911.
- Remind the family to alert appropriate people (e.g., teacher, school nurse, babysitter) of asthma and what to do during an attack.

EVALUATION

- Concerns and feelings of anxiety concerning managing asthma attack verbalized by Gina and her mother.
- Gina demonstrates proper use of peak flow monitor and accurately identifies her personal "green," "yellow," and "red" zones.
- Gina and mother accurately state symptoms of respiratory distress that warrant medical attention.
- Mother demonstrates proper administration of epinephrine with an EpiPen.

Instruct patients to perform and record peak flow measurement twice a day, once in the morning and once in the evening. Patients should take measurements before using any bronchodilators. Initially, the patient will determine his or her "personal best" (the highest peak flow measure that he or she obtains over a 2-week period during which the asthma was well controlled). Once this value is obtained, the following zones can be determined:

- Green zone—80% to 100% of personal best (asthma is well controlled; proceed on routine treatment plan)
- Yellow zone—50% to 80% of personal best (asthma is not well controlled, and treatment plan may need to be increased)
- Red zone—below 50% of personal best (take a fast-acting beta$_2$ agonist, and contact a healthcare provider immediately)

Refer to **Procedure 26-4** for detailed instruction outlining how to use a peak flow meter.

PROVIDING ADEQUATE HYDRATION

Inadequate moisture in the airways makes respiratory mucus thick and difficult to cough up. Sticky, tenacious sputum that coats the respiratory tract increases work of breathing for any patient and makes breathing especially difficult for those with chronic lung disease. Mucus that is hard to expectorate promotes infection because the bacteria it traps have time to multiply. Dried,

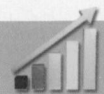
BACKGROUND

Ventilator-associated pneumonia (VAP) is defined as an airway infection that develops more than 48 hours after the patient is intubated. Preventing pneumonia is always an important goal in the acute care setting, but VAP is of particular concern. Approximately 10% to 20% of ventilated patients develop VAP. Patients who develop VAP have increased time spent on the ventilator, prolonged length of intensive care unit (ICU) stay, increased length of hospital stay after transfer from the ICU, and increased mortality (Klompas et al., 2014).

The ventilator bundle is a series of interventions designed to prevent VAP. Research suggests that when performed together, these interventions significantly improve outcomes compared to when they are performed individually.

KEY COMPONENTS

1. Elevation of the Head of the Bed

Elevating the head of the bed 30 to 45 degrees reduces the risk of aspiration. It is not clear whether it is gastrointestinal contents or oro-/nasopharyngeal contents that are not being aspirated. In addition, elevation of the head of the bed may improve the patient's ventilator efforts and may reduce the incidence of atelectasis.

NURSING IMPLICATIONS	
	◆ Use tracking mechanisms to ensure compliance with head-of-bed elevation.
	◆ Discuss compliance with head-of-bed elevation during interdisciplinary rounds.
	◆ Consider instituting degree levels on beds to ensure a minimum of 30-degree elevation.
	◆ Create an environment that encourages respiratory therapy to alert nursing when the head of bed is not at a minimum of 30 degrees. The respiratory therapists should be empowered to raise the head of bed to a minimum of 30 degrees after routine care.
	◆ Instruct the family about the importance of head-of-bed elevation. Educate the family to alert the nurse when the head of bed is not at a minimum of 30 degrees.

2. Daily Sedation Vacations with Assessment of Readiness to Extubate

Many ventilated patients are heavily sedated. Lightening of sedation allows for assessment of the need for ongoing ventilation. Removing mechanical ventilation when no longer needed reduces the risk of VAP. If patients are less sedated, they are more able to assist with their own ventilation and more likely to tolerate extubation.

NURSING IMPLICATIONS	
	◆ Establish a protocol to regularly lighten sedation to assess ventilation and readiness for extubation.
	◆ Consider performing the sedation vacation to coincide with a weaning trial.
	◆ Monitor closely during sedation vacations to prevent self-extubation.
	◆ Assess compliance with and outcome of sedation vacation each day during interdisciplinary care rounds.

3. Peptic Ulcer Disease Prophylaxis

Critically ill patients have a higher incidence of stress ulceration than other patients. Decreasing the pH of gastric contents may reduce the incidence of stress ulcers and protect against a greater pulmonary inflammatory response to aspiration of gastrointestinal contents. Aspiration causes pneumonia and may be worse if the gastrointestinal contents are acidic.

NURSING IMPLICATIONS	
	◆ Address peptic ulcer disease prophylaxis on admission to ICU.
	◆ Discuss peptic ulcer disease prophylaxis during interdisciplinary care rounds. If prophylaxis is not ordered, ensure a rationale is identified and documented.
	◆ Establish protocols that allow pharmacy to order peptic ulcer prophylaxis.

4. Deep Venous Thrombosis Prophylaxis

As with stress ulcers, deep vein thrombosis (DVT) occurs more commonly in critically ill patients. Administration of DVT prophylaxis reduces the risk of development of DVT.

NURSING IMPLICATIONS	
	◆ Address DVT prophylaxis on admission to ICU.
	◆ Discuss DVT prophylaxis during interdisciplinary care rounds; identify and document rationale if the patient is not receiving prophylaxis.
	◆ Consider sequential compression devices if the patient is not eligible for pharmacologic prophylaxis.
	◆ Establish protocols that allow pharmacy to order DVT prophylaxis if not already in place.

5. Chlorhexidine Oral Care

Mechanically ventilated patients are at increased risk for the development of dental plaque. This plaque may serve as a reservoir for organisms that may lead to VAP. Oral care, including oral rinse with 0.12% chlorhexidine, has been shown to reduce the incidence of VAP.

NURSING IMPLICATIONS	
	◆ Educate nursing and respiratory therapy staff about the benefits of performing good oral care in reducing VAP.
	◆ Perform daily oral care, including oral rinse with 0.12% chlorhexidine.
	◆ Address oral care during interdisciplinary rounds.
	◆ Add chlorhexidine to the medication administration record to ensure its application.

Source: Institute for Healthcare Improvement. (2014). Implement the IHI ventilator bundle. Retrieved from http://www.ihi.org/resources/Pages/Changes/Implement-theVentilatorBundle.aspx

sticky mucus also causes excessive coughing, which worsens pain in postoperative or trauma patients. Finally, mucous plugs in the airways can lead to atelectasis and decreased oxygenation.

The nurse can help maintain the mobility of mucus by encouraging fluids in all patients who are at risk for dried secretions. Fluid intake ideally should be 6 to 8 glasses of fluid, preferably water, every day. Caffeinated beverages (e.g., coffee, tea, cola) and alcohol can have a diuretic effect, thus dehydrating the patient. In some patients, milk products tend to thicken secretions, so these patients should avoid dairy products. Patients whose oral intake is restricted may require additional aerosol therapy to ensure secretion mobility.

POSITIONING AND AMBULATION

Changing positions and movement in general help to shift respiratory mucus into portions of the airways where it may generate a cough, making expectoration easier. Positioning and movement prevent mucus from pooling, which decreases the risk of bacterial colonization and infection. Mucus tends to pool in the airways of people with limited mobility. Immobile patients, patients experiencing pain, and patients with limited exercise tolerance (because of heart or lung disease) often retain secretions.

Encourage changing positions frequently. Whenever possible, position the patient with unilateral lung problems with the good lung down to promote optimal matching of ventilation and perfusion. Moving the patient from one side to another or assisting with ambulation when possible aids the lung's natural clearance mechanisms. Supine position has been associated with an increase in VAP and increased risk for aspiration, especially in patients receiving tube feedings.

Ambulation is difficult for some respiratory patients because of dyspnea with exertion. Whenever possible, help promote exercise tolerance by encouraging progressive ambulation. Additional benefits of increased exercise tolerance include decreased oxygen consumption and extra strength for effective coughing. Some patients may need portable oxygen during periods of ambulation.

 APPLY YOUR CRITICAL THINKING

You are caring for Mr. Jacob 1 day after his abdominal surgery. On your morning assessment, you obtain the following vital signs data: BP 142/80, pulse 84, respirations 14 and shallow, and temperature 38.2°C. Pain is well controlled on PCA morphine, breath sounds are diminished at the bases with a few crackles, and O_2 is at 94%. Based on this information, how will you individualize your plan of care for Mr. Jacob?

Check your answer in Appendix B.

DEEP BREATHING

Shallow breathing or an ineffective cough can lead to mucous plugging, atelectasis, hypoxemia, and pneumonia. Taking deep breaths helps to expand alveoli and promote an effective cough, which decreases the risk of atelectasis. Deep breathing is essential for the prevention of pulmonary complications in the at-risk patient. Pain, lung disease, muscle weakness, or neurologic impairment can hinder a patient's ability to breathe deeply. A major nursing task is to coach and encourage the patient in deep-breathing techniques. **Procedure 26-5** explains this technique.

Deep breathing is useful for all patients, especially after surgery. There are no contraindications to deep breathing: Anyone can do it at any time. Deep breathing may cause discomfort for the patient with an abdominal incision or broken ribs; this can be minimized by splinting the incision with a pillow. Deep breathing decreases the risk of atelectasis by opening collapsed alveoli. A deep breath also strengthens the cough and aids in moving mucus in the airways.

ASSISTING WITH INCENTIVE SPIROMETRY

The incentive spirometer motivates the patient to breathe deeply by offering the incentive of measuring progress. Models of incentive spirometers vary greatly, but all provide the patient with some observable indicator of how deep a breath he or she has taken. Some models use a bellowslike device that deflates as the patient inspires; others use ping-pong balls that float. Regardless of the device, the patient is visually motivated to take increasingly deeper breaths. The patient and nurse set realistic goals for each breathing session, and the patient works independently toward achieving each goal. Incentive spirometry motivates the patient to take responsibility for the progress of deep-breathing therapy. A reasonable therapy schedule is 8 to 10 breaths hourly during waking hours. To avoid hyperventilation, encourage the patient to perform the exercises slowly. **Procedure 26-6** explains the details of this technique. Document the results of the exercise in the medical record.

Nursing Interventions for Altered Respiratory Function

When atelectasis, excess secretions, or bronchoconstriction occurs, nurses can use many therapies to support the patient and improve oxygen status. Some of these techniques, such as coughing, are simple. Others, such as ventilators and tracheostomy care, are more complex and reserved for people with severe respiratory dysfunction.

COUGHING

Retained secretions increase the work of breathing and may contribute to atelectasis and hypoxemia. No single measure controls respiratory secretions more effectively than a strong cough that pushes secretions upward. To cough effectively, the patient must be able to take a deep breath and generate rapid airflow (see **Procedure 26-5**).

For many patients, producing a strong cough is difficult or impossible. The patient experiencing postoperative or trauma-related pain may be unable or unwilling to take the deep breath needed to cough. Patients with COPD are often unable to exhale quickly enough to generate an effective cough. Some patients are simply too weak to cough, and others do not understand how to produce an effective cough. Finally, a patient with a tracheostomy or endotracheal tube cannot cough with optimal efficiency because the glottis cannot close.

Deep Cough

Encourage the postoperative patient who does not have lung disease to cough deeply. Deep coughing will help to mobilize secretions and to open collapsed alveoli. The patient should inspire as deeply as possible and then hold the breath a second or so while closing the glottis. He or she should then release the air while suddenly opening the glottis.

The deep cough can cause pain around the incisional area in patients who have had abdominal or thoracic surgery. To help control the pain, the patient can support the incisional area with a pillow, using it as a splint to immobilize the wound. This is referred to as **splinting** the incision. For patients with severe incisional discomfort, scheduling coughing sessions after the patient has received pain medications may prove helpful.

Stacked Cough

Some patients find coughing painful even after having received pain medication. For them, a stacked cough may cause less pain and be almost as effective. Stacked coughing is the release of several short blasts of air instead of one deep cough. This type of cough prevents excessive stretching of the incisional area and also minimizes the airway collapse that may accompany deep coughing.

Low-Flow (Huff) Cough

A third type of cough is called low-flow or "huff" coughing. The low-flow cough is most effective for patients with COPD, whose airways tend to collapse with rapid exhalation. Slowing the airflow actually is more helpful in expelling secretions. Instruct the patient to inhale deeply. Instead of closing the glottis and generating high pressure, the patient says "huff" three or four times while exhaling.

Quad Cough

Patients with neuromuscular disease and quadriplegic patients often need direct assistance to generate an effective cough. The patient takes a deep breath, or the nurse provides a deep breath with a manual resuscitation bag. The patient then holds the deep breath for a moment. With your hands placed just below the patient's rib cage, assist the patient by quickly pushing in and upward, much like performing the Heimlich maneuver. The resultant rush of air acts as a cough by helping to dislodge mucus from the airways.

PURSED-LIP BREATHING

Pursed-lip breathing helps patients with obstructive lung diseases such as COPD or asthma by causing a back pressure in the airways, which eases exhalation and prevents air trapping.

To perform pursed-lip breathing, the patient takes a deep breath and holds it for a moment, then exhales slowly through lips held almost closed. By pushing the air against the small orifice made by the pursed lips, the patient builds pressure backward through the airways. This back pressure pushes the airways open throughout exhalation and prevents airway collapse. Thus, more air escapes during exhalation and helps prevent air trapping.

CHEST PHYSIOTHERAPY

Chest physiotherapy commonly is prescribed to help clear excessive bronchial secretions from airways. It is based on the premise that mucus can be shaken from the walls of the airways and helped to drain from the lungs. Chest physiotherapy can be useful for many patients with cystic fibrosis, COPD, lobar collapse, bronchiectasis, and mucous plugging. Contraindications are pneumonia (Yang et al., 2013), hemoptysis, and pneumothorax.

The primary techniques of this method of secretion mobilization are percussion, vibration, and postural drainage. Any of these physiotherapy techniques can be used alone, but they are most effective when used together. The patient's ability to tolerate these procedures may limit the vigor with which they are applied, so positioning and clapping techniques may need to be modified. Often, the respiratory therapist or physical therapist provides chest physiotherapy in the acute care setting.

Percussion

Percussion produces a mechanical wave of energy that is transmitted through the chest wall to the mucus-coated bronchial tubes. Strike the chest rhythmically with cupped hands over the area where secretions are located. Take care to avoid striking over the spine or kidneys, on female breasts, or on incisions or broken ribs. Pneumatic or electrical chest percussors are effective substitutes for manual percussion.

Vibration

Vibration works in much the same manner as percussion. In this technique, use your hands like a gentle jackhammer: Place them on the patient's chest and rapidly and vigorously vibrate them while the patient exhales. This technique may help dislodge secretions and stimulate a cough.

Oscillatory Positive Expiratory Pressure Therapy

Oscillatory positive expiratory pressure (PEP) therapy combines the resistive features of a PEP device with oscillations that produce vibration. Exhaling against resistance slows the expiratory phase of breathing and produces positive pressure that helps open peripheral airways (alveoli). PEP therapy can be performed independently by the patient and has outcomes equal to chest physiotherapy provided by the respiratory therapist or nurse. Indications and contraindication are the same as for chest physiotherapy.

Postural Drainage

Postural drainage uses gravity to assist in the movement of secretions. The patient is placed in various positions to facilitate mucus flow from different segments of the lung (Fig. 26-8). Placing a mucus-filled segment of the lung higher than the rest of the lung allows the mucus in that segment to flow more readily downward toward larger airways. In this way, coughing or suctioning more easily removes the mucus.

Postural Drainage Positions

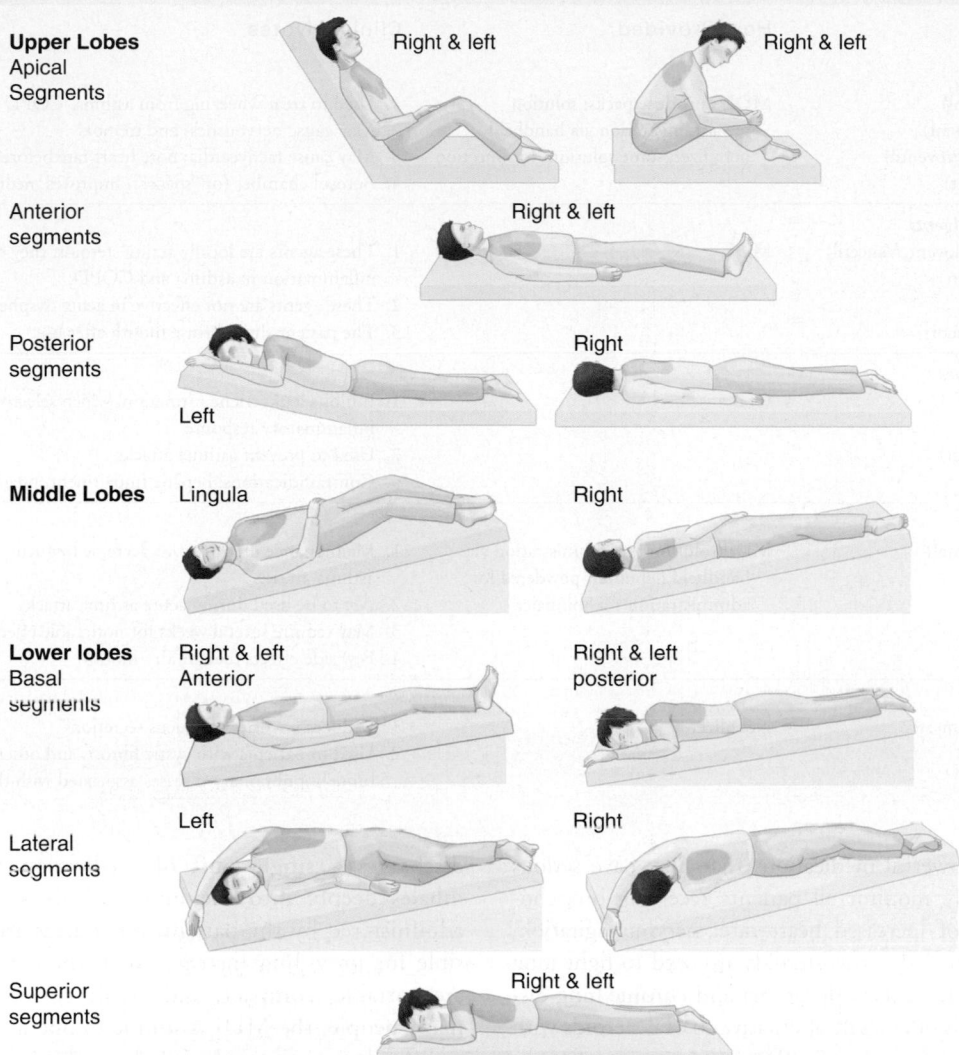

Upper Lobes
Apical
Segments

Right & left

Right & left

Anterior
segments

Right & left

Posterior
segments

Left

Right

Middle Lobes Lingula

Right

Lower lobes
Basal
segments

Right & left
Anterior

Right & left
posterior

Lateral
segments

Left

Right

Superior
segments

Right & left

FIGURE 26-8 Various postural drainage positions are used to mobilize secretions from specific lobes and segments of the lung.

Not all postural drainage positions are well tolerated by all patients. The Trendelenburg (head-down) position can increase shortness of breath in the patient with COPD because the abdominal organs limit diaphragm movement. Lying head down can increase intracranial pressure and is contraindicated for patients with acute head injuries. It can also be very stressful for patients with cardiac problems. The nurse or therapist who administers postural drainage may need to modify the treatment for patients who cannot tolerate the prescribed positions.

AEROSOL THERAPY

An aerosol is a suspension of microscopic liquid droplets in air or oxygen. Aerosol therapy may be given for any of the following reasons:

- To add moisture to oxygen delivery systems
- To hydrate thick sputum and prevent mucous plugging
- To administer various drugs to the airways

A large-volume nebulizer or an ultrasonic nebulizer will deliver a moist fog continuously to the airways. While absorbing the water, the mucous blanket loosens, which facilitates its removal. The watery mist also soothes inflamed airways. Heating the water in the nebulizer increases the amount of moisture delivered.

Check the reservoir frequently to ensure that it is filled with sterile water. Parts must be screwed together tightly to ensure full delivery of the prescribed level of oxygen. The large-bore tubing must be drained often to prevent buildup of condensation. Monitor the mist temperature to prevent possible injury. Finally, because aerosols loosen dried secretions, help the patient remove secretions by instructing the patient to cough or by suctioning.

Aerosol Medications

Various drugs are administered by aerosol. Bronchodilators reverse bronchospasm most quickly when administered directly to the lungs. Although commonly used and highly effective,

TABLE 26-5 COMMON MEDICATIONS FOR PATIENTS WITH RESPIRATORY CONDITIONS

Agent	How Provided	Clinical Notes
Bronchodilators Isoetharine (Bronkosol) Metaproterenol (Alupent) Albuterol (Ventolin, Proventil) Ipratropium (Atrovent)	MDI; unit-dose packs; solution for administration via handheld nebulizer; some solutions for injection	1. Used to treat wheezing from asthma, COPD 2. May cause nervousness and tremors 3. May cause tachycardia; note heart rate before and after treatment 4. Aerosol chamber (or "spacer") improves medication dispersal.
Anti-Inflammatory Agents Beclomethasone (Beclovent, Vanceril) Budesonide (Pulmicort) Fluticasone (Flovent) Triamcinolone (Azmacort)	MDI	1. These agents are locally acting steroids; they decrease inflammation in asthma and COPD. 2. These agents are not effective in acute dyspnea attacks. 3. The patient should rinse mouth after use.
Leukotriene Inhibitors Zafirlukast (Accolate) Zileuton (Zyflo) Montelukast (Singulair)	Oral	1. Inhibits leukotriene formation, which selectively decreases inflammatory response 2. Used to prevent asthma attacks 3. Contraindications: hepatic impairment, pregnancy
Antiasthmatic Agent Cromolyn sodium (Intal)	MDI; solution for administration via handheld nebulizer; powdered for administration via Spinhaler	1. Maintenance drug used to decrease frequency and intensity of asthma attacks 2. *Not* to be used during acute asthma attack 3. May require several weeks for noticeable effects 4. Few side effects (cough, dry mouth)
Mucolytic Agent Acetylcysteine (Mucomyst)	Nebulizer	1. Reduces viscosity of mucus secretions 2. Used in patients with cystic fibrosis and other acute or chronic bronchopulmonary diseases associated with thick mucus

these agents are powerful medications that may have serious side effects. Closely monitor all patients receiving bronchodilators for signs of increased heart rate, nervous agitation, and restlessness. Inhaled corticosteroids are used to fight lung inflammation. For patients with asthma and chronic lung disease, aerosol steroids offer a safe alternative to oral steroids with fewer long-term negative systemic effects. Other types of medications delivered by aerosol include cromolyn (Intal), which is used to prevent asthma attacks. Patients with cystic fibrosis can receive antibiotics delivered by aerosol to counter stubborn lung infections. Table 26-5 lists common respiratory medications.

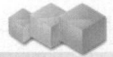 **Concept Mastery Alert**

Many patients with restrictive lung disease take bronchodilators as well as corticosteroids. Corticosteroids interfere with the pathways involved in the inflammatory process, relieving the symptoms of restrictive lung diseases over time. Bronchodilators do not affect inflammation. Instead, they relax the smooth muscle of the airway, decreasing resistance and improving airflow.

Metered-Dose Inhalers

Gas-powered, cartridge-type nebulizers called metered-dose inhalers (MDIs) provide the patient with a premeasured dose of aerosolized medication. Squeezing the gas cartridge

discharges a single puff of medication that the patient inhales deeply into the lungs. MDIs are ordinarily self-administered by the patient, but nurses are usually responsible for providing instruction in their use. These devices are portable, compact, and highly convenient to use. For many people, the MDI is simple to operate, but others find it difficult to activate the inhaler and inhale simultaneously. A chamber (or "spacer") that attaches to the MDI helps to minimize this problem and improves the MDI's efficiency. Figure 26-9 shows an MDI with a spacer, and Chapter 20 illustrates step-by-step guidelines for using an MDI to deliver medication.

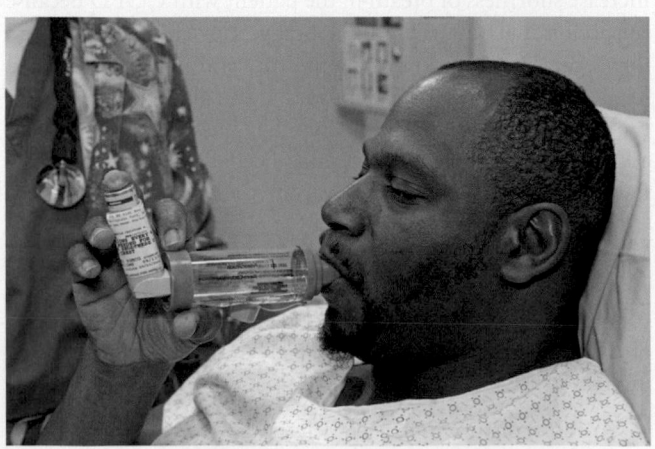

FIGURE 26-9 MDI with spacer.

Because MDIs can deliver different types of respiratory medication, patients may use several MDIs in their medication regimen. A complete understanding of each medication's actions and dosing schedule is essential for optimal management of respiratory symptoms. Instruct the patient to rinse the mouth with water after administration of an MDI; many drugs administered by this route may cause oral fungal infection (thrush).

Dry Powder Inhalers

An alternative to MDIs, a dry powder inhaler (DPI), delivers medication to the lungs in the form of a dry powder. DPIs come in different shapes and sizes. The device needs to be loaded or actuated and is breath activated. Once the dose is loaded, the patient places the mouthpiece of the device into the mouth and takes a deep breath. If the patient has an insufficient inhalation flow rate, the dose delivered may be incomplete. A minimum respiratory effort is needed for proper delivery; therefore, its use is reserved for older children and adults.

SAFETY ALERT

It is especially important to mark the MDI to be used in an emergency (fast-acting beta$_2$ agonist) because the long-acting medications are ineffective during an acute attack.

Handheld Nebulizers

Small-volume nebulizers (Fig. 26-10) offer an alternative to patients who are unable to operate MDIs. Instead of providing a full dose of medication in one or two breaths, the handheld nebulizer delivers a steady stream of aerosolized medicine that the patient breathes over the course of several minutes. The use of nebulizers eliminates the problem of trying to coordinate inspiration with cartridge activation. These devices are operated by means of a compressor or by oxygen at 4 to 5 L/min.

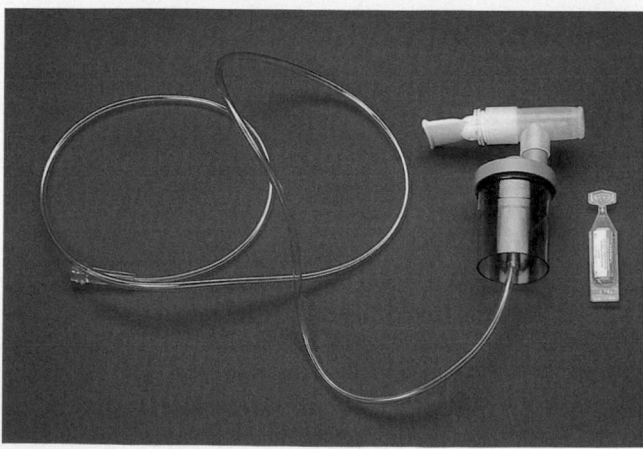

FIGURE 26-10 Handheld nebulizer.

The patient inhales deeply and holds each breath for a moment, which allows for more effective aerosol deposition into distant portions of the airways. The patient continues breathing slowly in this manner until the nebulizer is empty.

OXYGEN THERAPY

Some patients need oxygen therapy to maintain adequate arterial blood oxygen levels. Lung disease, cardiovascular problems, blood disorders such as anemia, and high metabolic demands of healing tissues can limit the body's oxygen supply.

Oxygen therapy is used primarily to reverse hypoxemia. It can help to accomplish three fundamental goals:

- Improved tissue oxygenation
- Decreased work of breathing in patients with dyspnea
- Decreased work of the heart in patients with cardiac disease

General Principles of Oxygen Administration

Oxygen is prescribed either in terms of flow or concentration, depending on the patient's needs and the delivery device's capabilities. Oxygen flow is expressed in liters per minute. Concentration is expressed as a percentage or as a fraction of inspired oxygen (FiO$_2$). A general rule for safe oxygen therapy is to use the lowest oxygen concentration or flow possible to achieve an acceptable blood oxygen level.

When administering oxygen, assess the patient's response regularly to determine the need for continuation or adjustment of therapy. The patient's color, alertness, heart rate, and breathing effort are general indicators of the effectiveness of oxygen therapy. **Arterial blood gas (ABG)** monitoring and pulse oximetry provide more specific information concerning patient response to oxygen therapy. For most patients, the aim of oxygen therapy should be to maintain the PaO$_2$ above 60 mm Hg or the SpO$_2$ above 93%. It is rarely necessary to exceed a PaO$_2$ of 90 mm Hg or an SpO$_2$ greater than 97%. Most often, patients use oxygen continuously for as short a time as possible until they can maintain satisfactory blood oxygenation without it. Most patients require relatively low concentrations of oxygen to correct hypoxemia. See **Procedure 26-7** for a general guide to administering oxygen.

Selection of Oxygen Systems

Various types of equipment are available to provide oxygen in a wide range of flows and concentrations (Fig. 26-11). Nurses should be familiar with the proper operation and capabilities of various oxygen devices.

The patient's oxygenation status determines which oxygen delivery device is most appropriate. Although comfort is also a factor, the best oxygen device for each patient is the one capable of providing his or her oxygen needs.

If a patient needs only a small amount of additional oxygen to maintain adequate oxygenation, he or she can use a cannula or low concentration Venturi-type mask. If the

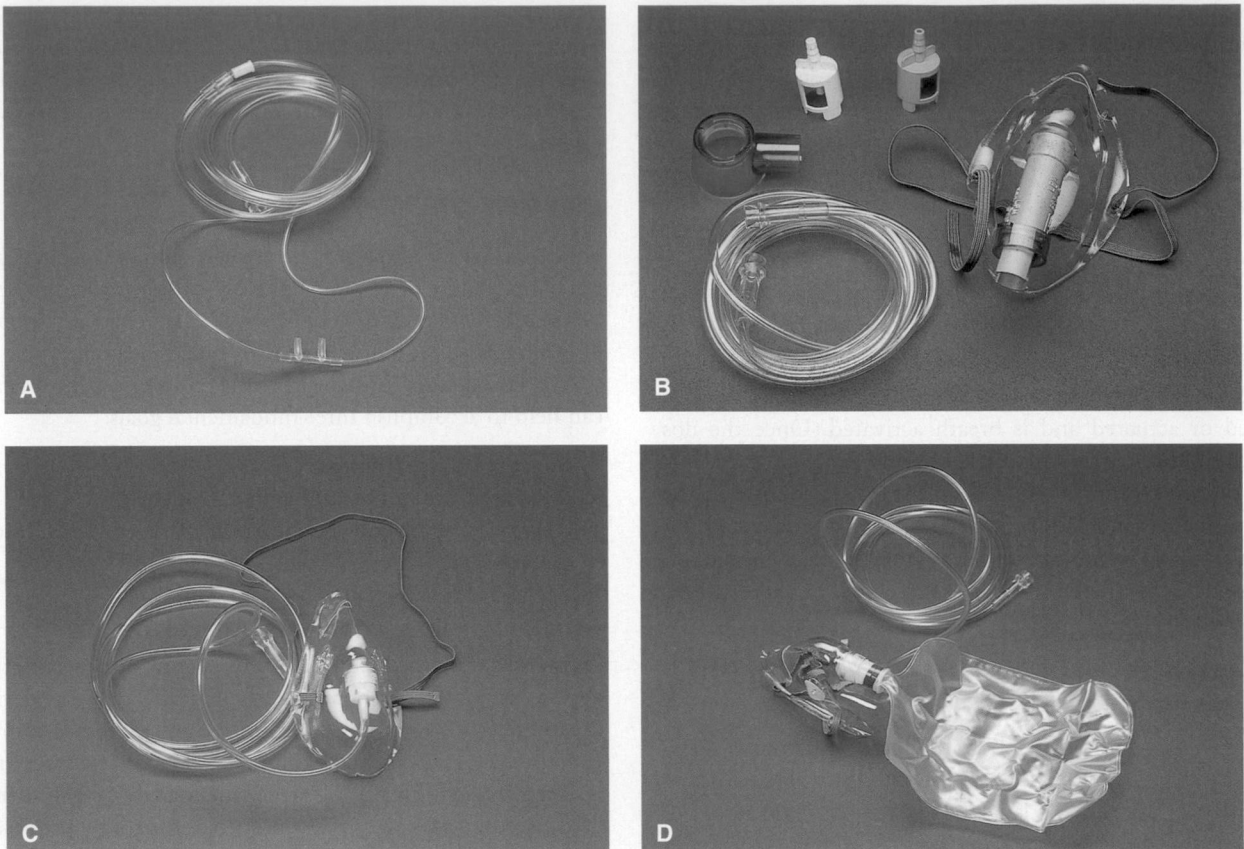

FIGURE 26-11 Common oxygen delivery devices. **A.** Cannula. **B.** Venturi mask. **C.** Simple oxygen mask. **D.** Reservoir mask.

patient requires a moderate amount of oxygen, a simple mask is suitable. When a patient needs a high concentration of oxygen, a reservoir-type mask, often called a nonrebreather mask, can be used. Although the reservoir bag does not need to be fully inflated, the oxygen flow rate should be set at 12-15 LPM. This valve and reservoir system reduces rebreathing of CO_2. Table 26-6 compares and contrasts various commonly used oxygen delivery systems. Patients who require more precise delivery of oxygen, along with assistance with ventilation, need a mechanical ventilator to regulate oxygen and breathing.

Orders for oxygen administration typically include parameters to maintain the patient's oxygen saturation at a certain level. For example, an order may read, "Administer oxygen per nasal cannula to maintain O_2 sat at ≥93%." The nurse will adjust the oxygen as needed, using the lowest flow rate or concentration possible to keep the O_2 saturation at the desired level. If high flow rates or concentrations are needed, the provider should be notified.

Transtracheal catheters, implanted surgically, are becoming more common. These catheters (12 French or smaller) are inserted through the patient's neck into the trachea. They are attached to a portable oxygen system. With this oxygen delivery device, less oxygen is wasted because the catheter enters the lung directly. The patient needs less oxygen to manage the condition well.

Safety Considerations

Because oxygen is a drug, its use requires a prescription. Policies and standing orders often permit the nurse to administer oxygen in emergency situations if the provider is not immediately available to write an order. Although oxygen is generally safe when used properly, certain precautions must be observed. As with all drugs, the potential exists for causing harm with misuse.

When a patient begins oxygen therapy, inform him or her of the importance of wearing the oxygen device.

> **SAFETY ALERT**
> When oxygen is administered in the home, a "no smoking" sign must be posted by the oxygen, and all visitors must be educated about the importance of not smoking. Although oxygen is not flammable, it greatly accelerates combustion and could cause a fire from a small spark.

Check the oxygen flow often to ensure that the prescribed amount is being delivered. If the patient is using a humidifier or nebulizer (to minimize the drying effect of oxygen on the airways), ensure that the reservoir is filled with water and is attached properly. A leak in the delivery system can prevent the patient from receiving the full amount of oxygen, so all connections must be tight.

TABLE 26-6 OXYGEN THERAPY EQUIPMENT

Device	Oxygen Capability	Nursing Considerations
Cannula (nasal prongs)	22%–44% when operated at 1–6 L/min	1. Most commonly used oxygen device because of convenience and patient comfort 2. Delivered oxygen concentration can vary with patient breathing pattern; "rule of four" used to estimate concentration: For each L/min of O_2, concentration increases by 4% (e.g., 1 L/min provides 22%, 2 L/min provides 26%) 3. Limit maximum O_2 flow to 6 L/min to minimize drying of nasal mucosa; use humidifier prn 4. Nasal passages must be patent for the patient to receive O_2: Mouth breathing does not appreciably diminish delivered O_2 5. Delivered O_2 concentration can vary depending on the patient's breathing pattern; relatively consistent O_2 delivery with quiet, steady breathing
Transtracheal catheter	0.5–2 L/min	1. Device is surgically implanted in trachea of O_2-dependent patient as alternative to cannula 2. Advantages: Efficient use of O_2 (no waste because all O_2 is delivered directly to lungs); practically invisible, so the patient feels less self-conscious 3. Suitable only for patients who can care for the device
Venturi (Venti) mask	24%–50% when operated at 3–8 L/min as specified by manufacturer	1. Provides precise and consistent O_2 concentration 2. Essential to adjust mask according to specifications to ensure accurate O_2 delivery 3. Noisy; like all masks, may cause claustrophobia
Simple mask	40%–60% when operated at 6–10 L/min	1. Most common midrange O_2 delivery device 2. Minimum of 5 L/min O_2 required to prevent the patient from rebreathing exhaled carbon dioxide 3. As with cannula, actual delivered O_2 concentration varies with breathing pattern 4. Not suitable for the patient with COPD because of potential for excessive oxygenation
Reservoir mask	Up to 90% + when operated at 10–15 L/min	1. Used for critically ill patient 2. Use sufficient flow to keep O_2 reservoir inflated
Large-volume pneumatic nebulizer	21%–100% when operated at 12–15 L/min	1. Used to deliver O_2 with continuous aerosol therapy; required by many patients with artificial airways (e.g., tracheostomies) 2. Temperature must be monitored and tubing must be drained frequently
Incubator	22%–40%+	1. Enclosure used for environmental control for newborn infants 2. Extremely imprecise O_2 delivery; accuracy varies each time unit is opened
Oxyhood	22%–90% + when operated at 7–12 L/min	1. Precise O_2 delivery for newborns and small infants 2. Minimum O_2 flow of 7 L/min flushes infant's exhaled carbon dioxide 3. Oxygen must be prewarmed and humidified to prevent infant heat loss 4. Frequent analysis needed to prevent excessive oxygenation
Oxygen tent	21%–30%+	1. Primarily used by small child unable to wear mask or cannula 2. Mainly used as "mist tent" to deliver high humidity to children with croup 3. Extremely inefficient O_2 delivery system; O_2 delivery fluctuates because leaks are common

prn, as needed.

Oxygen therapy has the potential for causing serious health consequences in some patients. Relatively low oxygen concentrations can damage the newborn's retina and result in blindness. For this reason, meticulously monitor all newborns receiving oxygen therapy.

High oxygen concentrations are toxic to lung tissue. Severely ill patients who require intense oxygen therapy for extended periods may suffer resultant lung damage. Although this concern is not serious for the average patient who uses a nasal cannula, oxygen toxicity poses a danger for the patient who needs intensive respiratory care.

In the past, concern has been raised that administering oxygen to patients with COPD may suppress the drive to breathe. In people with healthy lungs, the primary drive to breathe is hypercapnia. Some COPD patients chronically retain CO_2 and lose the hypercapneic incentive to breathe, relying on hypoxia as the motivation to breathe. Administering oxygen theoretically removes all drive to breathe; therefore, many people believe oxygen must be given with caution to all COPD patients. However, only some COPD patients retain CO_2. In addition, there is little evidence that oxygen administration reduces drive to breathe in any patient. If a patient with COPD needs oxygen, it should be given. As with all therapies, patients should be monitored closely. If the patient's condition deteriorates, further intervention is needed (Abdo & Heunks, 2012).

> **! SAFETY ALERT**
> Administration of oxygen to patients with COPD should be done cautiously. Target oxygen saturation for patients with COPD is 88% to 92%. Watch for possible signs of deterioration; provide additional respiratory support, including mechanical ventilation, if needed.

DYSPNEA MANAGEMENT

Effective treatment for dyspnea addresses both its physical and psychological components. Common interventions used to manage dyspnea include anxiety control, activity modification, and comfort measures that modify the patient's breathing pattern.

Regardless of its specific cause, dyspnea can be extremely frightening, both for the patient who is experiencing it and for the nurse who must treat it. To help the patient, remain calm while offering reassurance. Speak calmly and slowly, offering one simple direction at a time to minimize the patient's anxiety. Listening empathically and helping the patient relax are sometimes all that he or she needs to relieve dyspnea. When uncontrolled anxiety is the primary cause of a patient's dyspnea, the provider may prescribe mild antianxiety medication.

Comfort measures include the use of positioning. The patient usually is most comfortable sitting upright, which allows the diaphragm to move freely. If oxygen is ordered, see that it is operating as prescribed. Focus the patient's efforts on slowing the breathing rate. The patient should breathe through the nose if possible, using the diaphragm for inspiration. Assist by gently pushing down on the patient's shoulders; this discourages the inefficient use of accessory muscles. Usually, with gentle encouragement and reassurance, the patient's breathing rate will gradually decrease and the dyspnea will pass. Whenever dyspnea occurs, try to establish its immediate cause and its severity. Comfort measures are always appropriate, as is oxygen when a standing order is available. Most institutions have policies allowing nurses to begin oxygen therapy for the dyspneic patient while they are seeking a provider's order. When oxygen and comfort measures do not decrease dyspnea within a short period or when dyspnea appears suddenly and without warning, notify the provider.

HYPERVENTILATION MANAGEMENT

The patient who hyperventilates exhibits rapid breathing and symptoms such as dizziness and tingling sensations; ABG indicates a $PaCO_2$ below 35 mm Hg. The patient may experience subjective feelings of dyspnea. Direct nursing efforts at decreasing patient anxiety and getting the patient to breathe at a slower rate.

If simple encouragement cannot accomplish this, the patient may use a paper bag as a rebreathing device. The patient breathes in and out of the bag for several breaths. In the process of rebreathing the exhaled carbon dioxide from the bag, the patient's $PaCO_2$ can gradually slow the rate of breathing until it returns to normal. The dizziness and tingling sensations should disappear. As with dyspnea, a complete assessment of hyperventilation is needed, and referral to the provider may be required. Patients hyperventilating for medical conditions other than anxiety may delay needed treatment while breathing into a bag. Breathing into a bag should be performed only under the direct supervision of the nurse and under protocols or a provider's order; excessive breathing of CO_2 may increase the patient's panic.

ASSISTED VENTILATION

Bilevel positive airway pressure therapy uses a mechanical ventilator to assist inspiration. The patient's inspiratory effort triggers the ventilator, which pushes air into the lungs. The positive pressure helps to prevent and treat atelectasis by helping to open underinflated alveoli. Bilevel positive airway pressure delivers higher pressures during inspiration and lower pressures during expiration to keep airways open. Continuous positive airway pressure (CPAP) uses oxygen under constant pressure to accomplish this objective. CPAP is often used at night to decrease periodic hypoxemia associated with sleep apnea. CPAP is delivered via specially fitted masks or nasal prongs that are attached to a machine that delivers appropriate pressure. Many patients do not tolerate CPAP or bilevel positive airway pressure well because the equipment is claustrophobic and noisy. When these devices are used, the individual controls the respiratory rate and depth. It is important to note that bilevel positive airway pressure or CPAP does not breathe for the patient and never replaces a ventilator for a patient who requires ventilatory support. Patients using CPAP or bilevel positive airway pressure devices should always have the physical and cognitive ability to remove the mask in case of vomiting.

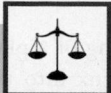

ETHICAL/LEGAL ISSUE

WITHDRAWAL OF VENTILATOR SUPPORT

You are working in an ICU, caring for an 18-year-old girl who was in a very serious automobile accident two nights ago. Prognosis is very poor because two electroencephalograms (EEGs) demonstrated no brain wave activity. She is being supported by a mechanical ventilator. The provider tells you that he plans to talk with her grieving parents about removing the ventilator and obtaining permission to donate the daughter's organs for transplantation.

CRITICAL THINKING CHALLENGE

- Try to identify factors that healthcare providers need to consider when requesting organs for transplantation.
- Visualize how you would feel if present with the provider and family at this time. Identify ways that you could be supportive.
- Do the parents have the right to refuse a request for organ transplantation? If so, how would you support them in this decision?
- How might consenting to organ transplantation assist this family in the grieving process?

To optimize the benefits, experienced personnel should administer positive pressure therapy. The nurse or respiratory care practitioner (RCP) must assess each patient's breathing needs and individualize treatment accordingly. Encourage all patients who use CPAP or bilevel positive airway pressure to bring their equipment to the hospital so that potential respiratory complications can be avoided.

SAFETY ALERT

Alarms should always be audible and never turned off.

ARTIFICIAL AIRWAYS

An artificial airway is a device inserted through the mouth, nose, or throat to provide direct access to the lungs. Oropharyngeal airways, nasopharyngeal airways ("nasal trumpets"), endotracheal tubes, and tracheostomy tubes are examples of artificial airways.

Oral or Nasal Pharyngeal Airways

These airways are used to bypass upper airway obstructions or to facilitate secretion removal (Fig. 26-12). Oropharyngeal airways (Fig. 26-12A) are simple to insert but are poorly tolerated

COLLABORATING WITH THE HEALTHCARE TEAM:
Consulting With Respiratory Therapy

You have just admitted Mr. Johnson, a 52-year-old man, from the postanesthesia care unit (PACU); he had gastric bypass surgery. After completing your assessment and reading his medical history, you feel that he is at high risk for respiratory complications and decide to consult with a respiratory therapist.

SITUATION: John (respiratory therapist covering your medical-surgical unit), I would like you to come up and assess Mr. Johnson and help us develop a plan to prevent respiratory complications during his postoperative recovery.

BACKGROUND: Mr. Johnson had gastric bypass surgery this morning. He has a BMI of 40 and a history of sleep apnea. His history states he has been noncompliant using his CPAP and did not bring it with him. He has a PCA for pain management since transfer from the PACU, he has rated his pain at 10, and he needed two extra pain medication boluses. His respiratory rate is 22 but shallow, and his oxygen saturation is 91% on 2 L/min via cannula.

ASSESSMENT: I am concerned that Mr. Johnson might experience atelectasis, pneumonia, or even respiratory depression considering his surgery, his obesity, his history of sleep apnea, and his requirement for large doses of medication to control his pain.

RECOMMENDATION: Please see Mr. Johnson today and evaluate whether he needs CPAP or a continuous oximetry to prevent and monitor respiratory depression. Also, let's individualize his plan to prevent postoperative respiratory complications.

CRITICAL THINKING CHALLENGE

- Discuss why Mr. Johnson's risk factors can cause respiratory complications postoperatively.
- Consider independent nursing actions that you can discuss with the respiratory therapist to add to Mr. Johnson's plan of care.
- Do you need an order to consult with respiratory therapy concerning Mr. Johnson? How would you find out if an order is required?
- Since CPAP and continuous oximetry are not frequently used on your medical-surgical unit, how could you familiarize yourself with this new equipment to be able to provide safe care for Mr. Johnson?

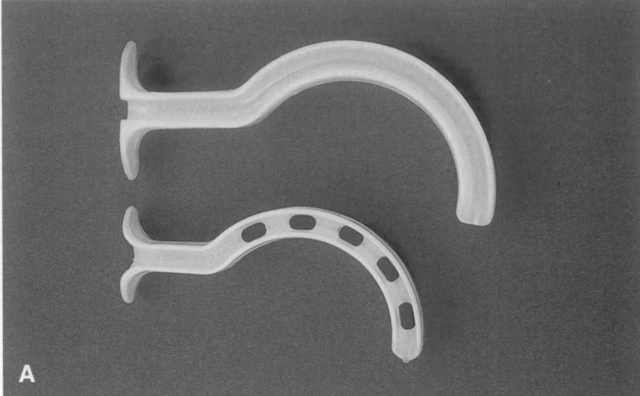

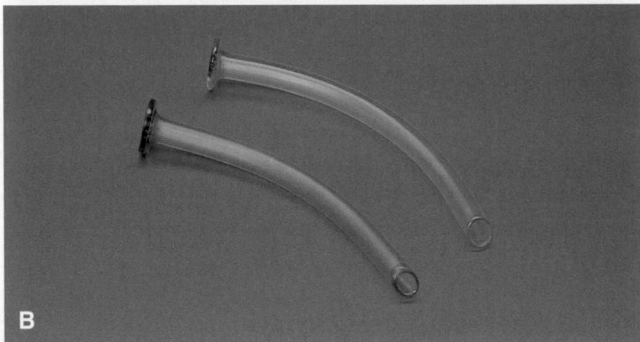

FIGURE 26-12 Artificial airways. **A.** Oral airways. **B.** Nasal trumpets.

by all but the comatose patient. The noncomatose patient is likely to gag on an oropharyngeal airway, so a nasal trumpet (Fig. 26-12B) is preferable. These airways should be well lubricated with water-soluble gel before they are inserted into the nose.

Endotracheal Tubes

An endotracheal tube is a plastic tube inserted through the nose or mouth into the trachea (Fig. 26-13). These airways are used to ventilate a patient during surgery or when mechanical ventilation is necessary. They are also used to protect the airway in a comatose person.

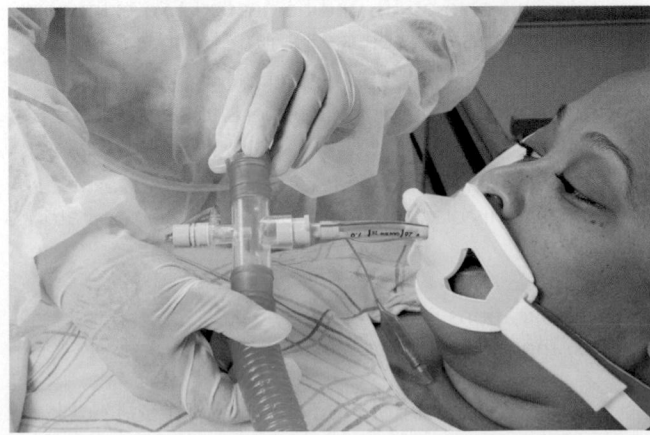

FIGURE 26-13 Endotracheal tube setup with ventilator tubing attached.

Tracheostomy

The **tracheostomy** is an artificial airway consisting of a plastic tube surgically implanted just below the larynx into the trachea; the tube bypasses the mouth and upper airway. The surgical procedure that establishes the artificial airway is called a tracheotomy; the resultant airway is a tracheostomy. This procedure is most often done as a temporary measure. Unlike a permanent laryngectomy, in which the entire larynx is removed, a tracheotomy leaves the structure of the airway intact. A patient may require this procedure to bypass a severe or recurrent upper airway obstruction. The patient who regularly aspirates food or stomach contents may need a tracheostomy to protect the airway. A few patients may need this type of airway to help with secretion control because a tracheostomy provides ready access for suctioning. Finally, the patient who requires long-term mechanical ventilation may need a tracheostomy to provide the safest and most stable artificial airway available. Many tracheotomized patients on the general nursing unit are former patients of the ICU or have had head and neck surgery.

Tracheostomy tubes come in various types. All tubes contain an outer cannula that fits into the trachea and a flange that rests against the neck and allows the tube to be fastened in place. An obturator is a guide that is inserted into the tracheostomy tube to ease insertion and is then removed. Some tracheostomy tubes contain an inner cannula that locks into place and can be removed for cleaning (Fig. 26-14). Cuffed tracheostomy tubes contain an inflatable cuff (or balloon) that is inflated to stabilize the tube in the trachea (Fig. 26-15). Advantages of a cuffed tracheostomy tube include decreased risk of aspiration, prevention of air leakage, and access to mechanical ventilation. Low-pressure cuffs are preferred to decrease the incidence of tracheal mucosal damage. Fenestrated tracheostomy tubes are tubes with holes in the outer cannula. When the patient is being ventilated, the inner cannula remains in place. When weaning is attempted, the inner cannula can be removed and the cuff deflated; this allows the patient to breathe around the tube and through the fenestration. Another advantage of the

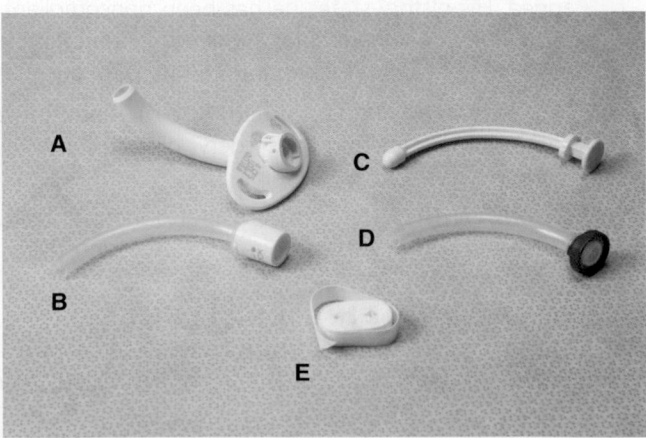

FIGURE 26-14 Uncuffed tracheostomy components. **A.** Outer cannula. **B.** Inner cannula. **C.** Obturator. **D.** Tracheostomy plug. **E.** Tracheostomy ties.

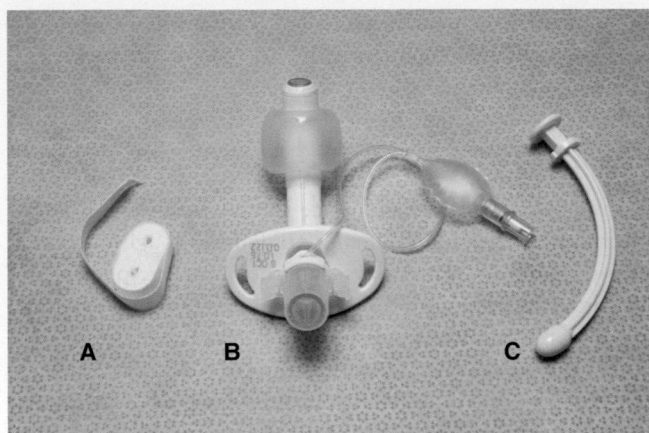

FIGURE 26-15 Cuffed tracheostomy components. **A.** Tracheostomy ties. **B.** Cuffed tracheostomy tube. **C.** Obturator.

fenestrated tube is that speaking is possible when the tracheostomy is plugged because the hole permits exhaled air to flow over the vocal cords.

SAFETY ALERT

The tube must never be plugged if the cuff is inflated because this could cause suffocation and possibly death.

Risks of a tracheostomy are numerous. Immediately after surgery, bleeding of the incision is common. Change dressings frequently during this period. Assess the extent of blood loss, and be prepared to call the surgeon if bleeding is excessive. Careful care of the stoma is necessary to keep it free from infection. Because the tracheostomy bypasses the defenses of the upper airway, the patient is at risk for pneumonia. Thus, during the postoperative hospitalization period, use sterile technique when cleaning the tracheostomy site and when suctioning the patient.

Patients who require a tracheostomy often have decreased breathing ability. Dried secretions can completely occlude the tube, creating a respiratory emergency. For this reason, tracheostomy patients must be well hydrated, and the air they breathe must be completely humidified by a nebulizer or high-output humidifier.

A tracheostomy also poses communication problems. Because the vocal cords are above the level of the tracheostomy tube, the patient cannot speak. A tablet and pencil can eliminate a great deal of frustration and confusion. Specialized tracheostomy tubes can be attached to a standard tracheostomy tube, making speech possible. Tracheostomy buttons are used temporarily to plug the tracheostomy so that the patient's ability to breathe through the natural airway can be assessed. When these buttons are in place, the patient can once again speak.

Body image is a potential problem for these patients. The patient may perceive the stoma as disfiguring and may be embarrassed by its bubbling secretions. Feelings of failure and depression may result from the inability to perform such a basic life function as breathing without assistance. The patient is also likely to feel fear and anxiety about the inability to speak. Refer to Chapter 38 for therapeutic interventions for altered body image.

SAFETY ALERT

Specialized tracheostomy tubes are appropriate for use only by the patient with strong spontaneous respirations. Follow the directions for each of these specialized devices. Improperly applied, they are unlikely to work and may cause complete airway blockage.

Tracheostomy care is necessary to decrease infection risk and to ensure that crusted secretions do not plug the tube. Remove dried mucus from around the incision site. The inner cannula may be cleaned; some tracheostomy tubes have a disposable inner cannula that is changed rather than cleaned. Change stoma dressings regularly. Commercially made tracheostomy dressings are available, or gauze may be folded to size. Do not cut dressings with scissors because threads from the gauze can cause an inflammatory reaction at the stoma. If the patient has large amounts of secretions, change tracheostomy dressings as often as necessary. If the tracheostomy produces few secretions, the dressing may need to be changed only once or twice a day. Well-established, dry tracheostomies may require no dressing. **Procedure 26-8** gives detailed instructions on tracheostomy care.

SAFETY ALERT

Take great care while changing the security ties that hold the tracheostomy tube in place because the patient can easily cough out an unsecured tube. To minimize the danger of accidental extubation, tracheostomy care often is best performed by pairs of nurses.

SUCTIONING

Atelectasis and pneumonia may develop in patients who cannot cough effectively to expectorate mucus. Excessive mucus can even cause the airway to occlude. To prevent this, the nurse may have to suction the airways. Suctioning is appropriate only when secretions are present in the upper airways, as indicated by coarse crackles, diminished breath sounds, increased inspiratory pressure, increased respiratory rate, or decreased oxygen saturation.

To suction the airways, insert a catheter through the nose, mouth, or tracheal tube. Attach the catheter to a portable or wall unit suction device, which provides the suction pressure for secretion removal. Effective suctioning can clear the oral cavity and nasopharyngeal areas of secretions. Secretions deep in the trachea are more difficult to remove, but the suctioning procedure is similar, regardless of where the secretions are found.

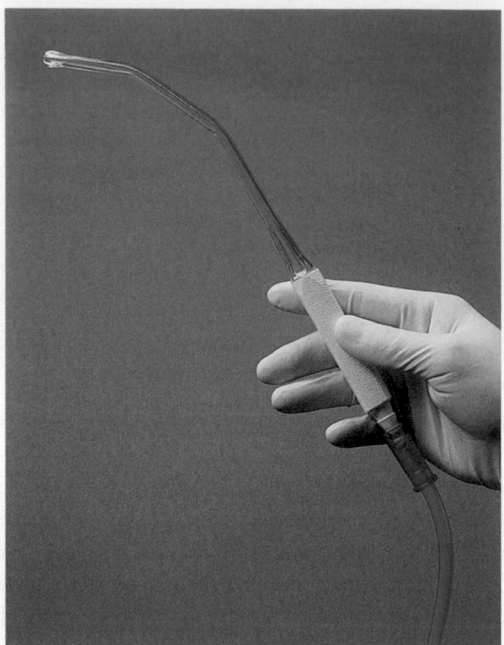

FIGURE 26-16 Tonsil-tip (Yankauer) suction catheter to clear oral cavity of excess secretions.

Procedure 26-9 gives complete instructions on secretion removal by suctioning.

Some patients produce excessive amounts of oral secretions. These patients can use a "tonsil-tip" (Yankauer) suction tube (Fig. 26-16) to evacuate excess saliva and thick mucus from the back of the throat. This suction catheter is also attached to wall or portable suction.

Patients with deep bronchial secretions may require deep suctioning. Properly performed, suctioning can greatly improve airflow in the lungs, which promotes oxygenation. However, the procedure carries several risks. Because oxygen, as well as mucus, is withdrawn from the airways, suctioning can cause temporary hypoxia.

> ! **SAFETY ALERT**
> Many studies over the last decade have demonstrated the significance of hyperoxygenation before each suctioning attempt to minimize hypoxemia and atelectasis (Lewis et al., 2014).

Apply suction intermittently to help minimize catheter damage to the trachea's delicate mucosal lining. Limit suctioning passes to three for each suctioning procedure, with 10 seconds as the recommended time limit for each suction attempt (Lewis et al., 2014). Usually, the suction regulator is set between 80 and 120 mm Hg for larger children and adults and between 60 and 80 mm Hg for infants.

In addition to causing hypoxia, suctioning can cause cardiac ysrhythmias, hypotension, and atelectasis. Because suctioning can stimulate a gag reflex, vomiting (with the potential for aspiration) is possible. Suctioning can greatly relieve the

dyspnea that accompanies excessive secretions, but the process is frightening and unpleasant for nearly all patients. Be prepared to offer a great deal of reassurance.

CHEST TUBES

A chest tube is a drainage device the physician places in the pleural space to drain fluid, air, or blood. Although the tube is placed and removed by a physician, the nurse is responsible for assisting with tube insertion and continually monitoring and assessing the status of a patient with a chest tube.

Normally, the pressure within the thoracic cavity is negative compared to atmospheric pressure. This negative pressure moves air into a person's lungs on inhalation. Any interruption in this negative pressure gradient may necessitate the need for a chest tube. The fluid buildup from a disease process may inhibit the lung's ability to expand normally; the fluid must be drained from the pleural space. An injury may result in blood in the pleural space (hemothorax). Surgery involving the chest wall almost always results in the collapse of a lung (pneumothorax); a chest tube is used to re-expand the collapsed lung and remove fluid. When a lung collapses spontaneously (spontaneous pneumothorax), a chest tube is used to remove air from the pleural space and re-expand the lung.

The physician inserts the chest tube into the intrapleural space. It is sutured in place and covered with an occlusive sterile dressing. The chest tube is connected to the collection/water seal system by a rubber tube that can be 2 to 4 feet long. Suction can be ordered if additional pressure is required to re-expand the lung. The water seal prevents air from entering the pleural space as the patient inspires. It is important to keep the extra tubing looped at the level of the patient; otherwise, fluid can accumulate in dependent loops.

The chest drainage systems currently used in the hospital are single-unit, disposable systems composed of a collection chamber, a water seal chamber, and a suction chamber (Fig. 26-17; **Procedure 26-10**). The collection chamber collects any fluid that drains from the chest tube. The chamber is composed of a series of graduated columns that fill sequentially. Because of this filling sequence, it is important to keep the chest collection system upright at all times. If the system is overturned, the drainage spills into all the collection columns. The nurse marks the amount of drainage accrued in the collection chamber during each shift.

The water seal chamber allows drainage and air to drain into the collection chamber without air entering the chest tube. The water seal chamber is filled with sterile water up to the mark identified by the manufacturer. Mild fluctuation in the water seal chamber is normal as the patient breathes. Bubbles in the water seal chamber when a patient coughs may indicate an intermittent air leak. Continuous bubbling in the water seal chamber indicates an ongoing air leak and should be reported to the physician.

When suction is ordered, the suction chamber is partially filled with sterile water and connected to suction. The physician orders the amount of suction to be used (usually 20 cm

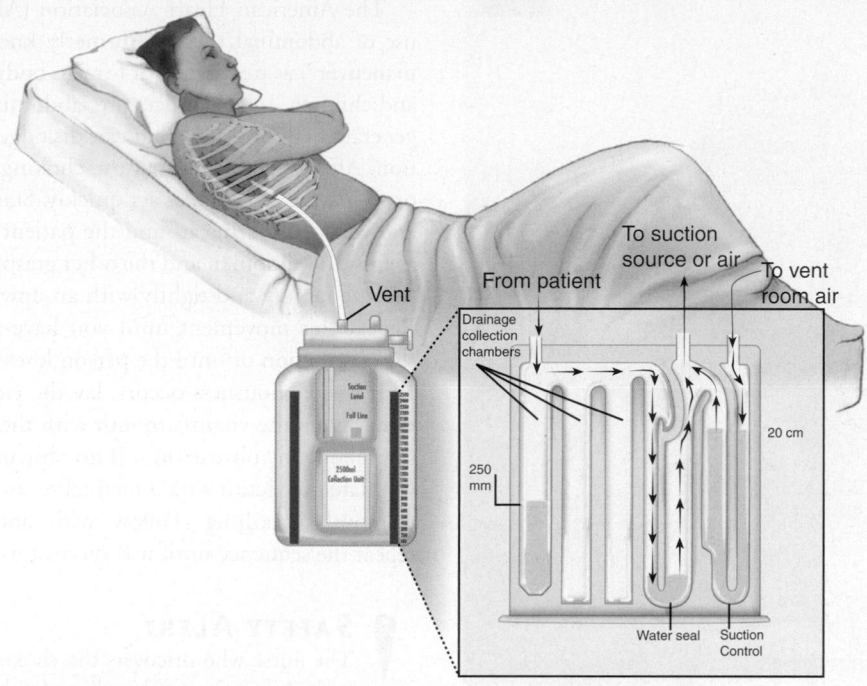

FIGURE 26-17 Chest drainage system (*From:* Smeltzer, S. C., & Bare, B. G. (2000). *Brunner & Suddarth's textbook of medical–surgical nursing* (9th ed.). Philadelphia, PA: Lippincott Williams & Wilkins.)

suction), and the suction chamber is adjusted so that there is gentle bubbling of the sterile water up to the line corresponding to the amount of suction ordered. The inclusion of suction in a chest drainage system establishes negative pressure to more readily reinflate a collapsed lung or encourage fluid removal from the pleural space. As a pneumothorax begins to reinflate, or if there is only minimal amount of fluid to be drained, a chest tube sometimes will be ordered to be disconnected from suction and attached just to water seal drainage. Refer to **Procedure 26-10** for details on monitoring a patient with a chest tube.

VENTILATORS

Ventilators are mechanical devices used to provide artificial breathing for patients who cannot breathe effectively. Until recently, these machines were used only in the ICU. Now, ventilator patients increasingly are cared for on some medical–surgical and rehabilitation units. Intermediate care facilities that deal exclusively with ventilator-dependent patients are becoming common, and the use of ventilators in the home is growing steadily.

Ventilators may be used to provide oxygen to patients, to assist with the mechanical breathing process, or both. Positive pressure ventilators deliver oxygen under pressure to patients who cannot breathe effectively. These machines range from simple pressure-limited devices to microprocessor-driven, volume-limited ventilators. Their uses range from full ventilatory support to simply assisting the patient who is too weak to maintain effective ventilation for long periods.

Ventilators require frequent monitoring by specially trained personnel. The person who is caring for a ventilator patient must become familiar with the ventilator's alarm system. The ventilator's alarms indicate changes in the patient's condition or possible machine malfunction.

More information on negative pressure ventilators can be found in the Home and Community Care section later in this chapter. For additional information on intensive ventilator care, consult texts on respiratory therapy or critical care nursing.

! SAFETY ALERT
Saline lavage, a practice commonly used to loosen thick secretions, can cause a significant (although temporary) drop in oxygenation. Although the research is inconclusive, there is no evidence that supports this practice (Caparros, 2014).

EMERGENCY AIRWAY MEASURES

Airway obstruction is a medical emergency requiring immediate attention. Because airway obstruction hinders breathing, the airway must be cleared to prevent suffocation and cardiorespiratory arrest. The neurologically impaired patient, such as the comatose patient or a person with a cerebrovascular, is most at risk for airway obstruction. Because the airway is only partially occluded, the person is able to breathe with effort. The partial obstruction is identified by loud snoring sounds as the patient inspires.

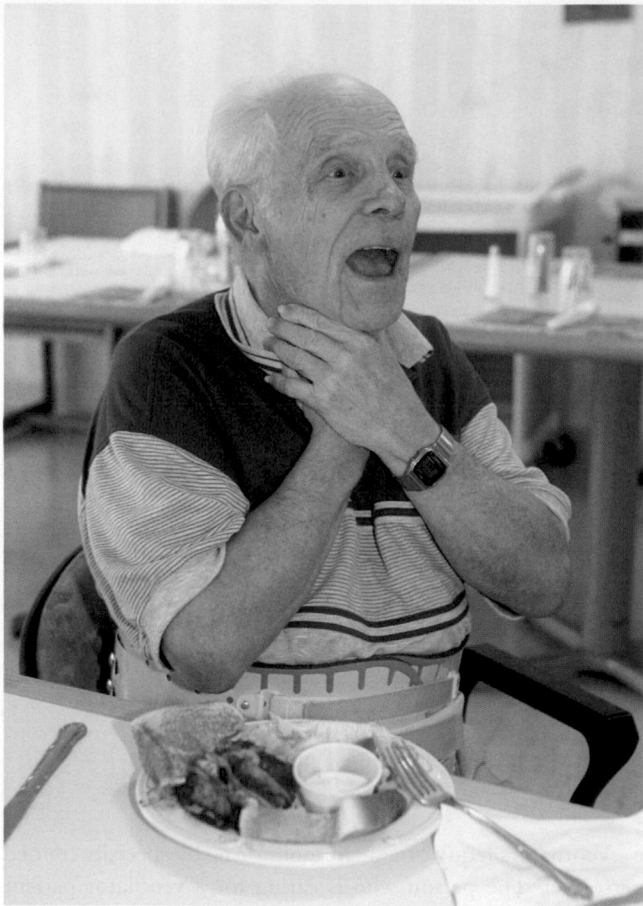

FIGURE 26-18 Grasping the throat is the universal sign for "I'm choking!"

The choking victim who has aspirated foreign matter such as food into the airway is in grave danger. Quickly assess the situation, and be ready to initiate steps to open the airway. On discovering the choking victim, quickly determine the relative extent of airway obstruction (Fig. 26-18). If the choking victim is coughing loudly and gasping for breath, the airway is only partially obstructed. In this case, allow the victim to cough with no assistance. The cough will be more effective than any other intervention. Do not slap the victim's back; it may lodge the obstructing material even more deeply in the airway.

If you hear high-pitched inspiratory stridor, the airway is near-totally obstructed. At best, the victim can produce only a very weak cough. If the victim cannot cough at all and makes no sounds, the airway is totally obstructed. In either case, treatment is as follows.

! SAFETY ALERT
The most common cause of airway obstruction is the tongue, which can fall back into the airway and interfere with ventilation and gas exchange. Positioning the patient on either side can relieve the obstruction. If such a position is undesirable or impractical, an oral or nasal airway may be needed.

The American Heart Association (AHA) recommends the use of abdominal thrusts (formerly known as the "Heimlich maneuver") as treatment for foreign body obstruction in adults and children. In this procedure, abdominal thrusts are used to generate high pressures that can dislodge an aspirated obstruction. After establishing that the choking person cannot cough or speak, the nurse must act quickly. Stand behind the person, and wrap your arms around the patient's waist. With one fist against the abdomen and the other grasping the opposite wrist, squeeze rapidly and tightly with an upward thrusting motion. Repeat this movement until you have successfully dislodged the obstruction or until the person loses consciousness.

If unconsciousness occurs, lay the victim in a supine position. Sweep the victim's mouth with the fingers in an attempt to pull out any obstruction. If no obstruction is evident, try to ventilate the victim with a manual resuscitator or with mouth-to-mouth breathing. Follow with abdominal thrusts, and repeat the sequence until it is successful.

! SAFETY ALERT
The nurse who discovers the choking victim should stay with the victim while calling for help. The nurse must then take immediate action to clear the obstruction by performing abdominal thrusts. The person arriving first to help will be ready to alert the cardiopulmonary resuscitation team, if necessary, and to offer other support.

Manual Resuscitation Bag and Mask

When the patient is unable to sustain adequate ventilation, use a manual resuscitation bag and mask until recovery occurs or an airway can be inserted and mechanical ventilation begun or death is pronounced. A manual resuscitation bag is a basic emergency equipment. This bag can also be used to hyperinflate the lungs just before suctioning and can be adapted to attach to a tracheostomy or endotracheal tube if the face mask is removed. (A resuscitation bag is pictured in Fig. 3 of **Procedure 26-7**.)

To deliver effective ventilation, tilt the patient's chin back and pull the jaw forward to open the airway. Hold the mask tightly over the patient's mouth and nose, maintaining a good seal with one hand as you use the other hand to compress the bag and deliver air into the lungs. The bag is self-inflating, and a one-way valve allows exhaled air to escape. A normal rate of inflations for an adult is 16 to 20 breaths per minute. The tidal volume delivered, as well as the amount of oxygen, can vary depending on the rate and technique used to compress the bag.

Home and Community Care

Most respiratory patients are managed in the community, except for those experiencing periods of acute respiratory dysfunction or who have exacerbation of a chronic respiratory condition. Home respiratory therapy can include peak flow monitoring, handheld aerosol treatments, chest physiotherapy, oxygen, or ventilator care. How much and what kind of home therapy the patient receives depends on many factors, including the patient's age, ability to learn procedures, family support, degree of impairment, and motivation. The nurse is often the one to assess these characteristics for the purpose of making recommendations to the provider. Often, the nurse is responsible for making home care arrangements and for much of the teaching involved.

INFECTION CONTROL

Patients are likely to use pieces of equipment normally considered disposable after 2 or 3 days in the hospital, such as cannulas or small-volume nebulizers, for much longer periods in the home. Hospital procedures performed under sterile conditions, such as tracheostomy care and suctioning, may be done using clean technique at home. Although cost considerations and limited facilities make sterilization difficult, infection control at home can be practically as effective as it is in the hospital.

Ensure that the patient clearly understands the importance of infection control because potentially lethal pneumonia may result from respiratory infection. Stress the importance of hand hygiene. Teach the patient effective cleaning of all equipment.

The patient must learn the signs of impending respiratory infection. Increased sputum production, change of sputum color to yellow or green, fever, and increasing difficulty in raising sputum often signal the onset of infection. If the patient has a standing order for antibiotics, it is appropriate to begin taking the medication when these signs appear. If there is no relief within a day or two, the patient should contact the provider. The patient should complete the full prescription of antibiotics to avoid fostering the development of drug-resistant organisms. He or she should immediately report appreciable amounts of blood in the sputum, a severe increase in shortness of breath, or any other severe symptoms to the provider.

MEDICATIONS

Home use of respiratory medications can be simplified by prepackaged unit-dose medications, but these are more expensive than stock bottles of medications. If the patient can learn to measure dosages, stock bottles may be more cost-effective. Teach the patient to recognize side effects of medications and to understand why they are dangerous. Stress the dangers of taking medications more frequently than ordered. If the medications provide no relief, the patient should call the provider.

HOME OXYGEN SYSTEMS

The respiratory equipment that patients use at home also differs from hospital equipment. At home, the patient can receive oxygen from high-pressure cylinders, liquid gas systems, or electrically powered concentrators. Compressed oxygen from high-pressure tanks is best for the patient who only occasionally requires supplemental oxygen. Liquid oxygen systems allow the patient to leave home. Portable "walkers" can be filled from a stationary unit at home. The walkers are small enough to be carried or wheeled in a small cart, yet they hold

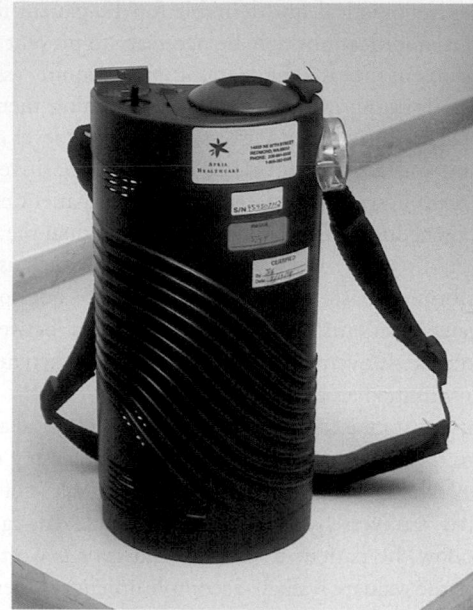

FIGURE 26-19 Portable oxygen walker—fill with liquid oxygen for longer period of ambulation.

an hour of oxygen (Fig. 26-19). A concentrator is a device that chemically separates oxygen from room air. It is an excellent choice for the patient who requires continuous oxygen in low concentrations.

Home ventilators are also quite different from those found in ICUs. Choices range from wraparound pulmonary-aid belts, which assist patients whose breathing is weak, to negative pressure chest shells and positive pressure portable ventilators that provide full ventilatory support.

The companies that rent these items or supply the oxygen should be well established and reliable. They should be able to provide service 24 hours every day. The patient should have the telephone numbers of the suppliers and must be able to get service whenever necessary. Suppliers often hire respiratory therapists to visit the patient routinely at home and to assess respiratory status and equipment function. The nurse or discharge planner coordinates these services.

ENERGY CONSERVATION

Respiratory dysfunction can seriously affect a patient's activities of daily living (ADLs), but with slight modifications, most patients can perform them. Energy conservation and the motivation to be independent are keys to success.

Make suggestions for modifying ADLs based on thoroughly assessing the extent to which respiratory dysfunction has affected each activity. For example, consider the following:

- If meal preparation is a problem, a referral to a Meals on Wheels program may be appropriate.
- If mobility is impaired, sponge baths may be a practical alternative to tub bathing.
- An elevated toilet seat may help decrease the work needed to rise from the toilet.

It is neither practical nor desirable for the patient to avoid activity, but modifications may be necessary to prevent activity from causing dyspnea. The patient may require assistance either in performing activities or in approaching them more efficiently. The nurse should assess the patient's level of ADL functioning and assist him or her to develop positive means for living with dyspnea and fatigue. Help the patient establish an activity schedule that allows for more time than the healthy person would require. Energy-saving measures such as sitting while performing basic tasks help to eliminate one source of breathlessness. Patients should space activities between rest periods to prevent overexertion and should limit activity for at least 1 hour immediately following meals.

Patients must take care not to exceed their physical abilities. Encourage them to work gradually toward increasing exercise tolerance. Helping the patient to set realistic goals is of utmost importance. Conversely, goals should provide enough challenge to allow the patient to feel the endeavor is worthwhile. Recognize the value of small accomplishments. Offer praise and encouragement because progress at building endurance is often slow.

FOSTERING SELF-ESTEEM

Like most people, the person with lung disease wants to be independent, contribute to society, feel self-reliant, and not burden others. The ability to get around independently and to do meaningful work can help foster these feelings. These activities are also essential to avoid the debilitating effects of depression.

The diagnosis of pulmonary disease does not mean the person is automatically unable to work. If the patient derives satisfaction from a job, he or she should continue to work for as long as possible. Frequent illness can make it difficult for the severely dyspneic patient to hold a demanding job; however, the Family and Medical Leave Act (FMLA) can assist with job security during periods of illness. Respiratory disease can severely inhibit both sexual desire and sexual performance. Chronic fatigue, shortness of breath, and embarrassment caused by excessive mucus or dyspnea are often reasons the patient with respiratory problems loses sexual function. The patient should use prescribed bronchodilators before beginning sexual relations because this will help the patient avoid dyspnea throughout sexual activity. Inform the patient that passive positions save energy. Finally, stress the importance of open communication between the patient and his or her partner, and help the patient recognize that adjustments will be necessary.

Offer suggestions for activities outside the home. Social outlets can help the patient to cope with the day-to-day frustrations of lung disease. The ALA sponsors classes and support groups for people with respiratory disease. Nurses, providers, or therapists often are guest speakers at such gatherings. Rehabilitation programs offer more structured activities. Their purpose is to increase the patient's ability to function with lung disease. Such programs may provide breathing retraining, exercise, and diet and occupational counseling.

EVALUATION

Work with the patient to develop goals and individualized outcome criteria depending on the patient's current breathing status.

Goal

The patient will demonstrate knowledge regarding prevention of respiratory dysfunction.

POSSIBLE OUTCOME CRITERIA

- After the teaching session, the patient demonstrates deep breathing or coughing techniques.
- After the teaching session, the patient discusses the physiologic effects of smoking.
- The patient joins and regularly attends meetings of a stop smoking program for 6 months.

Goal

The patient will demonstrate knowledge regarding optimal management of respiratory dysfunction.

POSSIBLE OUTCOME CRITERIA

- After the teaching session, the patient lists signs of respiratory infection and knows when to call the provider.
- After the teaching session about any medication administered for respiratory problems, the patient verbalizes the name, action, and side effects of the drug, dose to be taken, and any special considerations for administration.
- Before discharge, the patient demonstrates the safe use of home oxygen equipment.
- After teaching session, the patient demonstrates pursed-lip breathing.

Goal

The patient will mobilize pulmonary secretions.

POSSIBLE OUTCOME CRITERIA

- After the teaching session, the patient demonstrates proper coughing technique.
- Caregiver or parent demonstrates proper techniques of chest physiotherapy, including percussion, vibration, and postural drainage, by the next home visit.
- The patient demonstrates correct self-suctioning technique before discharge.

Goal

The patient will effectively cope with changes in self-concept and lifestyle.

PATIENT PLAN OF CARE
The Patient with Ineffective Airway Clearance

NURSING DIAGNOSIS
Ineffective Airway Clearance related to tracheobronchial infection as manifested by weak cough, adventitious breath sounds, and copious green sputum production.

PATIENT GOAL
The patient will mobilize pulmonary secretions.

PATIENT OUTCOME CRITERIA
- After teaching session, the patient demonstrates proper coughing techniques.
- The patient drinks at least six glasses of water per day while in hospital.
- The patient demonstrates correct self-suctioning technique before discharge.

NURSING INTERVENTION	SCIENTIFIC RATIONALE
1. Provide and teach the patient the importance of adequate hydration. **a.** Encourage fluids (2,000 to 3,000 mL per 24 hours) **b.** Monitor intake and output **c.** Avoid milk and milk products **d.** Ultrasonic nebulizer treatment	**1.** Adequate hydration thins secretions, which prevents mucus from plugging airways. **a.** Evaluate hydration status of the patient. **b.** Milk products tend to thicken secretions. **c.** Moisten and aid mobility of respiratory secretions.
2. Position and encourage the patient to cough to promote mobilization of secretions. **a.** Deep breathing every hour while awake **b.** Huff coughing **c.** Have the patient assume sitting position if possible	**2.** Open alveoli and prevent further atelectasis. **a.** Prevent airway collapse. **b.** Permit deep inspiration and forceful abdominal contractions necessary for coughing.
3. Administer analgesic before cough session if pain limits coughing effectiveness.	**3.** If the patient fears pain, he or she hesitates to breathe deeply and cough effectively.
4. Provide or teach the patient tracheal suctioning if he or she is unable to remove secretions with effective coughing. **a.** Hyperoxygenate with 100% O^2 before and after suctioning procedure. **b.** Suction for no longer than 10 seconds per suctioning attempt. **c.** Provide opportunities for the patient to practice and demonstrate suctioning technique if self-suctioning is necessary.	**4.** A weak, nonproductive cough causes secretions to be retained in airways and interfere with gas exchange. **a.** Hypoxemia, which can occur during the suctioning procedure, is prevented. **b.** Longer periods of suction can contribute to tissue trauma and hypoxemia. **c.** Suctioning is a complex motor skill that requires practice for skill acquisition and comfort.
5. Provide or teach postural chest physiotherapy as ordered. Have the patient or family members demonstrate when comfortable with skill mastery.	**5.** Secretions drain from major airways using the force of gravity.

POSSIBLE OUTCOME CRITERIA
- Within a week of diagnosis, the patient identifies support people to provide emotional strength.
- By the end of teaching session, the patient lists community agencies and services that he or she plans to use.
- Before discharge, the patient demonstrates oxygen-conserving measures, such as sitting while dressing and planning rest periods.

KEY CONCEPTS
- The primary functions of breathing are the delivery of oxygen to the blood, the removal of carbon dioxide from the blood, and the maintenance of acid–base balance.
- Although almost always effortless, the work required for breathing increases tremendously when the airways are obstructed by inflammation, bronchospasm, or excessive mucous secretions.

- Deep breathing and coughing are the two most important measures for preventing pulmonary complications such as atelectasis and pneumonia.

- Adequate hydration is essential to keep respiratory secretions moist and easily expectorated from the respiratory tract.

- Smoking is the single most important factor affecting pulmonary health.

- Common manifestations of respiratory dysfunction are cough, dyspnea, chest pain, and sputum production.

- Health promotion for respiratory health includes smoking cessation, peak flow monitoring, allergen reduction, and appropriate vaccination.

- Major nursing interventions for the respiratory patient are measures to promote airway patency, improve air distribution in the lungs, and promote oxygenation.

- Airway maintenance interventions include hydration, aerosol therapy, positioning, coughing, chest physiotherapy, suctioning, and management of artificial airways.

- Hyperinflation techniques, such as deep breathing, incentive spirometry, and intermittent positive pressure breathing or bilevel positive airway pressure, help prevent atelectasis and promote a strong cough.

- Oxygen therapy raises the amount of oxygen in the lungs, thereby making more oxygen available to the blood and tissues.

- Dyspnea, excessive mucous secretions, dried secretions, hyperventilation, and hypoventilation are common nursing problems of the respiratory patient.

- Home care must be individualized for the respiratory patient. Ability to perform ADLs and manage home procedures must be considered carefully before discharge.

PRACTICING FOR THE NCLEX

CHECK YOUR ANSWERS IN APPENDIX A.

1. A baby is born prematurely at 26 weeks requiring ventilatory support. The nurse caring for this neonate knows that this is because of which of the following?
   a. Lack of functioning alveoli
   b. Bronchospasm
   c. Ineffective cough
   d. Lack of surfactant

2. A nurse is caring for a patient with COPD. In performing his assessment, he finds rounded, enlarged finger tips. He realizes that this is which of the following symptoms?
   a. Cyanosis
   b. Dyspnea
   c. Clubbing
   d. Arthritis

3. An asthmatic patient is self-administering his MDI. The nurse notes that he is not able to time his inhalations with activation of the inhaler. Which of the following is most appropriate?
   a. Recommend additional puffs to meet the prescribed dosing.
   b. Insist on administering the MDI for the patient.
   c. Provide a spacer attachment with appropriate education.
   d. Administer supplementary oxygen.

4. A patient with COPD has an order to maintain his oxygen saturation at 90% or greater using nasal cannula. The patient is currently receiving 4 LPM of O_2 with a saturation of 95%. What should the nurse do first?
   a. Remove the supplementary oxygen and check the SpO_2 level.
   b. Switch the nasal cannula to a mask.
   c. Reduce the oxygen to 3 LPM and recheck the saturation in 30 minutes.
   d. Increase the oxygen to 5 LPM via nasal cannula.

5. A patient is having difficulty coughing up secretions, has rhonchi in the lungs, has respiratory rate of 28, and has dyspnea. The nurse recognizes these as symptoms of which nursing diagnosis?
   a. Ineffective Breathing Pattern
   b. Ineffective Airway Clearance
   c. Impaired Gas Exchange
   d. Impaired Deep Breathing

6. A patient has come to the clinic for a routine physical assessment reporting a history of asthma as a child and history of smoking one pack a day for the past 5 years. Which of the following interventions will the nurse perform to promote the health of this patient? Select all that apply:
   a. Encourage pursed-lip breathing.
   b. Teach proper use and care of oxygen equipment.
   c. Discuss smoking cessation at every visit.
   d. Provide positive encouragement to stop smoking.

7. A nurse is making a home health visit to a patient using oxygen for the diagnosis of COPD. Which of the following interventions would be considered the highest priority? Select all that apply:
   a. Post a "no smoking" sign by the oxygen.
   b. Discuss the latest evidence about COPD.
   c. Talk with spouse about role changes.
   d. Check the oxygen flow for tight connections.

8. A nurse is performing nasotracheal suctioning on a patient who has respirations of 30, audible respiratory secretions in the airway, and decreased breath sounds. Which order of steps is most appropriate?
   a. Put on the sterile gloves in the kit.
   b. Pour the sterile saline into the suction cup.
   c. Position the patient in a semi-Fowler's position.
   d. Attach the catheter to the suction tubing.

9. The nurse is caring for a patient with a tracheostomy tube. Great care is taken when changing the security ties that hold the tracheostomy in place for which of the following reasons?

   a. If the trach tube is plugged when the cuff is inflated, it could cause suffocation.

   b. The tracheostomy buttons may be improperly applied to the tie.

   c. Accidental saline lavage may cause a significant drop in oxygenation.

   d. The patient may accidentally cough out the tube, impairing the airway.

10. The nurse is teaching the patient about using the incentive spirometer for the first time. Which instructions will be included in the teaching?

   a. "Seal your lips tightly around the mouthpiece."

   b. "Observe the indicator for progress toward the goal."

   c. "Exhale slowly around the mouthpiece and breath normally."

   d. "Inhale deeply through the mouth and hold breath for 2 to 3 seconds."

REFERENCES

Abdo, W., & Heunks, L. (2012). Oxygen-induced hypercapnia in COPD: Myths and facts. *Critical Care, 16*(5), 323. doi: 10.1186/cc11475

Agency for Healthcare Research and Quality. (2008). AHCPR supported clinical practice guidelines. Treating tobacco use and dependence: 2008 update. Chapter 3 clinical interventions for tobacco use and dependence. Retrieved November 11, 2010, from www.ncbi.nlm.nih.gov/bookshelf/br.fcgi?book=hsahcpr&part=A28251#A29458

American Lung Association, Epidemiology and Statistics Unit. (2012). Trends in asthma morbidity and mortality. Retrieved from http://www.lung.org/finding-cures/our-research/trend-reports/asthma-trend-report.pdf

Caparros, A. (2014). Mechanical ventilation and the role of saline instillation in suctioning adult intensive care unit patients: An evidence-based practice review. *Dimensions of Critical Care Nursing, 33*(4), 246–253. doi:10.1097/DCC.0000000000000049

Centers for Disease Control and Prevention. (2010). Seasonal influenza (flu) vaccination. Retrieved from www.cdc.gov/vaccines/vpd-vac/flu/default.htm

Centers for Disease Control and Prevention. (2014a). E-cigarette use more than doubles among U.S. middle and high school students from 2011-2012. http://www.cdc.gov/media/releases/2013/p0905-ecigarette-use.html

Centers for Disease Control and Prevention. (2014b). New CDC study finds dramatic increase in e-cigarette-related calls to poison centers. http://www.cdc.gov/media/releases/2014/p0403-e-cigarette-poison.html

Centers for Disease Control and Prevention. (2014c). Youth and tobacco use. www.cdc.gov/tobacco/data_statistics/fact_sheets/youth_data/tobacco_use/index.htm

Centers for Disease Control and Prevention. (2014d). Use of 13-valent pneumococcal conjugate vaccine and 23-valent pneumococcal polysaccharide vaccine among adults aged ≥65 Years: Recommendations of the Advisory Committee on Immunization Practices. *MMWR Morb Mortal Wkly Rep, 63*(37), 822–825.

Czogala, J., Goniewicz, M., Fidelus, B., Zielinska-Danch, W., Travers, M., & Sobczak, A. (2014). Secondhand exposure to vapors from electronic cigarettes. *Nicotine & Tobacco Research, 16*(6), 655–662. doi:10.1093/ntr/ntt203

Davidson, E., Lui, J. J., & Sheikh, A. (2010). The impact of ethnicity on asthma care. *Primary Care Respiratory Journal, 19*(3), 202–208.

Herdman, T. H., & Kamitsuru, S. (Eds.). (2014). *Nursing diagnoses: Definitions and classifications. 2015-2017.* West Sussex, England: Wiley-Blackwell.

Institute for Healthcare Improvement. (2014). Implement the IHI ventilator bundle. Retrieved from http://www.ihi.org/resources/Pages/Changes/ImplementtheVentilatorBundle.aspx

Klompas, M., Branson, R., Eichenwald, E., Greene, L., Howell, M., Lee, G. et al. (2014). Strategies to prevent ventilator-associated pneumonia in acute care hospitals: 2014 update. *Infection Control and Hospital Epidemiology, 35*(8), 915–936. Retrieved from http://www.jstor.org/stable/10.1086/677144

Lewis, S., Dirksen, S., Heitkemper, M., & Bucher, L. (2014). *Medical surgical nursing: Assessment and management of clinical problems* (9th ed.). St. Louis, MO: Mosby.

Netuveli, G., Hurwitz, B., & Sheikh, A. (2007). Lineages of language and the diagnosis of asthma. *Journal of the Royal Society of Medicine, 100*(1), 19–24.

Suleman, A., Riaz, K., & Heffner, K. D. (2013). Exercise physiology. Retrieved November 11, 2010, from http://emedicine.medscape.com/article/88484-overview

Tabloski, P. (2013). *Gerontological nursing* (3rd ed.). Upper Saddle River, NJ: Pearson Prentice Hall.

Tammemagi, M. C., Berg, C. D., Riley, T. L., Cunningham, C. R., & Taylor, K. L. (2014). Impact of lung cancer screening results on smoking cessation. *Journal of the National Cancer Institute, 106*(6). doi: 10.1093/jnci/dju084

Widmaier, E. P., Raff, H., & Strang, K. T. (2013). *Vander's human physiology: The mechanisms of body function* (13th ed.). Boston, MA: McGraw-Hill.

Yang, M., Yan, Y, Yin, X., Want, B., Wu, T., Liu, G., et al. (2013). Chest physiotherapy for pneumonia in adults. *Cochrane Database Systematic Reviews*, (2), Art. No.: CD006338. doi: 10.1002/14651858.CD006338.pub3 (http://onlinelibrary.wiley.com/doi/10.1002/14651858.CD006338.pub3/abstract;jsessionid=B52ADA0C1CF69C49F3F0F651BB659507.f03t03)

Procedure 26-1 Monitoring With Pulse Oximetry

Purpose
1. Monitor arterial oxygen saturation (SpO_2) noninvasively.
2. Detect clinical hypoxemia promptly.
3. Assess the patient's tolerance to activity or tapering of oxygen therapy.

Equipment
Pulse oximeter
Nail polish remover, if needed

Assessment
- Identify patients at risk for hypoxemia (e.g., respiratory and cardiac disease) who would benefit from pulse oximetry.
- Identify indications for continuous or intermittent oximetry monitoring.
- Assess the patient's baseline respiratory status including vital signs, skin and nail bed color, breath sounds, dyspnea, alterations in breathing patterns, current oxygen supplementation, dysrhythmias, and tissue perfusion of extremities.
- Review laboratory hemoglobin values to identify anemic patients whose oxygen content in the blood may be low although their SpO_2 is within normal levels.
- To choose appropriate sensor, observe the patient's height, weight, and size, and note any allergies to adhesive.

Procedure

1. **Select appropriate type of sensor. Various sensors are available in sizes for neonates, infants, children, and adults. In addition, there are clip-on, adhesive, and disposable sensors. To select the appropriate sensor, consider the patient's weight, activity level, if infection control is a concern, tape allergies, and anticipated duration of monitoring.**

   Rationale: Proper sensor will increase accuracy of reading.

2. **Perform hand hygiene.**

   Rationale: Reduces microbe transmission.

3. **Identify the patient.**

   Rationale: Ensures correct patient receives proper assessment or treatment and reduces errors.

4. **Close door or bed curtains and explain the procedure to the patient and the family.**

   Rationale: Ensures patient privacy, increases patient compliance, reduces patient anxiety, and promotes learning.

5. **Instruct the patient to breathe normally.**

   Rationale: Consistent breathing prevents large fluctuations in minute ventilation and inaccurate reflections of SpO_2 levels.

6. **Select appropriate site to place sensor (Fig. 1). Avoid using lower extremities that may have compromised circulation and extremities receiving infusions or other invasive monitoring. If the patient has poor tissue perfusion due to peripheral vascular disease or is receiving vasoconstrictor medications, a nasal sensor or forehead sensor may be considered.**

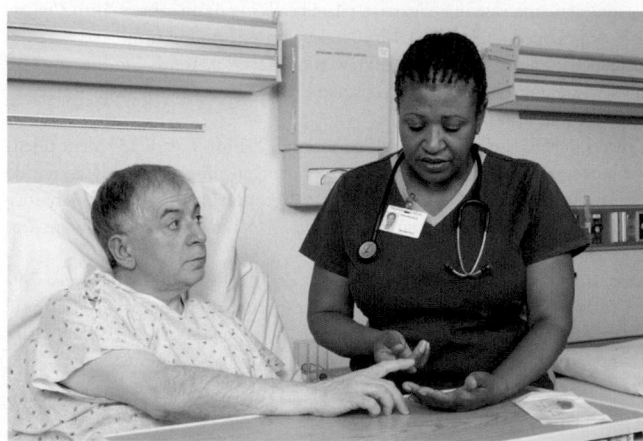

FIG. 1 Select appropriate site with good tissue perfusion.

7. **Remove nail polish or acrylic nail from digit to be used.**

   Rationale: Some nail polish (dark colors) and artificial nails can interfere with accurate measurements.

8. **Attach sensor probe (Fig. 2) and connect it to the pulse oximeter (Fig. 3). Make sure the photosensors are accurately aligned (Fig. 4).**

Procedure 26-1   *continued*

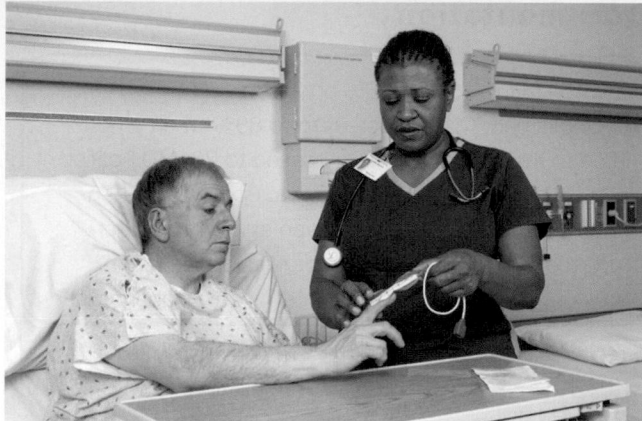

FIG. 2 Attach sensor probe.

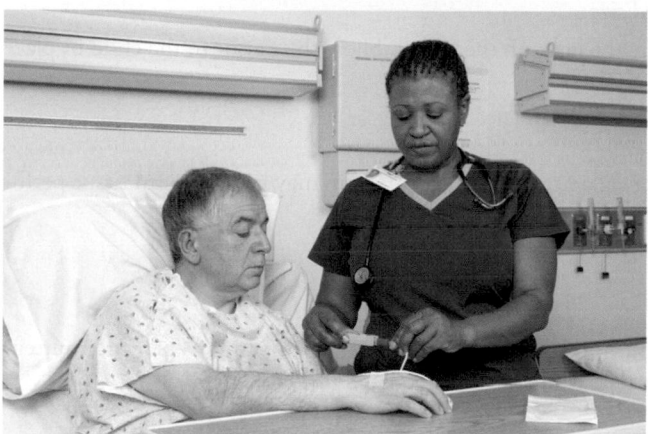

FIG. 3 Connect sensor probe to pulse oximeter.

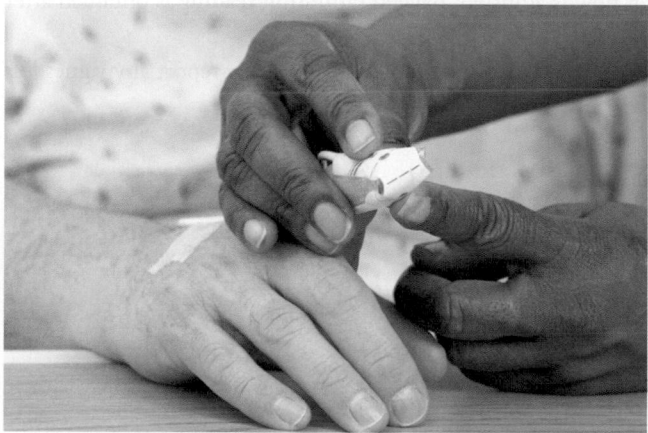

FIG. 4 Check proper alignment of photosensors.

Rationale: Proper alignment is essential for accurate SpO$_2$ measurement.

9. **Watch for pulse-sensing bar on face of oximeter to fluctuate with each pulsation and reflect pulse strength. Double-check machine pulsations with the patient's radial or apical pulse (Fig. 5).**

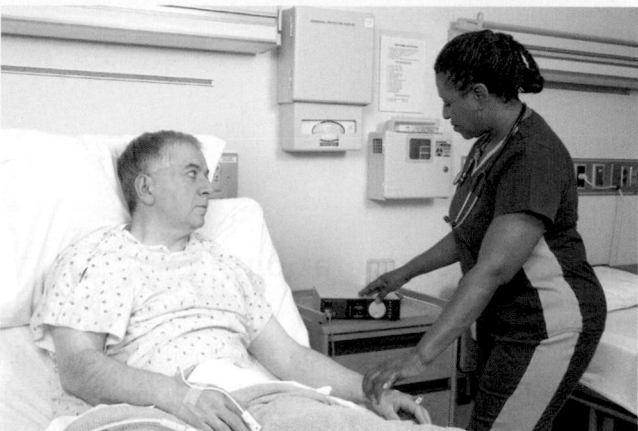

FIG. 5 Compare pulse oximeter pulsations with patient's radial pulse.

Rationale: A weak signal or missed pulsations will not produce an accurate measurement.

10. **If continuous pulse oximetry is desired, set the alarm limits on the monitor to reflect the high and low oxygen saturation and pulse rates. Ensure that the alarms are audible before leaving the patient. Inspect the sensor site every 4 hours for tissue irritation or pressure from the sensor.**

    Rationale: Ensure patient safety by prompt detection of low critical oxygen saturation values or tissue irritation.

11. **Read saturation on monitor and document as appropriate with all relevant information on patient's chart (Fig. 6). Report SpO$_2$ less than 93% to provider.**

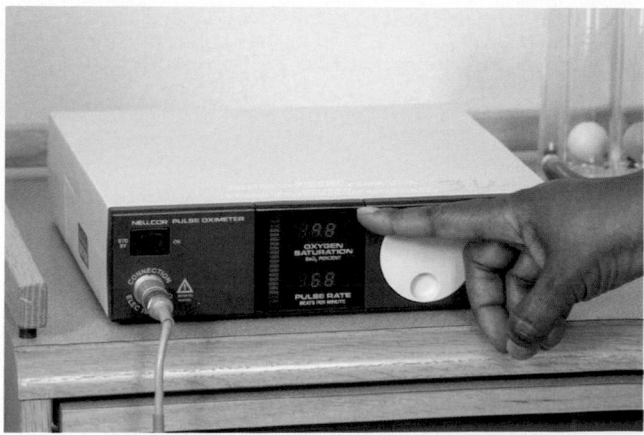

FIG. 6 Read oxygen saturation from machine.

Procedure 26-1   *continued*

Rationale: Ensure patient safety by prompt detection of low critical oxygen saturation values or tissue irritation.

12. **Document procedure.**

    Rationale: Maintains legal record and communicates with healthcare team.

Documentation

8/1/16: 14:00—O$_2$ sat 93% on 2 L/m via cannula while resting in bed, O$_2$ sat decreased to 88% when ambulated to the bathroom, RR increased to 26, MD notified and patient returned to bed. O$_2$ sat up to 93% when returned to bed and oxygen given at 2 L/m. Oxygen required during ambulation to prevent desaturation.

—S. Roberts, RN

Life Span Considerations

Infant and Child

● Use a sensor that is appropriate for the patient's weight and size.

● Young children may express fear of being burned or hurt by the light on the sensor. Show the sensor to the child or place it on Mom or Dad's finger before placing it on the child.

Older Adult

● Patients who have peripheral vascular disease or who smoke cigarettes or use nicotine gum may have reduced tissue perfusion. This can make monitoring difficult and interfere with the accuracy of the readings.

Home Care Modifications

● Because they are portable, pulse oximeters may be used in home care to monitor oxygen therapy. When intermittent monitoring is needed, the home nurse may assess pulse oximetry on each visit.

Collaboration and Delegation

● Consult a respiratory therapist to develop a plan for the patient with O$_2$ saturation below 93%. Frequently, respiratory therapists will titrate oxygen levels as needed. When oxygen flow is adjusted, oxygen saturation reading is obtained after 15 to 30 minutes to evaluate the patient's response.

● When delegating O$_2$ saturation monitoring to unlicensed nursing personnel, tell them to promptly report any values less than 93%. Validate any unusual values obtained.

Procedure 26-2 Obtaining a Sputum Specimen

Purpose	1. Obtain sputum specimen for laboratory examination.
Equipment	Sterile specimen cup Examination gloves
Assessment	• Assess the patient for presence of sputum. • Assess the patient for ability to assist with collection of specimen.

Procedure

1. **Verify the provider order.**
   Rationale: Prevents errors.

2. **Perform hand hygiene.**
   Rationale: Reduces microbe transmission.

3. **Identify the patient.**
   Rationale: Ensures correct patient receives proper assessment or treatment and reduces errors.

4. **Close door or bed curtains and explain the procedure to the patient (Fig. 1). Place the patient in semi- to high Fowler's position.**

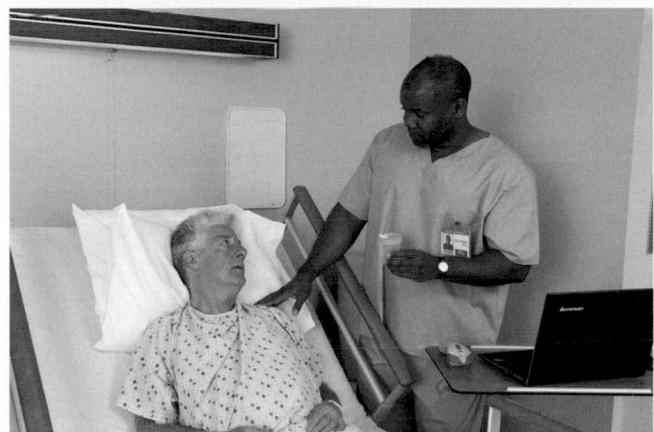

FIG. 1 Greet the patient and explain procedure.

Rationale: Ensures patient privacy, increases patient compliance, reduces patient anxiety, and promotes learning.

5. **Don clean examination gloves.**
   Rationale: Reduces microbe transmissions.

6. **Take the lid off the specimen container, maintain sterility of the inside of the cup (Fig. 2).**

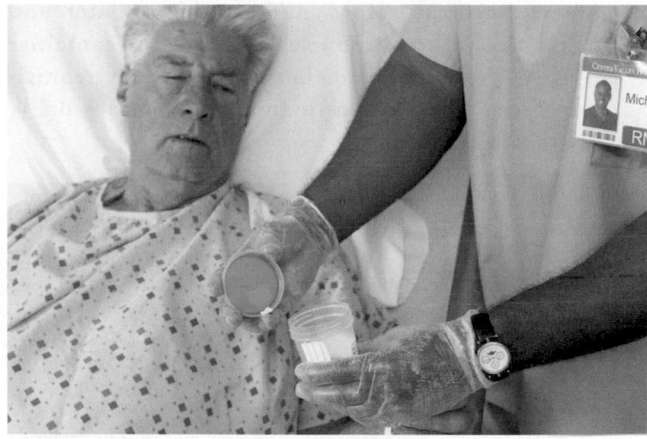

FIG. 2 Remove lid from specimen cup.

Rationale: Prevents introduction of microorganisms and ensures any organisms identified in the culture are not due to contamination.

7. **Instruct the patient to perform a deep cough to expel sputum into the cup (Fig. 3).**

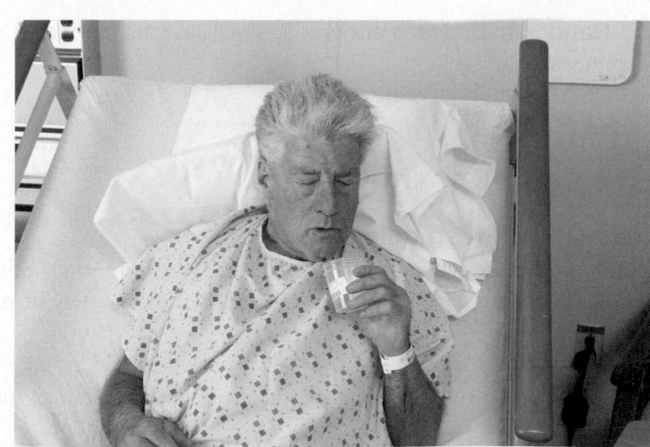

FIG. 3 Instruct the patient to expel sputum into cup.

Rationale: A deep cough increases likelihood that the specimen is sputum, not saliva.

Procedure 26-2   *continued*

8. **Inspect the sample to determine if it is most likely sputum (opaque, thicker) or saliva (thin, clear, watery). If the sample does not appear to be sputum, obtain another specimen.**

   Rationale: A specimen comprised of saliva is not adequate for diagnosis.

9. **If the patient is not able to produce a specimen immediately, the specimen cup may be left at the bedside. Ensure the patient understands the need to not touch the inside of the specimen container.**

10. **Replace the cap on the specimen container.**

    Rationale: Covers specimen to prevent contamination.

11. **Identify the patient with at least two identifiers (name, medical record number, birth date) and match this information to the label on the container (Fig. 4). Note date and time on laboratory requisition form. Place in plastic biohazard bag for delivery to the laboratory.**

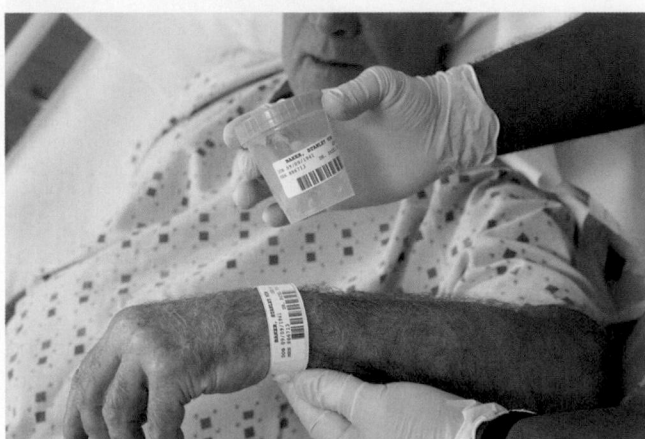

FIG. 4 Check label on specimen cup with patient's armband.

Rationale: Prevents errors; bagging prevents spread of microorganisms.

12. **Send specimen to laboratory immediately.**

    Rationale: Laboratory examination is needed as soon as possible to identify the quantity of microorganisms in the lungs rather than those that multiplied in the specimen cup.

13. **Remove gloves and perform hand hygiene.**

    Rationale: Prevents the transfer of microorganisms.

Documentation

2/17/16: 06:30—Deep sputum specimen obtained without difficulty and sent to lab for culture.
—S. Roberts, RN

Life Span Considerations

Toddler and Preschooler
Children in these age groups will need supervision during specimen collection to ensure a good sample and maintenance of sterility. More invasive techniques, such as suctioning, may be needed to acquire an adequate sample from children.

Older Adults
Frail older adults may have weak coughs and need assistance, such as pillow support, with coughing.

Collaboration and Delegation

Respiratory therapists often obtain sputum specimens, especially if suctioning is needed to obtain the specimen. Unlicensed assistive personnel may remind patients to collect the specimen, once the nurse or therapist has provided teaching.

Procedure 26-3 End-Tidal CO$_2$ (EtCO$_2$) Monitoring

Purpose
1. Assess adequacy of ventilation through measurement of exhaled CO$_2$.
2. Early detection of hypoventilation evidenced by decreased end-tidal CO$_2$ reading.

Equipment
EtCO$_2$ monitoring device
Nasal sampling equipment

Assessment
- Identify patients at risk for hypoventilation, such as those receiving patient-controlled analgesia.
- Assess respiratory system, including rate, depth, and rhythm of respirations; breath sounds; and SpO$_2$ level.

Procedure

1. **Verify the provider order and identify the patient.**
   Rationale: Prevents potential errors.

2. **Perform hand hygiene.**
   Rationale: Reduces microbe transmission.

3. **Identify the patient.**
   Rationale: Ensures correct patient receives proper assessment or treatment and reduces errors.

4. **Close door or bed curtains and explain the procedure to the patient and the family.**
   Rationale: Ensures patient privacy, increases patient compliance, reduces patient anxiety, and promotes learning.

5. **Set up the EtCO$_2$ device according to manufacturer's instructions (Fig. 1).**

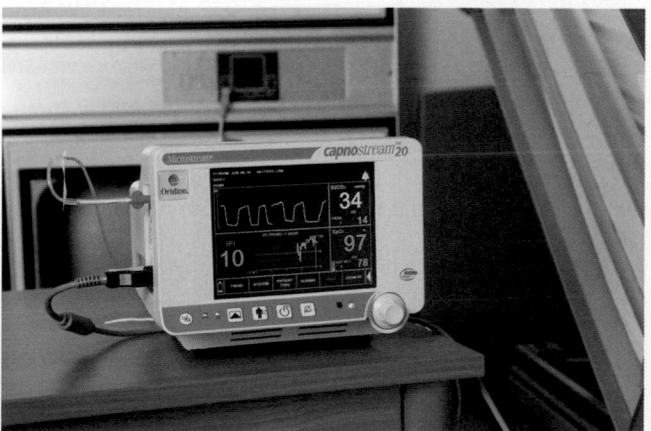

FIG. 1 Program the EtCO$_2$ device.

Rationale: Each device will have its own instruction manual; following manufacturer's instructions preserves safety features of device.

6. **Apply nasal sampling setup to the patient's face (Fig. 2). If strapped around ears, pad the tubing with gauze as needed.**

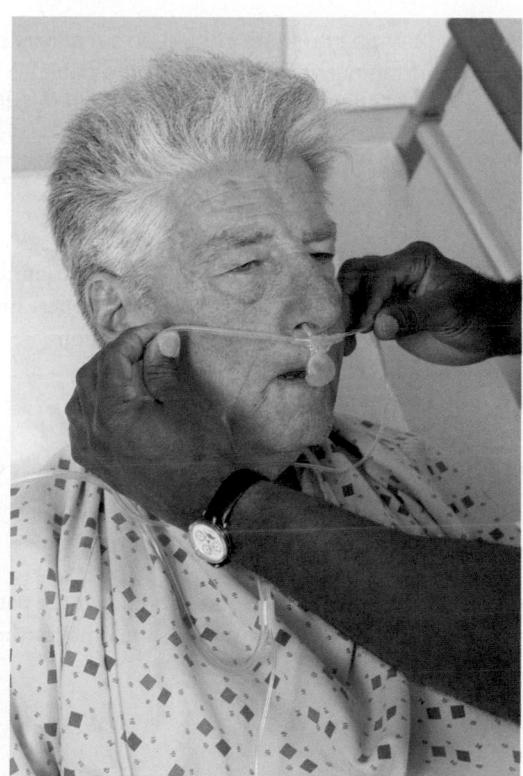

FIG. 2 Apply padded nasal sampling tubing to patient's face.

Rationale: Nasal sampling setup measures amount of CO$_2$ exhaled by the patient. Hypoventilation results in lower exhalation of CO$_2$. Padding the tubing around the ears protects against device-related pressure ulcers.

Procedure 26-3   *continued*

7. Ensure alarm settings on device are set at recommended or ordered parameters (Fig. 3).

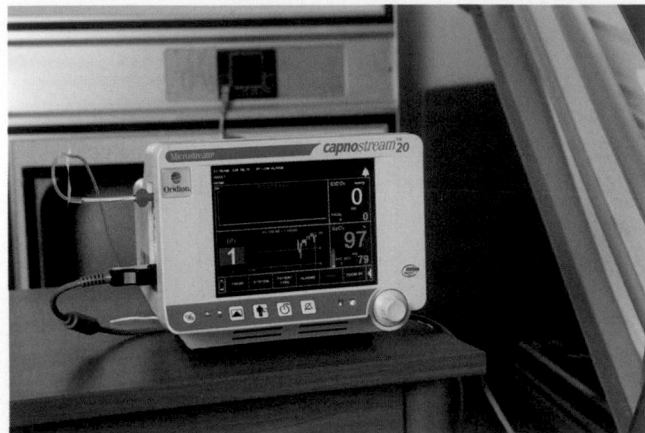

FIG. 3 Confirm alarm settings.

Rationale: Alarm parameters should be set at levels sufficient to alert the nurse to changes in the patient's condition without excessive alarms leading to alarm fatigue.

8. If the patient also requires oxygen therapy, determine if manufacturer produces tubing that allows measuring of $EtCO_2$ and simultaneous O_2 delivery with the same device.

Rationale: Performing both functions with the same tubing promotes comfort for the patient and reduces excess equipment on or near the patient.

Documentation

3/5/2016: 03:30—$EtCO_2$ level 30 mm Hg. Patient alert and oriented; respiratory rate 18. Nasal sampling device readjusted and $EtCO_2$ level rose to 40 mm Hg. Instructed patient to check placement of nasal device and to report problems to RN. Will reassess in 30 minutes or sooner if needed.

—S. Roberts, RN

Life Span Considerations

Explain equipment to children. Elicit their cooperation through play as appropriate. Apnea is a concern in children. $EtCO_2$ measurement may provide an early indicator of apnea. $EtCO_2$ levels will increase with apnea sooner than SpO_2 would drop, providing an earlier indication of lack of respirations.

Home Care Modifications

- Follow manufacturer recommendations for use of $EtCO_2$ monitors in the home.

Collaboration and Delegation

- Unlicensed assistive personnel should ensure patients are wearing the device. Unlicensed assistive personnel should never silence the $EtCO_2$ alarms; they should notify the RN.

Procedure 26-4 Monitoring Peak Flow

Purpose

1. Measure peak expiratory flow rate (PEFR), which is the point of highest air flow during maximal exhalation.
2. Better control asthma by quickly detecting subtle changes in airway diameter so that preventive interventions can be instituted.
3. Provide objective data to assess respiratory function.

Equipment

Peak flow meter
Charts to calculate green, yellow, and red zones based on personal best data
Daily log to record peak flow values obtained

Assessment

- Identify patients who would benefit from or have been prescribed peak flow monitoring (e.g., patients with asthma).
- Assess the patient's baseline oxygenation status including vital signs, skin and nail bed color, breath sounds, shortness of breath, alterations in breathing pattern, and cognitive changes.
- Note any subjective verbalizations regarding respiratory status (e.g., tightness in the chest, more difficult to breathe).
- Note new or recent exposure to factors that could alter airway diameter (e.g., smoke, chemicals, animal dander, pollens, and molds).
- Note any use of medications that could alter airway diameter (e.g., sympathomimetics, anticholinergics, corticosteroids).

Procedure

1. **Perform hand hygiene.**
   Rationale: Reduces microbe transmission.
2. **Identify the patient.**
   Rationale: Ensures correct patient receives proper assessment or treatment and reduces errors.
3. **Close door or bed curtains and explain the purpose of peak flow monitoring to the patient and the family (Fig. 1).**

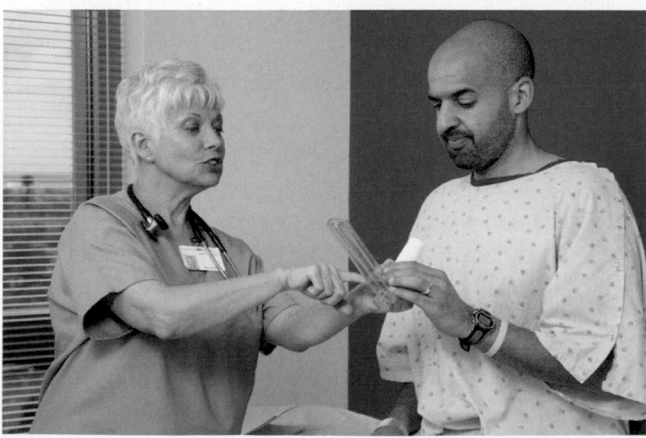

FIG. 1 Explain purpose of peak flow monitoring.

Rationale: Ensures patient privacy, increases patient compliance, reduces patient anxiety, and promotes

learning. Measurements taken before using bronchodilators will provide more accurate data regarding baseline airway diameter.

4. **Place indicator at the base of the numbered scale. Have the patient stand up.**
   Rationale: Having the indicator in the correct position will ensure accurate measurement of peak expiratory flow. Standing position allows full expansion of the lungs.
5. **Tell the patient to take a deep breath, then place the meter in his or her mouth (Fig. 2). The patient should close the lips around the mouthpiece. Remind the patient not to put his or her tongue in the hole.**

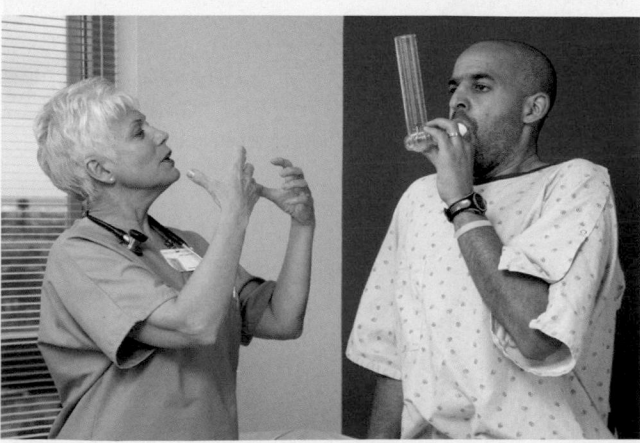

FIG. 2 Verbally encourage the patient to take a deep breath and place meter in mouth.

Procedure 26-4   *continued*

Rationale: A close fit around the mouthpiece and an unobstructed mouthpiece are necessary for proper measurement of exhaled air.

6. **Tell the patient to exhale as fast and as hard as he or she can, keeping a tight fit around the mouthpiece (Fig. 3).**

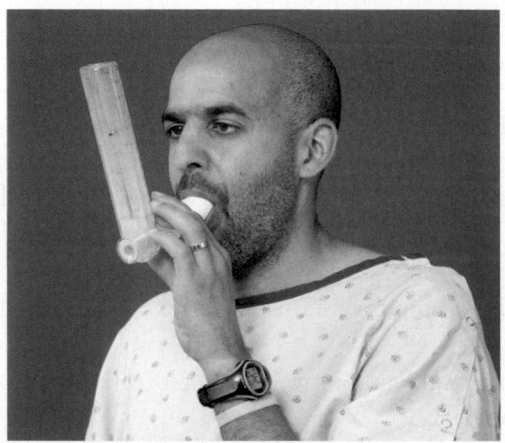

FIG. 3 The patient exhales fast and hard.

Rationale: Motivation and proper technique will obtain the highest peak flow.

7. **Repeat steps 4 through 6 twice more, and record the highest peak flow obtained in the three attempts (Fig. 4).**

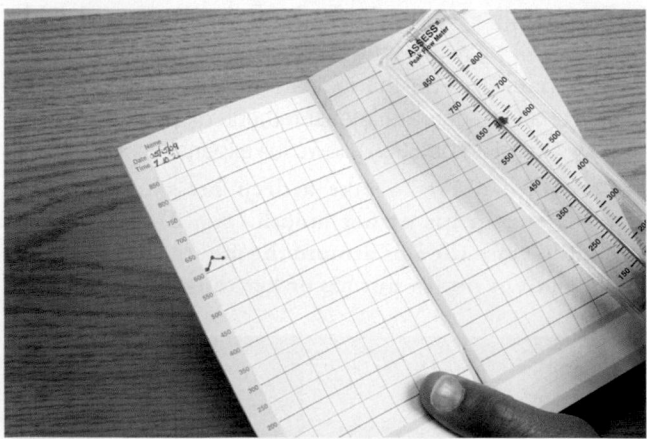

FIG. 4 Record highest peak flow obtained in three attempts.

Rationale: Peak flow varies from one attempt to another. The highest number represents the patient's best effort.

8. **To determine "personal best" when beginning peak flow monitoring, obtain peak flow measurements in the morning and again in the evening over a 2-week period of good asthma control (feeling good without any asthma symptoms). The patient should take measurements before using bronchodilators.**

Rationale: "Personal best" represents the patient's best effort during a period of good control. This will provide a baseline from which to predict green, yellow, and red zones.

9. **Healthcare provider will calculate zones based on percentage of personal best (green 80% to 100%, yellow 50% to 80%, red below 50%) and give instructions for what to do when in each zone.**

Rationale: Zones determine how well asthma is controlled and provide guidelines for the patient to adjust treatment or contact the healthcare provider.

10. **Encourage the patient to comply with twice-a-day (morning and evening) peak flow monitoring before bronchodilator therapy and follow healthcare provider's instructions for peak flows in each zone. Follow steps 4 through 7.**

Rationale: Consistent use of peak flow monitoring allows the patient to detect subtle changes in airway diameter and to institute appropriate therapy to avoid acute asthma exacerbations.

11. **Document procedure.**

Rationale: Maintains legal record and communicates with healthcare team.

Documentation

8/5/16: 09:00—
P: Health management of newly diagnosed asthma, hospitalized 2 weeks ago.
I: RT instructed use of peak flow meter and obtained baseline values, calculating green, yellow, and red zones.
E: Patient and wife could verbalize what to do when peak flows fell into each zone. Nursing will follow up at next appointment.

—S. Roberts, RN

Life Span Considerations

Child and Adolescent

- Peak flow monitoring is appropriate for children who are able to follow directions and use effective technique. Baseline values need to be recalculated every 6 months during growth spurts. Children may need reminders from family members and help keeping a daily log. Adolescents need to assume more responsibility and control over their asthma management.

Home Care Modifications

- Most peak flow monitoring is done in the home setting. Initial teaching is usually done in the clinic or provider's office. Follow-up is important. Home care nurses use peak flow logs to assess asthma control.

Collaboration and Delegation

- Respiratory therapists may be responsible for initial teaching of peak flow monitoring and calculation of zones.

Procedure 26-5 Teaching Deep Breathing and Coughing

Purpose

1. Facilitate respiratory functioning by increasing lung expansion and preventing alveolar collapse.
2. Encourage expectoration of mucus and secretions that accumulate in the airways after general anesthesia and immobility.

Equipment

Pillows for positioning and to splint incision

Assessment

- Assess patient's risk factors for development of respiratory complications (e.g., general anesthesia, history of pulmonary disease or smoking, chest wall trauma, cold or respiratory infection within past week).
- Assess quality, rate, and depth of respiration.
- Auscultate breath sounds.
- Inspect placement of incision and evaluate whether or not it interferes with chest expansion.
- Evaluate the patient's physical ability to cooperate and perform pulmonary exercises:
  - Level of consciousness
  - Language or communication barriers
  - Ability to assume Fowler's position
  - Pain level (medicate as ordered)

Procedure

1. **Perform hand hygiene.**

   Rationale: Reduces microbe transmission.

2. **Identify the patient.**

   Rationale: Ensures correct patient receives proper assessment or treatment and reduces errors.

3. **Close door or bed curtains and explain the procedure to the patient.**

   Rationale: Ensures patient privacy, increases patient compliance, reduces patient anxiety, and promotes learning.

Deep Breathing

4. **Assist the patient to Fowler's or sitting position.**

   Rationale: Upright position allows increased diaphragmatic excursion secondary to downward shift of internal organs from gravity.

5. **Have the patient place hands palm down, with middle fingers touching, along the lower border of the rib cage (Fig. 1).**

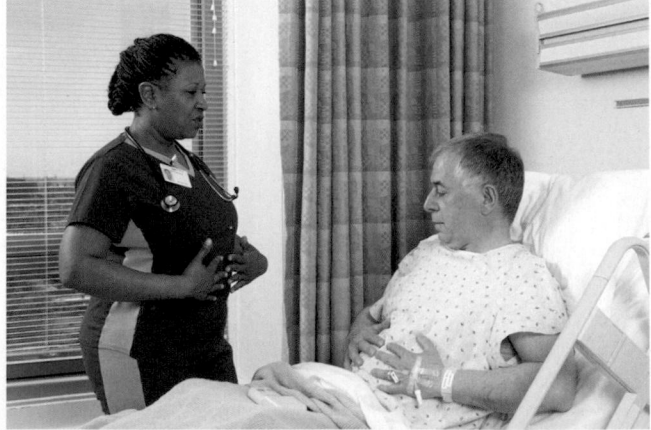

FIG. 1 Instruct the patient to place hands along the lower rib cage to feel diaphragm movement.

Rationale: This position allows the patient to feel movement of the diaphragm, indicating a deep breath.

6. **Ask the patient to inhale slowly through the nose, feeling middle fingers separate. Hold breath for 2 or 3 seconds (Fig. 2).**

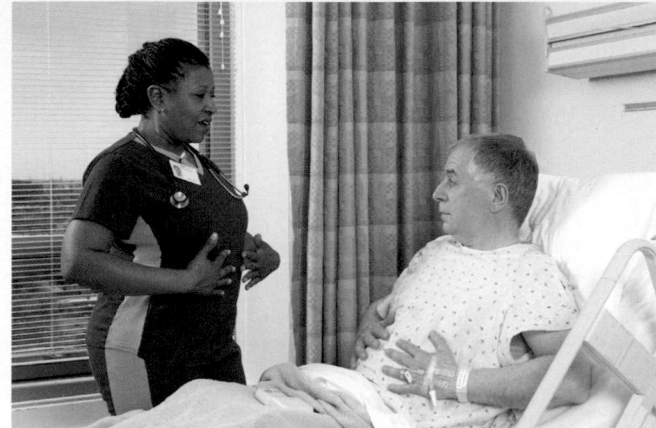

FIG. 2 Encourage the patient to inhale slowly and deeply through the nose, holding breath for 2 to 3 seconds.

Rationale: Inhaling through the nose allows air to be filtered, warmed, and humidified. Holding the breath allows the lungs to expand fully.

7. **Have the patient exhale slowly through mouth (Fig. 3). Repeat three to five times.**

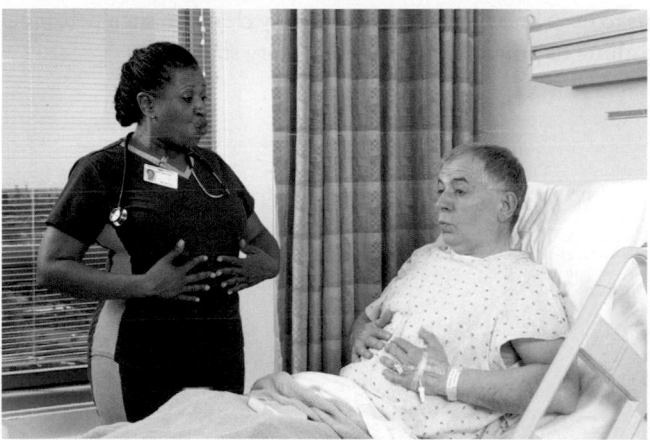

FIG. 3 Instruct the patient to exhale slowly through the mouth.

Rationale: Slow expulsion of air frequently initiates the coughing reflex, which facilitates expectoration of mucus and prevents hyperventilation.

Controlled Coughing

8. **If adventitious breath sounds or sputum is present, have patient take a deep breath, hold for 3 seconds, and cough deeply two or three times. Stand to the patient's side to ensure the cough is not directed at you. The patient must cough deeply, not just clear the throat.**

Rationale: Several consecutive coughs are more effective than one single cough at moving mucus up and out of the respiratory tract.

9. **If the patient has an abdominal or chest incision that will cause pain during coughing, instruct the patient to hold a pillow firmly over the incision (splinting) when coughing (Figs. 4 and 5).**

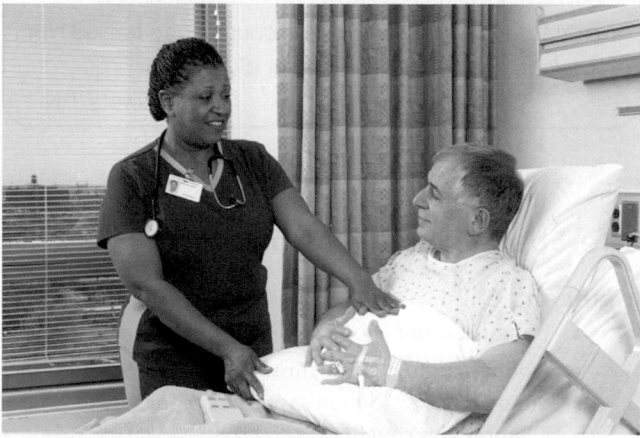

FIG. 4 Instruct the patient to hold pillow firmly over incision.

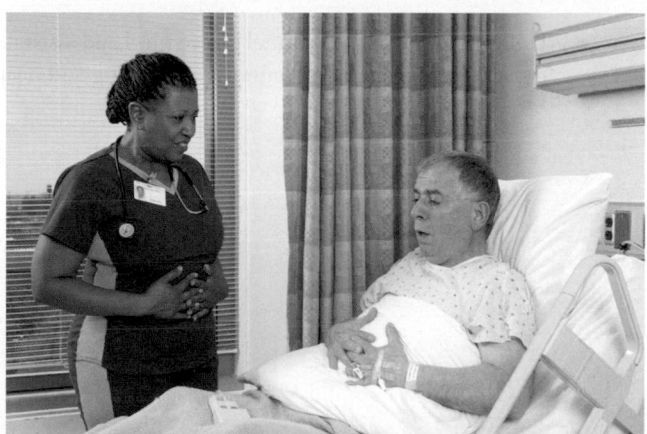

FIG. 5 Encourage the patient to splint with pillow during coughing to promote comfort.

Rationale: Coughing uses abdominal and accessory respiratory muscles, which may have been cut during surgery. Splinting supports the incision and surrounding tissues and reduces pain during coughing.

10. **Instruct, reinforce, and supervise deep breathing and coughing exercises every 2 to 3 hours postoperatively.**

Rationale: Performing these exercises every 2 to 3 hours will facilitate pulmonary ventilation and promote airway clearance without overtiring the patient.

11. **Document procedure.**

Rationale: Maintains legal record and communicates with healthcare team.

Procedure 26-5   *continued*

Documentation

> 8/5/2016: 17:00—Crackles and diminished breath sounds. Instruction on DB & C given, needs encouragement as respiration is shallow and has weak cough. Importance explained and wife encouraged to remind him to perform hourly. Will get order for IS.
>
>   —S. Roberts, RN

Life Span Considerations

Infant and Child

- Infants cannot cooperate with coughing and deep-breathing exercises, but crying is thought to hyperinflate the lungs.
- Young children learn through games and imitation. A preoperative game of "Simon Says" is one way to teach them lung exercises: "Simon says touch your nose," "Simon says stick out your tongue," "Simon says take a deep breath," and "Simon says cough."

Collaboration and Delegation

- Unlicensed nursing personnel can remind and assist patients to deep breathe and cough. Identify clearly to such personnel those patients who need aggressive coughing and deep breathing to promote optimal pulmonary status.

Procedure 26-6 Promoting Breathing With the Incentive Spirometer

Purpose
1. Provides incentives via visual clues to the patient regarding effective deep breathing.
2. Improves pulmonary ventilation and oxygenation, loosens respiratory secretions, and prevents or treats atelectasis by expanding collapsed alveoli.

Equipment
Incentive spirometer (flow oriented or volume oriented; type of incentive spirometer is usually determined by equipment available through respiratory therapy).

Assessment
- Identify patients at risk for atelectasis.
- Complete respiratory assessment (i.e., history of smoking, breath sounds, respiratory rate and rhythm, sputum production) (Fig. 1).

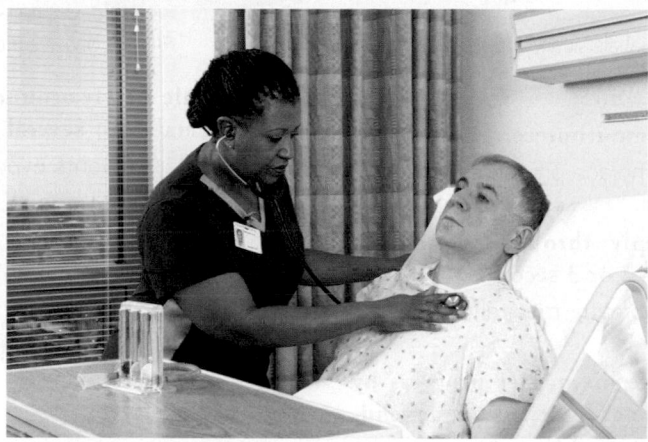

FIG. 1 Assess breath sounds.

Procedure

1. **Perform hand hygiene.**
   Rationale: Reduces microbe transmission.
2. **Identify the patient.**
   Rationale: Ensures correct patient receives proper assessment or treatment and reduces errors.
3. **Close door or bed curtains and explain the procedure to the patient.**
   Rationale: Ensures patient privacy, increases patient compliance, reduces patient anxiety, and promotes learning.
4. **Assist the patient to high Fowler's or sitting position.**
   Rationale: These positions facilitate optimal lung expansion.
5. **Determine the volume to set incentive spirometry goal based on calculated lung volumes. You may use chart or have respiratory therapy calculated. Set volume indicator. Explain goal to the patient (Fig. 2).**

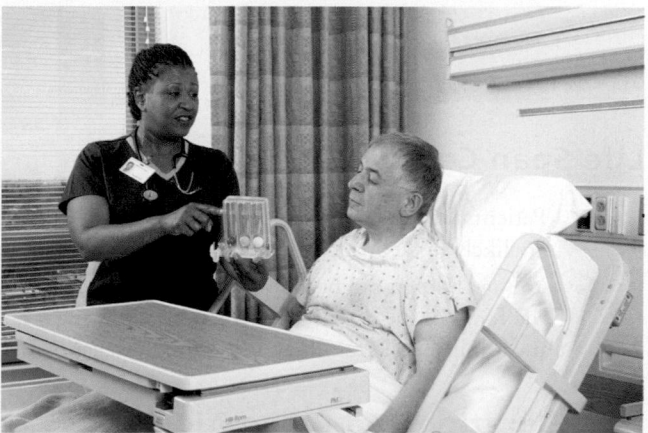

FIG. 2 Encourage the patient to reach goal.

Rationale: People of different sizes have different lung capacities. Individualize the preset goal to promote optimal lung inflation and provide realistic motivation.

Procedure 26-6 *continued*

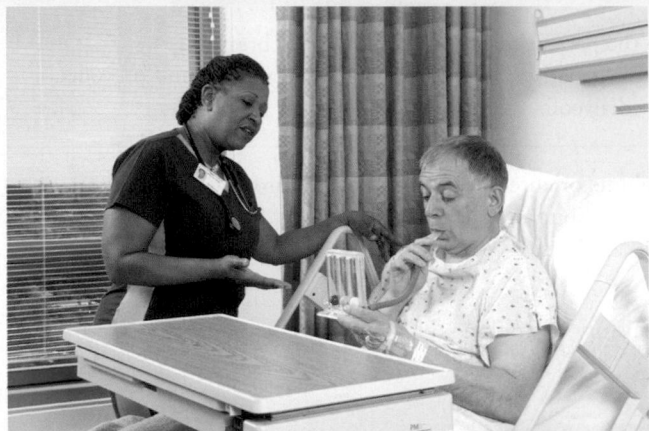

FIG. 3 Instruct the patient to inhale slowly and deeply.

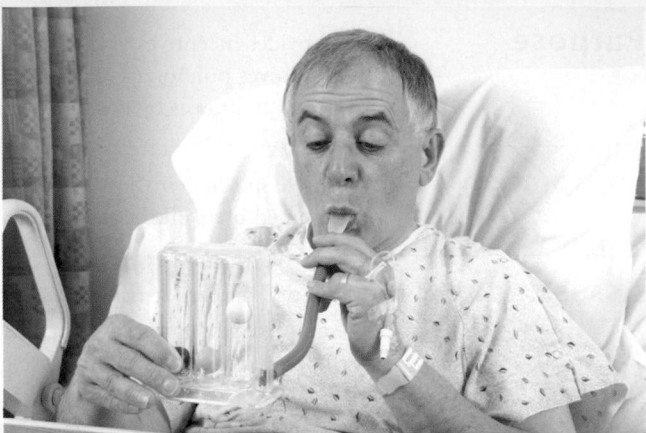

FIG. 4 Observe progress of elevating balls.

6. **Instruct the patient in procedure:**

   a. **Seal lips tightly around mouthpiece.**

      Rationale: A sealed mouthpiece prevents leakage of air around the mouthpiece.

   b. **Inhale slowly and deeply through the mouth (Fig. 3). Hold breath for 2 or 3 seconds.**

      Rationale: Holding the breath maintains maximal inflation of alveoli.

   c. **Have the patient observe his or her progress by watching the balls elevate or lights go on, depending on type of equipment used (Fig. 4).**

      Rationale: Observing progress provides visual feedback to the patient regarding depth of inspiration, which motivates the patient to breathe deeply.

   d. **Exhale slowly around the mouthpiece and breathe normally for several breaths.**

      Rationale: Prevents hyperventilation.

7. **Repeat procedure 5 to 10 times every 1 to 2 hours, per provider's orders.**

   Rationale: Frequent use will prevent alveoli collapse.

8. **Document procedure.**

   Rationale: Maintains legal record and communicates with healthcare team.

Documentation

> 8/1/16: 15:00—Using IS every hour while awake obtaining goal of 500 mL, lung sounds clear to auscultation.
>
> —S. Roberts, RN

Life Span Considerations

- Patients who are too young to follow directions, are cognitively impaired or malnourished, or lack necessary motor skills are likely to be unsuccessful at using incentive spirometry.
- Young children can be asked to blow up a balloon or pretend to blow out candles to accomplish the same goal. Although the focus of the activity is exhalation ("blowing") rather than the inhalation focus of the incentive spirometer, the child must inhale fully to achieve the strong exhalation.

Collaboration and Delegation

- Respiratory therapy often provides the initial instruction on how to use the incentive spirometer, calculating a realistic lung volume. For preoperative patients, try to coordinate teaching before surgery.

Procedure 26-7 Administering Oxygen by Nasal Cannula or Mask

Purpose	1. Deliver low to moderate levels of oxygen to relieve hypoxia.

Equipment	Appropriate oxygen delivery system (see Table 26-6) Oxygen source Flow meter "No smoking" sign for home use Humidifier and distilled water (for high-flow O_2 therapy)

Assessment/ Preparation

- Assess respiratory status (e.g., breath sounds, respiratory rate and depth, presence of sputum, ABG if available) (Fig. 1).

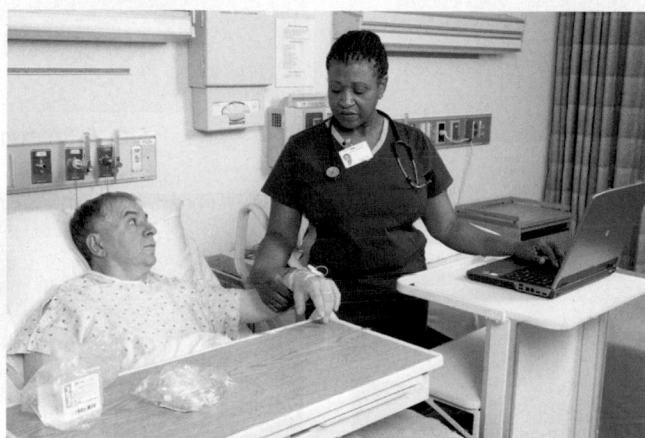

FIG. 1 Check the patient's identification against provider's order.

- Assess past medical history, noting COPD.
- Assess for clinical signs and symptoms of hypoxia: anxiety, decreased level of consciousness, inability to concentrate, fatigue, dizziness, cardiac dysrhythmias, pallor or cyanosis, and dyspnea.

Procedure

1. **Review provider's order for oxygen to ensure that it includes method of delivery, flow rate, and titration orders.**
   Rationale: Prevents errors.

2. **Perform hand hygiene.**
   Rationale: Reduces microbe transmission.

3. **Identify the patient.**
   Rationale: Ensures correct patient receives proper assessment or treatment and reduces errors.

4. **Close door or bed curtains and explain the procedure to the patient.**
   Rationale: Ensures patient privacy, increases patient compliance, reduces patient anxiety, and promotes learning.

5. **Proceed with the six rights of medication administration. Explain that oxygen will ease dyspnea or discomfort, and inform patient concerning safety precautions associated with oxygen use. If the patient is using the cannula, encourage him or her to breathe through the nose.**
   Rationale: Oxygen is a drug, and administering using the six rights avoids potential errors. Teaching helps ensure compliance with therapy.

6. **Assist the patient to semi- or high Fowler's position, if tolerated.**
   Rationale: These positions facilitate optimal lung expansion.

Procedure 26-7   *continued*

7. **Insert flow meter into wall outlet (Fig. 2). Attach oxygen tubing to nozzle on flow meter. If using a high O₂ flow, attach humidifier (Fig. 3). Attach oxygen tubing to humidifier (Fig. 4).**

8. **Turn on the oxygen at the prescribed rate (Fig. 5). Check that oxygen is flowing through the tubing (Fig. 6).**

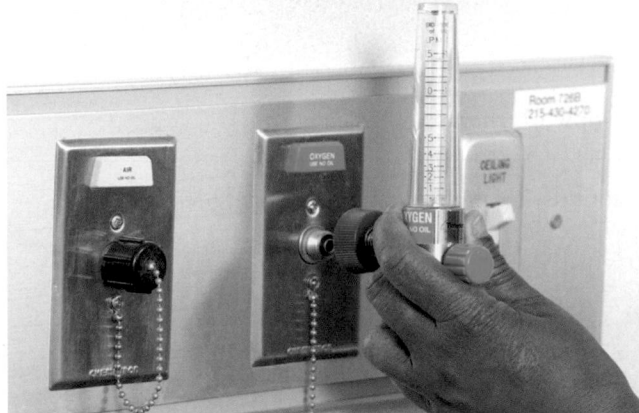

FIG. 2 Insert flow meter into wall unit.

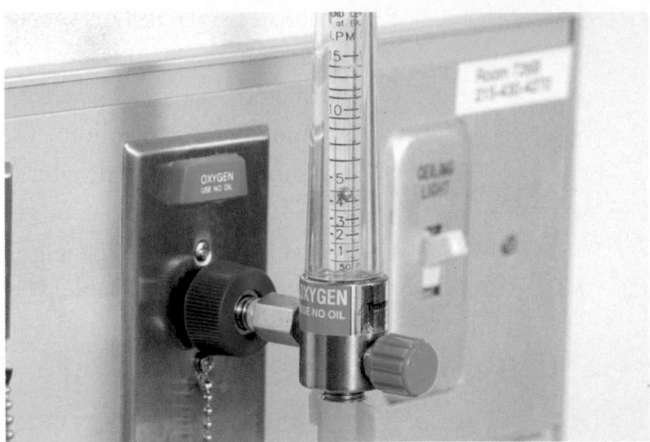

FIG. 5 Set oxygen to prescribed rate.

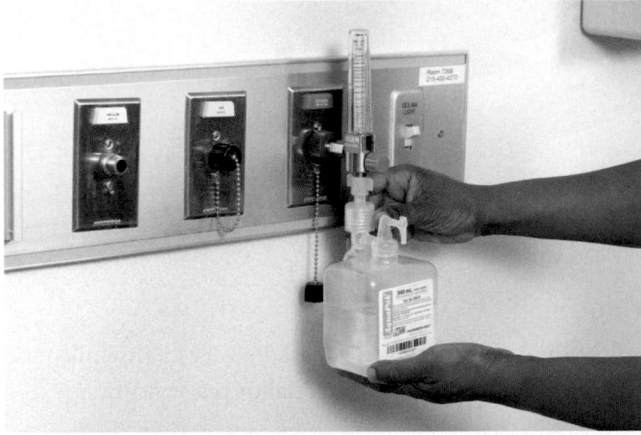

FIG. 3 Attach humidifier to flow meter.

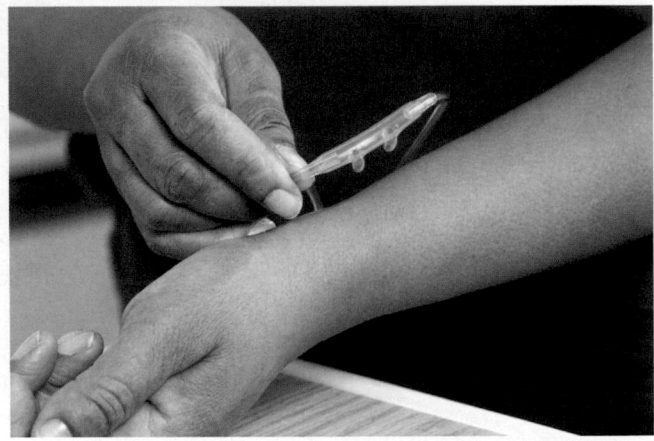

FIG. 6 Ensure the oxygen is flowing through the tubing.

Rationale: Oxygen must be administered as prescribed.

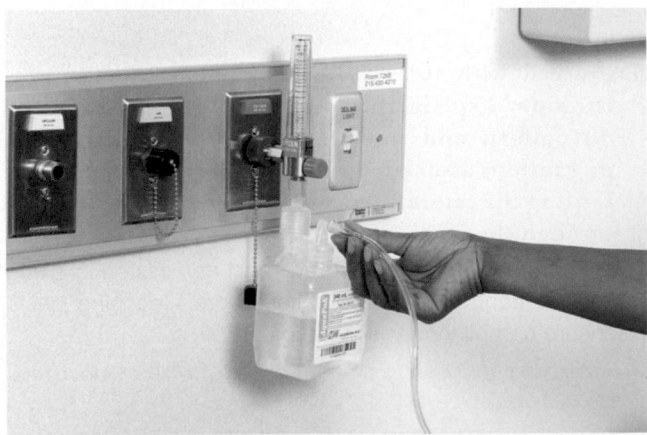

FIG. 4 Attach oxygen tubing to humidifier.

Rationale: Oxygen in high concentrations can be drying to the mucosa.

Procedure 26-7 *continued*

9. Cannula:

a. **Hold nasal cannula in proper position with prongs curving downward (Fig. 7).**

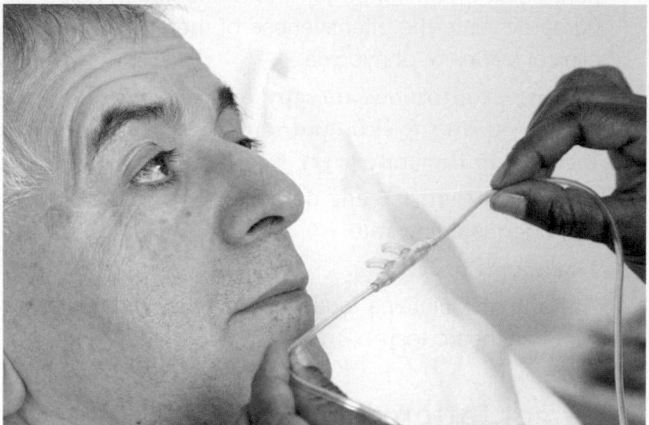

FIG. 7 Properly position nasal cannula with prongs curving downward.

b. **Place cannula prongs into nares (Fig. 8).**

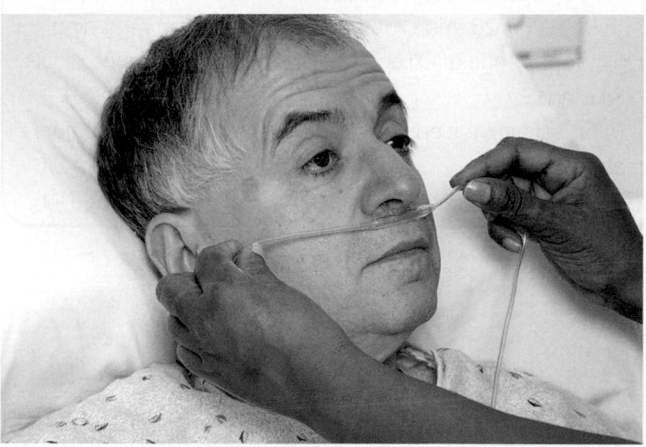

FIG. 8 Place cannula prongs into nares.

c. **Wrap tubing over and behind ears (Fig. 9).**

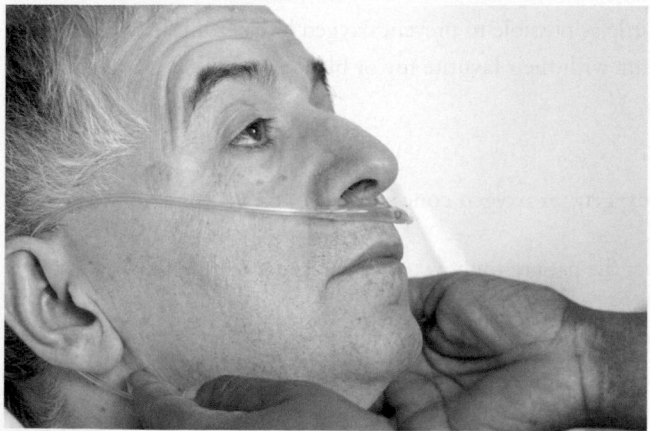

FIG. 9 Wrap tubing around ears.

d. **Adjust plastic slide under chin until cannula fits snugly (Fig. 10).**

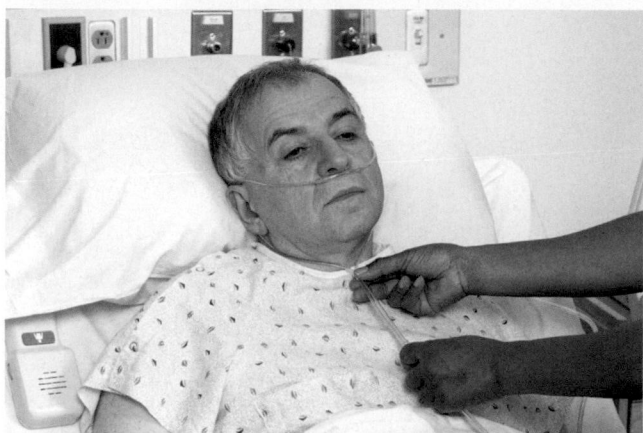

FIG. 10 Adjust plastic slide under chin until cannula fits snugly.

Rationale: Proper placement in nares ensures accurate administration. (*Note:* The cannula permits some freedom of movement and does not interfere with the patient's ability to eat or talk.)

e. **If tubing is noted padded over ears, place gauze at ear beneath tubing as necessary (Fig. 11).**

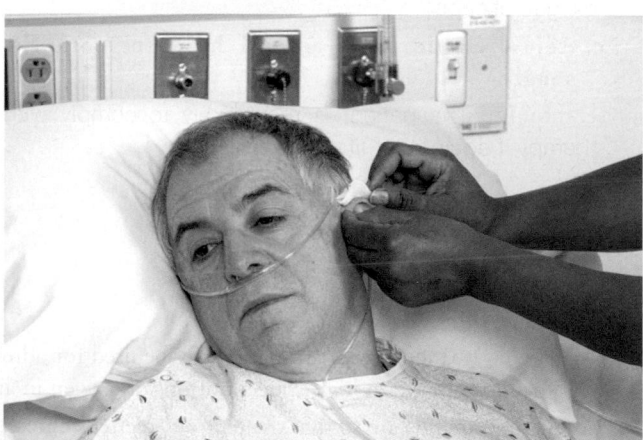

FIG. 11 Place gauze at ear to reduce irritation and promote comfort.

Rationale: Pressure from the tubing may cause device-related pressure ulcer.

f. **If prongs dislodge from nares, replace promptly.**

Rationale: Ensures correct oxygen delivery and prevents hypoxemia.

Procedure 26-7   *continued*

10. **Mask:**

   a. **Position mask on face, starting over the nose, then chin (Fig. 12).**

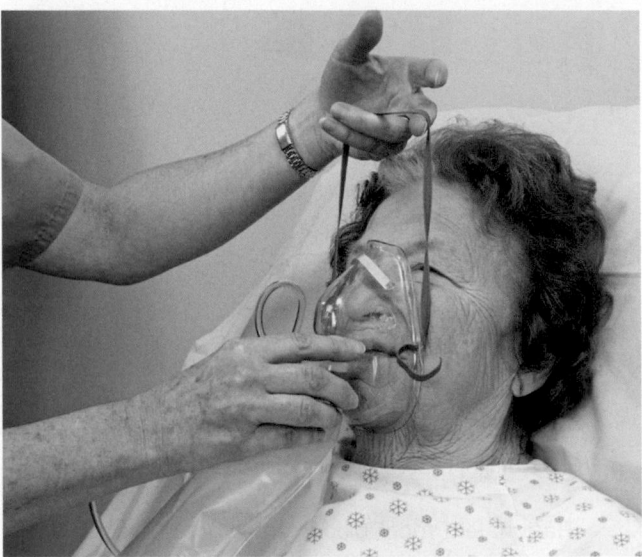

   FIG. 12 Position oxygen mask.

   b. **Adjust the metal rim over the nose and contour the mask to the face.**

   Rationale: When the mask fits the face properly, little oxygen escapes.

   c. **Adjust elastic band around head so mask fits snugly.**

   Rationale: The patient is more likely to comply with therapy if equipment fits comfortably.

11. **Assess for proper functioning of equipment and observe patient's initial response to therapy.**

   Rationale: Assessment of vital signs, oxygen saturation, color, breathing pattern, and orientation helps the nurse evaluate the effectiveness of therapy and detect clinical evidence of hypoxia.

12. **Monitor continuous therapy by assessing for pressure areas on the skin and nares every 2 hours and rechecking flow rate every 4 to 8 hours.**

   Rationale: Permits early detection of skin breakdown or inadequate flow rate.

13. **Document procedure.**

   Rationale: Maintains legal record and communicates with healthcare team.

Documentation

8/4/16: 08:00—
P: Impaired gas exchange.
I: O_2 at 2 L/m via cannula started because sats dropped to 91%. RR 26 and c/o of dyspnea. Teaching regarding the importance of O_2 and reinforced the importance of DB & using IS.
E: O_2 sats increased to 94%, RR18, states more comfortable.

—S. Roberts, RN

Life Span Considerations

Infant and Child

- Isolettes (incubators) and tents may be used for administering oxygen and humidity to infants and newborns. It is difficult to maintain high concentrations of oxygen in an isolette or tent, but it is nonintrusive and nonirritating.
- Plan nursing care so that the tent or isolette is entered as little as possible to prevent oxygen levels from dropping.
- Children frightened by the oxygen tent may feel more secure with their favorite toy or blanket.

Home Care Modifications

- In-home oxygen supply is delivered by cylinders, liquid oxygen, or oxygen concentrators. Portable oxygen systems are available to increase independence and social activities.
- The equipment vendor and home care nurse should instruct the patient on how to use home oxygen equipment and how often the equipment must be filled.
- Instruct the patient and family about the importance of not smoking in the area of oxygen use. A "no smoking" sign may be placed as a reminder.

- The patient should be informed about using an oxygen vendor whose services include the following:
  - Trained personnel to instruct the patient in use and maintenance of the equipment
  - 24-hour emergency service
  - Monthly follow-up visits for equipment maintenance and patient instruction
  - Vendor insurance billing
- Needing oxygen at home can be stressful for the patient. Patients should be encouraged to share their fears and concerns. A local support group of patients using home oxygen may help them to discuss their feelings.
- For insurance to cover home oxygen, patients must have oxygen saturation below 88% to 90% on room air.

Collaboration and Delegation

- Respiratory therapists often titrate oxygen concentrations per protocols using the patient's oxygen saturations.

Procedure 26-8 **Providing Tracheostomy Care**

Purpose

1. Maintain airway patency by removing mucus and encrusted secretions.
2. Promote cleanliness and prevent infection and skin breakdown at stoma site.

Equipment

Sterile tracheostomy care kit containing:

- Two basins
- Small brush or pipe cleaners
- 4″ × 4″ gauze
- Commercially available tracheostomy dressing
- Twill tape or tracheostomy ties

Hydrogen peroxide

Normal saline

Sterile gloves

Scissors

Tracheostomy suction supplies

Assessment

- Assess for excess peristomal secretions, excess intratracheal secretions, or soiled tracheostomy dressing and ties.
- Assess respiratory status: breath sounds, respiratory rate, skin color, labored breathing, flared nares or sternal retractions, and ABG.
- Identify factors that influence tracheostomy care:
- Inadequate nutritional status predisposes the patient to infection, poor healing, and weak cough reflex.
  - *Respiratory infection*: Pulmonary secretions increase in amount. Note color, amount, and odor.
  - *Fluid status*: Inadequate hydration increases tenaciousness of secretions. The patient may have difficulty coughing up thick secretions.
  - *Humidity*: Tracheostomy collars deliver humidified air to prevent dry, cracked membranes and thickened secretions.
- Identify type of tracheostomy tube used and if inner cannula is present. Identify if tracheostomy tube is cuffed and if the cuff is inflated.
- Assess the patient's ability to understand and perform independent tracheostomy care.

Procedure

1. **Verify the provider order.**
   Rationale: Prevents errors.
2. **Perform hand hygiene and don gloves.**
   Rationale: Reduces microbe transmission.
3. **Identify the patient.**
   Rationale: Ensures correct patient receives proper assessment or treatment and reduces errors.
4. **Close door or bed curtains and explain the procedure to the patient (Fig. 1). Place the patient in semi- to high Fowler's position.**

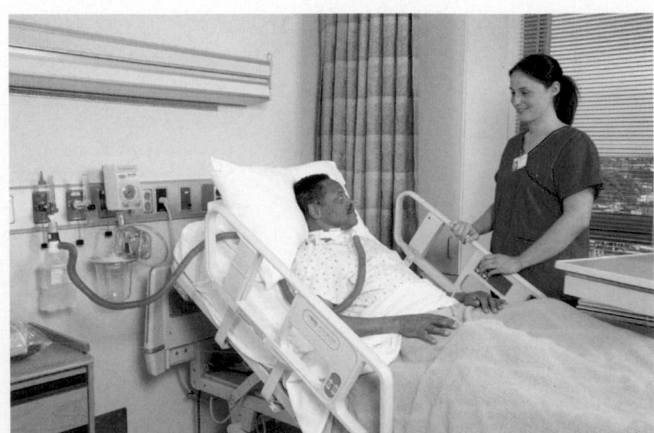

FIG. 1 Greet the patient and explain procedure.

Rationale: Ensures patient privacy, increases patient compliance, reduces patient anxiety, and promotes learning.

Procedure 26-8   *continued*

5. **Suction tracheostomy tube. Before discarding gloves, remove soiled tracheostomy dressing and discard with catheter inside glove.** (*Note:* **Follow Procedure 26-9, Suctioning Secretions From Airways. When suctioning through a tracheostomy tube, insert catheter about 10 to 12 cm [in an adult].**)

   Rationale: Removing secretions maintains a patent airway while doing tracheostomy cleaning.

6. **Replace oxygen or humidification source and encourage the patient to deep breathe as you prepare sterile supplies. Do not snap in place.**

   Rationale: Maintains good oxygenation status. Promotes easy removal prior to sterile procedure.

7. **Open sterile tracheostomy kit (Fig. 2). Pour normal saline into one basin and hydrogen peroxide into the second (Fig. 3). Don sterile gloves (Fig. 4). Open several sterile cotton-tipped applicators and one sterile precut tracheostomy dressing, and place on sterile field (Fig. 5).** (*Note:* **If kit does not contain sterile cotton-tipped applicators and dressing, open those items prior to donning sterile gloves.) If kit does not contain tracheostomy ties, cut two 15-inch pieces of twill tape and set aside.**

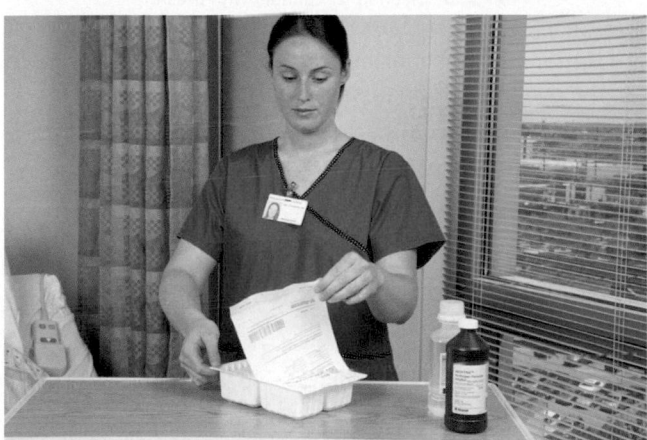

FIG. 2 Open sterile tracheostomy kit.

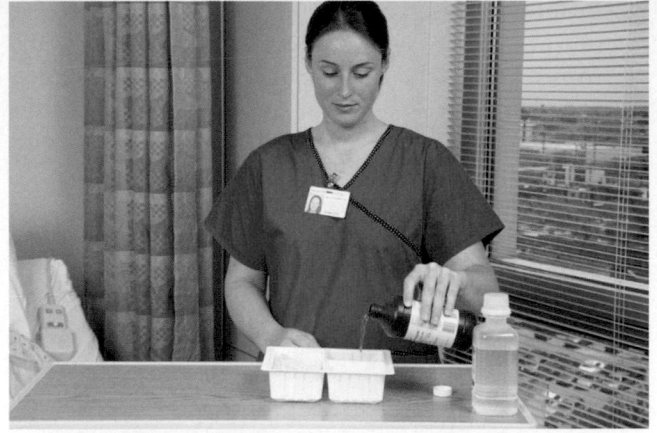

FIG. 3 Pour sterile hydrogen peroxide into basin.

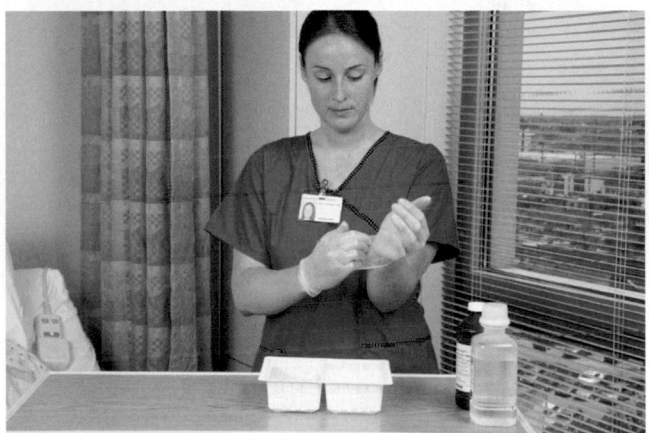

FIG. 4 Don sterile gloves.

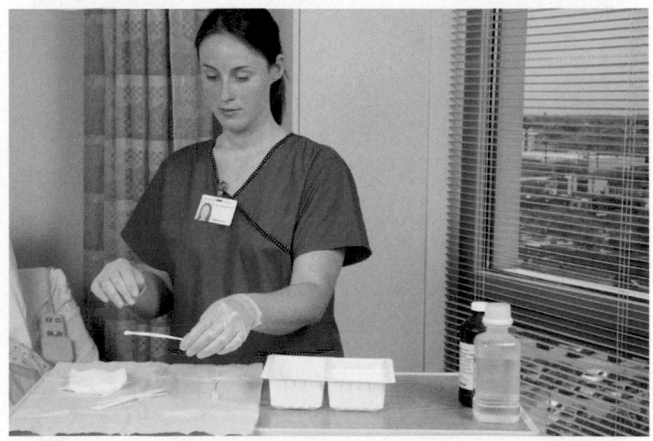

FIG. 5 Place items on sterile field.

Rationale: Preparing equipment allows for smooth, organized performance of tracheostomy care.

Procedure 26-8 *continued*

8. Remove oxygen source (Fig. 6). The hand that touches the oxygen source is no longer sterile. (*Note*: For tracheostomy tube with inner cannula, complete steps 7 to 25. For tracheostomy tube without inner cannula or plugged with a button, complete steps 15 to 26.)

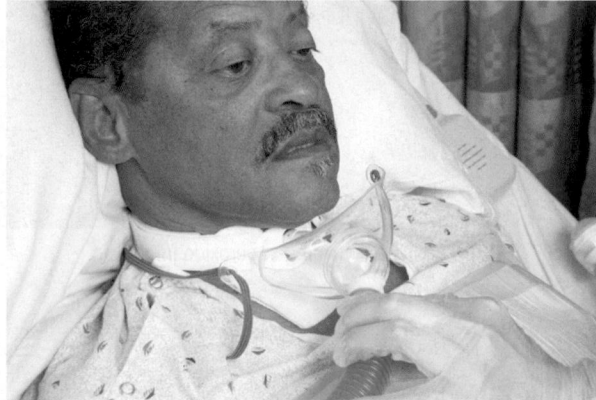

FIG. 6 Remove oxygen source.

Rationale: Prevents contamination of sterile gloves.

9. Unlock inner cannula by turning counterclockwise. Remove inner cannula (Fig. 7).

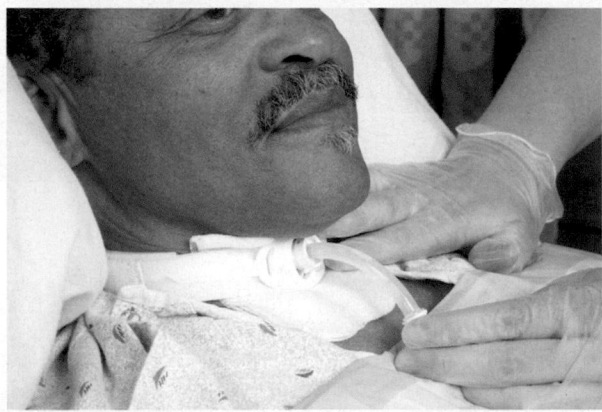

FIG. 7 Unlock inner cannula by turning counterclockwise.

10. Place inner cannula in basin with hydrogen peroxide (Fig. 8).

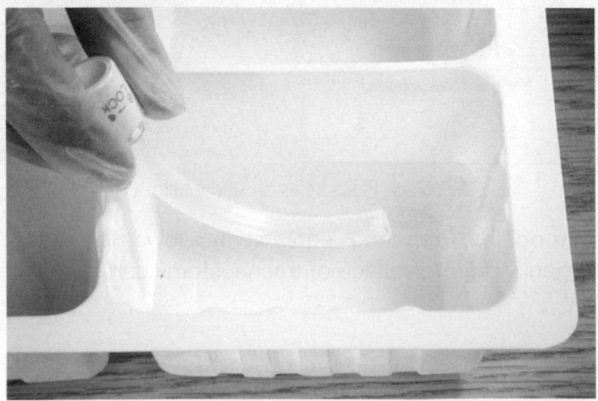

FIG. 8 Place inner cannula into basin with hydrogen peroxide.

Rationale: Hydrogen peroxide loosens and removes secretions from inner cannula.

11. Replace oxygen source over or near outer cannula.

Rationale: Maintains a constant supply of oxygen to prevent respiratory or cardiac distress. (*Note:* Not all patients require a constant oxygen supply during tracheostomy care.)

12. Clean lumen and sides of inner cannula using pipe cleaners or sterile brush (Fig. 9).

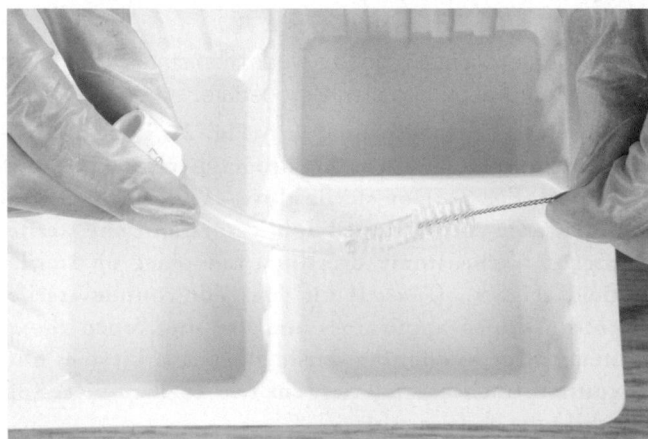

FIG. 9 Clean inner cannula with brush.

Rationale: Mechanical force and friction are needed to remove thick or dried secretions.

13. Rinse inner cannula thoroughly by agitating in normal saline for several seconds (Fig. 10).

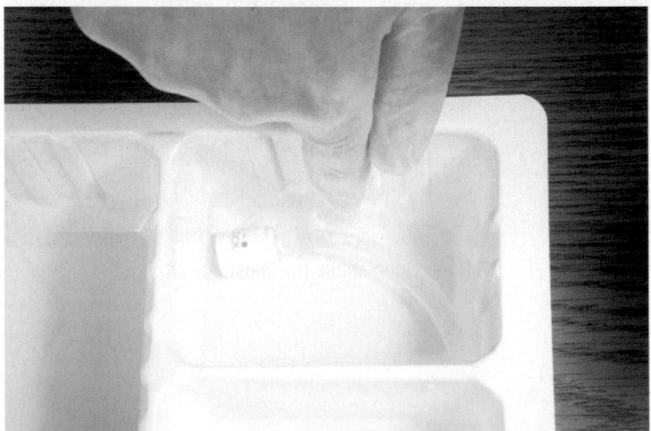

FIG. 10 Rinse inner cannula in normal saline.

Rationale: Rinsing and agitation remove secretions and water from the cannula and provide lubrication for easy reinsertion.

14. Remove oxygen source and replace inner cannula into outer cannula, then "lock" by turning clockwise until the two blue dots align (Fig. 11). Replace oxygen or humidity source.

Procedure 26-8   *continued*

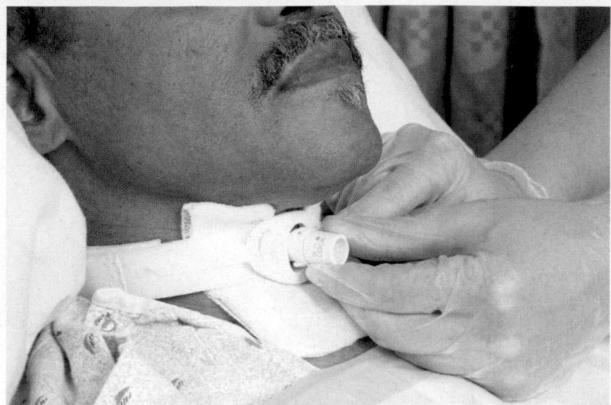

FIG. 11 Replace inner cannula, then lock into place.

Rationale: Oxygen is re-established to a secured inner cannula.

15. **Remove tracheostomy dressing from under face-plate (Fig. 12).**

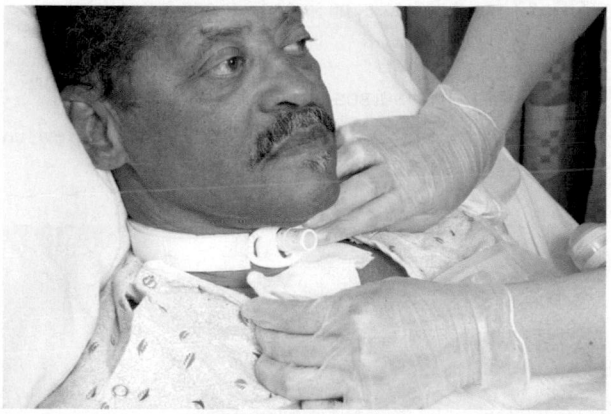

FIG. 12 Remove soiled tracheostomy dressing.

Rationale: The tracheostomy dressing is soiled and needs to be replaced.

16. **Clean stoma under faceplate with circular motion using normal saline–soaked cotton applicators. Clean dried secretions from all exposed outer cannula surfaces (Fig. 13).**

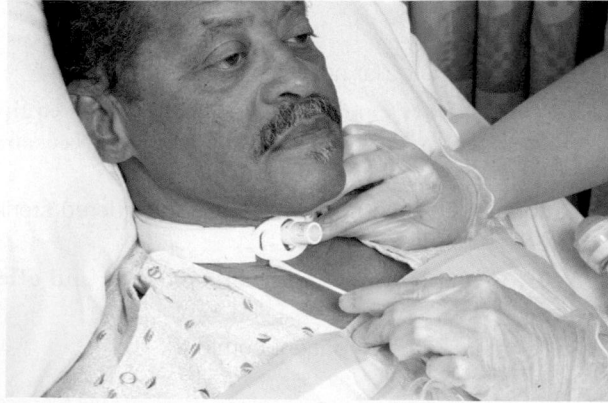

FIG. 13 Clean secretions from tracheostomy site with cotton applicator.

Rationale: Dried secretions are a good medium for bacterial growth.

17. **Pat moist surfaces dry with 4″ × 4″ gauze.**

Rationale: Moist surfaces support growth of microorganisms and skin excoriation.

18. **Place dry, sterile, precut tracheostomy dressing around tracheostomy stoma and under faceplate (Fig. 14). Do not use cut 4″ × 4″ gauze.**

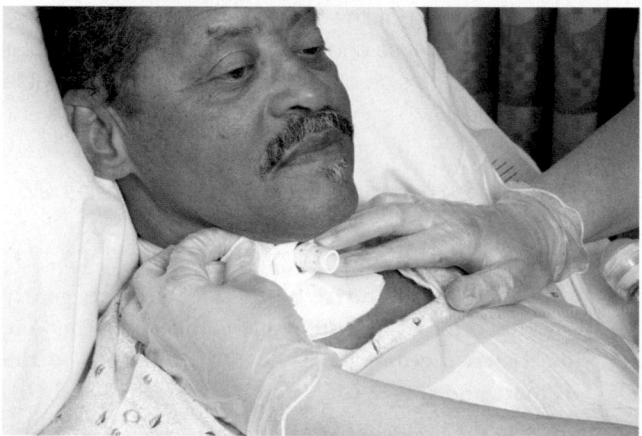

FIG. 14 Replace new precut tracheostomy dressing.

Rationale: Frayed cotton fibers from cut gauze could be aspirated into the trachea.

19. **If tracheostomy ties are to be changed, have an assistant don a sterile glove and hold the tracheostomy tube in place.**

Rationale: This action prevents accidental displacement of the tracheostomy tube if the patient moves or coughs when the ties are not secure.

For Tracheostomy Ties, Follow Steps 20 Through 24

20. **Cut a ½-inch slit approximately 1 inch from one end of both clean tracheostomy ties. This is easily done by folding back on itself 1 inch of the tie and cutting a small slit in the middle.**

Rationale: The slit makes room for the ties.

21. **Remove and discard soiled tracheostomy ties.**

Rationale: Ties need to be replaced.

22. **Thread end of tie through cut slit in tie. Pull tight.**

Rationale: The tie is secured to the faceplate without using knots. Knots are difficult to undo when ties become crusted with secretions.

Procedure 26-8   *continued*

23. Repeat step 22 with the second tie.

24. Bring both ties together at one side of the patient's neck. Assess that ties are tight enough to allow only one finger between tie and neck. Use two square knots to secure the ties. Trim excess tie length. (*Note*: Assess tautness of tracheostomy ties frequently in patients whose neck may swell from trauma or surgery.)

Rationale: Ties must be taut enough to prevent accidental dislodging of the tracheostomy tube but loose enough not to cause choking or pressure on the jugular veins. Ties at the side of the neck are more comfortable for the patient.

For Tracheostomy Collar, Follow Steps 25 Through 27

25. While an assisting nurse holds the faceplate, gently pull the Velcro tab and remove the collar on one side. Insert the new collar into the opening on the faceplate and secure the Velcro tab (Figs. 15 and 16).

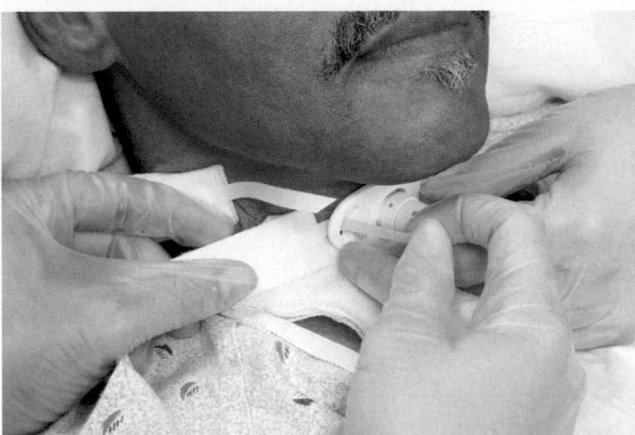

FIG. 15 Insert new collar into opening on faceplate.

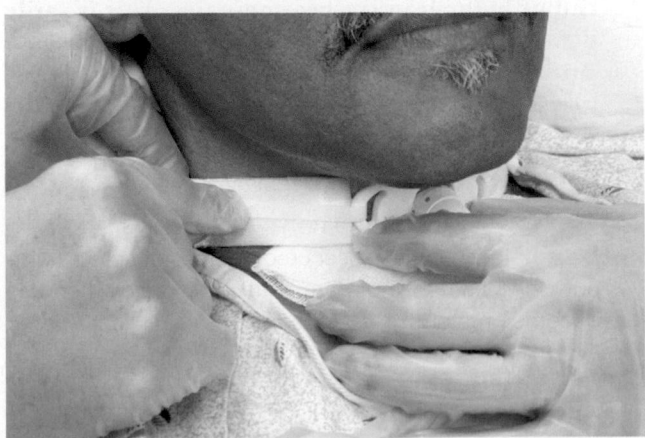

FIG. 16 Secure Velcro tab.

Rationale: The Velcro secures the faceplate.

26. Hold faceplate in place as the assisting nurse repeats step on the second side (Fig. 17).

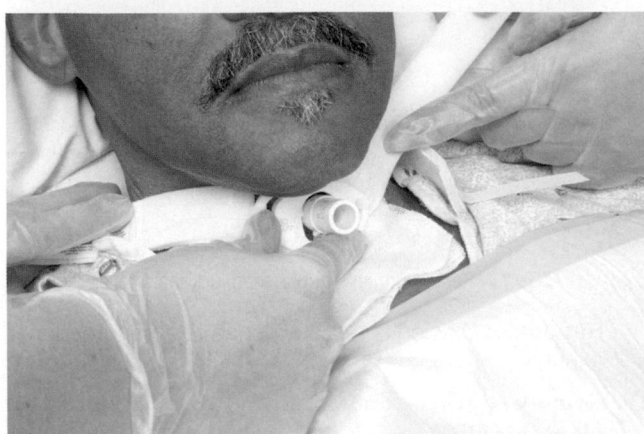

FIG. 17 Insert new collar on second side and secure Velcro tab.

Rationale: Two nurses are important for safety.

27. Remove the old collar and ensure that the new collar is securely in place (Fig. 18).

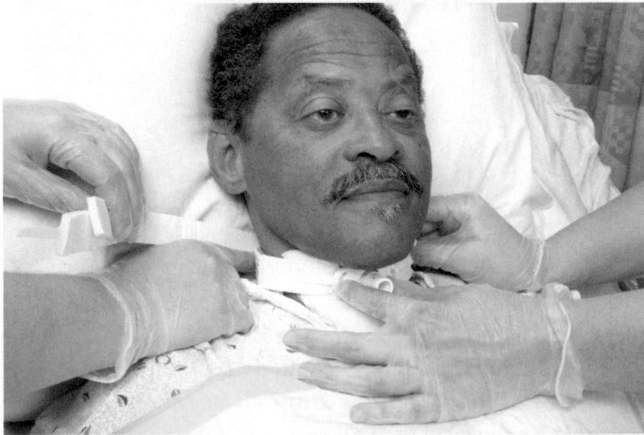

FIG. 18 Discard soiled collar, and ensure new collar is securely in place.

Rationale: The collar needs to be secure.

28. Remove gloves and discard disposable equipment. Label with date and time, and store reusable supplies.

Rationale: Opened normal saline is considered sterile for 24 hours.

29. Assist the patient to comfortable position and offer oral hygiene.

Rationale: Promotes patient comfort.

Procedure 26-8   *continued*

30. **Perform hand hygiene.**

    Rationale: Maintains infection control and communicates with other healthcare team members.

31. **Document procedure.**

    Rationale: Maintains legal record and communicates with healthcare team.

Documentation

9/1/16: 09:00—
P: Impaired airway clearance.
I: Trach care—large amount of thick secretions cleansed from inner cannula, skin around trach is intact but slightly red. The patient is able to expectorate secretions when encouraged to do so. Mist collar in place to maintain humidification.
E: Increase fluids and encourage pulmonary hygiene and mobility to decrease pooling of secretions.
—S. Roberts, RN

Life Span Considerations

Infant and Child

- Additional assistants may be necessary during tracheostomy care to prevent active children from dislodging or expelling their tracheostomy tubes.
- Encourage parents to participate with the procedure in an effort to comfort the child and promote patient teaching.

Home Care Modifications

- Teach the patient or caregiver the following:
  - That handwashing is the most important step before touching the tracheostomy
  - The function of each part of the tracheostomy tube
  - To remove, change, and replace the inner cannula
  - To clean the inner cannula two or three times a day
  - To clean the tracheostomy stoma
  - To suction tracheal secretions
  - To assess for symptoms of infection (e.g., increased temperature, increased amount of secretions, change in color or odor of secretions)
  - To use a mirror for better visualization
- A vaporizer may be used in the home to replace moisture into the air.
- The patient may wear a scarf or 4″ × 4″ over the tracheostomy if the air is dusty.
- Home care may be a clean, rather than sterile, procedure:
  - Plain, single-use paper cups may be used for soaking the inner cannula.
  - Tap water may be used to rinse secretions from the inner cannula.
  - Gloves need not be worn, but thorough handwashing is imperative.
- A list of needed supplies and equipment and the names of medical supply houses are useful.
- Names and telephone numbers of healthcare professionals who are available for emergencies or advice 24 hours a day should be readily available.

Collaboration and Delegation

- Respiratory therapists are responsible for tracheostomy care in some agencies. Communicate with therapists if secretions are excessive or crusted so that they provide tracheostomy care promptly to prevent airway occlusion.

Procedure 26-9 Suctioning Secretions From Airways

Purpose	1. Remove excess mucus secretions to maintain patent airway.
	2. Collect sputum or secretions for diagnostic testing.

Equipment

Portable or wall suction apparatus with tubing and reservoir

Sterile suction kit containing:

– Appropriate-sized catheter: infants, 5 to 8 French; children, 8 to 10 French; and adults, 12 to 18 French

– Pair of gloves

– Container for saline to flush and lubricate catheter

Sterile saline (may be provided in kit)

Water-resistant disposal bag

Facial tissues

Towel (optional)

Assessment/ Preparation

- Assess respiratory system:
  - Note rate, depth, and rhythm of respirations.
  - Note noisy, wet, or gurgling respirations.
  - Auscultate breath sounds.
- Assess the patient's ability to cough. Note amount and character of sputum.
- Assess vital signs. Compare to baseline vital signs. Note an elevation in temperature.
- Assess level of consciousness and ability to protect airway (i.e., cough reflex). Note any drainage from the mouth.

Procedure

1. **Verify the provider order and identify the patient.**

   Rationale: Prevents potential errors.

2. **Perform hand hygiene.**

   Rationale: Reduces microbe transmission.

3. **Identify the patient.**

   Rationale: Ensures correct patient receives proper assessment or treatment and reduces errors.

4. **Close door or bed curtains and explain the procedure to the patient and the family.**

   Rationale: Ensures patient privacy, increases patient compliance, reduces patient anxiety, and promotes learning.

5. a. **Position the conscious patient with an intact gag reflex in a semi-Fowler's position.**

   Rationale: The semi-Fowler's position helps prevent aspiration of secretions.

   b. **Position the unconscious patient in a side-lying position facing you.**

   Rationale: A side-lying position facilitates drainage of secretions by gravity and prevents aspiration.

6. **Turn on suction device and adjust pressure: infants and children, 50 to 75 mm Hg, and adults, 100 to 120 mm Hg (Fig. 1).**

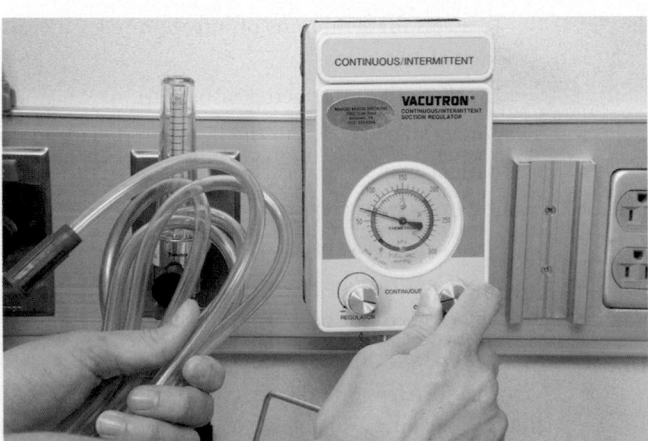

FIG. 1 Adjust suction to appropriate pressure.

Rationale: Excessive negative pressure traumatizes mucosa and can induce hypoxia.

Procedure 26-9 *continued*

7. **Open and prepare sterile suction catheter kit (Fig. 2):**

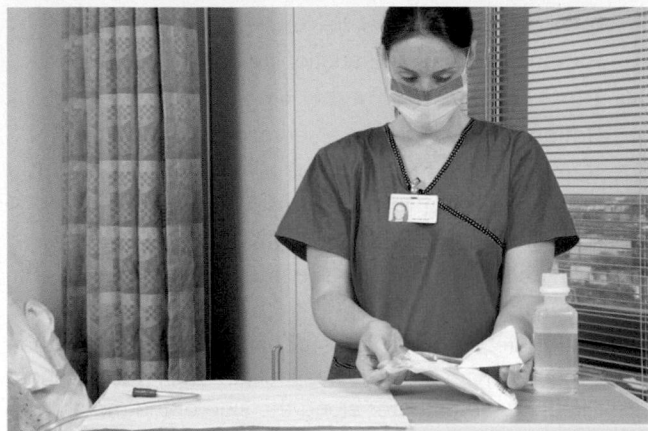

FIG. 2 Open and prepare sterile suction catheter kit.

   a. **Unfold sterile cup, touching only the outside. Place on bedside table.**

   b. **Pour sterile saline into cup.**

    Rationale: Sterile technique is maintained.

8. **Preoxygenate the patient with 100% oxygen; hyperinflate with manual resuscitation bag (Fig. 3).**

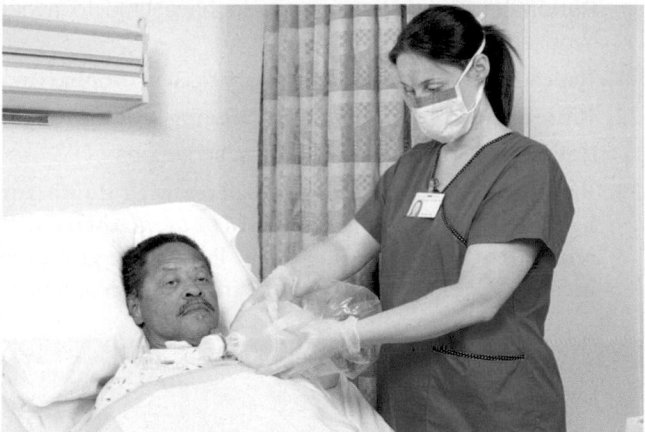

FIG. 3 Preoxygenate and hyperinflate before suction.

   Rationale: Preoxygenation helps prevent hypoxia; hyperinflation decreases atelectasis caused by suctioning.

9. **Don sterile gloves. If kit provides only one glove, place on dominant hand.**

   Rationale: Dominant hand will remain sterile. You may use a clean disposable glove on the nondominant hand to protect yourself from exposure to mucous membranes and sputum.

10. **Pick up catheter with dominant hand. Pick up connecting tubing with nondominant hand. The nondominant hand is now considered clean rather than sterile. Attach catheter to tubing without contaminating sterile hand (Fig. 4).**

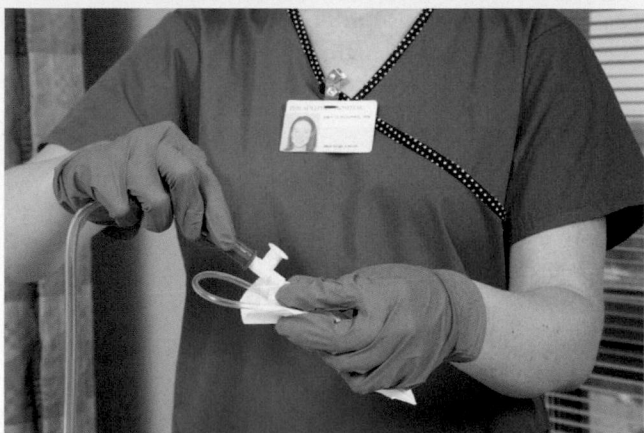

FIG. 4 Attach catheter to suction tubing.

Rationale: Keeps the dominant hand sterile.

11. **Place catheter end into cup of saline. Test functioning of equipment by applying thumb from nondominant hand over open port to create suction (Fig. 5). Apply nonpetroleum–based lubricant if suctioning through nostril.**

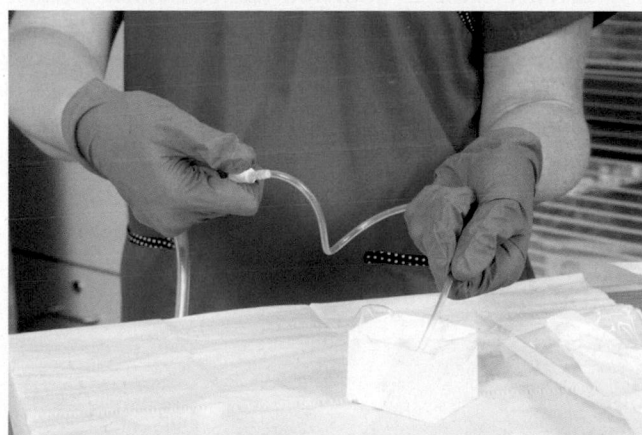

FIG. 5 Flush saline through catheter, occluding Y-port to test suction.

Rationale: Lubrication makes catheter insertion easier and ensures proper functioning of suction equipment.

Procedure 26-9   *continued*

12. **Insert catheter into the trachea through the nostril, nasal trumpet, or artificial airway during inspiration and without suction (Fig. 6).**

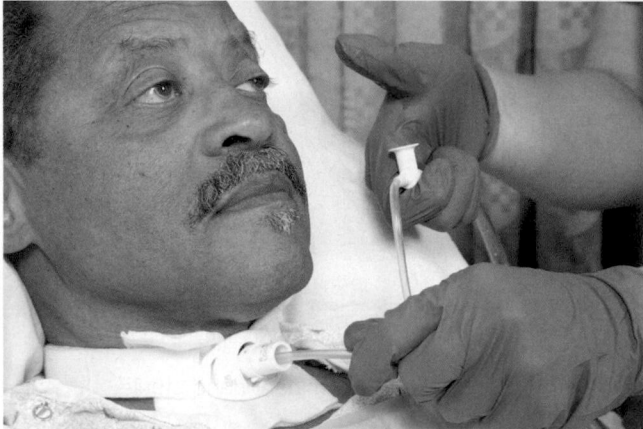

FIG. 6 Insert catheter into trachea without applying suction.

Rationale: Inspiration opens the epiglottis and facilitates catheter movement into the trachea.

13. **Advance catheter until you feel resistance. Retract catheter 1 cm before applying suction. (*Note*: The patient usually will cough when catheter enters the trachea.)**

Rationale: Retracting the catheter slightly prevents mucosal damage.

14. **Apply suction by placing thumb of nondominant hand over open port, then rotate the catheter with your dominant hand as you withdraw the catheter (Fig. 7). This should take 5 to 10 seconds.**

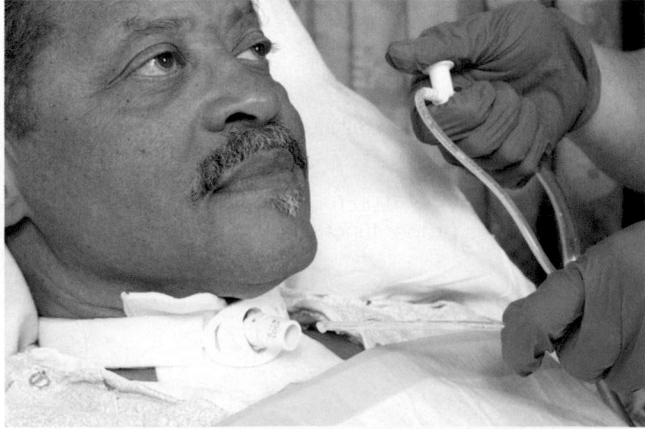

FIG. 7 Apply suction as you withdraw catheter.

Rationale: Rotation of the catheter prevents trauma to the mucous membranes from prolonged suctioning of one area. Limiting the suction time to 10 seconds or less prevents hypoxia.

15. **Hyperoxygenate and hyperinflate using manual resuscitation bag for a full minute between subsequent suction passes. Encourage deep breathing.**

Rationale: Prolonged suctioning can induce hypoxia.

16. **Rinse catheter thoroughly with saline.**

Rationale: Rinsing clears secretions from catheter.

17. **Repeat steps 11 to 15 until airway is clear, limiting each suctioning to three passes.**

18. **Without applying suction, insert the catheter gently along one side of the mouth. Advance to the oropharynx.**

Rationale: Suction the oropharynx after the trachea because the mouth is less clean than the trachea. Directing the catheter along the side of the mouth prevents stimulation of the gag reflex.

19. **Apply suction for 5 to 10 seconds as you rotate and withdraw the catheter.**

Rationale: Rotation of the catheter prevents trauma to the mucous membranes. Be sure to remove secretions that pool beneath the tongue and in the vestibule of the mouth.

20. **Allow 1 to 2 minutes between passes for the patient to ventilate. Encourage deep breathing. Replace oxygen if applicable.**

Rationale: The patient needs to have time to avoid hypoxemia.

21. **Repeat steps 17 and 18 as necessary to clear oropharynx.**

22. **Rinse catheter and tubing by suctioning saline through.**

Rationale: Rinsing removes thick secretions.

23. **Remove gloves by holding catheter with dominant hand and pulling glove off inside out. Catheter will remain coiled inside the glove. Pull other glove off inside out (Fig. 8). Dispose of in trash receptacle.**

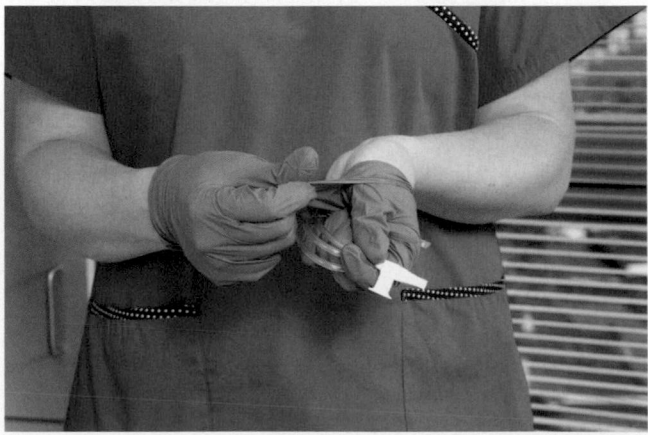

FIG. 8 Remove glove, pulling it over the catheter in other hand.

Rationale: Contains patient secretions inside the gloves to reduce the transmission of microorganisms.

Procedure 26-9   *continued*

24. **Turn off suction device. Assist the patient to comfortable position. Offer assistance with oral and nasal hygiene. Replace oxygen device if used.**

    Rationale: Accumulated respiratory secretions irritate the mucous membranes and are unpleasant for the patient.

25. **Perform hand hygiene.**

    Rationale: Reduces microbe transmission.

26. **Ensure that sterile suction kit is available at head of bed.**

    Rationale: Provides immediate access to suction equipment when needed.

27. **Document procedure.**

    Rationale: Maintains legal record and communicates with healthcare team.

Documentation

9/2/16: 08:00—
P: Impaired airway clearance.
I: Suctioned × 3 with preoxygenation, encouraged patient to deep breathe, cough, and increase fluid intake, mist collar on room air in place, O_2 sats remain above 92%.
E: Copious thick secretions obtained, will need resuctioning every 2 hours as cough is weak and secretions copious.

—S. Roberts, RN

Life Span Considerations

Infant and Child

- Infants and young children have airways that are easily occluded by a small amount of secretions. The nasal airway is smaller in diameter, the epiglottis is higher, and the tongue is proportionately larger.
- A bulb syringe is often used to aspirate secretions from an infant's nasal and oral cavities. This procedure is clean, rather than sterile, because the trachea is not entered.

Home Care Modifications

- Patients may need to learn to suction their secretions if they have difficulty coughing them effectively. Maintaining adequate hydration thins secretions and facilitates their removal.
- The type and number of microorganisms available to contaminate the respiratory system are different at home than in the acute care setting. Teach the patient or caregiver to use plain paper cups for suctioning, not a sterile basin. Keep the cups in a sealable package. The patient or caregiver should remove a clean cup from the bottom of the package for each suctioning effort and reseal the package between uses.
- Suction catheters can be clean, not sterile. They should be washed in soapy water, rinsed well, and soaked in a vinegar and water solution.
- To decrease expense, saline solution can be made by boiling water and adding salt.

Collaboration and Delegation

- Respiratory therapists frequently suction patients in the acute care setting. Nurses need to maintain skill in suctioning so that suctioning can occur quickly to maintain a patent airway if a respiratory therapist is unavailable.

Procedure 26-10 Monitoring a Patient With a Chest Drainage System

Purpose	1. Monitor respiratory status of a patient with a chest tube. 2. Ensure chest drainage system is functioning adequately to promote lung expansion.
Equipment	Occlusive sterile dressing (if needed) Chest tube Chest tube drainage system
Assessment	• Assess respiratory status (e.g., watch symmetrical expansion of thoracic cage; auscultate breath sounds; assess quality, depth, and rate of breaths; obtain pulse oximetry). • Assess for clinical signs and symptoms of hypoxia: anxiety, decreased levels of consciousness, inability to concentrate, fatigue, dizziness, cardiac dysrhythmias, pallor or cyanosis, and dyspnea. Notify physician immediately of any significant changes in patient's respiratory status.

Procedure

1. **Confirm physician's order including amount of suction.**
   Rationale: Prevents potential errors.

2. **Perform hand hygiene.**
   Rationale: Reduces microbe transmission.

3. **Identify the patient.**
   Rationale: Ensures correct patient receives proper assessment or treatment and reduces errors.

4. **Close door or bed curtains and explain the procedure to the patient.**
   Rationale: Ensures patient privacy, increases patient compliance, reduces patient anxiety, and promotes learning.

5. **Assist the patient to semi- or high Fowler's position.**
   Rationale: These positions assist with optimal lung expansion.

6. **Assess insertion site of chest tube. Note and document amount and color of drainage on dressing around insertion site. Feel insertion site for crepitus—air leaking into the subcutaneous tissue (Fig. 1). Document any crepitus found. Reinforce insertion dressing as needed.**

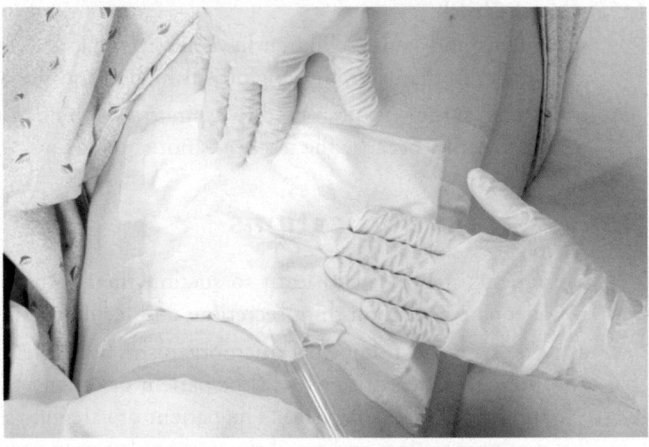

FIG. 1 Palpate insertion site of chest tube.

Rationale: Excessive drainage around the insertion site can indicate bleeding. The insertion site dressing may need to be changed by the surgeon who inserted the chest tube. Development of crepitus can indicate a small air leak into the subcutaneous tissue. Crepitus may indicate a need for the surgeon to adjust the chest tube placement.

7. **Assess status of chest tubing. Be sure tubing remains at the level of the patient and no dependent loops are present. Assess that there are no visible clots in the tubing. You may gently "milk" (compress tubing with fingers) the clots to encourage movement into the drainage system, but you never want to strip chest tubing.**
   Rationale: Dependent loops of tubing may collect fluid and prevent drainage of fluid from the chest cavity. Stripping chest tubing can create dangerous intrathoracic negative pressure, injuring the patient.

Procedure 26-10   *continued*

8. **Assess the drainage collection chamber (Fig. 2). Be sure to keep chest drainage system upright. Assess for amount, color, and character of drainage. Mark the collection chamber to accurately reflect the amount of drainage accumulated during your shift (Fig. 3). Note any significant increase in the amount of drainage.**

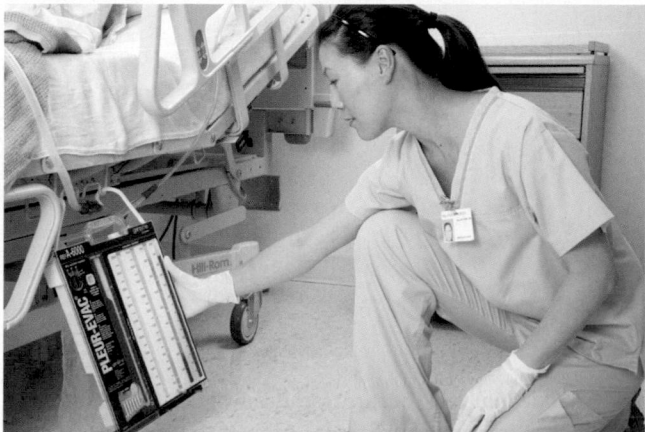

FIG. 2 Assess drainage collection chamber.

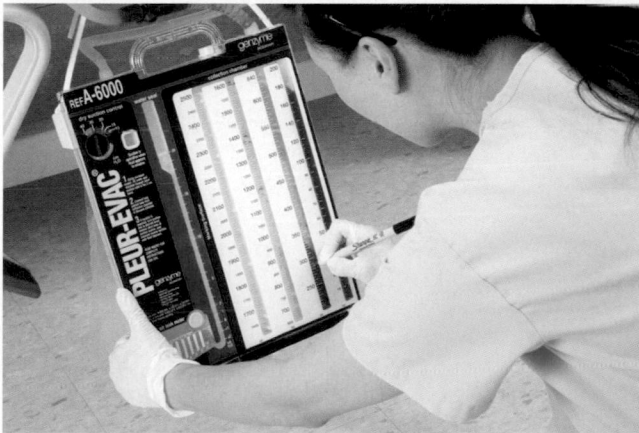

FIG. 3 Mark collection chamber.

Rationale: Keeping the drainage system upright will maintain a water seal and ensure proper sequential filling of the collection chambers. Marking the collection chamber at the end of each shift will allow the evaluation of output to detect excessive bleeding or healing.

9. **Assess suction chamber. Make sure the water level in the suction chamber is at the prescribed amount of suction and that it is connected to the wall suction that is turned on to continuous suction (Fig. 4). Usually, the suction on the device is set at 10 to 20 mm Hg. The suction on the wall or portable suction unit should be set to 80 to 120 mm Hg. The drainage collection device may have an indicator that shows if the amount of suction generated is sufficient.**

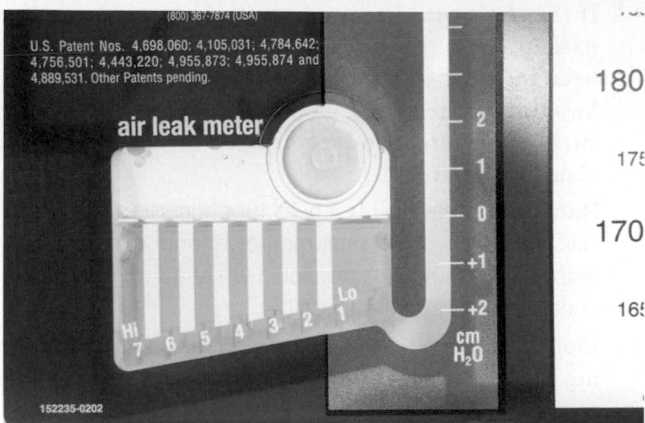

FIG. 4 Assess water level in suction chamber.

Rationale: The amount of suction is determined by the water level in the suction chamber rather than the suction setting on the wall unit. Gentle bubbling is normal in the suction chamber.

10. **Assess the system for any air leaks. Check all external connections (i.e., the chest tube's connection to the drainage system, the suction tubing's connection to the drainage system). Examine the water seal chamber as the patient breathes normally and as he or she coughs.**

Rationale: A chest drainage system needs to be a continuously closed system to maintain the negative pressure necessary for normal respiratory function. Any air leak interrupts this closed system. Bubbling in the water seal chamber may indicate an intermittent or continuous air leak. Bubbling when a patient coughs indicates an intermittent air leak. Ongoing bubbling in the water seal chamber indicates a continuous air leak. New air leaks need to be reported to the physician.

11. **Encourage the patient to cough, deep breathe, and use an incentive spirometer frequently. Provide analgesics as necessary.**

Rationale: Coughing and deep breathing will increase intrapleural pressure, facilitating fluid drainage from the pleural space and enhancing lung expansion. Analgesics will assist with pain control as the patient coughs, deep breathes, and uses an incentive spirometer.

12. **Clamping chest tubes is no longer recommended.**

Rationale: Clamping can result in sudden accumulation of air in the pleural space, which can cause a tension pneumothorax, resulting in tension on the heart and great vessels that can be life threatening. Momentary clamping—for example, when changing the drainage collection device—is acceptable.

Procedure 26-10 *continued*

13. **If the chest tube becomes expelled, do not leave the patient. Cover the opening where the chest tube had been inserted with plain sterile 4 × 4 gauze or with Vaseline-impregnated gauze, and keep direct pressure on the site. Send a colleague to call the physician immediately.**

    Rationale: Leaving the chest tube insertion site open will create an open pneumothorax and can result in respiratory distress. A physician will need to replace the chest tube as soon as possible.

14. **Document chest tube drainage, chest tube patency, air leak, amount of suction, pain level, dressing status, and respiratory status.**

    Rationale: Maintains legal record and communicates with healthcare team.

Documentation

8/4/16: 23:00—Chest tube to 20 mm Hg pressure, minimal drainage and no air leak. Anticipate CT removal in the AM.

—S. Roberts, RN

Collaboration and Delegation

- Notify the physician immediately if the chest tube dislodges, a sudden air leak occurs, significant unexpected drainage occurs, or the patient is experiencing dyspnea. Caution all personnel to maintain upright position of the chest tube drainage system and to keep it stable, often hooked to the bed. Take care that system does not get under the bed, where it could be accidentally cracked if the bed position were lowered.

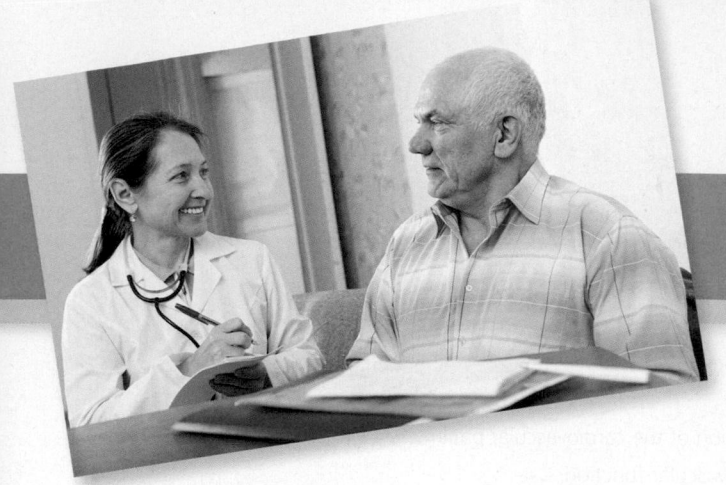

CHAPTER 27

Cardiac Function

Tamara Cyhan Cunitz

Case Scenario

A 59-year-old patient comes in for his yearly physical examination. His family history is positive for cardiac disease, and his father died at 60 years of age of a massive myocardial infarction (MI). The patient has been under stress lately at work (a very important legal trial) and at home (his 24-year-old daughter has returned home with two young children after a recent divorce). He used to play golf twice a week but recently has not had time to exercise. A physical examination reveals blood pressure (BP) of 178/94 mm Hg (last BP a year ago 184/96 mm Hg), pulse 94 beats per minute, and respirations 14 per minute. When you tell your patient his vital signs, he states, "Now don't you start yelling at me about my blood pressure. I'm as healthy as they come, and I am not about to go on any crazy vegetarian diet." He travels frequently and eats often at fast-food restaurants. He has gained 25 lb in the last 6 months, and his body mass index (BMI) is now between 28 and 29. He is a nonsmoker and drinks one to two beers a week.

Once you have completed this chapter and have incorporated cardiac function into your knowledge base, review the above scenario and reflect on the following areas of Critical Thinking:

1. Evaluate the risk factors that negatively affect this patient's cardiovascular health. How can the patient change these risk factors?

2. Describe some health promotion measures that can be implemented to improve this patient's health.

3. Discuss the impact of his lifestyle on his cardiovascular health.

4. Plan two possible approaches to encourage the patient's identification of healthy lifestyle changes.

5. Reflect on how you as a nurse would feel if a patient were reluctant to make positive lifestyle changes.

KEY TERMS

angina
automaticity
cardiac biomarkers
cardiac output (CO)
contractility
diastole
dysrhythmia
endocardium
epicardium
intermittent claudication
ischemia
metabolic syndrome (syndrome X)
myocardial infarction (MI)
myocardium
perfusion
sequential compression devices (SCDs)
shock
stroke
stroke volume
syncope
systole
telemetry
thrombus
transient ischemic attack (TIA)

Upon completion of this chapter, you will be able to do the following:

1. Discuss factors that contribute to normal cardiac output and tissue perfusion.
2. Discuss cardiovascular changes that occur across the life span.
3. Describe the causes of altered cardiovascular function.
4. Describe how altered cardiovascular function can affect normal activities.
5. Perform a basic nursing assessment of cardiovascular function.
6. Identify common procedures and diagnostic tests used in the evaluation of the cardiovascular patient.
7. Discuss nursing measures directed at promoting and restoring cardiovascular function.

The primary function of the cardiovascular system is to transport oxygen and nutrients to the body tissues and to deliver the waste products to appropriate organs for their excretion. The heart acts as a pump to deliver blood through the blood vessels. The proper function of every organ and tissue depends on the efficiency and effectiveness of the cardiovascular system. This chapter focuses on the importance of the cardiovascular system in the maintenance of health.

NORMAL CARDIOVASCULAR FUNCTION

Structure of the Cardiovascular System

The heart and blood vessels are part of the cardiovascular system. The system is a closed circuit with two major divisions: the pulmonary circulation and the systemic circulation. It is really a double pump, with the right side going to the lungs and the left side going to the body. The pulmonary circulation carries blood through the lungs, where carbon dioxide is released and oxygen is absorbed. The systemic circulation then transports oxygenated blood and nutrients to all body tissues (Fig. 27-1).

HEART

The heart is a hollow, muscular pump that is a little larger than a fist. It is an amazing organ, pumping about 5 quarts of blood per minute. Each day, the average heart beats 100,000 times and pumps about 2,000 gallons of blood (American Heart Association, 2014b).

Heart Layers

The heart consists of three layers. The innermost layer of the heart, the **endocardium**, is made of tissue that lines the heart. The thick muscular middle layer is called the **myocardium**. It produces the muscular contraction of the heart. The outer layer of the heart, or **epicardium**, is a thin-walled sac that surrounds the heart and attaches it to the diaphragm and sternal wall of the thorax (Fig. 27-1).

Heart Structure

The heart has two main walls that divide it into four chambers. A strong muscular wall, or septum, divides the heart into left and right halves. These halves are further divided crosswise into upper chambers (atria) and lower chambers (ventricles).

The muscle on the left side of the heart is much thicker than the muscle on the right because the left side of the heart must generate higher pressures to pump blood to all body tissues. The right side of the heart serves the lower-resistance pulmonary system.

Conduction System

The heart is unique because of its property of **automaticity**. Automaticity means that the heart is capable of generating its own electrical impulse, which is then conducted through specialized conduction cells (i.e., pacemaker cells). Impulses that stimulate contraction normally originate in these specialized cells (sinoatrial [SA] node) near the top of the right atrium. Through the atria, the impulse is channeled into the atrioventricular (AV) junction, and then to the bundle of His, and into its right and left bundle branches. It finally enters the many Purkinje fibers that extend throughout the ventricular muscle (Fig. 27-2).

Valves

The heart has four valves that allow blood to flow in one direction, maximizing efficiency and preventing the backflow of blood. Two AV valves separate the atria from the ventricles. The tricuspid valve separates the right atrium from the right ventricle; the mitral valve separates the left atrium from the left ventricle (Fig. 27-1).

The other two valves separate the ventricles from the large blood vessels they fill. The pulmonic valve separates the right ventricle from the pulmonary system, and the aortic valve separates the left ventricle from the aorta. These valves are called semilunar valves because of the half-moon shape of their leaflets.

BLOOD VESSELS

Circulation through the coronary blood vessels provides the heart muscle with oxygenated blood. The right and left coronary arteries come off the aorta, and their multiple branches

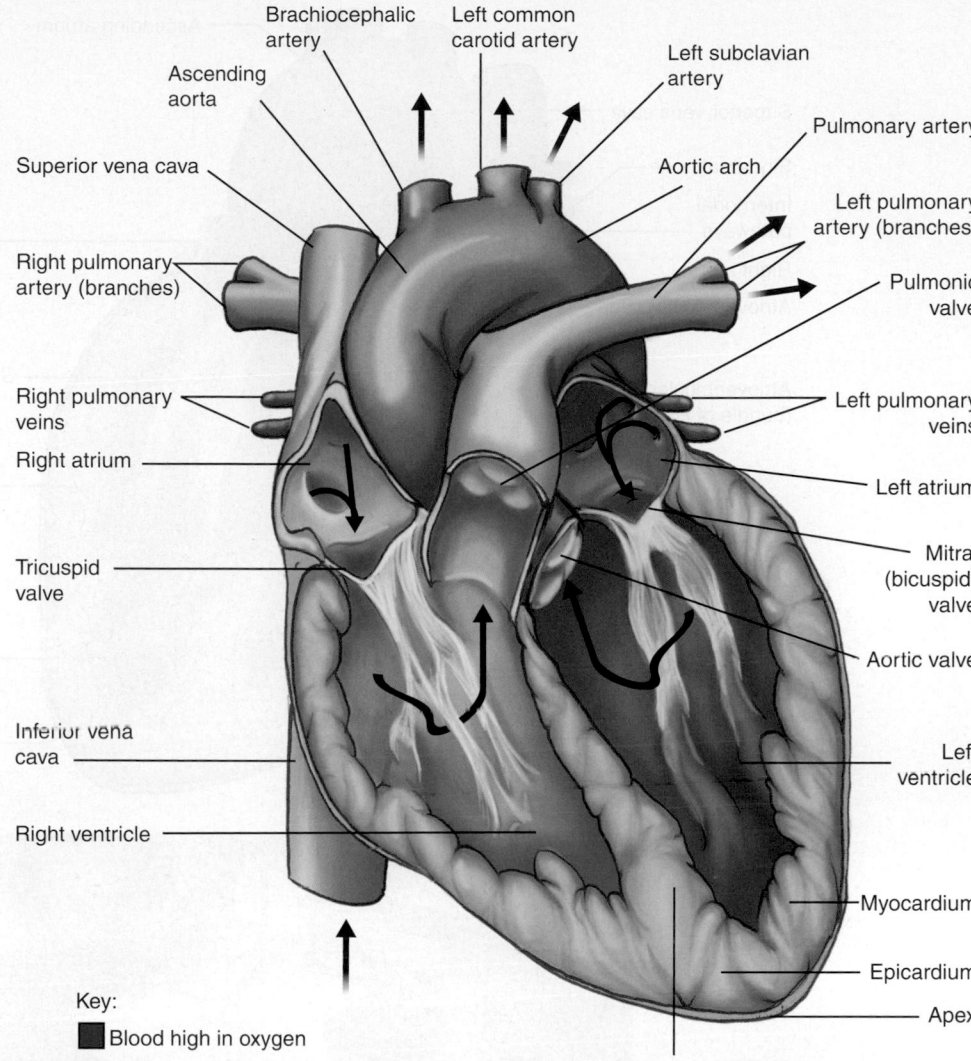

Brachiocephalic artery
Left common carotid artery
Left subclavian artery
Ascending aorta
Superior vena cava
Aortic arch
Pulmonary artery
Left pulmonary artery (branches)
Right pulmonary artery (branches)
Pulmonic valve
Right pulmonary veins
Left pulmonary veins
Right atrium
Left atrium
Mitral (bicuspid) valve
Tricuspid valve
Aortic valve
Inferior vena cava
Left ventricle
Right ventricle
Myocardium
Epicardium
Apex
Intraventricular septum

FIGURE 27-1 Heart chamber, valves, and circulation.

Key:
■ Blood high in oxygen
■ Blood low in oxygen

deliver fresh blood to all layers of the heart. One artery serves the right side of the heart; the other serves the left. Because the left side of the heart is more muscular, it has a greater blood supply. These coronary blood vessels fill when the heart relaxes.

Function of the Cardiovascular System

The heart's effectiveness as a pump depends on several factors. Among the most important factors are its ability to generate and conduct electrical impulses, its ability to fill and empty properly, and the strength with which it contracts.

HEART

The normal heartbeat is a rhythmic cycle of contraction and relaxation. The cardiac cycle begins with the generation of a small electrical impulse in the SA node. This impulse spreads throughout the heart, which causes muscle contraction, creating a pumping motion. With each contraction, called **systole**,

the ventricles eject blood into the aorta. The blood moves through the aorta to the arteries and into the capillaries, where exchange of oxygen and carbon dioxide occurs before the blood travels back to the heart through the veins. The period between contractions, called **diastole**, is twice as long as systole. This extra time allows the heart muscle to relax and its chambers to fill with blood (Fig. 27-3).

Impulse Conduction

In the SA node, small but significant changes in the concentrations of potassium, sodium, and calcium generate a small electrical impulse. This impulse (depolarization) travels through special conduction tissue and normally causes the muscles to contract. After the impulse has passed through the cells, their ionic concentrations return to previous levels (repolarization), and the muscle relaxes. Because the SA node establishes impulses that determine the rate at which the heart beats, it is often called the pacemaker of the heart.

When the impulse reaches the lower portion of the atria, it is delayed briefly at the AV junction before it continues into the

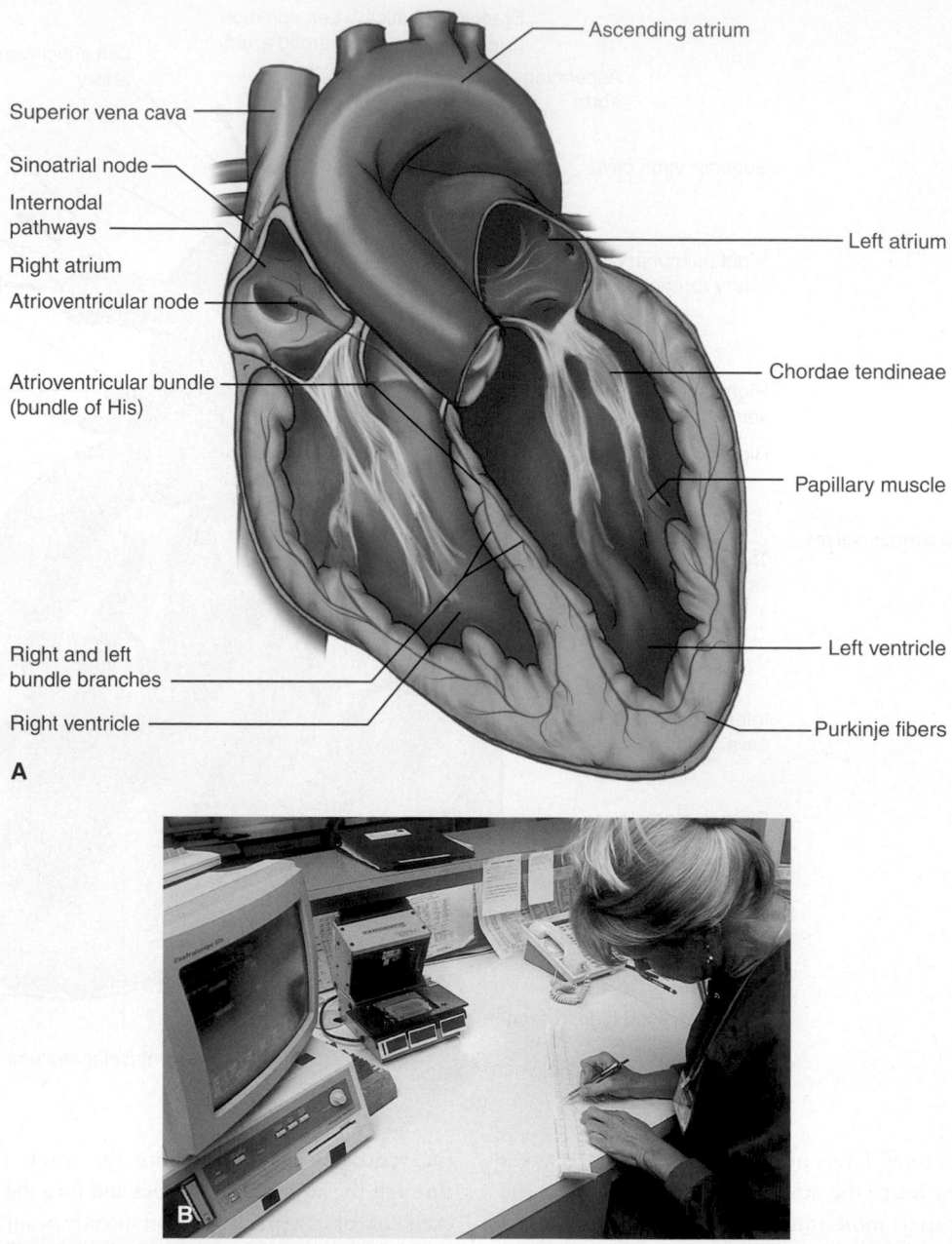

FIGURE 27-2 A. The electrical conduction system of the heart. **B.** Nurse evaluating ECG tracing in the coronary care unit to promptly detect dysrhythmias.

ventricles. This delay allows time for the atria to contract fully. In this way, the atria can add 30% more blood volume to the ventricles before the ventricles contract (Porth & Grossman, 2013). This is known as "atrial kick."

As the impulse spreads through special conduction tissue in the ventricles (bundle of His, bundle branches, and Purkinje fibers), the ventricular myocardial cells normally contract. In the healthy adult, the heart beats rhythmically, with an equal time interval between each beat. Also, every beat is normally the same strength or intensity as all other beats. The normal heart rate is 60 to 100 beats per minute (bpm), although it can vary greatly from person to person.

Blood Flow Through the Heart

The coordinated contraction of all muscle fibers is essential for maximum cardiac pumping power. The contraction of the muscle squeezes blood from inside the heart out into the blood vessels.

Between heartbeats, the heart is at rest. During this time, the atria fill passively, receiving blood from the venae cavae (on the right side of the heart) and the pulmonary veins (on the left). When the atrial muscle cells contract, pressure builds within the atrial chambers. The pressure forces the AV valves to open, and the blood is pushed into the ventricle below each atrium.

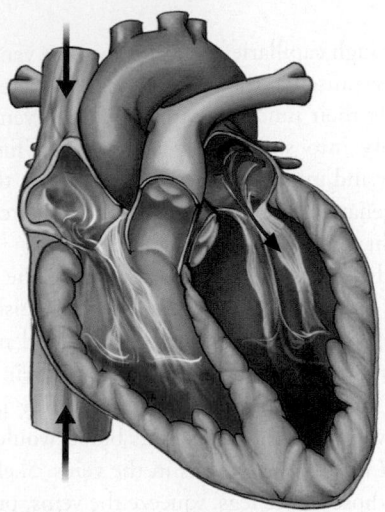

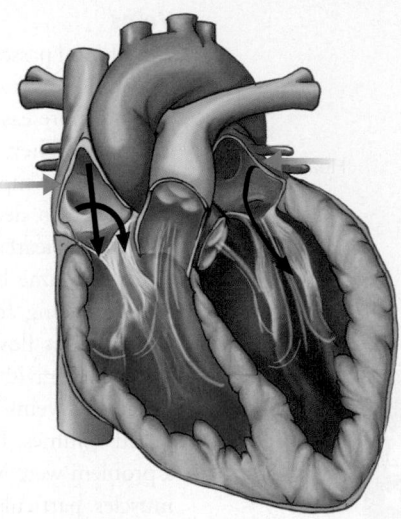

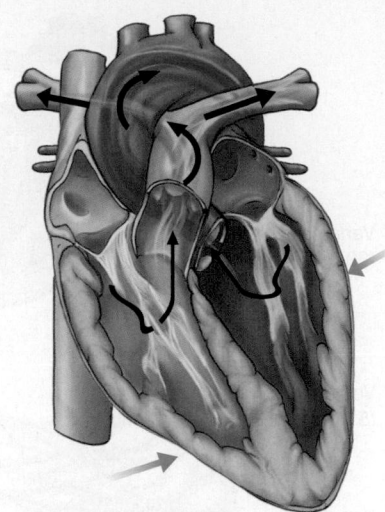

Diastole
Atria fill with blood, which begins to flow into ventricles as soon as their walls relax.

Atrial Systole
Contraction of atria pumps blood into the ventricles.

Ventricular Systole
Contraction of ventricles pumps blood into aorta and pulmonary arteries.

FIGURE 27-3 Pumping cycle of the heart.

After a brief pause at the AV junction, the ventricular muscle cells begin to contract. The rising pressure within the ventricles forces the AV valves to close and the valves to the pulmonary artery and the aorta to open. The blood from the right ventricle is ejected into the pulmonary artery for gas exchange, and the blood from the left ventricle enters the aorta for transport to body tissues.

Proper valve function is another essential element of effective pumping. The unidirectional action of the valves allows the heart chambers to pump forcefully. This is necessary to ensure that blood is ejected with sufficient pressure to reach the farthest tissues of the body.

Cardiac Output

Cardiac output (CO) refers to the amount of blood pumped by the heart each minute. In the normal resting adult, CO is approximately 3.5 to 8 L per minute (Porth & Grossman, 2013). The healthy person is able to increase CO to several times this amount in response to changing metabolic demands, such as with exercise.

CO is a function of two factors: heart rate (HR) and **stroke volume** (SV). CO = HR × SV. Heart rate is simply the number of times the heart beats each minute. Stroke volume refers to the amount of blood the heart ejects with each beat. An increase or decrease in either of these factors may change CO.

Heart rate is primarily determined by the heart's pacemaker, the SA node. This tissue receives information constantly from the autonomic nervous system. The parasympathetic branch via the vagus nerve slows the heart rate; the sympathetic branch increases it. Increased metabolic activity (e.g., vigorous exercise) produces cardiac-stimulating metabolites; it also stimulates the sympathetic nervous system. Therefore, CO increases under these conditions to meet the extra demands of the tissues.

Stroke volume depends on three factors. First, the amount of blood that enters the heart determines how much the heart can pump out. Healthy heart muscle is usually able to stretch to accommodate the volume of blood returning to it. Second, stroke volume depends on the natural strength of the heart muscle, or its **contractility**. Like any muscle, the healthy, well-exercised heart is stronger and more efficient than the weak and (flabby) heart, so it is able to eject a larger volume of blood with each beat. Finally, stroke volume depends on the resistance to blood flow in the circulatory system. The main resistance is in the diameter of the arterial system, which is measured by BP. If the BP (resistance) is high, the stroke volume will decrease (Porth & Grossman, 2013).

BLOOD VESSELS

The heart empties its contents into an interconnected network of arteries, arterioles, capillaries, venules, and veins. Collectively, the members of this network are called the blood vessels. These vessels range from more than 1 inch in diameter to microscopic in size. Arteries and arterioles carry blood away from the heart to the tissues; venules and veins carry blood from the tissues back to the heart. The capillaries, which are the smallest vessels, link arteries and arterioles together with venules and veins (Fig. 27-4). Arteries, capillaries, and veins are dynamic structures that are essential for adequate distribution and **perfusion** of blood to body tissues.

Distribution of Blood Flow

As the heart ejects blood, the thick, muscular walls of the arteries stretch slightly and then rebound. This is important to ensure that the blood has enough force to reach the tissues. The pressure generated in the arterial system is called *blood pressure* (BP). According to the (American Heart Association, 2014d), normal adult BP is less than 120 mm Hg systolic and less than 80 mm Hg diastolic.

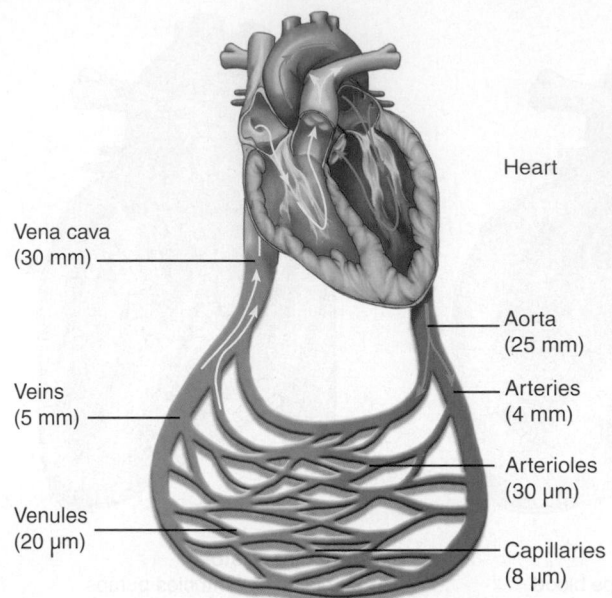

Heart

Vena cava
(30 mm)

Aorta
(25 mm)

Veins
(5 mm)

Arteries
(4 mm)

Arterioles
(30 μm)

Venules
(20 μm)

Capillaries
(8 μm)

FIGURE 27-4 Systemic circulation with blood traveling from the heart through the aorta, arteries, arterioles, capillaries, venules, and veins. Blood returns to the heart in the vena cava.

Arteries

Arteries are relatively thick-walled, muscular vessels. This characteristic provides them with strength and elasticity, which allows them to withstand the high pressure of blood that the heart constantly forces into them. The smallest arteries, called arterioles, connect to the capillaries and regulate blood flow into them. The arterioles contain smooth muscle cells, so they can expand (vasodilate) and contract (vasoconstrict). The arterioles are the primary regulators of blood flow, and they play a key role in the moment-to-moment regulation of BP. These tiny vessels are able to increase or decrease their diameter to meet local tissue needs. For example, a jogger's active leg muscles require more oxygen and nutrients than do the digestive tract organs. Metabolites from the working leg muscles, rapid depletion of the local muscle oxygen supply, and the autonomic nervous system cause the arterioles serving the leg muscles to dilate. By opening wider, the vessels allow more blood to flow into the legs to meet the tissue needs. At the same time, arterioles within the digestive tract may actually constrict, limiting the amount of blood entering it. Thus, the body is able to direct blood flow to where it is needed most.

Capillaries

These microscopic vessels run through all of the body's tissues. Their thin endothelial walls are permeable, which allows for the exchange of nutrients and waste products between the blood and tissues. By the time blood enters the capillaries, its pressure and velocity have decreased greatly. The slower flow rate of blood through the single-layered epithelium of capillaries is necessary to allow sufficient time for tissues to extract oxygen and nutrients. The slow flow also allows the tissues adequate time to deposit their wastes into the blood for removal.

Veins

After blood passes through capillaries, it drains into the venules and veins. Veins are less muscular than are arteries and therefore expand more easily. At their junction with capillaries, venules are small. They empty into successively larger veins, finally ending in the superior and inferior venae cavae. Together, these vessels return deoxygenated blood from the systemic circulation to the heart's right atrium.

By the time blood reaches the venules and veins, the initial propelling force of the heartbeat is greatly diminished, and blood is flowing slowly. In addition, venous blood must overcome gravity in the upright person. Because of their distensibility, veins can stretch to accommodate relatively large blood volumes. Backward flow of the venous blood would be a problem were it not for one-way valves in the veins. Skeletal muscles, particularly those of the legs, squeeze the veins, pushing blood forward and opening the valves; as the muscles relax, the valves of the veins close, preventing backflow (Porth & Grossman, 2013).

Tissue Perfusion

To maintain life, all living body cells must receive a constant supply of oxygen and nutrients. The flow of blood through the body tissues is called tissue perfusion.

Individual cells and tissues receive oxygen, glucose, and various ions through the walls of capillaries. At the arterial end of the capillary, the forward force of the blood helps to push fluid and soluble particles out of the vessel. This fluid surrounds the cells, and nutrients are exchanged for wastes. Oxygen and other molecules enter the cells primarily by diffusion, moving from an area of higher concentration (the fluid) to an area of lower concentration (the cell). Metabolites such as carbon dioxide diffuse from the cell into the fluid, also in response to a concentration difference.

At the venous end of the capillary, tissue hydrostatic pressure forces some fluid back into the vessel. Large protein molecules in the plasma pull the remaining fluid into the capillary. This spongelike action of the plasma proteins is called oncotic pressure.

The vital organs require continuous perfusion for their optimal function. The brain relies on a sophisticated network of neural receptors to guarantee a near-constant level of perfusion. These receptors, located in the major arteries leading to the brain, are sensitive to variations in BP. When pressure increases, the receptors cause arterial constriction. This reflex action protects the brain's delicate capillaries from possible injury caused by a sudden rise in pressure. If BP drops, the arteries dilate, thus ensuring a consistent flow of blood through the brain, despite a possible momentary decrease elsewhere (Porth & Grossman, 2013).

The coronary arteries that nourish the heart tissue are perfused primarily during the resting portion of the cardiac cycle (diastole). At increased heart rates, time in diastole shortens, and sufficient time may be unavailable for the coronary arteries to fill completely. Adequate coronary perfusion also depends on adequate CO.

The kidneys must receive a steady flow of blood to effectively filter and cleanse it. An adequate BP is needed to keep the renal arteries open and to ensure continuous blood flow and urine production.

BLOOD

The blood carries essential nutrients to the cells, but it can only do so effectively if its composition is normal and its volume is sufficient to fill the cardiovascular system. The red blood cells are responsible for delivering oxygen, which is carried on the hemoglobin portion of the cell. Plasma, which is the liquid portion of the blood, carries electrolytes, trace minerals, and nutrients (e.g., glucose) to the cells. To function optimally, the cardiovascular system must maintain a relatively constant fluid volume and viscosity (thickness) of blood.

Life Span Considerations

NEWBORN AND INFANT

The newborn's heart rate is normally 130 to 160 bpm, and its rhythm is commonly irregular. A heart rate of less than 100 bpm in a newborn is cause for alarm. As babies mature, the heart rate slows and becomes more rhythmic, but it can easily increase during activity or when the baby cries. In infancy, heart rate ranges between 80 and 150 bpm (Weber & Kelley, 2014).

BP is lowest during the newborn period, with a systolic pressure in the mid-40s. It is not routinely assessed in the infant. By 1 month of age, average systolic pressure is 80 to 90 mm Hg, with diastolic pressure ranging from the mid-40s to 60 mm Hg.

TODDLER AND PRESCHOOLER

By the end of the toddler period, the heart rate has decreased to a resting rate of about 70 to 110 bpm (Weber & Kelley, 2014). After 3 years of age, BP should be measured annually (Kyle & Carman, 2013). Using an appropriate cuff size (as described in Chapter 18) is important to obtain an accurate reading. Standardized BP tables can be used to evaluate if the child's BP is above the 95th percentile, which requires a follow-up evaluation for hypertension.

CHILD AND ADOLESCENT

As the heart increases in size, its rate continues to decline (Fig. 27-5). BP changes are gradual and slight during this period. Boys will generally have a slightly higher BP and lower heart rate than girls. By the age of 19 years, heart rate and BP have stabilized at the adult values of 60 to 80 bpm and 120/80 mm Hg, respectively (Weber & Kelley, 2014).

Developing healthy eating habits and exercise routines are important during childhood and adolescence to foster lifelong habits that will promote healthy heart function. Childhood obesity has increased greatly in the last few decades, which will greatly impact the heart health of these children when they are adults. Educational programs regarding the impact of smoking on cardiac function are important to decrease smoking among preadolescents and adolescents.

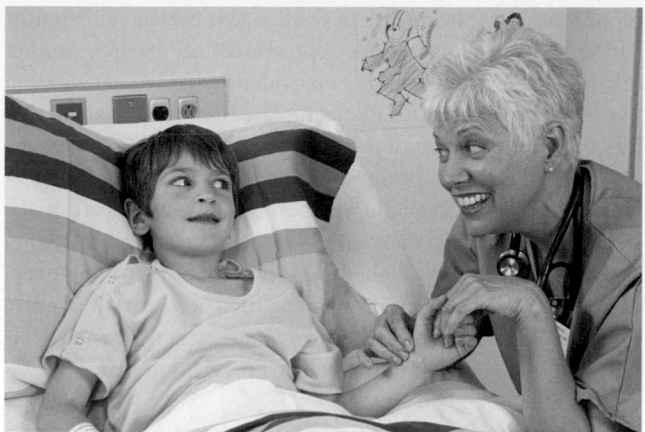

FIGURE 27-5 Assessing the radial pulse of a child.

ADULT AND OLDER ADULT

As individuals mature throughout adulthood, changes in the cardiovascular system may lead to decreased activity tolerance and decreased endurance. Along with natural aging, diet, stress, smoking, and other lifestyle factors may contribute to the processes of calcification, fatty degeneration, and diminished elasticity of the blood vessels. These processes are likely to account for increases in BP as adults grow older. Heart rate is also slightly higher in the older adult than in the younger adult due to the added workload of pumping blood through resistant vessels.

Cultural Considerations

Both genetics and lifestyle factors influence the incidence of cardiovascular disease among different socioeconomic and cultural groups. For example, the incidence of hypertension is much higher in non-Hispanic Black men and women than Caucasian men and women of the same age (Go et al., 2014). The incidence of risk factors such as obesity and diabetes is higher in areas of the country where the regional diet is focused on fried or salty foods and more individuals live a sedentary lifestyle. Education about healthy food choices that remain within a patient's particular ethnic cuisine may increase the chances that proper nutrients are consumed and unhealthy foods are avoided. Unfortunately, fresh fruits and vegetables may be less accessible in poorer urban neighborhoods. Health beliefs also vary among cultural groups; for example, certain groups may believe that seeing a healthcare professional is necessary only when someone is sick or dying, not for regular health screening. Thus, hypertension may go undiagnosed and untreated for many years. These particular examples illustrate the health disparities existing between different socioeconomic and cultural groups.

Gender Differences

There are noteworthy distinctions in cardiovascular functioning between men and women. Women generally have a smaller stature than men and therefore have a smaller heart and smaller blood vessels. Heart disease in women also presents differently. Although women are underrepresented in research studies (Shen & Melloni, 2014), there is evidence that women develop hypertension and cardiovascular disease later in life than men. A link between the onset of menopause and cardiovascular events and heart failure has been established (Ebong et al., 2014). A woman's risk for developing diabetes following a heart attack is three times higher than that of a man, and death following a heart attack is 50% higher in women than men (Solimene, 2010). Knowledge of these gender differences alerts the nurse to complete a very thorough history and assessment and to follow up closely with an individualized prevention plan.

FACTORS AFFECTING CARDIOVASCULAR FUNCTION

A host of risk factors can influence cardiovascular function. These risk factors can be stratified into nonmodifiable and modifiable risks. The nonmodifiable risk factors such as age, gender, and heredity are important in collecting a thorough patient history, but these cannot be altered. Modifiable risk factors include such things as cigarette smoking, diet, inactivity, and stress (Box 27-1). Although a diagnosis of diabetes, identified as a modifiable risk factor, most likely cannot be changed, the control of the disease is modifiable—that is, diabetes may be poorly or well controlled. Reducing multiple risk factors provides the most substantial benefit. Nurses can help improve the lives of their patients through education about healthier lifestyle choices, thereby addressing those modifiable risks.

Cigarette Smoking

Cigarette smoking is extremely harmful and has caused more deaths from cardiovascular disease than lung cancer or chronic obstructive pulmonary disease. It increases the heart rate and

---

BOX 27-1 Coronary Heart Disease Risk Factors

Nonmodifiable Risk Factors
- Family history of heart disease
- Gender (risk increases for men and for women after menopause)
- Increased age (risk increases with age)
- African American ethnicity

Modifiable Risk Factors
- High BP
- Cigarette/tobacco use
- High blood cholesterol
- Physical inactivity
- Obesity
- Diabetes
- Stress in daily living

BP, constricts arterioles, and may cause an irregular cardiac rhythm. It enhances the process of atherosclerosis and is the major cause of peripheral vascular disease. Smoking also limits the blood's oxygen-carrying capacity by displacing oxygen with carbon monoxide (Emerson, 2010).

Smokers who quit smoking reduce their risk of cardiovascular disease by 50% (Gellert, Schottker, & Brenner, 2012). The risk reduces to that of a nonsmoker within 3 to 4 years of smoking cessation.

High Blood Pressure

High BP is undoubtedly the most common manifestation of altered blood flow, affecting 33% of the adult population (Go et al., 2014). The highest rates of hypertension occur in individuals who are middle-aged, overweight, or obese and lead a sedentary lifestyle. Specific BP parameters have been set by the AHA in order to monitor patients who may be at increased risk (Table 27-1).

High BP may result from an increased level of circulating vasoactive substances or increased sympathetic nervous system activity. Changes in sodium excretion in the kidneys or in arterial smooth muscle contractility caused by changes in calcium absorption can also cause high BP.

High BP is unique in that it is a manifestation of cardiovascular dysfunction and, in turn, a cause of further dysfunction, resulting in severe tissue and organ damage. High BP can affect anyone, but in the United States, there are health disparities among specific groups for hypertension. High BP occurs more often in younger men than women, but after age 65 years, hypertension affects more women than men (Lloyd-Jones et al., 2010). Certain ethnic groups also present with higher rates of high BP. African Americans disproportionately suffer from hypertension (Go et al., 2014). Further research needs to be conducted to define and address these particular health disparities.

Nutrition

The relationship between diet and cardiovascular problems is complex. Assessing a patient's nutritional status and dietary practices is a crucial part of assessing risk factors for cardiovascular disease. A healthy diet low in fats, cholesterol, salt, and sugar and high in fiber helps fight cardiovascular disease, but a diet high in total fat and saturated fat is strongly associated with the risk of heart disease (Mozaffarian et al., 2012). Cholesterol is the primary component of the plaque (fatty lesion) that gradually occludes arteries. There are two primary types of cholesterol: high-density lipoprotein (HDL), or "good" cholesterol, and low-density lipoprotein (LDL), or "bad" cholesterol. High levels of LDL cholesterol lead to peripheral vascular disease and hypertension, which greatly increases the chance of a heart attack, or **myocardial infarction (MI)** (American Heart Association, 2014a).

Salt also plays a large role in cardiovascular health. A diet that is high in salt can increase blood volume and CO and thus aggravate chronic hypertension or heart failure. Increased

TABLE 27-1 AMERICAN HEART ASSOCIATION CLASSIFICATION OF HYPERTENSION

BP Category	Systolic mm Hg (upper number)		Diastolic mm Hg (lower number)
Normal	<120	and	<80
Prehypertension	120–139	or	80–89
High BP (hypertension) stage 1	140–159	or	90–99
High BP (hypertension) stage 2	160 or higher	or	100 or higher
Hypertensive crisis (emergency care needed)	Higher than 180	or	Higher than 110

From: Pickering, T. G., Hall, J. E., Appel, L. J., Falkner, B. E., Graves, J., Hill, M. N., et al. (2005). Recommendations for blood pressure measurement in humans and experimental animals: Part 1: Blood pressure measurement in humans: A statement for professionals from the Subcommittee of Professional and Public Education of the American Heart Association Council on High Blood Pressure Research. *Hypertension*, 45(1), 142–161.

sodium intake in sodium-sensitive people can increase the incidence of hypertension. Preserved foods and foods purchased from convenience or fast-food venues often contain a large amount of sodium.

Sugar overconsumption exists in epidemic proportions in the United States. High amounts of sugar intake increase the risk of coronary artery disease by increasing triglyceride levels. Increased sugar consumption has also been linked to hypertension, diabetes, and obesity.

Fiber and whole grains are important elements of cardiovascular health, and a diet high in fiber has been linked to heart health since it helps reduce blood cholesterol. In addition, whole grains contain nutrients essential to red blood cell formation and transport (American Heart Association, 2014e). A diet high in whole grains is an essential part of overall cardiovascular health. The AHA has established recommended guidelines for a healthy diet, which can be found on their website.

Sedentary Lifestyle

Engaging in regular physical activity to promote a nonsedentary lifestyle has protective effects on the heart. Just as regular exercise strengthens leg and arm muscles, it can improve the heart's pumping ability and efficiency. Increased blood circulation also helps prevent the formation of thrombi and atherosclerotic plaques by decreasing platelet stickiness. Exercise promotes weight reduction and protects the cardiovascular system by raising the "good" (HDL) cholesterol and reducing triglycerides, BP, and resting heart rate. A well-conditioned person has a lower risk of heart or circulatory problems than a person who does not exercise regularly. Engaging in regular physical activity decreases the risk of coronary artery disease. The AHA recommends that individuals between the ages of 18 and 65 years engage in aerobic activity of moderate intensity for a duration of 30 minutes five times a week. Adults should also maintain muscle strength by engaging the muscles of the body in activity at least twice a week.

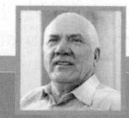

Cardiac PICO

Shawn is providing teaching about heart health to the patient from the chapter-opening scenario. The patient realizes after talking to the doctor that he needs to make some changes in his lifestyle to improve his BP or be put on meds. He informs Shawn that he is not happy about the dietary changes, especially cutting down on the salt. The patient questions if this is just another fad diet or if this change will really help improve his BP. Shawn decides to look for evidence before answering the patient. He searches the Cochrane database with a PICO question: *In adults, does reducing salt intake, compared to no change in salt intake, lower blood pressure?*

> **P**opulation = Adults
> **I**ntervention = Reducing salt intake
> **C**omparison = No change in salt intake
> **O**utcome   = Lower blood pressure

Shawn finds a meta-analysis article that reviewed 34 trials, which included 3,230 participants. The study examined randomized control trials that indicated decreasing a moderate amount of salt intake resulted to decreased BP. In fact, the study also showed regardless of sex or ethnic group, reducing salt intake for 4 weeks or more could lower BP in both hypertensive and normotensive population. Shawn is eager to discuss the evidence with the patient and help find ways to cut salt in the patient's diet.

REFERENCE:

He, F. J., Li, J., & MacGregor, G. A. (2013). Effect of longer-term modest salt reduction on blood pressure. *Cochrane Database of Systematic Reviews*, (4):CD004937. DOI: 10.1002/14651858.CD004937.pub2.

Diabetes

Diabetes predisposes people to cardiovascular disease due to increased risks of hypertension, hyperlipidemia, obesity, and elevated blood sugar. In addition, cardiovascular disease is the leading cause of death in diabetic individuals (American Heart Association, 2013b). Preventing diabetes-related cardiovascular disease requires education about modifiable risk factors. Encouraging patients to modify diet and physical activity levels can help decrease their chance of cardiovascular-related injury or death.

Obesity

Excessive weight places increased demands on the cardiovascular system. The extra adipose tissue must be supplied with blood to meet its metabolic requirements. To perform the additional work of pumping blood to these tissues, the heart may become enlarged. BP also increases, but perfusion may decrease. Obesity is a major risk factor for cardiovascular disease because it raises BP, cholesterol, and triglycerides (American Heart Association, 2014c). Body fat can be measured using a simple formula to calculate body mass index (BMI) (see Chapter 29). The numeric value can be broken down into categories of identification. This system of categorization is only one method of assessing obesity, but it may be used as a reference or to plan treatment. Additional lifestyle factors need to be considered.

Medical and Family History

Although it is clear that many cardiovascular problems have modifiable causes, genetics may play a role in certain disorders. Some patients may report a family history or pattern of disease manifestation (e.g., a high number of close relatives having experienced strokes or heart attacks). Hypertension can also have a familial link. **Metabolic syndrome (syndrome X)** is a genetic metabolic disorder involving diabetes, hypertension, atherosclerosis, centrally distributed obesity, and elevated blood lipids (Porth & Grossman, 2013; Box 27-2). These factors together greatly increase the risk of cardiovascular disease.

BOX 27-2   Metabolic Syndrome (Syndrome X)

Metabolic syndrome is a grouping of features related to glucose and fat metabolism that significantly increases the risk for cardiovascular disease.

- Triglyceride levels greater than 150 mg/dL
- HDL cholesterol levels less than 50 mg/dL for women or less than 40 mg/dL for men
- Abdominal obesity, waist circumference greater than 40 inches for men or greater than 35 inches for women
- BP greater than 130/85 mm Hg
- Fasting glucose greater than 110 mg/dL

Therefore, a positive family history for cardiovascular disease must be considered during assessment.

Medications and Drug Use

Many over-the-counter or prescription medications may affect CO and BP. For example, asthma medications and some cold remedies can substantially increase heart rate and BP. Diuretics can decrease blood volume and alter electrolyte balance, causing potentially dangerous changes in heart rhythm. Birth control pills significantly enhance the process of blood clotting and increase the risk of **thrombus** formation.

Herbal remedies, such as garlic, may be used by some to lower cholesterol and BP, but herbal medications may have serious cardiovascular side effects. For example, some "natural" weight-loss remedies contain ephedrine, which can cause **dysrhythmias**. Ephedrine can interact with BP medications or antidepressants to dangerously elevate BP and heart rate.

Coffee can also increase heart rate and BP and cause palpitations. Excessive alcohol intake has been associated with hypertension, increased cardiovascular risk, and cardiomyopathy (Awtry & Philippides, 2010). A thorough review of the patient's daily medications and supplements allows practitioners to be aware of possible medication interactions and side effects.

The use of illicit drugs can have serious cardiovascular complications. Intravenous (IV) use of any drug provides a portal of entry for bacteria into the bloodstream and puts the user at high risk for infection, such as endocarditis. Impurities in the injected drug can cause cardiac inflammation and may form the nucleus of an embolism. Repeated IV injections in the same vessel can result in its eventual destruction. Cocaine use has been increasingly associated with sudden cardiac arrest, vascular abnormalities, and cardiomyopathy (Awtry & Philippides, 2010). Overdoses of opiates (e.g., heroin, morphine) can cause severe hypotension and respiratory arrest and can induce pulmonary edema.

Stress

Stress is often mentioned as a cause of high BP, **angina**, and MI. Stress elevates serum lipids, increases blood coagulation, elevates BP, and can cause myocardial **ischemia**. People with preexisting cardiac problems who encounter extraordinary or protracted periods of business, family, or personal stress may be at added risk for exacerbations of these problems. Depression and lack of quality social support have also been linked to increased cardiovascular risk.

Personality Types

Much has been written about personality types and their predisposition toward heart disease. The hard-striving, competitive, highly assertive person with the "type A" personality is believed to experience a higher incidence of heart attacks than the easygoing, relaxed, more cooperatively oriented "type B" personality. Anger and hostility have been identified as risk factors for cardiovascular disease.

Recent research has also focused on another personality type linked to increased risk for cardiac disease: "type D" or "distressed" personality. Type D personality traits include negativity and lack of involvement in close social relationships and situations (Jokela, Pulkki-Raback, Elovainio, & Kivimaki, 2014). The links between personality types and heart disease have not been clearly defined, but assessing a patient's stress level and coping responses can help nurses identify areas of risk when developing a plan of care.

Community Factors

In addition to a focus on factors affecting the individual patient, much focus has been placed on assessing and improving the community and population. The individual, for example, may face barriers to good cardiovascular health such as poor nutrition, obesity, genetics, stress, and lack of access to medical care. A specific community or population may face barriers as a group, such as lack of access to nutritional foods, poor economic conditions, and high unemployment. These factors contribute to disease within the population and therefore contribute to poor public health.

ALTERED CARDIOVASCULAR FUNCTION

The cardiovascular system needs to be working properly for adequate tissue oxygenation to occur. Alterations in the conduction system, improper opening or closing of the valves, or damage to cardiac muscle fibers can diminish the heart's effective pumping ability. Changes in the blood vessels and in the blood itself can also create the potential for altered function.

Manifestations of Altered Cardiovascular Function

Altered cardiovascular function has a wide range of symptoms. Vital signs are typically negatively affected. Hypertension, abnormal heart rates, and decreased oxygenation status may occur. When cardiovascular changes cause tissue ischemia, common indicators of inadequate tissue perfusion include pain, skin changes, and changes in cognition. Edema and thrombus (clot) formation are manifestations of alterations in blood flow. Finally, multiple organ dysfunction and possible failure are manifestations of altered cardiovascular status.

CHANGES IN VITAL SIGNS

Blood Pressure

BP may fluctuate with changes in CO and fluid volume. Abnormally low BP (less than 90 mm Hg systolic), when accompanied by other indicators of diminished oxygenation, is a serious sign of decreased CO. This may lead to decreased circulating blood volume or increased venous pooling and may be evidenced by orthostatic hypotension. Alternatively, high BP leads to multiple complications over time such as arterial hardening and heart enlargement and should be treated with medication and lifestyle modifications.

Pulse Character

Diminished or absent pulses may indicate inadequate blood flow to an area. Although the pulse normally diminishes as the distance from the heart increases, absence of pulse may indicate vessel occlusion. Complete vessel occlusion is most often associated with other signs, such as skin changes and pain. In some people, the most distal peripheral pulses (the dorsalis pedis and posterior tibial) may not be palpable but can be confirmed with the use of a Doppler instrument (Hogan-Quigley, Palm, & Bickley, 2012).

Heart Rate

The heart rate increases in response to increased oxygen demand and decreases at rest when oxygen demands are low. A heart rate of greater than 100 bpm at rest may indicate problems with CO if known contributing factors (e.g., fever, pain, medications, anxiety) are absent. An increase in heart rate of more than 20 bpm during mild activity (e.g., walking, moving to the commode) may indicate that decreased CO is contributing to activity intolerance. Conversely, a heart rate that does not increase with exercise may indicate that the heart is unable to adjust to changing oxygen demands. Heart rate should be monitored before, during, and after activity to allow for complete assessment of heart function.

Respiration

Respiratory rate and effort often increase in individuals with cardiovascular dysfunction. Decreased CO or diminished blood flow limits the amount of oxygen available to the tissues. As activity increases and tissues demand more oxygen, respirations increase to supplement blood oxygenation. Shortness of breath can occur in a person with heart or circulatory problems with even slight activity because the cardiovascular system is unable to meet the added oxygen demand. In extreme cases, a person may experience shortness of breath at rest or when lying down. A productive cough producing frothy sputum is a common manifestation of heart failure (Hogan-Quigley et al., 2012).

CHANGES IN THE SKIN

Changes in skin color indicate a change in the level of blood oxygenation and adequacy of local blood flow. Because skin color varies greatly among individuals, it is helpful to assess uniformity of color and compare differences between sides of the body. The mucous membranes of normal, healthy individuals are generally pink. Assess the inner linings of the lips and mouth and the inner lining of the eyelids. Variations from normal may indicate poor perfusion.

Rubor is a term for red skin discoloration caused by hyperemia, or increased blood flow. Temporary increases in skin perfusion cause flushing, as is evident during fever or times of embarrassment. Skin temperature rises with increased blood flow to the skin; vascular constriction or poor perfusion cools the skin. If the sympathetic nervous system has caused constriction (e.g., in **shock**), sweat glands may become activated, and the patient's skin may feel clammy to the touch. Cyanosis, a bluish appearance of skin and mucous membranes, occurs when hemoglobin is not carrying an adequate amount of oxygen. Peripheral cyanosis (of the fingers, toes, and earlobes) occurs when blood flow is restricted. Central cyanosis is a serious sign of decreased oxygenation. It appears around the lips and tissues of the oral cavity (Hogan-Quigley et al., 2012).

Changes in skin character also occur with alterations in perfusion. Chronic poor perfusion may result in hair loss in the affected area, discolored skin, thickened nails, and shiny, dry skin indicative of inadequate tissue nutrition. Some people with chronic heart disease may also have clubbed fingers and toes (Hogan-Quigley et al., 2012).

Skin lesions, dermatitis, and ulcerations can develop readily in patients with compromised skin perfusion. Chronically limited arterial flow to an area can cause skin breakdown, with possible tissue necrosis and gangrene. Disrupted venous flow or congestion can cause stasis ulcers to form.

DECREASED CARDIAC OUTPUT

Muscle damage, valve dysfunction, or conduction problems can decrease the heart's ability to pump blood effectively, resulting in heart pump failure.

Muscle Damage

The heart requires a constant supply of oxygen and nutrients. If blood flow decreases through the coronary arteries, the active muscle becomes hypoxic (without oxygen) and ischemia occurs. Unless blood flow is restored, portions of the heart muscle can die, causing an MI, or heart attack. The person who survives a heart attack may have areas of scar tissue replacing healthy heart muscle tissue.

A second cause of cardiac muscle damage or weakening is severe overwork of the heart. The normal heart responds to extra work by enlarging. Eventually, excessive demands stretch the heart to its limits. It finally weakens and fails. Increased vascular resistance (e.g., with high BP), excessive blood volume, and alterations in blood viscosity are common contributing factors in the development of heart failure. Other possible causes of heart muscle damage are infections, inflammatory or metabolic diseases, nutritional deficiencies, traumas, and substance abuse.

Valve Dysfunction

The four valves of the heart must be able to open fully and close tightly to guarantee forward blood flow. Heart valves may be damaged by inflammation, infection, or trauma, or they may be congenitally malformed. Generally, valve damage results in stenosis (narrowing) or regurgitation (not completely closing resulting in backflow of blood). These conditions can limit stroke volume and force the heart to work much harder than normal to maintain an adequate CO. Heart failure inevitably occurs.

Conduction Problems

Proper function of the conduction system ensures the orderly contraction of myocardial muscle fibers. This results in a coordinated, concerted pumping action, with all muscle fibers operating as a unit. If the conduction system is damaged or malfunctions, the electrical impulses it generates do not spread sequentially through the muscle. The fibers that normally contract together may do so out of sequence or may contract independently of each other. This discordant fiber contraction affects the heart's inherent rhythm and may impair its ability to pump effectively.

A dysrhythmia (sometimes referred to as an arrhythmia) is an abnormality in heart rhythm. Dysrhythmias range from minor, clinically insignificant abnormalities to life-threatening conditions. Dysrhythmias may be caused by damage to the heart muscle or conduction system, diminished coronary blood flow, decreased blood oxygen levels, medications, alterations in serum electrolytes (e.g., potassium, calcium), stress (e.g., from exercise, fever, emotional stress), or overstretching of the heart muscle.

ALTERED BLOOD FLOW

Conditions that affect the blood and blood vessels can alter tissue perfusion and CO.

Alterations in the Blood

Alterations in the red blood cells or plasma or changes in circulating blood volume or consistency can affect cardiovascular function. An insufficient number of red blood cells (as in anemia) or damage to the hemoglobin molecules results in tissue hypoxia. Hypoxia affects all tissues, but the brain and heart are particularly sensitive to oxygen deprivation. Changes in the normal levels of serum electrolytes or pH can also cause alterations in cardiovascular function. For example, slight changes in serum potassium levels can cause serious dysrhythmias. Increased sodium intake can cause an increase in blood volume, which increases cardiac work. An acidotic blood pH can decrease the ability of hemoglobin to carry oxygen.

Dehydration or hemorrhage can cause a decrease in circulating volume. Because tissue perfusion depends on a sufficient volume of circulating blood, any decrease in volume can lead to tissue hypoxia. This occurs in the condition commonly called hypovolemic shock.

Excessive fluid volume occurs in people with heart failure and kidney failure and after overload from IV therapy. The heart must work harder than normal to pump the additional blood through the vascular system. The additional blood volume and pressure also overload capillaries, causing edema. If fluid overload occurs in the lungs, air sacs fill with fluid, causing pulmonary edema and decreasing oxygenation.

Thinner, less viscous blood flows more quickly than normal blood through the vessels. Increased blood flow increases venous return to the heart. This usually forces the heart to pump faster to empty itself. The opposite condition, called *polycythemia*, results in thicker, more viscous blood. Polycythemia results in blood flowing too slowly through the vessels. To pump this thicker blood through the system, the heart must work harder than usual.

Arterial Dysfunction

Atherosclerosis is the most common cause of arterial occlusion. It is seriously compounded in patients with risk factors such as hypertension, genetic predisposition, diabetes, and smoking. This condition is characterized by fatty deterioration of the arterial smooth muscle walls. With time, the lumen of the arteries narrows as the arterial walls absorb increasing amounts of circulating fat particles, or lipids. Affected vessels also become stiff and fibrinous and eventually may close completely. The resultant change in the walls of the vessel causes plaques to form. This degenerative process occurs gradually, over a period of years. Hypertension, high serum lipid levels, and cigarette smoking are those modifiable lifestyle risk factors contributing to atherosclerosis that require patient education by the nurse.

Additional important causes of arterial occlusion include infection, inflammation, and trauma to the arteries. Arteries also can have increased smooth muscle tone as a result of increased sympathetic nervous system stimulation (Porth & Grossman, 2013).

An aneurysm is an outpouching of a blood vessel with a weakened vessel wall and can occur anywhere within the vasculature, especially places with increased blood flow and pressure or where vessels bifurcate or branch off into other parts. A specific type, abdominal aortic aneurysm (AAA), increases with age, and 5% of men older than 50 years are affected. Risks are higher for individuals with coronary artery disease and those who smoke (Durieux et al., 2014). The danger is that the aneurysm will burst, causing major bleeding and reduced blood flow to the kidneys. Abdominal or low back pain may signal the beginning of rupture. Sudden severe back pain, shock, and pulsatile palpable abdominal mass are classic symptoms during rupture. The patient in shock requires emergency surgery.

Capillary Dysfunction

Problems within the arteries, veins, and surrounding tissues affect the capillaries because they are passive structures. Capillaries can become leaky and can cause or contribute to tissue edema. Increased BP or venous congestion can excessively stretch the walls of the capillaries, allowing fluid to leak out into interstitial tissues. Toxins, trauma, and inflammation can increase capillary permeability, promoting fluid leakage. Capillaries can leak if plasma proteins are deficient because these substances are responsible for exerting the osmotic pressure that retains fluid in the blood vessels.

Swollen tissues may compress capillaries and smaller arteries, limiting blood flow and causing ischemia. Possible causes of such swelling include edema, bruising, and tumors. Often, swelling results from venous pooling caused by heart failure or incompetent venous valves. The resultant edema can cause pain by compressing local nerves (Emerson, 2010). Compression of vessels from edema may lead to skin breakdown.

Venous Dysfunction

Decreased venous blood flow can aggravate hypertension and cause ischemia. Unless blood moves steadily through the veins, tissue edema or clot formation may occur. Causes of venous pooling include right-sided heart failure and ineffective venous valves.

Trauma or vein inflammation (phlebitis) can cause venous valve incompetency. More often, however, gravity and muscle inactivity are responsible. In the upright person, gravity hinders venous return, thereby promoting the gradual collection of blood in the veins of the lower leg. A person who must stand or sit for long periods (or who is immobile, such as a patient confined to bed) does not have the benefit of regular muscle compression against the veins. As more blood collects in the leg veins, the veins can become dilated, and distorted varicosities may develop. The valves become so overstretched that their edges cannot approximate, so blood moves backward and forward through the incompetent valves.

An additional effect of venous pooling is increased myocardial work. Because stroke volume depends on the amount of blood entering the heart, venous pooling limits venous return. To maintain normal output, the heart must beat faster. This added work is compounded because increased venous pressure causes increased vascular resistance (Emerson, 2010).

DECREASED TISSUE PERFUSION

Decreased tissue perfusion causes tissue hypoxia because less oxygen is available for metabolism. Compromised blood flow provides fewer nutrients and contributes to abnormalities resulting from the buildup of waste products. This condition of inadequate perfusion and its consequences is called ischemia. The manifestations of ischemia include pain and organ dysfunction.

A thrombus, a solid mass or clot that can develop in arteries or veins and steadily increase in size until it occupies the entire lumen of the vessel, can cause ischemia. The thrombus halts blood flow because the mass or clot becomes a barrier to blood. Wherever a clot blocks a vessel, ischemia, infarction, and tissue necrosis can occur.

Thrombi can form in any blood vessel, but they are most likely to form in the deep veins of the legs. The surgical patient, the immobile patient, and those with added risk for clot formation are the most susceptible to thrombus formation. Blood disorders, infection, malignancy, pregnancy, and oral contraceptives greatly increase the risk of clot formation (Emerson, 2010).

An embolus occurs when a thrombus breaks loose and travels in the circulation. Plaque or fat from bone also can cause emboli. If an embolus or thrombus lodges in the pulmonary artery, it is called a pulmonary embolism. Pulmonary emboli disrupt blood flow to the affected portion of the lung, disrupt gas exchange, and, if large enough, can cause death. If the thrombus or embolus lodges in the brain, it can cause a **stroke**.

Pain

Pain occurs commonly with ischemia when tissues are deprived of oxygen. The exact mechanism by which it results is not fully understood. Pain that is not lessened by rest or by measures to improve blood flow and oxygenation may signal tissue infarction. Angina is chest pain associated with decreased coronary blood flow. **Intermittent claudication** is limb pain caused by poor blood flow.

> ! **SAFETY ALERT**
> Teach patients never to ignore chest pain or discomfort and to report such unrelieved symptoms to medical personnel immediately.

Organ Dysfunction and Failure

The body's vital organs require consistent, normal CO and perfusion for optimal function. High BP or ischemia can have serious consequences for the brain, kidneys, and other vital organs. The more impairment of perfusion present, the greater the possibility of permanent damage and organ failure. The kidneys are commonly affected. If the kidneys do not receive a good blood supply, they will cease to function, be unable to filter the blood, and cause waste products to accumulate. Urine will not be produced, and additional fluid will build up, causing heart failure (Porth & Grossman, 2013).

Cognitive Dysfunction

The brain is extremely sensitive to any alterations in blood flow. If cerebral blood supply diminishes even slightly, changes in cognition occur. Most commonly, the patient becomes restless and anxious. Confusion, fatigue, listlessness, and slurred speech may occur with a prolonged decrease in cerebral blood flow and oxygenation to the brain, as in shock. Chronic brain ischemia limits cognitive function.

When the blood supply to the brain is acutely diminished or completely interrupted (as when the vessels to the brain are blocked or when CO is abnormally low), dizziness and loss of consciousness may result. A **transient ischemic attack (TIA)** is a temporary decrease in blood flow to the brain caused by thrombi or atherosclerosis. There can be brief disturbances in speech, vision, and mobility; confusion; and numbness felt on one half of the body. TIAs are important warning signs of an impending stroke. Complete lack of blood flow to specific areas of the brain causes tissue infarction, resulting in a stroke, or cerebrovascular accident (CVA). Stroke is a medical emergency, and fast action is imperative to prevent irreversible brain injury. Collaborative communication with health team members is essential so that medical interventions can be implemented promptly and morbidity and mortality limited.

Think back to the patient with high BP and family history of cardiac disease in the case scenario. Recall that the patient had gained a significant amount of weight recently and eats often at fast-food restaurants. Use the concept map (Fig. 27-6) to help understand the patient's situation and to plan for his care.

ASSESSMENT

The extent and timeliness of the cardiovascular assessment vary depending on the patient's immediate condition. All patients require a thorough and methodical assessment, which is easiest to perform in patients with stable or chronic cardiovascular conditions. Acutely ill patients who are experiencing severe chest pain or other acute symptoms must be assessed rapidly and on a moment-to-moment basis. In such cases, intervention begins immediately, and evaluation is ongoing.

Normal Pattern

The nurse can gain information about the patient's normal functional pattern by assessing activity tolerance. The ability to perform a normal range of activities of daily living and to tolerate a reasonable level of physical exertion strongly indicates good cardiovascular health. Healthy people experience no chest pain or other remarkable discomfort while at rest or while engaged in moderate activity.

Most people are aware that strenuous work or exercise causes the heart to beat faster and more forcefully. Although these changes are noticeable, few people would describe them as painful or uncomfortable. Consequently, complaints of chest pain with activity always warrant a full investigation. People with cardiovascular problems often experience discomfort, pain, or other symptoms at a lower level of activity than do healthy individuals. This tendency usually leads to self-imposed activity restriction as the patient adjusts to the condition.

Risk Identification

Many factors contribute to the development of cardiovascular problems. Question the patient concerning past cardiovascular conditions, such as previous circulatory difficulties, invasive procedures such as cardiac catheterization or cardiac surgery, MI, or stroke. Determine any functional deficits that resulted from these conditions and the management program the patient is using. Also determine if there are any nonmodifiable risk factors such as a family history of strokes, heart attacks, or high BP.

Question the patient regarding modifiable risk factors because those may involve lifestyle changes for the patient. Assess the patient for a history of smoking. The number of packs of cigarettes smoked daily and the number of years smoked (pack-per-year history) are important measures of the patient's total exposure.

Assess dietary intake of saturated fats, cholesterol, and sodium. Ask patients directly about cooking habits and dietary patterns. Many people are unaware of the fat, cholesterol, and sodium content of specific foods. It may help to ask the patient to describe a normal day's intake and ask for an estimate of specific high-risk foods (e.g., "How many fried foods do you eat per week?" "How often do you eat red meat or eggs?"). Despite an increased emphasis on health, many prepackaged supermarket foods and fast-food options contain an extremely

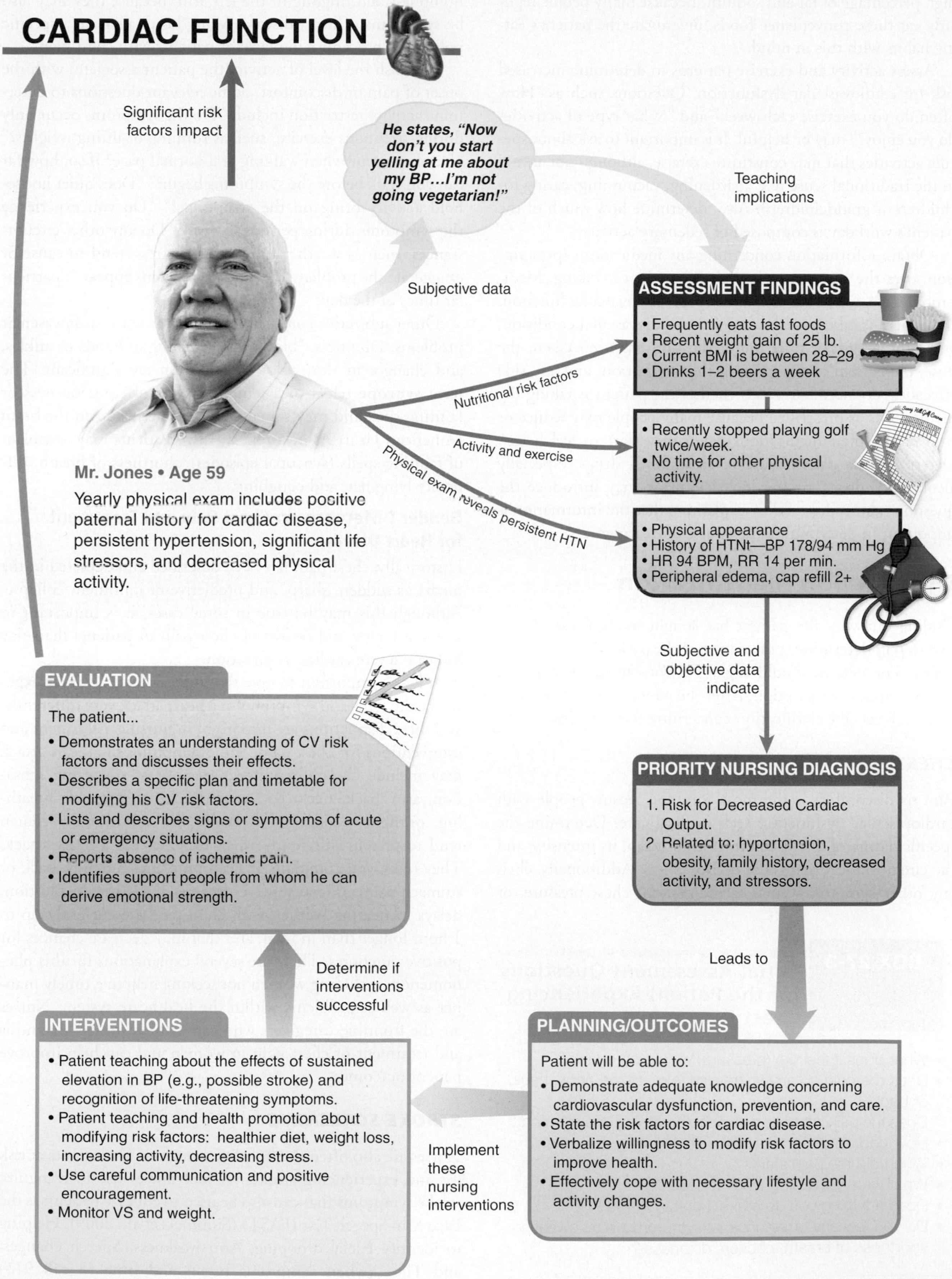

CARDIAC FUNCTION

Significant risk factors impact

He states, "Now don't you start yelling at me about my BP...I'm not going vegetarian!"

Teaching implications

Subjective data

Mr. Jones • Age 59

Yearly physical exam includes positive paternal history for cardiac disease, persistent hypertension, significant life stressors, and decreased physical activity.

Nutritional risk factors

Activity and exercise

Physical exam reveals persistent HTN

ASSESSMENT FINDINGS

- Frequently eats fast foods
- Recent weight gain of 25 lb.
- Current BMI is between 28–29
- Drinks 1–2 beers a week

- Recently stopped playing golf twice/week.
- No time for other physical activity.

- Physical appearance
- History of HTNt—BP 178/94 mm Hg
- HR 94 BPM, RR 14 per min.
- Peripheral edema, cap refill 2+

Subjective and objective data indicate

PRIORITY NURSING DIAGNOSIS

1. Risk for Decreased Cardiac Output.
2. Related to: hypertension, obesity, family history, decreased activity, and stressors.

Leads to

EVALUATION

The patient...

- Demonstrates an understanding of CV risk factors and discusses their effects.
- Describes a specific plan and timetable for modifying his CV risk factors.
- Lists and describes signs or symptoms of acute or emergency situations.
- Reports absence of ischemic pain.
- Identifies support people from whom he can derive emotional strength.

Determine if interventions successful

INTERVENTIONS

- Patient teaching about the effects of sustained elevation in BP (e.g., possible stroke) and recognition of life-threatening symptoms.
- Patient teaching and health promotion about modifying risk factors: healthier diet, weight loss, increasing activity, decreasing stress.
- Use careful communication and positive encouragement.
- Monitor VS and weight.

Implement these nursing interventions

PLANNING/OUTCOMES

Patient will be able to:

- Demonstrate adequate knowledge concerning cardiovascular dysfunction, prevention, and care.
- State the risk factors for cardiac disease.
- Verbalize willingness to modify risk factors to improve health.
- Effectively cope with necessary lifestyle and activity changes.

FIGURE 27-6 Concept map for cardiac function.

high percentage of fat and sodium. Because many people regularly eat these convenience foods, investigate the patient's eating habits with this in mind.

Assess activity and exercise patterns to determine increased risk for cardiovascular dysfunction. Questions such as "How often do you exercise each week" and "What type of activities do you enjoy?" may be helpful. It is important to ask about specific activities that may constitute exercise, although not always in the traditional sense (e.g., gardening, vacuuming, caring for children or grandchildren). Also, determine how much of the patient's workday is composed of sedentary activity.

Obtain information concerning any medications (prescription, over the counter, or herbal) the patient is taking. Medications have side effects that can impact cardiovascular function. If a patient is taking medication for a cardiovascular condition, assess the length of time the medication has been taken, the dose, the patient's knowledge of the medication, and any side effects experienced. Also ask whether the patient is taking the medications as prescribed because many people may reduce or stop taking their medications when they start to feel better. Determine the patient's use of recreational drugs, especially alcohol, IV drugs, or cocaine. The nurse may introduce the questions about drug use by explaining that the information is important in determining the course of treatment.

Dysfunction Identification

Finding out why the patient has sought medical care is the first step in determining the nature of the patient's health complaint. The patient should explain reasons in his or her own words without interruption. After the patient's initial explanation, seek specific clarification concerning the problem.

CHEST PAIN

Pain or discomfort is the most common reason people with cardiovascular dysfunction seek medical care. Determine the specific nature of the discomfort: its location, its intensity, and the circumstances that cause it (Box 27-3). Additionally, elicit any other symptoms, such as indigestion, chest pressure, or

---

BOX 27-3	**Initial Assessment Questions for the Patient Experiencing Chest Discomfort**

- What does it feel like (pressure, weight on chest)?
- Does the pain go anywhere else (e.g., to the arms, neck, or back)?
- Does the pain increase with deep breathing or movement?
- How bad is it (0 to 10 scale, with 10 being the worst)?
- When did the pain start?
- What were you doing when it began?
- Does anything you do make it better/worse?
- Do you feel any other unusual symptoms (e.g., sweating, shortness of breath, nausea, dizziness)?

---

numbness and tingling in the left arm, because they may also be symptoms of heart disease. Many hospitals have a specific policy and procedure in place for patients with chest pain.

Establish the level of activity the patient associates with the onset of pain or discomfort. Some relevant questions to determine activity restriction include "Do the symptoms occur only during strenuous exercise, such as running or lifting weights?" "Do they occur when walking at a normal pace? If so, how far can you walk before the symptoms begin?" "Does quiet household activity bring on the symptoms?" "Do you experience the symptoms during periods of rest?" "Do any other circumstances, such as weather or emotional stress, tend to cause or exaggerate the problem?" "Do the symptoms appear at particular times of the day?"

Other subjective complaints may occur with cardiovascular problems. Dizziness, "blackouts," swelling of hands or ankles, and changes in skin color or sensation are significant. The term **syncope** refers to a temporary loss of consciousness or fainting spell and may signal decreased perfusion to the brain (American Heart Association, 2012b). Patients may complain of fainting spells (syncopal episodes), shortness of breath, difficulty lying flat, and coughing.

Gender Differences in Chest Pain and Treatment for Heart Disease

Historically, chest pain has been described and depicted in the media as sudden, sharp, and predictive of imminent collapse. Although this may be true in some cases, it is important to assess any type and degree of chest pain in patients that may indicate severe cardiac dysfunction.

It is also important to note that men and women may experience the signs and symptoms of a heart attack very differently, and these distinctions are important in nursing assessment and interventions for chest pain. Some symptoms of a heart attack may include chest discomfort; pressure or squeezing sensation; arm, back, neck, jaw, or stomach pain; trouble breathing; or light-headedness. Research has shown that women tend to present differently when experiencing a heart attack. They often will complain of sleep problems, lethargy, back or stomach pain, and nausea (Lichtman et al., 2015). In addition, delays in treating women with chest pain are currently up to 1 hour longer than in men, and that may decrease chances for positive outcomes. There are several explanations for this phenomenon, including women not seeking help in a timely manner as well as problems within the healthcare system. Nurses are the frontline caregivers who can assist in timely diagnosis and treatment of chest pain in women and can help improve patient outcomes.

STROKE SCREENING

Nurses are also often the frontline caregivers for patients at risk for and experiencing strokes. A tool nurses use to recognize stroke symptoms that can also be used to educate patients is the Face Arm Speech Test (FAST) (Summers et al., 2009). Helping to identify **F**acial drooping, **A**rm weakness, **S**peech changes, and **T**ime (when symptoms began and time to call 911) can get a person experiencing a stroke the care needed in a timely manner. Nurses must also be able to categorize stroke severity. The National Institutes of Health Stroke Scale (Lyden et al., 2009) is an evidenced-based tool used to standardize the evaluation of neurologic deficits in the acute stroke patient. It also provides a baseline to compare subsequent assessments. It is the most widely used instrument available for clinical assessment in stroke patients. Five areas of patient function—wakefulness (level of consciousness), vision, movement, sensation, and language and speech—are evaluated and scored. The test is administered at the bedside, and each item is given a numeric value; when the values are summed, the total score allows the nurse to evaluate the severity of the patient's deficits and develop a care plan.

Physical Assessment

INSPECTION

Observing the patient's general behavior and appearance yields significant information about tissue perfusion and CO. Decreased CO, vascular disease, or both can change cognitive and perceptual function. Because the brain is extremely sensitive to any decrease in blood flow, assessment of cognition and level of consciousness provides clues about cerebral perfusion.

Cognition is often the first indicator of perfusion to be assessed as the nurse initially interacts with the patient. People with normal cerebral perfusion usually speak in a normal cadence; answer questions quickly and appropriately; are oriented to person, place, and time; and are able to follow directions. Note if a patient's speech is slow or if there are overt difficulties with speaking. Inappropriate responses to questions or statements, confusion, apathy, decreased understanding, disorientation, restlessness, and anxiety are all possible signs of decreased cerebral perfusion. Level of consciousness is indicated by the patient's alertness. The patient who requires much stimulation to arouse him or her may have diminished cerebral blood flow.

Because skin color can roughly indicate blood flow adequacy, examine the patient for central and peripheral cyanosis. Note localized skin discolorations, such as bruises, redness, or mottling. Dependent edema (in the hands, sacrum, or ankles) indicates possible circulatory problems. Neck veins should be relatively flat; engorgement of these veins implies inefficient right-sided heart pumping.

Inspect the legs and arms for changes in hair distribution, skin color, shiny skin, ulcerations, edema, and venous distention. Note any varicosities. Toenails and fingernails should be smooth; ridged, thickened, hornlike nails indicate decreased peripheral perfusion. Digits are normally round in shape; clubbed fingertips are associated with oxygenation problems from lung or cardiovascular disease.

PALPATION

The patient with adequate perfusion is warm and dry to the touch. Although cool extremities are normal in many people, chronically cold fingers and toes often indicate poor circulation.

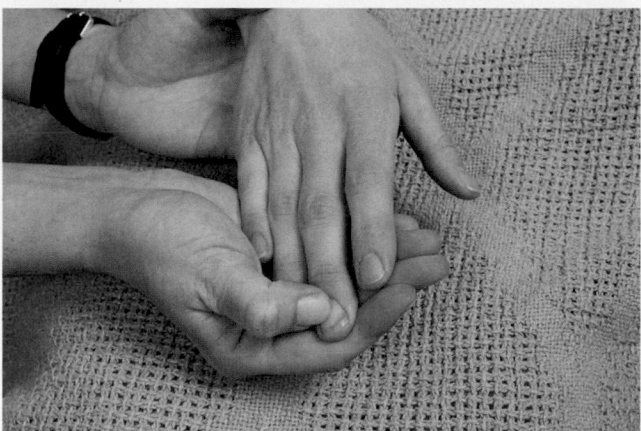

FIGURE 27-7 Test for capillary refill time. Pressure is applied to the nail bed and then released. Time for the nail to regain color is noted.

Palpate the pulse for quality and rate. Note regularity of rhythm, pulse intensity, and the number of beats per minute. Assess peripheral circulation by checking femoral (groin), popliteal (behind the knee), posterior tibial (ankle), and dorsalis pedis (foot) pulses for equal intensity in both legs. If an irregular pulse is detected, assess the apical and radial pulses simultaneously to determine whether all heartbeats are being perfused to distant pulse sites (Hogan-Quigley et al., 2012).

Capillary refill time, which reflects peripheral tissue perfusion and CO, is determined by pressing a nail bed until it blanches (Fig. 27-7). Pressure is released, and the time it takes for the nail to return to its original color is noted. This capillary refill time is ordinarily less than 3 seconds. A longer refill time indicates narrowing of the blood vessels, decreased circulating blood volume, or otherwise decreased CO (Hogan-Quigley et al., 2012).

Palpate for edema and note its extent (Fig. 27-8). Edema has traditionally been described in terms of a scale ranging from 0 (no edema present) to 4 (severe, pitting edema). This scale offers a subjective but moderately useful means for indicating the amount of edema present (Hogan-Quigley et al., 2012).

More accurate means of measuring edema include serial girth measurements of the affected extremities or abdomen (for ascites). Daily weight assessment can also indicate the extent of edema. One liter of fluid weighs one kilogram. A patient gaining more than about 11 kg in a week needs to be assessed by a physician because this may indicate an exacerbation of heart failure.

AUSCULTATION

A stethoscope is used to determine BP, count the apical pulse, and identify normal and abnormal heart sounds. Auscultate the apical pulse to establish its rate and character. This simple measurement is essential for complete assessment of the patient who has a pulse that is difficult to palpate or an irregular heart

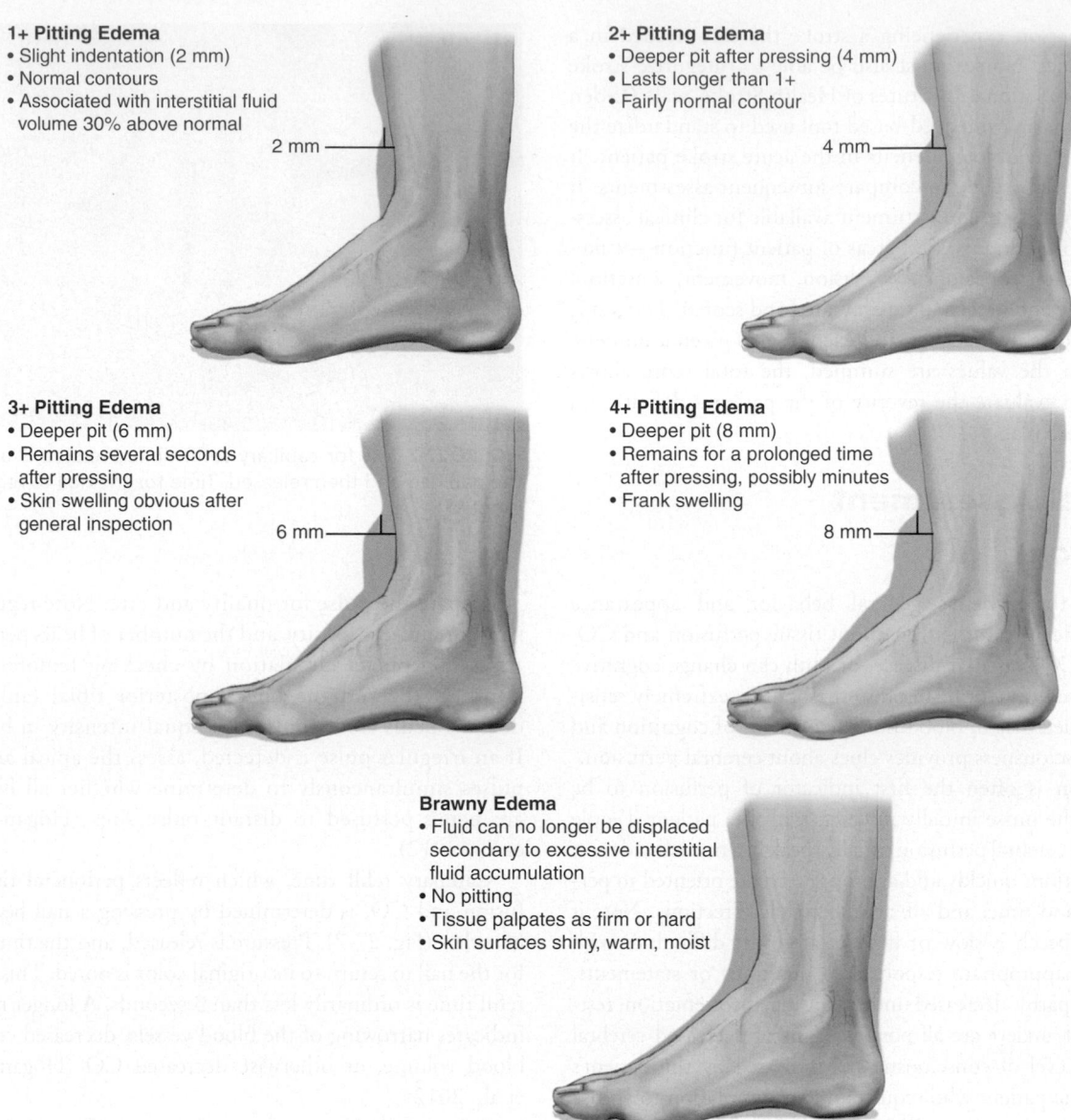

1+ Pitting Edema
• Slight indentation (2 mm)
• Normal contours
• Associated with interstitial fluid volume 30% above normal

2 mm

2+ Pitting Edema
• Deeper pit after pressing (4 mm)
• Lasts longer than 1+
• Fairly normal contour

4 mm

3+ Pitting Edema
• Deeper pit (6 mm)
• Remains several seconds after pressing
• Skin swelling obvious after general inspection

6 mm

4+ Pitting Edema
• Deeper pit (8 mm)
• Remains for a prolonged time after pressing, possibly minutes
• Frank swelling

8 mm

Brawny Edema
• Fluid can no longer be displaced secondary to excessive interstitial fluid accumulation
• No pitting
• Tissue palpates as firm or hard
• Skin surfaces shiny, warm, moist

FIGURE 27-8 Edema can be graded by gently pressing the edematous area with the fingers for up to 5 seconds.

rate. It also is necessary to auscultate the apical pulse for 1 full minute when administering certain medications, notably cardiac glycosides and beta-blockers (e.g., digoxin, metoprolol) in order to establish beats per minute with certainty and to assess the character of the heartbeat.

Normal heart sounds, murmurs, and other abnormal sounds also are audible by stethoscope. S_1 and S_2 are the "lub" and "dub" that are normally heard as the heart valves close. They are discussed in Chapter 17 along with abnormal heart sounds, such as murmurs and gallops, and normal heart sounds. Interpretation of these sounds takes a considerable amount of practice and a strong understanding of their underlying physiology.

Assess BP to establish the presence of hypotension, high BP, and positional differences. (For a detailed discussion of pulse and BP assessment, see Chapter 18.)

Diagnostic Tests and Procedures

The most common tests and procedures are described briefly here. Table 27-2 lists selected tests and diagnostic procedures used to assess cardiovascular function. The diagnoses of MI or heart failure are made after interpreting the results of several comprehensive tests. A patient having a cardiac workup may require several of the following studies.

LABORATORY STUDIES

Several laboratory tests that provide useful information concerning cardiovascular function range from basic blood assessment to highly sophisticated assays.

The complete blood count (CBC) provides information on white blood cells, platelets, and sedimentation rate. In

TABLE 27-2 SELECTED TESTS AND PROCEDURES USED TO ASSESS CARDIOVASCULAR FUNCTION

Test/Procedure	Purpose
CBC	Yields information on platelets, presence or absence of infection, oxygen-carrying capacity; used to diagnose anemias, nutritional deficiencies, and selected metabolic disorders
Blood chemistry tests	Determines serum electrolyte and lipid levels; also determines creatinine and BUN levels to assess kidney function
Cardiac biomarkers	Rules out or confirms MI
ECG	Identifies dysrhythmias; determines types and extent of heart damage from MI
Stress ECG (treadmill)	Identifies cardiac abnormalities not evident on resting electrocardiogram
Echocardiography	Measures heart size and thickness; observes valve function; measures CO
Heart catheterization	Measures pressure within heart chambers to determine heart strength, valve competency, CO, and fluid volume status
Angiography	Outlines blood flow through vessels to identify blockages and aneurysms
Electrophysiology	Identifies arrhythmias and effectiveness of antiarrhythmic treatment

addition, the CBC determines the number of red blood cells, hemoglobin, and hematocrit. These latter measures are important indicators of the blood's oxygen-carrying capability.

Cardiac biomarkers, previously referred to as cardiac enzymes, are proteins that are released from cells when tissue damage occurs. Some of the biomarkers are general to muscles of the body, while others are specific to the heart muscle. Serum levels of specific biomarkers (e.g., myoglobin, creatine kinase-MB [CK-MB], and troponin) are drawn and assessed to confirm a suspected MI.

B-type natriuretic peptide (BNP) is another diagnostic lab value that is specifically used to diagnose heart failure. BNP is a hormone naturally produced in the heart's muscle cells. It acts to dilate the blood vessels and improve the excretion of sodium and water from the kidneys, in turn decreasing the workload of the heart. BNP greatly increases when the cardiac muscle is overstretched, such as in heart failure.

Kidney function studies can indicate problems with perfusion. Blood urea nitrogen (BUN) and creatinine may be elevated in patients with hypoperfusion of the kidneys. Changes in kidney function can also affect acid–base and fluid or water balance. Deviations from normal levels of serum electrolytes

can adversely affect cardiovascular function. Dysrhythmias can result from potassium, calcium, and magnesium imbalances. Diuretics and other medications that affect cardiac function influence serum electrolyte levels.

Elevated lipoprotein levels indicate an increased risk for cardiovascular disease. Two of the main blood cholesterol carriers are LDLs and HDLs. LDL is commonly called the "bad" cholesterol because high levels in the bloodstream are associated with plaque formation contributing to coronary artery disease. Conversely, HDL is the "good" cholesterol that helps mobilize and remove those plaques that cause atherosclerosis. High levels of HDL and low levels of LDL offer the best protection from increased plaque formation leading to coronary artery disease (American Heart Association, 2013a, 2013b). A total cholesterol at or below 180 mg/dL is considered optimal. In 2013, the AHA and American College of Cardiology released new guidelines for prevention of cardiovascular disease that incorporate more than just cholesterol values. A CV risk calculation tool was developed to calculate 10-year and lifetime risk of atherosclerotic cardiovascular disease. They identified four key areas of focus for optimal treatment: assessment of risk, obesity, cholesterol, and lifestyle (Goff et al., 2013). Nurses should be ready to provide patient education about prevention as well as about use of medications such as statins.

DIAGNOSTIC PROCEDURES

Diagnostic procedures can yield information about cardiac function or blood flow. Tests relating to the heart include those that measure its electrical conductivity (e.g., electrocardiography [ECG], exercise testing) and those that measure its size and mechanical ability (e.g., chest radiography, echocardiography, cardiac catheterization). Angiography and hemodynamic monitoring provide precise information concerning blood flow.

Radiography

Chest radiography, which can establish the size and shape of the heart and aorta and detect pulmonary congestion or edema, is used to confirm correct placement of indwelling heart catheters and pacemakers.

Electrocardiography

ECG records the heart's electrical impulse conduction. Electrodes are placed on specific areas of the patient's limbs and chest. The electrodes are connected to a highly sensitive voltmeter, which controls a delicate pen. As the electrodes detect electrical impulses, the pen scribes a tracing on a moving strip of paper. The various deflections of the ECG tracing correspond to the individual events of the cardiac conduction cycle (Fig. 27-9).

Electrodes are placed on several areas of the limbs and chest to provide several "views" of cardiac impulses. Many views (called "leads") are needed to differentiate among the various conditions that can affect the heart because abnormalities may not appear in all leads. Single-lead electrocardiograms

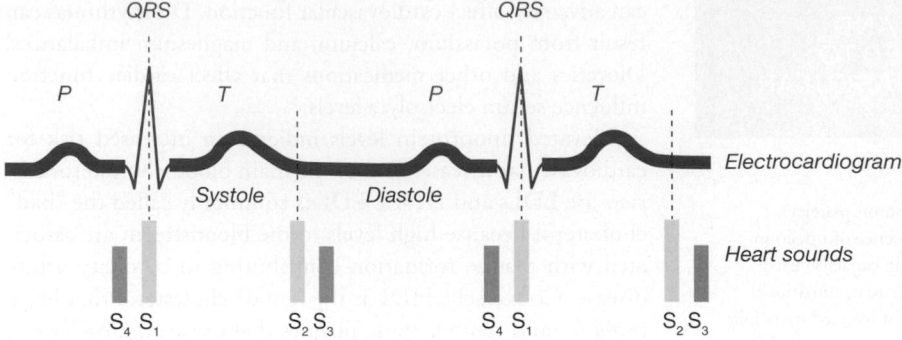

FIGURE 27-9 An electrocardiogram provides valuable information about the heart's ability to conduct impulses.

(**telemetry**) are useful for continuous monitoring of a patient, but the standard 12-lead electrocardiogram is needed for a thorough evaluation of the heart's electrical conductivity. When properly interpreted, the electrocardiogram can detect myocardial damage, cardiac ischemia, alterations from normal heart rhythm, changes in heart position or size, or problems within the conduction system.

Exercise Testing

Exercise testing can assess a person's response to cardiovascular stress. In some people, problems of cardiac ischemia are not detectable with conventional resting ECG because ischemia occurs only during periods of activity. The test involves the use of a treadmill with adjustable speed and slope. The patient begins walking at a normal pace on the treadmill. The electrocardiogram and BP are monitored continually while the speed and slope of the treadmill are gradually increased. The test usually lasts about 15 minutes, unless it is terminated because of ECG or BP changes or by the patient's fatigue, pain, or shortness of breath. Exercise testing allows practitioners to determine with some precision the degree of the person's functional ability.

Echocardiography

Echocardiography uses ultrasonic waves to diagnose structural heart defects. A penlike probe sends high-frequency sound waves through the chest wall. The waves produce echoes as they bounce off the heart, and the echo pattern is recorded. Using these patterns, cardiologists can obtain an accurate view of the heart without performing potentially dangerous invasive procedures, such as cardiac catheterization. Echocardiography can detect myocardial thickness and motion, structure and motion of the valves, the size of the chambers, and fluid around the heart.

Blood Flow Studies

Blood flow studies determine the patency and shape of blood vessels and the direction and volume of blood flow through them. The simplest and least expensive test of this type is Doppler examination. It is commonly used to monitor blood flow in the extremities and the brain. Doppler instruments enhance the turbulent sounds the blood makes as it circulates through the heart or vessels. Using ultrasound technology, the Doppler instrument produces a graphic representation of the course of blood flow.

Cardiac Catheterization

Catheterization of the heart and large vessels is used to determine precise information concerning valve function and cardiac muscle strength. This type of procedure is more invasive than the previously discussed tests. Various types of catheters can be inserted through a vein or artery in the arm or leg and directed (under fluoroscopy) into the heart's chambers. The catheter is able to measure the pressure generated within each chamber and to establish how efficiently the heart is pumping.

Some types of cardiac catheters also can measure CO and pressures within the pulmonary vascular system. Because they furnish information about vascular pressures, indwelling catheters are valuable tools in fluid and BP management. Pulmonary artery pressure, mixed venous oxygen (SVO_2), and central venous pressure catheters are used for this purpose. Arterial catheters allow the nurse to monitor arterial BP closely and to draw blood for evaluation of oxygenation and acid–base status. Arterial and other indwelling vascular catheters are used only when constant monitoring is possible, usually in an intensive care setting.

Angiography

Cardiac catheterization can also visualize the coronary arteries and possible narrowing of the arteries. Angiography uses a radiopaque dye to outline blood vessels and to confirm or rule out vessel blockage. This technique also is used to detect aneurysms. Radionuclide examinations use radioactive substances to detect decreased myocardial blood flow.

Electrophysiology

Electrophysiology is a study done to determine whether problems exist with electrical conduction or automaticity in the heart. Specialized wires are threaded through large veins and arteries, and attempts are made to stimulate the dysrhythmia. Patients are treated with medication or devices, and testing may be done to evaluate whether the treatment is effective.

Radiofrequency ablation is the process of ablating or burning the cardiac tissues where dysrhythmias (atrial fibrillation, supraventricular tachycardia) originate so that the abnormal pathways are destroyed. Initially, a known dysrhythmia is induced in the laboratory via electrical stimulation or medications and the abnormal pathway is identified. Small radiofrequency burns are then applied to that area in order to destroy the pathway and halt the dysrhythmia.

NURSING DIAGNOSES

The two primary NANDA-International (Herdman & Kamitsuru, 2014) nursing diagnoses that specifically address problems of cardiovascular function are Decreased Cardiac Output and Ineffective Peripheral Tissue Perfusion. Activity Intolerance also is a significant problem for many patients with cardiovascular dysfunction, although it is not exclusively a cardiovascular problem. Additional nursing diagnoses identify risk for ineffective perfusion by body area: cardiac, cerebral, or peripheral. See Table 27-3 for a summary of nursing diagnoses, outcomes, and interventions for cardiac problems.

OUTCOME IDENTIFICATION AND PLANNING

Outcome identification depends greatly on the patient's level of cardiac dysfunction as well as the patient's needs. In healthy patients, the nurse should focus on prevention of cardiovascular disease by increasing awareness of modifiable risk factors. Outcomes pertinent to the patient who is admitted with an acute problem focus on recovery from the cardiovascular problem without residual complications. Realistic outcomes for the patient with chronic cardiovascular disease focus on helping the patient to live within limitations imposed by the disease and to

improve acceptance of changes in lifestyle and self-concept. In cases of terminal cardiovascular disease, the nurse should center on maintenance of adequate comfort and, if critical, provide a timely assessment of current status and honor the end-of-life care wishes of the patient and family.

Goals are individualized based on the patient's health status. In general, the following are appropriate goals for the patient with cardiovascular dysfunction:

- The patient will demonstrate adequate knowledge concerning cardiovascular dysfunction, prevention, or care.
- The patient will maintain adequate CO.
- The patient will demonstrate adequate tissue perfusion with adequate oxygenation of body tissue.
- The patient will cope effectively with resulting changes in self-concept and lifestyle.

IMPLEMENTATION

Health Promotion

MODIFYING RISK FACTORS

Primary prevention of cardiovascular disease begins with understanding its causes. Healthcare providers teach in the areas of smoking cessation, nutrition, and a healthy lifestyle

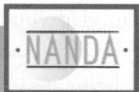

Table 27-3 SELECTED NANDA-I NURSING DIAGNOSES INVOLVING CARDIAC FUNCTION

Nursing Dx	Related Factors	Diagnosis Statement	NOC*	NIC†
Decreased Cardiac Output—inadequate blood pumped by the heart to meet metabolic demands of the body	High B/P, high cholesterol, smoking, sedentary lifestyle, increased cardiac workload	Decreased Cardiac Output R/T hypertension, obesity, stress AEB edema, tachycardia, and oliguria	Knowledge: Lipid Disorder Management, Healthy Lifestyle, and Treatment Regimen; Activity Tolerance; Cardiac Disease Self-Management; Cardiac Pump Effectiveness; Energy Conservation	Teaching: Disease Process, Diet, Activity/Exercise, Medication; Smoking Cessation; Medication Management; Vital Signs Monitoring; Oxygen Therapy
Ineffective Peripheral Tissue Perfusion—decrease in oxygen resulting in failure to nourish tissues at the capillary level	Hypovolemia, reduction in arterial and venous flow	Ineffective Peripheral Tissue Perfusion R/T hypovolemia post surgery AEB weak, thready pulse; BP <80/50; confusion	Tissue Perfusion: Cerebral; Urinary Elimination; Fluid Balance; Vital Signs	Bleeding Reduction; Fluid Monitoring and Management; Blood Administration; Shock Management; Vital Signs Monitoring; Oxygen Therapy
Activity Intolerance—insufficient physiologic or psychological energy to endure or complete required or desired daily activities	Imbalance between oxygen supply and demand, bed rest, sedentary lifestyle, obesity, deconditioned status	Activity Intolerance R/T Sedentary Lifestyle and deconditioned status AEB dyspnea and tachycardia with activity	Activity Tolerance; Knowledge: Prescribed Activity; Vital Signs	Exercise Promotion; Nutrition Management; Teaching: Prescribed Activity/Exercise; Weight Reduction Assistance

Dx, diagnosis; R/T, related to; AEB, as evidenced by.
*From: Moorhead, S., Johnson, M., Maas, M., & Swanson, E. (2013). *Nursing outcomes classification (NOC): Measurement of health outcomes* (5th ed.). St. Louis, MO: Elsevier.
†From: Bulecheck, G., Butcher, H., Dochterman, J., Wagner, C. (2013). *Nursing interventions classification (NIC)* (6th ed.). St. Louis, MO: Elsevier.
From: Herdman, T. H., & Kamitsuru, S. (Eds.). (2014). *Nursing diagnoses: Definitions and classifications, 2015–2017.* West Sussex, England: Wiley-Blackwell.

THERAPEUTIC DIALOGUE: CARDIAC SURGERY

SCENE FOR THOUGHT

Jean Norman is a 77-year-old woman lying in her bed in the intensive care unit with tubes and beeping monitors around her. She turns to the nurse, who approaches with an extra blanket that she had requested.

LESS EFFECTIVE	
Jean:	Thank you for the blanket, dear. I'm so cold here. (*Speaks softly and weakly.*)
Nurse:	How are you feeling otherwise, Ms. Norman? (*Arranges the blanket over her.*)
Jean:	Very tired and sore. I guess a bypass operation takes a lot out of you. (*Smiles weakly.*) But I'm sure it will turn out fine. (*Doesn't maintain eye contact.*)
Nurse:	You seem to be doing just great—your vital signs are normal, your incisions are healing well, and everything else looks good. I don't think I've seen too many people recover from surgery this fast, honestly. Are you in much pain right now? (*Stands quietly by the bed and holds the patient's hand.*)
Jean:	A little. If you have some time perhaps you could get me something? (*Still smiling.*)
Nurse:	Right away, Ms. Norman. You only have to let me know. (*Smiles and gives her hand a warm squeeze.*)
Jean:	Thank you, dear. I appreciate it. (*Squeezes back.*)

MORE EFFECTIVE	
Jean:	Thank you for the blanket, dear. I'm so cold here. (*Speaks softly and weakly.*)
Nurse:	How are you feeling otherwise, Ms. Norman? (*Arranges the blanket over her.*)
Jean:	Very tired and sore. I guess a bypass operation takes a lot out of you. (*Smiles weakly.*) But I'm sure it will turn out fine. (*Doesn't maintain eye contact.*)
Nurse:	Tell me more about that. (*Stands at the bedside, looking at her.*)
Jean:	What do you mean, dear?
Nurse:	You sound a little worried.
Jean:	(*Her eyes fill with tears, and she looks toward the hallway where her husband is sitting.*) Yes. I'm really worried if I'll be able to be as active as I was. (*Cries.*)
Nurse:	(*Holds her hand, stands quietly by the bed.*)
Jean:	I know I'm being silly. People go through this operation all the time. (*Dries her eyes.*)
Nurse:	It's usual for people to be worried. I'm glad you decided to share that worry with me.
Jean:	Do you think so? You don't think I'm being neurotic about this?
Nurse:	I'm not sure what you mean by neurotic, but I know that you seem fearful, and sometimes, talking about fears helps them become more manageable.
Jean:	That's true. (*She begins to talk about her fear of becoming an invalid and not being able to golf with her husband.*)

CRITICAL THINKING CHALLENGE

- Both nurses cared for Ms. Norman's needs. Compare and contrast the dialogues.
- What made the first dialogue less effective?
- Consider how the nursing assessment, diagnoses, and interventions differ between the first and second dialogues.
- Discuss which nursing outcome would be most effective in Ms. Norman's care.

including physical activity. Presenting information concerning risk factors in an objective manner can help patients choose appropriate behavior modification measures.

Nurses help patients who are seeking to modify their risks for cardiovascular disease by being knowledgeable about local support groups and classes that focus on modification. The recent proliferation of self-help programs, fitness clubs, and

aggressively advertised diets has provided the public with many options. Offer guidance in program selection and help the patient identify and avoid programs that promise overly simplistic or unrealistic or unsafe means to cardiovascular health.

The patient may need to become aware of appropriate supervised physical activity programs. If the patient has a known medical problem or is older than 35 years of age, recommend a complete physical examination before the patient starts an intensive exercise regimen. Various classes or support groups may be available to help the patient alter unhealthy lifestyle habits. Clinics, hospitals, and other local agencies often sponsor diet management, smoking cessation, and stress management programs. Group formats that offer an opportunity to share experiences can be effective, especially for social individuals who enjoy sharing. Nurses can be instrumental in developing and implementing such programs in the workplace. Electronic applications (apps) can help patients track success and stay motivated.

Education about food purchasing may be helpful for some patients. Selecting more fresh or frozen fruits and vegetables as opposed to canned ones can decrease sodium and sugar intake and increase fiber intake.

PREVENTING VENOUS STASIS

Venous stasis in the patient with limited mobility may result in edema and the formation of DVT. More emphasis has been directed toward preventive strategies for high-risk patients, including the prophylactic use of anticoagulation medications. By taking measures to improve the return of blood to the heart, nurses help to reduce the risk of dangerous clot formation. Leg exercises, antiembolism stockings, **sequential compression devices (SCDs)**, and avoidance of constriction help to prevent venous stasis.

Avoiding Constriction

Immobilized and inactive patients must be warned against venous constriction. Any article of clothing that exerts excessive pressure on the calves or thighs may constrict the veins, diminishing venous return and promoting the formation of clots and varicosities. Patients should avoid socks with tight elastic bands around the tops and short-legged pants with tight elastic or belted bottoms.

In addition to garments, orthopedic casts made of plaster or other materials can tighten and restrict blood flow. Warm fingers or toes indicate sufficient blood flow, but cool extremities, numbness or tingling, or limited capillary refill may indicate a need for recasting.

SAFETY ALERT

Report any changes in circulation, movement, or sensation (CMS) to the physician immediately.

Advise patients to avoid the crossing of legs, which creates pressure points against veins. Patients who must sit for extended periods (e.g., at work or on airplanes) should be careful not to create venous constriction by sitting too far back in chairs. The back of the calves should not rest against the edge of the chair because this compresses the veins. Teach these patients to flex their leg muscles periodically and to stand and walk frequently to encourage venous return.

Assisting with Leg Exercises

Nurses commonly teach leg exercises to patients before surgery to prevent postoperative circulatory complications. These simple exercises are helpful for any patient with impaired mobility, especially those confined to bed rest. Leg exercises are also recommended for people traveling on long airplane flights.

Leg exercises alternately contract and relax the muscles of the lower extremity. Contraction of these muscles helps promote the flow of blood back to the heart. Three separate leg movements can be encouraged (Table 27-4). First, have the patient perform calf-pumping exercises, which involve alternate dorsiflexion and plantar flexion of the feet. Second, have the patient bend one knee, sliding the foot up as far as possible along the mattress and back again. The patient should repeat this process with the other leg. Finally, have the patient alternately raise and lower each straight leg off the mattress as far as comfort allows.

Leg exercises should begin as soon as the patient returns from surgery or whenever the patient is immobile. The patient should perform exercises at least once every 1 to 2 hours while awake. If the patient is not able to perform leg exercises independently because of decreased strength or neurologic impairment, assist with passive leg exercises, encouraging as much patient participation as possible.

Applying Antiembolism Stockings

Immobility deprives the bedridden patient of the circulatory benefit of muscular contraction against the veins. Venous engorgement can be offset in these patients by the use of antiembolism stockings. Antiembolism stockings are made of strong elastic material. They are not the same as support hose because they provide varying degrees of compression at different areas of the leg. When correctly fitted and applied, they exert external pressure, decreasing venous blood from pooling in the extremities. The stockings promote venous return in much the same manner as the leg muscles, using continuous instead of intermittent pressure.

To do their job effectively, antiembolism stockings must fit properly. Stockings that are too large for the patient cannot provide sufficient vein compression, and stockings that are too tight obstruct blood flow to the legs. Guidelines for proper measurement and size selection of antiembolism stockings are available from the manufacturer and should be followed instead of estimating stocking size by the height or weight. Wrinkles and poorly made seams can lead to pressure ulcer development. **Procedure 27-1** provides instructions on application of antiembolism stockings.

Antiembolism stockings are usually removed for 30 minutes once every 8 hours. When they are in place, the patient's toes should remain warm, and the stockings should cause no obvious constriction or excoriation. They should be applied in the morning, before the patient has gotten out of bed, in order for them to be fitted while the patient's legs are least edematous.

SAFETY ALERT

Inspect the patient's legs and feet regularly to ensure that antiembolism stockings do not impair circulation.

TABLE 27-4 LEG EXERCISES TO PROMOTE CIRCULATION

Calf Pumping
Point toes of both feet toward the foot of the bed.

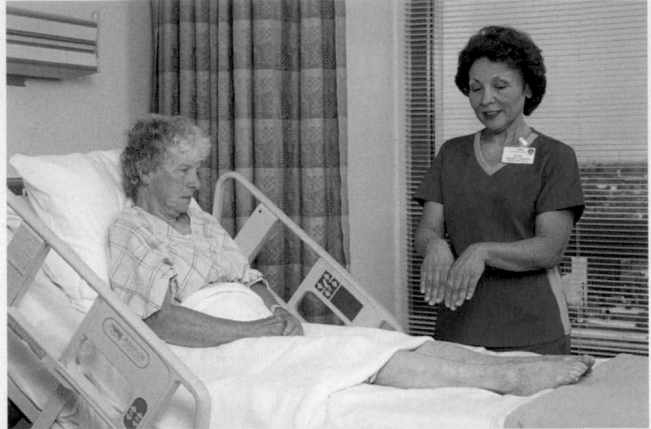

Relax. Then, pull toes toward the chin.

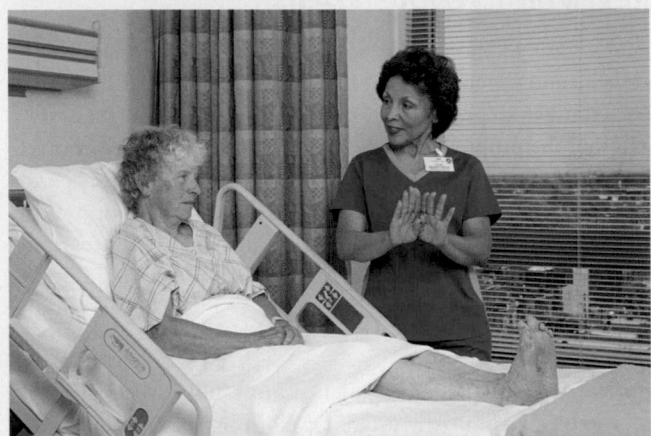

Make circles with both ankles in one direction and then in the other.

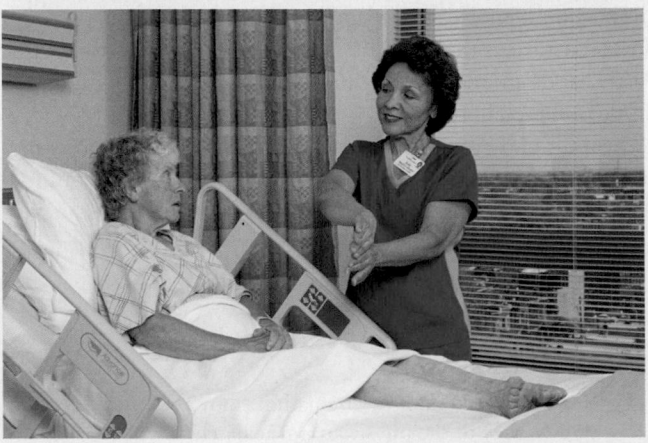

TABLE 27-4 LEG EXERCISES TO PROMOTE CIRCULATION (*Continued*)

Knee Flexion and Extension

Start with knees in flexed position with feet flat on the bed.

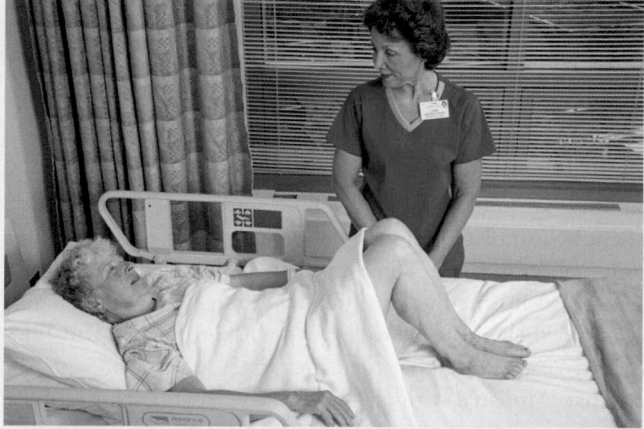

Slide feet forward as far as possible. Slide feet back to repeat flexed position.

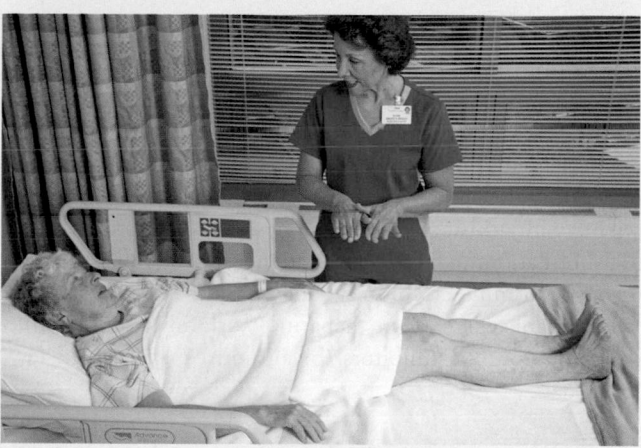

Raising and Lowering Leg

Raise and lower each leg alternately. Raise as far as comfort allows without straining.

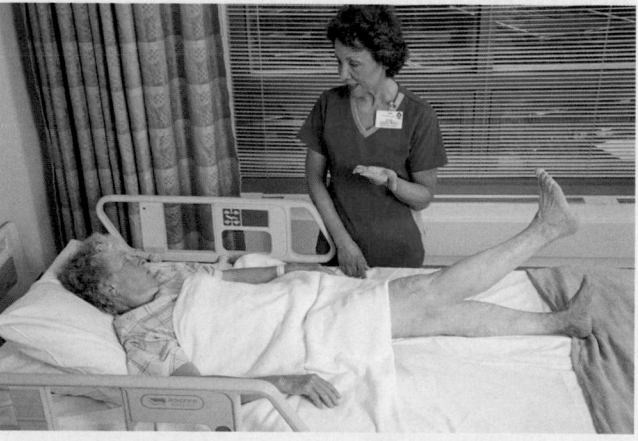

Using Pneumatic Compression Devices

Intermittent compression devices improve venous return by use of alternating pressure exerted against the extremity by inflation and deflation of plastic sleeves that are wrapped around the leg. The pneumatic compression device consists of an air pump, extremity sleeves, and connecting tubing. Pneumatic compression devices are of two types: intermittent and sequential. Intermittent devices turn chambers off and then on. SCDs sequentially compress various chambers within the extremity sleeve to promote venous return. A complete cycle can take 75 seconds to 5 minutes. Each of these devices is attached to an air pump that alternates inflation and deflation of the sleeve. Pneumatic compression devices should not be used for patients with arterial occlusive disease, severe edema, cellulitis, or infection of the extremity.

Frequently, SCDs are ordered for surgical patients who have mobility restrictions or for any immobilized patient. Patients often wear antiembolism hose underneath the plastic sleeves to decrease irritation from the plastic and provide extra support. When the patient gets up to ambulate, the devices are removed; once normal ambulation has resumed, the use of the SCD is usually discontinued. Refer to **Procedure 27-2** for application of SCDs.

Impulse Foot Pump

Impulse foot pumps improve venous return in the immobile patient by stimulating the venous plantar plexus, the large vein on the sole of the foot. When a person is walking, the plexus is squeezed each time the foot hits the ground, pumping blood back into the veins that will eventually return blood to the heart. On each foot, the patient wears a foot sleeve with a rigid base that is inflated with air and then deflated. Each sleeve is attached via a hose to a controller that controls the inflation and deflation (Fig. 27-10).

Anticoagulation Prophylaxis

High-risk individuals may receive anticoagulation drugs to prevent DVT or pulmonary embolism. High-risk groups include patients undergoing orthopedic or gynecologic surgical procedures; patients on bed rest for more than 5 days; patients with a history of major illnesses such as stroke, MI, atrial fibrillation, or DVT; and patients undergoing a percutaneous transluminal coronary angioplasty. Low-dose heparin, low-molecular-weight heparin, warfarin (Coumadin), or direct thrombin inhibitors (bivalirudin) may be used for prophylaxis.

Nursing Interventions for Altered Cardiovascular Function

Quality of life for the patient with altered cardiovascular function often depends on teaching and support. Important areas for instruction include medication management, edema reduction, pain management, and energy conservation. The nurse must also be skilled at recognizing life-threatening cardiac

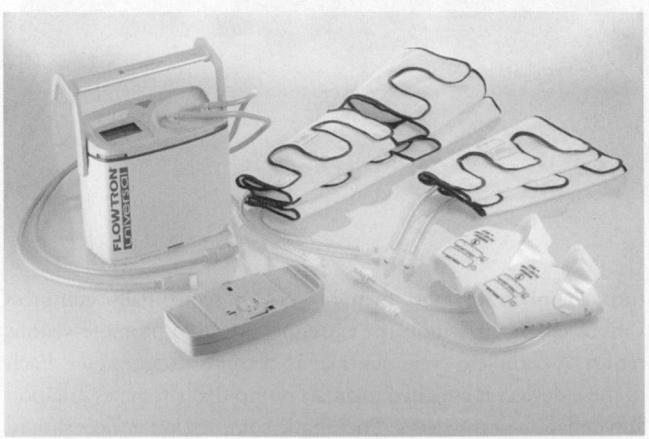

FIGURE 27-10 Impulse foot pumps improve venous return.

situations so that the medical emergency or rapid response team (MET or RRT) can be called. If the patient is found pulseless, a code is called and cardiopulmonary resuscitation (CPR) started.

PATIENT TEACHING

Teach the patient with altered cardiovascular disorders to recognize warning signs of decreased CO or decreased perfusion. Signs and symptoms that indicate the need for medical help are listed in Box 27-4. Instruct the patient on how to promote blood flow and reduce edema, promote skin integrity, and avoid fatigue.

MEDICATIONS

The patient with cardiovascular disease must often take numerous medications. The quality of the nurse's teaching can help promote patient compliance with the medication regimen. Cardiovascular drugs are complex and may be confusing to the patient. Therefore, it is beneficial to include the patient's spouse or significant other in discussions concerning medications. Explain clearly the reasons for taking prescribed medications and provide written information. Explain drug effects, side effects, and special considerations to the patient. Written information and schedules are also helpful so that patients have a reference if problems arise.

Simple, yet accurate, descriptions of each medication's action help the patient appreciate and remember the importance of complying with the medication regimen. Also stress the importance of taking medications as ordered. Warn the patient against missing doses or stopping a medication without consulting the physician. Be certain that the patient understands how and when to take medications, whether to avoid any foods or other substances (to prevent interactions), and what side effects to expect. Also teach the patient to recognize signs of toxicity and when to contact the physician. After teaching, assess the patient's knowledge and understanding by having him or her repeat the key concepts back to you. This will aid in your assessment and also help the patient solidify his or her knowledge.

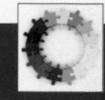

COLLABORATING WITH THE HEALTHCARE TEAM
Requesting Medical Emergency Team Assistance

You decide to call the MET* to evaluate Mrs. Chin. Your morning assessment revealed a sudden decrease in her neurologic status.

SITUATION: I am concerned because Mrs. Chin's neurologic status has suddenly deteriorated.

BACKGROUND: Her recent history includes fainting in church with slurred speech and confusion and a medical history of AFib and heart failure. She had a negative CT scan in the ED but my neuro assessment includes pupils slow to react and right-sided weakness. VS: 198/112, 98, 20.

ASSESSMENT: I am concerned that Mrs. Chin's neurologic deterioration signals a stroke.

RECOMMENDATION: Come to the bedside immediately for a patient evaluation.

CRITICAL THINKING CHALLENGE

- How does a nurse decide that the MET should be called? Many agencies have MET criteria. Identify some possible MET criteria.
- How might communication with the MET be different from communicating with the primary care physician?
- How might you communicate with the family about the MET and Mrs. Chin's status?
- What are some of the advantages, for you as a nurse, to have the MET at your hospital?

*The MET or RRT is a team that has been formed in many acute care facilities to better care for patients who suddenly become unstable, requiring immediate medical intervention. Members often include a physician (frequently a hospitalist), a respiratory therapist, and a critical care nurse. When called, they evaluate the patient, order appropriate medical interventions, decide whether the patient should be transferred to a higher level of care, and provide nursing support. Successful interventions by METs have decreased the number of cardiac and respiratory arrests in many hospitals.

Often, multiple medications are necessary, and regimens are complex and difficult to follow. More cardiovascular medications are being formulated as combination drugs (e.g., containing an angiotensin-converting enzyme [ACE] inhibitor and a diuretic in one tablet) or long-acting drugs to simplify medication management. To help with organizing, a small box with multiple compartments can be used to "load" in the day's or week's supply of medications. Side effects can be unpleasant and potentially serious, at times making compliance difficult. Table 27-5 lists some drug classes that are commonly used to treat cardiovascular problems.

TABLE 27-5 MEDICATIONS AFFECTING CARDIAC FUNCTION AND TISSUE PERFUSION

Medications	Example	Drug Action	Side Effects
Cardiac glycoside	Digoxin	Increases cardiac contractility; decreases heart rate	Bradycardia, arrhythmias
Antihypertensive agents: • Beta-adrenergic blockers • Calcium channel blockers • Vasodilators • ACE inhibitors • Angiotensin receptor blockers (ARBs)	Atenolol Nifedipine Apresoline Captopril Losartan	Decreases BP	Low BP, dizziness, syncope
Vasopressors	Norepinephrine	Increases BP	High BP
Antiarrhythmics	Amiodarone	Regulates heart rhythm	Hypotension, dizziness
Nitrates	Nitroglycerin	Relieves angina via peripheral vasodilation	Hypotension, headache
Antilipid agents	Lovastatin	Decreases cholesterol levels, reducing atherosclerosis risk	Nausea, bowel changes
Diuretics	Lasix	Reduces edema and fluid volume by increasing urinary output	Electrolyte imbalance (hypokalemia), volume depletion
Anticoagulants	Heparin Coumadin	Decreases potential for clot formation	Bleeding

ARBs, angiotensin receptor blockers.

SAFETY ALERT

Many cardiovascular medications (e.g., antihypertensive agents, nitrates) can cause postural hypotension, potentially resulting in a fall or injury. Caution patients to get out of bed slowly and to avoid hot baths, which could increase vasodilation and syncope.

EDEMA REDUCTION

Peripheral edema can impede blood flow to the tissues. It is unsightly and often uncomfortable or painful for the patient. Control of edema is an important nursing priority (Fig. 27-11).

Elevation of Limbs

One of the simplest measures for reducing edema is to elevate affected limbs. Limb elevation allows gravity to assist venous return to the heart and helps to decrease venous pressure, reducing fluid leakage from vessels and promoting its reabsorption. Vessels can reopen, and perfusion is improved.

Avoid causing venous constriction when elevating edematous limbs. The legs should be fully supported when elevated, and there must be no pressure points. Do not raise the patient's leg so high that a constriction occurs at the groin. Do not elevate the hospital bed at the knees because this restricts venous flow behind the knee.

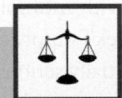

ETHICAL/LEGAL ISSUE

PATIENT'S REFUSAL OF TREATMENT

Mrs. Anderson, a competent 74-year-old patient, lives in a retirement center. She has had heart failure for the past 12 years. Her feet become swollen and painful when she walks. Difficult breathing from the heart failure limits her activity tolerance. When you enter her room to give her a diuretic, she states, "I don't want to take it anymore." You explain that the water pill is necessary to help her kidneys excrete the excess fluid. Her response is, "When I take it, I wet on myself. I would rather have my dignity than have that happen." Over the course of several days, her condition worsens to the point where she needs the diuretic to live. She continues to state that she would rather die with dignity than take the diuretic.

CRITICAL THINKING CHALLENGE

- Identify the important issues in this case.
- Explore how your own feelings, values, and beliefs are the same or different from those of Mrs. Anderson.
- Consider your position. What is your role as a nurse in this situation?
- Target ways to work with the patient to help her make choices about her healthcare and the outcomes.

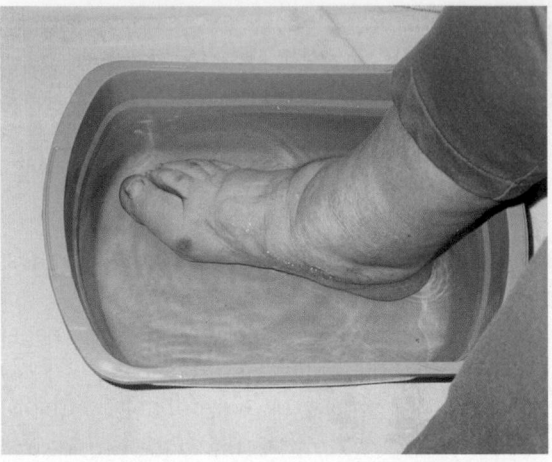

FIGURE 27-11 Foot care is very important for the patient with edema or peripheral vascular disease. Note the edema and reddened areas that could easily break down.

Reducing Sodium Intake

The patient with fluid retention problems usually benefits from a low-sodium diet, with daily sodium intake less than 2.5 g. Because sodium molecules attract water, limiting salt intake helps to control edema. Limiting the use of table salt is a logical first step in a sodium-restricted diet, but the patient also must understand "hidden" sodium content. Teach the patient to look for sodium content on the labels of beverages, health products, over-the-counter medicines (especially antacids), and foods. Canned vegetables generally contain more sodium than do frozen ones. The patient should avoid highly processed convenience foods. Spices and herbs can be used as a replacement for salt in cooking. Finally, encourage the patient to discuss possible salt substitutes with the physician, although salt substitutes contain potassium and should not be used by patients with renal failure.

Fluid Restriction

Patients who have fluid volume excess may restrict fluid intake until balance is restored. Monitor intake and output carefully to assess fluid status. An output of more than 2 L (2,000 mL) greater than intake suggests fluid retention. Weigh the patient daily, preferably at the same time and ideally before breakfast. Weight should not vary by more than 1 kg (2.2 lb) per day.

POSITIONING

Body position affects cardiac work and tissue perfusion. The heart works harder in the supine position than in the upright position. Lying flat promotes venous return. Because all vessels are at the same level of the heart, gravity's effect on the blood is minimized. Blood can flow more freely into the venae cavae. The increased volume of blood entering the atria increases stroke volume and workload of the heart. Those with healthy hearts easily tolerate the enhanced venous return in the supine position.

Recommended positioning for a hypotensive patient is with legs elevated 20 to 30 degrees (6 to 12 inches) to improve venous return and blood perfusion to vital organs. During this period, the hypotensive patient must also receive specific treatment for the cause of the hypotension to ensure restoration of perfusion to all vital organs.

On a smaller scale, positioning can be used to improve blood flow to selected underperfused areas. Gravity enhances arterial flow. Allowing ischemic hands or feet to hang in dependent positions may improve perfusion; however, this measure is contraindicated in the patient with edema.

PAIN MANAGEMENT

Some patients with cardiovascular problems experience infrequent, relatively slight discomfort; others have constant debilitating pain. Patients may report chest tightness, pressure, or numbness and tingling in the neck and arm. Helping these patients manage their ischemia is an essential nursing skill.

Chest Pain

When acute chest pain is evident, the patient should stop all activity and rest, sitting comfortably; lying flat inhibits full chest expansion and limits gas exchange in the lung, so the patient should avoid this position. Chest pain may be a life-threatening situation, and help should be obtained to evaluate it. Document the duration, activity during onset, and vital signs during the episode of pain. Report this information to the physician. Careful attention should be paid to pain relief to avoid increasing myocardial oxygen demand through increased heart rate, contractility, and arrhythmias.

> ### ! SAFETY ALERT
> Never ignore any patient's complaints of chest pain or discomfort. Such feelings have many causes, but unless proven otherwise, chest pain in the cardiac patient must be assumed to be a serious sign of cardiac hypoxia. As a student, chest pain is a situation in which you will want to get help right away.

In hospitals, a stat 12-lead ECG should be ordered in an attempt to record an ischemic event or infarction (American Heart Association, 2012a). Once the ECG is read, measurements are made to determine the extent of the cardiac event, and a reperfusion treatment (stent, angioplasty) within 90 minutes if clinically indicated is the standard of care. Oxygen should be started immediately, the patient should maintain bed rest, and sublingual nitroglycerin should be given. Administer sublingual nitroglycerin while the patient is sitting or lying down. Assess BP 5 minutes after giving this medication because nitroglycerin is a vasodilator, and the BP may fall. For a patient at home, if the pain is new and not relieved after one dose of nitroglycerin, the family should call 911 or emergency services.

Patients with chronic angina can be helped primarily by assistance with activity management. They should learn to monitor their pulse rate and to pace activities to prevent increases of more than 20 bpm above the baseline rate. They should perform activities on an empty stomach whenever possible to avoid acute angina. Because blood is diverted to the gut after eating, less oxygen is available to the muscles, including the heart. For this reason, the nurse should not schedule procedures or activities, such as bathing or walking, immediately after meals. If sublingual nitroglycerin is ordered, the patient may take a dose before performing an activity that has previously produced pain.

Claudication and Peripheral Ischemic Pain

Claudication and pain are present in acute and chronic arterial disease. If the pain is new, the physician should be notified because it indicates worsening status. Chronic disease, cold surroundings, cigarette smoking, or activities that exceed individual tolerance may precipitate pain. Nursing measures to prevent such pain are directed at enhancing oxygen delivery to tissues by improving blood flow or decreasing oxygen demand. Planned exercise with rest periods reduces symptoms of claudication and can be an appropriate nursing intervention.

When a heating pad is used, it should be covered with a towel

> ### ! SAFETY ALERT
> Chronically impaired perfusion of extremities can cause impaired perception of the sensation of heat. For this reason, the patient with vascular disease is prone to burns. Exercise great care to avoid excessively hot soaks or compresses. Their temperature should not exceed 95.8°F to 100.8°F (35.8°C to 38.8°C).

or pillowcase and not allowed to come into direct contact with the skin. Heating pads should not be used by people with impaired sensation or cognitive function because of the danger of burns.

INCREASED ACTIVITY

As part of rehabilitation after a heart attack or cardiovascular problem, activity begins slowly and progresses gradually. Initially, the patient is sedentary, ambulating to the bathroom and or for short distances in the room. The patient performs lower and upper range-of-motion exercises to maintain muscle tone and joint movement. He or she then progresses to sitting in the chair for meals and walking around the room. A sitting shower and short walk (100 to 250 feet) are done if the patient has tolerated previous activity. A chair may be placed nearby for safety. Finally, the patient can perform independent activities; walking 100 to 250 feet three to four times daily is recommended. Monitor the patient for ability to climb stairs without difficulty. Warn the patient about the potential for light-headedness with showering, especially with very warm water.

At home, healthcare providers and family members should encourage the patient to start a walking program of 10 minutes per day at a slow, regular pace. Instruct the patient to accommodate for hills because they necessitate increased effort. Also, reinforce the concept that the patient should plan to allow 5 minutes away and then 5 minutes back. He or she should increase time for walking, as tolerated, to 1 hour. Within 2 to 3 weeks after the event, an outpatient cardiac rehabilitation program is recommended; at this type of facility, the patient will encounter physical therapists and others who monitor more vigorous physical exertion and weight training.

ENERGY CONSERVATION

Pain can occur when the patient exceeds normal activity tolerance. Effective conservation of energy can promote activity tolerance and thus can help prevent pain.

Patients with newly diagnosed MI should avoid repeated movement of the upper arms. This movement increases the metabolic demands of the arm muscles and forces the heart to pump harder for the blood to overcome gravity.

Activities involving lifting or pushing heavy objects and straining during bowel movements often involve Valsalva's maneuver. Instruct the cardiac patient to avoid the stress this places on the heart by consciously maintaining a steady breathing pattern or exhaling slowly during such activities. Remind cardiovascular patients to avoid isometric (static strength training) exercises, which tend to cause changes in BP and heart rate.

SAFETY ALERT

Warn the patient against using Valsalva's maneuver, which occurs during bearing down.

The most important energy conservation measure for the patient with acute cardiovascular problems is regular rest. Breathlessness or increased heart rate lasting for longer than 10 minutes after exercise indicates a need to go slower in the rehabilitation effort. Nocturnal insomnia or daytime fatigue also may mean that the previous day's exercise has been too strenuous. The patient should rest undisturbed for 1 hour after meals. Encourage rest before and after activities such as bathing or when lengthy treatments are scheduled. Space out activities to avoid fatigue. Periods of work should alternate with rest or lighter activity. During activities, the patient should sit whenever possible to avoid cardiovascular strain. When activities or tasks require gathering several materials, good planning is essential to eliminate unnecessary and inefficient or wasted effort. The patient should immediately stop any activity that produces fatigue, breathlessness, pressure, or pain.

CARDIOPULMONARY RESUSCITATION

Cardiac arrest is the most serious emergency that can occur. When a patient's heart stops, acute hypoxia begins to destroy all tissues. Unless oxygenation is restored quickly, the victim will die. CPR is a means of artificially supporting circulation and oxygenation until the victim's heart begins beating on its own.

Healthcare agencies usually require most or all personnel to be trained in basic life support (BLS). The Red Cross, the AHA, and other agencies offer classes for BLS certification. These courses can be completed in 1 day, often through the employing agency. Recertification is usually required every 2 years to keep skills updated. The AHA modified its teaching in 2010 to promote CAB (circulation, airway, breathing) as the order of care, promoting chest compressions as the first-line and most important treatment for victims of cardiac arrest (Hazinski, 2010). Defibrillation with an automatic external defibrillator (AED) has also become part of the training (CAB "D"). In a lethal,

nonperfusing rhythm (e.g., ventricular fibrillation), without prompt defibrillation, a patient will not survive.

Advanced cardiac life support (ACLS) requires extensive training and rigorous testing. People certified in ACLS are trained in electrocardiogram interpretation and advanced airway management. They are qualified to administer emergency drugs or electrical shock (defibrillation) as needed.

Hospital resuscitation is often referred to as a "code" as cardiac arrest is often announced as "code blue." The code team consists of physicians, nurses, pharmacists, and respiratory therapists. All members of the code team should have specialized training, which may include ACLS.

The nurse may be the first person to discover a patient in cardiac arrest. Along with the techniques of CPR, nurses must be proficient in handling many duties at the scene of a cardiac arrest. The following sections focus on some important nursing aspects of CPR efforts in an agency with emergency equipment and trained responders. Each healthcare agency establishes specific cardiac arrest protocols. It is every nurse's responsibility to be familiar with these protocols.

Initial Management

After quickly establishing that an arrest has occurred, shout for help and press the emergency button (if available). If you are working alone in the home or community setting, establish that the patient is unresponsive and then call the emergency response operator. Do not hang up until instructed to do so by the operator. Initiate and continue CPR until the rescuers arrive. If a facility emergency response is available, alert the hospital operator. Dial the emergency number and announce to the operator, "There is a cardiac arrest on (location), room (number)." The operator can summon help using the paging system.

The nurse's first calls for help should bring other nurses to the room. They bring the emergency supplies ("crash cart") while the first nurse begins preparations for CPR (Fig. 27-12). Whether or not assistance comes immediately, the discovering nurse must stay with the victim and continue to call for help until it arrives.

If the patient has been sitting upright, lower the bed to a flat position. Move extra equipment away from the bed for easy access to the patient. Remove the pillow from under the patient's head. If the bed is elevated to stretcher level, lower it. Put the board or other hard surface under the patient's chest; alternatively, some mattresses can be inflated so that they provide a hard surface. All of these adjustments must be made as quickly as possible, and CPR must be initiated immediately. Other nurses can move the furniture from around the bed to make room for the crash cart, defibrillator, and ECG machine. As soon as the defibrillator arrives, it should be connected to the patient so that a rhythm can be assessed and the proper treatment initiated, including prompt defibrillation.

The Code Team

Management of a cardiac arrest usually requires a team of people. Every hospital's code team may differ slightly, but they are striving to achieve the same end goal: restoring the patient's health. Three critical components have been identified to increase the odds of a favorable patient outcome: planning, establishing

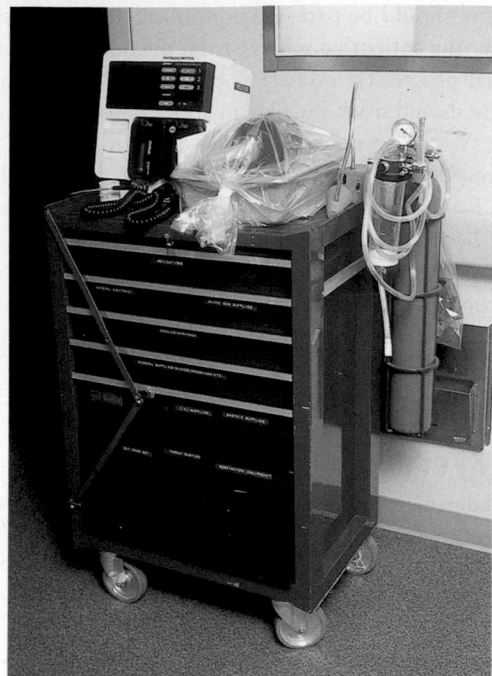

FIGURE 27-12 A crash cart contains emergency supplies and medications to manage a cardiac arrest.

leadership, and effective open communication (Castelao et al., 2013). Usually, a code leader (perhaps an attending physician or resident) is identified who will lead the code and give orders. Other members of the team are responsible for such roles as establishing and managing the patient's airway, performing chest compressions to maintain circulation, and establishing IV lines or central line access as needed. Other key roles include performing defibrillation if needed and administering medications as well as maintaining an accurate record of medications and interventions and retrieving needed supplies. Team members may switch roles during the resuscitation effort and take turns at compressions, which are especially fatiguing. Code drills or practice often can be arranged so that code team members can become proficient and work well as a team. These code drills reiterate the importance of planning, reinforce leadership skills, and foster open communication in a simulated setting.

After Resuscitation Begins

Once the code team has taken charge, the nurse who discovered the person should remain with the team to provide essential information. The circumstances under which the person was found, the patient's status before the arrest, primary diagnoses, recent medications, and recent laboratory data are relevant. The nurse also may be needed to assist with procedures. The person in charge assigns specific duties to members of the code team. Those who are not actively participating in the resuscitation efforts should leave the room and care for other patients.

Consideration of privacy is important. If another patient shares the room, he or she should be moved elsewhere if possible. If moving the roommate is not practical, the curtain should be drawn, and a nurse should stay with the roommate. This patient may be anxious; answer his or her questions honestly.

Finally, one of the most difficult tasks for the nurse is dealing with the sorrow and fears of the patient's loved ones. Provide emotional support during and after the resuscitation. Provide honest, up-to-date information, but do not speculate on the patient's condition. Recent studies have demonstrated the positive benefit of having family members present during resuscitation efforts (Jabre et al., 2014). Family presence during invasive procedures and resuscitation has been endorsed by the Emergency Nurses Association based on this research, and the American Association of Critical-Care Nurses (2010) issued a practice alert about this topic. Although research supports family presence, only a small number of hospitals have instituted policies and procedures regarding this practice to date. Check with your agency policy regarding this practice.

Home and Community Care

Most cases of chronic cardiovascular disease are managed in the community. Hospital stays for acute episodes, such as MI or open heart surgery, have decreased dramatically in length during the last decade. Many other less acute problems are diagnosed in ambulatory settings and completely managed at home.

Community-based care often focuses on prevention, especially among high-risk people. On routine examination, if a patient is found to be overweight, to be sedentary, to smoke, or to have high cholesterol levels, lifestyle modification education is appropriate. Often, detection of elevated cholesterol or hypertension is significant motivation for making necessary changes. Follow-up is important for these patients (Fig. 27-13).

CARDIAC REHABILITATION

For many patients, cardiovascular problems need not permanently prevent them from enjoying a normal lifestyle. The purpose of rehabilitation is to help the cardiovascular patient restore or improve lost function. This goal depends on physical endurance, which is improved by graded physical activity. Therefore, although rest is an essential part of the management

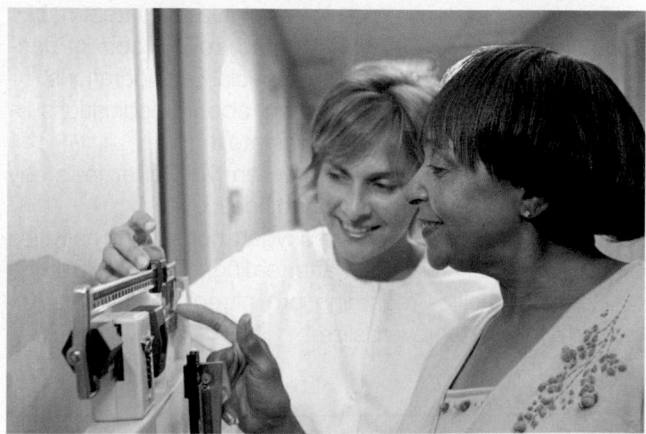

FIGURE 27-13 Weight management and follow-up care are important aspects of care for patients with cardiovascular problems.

APPLY YOUR CRITICAL THINKING

You are a home health nurse visiting Mr. Brown. He has recently had a heart attack, followed by emergency open heart surgery for blocked coronary arteries. He tells you that he has been feeling tired lately. He has been trying to eat right, remember his medications, and walk. Every time he tries to move, his chest is painful. His wife says that he has stopped buttering his bread and is taking naps frequently during the day. Explain what you will do next, and provide your rationale.

Check your answer in Appendix B.

---

of cardiovascular problems, activity also must play a part. Exercise is an important intervention because it reduces BP and produces improvements in the lipid profile.

Promotion of activity tolerance starts after the medical problem has been identified and treated. Next, a functional assessment of the patient is conducted. Only after the patient's physical, mental, and emotional readiness for rehabilitation have been thoroughly assessed can appropriate measures be implemented.

Exercise should be part of a continuing rehabilitation program after the patient's discharge from the hospital. A program of gradual progressive exercise is prescribed by the physician. The nurse should teach the patient about safe exercise practices at home. Warm-up exercises prevent sudden demands on the heart; cool-down exercises help prevent pooling of blood in the legs. Patients should not exercise in extremes of weather or within 1 hour after a meal.

Instruct the patient to recognize untoward symptoms of overexertion, such as palpitations or fluttering in the chest, racing pulse, pain, and pressure. Teach the patient how to take his or her pulse using the carotid or radial sites.

❗ SAFETY ALERT

The patient should stop activity if the pulse rate exceeds the specified target zone prescribed by the provider. If the pulse lowers with activity or becomes irregular, or if the heart rate does not return to its resting level within 10 minutes after exercise, the patient should contact the physician.

Patience is essential for the patient and the nurse; neither should try to hurry the rehabilitation process. Exercise must

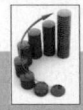

OUTCOME-BASED TEACHING PLANS

George Porter, a 54-year-old executive, is being discharged from the telemetry unit following an MI. He and his wife have both expressed concern that an emergency could arise when they return home. They want to be prepared to handle such an emergency.

OUTCOME

Mr. and Mrs. Porter can verbalize how to recognize and treat anginal pain.

STRATEGIES

- Provide a handout explaining angina and its treatment.
- For each new medication ordered, review correct dosage, when to take it, and any special considerations.
- Provide the above information about medications in writing and have the patient restate it.
- Stress the necessity for rest when Mr. Porter feels any pain or pressure to see if it subsides.
- Instruct Mr. Porter to space oxygen-consuming activities (e.g., don't exercise right after eating).
- Review specifics regarding prn nitroglycerin. Have Mr. and Mrs. Porter reverbalize.

OUTCOME

Mrs. Porter can verbalize when to call 911 and develop a plan to become proficient in CPR.

STRATEGIES

- Discuss with Mr. and Mrs. Porter their plan for handling a cardiac emergency (unrelieved chest pain and cardiac arrest).
- Explore Mrs. Porter's comfort with performing CPR on her husband if needed.
- Assess Mrs. Porter's specific plans for taking a community course to learn CPR.
- Provide a written list of when to call 911 (unrelieved chest pain; new onset of rapid, irregular, or very slow heart rate, especially if accompanied by severe fatigue or dizziness; fainting or loss of consciousness).
- Provide a sticker with emergency numbers for the Porters to keep on the phone.

EVALUATION

5/1/17: 08:30—The Porters were able to describe the cause and treatment of angina and verbalized an appropriate plan for dealing with a cardiac emergency. Mrs. Porter is planning to sign up for a CPR class and research the cost of a home defibrillator.

—M. Klim, RN

be graduated, with more strenuous activities being added to the regimen only as patient tolerance allows. Warn the patient against thinking, "If this much exercise is good, twice as much will cure me in half the time." Exercise can provide several valuable physiologic and psychological benefits to the patient with cardiovascular disease. Exercise is one facet of a holistic approach to regaining health. Adherence to prescribed medical therapies, reduction of stress, and modification of lifestyle risk factors are vital parts of any successful rehabilitation program.

A common area of concern for the patient during rehabilitation is the possible impact such limitations may have on sexual function. After cardiac surgery or an MI, sexual activity may be limited for about 6 to 8 weeks, until recovery permits more strenuous activity. Another common concern is the fear that another serious cardiac episode may occur during sexual activity. This can create much stress for the patient and his or her sexual partner. Instruct the patient to use positions that require less energy expenditure (e.g., side lying, supine), to participate when well rested, to avoid sexual activity after a large meal or heavy consumption of alcohol, and to stop and rest if any chest pain occurs.

> **! SAFETY ALERT**
> If the chest pain persists after nitroglycerin administration, the patient or a family member should notify 911 or emergency community services. The patient should not attempt to drive to the hospital.

EMERGENCIES

The patient and family members need to be knowledgeable concerning emergency situations. In patients with a history of pain, nitroglycerin should always be available so that it can be quickly administered if chest pain occurs. Nitroglycerin breaks down over time and with exposure to light. It should tingle when placed under the tongue. The prescription should be refilled whenever it has passed the expiration date to ensure potency in case an emergency occurs. All family members and caregivers should complete a BLS course and be able to administer CPR.

EVALUATION

Patients with cardiovascular dysfunction show widely variable rates of progress. For this reason, specific goals for these patients must be individualized. Together, the nurse and patient can establish realistic goals with appropriate outcome criteria for measuring goal attainment.

Goal

The patient will demonstrate adequate knowledge concerning cardiovascular dysfunction prevention or care.

POSSIBLE OUTCOME CRITERIA

The following should occur by the end of the teaching session:

- The patient demonstrates an understanding of cardiovascular risk factors by reciting those that apply and discussing their physiologic effects.
- The patient describes a specific plan and timetable for modifying his or her cardiovascular risk factors.
- The patient states the following for any medication administered for cardiovascular problems: name, action, and side effects of the drug; dose to be taken; and any special considerations for administration.
- The patient describes the rationales for prescribed therapies.
- The patient lists and describes signs or symptoms of acute or emergency situations.

Goal

The patient will demonstrate adequate tissue perfusion with adequate oxygenation of body tissue.

PATIENT PLAN OF CARE
The Patient with Activity Intolerance

NURSING DIAGNOSIS
Activity Intolerance related to an imbalance between oxygen supply and demand manifested by verbal reports of fatigue or weakness, abnormal heart rate or BP response to activity, exertional discomfort or dyspnea.

PATIENT GOAL
Patient will balance activity with physical limitations.

PATIENT OUTCOME CRITERIA
- Patient's heart rate has regular rhythm and remains between 60 and 100 bpm at rest. (Values may require adjustment for patients with chronic cardiovascular or pulmonary problems.)
- Patient's heart rate rises in proportion to level of activity and does not exceed an increase of 20 bpm.
- Patient's BP remains within normal limits for age group; fluctuations with position change are minimal.

(Continued)

PATIENT PLAN OF CARE (*Continued*)
The Patient with Activity Intolerance

NURSING INTERVENTION	SCIENTIFIC RATIONALE
1. Limit activity 1 hour after meals.	**1.** Blood flow is directed to digestive tract to aid digestion; increases workload on the heart.
2. Plan heavy activities (e.g., morning hygiene, ambulation) to alternate with rest period of 1 to 2 hours.	**2.** Careful scheduling allows for uninterrupted rest period. Spacing activity conserves energy and avoids activity intolerance.
3. Offer prescribed nitroglycerin before activity or when pain develops with activity.	**3.** Nitrates vasodilate, decreasing venous return and decreasing cardiac workload.
4. Monitor pulse, BP, and respiratory rate before, during, and after activity.	**4.** Sudden changes in vital signs indicate activity intolerance and provide a parameter for scheduling activity.
5. Gradually increase activity within physician's activity order.	**5.** Gradual increase in activity level helps the patient build endurance and better tolerate increased activity.

EVALUATION

4/14/17: 09:30—Ambulated in hall, approximately 200 yards with no c/o of dizziness or dyspnea. HR 94 post activity—remained within 20 beats/min of baseline and oxygen sat at 93%. Continue with progress activity monitoring tolerance.

—M. Kim, RN

PATIENT GOAL

The patient will effectively cope with necessary lifestyle and activity changes.

PATIENT OUTCOME CRITERIA

- The patient demonstrates energy-conserving measures, as evidenced by sitting while dressing and planning rest periods during hospital stay.
- The patient discusses realistic plans concerning return to work and other normal activities by end of hospital stay.

NURSING INTERVENTION	SCIENTIFIC RATIONALE
1. With the patient, establish a plan for the day's activity schedule.	**1.** Offering an opportunity to plan activity periods increases patient's feeling of control.
2. Educate patient regarding signs of activity intolerance (e.g., shortness of breath, increased heart rate).	**2.** Knowledge of symptoms of activity intolerance helps patient identify activity tolerance and manage own activity level.
3. Encourage goal setting for future activity periods (i.e., "Next time, what would you hope to be able to do for yourself?").	**3.** The goal-directed patient is in greater control of the situation. Communicates confidence that progress will occur
4. Explore with the patient inventive ideas to conserve energy (e.g., doing tasks from a chair rather than standing; sitting in shower).	**4.** Conservation of energy increases energy available for other, more important activities and increases independence.

EVALUATION

4/14/17: 10:00—Worked with OT (occupational therapy) for AM care this morning. Was able to demonstrate and verbalize how to conserve energy by sitting during activity and keeping arms at waist level. Will continue to work with OT.

—M. Jones, RN

POSSIBLE OUTCOME CRITERIA

The following will occur within 48 hours after initiation of nursing interventions:

- The patient reports absence of severe ischemic pain and improvement in comfort.
- The patient demonstrates improved color and temperature of extremities.
- The patient demonstrates improved activity tolerance by experiencing decreasing pain with ambulation.

Goal

The patient will effectively cope with changes in self-concept and lifestyle.

POSSIBLE OUTCOME CRITERIA

The following will occur by the second home visit:

- The patient verbalizes how his or her cardiovascular condition has caused life changes.
- The patient identifies support people from whom he or she can derive emotional strength.
- The patient demonstrates energy conservation measures, evidenced by sitting while dressing and planning rest periods.
- The patient discusses realistic plans concerning return to work and other normal activities.

KEY CONCEPTS

- Good cardiovascular function depends on a healthy heart to pump blood, an adequate blood volume, and healthy blood vessels to distribute blood to tissues.
- Tissue perfusion, or the flow of blood through the tissues of the body, is essential for cell viability. Tissue perfusion depends on adequate functioning of the cardiovascular system to supply body tissues with oxygen and to remove waste products.
- Cardiovascular function is affected by modifiable and non-modifiable factors. Nonmodifiable factors include age, gender, ethnicity, and family history. Modifiable factors include activity level, BP, smoking, nutrition, and obesity.
- Altered cardiovascular function can occur when the heart is less effective as a pump (e.g., dysrhythmias, muscle damage, valve dysfunction), when the blood vessels are not able to deliver blood adequately to the tissues (e.g., atherosclerosis, vein problems, clots, emboli), or when abnormalities occur within the blood (anemia, low blood volume).
- Manifestations of altered cardiovascular function include changes in vital signs, changes in the color or temperature of the skin, decreased CO, altered blood flow to vital organs, and decreased tissue perfusion.
- Cardiovascular dysfunction can have a great impact on a person's ability to perform activities of daily living and may necessitate lifestyle changes.

- The nurse is instrumental in promoting optimal cardiovascular health by teaching cardiovascular risk factor modification for the general public.
- Nursing measures that can help maximize cardiovascular health and prevent complications include improving modifiable risks, prevention of venous stasis, patient teaching, edema reduction, positioning, pain management, appropriate activity, and energy conservation.
- Cardiac arrest is a medical emergency for which CPR must be quickly and effectively performed to prevent morbidity and mortality.

PRACTICING FOR THE NCLEX

CHECK YOUR ANSWERS IN APPENDIX A.

1. A patient with renal failure is found to have an elevated potassium of 6.0 mEq/L. The effect of the high potassium is problems with conduction resulting in abnormal cardiac rhythm. Which of the following describes this type of abnormality?
   a. Mitral regurgitation
   b. MI
   c. Low CO
   d. Dysrhythmia

2. A 65-year-old male patient is seen in an internal medicine clinic for an annual exam. Which of his conditions or risk factors increases his risk for atherosclerosis? Select all that apply:
   a. Hypertension
   b. Hyperlipidemia
   c. Cigarette smoking
   d. Depression

3. The patient described in question 2 is told to modify his lifestyle factors to decrease his risk. Which would be the most important modification to emphasize?
   a. Quit smoking.
   b. Start taking anticoagulant medication.
   c. Reduce salt intake.
   d. Decrease fluid consumption.

4. A nurse finds the following signs on assessment of his patient: 3 + ankle edema, feet cool to the touch, heart rate 116 bpm, distended neck veins. Which diagnosis is best supported by these findings?
   a. Endocarditis
   b. Right-sided heart failure
   c. Atrial fibrillation
   d. Postoperative fluid overload

5. A patient admitted with coronary artery disease as a result of diabetes mellitus type 2 is best classified using which nursing diagnosis?
   a. Risk for Decreased Cardiac Output
   b. Self-Care Deficit
   c. Activity Intolerance
   d. Infection

6. A new mother is found to have a BP of 70/49 mm Hg and heart rate of 126 bpm immediately postpartum. Which nursing diagnosis is highest priority?
   a. Ineffective Tissue Perfusion
   b. Activity Intolerance
   c. Risk for Infection
   d. Ineffective Childbearing Process

7. Which of the following outcomes is highest priority for an end-stage renal disease (ESRD) patient on hemodialysis at risk for fluid overload? Select all that apply:
   a. Knowledge: treatment regimen
   b. Respiratory status: ventilation
   c. Urinary continence
   d. Electrolyte balance

8. A nurse is assessing the feet of a patient on bed rest wearing antiembolism stockings. She finds edema present with deep creases from the stockings and the toes cold to the touch. What is the best nursing intervention?
   a. Apply SCDs.
   b. Remove antiembolism stockings.
   c. Perform calf-pumping exercises.
   d. Call the physician for anticoagulation medication.

9. A patient with a history of anxiety reports pain in her chest. Which response by the nurse is most appropriate?
   a. "Let me see if I can give you your pain medication yet."
   b. "Try to relax. I'll dim the lights and give you a backrub.
   c. "When did the pain start? What were you doing when it started?"
   d. "I will call a code, this is an emergency!"

10. The nurse walks into a patient's room and finds him unresponsive and pulseless sitting up in bed. She calls a code blue using the emergency button in the room. Which of the following should she do first?
   a. Retrieve crash cart
   b. Begin CPR
   c. Lower head of bed
   d. Remove furniture from room

REFERENCES

American Heart Association. (2013a). Cardiovascular disease and diabetes. Retrieved from http://www.heart.org/HEARTORG/Conditions/Diabetes/WhyDiabetesMatters/Cardiovascular-Disease-Diabetes_UCM_313865_Article.jsp

American Association of Critical Care Nurses. (2010). AACN Practice Alert: Family presence during resuscitation and invasive procedures. Retrieved from http://www.aacn.org/wd/practice/docs/practicealerts/family-presence-during-resuscitation-invasive-procedures.pdf

American Heart Association. (2012a). *Mission: Lifeline component summary table.* Retrieved from http://www.heart.org/HEARTORG/HealthcareResearch/MissionLifelineHomePage/Mission-Lifeline-Component-Summary-Table_UCM_307832_Article.jsp

American Heart Association. (2012b). *Syncope.* Retrieved from http://www.heart.org/HEARTORG/Conditions/Arrhythmia/SymptomsDiagnosisMonitoringofArrhythmia/Syncope_UCM_430006_Article.jsp

American Heart Association. (2013b). *Cardiovascular disease and diabetes.* Retrieved from http://www.heart.org/HEARTORG/Conditions/Diabetes/WhyDiabetesMatters/Cardiovascular-Disease-Diabetes_UCM_313865_Article.jsp

American Heart Association. (2014a). *About cholesterol.* Retrieved from http://www.heart.org/HEARTORG/Conditions/Cholesterol/AboutCholesterol/About-Cholesterol_UCM_001220_Article.jsp

American Heart Association. (2014b). *Heart, how it works.* Retrieved from http://www.heart.org/HEARTORG/Conditions/CongenitalHeartDefects/AboutCongenitalHeartDefects/How-the-Healthy-Heart-Works_UCM_307016_Article.jsp

American Heart Association. (2014c). *Obesity information.* Retrieved from http://www.heart.org/HEARTORG/GettingHealthy/WeightManagement/Obesity/Obesity-Information_UCM_307908_Article.jsp

American Heart Association. (2014d). *Understanding blood pressure readings.* Retrieved from http://www.heart.org/HEARTORG/Conditions/HighBloodPressure/AboutHighBloodPressure/Understanding-Blood-Pressure-Readings_UCM_301764_Article.jsp

American Heart Association. (2014e). *Whole grains and fiber.* Retrieved from http://www.heart.org/HEARTORG/GettingHealthy/NutritionCenter/HealthyDietGoals/Whole-Grains-and-Fiber_UCM_303249_Article.jsp

Awtry, E. H., & Philippides, G. J. (2010). Alcoholic and cocaine associated cardiomyopathies. *Progress in Cardiovascular Disease*, 52, 289–299.

Castelao, E. F., Russo, S. G., Riethmuller, M., & Boos, M. (2013). Effects of Team Coordination during cardiopulmonary resuscitation: A systematic review of the literature. *Journal of Critical Care*, 28(4), 504–521.

Durieux, R., Van Damme, H., Labropoulos, N., Yazici, A., Legrand, V., Albert, A., et al. (2014). High prevalence of abdominal aortic aneurysm in patients with three-vessel coronary artery disease. *European Journal of Vascular and Endovascular Surgery*, 47(3), 273–2778. doi:10.1016/j.ejvs.2013.12.011

Ebong, I. A., Watson, K. E., Goff, D. C., Bluemke, D. A., Srikanthan, P., Horwich, T., et al. (2014). Age at menopause and incident heart failure: The Multi-Ethnic Study of Atherosclerosis. *Menopause*, 21(6), 585–591. doi:10.1097/GME.0000000000000138

Emerson, R. J. (2010). Alterations in blood pressure. In L. C. Copstead, & J. L. Banasik (Eds.), *Pathophysiology: biological and behavioral perspectives* (4th ed.). Philadelphia, PA: W. B. Saunders.

Gellert, C., Schottker, B., & Brenner, H. (2012). Smoking and all-cause mortality in older people: Systematic review and meta-analysis. *JAMA Internal Medicine*, 172(11), 837–844. doi:10.1001/archinternmed.2012.1397

Go, A. S., Mozaffarian, D., Roger, V. L., Benjamin, E. J., Berry, J. D., Blaha, M. J., et al. (2014). Heart disease and stroke statistics—2010 update: A report from the American Heart Association. *Circulation*, 129, e28–e292. doi:10.1161/01.cir0000441139.01012.80

Goff, D., Lloyd-Jones, D., Bennet, G., Coady, S., D'Agostino, R.., Gibbons, R., et al. (2013). ACC/AHA Guideline on the Assessment of Cardiovascular Risk: A report of the American College of Cardiology/American Heart Association Task Force on Practice Guidelines.

Hazinski, M. (Ed.). (2010). Highlights of the 2010 American Heart Association Guidelines for CPR and ECC. Retrieved from http://www.heart.org/idc/groups/heart-public/@wcm/@ecc/documents/downloadable/ucm_317350.pdf

Herdman, T. H., & Kamitsuru, S. (Eds.). (2014). *Nursing diagnoses: Definitions and classifications, 2015–2017.* West Sussex, England: Wiley-Blackwell.

Hogan-Quigley, B., Palm, M. L., & Bickley, L. S. (2012). *Bates' guide to physical examination and history taking.* Philadelphia, PA: Lippincott Williams & Wilkins.

Jabre, P., Tazarourte, K., Azoulay, E., Borron, S. W., Belpomme, V., Jacob, L., et al. (2014). Offering the opportunity for family to be present during cardiopulmonary resuscitation: 1-year assessment. *Intensive Care Medicine*, 40, 981–987. doi:10.1007/s00134-014-3337-1

Jokela, M., Pulkki-Raback, L., Elovainio, M., & Kivimaki, M. (2014). Personality traits as risk factors for stroke and coronary heart disease morality: Pooled analysis of three cohort studies. *Journal of Behavioral Medicine*, 37, 881–889. doi:10.1007/s10865-013-9548-z

Kyle, T., & Carman, S. (2013). *Essentials of pediatric nursing* (2nd ed.). Philadelphia, PA: Lippincott Williams & Wilkins.

Lichtman, J., Leifheit-Limson, E., Watanabe, E., Allen, N., Garavalia, B. Garavalia, L., et al. (2015). Symptom recognition and healthcare experiences of young women with acute myocardial infarction. *Circulation: Cardiovascular Quality and Outcomes*, 8, 531–538. doi:10.1161/CIRCOUTCOMES.114.001612

Lloyd-Jones, D., Adams, R. J., Brown, T. M., Carnethon, M., Dai, S., DeSimone, G., et al. on behalf of the American Heart Association Statistics Committee and Stroke Statistics Subcommittee. (2010). Heart disease and stroke statistics—2010 update: A report from the American Heart Association. *Circulation*, 121, e46–e215.

Lyden, P., Raman, R., Liu, L., Emr, M., Warren, M., & Marler, J. (2009). National Institutes of Health stroke scale certification is reliable across multiple venues. *Stroke*, 40, 2507–2511.

Mozaffarian, D., Afshin, A., Benowitz, N., Bittner, V., Daniels, S., Franch, H., et al. (2012). Population approaches to improve diet, physical activity, and smoking habits: A scientific statement from the American Heart Association. *Circulation*, 126, 1514–1563. doi:10.1161/CIR.0b013e318260a20b

Porth, C., & Grossman, S. (2013). *Pathophysiology: Concepts of altered health states* (9th ed.). Philadelphia, PA: Lippincott Williams & Wilkins.

Shen, L., & Melloni, C. (2014). Representation of women in randomized clinical trials of cardiovascular disease prevention. *Current Cardiovascular Risk Reports*, 8, 390. doi:10.1007/s12170-014-0390-9 Accessed 10/18/2014

Solimene, M. (2010). Coronary heart disease in women: A challenge for the 21st century. *Clinics*, 65(1), 99–106.

Summers, D., Leonard, A., Wentworth, D., Saver, J., Simpson, J., Spilker, J., et al. (2009). Comprehensive overview of nursing and interdisciplinary care of the acute ischemic stroke patient: a scientific statement from the American Heart Association. *Stroke*, 40, 2911–2944.

Weber, J., & Kelley, J. (2014). *Health assessment in nursing* (5th ed.). Philadelphia, PA: Lippincott Williams & Wilkins.

Procedure 27-1 **Applying Antiembolic Stockings**

Purpose	1. Promote supplementing the action of muscle contraction by venous return from the legs. 2. Prevent DVT in the immobile or postoperative patient.
Equipment	Stockings (available in knee-high and thigh-high lengths) Measuring tape to assess correct size of stocking Baby powder or talcum powder Towel or waterproof pad if applying powder
Assessment	• Identify patients at high risk for DVT (e.g., long-term bed rest, cardiovascular disease, surgical patients). • Obtain physician order.

Procedure

1. **Perform hand hygiene.**

   Rationale: Reduces microbe transmission

2. **Identify the patient.**

   Rationale: Ensures correct patient receives proper assessment or treatment and reduces errors

3. **Close door or bed curtains and explain the procedure to the patient.**

   Rationale: Ensures patient privacy, increases patient compliance, reduces patient anxiety, and promotes learning

4. **Position the patient in supine position for a half hour before applying stockings.**

   Rationale: Veins should not be distended with blood when stockings are applied.

5. **Measure for proper fit before first application. Measure length (heel to groin) and width (calf and thigh) and compare to manufacturer's printed material to ensure proper fit (Fig. 1).**

Rationale: Stockings that are too tight can lead to venous occlusion, and stockings that are too loose do not promote venous return. Estimating the size rather than measuring often results in errors.

6. **Make sure legs are dry or apply a light dusting of powder (Fig. 2).**

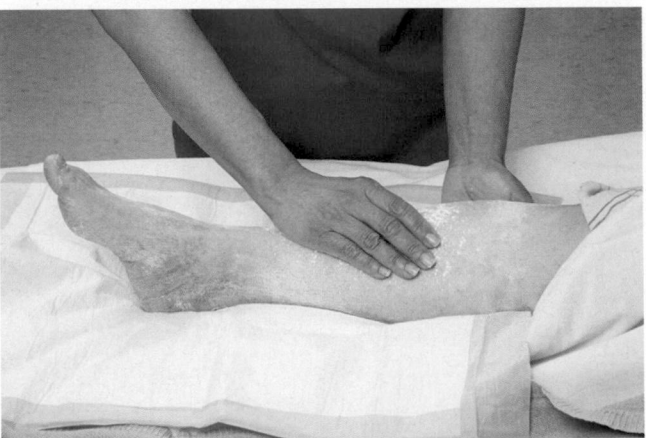

FIG. 2 Powder skin lightly unless contraindicated.

Rationale: Dry legs ease application.

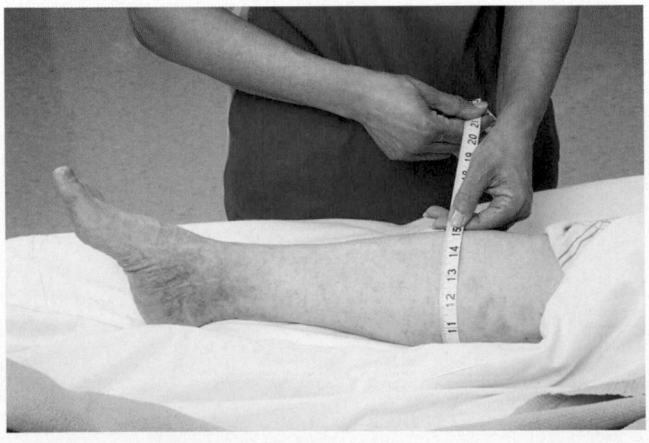

FIG. 1 Measure to ensure proper fit.

Procedure 27-1   *continued*

7. **Turn the stocking inside out, tucking the foot inside (Fig. 3).**

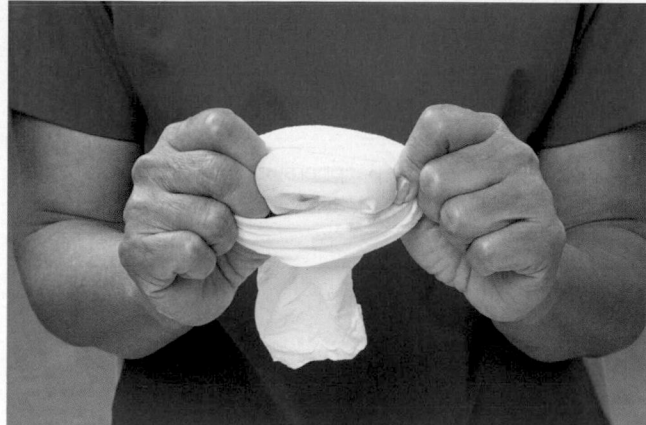

FIG. 3 Turn stocking inside out, tucking heel inside.

Rationale: Inside-out method allows for easier application of the stocking because the stocking is not bunched up.

8. **Ease foot section over the patient's toe and heel, adjusting as necessary for proper smooth fit (Fig. 4).**

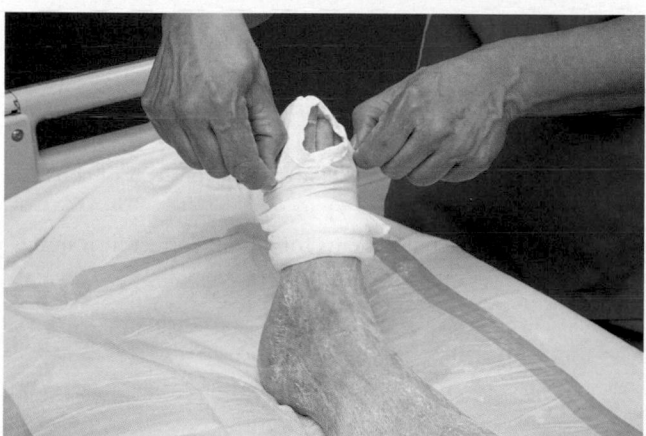

FIG. 4 Ease foot section over toe and heel.

Rationale: Minimize wrinkles that impede circulation.

9. **Gently pull the stocking over the leg, removing all wrinkles (Figs. 5 and 6).**

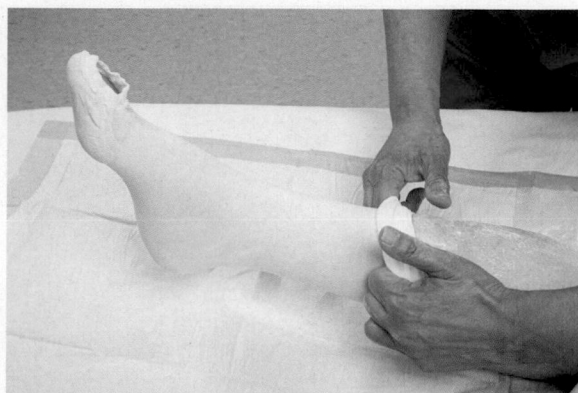

FIG. 5 Pull stocking over leg.

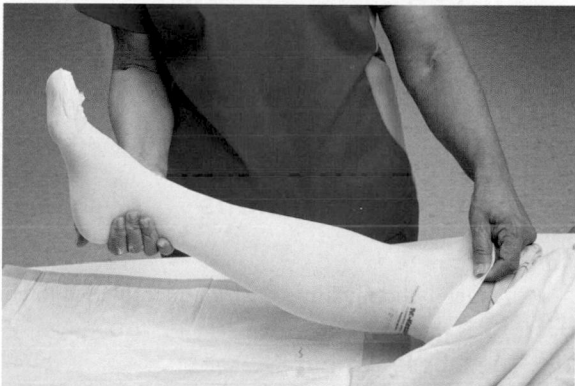

FIG. 6 Stretch stocking over knee. Smooth to remove wrinkles.

Rationale: Irregularities in fit may cause pressure areas.

10. **Assess the toes for circulation and warmth (Fig. 7). Check the area at the top of the stocking for binding.**

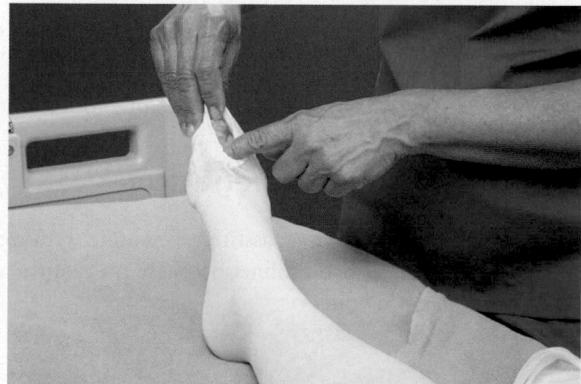

FIG. 7 Assess for skin color, temperature, sensation, swelling, and the ability to move.

Rationale: Constriction and rolling down of stockings during wear are the result of poor fit and can impede circulation and cause thrombosis.

Procedure 27-1   *continued*

11. **Antiembolic stockings should be removed at least twice daily (Fig. 8).**

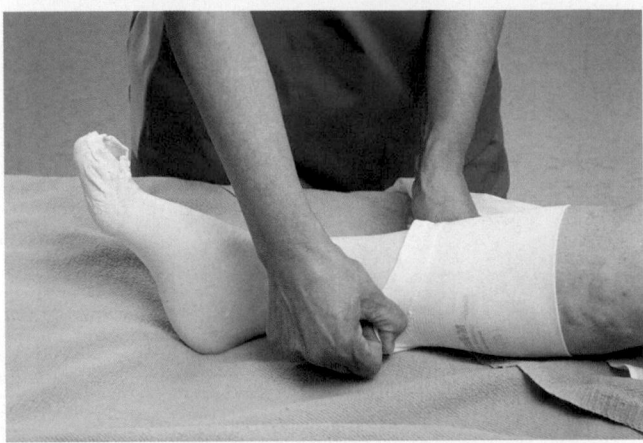

FIG. 8 Grasp stockings and smoothly pull off inside out.

Rationale: Allows for washing of the skin and assessment for edema or irritation.

Documentation

4/12/17: 09:00—
P: Impaired peripheral circulation secondary to bed rest
I: Measured for antiembolic stockings, medium hose applied, taught regarding importance of stocking in preventing blood stasis and clots.
E: Continue to monitor peripheral circulation, and remove stocking every shift to inspect skin for areas of breakdown.
—S. Roberts, RN

Life Span Considerations

Child
• Antiembolic stockings are infrequently used in children.

Adult: The Obese Patient
• Proper fitting of antiembolic stockings is difficult in the obese patient and requires special attention for areas of constriction and binding.
• Elastic (Ace) bandages may be an alternative to provide antiembolic protection in patients for whom correct fit is impossible with standard stocking sizes.

Home Care Modifications

• Instruct patients to apply stockings before getting out of bed.
• Instruct patients to remove stockings regularly for skin inspection and cleansing.
• Be sure patients understand that commercial support stockings are not a substitute for medical antiembolic stockings.

Collaboration and Delegation

• Frequently, unlicensed assistive personnel remove and replace antiembolic stockings while performing hygiene care. Ensure that such personnel do these procedures at least twice every day and that they report any signs of pressure or breakdown to you.

Procedure 27-2 Applying a Sequential Compression Device

Purpose
1. Promote venous return from legs to decrease the risk of DVT and pulmonary embolism in patients with reduced mobility.

Equipment
Measuring tape
Compression sleeves
Inflation unit
Antiembolism stockings (optional)

Assessment
- Identify patients at increased risk for development of DVT.
- Assess skin integrity and identify any existing leg condition that would be exacerbated by use of the plastic sleeve or compression device. Clinical examples in which use of SCD is contraindicated are as follows:
  - Dermatitis, cellulitis
  - Postoperative vein ligation
  - Gangrene
  - Recent skin graft
  - Massive edema of legs
  - Extreme deformity of legs
  - Suspected or existing deep vein thrombus
- Verify physician order.

Procedure

1. **Perform hand hygiene.**
   Rationale: Reduces microbe transmission

2. **Identify the patient.**
   Rationale: Ensures correct patient receives proper assessment or treatment and reduces errors

3. **Close door or bed curtains and explain the procedure to the patient.**
   Rationale: Ensures patient privacy, increases patient compliance, reduces patient anxiety, and promotes learning

4. **Measure leg to ensure proper sleeve sizing. (*Note:* Knee length, one size fits all; thigh length, measure length of leg from ankle to popliteal fossa.) Measure circumference of thigh at the gluteal fold. Use the correct sleeve size, as follows: extra small (circumference, 22 inches; length, 16 inches), regular (circumference, 29 inches; length, 16 inches), extra large (circumference, 35 inches; length, 16 inches).**
   Rationale: Proper sleeve size ensures proper fit and function of the sleeve.

5. **Apply antiembolism stockings. Ensure that there are no wrinkles or folds (see Procedure 27-1). (*Note:* Stockinette or Ace wraps are recommended options if patient cannot be fitted with antiembolism stockings.)**
   Rationale: Wearing stockings decreases the risk of skin irritation and diaphoresis under the plastic sleeves.

6. **Place patient in supine position.**
   Rationale: Proper positioning makes it easier to secure the plastic sleeve.

7. **Place a plastic sleeve under each leg so that the opening is at the knee (Fig. 1). If only one sleeve is required, leave the other sleeve in package and connect to control unit.**

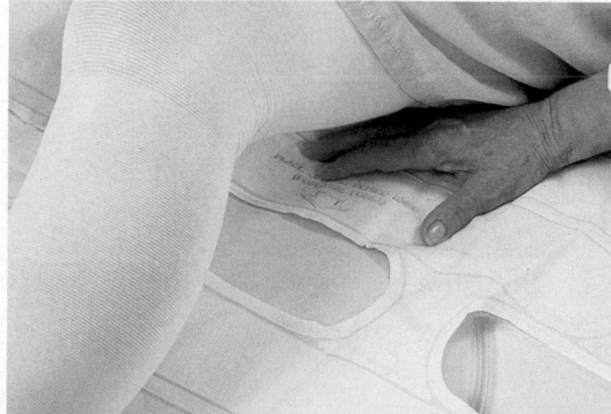

FIG. 1 Place plastic sleeve under leg.

Rationale: The unit will not reach proper pressure if the single sleeve is left to inflate in an unconfined area.

Procedure 27-2 *continued*

8. Fold the outer section of the sleeve over the inner portion and secure with Velcro tabs (Fig. 2). Check sleeve fit. Two fingers should fit between the sleeve and leg.

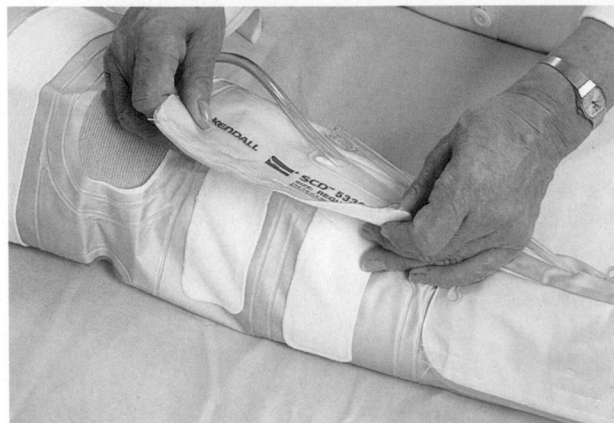

FIG. 2 Secure plastic sleeve around leg.

Rationale: Proper fit prevents irritation to the leg and allows the unit to reach adequate inflation pressure.

9. Connect the tubing to the control unit (Fig. 3). The premarked arrows on the tubing from the sleeve and from the controller must be aligned to make adequate connection. Turn machine on (Fig. 4).

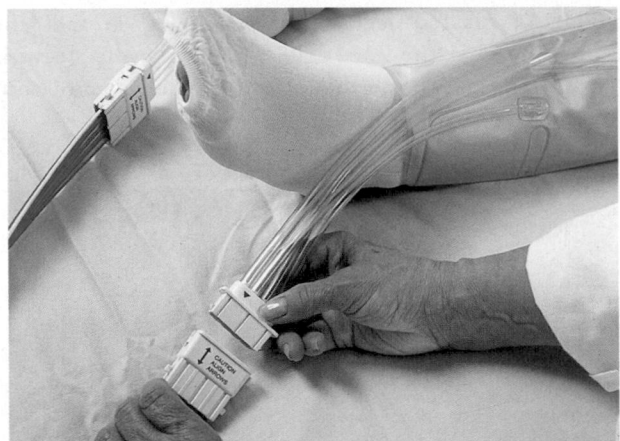

FIG. 3 Connect tubing to control unit.

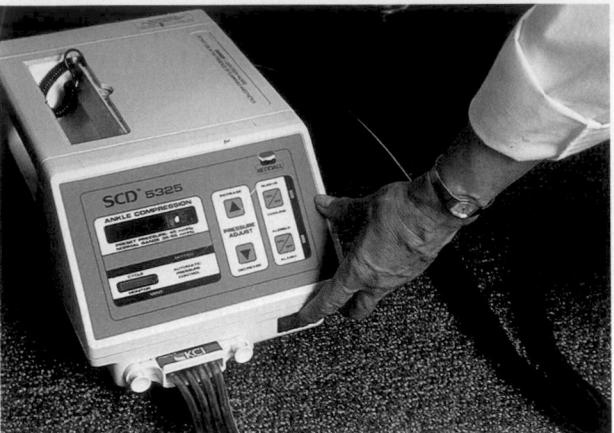

FIG. 4 Turn on control unit.

Rationale: The control unit performs a system self-check.

10. Adjust control unit settings as necessary. Unit control is preset with sleeve cooling in "off" position and audible alarm in "on" position. Sleeve cooling should be in "on" position at all times except during surgery. Ankle pressure should be set at 35 to 55 mm Hg.

Rationale: Plastic sleeves can become warm and uncomfortable if cooling is in the "off" position. The skin and stocking under the sleeve can become wet with diaphoresis, which increases the risk for impaired skin integrity. Cooling may be turned "off" during surgery to preserve warmth for the patient.

11. Recheck control unit settings whenever the unit has been turned off.

Rationale: The unit will convert to preset mode.

12. Respond to and promptly correct all "fault" indicator alarms. (*Note:* The control unit will sense and indicate four pressure "fault" conditions: (a) pressure failed to drop to zero during the cycle; (b) the ankle pressure failed to reach 20 mm Hg for five consecutive cycles; (c) the ankle pressure exceeded 90 mm Hg; (d) an internal diagnostics error has occurred.)

Rationale: Alarms will allow prompt detection and correction of problems.

13. Document time and date of application. If SCD is applied to only one leg, document reason.

Rationale: Maintains legal record and communicates with health team members

14. Assess and document skin integrity every 8 hours.

Rationale: Frequent assessment of skin integrity is necessary to prevent and provide early intervention in case of skin irritation.

15. Remove the sleeves and notify the physician if the patient experiences tingling, numbness, or leg pain.

Rationale: These findings may indicate nerve compression.

Procedure 27-2 *continued*

Documentation

> 7/1/17: 13:00—
> P: Impaired peripheral circulation
> I: SCDs off to ambulate, c/o of having to wear SCDs, teaching included the importance of SCDs to prevent blood clots and the need to use whenever in bed until he is ambulating 3 to 4 hours per day. Statistics cited re number of deaths due to pulmonary emboli.
> E: Agrees to comply with therapy and try to ambulate more. Toes warm, no calf swelling or discomfort, continue to encourage ambulation and continual use of SCDs while in bed or in the chair.
>
> —S. Roberts, RN

Collaboration and Delegation

- Unlicensed assistive personnel frequently remove and then reapply SCDs as they help patients ambulate or shower. Check to ensure that SCDs are reapplied and the unit is "on" so that patients do not experience long periods without the SCD in place to promote circulation.

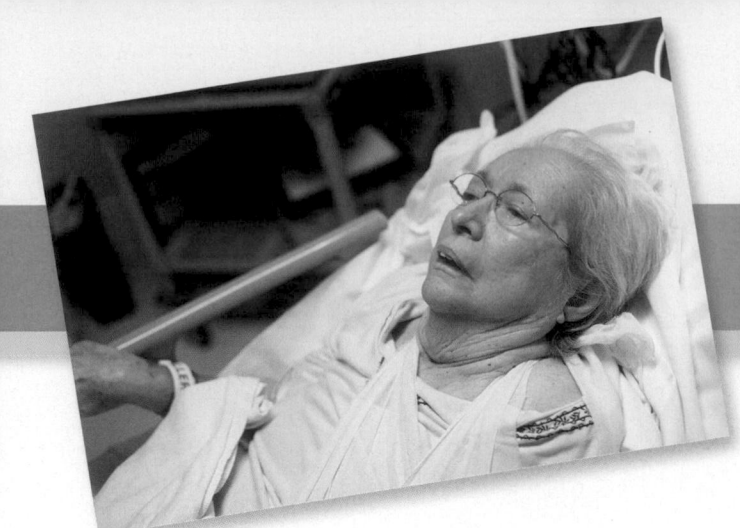

CHAPTER 28

Fluid, Electrolytes, and Acid–Base

Christine M. Henshaw

Case Scenario

You are a nursing student working on a medical unit. One of your assigned patients has a diagnosis of pneumonia. During shift change, you are told that the patient has had diarrhea for the last 4 days, accompanied by a 2-kg weight loss. She has been experiencing fever and chills, and she has had 150 mL of urine output during the last shift. The laboratory called with the following results: serum Na$^+$ 128 mEq/L, serum K$^+$ 4.1 mEq/L, blood urea nitrogen 28 mg/dL, and blood glucose 326 mg/dL. What is your patient's fluid balance status? What tentative nursing diagnoses would you make? What further data should you collect to confirm or alter your tentative diagnoses? What nursing interventions may be indicated?

Once you have completed this chapter and have incorporated fluid, electrolytes, and acid–base into your knowledge base, review the above scenario and reflect on the following areas of Critical Thinking:

1. Summarize the information about this patient's extracellular fluid (ECF) volume status, water balance, and electrolyte balance.

2. Based on this information, make a tentative nursing diagnosis for each of the following: ECF volume status, water balance, and electrolyte balance. Describe what additional data for each you need to confirm or correct your nursing diagnoses.

3. Propose types of oral fluids you would offer this patient to drink, and give your reasons.

4. Discuss your safety concerns for this patient, and outline how you would plan her care to ensure safety.

5. Plan what teaching you would do today and before the patient is discharged.

KEY TERMS
acid
active transport
anions
ascites
baroreceptors
base (or alkali)
buffers
cations
diffusion
electrolytes
extracellular fluid
filtration
hyperosmolar
hypertonic
hypoosmolar
hypotonic
interstitial fluid
intracellular fluid
intravascular fluid
ions
milliequivalent
osmolality
osmolarity
osmosis
osmotic pressure
tonicity

Upon completion of this chapter, you will be able to do the following:

1. Describe physiologic factors that affect fluid, electrolyte, and acid–base homeostasis.
2. Discuss common alterations in fluid, electrolyte, and acid–base balance.
3. Explain the impact of age on fluid, electrolyte, and acid–base status.
4. Describe assessment parameters for the patient with potential or actual imbalances.
5. Identify appropriate nursing diagnoses for patients with imbalances.
6. Implement appropriate patient teaching to prevent or manage fluid, electrolyte, and acid–base imbalances.

Health and normal body functioning depend on fluid, electrolyte, and acid–base balance. Most body fluid is found in three locations: inside blood and lymph vessels (vascular fluid), between cells (interstitial fluid), and within cells (intracellular fluid [ICF]). Vascular fluid is essential for the maintenance of adequate blood volume, blood pressure, and cardiovascular system functioning. Interstitial fluid, which surrounds the body's cells, is important for the transportation of oxygen, nutrients, hormones, and other essential chemicals between the blood and the cell cytoplasm. Vascular and interstitial fluids also are important for waste removal. ICF is critical for maintaining cell size and function. Optimal cell function depends on maintaining the volume and composition of body fluids within a narrow, normal range.

The balance of fluids, electrolytes, acids, and bases within the body is regulated by physiologic control mechanisms. Common activities, such as participating in vigorous exercise, require continuous adaptation to maintain this balance. Healthy adults and children are able to compensate for such physiologic challenges. For example, on a hot summer day, most people increase their fluid intake as a result of thirst, and their urine volume decreases. At the same time, changes in respiratory rate and urine composition play an important role in regulating acid–base balance.

Problems such as vomiting and diarrhea, or therapies such as surgery, can temporarily disrupt fluid, electrolyte, and acid–base homeostasis despite general good health. Sustained vomiting or diarrhea, for example, may require intervention by a healthcare professional to replace lost fluid and electrolytes. Diseases such as heart failure, kidney impairment, or liver dysfunction seriously disrupt the body's ability to maintain fluid, electrolyte, and acid–base balance. People with such medical problems are in constant danger of potentially life-threatening excesses or deficits.

Nurses play a vital role in promoting normal fluid, electrolyte, and acid–base balance and in preventing life-threatening imbalances. Patient teaching about the importance of adequate food, fluid, and electrolyte intake, and about managing common problems such as fever, vomiting, and diarrhea, can aid in preventing imbalances. Nursing assessment of fluid, electrolyte, and acid–base balance is essential for early detection of imbalances so that appropriate interventions can begin promptly. Interventions such as promoting appropriate oral fluid intake, assisting with eating, monitoring intravenous (IV) infusions, and administering medications can all help to maintain fluid, electrolyte, and acid–base balance.

NORMAL FLUID AND ELECTROLYTE BALANCE

Body fluid is water containing chemical compounds called electrolytes plus blood cells and other soluble molecules. Within the body, this fluid is contained within compartments or spaces. The body monitors and controls two aspects of body fluid balance:

- The volume of fluid in the extracellular space, particularly vascular volume
- The concentration of solutes (osmolality) of all body fluids, which influences the volume of ECF and ICF

People can experience an excess or deficit of either or both of these aspects of body fluid balance.

Fluid Compartments

Approximately 45% to 80% of body weight is fluid. This percentage varies depending on age, body fat, and gender (Table 28-1).

TABLE 28-1 VARIATIONS IN TOTAL BODY FLUID ACCORDING TO AGE AND GENDER

Age	Total Body Fluid (% Body Weight)
Newborn (premature)	90%
Newborn (full-term)	70%–80%
Child (1–12 y)	64%
Puberty–39 y	*Male:* 60% *Female:* 52%
40–60 y	*Male:* 55% *Female:* 47%
Older than 60 y	*Male:* 52% *Female:* 46%

From: Metheny, N. M. (2012). *Fluid and electrolyte balance: Nursing considerations* (5th ed.). Sudbury, MA: Jones & Bartlett.

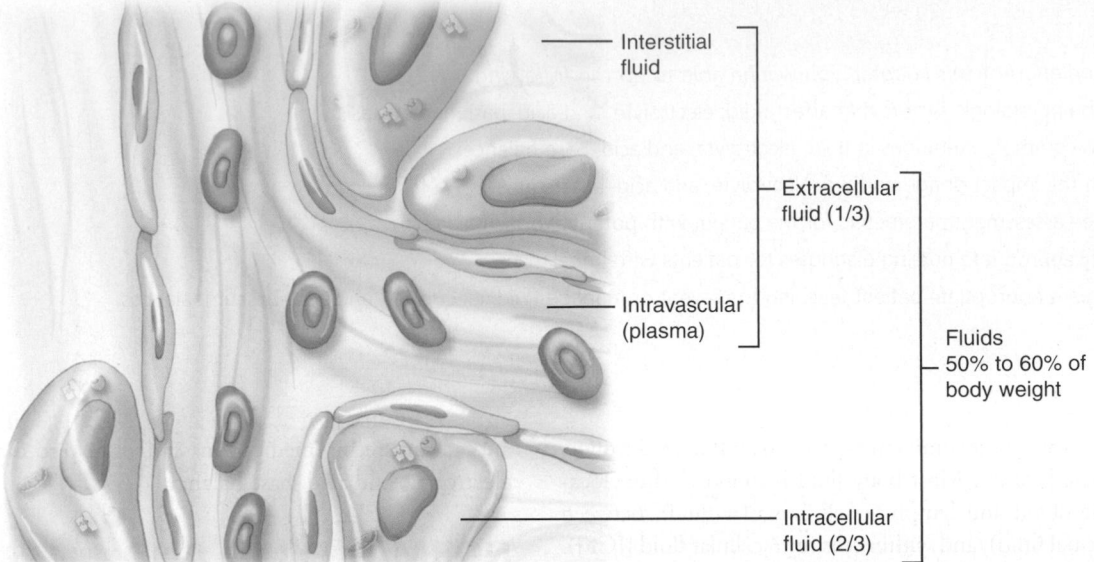

FIGURE 28-1 Fluid compartments showing ICF and ECF (which includes intravascular and interstitial fluid). Total body fluids are 50% to 60% of body weight.

Fat contains proportionately less fluid than does muscle, so heavier people have relatively less fluid than do leaner people. Women have a lower fluid content because they have more adipose tissue than do men. Fluid accounts for 46% to 52% of body weight in adult women and 52% to 60% of body weight in adult men.

There are two main types of body fluid: **intracellular fluid**, located within the cells, and **extracellular fluid**, comprising all fluid outside the cells. Each of these types of body fluid varies in electrolyte composition (see later discussion) and in location. The primary intracellular electrolytes are potassium, phosphate, and sulfate. The primary ECF electrolytes are sodium, chloride, and bicarbonate. Adults have about two thirds of their total fluid within the ICF and one third in the ECF (Fig. 28-1).

ECF includes **intravascular fluid**, the fluid inside the blood and lymphatic vessels, and **interstitial fluid**, the fluid between the cells. The maintenance of the proportional distribution of ECF between the vascular and interstitial spaces depends on three factors:

- Protein content of the blood (serum proteins, mainly albumin and globulin)
- Integrity of the vascular endothelium (the layer of cells lining blood vessels)
- Hydrostatic pressure inside the blood vessels

The protein content of the blood and an intact vascular endothelium function to keep fluids within the blood vessels, whereas the hydrostatic pressure tends to force fluid out of the vessels. In healthy people, these forces are equally balanced so that approximately one third of the ECF volume is intravascular and two thirds is interstitial.

EXTRACELLULAR FLUID VOLUME

The volume of ECF, particularly vascular volume, is the most important and regulated aspect of fluid balance. Without adequate vascular volume, blood pressure cannot be maintained. Prolonged periods of very low blood pressure can result in shock, a potentially lethal condition. **Baroreceptors**, located in major arteries and veins, respond to stretching of arteries and monitor vascular volume. The renin–angiotensin–aldosterone and natriuretic peptide hormone systems regulate the volume within narrow limits by adjusting fluid intake and the urinary excretion of sodium, chloride, and water.

Decreased arterial blood pressure, decreased renal blood flow, increased renal sympathetic nerve activity, or low blood sodium levels can stimulate renin release. Renin, an enzyme secreted by cells in the kidney, splits angiotensinogen, produced by the liver and circulating in the blood, into angiotensin I. Converting enzymes in the lungs and other vascular beds convert angiotensin I into angiotensin II, a potent vasoconstrictor. Angiotensin II stimulates secretion of aldosterone. Aldosterone, produced by the adrenal cortex, regulates sodium reabsorption in the distal tubules and collecting ducts of the kidney. Chloride and water passively accompany the reabsorbed sodium, resulting in the reabsorption of saline, a 0.9% solution of sodium chloride, which is the same concentration as ECF.

Natriuretic peptides are produced by the cardiac atria (ANP), ventricles (discovered first in the brain and called BNP, now referred to as B-type natriuretic peptide), and other body parts in response to changes in ECF volume. When atrial pressure is increased, ANP acts on the nephron to increase sodium excretion. Low atrial pressures inhibit release of ANP.

INTRACELLULAR FLUID VOLUME

The volume in the intracellular space is closely regulated. Although water moves freely across the cell membrane, many electrolytes move only with active transport. Intracellular organs require an appropriate balance of water and electrolytes to function adequately. Cells with too much water in them swell and burst if stretched too far. Cells with too little water, however, also cease to function and shrivel and die. Forces that regulate movement of water and molecules across the cell wall are described later in this chapter.

Water Concentration (Osmolality) of Body Fluid

The second regulated aspect of body fluid balance is osmolality. **Osmolality** refers to the proportion of dissolved particles (solute) in a given weight of fluid (e.g., a kilogram). **Osmolarity** refers to the concentration of dissolved substances in a given volume of fluid (e.g., a liter). Osmolality is expressed in milliosmoles per kilogram (mOsm/kg), whereas osmolarity is expressed in milliosmoles per liter (mOsm/L). Because body fluids are very dilute, these terms are often used interchangeably. The normal range for serum osmolality is from 280 to 300 mOsm/kg. Whereas body fluids are measured in osmolality, other fluids, such as IV fluids, are measured in osmolarity.

Cells in the hypothalamus of the brain monitor changes in body fluid osmolality. They respond by varying the secretion of antidiuretic hormone (ADH) from the posterior pituitary. Some clinicians identify disorders of body osmolality as disorders of body water balance, whereas others refer to these imbalances as *hyponatremia* or *hypernatremia* because an excess or deficit of water directly influences the concentration of sodium. Sodium, its accompanying anions, and glucose are the predominant osmotically active particles in ECF.

ADH is produced in the hypothalamus. It passes down axons into the posterior lobe of the pituitary, where it is stored. When plasma osmolality increases and activates the hypothalamic osmoreceptors, ADH is released into systemic circulation. ADH maintains the blood's osmolality within normal limits by adjusting the amount of water excreted in the urine. The hormone acts by causing molecules to be inserted into the membranes of the distal and collecting tubules in the kidney that act like pores, allowing water to pass through. This increased permeability allows more water reabsorption and serves to conserve water in the body. When ADH is increased, the urine becomes more concentrated. Conversely, if plasma osmolality is decreased due to an excess of water in relation to solute, ADH release is inhibited. Water permeability of the distal tubules and collecting ducts is decreased. Less water is reabsorbed, causing the urine to be more dilute. Water is lost from the body, subsequently causing plasma osmolality to increase.

When vascular volume is normal, changes in plasma osmolality control ADH release. However, when arterial blood pressure is markedly diminished (e.g., heart failure, shock), ADH is released regardless of plasma osmolality in response to input from the vascular baroreceptors (Imamura et al., 2014).

Electrolytes

Electrolytes are chemical compounds that partially separate in solution. These particles carry electrical charges and are known as **ions**. Positively charged ions are referred to as **cations**, and negatively charged ions are **anions**. Biologically important cations include sodium (Na^+), potassium (K^+), calcium (Ca^{++}), and magnesium (Mg^{++}). Chloride (Cl^-), phosphate (HPO_4^- and $H_2PO_4^-$), sulfate (SO_4^-), and bicarbonate (HCO_3^-) are common anions. As mentioned previously, the concentration of each of these electrolytes is very different in the ICF and ECF compartments. The most common extracellular electrolytes are sodium, chloride, and bicarbonate, whereas potassium, phosphate, and sulfate are the most common intracellular electrolytes.

Electrolyte concentrations are expressed in terms of their combining power, or the ability of cations to combine with anions. The **milliequivalent** is the measure of this chemical activity. The amount of electrolyte in a solution is most commonly expressed in terms of milliequivalents per liter (mEq/L). Maintaining electrolyte balance refers to keeping the concentration of each electrolyte in the serum within normal limits. Electrolyte imbalance refers to an increase or decrease of the concentration of ions within the serum. Because the concentration of cellular electrolytes (ICF) cannot be measured clinically, the nurse relies on changes in the serum levels (ECF) to reflect body electrolyte imbalance. Normal serum electrolyte ranges for the adult are given in Table 28-2. Normal values vary slightly between laboratories. Whenever possible, monitoring of trends in electrolyte concentration over time provides more information about a patient's status than does a single laboratory value.

SODIUM

Sodium is the most abundant cation in the ECF. Normal serum sodium levels range from 135 to 145 mEq/L. Interestingly, changes in the serum sodium level reflect changes in body water balance or osmolality more than reflecting sodium intake and output directly. Usually, where sodium goes, water will follow. If the sodium is high, this means that there is not enough water to follow. If the sodium is low, this means that there is too much water. Sodium along with chloride and a proportionate volume of water (which is normal saline) are regulated by the renin–angiotensin–aldosterone system and natriuretic peptides.

TABLE 28-2 NORMAL SERUM ELECTROLYTE VALUES	
Electrolyte	Serum Value
Cations	
Sodium (Na^+)	135–145 mEq/L
Potassium (K^+)	3.5–5.0 mEq/L
Calcium (Ca^{++}) (8.9–10.1 mg/dL)	4.3–5.3 mEq/L
Magnesium (Mg^{++}) (1.8–2.3 mg/dL)	1.5–1.9 mEq/L
Anions	
Chloride (Cl^-)	95–108 mEq/L
Bicarbonate (HCO_3^-)	22–26 mEq/L
Phosphate (HPO_4^-, $H_2PO_4^-$) (2.5–4.5 mg/dL)	1.7–2.6 mEq/L

Note: Normal value ranges may vary slightly from laboratory to laboratory.

Sodium is found in table salt (sodium chloride), dairy products, meat, eggs, and certain vegetables; food processing also tends to add salt in the preserving process. Food labels list the number of milligrams of sodium in a serving of product.

POTASSIUM

Potassium is essential for normal cardiac, neural, and muscle function and contractility of all muscles. Normal serum potassium ranges from 3.5 to 5.0 mEq/L.

Two hormones exert major control over the extracellular concentration of potassium: insulin and aldosterone. Insulin, a pancreatic hormone, promotes the transfer of potassium (and also glucose) from the ECF into skeletal muscle and liver cells. Aldosterone enhances renal excretion of potassium. An increase in serum potassium stimulates the release of aldosterone to lower the concentration of the ion. Conversely, a decrease in serum potassium inhibits the release of aldosterone to reduce excretion of the ion.

A person loses approximately 30 mEq of potassium per day, while a typical Western diet contains about 100 mEq/day. The kidneys play the major role in the maintenance of potassium balance, varying excretion with daily intake. Potassium also is excreted from the body in stool and perspiration.

CALCIUM

Normal total serum calcium levels range between 8.9 and 10.1 mg/dL. Approximately 99% of the body's calcium is found within the bones and teeth. The remainder is in the serum. Calcium is present in the blood primarily in two states: ionized and bound to protein. Approximately 50% is ionized, with the remainder bound to proteins, mainly albumin. The level of ionized calcium determines physiologic function, and only changes in the ionized calcium levels can cause signs and symptoms associated with calcium imbalances. Because a large portion of calcium is bound to albumin, serum albumin levels should be checked when laboratory data are evaluated. If serum albumin levels are decreased, which may happen with liver disease or wasting, the total calcium level probably also will be decreased, but the ionized calcium level may be within normal limits. Measurement of the ionized calcium level, normally 4.0 to 4.9 mg/dL, is required to determine whether calcium replacement is required (Popovtzer, 2010). Calcium usually has a reciprocal relationship with phosphorus.

Calcium is indispensable for healthy functioning. The cell membrane structure depends on calcium, which promotes cell-to-cell adhesion. Calcium also is important in wound healing, synaptic transmission in nervous tissue, membrane excitability, muscle contractility, and teeth and bone structure. Calcium is essential for blood clotting and is critical in metabolic reactions involved in energy production (glycolysis).

Parathyroid hormone (PTH), vitamin D, and, to some extent, calcitonin regulate calcium and phosphate balance. PTH causes serum calcium levels to increase by increasing intestinal and renal reabsorption of calcium and releasing calcium from bone. PTH increases calcium levels but decreases serum phosphate levels. Conversely, decreased secretion of PTH lowers serum calcium levels and increases the serum phosphate concentration (Popovtzer, 2010).

The number of good dietary sources for calcium is limited. Dairy products (e.g., milk, cheese, and yogurt) are excellent sources. Sardines, whole grains, and leafy green vegetables also contribute calcium. Food labels indicate the percentage of the daily value of calcium contained in a serving.

MAGNESIUM

The normal serum magnesium level ranges from 1.4 to 1.75 mEq/L. Fifty to sixty percent of magnesium is in bone; much of the rest is in soft tissue and body fluids. Like potassium, magnesium is primarily an intracellular ion, with only 2% in the ECF (Spiegel, 2010). Magnesium is important in regulating neuromuscular function and cardiac activity. Alterations in magnesium are often paralleled by changes in potassium, and the signs and symptoms of a deficit of either ion are similar. In addition, a magnesium deficiency often is accompanied by hypocalcemia (Spiegel). The kidney regulates magnesium levels by reabsorbing the ion when serum levels are low and excreting it when serum levels are high. No hormones have been identified that regulate body magnesium levels. Good dietary sources of magnesium include green leafy vegetables, legumes, citrus fruit, peanut butter, and chocolate.

PHOSPHORUS

The normal serum phosphorus level in adults ranges from 2.5 to 4.0 mg/dL (Popovtzer, 2010). Serum levels are higher in children and even higher in infants. Approximately 85% of phosphorus is in bone, 14% is in the ICF, and only 0.1% is in the ECF (Popovtzer). Blood levels of phosphorus are controlled by the regulation of renal excretion under the influence of vitamin D and PTH. Phosphorus is important in energy metabolism, structure of bones and membranes, and synthesis of nucleic acids (RNA and DNA). There is often, but not always, a reciprocal relation between body phosphorus and calcium levels. Good dietary sources of phosphorus include dairy products, meats, vegetables, fruits, and cereals.

Fluid and Electrolyte Distribution

Movement of fluid, electrolytes, nutrients, and waste products between body fluid compartments is constant. The membranes of individual cells, the vascular capillary walls, and the lymphatic capillary walls are semipermeable. Water and some electrolytes move easily across these semipermeable membranes. Larger molecules, such as proteins, are less able to move across capillary walls. Fluid movement occurs primarily by osmosis and filtration. Electrolytes and other dissolved particles move by means of diffusion, filtration, and active transport. Hydrostatic pressure and oncotic pressure are important determinants of fluid filtration between the ECF and ICF spaces.

PROCESSES OF FLUID AND ELECTROLYTE MOVEMENT

Diffusion

Diffusion is the movement of a solvent or solutes (molecules) from an area of higher solvent or solute concentration to an area of lower solvent or solute concentration. Molecules are in constant motion. If a drop of highly concentrated solution is placed in one side of a container of fluid, the molecules will bounce off each other until they are equally distributed throughout the solution.

Osmosis

Osmosis refers to the movement of a fluid through a semi-permeable membrane. A semipermeable membrane allows some substances to cross it but not others. Osmosis can occur if a semipermeable membrane separating two fluid compartments is permeable to water and if one compartment contains a greater concentration of a dissolved substance (**hyperosmolar**) than does the other compartment (**hypoosmolar**). Water passes through the membrane to the area of greater concentration of the dissolved substance. Capillary vessel walls and cell walls are semipermeable membranes.

Active Transport

Active transport is the process by which ions and other molecules are moved across membranes from an area of lesser concentration to an area of greater concentration. Energy is required to move ions against a concentration gradient. Enzymes, such as sodium–potassium adenosine triphosphatase (Na, K-ATPase), are involved in active transport.

The process of active transport can be illustrated by the functioning of the body's sodium–potassium pump (Fig. 28-2).

A higher concentration of sodium ions is present in ECF (135 to 145 mEq/L), whereas the concentration of sodium in the ICF is lower (10 mEq/L). Although cell membranes are relatively impermeable to sodium ions, a small number of ions continuously diffuse across the cell membrane into the cell down this concentration gradient. Without the sodium–potassium pump or Na, K-ATPase, intracellular sodium would continue to rise and cell function would be disrupted. This pump prevents sodium from accumulating inside cells by actively transporting sodium out of cells. The difference in concentration between sodium and potassium in intracellular and extracellular compartments is essential for the resting membrane potential, action potential initiation, nerve impulse propagation, and muscle contraction.

Filtration

Filtration involves the transfer of water and dissolved substances through a permeable membrane from a region of high pressure to a region of low pressure. Hydrostatic pressure, or the pressure exerted by fluid against the walls of its container, promotes the flow of fluid out of the capillaries (Fig. 28-3). Filtration occurs within the kidney's glomerular capillaries and in blood capillaries.

PRESSURES AFFECTING FLUID AND ELECTROLYTE MOVEMENT

Osmotic Pressure and Tonicity

Osmotic pressure, the force of attraction for water by undissolved particles, helps to keep fluid within blood vessels, opposing net flow outward. Plasma proteins contribute to

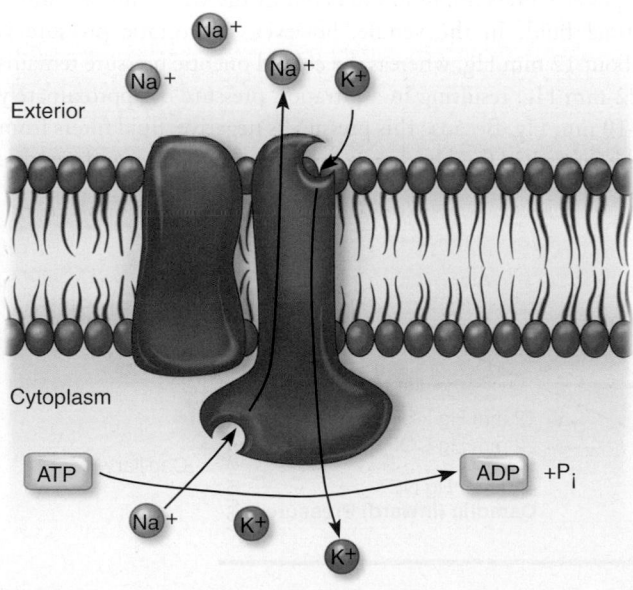

FIGURE 28-2 Sodium–potassium pump. Energy provided by ATP causes sodium to move to the outside of the cell and potassium to move to the inside of the cell. For every molecule of ATP, three molecules of sodium are transported out and two molecules of potassium move into the cell.

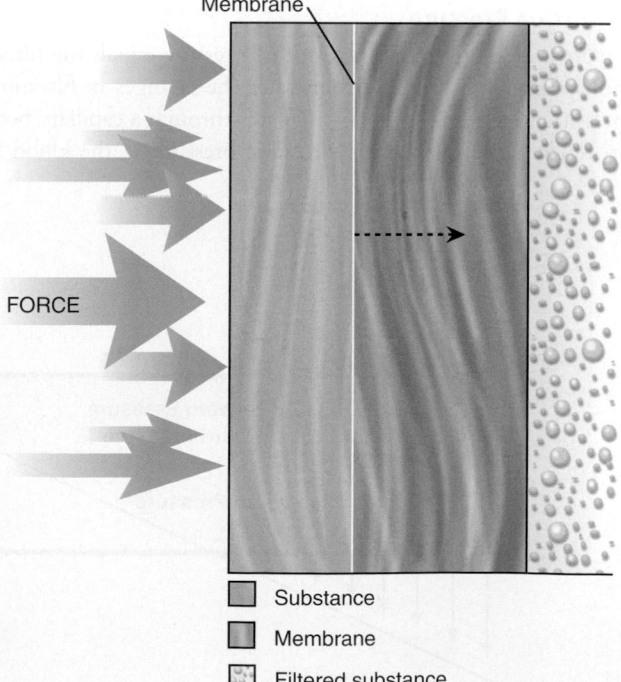

FIGURE 28-3 Filtration. A mechanical force pushes a substance through a membrane.

the osmotic pressure because they attract water. The term for the osmotic pressure that is produced by plasma proteins is *colloid oncotic pressure*. Osmotic pressure depends on the solution's osmolality.

Fluids can differ in osmolality, depending on the concentration of their solutes. The major extracellular substances that contribute to the movement of water between the ECF and cell cytoplasm are sodium, chloride, and glucose. A solution that has the same osmotic pressure or osmolality as blood plasma is called iso-osmotic.

Solutions are also categorized in relation to their **tonicity**, a term that refers to the fluid's effect on cell size. When an isotonic solution enters the circulation, there is no net movement of water across membranes, so cells retain their normal size. Normal saline (0.9% NaCl) is an isotonic solution. A **hypotonic** solution has a concentration of solute that is less than that of blood plasma. When a hypotonic solution (e.g., water) surrounds cells, water crosses the membrane into the cells, causing them to swell, which explains why pure water is never used as an IV fluid. The opposite is true for a hypertonic solution. In a **hypertonic** solution, the effective concentration of solute is greater than that of the blood plasma. When a hypertonic solution such as 3% sodium chloride (hypertonic saline) is infused, water leaves the cells, causing them to decrease in size (Fig. 28-4).

Hydrostatic Pressure

Hydrostatic pressure causes filtration of fluid from an area of higher pressure to an area of lower pressure, such as from the blood vessels into the interstitial fluid compartment. Factors that influence hydrostatic pressure include the arterial blood pressure (the force with which the heart pumps blood), the rate of blood flow, and the venous pressure.

Filtration Pressure

Hydrostatic pressure minus osmotic pressure equals the filtration pressure. Figure 28-5 illustrates the changes in filtration pressure that occur as blood circulates through a capillary bed. In normal arterioles, the hydrostatic pressure of the blood is

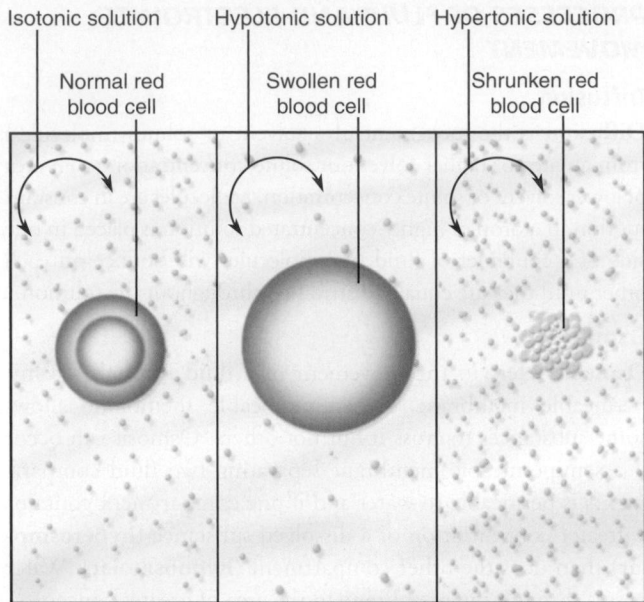

FIGURE 28-4 Osmosis. Water molecules moving through a red blood cell membrane in three different concentrations of fluid. **Left:** The normal saline solution has a concentration nearly the same as that inside the cell, and water molecules move into and out of the cell at the same rate. **Center:** The dilute solution causes the cell to swell and eventually hemolyze (burst) because of the large number of water molecules moving into the cell. **Right:** The concentrated solution causes the water molecules to move out of the cell, leaving it shrunken.

about 32 mm Hg, and the colloid oncotic pressure is approximately 22 mm Hg. The filtration pressure is the difference between them, or approximately +10 mm Hg. Because this is a positive pressure, fluid filters out of the vessel into the interstitial fluid. In the venule, however, hydrostatic pressure is about 12 mm Hg, whereas the colloid oncotic pressure remains 22 mm Hg, resulting in a filtration pressure of approximately –10 mm Hg. Because this pressure is negative, fluid filters from the interstitial fluid back into the venous capillaries and venules.

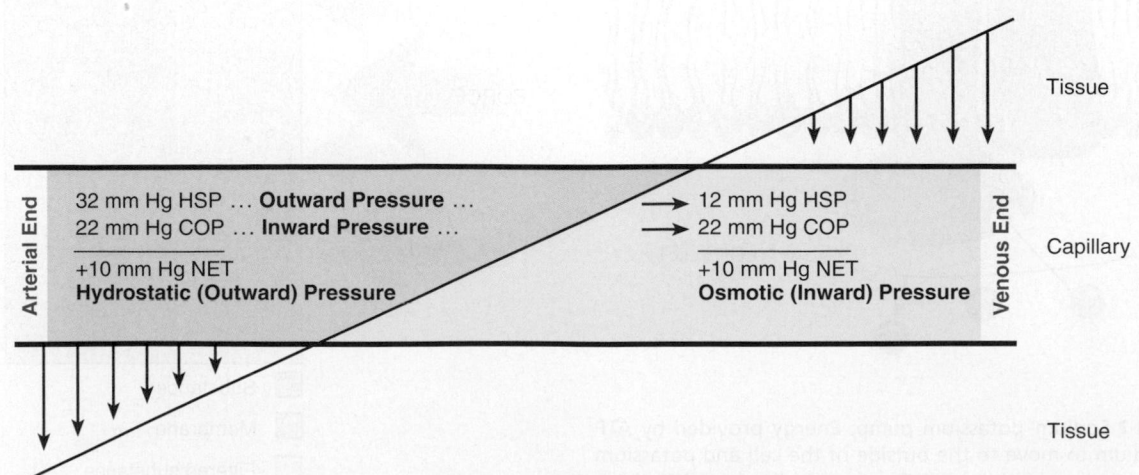

FIGURE 28-5 Filtration pressure in a capillary. In the arterial end of a capillary, fluid is pushed out into the tissues; in the venous end, fluid is absorbed back into the circulation.

This process of fluid leaking out of the arterioles, only to be reabsorbed in the venules, is continuous. It is also the manner by which the body is able to transport oxygen and other nutrients to the cells and remove waste products. In the healthy person, this process is balanced so that almost all filtered fluid is returned to the vascular space. The lymphatic vessels return excess fluid to the circulation through the thoracic duct and, at the same time, carry cells and proteins from the periphery through the lymph nodes. Movement of fluid and white blood cells through the lymphatic vessels is key to the ability of the body's inflammatory and immune systems to screen continuously for injury and infection. If the hydrostatic pressure is greatly increased or the colloid oncotic pressure is greatly reduced, some of the filtered fluid remains in the interstitial space. This accumulation is called edema. Blockage of lymph drainage or removal of lymph nodes can also produce edema. A fourth mechanism of edema is increased capillary permeability. Table 28-3 identifies these four primary mechanisms of edema and several causes of each.

Life Span Considerations

Age is a significant factor in fluid and electrolyte balance. The very young and older adults are at greatest risk for fluid or electrolyte imbalances. An understanding of age-related differences is important for the prevention, identification, and management of fluid and electrolyte problems.

NEWBORN AND INFANT

Infants have a proportionately larger percentage of total body weight as water (70% to 80%) than do adults (60%). Preterm infants have an even greater amount of body fluid, possibly as much as 90%. A greater amount of the fluid is contained within the ECF compartment in infants than within that of adults. Because infants also have a greater surface area in relation to weight, they can lose a proportionately larger volume of fluid through the skin.

TABLE 28-3	CAUSES AND MECHANISMS OF EDEMA
Mechanism	**Cause**
Increased hydrostatic pressure	Elevated blood pressure Fluid overload Decreased cardiac output with backup of blood, e.g., heart failure
Decreased colloid oncotic pressure (decreased plasma proteins)	Malnutrition Liver failure Nephrosis
Blockage or removal of lymph nodes	Mastectomy Lymphoma
Increased capillary permeability	Allergies Septic shock Pulmonary edema

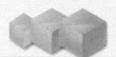
Concept Mastery Alert

Infants have a far greater volume of total fluid as a percentage of body weight than do older individuals. However, this high percentage of fluid does not give infants a greater reserve against fluid deficit. Instead, it creates a vulnerability to fluid deficit due to the high percentage of fluid required for homeostasis.

Fluid requirements vary according to age, as does normal urine output. The infant's kidneys are immature and lack the ability to concentrate urine fully. Metabolic and respiratory rates are high in infants, contributing to increased insensible fluid loss. Fluid loss can occur very rapidly in this age group. The nurse should teach parents and caregivers about how serious vomiting or diarrhea can be for infants, urging them to contact their healthcare providers and to provide appropriate fluid replacement, with sodium and water, rather than just water, if these symptoms occur.

! SAFETY ALERT

Carefully monitor infants when they are losing or being given fluid. Kidney immaturity and increased body surface area in relation to body size place infants at greater risk than older children or adults for fluid and electrolyte imbalances.

TODDLER AND PRESCHOOLER

Approximately 62% of the toddler's weight is water. Fluid requirements vary but are generally 1,000 to 1,200 mL over a 24-hour period. Urine output increases from approximately 500 to 700 mL/day at 2 years to 600 to 850 mL/day at 5 years. Water loss through the skin, respiration, urine, and stools is proportionately greater for young children than for adults.

CHILD AND ADOLESCENT

The ratio of total body water to total body weight decreases throughout childhood and adolescence. By the time a child is 12 years old, the percentage of body water to body weight is approximately the same as in adults. Children in this age group often drink soda or sugared beverages to supply their fluid needs. Research has shown that childhood obesity is linked with the intake of this type of sweetened drink (Seo et al., 2014). Part of the nurse's teaching would include encouraging water and other, more nutritious fluids, such as milk or tomato juice.

Another aspect of the nurse's teaching would be to caution children and adolescents against the potential dangers of excessive exercise without adequate fluid replacement, especially in hot weather, because muscle damage (rhabdomyolysis) and fluid and electrolyte imbalances can occur. Balanced dietary intake is important to promote normal electrolyte balance. Dietary intake may be erratic in adolescents. Fad diets or purging to lose weight can cause severe fluid and electrolyte imbalances.

ADULT AND OLDER ADULT

After age 25 years, the number of nephrons in the kidney begins to decrease. During middle age (after age 40 years), adipose tissue tends to increase, resulting in a continual decline in the percentage of body weight that is fluid. There are decreases in kidney mass, blood flow, and glomerular filtration rate (10% decrement per decade after age 30 years). Drug clearance is also reduced, placing the elderly at risk for adverse drug events (Hartford Institute for Geriatric Nursing, 2012).

Adults are most likely to experience fluid and electrolyte imbalances after an acute illness or elective surgery. Older adults often experience alterations in fluid and electrolyte status secondary to chronic disease (e.g., renal failure, heart failure). Diuretics, commonly given to treat high blood pressure and heart failure, can cause an ECF deficit or loss of electrolytes, including potassium, calcium, and magnesium. Excessive use of laxatives can reduce gastrointestinal absorption of potassium, promoting hypokalemia and loss of ECF. Some older people may choose to restrict their fluid intake either in the evening to minimize the need to urinate in the middle of the night or during the day so that they will not need to urinate while they are away from home. Although calcium levels are typically normal in older adults, there is a gradual loss of bone calcium over time, predisposing the elderly to osteoporosis and consequently to fractures when falls occur.

Older adults are at increased risk for electrolyte imbalances during and after bowel preparation for procedures such as a colonoscopy or barium enema. Research has shown that bowel preparation solutions in patients over 65 years old are associated with vascular volume deficit, hyperphosphatemia, hypokalemia, and hypocalcemia (Parra-Blanco et al., 2014); Patients over 65 require careful assessment prior to administration of bowel preparation solutions. Use of low-volume preparations may avoid some of the fluid and electrolyte problems associated with high-volume preparation.

Cultural Considerations

The incidence and mortality of chronic kidney disease are disproportionately higher in African Americans compared to Whites (Fox et al., 2011). African Americans' risk for kidney disease is almost three times higher than that of Whites. High rates of hypertension, diabetes, and obesity in the middle-aged African American population contribute in part to the racial difference. Persons with hypertension, diabetes, and chronic kidney disease, as well as middle- and older-aged persons and African Americans, tend to be more sensitive to sodium than do healthier, younger Whites. Genetic factors also influence the blood pressure response to sodium. There are 14 identified genes that affect blood pressure and renal sodium handling (Report of the DGAC on the Dietary Guidelines for Americans, 2010).

NORMAL ACID–BASE BALANCE

For cells to operate with maximum efficiency, they need oxygen, nutrients, electrolytes, and a controlled temperature to produce a stable environment. Another important component of cellular environment is the hydrogen ion concentration ($[H^+]$), which is regulated within extremely narrow limits. The maintenance of this narrow concentration range is called acid–base balance. Vital functions such as nerve conduction, hormonal activity, and cardiac rhythm depend on a stable acid–base environment. Significant deviations from normal blood $[H^+]$ are life threatening.

Acids, Bases, and pH

Any substance that can donate free H^+ ions to a solution is called an **acid**. By contrast, any substance that can decrease $[H^+]$ in a solution is a **base** (also called an **alkali**).

Acids and bases can be categorized as either strong or weak. Hydrochloric acid (HCl), which is secreted by cells in the stomach lining, is an example of a strong acid. Solutions that contain more acid than base are described as acidic, whereas solutions containing relatively more base are termed basic (or alkaline).

The number of H^+ ions in any solution is indicated indirectly by means of the pH scale; pH describes the degree of acidity or alkalinity of solutions (Fig. 28-6). The pH scale ranges from 1 to 14, with 7 representing a neutral solution that is neither acidic nor alkaline. A solution with a pH between 1 and 7 is acidic. Weak acids have a pH only slightly below 7, whereas the strongest acids have pH values closer to 1. Similarly, bases have pH values above 7, with higher pH values indicating increasingly strong bases.

Acids and Bases in the Blood

The pH of the ECF is normally between 7.35 and 7.45. This very narrow pH range is maintained by buffers that limit pH changes in the body fluids and by elimination of acids from the body through the lungs (carbon dioxide) and kidneys. The kidneys can also excrete excess base if the body is in an alkalotic state (pH greater than 7.45).

A very important acid in the body is carbonic acid. Together, carbonic acid and bicarbonate ion form what is known as a *buffer pair*. Although other buffer systems (see below) participate in maintaining acid–base balance, the bicarbonate–carbonic acid buffer system is the most important in clinical practice for two reasons. First, because all the buffer systems are in equilibrium, changes in the bicarbonate–carbonic acid system mirror changes in all other systems. Second, the body regulates the carbon dioxide level by changes in the respiratory rate (ventilation) and bicarbonate level by adjustments in the amount of bicarbonate lost in the urine or the amount regenerated by the kidneys. The bicarbonate–carbonic acid buffer system can be expressed as an equation:

$$H^+ + HCO_3^- \rightleftarrows H_2CO_3 \rightleftarrows H_2O + CO_2$$

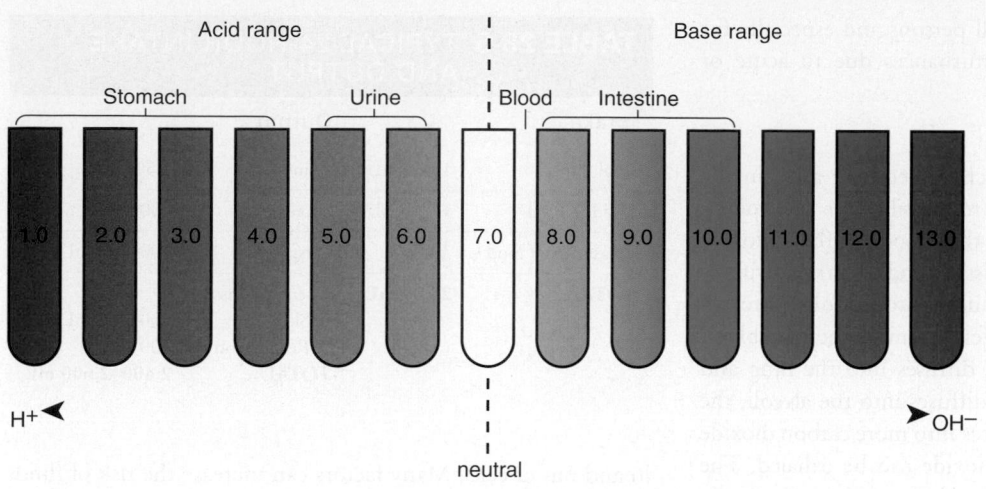

FIGURE 28-6 The pH scale measures the degree of acidity or alkalinity.

The components of this equation combine and disassociate and combine again to maintain acid–base balance. The body continually produces carbon dioxide, a cellular waste product, as it uses oxygen to metabolize glucose. The bicarbonate–carbonic acid buffer system helps the body manage this carbon dioxide.

Acid–Base Balance Regulation

Hydrogen ion balance is closely regulated. Compared with electrolytes in the plasma, the concentration of H$^+$ in the blood is normally 1 million times smaller. Death usually results if blood pH falls below 6.8 or increases above 7.8. Because metabolism continually produces acids, maintenance of the pH within these incredibly narrow limits depends on two processes: buffering and compensation. Buffers allow acids or bases to be transported from where they are produced to where they are excreted without causing large swings in pH, and with compensation the body either excretes or retains acids or bases to compensate for losses. Acid–base balance is commonly evaluated by measuring arterial blood gases (Table 28-4).

BUFFERING

Buffers are substances that help to prevent large changes in pH by absorbing or releasing H$^+$ ions. When the blood has excess acid, successful buffering prevents a large drop in pH despite the influx of extra H$^+$ ions into the blood. In such cases, buffers combine with additional H$^+$ ions the acid releases, minimizing the potentially damaging effect of extra free H$^+$ ions in the blood. Similarly, a deficit of blood acid or excess of base can result in a serious increase in pH. Successful buffering causes extra H$^+$ ions from the weak acids of the buffer pairs to be released into the blood.

COMPENSATION

The respiratory and renal systems excrete acids and bases from the body and thus are usually able to compensate for any imbalances. The lungs handle moment-to-moment maintenance of acid–base status because they react almost instantly to minute changes in blood pH. The kidneys are slower than the lungs to react to changes, taking hours to days to respond. Failure or impairment of either system can lead to life-threatening acid–base imbalances. Therefore, preservation of optimal lung

TABLE 28-4 NORMAL ARTERIAL BLOOD GAS VALUES

Abbreviation	Normal Range	Definition
pH	7.35–7.45	Reflects the hydrogen ion concentration of arterial blood *Acidosis:* <7.35 *Alkalosis:* >7.45
PaCO$_2$	35–45 mm Hg	Reflects partial pressure of carbon dioxide in arterial blood *Hypocapnia:* Low partial pressure of carbon dioxide in arterial blood, <35 mm Hg *Hypercapnia:* High partial pressure of carbon dioxide in arterial blood, >45 mm Hg
PaO$_2$	80–100 mm Hg	Partial pressure of oxygen in arterial blood
HCO$_3^-$	22–26 mEq/L	Amount of bicarbonate in arterial blood

and renal function is crucial for all persons and especially for patients at risk for acid–base disturbances due to acute or chronic disease states.

Respiratory Compensation

The lungs, under the control of chemoreceptor areas in the brainstem respiratory center, are responsible for controlling the amount of carbon dioxide in the blood. Carbon dioxide diffuses into the blood from the tissues and is carried primarily as carbonic acid, bicarbonate, and hydrogen ions (through the bicarbonate–carbonic acid buffer system). When the blood reaches the lungs, carbon dioxide diffuses into the lung and is exhaled. As the carbon dioxide diffuses into the alveoli, the carbonic acid in the blood dissociates into more carbon dioxide and water so that more carbon dioxide can be exhaled. The lungs in collaboration with the respiratory center normally maintain the carbon dioxide level in the arterial blood ($PaCO_2$) at a pressure of 35 to 45 mm Hg.

When the tissues produce carbon dioxide during metabolism, the lungs respond to input from the chemoreceptors and increase the rate and depth of ventilation, which increases the rate at which this acid is excreted and prevents any significant change in pH. The respiratory system reacts oppositely if carbon dioxide production decreases. Because breathing also is needed to supply oxygen to the blood and to regulate carbon dioxide, people are able to decrease ventilation only to a limited extent.

Renal Compensation

The kidneys influence the maintenance of the normal acid–base balance by changing the rate of excretion or retention of H^+ and HCO_3^- ions. The kidneys handle increases in blood acids in two ways: They increase excretion of H^+ ions into the urine and return HCO_3^- ions to the blood. Additional serum bicarbonate is thus made available to absorb more free H^+ ions, and normal pH can be reestablished. The kidneys balance a gradual loss of blood acid (or excess of blood base) by increasing retention of H^+ ions and increasing the excretion of HCO_3^- ions into the urine. In this way, they prevent a rise in pH by keeping the relative concentration of bases and acids in the correct ratio. The kidneys' response takes several hours, and it may be as long as 2 days before fully functioning. For this reason, the kidneys are slower than the lungs to compensate for changes in acid–base status.

FACTORS AFFECTING FLUID, ELECTROLYTE, AND ACID–BASE BALANCE

Homeostasis requires a balanced fluid, electrolyte, and acid–base status. Normally, fluids and electrolytes lost from the body are replenished through adequate intake. Hormonal controls and kidney function regulate this process; Table 28-5 shows a typical adult fluid intake and output pattern for a 24-hour period. Hormones also influence the movement of electrolytes

TABLE 28-5 TYPICAL 24-HOUR INTAKE AND OUTPUT			
Intake		**Output**	
Oral fluids	1,300 mL	Urine	1,500 mL
Fluid in food	1,000 mL	Feces	200 mL
Oxidation of food	300 mL	Perspiration	100–200 mL
TOTAL	**2,600 mL**	Insensible loss:	
		Skin	300–400 mL
		Respiration	300 mL
		TOTAL	**2,400–2,600 mL**

in and out of cells. Many factors can increase the risk of fluid, electrolyte, or acid–base imbalances, including inadequate oral intake, excessive loss of fluid or electrolytes, stress, chronic illness, and surgery.

Fluid and Food Intake

Water is usually taken in orally, about two thirds in the form of water or other beverages and the remainder from foods. The body produces an additional small amount of water as it oxidizes hydrogen during food metabolism. An average daily intake for an adult is 1,300 mL of water (about six glasses). An additional 1,000 mL of water is obtained from foods, especially fruits and vegetables, which are 80% to 90% water. About 300 mL of water is obtained through food oxidation.

The thirst mechanism helps to regulate fluid intake. The thirst center, located in the hypothalamus, is usually stimulated by an increase in plasma osmolality; in cases of prolonged fluid intake deficit, it can also be stimulated by a decrease in blood volume (ECF deficit). Psychological factors or a dry mouth also may stimulate thirst. Adequate intake of fluids usually will satisfy thirst if osmolality returns to normal or, if there has been an ECF deficit, when blood volume is restored. The level of serum osmolality at which people begin to experience thirst has been shown to be decreased during pregnancy and elevated in older adults.

Food also provides the body with electrolytes. Calcium is abundant in dairy products. Sodium is found in salt, processed meats and foods, bread products, and dairy products. Bananas, melons, oranges, apricots, broccoli, raisins, and dates are all good sources of potassium. A well-balanced diet contains all of the necessary electrolytes for the body to maintain homeostasis.

Various common circumstances can affect the ability to achieve adequate fluid intake. Fluids and food must be readily accessible. Older adults may be unable to shop for or prepare a well-balanced diet, and as a result, they may decrease their intake of needed fluids and electrolytes. People in bed may be too weak to reach for and drink fluids or too fatigued to consume entire meals. People with difficulty communicating, including those with dementia, brain injury/trauma, or stroke, may be unable to indicate that they are thirsty or hungry.

Psychological factors, such as depression or confusion, also may contribute to decreased oral food or fluid intake. Some people purposely limit oral intake to lose weight or decrease the number of times they must void. Lack of knowledge regarding the consequences of these actions may contribute to such behavior. Physiologic factors such as nausea can limit oral intake. In addition, the ability to swallow may be impaired after a stroke or by the discomfort of a sore throat.

Fluid and Electrolyte Output

Water and electrolytes can be lost from the body in four ways:

- From the kidneys as urine
- From the skin as perspiration
- From the gastrointestinal tract in stool or vomit
- From the lungs as insensible water loss

The kidney is the main organ regulating fluid balance. Glomerular filtration and tubular reabsorption permit the kidneys to conserve or excrete water and electrolytes as necessary to maintain homeostasis. The hormones discussed previously regulate these processes. Normal urine output for 24 hours is approximately 1,500 mL if intake is normal (see Table 28-5). Loss of fluid through the skin as perspiration accounts for an average daily loss of 100 to 200 mL of fluid. In addition to perspiration, insensible fluid loss through the skin amounts to about 300 to 400 mL/day. Insensible water loss occurs when water molecules move from an area of higher concentration (the body) to an area of lower concentration (the atmosphere). Insensible water loss differs from perspiration, during which sweat glands actively expel water through the skin. Loss of fluid through the gastrointestinal system in the form of feces is usually minimal (approximately 200 mL). The final route for fluid loss is through the lungs during respiration. Exhalation contains not only carbon dioxide but also water vapor. The loss of water through respiration is approximately 300 mL/day. As body temperature increases with fever, the amount of fluid lost as perspiration, as insensible water loss, and from the lungs with respiration increases proportionally.

Fluid, electrolyte, and acid–base imbalances can occur when a person experiences abnormal loss of fluid or electrolytes. Vomiting, diarrhea, diaphoresis, or increased urine output secondary to the administration of diuretics can cause such a loss. Not all losses result in imbalances; however, when losses do occur, your assessment needs to include vigilant observation for any signs or symptoms of an imbalance.

VOMITING

If sufficient gastric juice (ECF with additional acid) is lost from the stomach, hydrogen, sodium, and chloride ions are depleted, increasing the risk of ECF volume deficit and/or metabolic alkalosis. Gastric fluid also is high in potassium, and excessive losses may contribute to hypokalemia. Vomiting compounds fluid and electrolyte problems because the ability to maintain adequate intake is reduced.

DIARRHEA

Intestinal secretions contain bicarbonate. For this reason, diarrhea may result in metabolic acidosis due to depletion of base. Intestinal contents also are rich in sodium, chloride, water, and potassium, possibly contributing to an ECF volume deficit and hypokalemia. The development and promotion of oral rehydration fluids, which replace the fluid and electrolytes lost in diarrhea, have significantly reduced worldwide death rates from diarrheal disease, particularly among infants (UNICEF/WHO, 2009).

DIAPHORESIS

Diaphoresis, or excessive sweating, can occasionally increase the loss of fluid and electrolytes. Sweat is a hypotonic fluid containing sodium, potassium, and chloride. Diaphoresis can occur with increased and/or prolonged physical activity, fever, or exposure to elevated environmental temperatures.

USE OF DIURETICS

Diuretics are prescribed to increase the excretion of sodium, chloride, and water in patients with high blood pressure or with chronic heart, renal, or liver problems. At times, the medications may remove too much ECF from the body, resulting in a deficit. Diuretics, except for the potassium-sparing diuretics, also promote the excretion of potassium and magnesium from the body, increasing the risk of electrolyte deficits as well.

STRESS

Stress caused by many factors, such as physical trauma, anxiety, and pain, can affect fluid and electrolyte balance. When stress occurs, aldosterone production is increased, causing ECF retention. Stress also increases ADH production, resulting in decreased renal excretion of water.

CHRONIC ILLNESS

Many chronic medical problems adversely affect a person's ability to maintain normal fluid, electrolyte, and acid–base homeostasis. Imbalances commonly accompany chronic renal, heart, liver, and respiratory problems. Other disease states such as cancer and diabetes mellitus also result in fluid and electrolyte imbalances. Adverse effects on fluid, electrolyte, and acid–base balance also may accompany treatments such as chemotherapy for cancer.

RENAL FAILURE

As kidney function decreases due to damaged or dying nephrons, there may be an abnormal loss or accumulation of sodium, chloride, potassium, and fluid in the body, resulting in ECF and water excesses or even deficits. The kidneys are less able to regulate electrolyte excretion, so abnormal levels may occur. Hyperkalemia and hypocalcemia are common. Because metabolism results in acidic by-products, metabolic acidosis occurs when the kidneys fail.

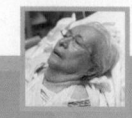

Fluid, Electrolyte, and Acid–Base PICO

The nursing student from the chapter-opening scenario is taking care of the patient from that scenario. During report, the student hears that the patient continues to have diarrhea and the provider is considering putting her on antibiotics. The off-going nurse is concerned that the patient may have *Clostridium difficile* (*C. difficile*). The student nurse remembers learning about probiotics in the classroom and their effect on the digestive system. She asks her nurse preceptor, Kyle, if probiotics would be a good option to ask the provider about. Kyle encourages her to look for evidence about it and then bring it up during patient rounds. The student nurse turns to the Cochrane Library with the inquiry. The following PICO statement is used to guide the search: *In adults, how do probiotics compared to no probiotic treatment prevent Clostridium difficile?*

P = adults

I = probiotic

C = no probiotics

O = prevent *Clostridium difficile*

The student nurse finds a systematic review and meta-analysis, which looked at 31 randomized controlled trials with 4,492 participants. Twenty-three studies assessed the benefit of taking probiotics while taking antibiotics. The results did not show a statistically significant reduction in the rates of occurrence in C-diff *infections*. However, the meta-analysis did demonstrate a decrease of 64% in C-diff–associated diarrhea. Furthermore, common adverse effects, such as abdominal cramping, nausea, fever, soft stools, flatulence, and taste disturbance, were reduced by 20% in the probiotic trial group.

The student nurse is eager to share this information during patient rounds.

REFERENCE

Goldenberg, J. Z., Ma, S. S. Y, Saxton, J. D, Martzen, M. R., Vandvik, P. O., Thorlund, K., et al. (2013). Probiotics for the prevention of *Clostridium difficile-*associated diarrhea in adults and children. *Cochrane Database of Systematic Reviews*, (5), Art. No.: CD006095. doi: 10.1002/14651858.CD006095.pub3

HEART FAILURE

As the heart fails to pump effectively, blood pressure falls. The secretion of aldosterone and ADH is stimulated, often resulting in ECF volume and water excesses. This fluid collects in the lungs, increasing the risk of pulmonary edema, and in the rest of the body, where it appears as pitting or dependent edema. Fluid volume excess is complicated by the fact that as the heart pumps less effectively, blood flow to the kidneys decreases, resulting in decreased fluid excretion.

LIVER FAILURE

Liver failure influences ECF and water balance. People with liver failure frequently present with a water excess thought to be related to increased plasma levels of ADH (Berl & Schrier, 2010). In addition, as the liver fails, plasma levels of albumin decrease, so the distribution of ECF changes, vascular volume decreases, and interstitial volume increases. **Ascites**, an abnormal collection of fluid within the peritoneal cavity, commonly accompanies liver failure.

RESPIRATORY FAILURE

Chronic respiratory problems disrupt acid–base balance. Progressive destruction of alveoli limits the lungs' functional ability to excrete carbon dioxide (carbonic acid). The pH of the blood falls, and chronic respiratory acidosis occurs.

SURGERY

Many preoperative and postoperative factors influence the surgical patient's fluid, electrolyte, and acid–base status. Before surgery, the patient may not be allowed food or fluids by mouth (NPO) and may receive enemas. During surgery, increased insensible water loss occurs as the internal body structures are exposed to air, and blood also is lost. The amount lost depends on the type of surgery. Potassium levels frequently fall after surgery because of cellular trauma and inadequate intake. As cells are destroyed, potassium is released from inside the cell, which may cause a temporary increase in serum potassium. As this potassium is excreted in the urine, serum potassium can become reduced, and supplemental potassium may be necessary. Some patients are NPO or on a restricted diet for a period after surgery. Drainage from nasogastric tubes or surgical drains increases the potential for loss of fluids, electrolytes, and acid. Emotional stress, pain, nausea, and vomiting are common after surgery and can contribute to fluid, electrolyte, and acid–base imbalances.

PREGNANCY

Physiologic changes occur during pregnancy that can alter fluid, electrolyte, and acid–base status. Acid–base balance is altered. Higher progesterone levels cause hyperventilation and may result in alkalosis as $PaCO_2$ decreases. Pregnancy is a state of compensated respiratory alkalosis. Glomerular filtration rate increases in early pregnancy, caused by an increase in blood volume, posture, activity, and nutrition. Additional sodium is retained through tubular reabsorption. In late pregnancy, fluid pools in the legs, renal blood flow is decreased, and edema may result.

ALTERED FLUID, ELECTROLYTE, AND ACID–BASE BALANCE

Disruptions in homeostasis and disease states can affect fluid, electrolyte, or acid–base balance. Fluid imbalances include ECF volume excess or deficit and water excess or deficit. Electrolyte imbalances include excesses or deficits of potassium, calcium, magnesium, or phosphate. Acid–base imbalances are referred to as respiratory acidosis, respiratory alkalosis, metabolic acidosis, or metabolic alkalosis.

Frequently, more than one imbalance occurs at a time. For simplicity, each imbalance is discussed separately here. Refer to a medical–surgical nursing text for more information on complex problems of fluid, electrolyte, and acid–base imbalance.

Fluid Imbalances

A state of fluid imbalance can occur if too much (excess) or too little (deficit) fluid is in any fluid compartment. The two major categories of fluid balance problems are ECF volume balance problems and water or osmolality balance problems. A patient may present with any of eight possible combinations of fluid balance problems: ECF volume excess or deficit, water excess or deficit, or a combination of an ECF and a water balance problem. To simplify and organize assessment and diagnosis, first assess ECF volume balance and then water balance. Once you have a diagnosis for ECF and water balance (normal, excess, or deficit for each), then you can integrate the information to make management decisions and to evaluate the appropriateness of ordered fluid replacement. Changes in ECF volume influence only the volume of fluid in the vascular and interstitial spaces, whereas changes in serum osmolality or water imbalance influence the volume of all body fluids, intracellular and extracellular. There is no physiologic possibility that there can be a change in intracellular volume alone.

EXTRACELLULAR FLUID VOLUME IMBALANCE

ECF is a 0.9% solution of sodium, chloride, and water. Because cell membranes are relatively impermeable to the sodium ion and also because sodium is actively pumped out of cells (with chloride and water following passively), changes in ECF volume influence only the vascular and interstitial compartments of body fluid. Baroreceptors that sense the volume of fluid in the blood vessels monitor ECF volume status of the body. There is no change in cell volume with ECF volume imbalances because there is no change in the osmolality or concentration of body fluid. The most critical ECF volume imbalance is an ECF deficit because it can lead to low blood pressure, shock, and death.

Extracellular Fluid Volume Deficit

ECF volume deficit involves the loss of ECF, which contains primarily sodium, chloride, bicarbonate, and water in the same concentrations as plasma. Loss of this isotonic fluid results in a decrease in the volume of the ECF compartment. There are two subdivisions of the ECF: the vascular volume (fluid inside the blood and lymphatic vessels) and the interstitial volume (fluid between the cells). Other terms that are used for ECF volume deficit include *hypovolemia, saline deficit,* and *isotonic dehydration.* ECF volume deficit can occur because of inadequate intake, abnormal losses (such as vomiting or diarrhea), or both.

A special type of ECF volume balance problem is sometimes called *third spacing.* It occurs when fluid leaves the vascular volume and is trapped within the interstitial fluid in a given body area (Metheny, 2012). A "third space" is any area in which fluid accumulates that is physiologically unavailable to return to its appropriate compartment. For example, collection of fluid in the peritoneal cavity is known as ascites. There is no actual third space, and the retained fluid is within the interstitial space. More appropriate terms for this imbalance would be *vascular volume deficit* and *interstitial volume excess.*

The signs and symptoms of an ECF volume deficit reflect decreases in fluid volume in the vascular and interstitial spaces. The signs and symptoms of a decrease in *vascular volume* include orthostatic or postural changes in pulse rate and blood pressure (i.e., an increase in pulse rate and decrease in blood pressure when the person moves from a lying to a standing position); weak, rapid pulse; decreased urine output; and slow-filling peripheral veins. Infants may need fewer diaper changes and may not produce tears when crying. The signs and symptoms of decreased *interstitial volume* include dry mucous membranes and poor skin turgor. Serum sodium values do not change noticeably because the fluid that is lost has the same concentration of electrolytes as the serum. Thirst occurs due to the loss of fluid from the vascular and interstitial spaces. Weight loss occurs if the fluid is lost from the body. Third spacing would result in a stable weight, or an increase in weight if additional fluid is retained to replace the fluid that has moved into the interstitial space.

Treatment for ECF volume deficit includes either oral or IV replacement of sodium, chloride, and water in the same concentrations found in body fluid. Use oral rehydration fluids, salty liquids such as broth and tomato juice, or IV normal saline (0.9% sodium chloride). Protect the patient from injury that could result from dizziness and weakness secondary to postural hypotension.

> ### ❗ SAFETY ALERT
>
> Monitor postural heart rate and blood pressure when getting patients with ECF deficit out of bed. Have them take several minutes to get up, going in slow steps from a lying to a sitting to a standing position. Be sure someone is present when they get out of bed.

THERAPEUTIC DIALOGUE: EDEMA IN PREGNANCY

SCENE FOR THOUGHT

Eileen Watkins is 35 years old and happily pregnant for the second time. Her first child, Katie, is 4 years old. Eileen and Katie are in the clinic for Eileen's 6-month checkup.

LESS EFFECTIVE

Nurse: Hello. How are you today?

Eileen: Hi, Cindy. We're doing just fine. Right, Katie?

Nurse: Let me get some weight and blood pressure readings on you, Eileen. *(Does so, and Katie gets her weight read, too.)* You know, I think your blood pressure is a little high this month, Eileen. Have you noticed anything different?

Eileen: *(Looks worried.)* What do you mean different?

Nurse: Have you had headaches, feet swelling, feeling extra tired? *(Good eye contact.)*

Eileen: *(Looks down at her feet.)* A little, right around the ankles and over the instep. *(Looks at the nurse.)* Is there a problem? *(Katie looks over at her mother.)*

Nurse: *(Reaches down to assess the edema—2+ pitting over the ankle.)* Nothing unusual for most pregnant women. If I remember, you had some swelling when you were pregnant with Katie, right?

Eileen: Yes, but not this early; it was in the eighth month, I think.

Nurse: Yes, it's a little earlier than last time, Eileen, but you're 4 years older, you're working harder now with Katie and your job, and besides, it's summertime! Edema is always worse in the summer. *(Pats Eileen's hand.)* Don't worry. You're fine. Let me give you some information on salt in food that might be hidden in stuff like biscuit mix. This is a really good pamphlet.... *(Continues to talk about hidden sodium and resting throughout the day in a reassuring tone.)*

Eileen: *(Listens carefully and anxiously, holds Katie close.)*

MORE EFFECTIVE

Nurse: Hello. How are you today?

Eileen: Hi, Sarah. We're doing just fine. Right, Katie?

Nurse: Let me get some weight and blood pressure readings on you, Eileen. *(Does so, and Katie gets her weight read, too.)* You know, I think your blood pressure is a little high this month, Eileen. Have you noticed anything different?

Eileen: *(Looks worried.)* What do you mean different?

Nurse: Have you had headaches, feet swelling, feeling extra tired? *(Good eye contact.)*

Eileen: *(Looks down at her feet.)* A little, right around the ankles and over the instep. *(Looks at the nurse.)* Is there a problem? *(Katie looks over at her mother.)*

Nurse: *(Reaches down to assess the edema—2+ pitting over the ankle.)* Nothing unusual for most pregnant women. If I remember, you had some swelling when you were pregnant with Katie, right?

Eileen: Yes, but not this early; it was in the eighth month, I think.

Nurse: *(Checks the chart.)* That's right. This seems to worry you. *(Good eye contact.)*

Eileen: Yes. I guess I thought everything was going to be the same as last time—no problems. *(Smiles at Katie, a little sadly.)*

Nurse: Does something particularly worry you?

Eileen: I didn't tell you last time; my mother lost a baby after her blood pressure got really high and her legs swelled up. It happened when I was about 10, and it really scared me. I was so glad when my pregnancy was so easy.

Nurse: I can hear that this concerns you. Let's talk more about it. *(Continues to listen to Eileen's concerns and explore current condition.)*

CRITICAL THINKING CHALLENGE

- Relate anxiety to the ability to hear and learn.
- Detect what Cindy did to deal with Eileen's anxiety about the pedal edema.
- Analyze how you could tell that one nurse was more effective than the other by observing body language.
- Determine what emotions you would assess on Eileen's next checkup.
- Describe how you would assess for them if you were Sarah and then if you were Cindy.

Extracellular Fluid Volume Excess

ECF volume excess, an increase in interstitial or vascular volume, often occurs in persons with cardiac failure, renal failure, or liver disease. When excess fluid cannot be eliminated, hydrostatic pressure forces some of it into the interstitial space, where it is observable as edema. A significant increase in ECF volume has to occur before edema is visible.

Rapid weight gain (more than 0.5 kg/day) is the most significant symptom indicating ECF volume excess. A weight gain of 1 kg reflects retention of 1 L of ECF. Other symptoms may include increased blood pressure, bounding pulse, and fullness of neck veins; however, because the veins are very distensible, large volumes of fluid can be retained without any increase in blood pressure. Although urine output might be expected to increase when there is ECF volume excess, it often decreases because of the underlying cause (e.g., heart or renal failure). As venous pressures increase, excess ECF volume can filter across the alveoli into the lungs, causing pulmonary edema, manifested by dyspnea, orthopnea (difficulty breathing when supine), and crackles (rales). As with ECF volume deficit, serum sodium values are within normal limits unless the patient also has a water balance problem.

Medical management of ECF volume excess typically involves restriction of sodium and saline intake (low sodium diet) and administration of diuretics. The underlying pathology is identified and treated.

WATER OR OSMOLALITY IMBALANCE

Water or osmolality balance problems occur when water intake is increased or decreased markedly or when water is retained or excreted excessively. To determine if a patient has a water balance problem, measure or estimate the serum osmolality. Osmolality is the number of dissolved particles in solution. Body fluid osmolality can be approximately determined by estimating the number of particles per kilogram of body fluid. Making this estimate is simplified by the fact that the most abundant osmotically active extracellular particles are the sodium ions, each one of which has an accompanying anion, either chloride or bicarbonate. Glucose is the only other molecule that makes a contribution to serum osmolality that influences the distribution of body fluid. (Other molecules, such as urea, also contribute to serum osmolality, but because they move easily across cell membranes, they have no net effect on body fluid volume distribution.)

Because water moves freely across almost all cell membranes, the serum osmolality indicates ICF osmolality except for relatively brief periods, when changes in one fluid compartment have not yet had time to equilibrate with the other.

Water moves down its concentration gradient from areas of higher concentration to areas of lower concentration. For example, if a patient is given a hyperosmotic IV solution (e.g., 2× normal saline), the osmolality of the ECF will increase, and water will move from the cells into the ECF until the osmolality of both compartments is the same. Conversely, if a patient takes in too much water, the osmolality of the ECF will decrease, and water will move from the ECF into the cells. When patients receive an IV infusion of dextrose 5% in water, which initially has an osmolality close to that of blood, the glucose is subsequently metabolized and actively transported into cells, leaving the water behind in the ECF. This water then distributes one third into the ECF and two thirds into the ICF, resulting in a decreased osmolality of all body fluids.

Water Deficit or Hyperosmolality

A water deficit or serum hyperosmolality occurs when there is a decrease in water intake, an increase in water loss, or an excess intake of solute. The estimated serum osmolality is greater than 300 mOsm/kg, and the serum sodium may be greater than 145 mEq/L, depending on the glucose level. As serum osmolality increases, water is drawn from the ICF compartment, causing cellular shrinking. As fluid is pulled from the cells of the brain, confusion, agitation, convulsions, coma, and death may result. If a water deficit develops slowly, brain cells have some capacity to adapt by creating so-called idiogenic osmoles that prevent excessive cell shrinkage. There is, however, a risk of long-term neurologic dysfunction, particularly if the water deficit occurs acutely (Berl & Schrier, 2010). Other symptoms of a water deficit may include decreased urine output with an increase in urine concentration, thirst, and dry mucous membranes. Other terms used for water deficit include *hypernatremia, hypertonic dehydration,* and *hypertonicity.*

The medical management of a water deficit involves giving water either orally, if feasible, or intravenously in the form of 5% dextrose in water. Because of the brain cell adaptation that can occur with a water deficit, it is recommended that the rate at which the serum sodium is returned toward normal should be no greater than 2 mEq/L/h in adults and 0.5 mEq/L/h in children. An excessive rate of correction has been associated with seizures, permanent brain damage, and death (Berl & Schrier, 2010).

Water Excess or Hypoosmolality

A water excess or body fluid hypoosmolality occurs when there is an increase in water intake, abnormal secretion of ADH, or decreased urinary output of water. The estimated serum osmolality is less than 275 mOsm/L, and the serum sodium is less than 135 mEq/L, depending on the glucose level. As serum osmolality decreases, water diffuses down its concentration gradient into cells. The major impact is on the cells of the central nervous system because the swollen cells are encased with the rigid skull. The resulting symptoms include lethargy, irritability, confusion, personality changes, seizures, coma, and eventually death if there is no treatment or treatment is ineffective. If water excess develops quickly, there is risk of permanent brain damage; if it develops slowly, the brain cells are able to adapt by extruding osmolytes by a process that is not yet well understood (Berl & Schrier, 2010). Additional symptoms include anorexia, nausea, vomiting, weakness, and cramps. Other terms used for water excess include *hypotonic disorder, hyponatremia,* and *hypotonicity.*

! SAFETY ALERT

If an unexplained change occurs in the patient's level of consciousness, estimate serum osmolality or request a serum osmolality blood sample for analysis if current results are unavailable. Water excess or deficit can cause such changes.

Management of water excess typically involves free water restriction. Limited fluids include water, coffee, tea, and simple fruit juices such as apple juice. More concentrated fluids such as milk, broth, or tomato juice may be given. Patients experiencing confusion or seizures related to water excess may be given a hypertonic IV solution such as 3% sodium chloride.

Electrolyte Imbalances

Electrolyte balance is necessary for maintaining normal physiologic functioning. Table 28-6 summarizes the major imbalances.

Acid–Base Imbalances

An arterial pH between 7.35 and 7.45 is necessary for efficient cellular metabolism. A person is said to be acidotic when the arterial pH is less than 7.35 and alkalotic when the pH is greater than 7.45. Specific normal values vary slightly by institution and are also influenced by altitude, gender, and age. Acidosis and alkalosis can be categorized as either respiratory or metabolic, depending on the underlying cause. Disturbances in acid–base balance can influence blood oxygen transport, neurologic function, and cardiac rhythmicity. The degree of impairment varies with the severity, speed of onset, and type of acid–base imbalance.

RESPIRATORY ACIDOSIS

Respiratory acidosis is indicated by a low pH accompanied by an increased arterial concentration of carbon dioxide, which often is clinically defined as a $PaCO_2$ of greater than 45 mm Hg.

TABLE 28-6 ELECTROLYTE IMBALANCES

Imbalance	Causes	Signs and Symptoms	Treatment*
Hyperkalemia (serum potassium >5.0 mEq/L)	Most often accompanies kidney failure (renal impairment prevents proper excretion of excess potassium). Also associated with cellular damage (potassium released into ECF when cells are destroyed), insulin deficiency (less potassium moves into cells), adrenal deficiency (less aldosterone produced), and rapid IV infusion of potassium	Resultant increase in cell membrane responsiveness to stimuli with changes in skeletal, smooth, and cardiac muscle activity: anxiety, irritability; gastrointestinal hyperactivity (diarrhea and intestinal cramping); tall, peaked T waves on electrocardiogram and cardiac dysrhythmias Resultant decrease in cell membrane responsiveness if serum potassium is elevated (>8 mEq/L) with symptoms similar to those of hypokalemia: cardiac arrest (especially if serum levels increase rapidly)	Depends on severity of elevation and onset *If levels very high:* Administer IV calcium gluconate to oppose potassium's effect on the membrane potential of excitable cells. Infuse insulin and glucose to move potassium into the cell. Remove potassium from body by dialysis or administration of ion exchange resins such as Kayexalate. *If levels moderately elevated:* Administer diuretics and potassium exchange resins. Identify and treat the underlying cause.
Hypokalemia (serum potassium <3.5 mEq/L)	Abnormal loss of potassium; inadequate replacement; increased movement into cells (possible when insulin given)	Resultant decreased responsiveness of cellular membranes to stimuli and lack of responsiveness to stimuli leading to characteristic skeletal muscle, smooth muscle, renal, and cardiac (symptoms usually appearing when serum potassium is below 3 mEq/L): muscle weakness (begins in lower extremities and moves up trunk to upper extremities); fatigue; impaired respiratory muscle function (if level severely low); abdominal distention, nausea, vomiting, constipation, and paralytic ileus (from decreased gastrointestinal responsiveness); increased urination (polyuria) and thirst (polydipsia); dysrhythmias and flattened T waves on electrocardiogram; elevated blood glucose levels (from suppression of insulin release)	Increase intake of potassium: encourage potassium-rich foods in diet; administer oral potassium supplements; use potassium-sparing diuretics; and administer IV potassium (if level very low). Identify and treat underlying cause. Administer oral phosphate replacement if indicated.
Hypophosphatemia (serum level <2.5 mg/dL)	*Redistribution:* Increased carbohydrate calories; respiratory alkalosis *Depletion:* Alcoholism; uncontrolled diabetes mellitus; renal phosphate wasting	Neuromuscular dysfunction; weakness, especially respiratory muscles; fatigue; myocardial depression; ventricular dysrhythmias; rhabdomyolysis; confusion; coma; decreased oxygen delivery to tissues; renal loss of bicarbonate, calcium, magnesium, and glucose; bone changes (osteomalacia); endocrine changes (insulin resistance)	Identify and treat underlying cause. Encourage foods high in phosphorus. Administer oral phosphate replacement if indicated.

*Most treatments require a physician's order.

When lung disease (e.g., asthma, emphysema) or depressed neural or muscular function (as with opioid overdose, head trauma, or motor neuron disease) compromises breathing ability, carbon dioxide accumulates in the blood. As the carbonic acid level increases, free [H+] increases, causing pH to drop. With time, the kidneys compensate for this acid buildup by increasing the excretion of H+ ion into the urine and the return of HCO_3^- ion to the blood. Normal pH can be reestablished only if the original problem can be reversed. People with damaged lungs may have chronic respiratory acidosis.

METABOLIC ACIDOSIS

Metabolic acidosis occurs either when excess acid is ingested or created (diabetic ketoacidosis) or when the kidneys are unable to retain enough bicarbonate ions to buffer free hydrogen ions in the blood. Metabolic acidosis is characterized by a pH lower than 7.35 and a plasma HCO_3^- concentration lower than 22 mEq/L. It can occur with loss of bicarbonate, as may happen with severe diarrhea, or with acid accumulation (e.g., ketoacids formed in uncontrolled diabetes mellitus or lactic acids produced by oxygen deprivation).

The respiratory system compensates for metabolic acidosis by increasing ventilation, thus increasing the rate of carbonic acid excretion, resulting in a fall in $PaCO_2$. This respiratory compensation occurs relatively rapidly but cannot alone return the acid–base balance to normal limits. Renal compensation with the excretion of H+ ion and retention of HCO_3^- takes from hours to days to occur and can, in conjunction with respiratory compensation, return the pH to within normal limits. Renal compensation cannot occur if the kidneys are the cause of the metabolic acidosis.

RESPIRATORY ALKALOSIS

Hyperventilation causes respiratory alkalosis, which is present when a high pH is accompanied by a blood carbon dioxide concentration lower than 35 mm Hg. Hyperventilation, commonly caused by anxiety, fever, pain, high altitude, or asthma, increases carbon dioxide (carbonic acid) excretion, leading to a relative excess of blood base and an increase in pH. To compensate, the kidneys increase the excretion of HCO_3^- to the urine, and pH returns toward normal. Intervention, mainly treatment for the causative underlying disorder, may be required to reduce the hyperventilation.

METABOLIC ALKALOSIS

Metabolic alkalosis occurs when there is excessive loss of body acids or with unusual intake of alkaline substances. It can also occur in conjunction with an ECF deficit or potassium deficit (known as contraction alkalosis). Vomiting or vigorous nasogastric suction frequently causes metabolic alkalosis. Endocrine disorders and ingestion of large amounts of antacids are other causes. The loss of stomach acid or taking in of base causes H+ shifts in the blood, and pH increases.

Compensation for metabolic alkalosis includes a decrease in ventilation, which allows the blood carbon dioxide concentration to rise. The kidneys respond to metabolic alkalosis by retaining acid and excreting HCO_3^-. Renal compensation for metabolic alkalosis is impaired if the person has an ECF volume deficit or hypokalemia.

Manifestations of Fluid, Electrolyte, or Acid–Base Imbalances

Although each fluid, electrolyte, or acid–base imbalance has specific symptoms, groups of symptoms frequently accompany states of imbalance. The degree of the imbalance, the suddenness with which it occurs, and the patient's age influence symptom severity. When evaluating manifestations, check to see whether all of the data support the same conclusion. Suspect a fluid, electrolyte, or acid–base imbalance in any patient who presents with the following signs or symptoms.

IMBALANCE OF INTAKE AND OUTPUT AND BODY WEIGHT

Intake and output should be approximately equal for a 24-hour period. When output is significantly greater or less than intake, suspect a fluid balance problem. Because mistakes are common, make certain that the intake and output record is accurate. Comparison of daily body weights is the best way to confirm apparent discrepancies in intake and output. Normally, urine output is approximately 1,500 mL in a 24-hour period, but a wide range of variation is normal, depending on many factors, particularly input. A decrease in body weight may indicate an ECF volume deficit or a water deficit; an increase may indicate an ECF volume excess or a water excess.

When evaluating trends in intake, output, and weight, consider at least the last 48 hours or longer for some chronic health problems. Look for a pattern of imbalance between intake and output or increases or decreases in weight.

CHANGES IN MENTAL STATUS

Level of consciousness is a person's state of awareness and arousal. Changes in level of consciousness can occur with changes in serum osmolality (water balance). At first, changes are minor and may not be very apparent unless the nurse knows the patient well. The patient may simply report feeling fatigued, restless, or apprehensive. Confusion can occur as the imbalances become more severe. Changes in level of consciousness can vary from excessive excitability to lethargy. Lethargy can progress to coma and eventually death. Abruptness of onset of the imbalance results in increased severity of symptoms.

> ! **SAFETY ALERT**
> Subtle changes in a person's ability to understand and relate to his or her environment can be the earliest indications of a fluid or electrolyte imbalance.

CHANGES IN VITAL SIGNS

Respiratory Rate and Depth

Deep, labored respirations may occur to compensate for metabolic acidosis, whereas shallow respirations may be present in alkalosis. In ECF volume excess, fluid can accumulate in the lungs, decrease oxygenation, and be accompanied by dyspnea. Lung auscultation can detect crackles (rales), a subtle sign of fluid excess, before dyspnea is observable.

Heart Rate and Rhythm

The quality of the pulse depends in part on vascular volume. With ECF volume excess, the pulse may be strong, full, and bounding, whereas with ECF volume deficit, the pulse is usually weak, thready, and rapid. Irregular heart rhythms are common with potassium, calcium, and magnesium imbalances.

Postural Pulse Rate and Blood Pressure

An increase in pulse rate and perhaps a decrease in blood pressure will occur in ECF volume deficit. To assess for an ECF volume deficit, determine the effect that position change has on pulse rate and blood pressure. The pulse and blood pressure are first measured in the supine position and then with the patient standing (postural vital signs).

An increase in pulse rate of more than 20 beats per minute is a more sensitive indicator of ECF volume deficit than is a decrease in blood pressure. A drop of more than 15 mm Hg in systolic pressure or 10 mm Hg in diastolic pressure with an increase in pulse rate frequently means the patient is experiencing ECF volume depletion. Postural pulse and blood pressure readings are a useful assessment tool with all patients at risk for ECF volume depletion (e.g., after surgery).

> ! **SAFETY ALERT**
> Because patients who have a marked ECF volume deficit may become faint or dizzy when they stand, have help available and be vigilant to prevent patient injury when taking postural vital signs.

ABNORMAL TISSUE HYDRATION

When ECF volume or water imbalances occur, tissues can retain excess fluid, appearing edematous (turgid), or lose fluid, appearing dry and shriveled. Tissue hydration can be noted in the mouth and tongue, where the mucous membranes and tongue can appear dry with ridges in the tongue due to lack of moisture, or by pinching the skin usually over the sternum. Fluid imbalance affects tissue turgor, or the skin's ability to return to normal position immediately after being pinched. Poor tissue turgor occurs in ECF volume deficit or when elasticity is lost from the skin during normal aging.

Edema is not observable in most patients until 2.5 to 3.0 L of fluid has been retained. Edema is most noticeable in dependent areas of the body (e.g., the legs when sitting or standing,

the back and sacral area when supine in bed). When edema is severe, an indentation remains when a finger is pressed into edematous tissue ("pitting edema").

ABNORMAL MUSCLE TONE OR SENSATION

Changes in muscle tone and muscle irritability frequently accompany imbalances, as described in Table 28-6. Increased or decreased neuromuscular excitability manifests as increasing irritability, muscle weakness, twitching, or cramping. Changes in gastrointestinal neuromuscular tone result in anorexia, nausea, constipation, and vomiting. Patients with electrolyte imbalance may experience tingling and other paresthesias. Observe patients for seizure activity, which can occur with severe or rapid-onset imbalances.

Recall the patient in the case scenario at the beginning of the chapter. Use the concept map (Fig. 28-7) to help understand and manage the patient's situation and to plan for his care.

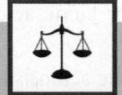 **ETHICAL/LEGAL ISSUE**

DECISIONS REGARDING TREATMENT

You have been assigned to care for Mr. Lane, 72 years old, who has heart failure and emphysema that are no longer responding to treatment. Earlier in the disease process, Mr. Lane participated in planning for end-of-life care, deciding to remain as comfortable as possible until his death. Mr. Lane's family seemed to agree with the physician's prognosis and the end-of-life treatment plan to discontinue further active treatment. Mr. Lane's youngest son, who lives at a distance, is disturbed by this decision. He believes that IV therapy should be started and that Mr. Lane should receive vitamins and fluids. He doesn't think that they would hurt Mr. Lane and might even help him. Another nurse in the unit is protesting this treatment, expressing her view that it is utterly useless and offers false hope. The family at Mr. Lane's bedside is disturbed by this difference in opinion between their sibling and the healthcare provider.

CRITICAL THINKING CHALLENGE

- Describe the feelings that you have after reading this situation. How would you feel if you were the youngest son? The nurse? Another family member?
- Identify any concerns you have regarding your nurse's role in this situation.
- Identify possible approaches to assisting the patient's family in resolving the dilemma.
- Recognizing the patient's rights, the family's rights, and the healthcare provider's advice, define what you see as your ethically appropriate behavior.

FLUID, ELECTROLYTES, AND ACID-BASE BALANCE

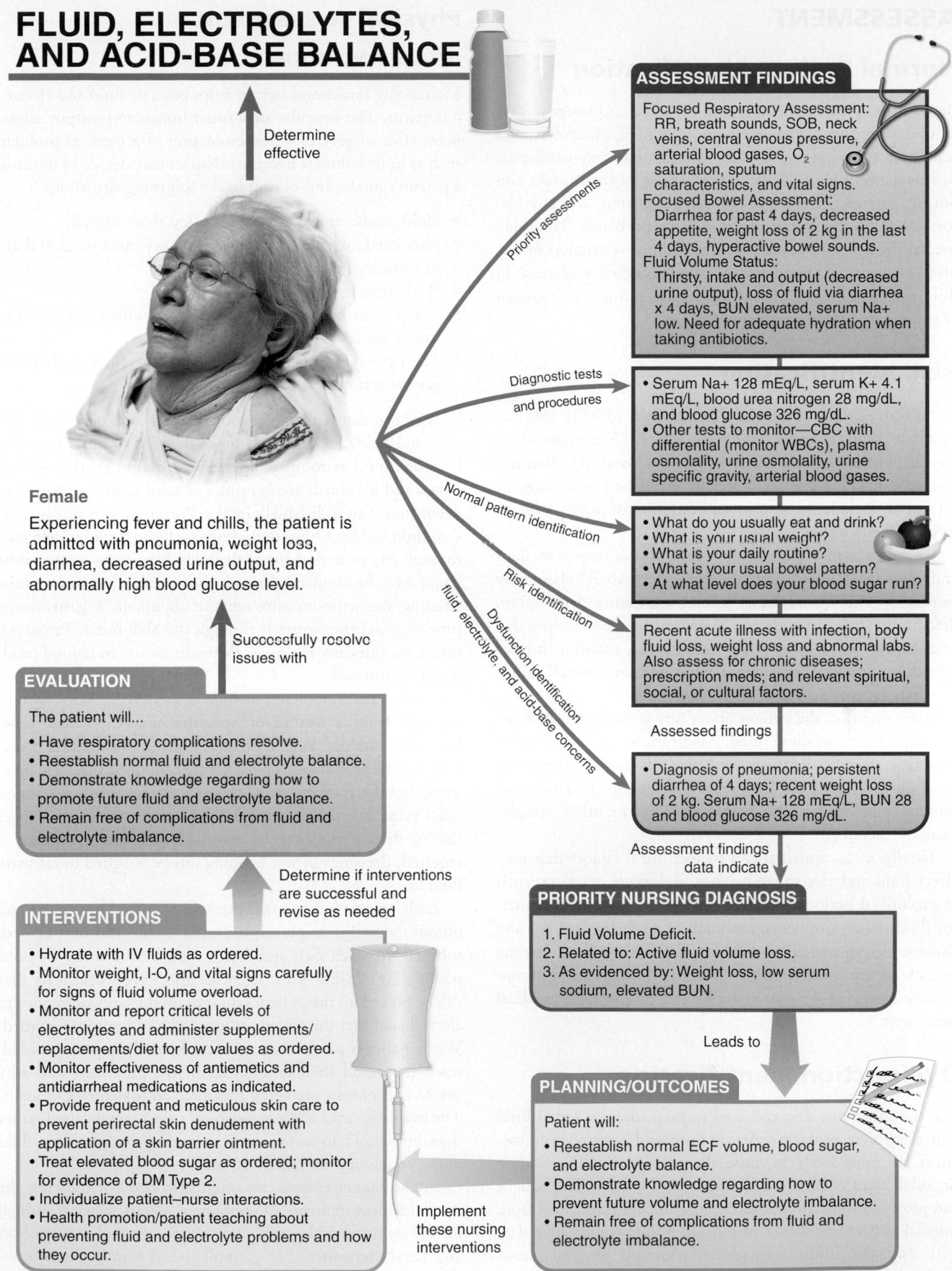

Determine effective

Female

Experiencing fever and chills, the patient is admitted with pneumonia, weight loss, diarrhea, decreased urine output, and abnormally high blood glucose level.

Successfully resolve issues with

EVALUATION

The patient will...

• Have respiratory complications resolve.
• Reestablish normal fluid and electrolyte balance.
• Demonstrate knowledge regarding how to promote future fluid and electrolyte balance.
• Remain free of complications from fluid and electrolyte imbalance.

Determine if interventions are successful and revise as needed

INTERVENTIONS

• Hydrate with IV fluids as ordered.
• Monitor weight, I-O, and vital signs carefully for signs of fluid volume overload.
• Monitor and report critical levels of electrolytes and administer supplements/replacements/diet for low values as ordered.
• Monitor effectiveness of antiemetics and antidiarrheal medications as indicated.
• Provide frequent and meticulous skin care to prevent perirectal skin denudement with application of a skin barrier ointment.
• Treat elevated blood sugar as ordered; monitor for evidence of DM Type 2.
• Individualize patient–nurse interactions.
• Health promotion/patient teaching about preventing fluid and electrolyte problems and how they occur.

ASSESSMENT FINDINGS

Priority assessments

Focused Respiratory Assessment:
RR, breath sounds, SOB, neck veins, central venous pressure, arterial blood gases, O₂ saturation, sputum characteristics, and vital signs.
Focused Bowel Assessment:
Diarrhea for past 4 days, decreased appetite, weight loss of 2 kg in the last 4 days, hyperactive bowel sounds.
Fluid Volume Status:
Thirsty, intake and output (decreased urine output), loss of fluid via diarrhea x 4 days, BUN elevated, serum Na+ low. Need for adequate hydration when taking antibiotics.

Diagnostic tests and procedures

• Serum Na+ 128 mEq/L, serum K+ 4.1 mEq/L, blood urea nitrogen 28 mg/dL, and blood glucose 326 mg/dL.
• Other tests to monitor—CBC with differential (monitor WBCs), plasma osmolality, urine osmolality, urine specific gravity, arterial blood gases.

Normal pattern identification

• What do you usually eat and drink?
• What is your usual weight?
• What is your daily routine?
• What is your usual bowel pattern?
• At what level does your blood sugar run?

Risk identification

Dysfunction identification

fluid, electrolyte, and acid-base concerns

Recent acute illness with infection, body fluid loss, weight loss and abnormal labs. Also assess for chronic diseases; prescription meds; and relevant spiritual, social, or cultural factors.

Assessed findings

• Diagnosis of pneumonia; persistent diarrhea of 4 days; recent weight loss of 2 kg. Serum Na+ 128 mEq/L, BUN 28 and blood glucose 326 mg/dL.

Assessment findings data indicate

PRIORITY NURSING DIAGNOSIS

1. Fluid Volume Deficit.
2. Related to: Active fluid volume loss.
3. As evidenced by: Weight loss, low serum sodium, elevated BUN.

Leads to

PLANNING/OUTCOMES

Patient will:

• Reestablish normal ECF volume, blood sugar, and electrolyte balance.
• Demonstrate knowledge regarding how to prevent future volume and electrolyte imbalance.
• Remain free of complications from fluid and electrolyte imbalance.

Implement these nursing interventions

FIGURE 28-7 Concept map of fluid, electrolyte, and acid–base.

ASSESSMENT

Normal Pattern Identification

Begin with obtaining or reviewing the patient's history to gain an understanding of the person's normal fluid, electrolyte, and acid–base status, along with any factors that may predispose to imbalance. Question the patient about normal intake and output, any recent changes that have occurred, and any history of fluid, electrolyte, or acid–base problems. Note any special dietary restrictions, such as sodium restriction or use of salt substitutes. Reported increased thirst or a decrease in fluid intake also is significant. Assess the amount and pattern of urine output along with any changes.

Risk Identification

Collection of subjective data also can help identify risk factors that could contribute to an imbalance. Elicit information concerning recent acute illnesses. Nausea, vomiting, diarrhea, and severe diaphoresis are especially important to document. Be sure to include the severity and duration of these problems in your documentation.

Certain chronic diseases also predispose a person to fluid and electrolyte imbalance. Question the patient about any history of renal failure, heart failure, respiratory dysfunction, diabetes mellitus, liver disease, Addison disease, Cushing disease, or thyroid disease. If any are present, question further regarding individualized management and any complications that may have occurred.

Also, question the patient about any prescription or nonprescription medications used. Medications such as insulin, diuretics, steroids, laxatives, and antacids can contribute to fluid and electrolyte disturbances. Note the use of vitamin and mineral supplements plus herbal remedies or other complementary therapies.

Finally, assess spiritual and sociocultural factors that may affect fluid and electrolyte balance. Religious practices, such as prolonged periods of fasting, could increase the potential for fluid deficit problems, especially if an individual has any chronic diseases such as diabetes mellitus. A fixed income or lack of transportation may make it difficult for a person to buy medicine or special foods to comply with medical treatment.

Dysfunction Identification

Use the subjective data collected to help identify actual fluid and electrolyte problems. Actual fluid and electrolyte imbalances are most likely to cause altered cognitive functioning or imbalances of intake and output and weight. The patient can provide information regarding significant differences from normal patterns of intake or output. Validate subjective data with objective information gained through physical assessment and evaluation of laboratory test results before making an actual diagnosis.

Physical Assessment

INTAKE AND OUTPUT

Monitoring intake and output helps evaluate fluid and electrolyte status. The provider may order intake and output assessment after surgery or when evaluation of a medical problem such as heart failure is necessary. Nurses may decide to monitor a patient's intake and output in the following situations:

- Fluid intake or urinary output is less than normal.
- Abnormal losses are occurring, such as from a surgical drain or vomiting.
- IV therapy is being administered.
- The patient has medical problems that affect fluid or electrolyte status.
- The patient is not physiologically stable, such as after surgery or trauma.

Intake measurements include all oral and parenteral fluids. Oral fluids include any liquids ingested or any foods that become liquid at room temperature. Gelatin, sherbet, frozen treats, and ice cream are examples of solid foods to include in determining an individual's intake. Pureed food is not considered fluid intake. Other oral intake includes feedings delivered through any tube that enters the body (e.g., a nasogastric tube going into the stomach through the nose, a jejunostomy tube entering the jejunum through the abdomen, a gastrostomy tube entering the stomach through the abdomen). Parenteral intake includes any IV fluids, IV medications, and blood products administered.

Output measurements include urine, liquid stool, vomit, drainage from a wound or operative site (e.g., chest tube, Hemovac drain), and drainage from a nasogastric tube. Diaphoresis or drainage on a dressing cannot be precisely measured, but if it is excessive, its presence can be noted without an exact value stated. For example, the number of linen changes due to diaphoresis may be recorded. If greater precision is required, dressings or wet bedding can be weighed to estimate fluid loss.

Each agency has its own method of recording intake and output. Most forms permit listing of intake and output with subtotals for each shift and then a total for the entire 24-hour period (Fig. 28-8). Some agencies also have worksheets that can be posted on the patient's door or on the bathroom door to alert all staff that the patient needs intake and output recorded. When patients are having their intake and output recorded, teach them and their families about the procedure and why intake and output are being measured so that they can assist. The milliliter (mL) is the standard of measurement used rather than household measures such as cups or ounces. One fluid ounce equals approximately 30 mL.

Intake measurements are often obtained by knowing the standard measurements of containers. Often, what is normal for the agency may be printed on the intake and output sheet as a handy reference. For example, when a milk carton contains 240 mL and the patient drinks half of the milk, 120 mL is recorded. All intake must be included. Sips of water taken

Intake and Output Documentation Form

			BED			DATE		

INTAKE			OUTPUT					
TIME	PO/NG	AMOUNT	TIME	URINE	STOOL	EMESIS/GASTRIC	OTHER	OTHER
NIGHT								
NIGHT TOTAL			NIGHT TOTAL					
DAY								
DAY TOTAL			DAY TOTAL					
EVENING								
EVENING TOTAL			EVENING TOTAL					

FIGURE 28-8 Example of an intake–output form.

during the day can add up to significant intake, as can oral medications (e.g., antacids) that are given frequently. Ice chips should be recorded as approximately half their volume.

Urine output is measured every time the patient voids. To obtain an accurate measurement, keep toilet paper separate from the urine. If the patient voids in a bedpan or a commode, transfer the urine into a calibrated container for measurement (Fig. 28-9). If the patient is able to use the toilet, place a measuring device (sometimes called a hat) between the toilet seat and the toilet to collect the urine (Fig. 28-10). If a voiding cannot be measured, indicate it on the intake and output record

(e.g., "320 mL plus incontinent × 2"). If the patient has a Foley catheter, empty the collection bag and measure the urine at the end of each shift, unless the bag becomes full sooner. Other drainage also is usually emptied and measured at the end of each shift, or more frequently if indicated.

In addition to measuring and recording intake and output, also evaluate patterns and values that are outside the normal range. Intake and output should be roughly equal. When a person has other significant losses (e.g., vomiting, diarrhea), urinary output also may be affected. Urine output of less than 30 mL/hour indicates possible impending renal failure

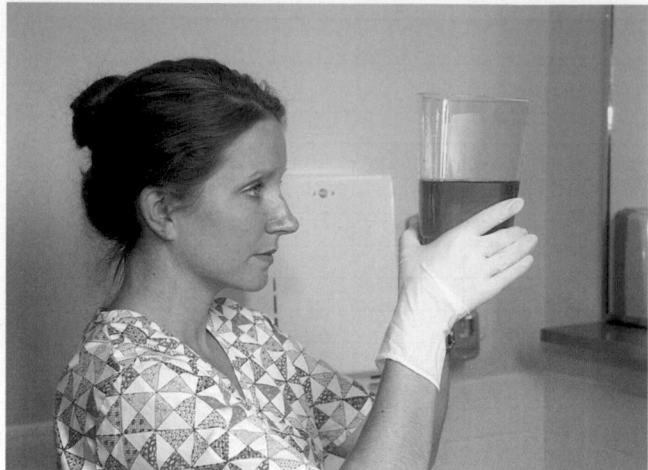

FIGURE 28-9 Measuring urinary output using a calibrated container.

or marked ECF deficit. If large discrepancies occur between intake and output, ascertain the accuracy of the data collected. Because many people may be responsible for recording intake and output, some values could have inadvertently not been recorded.

BODY WEIGHT

Assessing weight provides data concerning fluid balance. Rapid changes in weight indicate body fluid changes. Each kilogram of weight lost or gained equals approximately 1 L of fluid. The greater the weight loss, the greater the severity of the deficit. Note that ECF and water weigh the same, so a complete assessment is necessary to determine whether the weight that is gained or lost is due to an accumulation or loss of ECF or water or both.

Daily weights are often ordered for patients who are at risk for ECF volume problems. Obtain weights at the same time of day (preferably in the morning before breakfast), with the patient wearing the same clothing, using the same scale to ensure accuracy. If a patient is too ill or too weak to stand, use a bed scale, which is a portable scale on wheels onto which

the patient can be transferred and weighed. Data from intake and output and daily weight are used together to evaluate for an ECF imbalance. A decreasing output in conjunction with an increasing weight indicates ECF volume retention. A sudden weight loss with low urine output may indicate ECF volume deficit.

INTEGUMENTARY ASSESSMENT

Changes in the skin and mucous membranes can indicate fluid imbalance. The skin's general appearance is important to note. Flushed, dry skin may signal a fluid volume deficit. Lack of tearing or perspiration also is important to note. Skin turgor should be assessed (Fig. 28-11). Variations in tissue turgor have been discussed.

Edema, or excessive accumulation of interstitial fluid, also can be detected when examining the skin. Interstitial fluid can collect in various body parts, such as around the eyes, around the sacrum, and in the extremities. Pressing a finger into tissue over a bony prominence (e.g., lower tibia) best assesses edema. Pitting edema occurs when an indentation remains in the skin (often for 15 to 30 seconds) after a finger presses into edematous tissue. Pitting edema is not apparent until there is approximately a 10% increase in body weight. Historically, edema has been quantified clinically by the use of plus (+) signs with a range from 0 to 4+.

- A measurement of 0 indicates no edema.
- A measurement of 1+ indicates edema that is just perceptible (2 mm).
- A measurement of 2+ indicates moderate edema (4 mm).
- A measurement of 3+ is deeper (6 mm).
- A measurement of 4+ indicates severe edema (8 mm or more).

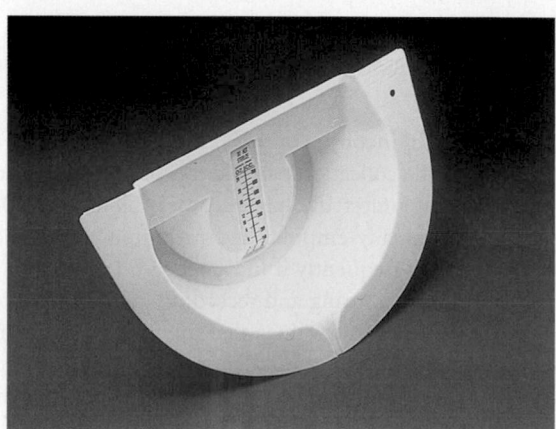

FIGURE 28-10 Urinary "hat" for measuring urine.

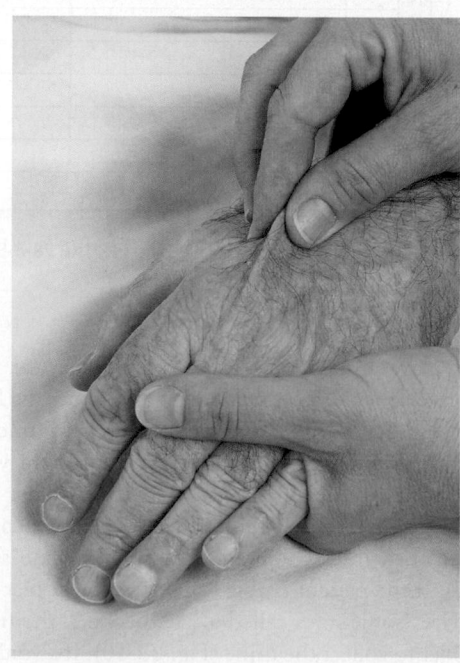

FIGURE 28-11 Testing skin turgor.

Edema may be more precisely evaluated by measuring the circumference of body parts (e.g., leg, abdomen). If the circumference is measured at the same location with the same technique, an increase in circumference indicates increased fluid in the interstitial space. Accumulation of fluid in the abdominal cavity (ascites) can also be evaluated in this way. If it is acceptable to the patient, the measurement location could be marked with a felt pen so that each measurement will be made in the identical location.

VITAL SIGNS

Vital signs are important parameters to monitor and detect potential fluid, electrolyte, and acid–base imbalances. Variations in vital signs have been discussed.

NECK VEINS

Distention of neck veins accompanies ECF excess. The jugular veins are visible in the neck. Changes in jugular vein distention can indicate alterations in ECF volume. To assess jugular vein distention, place the patient in a sitting position with the head elevated to approximately 45 degrees (Fig. 28-12). The neck should be straight in alignment with the body. With the patient in this position, the distention within the jugular vein should not extend more than 2 cm above the sternal angle. An increase in ECF volume may be indicated by distention of the neck veins from the top portion of the sternum to the angle of the jaw. Neck vein distention occurs in heart failure because of fluid retention.

CENTRAL VENOUS PRESSURE

Measurement of central venous pressure is a more accurate method of evaluating fluid status than is visual inspection of neck vein distention. The central venous pressure is the pressure in the right atrium or vena cava and can be measured by adding a transducer to a central venous catheter. The transducer converts the pressure into a waveform that can be measured.

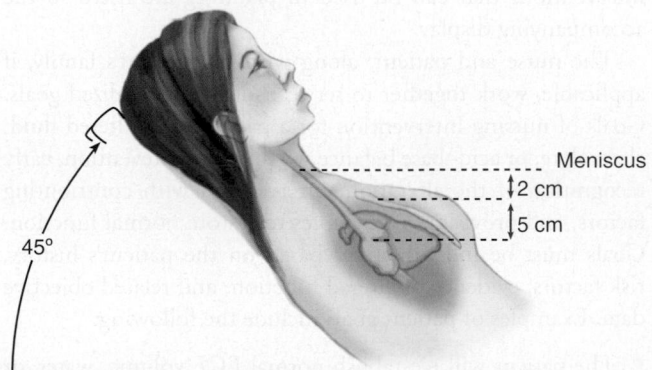

FIGURE 28-12 Measuring jugular venous distention. Place the patient with the head of the bed elevated at approximately a 45-degree angle so that the sternal angle is approximately 5 cm above the right atrium. Then, measure the vertical distance in centimeters from the sternal angle to the level at the highest point where you see visible pulsation of the neck veins. The distention should not extend more than 2 cm above the sternal angle.

The normal pressure is approximately 4 to 11 cm H_2O. An increase in the pressure may indicate an ECF volume excess or heart failure. A decrease in pressure may indicate an ECF volume deficit.

BOWEL ASSESSMENT

Bowel elimination is important to consider when detecting fluid and electrolyte imbalances. Because diarrhea predisposes a person to ECF volume and electrolyte disorders, any diarrhea should be evaluated carefully. Bowel sounds should be assessed, with any hypoactivity or hyperactivity noted. Abdominal distention, hypoactive bowel sounds, or a paralytic ileus can accompany a potassium deficit, whereas constipation commonly occurs in persons with hypercalcemia.

Laboratory and Diagnostic Tests

Laboratory data assist in the early identification and continuous monitoring of fluid and electrolyte imbalances. Trends revealed in laboratory data are more significant than is any single value. Be familiar with serum electrolyte, serum or urine osmolality, urine specific gravity, and arterial blood gas values. Information from these laboratory tests can help the nurse individualize the patient's plan of care.

SERUM ELECTROLYTES

Monitoring of serum electrolyte values provides information about trends and helps to evaluate whether electrolyte imbalances are developing, improving, or worsening. Electrolytes are usually obtained and evaluated in groups rather than singularly. Standard electrolytes include serum sodium, potassium, chloride, and serum carbon dioxide. A more comprehensive chemistry profile would include serum calcium, magnesium, glucose, blood urea nitrogen, creatinine, and protein (total, albumin, and globulin values) and can be helpful when evaluating total fluid and electrolyte status.

PLASMA OSMOLALITY

Obtain plasma osmolality with a venous blood sample. Normal osmolality is 280 to 300 mOsm/kg. Plasma osmolality decreases in water excess and elevates in water deficit.

URINE OSMOLALITY

Urine osmolality measures the urine's solute concentration. Increased amounts of nitrogenous wastes (e.g., urea, creatinine, uric acid) increase urinary osmolality. Additionally, the circulating amount of ADH affects urine osmolality. Normal urine osmolality ranges from 50 to 1,200 mOsm/kg. The more concentrated the urine, the greater its osmolality. Comparison of plasma and urine osmolality can be informative. If the kidneys are functioning normally, urine osmolality should be elevated when plasma osmolality is elevated and decreased when plasma osmolality is decreased. That is, the kidneys should be retaining water when plasma osmolality is increased and losing

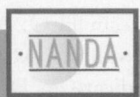

TABLE 28-7 SELECTED NANDA-I NURSING DIAGNOSES INVOLVING FLUID, ELECTROLYTE, AND ACID–BASE BALANCE

Nursing Dx	Related Factors	Diagnostic Statement	NOC*	NIC†
Deficient Fluid Volume—decreased intravascular, interstitial, and/ or ICF	Prolonged or marked loss of body fluids Hypoaldosteronism Prolonged decrease in intake of fluids Diuretic use	Deficient Fluid Volume R/T vomiting AEB decreased BP, skin turgor, urine output, weight loss, thirst, and dry mucous membranes	Fluid Balance, Hydration, Hypotension Severity, Vital Signs, Weight, Delirium Level	Fluid Management Hypovolemia Management Shock Management
Excess Fluid Volume—increased isotonic fluid retention	Excess fluid intake Excess sodium intake Compromised regulation of fluid	Excess Fluid Volume R/T heart failure AEB decreased breath sounds, edema, weight gain, and jugular venous distinction	Electrolyte and Acid/Base Balance, Fluid Balance, Hydration	Fluid Management Fluid Monitoring (e.g., weight and intake/ output)

Dx, diagnosis; R/T, related to; AEB, as evidenced by; BP, blood pressure.
*From: Moorhead, S., Johnson, M., Maas, M., & Swanson, E. (2013). *Nursing outcomes classification (NOC): Measurement of health outcomes* (5th ed.). St. Louis, MO: Elsevier.
†From: Bulecheck, G., Butcher, H., Dochterman, J., Wagner, C. (2013). *Nursing interventions classification (NIC)* (6th ed.). St. Louis, MO: Elsevier.
From: Herdman, T. H., & Kamitsuru, S. (Eds.). (2014). *Nursing diagnoses: Definitions and classification, 2015–2017*. West Sussex, England: Wiley-Blackwell.

water when the blood is hypoosmotic. If the urine concentration is not what one would predict from the plasma osmolality, the patient may have a renal problem.

URINE SPECIFIC GRAVITY

Urine specific gravity measures the weight of a substance compared with an equal part of water. The specific gravity of water is 1.000. With normal fluid intake, urine specific gravity is usually 1.010 to 1.020. A higher specific gravity is obtained when the urine is concentrated, and a lower specific gravity is obtained when the urine is dilute. The urine specific gravity and osmolality are correlated. A urine specific gravity of 1.010 is equivalent to a urine osmolality of 300 mOsm/kg.

ARTERIAL BLOOD GASES

Arterial blood gases include the pH, partial pressure of carbon dioxide ($PaCO_2$), partial pressure of oxygen (PaO_2), bicarbonate (HCO_3^-), and oxygen saturation of hemoglobin (O_2 sat). These blood gases are used to evaluate acid–base balance and pulmonary function. A pH lower than 7.35 indicates acidosis, whereas a pH greater than 7.45 indicates alkalosis. Normal ranges for other blood gas values are given in Table 28-3.

NURSING DIAGNOSES

Information gathered in the assessment helps identify actual or potential fluid and electrolyte problems. NANDA-International (Herdman & Kamitsuru, 2014) has four diagnoses related to fluid disturbances: Deficient Fluid Volume, Excess Fluid Volume, Risk for Deficient Fluid Volume, and Risk for Imbalance of Fluid Volume. To make them more usable, these diagnoses have been expanded here to ECF Volume Excess or

Deficit and Water Excess or Deficit. These fluid imbalances also can be actual or potential, and a patient can present with an ECF volume and a water balance problem. These diagnoses are more useful than are those offered by NANDA-I because they reflect the ways in which the body monitors and regulates body fluid balance and, most importantly, how the problem should be managed. Refer to Table 28-7.

OUTCOME IDENTIFICATION AND PLANNING

After nursing diagnoses and related factors have been identified, the nurse and patient can plan outcomes and interventions. In many situations, the nurse will also include the patient's family or support people in this planning process. Examples of some interventions that can be used in planning are listed in the accompanying display.

The nurse and patient, along with the patient's family, if applicable, work together to set realistic, individualized goals. Goals of nursing intervention for a patient with altered fluid, electrolyte, or acid–base balance will focus on prevention, early recognition of the alteration, intervention with contributing factors, and provision of therapies to restore normal function. Goals must be individualized based on the patient's history, risk factors, evidence of altered function, and related objective data. Examples of patient goals include the following:

- The patient will reestablish normal ECF volume, water, or electrolyte balance.
- The patient will demonstrate knowledge regarding how to promote (or prevent) future ECF volume, water, or electrolyte balance.
- The patient will remain free from complications from fluid or electrolyte imbalance.

The nurse and patient together can determine specific outcome criteria to individualize the plan of care. Short-term goals (e.g., "The patient will increase fluid intake to 2,000 mL in 24 hours") may be easy to reach within a short period. Other goals may involve changes in long-established dietary patterns, and these goals will take longer to accomplish.

APPLY YOUR CRITICAL THINKING

Your patient, Ms. Simpson, a 24-year-old woman requiring fluid restriction, has an IV line in her left arm and is allowed nothing by mouth. She has been irritable and impatient with the staff this morning, and now she has her call light on again. When you ask her what you can do for her, she says that she wants a drink. "I'm so thirsty, my mouth feels like cotton balls." How should you intervene?

Check your answer in Appendix B.

IMPLEMENTATION

Health Promotion

Teaching is an important nursing role in preventing fluid and electrolyte problems. Nurses can help people understand how fluid and electrolyte imbalances occur and how people can prevent them. The type of fluid replacement that the patient uses should be matched to the type of fluid that is being lost. If there is a deficit of ECF volume, consumption of mildly salty solutions, such as chicken broth or oral rehydration fluid, is appropriate. The risk of water excess or hyponatremia increases in people who participate in strenuous athletic competitions. Exercise-associated hyponatremia occurs because of inadequate suppression of ADH. Excessive water intake compounds the problem, and extremes of temperature (very hot or very cold) also contribute (Urso, Brucculeri, & Caimi, 2014).

Teaching can occur in various settings and with any age group. When interacting with new parents, stress the fluid needs of newborns; how quickly serious problems can develop if vomiting, diarrhea, or a fever occurs in an infant; and symptoms that warrant contacting a provider. Follow-up teaching, explaining normal fluid requirements and dietary patterns, can occur as children grow. When children are ill, explain measures to help parents adequately replace fluid that is lost. Balanced electrolyte solutions are available commercially. Because the commercial solutions are relatively costly, a homemade solution of 1 L of boiled or clean water containing 12 teaspoons of salt and 8 teaspoons of sugar is an inexpensive substitute for short-term fluid loss; however, it does not contain potassium or bicarbonate. Fruit juices (except tomato juices), sodas, and other sugary drinks can also be considered the equivalent of water. In addition, ice pops and other frozen treats may help to encourage fluid intake by reluctant children.

School nurses can reinforce teaching in health classes. Many school-age children participate in sports activities. Encouraging adequate water and electrolyte intake before, during, and after strenuous exercise is important, particularly in hot weather. Discuss the dangers of fad diets, excessive training for sports, and eating disorders, especially with adolescents.

Nurses who work in industry should be aware of working conditions that could affect fluid and electrolyte balance. When employees must work in hot, humid environments and perform strenuous exercise, they should schedule periodic breaks so that adequate fluid and electrolyte replacement is possible. Nurses can be influential in supporting policies and legislation to ensure such practices.

Health teaching is especially important among older adults because older people often take medications such as diuretics that can increase the risk of fluid and electrolyte imbalance. Teaching is important to ensure patient compliance and to help prevent any problems that can occur with treatment. Teach patients how to detect signs of fluid and electrolyte imbalance, such as rapid weight gain or loss, swelling, changes in normal urine output, muscle weakness, or abnormal skin sensation, and give them guidelines for when to notify a provider. Senior citizen centers or community agencies can offer classes to reinforce good diet and appropriate fluid intake.

Nursing Interventions for Altered Fluid, Electrolyte, and Acid–Base Status

ORAL FLUIDS

Depending on the patient's current status, oral fluids may need to be regulated. If a potential or actual ECF volume or water deficit has been identified, institute a plan to increase oral intake of mildly salty fluids, oral rehydration fluids, sports drinks, or water. If the nursing diagnosis involves potential or actual ECF volume or water excess, curtail oral intake of salt and salty fluids or water. Providers also may order that fluids be either restricted or encouraged.

Increasing Oral Fluids

Instructions to *force fluids* or *push fluids* are general terms indicating that increased fluid intake is required. Individual goals should be set for each patient, depending on current fluid status. To enhance compliance, explain why the increased fluid intake is desirable and involve the patient in setting goals for fluid intake. Patient teaching and goal setting may include the family if the patient is unable or reluctant to drink fluids independently. Encourage the family members to offer fluids frequently during their visits, and teach them how to record intake and output.

Ensure that fluids are placed and kept within the patient's reach. Determine what water temperature the patient prefers, and change the water pitcher as often as needed to maintain that temperature. If the patient is unable to drink independently, ensure that you and your support staff offer fluids and encouragement to drink during every patient interaction. Some

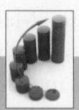

OUTCOME-BASED TEACHING PLANS

Mrs. Kern, a recent widow with a history of chronic bladder infections, comes to the clinic for a routine checkup. During your assessment, you discover she also has a problem with urinary frequency, which she controls by limiting her fluid intake. Mrs. Kern tells you that she drinks only one cup of tea at breakfast, lunch, and dinner, then nothing after dinner. That way, she does not have to worry about her urinary urgency problem.

OUTCOME

Mrs. Kern will verbalize a realistic plan to increase fluid intake.

STRATEGIES

- Discuss the reasons an increased fluid intake is desirable (e.g., decreased risk of kidney stones, decreased risk of bladder cancer).
- Explore Mrs. Kern's feelings about her pattern of urinary urgency.
- Discuss possible evaluations and assessments that could help Mrs. Kern discover the cause and resulting treatment for her urinary urgency.
- Review her daily pattern of fluid intake. Discuss other sources of fluid in addition to water. Question Mrs. Kern about her likes and dislikes regarding fluids.

- Problem-solve with Mrs. Kern a plan for increased fluid intake that she feels most inclined and motivated to follow.
- Encourage Mrs. Kern to increase her fluid intake with fluids she prefers throughout the day as a preventive measure for recurrent bladder infection.
- Have Mrs. Kern set up six to eight glasses of water in her refrigerator. Remind her to drink them throughout the day and to consume them all before she goes to bed at night. Encourage her to place a reminder sheet and checklist on the refrigerator door to aid in monitoring and adhering to the plan.
- Provide phone call follow-up to assess and provide encouragement for increasing Mrs. Kern's daily fluid intake.

EVALUATION

8/15/16: 11:00—Made follow-up phone call. Mrs. Kern is taking in 8 glasses of water daily. She prefers to take these prior to dinner to avoid urinating at night. She is following a regular voiding pattern every two hours to avoid her pattern of urgency. Follow up in the clinic in 2 weeks.

—S. Roberts, RN

---

patients may verbally refuse fluids, but when the straw or glass is respectfully and gently placed in their mouth and encouragement is given, they may decide to drink. Providing fluids that the patient especially likes may increase intake. Consider any dietary restrictions when providing patients with additional fluids. For example, a patient on a potassium-restricted diet should not be offered fluids high in potassium, such as orange juice. You and your support staff can also encourage foods that have a high fluid content, such as custards, soups, and ice creams.

When a specific fluid order is given (e.g., "Increase fluids to 2,000 mL per 24 hours"), plan how much the patient should consume in each shift (or equivalent period for patients at home). Usually, the largest volume is consumed during the daytime and early evening. Large amounts taken near bedtime may necessitate having to go to the bathroom during the night, thus interrupting sleep, and should be avoided.

Adequate fluid replacement also is necessary for patients who are receiving tube feedings. These patients may need additional water to prevent water deficit. They often cannot independently drink when they are thirsty or even notify a nurse or family member of their thirst. For this reason, carefully assess the fluid needs of patients receiving tube feedings, and administer water as needed.

Restricting Oral Fluids

Oral fluids may need to be restricted when ECF volume excess or water excess is present or when a patient has certain medical conditions, such as heart failure or renal failure. Assisting the patient to comply with limited fluid intake despite thirst can be a challenge.

The provider's orders for fluid restriction will include the number of milliliters of fluid to be taken every 24 hours. Most fluid restrictions include all fluids ingested. When a free water restriction is ordered, mainly free water is restricted; other fluids, such as tomato juice or milk, which contain at least 150 mEq/L of sodium, can be given in moderate amounts because they would not contribute to a water excess.

Plan with the patient and family how best to allocate the allotted fluid during a 24-hour period. Some patients prefer to drink with their meals, whereas others prefer to save the fluid and drink it between meals. Most fluids are designated for day and evening, with about 100 mL remaining for nighttime, in case the patient has to take medication or wants a drink. Ice chips may help people on fluid restriction. Ice melts to one half its volume and should be noted as such on the intake and output record. If necessary, remove any water containers from the room and offer water in small cups to avoid the temptation of drinking too much at one time. Diversional activities also may help the patient focus less on the thirst that he or she is experiencing.

To minimize thirst for patients on fluid restriction, avoid salty or very sweet fluids. Gum and hard candy may temporarily relieve thirst by drawing fluid into the oral cavity because the sugar content increases oral tonicity. Fifteen to 30 minutes later, however, oral membranes may be even drier than before. To avoid this rebound effect, sugar-free candy and gum may help. Dry foods, such as crackers and bread, also may increase the patient's feeling of thirst. Allowing the patient to rinse his or her mouth frequently may decrease thirst. The patient takes a sip of water, swishes it around the oral cavity, and then spits it out before swallowing. Avoid giving mouthwashes that contain alcohol because they have a drying effect. Frequent oral care is necessary for anyone on fluid restriction. Moisten the patient's lips with a water-soluble gel to prevent drying and cracking.

ELECTROLYTE REPLACEMENT

Diet Teaching

After the potential for an electrolyte imbalance has been identified, an individualized dietary teaching plan is needed. Provide the patient with a list of foods that are high or low in the identified electrolyte (Table 28-8). Give some guidelines for the amount to consume each day. For example, for the patient who has recently been prescribed a potassium-depleting diuretic, indicate the importance of eating at least one banana or other potassium-rich food each day. Also, teach the patient about the signs and symptoms of hypokalemia so that he or she can monitor and report if any occur.

TABLE 28-8	SELECTED DIETARY SOURCES FOR ELECTROLYTES
Electrolyte	**Dietary Source**
Sodium	Salt (sodium chloride), monosodium glutamate (MSG), soy sauce, dairy products (milk, cheese), processed food (luncheon meats, bacon), snack foods (peanuts, chips, pretzels), bouillon, canned or packaged soup, pickles, olives, sauerkraut, tomato juice
Potassium	Fruits (banana, cantaloupe, apricots, peaches, dates, raisins), vegetables (avocado, navy beans, potatoes, squash, carrots, cauliflower), orange juice, tomato juice
Calcium	Dairy products (milk, cheese, yogurt, ice cream), dark green vegetables (broccoli, spinach, greens), sardines, salmon, oysters, tofu
Magnesium	Nuts and peanut butter, egg yolk, milk, whole grain cereals, bananas, citrus fruit, dark green vegetables, legumes, seafood, chocolate
Phosphorus	Dairy products, meats, fish, bran and wheat cereals, nuts

Electrolyte Supplements

When normal dietary intake is insufficient, electrolyte supplements may be administered orally or intravenously. Liquid oral potassium supplements taste unpleasant and can be mixed with juice to promote compliance. IV administration is most commonly used for patients with severe electrolyte imbalances and for those who are unable to take anything orally. IV preparations of potassium must be administered carefully because a concentrated infusion can irritate the veins and also may cause rebound hyperkalemia, which is potentially lethal.

> **❗ SAFETY ALERT**
> Monitor patients receiving IV potassium carefully. Make sure the infusion rate does not exceed 10 to 20 mEq/hour, unless otherwise ordered.

INTRAVENOUS THERAPY

IV therapy is used to prevent or treat fluid and electrolyte imbalances. In hospitals, nurses are responsible for initiating, monitoring, and discontinuing IV infusions. Providers order the type and amount of IV fluid and electrolyte replacement. When IV fluid therapy is provided in the home, family members or visiting nurses assist with monitoring (see Chapter 3).

Home and Community Care

Many patients continue treatment for fluid and electrolyte imbalances at home, which may require dietary changes. Certain restrictions may be enforced, or certain foods may need to be encouraged. Give patients appropriate lists of foods, and work out a plan as to who will shop for and prepare meals. These tasks may tire patients who are weak from fluid or electrolyte imbalances.

Patients with fluid or electrolyte imbalances may take various medications. For each medication, emphasize its purpose, dosage, frequency, precautions, and potential side effects and complications. If the patient has a prescription for a medication (e.g., diuretic), explain the signs and symptoms of potential electrolyte imbalance and methods for circumventing the problem. For example, if the patient is taking a diuretic that enhances potassium excretion, reinforce the importance of the patient's replacing potassium by taking ordered supplements and making necessary dietary changes (e.g., eating bananas, dried apricots, and other fruits daily).

Teach patients with restricted sodium intake how to read food labels. Be sure that the patient understands that 1 g contains 1,000 mg because the food labels report sodium content in milligrams, whereas diet restrictions are usually given in g., for example, 2-g sodium diet. Also, have the patient or family member who does the cooking check the content of spices because many spice mixtures contain sodium chloride. Check with the provider before suggesting salt substitutes because many contain potassium, which may also need to be restricted.

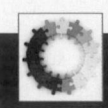

COLLABORATING WITH THE HEALTHCARE TEAM
The Home Health Nurse Calling a Provider for Fluid Issues in the Home

Mr. Jefferson, 87, has had diarrhea and some mild dizziness and nausea.

SITUATION: This is Maria Smith, the home health nurse for Mr. Jefferson, who was released from the hospital 2 days ago after treatment for community-acquired pneumonia.

BACKGROUND: Mrs. Jefferson, 85, is quite active and has provided good care for her husband but says that since discharge from the hospital, he hasn't been thirsty and hasn't eaten much. He has had diarrhea for the last day, with four liquid stools. He has been increasingly unsteady on his feet and not as bright and responsive as he was yesterday. I have assessed that Mr. Jefferson has poor skin turgor, his blood pressure demonstrates postural hypotension with dizziness and unsteadiness, and he seems a little lethargic.

ASSESSMENT: I am concerned that he is fluid depleted and that this might increase his risk for falls.

RECOMMENDATION: Would you order a bolus of IV fluids for Mr. Jefferson? Then, we can determine if adequate fluids will take care of this situation.

CRITICAL THINKING CHALLENGE
- Discuss the reasons why Mr. Jefferson may have a water deficit.
- What other suggestions could you make to Mrs. Jefferson to help her manage his fluid deficit?
- What support does Mrs. Jefferson need in this situation? Mr. Jefferson?

Because fluid and electrolyte imbalances can cause poor coordination, weakness, confusion, and altered gait, emphasize the need for a safe home environment. Such teaching may include assistance with ambulation or suggestions for safety features in the home (e.g., installing night-lights, removing throw rugs).

Explaining signs and symptoms that need to be relayed to the provider is an important part of patient teaching. For example, some providers want to know if the patient gains more than 5 lb or has an episode of vomiting or diarrhea that lasts for more than 1 day. The goal of patient teaching is to prevent or minimize future occurrences of fluid and/or electrolyte imbalances.

EVALUATION

Evaluation is important to ensure that the goals of promoting optimum fluid and electrolyte balance, preventing complications of imbalance, and increasing the patient's knowledge are achieved. Modifications or more realistic outcome criteria may be necessary if the goals are not attained.

Goal

The patient will reestablish normal fluid and electrolyte balance.

POSSIBLE OUTCOME CRITERIA

- The patient maintains equal intake and output within 300 mL in 24 hours.
- By discharge, the patient demonstrates weight within 2 kg of baseline weight (give specific amount to be lost or gained).
- The patient does not experience an increase or decrease in weight of more than 1 kg/day.

- By discharge, the patient has reestablished electrolyte values within normal limits.
- The patient experiences a decrease in postural pulse and blood pressure changes.
- By discharge, the patient verbalizes that he or she does not have excessive thirst.
- By discharge, the patient exhibits no signs or symptoms of edema.
- By discharge, the patient does not have concentrated urine.

Goal

The patient will demonstrate knowledge regarding how to promote future fluid and electrolyte balance.

POSSIBLE OUTCOME CRITERIA

- By the conclusion of the teaching session, the patient verbalizes the importance of drinking six to eight glasses of water per day.
- By the conclusion of the teaching session, the patient lists foods that are high in sodium and verbalizes needed modifications in diet.
- By the conclusion of the teaching session, the patient lists foods high in potassium.
- By the conclusion of the teaching session, the patient demonstrates an ability to read and understand a food label.
- The patient maintains a daily record of weight for the next month.
- The patient notifies the physician of any weight gain greater than 1 kg/day.
- By the conclusion of the teaching session, the patient verbalizes a plan to cope with temporary problems of diarrhea or vomiting.

PATIENT PLAN OF CARE
The Patient with Extracellular Fluid Volume Deficit

NURSING DIAGNOSIS

ECF Volume Deficit related to inadequate oral intake as manifested by concentrated urine, decrease in urine output, dry mucous membranes, postural hypotension, and change in postural tachycardia.

PATIENT GOAL

Patient will reestablish normal fluid and electrolyte balance.

PATIENT OUTCOME CRITERIA

Patient has urine output greater than 30 mL/hour and no more postural tachycardia or hypotension.

NURSING INTERVENTION	SCIENTIFIC RATIONALE
1. Monitor intake and output.	**1.** Observation of trends in intake and output provides essential data regarding patient's fluid and electrolyte status and guides interventions. Intake should approximately equal output, but observing for trends and significant increase or decrease is more important than specific numbers.
2. Monitor serum electrolytes, serum osmolality, and urine specific gravity	**2.** Monitoring these common laboratory values provides essential data regarding patient status and guides interventions.
3. Increase oral fluid intake to at least 2,000 mL/24 h of mildly salty solutions or as ordered by physician.	**3.** Increased intake of fluids (and high fluid–content foods) helps correct fluid volume deficit and maintain adequate hydration.
4. Monitor IV fluid therapy as prescribed.	**4.** Fluids must be provided when patient cannot obtain adequate intake by oral intake alone. Monitoring ensures infusion at prescribed rate and allows early detection of complications.
5. Assess fluid preferences.	**5.** Patient is more likely to increase fluid intake with fluids that are appealing.
6. Ensure optimal access to preferred fluids, and assist as needed.	**6.** Availability and assistance are necessary to ensure increased fluid intake.
7. Give positive reinforcement or verbal cueing as necessary.	**7.** Reinforcement helps to increase compliance for patients who may be forgetful or disinterested.

EVALUATION

8/15/16: 09:30—Patient intake 1,600 mL and output 1,200 mL. Weight has increased by 1 kg. Serum sodium, potassium, and calcium are within normal limits. BUN: creatinine ratio normal. Prefers cranberry juice instead of water. Provided positive feedback for attempts to increase fluids. Will leave juice at bedside and remind to drink every hour.

—S. Roberts, RN

Goal

The patient will remain free from complications of fluid or electrolyte imbalance.

POSSIBLE OUTCOME CRITERIA

- The patient stands and walks without dizziness or falling.
- The skin remains intact despite edema until edema is reduced.

KEY CONCEPTS

- Homeostasis of body fluids, electrolytes, and pH is necessary for cellular function and health maintenance. Processes such as diffusion, osmosis, active transport, and filtration that facilitate fluid or electrolyte movement maintain homeostasis.
- ICF refers to the fluid within the cells of the body; ECF refers to fluid outside the cell and includes the intravascular fluid and the interstitial fluid.

■ Cations are positively charged electrolytes (sodium, potassium, calcium, and magnesium); anions are negatively charged electrolytes (chloride, phosphate, sulfate, and bicarbonate). Balance between anions and cations is a dynamic process that is necessary to maintain neutrality. The electrolyte composition of ICF and ECF is different although the osmolality is the same in all body fluids.

■ Inadequate intake; excessive loss through vomiting, diarrhea, diaphoresis, or use of diuretics; stress; and chronic illness such as renal, cardiac, or respiratory failure, surgery, or pregnancy can increase the potential for altered fluid, electrolyte, and acid–base balance.

■ States of altered fluid balance include ECF volume excess or deficit and water excess or deficit.

■ States of electrolyte imbalance include hyperkalemia, hypokalemia, hypercalcemia, hypocalcemia, hypermagnesemia, hypomagnesemia, hyperphosphatemia, and hypophosphatemia.

■ States of altered acid–base balance include respiratory acidosis, metabolic acidosis, respiratory alkalosis, and metabolic alkalosis.

■ Alterations in normal fluid, electrolyte, or acid–base balance are manifested by imbalances in intake and output, weight gain or loss, changes in mental status, changes in vital signs, abnormal states of tissue hydration, or abnormal neuromuscular status.

■ Intake and output, weight, edema, tissue turgor, neck vein and hand vein engorgement, and vital signs are important objective data to collect to identify actual problems in fluid and electrolyte status. Laboratory data, such as serum electrolytes, serum osmolality, urine specific gravity, and arterial blood gases, also provide important information for identifying potential disruption in fluid and electrolyte status.

■ Important nursing interventions include preventive health teaching; regulating oral fluids; assisting with electrolyte replacement; initiating, regulating, and monitoring IV therapy; and monitoring blood transfusions.

PRACTICING FOR THE NCLEX
CHECK YOUR ANSWERS IN APPENDIX A.

1. A nurse is caring for a 65-year-old patient with pneumonia. The arterial blood gases come back as pH 7.25, $PaCO_2$ 52 mm Hg, HCO_3^- 24 mEq/L, and PaO_2 66 mm Hg. The nurse interprets these blood gases as:
   a. Respiratory alkalosis
   b. Respiratory acidosis
   c. Metabolic alkalosis
   d. Metabolic acidosis

2. A patient has pitting edema in the extremities and generalized edema throughout the body. The nurse recognizes that these are symptoms of:
   a. Extracellular volume excess
   b. Extracellular volume deficit
   c. Intracellular volume excess
   d. Intracellular volume deficit

3. A patient has had 3 days of nausea, vomiting, and diarrhea. The nurse expects the following abnormal findings. Select all that apply.
   a. Hypokalemia
   b. Peripheral edema
   c. Low blood pressure
   d. Diaphoresis

4. A nurse is caring for a group of patients. Which of the following patients is highest priority for an intervention related to fluid and electrolyte imbalance? A patient with:
   a. Pulse 60, nausea
   b. Blood pressure 88/50, dizziness
   c. Respirations 20, pain
   d. Temperature 37.4°C, warm

5. A nurse is interacting with a new parent of a newborn who has vomiting, diarrhea, and fever. Which of the following topics is most important to include in patient teaching?
   a. Commercial solutions are relatively costly.
   b. Serious problems can develop quickly.
   c. Fluid needs of infants are different from those of adults.
   d. New parents may be overly concerned.

6. A patient in the hospital has an intake of 450 mL, output of 1,200 mL, thirst, dry mouth, and poor skin turgor. Which of the following interventions are indicated? Select all that apply:
   a. Ensure that fluids are kept within the patient's reach.
   b. Assess which juices the patient prefers.
   c. Monitor daily weight at the same time every day.
   d. Assess electrolytes for elevated serum sodium.

7. A nurse is visiting a patient in the home setting. The patient has a weight gain of 2.5 kg in 1 day, has 3+ peripheral edema, and has crackles in the bases of the lungs. The patient is also noting that her rings are tight and that she is having some shortness of breath. Which of the following is the most important intervention?
   a. Consult with the dietician about nutritional supplements.
   b. Instruct the patient to take periodic rest breaks during the day.
   c. Contact the physician to further evaluate a treatment plan.
   d. Teach the patient to increase potassium in the diet.

8. Which nursing statement is most appropriate when a patient has been on fluid restriction for 2 days?
   a. "It might help to rinse your mouth frequently."
   b. "I will get you some mouthwash to swish in your mouth."
   c. "I will get you some cranberry and orange juice."
   d. "Have your partner bring in some lemon drops."

9. A patient with dehydration is having his electrolyte values drawn by the laboratory each morning. The patient asks the nurse, "Why are you drawing my blood so much?" The nurse's best response is:
   a. "The physician ordered it for you"
   b. "I don't know; I'll find out"
   c. "It shows the balance of protein"
   d. "To see if you need any replacements"

10. A 78-year-old patient is admitted to the hospital. The nurse expects the patient to respond to treatment based upon which of the following principles? Select all that apply:
   a. Older adults often experience imbalances due to chronic disease.
   b. The use of medications such as diuretics or laxatives can cause an ECF deficit.
   c. Electrolyte imbalances may occur due to bowel preparation for a procedure.
   d. An acute illness often predisposes an older adult to fluid imbalances.

REFERENCES

Berl, T., & Schrier, R. W. (2010). Disorders of water homeostasis. In R. W. Schrier (Ed.), *Renal and electrolyte disorders* (7th ed., pp. 1–44). Philadelphia, PA: Lippincott Williams & Wilkins.

Fox, E. R., Benjamin, E. J., Sarpong, D. F., Nagarajarao, H., Taylor, J.K., Steffes, M. W., et al. (2011). The relation of C-reactive protein to chronic kidney disease in African Americans: The Jackson Heart Study. Retrieved July 28, 2011, from http://cme.medscape.com/viewarticle/717453

Hartford Institute for Geriatric Nursing. (2012). Normal aging changes. Retrieved from http://consultgerirn.org/topics/normal_aging_changes/want_to_know_more#item_6

Herdman, T. H., & Kamitsuru, S. (Eds.). (2014). *Nursing diagnoses: Definitions and classification, 2015–2017.* West Sussex, UK: Wiley-Blackwell.

Imamura, T., Kinugawa, K., Hatano, M., Fujino, T., Inaba, T., Maki, H., et al. (2014). Low cardiac output stimulates vasopressin release in patients with stage D heart failure: Its relevance to poor prognosis and reversal by surgical treatment. *Circulation Journal, 78*(9), 2259–2267. doi: http://dx.doi.org/101253/cirj.CJ-14-0368

Metheny, N. M. (2012). *Fluid and electrolyte balance: Nursing considerations* (5th ed.). Sudbury, MA: Jones & Bartlett.

Parra-Blanco, A., Ruiz, A., Alvarez-Lobos, M., Amoros, A., Gana, J., Ibanez, P., et al. (2014). Achieving the best bowel preparation for colonoscopy. *World Journal of Gastroenterology, 20*(47), 17709–17726. doi: 10.3748/wjg.v20.i47.17709

Popovtzer, M. M. (2010). Disorders of calcium, phosphorus, vitamin D and parathyroid hormone activity. In R. W. Schrier (Ed.), *Renal and electrolyte disorders* (7th ed., pp. 166–228). Philadelphia, PA: Lippincott Williams & Wilkins.

Report of the DGAC on the Dietary Guidelines for Americans. (2010). Part D. Section 6: Sodium, potassium and water. Retrieved from www.cnpp.usda.gov/Publications/DietaryGuidelines/2010/DGAC/Report/D-6-SodiumPotassiumWater.pdf

Seo, D., King, M., Kim, N., Sovinski, D., Meade, R., & Lederer, A. (2014). Predictors for persistent overweight, deteriorated weight status, and improved weight status during 18 months in a school-based longitudinal cohort. *American Journal of Health Promotion.* doi: http://dx.doi.org/10.4278/ajhp.131118-QUAN-585

Spiegel, D. (2010). Normal and abnormal magnesium metabolism. In R. W. Schrier (Ed.), *Renal and electrolyte disorders* (7th ed., pp. 229–250). Philadelphia, PA: Lippincott Williams & Wilkins.

UNICEF/WHO. (2009). *Diarrhoea: Why children are still dying and what can be done.* New York, NY: UNICEF.

Urso, C., Brucculeri, S., & Caimi, G. (2014). Physiopathological, epidemiological, clinical and therapeutic aspects of exercise-associated hyponatremia. *Journal of Clinical Medicine, 3*(4), 1258–1275. doi:10.3390/jcm3041258

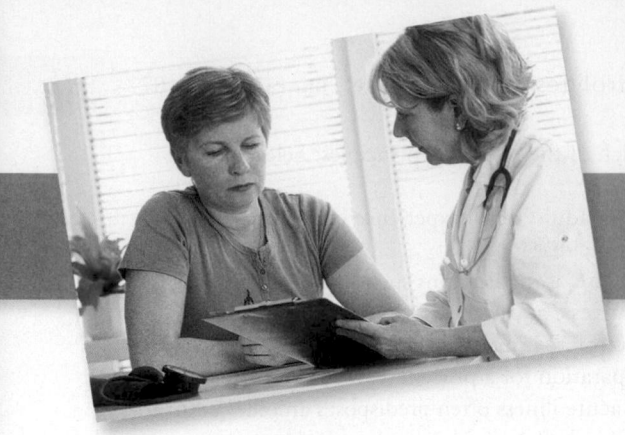

CHAPTER 29

Nutrition

Judith L. St. Onge

Case Scenario

You are a nurse working in a wellness clinic. Your next patient is a 42-year-old woman who expresses a desire to lose weight. She has tried numerous diet programs and was able to lose weight for a short while but always gained the weight back plus some. Her body mass index (BMI) is 28. She states that she usually does not eat breakfast in the morning but has a diet soda to keep her energy up. For lunch, she eats a fast-food sandwich and a salad, and for dinner, she eats with her family. How will you respond to this patient, addressing both her nutritional needs and weight management?

Once you have completed this chapter and have added the many facets of nutrition to your knowledge base, return to the above scenario and reflect on the following areas of Critical Thinking:

1. Describe your immediate impressions, and identify the knowledge and values that led you to them.
2. Determine what you would focus on for people beginning a weight loss program.
3. Describe how being overweight or obese can affect one's health.
4. Contrast and compare your assessments for possible biologic and psychological factors related to weight.
5. Describe the essential components of weight loss and weight maintenance programs for people at the wellness clinic.

KEY TERMS

absorption
anorexia
anorexia nervosa
basal metabolism
calorie (kilocalorie)
carbohydrates
complete proteins
digestion
disaccharide
fats
fiber
gastric residual volumes (GRVs)
glycogenesis
incomplete proteins
macronutrients
metabolism
micronutrients
monosaccharide
monounsaturated fatty acid (MUFA)
nutrients
obese
overweight
partially complete proteins
polysaccharide
polyunsaturated fatty acid (PUFA)
proteins
saturated fats
small-bore feeding tubes
trans fatty acids
trace elements
underweight
unsaturated fats
vitamins

LEARNING OBJECTIVES

Upon completion of this chapter, you will be able to do the following:

1. Identify essential nutrients and examples of good dietary sources for each.
2. Describe normal digestion, absorption, and metabolism of carbohydrates, fats, and proteins.
3. Discuss nutritional considerations across the life span.
4. List factors that can affect dietary patterns.
5. Describe manifestations of altered nutrition.
6. Explain nursing interventions to promote optimal nutrition and health.
7. Discuss nursing responsibilities for interventions used to treat altered nutritional states.

As part of a holistic approach to good health, a nutritionally adequate diet is vital for promoting normal growth and development and preventing deficiency states. Optimal nutrition is essential to maintain health and to prevent disease. An adequate diet is necessary to maintain bodily functions, healthy tissues, and body temperature; to promote healing; and to build resistance to infection.

Nutrients are biochemical substances obtained from ingested food and fluids. **Carbohydrates**, **proteins**, and fats are nutrients that supply the body with energy. **Vitamins**, minerals, **trace elements**, and water are not sources of energy but are important in regulating body processes.

The body cannot synthesize essential nutrients in adequate amounts; therefore, the body must receive them through the diet. Dietary intake of nonessential nutrients is not required because the body can synthesize such nutrients in adequate amounts or does not require them for body functioning.

Nurses are in key positions to assess, monitor, and promote good nutrition. In many settings (e.g., health fairs, classes in schools and community centers, and interactions with families during health screening), they can teach principles of normal nutrition. Nurses can participate in educating individuals and groups to reverse the growing number of illnesses related to obesity and sedentary lifestyles. Nurses also screen for altered nutritional states to detect obesity, **overweight**, malnutrition, and **anorexia**. Nutritional assessment is important for all preoperative patients. Nurses teach patients and family members how to adapt to dietary prescriptions or restrictions, especially when special diets are necessary. Nurses also are responsible for monitoring nutritional therapies, such as enteral tube feedings or parenteral nutrition, which may be necessary to maintain optimal nutrition in patients with significant impairments.

INTRODUCTION TO NUTRITION

The body uses nutrients to build and maintain body tissues, furnish energy, and regulate body processes. Cellular composition is constantly changing. Cells need nutrients to supply building materials, such as calcium for teeth and bones and fat for padding and support of vital organs. Each cell requires energy to fulfill its daily tasks. Chemicals in the form of nutrients act and react to regulate body processes, which can be as basic as breathing or as circumstantial as wound healing. Water, which makes up one half to two thirds of adult weight, is an important regulator in body processes.

The body breaks down ingested nutrients into a form that it can absorb and use. **Metabolism** is the process by which cells use or store energy from nutrients. Anabolic processes build up substances and body tissues; catabolic processes break down substances or body stores. The body uses stored energy when the person is not eating, as in a serious illness, or when there is an increased need for nutrients, such as following trauma or during pregnancy.

Energy obtained from food is measured in large calories (kilocalories, abbreviated kcal or Cal). The large **calorie (kilocalorie)** is the amount of heat required to raise 1 kg of water 1°C.

NUTRIENTS

Nutrients, or food containing elements for normal body functioning, are divided into six categories: carbohydrates, proteins, fats, vitamins, minerals, and water. The first three are called **macronutrients** because the body uses them in relatively large amounts. The next two are **micronutrients**, or substances used by the body in small quantities. A subgroup of minerals is called trace elements. The metabolism of carbohydrates, fats, and protein provides energy. Water is essential to maintain normal fluid balance and promote normal **digestion**, **absorption**, and metabolism of food. Vitamins and minerals are organic and inorganic compounds important for normal body processes.

At one time, public health professionals were more concerned about people with nutrient deficiencies, and guidelines were written to help prevent these deficiencies. Current concerns, however, are related to avoiding excesses for possible prevention of chronic diet-related diseases. A discussion of normal nutrition and advice for healthy eating follows. Because no single food supplies all essential nutrients, people should eat various foods.

Types of Nutrients

CARBOHYDRATES

Carbohydrates are simple sugars (**monosaccharides** and **disaccharides**) and complex sugars (**polysaccharides**). They are composed of carbon, hydrogen, and oxygen. Sugars, syrups, molasses, honey, fruit, and milk are excellent sources of simple carbohydrates. Bread, cereal, potatoes, rice, pasta, crackers, flour products, and legumes contain complex carbohydrates.

The main function of carbohydrates is to provide energy. Each gram of oxidized carbohydrate yields about 4 kcal. Carbohydrates also are important for oxidizing fats in normal fat metabolism; promoting desirable bacterial growth in the gastrointestinal (GI) tract, which contributes to the synthesis of vitamin K and small amounts of vitamin B_{12}; producing the carbon component in the synthesis of nonessential amino acids; and producing other essential body acids and compounds.

Polysaccharides not digested in the GI tract are one of the main components of dietary **fiber**. Dietary fiber is a minimal source of energy but plays an essential role in stimulating peristalsis and maintaining normal bowel elimination. Another characteristic of carbohydrates is their protein-sparing action. Protein sparing occurs when the body uses carbohydrates, rather than protein, as a source of energy, thus sparing protein for the vital function of tissue building.

The circulation of blood supplies glucose to the cells as a source of energy and for the production of vital substances. The blood glucose level is maintained within relatively narrow limits (about 80 to 110 mg per deciliter or 3.9 to 6.1 mmol per liter). In the fasting state, the blood glucose level is about 60 to 80 mg per deciliter, but if measured 2 hours after a meal, it can rise to 140 to 180 mg per deciliter, depending on the person's age. Hyperglycemia, in which the blood glucose level is higher than normal due to impaired production or use of insulin, occurs in diabetes mellitus. Hypoglycemia, in which the blood glucose level is lower than normal, can be symptomatic of liver or pancreatic abnormalities.

PROTEINS

Proteins are organic compounds composed of polymers of amino acids connected by peptide bonds. They contain carbon, hydrogen, oxygen, and nitrogen. Depending on the specific amino acids of which they are composed, proteins also may contain trace elements such as iron or copper. The body synthesizes these proteins for specific functions, including hemoglobin for carrying oxygen to tissues, insulin for blood glucose regulations, and albumin for regulating osmotic pressure in the blood. These functions generally cannot be performed by another body protein.

Proteins are vital to growth, development, and normal functioning of almost all body systems. They are major constituents of most living cells and body fluids, including bones, skin, teeth, muscle, hair, blood, and serum. The main functions of proteins include growth, regulation of body functions and processes, replacement of cellular proteins, and energy. Protein catabolism supplies 4 kcal per gram. Protein also plays an important role in regulatory functions and in the body's immune system. Catalytic enzymes derived from proteins function in the regulation of digestion, absorption, metabolism, and catabolism.

Dietary proteins can be classified as complete, partially complete, or incomplete. **Complete proteins** contain sufficient amounts of the essential amino acids to maintain body tissues and to promote growth. The diet must supply essential amino acids because the body cannot synthesize them at a rate sufficient to meet its needs. The body can synthesize nonessential amino acids from available sources. An adequate diet contains a good supply of essential and nonessential amino acids. Good sources of complete proteins are meat, fish, poultry, milk, cheese, and eggs.

Partially complete proteins contain sufficient amounts of amino acids to maintain life but do not promote growth. **Incomplete proteins** do not contain sufficient amounts of all essential amino acids to maintain life, build tissue, or promote growth. By themselves, incomplete proteins are not compatible with maintaining life. Sources of incomplete protein are dried peas and beans, peanut butter, seeds, fruits and vegetables, bread, cereal, rice, and pasta.

Protein requirements depend on a person's state of health, age, body weight, nutritional state, stress level, activity level, and other factors. One measure of protein requirement is the state of nitrogen balance. Nitrogen equilibrium, the normal state for a healthy adult, exists when the amount of nitrogen taken in equals the amount of nitrogen excreted. A state of positive nitrogen balance exists when the intake of nitrogen is greater than the amount excreted. This situation exists when new tissues are being synthesized, as in recovery from illness, athletic training, pregnancy, and childhood growth. A negative nitrogen balance exists when the excretion of nitrogen exceeds the intake. This undesirable condition may exist when a disease or treatment is causing excessive tissue breakdown or when the diet is inadequate in protein, calories, or both.

FATS

Fats, also called lipids, include neutral fats, oils, fatty acids, cholesterol, and phospholipids. Fats are organic substances composed of carbon, hydrogen, and oxygen. They are a significant component of the North American diet.

Fat is a component of all body cells and ideally makes up approximately 20% of the body weight of healthy, nonobese people. Fat performs many important functions, including cellular transport, insulation, protection of vital organs in the form of padding, provision of energy, energy storage of adipose tissue, vitamin absorption, and transport of fat-soluble vitamins (vitamins A, D, E, and K).

The energy value of fats is significant. Fats supply 9 kcal per gram of oxidized fat, which is more than twice as much energy per gram provided by oxidation of an equal amount of proteins and carbohydrates. Fats provide taste, consistency, and stability and have a significant satiety value—they provide a feeling of fullness because they remain in the stomach longer than do carbohydrates and proteins.

Based on chemical differences, fats are classified as saturated or unsaturated. Chemically, **saturated fats** have two hydrogen atoms attached to each of the carbon atoms in the carbon atom chain. **Unsaturated fats** have a single hydrogen atom missing from each of two side-by-side carbon atoms; as a result, a double bond forms between the two carbon atoms. This bond is an "unsaturation," and this fatty acid is called **monounsaturated fatty acid (MUFA)**. With two or more carbon-to-carbon double bonds present, this fatty acid is called **polyunsaturated fatty acid (PUFA)**. Unsaturated fat molecules with an unusual configuration around the double carbon bond(s) (i.e., trans location vs. cis location on the carbon chain) are called trans fats or **trans fatty acids**. These trans fats are found in nature as a result of fermentation in grazing animals and can form during hydrogenation (addition of hydrogen). These differences are significant in terms of the physical characteristics of the fats, including such factors as melting point, hardness, the ability to form an emulsion, and body response to these different fats.

Most sources of fat contain a combination of saturated and unsaturated fatty acids. Sources of animal fats, especially beef and lamb, generally contain a higher percentage of saturated fatty acids and are harder than vegetable sources of fatty acids. Coconut oil, palm oil, and palm kernel oil also are highly saturated. Chicken fat contains a significantly higher percentage of unsaturated fatty acids and is measurably softer than beef or lamb fat. Fish and vegetable sources are classified as unsaturated because they contain a higher percentage of unsaturated fatty acids and are generally softer than animal fats. Fried and baked goods often have trans fats.

VITAMINS

Vitamins are organic compounds that are essential to the body in small quantities for growth, development, maintenance, and reproduction (see Appendix D for the Summary of Vitamins).

They do not supply energy, but they assist in the use of energy nutrients. Most vitamins cannot be synthesized by the body and must therefore be supplied by the diet. Dietary Reference Intakes (DRIs) are expanded standards for nutrient intake; DRIs are discussed in detail in the Nutritional Guidelines section later in the chapter. Appendix D offers current clinically useful DRI values. Vitamins are present in small quantities in food. In varying degrees, exposure to light, air, heat, and some types of food preparation can destroy them. For this reason, fresh foods are usually the best source of vitamins. Some foods, such as fortified milk or cereals, have extra vitamins added. The widespread use of vitamin supplements has recently been questioned by nutrition professionals suggesting that well-nourished adults do not need them (Guallar, Stranges, Mulrow, Appel, & Miller, 2013). Other experts support vitamin supplementation by pointing out that most Americans do not get sufficient quantities of essential vitamins in their diets (Linus Pauling Institute, 2014). More evidence is needed on this important debate. Vitamins are classified as fat soluble or water soluble.

Fat-Soluble Vitamins

Fat-soluble vitamins (A, D, E, and K) are absorbed with fat into the circulation. A deficiency of fat-soluble vitamins can occur when fat digestion or absorption is altered. Excess fat-soluble vitamins are stored in the liver or adipose tissue; therefore, excessive intake of vitamins A and D can cause toxicity.

Vitamin A. Vitamin A is important in the following:

- Maintenance of normal vision, especially in dim light
- Maintenance of healthy epithelium
- Promotion of normal skeletal and tooth development
- Promotion of normal cellular proliferation

The effects of vitamin A deficiency are significant, and in many countries, vitamin A deficiency is the most prevalent vitamin deficiency. Signs of vitamin A deficiency:

- Night or total blindness
- Epithelial changes, such as keratinization (progressive degeneration of the cells that may lead to infections in the eyes, ears, or nasal passages)
- Follicular hyperkeratosis (skin changes leading to rough, dry, and scaly skin)
- Dryness of the eyes (xerophthalmia)
- Inadequate tooth and bone development

Vitamin A is stored in the liver, and excessive intake can be toxic.

Vitamin D. Vitamin D is changed to an active form by exposure of the skin to ultraviolet light. The liver and kidney also play a role in vitamin D metabolism. Vitamin D is important in the following:

- Intestinal absorption of calcium
- Mobilization of calcium and phosphorus from bone
- Renal reabsorption of calcium

These effects increase the blood levels of calcium and phosphorus, allowing for normal mineralization of bone and cartilage and maintenance of calcium in extracellular fluid for normal muscle contraction.

A deficiency in vitamin D intake is significant because it leads to inadequate absorption of calcium and phosphorus and a deficiency of mineralization in bones and teeth. The bones become soft and cannot bear weight, resulting in skeletal deformities. Signs of vitamin D deficiency:

- Rickets in children
- Poor dental health
- Tetany (muscle twitching and convulsions caused by low serum calcium)
- Osteomalacia (soft bones and a tendency toward spontaneous fractures secondary to vitamin D and calcium deficiency)

Excessive amounts can be toxic. Some older adults may exhibit poor vitamin D status.

Vitamin E. The physiologic effects of vitamin E are not well understood. A major function is its role as an antioxidant, in which vitamin E assists in maintaining the integrity of cellular membranes and protecting vitamin A from oxidation. Vitamin E deficiency is rare, but signs of severe deficiency are increased hemolysis of red blood cells, poor reflexes and impaired neuromuscular functioning, and anemia.

The body does not store vitamin E to any appreciable extent, and toxicity is rare.

Vitamin K. An adequate intake of vitamin K is needed in the liver for the formation of prothrombin and other clotting factors. The major physiologic effect of vitamin K appears to be its role in blood coagulation.

Vitamin K deficiencies are manifested in two ways: an increased tendency to hemorrhage (prolonged clotting time) and hemorrhagic disease of the newborn, which is most common in premature or anoxic newborns.

Approximately half of the body's requirement of vitamin K is synthesized by bacteria in the lower intestinal tract. The body does not store vitamin K to an appreciable extent. Large amounts are not usually toxic, except in newborns.

Water-Soluble Vitamins

The water-soluble vitamins are the B-complex vitamins and vitamin C. Water-soluble vitamins are not stored in the body, although some body tissues can hold limited amounts. Adequate daily intake of water-soluble vitamins is recommended to prevent deficiencies. When the intake of water-soluble vitamins exceeds the amount absorbed by the tissues, the excess is excreted in the urine.

B-Complex Vitamins. Each B-complex vitamin has its own function and DRI value set. Vitamin B_1 (thiamine) functions in carbohydrate metabolism, and adequate thiamine intake results in healthy nerve functioning and normal appetite and digestion. Deficiency symptoms include poor appetite, apathy, mental depression, fatigue, constipation, edema, cardiac failure, and neuritis. The disease associated with inadequate thiamine intake is beriberi. Acute beriberi adversely affects the cardiac, nervous, and GI systems. Death can result from cardiac failure.

Vitamin B_2 (riboflavin) functions in protein and carbohydrate metabolism and contributes to healthy skin and normal vision. Deficiency symptoms are cheilosis (cracking and fissures at the corners of the mouth), dermatitis, increased vascularization of the cornea, and other vision irregularities.

Vitamin B_3 (niacin) is involved in glycogen metabolism, tissue regeneration, and fat synthesis. The niacin deficiency disease is pellagra; its symptoms are fatigue, headache, loss of appetite and weight loss, abdominal pain, diarrhea, dermatitis, and neurologic deterioration.

Vitamin B_{12} (cyanocobalamin) functions in the formation of mature red blood cells and in the synthesis of DNA and RNA. It requires intrinsic factor, a substance produced in the stomach, for absorption. A vitamin B_{12} deficiency leads to pernicious anemia, other forms of anemia, and neurologic deterioration. This vitamin is found only in animal foods (meats, fish, poultry, milk, and eggs).

Folic acid functions as a coenzyme in protein metabolism and cell growth. Folic acid is necessary for red blood cell formation. Folic acid has been suggested to prevent vascular clots in the hearts or brains of people with high circulating levels of homocysteine, an amino acid. Deficiency signs include glossitis, diarrhea, macrocytic anemia, and birth defects. Although recent evidence suggests that most Americans consume adequate folic acid, certain groups are at risk for deficiency. These groups include women of childbearing years, non-Hispanic Black women, people with alcohol dependence, and individuals with malabsorption disorders (NIH, 2012). Folic acid deficiency in pregnant women can lead to neural tube deficits (e.g., spina bifida) in the fetus. Because fetal neural development begins so early in pregnancy, women in their childbearing years must have adequate folic acid intake. Folic acid occurs in most foods, particularly dark leafy green vegetables, fruits, nuts, beans, peas, meat, eggs, seafood, and grains (NIH, 2012).

Other important B vitamins are vitamin B_6, pantothenic acid, and biotin. Deficiencies are rare.

Vitamin C. Vitamin C is important in the following:

- Protection against infection
- Adequate wound healing
- Collagen formation
- Iron absorption
- Metabolism of several important amino acids

Vitamin C is an antioxidant that protects vitamins A and E from excessive oxidation. Signs of vitamin C deficiency are inadequate formation of collagen (poor wound healing), increased susceptibility to infection, retardation of growth and development, joint pain, and anemia. Scurvy, although rare, is associated with a deficiency of vitamin C from a lack of fresh fruits and vegetables, particularly citrus fruits in the diet. The body stores little vitamin C, so a daily supply is needed. Although large doses of vitamin C (30 to 100 times the recommended

allowances) have not proved toxic, excessive doses are not advised because of the possibility of kidney stone formation and GI disturbances.

MINERALS

Minerals are inorganic substances found in nearly all body tissues and fluids. When plant or animal tissue is burned, what remains is ash or mineral matter. Minerals help build body tissues and regulate metabolism. There are more than 25 known minerals in the adult body; the most notable are described here and in Appendix D, which shows current clinically useful DRI values.

Calcium

Almost all of the calcium in the body is found in the bones and teeth. The bones provide the framework for the body and are a storage area that keeps the plasma concentration of calcium relatively constant. Calcium, the most abundant mineral in the body, is important in the following:

- Conversion of prothrombin to thrombin and other steps of the coagulation process
- Nerve impulse transmission by participating in the formation of acetylcholine
- Regulation of materials in and out of cells
- Contraction and relaxation of muscles, most notably the heart muscle

Calcium is absorbed mainly from the duodenum by active transport. Calcium is also passively diffused across the intestinal mucosa from the jejunum and the ileum. The amount of calcium absorbed is determined mainly by the body's need. About 30% to 40% of dietary calcium is absorbed in the healthy adult. Children, adolescents, and pregnant and lactating women absorb a greater percentage of their dietary calcium because of their increased need. Some ingested calcium forms insoluble salts, which cannot be absorbed.

Adequate amounts of vitamin D, parathyroid hormone, ascorbic acid, lactose, several other amino acids, and physical activity assist in calcium absorption. Inadequate amounts of vitamin D, insufficient exposure to sunlight, decreased amounts of ascorbic acid, decreased physical activity, and emotional stress may decrease calcium absorption. Other factors, such as a high consumption of dietary fiber and excessive phosphorus intake, impair the absorption of calcium. These factors are still being researched.

The effects of calcium deficiency can be profound. Rickets, a disease of infants and children caused by inadequate calcium and vitamin D, involves the inadequate deposition of calcium and phosphorus in the bone. Symptoms include soft bones, enlarged joints, enlarged skull secondary to delayed closure of the cranial fontanelles, bowed legs, and spinal and chest deformities. Osteomalacia, the adult form of rickets, results from inadequate intake of calcium, phosphorus, and vitamin D. The mineral content of the bone is reduced, but the bone stays the same size.

Osteoporosis involves a reduction in bone mass. It is commonly seen in postmenopausal women and in elderly men. Factors contributing to the development of osteoporosis may include a chronically insufficient calcium intake, decreased estrogens, hereditary factors, smoking, race, and decreased physical activity. Symptoms vary in severity and may include reduced bone mass, leading to poor posture; increased fragility of bones, leading to an increase in bone fractures; and delayed healing of fractures. Malabsorption syndromes can lead to problems in calcium absorption, and osteoporosis can develop. Low dietary intake of calcium also has been associated with hypertension.

Iron

Most iron in the body is found in hemoglobin, the red-pigmented, iron-containing protein. Hemoglobin carries oxygen from the lungs to the tissues and helps transport carbon dioxide to the lungs. Iron is also found in the body's myoglobin, an iron–protein deficiency compound in the muscle that is an oxygen storage system for the muscles.

Iron deficiencies may manifest themselves in iron deficiency anemia. This form of anemia is not uncommon, especially in infants, adolescents, and menstruating women. In anemia, circulating hemoglobin is reduced, and the blood cannot provide for the oxygen needs of the tissues. Iron deficiency anemia may result from a diet chronically deficient in iron. Other factors that may lead to iron deficiency anemia are blood loss, chronic disease, pregnancy and lactation, diarrhea, and other nutritional deficiencies (protein and calorie). Symptoms of iron deficiency anemia are excessive fatigue, lethargy, and poor resistance to infection. Because obtaining sufficient iron to combat anemia by dietary measures alone is impractical, recommended treatment includes taking iron salts (ferrous sulfate or gluconate) along with a well-balanced diet.

Sodium

Sodium is found primarily in the extracellular fluid in the body. As an ion, it helps maintain fluid and acid–base balance. The average diet contains more sodium than the body requires, and sodium deficiencies (except rarely) have not been identified. Many people would benefit from eating less sodium, and sodium restriction is important for people with heart disease, hypertension, edema, renal disorders, liver disease, or pregnancy-induced hypertension. Only 12% of dietary sodium intake is from natural food sources. More than 75% of the sodium Americans eat is from restaurant, packaged, and processed foods, and 11% is added during cooking or at the table (CDC, 2012).

Potassium

Potassium is found primarily in the body's intracellular fluid. It functions in protein synthesis, in fluid balance (as an ion), and in regulation of muscle contraction. The adequate intake (AI) level of potassium for males and females aged 14 years and older is 4.7 g/day; for lactating females, the value is 5.1 g/day. The AI for children aged 1 to 3 years is 3.0 g/day; 4 to 8 years, 3.8 g/day; and 9 to 13 years, 4.5 g/day. No upper intake levels (ULs) are set, and deficiencies have not been identified, except in cases such as severe vomiting, diarrhea, use of non–potassium-sparing diuretics, and diabetic acidosis. Potassium restriction is indicated for patients with renal impairment or renal failure. Potassium is present in many foods, including protein-rich foods, bread, cereal, fruits, and vegetables.

Iodine

Although iodine is a trace element, it is an important mineral. The primary location of iodine in the body is the thyroid gland. Iodine is a component of the thyroid hormones thyroxine and triiodothyronine. These hormones help regulate energy metabolism, nervous and muscle cell functioning, and mental and physical growth.

A chronic deficiency of iodine can lead to endemic goiter. The major initial symptom is an enlarged thyroid gland. This condition is especially significant in pregnant women because it can lead to physical and mental retardation in the fetus. In its severe form, this condition in the infant is known as cretinism. Cretinism is rare in the United States but remains a problem in certain areas of Central and South America, Africa, and Asia. Characteristics of cretinism are muscle flabbiness, weakness, dry skin, thick lips, skeletal retardation, and severe mental retardation. Thyroid hormone given early to infants can be of some value, but certain physical and mental deficiencies are irreversible. Everyone, especially pregnant women, should eat a diet sufficient in iodine.

Fluoride

Fluoride, another trace element, is found primarily in the bones and teeth. It maintains bone structure and reduces tooth decay by strengthening tooth enamel. Fluoride is found in the diet, in water, and in soil in generally safe and adequate amounts. In many areas in the United States and Canada, fluoride, a fluorine compound, has been added to the water in amounts equivalent to the normal soil concentration (1 part fluoride per 1 million parts water or soil).

Water

Water is necessary to maintain normal cell function. Water is obtained by drinking fluid and eating foods with a high water content (fresh fruits and vegetables) and by the oxidation of food. Generally, thirst signals the need for water and encourages a person to drink. This sensation often is diminished in the aged. Fluid balance is discussed in Chapter 28.

NUTRITIONAL GUIDELINES

The United States and many other countries have developed nutritional guidelines for their populations. The United States has established DRIs and the ChooseMyPlate.gov guide (which are described later in this section). The World Health

TABLE 29-1 PERCENTAGE OF ADULTS WHO SELF-REPORT MEETING FEDERAL AEROBIC AND MUSCLE STRENGTHENING ACTIVITIES GUIDELINES FOR AMERICANS*

Characteristic	Percentage Meeting Guidelines
Total	20.7
Sex	
Men	24.6
Women	17.1
Age Group (years)	
18–44	25.7
45–64	17.2
65–74	14.8
≥75	7.9
Educational Level	
Less than high school graduate	7.6
High school graduate	12.3
Some college	19.8
College graduate	29.5

*At least 150 minutes per week of moderate activity such as brisk walking or 75 minutes of brisk activity such as jogging, plus 2 or more workouts per week to strengthen major muscle groups

From: Blackwell, D., Lucas, J., & Clarke, T. (2014). Summary health statistics for U.S. adults: National Health Interview Survey, 2012. *National Center for Health Statistics. Vital Health Statistics 10(260)*. Washington, DC: U.S. Government Printing Office.

Organization (WHO), together with the Food and Agriculture Organization of the United Nations, developed nutritional guidelines for worldwide use. Factors within various countries and the opinions of scientists vary, explaining slight differences in recommendations among countries. The U.S. government has also developed aerobic and muscle strengthening activities guidelines intended to complement dietary recommendations. See Table 29-1 for the percentage of adults who self-report meeting these guidelines.

Dietary Reference Intakes

The Food and Nutrition Board of the Institute of Medicine (IOM)/National Academy of Sciences has published dietary standards for common nutrients (IOM, 2005). In place of the single recommended dietary allowance (RDA) for each nutrient that was used in the past, the current DRIs have multiple recommended values for nutrients based upon age groups, physiologic states, and gender. The DRIs include estimated average requirements (EARs), RDAs, AIs, and tolerable ULs:

- The EAR level is the average dietary nutrient intake value estimated to meet the needs of 50% of healthy people in a selected age and gender group.
- The RDA level is the average dietary nutrient intake level that meets the nutritional requirement of almost all (97% to 98%) healthy people in a selected age and gender group.
- The AI level is the average dietary nutrient value set as a goal for nutrients that do not have an RDA.
- The UL level is the highest average value of a nutrient that is likely not to pose a risk of adverse health effects for almost all people in the general population.

The relationship of these values to one another is shown in Figure 29-1. Published levels have multiple uses, including assessment, planning, and education. These values do not consider factors that may significantly increase metabolic demands (e.g., exercise, hypermetabolic states). Because nutritional requirements vary with age, gender, pregnancy, and lactation, separate values are given for each category. A common mistake is to think that the "D" in RDA and DRI stands for "daily" rather than "dietary."

The ChooseMyPlate.gov Food Guide

The U.S. Department of Agriculture (USDA) provides a guide for planning balanced, nutritious, and appetizing meals. It is entitled ChooseMyPlate.gov, a web-based food guidance system that demonstrates the desired amounts of the food

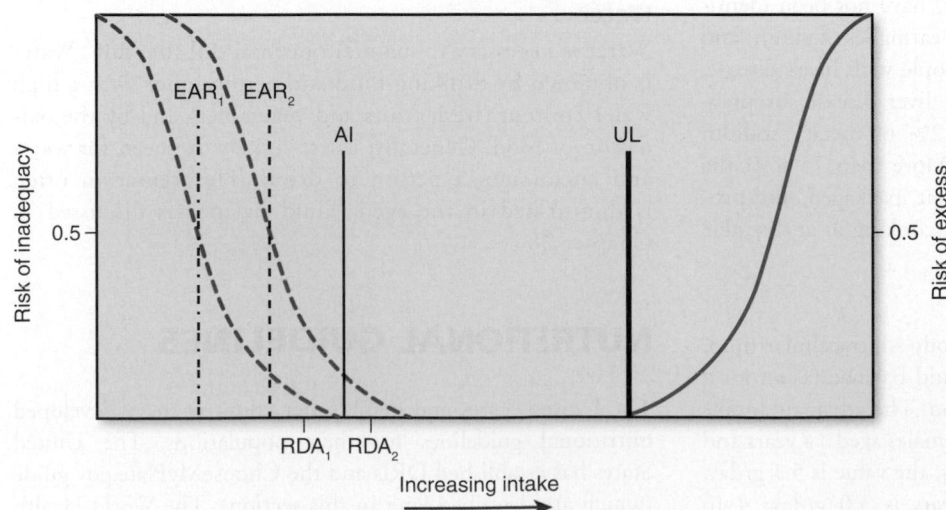

FIGURE 29-1 Relationships among reference values and several points key to intake amounts (AIs, EARs, RDAs, and ULs).

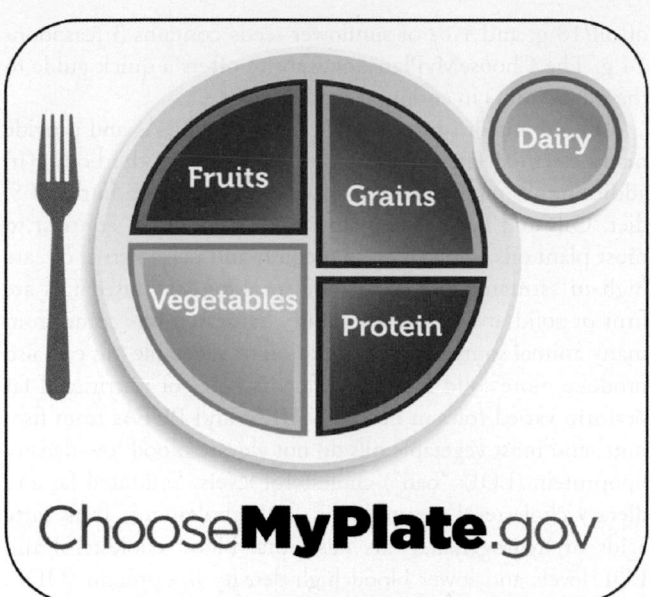

FIGURE 29-2 The USDA's ChooseMyPlate.gov.

groups by means of portions on a plate (USDA, 2013). A guide to portion size is an effort to illustrate how to divide healthy food choices in a more easily understood way (Fig. 29-2). It also provides comprehensive information to aid in making choices about each of the major food groups. It emphasizes food intake moderation, proportionality of foods chosen, and variety across the food groups. Different-sized wedges of color on ChooseMyPlate.gov represent the major food groups:

- *Orange*: Grains
- *Green*: Vegetables
- *Red*: Fruits
- *Blue*: Dairy
- *Purple*: Protein

ChooseMyPlate.gov features selected messages to help consumers focus on key food behaviors. Selected messages include the following (USDA, 2013):

- Enjoy your food, but eat less quantity.
- Avoid oversized portions of any food.
- Make half your plate fruits and vegetables.
- Switch to fat-free or low-fat (1%) milk.
- Make at least half your grains whole grains.
- Compare sodium in foods like soup, bread, and frozen meals, and choose foods with lower numbers.
- Drink water instead of sugary drinks.

GRAINS GROUP

A grain product is a food made from wheat, rice, oats, cornmeal, barley, or other cereal grain. Grains may be classified as whole or refined. Whole grains contain the entire kernel (i.e., endosperm, germ, and bran). Products that list ingredients as "whole grain" or "whole wheat" would contain whole grain. At least half of all grains eaten should be whole.

Refined grains have undergone a process that removes the germ and bran from the product. This process also removes dietary fiber, iron, and many B vitamins. If a product is listed as "enriched," then selected B vitamins and iron have been added to replace those lost during milling.

For sedentary adults, recommended intake from the grains group is from 5 to 8 oz (150 to 240 mL) equivalents per day. In general, a slice of bread, 1 cup of ready-to-eat cereal, or ½ cup cooked rice, cooked pasta, or cooked cereal would be a 1 oz equivalent from this food group. Detailed intake recommendations have been replaced by suggested portions on the plate. With increased activity, the amount needed would increase.

Enriched breads and cereals are good sources of thiamine, iron, niacin, and riboflavin. Whole grains also are excellent sources of zinc, copper, B-complex vitamins, vitamin E, and fiber. These foods are a good source of carbohydrates, calories, and incomplete proteins, and they are low in fat.

VEGETABLES GROUP

Vegetables and 100% vegetable juice make up this group. The current guidelines outline five vegetable categories: dark green vegetables, orange vegetables, dry beans and peas, starchy vegetables, and other vegetables. Vegetables can be fresh, frozen, canned, dried or dehydrated, whole, cut, or mashed. The ChooseMyPlate.gov guide recommends the portion of vegetables that should occupy the meal plate. Vegetables and fruits should compose about 50% of the plate portions.

Vegetables provide vitamins A and C, folate, and minerals such as iron and magnesium. Because they are low in fat and provide fiber, they are excellent for human nutrition.

FRUITS GROUP

Fruits and 100% fruit juice make up this group. Fruits can be fresh, frozen, canned, dried or dehydrated, whole, cut, or mashed. Various fruits are recommended. Fruit juices should be limited, in part, because they have little or no fiber content. The ChooseMyPlate.gov guide recommends the portion of fruits that should occupy the meal plate. Fruits and vegetables should compose about 50% of the plate portions.

In addition to being important sources of vitamins A and C, potassium, and fiber, most fruits are low in fat, sodium, and calories. As a group, these foods have high water content and are generally low in calories and protein. They contain no cholesterol. People should avoid fruits canned in heavy syrups and sweetened fruit drinks.

DAIRY GROUP

The dairy group includes liquid milk products and foods made from milk that retain their calcium content. Choices from this group should be fat-free milk, yogurt, or low-fat cheese. According to these guidelines, if a person eats milk products with additional fat, the fat amount counts in the discretionary calorie allowance. The recommended amount in the milk group is age related. Regardless of activity, recommended intake from the milk group is 3 cups per day for people aged 9 years and older. One cup in this group equals a cup of milk or yogurt (8 oz; 240 mL), 1½ cups of ice cream, 1½ oz of natural cheese, or 2 oz of processed cheese.

Milk is an excellent source of calcium, phosphorus, and riboflavin. It is also fairly rich in sodium, potassium, magnesium, vitamin A, thiamine, vitamin B_6, vitamin B_{12}, niacin, and vitamin D. Milk is an excellent source of protein, but it has little iron. The fat content of milk depends on the type of product.

The nutritional characteristics of cheese are similar to those of milk, depending on the type of cheese. One noteworthy difference (which could be important for people with lactose intolerance) is that cheese contains only a trace amount of lactose.

PROTEINS GROUP

Meat, poultry, fish, dry beans and peas, eggs, nuts, and seeds make up this food group. "Lean" is the key to food selection in this group. Fish, nuts, and seeds bring healthy oils to the diet. Balancing the amount of meat with fish, nuts, and seeds can enhance intake of various nutrients within this food group. Regular substitution of foods within this group, rather than the addition of foods such as nuts or seeds to meat or fish portions, can provide variety and maintain levels within serving guidelines. Fish rich in omega-3 fatty acids include salmon, trout, and herring. Sunflower seeds, almonds, and hazelnuts are rich in vitamin E.

The proteins group is an excellent source of protein and a good source of B-complex vitamins and minerals (iron and zinc). Other foods in the group similarly provide protein and most vitamins and minerals. This group can contain a large amount of fat, depending on the cut of the meat, the type of meat, and the method of processing and preparation. Animal foods can contain a significantly larger amount of cholesterol and saturated fat than do plant foods, but fish is generally lower in cholesterol and saturated fat. Egg yolks contain a large amount of cholesterol, whereas egg whites are cholesterol free.

OILS GROUP

The oils group replaces the fats, oils, and sweets groups in the old food pyramid and is not shown on the ChooseMyPlate. gov illustration. Oils are considered an additional group or factor that need to be considered in the diet. Oils are fats that are liquid at room temperature. They come from fish and plants. Olive oil, canola oil, and safflower oil are examples of vegetable oils. The amount of oil eaten should balance with activity. For sedentary adults, recommended intake from the oils group is from 5 to 7 teaspoons per day. Most people in the United States ingest enough oil daily through foods such as nuts, fish, cooking oil, or salad dressing. Calculation of oil amount in foods may require some conversions. For example, half a medium avocado contains 3 teaspoons of oil/15 g; 1 tablespoon of soft (trans fat free) margarine contains 2½ teaspoons of oil/11 g; 1 oz of hazelnuts contains 4 teaspoons

of oil/18 g; and 1 oz of sunflower seeds contains 3 teaspoons 14 g. The ChooseMyPlate.gov website offers a quick guide to the oil amounts in common foods.

Oils are major sources of MUFAs and PUFAs and provide many essential fatty acids (those not made by the body). In addition, oils represent a good source of vitamin E in the U.S. diet. Oils and fats are also sources of calories. In contrast to most plant oils, a few, such as coconut and palm kernel oil, are high in saturated fats. Generally speaking, saturated fats are firm or solid at room temperature. Saturated fats come from many animal sources. Hydrogenation of vegetable oils can also produce more solid fat. The different types of nutritional fat perform varied roles in health. MUFAs and PUFAs from fish, nuts, and most vegetable oils do not elevate blood low-density lipoprotein (LDL; "bad") cholesterol levels. Saturated fat and dietary cholesterol elevate blood LDL cholesterol. Trans fatty acids or hydrogenated fats raise total blood cholesterol and LDL levels and lower blood high-density lipoprotein (HDL; "good") cholesterol levels.

THE DIGESTIVE SYSTEM

Structure of the Digestive System

The digestive system consists of the organs of the GI tract (mouth, pharynx, esophagus, stomach, small intestine, and large intestine), through which food enters, travels, and exits the body, and accessory organs that play a role in the process of digestion (tongue, salivary glands, teeth, liver, pancreas, and gallbladder).

The mouth is lined with mucous membrane. The tongue is composed of skeletal muscle and is covered with mucous membrane. The papillae, which are the elevations on the tongue, contain the taste buds. The salivary glands are sublingual (the interior part of the mouth under the tongue), submandibular (the posterior part of the floor of the mouth), and parotid (near the temporomandibular joint). The salivary glands secrete saliva, which contains fluid and the salivary enzymes. Mastication includes chewing, reducing the size of food particles, and mixing the food with saliva. The pharynx extends from the base of the skull to the esophagus and is composed of muscle lined with mucous membrane. Food and air pass through this structure before reaching the appropriate outlet (the epiglottis for food and the trachea for air). The epiglottis closes off the airway during swallowing. The esophagus extends from the pharynx to the stomach and transports food from the mouth to the stomach. It is a long, collapsible tube composed of muscular walls lined with mucous membrane.

The stomach lies in the midline and left upper portion of the abdominal cavity. It is connected to the esophagus at the upper end and to the duodenum at the lower end. The stomach varies in size according to body size, sex, and distention. The stomach is lined with mucous membrane and has a muscle layer and an outer fibroserous layer.

The small intestine lies in the abdominal cavity and measures about 1 inch (2.5 cm) in diameter and 20 feet (6 meters) in length. It has a mucous lining, two muscle layers, and an outer visceral peritoneal layer. The small intestine consists of the duodenum, the jejunum, and the ileum.

The large intestine, located at the lower end of the GI tract, is about 2 to 3 inches (5 to 7.5 cm) in diameter and 6 feet (1.8 meters) long. It has a mucous lining, two muscle layers, and, over some sections, an outer visceral peritoneal layer. The large intestine consists of the cecum, the colon (ascending, transverse, descending, and sigmoid), and the rectum.

The accessory organs of digestion are located outside the GI tract, but their secretions are conveyed there by ducts. The liver, the largest gland in the body, lies in the right upper quadrant of the abdominal cavity. Bile produced in the liver is transported through the hepatic duct and the cystic duct to the gallbladder, where it is stored and concentrated. The common bile duct transports bile to the duodenum, where it participates in digestion. The pancreas is located behind the stomach and lies in the curvature of the duodenum. Pancreatic enzymes are transported to the duodenum through the pancreatic ducts.

Function of the Digestive System

The digestive system is primarily responsible for converting food into substances that the body's cells can absorb and use. It also plays a role in immunologic response.

CONVERSION OF FOOD

Conversion involves the processes of digestion, absorption, metabolism, and excretion.

Digestion

Digestion is the process by which foods are broken down for the body to use in growth, development, healing, and prevention of disease. Digestion includes the mechanical and chemical processes necessary to convert foods into their physically absorbable states.

Mechanical Process. The mechanical process of digestion consists of the following events:

1. Mastication takes place in the mouth. Food particles are reduced in size and mixed with enzymes in saliva.
2. Deglutition (swallowing) begins in the mouth and continues in the pharynx and the esophagus.
3. Churning movements and peristalsis mix and move the ingested material through the stomach and into the duodenum.
4. In the small intestine, the ingested material is further churned and mixed with many digestive enzymes. It comes in contact with the intestinal mucosa to allow for absorption.
5. Peristalsis moves the ingested material into the large intestine.
6. Further churning, peristalsis, and absorption help move the residual ingested mass along the full length of the large intestine, where it is stored until it is evacuated from the body.

Chemical Process. The chemical process of digestion changes the composition of ingested material. Most carbohydrates and all fats and proteins must be chemically reduced for absorption.

Carbohydrate digestion involves the hydrolysis of polysaccharides (with the exception of cellulose and other fibers) into disaccharides by the amylase enzymes found in saliva and pancreatic juices. Hydrolysis is a chemical process between a compound and water that results in the division of the compound into simpler components. A polysaccharide is a carbohydrate compound containing three or more saccharide groups, a disaccharide contains two saccharide groups, and a monosaccharide contains only one saccharide group. Disaccharides are further hydrolyzed into monosaccharides by the enzymes sucrase, maltase, and lactase secreted by the intestines.

Fat digestion is accomplished by emulsification of fats, which is facilitated by bile. Emulsification involves breaking down fats into smaller fat droplets and dispersing these droplets into solution. The pancreatic enzyme lipase hydrolyzes the small fat droplets into fatty acids and glycerol.

Protein digestion involves the hydrolysis of the larger protein compounds into amino acids. This is done by the protease enzymes, which include pepsin from the gastric fluid, trypsin and other proteases from the pancreatic fluid, and peptidases from the intestinal fluid.

Absorption

Absorption is the process by which the digested proteins, fats, carbohydrates, vitamins, minerals, and water are actively and passively transported through the intestinal mucosa into the blood or lymphatic circulation. The proteins, such as amino acids, and the digested carbohydrates and simple sugars, in the form of monosaccharides, are absorbed into the bloodstream through the intestinal capillaries. The fats, in the form of glycerol and fatty acids, are absorbed into the lymphatic system through the lymphatic capillaries in the intestinal villi. Some finely emulsified neutral fats are absorbed undigested into the capillaries.

Metabolism

After ingested food is digested and absorbed, the products are ready to be metabolized. Metabolism is the complex chemical process that occurs in the cells to allow for energy use and for cellular growth and repair. Metabolism involves catabolic and anabolic processes: catabolic processes break down complex substances into simpler substances (e.g., tissue breakdown), and anabolic processes convert simple substances into more complex ones (e.g., tissue repair).

Carbohydrate Metabolism. The liver cells change short-term glucose excesses into glycogen in the presence of insulin; this anabolic process is called **glycogenesis**. Glycogen is stored in the liver and skeletal muscles until needed and is then converted back into glucose by a catabolic process called glycogenolysis.

Longer-term storage of glucose in the presence of insulin takes the form of fat deposits (adipose tissue). When the amount of glucose entering the cells is not enough to meet cellular demands, gluconeogenesis (the formation of glucose from protein and fat in the liver) occurs. This catabolic process yields about 4 kcal of energy per gram of oxidized carbohydrate.

Fat Metabolism. Fats are converted to adipose tissue and stored in the body's fat deposits if they are not immediately needed. Stored fat deposits make up the body's largest reserve energy source. The catabolism of fats involves the hydrolysis of fat into glycerol and fatty acids. The fatty acids are then converted by a series of chemical reactions known as ketogenesis into ketone bodies. In the tissue cells, ketones are converted by the citric acid cycle into energy, carbon dioxide, and water. Glycerol is converted by gluconeogenesis into glucose. Fats are a more concentrated source of energy than carbohydrates, yielding 9 kcal of energy per gram of catabolized fat.

Protein Metabolism. Protein anabolism builds tissues, produces antibodies, replaces blood cells, and repairs tissues. Temporary excesses of protein are stored in the liver and in skeletal muscle or converted to fat. Protein catabolism involves the hydrolysis of cellular proteins into amino acids in the tissue cell. It also involves the deamination process of amino acids, in which an amino group is split off from an amino acid to form ammonia and keto acid. This process takes place in the liver cell to form glucose and urea.

Excretion

The excretory organs (kidneys, sweat glands, skin, lungs, and intestines) remove waste products from the body. Water, toxins, salts, and nitrogen wastes are excreted through the kidneys, skin, and sweat glands. Carbon dioxide and water are excreted through the lungs. Digestive wastes are excreted through the intestines and rectum.

IMMUNOLOGIC FUNCTION

The GI tract is a major immunologic organ and plays a significant role in the body's immune response. The GI tract contains 70% to 80% of all immune-secreting cells. Also, 25% of the GI tract is lymphoid tissue. Since many microorganisms that threaten the body enter through the nose and mouth, maintaining the integrity and health of the GI tract helps prevent complications and speed recovery. Enteral (through the digestive tract) nutrition stimulates a complex response that promotes immunologic integrity (Bristrian & Driscoll, 2012). An intact and active GI tract plays an important role as a first line of defense against infection.

Characteristics of Normal Nutrition

Normal nutrition involves a balanced intake of food to meet the energy requirements necessary for organ function, body movement, and work. Adequate food intake also provides raw materials for the production of enzymes and the production of cells necessary for growth, replacement of tissues, and tissue repair.

NUTRIENT DENSITY

The concept of nutrient density can be used to evaluate the nutritional quality of foods. Foods that provide more nutrient value than just kilocalories are called "nutrient-dense" foods. Foods with low nutrient density (e.g., sugar, alcohol) provide energy but usually lack essential nutrients. Foods that are nutrient dense are preferred to promote optimal nutrition.

DIETARY GUIDELINES FOR AMERICANS

The USDA and U.S. Department of Health and Human Services establish new dietary guidelines every 5 years (USDA, 2010). Because many Americans overeat and lead sedentary lives, the number of people with cardiovascular problems, diabetes, and cancer has risen significantly. To help reverse this trend, recent guidelines place an increased emphasis upon calorie control and exercise. Box 29-1 compares current with previous guidelines.

Key recommendations can be grouped into eight mutually dependent categories and one category on food safety. These categories include adequate nutrients within caloric needs; weight management; physical activity; food groups to encourage; fats, carbohydrates, sodium, and potassium; and alcoholic beverages. To summarize, most Americans can ingest fewer calories, become more active, and make wiser food choices.

ENERGY BALANCE

Dietary patterns should be adjusted to maintain a balance between caloric intake and energy expenditure. **Basal metabolism** is the amount of energy required to carry out involuntary activities at rest (e.g., breathing, circulating blood, maintaining body temperature). Men usually have a higher basal metabolic rate (BMR) than do women because of their proportionally greater muscle mass. Other factors, such as growth, infection, fever, stress, and extreme environmental temperatures, can increase BMR. Decreased BMR can occur as a result of aging, prolonged fasting, and sleeping. Increased physical exercise creates caloric demands above basal requirements.

To maintain body weight, dietary intake of calories must equal caloric expenditures. When caloric intake is greater than energy expended, weight gain occurs because energy is stored in body fat. When caloric intake is less than energy expended, weight loss occurs because body stores of energy are depleted. For an average person, a daily deficit of 500 kcal (3,500 kcal per week) will result in the loss of 1 lb (0.37 kg) per week.

Caloric requirements can be calculated by estimating how much energy is required for basal activities and adding the calories needed for voluntary muscular activity. Box 29-2 shows one method for calculating kilocalorie energy output for BMR and voluntary muscular activity.

NUTRITIONAL STATUS

There are many assessment criteria used to determine nutritional status.

Body Mass Index

BMI is the measure that describes a person's relative weight for height and is recognized as a predictive measure for morbidity and mortality. BMI is calculated as weight (in kilograms) divided by the height (in meters) squared. If pounds and inches are being used, the formula is BMI = [(weight in pounds) ÷ (height in inches squared)] × 703. The BMI correlates with total body fat content and is considered a useful tool to track weight changes and to identify weight categories that may lead to health problems (CDC, 2011).

BOX 29-1 Changes in American Dietary Guidelines: The Need for Wiser Choices

Calories

Current Guidelines: Balance calories from foods and beverages you eat with the amount of energy you burn. For moderately active people between 31 and 50 years, daily calories recommended for women would be 2,000; for men, 2,400 to 2,600.

Previous Guidelines: Aim for a healthy weight, based on BMI.

Physical Activity

Current Guidelines: 30 minutes per day of exercise is the minimum level; 60 minutes per day to maintain weight and prevent weight gain; 60 to 90 minutes per day to maintain weight loss.

Previous Guidelines: Be physically active every day, accumulating approximately 30 minutes of exercise per day.

Nutrition

Current Guidelines: Eat various foods that are high in nutrient value and low in saturated and trans fats, cholesterol, added sugars, and salt.

Previous Guidelines: Let the pyramid guide your food choices, and pick various grains, especially whole grains, and fruits and vegetables.

Fruits and Vegetables

Current Guidelines: Eat at least 2 cups of fruits and 2½ cups of vegetables a day if you are eating 2,000 calories. Eat more or less than that depending on the caloric level.

Previous Guidelines: Eat 3 or 4 servings of vegetables and 2 to 4 servings of fruit every day.

Carbohydrates

Current Guidelines: Eat fiber-rich whole grains, whole fruits, and vegetables often. Eat and drink little added sugar or caloric sweeteners.

Previous Guidelines: Choose various grains, especially whole grains, and various fruits and vegetables daily. Choose food and drinks to moderate sugar intake.

Fat

Current Guidelines: Keep trans fats as low as possible. Get no more than 10% of your calories from saturated fat and no more than 300 mg of cholesterol daily.

Previous Guidelines: Keep your diet low in saturated fat and cholesterol and moderate in total fat.

Sodium and Potassium

Current Guidelines: Limit sodium (salt) to less than 2,300 mg (about 1 level teaspoon) per day; eat potassium-rich foods, such as fruits and vegetables.

Previous Guidelines: Eat and prepare foods with less salt.

Alcohol

Current Guidelines: If you drink alcohol, do it sensibly and in moderation—about 1 drink per day for women and 1 drink per day for men.

Previous Guidelines: Same.

Food Safety

Current Guidelines: Actions can be taken to avoid microbial foodborne illness—these include cleanliness; separation of raw, cooked, and ready-to-eat foods; cook to safe temperature; chill and defrost foods promptly and properly; and avoid unpasteurized milk and milk products and raw or undercooked foods.

Previous Guidelines: None.

From: U.S. Department of Agriculture and U.S. Department of Health & Human Services. (2010). *Dietary guidelines for Americans*, 2010 (7th ed.). Washington, DC: U.S. Government Printing Office.

Ideal Body Weight

Normal nutritional intake usually results in body weight appropriate for a person's height and frame. Ideal body weight (IBW) is the estimated optimal weight for body functioning and health. Ranges for IBW according to height and body frame are listed in standardized tables. Such information can be misleading because it does not always reflect accurately the amount of body fat present. For example, a bodybuilder may be heavier than the IBW listed but may have a less than average amount of body fat.

A rule of thumb for estimating IBW is that a woman who is 5 feet (152 cm) tall should weigh about 100 lb (45.4 kg), and 5 lb (2.26 kg) should be added for each additional inch (2.5 cm). The IBW for a 5-foot (152 cm) man is 105 lb (47.6 kg), to which 6 lb (2.72 kg) should be added for each additional inch (2.5 cm).

Physical Status

Normal nutrition is apparent in the appearance of many parts of the body. General appearance should reflect alertness and responsiveness. The skin should have normal tone and good turgor. The mouth, gums, and lips should appear moist, pink, and free from cracks and lesions. Hair and nails should appear healthy. Bones should hold the body erect, and muscles should maintain good tone. Normal reflexes should be apparent. The abdomen should appear flat and without distention.

Normal Laboratory Values

Laboratory values are usually within normal ranges in healthy people. Normal hematocrit and hemoglobin values suggest adequate iron stores if hydration status is normal. Plasma protein values (e.g., serum prealbumin, albumin) are often used as a reflection of normal adequate protein intake.

Life Span Considerations

PREGNANCY AND LACTATION

The pregnant woman's diet should include a substantial increase in calories, protein, calcium, folic acid, and iron (Fig. 29-3). Usually, a prenatal multivitamin and mineral supplement is

BOX 29-2   Estimating Energy Requirements for Adults

ChooseMyPlate.gov and other web-based calculators estimate the energy in calories that a body uses, based upon height, weight, degree of physical activity, and age. The following formula may also be used to estimate daily calorie requirements for nonpregnant, nonlactating, healthy adults. It includes factors for basal metabolism and physical activity in its calculations. Total daily estimated energy requirements (EER) are calculated as follows:

1. *Change weight in pounds to kilograms (kg)*: pounds ÷ 2.2 = weight in kilograms.
2. *Calculate basal metabolic rate (BMR)*:
   Males: Multiply weight in kg by 1 kcal per kilogram body weight per hour × 24 hours per day.
   Females: Multiply weight in kg by 0.9 kcal per kilogram body weight per hour × 24 hours per day.
3. Estimate activity level that best describes individual lifestyle:

Physical Activity Level	Males	Females
Sedentary (little to no exercise; mostly sitting)	25%–40%	25%–35%
Lightly active (some walking or moving around; light lifting)	50%–70%	40%–60%
Moderately active (physically active work plus intentional exercise 4–5 days per week)	65%–80%	50%–70%
Heavily active (great deal of physical labor or intentional exercise)	90%–120%	80%–100%
Exceptionally active (athletic training; arduous work and play)	135%–145%	110%–130%

4. **Calculate kcal needed for daily activity**: Multiply the BMR times lowest and highest percentage numbers from table. This will provide the approximate range of kcal used per day.
5. **Calculate range of total daily energy needs**: Add BMR + kcal needed for daily activities to obtain daily estimated energy requirements (EER).

Example:
The calculation for a 175-lb male with a lightly active lifestyle is as follows:

a. 175 lb ÷ 2.2 lb per kilogram = 79.5 kg
b. 1 kcal per kilogram body weight per hour × 79.5 kg × 24 hours per day = 1,909 kcal per day BMR
c. 1,909 kcal per day × 50% = 955 kcal per day
d. 1,909 kcal per day × 70% = 1,336 kcal per day
e. 1,909 kcal per day + 955 kcal per day = 2,864 kcal per day
f. 1,909 kcal per day + 1,336 kcal per day = 3,245 kcal per day

To maintain present weight, this man requires 2,864 to 3,245 kcal per day, based upon age, body build, and other personal factors.

Source: Thompson J., & Manore M. (2012). *Nutrition: An applied approach* (3rd ed., p. 380). Boston, MA: Pearson.

prescribed. The pregnant woman should gain weight throughout her pregnancy, as prescribed and monitored by her healthcare professional. Pregnant women at particular risk for nutritional deficiencies are adolescents, **underweight** women, **obese** women, women with chronic nutritional problems, women who smoke or ingest alcohol or drugs, low-income women, and women with chronic illnesses such as diabetes or anemia.

The lactating woman also has special needs. Minor deficiencies in the lactating woman's diet are more likely to influence her nutritional state than the nutritional quality of her milk. Major deficiencies in the woman's diet may result in a decrease in the nutritional quality and quantity of her milk. Lactating women need to increase their intake of calcium, protein, fluid, and calories. These increases are important because the quality and quantity of breast milk produced directly affects the adequacy of the breast-feeding infant's diet.

NEWBORN AND INFANT

Adequate nutrition during infancy is important because the infant's growth and development are more rapid during the first year of life than at any other time. Birth weight usually doubles within the first 4 to 6 months and triples by 12 months of age. Newborns need more calories per pound of body weight because their BMR is so high. The infant's growth and development also are influenced by genetic characteristics and by the quality of prenatal nutrition and care.

Milk is the food of choice for newborns. Breast-feeding should begin as soon after birth as possible. For the first 3 days after birth, the mother's breasts produce colostrum, a thin, watery fluid. The breasts produce milk, which contains about 20 cal per ounce (30 mL), after the 3rd day. Weight gain may be less rapid in breast-fed infants. Feedings are usually frequent (e.g., every 2 to 3 hours) because breast milk is easily digested. Breast milk provides infants with immunity against some bacte-

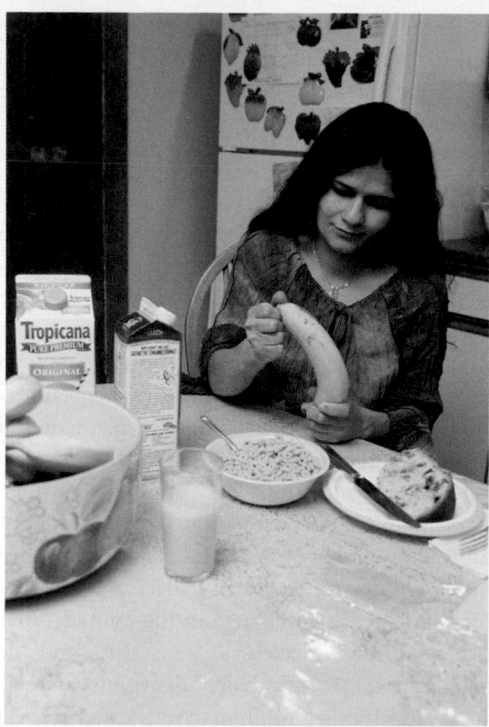

FIGURE 29-3 Pregnant women should adjust their dietary intake to increase calories and important nutrients.

ria and viruses, results in different intestinal flora than with artificial formula, decreases the incidence of allergies, and provides a well-balanced and ideal source of nutrition. Breast-feeding mothers should avoid taking drugs because small amounts can be transferred to the breast milk and ingested by the infant. In addition, infants may not tolerate products from some foods, such as citrus foods, some vegetables, and spicy foods.

Formula is a safe and nutritious substitute for mothers who cannot or choose not to breast-feed. Iron-fortified commercial formulas should be used until the infant is at least 1 year old. Most formulas are modified cow's milk that has been heat treated to aid digestion. Soy formulas and predigested formulas also are available. Foods (e.g., juices, fruits, vegetables, iron-fortified cereals) are gradually added to the diet to provide additional nutrition and to begin to accustom infants to foods of different textures, flavors, and consistencies. The age at which to introduce these foods varies according to the infant's need, the practices of the healthcare provider, and the influence of the infant's culture and environment. Cereals, fruits and vegetables, and egg yolk are added at about 4 to 6 months. When teeth begin to erupt at about 6 months, crackers and teething biscuits are often added. Parents and caregivers should introduce new foods one at a time so that any offending food can be identified if allergies develop. By the second half of the first year, motor development has improved so that the infant can begin to sit up, eat finger foods, and drink from a cup.

TODDLER AND PRESCHOOLER

Adequate nutritional intake is important between the ages of 1 and 5 years because this is a period of rapid physical growth and development. Variations among toddlers necessitate some

differences in their diets. During this period, the growth rate begins to decline, and the appetite decreases as children need less food to meet normal metabolic demands. Children's appetites may be erratic during these years. Teeth continue to erupt into the second and sometimes the 3rd year. Muscle mass and bone density increase. These developments necessitate adequate protein, calcium, and phosphorus in the diet. Energy levels remain high, requiring adequate caloric intake.

Independence in feeding greatly increases as coordination and ability to use eating utensils develop. Many children can feed themselves by 2 years of age. Mental abilities and language development are increasing, so children are better able to communicate food likes and dislikes. Values and attitudes about eating develop during these stages. Parents and other caregivers must learn the importance of not using food to punish, reward, bribe, or convey love. Some children may become picky eaters, especially when refusal to eat gains them attention from their families.

Maintaining adequate dietary habits for toddlers and preschoolers is important because good habits are established at an early age. The most common dietary deficiency in this age group is iron deficiency, which leads to iron-deficiency anemia. A diet that includes iron-rich foods is indicated, and iron supplements may be necessary. Vitamins A and C also may be deficient in the diets of toddlers and preschoolers, so they must eat foods rich in these vitamins. Active children in this age group benefit from appropriately spaced, nutritious, between-meal snacks.

SAFETY ALERT

Remind parents and other caregivers to keep hot liquids away from toddlers or confused patients who may accidentally spill them or burn themselves.

CHILD AND ADOLESCENT

Children's growth rates vary greatly during the school years. The digestive system matures, and permanent teeth erupt. Children can eat larger meals less frequently, requiring fewer calories per unit of body weight. Adolescence is a period of rapid growth and sexual maturation. Macronutrients and micronutrients are needed to support body tissue growth during this time.

A diet that includes adequate carbohydrates and the recommended allowances of protein, vitamins, and minerals for the individual's age group, physical status, and developmental level is necessary for optimal health. Nutritional deficiencies that are most common during childhood and adolescence are those of iron, calcium, zinc, and vitamin A. Adequate amounts of these minerals and vitamins must be included in the diet. Health problems that respond well to nutritional intervention during this age include dental caries, anemia, and obesity.

School lunch programs play an important role in providing nutritionally balanced, low-cost meals (Fig. 29-4). Some schools also have breakfast programs and snack programs.

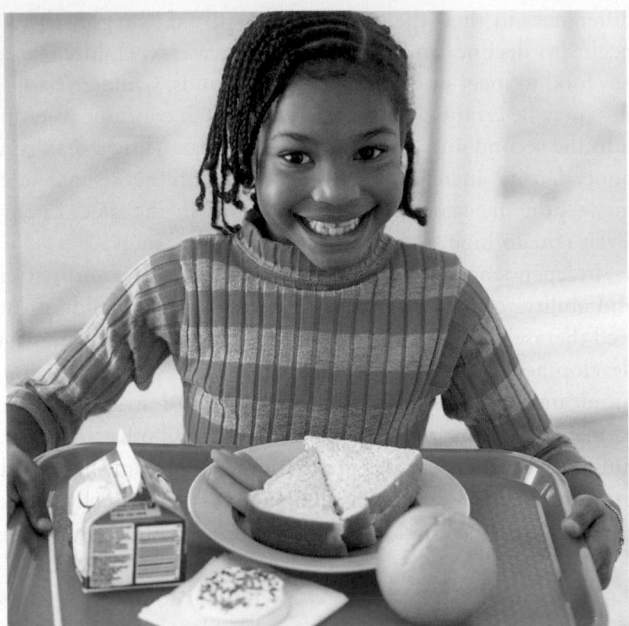

FIGURE 29-4 Children can receive well-balanced meals through a school lunch program.

These programs usually are available free or at a reduced cost for needy children. In addition to providing a substantial part of the daily nutrition needs for children, these programs make a valuable contribution in terms of nutrition education and development of good nutrition habits.

Social pressure and emotional stress can have adverse effects on a young person's efforts to maintain a nutritionally adequate diet. Peers may dictate dietary choices. Children may eat fewer meals at home than in earlier years; fast food, soda, and candy are often favorites. Smoking, drinking, and substance abuse also can affect nutritional status. Children or adolescents may experience an unbalanced pattern of activity or rest. Increased participation in sports requires additional caloric intake. Weight gain is common during the preadolescent period as the body prepares for rapid growth. If the child leads a sedentary life and eats a high-calorie diet, weight gain can be excessive and can contribute to obesity. On the other hand, weight consciousness, especially among adolescent girls, can lead to fad diets, **anorexia nervosa**, and bulimia.

ADULT

Growth stops and metabolism declines during adulthood, so adults require fewer calories. Weight gain is common, especially if physical activity is limited. Calcium deficiency and osteoporosis can be concerns for adults, especially postmenopausal women. Adults should maintain calcium intake throughout adulthood. Adequate intake of calcium is especially important before 30 years of age, when peak bone mass is being attained. Among adult Americans, nutritional excesses of fats, carbohydrates, and proteins are more common than deficiencies.

Inadequate nutritional intake during this time may result from increased daily demands that decrease the time and energy available for buying, cooking, and eating food. Dietary patterns can be affected when both parents in a family work. Some adults lack adequate resources or knowledge about good nutrition. Pregnancy and lactation, as discussed previously, greatly alter nutritional requirements.

OLDER ADULT

Physiologic changes that have a major impact on nutrition occur in later years. The metabolic rate continues to decline. Although the need for calories decreases, the need for vitamins and most minerals remains high; however, a woman's need for iron decreases after menopause. The diets of many older adults are deficient in whole grains, fruits, vegetables, low-fat milk/milk products, and dietary oils (in place of solid fats), often due to financial concerns (Federal Interagency Forum on Aging-Related Statistics, 2012). Adequate fiber intake is necessary to prevent constipation, a common problem in older adults. The senses of taste and smell diminish; this can affect enjoyment of eating and cause decreased intake of food. Digestion is affected by a change in the contents of bile and pancreatic secretions, decreased peristalsis, and decreased blood flow to the GI tract. Impaired dentition can make chewing difficult, and food–drug interactions can affect digestion. A growing concern in the older adult population is obesity. In the last decade, U.S. rates of obesity in elders have more than doubled. Now more than 70% of people between 65 and 74, and over 60% of individuals over 75, are overweight or obese (Thompson & Manore, 2012).

For older adults, socioeconomic factors can contribute to inadequate nutrition. Transportation for shopping and carrying of groceries can be problems for the older person with impaired mobility. Older adults may have trouble using cooking appliances because of failing eyesight or because of the complexity of modern appliances. Selecting economical, nutritious foods can be difficult for the older shopper because of the various products available.

Social isolation can also affect nutrition. Those who have lost friends and live far from relatives may become lonely and depressed, which can affect eating habits (Dudek, 2014).

Several community resources have been developed to help older adults continue living at home by combating the problems mentioned previously. Programs for home-delivered meals (e.g., Meals on Wheels) provide nutritious, low-cost meals for older, homebound people. This program is able to remain low in cost partly because of a volunteer staff. Food stamps and food banks are useful to older adults. Another excellent resource for older adults is local senior centers, which can provide meals, health screening and medication assistance, transportation assistance, dietary counseling, recreational activities, and assistance and referral for economic and legal problems.

Cultural Considerations

Definitions of normal nutrition vary widely among cultures. Each culture defines life, health, and the meaning of each in society (Kittler & Sucher, 2011). Many cultures identify certain foods or drinks as being comforting or medicinal. Some cultures equate thinness with health, while others view being overweight as a sign of health and prosperity (Kittler & Sucher, 2011).

Culture plays a significant role in the type of food eaten and feelings about diet and nutrition. Food can be a way of saying "this is home," a form of communication, and an identity itself. Staple products vary among cultural groups; for example, Asians may eat rice with most meals, and Italians may prefer pasta. Spices and methods of cooking also vary.

Some religions dictate when or whether certain foods can be eaten and how foods are to be prepared. An example of this is the Jewish dietary law, which restricts (among other things) eating dairy and meat products at the same time. Religions may restrict intake of all meats or of particular meats such as pork or beef. Some religions require fasting during certain seasons. In addition, most religions have special foods that are traditional for specific observances (Kittler & Sucher, 2011).

FACTORS AFFECTING NUTRITION

Physiologic Factors

Healthy body functioning promotes normal digestion and absorption of food. Healthy teeth and gums or well-fitting dentures are important for chewing, which is necessary to break up food particles to facilitate digestion. The GI system must function properly for optimal use of ingested nutrients. Hormone production of insulin and pancreatic digestive enzymes is also important for food use.

INTAKE OF NUTRIENTS

Ability to Acquire and Prepare Food

Physical factors can affect a person's ability to buy, transport, cook, and eat food. Physical mobility and energy are necessary for shopping, cooking, and eating. Being able to read and understand food labels can help with healthy food choices.

People who are unable to purchase, transport, and prepare food may have inadequate intake unless other people or agencies can be found to fulfill such needs. In third world countries, starvation is common due to drought and famine. Starvation or malnutrition also can occur in developed nations when people lack the resources to obtain adequate food. Confused or disoriented persons may forget to eat or may be unable to organize the complex tasks of buying and cooking food independently.

Knowledge

Some people may not eat a balanced diet because they lack information about nutrition. People are likely to eat only what tastes good or what is convenient if they do not know or care that such eating patterns can be unhealthy. The consequences of poor nutrition are not immediately observable, so motivation to change poor eating patterns may be weak.

Swallowing Impairment

People who have difficulty swallowing may be unable to ingest sufficient nutrients to meet daily requirements. Swallowing impairment can occur when the gag reflex is absent due to neurologic dysfunction (e.g., cerebrovascular accident [CVA]) or muscle weakness. Obstruction of the oropharyngeal cavity secondary to a tumor or edema also can impair swallowing.

Discomfort During or After Eating

When people experience discomfort during or after eating, they may decrease their food intake. A sore throat, a tonsillectomy, a mouth lesion, and ill-fitting dentures are possible causes.

Anorexia

Anorexia, or loss of appetite, occurs for various reasons. Depression, GI dysfunction, infections, illnesses, malignancies, and side effects of many medications can cause anorexia, resulting in decreased food intake.

Nausea and Vomiting

Nausea and vomiting interfere with normal food intake. They may be caused by motion sickness, viral or bacterial infections of the GI tract, gallbladder disease, general anesthesia, disruption of inner ear function, side effects of various medications, or pregnancy. Some people may feel nauseated or vomit from unpleasant smells, sensations, or sights.

Excessive Intake of Calories and Fat

Caloric intake in excess of daily energy requirements results in storage of energy in the form of increased adipose tissue. As the percentage of stored fat increases, a person becomes overweight or obese. Figure 29-5 presents U.S. self-reported obesity rates by state. No state has less than 20% obesity in its population. Obesity rates range from 20.5% to 34.7%. Higher obesity rates

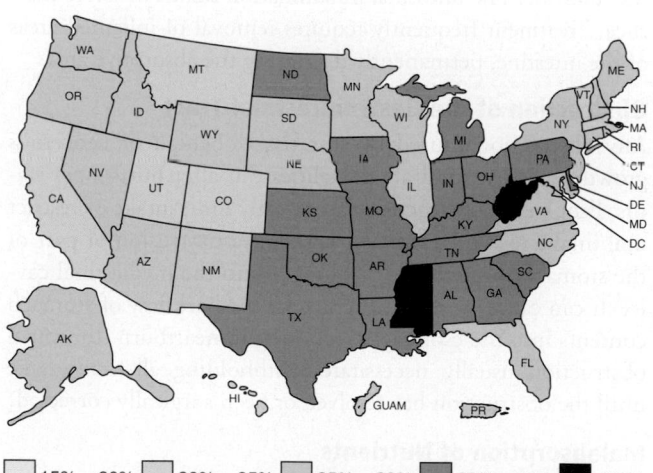

15%–<20%   20%–<25%   25%–<30%   30%–<35%   35%

FIGURE 29-5 Prevalence of self-reported obesity among U.S. adults. (*Source:* Behavioral Risk Factor Surveillance Systems, CDC. Prevalence estimates reflect BRFSS methodological changes started in 2011. These estimates should not be compared to prevalence estimates before 2011; (U.S. Centers for Disease Control and Prevention. (2013). *Behavioral Risk Factor Surveillance System (BRFSS)*. Retrieved from www.cdc.gov/obesity/data/adult.html)

are found in the Midwest and the South; lower rates are found in the Northeast and the West (CDC, 2014).

Excess weight increases stress on body organs and predisposes people to chronic health problems, such as diabetes mellitus and hypertension. Excessive caloric intake does not ensure adequate intake of essential nutrients: obese persons may be malnourished in some areas due to a lack of elements such as essential vitamins or particular nutrients.

Americans have a higher percentage of fat in their diets than do people in many other countries. Excess fat intake has been related to obesity; increased risk of coronary artery disease (especially increased intake of saturated and trans fats); and several forms of cancer, including breast, colon, and uterine cancer. Dietary modifications can lower fat and cholesterol intake.

ABILITY TO USE INGESTED NUTRIENTS

Inflammation of the Gastrointestinal Tract

Inflammation of the lining of the GI tract causes discomfort and interferes with nutrient absorption. Esophagitis, an inflammation of the esophagus, can result from burns, poisons, infections, or chronic vomiting. It causes discomfort and impairs swallowing. Gastritis is characterized by inflammation of the mucosal layer of the stomach, which can proceed to ulceration if untreated.

Cholecystitis is an inflammation of the gallbladder; it is usually caused by gallstones. Inflammation and stones cause pain after ingestion of a meal that is high in fat because the gallbladder spasms as it attempts to release bile to assist with fat digestion.

Inflammatory bowel disease (i.e., Crohn disease or ulcerative colitis) greatly affects absorption of nutrients and water from the intestine. The intestinal inflammation results in severe diarrhea. Treatment frequently requires removal of inflamed areas of the intestine, permanently decreasing the absorptive area.

Obstruction of the Gastrointestinal Tract

Any obstruction caused by scar tissue, benign or cancerous growths, or structural abnormalities can alter nutritional status. Esophageal obstruction can severely limit intake or restrict oral intake to fluids. A hiatal hernia is a protrusion of part of the stomach through the diaphragm into the mediastinal cavity. It can cause esophageal reflux, or the backflow of stomach contents into the esophagus, resulting in heartburn. Intestinal obstruction usually necessitates withholding all oral intake until the obstruction has resolved or been surgically corrected.

Malabsorption of Nutrients

The inability to tolerate certain foods can cause malabsorption syndromes. An intolerance to gluten, which is found in wheat, rye, oats, and barley, can cause mucosal villi to atrophy, decreasing their absorptive abilities. Lactose intolerance occurs when there is a deficiency of lactase, a digestive enzyme that breaks down the sugar found in milk.

A decrease in pancreatic enzyme production occurs in some pancreatic disorders, resulting in altered digestion of fats

and protein. In cystic fibrosis, an inherited disorder, excessive mucus plugs pancreatic ducts, leading to altered protein, carbohydrate, and fat digestion.

Malabsorption also can occur secondary to surgical intervention. Gastric or intestinal resection removes large areas of the GI tract normally involved in absorption of nutrients. Decreased blood flow to the GI tract can decrease the rate of nutrient absorption.

Diabetes Mellitus

Diabetes mellitus is a chronic condition in which the body produces insufficient amounts of insulin or cannot effectively use circulating insulin. Insulin is a hormone essential for proper metabolism of fats, proteins, and carbohydrates. When adequate insulin is unavailable, transfer of glucose into the cell is impaired, and the glucose level of the blood rises. Thus, cells cannot use glucose to produce energy. **Procedure 29-1** discusses monitoring blood glucose.

METABOLIC DEMAND

Certain conditions increase the body's nutritional requirements, potentially affecting nutritional status:

- Periods of rapid growth (infancy, adolescence, pregnancy)
- Conditions that increase the BMR (infection, exercise, hyperthyroidism)
- Stress (from emotional distress, fear, trauma, surgery, or illness)
- Wasting diseases such as cancer and AIDS (from reduced energy and protein intake, malabsorption, and metabolic disturbances)

Lifestyle and Habits

Eating patterns are highly individualized and greatly determined by personal preference. Food patterns and eating habits are often set during childhood and may be passed from one generation to the next. Some families love trying new recipes; others prefer having specific meals prepared exactly the same way repeatedly. If children are raised in families that eat throughout the day, rather than at three distinct meals, this pattern will seem normal and will probably influence their lifelong eating patterns. Early experience also helps determine the amounts and types of food eaten. While children are young, parents play a role in reducing unhealthy food choices (Salvy et al., 2011). But, if children are fed large servings and rewarded with desserts, overeating may become a problem later. There is evidence that families that regularly eat meals together are more likely to eat healthier, higher quality meals through adulthood (Berge et al., 2012). The atmosphere at mealtimes also subtly affects feelings about food and eating.

Peer pressure and gender differences can affect eating patterns. During adolescence, girls often select healthy choices when eating with their friends, whereas boys have not been found to alter eating habits according to social context (Salvy et al., 2011). It is not known whether these patterns extend into adulthood. There is also evidence that websites and social media can affect individual perceptions of appropriate body weight and food intake (Juarez, Soto, & Pritchard, 2012).

Food fads also can affect dietary patterns. Some foods and nutritional supplements can be linked with beliefs about health that are not grounded in scientific fact.

Professional persons who work long hours and are single may not have enough time to shop for and cook food. Families with two working parents may eat out often for the same reason. Some single older adults may have limited motivation or energy to cook and eat meals alone. People who lead active lives with strenuous physical exertion may need more frequent meals and more calories to meet their minimal nutritional requirements. On the other hand, sedentary people who spend hours in front of the television may gain weight from decreased physical activity and increased snacking.

Economic Resources

An adequate diet may be related to a person's finances. Money is necessary to buy and transport food and to obtain and maintain the equipment needed to cook and store food safely. The lower a person's economic level, the less likely it is that the diet will be nutritionally adequate. Low-income areas usually have fewer grocery stores, with fewer selections and higher prices. People with low incomes may lack transportation to shop outside their neighborhoods. More affluent people can stock up when items are on sale, stretching their food budget.

Low-income families may sacrifice their food budgets to leave enough money for other bills. The result may be less expensive meals that are low in protein and high in starch. Sources of protein, such as meat and dairy products, are usually expensive and require refrigeration.

Drug and Nutrient Interactions

Specific foods may interact with medications, altering the effectiveness of the drug. This consideration is particularly important with long-term drug treatments, use of multiple drugs, or alterations in nutritional status. For example, a high sodium intake decreases the effectiveness of lithium, a commonly used psychiatric medication. Vegetables high in vitamin K decrease the effectiveness of the commonly used anticoagulant Coumadin. References are available that detail specific interactions among food and drugs (Pronsky et al., 2012).

Gender

Nutritional requirements vary slightly between men and women. Men usually need more calories and protein to maintain a larger muscle mass. Women have proportionally more adipose tissue and need fewer calories to maintain body weight. To prevent anemia, women need more dietary iron to offset losses from menstruation. The DRI value sets and ChooseMyPlate.gov outline nutritional standards for each gender by age group.

Surgery

Surgery greatly increases the risk of nutritional deficits. Increased metabolic demands related to the stress of surgery and wound healing, along with inadequate postoperative intake, compound nutritional deficits. Many surgical patients are nutritionally depleted at the time of surgery due to chronic illness, GI problems, or prior medical procedures.

Cancer and Cancer Treatment

Cancer greatly increases the body's metabolic demands, and cancer cells compete with normal cells for nutrients. Patients with cancer may experience anorexia, nausea, vomiting, and depression, all of which can decrease food consumption. Radiation or chemotherapy also can alter nutrition because loss of appetite, nausea, and vomiting are commonly associated with such treatments. Mouth lesions (known as stomatitis) may occur with chemotherapy, causing pain and difficulty in chewing. Chemotherapy and radiation cause fatigue, decreasing the amount of energy available for cooking and eating.

Alcohol and Drug Abuse

Excessive, chronic ingestion of alcohol can impair nutrition. Excessive alcohol intake may limit the necessary intake of calories and nutrients. People who abuse alcohol may use money normally spent on food to buy alcohol. Deficiencies of B-complex vitamins (thiamine, folate, niacin, and B_6) are common because these vitamins are necessary to metabolize alcohol. Alcohol's toxic effect on the intestinal mucosa can impair the normal absorption of nutrients. Chronic alcohol use also can cause irreversible changes to liver cells, affecting the liver's role in metabolic pathways.

Drug abuse also can affect nutrition. Addiction to heroin or cocaine can decrease the user's desire for food because preoccupation with buying drugs disrupts normal routines. Other drugs, such as amphetamines and barbiturates, can result in increased or decreased food intake.

Psychological State

Psychological state can affect a person's desire to eat. Anxiety causes some people to increase their food intake; others eat less when they feel anxious. Depression often decreases a person's appetite and depletes the energy available for cooking and eating. Some people willingly alter eating patterns to help achieve weight loss. Rather than changing eating patterns, some people seek rapid weight loss through crash diets. Anorexia nervosa is an eating disorder in which the person refuses to eat due to a fear of becoming overweight, even with normal or less than IBW.

ALTERED NUTRITIONAL FUNCTION

The body undergoes constant renewal. If proper nutrition is not provided, body tissues will not be adequately maintained, energy will not be adequate for activities, and normal body

TABLE 29-2 SIGNS OF POOR NUTRITION AND POSSIBLE NUTRIENT DEFICIENCY

Signs	Possible Lacking Nutrient
Hair: Thin, coarse, lacking luster, breaks easily	Protein
Skin: Excessive bruising, bleeding	Vitamin K
Skin: Pressure sores, poor wound healing	Vitamin C and protein
Gums: Swollen, bleeding	Vitamin C
Muscles: Wasting	Protein
Lack of growth	Protein, calories
Skeletal: Poor posture, painful joints, bowed legs, increase in bone fractures	Calcium, vitamin D, vitamin C, protein
Mental: Confusion, motor weakness	Thiamine, niacin, B complex

processes will suffer. Indications of altered nutrition are overweight; obesity; underweight; recent significant weight loss or gain; decreased energy levels; altered bowel patterns; and altered appearance of the skin, hair, teeth, and mucous membranes (Table 29-2). If the patient's weight varies significantly from ideal body weight, a nutrition problem is likely.

Overweight

A person is said to be overweight if the BMI is between 25 and 29.9 kg per meters squared (BMI = kg/m²) (CDC, 2014). A person gains weight when he or she takes in more calories than the body needs.

Obesity

A person is obese if the BMI is 30 kg per meters squared or more. Obesity is present in greater than 34.9% of adults in the United States (Ogden et al., 2014). Obesity-related health conditions include heart disease, some types of cancer, and type 2 diabetes (CDC, 2014). Of obese individuals, 6.6% are extremely or morbidly obese, which is defined as a BMI greater than 40 kg per meters squared (Sturm & Hattori, 2013). In addition to health consequences, morbid obesity can significantly interfere with normal daily functioning in areas such as job performance, self-care, mobility, and breathing.

Underweight

A person is said to be underweight if he or she is below the ideal BMI of 20 to 25 kg per meters squared and is extremely underweight with a BMI less than 18.5 kg per meters squared. Underweight occurs when caloric intake is insufficient to meet the body's nutritional requirements. Approximately 1.7% of

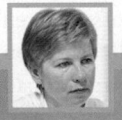

Nutrition PICO

Logan is calling the patient from the chapter-opening scenario with her lab results. During the conversation, the patient discloses that she has been taking chromium supplements for weight loss. The patient goes on to explain that her neighbor from Europe recommended this course of action and swears that it works. The patient is asking Logan what he thinks about the supplements. He informs the patient that he has heard of chromium but does not know how it affects weight loss. He tells the patient he will need to research it further and discuss it with the patient's nurse practitioner. Logan utilizes the Cochrane Library for his search and uses the following PICO question: *In overweight patients, how do Chromium supplements compared to no supplements help with weight loss?*

P = Overweight patients

I = Chromium supplements

C = other supplements

O = weight loss

Logan finds a meta-analysis that compared chromium supplements with a placebo. The study reviewed nine randomized controlled trials (RCTs) with 622 participating patients. A few of the RCT even compared using weight training with both the chromium supplement and placebo. Various doses of the chromium supplement were trialed to understand both efficacy and safety factor. Unfortunately, there was not clear statistical evidence that indicated that chromium supplements were beneficial in achieving weight loss safely. Logan informed the provider about the patient's inquiry and his findings. After reviewing the study, the nurse practitioner agreed with Logan that chromium supplements might not be the best recommendation for the patient.

REFERENCE:

Tian, H., Guo, X., Wang, X., He, Z., Sun, R., Ge, S., & Zhang, Z. (2013). Chromium picolinate supplementation for overweight or obese adults. *Cochrane Database of Systematic Reviews*. Issue 11. Art. No.: CD010063. DOI: 10.1002/14651858.CD010063.pub2

U.S. adults are underweight (Fryar & Ogden, 2012). Being underweight can increase the risk for infections, osteoporosis, and other health conditions. In the United States, common causes of being underweight include heavy smoking, an underlying disease such as cancer, or certain eating disorders (Thompson & Manore, 2012).

Recent Significant Weight Gain or Loss

Minor fluctuations in weight occur on a day-to-day basis due to fluid losses and gains, but changing weight patterns over weeks or months may indicate altered nutrition. A significant weight gain (5% in 1 month or 10% in 6 months) can occur when a person eats more than the body needs for energy expenditure. This can happen when a person becomes less active or when the intake of food is increased from, for example, stress or boredom. Significant weight loss, especially when intake has remained constant, can indicate hypermetabolic states, such as cancer or hyperthyroidism, or an inability to use ingested nutrients.

Decreased Energy

Food provides the body with energy to perform normal cellular processes and to carry out normal movement and activities. When nutritional deficits occur, adequate energy may be unavailable. Fatigue and activity intolerance are common manifestations of altered nutrition. The patient may report feeling tired or weak.

Altered Bowel Patterns

Inadequate dietary intake may affect bowel function and regularity. Constipation can occur when fiber or fluid intake is inadequate. Diarrhea may result when patients eat large quantities of fresh fruits. With food intolerance (e.g., lactase deficiency) or malabsorption syndrome, GI distress occurs. When a patient's bowel regularity changes, nutritional deficits must be ruled out as a causative factor.

Altered Skin, Teeth, Hair, and Mucous Membranes

Skin, nails, hair, and mucous membranes are rapidly growing tissues that continuously require adequate nutrition for growth. Protein is especially important in this process. Vitamin deficiencies are often manifested by altered development and growth of skin, teeth, hair, and mucous membranes. When protein is lacking, hair may become thin, lack luster, and break easily. Skin heals slowly and may appear thin and fragile when nutrition is inadequate. Mucous membranes may develop sores and bleed easily. Teeth and gums are more prone to disease.

Recall the patient in the case scenario at the beginning of the chapter. Use the concept map (Fig. 29-6) to help understand and manage the patient's situation and to plan for her care.

ASSESSMENT

Normal Pattern Identification

Ask questions to determine the patient's normal eating patterns and food preferences. The patient should describe his or her appetite as good, fair, or poor and discuss whether eating is usually pleasant.

Asking patients to describe food and fluid intake on a typical day provides a sense of what is normal for them. One of two surveying methods usually is used: the 24-hour recall or the food diary. In the 24-hour recall, the patient recalls and records the type, quality, and method of preparation of all food eaten within a 24-hour period. In the food diary, the patient keeps an ongoing log of the amount, time, and manner of preparation for all food consumed within a specific period. This time period can vary but is often 3 days to 1 week. The food diary ensures that the evaluation is affected less by "one time only" dietary indiscretions. Both surveying methods are subject to recall and recording errors.

Patients need to discuss food likes and dislikes, normal timing of meals, and routine snacks. Does the patient follow a special diet for any reason, have food allergies, or limit the intake of certain foods? How do cultural or religious concerns or practices influence the diet? For some patients, it is important to inquire how stress affects eating patterns. Some people under stress limit their food intake, but others increase the amount and frequency of food consumption.

Find out who in the family is responsible for shopping and cooking or whether family members share such responsibilities. Determine whether patients use prepackaged, prepared foods and how many times per week they eat at restaurants.

Risk Identification

Nutritional assessment helps to identify patients at risk for nutritional deficits. Determine a patient's knowledge and values related to nutrition by asking questions such as, "Do you believe your diet helps promote health?" and "What (if any) changes in your diet do you believe might be beneficial?" If the patient is following a specific diet, ask which foods are important to include or to avoid. Doing so can help assess the patient's understanding of the dietary restrictions. Who prescribed the diet? Was it a neighbor or a nutritionist?

Identify anorexia, chewing problems, sore mouth, dysphagia, nausea, and vomiting, and, if food intake has been affected, for how long. Note any chronic or acute health problems affecting the GI tract (e.g., ulcers, gallbladder disease, inflammatory bowel disease). Document chronic health conditions and their treatments (e.g., diabetes mellitus, cancer, renal disease, heart disease, lung disease), and assess their effect on appetite and food intake. Note any condition that impairs swallowing (e.g., a neurologic impairment) and its specific deficits.

Assessing socioeconomic factors helps determine possible nutritional deficits. Does the patient have money and transportation to buy nutritious food? Are safe storage and adequate cooking facilities available? Does the patient or caregiver have the energy to shop for and prepare meals?

NUTRITION

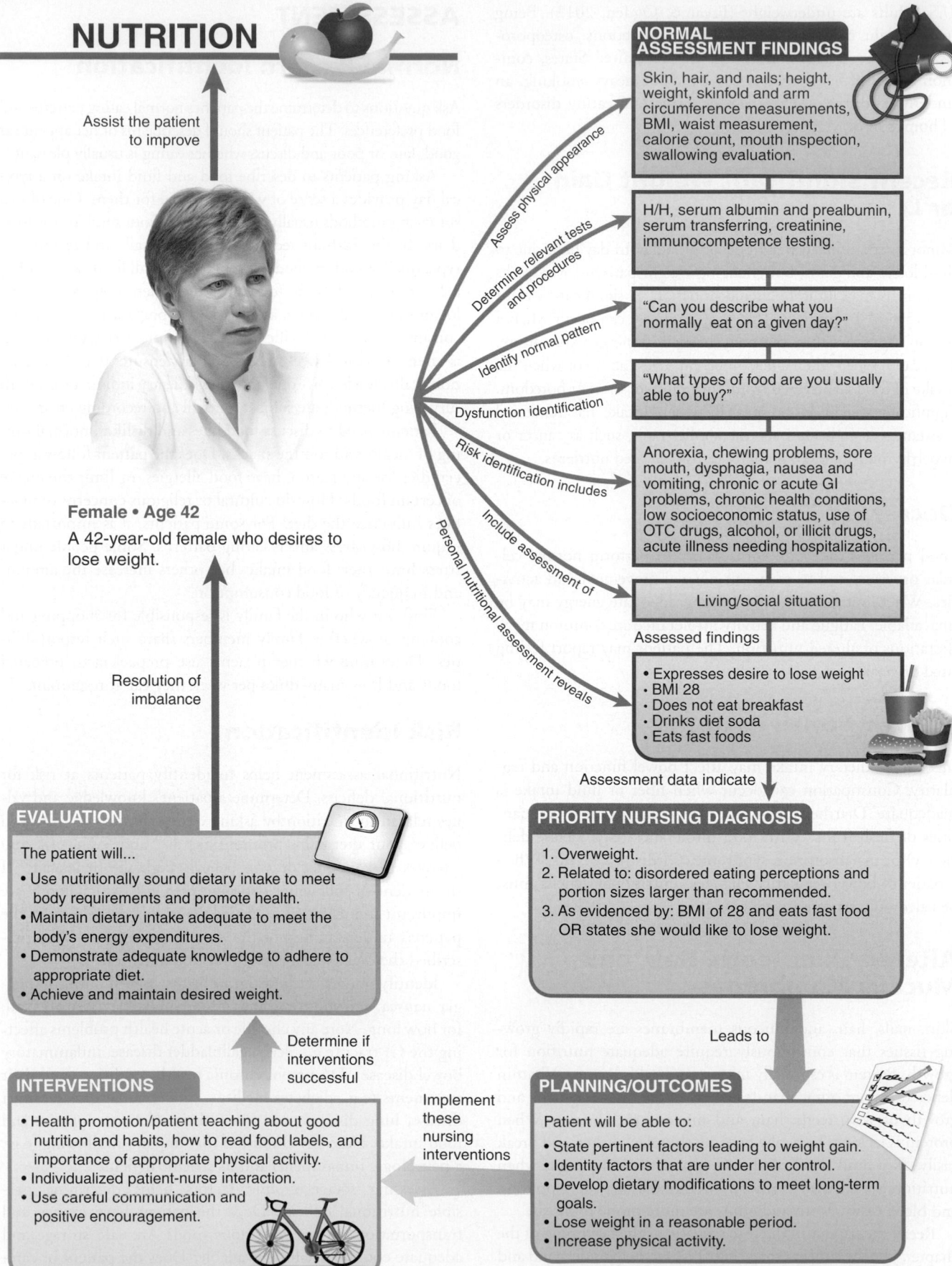

Assist the patient to improve

Female • Age 42

A 42-year-old female who desires to lose weight.

Resolution of imbalance

NORMAL ASSESSMENT FINDINGS

Assess physical appearance → Skin, hair, and nails; height, weight, skinfold and arm circumference measurements, BMI, waist measurement, calorie count, mouth inspection, swallowing evaluation.

Determine relevant tests and procedures → H/H, serum albumin and prealbumin, serum transferring, creatinine, immunocompetence testing.

Identify normal pattern → "Can you describe what you normally eat on a given day?"

Dysfunction identification → "What types of food are you usually able to buy?"

Risk identification includes → Anorexia, chewing problems, sore mouth, dysphagia, nausea and vomiting, chronic or acute GI problems, chronic health conditions, low socioeconomic status, use of OTC drugs, alcohol, or illicit drugs, acute illness needing hospitalization.

Include assessment of → Living/social situation

Personal nutritional assessment reveals

Assessed findings

- Expresses desire to lose weight
- BMI 28
- Does not eat breakfast
- Drinks diet soda
- Eats fast foods

Assessment data indicate

PRIORITY NURSING DIAGNOSIS

1. Overweight.
2. Related to: disordered eating perceptions and portion sizes larger than recommended.
3. As evidenced by: BMI of 28 and eats fast food OR states she would like to lose weight.

Leads to

EVALUATION

The patient will...

- Use nutritionally sound dietary intake to meet body requirements and promote health.
- Maintain dietary intake adequate to meet the body's energy expenditures.
- Demonstrate adequate knowledge to adhere to appropriate diet.
- Achieve and maintain desired weight.

Determine if interventions successful

INTERVENTIONS

- Health promotion/patient teaching about good nutrition and habits, how to read food labels, and importance of appropriate physical activity.
- Individualized patient-nurse interaction.
- Use careful communication and positive encouragement.

Implement these nursing interventions

PLANNING/OUTCOMES

Patient will be able to:

- State pertinent factors leading to weight gain.
- Identity factors that are under her control.
- Develop dietary modifications to meet long-term goals.
- Lose weight in a reasonable period.
- Increase physical activity.

FIGURE 29-6 Concept map for nutrition.

Document intake of over-the-counter drugs, alcohol, and illicit drugs, such as cocaine or heroin. Note the use of vitamin and mineral supplements and prescription medications, such as insulin, antacids, chemotherapeutic agents, and steroids. Assess any impact of such substances on nutrition.

Acute illness and hospitalization often affect the ability to take food orally. Many tests and procedures (e.g., endoscopy or interventional radiology procedures), as well as critical and acute illness, require "nothing by mouth," or NPO status. Specialized nutritional support (SNS) is a way to provide adequate nutrition to individuals with an actual or anticipated nutritional deficit. SNS may also be called nutritional support therapy or artificial nutrition therapy. The American Society for Parenteral and Enteral Nutrition (ASPEN) recommends SNS for patients based upon length of anticipated nutritional deficit and patient nutritional status prior to acute illness (Malone, 2014). SNS may deliver nutrients by tube through the GI tract (enteral nutrition) or intravenously (total parenteral nutrition [TPN]). ASPEN recommends the enteral route as the preferred method. The use of parenteral nutrition should be reserved for situations in which neither oral intake nor enteral feedings are feasible for at least 7 days (Malone, 2014).

Dysfunction Identification

Nutrition may be impaired when the patient cannot buy and prepare food, is unwilling or unable to eat, eats excessively, or cannot use ingested nutrients. Such dysfunctions are often determined by asking questions. Nutritional alterations can be identified if the patient's BMI is higher than 25 or lower than 20 kg per meters squared.

Reports of significant recent weight loss without altered diet indicate an inability to meet normal nutritional requirements. A dietary intake that supplies significantly less than RDAs or DRIs also helps identify deficits. Look for signs and symptoms of nutritional dysfunction, such as fatigue, muscle wasting, and obesity.

Physical Assessment

GENERAL OBSERVATIONS

General observation provides important information on nutritional status. An adequately nourished person appears robust, vital, and energetic and has erect posture. Skin, hair, and nails appear healthy (Box 29-3).

ANTHROPOMETRIC MEASUREMENTS

Anthropometric measurements include height and weight, waist measurement, skinfold measurements, and arm circumference measurements. Accurate skinfold and arm circumference measurements take practice and skill to achieve.

Height and weight are compared with findings in a table of standard measurements grouped by age, sex, and body frame. Estimate small, medium, or large body frame. Ask what the person thinks is his or her IBW; this may vary from standardized tables. BMI is calculated by height and weight values.

BOX 29-3 | Characteristics of a Well-Nourished Person

- Normal weight and height for age, body build, and developmental stage
- Adequate appetite
- Active, alert, and able to maintain adequate attention span
- Firm, healthy skin and mucous membranes
- Erect posture, with straight arms and legs
- Well-developed muscles without excess body fat
- Normal schedule of tooth eruption and healthy teeth and gums
- Normal urinary and bowel elimination patterns
- Normal sleep patterns
- Normal hemoglobin, hematocrit, and serum protein levels
- Absence of diet-related abnormalities

Waist measurement is taken just above the top of hip bones (iliac crest) and is a clinical measure of abdominal fat cells. A waist measure higher than 42 inches in women or 47 inches in men has been associated with higher risk for health problems such as heart disease, diabetes, hypertension, and dyslipidemia. In addition, recent evidence suggests that very large waist sizes may also increase the risk of certain cancers (American Cancer Society, 2010).

Skinfold measurements are used to help determine fat stores in the body. The triceps skinfold and the subscapular skinfold are most commonly used. A caliper measures the fold of skin, which includes the subcutaneous tissue but not the underlying muscle. Measurements are compared with a table of standards grouped by age and sex to detect excess fat.

Midarm circumference measurements are taken of the upper arm to provide information about the muscle mass. Because muscles are the major protein stores, measuring arm circumference helps evaluate protein status. Again, measurements are compared with a table of standards.

CALORIE COUNT

When inadequate intake is suspected, calories can be counted. The percentage of calories eaten of each food served must be recorded. The dietitian uses this information to calculate the calories consumed and to evaluate whether the caloric intake is adequate. Computer programs are also available to aid in calculations.

MOUTH INSPECTION

Observe the condition of the teeth, gums, and mucous membranes. Mucous membranes should be moist, and adequate saliva should be present. Note any caries, excessive plaque, and gingivitis. If the patient uses dentures, evaluate proper fit and condition. Detect any lesions of the oral cavity (canker sores, stomatitis, *Candida* infections), and treat them promptly. Discomfort associated with such lesions can alter food intake.

SWALLOWING EVALUATION

A swallowing evaluation is necessary when potential difficulty in swallowing is suspected. Usually, patients are referred to speech therapists for swallowing evaluations, but nurses may need to evaluate swallowing abilities to determine whether feeding is safe. A swallowing evaluation includes assessment of motor function of the facial, oral, and tongue muscles; cough reflex; swallowing reflex; and gag reflex.

Assess motor function by observing the face, jaw, and tongue for symmetry and strength during normal movements. Asking the patient to cough permits evaluation of the briskness and strength of the cough reflex, which is necessary to clear aspirated food from the airway. Evaluate ability to swallow by placing the index finger and thumb on the patient's laryngeal protuberance and asking the patient to swallow. As the patient with an intact swallowing reflex swallows, the nurse will feel the larynx elevate. Finally, evaluate the gag reflex by stroking the patient's right or left pharyngeal wall with a tongue blade.

SAFETY ALERT

When ability to swallow is questionable, never give oral food or fluids until a complete evaluation is done.

Diagnostic Tests and Procedures

Biochemical data can help establish a diagnosis, determine the necessary dietary modifications, or identify specific nutritional deficiencies before clinical signs appear. Evaluation of blood and urine is most useful when analyzing a patient's nutritional state. The most common laboratory data used are hematocrit, hemoglobin, serum albumin, prealbumin, serum transferrin, and total lymphocyte count. Anergy testing can be done to identify severe nutritional deficits.

HEMATOCRIT AND HEMOGLOBIN

Hematocrit is the percentage of red blood cells found in 100 mL of blood. This measure of size and number of cells in the blood, combined with the hemoglobin value, aids in determining the presence and severity of anemia.

A hemoglobin count measures the blood's oxygen- and iron-carrying capacity. A decreased hemoglobin value indicates decreased iron intake or decreased iron reserves, conditions that often are present in anemia.

SERUM ALBUMIN AND PREALBUMIN

Serum albumin and prealbumin are protein markers that help assess nutritional status. Serum albumin accounts for more than half of the body's total serum protein. Serum albumin values reflect protein intake or absorption. Values less than 3.5 g per deciliter (35 g per liter) may indicate nutritional deficits. Such protein changes take more than 2 weeks to appear in serum albumin values because the half-life of albumin is about 18 days.

A low albumin level also can be related to overhydration and may not necessarily indicate malnutrition. Prealbumin has a half-life of 2 days and accurately assesses protein synthesis and nitrogen balance. It is considered a very sensitive and specific marker for nutritional status (Dudek, 2014).

SERUM TRANSFERRIN

Transferrin, a blood protein that binds with iron and is important in its transport, is considered a sensitive indicator of protein deficiency. Transferrin, which is synthesized in the liver, increases when iron stores are low and decreases when iron stores are high. Changes in protein intake or visceral protein stores are more rapidly reflected in serum transferrin levels than in serum albumin levels.

CREATININE EXCRETION

The rate of creatinine formation is proportional to total muscle mass. Creatinine is released during skeletal muscle metabolism and is excreted from the body through the kidneys. Creatinine excretion usually is measured by collecting and measuring creatinine in all voided urine during a 24-hour period. As muscles atrophy during malnutrition, creatinine excretion decreases.

IMMUNOCOMPETENCE TESTING

Nutritional status affects immunity. In severe nutritional depletion, patients may be unable to mount an immune response (anergy). Commonly, this is seen as the lymphocyte count decreases with protein depletion. Skin testing also may be performed to evaluate the impact of nutritional deficits on immune function. Antigen skin tests (e.g., tuberculosis, *Candida*, mumps) can be used to evaluate the patient's response to antigens to which he or she has already been sensitized. If no skin response is observed after 48 hours, anergy is present. Anergy indicates the need for aggressive nutritional support.

NURSING DIAGNOSES

NANDA-International (NANDA-I, 2014) nursing diagnoses that have been identified in the area of nutrition include Imbalanced Nutrition: Less Than Body Requirements; Obesity; Overweight; and Impaired Swallowing. Selected nursing diagnoses along with Nursing Outcomes Classification (NOC) and Nursing Interventions Classification (NIC) are presented in Table 29-3.

OUTCOME IDENTIFICATION AND PLANNING

After the nursing diagnoses and related factors have been identified, patient goals and nursing interventions are planned. Patient goals for nutrition include ensuring adequate

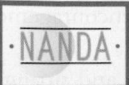

Table 29-3	SELECTED NANDA-I NURSING DIAGNOSES INVOLVING NUTRITION			
Nursing Dx	**Related Factors**	**Dx Statement**	**NOC***	**NIC†**
Imbalanced Nutrition: Less Than Body Requirements—intake of nutrients insufficient to meet metabolic needs	Biologic, economic, and psychological factors; inability to absorb nutrients; inability to digest or ingest food	**Imbalanced Nutrition:** R/T lack of food AEB loss of weight, pale mucous membranes, poor muscle tone, and food intake less than RDA	Appetite Compliance Behavior Nutritional Status: Nutrient Intake Tissue integrity Weight: Body Mass	Behavior Modification Energy Management Health Screening Nutritional Monitoring Nutritional Status: Nutrient Intake Teaching: Prescribed Diet Weight Gain Assistance
Overweight—intake of nutrients that exceeds metabolic needs	Excessive intake in relation to metabolic need	**Overweight**—R/T excessive caloric intake AEB weight 20% over ideal, sedentary activity level, and dysfunctional eating patterns	Body Image; Knowledge: Diet Weight: Body Mass Weight control	Body Image Enhancement Behavior Modification Eating Disorders Management Health Screening Nutrition Management Nutritional Status: Nutrient Intake NANDA-International (NANDA-I, 2009). Weight Reduction Assistance Weight Management

From: Moorhead, S., Johnson, M., Maas, M., & Swanson, E. (2013). *Iowa outcomes project: Nursing outcomes classification (NOC)* (5th ed.). St. Louis, MO: C. V. Mosby.
†*From:* Bulecheck, G., Butcher, H., Dochterman, J., & Wagner, C. (2013). *Iowa intervention project: Nursing interventions classification (NIC)* (6th ed.). St. Louis, MO: C. V. Mosby.
Dx, diagnosis; R/T, related to; AEB, as evidenced by; RDA, recommended dietary allowance.
From: NANDA-Association International (NANDA I). (2014). *Nursing diagnoses: Definitions and classification, 2015–2017.* West Sussex, England: Wiley-Blackwell.

nutritional intake and understanding and complying with dietary modifications. Common goals in nutrition include the following:

- The patient will use nutritionally sound dietary intake to meet body requirements and to promote health.
- The patient will maintain dietary intake balance to meet the body's energy expenditures.
- The patient will demonstrate adequate knowledge to adhere to dietary prescription or therapies to promote health.
- The patient will achieve and maintain desired weight.

Cooperation from patients is necessary to plan and to set goals because patients are responsible for their own nutrition (unless others plan meals for them). Planning revolves around each patient's motivation and abilities. If the patient is unable to shop or to prepare food, a support person must be included in the planning. Many nursing interventions for healthy nutritional balance are educational. Examples of nursing interventions commonly used in planning for nutritional education and support are discussed in the next section of this chapter.

IMPLEMENTATION

Health Promotion

Collaborating with the healthcare team, nurses are responsible for promoting optimal nutrition through teaching. Promoting optimal nutrition, providing assistance, and creating an atmosphere that encourages healthy eating are important nursing roles.

PROVIDING PATIENT TEACHING

Nurses actively promote good nutrition in various settings: health fairs, schools, prenatal classes, health screening visits, and homes. The goal of such education is to encourage good nutrition by increasing understanding of the importance of a healthy diet (see dietary guideline comparison in Box 29-1 earlier in this chapter).

Although knowledge about nutrients does not guarantee healthy eating, patients with greater nutritional knowledge generally choose more healthy diets. In the early 1990s, food labels were introduced to assist consumers in choosing healthier foods. This label has been revised to include trans fats levels (USDA, 2013) (Fig. 29-7). The U.S. Food and Drug administration is proposing additional evidence-based changes in the label to further promote health. One important proposed change, in part to combat the obesity epidemic, is to change serving sizes that are listed on food labels (U.S. Food and Drug Administration, 2014). Helping consumers and patients incorporate this information into eating patterns can have lasting effects. Nurses can refer at-risk people to appropriate private and community resources, including USDA websites.

Some hospitalized patients are receptive to nutrition teaching. When working with such patients, direct your statements toward actions that the patient can take immediately (e.g., "While your incision is healing, it's important to eat enough protein."). Informal diet instruction can occur when helping patients make menu selections. Praise food choices, emphasizing the importance of each food in maintaining health. Gently encourage patients to improve diet selections (e.g., "Have you tried 1% milk rather than 2% milk? Many people don't notice the difference, and it's a good way to reduce your fat intake.").

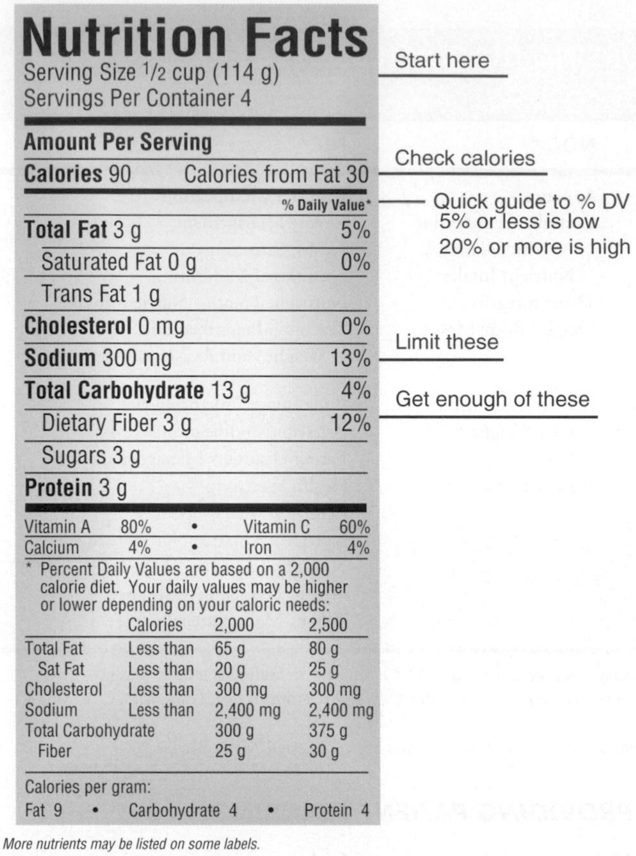

Nutrition Facts

Serving Size ¹/₂ cup (114 g)
Servings Per Container 4

Amount Per Serving

Calories 90   Calories from Fat 30

	% Daily Value*
Total Fat 3 g	5%
Saturated Fat 0 g	0%
Trans Fat 1 g	
Cholesterol 0 mg	0%
Sodium 300 mg	13%
Total Carbohydrate 13 g	4%
Dietary Fiber 3 g	12%
Sugars 3 g	
Protein 3 g	

Vitamin A	80%	•	Vitamin C	60%
Calcium	4%	•	Iron	4%

* Percent Daily Values are based on a 2,000
calorie diet. Your daily values may be higher
or lower depending on your caloric needs:

	Calories	2,000	2,500
Total Fat	Less than	65 g	80 g
Sat Fat	Less than	20 g	25 g
Cholesterol	Less than	300 mg	300 mg
Sodium	Less than	2,400 mg	2,400 mg
Total Carbohydrate		300 g	375 g
Fiber		25 g	30 g

Calories per gram:
Fat 9   •   Carbohydrate 4   •   Protein 4

Start here

Check calories

*Quick guide to % DV
5% or less is low
20% or more is high*

Limit these

Get enough of these

* More nutrients may be listed on some labels.

FIGURE 29-7 Example of a food label and its nutritional information.

Patients often question nurses about nutrition or ask for suggestions for altering their diet. For example, an overweight patient may ask the nurse's opinion of a new diet that a friend has recommended. Many magazines highlight food in each issue. Provide patients with accurate information, encouragement, praise, and referral to appropriate resources. Tips relating to each food group are part of the ChooseMyPlate.gov information (USDA, 2013).

PROMOTING OPTIMAL INTAKE

Illness often affects eating, and nurses play a role in encouraging optimal nutrition for patients. Rooms where eating will take place should be clean, well ventilated, and free from strong odors. The atmosphere should be relaxing. Interruptions, such as treatments and procedures, should not occur during mealtimes. Oral care before eating promotes comfort and taste. Timing administration of medications to control nausea and pain will help patients achieve optimal relief at mealtimes.

Food should be served in an attractive, appetizing manner and at the right temperature. Microwave ovens can rewarm cooled food. Food preferences should be considered. Small servings are preferable because they do not overwhelm patients. Family members can bring favorite foods from home, as long as such food is permitted in the patient's diet.

Pleasant company can improve the incentive for eating for some patients, but conversation should not distract the patient.

Staff or relatives can provide verbal cues and encouragement during eating for confused or reluctant patients.

It is preferable for patients to be out of bed and sitting in chairs for meals. This position facilitates chewing and swallowing and prevents reflux of stomach contents. Some patients may need assistance in cutting food, opening packages, or eating. **Procedure 29-2** suggests methods for assisting patients with feeding.

> **SAFETY ALERT**
>
> When feeding patients, maintain foods at proper temperature, including recommended temperature when cooking, to minimize microbial contamination.

Nursing Interventions for Altered Nutritional Function

WITHHOLDING FOOD

The term *NPO*, or nothing by mouth (Latin, *non per os*), is used when ingestion of food or fluids orally is contraindicated. Withholding food may be indicated in the following situations:

- To rest the GI tract to promote healing
- To clear the GI tract of contents before surgery or diagnostic procedures
- To prevent aspiration during surgery or in high-risk patients
- To give normal intestinal motility time to return
- To treat severe vomiting or diarrhea
- To treat medical problems, such as bowel obstruction or acute inflammation of the GI tract

Well-nourished patients can go without food for a few days, but they must receive fluids to prevent fluid and electrolyte disturbances. Some patients find being unable to eat difficult. The following nursing measures can promote comfort during this period:

- Provide frequent oral hygiene.
- Give ice chips, hard candy, and gum or mouth rinses if permitted.
- Avoid exposing patients to others who are eating, to food odors, or to advertisements for food.

If the NPO period is longer than 5 to 7 days, or if certain patient conditions exist, specialized nutritional support, such as enteral tube feeding, is recommended. If enteral feedings are not feasible, parenteral routes may be considered. ASPEN has published guidelines for patient selection and for safe, appropriate administration of nutritional support (Malone, 2014).

USING SPECIAL DIETS

When a patient can eat any food, the diet is called general or regular. A regular diet is well balanced and supplies the metabolic requirements for a sedentary person (about 2,000 cal per day).

Menus allow patients to select from various choices, but all offerings are nutritionally planned to supply recommended daily allowances. In hospital or long-term care settings, special requests or preferences (e.g., vegetarian diet, kosher diet) and food allergies should be reported to the dietary department when the patient is admitted.

Often, dietary intake must be altered to promote healing and to restore health. Some objectives of dietary treatment are to increase or decrease weight, to allow an organ to rest, to remedy nutritional deficits, to promote healing, and to provide nutrients the body can metabolize.

Modifying a diet's texture, consistency, calories, or other nutrients may be necessary for patients who have had surgery or have a medical condition that requires an altered diet. Examples of types of diets with different textures and consistencies are clear liquid, full liquid, soft, and mechanical soft.

Clear Liquid

This diet includes only liquids that lack residue, such as juices without pulp (e.g., apple, cranberry), tea, gelatin, soda pop, and clear broth. The clear liquid diet is used as a first diet after surgery, before some diagnostic tests, and after an acute episode of vomiting or diarrhea.

Full Liquid

A full liquid diet includes all fluids and foods that become liquid at room temperature (e.g., ice cream, sherbet). This diet may be ordered after surgery after a clear liquid diet has been well tolerated or for patients who cannot chew food adequately.

Soft

Soft diets include soft foods and those with reduced fiber content, which require less energy for digestion. Soft diets are appropriate for patients who have difficulty chewing or no teeth. Mechanical soft diets include similar foods that are further chopped or pureed for those with difficulty chewing. They also may be used after surgery as the diet progresses.

Diet as Tolerated

Diet as tolerated is ordered when a patient's ability to tolerate certain foods will change, such as after surgery or after GI distress. Nurses order such diets based on the patient's appetite, ability to eat, and food tolerance. For example, on the first postoperative day, a patient may receive a clear liquid diet. If no nausea occurs, normal intestinal motility returns, and the patient feels like eating, the diet may advance to a regular diet.

Restrictive Diets

Diets may be ordered to fulfill a special requirement in patients with chronic disease or altered metabolism. For example, patients with cardiac problems may need to limit sodium and types of dietary fat, obese patients may need to restrict calories, and patients with diabetes may need to follow a prescribed American Diabetes Association diet. Any food or fluid given must fit the dietary restrictions. Examples of such dietary modifications are given in Table 29-4.

TABLE 29-4 DIETARY MODIFICATIONS FOR DISEASES

Disease	Modification
Renal disease	Restrict intake of sodium, potassium, protein, and possibly fluids.
Liver disease (cirrhosis)	Restrict intake of sodium; increase intake of protein, unless hepatic coma is pending, at which time protein is virtually eliminated.
Congestive heart failure	Restrict intake of sodium and calories.
Coronary artery disease	Restrict intake of sodium, calories, and fats (saturated fats and cholesterol).
Burns	Increase intake of calories, protein, vitamin C, and the B-complex vitamins.
Respiratory (emphysema)	A soft, high-calorie, high-protein diet is recommended.
Tuberculosis	Increase intake of protein, calories, calcium, and vitamin A.
Hypertension	Restrict sodium intake; lose weight, if appropriate.

When patients are placed on restrictive diets, teaching must promote necessary dietary changes. Dietitians may do initial teaching, and nurses reinforce such teaching. Written materials are available to assist in such education. Changing long-established eating patterns is difficult for many patients, and goals should be realistic, mutually set, and individualized.

USING NUTRITIONAL SUPPLEMENTS

Nutritional supplements, in the form of formulas or vitamins and minerals, may be added to prescribed diets to provide necessary nutrients, especially during periods of increased metabolic demand. Nurses can request supplements, which physicians order. Supplements are typically milkshake-type drinks given between meals three or four times a day to increase calorie and/or protein intake. Malnourished patients and patients with excessive metabolic demands from trauma, fever, infection, surgery, or cancer benefit from such "power-packing" therapy.

ADMINISTERING ENTERAL TUBE FEEDINGS

Enteral nutrition involves the direct delivery of nutrients into the GI system, bypassing the mouth. Tube feedings contain nutritionally balanced, commercial formulas given through a tube directly into the stomach, duodenum, or jejunum. Access to the GI system can be achieved by inserting a tube through the nose into the stomach or intestine or percutaneously through the abdominal wall into the stomach or intestine.

Tube feedings provide nutrition to patients with functional GI systems who have difficulty with swallowing or have disease states that contribute to malnutrition. Obstruction can occur secondary to edema from head or neck surgery, tumor, or trauma (e.g., swallowing caustic substances, inhaling smoke). Tube feedings are indicated when decreased level of consciousness prevents safe eating. Tube feedings are used as adjunctive therapy for patients who can eat but who cannot consume adequate nutrients to meet the body's nutritional demands (e.g., patients who have cancer or severe pancreatitis). Premature newborns who have an inadequate sucking reflex or lack of strength to feed also can be fed this way. Tube feedings are appropriate only when nutrients can be absorbed from the GI tract.

Types of Tubes

The type of tube used to deliver enteral feedings depends on how long, where, and how the feeding is delivered. Flexible, **small-bore feeding tubes** have been developed for use when tube feeding is indicated for a short period of time. These tubes vary in size from 8 to 10 French and are composed of polyurethane, silicon, or polyvinyl chloride. Most have weighted distal tips and are placed transnasally with the use of a removable stylet. The tubes are radiopaque so that radiographic examination can confirm tube placement.

Tube Placement

Enteral access devices are selected based upon patient-specific factors. Nasal and oral routes are usually placed for short-term use in the hospitalized patient. Gastric feedings rely upon a stomach that is free from fistula, obstruction, or delayed gastric emptying. Tubes may be placed into the small bowel for patients who cannot tolerate gastric feedings due to intolerance, reflux, or stomach disorders (Bristrian & Driscoll, 2012). Tube feedings should never be started without an abdominal x-ray to confirm placement of the tube (Simons & Abdallah, 2012).

Transnasal feeding tubes are secured to the bridge of the nose with tape. Care is taken to anchor the feeding tube so that rubbing against the naris is minimized. Skin integrity is assessed each shift to ensure that pressure ulcers are prevented.

Enteral feeding tubes inserted percutaneously through the abdominal wall can be placed into the stomach (gastrostomy) or intestine (jejunostomy). They are larger in diameter and are made of soft biocompatible material. The procedure for gastrostomy placement is called percutaneous endoscopic gastrostomy (PEG). PEG involves endoscopic percutaneous insertion of a specially designed catheter into the stomach (Fig. 29-8). Although urinary catheters or other devices have been used in some settings due to convenience and low cost, this practice can lead to dislodgement, balloon rupture, and possible increases in infections (Ojo, 2014). PEG placement may be done under moderate sedation or general anesthesia and can sometimes be done on an ambulatory basis. An internal or external fixation device is placed over the tube during the insertion procedure and against the abdominal wall to avoid migration of the tube.

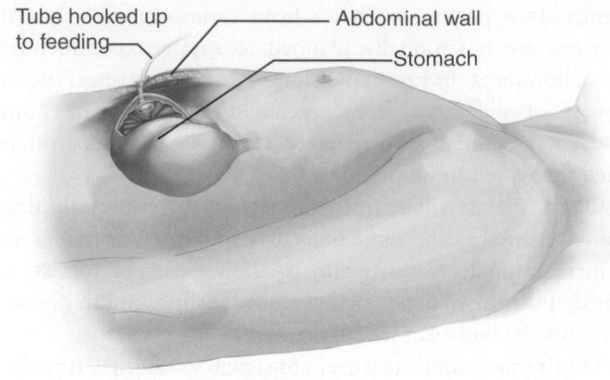

A

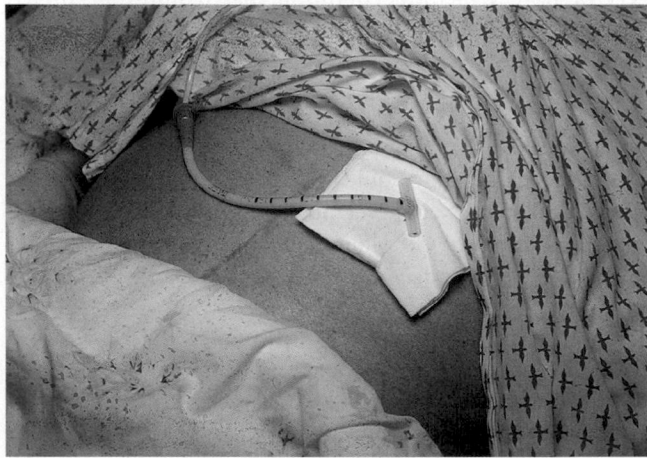

B

FIGURE 29-8 PEG. **A.** Tube is placed in the stomach for feedings. An internal fixation device prevents dislodgement. **B.** Dressing over the tube on the abdomen protects the PEG tube site.

Skin care at the insertion site includes cleaning the site with warm soap and water, intermittent use of hydrogen peroxide, and careful drying to decrease skin breakdown. A clean drain dressing may be placed under the bolster for comfort if the patient desires.

A dual-lumen gastrostomy/jejunostomy tube (PEG/J tube) can be inserted if the patient needs simultaneous gastric decompression and small bowel feedings. This tube allows feedings to enter the jejunum through one lumen while the second lumen drains the stomach (Chan & Burakoff, 2012).

Enteral Formulas

Enteral feedings consist of nutritionally balanced formulas. Many brands are available commercially; they vary in relative proportions of nutrients and calories, osmolarity, and ease of digestibility and absorption. Most formulas can be stored unrefrigerated until opened, but after opening, they should be refrigerated to limit microbial growth. To minimize bacterial contamination, ready-to-use formula should be discarded within 24 hours after opening, or according to manufacturer direction. Reconstituted formulas should be used or discarded within 4 hours (Ojo & Bowden, 2012).

Intermittent Versus Continuous Feedings

Enteral feedings may be given intermittently or continuously, as summarized in **Procedure 29-3**. The physician or registered dietitian orders the rate of infusion and the formula to use. Continuous feedings are permitted to flow in at the prescribed rate by the gravitational drip method, or they are monitored by an infusion pump. For patients who are eating, feedings may be ordered to infuse continuously during the night and may be discontinued a few hours before breakfast to stimulate the appetite.

Intermittent feedings are given at specific intervals, often corresponding to mealtimes. Intermittent feedings may be given over a long (e.g., hours) or shorter (e.g., minutes) period, depending on factors such as tube placement, feeding volume, and number of feedings per day. A syringe, gravity flow, or a pump is used. When feedings are alternated with nonfeeding times, such a schedule may also be called cyclic.

Hazards and Complications

Nursing responsibilities for patients receiving tube feedings include prevention and assessment of complications, such as nausea, vomiting, aspiration, fluid and electrolyte imbalance, diarrhea, intestinal cramping, tube occlusion, and hyperglycemia. Nausea, vomiting, cramping or bloating, and diarrhea can occur when the feeding is administered at a rate faster than the formula can be absorbed. It is important to watch for these symptoms and adjust the rate according to tolerance, always notifying the physician or registered dietitian of clinical symptoms associated with feeding intolerance. **Gastric residual volumes (GRVs)** are sometimes requested as a way to assess tolerance of enteral feeding. This is usually done by inserting a catheter tip or Luer-lock syringe into the proximal end of the feeding tube and aspirating gastric contents. There is conflicting data supporting a correlation of GRVs with regurgitation or aspiration, and they cannot be relied upon as the sole means of protecting patients against aspiration pneumonia (Simons & Abdallah, 2012). Feedings should generally not be stopped for GRVs of more than 400 to 500 mL unless the patient exhibits signs of intolerance. Patients at high risk for aspiration should be monitored based on their disease process, not solely on their GRVs. Physical findings suggesting paralytic ileus (clinical findings can be abdominal distention, nausea, or vomiting) or overt aspiration or regurgitation require timely intervention and close monitoring and surveillance.

SAFETY ALERT

Always use an oral syringe (one with catheter or tapered tip) when administering food or medicines by mouth or enteral tube. A parenteral syringe (one with a Luer-lock end) can accidentally be connected to an intravenous (IV) line resulting in IV administration of food or oral medications (Institute for Safe Medication Practices, 2014).

Increased risk of aspiration should be anticipated in patients with altered mental status. Jejunal feeding tube placement is recommended for patients at risk for aspiration to enhance feeding safety.

Minimize the risk of aspiration by checking proper tube placement before initiating feedings and at frequent intervals and by keeping the patient in Fowler's position (head of bed elevated at least 30 to 45 degrees) at all times when feedings are infusing and for 30 minutes after completion of intermittent or continuous feeding.

SAFETY ALERT

Always check proper tube placement before beginning tube feedings to prevent accidental aspiration of feedings.

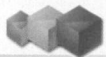

Concept Mastery Alert

For patients receiving enteral feedings, elevating the head of the bed to a height of 30 to 45 degrees is a bare minimum, not the optimal range. Ideally, to provide the best protection against aspiration, the nurse should elevate the patient's head of the bed at 90 degrees, or as close to this high Fowler's position as possible.

Feeding tubes inserted transnasally should be marked clearly at the level of naris insertion once an abdominal x-ray has verified correct placement. This allows the nurse to tell at a glance whether the tube has migrated out during feeding and decreases the risk of aspiration.

Nursing documentation of transnasal small-bore feeding tube placement should always include the patient's tolerance of the tube insertion procedure, x-ray confirmation, and depth of feeding tube insertion in centimeters (printed on the outside of the small-bore feeding tube). In the past, methylene blue dye was added to enteral feedings as a way to track aspiration; however, this dye has been implicated in serious liver and GI damage and has also been shown to precipitate toxic mitochondrial activity. This dye is unsafe and should not be used (Metheny, 2009).

Diarrhea, intestinal cramping, and fluid loss can occur when high-osmolarity formulas are used. Slow administration of room temperature feedings helps limit GI intolerance. Giving the patient adequate hydration via the feeding tube (e.g., 200 mL of free water every 6 hours) may prevent severe osmotic shifts and is generally an important part of the feeding regimen.

Feeding tubes, especially those with small-bore lumens, clog easily. Tube occlusion should be avoided. Prevent clogging by flushing the tube with 30 to 60 mL of warm water before and after giving medications and when disconnecting tube feedings. For a clogged feeding tube, instill a solution of meat tenderizer and water (1 tablespoon in 30 mL of warm water). Let the solution sit for 5 minutes in the feeding tube to dissolve particles formed by proteins in the formula. Follow up with a warm water flush.

Hyperglycemia may occur in patients who cannot produce enough insulin to deal with the carbohydrate load in the formula. For patients with diabetes and others considered to be at high risk, blood glucose monitoring at least two and possibly four times a day permits careful regulation of increased insulin need.

APPLY YOUR CRITICAL THINKING

Gina Round has a gastrostomy tube in place and is receiving full-strength Isocal formula at 80 mL/hour. Isocal comes in cans containing 240 mL. How would you prepare this tube feeding? What assessments and nursing considerations are important for patients who receive tube feedings?

Check your answer in Appendix B.

Home and Community Care

Nutrition is an important consideration in independent home management. Patients must be able to buy, store, prepare, and eat food independently to function at home; many patients need assistance with shopping or cooking. Family and friends

ETHICAL/LEGAL ISSUE

ENDING TUBE FEEDING

Mr. Camper (47 years old) was admitted to a long-term care facility 6 months ago, following a motorcycle accident. He experienced severe head injuries that left him comatose. He requires total physical care, including tube feedings for nutrition. Mr. Camper has started to develop increasing joint stiffness and contractures and has not shown any signs of responsiveness. Mr. Camper's physician and family have been conferring on his prognosis and plans for care. They have decided together that it would be best to end the tube feedings and "let nature take its course." As the nurse on the unit, Ms. Goldmark has been asked to remove the gastrostomy tube and stop the feedings. Ms. Goldmark believes that removing the tube feedings will actually add to Mr. Camper's discomfort. She is reluctant to carry out this order and is also reluctant to require another nurse to do it, which would not erase her moral objection to the procedure.

CRITICAL THINKING CHALLENGE

- Explore your feelings in this situation. Do you agree or disagree with Ms. Goldmark?
- Identify any concerns that Ms. Goldmark has not mentioned that you have about this situation.
- Identify possible approaches to seeking additional information and resolving the dilemma.
- Recognizing the patient's rights, the family's rights, and the physician's order, define what you see as Ms. Goldmark's ethically appropriate behavior.

may be available to help. The plan of care should reflect the patient's needs and available support. Nurses can enlist the help of others to provide services if necessary.

Patients with chronic health problems may face great nutritional challenges. Many local and national agencies (e.g., American Cancer Society, American Heart Association, American Diabetes Association) and governmental agencies (e.g., USDA, USDA Food and Nutrition Center, National Institutes of Health) publish pamphlets that provide dietary guidance and realistic suggestions. Malnourished patients and those at risk for nutritional deficits may be referred to community health agencies.

When new restrictive diets are ordered for patients, teaching should start as soon as possible. Dietitians sometimes begin such teaching. Patients should receive written materials outlining foods to include and those to exclude from the diet. Help patients determine how best to incorporate dietary changes into their lives. Including the persons who will actually prepare the food in these teaching sessions is essential.

Nutritional support technologies, such as tube feedings or parenteral nutrition, are sometimes managed at home. In many instances, nurses teach patients and their caregivers how to administer such therapies. Teaching should begin early in the hospitalization by explaining the special feedings as they are performed. Before discharge, the patient or caregiver should be able to demonstrate necessary administration techniques and to solve problems that may arise. Arrangements for equipment and supplies should be made before discharge, and patients should receive the name of the vendor.

Governmental and private voluntary programs have been developed for people who need dietary enhancement and nutrition education. Nurses are actively involved in providing education and care through such programs. Community-based programs include the following:

- Senior center services
- Home-delivered meals
- Supplemental Nutrition Assistance Program (SNAP), a program that offers assistance in purchasing food to eligible, low-income individuals and families (formerly called Food Stamps)
- Missions and shelters
- Women, Infants, and Children (WIC), a nutrition and healthcare program for pregnant women, new mothers, infants, and children
- Child care centers
- School lunch programs

In addition to providing food for groups at risk, many of these services also provide education and counseling. The USDA's Nutrition Education and Training Program has been developed to help public schools in state and local communities incorporate nutrition education in their curricula.

Community resources also include the nutritional services of public health nurses, nutritionists, home health caregivers, and welfare agency workers. These people teach, assist with meal

OUTCOME-BASED TEACHING PLANS

When Mr. Lyman, a recent widower, comes to the clinic for a routine checkup, data reveal that he has lost 15 lb since his wife's death 6 months ago. He is 6 feet tall and currently weighs 160 lb. During your assessment, you discover that he usually eats cereal for breakfast, a sandwich for lunch, and skips dinner or has some soup. He states, "My wife always took care of the cooking. Since she died, nothing tastes good anymore." He has one son who lives 300 miles away and lots of friends in the area, but he doesn't feel comfortable hinting for dinner invitations. He asks you to help him develop a plan that he feels inclined and motivated to follow.

OUTCOME

Mr. Lyman will verbalize a realistic plan to increase food intake, which will permit him to maintain his present weight.

STRATEGIES

- Explore Mr. Lyman's feelings about his recent weight loss and desire to reverse weight loss trend.
- If Mr. Lyman is motivated to maintain or gain weight, discuss his eating pattern before his wife's death, including food likes and dislikes.
- Have Mr. Lyman keep a food diary.

- Discuss possible community agencies that could support his efforts (e.g., Meals on Wheels; senior program at the community center).
- Discuss foods that are dense in calories and protein.
- Suggest protein supplements between meals to boost caloric intake.
- Discuss easy-to-prepare frozen dinners that can be microwaved.
- Provide home health follow-up to assess and provide encouragement for weight gain and good nutrition.
- Refer Mr. Lyman to a nutritionist if he continues to lose weight despite the above efforts.

EVALUATION

2/23/17: 16:30—Examples of progress toward his goal as evidenced by:
- Mr. Lyman has identified a list of favorite foods to begin his program to gain weight.
- Mr. Lyman's food diary indicates that he has increased his protein and calorie intake to levels recommended by his physician for weight gain.
- Mr. Lyman reports increased mealtime pleasure since joining the local senior meal program.
- Mr. Lyman has gained 3 lb in the past month.
—J. Woodman, RN

planning and food buying, consult, make referrals, and conduct research. Library and online resources also provide evidence-based guidance for nurses helping patients meet their nutritional goals, as illustrated in the application example in the box above.

International agencies promote health and nutritional adequacy on a worldwide level. Programs include the Food and Agriculture Organization of the United Nations, the WHO, and the United Nations Children's Fund.

EVALUATION

Nursing interventions related to nutrition are helpful if the nurse and patient agree that progress has been made toward identified outcomes. Progress is measured by outcome criteria established in the planning phase. The following general goals were identified previously in this chapter with outcome criteria for patients, although goals and outcome criteria are always individualized. After reaching conclusions, the nurse and patient can decide whether to readjust previous goals, establish new goals, or terminate goals.

Goal

The patient will use nutritionally sound dietary intake to meet body requirements and to promote health.

POSSIBLE OUTCOME CRITERIA

- Within 24 hours, the patient describes a diet that provides his or her nutritional requirements using the appropriate USDA ChooseMyPlate.gov information.
- Within 3 days, the patient verbalizes use of proper daily food selection from the appropriate USDA ChooseMyPlate.gov information.
- The patient ingests healthy diet by limiting intake of trans and saturated fats, refined sugar, and sodium, as witnessed by the caregiver at five meals during the next 5 days.
- The patient's skin and nails demonstrate absence of clinical signs of nutritional deficiency or excess.
- During hospitalization, the patient's weight, blood glucose, albumin, and other values remain within normal limits as shown in laboratory tests.

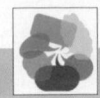

THERAPEUTIC DIALOGUE: NUTRITION

SCENE FOR THOUGHT

Mr. Rose, an 83-year-old man with squamous cell cancer of the left jaw, had a radical left composite resection surgery and placement of tracheostomy and nasogastric tube. On admission, his weight was 150 lb (height 69 inches). Enteral feedings are to be his sole nutritional source for at least 3 weeks after discharge. His 80-year-old wife stays with him during the day and will care for him upon discharge, scheduled tomorrow.

LESS EFFECTIVE	MORE EFFECTIVE
Nurse: Good morning, Mr. Rose. I am Wilma Brown, your nurse. I understand you're going home tomorrow.	**Nurse:** Good morning, Mr. and Mrs. Rose. I am Jeff Wilcox. I will be your nurse today. How are you both feeling?
Mrs. Rose: That's what they said, but I don't know if I can manage, especially the tube feedings.	**Mrs. Rose:** He's getting better, but the doctors said he's going home tomorrow. Do you think he'll be ready? *(Mr. Rose is alert and follows the discussion but cannot talk because his tracheostomy has not yet been plugged.)*
Nurse: *(Looks at Mrs. Rose.)* Did you care for him before he came into the hospital? *(Acknowledges wife seeks some information.)*	**Nurse:** There are things you will need to know how to do. Can we talk about them? *(Acknowledges reality gives choice.)*
Mrs. Rose: He was well until this surgery, and always cared for himself.	**Mrs. Rose:** I don't know if I'm going to be able to do everything you do. *(Sounds anxious.)*
Nurse: I'm going to get his morning feeding ready now. Watch what I'm doing, and let me know if you have any questions. *(Requires wife to initiate questions.)*	**Nurse:** What we can do is identify the most important things and have you help me with those today. Would you be willing? *(Looks at them both for affirmation sets priorities, asks permission.)*
Mrs. Rose: I'm so worried I won't be able to do all the things that you do. What happens if I do something wrong? *(Looks to Mr. Rose and asks him if he can remember the procedure used with his tube feeding. He responds by writing "yes" on a notepad.)*	**Mrs. Rose:** I've sort of watched what happens when they start his feedings, but I don't know if I can remember everything. What if I do something wrong?
Nurse: Between the two of you, this procedure should go fairly smoothly. *(Minimizes the complexity of a new skill that includes both knowledge and physical dexterity.)*	**Nurse:** Mrs. Rose, are you afraid you might hurt your husband? *(Seeks clarification.)* Mr. Rose, I'm going to start your feeding now. Let me get two copies of a paper that lists all the steps for the tube feedings. I'll tell you both what I'm doing, and you can follow along with the list. *(Includes both Mr. and Mrs. Rose.)* Then, Mrs. Rose, you can help me flush the tube and disconnect the tubing when the feeding is finished.
	Mrs. Rose: I do better when I have a checklist to follow. Will you stay while I work with the feeding tube?
	Nurse: Yes, I will. I know this is new for you both. I want to be with you when you are learning what is safe, and not safe. *(Acknowledges unfamiliarity of situation and establishes boundaries.)*

CRITICAL THINKING CHALLENGE

- Discuss the factors affecting the amount and type of nutrients that Mr. Rose needs.
- Identify questions this scenario raises about the concerns of Mrs. Rose.
- What success do you think each nurse will have in helping this couple successfully manage the tube feedings? Explain reasons for your feelings.
- What clues did Jeff notice that Wilma ignored?

PATIENT PLAN OF CARE
The Patient with Imbalanced Nutrition

NURSING DIAGNOSIS

Imbalanced Nutrition: Less Than Body Requirements, as manifested by being underweight and having a low hematocrit and inadequate intake of calcium, iron, protein, vitamin A, and vitamin C

PATIENT GOAL

The patient will construct a diet that meets the appropriate USDA ChooseMyPlate.gov guide and DRI standards, is psychologically satisfying, can be readily understood, and is relatively easy to prepare or obtain.

Patient Outcome Criteria

- The patient obtains correct, useful information in which he or she expresses confidence.
- The patient describes the basic function of nutrients.
- The patient uses a diet that contains adequate amounts of all nutrients to meet the appropriate USDA ChooseMyPlate.gov guide and DRI standards.
- The patient reports satisfaction with the diet and an increased energy level.
- The patient increases weight within the normal range for height, age, and sex.

NURSING INTERVENTION	SCIENTIFIC RATIONALE
1. Assess the patient's laboratory values (hematocrit, hemoglobin, serum prealbumin) and physical parameters (height, weight, BMI, skinfold measurements).	**1.** Noting deviations from baseline and normal standards can help begin measures that correct deficiencies.
2. Assess the patient's ability to obtain food.	**2.** Minimize or prevent financial or physical limitations from contributing to inadequate diet.
3. Assess the patient's motivational level and ability to learn and follow the new diet prescription.	**3.** Prevent motivational or learning difficulties from interfering with obtaining a nutritionally adequate diet.
4. Instruct the patient in the new diet prescription, and assess understanding (increased intake of protein, calcium, iron, vitamins A and C, and calories).	**4.** Encourage an improved intake of nutrients, especially those that had been determined to be low.
5. Provide the patient with written information on the basic functions of the major nutrients; discuss this information and assess understanding.	**5.** Written format assists the patient in retaining the information.
6. Answer patient's questions; discuss areas of concern; provide the patient with additional reference material as necessary.	**6.** Assist the patient toward increased knowledge; relieve uncertainties; improve knowledge of self-care activities.
7. Assess the patient's family history of diabetes and predisposing characteristics toward possible development of diabetes.	**7.** Establish a baseline of information to prevent potential problems or detect them early or treat promptly.

EVALUATION

2/23/17:16:00—The patient confidently describes his understanding of the basic function of nutrients.

- The patient expresses satisfaction with the prescribed diet as demonstrated by his meal intakes and his resulting increased energy level.
- The patient's weight has increased at expected amount this week.

—J. Woodman, RN

Goal

The patient will maintain dietary intake adequate to meet the body's energy expenditures.

POSSIBLE OUTCOME CRITERIA

- Within 24 hours, the patient or caregiver describes dietary changes necessary to meet adequate caloric intake when demand is increased (e.g., pregnancy, lactation, adolescence, trauma, surgery).
- The patient exercises daily for 30 to 90 minutes.
- For 1 month, the patient uses nutritional supplements (e.g., protein supplement, vitamins) during periods of increased demand.

Goal

The patient will demonstrate adequate knowledge to adhere to dietary prescription or therapies to promote health.

POSSIBLE OUTCOME CRITERIA

- After a teaching session, the patient lists foods to avoid on the special diet (e.g., foods high in sodium and fat).
- Before discharge, the patient describes how to alter his or her lifestyle (eating in restaurants, preparing food) to comply with dietary restrictions.
- Before discharge, the patient discusses realistic use of family and community support groups to ensure adequate nutrition after discharge.
- Before discharge, the patient or caregiver demonstrates how to safely administer tube feedings or TPN.

Goal

The patient will achieve and maintain desired weight.

POSSIBLE OUTCOME CRITERIA

- By mutual goal setting with the patient, a specific weight to achieve is set.
- The patient expresses satisfaction with meals.
- If overweight, the patient achieves a 10% reduction in body weight by 6 months.
- The patient loses weight at a rate of about 1 to 2 lb (0.45 to 0.9 kg) per week for 6 months.
- The patient combines a lower-calorie healthy diet, increased physical activity, and behavior therapy into his or her lifestyle.
- If underweight, the patient gains weight to a specific goal by a set time period.
- The patient is able to ingest food without pain or discomfort.

KEY CONCEPTS

- Adequate nutritional intake is important to maintain body functions, healthy tissues, and body temperature; to promote healing; and to build resistance to infection.

- Essential nutrients are carbohydrates, protein, fat, vitamins, minerals, and water.
- The complex processes of digestion, absorption, and metabolism permit the body to break down food and use it as energy.
- Great variations exist in dietary intake among people, but guidelines are useful when evaluating adequate intake.
- Manifestations of altered nutrition include body weight that is less or greater than the IBW; recent significant weight gain or loss; decreased energy; altered bowel patterns; and altered skin, teeth, hair, or mucous membranes.
- A nutritional health assessment includes collecting subjective data about normal eating patterns, risk factors for nutritional deficits, and altered nutrition.
- Accurate anthropometric measurements (height and weight, BMI, skinfold measurements, and arm circumference), calorie counts, and swallowing evaluation provide objective data to help assess a patient's nutritional state.
- NANDA-I nursing diagnoses in the area of nutrition are Imbalanced Nutrition: Less Than Body Requirements; Imbalanced Nutrition: More Than Body Requirements; Readiness for Enhanced Nutrition; Overweight; Obesity; and Impaired Swallowing.
- Health promotion for optimal nutrition includes patient teaching, measures to encourage healthy eating habits, and physical activity.
- Therapeutic diets are used to promote health, manage disease, or encourage healing.
- Various community programs are useful for patients who have nutritional needs.

PRACTICING FOR THE NCLEX

CHECK YOUR ANSWERS IN APPENDIX A.

1. You are taking care of an elderly patient with osteoporosis. Which dietary supplements would be most appropriate as a treatment regimen?
    a. Iron and calcium
    b. Calcium and vitamin D
    c. Vitamin K and B-complex vitamins
    d. Fluoride and iron

2. Impaired liver function related to chronic alcohol use may result in inadequate digestive function. Which of the following processes would be impacted? Select all that apply:
    a. Digestion
    b. Absorption
    c. Metabolism
    d. Excretion

3. The following groups must increase their calcium, protein, and iron intakes to prevent nutritional deficits:
    a. Pregnant women
    b. Lactating women
    c. Older adults
    d. Newborns

4. You are providing patient education for a patient with anemia. Which of the following foods should you recommend that the patient includes in her regular diet? Select all that apply:
   a. Beef
   b. Spinach
   c. Milk
   d. Enriched whole wheat bread

5. In caring for a patient with a history of alcohol abuse, you administer thiamine, niacin, folate, and IV TPN with lipids. Your patient education should consist of which of the following? Select all that apply:
   a. "B-complex vitamin supplements are quickly used up in alcohol metabolism, leaving your body at a deficit."
   b. "Liver damage impairs your ability to metabolize fats and nutrients."
   c. "Nutrient absorption in the intestines is impaired by alcohol's effects on the mucosa."
   d. "Your appetite and oral intake is excellent; I'll talk to the physician about canceling these supplements."

6. You hear in report that your elderly patient was admitted for malnutrition. In planning for discharge to home, you discuss which of the following issues with the social worker? Select all that apply:
   a. Local food availability
   b. History of depression
   c. Poor-fitting dentures
   d. Impaired mobility

7. Your physical assessment findings include poor blood clotting, muscle weakness, and delayed fracture healing. Which of the following nutritional deficits is most likely based on these findings?
   a. Protein deficiency
   b. Calcium deficiency
   c. Iron deficiency
   d. B-complex deficiency

8. Your patient reports that he just started a new diet including spinach salads daily for lunch and kale, chard, or broccoli for dinner. He has been taking Coumadin for a history of deep vein thrombosis. Which of the following symptoms would be most concerning?
   a. Leg pain and swelling
   b. Bleeding gums
   c. Serum iron within normal limits
   d. International normalized ratio (INR) 2.6

9. You suspect that your patient is experiencing acute malnutrition. Which lab would give you the best indication of the patient's current nutritional status?
   a. Low albumin
   b. Low prealbumin
   c. Elevated white blood cell count
   d. Elevated cholesterol

10. You are monitoring a tube feeding for a patient with altered mental status following a CVA. Which of the following would you do to prevent aspiration?
    a. Maintain the head of the bed greater than 30 degrees.
    b. Check residual volumes hourly.
    c. Hold tube feeding if residual volumes are greater than 100 mL.
    d. Monitor blood glucose two to four times per day while on tube feeding.

REFERENCES

American Cancer Society. (2010). *Study: Large waist size increases health risk.* American Cancer Society News Center. Retrieved May 21, 2014, from www.cancer.org/cancer/news/larger-waist-size-increases-health-risks

Berge, J., Wickel, K., & Doherty, W. (2012). The individual and combined influence of the "quality" and "quantity" of family meals on adult body mass index. *Families, Systems & Health, 30*(4), 344–351.

Bristrian, B., & Driscoll, D. (2012). Chapter 76. Enteral and parenteral nutrition therapy. In D. Longo, A. Fauci, D. Kasper, S. Hauser, J. Jameson, & J. Loscalzo (Eds.), *Harrison's principles of internal medicine* (18th ed.). New York: McGraw-Hill.

Centers for Disease Control and Prevention (CDC). (2011). *Healthy weight—it's not a diet, it's a lifestyle!* Retrieved May 20, 2014, from www.cdc.gov/healthyweight/assessing/bmi/adult_bmi/index.html

Centers for Disease Control and Prevention (CDC). (2012). *Get the facts: Sources of sodium in your diet.* Retrieved May 22, 2014, from www.cdc.gov/salt/pdfs/sources_of_socium.pdf

Centers for Disease Control and Prevention (CDC). (2014). *Overweight and obesity: Adult obesity facts.* Retrieved May 20, 2014, from www.cdc.gov/obesity/data/adult.html

Chan, W., & Burakoff, R. (2012). Chapter 18. Disorders of gastric and small bowel motility. In H. Greenberger, R. Blumberg, & R. Burakoff (Eds.), *Current diagnosis and treatment: gastroenterology, hepatology, and endoscopy.* New York: McGraw Hill.

Dudek, S. (2014). *Nutrition essentials for nursing practice* (7th ed.). Philadelphia, PA: Wolters Kluwer Health | Lippincott Williams & Wilkins.

Federal Interagency Forum on Aging-Related Statistics. (2012). *Older Americans 2012: Key indicators of well-being.* Washington, DC: U.S. Government Printing Office.

Fryar, C., & Ogden, C. (2012). *Prevalence of underweight among adults aged 20 years and over: United States, 1960–62 through 2007–2010.* Retrieved May 21, 2014, from www.cdc.gov/nchs/data/hestat/underweight_adult_07_10/underweight_adult_07_10.htm

Guallar, E., Stranges, S., Appel, L., & Miller, E. (2013). Enough is enough: Stop wasting money on vitamin and mineral supplements. *Annals of Internal Medicine, 159*(12), 850–851.

Institute of Medicine. (2005). Dietary reference intakes for energy, carbohydrate, fiber, fat, fatty acids, cholesterol, protein, and amino acids. Food and Nutrition Board. Washington, DC: National Academy Press.

Institute for Safe Medication Practices. (2014). *Oral syringes: A crucial and economical risk-reduction strategy that has not been fully utilized.* Retrieved May 21, 2014, from www.ismp.org/Newsletters/acutecare/articles/20091022.asp

Juarez, L., Soto, E., & Pritchard, J. (2012). Drive for muscularity and drive for thinness: The impact of pro-anorexia websites. *Eating Disorders, 20*(2), 99–112.

Kittler, R., & Sucher, K. (2011). *Food and culture* (6th ed.). Belmont, CA: Thomson Wadsworth.

Linus Pauling Institute. (2014). The case is far from closed for vitamin and mineral supplements. *The Linus Pauling Institute Research Newsletter*, Spring/Summer, 7.

Malone, A. (2014). Clinical guidelines from the American Society for Parenteral and Enteral Nutrition: Best practice recommendations for patient care. *The Art and Science of Patient Care, 37*(3), 179–184.

Metheny, N. (2009). *AACN practice alert: Dye in enteral feeding*. Retrieved June 2, 2014, from www.aacn.org/WD/Practice/Docs/PracticeAlerts/Dye_in_Enteral_Feeding_4-2005.pdf

National Institutes of Health. (2012). *Folate: Dietary supplement fact sheet. NIH Office of Dietary Supplement*. Retrieved May 20, 2014 from http://ods.od.nih.gov/pdf/factsheets/Folate-HealthProfessional.pdf

North American Nursing Diagnosis Association International (NANDA-I). (2014). *Nursing diagnoses: Definitions and classification, 2015–2017*. West Sussex, England: Wiley-Blackwell.

Ogden, C., Carol, M., Kit, B., & Flegal, K. (2014). Prevalence of childhood and adult obesity in the United States, 2011–2012. *Journal of the American Medical Association, 311*(8), 806–814.

Ojo, J. (2014). Problems with use of a Foley catheter in enteral tube feeding. *British Journal of Nursing, 23*(7), 360–364

Ojo, O., & Bowden, J. (2012). Infection control in enteral feed and feeding systems in the community. *British Journal of Nursing, 21*(18), 1070–1075.

Pronsky, Z., Crowe, J., Elbe, D., Epstein, S., Roberts, W., Young, V., & Ayoob, K. (2012). *Food and medication interactions* (17th ed.). Birchrunville, PA: Food Medication Interactions.

Salvy, S., Elmo, A., Nitecki, L., Kluczynski, M. & Roemmich, J. (2011). Influence of parents and friends on children's and adolescents' food intake and food selection. *American Journal of Clinical Nutrition, 98*(1), 87–92.

Simons, S., & Abdallah, L. (2012). Bedside assessment of enteral tube placement: Aligning practice with evidence. *American Journal of Nursing, 112*(2), 40–48.

Sturm, R., & Hattori, A. (2013). Morbid obesity rates continue to rise rapidly in the United States. *International Journal of Obesity, 37*(6), 889–891.

Thompson, J., & Manore, M. (2012). *Nutrition: An applied approach* (3rd ed.). Boston, MA: Pearson.

U.S. Department of Agriculture and U.S. Department of Health and Human Services. (2010). *Dietary guidelines for Americans, 2010* (7th ed.). Washington, DC: U.S. Government Printing Office..

U.S. Department of Agriculture. (2013). *ChooseMyPlate.gov*. Retrieved May 20, 2014, from www.ChooseMyPlate.gov

U.S. Food and Drug Administration. (2014). *How to understand and use the nutrition facts label*. Retrieved May 21, 2014, from www.fda.gov/food/ingredientspackaginglabeling/labelingnutrition/ucm274593.htm

Procedure 29-1 Measuring Blood Glucose by Skin Puncture

Purpose
1. Monitor blood glucose levels for patients who are at risk for hypoglycemia or hyperglycemia.
2. Monitor the effectiveness of insulin administration.

Equipment
Alcohol swab
Sterile lancet or Autolet
Cotton balls
Blood glucose reagent strip
Glucose testing meter
Disposable gloves

Assessment
- Assess the patient's medical history to determine risk for complications from skin punctures (e.g., bleeding disorders, anticoagulant therapy, low platelet count).
- Assess the skin area to be used for puncture (fingers, toes, heels). Avoid areas with open lesions or ecchymosis.
- Assess the patient's understanding of the purpose of the procedure and his or her physical and emotional ability to learn and perform the procedure independently.

Procedure

1. **Review the provider's orders to determine the type and frequency of glucose monitoring. (*Note*: The procedure should be performed before meals because carbohydrate ingestion alters blood glucose levels.)**
   Rationale: Prevents errors.

2. **Perform hand hygiene.**
   Rationale: Reduces microbe transmission.

3. **Identify the patient.**
   Rationale: Ensures correct patient receives proper assessment or treatment and reduces errors.

4. **Close door or bed curtains and explain the procedure to the patient.**
   Rationale: Ensures patient privacy, increases patient compliance, reduces patient anxiety, and promotes learning.

5. **Have the patient wash hands with soap and warm water.**
   Rationale: The fingertips are the most common skin puncture sites in adults. Washing not only decreases the chances of infection but, due to the warm water, promotes vasodilation of the puncture site.

6. **Position the patient comfortably.**
   Rationale: Ensures the patient's comfort during the procedure.

7. **Remove the test strip from the container and handle according to the manufacturer's instructions.**
   Rationale: The glucose meter may need recalibration or "re-zeroing."

8. **Place the test strip with test pad up on a dry surface.**
   Rationale: Moisture on the test pad could alter the final test results.

9. **Don gloves.**
   Rationale: Part of Standard Precautions against transfer of microorganisms.

10. **Choose the finger to be punctured, massage gently, and hold in a dependent position (Fig. 1).**

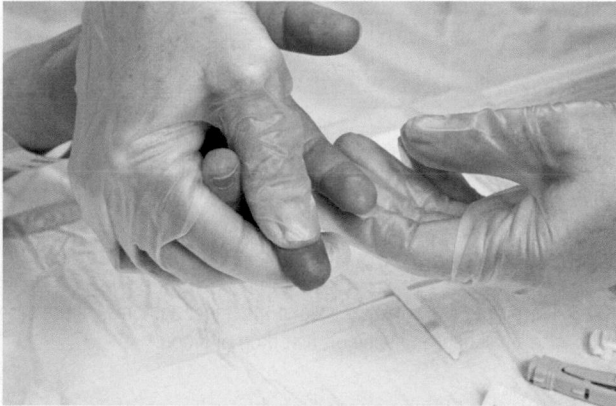

FIG. 1 Massage the finger that will be punctured.

Rationale: The dependent position and stimulation will help increase circulation to the puncture site.

Procedure 29-1   *continued*

11. **Wipe the puncture site with alcohol (Fig. 2). Allow the site to dry completely.**

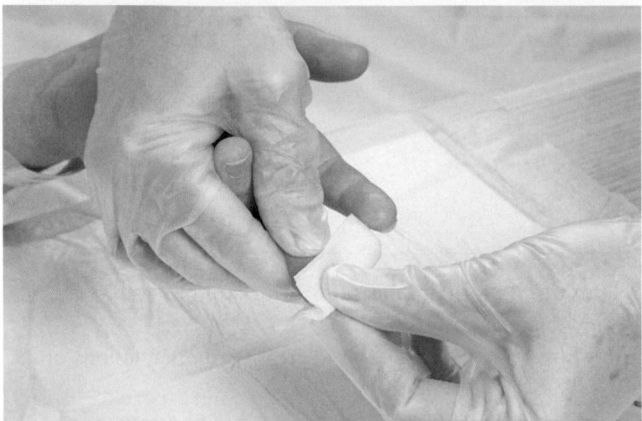

FIG. 2 Clean puncture site with alcohol wipe.

Rationale: If tracked into the puncture site, alcohol may cause stinging and could hemolyze or dilute the blood sample, giving an inaccurate reading.

12. **Remove the cover of the lancet or Autolet. Place the Autolet against the side of the finger and push the release button (Fig. 3). If using a lancet, hold it perpendicular to the site and pierce the site quickly.**

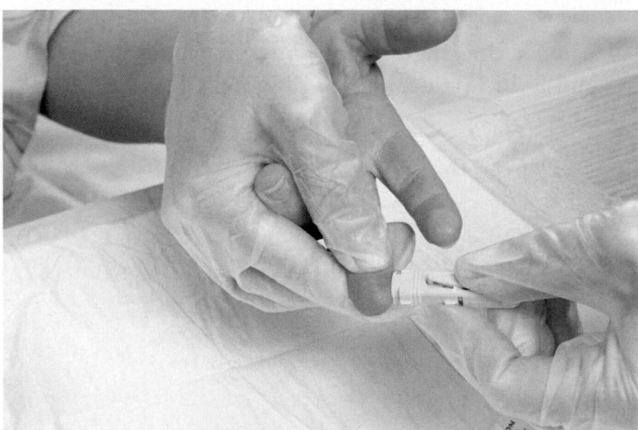

FIG. 3 Place Autolet against the side of the finger and press the release button. Use small gauze to wipe off first drop of blood.

Rationale: Quick puncture of skin is less painful.

13. **Squeeze the finger gently or milk the skin toward the puncture site. Use a small gauze to wipe off first drop of blood that appears. Continue gently milking to obtain a large drop of blood. Hold the test strip next to the drop of blood and allow the blood to cover the test pad completely (Fig. 4). Do not smear the blood. In some meters, bring the finger to the test site on the meter and allow blood to drop and wick along the test strip, covering the test strip area.**

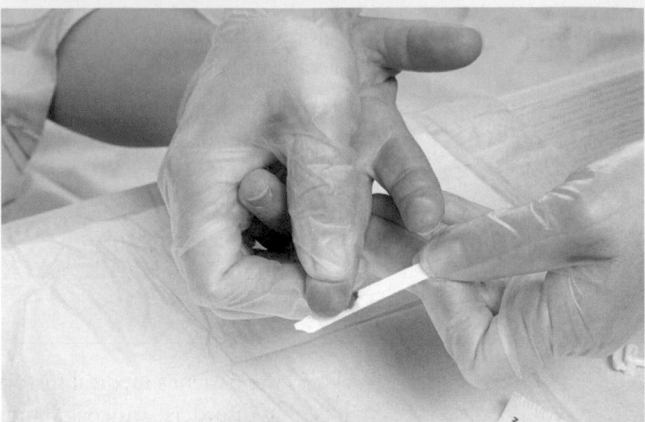

FIG. 4 Collect drop of blood on test strip.

Rationale: Smearing or incomplete coverage of the test pad will lead to inaccurate glucose readings.

14. **Start the timing (usually less than 60 seconds) using the glucose meter, or use a watch if the meter is not available.**

Rationale: Blood must be in contact with the test pad for the time required by the manufacturer to ensure accurate results.

15. **Insert the test strip into the glucose meter (Fig. 5). After the recommended period, read the results. For meters on which blood is placed directly, read the results at the designated time. If a glucose meter is not available, compare the color of the test pad with the color strip on the side of the reagent strip container.**

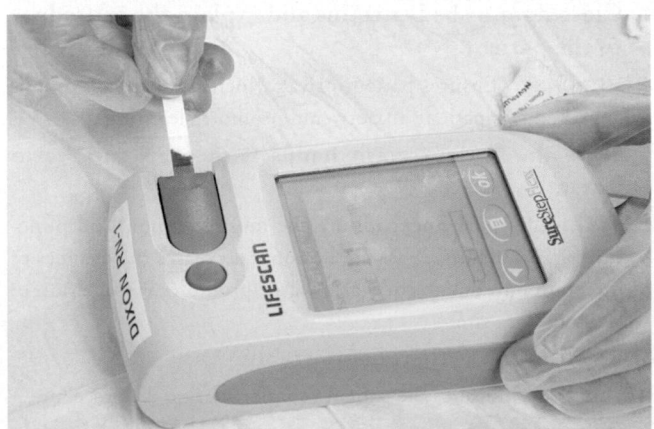

FIG. 5 Insert test strip into glucose meter.

Rationale: Accurate timing of the test ensures a correct reading of the glucose level.

16. **Turn off the glucose meter. Dispose of used equipment in the appropriate manner.**

Rationale: Avoids inadvertent punctures.

Procedure 29-1   *continued*

17. **Share test results with the patient and record obtained values in the patient's chart.**

    Rationale: Encourages the patient's participation and maintains appropriate documentation.

18. **Document procedure.**

    Rationale: Maintains legal record and communicates with healthcare team.

Documentation

10/8/17: 07:30—Performed fingerstick blood glucose test on the patient. Fasting blood glucose level is 92, within target range.

—J. Lawrence, RN

Life Span Considerations

Infants

- The heel is the most common site for skin puncture. Use a heel-warming device or wrap a warm, moist towel around the foot before the skin puncture is done to promote vasodilation.

Children

- Children may be especially apprehensive about skin puncture. Use distraction techniques and allow parents to be present to increase the child's cooperation with the procedure.

Home Care Modifications

- Handwashing alone before skin puncture is sufficient to cleanse the skin when the test is performed at home.
- Instruct the patient to keep a log of all blood glucose readings.

Collaboration and Delegation

- Collaboration between the healthcare provider and the registered nurse (RN) assures that an appropriate plan of care is in place to manage deviations of blood glucose from target range (hypoglycemia and hyperglycemia protocols).
- The fingerstick blood glucose test may be delegated to trained assistive personnel. The professional nurse correlates test results with clinical signs and symptoms and implements the plan of care when findings deviate from target range.
- Involvement of the family and nutritionist is essential in managing patients with diabetes and other conditions that affect blood glucose. Other resources, such as a diabetes team, may also be available to provide expert consultation.

Procedure 29-2 Assisting an Adult with Feeding

Purpose	1. Maintain nutritional status. 2. Provide a time for socialization.
Equipment	Personal hygiene supplies for the patient to wash hands Glasses, if necessary Special devices (splints, prostheses, spoons, cups) Meal tray Oral hygiene equipment
Assessment	• Assess the patient's physical and emotional ability to feed self (i.e., motor function, coordination, level of consciousness, vision, interest, depression). • Assess the patient's eating habits and food preferences; cultural and religious beliefs may eliminate certain food from the diet. • Review history for food allergies. • Assess ability of the GI tract to absorb and digest oral nutrition (i.e., bowel sounds, regular bowel movements, history of GI disorders, Crohn disease, duodenal ulcers, pancreatitis, cholecystitis, ulcerative colitis).

Procedure

1. **Review physician's orders for type of diet.**
   Rationale: Prevents errors.

2. **Identify the patient.**
   Rationale: Ensures correct patient receives proper assessment or treatment and reduces errors.

3. **Close door or bed curtains and explain the procedure to the patient and patient's family.**
   Rationale: Ensures patient privacy, increases patient compliance, reduces patient anxiety, and promotes learning.

4. **Prepare the patient's environment for meal:**
   a. **Remove urinals, bedpans, dressings, trash.**
   b. **Ventilate or aerate room for unpleasant odors.**
   c. **Clean overbed table.**
      Rationale: A clean, uncluttered environment enhances appetite.

5. **Prepare the patient for meal:**
   a. **Help the patient urinate or defecate.**
   b. **Help the patient wash face and hands.**
   c. **Assist with oral hygiene.**
   d. **Help the patient apply dentures, glasses, or special appliances.**
   e. **Assist the patient to upright position in bed or chair.**
      Rationale: Comfort and optimal physical condition stimulate appetite and help the patient ingest the meal.

6. **Perform hand hygiene.**
   Rationale: Reduces microbe transmission.

7. **Check the patient's tray against diet order and with the patient's identification.**
   Rationale: Diets are prepared for specific patients.

8. **Place tray on overbed table and move in front of the patient.**

9. **Place a napkin or towel under the patient's chin, and cover clothing. Prepare tray. Open cartons, remove lids, season food, cut food into bite-size pieces (Fig. 1).**

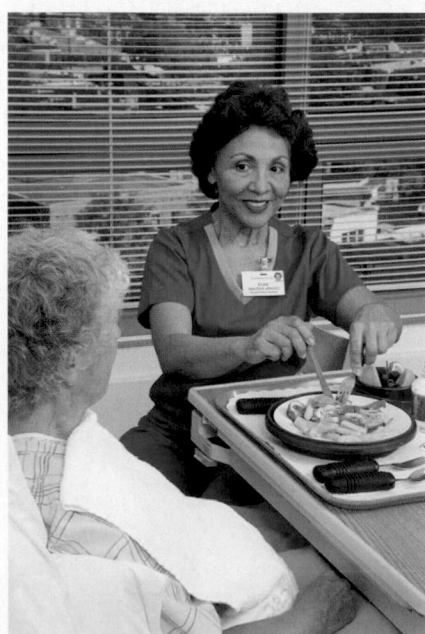

FIG. 1 Prepare meal by cutting food into bite-size portions.

Rationale: Patients with impaired physical or cognitive function may be unable to prepare food for eating.

Procedure 29-2 *continued*

10. **If the patient can feed self, you may leave at this point, assuring that call light is within reach. Return after 10 to 15 minutes to determine whether the patient is tolerating diet. Do not leave patients with overly hot liquids or food unless they are fully independent with feeding.**

    Rationale: Self-care enhances feelings of independence and positive self-esteem. Decreased sensation or lack of motor coordination could result in burns from hot foods or liquid. The call light enables the patient to summon help if needed.

11. **Assist patients who cannot feed themselves. If the patient can sit in a chair but needs help to eat, sit in chair facing the patient. If the patient must remain in bed, sit in chair (depending on chair height) or stand to feed the patient.**

    Rationale: Allows the nurse to comfortably assist the patient.

12. **Allow the patient to choose the order he or she would like to eat. If the patient is visually impaired, identify the food on the tray.**

    Rationale: Promotes a sense of control and participation.

13. **Warn the patient if food is hot or cold. Allow enough time between bites for adequate chewing and swallowing (Fig. 2).**

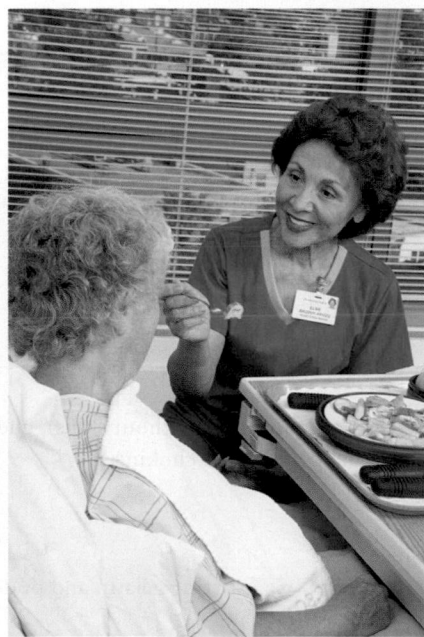

FIG. 2 Pause between offering bites of food, allowing the patient sufficient time to chew and swallow.

    Rationale: Helps digestion.

14. **Offer liquids as requested or between bites (Fig. 3). Use a straw or special drinking cup if available.**

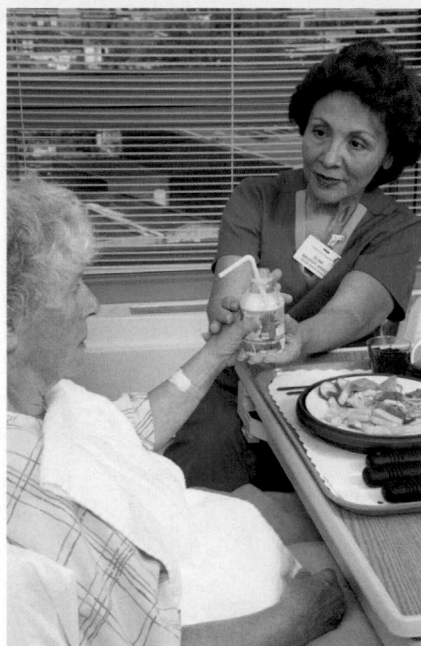

FIG. 3 Offer liquid between bites or at regular intervals.

    Rationale: Liquids assist in swallowing.

15. **Provide conversation during meal (Fig. 4). Choose topic of interest to the patient. Reorient to current events, or use meal as an opportunity to educate on nutrition or discharge plans. However, do not talk to patients who are relearning swallowing techniques; they need to concentrate.**

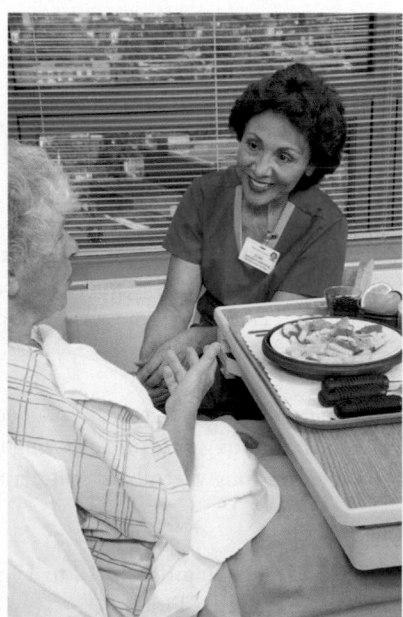

FIG. 4 Provide conversation because mealtimes are usually social occasions.

    Rationale: Conversation makes mealtime more enjoyable for the patient.

Procedure 29-2   *continued*

16. Remove and dispose of tray. Help the patient wash hands and face and perform oral hygiene after meal (Fig. 5).

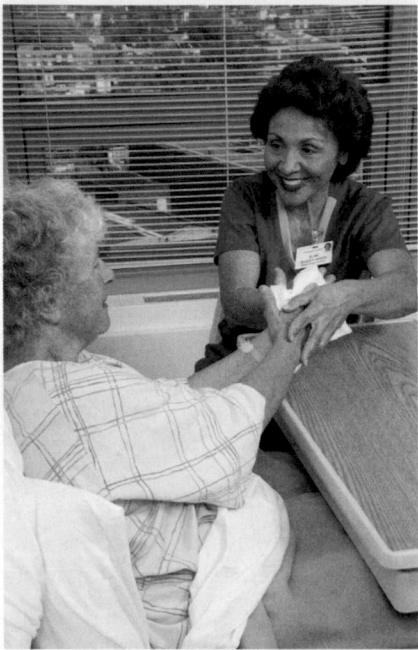

FIG. 5 Assist the patient to clean the hands.

Rationale: Prevents transfer of microorganisms.

17. **Assist the patient to comfortable position, and allow rest period. (*Note*: If the patient is at risk for aspiration, leave the head of the bed elevated for 30 minutes after eating.)**

Rationale: Elevating the head of the bed reduces the risk of aspiration.

18. **Perform hand hygiene.**

Rationale: Prevents transfer of microorganisms.

19. **Document fluids and amount of meal consumed, if ordered.**

Rationale: Allows monitoring of fluids and nutritional status.

Documentation

7/8/17: 12:30—Assisted patient with feeding. The patient finished three quarters of her chicken and rice, entire serving of carrots, and 12 oz of water. She verbalized satisfaction with the meal. She did not experience any difficulty chewing or swallowing.

—J. Lawrence, RN

Life Span Considerations

Infant

- Infants do not usually need food other than breast milk or formula until 4 to 6 months of age. Strained or blended foods may be introduced at that time.
- Infant cereal is recommended as the first solid because of its iron content and low incidence of intolerance.
- At 6 months of age, infants are interested in self-feeding with a spoon or teething crackers.

Toddler

- Toddlers are often independent and insist on feeding themselves.
- Appropriate "finger foods" include meatballs, hard-boiled eggs, cooked carrots, fruit slices (without skins), cheese pieces, dry cereal, and crackers. Avoid whole grapes, hard candy, and other foods that could cause choking.

Preschooler

- This is a period of slower growth, so a decrease in appetite is not unusual.
- Using foods in color games and allowing the child to help with food preparation (e.g., stirring gelatin and pudding, peeling oranges, washing vegetables) stimulate the child's interest and teach good eating habits.

Adolescent

- Ages 10 to 11 years in girls and 12 to 13 years in boys are periods of rapid growth. These children need larger consumption of nutrients and calories.
- Girls beginning menstruation need increased iron in the diet.
- Many adolescent diets are low in calcium, iron, vitamin A, and protein.

Procedure 29-2   *continued*

Older Adult

- Older adults may have diminished appetites from loss of taste and smell and decreased number of taste buds.
- Many older adults wear dentures. Poorly fitting dentures can impair their ability and desire to eat properly.
- People in this age group usually need fewer calories because of decreased activity and slowing metabolism.
- Calcium intake is often much lower than DRIs for both men and women.

Home Care Modifications

- Loneliness and poverty may decrease a patient's ability or interest in eating balanced meals at home.
- Federal programs, such as food stamps and supplemental security income, can increase the food-buying power for patients at home.
- In 1972, a federally funded nutrition program for older adults was instituted that provides low-cost, nutritious meals served in community settings. These programs, and similar private programs, also provide socialization for lonely older adults.
- Meals on Wheels is available in many communities to deliver nutritious meals to patients in their homes.

Collaboration and Delegation

- Patient diets are ordered by the healthcare provider in collaboration with the professional nurse who often best understands the patient's preferences, eating habits, and skills.
- Feeding a patient is often delegated to properly trained assistive personnel. It is important that these individuals understand the special precautions and observations required for each patient as well as situations requiring consultation with the healthcare provider or professional nurse.
- For special patient needs, consultations with the patient's family, the dietician, the speech therapist (for swallowing difficulties), and the occupational therapist enhance the healthcare team's ability to provide nutrition and to promote self-care in feeding.

Procedure 29-3 Administering Specialized Nutritional Support Via Small-Bore Nasogastric, Gastrostomy, or Jejunostomy Tube

Purpose
1. Provide enteral nutrition for patients who cannot swallow or who have an esophageal obstruction.
2. Provide nutrition to comatose or semiconscious patients.
3. Provide additional nutrients for patients who cannot orally consume adequate calories.

Equipment
Gloves
Formula
Feeding bag and tubing
60-mL catheter tip (feeding) syringe
Infusion pump
Water
Measuring container

Assessment
- Assess the patient's nutritional status, and identify need for tube feedings:
  - Impaired swallowing
  - Decreased level of consciousness
  - Head, neck, or facial surgery or trauma
  - Extraordinary caloric requirements
- Assess the patient's GI system:
  - Assess for nausea, vomiting, abdominal distention, or tenderness
  - Auscultate bowel sounds
  - Determine time of last bowel movement
  - Assess for existing feeding tube

Procedure

1. **Review chart for food allergies and provider's order for type, amount, rate, route, and frequency of feeding.**
   Rationale: Prevents errors.

2. **Perform hand hygiene and don gloves.**
   Rationale: Reduces microbe transmission.

3. **Identify the patient.**
   Rationale: Ensures correct patient receives proper assessment or treatment and reduces errors.

4. **Close door or bed curtains and explain the procedure to the patient.**
   Rationale: Ensures patient privacy, increases patient compliance, reduces patient anxiety, and promotes learning.

5. **Help the patient to Fowler's position by elevating the head of the bed at least 30 to 45 degrees or assisting to a chair. If an upright position is contraindicated, help the patient to a right side-lying position with the head elevated 30 degrees.**
   Rationale: These positions reduce the chance of aspiration of formula into the lungs and facilitate flow of the feeding into the gut.

6. **Confirm placement of tube. Following initial tube insertion, placement is confirmed by x-ray. At that time, tube is marked where it exits naris with tape or indelible marker. External portion is also measured and documented. At each feeding, tube must be examined to assure that marked portion remains in place and that length of remaining tube has not changed. Routine x-rays of the abdomen and chest should also be reviewed. If available, test pH of aspirate per facility protocol.**
   Rationale: Auscultation is not a reliable indicator of tube placement. Incorrect placement creates risk for complications including aspiration of feeding.

7. **Check GRVs.**
   Rationale: Gastric residuals are checked to evaluate if gastric emptying is adequate.
   a. **If GRVs are requested, note amount aspirated in documentation. Notify provider if GRV exceeds 500 mL.**
   b. **Replace all gastric contents after residual check.**
      Rationale: Gastric content is rich in electrolytes. Electrolyte imbalance could occur if residuals are discarded.

Procedure 29-3 *continued*

8. **Prepare correct amount and strength of formula. Formula should be room temperature.**

   Rationale: Amount and strength of formula are gradually increased to prevent diarrhea and gastric intolerance. Formula should be at room temperature because it will not be warmed or cooled by the oral and esophageal mucosa as occurs in normal swallowing. Cold formula can cause abdominal cramping and discomfort; hot formula can burn the stomach.

9. **Select steps 10a through 16a below for bolus or intermittent feeding or steps 10b through 18b below for continuous feeding.**

Bolus or Intermittent Feeding

10a. **Remove plunger from irrigation syringe. Clamp gastric tubing and attach syringe or feeding bag. If using a feeding bag, prime the tubing and attach feeding bag and tubing to the patient's feeding tube.**

   Rationale: Clamping tubing prevents air from entering the stomach and prevents stomach contents from leaking out.

11a. **Fill syringe or feeding bag with formula (Fig. 1). Allow feeding to flow in slowly (10 to 15 minutes). If using syringe, raise or lower syringe to adjust flow rate by gravity. Refill syringe as needed without disconnecting, avoiding airspaces in tubing. If a feeding bag is used, hang bag on IV pole, and adjust flow rate with clamp on tubing. Stop feeding if the patient shows signs of intolerance.**

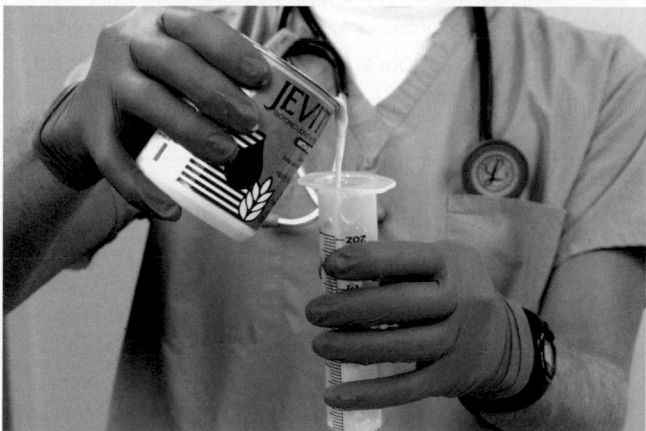

FIG. 1 Pour formula into syringe.

Rationale: Feedings given too rapidly cause nausea, vomiting, flatus, and abdominal cramps. Intolerance can also be a sign of tube displacement.

12a. **Clamp tubing just as feeding is completing. Rinse tube with 30 to 60 mL warm tap water. Do not allow air to enter tubing.**

   Rationale: Clamping tubing prevents air from entering the stomach and thus reduces bloating or cramps. Rinsing with water clears the gastric tube to prevent blockage and bacterial growth.

13a. **Clamp gastric tube, and disconnect from syringe or feeding bag.**

14a. **Have the patient remain in Fowler's or elevated side-lying position for 30 to 60 minutes after feeding.**

   Rationale: Decreases the risk of aspiration.

15a. **Wash any reusable equipment with soap and water. Change equipment every 24 hours or according to agency policy.**

   Rationale: Clean equipment prevents inadvertent administration of spoiled or contaminated feeding.

16a. **Perform hand hygiene.**

   Rationale: Prevents the spread of microorganisms.

Continuous Feeding

10b. **Connect feeding bag and tubing to the patient's feeding tube.**

   Rationale: Allows formula to be administered.

11b. **Pour in desired amount of formula (Fig. 2). (*Note*: Usually, hang amount of formula to infuse in 3 to 4 hours; check manufacturer's recommendations and agency policy.) Place label on bag with the patient's name, date, and time feeding was initiated (Fig. 3).**

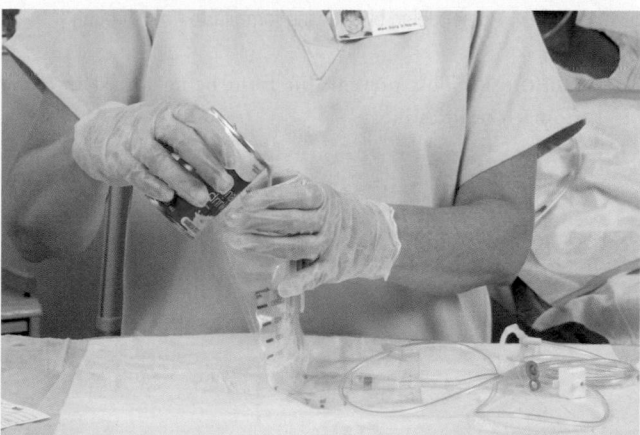

FIG. 2 Pour formula into bag.

Rationale: Formula that is no longer in a sealed container or the refrigerator must generally be infused within 3 to 4 hours to prevent spoiling.

Procedure 29-3   *continued*

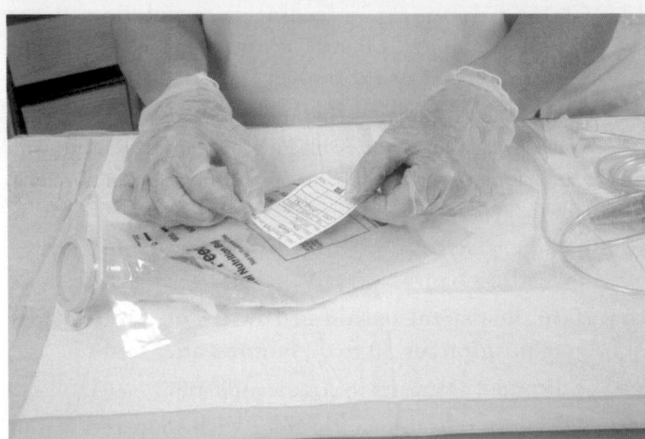

FIG. 3 Attach label to bag.

12b. Hang feeding bag on IV pole. Allow formula to flow through bag (Fig. 4).

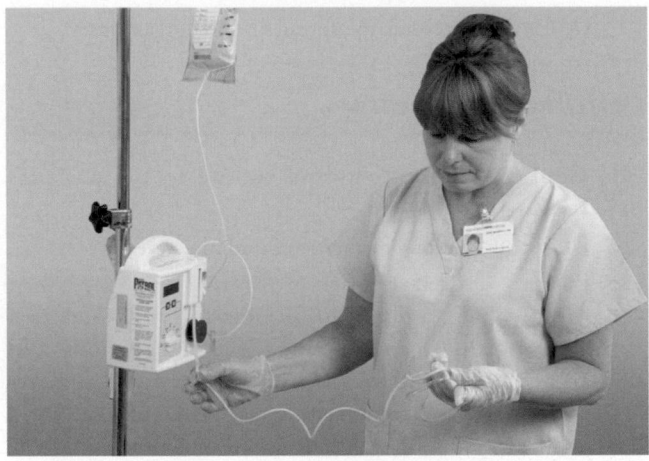

FIG. 4 Prime tubing by allowing formula to flow through.

Rationale: This prevents air from being forced into the stomach or intestine.

13b. Connect tubing to infusion pump and set rate ordered by provider (Fig. 5).

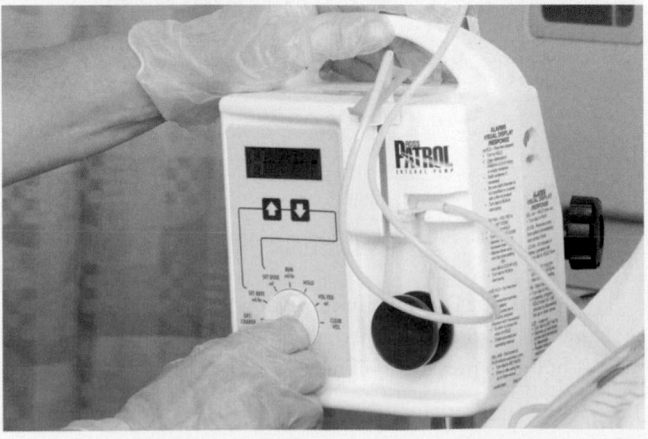

FIG. 5 Turn on infusion pump and set rate.

Rationale: If feeding is infused too rapidly, vomiting and cramps may result.

14b. Patients receiving continuous feedings should have gastric residuals checked every 4 to 6 hours, according to agency policy. After checking residual and replacing stomach contents, flush the tubing with 30 to 60 mL of warm water.

Rationale: Checking for gastric residual (GRV) assesses for adequate absorption of feeding and verifies correct placement of tube. Flushing with warm water ensures patency of tubing and discourages bacterial growth.

15b. Have the patient remain in Fowler's or in slightly elevated side-lying position.

Rationale: Decreases the risk of aspiration.

16b. Wash any reusable equipment with soap and water. Change equipment every 24 hours or according to agency policy.

Rationale: Clean equipment decreases the possibility of inadvertent administration of a spoiled or contaminated feeding.

17b. Perform hand hygiene.

Rationale: Reduces microbe transmission.

18b. Document appropriately.

Rationale: Maintains legal record and communicates with healthcare team.

Documentation

6/16/17: 10:30—Small-bore NG feeding tube inserted, placement verified by radiology. 250 mL of formula hung and pump set for ordered milligrams per hour. The patient understands the purpose of the feeding tube and is fully alert and cooperative.

—D. Hale, RN

Life Span Considerations

Infant and Child

- Intermittent feeding and reinsertion of the nasogastric feeding tube at each feeding are recommended in children. There is significant risk of stomach perforation, nasal airway obstruction, and ulceration and irritation of the mucous membrane if a nasogastric feeding tube is left in continuously.

Home Care Modifications

- Encourage patients to participate in the preparation and procedure of tube feeding if possible to increase their feelings of independence and self-esteem.
- Instruct the patient or caregiver in correct techniques and rationales as stated previously.
- Feedings can be provided from commercially prepared formulas or home-blended foods. Formulas may be thinned with juice, milk, or water.
- Teach the caregiver proper storage of extra formula:
  - Seal and store commercially prepared formulas in the refrigerator once the container is open. Use within 24 hours.
  - Tightly seal, date, and refrigerate home-blended feedings. Use within 24 hours after preparation.
- Tube-fed patients may feel isolated or may have altered self-esteem and body image from the loss of sensory and social stimulation associated with eating. Encourage caregivers to schedule feedings with family mealtimes.
- If medically permitted, the patient can consume some favorite foods orally. If swallowing is contraindicated, it may be possible for the patient to chew and taste a few favorite foods, then spit them out.
- Follow-up and consultation with a home health nurse often allow patients and caregivers to arrange creative solutions to problems or concerns that arise.

Collaboration and Delegation

- Collaboration between the healthcare provider and the RN is essential for safe administration of adequate nutrition.
- Enteral feedings are generally given by professional nurses, but in some circumstances, other personnel may be trained to perform this skill.
- Including the dietitian in planning and evaluating tube feeding programs is essential.

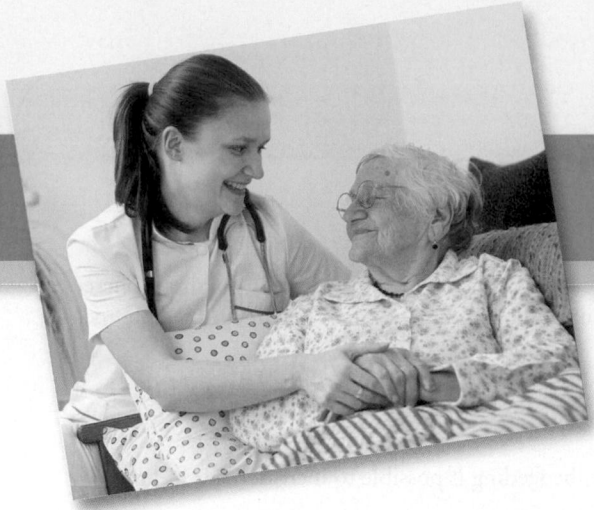

CHAPTER 30

Skin Integrity and Wound Healing

Debra Beauchaine

Case Scenario

You are a home health nurse making visits twice a week to a patient with a stage III pressure ulcer. The patient is recovering from a stroke and receives regular visits from a physical therapist for mobility training. The patient's husband is actively involved in her care. You are planning today's care.

Once you have completed this chapter and have incorporated skin integrity and wound healing into your knowledge base, review the above scenario and reflect on the following areas of Critical Thinking:

1. Describe assessments you will make today and on subsequent visits.
2. Summarize factors that could affect the rate of wound healing in this patient.
3. Outline teaching you will provide to help prevent further occurrence of pressure ulcers.
4. List the primary nursing diagnoses that will guide your care and related nursing diagnoses that might apply in this situation.
5. Explore how you would collaborate with the patient, family, and other healthcare providers to promote effective wound healing.

KEY TERMS

abscess
abrasion
approximated
binders
deep tissue injury (DTI)
debridement
dehiscence
dermatitis
dermis
desquamation
epidermis
epithelialization
evisceration
fistula
friction
granulation tissue
hematoma
incision
induration
laceration
macerated
MARSI (Medical Adhesive-Related Skin Injury)
necrotizing fasciitis
negative-pressure wound therapy (NPWT)
periwound
pressure ulcer
purulent
sanguineous
serosanguineous
serous
shear
subcutaneous tissue
tunneling
undermining

LEARNING OBJECTIVES

Upon completion of this chapter, you will be able to do the following:

1. Describe the structure and function of the integumentary system.
2. Identify factors affecting integumentary function and the manifestations of impaired function.
3. Identify the components of nursing assessment of skin integrity.

4. Describe normal wound healing.
5. Describe the scientific principles of moist wound healing.
6. Discuss nursing interventions to promote skin integrity.
7. Explain scientific principles in the application of heat and cold to injured areas.
8. Describe the categories and function of wound dressings and how to select the appropriate dressing for wound healing.

Skin, also called integument, is the body's external covering. It is the body's largest organ, providing protective, sensory, and regulatory functions. Disruptions in skin integrity can interfere with these important functions.

A wound is a break in skin integrity. Wounds can occur when the skin is exposed to extremes in temperature, pH, caustic chemicals, excessive pressure, moisture, friction, trauma, or radiation. An incision is a type of acute wound created intentionally as part of surgical treatment. A chronic wound persists beyond the expected amount of time for usual wound closure. The body responds to an acute or chronic wound through a complex restorative process called wound healing.

Nurses play a significant role in preventing impaired skin integrity and promoting optimal healing when disruptions in the skin or underlying structures occur. Nurses also teach patients how to avoid accidental injury, maintain skin integrity, and promote optimal healing.

NORMAL INTEGUMENTARY FUNCTION

The body's ability to protect itself from the environment depends largely on the integrity of the integumentary system. The skin contributes to metabolic activities and is a key part of maintaining homeostasis. A review of the skin's structure and function provides a framework for understanding the importance of nursing care of skin and wounds.

Structure of the Skin

SKIN LAYERS

The skin has two major tissue layers: epidermis and dermis (Fig. 30-1). The **epidermis**, the skin's outer layer, is avascular and composed of layers of stratified squamous epithelial cells. The epidermis specializes to form the hair, nails, and glandu-

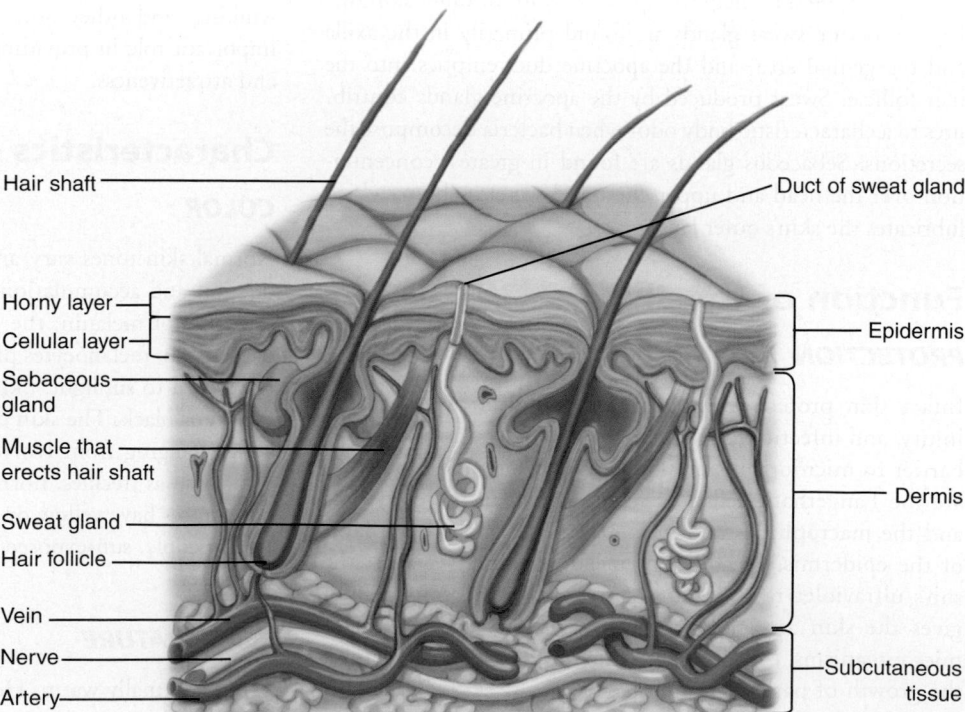

FIGURE 30-1 Cross section of skin and underlying structures.

Hair shaft

Horny layer
Cellular layer
Sebaceous gland
Muscle that erects hair shaft
Sweat gland
Hair follicle
Vein
Nerve
Artery

Duct of sweat gland
Epidermis
Dermis
Subcutaneous tissue

lar structures. The epidermis relies on the dermis for its nutrition. The thin, outermost layer of the epidermis (the stratum corneum or horny layer) is continuously shed in a process called **desquamation**. The major cell of the epidermis is the keratinocytes, producing keratin, the primary material in the shed layer of cells. Basal layers of the epidermis contain melanocytes, which produce melanin, the substance responsible for skin pigmentation.

The **dermis**, which underlies the epidermis, is the thickest skin layer and is composed of tough connective tissue. This dermal matrix supports and nourishes the constantly changing epidermis. The major cell of the dermis, the fibroblast, produces the proteins collagen and elastin. The dermis is well vascularized and contains lymphatic vessels and nerve tissues. **Subcutaneous tissue** underlies the skin. It consists primarily of fat and connective tissues that support the skin.

A partial-thickness wound involves the loss of epidermis and possibly partial loss of the dermis. A full-thickness wound extends through the dermis to involve subcutaneous tissue and possibly muscle and bone (Bryant & Nix, 2012).

SKIN APPENDAGES

The enfolding of the epidermis into the underlying dermis forms the skin appendages (hair, nails, eccrine sweat glands, apocrine sweat glands, and sebaceous glands). Hair consists of keratinous fibers; it grows on the entire skin surface, except for the palms and soles. Nails are formed by rapidly dividing epidermal cells in the nail bed. Both hair and nails have no nerve endings or blood supply. The eccrine and apocrine glands are sweat glands. Eccrine glands, which are widely distributed throughout the skin, help transport sweat to the outer skin surface. Apocrine sweat glands are found primarily in the axilla and the genital area, and the apocrine duct empties into the hair follicle. Sweat produced by the apocrine glands contributes to a characteristic body odor when bacteria decompose the secretions. Sebaceous glands are found in greatest concentration over the head and upper chest and secrete sebum, which lubricates the skin's outer layer.

Function of the Skin

PROTECTION

Intact skin protects the body from physical and chemical injury, and infection is less likely when intact skin provides a barrier to microorganisms. The cells that provide protection are the Langerhans cells and keratinocytes in the epidermis and the macrophages and mast cells beneath the basal layer of the epidermis. In addition, melanin protects against the sun's ultraviolet rays. Sebum, secreted by sebaceous glands, gives the skin an acidic pH, which retards the growth of microorganisms. Additionally, microorganisms that inhibit the growth of pathogens are present on the skin. These resident skin floras include *Staphylococcus*, *Streptococcus*, yeast, and others.

THERMOREGULATION

Through dilation and constriction of the blood vessels in the dermis, the skin helps to regulate body temperature and adjust to external temperature changes. Vasoconstriction produces shivering, which helps the body maintain its temperature in cool environments. Sweating cools the body through evaporation of fluid and dissipation of heat. Large volumes of fluid can be lost through profuse sweating during exercise or warm external temperatures. Loss of large areas of skin due to burns or other injury can significantly impair the body's ability to maintain temperature and fluid regulation.

SENSATION

The skin contains networks of nerves that are sensitive to pain, touch, itch, vibration, heat, and cold. These nerve endings are contained within the dermis, and some extend into the epidermis. The fine hair on body surfaces also provides sensation because of the sensory nerves that surround the hair follicles.

METABOLISM

From the sun's ultraviolet rays, the skin synthesizes vitamin D. Vitamin D is necessary for efficient absorption of calcium and phosphorus.

COMMUNICATION

The skin provides a means of communication through facial expression and physical appearance. Facial skin and underlying muscles produce expressions, such as frowning, blinking, winking, and other nonverbal messages. The skin plays an important role in providing some aspects of body appearance and attractiveness.

Characteristics of Normal Skin

COLOR

Normal skin tones vary among races, depending on the production and accumulation of melanin. The greater the accumulation of melanin, the darker the skin tone. In races with darker skin, melanocytes produce more melanin when the skin is exposed to sunlight. Skin tones can range from tan to dark brown or black. The skin color of lighter-pigmented races also varies, ranging from ivory to pink. Areas of hyperpigmentation, such as freckles, normally occur in light-skinned people. Some races have yellow or olive undertones to their skin color. In all people, sun-exposed areas, such as the face or arms, can be darker.

TEMPERATURE

Skin is normally warm. However, peripheral areas, such as the feet or hands, may be cool if vasoconstriction in the skin has occurred.

MOISTURE

Normally, the skin is dry to the touch, but moisture can accumulate in skin folds. Anxiety can increase the moisture normally detected in the axillae or palms of the hands.

TEXTURE AND THICKNESS

The texture of unexposed skin usually is smooth. Areas exposed to friction (e.g., soles of the feet, palms of the hands) may become rough and hypertrophied. Sun exposure, aging, and smoking also make skin less smooth. Skin thickness varies depending on the body location. The skin on the soles of the feet may be 0.25 inch thick, but the skin covering the eyelids may be only 0.02 inch thick.

Normally, skin has good elasticity, rapidly returning to its normal shape when pinched between the thumb and forefinger, a quality called skin turgor. As a person ages, skin turgor normally decreases. Another factor that decreases skin turgor is fluid loss caused by dehydration.

ODOR

Skin is usually free from odor. Stress, exercise, or warm external temperature can increase sweat gland production, which can increase odor.

Life Span Considerations

Skin changes during the life span. The greatest variations occur in the very young and in older adults.

NEWBORN AND INFANT

The skin of newborns is thinner and more sensitive than that of older infants. Superficial blood vessels are so prominent that they give newborn skin a characteristic red color. Only the sebaceous glands are active during early infancy. Milia—sebaceous retention cysts seen as white, opalescent spots around the chin and nose—appear during the first few weeks of life and disappear spontaneously. Fine hair called lanugo covers the newborn's body. Lanugo is lost during the first weeks of life and is replaced by hair of a different color and texture. Infants characteristically have long, thin fingernails and toenails that often scratch their delicate skin.

Infant skin is susceptible to blistering, chafing, and rashes from friction or irritation. Exposure to a warm, humid environment can lead to prickly heat, and frequent bathing can cause dryness, leading to other skin problems. Exposure to cold environmental temperatures may produce hypothermia because infants have a decreased ability to thermoregulate. Irritant contact dermatitis and bacterial infections can occur from exposure to soiled diapers.

Other common skin disorders of infancy are diaper rash and eczema. Parents and caregivers can prevent diaper rash by keeping infants clean and dry. Eczema may be an allergic response to foods, soaps, or other stimuli, so parents should introduce new foods one at a time into their babies' diets.

TODDLER AND PRESCHOOLER

After the first year of life, skin normally shows few changes until puberty. As motor skills develop, children are more prone to accidents, which may result in lacerations or abrasions. Many children spend extensive time outdoors, and sunscreen is necessary to protect against damage caused by ultraviolet rays.

Toddlers and preschoolers are susceptible to burns. Keeping hot liquids out of their reach and keeping children away from heaters, barbecue grills, stoves, and fires are necessary safety measures. Capping electrical outlets with protective covers helps prevent accidental electrical burns.

SCHOOL-AGE CHILD AND ADOLESCENT

Although the skin remains stable until adolescence, communicable illnesses, such as impetigo, scabies, and head lice, commonly affect skin integrity and may necessitate absence from school. As children become older, they are more aware of their bodies and are concerned when rashes or scars affect their appearance. Therefore, identifying rashes and instituting measures to avoid spread of infectious diseases that impair skin integrity are important. Provide emotional support for parents and children when such conditions appear so that the children are better able to cope with the stress and discomfort of skin disruptions.

During adolescence, pubic, axillary, and other body hair appear. The most common skin disorder of adolescence is acne vulgaris. As the sebaceous glands enlarge at puberty, production of sebum increases. Acne lesions result from plugging of pilosebaceous glands. Lesions form primarily on the face, neck, back, chest, and shoulders. Because adolescence is a time when physical appearance is important to self-concept, severe acne can be emotionally disturbing to an adolescent.

Adolescents engage in many leisure activities that involve sun exposure (e.g., swimming, outdoor sports, sunbathing). Because excessive sun exposure has been linked to skin cancer, discourage tanning bed use and teach teens to protect their skin by using effective sunscreen products when outdoors.

ADULT AND OLDER ADULT

Skin changes are part of normal aging. As skin ages, it generally becomes thinner because it loses dermal and subcutaneous mass. Because sebaceous and sweat glands are less active, dry skin is more common. Wrinkling and poor skin turgor result from loss of elastic fibers and collagen changes in the dermal connective tissue. Circulation to the skin is reduced, and healing is slower. The nails may become thicker and more brittle, and hair may lose pigment and turn gray. Pruritus (itching) commonly occurs in older adults and is caused mainly by dry, scaling skin.

The size and number of benign skin growths markedly increase in older adults. Skin tags, which are loose flaps of skin, occur mainly around the neck, eyelids, and axillae. Keratoses are horny, slow-growing proliferations of the keratinizing cells of the epidermis. They may itch and bleed if traumatized. Senile lentigines, also called age or liver spots, are pigmentation changes that occur on sun-exposed areas. Although many skin changes are benign, adults must self-examine their skin to enhance early detection of abnormalities such as melanoma, a type of skin cancer.

Cultural Considerations

Nursing assessment of skin and wounds requires sensitivity to variations in skin color among people. For example, stage I pressure ulcers and suspected deep tissue injuries will present with subtle changes and variations of skin color in persons with darkly pigmented skin.

Traditional Western medicine advocates a scientific-based approach to wound healing. However, several modalities that complement scientific wound management are available. Many cultures have historical preferences for the use of botanicals or herbal remedies for wound care. Lotions and gels containing aloe vera are widely accepted as adjuvants to standard medical topical treatments for wounds, especially minor burns, insect bites, dermatitis, and dry skin. Chamomile, lavender, and tea tree oils are commonly used for healing wounds. Witch hazel is an herbal remedy for minor burns and abrasions.

A culturally competent nurse respects the traditions of his or her patients. Native American tribes often recognize an elder who specializes in specific healing rituals, which may include herbal or spiritual therapy to heal wounds. Asian cultures frequently use acupuncture to stimulate wound healing. Specific cultural differences were identified in a study regarding wound-related pain experiences. French participants expressed concern about body image, British participants were concerned about medication use, and Canadian participants were anxious about financial considerations related to wound care (Mudge, Meaume, Woo, Sibbald, & Price, 2008).

FACTORS AFFECTING INTEGUMENTARY FUNCTION

Circulation

Adequate blood flow to the skin is necessary for healthy, viable tissues. Adequate skin perfusion requires four factors:

- The heart must be able to pump adequately.
- The volume of circulating blood must be sufficient.
- Arteries and veins must be patent and functioning well.
- Local capillary pressure must be higher than external pressure.

Alterations in any of these factors can lead to skin that has abnormal color, texture, thickness, moisture, or temperature or that becomes ulcerated.

Leg and foot ulcers occur from various causes, but the most common are ulcers secondary to venous insufficiency, arterial insufficiency, and peripheral neuropathy. Impaired arterial or venous function in the lower extremities can produce ulcerations that are refractory to healing unless the underlying disorder is treated.

Venous dermatitis results from impaired venous return secondary to venous insufficiency or structural alterations in the legs. Pooling of blood leads to edema, vasodilation, and plasma extravasation, all of which result in inflamed skin. See Table 30-1, Lower Extremity Chronic Wounds, for a comparison of the etiology, manifestation, and treatment options for LEAD (lower extremity arterial disease), LEVD (lower extremity venous disease), and LEND (lower extremity neuropathic disease).

Nutrition

A well-balanced diet promotes healthy skin. With a deficiency of protein or calories, hair becomes dull and dry and may fall out. Skin also becomes dry and flaky. Adequate intake of vitamins A, B_6, C, and K; niacin; and riboflavin is important to prevent abnormal skin changes. Adequate intake of iron, copper, and zinc is important to prevent abnormal pigmentation and changes in nails and hair.

Condition of the Epidermis

To maintain its protective function against invading microorganisms, the epidermis must be free from any breaks. Maintenance of the skin's natural moisture is necessary because abnormal drying can cause microscopic cracks. Excessive moisture can predispose the skin to breakdown. Skin that is continually exposed to moisture softens and becomes macerated, increasing its susceptibility to trauma and infection. **Macerated** tissue appears wrinkled and is lighter in appearance than healthy tissue. Fecal and urinary incontinence increase an individual's risk for maceration. Diaphoresis or inadequate drying after hygiene, especially in skin folds, can increase moisture and encourage the growth of yeast, leading to rashes.

Allergy

Allergic reactions and skin inflammation are responses to injury mediated by histamine release. External or internal irritants can cause the reactions. The irritants may be chemical (e.g., skin creams, latex gloves, detergents, plants such as poison ivy or poison oak) or mechanical (e.g., rubbing against an irritant, such as wool). Foods and medications also may cause skin reactions. **Dermatitis**, an inflammation of the skin, most often produces epidermal and dermal damage or irritation, possibly accompanied by pain, itching, redness, and blisters. Chronic dermatitis produces changes in the epidermis, including thickening, scaling, and increased pigmentation. Treatment focuses on eliminating exposure to the allergen and may include lubrication of the skin and application of topical medications.

TABLE 30-1 CHRONIC LOWER EXTREMITY WOUNDS

	Lower Extremity *Arterial* Wounds	Lower Extremity *Venous* Wounds	Lower Extremity *Neuropathic* Wounds
Etiology	Decreased arterial blood flow and perfusion	Venous insufficiency	Peripheral neuropathy usually caused by diabetes and/or peripheral vascular disease
Location	Tips or phalangeal heads of toes Between the toes Bony prominences, such as, midtibial (shin) or lateral malleolus	Between knee and area above the medial malleolus; usually anterior	Located on the pressure areas of the plantar, medial, or lateral aspect of the foot. The majority are on the plantar surface of the 1st metatarsal head.
Wound Characteristics	Rounded smooth edges with punched out appearance Dry, pale wound bed with minimal exudate Gangrene or necrotic areas may be present.	Shallow with irregular borders Wound bed is pale red often mixed with yellow loose slough. Exudate may be moderate or profuse.	Repeated pressure or shear in an insensate foot causes a callus to form with ulcer underneath. An open wound is often round, surrounded by callus. Wound bed may be necrotic, pink, or pale. Minimal exudate
Associated Assessment Findings	Diminished peripheral pulses, cool feet, thick toenails, decreased hair growth on legs Intermittent claudication progressing to rest pain. Legs are pale when elevated 60 degrees but rubor when legs lowered to dependent position.	Lower extremity edema. Hyperpigmentation of surrounding tissue due to hemosiderin staining. Scaling, crusting, maceration, and weeping of the lower legs may be present.	History of diabetes along with decreased sensation in the toes and feet Foot deformities, such as hammertoes or prominent metatarsal heads. Abnormal gait or limited joint mobility Footwear may reveal abnormal wear patterns
Treatment Goal	Improve perfusion. Attain or maintain intact skin. Reduce pain. Optimize wound healing.	Improve venous return and optimize wound healing.	Off-load pressure on feet and optimize wound healing.
Nursing Wound Care Treatment Plan	Cleanse open wounds with noncytotoxic cleansers only. Maintain stable or dry eschars (do not moisten arterial eschars)	Cleanse wounds at every dressing change. Avoid use of tapes or adhesives on the skin. Protect periwound skin from contact with exudate Use dressings that absorb drainage, such as foam or calcium alginates	Inspect feet carefully for any open lesions, cuts, or scratches. Cleanse open wounds at every dressing change. Use dressings that maintain a moist wound bed. Maintain stable or dry noninfected eschars.
Collaborative Treatment Plan	Manage hypertension and diabetes. Smoking cessation Improve nutrition ABI measurements Local or surgical debridement only if perfusion is adequate Surgical procedures to increase blood flow	Elevate legs. Compression therapy if ABI (ankle brachial index) is >0.8. Identify and treat wound infections. Improve nutrition.	Protect feet from trauma. Podiatry for callus debridement; sharp or surgical debridement of avascular tissue Biologic wound dressings Therapeutic, custom-fit shoes Off-load pressure—total contact casting Glycemic control Nutrition counseling Assess for osteomyelitis.

Infections

Bacterial, viral, or fungal infections can affect skin integrity. Streptococcal and staphylococcal organisms are responsible for most bacterial skin infections. Impetigo, which usually is caused by beta-hemolytic streptococci, is a common bacterial skin infection. An **abscess** is a localized collection of white blood cells and cellular debris (pus) that appears swollen and inflamed. An abscess can occur on or under the skin. Group A strep bacteria usually cause mild skin infections but can also be the cause of a rare but serious infection called **necrotizing fasciitis**. Toxins made by the bacteria destroy the soft tissue they infect, causing it to die. "Necrotizing" means "causing the death of tissues." Accurate diagnosis and prompt treatment with intravenous antibiotics and surgery to remove the dead tissue are important (CDC, 2013).

Cutaneous warts caused by the papillomavirus are another common disease of the skin, with hands and feet most typically affected. Herpes virus infections can cause skin disruption of the lips, face, mouth, and genitals. Many communicable childhood illnesses of viral origin cause rashes. Pruritus usually accompanies these rashes and may lead to secondary infection.

Fungal infections can infect nonhairy skin, the scalp, the genital region, nails, and, most commonly, the feet. Candidal fungal infections, occurring most often in the mouth, genital area, or in skin folds, frequently occur when normal body flora is disrupted secondary to antibiotic therapy or immunosuppression.

Abnormal Growth Rate

When the skin is produced at an abnormal rate by malignant or nonmalignant processes, normal integrity can be disrupted. Psoriasis is a nonmalignant, chronic disorder that greatly increases the rate of skin production: The normal epidermal turnover rate of 14 to 20 days accelerates to 3 to 4 days. Certain forms of psoriasis characteristically occur in children and young adults. The elbows, knees, scalp, and soles of the feet are common sites for psoriasis. Periods of remission are followed by exacerbations, which can be triggered by stress, infection, or environmental factors.

Benign or malignant neoplasms also can affect skin integrity. Most benign neoplasms result from viral infections or normal aging. Most malignant skin lesions result from prolonged exposure to ultraviolet radiation.

Systemic Diseases

Many chronic diseases can produce skin abnormalities and ulceration. Inflammatory bowel disease, pemphigus, and diabetes are examples of diseases that can produce impaired skin integrity. Peripheral neuropathy is a common complication of diabetes and the leading cause of lower extremity neuropathic wounds. See Table 30-1 for a comparison of the common lower extremity wounds, including neuropathic wounds. Interventions to treat skin problems caused by systemic disease need to treat and control the underlying disorder in order for wound healing to occur.

Trauma

Any trauma to the skin, such as a wound, creates a risk for altered skin function. Wounds can be divided into broad categories of accidental and surgical (Table 30-2).

ACCIDENTAL WOUNDS

Common accidental wounds include abrasions, lacerations, and puncture wounds. An **abrasion** results when skin rubs against a hard surface. Friction scrapes away the epithelial layer, exposing the epidermal or dermal layer. Falls onto hands, elbows, or knees cause most abrasions. A **laceration** is an open wound or cut. Most lacerations affect only the upper layers of skin and subcutaneous tissue underneath. Permanent damage may result, however, if injury occurs to internal structures such as muscles, tendons, blood vessels, or nerves. Accidents involving automobiles, machinery, or knives may result in lacerations. A puncture wound is made when a sharp, pointed object penetrates tissue. Damage to underlying structures or gross contamination with debris and pathogens may result. Nails, pins, tacks, and other sharp objects are common causes.

SURGICAL WOUNDS

Surgical wounds vary from simple and superficial (e.g., a thyroidectomy incision) to deep and contaminated (e.g., an abdominal incision done for septic peritonitis). They may be

TABLE 30-2 TYPES OF WOUNDS

Wound	Description
Broad Categories	
Acute	Injury, such as knife, gunshot, burn, or surgical incision; heals within 6 months
Chronic	Wound that persists beyond usual healing time (>6 months) or recurs without new injury to the area
Open	Break present in the skin; tissue damage present
Closed	No break seen in the skin, but soft tissue damage evident
Descriptors	
Abrasion	Wound involving friction of skin; superficial; dermatologic procedure for scar tissue removal
Puncture	Intentional or unintentional penetrating trauma by sharp or pointed instrument that penetrates skin and underlying tissue
Laceration	Cut in the skin; wound edges may be smooth or jagged; depth may be shallow or deep; object possibly contaminated; infection risk
Contusion	Closed wound; bleeding in underlying tissues from blunt blow; bruising
Classifications of Surgical Wounds	
Clean	Closed surgical wound that did not enter gastrointestinal, respiratory, or genitourinary systems; low infection risk
Clean/contaminated	Wound entering gastrointestinal, respiratory, or genitourinary systems; infection risk
Contaminated	Open, traumatic wound; surgical wound with break in asepsis; high infection risk
Infected	Wound site with pathogens present; signs of infection

divided into several categories. The wound's severity influences healing time, degree of pain, probability of complications, and presence of any tubes, drains, or suction devices.

Ostomies are surgical openings in the abdominal wall that allow part of an organ to open onto the skin. Medical conditions, such as cancer of the intestine or urinary bladder or inflammatory bowel disease, may require an ostomy. Because the skin surrounding the opening (stoma) may be continuously exposed to feces, urine, or intestinal secretions, skin irritation may develop if appropriately fitted ostomy pouches and products are not used.

Burns

Exposure to excessive heat, electricity, caustic chemicals, or radiation can result in tissue damage and burns. Burns range from minor injuries, such as simple sunburn, to major insults that cause significant life disruptions. The degree of damage depends on the type of burn, its extent and depth, and the patient's state of health before the burn.

Partial-thickness burns may be superficial or moderate to deep. A superficial partial-thickness burn (first degree; epidermal) is pinkish or red with no blistering; a mild sunburn is a good example. Moderate to deep partial-thickness burns (second degree; dermal or deep dermal) may be pink, red, pale ivory, or light yellow-brown. They are usually moist with blisters. Exposure to steam can cause this type of burn.

A full-thickness burn (third degree) may vary from brown or black to cherry red or pearly white. Thrombosed vessels and blisters or bullae may be present. The full-thickness burn appears dry and leathery. Sometimes, when fascia, muscle, or bone is extensively damaged, the injury is called a fourth-degree burn.

Thermal burns, the most common type, are caused by contact with various heat sources, including flames, hot liquids, hot surfaces, and steam. Chemical burns are caused by contact with noxious substances. The amount of tissue damaged as a result of chemical injury depends on the concentration of the chemical and the length of exposure. The severity of an electrical burn depends on the current's type and voltage, the pathway the current takes through the body, and the duration of contact. Radiation burns can occur when a person is accidentally exposed to radiation or when radiation is used as a form of therapy.

Mechanical Forces

Forces applied to the skin such as friction, shear, and pressure can create skin damage.

FRICTION

Friction occurs when two surfaces rub together. When skin rubs against a firm surface, such as wrinkled bedding, small abrasions may occur. Adequate lubrication of the skin and care during handling, moving, and washing patients can limit the negative effect of friction. The skin damage is usually very shallow, involving the epidermis.

SHEAR

Shear force occurs when tissue layers move on each other, causing blood vessels to stretch as they pass through the subcutaneous tissue (Fig. 30-2). Most commonly, this occurs when patients slide down in bed or are pulled up in bed. The patient's skin remains relatively immobile because friction anchors it to the sheets, but deeper structures, such as fascia, move with the patient because they are attached to the bone. In the process, capillaries in the underlying tissue are stretched and often torn, increasing the risk of ulcer formation. This force intensifies the destructive effects of pressure on the skin.

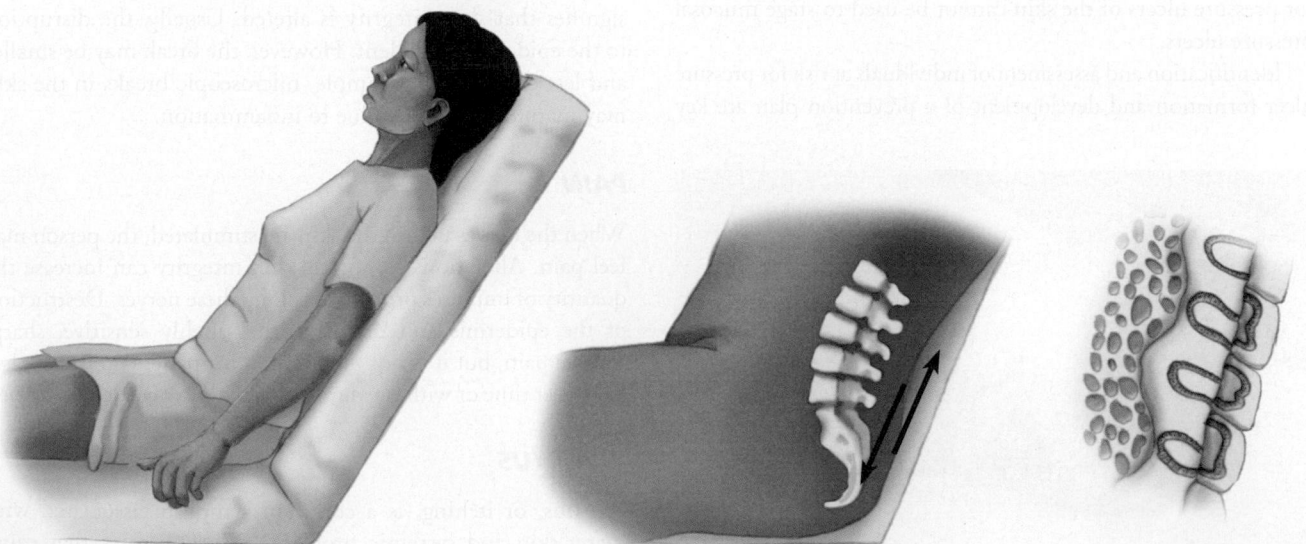

FIGURE 30-2 Shearing force contributes to pressure ulcer development when opposing forces cause capillaries to stretch and tear as the patient slides down in bed.

SAFETY ALERT

Move and reposition immobile patients carefully to prevent injury to the skin as a result of shearing force.

PRESSURE

Pressure is the major factor in pressure ulcer formation. The intensity and duration of pressure along with tissue tolerance influence the effects of pressure on the skin. Both low-intensity pressure for a long period of time and high-intensity pressure for a short period of time can lead to tissue damage.

A **pressure ulcer** is localized injury to the skin and/or underlying tissue, usually over a bony prominence, as a result of pressure or pressure in combination with shear (European Pressure Ulcer Advisory Panel and National Pressure Ulcer Advisory Panel, 2009). This pressure decreases the blood flow, impairing the supply of nutrients and oxygen to the skin and underlying tissues. Cells die and decompose, and an ulcer forms. Pressure ulcers usually occur over bony prominences, such as the coccyx, ischial tuberosities, trochanters, and heels (Fig. 30-3). Pressure ulcers are classified based on their depth of tissue destruction using a staging system (Box 30-1). If a pressure ulcer is covered with nonviable tissue and the base of the wound is obscured, staging is not possible until the dead tissue is removed.

Medical devices can be the source of the pressure causing a pressure ulcer. Oxygen tubing or masks, tracheostomy plates or ties, splints or braces, compression stockings, and bedpans are examples of devices potentially causing pressure ulcers. The tissue injury under the device often matches the shape or contour of the device.

A mucosal pressure ulcer is a type of pressure ulcer found on mucous membranes with a history of a medical device in use at the location of the ulcer. Types of medical devices associated with mucosal pressure ulcers include endotracheal tubes, nasogastric tubes, or fecal management tubes. The staging system for pressure ulcers of the skin cannot be used to stage mucosal pressure ulcers.

Identification and assessment of individuals at risk for pressure ulcer formation and development of a prevention plan are key

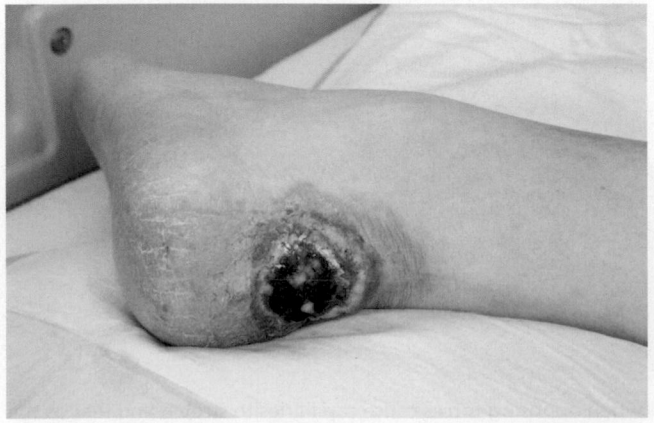

FIGURE 30-3 A pressure ulcer on the upper aspect of the heel.

to preventing pressure ulcers. Identifying high-risk settings and patients allows the nurse to target prevention efforts. Decreased mobility, decreased activity, and decreased sensory/perceptual ability increase the risk of pressure ulcers. Therefore, an individual who cannot move independently or who will be immobilized is at increased risk. In addition, patients with neuropathy or paralysis are at increased risk because of impaired sensation.

Extrinsic factors that decrease tissue tolerance and increase the likelihood of pressure ulcer development include moisture and shearing force. Other contributing factors are malnutrition, age, and low arteriolar pressure. Often, the relationship among risk factors ultimately causes a pressure ulcer to develop.

Impaired nutritional status increases the risk of pressure ulcer development. In patients who are nutritionally depleted, capillaries become more fragile, and as they break, blood flow to the skin can be impaired. Patients who are malnourished may have weight loss, decreased serum proteins, and reduced immune function. Loss of subcutaneous tissue and muscle mass affects the amount of protective padding between skin and bone and increases the risk of pressure ulcers.

Structured assessment tools are available to assist in the prediction of patients at increased risk for pressure ulcers. The two risk assessment tools that have been tested extensively are the Braden Scale (Box 30-2) and the Norton Scale. These scales provide a numeric score to rate the individual patient's level of risk.

ALTERED INTEGUMENTARY FUNCTION

Manifestations of Altered Integumentary Function

Disruption in normal skin integrity can manifest as pain, pruritus, rashes, lesions, or open wounds; usually, more than one symptom is present. Any break in the skin's epidermal layer signifies that skin integrity is altered. Usually, the disruption to the epidermis is evident. However, the break may be smaller and less obvious. For example, microscopic breaks in the skin may manifest as redness due to inflammation.

PAIN

When the nerves within the skin are stimulated, the person may feel pain. Alterations to normal skin integrity can increase the quantity of impulses propagated along these nerves. Destruction of the epidermis and dermis creates highly sensitive, sharp, intense pain, but it is not uncommon for patients to report less pain over time or with pressure ulcers that involve deeper tissues.

PRURITUS

Pruritus, or itching, is a common symptom associated with many skin and systemic problems. Most diseases that cause itching are inflammatory or allergic. Pruritus is often the cause of secondary lesions because scratching breaks the skin surface.

BOX 30-1   Pressure Ulcer Staging

Stage I

Intact skin with nonblanchable redness of a localized area, usually over a bony prominence. Darkly pigmented skin may not have visible blanching; its color may differ from the surrounding area. The area may be painful, firm, soft, warmer, or cooler as compared to adjacent tissue. Stage I may be difficult to detect in individuals with dark skin tones. May indicate "at-risk persons" (a heralding sign of risk) (EPUAP & NPUAP, 2009).

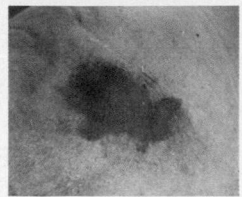 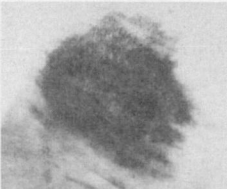

Stage II

Partial-thickness loss of dermis presenting as a shallow open ulcer with a red-pink wound bed, without slough. May also present as an intact or open/ruptured serum-filled blister. Presents as a shiny or dry shallow ulcer without slough or bruising (bruising indicates suspected **deep tissue injury [DTI]**). This stage should not be used to describe skin tears, tape burns, perineal dermatitis, maceration, or excoriation (NPUAP, 2007).

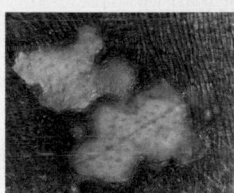 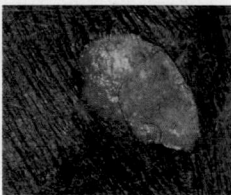

Stage III

Full-thickness tissue loss. Subcutaneous fat may be visible, but bone, tendon, or muscle is not exposed. Slough may be present but does not obscure the depth of tissue loss. May include undermining and tunneling. The depth of a stage III pressure ulcer varies by anatomic location. The bridge of the nose, ear, occiput, and malleolus do not have subcutaneous tissue, and stage III ulcers can be shallow. In contrast, areas of significant adiposity can develop extremely deep stage III pressure ulcers. Bone/tendon is not visible or directly palpable (NPUAP, 2007).

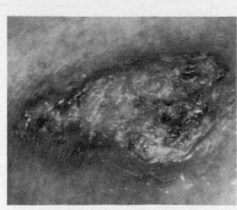 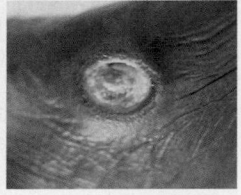

Stage IV

Full-thickness tissue loss with exposed bone, tendon, or muscle. Slough or eschar may be present on some parts of the wound bed. Often includes undermining and tunneling. The depth of a stage IV pressure ulcer varies by anatomic location. The bridge of the nose, ear, occiput, and malleolus do not have subcutaneous tissue, and these ulcers can be shallow. Stage IV ulcers can extend into muscle and/or supporting structures (e.g., fascia, tendon, or joint capsule), making osteomyelitis possible. Exposed bone/tendon is visible or directly palpable (NPUAP, 2007).

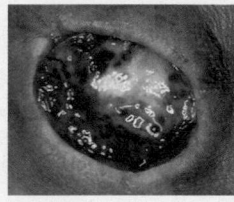 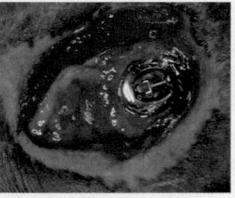

Unstageable

Full-thickness tissue loss in which the base of the ulcer is covered by slough (yellow, tan, gray, green, or brown) and/or eschar (tan, brown, or black) in the wound bed. Until enough slough or eschar is removed to expose the base of the wound, the true depth, and therefore stage, cannot be determined. Stable (dry, adherent, intact without erythema or fluctuance) eschar on the heels serves as "the body's natural (biologic) cover" and should not be removed (NPUAP, 2007).

Suspected Deep Tissue Injury

Purple- or maroon-localized area of discolored intact skin or blood-filled blister due to damage of underlying soft tissue from pressure and/or shear. The area may be preceded by tissue that is painful, firm, mushy, boggy, warmer, or cooler as compared to adjacent tissue. DTI may be difficult to detect in individuals with dark skin tones. Evolution may include a thin blister over a dark wound bed. The wound may further evolve and become covered by thin eschar. Evolution may be rapid, exposing additional layers of tissue even with optimal treatment (NPUAP, 2007).

Photos from: Calrenno, C. (2000). Assessing and preventing pressure ulcers. *Advances in Skin and Wound Care, 13*(5), 245.

BOX 30-2 **Braden Scale for Predicting Pressure Ulcer Sore Risk**

Sensory Perception: Ability to Respond Meaningfully to Pressure-Related Discomfort

1. **Completely Limited**: Unresponsive (does not moan, flinch, or grasp) to painful stimuli, due to diminished level of consciousness or sedation, OR limited ability to feel pain over most of body surface.
2. **Very Limited**: Responds only to painful stimuli. Cannot communicate discomfort except by moaning or restlessness, OR has a sensory impairment that limits the ability to feel pain or discomfort over half of body.
3. **Slightly Limited**: Responds to verbal commands but cannot always communicate discomfort or need to be turned, OR has some sensory impairment that limits ability to feel pain or discomfort in one or two extremities.
4. **No Impairment**: Responds to verbal commands. Has no sensory deficit that would limit ability to feel or voice pain and discomfort.

SCORE

Moisture: Degree to Which Skin is Exposed to Moisture

1. **Constantly Moist**: Skin is kept moist almost constantly by perspiration, urine, etc. Dampness is detected every time the patient is moved or turned.
2. **Very Moist**: Skin is often but not always moist. Linen must be changed at least once a shift.
3. **Occasionally Moist**: Skin is occasionally moist, requiring an extra linen change approximately once a day.
4. **Rarely Moist**: Skin is usually dry; linen requires changing only at routine intervals.

SCORE

Activity: Degree of Physical Activity

1. **Bedfast**: Confined to bed.
2. **Chairfast**: Ability to walk severely limited or nonexistent. Cannot bear own weight and/or must be assisted into chair or wheelchair.
3. **Walks Occasionally**: Walks occasionally during the day, but for very short distances, with or without assistance. Spends most of each shift in bed or chair.
4. **Walks Frequently**: Walks outside the room at least twice a day and inside room at least once every 2 hours during waking hours.

SCORE

Mobility: Ability to Change and Control Body Position

1. **Completely Immobile**: Does not make even slight changes in body or extremity position without assistance.
2. **Very Limited**: Makes occasional slight changes in body or extremity position but unable to make frequent or significant changes independently.
3. **Slightly Limited**: Makes frequent though slight changes in body or extremity position independently.
4. **No Limitation**: Makes major and frequent changes in position without assistance.

SCORE

Nutrition: Usual Food Intake Pattern

1. **Very Poor**: Never eats a complete meal. Rarely eats more than one third of food offered. Eats two servings or less of protein (meat or dairy products) per day. Takes fluids poorly. Does not take a liquid dietary supplement, or is NPO and/or maintained on clear liquids or IV for more than 5 days.
2. **Probably Inadequate**: Rarely eats a complete meal and generally eats only about half of any food offered. Protein intake includes only three servings of meat or dairy products per day. Occasionally will take a dietary supplement, OR receives less than optimum amount of liquid diet or tube feeding.
3. **Adequate**: Eats over half of most meals. Eats a total of four servings of protein (meat, dairy products) each day. Occasionally will refuse a meal but will usually take a supplement if offered, or is on a tube feeding or TPN regimen, which probably meets most of nutritional needs.
4. **Excellent**: Eats most of every meal. Never refuses a meal. Usually eats a total of four or more servings of meat and dairy products. Occasionally eats between meals. Does not require supplementation.

SCORE

BOX 30-2 Braden Scale for Predicting Pressure Ulcer Sore Risk *(Continued)*

Friction and Shear

1. **Problem**: Requires moderate to maximum assistance in moving. Complete lifting without sliding against sheets is impossible. Frequently slides down in bed or chair, requiring frequent repositioning with maximum assistance. Spasticity, contractures, or agitation leads to almost constant friction.
2. **Potential Problem**: Moves feebly or requires minimum assistance. During a move, skin probably slides to some extent against sheets, chair, restraints, or other devices. Maintains relatively good position in chair or bed most of the time but occasionally slides down.
3. **No Apparent Problem**: Moves in bed and in chair independently and has sufficient muscle strength to lift up completely during move. Maintains good position in bed or chair at all times.

SCORE

Braden Scale Scores

1 = Highly Impaired
3 or 4 = Moderate to Low Impairment
Total Points Possible: 23
Risk Predicting Score: 16 or Less

Total SCORE

RASH

Many conditions, such as excessive heat, communicable disease, allergy, or emotional distress, can cause a *rash*, a general term for a temporary skin eruption. A rash is described according to its characteristics and distribution on the body's surface. A macular rash is level with the skin surface; a papular rash involves solid elevations above the skin surface. A generalized rash covers most body areas, whereas a localized rash is limited to specific areas. Pruritus may accompany a rash.

LESIONS

A lesion involves the loss of structure or function of normal tissue. Lesions vary in size from a fraction of a millimeter to many centimeters in diameter. Lesions also are described by their shape, arrangement, and distribution (Table 30-3). Primary lesions arise in previously normal skin, and secondary lesions develop from primary lesions. Examples of secondary lesions include scales, crusts, and fissures. In the acute form of dermatitis, vesicles develop, burst, and ooze, and crusts form.

Wound Healing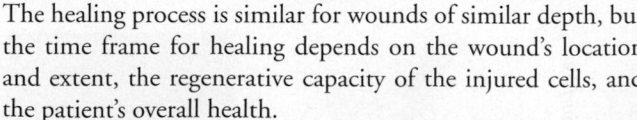

The healing process is similar for wounds of similar depth, but the time frame for healing depends on the wound's location and extent, the regenerative capacity of the injured cells, and the patient's overall health.

PHASES OF WOUND HEALING

Wounds heal through a systematic four-phase process: hemostasis, inflammatory phase, proliferative phase, and maturation. This process begins at the moment of injury and under normal conditions is completed in 12 to 24 months. Many cells are involved in wound healing, several of which produce and release chemical messengers called growth factors. Growth factors play an important role in the healing process and are being studied for possible use in optimizing wound repair.

The first phase of hemostasis begins immediately upon wounding with the onset of vasoconstriction, platelet aggregation, and clot formation. Next is the inflammatory phase, which lasts up to about 3 days. This phase is marked by vasodilation and phagocytosis as the body works to clean the wound to begin the repair process.

At this point, the healing process differs depending on whether the wound is partial or full thickness, but the four phases remain the same. In partial-thickness wounds, in the third phase, the proliferative phase, epidermal cells, which appear pink, reproduce and migrate across the surface of the wound in a process called **epithelialization**. When epithelial cells have covered the base of the wound, cells continue to replicate, increasing the number of cellular layers in the epidermis to assume the thickness of normal healthy epidermis.

In a full-thickness wound, the proliferation phase begins with the development of **granulation tissue**, which appears as beefy, red, and granular and consists of a matrix of collagen embedded with macrophages, fibroblasts, and capillary buds. As it is produced, it fills the wound with connective tissue. Open full-thickness wounds (other than those primarily closed) undergo contracture and epithelialization during this phase of healing. Contracture can be identified by its effect of pulling the wound inward, leading to a decrease in depth and dimension of the wound. The proliferative phase lasts from day 4 after injury to about day 21 in a normally healing full-thickness wound.

Maturation is the final stage of full-thickness wound healing. It begins about 3 weeks after the injury and

TABLE 30-3   BASIC TYPES OF SKIN LESIONS WITH EXAMPLES

Primary Lesions (May Arise From Previously Normal Skin)

Circumscribed, Flat, Nonpalpable Changes in Skin Color

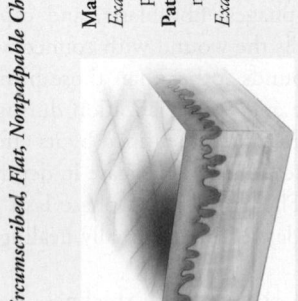

Macule—small spot
Examples: Freckle, petechia
Patch—larger than macule
Example: Vitiligo

Palpable Elevated Solid Masses

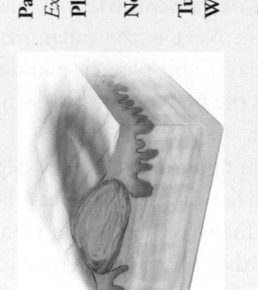

Papule—up to 0.5 cm
Example: Elevated nevus
Plaque—flat, elevated surface larger than 0.5 cm, often formed by the coalescence of papules
Nodule—larger than 0.5 cm; often deeper and firmer than a papule
Tumor—large nodule
Wheal—somewhat irregular, relatively transient, superficial area of localized skin edema.
Examples: Mosquito bite, hive

Circumscribed Superficial Elevations of the Skin Formed by Free Fluid in a Cavity Within the Skin Layers

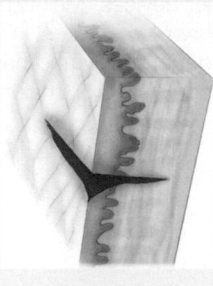

Vesicle—up to 0.5 cm; filled with serous fluid
Example: Herpes simplex
Bulla—>0.5 cm; filled with serous fluid
Example: Second-degree burn
Pustule—filled with pus
Examples: Acne, impetigo

Secondary Lesions (Result From Changes in Primary Lesions)

Loss of Skin Surface

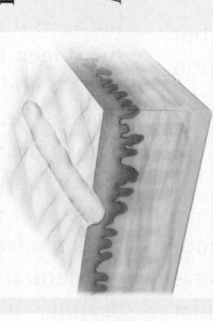

Erosion—loss of the superficial epidermis; surface moist but does not bleed
Example: Moist area after the rupture of a vesicle, as in chickenpox

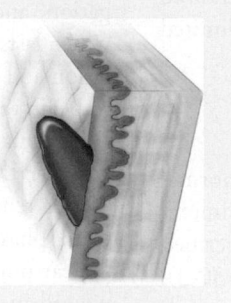

Ulcer—deeper loss of skin surface; may bleed and scar
Examples: Stasis ulcer of venous insufficiency; syphilitic chancre

Fissure—linear crack in the skin
Example: Athlete's foot

Material on Skin Surface

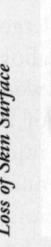

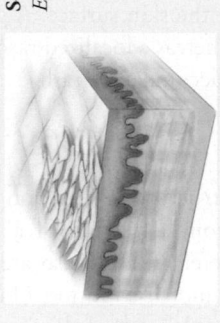

Crust—dried residue of serum, pus, or blood
Example: Impetigo

Scale—thin flake of exfoliated epidermis
Examples: Dandruff, dry skin, psoriasis

Miscellaneous Lesions

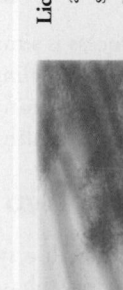

Lichenification—thickening and roughening of the skin with increased visibility of the normal skin furrows
Example: Atopic dermatitis

Atrophy—thinning of the skin with loss of the normal skin furrows; the skin looks shinier and more translucent than normal
Example: Arterial insufficiency

Excoriation—abrasion or scratch mark; may be linear, as illustrated, or rounded, as in a scratched insect bite

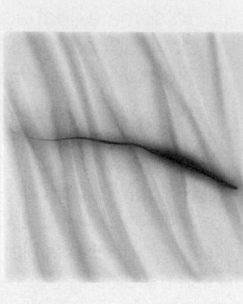

Color photographs from: Sauer, G. C. (1996). *Manual of skin diseases* (6th ed.). Philadelphia, PA: Lippincott-Raven.

THERAPEUTIC DIALOGUE: SKIN INTEGRITY AND WOUND HEALING

SCENE FOR THOUGHT

Mrs. Cook is a 72-year-old woman who is active in the retirement community where she lives. The community health nurse frequently visits the retirement community. Today, Mrs. Cook wants to see the nurse about "a mole."

LESS EFFECTIVE

Nurse: Hi, Mrs. Cook. What can I do for you?

Mrs. Cook: I need to show you this mole. It's been bleeding when it rubs against my collar *(Looks worried.)*

Nurse: *(Examines the mole carefully.)* I don't see any problem right now, Mrs. Cook, but I think you need to see your primary care provider. Shall I make the appointment for you? *(Looks up the physician's number in the card file.)*

Mrs. Cook: No, no. I'll do it myself. I'll use the one who removed my husband's skin cancer. *(Still looks worried.)*

Nurse: That sounds like a good plan. At least the physician will be familiar. Anything else?

Mrs. Cook: No, that's okay. Have a good week. *(Leaves the office with mouth set grimly.)*

MORE EFFECTIVE

Nurse: Hi there, Mrs. Cook. How are you?

Mrs. Cook: Hi, Rhonda. I'm so glad to see you. I was worried you wouldn't be here today. *(Looks concerned and a little scared.)*

Nurse: Here I am. What can I help you with?

Mrs. Cook: I'm worried about this mole I have on the back of my neck. It rubs against my collar, and yesterday, I found blood on the collar in the same place as the mole. Could you look at it? *(Shows the nurse, who finds a small amount of dried blood on the mole.)*

Nurse: How long have you had the mole?

Mrs. Cook: Years and years. I never noticed anything about it until now, though. *(Continues to look worried.)*

Nurse: What worries you about this, Mrs. Cook?

Mrs. Cook: Cancer. My husband had a lot of these removed, and both my parents had skin cancer. Could it be cancer? *(Her body stiffens as she awaits the answer.)*

Nurse: It could be, but it may not. Your primary care provider needs to see it and will possibly remove it in the office. Then, it'll go to the pathologist for examination of the cells. You should know if it's cancer or not within a week. What do you think?

Mrs. Cook: I think I'd better make the appointment today. I want to know as soon as possible. Thanks, Rhonda.

CRITICAL THINKING CHALLENGE

- Analyze what the second nurse did that the first did not do.
- Detect what clue the first nurse missed and what difference it made.
- In both instances, Mrs. Cook will call the primary care provider to be seen, evaluated, and helped. Compare and contrast the nursing care that each nurse supplied.
- Infer how Mrs. Cook would seek care in the future from both nurses.

---

may last as long as 2 years. The number of fibroblasts decreases, collagen synthesis stabilizes, and collagen fibrils become increasingly organized, resulting in greater tensile strength of the wound. The tissue usually reaches maximum strength in 10 to 12 weeks, but even after complete healing, only 70% to 80% of the original strength can be expected.

TYPES OF WOUND HEALING

Wounds heal differently, depending on whether tissue loss has occurred. The major types of wound healing are classified as primary, secondary, and tertiary intention (Fig. 30-4).

Primary Intention

Wounds with minimal tissue loss, such as clean surgical incisions or shallow sutured wounds, heal by primary intention. The edges of the primary wound are **approximated** or lightly pulled together. Granulation tissue is not visible, and scarring is usually minimal. Infection risk is lower when a clean, surgical wound heals by primary intention.

Secondary Intention

Wounds with full-thickness tissue loss, such as deep lacerations, burns, and pressure ulcers, have edges that do not readily approximate. They heal by secondary intention. The open wound gradually fills with granulation tissue. Eventually, epithelial cells migrate

Primary Intention (Primary Union)

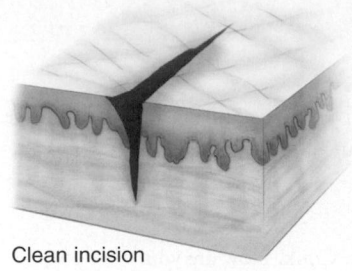

Clean incision

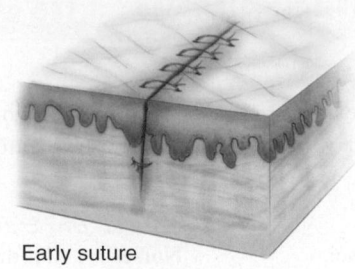

Early suture

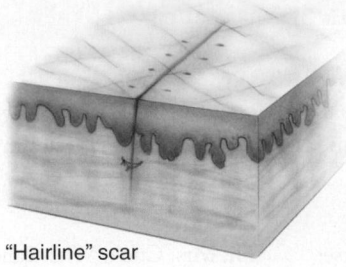

"Hairline" scar

Secondary Intention (Contraction and Epithelialization)

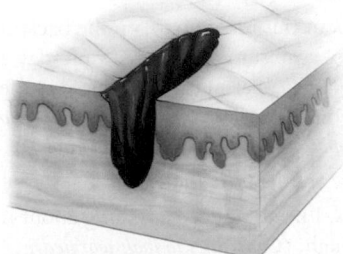

Gaping irregular wound

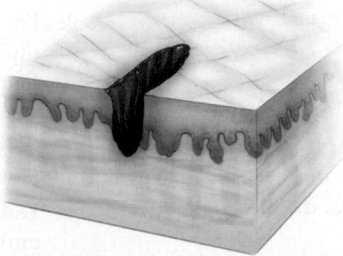

Granulation

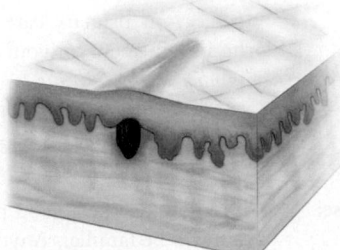

Epithelium grows over scar

Tertiary Intention (Delayed Closure)

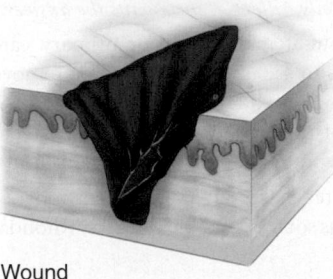

Wound

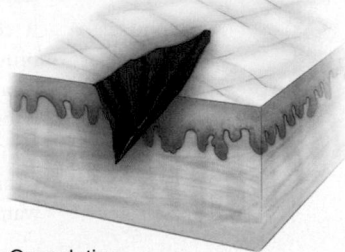

Granulation

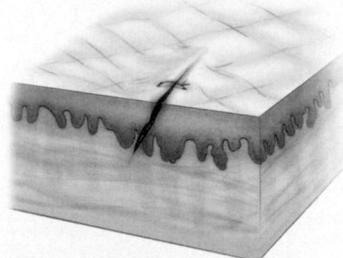

Closure with wide scar

FIGURE 30-4 Wound healing by primary, secondary, and tertiary methods.

across the granulation base, completing the cycle. Scarring is more prevalent. Because the wound is open for a longer time, it becomes colonized with microorganisms that may lead to infection.

Tertiary Intention

Healing by tertiary intention occurs when a delay ensues between injury and wound closure. This type of healing also is referred to as delayed primary closure. It may happen when a deep wound is not sutured immediately or is purposely left open until there is no sign of infection and then closed with sutures. When a wound heals by secondary or tertiary intention, a deeper and wider scar is common.

FACTORS AFFECTING WOUND HEALING

Many variables can enhance or delay wound healing. Systemic factors include nutrition, circulation, oxygenation, and immune cellular function. Individual factors include age, obesity, smoking history, and drug therapy. Local factors include the nature and location of the injury, infection, and the type of wound dressing used.

Systemic Factors

Nutrition. Sound nutrition is essential for optimal wound healing. Nutritional deficiencies can retard wound healing by inhibiting collagen synthesis and epithelialization and by reducing the activity of cells that are important to the healing process. Nutritional requirements increase with physiologic stress, which may contribute to protein deficiencies. Patients with sepsis or burns and those undergoing surgery (especially major abdominal surgery) are susceptible to protein deficiency. Patients with protein deficiencies are most likely to experience wound infections because they have decreased leukocyte functions (e.g., phagocytosis, immunogenesis).

Vitamins A, C, and E, protein, arginine, zinc, and water are especially important in wound healing. Carbohydrates, glucose, and fats also play key roles. Fats are essential because they are the building blocks for the cell membranes being formed. Many vitamins and minerals (micronutrients) are important in wound healing and should be part of a comprehensive wound management program (Kaminski & Drinane, 2014).

Circulation and Oxygenation. Circulation to the involved wound and oxygenation of the tissues greatly influence wound healing. Wound healing slows whenever local blood flow is reduced, which is why ulcers secondary to venous insufficiency and pressure ulcers are so difficult to heal. Decreased arterial oxygen tension alters both collagen synthesis and formation of epithelial cells. When hemoglobin levels are reduced by more than 15%, such as in severe anemia, oxygenation is reduced, and tissue repair is altered. Anemia may combine with preexisting states, such as diabetes or arteriosclerosis, to impair oxygenation further and retard wound healing. Elevated blood glucose found in patients with uncontrolled diabetes has been associated with delayed wound closure and increased susceptibility to infection. A comprehensive literature review concluded that patients with diabetes had almost a two-fold increased risk of surgery-related pressure ulcers (Lie, He, & Chen, 2012).

Immune Cellular Function. Drugs and therapies can affect immune cellular function and, subsequently, wound healing. Immunosuppressive drugs, such as corticosteroids, which may be given to prevent rejection of a transplanted organ, also depress the natural defenses against infection and mask the inflammatory response. Immunosuppressive agents also usually suppress protein synthesis, wound contraction, and epithelialization.

Patients with cancer are at risk for delayed wound healing and infection. Some patients have deficient or defective circulating antibodies. Chemotherapy and radiation treatments retard wound repair. Chemotherapeutic agents, such as 5-fluorouracil, inhibit fibroblast replication and collagen synthesis, whereas vincristine suppresses antibody production. Radiation therapy negatively affects fibroblastic activity.

Individual Factors

Age. Changes that are part of the normal aging process can hinder wound healing. Circulation slows slightly, compromising oxygen delivery to the wound. Changes occur in the clotting process, and the inflammatory response and phagocytosis are impaired, increasing the risk of infection. Fibroblastic activity and collagen synthesis decrease with age, so cell growth, differentiation, and reconstruction are slower.

Obesity. Wound healing may be decreased in obese patients. Because adipose tissue is relatively avascular, it provides only a weak defense against microbial invasion and impairs delivery of nutrients to the wound. Obese patients are at increased risk for complications and are often advised to lose weight before elective surgery. In general, surgery on an obese person takes longer, and suturing of adipose tissue can be difficult. The potential for wound dehiscence and infection also is greater in obese patients.

Smoking. Physiologic changes that hinder wound healing occur in smokers. Functional hemoglobin levels decrease, vasoconstriction occurs, and tissue oxygenation is impaired. Long-time smokers have an increased number of platelets, which are also more adhesive. This hypercoagulability leads to the formation of thrombi, which may block small vessels.

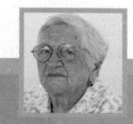

Skin Integrity and Wound Healing PICO

Victoria is the wound nurse consulting on the patient from the chapter-opening scenario. The husband is very concerned that his wife's pressure ulcer is not healing. He asks Victoria if adding nutritional supplements such as protein drinks or vitamin C to her diet will help heal the pressure ulcer. Victoria looks for the latest evidence in the Cochrane Library. She uses the following PICO statement to begin her search: *In bedridden patients, how does using nutritional supplements compare to regular dietary intake affect pressure ulcers?*

P = Bedridden patients
I = Nutritional supplement
C = Regular diet
O = Affect pressure ulcers

Victoria finds a study that examined 23 randomized controlled trials. A meta-analysis was done on eight trials with 6,062 participants to see if pressure ulcer developed when combining nutritional supplements with regular hospital diets. Fourteen trials examined the effects of proteins, zinc, and ascorbic acid on existing pressure ulcers. The review showed no evidence that adding nutritional supplements would be effective in preventing or healing pressure ulcers.

Victoria shares the results with the husband, who is very disappointed. However, Victoria points out that it is important to eat a balanced diet to promote healing, and there are other proven measures to help treat pressure ulcers.

REFERENCE

Langer, G., & Fink, A. (2014). Nutritional interventions for preventing and treating pressure ulcers. *Cochrane Database of Systematic Reviews*, (6). Art. No.: CD003216. doi: 10.1002/14651858.CD003216.pub2.

Medications. Many drugs, in addition to those that directly affect the immune response, affect wound healing. Anticoagulants, given to decrease potential thrombus formation, increase the potential for bleeding into the wound. Even over-the-counter drugs, such as aspirin and nonsteroidal anti-inflammatory drugs, decrease platelet aggregation and prolong bleeding time. Antibiotics may be prescribed preoperatively for certain surgeries that carry a high risk for postoperative infection. The use of anti-inflammatory medications such as prednisone can contribute to delayed wound closure and increased risk for skin injury.

Stress. Physical and emotional stress triggers the release of catecholamines, causing vasoconstriction and ultimately decreasing blood flow to the wound. Trauma, pain, and acute or chronic illness can cause stress.

Local Factors
Nature of the Injury. Usually, a surgical incision made with strict aseptic technique heals faster than, for instance, a deep wound embedded with debris from a traumatic accident. The deeper the wound and the more extensive the tissue loss, the longer the wound will take to heal. Even the wound's shape has an effect: The greater the irregularity, the more prolonged the wound healing process. If trauma or surgery has caused hematomas (blood clots) to form, this also can impede healing.

Infection. Although most open wounds quickly become colonized with diverse microbial flora, healing usually progresses. When sufficient quantities of pathogens are present to produce clinical infection, wound healing is delayed. This is especially true with pressure and leg ulcers. Inadequate handwashing and poor dressing-change techniques may introduce infection. Infection may also result from surgery, especially if a contaminated area, such as the gastrointestinal or genitourinary tract, is the operative site. Infection is more likely to occur in wounds that contain foreign particles or necrotic tissue.

Local Wound Environment. Many factors in the local wound environment affect healing. The pH, which should be between 7.0 and 7.6, can be altered by drainage, which may need to be contained or siphoned away for proper healing.

Bacterial growth must be controlled because infection slows the healing process. The elimination of all microorganisms is neither required nor desirable because normal flora helps to regulate some events that occur in wound healing. Although excess debris and drainage can slow the healing process, a moist surface is essential to the activity of the cells (platelets, leukocytes, fibroblasts, and epithelial cells) that work to heal the wound.

Tension or stress on the wound is a factor in healing. Any activity that puts tension on the wound during healing can cause stress. Vomiting, coughing without splinting, and abdominal distention can place tension on an abdominal incision, potentially interfering with wound healing.

COMPLICATIONS OF WOUND HEALING
Hemorrhage and Interstitial Fluid Loss
After the initial trauma, bleeding is expected, but within several minutes, hemostasis occurs as part of the first phase of wound healing. If large blood vessels are severed or the patient has poor clotting ability, however, bleeding may continue. Hemorrhage can occur later in the postoperative period if a suture slips, a clot dislodges, erosion through a blood vessel occurs, or abnormal stress or trauma is applied to the wounded area.

Hemorrhage may occur internally or externally. External bleeding is obvious: Bloody drainage, more than normally expected, is visible from the wound. Internal bleeding is less observable and may be indicated by swelling of the affected area, an abnormal amount of bloody drainage from a catheter or drain, an increase in pain, or abnormal vital signs.

Electrolyte-rich fluids may be lost in significant amounts in certain types of wounds, such as burns and other large open wounds. Patients with large draining wounds or loss of a large amount of skin require careful monitoring of fluid balance, with appropriate fluid replacement as indicated.

Hematomas
A **hematoma** is a localized collection of blood. It appears as a swelling or mass underneath the skin surface, often with a bluish color. Small hematomas are readily absorbed into the systemic circulation as debris from the wound. Larger hematomas may take weeks to reabsorb, creating dead space and dead cells that inhibit healing. Large hematomas may require evacuation or surgical removal to promote optimal wound healing.

Infection
A break in skin integrity, whether caused by a surgical incision or by trauma, gives microorganisms a portal for entry into the body. Bacterial contamination of a wound can result in infection if the patient's defenses are inadequate. The incidence of wound infection depends on the following:

- *Local factors*: Contamination, degree of closure, and foreign bodies
- *Treatment factors*: Surgical technique and environmental conditions
- *Host factors*: The patient's age, nutritional status, and chronic health problems
- Virulence of the organism

Chapter 31 explores these concepts in more depth.

Symptoms of an infected wound are purulent drainage, an inflamed incisional area, fever, and an elevated leukocyte count. Wound infections greatly increase the cost of medical care and can substantially lengthen recovery time.

Dehiscence
Dehiscence is a total or partial disruption in wound edges (Fig. 30-5). Wound separation, synonymous with dehiscence, is most commonly used to describe surgical incisions in which the skin has separated but underlying subcutaneous tissue has not parted. As wound edges separate, an increase in drainage

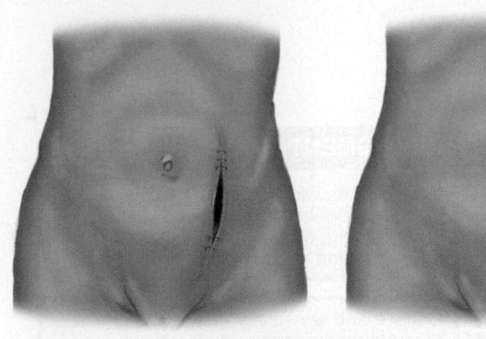

Dehiscence   Evisceration

FIGURE 30-5 *Dehiscence* is the disruption of wound edges. *Evisceration* is the protrusion of viscera through that wound opening.

usually occurs. Dehiscence most commonly occurs before collagen formation is complete in high-risk patients (3 to 14 days after injury). Obesity, poor nutritional status, and increased stress on the incisional area increase the risk of dehiscence. Patients often report feeling that their incision has "given way" after activities, such as coughing or vomiting, that increase the pressure on the incision. Dehiscence also may occur if sutures or staples are removed before the wound is healed adequately. Although not a medical emergency, the physician should be notified and the open areas protected with a saline-moistened dressing until a wound treatment plan based on the wound assessment is developed. Monitor postoperative wounds carefully and prevent undue stress to the wound by supporting the wound during coughing or vomiting.

Evisceration

Evisceration is the protrusion of viscera through an abdominal wound opening (see Fig. 30-5). Evisceration can follow dehiscence if the opening extends deeply enough to allow the abdominal fascia to separate and internal organs to protrude.

> **SAFETY ALERT**
> Evisceration is considered a medical emergency, and the nurse should notify the surgeon and place the patient in a supine position, minimize activity, and cover the exposed tissue and wound with saline-moistened gauze and a cover dressing to secure.

FISTULA

A **fistula** is an abnormal tubelike passageway that forms between two organs or from one organ to outside the body. Fistula tracts can be the result of poor wound healing after tissue injury from surgery. Fistulas also may result from illness, such as inflammatory bowel disease. The name of the fistula designates the site of the abnormal communication. For example, a rectovaginal fistula is an abnormal opening between the rectum and the vagina that permits feces to enter the vagina.

Protection of surrounding skin is essential if the fistula output is caustic. Pouches, drainage tubes, and dressings may be used to manage output until the fistula is closed. Fistulas may be managed conservatively with good nutrition and bowel rest, or they may require surgical closure.

ASSESSMENT

Interviewing the patient allows the nurse to gather data about the patient's normal skin status, history of skin problems, and risk factors that can increase the potential for altered skin integrity or affect wound healing. Assessment also provides detailed information on the development of actual skin or wound problems.

Risk Identification

The interview helps identify patients at risk for problems with skin integrity or delayed wound healing. The interview should include the following elements:

- *Allergy history*: Identify allergen and allergic response.
- *History of past skin conditions*: Describe the problem and past treatment.
- Recent exposure to factors that can cause skin trauma, rash, or lesions.
- Factors that may delay wound healing, such as malnutrition, impaired circulation, immunosuppression, obesity, smoking, diabetes mellitus, or infection.
- Risk for pressure ulcer formation using the Braden or Norton pressure ulcer risk scales (see Box 30-2).

Dysfunction Identification

If any skin problems (rashes, wounds, lesions) are present, obtain additional information about the problem, its duration, what it looked like when it first appeared, if and how it spread, and any associated symptoms. Also, ask whether the patient has used any treatments, including medical advice and therapies, home remedies, and over-the-counter preparations.

If an injury has resulted in a wound, burn, or other problem, evaluate the nature of the events leading to the trauma. If the patient gives vague or suspicious explanations, obtain a follow-up evaluation to determine the possibility of abuse. Note any contamination of the area with dirt or debris, and for all accidental wounds, even minor ones, ask about the status of the patient's tetanus immunization and update it if necessary.

Interview questions also can help assess the impact a skin condition or wound has on activities of daily living. Such conditions can affect self-concept, causing patients to withdraw from social interaction. Watching nonverbal cues helps nurses assess the psychological impact of the skin impairment.

Recall the patient with the stage III pressure ulcer in the case scenario at the beginning of the chapter. Use the concept map (Fig. 30-6) to help understand and manage the patient's situation and to plan for his care.

SKIN INTEGRITY & WOUND HEALING

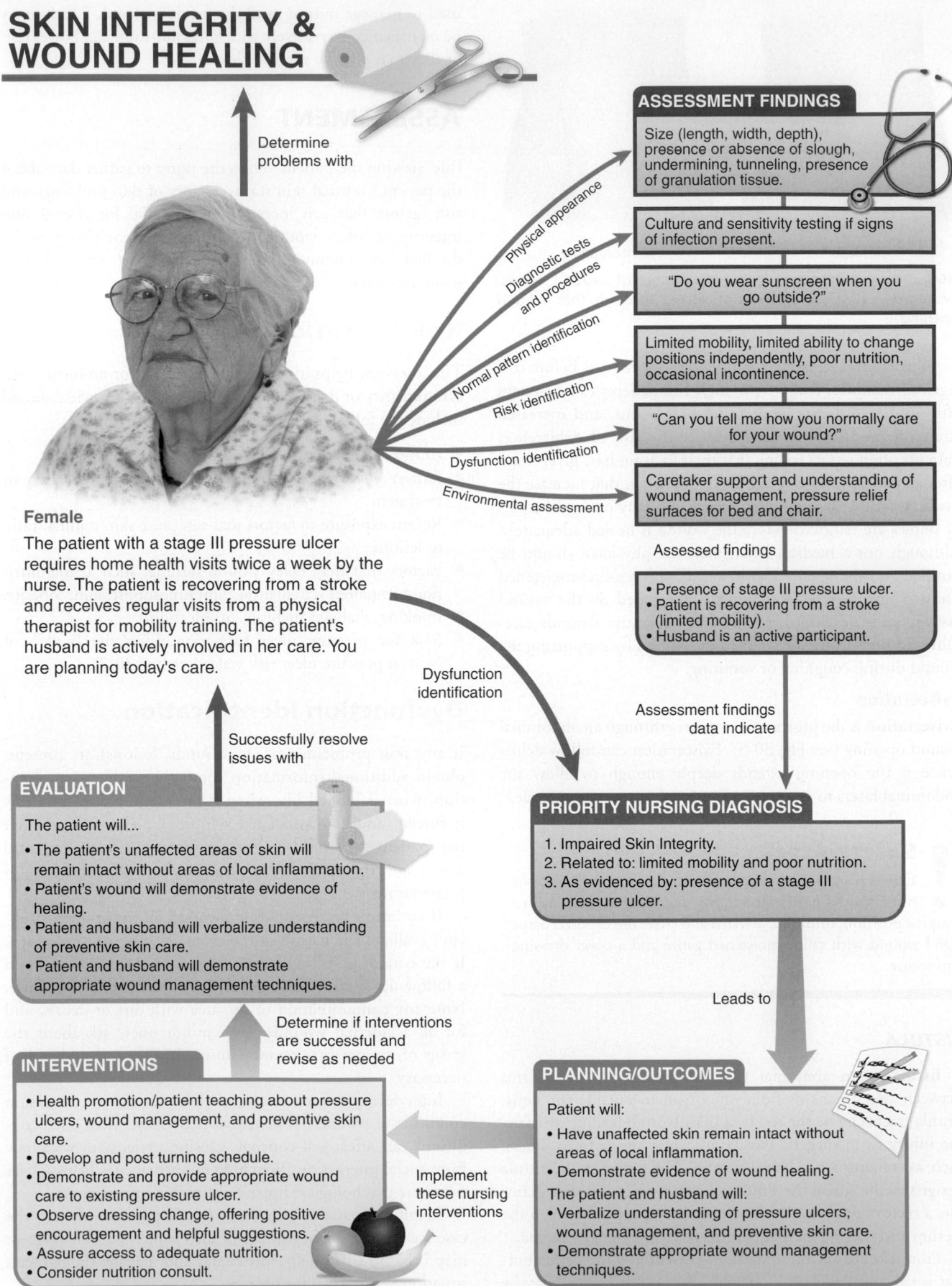

ASSESSMENT FINDINGS

Determine problems with

Physical appearance

Size (length, width, depth), presence or absence of slough, undermining, tunneling, presence of granulation tissue.

Diagnostic tests and procedures

Culture and sensitivity testing if signs of infection present.

Normal pattern identification

"Do you wear sunscreen when you go outside?"

Risk identification

Limited mobility, limited ability to change positions independently, poor nutrition, occasional incontinence.

"Can you tell me how you normally care for your wound?"

Dysfunction identification

Environmental assessment

Caretaker support and understanding of wound management, pressure relief surfaces for bed and chair.

Female

The patient with a stage III pressure ulcer requires home health visits twice a week by the nurse. The patient is recovering from a stroke and receives regular visits from a physical therapist for mobility training. The patient's husband is actively involved in her care. You are planning today's care.

Assessed findings

- Presence of stage III pressure ulcer.
- Patient is recovering from a stroke (limited mobility).
- Husband is an active participant.

Dysfunction identification

Assessment findings data indicate

EVALUATION

Successfully resolve issues with

The patient will...

- The patient's unaffected areas of skin will remain intact without areas of local inflammation.
- Patient's wound will demonstrate evidence of healing.
- Patient and husband will verbalize understanding of preventive skin care.
- Patient and husband will demonstrate appropriate wound management techniques.

PRIORITY NURSING DIAGNOSIS

1. Impaired Skin Integrity.
2. Related to: limited mobility and poor nutrition.
3. As evidenced by: presence of a stage III pressure ulcer.

Leads to

Determine if interventions are successful and revise as needed

INTERVENTIONS

- Health promotion/patient teaching about pressure ulcers, wound management, and preventive skin care.
- Develop and post turning schedule.
- Demonstrate and provide appropriate wound care to existing pressure ulcer.
- Observe dressing change, offering positive encouragement and helpful suggestions.
- Assure access to adequate nutrition.
- Consider nutrition consult.

Implement these nursing interventions

PLANNING/OUTCOMES

Patient will:

- Have unaffected skin remain intact without areas of local inflammation.
- Demonstrate evidence of wound healing.

The patient and husband will:

- Verbalize understanding of pressure ulcers, wound management, and preventive skin care.
- Demonstrate appropriate wound management techniques.

FIGURE 30-6 Concept map for skin integrity and wound healing.

Physical Examination

INSPECTION OF THE SKIN

A general inspection of the skin is followed by a more detailed examination of any abnormalities noted, comparing for symmetry in contralateral areas. Examine for the following:

- Color
- Vascularity
- Turgor
- Texture
- Presence or absence of lesions; note size, shape, pattern of distribution, and color

Skin color varies from one person to another, from one body part to another, and according to race. Some pigment variations are normal. Other changes in skin color may be evidence of systemic disease.

Skin texture refers to the palpable and visible surface structure; the fineness or coarseness of the skin; and whether it is scaly, crusted, or macerated. Skin may appear thick and tough or thin and friable. Note any edema and presence or absence of peripheral pulses when assessing patients with ulcers or wounds of the extremities.

Examine the patient's hair and nails. Inspect the hair for distribution, quantity, and quality. Absence of hair growth on lower extremities can indicate decreased peripheral circulation. Nutritional deficits or impaired circulation may cause thin and brittle nails.

WOUND ASSESSMENT

Inspection permits nurses to evaluate wound healing and to detect possible complications. Clean surgical incisions are usually closed with sutures, staples, or clips so that the skin edges are well approximated to promote healing. Initially, the incision may appear slightly swollen or red due to normal inflammation. Usually within 1 week after surgery, the wound edges heal together and swelling subsides. If staples have been in place for a prolonged period, they may rise and show signs of inflammation where they enter the skin. See Box 30-3 for instructions on how to measure a wound.

> **! SAFETY ALERT**
>
> Use gloves when examining the skin when drainage is present to avoid exposure to infectious agents.

The parameters of a thorough wound assessment should include the following:

- *Wound type*: Surgical versus nonsurgical; acute versus chronic.
- *Wound location*: Use proper anatomic terminology ("trochanter" instead of "hip").
- *Wound size*: Measure the length, width, and depth in centimeters.
- *Wound classification*: Partial versus full thickness; stage only if a pressure ulcer.

BOX 30-3   How to Measure a Wound: Using the Linear Measurement "Clock" Method

Supplies
- Measuring guide in centimeters (cm)
- Cotton tip applicators
- Normal saline
- Gauze
- Gloves

Process
1. Wash your hands and then don gloves. Remove old dressings and cleanse the wound well using normal saline. Pat dry using the gauze.
2. Start by measuring the longest length (up and down) using your measuring guide. Your ruler should be placed over the wound on the longest length using the clock face. The head is always at 12 o'clock and the feet are always at 6 o'clock.
3. Next, measure the greatest width (side to side) using your measuring guide. Place your measuring guide over the widest aspect of the wound and measure.

4. Measure the greatest depth (bottom of the wound) using your cotton tip applicator. Measure the deepest portion of the wound bed. Grasp the swab with your fingers to the level of the skin. Remove the cotton tip applicator and place against the measuring guide: Measure the distance from your fingers on the cotton tip applicator to the end of the swab to determine the depth. If necrotic tissue comes up close to the skin surface, then document "depth unknown."
5. Using a new cotton tip applicator, assess wound bed edges for any undermining (wound not attached to wound bed) or tunneling (channel or pathway that extends from the wound). Follow step 4 instructions on how to measure. Undermining and tunneling findings should be documented using the clock system, for example, tunneling at 2 o'clock measuring 3.4 cm or undermining located from 4 o'clock through 8 o'clock measuring 4.2 cm.

Reminder: Measure a minimum of every 7 days.

Nancy Angulo, RN, BSN, CWOCN. 2014. Cancer Treatment Centers of America.

- *Wound base* (percentage of viable vs. nonviable tissue): Viable, healthy tissue appears pink to red; nonviable or necrotic tissue is white to yellow (slough) or brown to black (eschar).
- *Wound drainage* (color, amount, consistency, and odor):
  - Attempt to quantify the amount of drainage by noting the number of dressings that were saturated and the number of times the dressing required changing. If the dressing is not being changed (as in a fresh postoperative wound), drainage is sometimes circled on the dressing and marked with a date and time.
  - **Serous** drainage is pale yellow, watery, and like the fluid from a blister.
  - **Sanguineous** drainage is bloody, as from an acute laceration.
  - **Serosanguineous** drainage is pale pink-yellow and thin and contains plasma and red cells.
  - **Purulent** drainage contains white cells and microorganisms and occurs when infection is present. It is thick and opaque and can vary from pale yellow to green or tan, depending on the offending organism.
- *Undermining/tunneling*: Assess the wound edges to check for dead space or a sinus tract.
- *Tubes/drains*: Check patency and stabilization.
- *Signs and symptoms of infection*: Local (pain, redness, swelling, **induration** [underlying firmness], or purulent drainage) or systemic symptoms (fever, elevated leukocyte count). (Refer to Chapter 31 for a detailed discussion.)
- *Condition of the surrounding skin*: Palpate to assess for swelling, warmth, tenderness, and induration (firmness). Observe for redness, irritation, or fragility.
- *Pain*: Use an objective pain assessment tool.

Diagnostic Tests and Procedures

Laboratory and diagnostic tests may be performed to confirm the cause of a skin or wound abnormality. Most commonly, culture and sensitivity testing is done to identify infectious organisms that can cause a skin lesion or infect a wound. Refer to Chapter 31 for a detailed description of tests used to diagnose infection. A biopsy may be done to rule out or stage cancer.

NURSING DIAGNOSES

Impaired Skin Integrity, Impaired Tissue Integrity, and Risk for Pressure Ulcer are NANDA-International (Herdman & Kamitsuru, 2014) diagnoses used to identify problems with skin breakdown and healing. Impaired Skin Integrity is used to identify disruption of the skin's surface. Impaired Tissue Integrity is used when the damage involves mucous membrane, cornea, skin, or subcutaneous tissue. Risk for Impaired Skin Integrity, Risk for Trauma, and Risk for Pressure Ulcer are used when the patient's skin is at risk due to extremes in tem-

perature, mechanical trauma, immobility, patient behaviors, or other factors. Table 30-4 outlines these diagnoses with appropriate Nursing Outcomes Classification (NOC) and Nursing Interventions Classification (NIC).

OUTCOME IDENTIFICATION AND PLANNING

Data gathered in the assessment, resulting nursing diagnoses, and outcome identification form the basis for planning nursing interventions to prevent and treat skin integrity problems. Patient-centered goals for skin and tissue integrity involve promoting skin integrity, preventing damage, and promoting optimal healing of damaged tissues:

- The patient's skin will remain intact without areas of local inflammation.
- The patient's wounds will demonstrate evidence of healing.
- The patient will verbalize understanding of preventive skin care.
- The patient or family will demonstrate appropriate wound management techniques.

These goals must reflect the specific and individualized needs of the patient and family.

IMPLEMENTATION

Health Promotion

There are several basic principles of skin care (Box 30-4). One of the most important involves maintaining intact skin because skin is the body's first line of defense against trauma and infection. Measures to prevent irritation or injury are imperative. Avoiding mechanical irritation from rubbing or friction can prevent skin breakdown. Removing tape carefully, judicious use of skin sealants, and patting skin dry prevent traumatization of delicate skin. To minimize chemical irritation, use mild soap, plain water, or products that contain emollients. Patients who are very young, old, emaciated, or obese may have particularly sensitive skin that is more prone to chemical irritation and dryness.

Maintaining adequate hydration of the skin also contributes to healthy function. Because very dry skin is susceptible to breakdown, avoid using drying agents, such as alcohol, and instead use lotions or creams. Patients with dry skin should bathe only once or twice a week. However, exposure to excessive moisture for prolonged periods can lead to bacterial growth and irritation. Patients who are incontinent of urine or stool or who perspire excessively need prompt, thorough, and frequent cleansing and adequate drying of skin, followed by application of a skin barrier product. Many pH-balanced no-rinse cleansing agents are available for frequent perineal cleans-

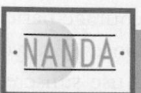

Table 30-4 SELECTED NANDA-I NURSING DIAGNOSES INVOLVING SKIN INTEGRITY

Nursing Dx	Related Factors	Dx Statement	NOC*	NIC†
Risk for Impaired Skin Integrity—at risk for alterations in epidermis and/or dermis	*External:* Chemicals, hyperthermia, hypothermia, shearing force, pressure, secretions, moisture *Internal:* Impaired circulation, imbalanced nutrition, impaired sensation, medications	Risk for Impaired Skin Integrity R/T immobility, poor nutrition, age, and incontinence	Tissue Integrity: Skin & Mucous Membranes, Body Positioning: Self-Initiated, Nutritional Status: Nutrient Intake, Urinary Continence	Skin Surveillance, Pressure Ulcer Prevention, Positioning, Pressure Management, Skin Care: Topical Treatments
Impaired Skin Integrity—altered epidermis and/or dermis	*External:* Chemicals, hyperthermia, hypothermia, shearing force, pressure, secretions, moisture *Internal:* Impaired circulation, imbalanced nutrition, impaired sensation, medications	Impaired Skin Integrity R/T immobility, poor nutrition, age, and incontinence AEB a 3-cm × 4-cm stage II sacral pressure ulcer	Tissue Integrity: Skin & Mucous Membranes, Body Positioning: Self-Initiated, Nutritional Status: Nutrient Intake, Urinary Continence	Pressure Ulcer Care, Wound Care, Skin Care: Topical Treatments, Infection Control, Skin Surveillance, Pressure Ulcer Prevention, Positioning, Pressure Management
Impaired Tissue Integrity—damage to mucous membrane, corneal, integumentary, muscle, tendon, bone, cartilage, or ligament.	Altered circulation, chemical irritants, fluid imbalance, impaired physical mobility, pressure, shear, friction, temperature extremes, radiation, nutritional deficits	Impaired Tissue Integrity R/T infected surgical wound, diabetes, steroids, poor nutrition AEB large abdominal dehiscence	Wound Healing: Secondary Intention, Tissue Integrity: Skin & Mucous Membranes, Nutritional Status: Nutrient Intake, Infection Severity	Wound Care, wound drainage: closed system, Medication Management
Risk for Pressure Ulcer	Adult Braden score <18 (child <16), altered cognition or sensation, decreased mobility, pressure over bony prominence, decrease tissue oxygenation or perfusion, incontinence, inadequate nutrition	Risk for Pressure Ulcer R/T Braden score 13, immobility, inadequate nutrition	Tissue Integrity: Skin & Mucous Membranes, Body Positioning: Self-Initiated, Nutritional Status: Nutrient Intake, Urinary Continence	Skin Surveillance, Pressure Ulcer Prevention, Positioning, Pressure Management, Skin Care: Topical Treatments

Dx, diagnosis; R/T, related to; AEB, as evidenced by.

From: Moorhead, S., Johnson, M., Maas, M., & Swanson, E. (2013). *Iowa outcomes project: Nursing outcomes classification (NOC)* (5th ed.). St. Louis, MO: C.V. Mosby.

†*From:* Bulecheck, G., Butcher, H., Dochterman, J., & Wagner, C. (2013). *Iowa Intervention Project: Nursing Interventions Classification (NIC)* (6th ed.). St. Louis, MO: C.V. Mosby.

From: Herdman & Kamitsuru, S. (Ed.). (2014). *NANDA International. Nursing diagnoses: Definitions and classifications 2015–2017.* West Sussex, UK: Wiley-Blackwell.

BOX 30-4 Principles of Skin Care

- Intact skin is the body's first line of defense against trauma and infection.
- Breakdown of the skin's integrity must be prevented.
- Skin must be adequately hydrated.
- The body's cells must be adequately nourished.
- Adequate circulation is needed to maintain cells.
- Skin hygiene is necessary.
- Skin sensitivity varies among people and according to their health status.

ing. Repeated use of soap that has an alkaline pH decreases the skin's acidity and its protective function.

Areas where skin lies in folds, such as under the breasts and in the groin and gluteal areas, can collect moisture and require special attention. A gauze pad or light absorbent cloth or towel may help prevent moisture buildup in skin folds. A silver-impregnated textile may be prescribed for treatment of fungal or yeast infections in skin folds.

Adequate nutrition is essential for normal skin integrity. Adequately nourished cells are better able to resist injury and disease. A diet with appropriate vitamins, minerals, and protein is essential. A patient who has poor absorption of nutrients, excessive losses of protein, or inadequate food and fluid intake may need additional nutritional support (e.g., high-protein enteral or parenteral supplements) to prevent skin breakdown and to promote healing.

Adequate circulation also is needed to maintain cell life. Inadequate blood flow to the skin results in ischemia and tissue breakdown. Exercising adequately and avoiding constrictive clothing can help ensure optimal blood flow. Frequent turning and repositioning also can prevent localized obstruction of blood flow caused by increased pressure.

Patient Teaching

HYGIENE

Hygiene is important in maintaining skin integrity. The frequency of cleaning and choice of cleaning product can have an effect on pH, resident flora, and hydration of the skin. Because patients with impaired sensation from neuropathies or paralysis are less able to sense injury to the skin, teach them to inspect skin surfaces (especially the feet) routinely for signs of breakdown.

 APPLY YOUR CRITICAL THINKING

Gwen Nelson, 66 years old, is in the clinic for a follow-up visit related to her diabetes mellitus. While she is there, she mentions to you that she has a discolored spot on her foot. She thought she would just soak it and use an emery board to remove it. She stated that it didn't have any feeling anyway, so removing it in this fashion shouldn't hurt.

What assessment data do you need to collect at this point? Discuss how you will help to maintain skin integrity for this patient.

Check your answer in Appendix B.

Instruct patients to avoid going without shoes or wearing ill-fitting shoes, and advise them to check frequently for irritation and blisters when they are wearing new shoes. Encourage patients to turn down the temperature of water heaters to avoid accidental burns to children and individuals with impaired temperature discrimination.

Hygiene teaching for the parents of newborns should include how to prevent skin trauma. Reassure parents about normal skin changes or congenital skin lesions.

Education about trauma prevention is important. See Chapter 23 for more information on safety.

PROTECTION FROM THE SUN

All patients should learn the importance of limiting exposure to ultraviolet radiation (sunlight and artificial tanning lights). The use of clothing, wide-brimmed hats, and sunglasses to protect frequently exposed areas is most practical. Discourage patients from using tanning machines for cosmetic purposes. Everyone except infants younger than 6 months should use sunscreen, which protects against both UVA and UVB radiation, with a minimum sun protection factor of 30 or higher daily.

PRESSURE ULCER PREVENTION

A pressure ulcer is a localized injury to the skin and/or underlying tissue and usually occurs over a bony prominence as a result of pressure or pressure in combination with shear (EPUAP & NPUAP, 2009). Most, but not all, pressure ulcers are avoidable (Edsberg, Langemo, Baharestani, Posthauer, & Goldberg, 2014). Many stage I ulcers resolve with pressure reduction interventions. Prevention is less costly than treatment, and ulcers can be prevented through patient assessment, the use of risk factor predictors, and nursing interventions aimed at compensating for those identified risk factors. Once a patient is determined to be at risk for a pressure ulcer, nursing measures to manage and reduce those risk factors must be implemented (Box 30-5).

Support Surfaces for Pressure Management

One aspect of pressure ulcer prevention is the use of pressure redistribution support surfaces—products that distribute load over the contact areas of the patient's body throughout the support surface of the bed or chair. Various beds, mattresses, and cushions are available. The primary goal for any of these products is to prevent and/or manage pressure-related skin breakdown. Choosing a particular support surface for a patient requires consideration of product efficacy, desired effect, anticipated duration of treatment, patient preferences, cost, upkeep, and impact on patient mobility.

The support surfaces used for pressure ulcer prevention and care can be broadly categorized as nonpowered or powered (connected to an external power source) and reactive or active. Self-adjusting foam mattresses, overlay mattresses, mattress replacement systems, and specialty integrated bed systems with bed frame and support surface combined into a single unit are among the options. Bariatric beds provide a sleep surface for patients who weigh more than 300 to 400 lb. The bed frames are available with a nonpowered pressure redistribution surface or with more specialized powered pressure redistribution properties.

Given the various available support surfaces, deciding which product will best meet the needs of individual patients can be complex. Most acute care facilities have a nonpowered pressure redistribution mattress on hospital bed frames. However, to standardize the selection of more specialized support surfaces for high-risk patients, many facilities create algorithms to guide selection of rental support surfaces. Algorithms are typically designed to guide pressure ulcer prevention strategies of moisture and/or impaired mobility management. When a powered pressure redistribution surface is in use, it is important for the nurse to determine that the support system is functioning properly.

BOX 30-5   Pressure Ulcer Prediction and Prevention

Risk Prediction
- Identify patients at risk and the specific factors placing them at risk.

Skin Care
- Maintain and improve tissue tolerance to pressure to prevent injury. Inspect pressure points at least once a day; document all findings.
- Cleanse skin regularly and whenever soiled, using a mild cleansing agent and warm, not hot, water.
- Minimize factors that dry the skin. Treat dry skin with moisturizers.
- Do not massage bony prominences.
- Minimize exposure of skin to incontinence, perspiration, or wound drainage.
- Protect skin from friction and shear.
- Provide adequate calories and nutrients.
- Maintain or improve mobility, activity level, and range of motion.

Pressure Reduction for At-Risk Patients
- Reposition every 2 hours. Use a 30-degree sidelying position when the patient is lateral to avoid excessive pressure on the trochanter.
- Use pillows to keep bony prominences from rubbing against each other.
- Keep heels from pressing on the bed if the patient is completely immobile.
- When the patient is on his or her side, avoid positioning directly on the trochanter.
- Limit the time the head of the bed is elevated.
- Lift, do not drag, patients to move them up in bed. Use ceiling lifts if available.
- Place patients on a pressure redistribution mattress when in bed (may or may not be a powered surface).
- Avoid prolonged sitting. Reposition or shift the patient's weight every hour.
- For chairbound patients, place a pressure redistribution device on the chair that maintains good postural alignment, balance, and stability.
- Use a written plan regarding the use of positioning devices and repositioning schedules.

Education
- Provide structured education about pressure ulcer prevention to healthcare providers, patients, and family or caregivers.

Nonpowered Mattresses. Healthcare facilities usually purchase mattresses with some level of pressure redistribution technology as the "standard" facility mattress. Various manufacturers offer a foam mattress that allows air to adjust within the mattress via a system of valves or other technology in reaction to a specific applied load (the patient's body). The weight of the patient's body is distributed over more of the mattress surface, thereby minimizing pressure on a single body part. The pressure redistributes whenever the patient shifts weight or changes position. Mattress covers are made from durable fabric that is easy to clean and disinfect and is semipermeable or "breathable" to better manage body heat and moisture.

Mattress Overlays. An overlay is an additional support surface that is placed directly on top of an existing bed mattress. Overlays can be made of viscoelastic foam (memory foam) or filled with air, gel, or water. Foam and gel overlays are usually nonpowered and reactive mattresses. Air-filled overlays, the most common type of specialty surface, are usually powered (connected to an external power source). They are also considered active support surfaces (i.e., able to change load distribution properties with or without a patient on the support surface—as long as the surface is powered "on"). The pressure redistribution occurs via cyclic changes in loading and unloading or "alternating pressure" throughout the support surface (NPUAP, 2007b). These surfaces also usually include a low air loss feature—a series of very small holes in the mattress surface—that provides a flow of air to assist in managing body heat and moisture (microclimate). An overlay mattress adds height to the overall mattress on the bed frame, thereby decreasing effective side rail height. Avoid using an overlay mattress for a confused patient related to increased fall risk; choose a mattress replacement system instead for confused or otherwise restless patients.

Replacement Mattresses. Replacement mattresses fit on a standard bed frame after removal of the original mattress. Replacement mattresses are usually powered, alternating pressure, low air loss support surfaces. These types of powered support surfaces are active—providing pressure redistribution as long as the power source is on.

Specialty Beds
Specialty beds include integrated bed systems using air-fluidized or fluid immersion therapy. An integrated bed system is one where the bed frame and support surface are combined into a single unit; the support surface cannot function separately. Air-fluidized support surfaces use a high flow rate of air or air in combination with fine particles of silicone microspheres within a protective cover. The resulting support surface behaves like a liquid and feels similar to a waterbed. Shear and friction is virtually eliminated. Air-fluidized therapy is used for complex stage IV pressure ulcers or during the immediate postoperative period for fragile skin flap repairs.

Another type of integrated bed system is a rotational or kinetic bed. These surfaces turn a patient automatically in a side-to-side rotation of 40 degrees or more. Some beds can turn a patient from supine to a prone position. In addition,

JUDGMENT OF THE PATIENT'S SELF-CARE

Jim Neal, a 35-year-old man, is paraplegic as a result of a motorcycle accident 7 years ago. He lives at home, and home care assistants help him sporadically. He is frequently readmitted to acute care for treatment for recurrent pressure ulcers. Healthcare providers have repeatedly advised him about appropriate care for these lesions and the need to relieve pressure on his buttocks regularly. He is now an inpatient, with more problems with his pressure ulcers. You overhear two nurses talking:

"I'm so sick of taking care of this man over and over!"
"I agree. He won't help himself and keeps doing all the wrong things for his pressure ulcers. He should just have to live with the consequences of his choices!"

CRITICAL THINKING CHALLENGE
- Identify your concerns about Mr. Neal and his situation.
- Describe your feelings in light of what you overheard the nurses say. How do their attitudes contribute to your reaction?
- Identify possible approaches to this situation.
- Recognizing the patient's dysfunction, define what you see as your ethically appropriate behavior.

there is a bed that can both rotate side to side and also prone a patient. These specialty beds are most often used for trauma patients and/or patients with severe respiratory symptoms. The side-to-side rotation that occurs with pulmonary rotational bed surfaces is effective in improving respiratory outcomes but is insufficient to prevent pressure ulcers. Proning beds for ARDS (acute respiratory distress syndrome) require protective padding over high-risk body parts—for example, face, chest, and bilateral shins to prevent pressure ulcer development.

Nursing Interventions for Skin Impairment

Multidisciplinary care planning—including nurses, physicians, surgeons, nursing assistants, nutritionist, and physical therapist—may be necessary for patients with skin impairment.

THE WOUND OSTOMY CONTINENCE NURSE

The wound ostomy continence nurse (WOCN)—who specializes in the care of patients with wound, ostomy, or continence disorders—is often consulted for complex wound issues. The WOCN has additional education and training in the treatment for pressure ulcers and other chronic wounds that result from lower extremity arterial disease, venous disease, neuropathic disease, fistulas, and surgical wounds (Wound, Ostomy and Continence Nurses Society, 2010). WOCNs collaborate with other healthcare providers and make recommendations for the prevention of and treatment for wounds. These nurses provide education to patients, family, and nursing staff about prevention measures or techniques to optimize wound healing (Wound, Ostomy and Continence Nurses Society, 2010). WOCNs practice across healthcare settings, including acute care, long-term care, home care, and outpatient clinics; many are independent healthcare providers. WOCNs are a valuable resource for patients, families, nurses, and other healthcare professionals.

Nursing interventions to encourage independence, reinforce patient accomplishments, and teach patients and families to achieve optimal self-care are important. Nurses can help patients with chronic wounds learn ways to minimize factors that impair wound healing. Heat and cold also can be used as therapeutic modalities to promote healing and provide pain relief. Nurses help select topical therapies that will cleanse, debride, and protect the wounded area during healing.

PRURITUS RELIEF

Pruritus often accompanies skin problems. Nursing management aims at relieving the situations that cause pruritus, decreasing the associated discomfort, and preventing additional trauma to the skin.

Excessive drying of the skin often causes pruritus, especially in older patients. Applying lotions and moisturizing creams regularly promotes rehydration of dried areas. Limiting bathing prevents excessive drying of the skin. If patients use soap, instruct them to rinse it thoroughly from the skin.

! SAFETY ALERT
Urge patients to take extra care if they add oil to bathwater because oil makes the bathtub slippery and may cause a fall.

Patients should use warm (not hot) water and should gently pat the skin dry to decrease skin irritation. Explaining the importance of not scratching may increase compliance for adults, but such cautions rarely work for young children. Keeping children's fingernails cut short and having them wear cotton gloves may help to decrease skin trauma. Diversional activities also may help focus a child's attention away from unpleasant sensations.

Cool baths and moist, cool compresses promote vasoconstriction and provide relief. Prescriptive medications may be required. Antihistamines and sedatives, although commonly used, have systemic side effects. Topical medications, such as corticosteroids or antibiotics, can decrease inflammation or treat infection.

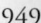

COLLABORATING WITH THE HEALTHCARE TEAM
Consulting with a WOCN

You are a nursing student assigned to care for Mrs. Johnson, a 78-year-old widow who had a stroke 5 days ago. She was found on the floor of her bedroom by her son when he returned from a trip. You provide the following SBAR report to Mrs. Johnson's RN, Emily.

SITUATION: Emily, I am concerned that Mrs. Johnson may be developing pressure ulcers.

BACKGROUND: Mrs. Johnson had a stroke 5 days ago and laid on the floor overnight before she was found by her son. She has right-sided hemiparesis and has been incontinent of urine. When bathing her, I notice a shallow 3-cm area of breakdown on her sacrum and her heels appear bruised and mushy. Her Braden score is 12. When I checked her chart, no abnormal skin assessment was documented.

ASSESSMENT: I am concerned that Mrs. Johnson may have a stage 2 sacral pressure ulcer and a possible deep tissue injury on her heels. Her Braden score indicates she is at high risk for pressure ulcers.

RECOMMENDATION: I think we may want Ken, the WOCN, to assess her and develop a treatment plan. I think it is important to start interventions soon before things get worse.

CRITICAL THINKING CHALLENGE
- Describe Mrs. Johnson's risk factors for pressure ulcers.
- Is it appropriate in the situation to consult the WOCN or should the nurse try to develop a plan independently and see if it works?
- Reflect on the courage it takes as a student to recommend what you think should be done. Remember others may not always agree with your plan but often they provide the rationale for a different plan, which assists your learning.

FIRST AID FOR MINOR WOUNDS

Basic principles in caring for minor wounds include promoting hemostasis, cleansing the wound, and protecting it from additional injury. Initial bleeding may help remove dirt and contaminants from the wound, and prolonged bleeding can be controlled by putting direct pressure on the wound or by elevating the affected part.

Cleansing the wound removes potential sources of infection, such as dirt or cinders. For most minor wounds, running water as an irrigating solution and mild soap as a cleansing agent are recommended. Any patient with a wound that requires more extensive treatment should be referred for immediate care.

After bleeding has subsided and the area has been cleansed, protect the wound with a sterile or clean dressing that promotes the principle of moist wound healing.

Assess the wound closely for potential complications. Signs of infection usually take as long as 24 hours to develop. Exudate, fever, redness, or swelling indicates that the wound needs medical attention. If excessive bleeding occurs, sutures are usually necessary to ensure healing by primary intention.

FIRST AID FOR MINOR BURNS

The type of burn dictates the appropriate first aid measures. In all cases, it is important to halt the burning process, prevent additional damage, and take emergency measures to promote adequate airway, breathing, and circulation. Burn-related complications can develop quickly and warrant medical evaluation in an emergency room or burn/trauma center.

In the case of thermal burns, first remove the heat source. If someone is on fire, the immediate action should be to get the person to stop, drop, and roll. After the heat source has been removed, the burned area should immediately be flushed with copious amounts of cool water. If done quickly, this action halts the burning process by speeding heat dissipation. It also helps to relieve pain. Remove any of the patient's clothing and jewelry in the affected area because clothing and metal can retain heat. If clothing sticks to the burned area, cut around it rather than pulling it, which may traumatize underlying burned tissues. Avoid ointments and home remedies because they can complicate burn healing.

The treatment for chemical burns is similar to that for thermal burns. The first step is to remove the patient's clothing and flush the burned area with water, which dilutes the chemical and halts the burning process. If a large area has been exposed, placing the patient in a shower may be the easiest way to flush the burned area. Brush powdered chemicals off the area before irrigating. Avoid splashing any of the irritant because exposure to even dilute forms of some chemicals can result in burns or irritation of mucous membranes. Some chemicals (e.g., alkali powders) react with water to produce heat, so industrial nurses should be knowledgeable about the chemicals used in their workplaces.

Before an electrical burn can be treated, the victim must be freed from the electrical source. If the person is still in contact with the electrical current, it must be turned off at its source. Removing the victim from the source of current requires special training and equipment. Once the victim has been freed from the current, if the injury site or clothing is smoldering, douse it with water to dissipate the heat. Cardiopulmonary resuscitation may be necessary because ventricular fibrillation or cardiac arrest often occurs with electrical burns.

TREATMENT FOR MOISTURE-ASSOCIATED SKIN DAMAGE

Moisture-associated skin damage (MASD) is inflammation and erosion of the skin caused by prolonged exposure to various sources of moisture, including urine or stool, perspiration, wound exudate, mucus, or saliva (Gray et al., 2011). If it occurs on the buttocks or perineal area, it is often a result of urinary or fecal incontinence–associated dermatitis. The most important factor leading to skin healing in MASD is resolution of the underlying problem. The reasons for incontinence must be investigated and treated. Treatment options for the skin include cleansing the skin of irritants and protecting skin from incontinent urine or stool with protective barrier ointments or skin sealants. Underpads that wick moisture into the pad and away from skin, and urinary or fecal management systems, can also be helpful. Male patients may benefit from external catheters temporarily for urinary incontinence. While the skin is protected, take measures to resolve the underlying cause of the incontinence.

WOUND SUPPORT

Keeping wounds supported and the wound edges close together will foster healing. Steri-Strips, staples, sutures, cyanoacrylate glue, and binders can be used to support a wound.

Steri-Strips

Steri-Strips are commercially prepared adhesive strips that come in various widths and can be applied to wounds to approximate wound edges and promote healing. One edge is placed on the skin and pulled until wound approximation is achieved, and then, the other adhesive side is placed on the skin. On small wounds, Steri-Strips may eliminate the need for sutures. Skin sealant or other barrier film may be applied to the skin before application of Steri-Strips to help them adhere longer.

Sutures, Staples, and Clips

Support is provided in a surgical incision by use of sutures, surgical staples, or surgical clips to hold the incision together until healing occurs. The type of material used for wound closure affects wound healing.

A suture, the material used to sew an incision together, can be absorbable (e.g., catgut, chromic) or nonabsorbable (e.g., nylon, silk, polypropylene). The type of suture used depends on the wound's size and location, how strong the suture material needs to be, the desired cosmetic effect, and the provider's preference. Usually, the least amount and smallest size of suture result in optimal wound closure.

Skin staples are made of stainless steel and are minimally reactive to the body as a foreign substance. Usually, when skin staples are used, absorbable sutures are used to close viscera and underlying tissue layers. Staples decrease the risk of infection and reduce tissue handling because they allow faster wound closure. Larger stainless steel clips also may be used to approximate wound edges.

Inspect sutures, staples, or clips when dressings are changed. The provider determines how long they must remain in place. Sutures are usually removed 7 to 10 days after surgery if wound edges are well approximated and healing appears normal, but larger retention sutures may remain in place longer. Skin staples are usually removed in 5 to 7 days. Sometimes, the provider orders removal of every other staple or suture to ensure that adequate healing has occurred and to avoid dehiscence. Most surgical patients also have absorbable sutures in place holding deeper layers of tissue or fascia together.

Staples are removed with a staple remover (Fig. 30-7); it is inserted under each staple, and the handle is compressed. The pressure causes the staple to bend in the middle, and the edges pop out of the skin. The patient may experience minor discomfort as the staples are removed. Steri-Strips are usually

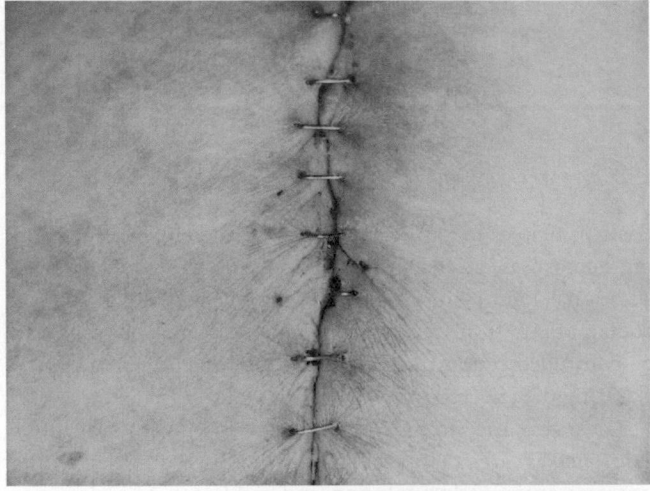

A

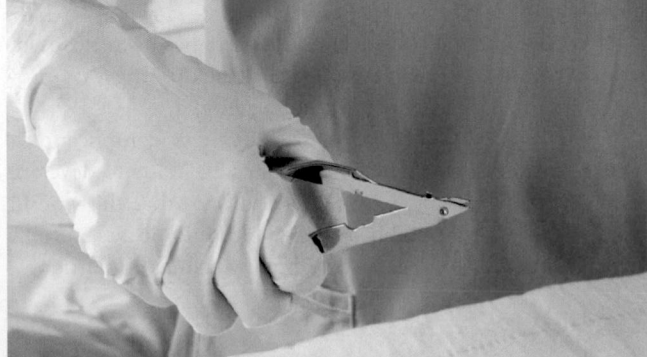

B

FIGURE 30-7 A. Skin staples. **B.** Staple remover.

applied after the staples are removed to keep skin edges approximated until healing is more complete.

Sutures are removed with forceps and scissors. The suture is cut close to the skin, and the forceps is used to remove the suture. Care is essential to avoid pulling the visible portion of the suture through underlying tissue because this can contaminate the incisional area and contribute to an infection. Sutures may be intermittent or continuous, and the nurse must discern the suturing technique before removing the sutures. As with staples, Steri-Strips are often applied after suture removal.

Cyanoacrylate Glue

An adhesive glue for human skin is available and may be used to close acute wounds in certain situations. The wound must be easily approximated and on a part of the body that will not be subject to tension or stretching. Keep the wound dry; do not apply any ointments over the wound until the wound has completely healed. The adhesive material gradually sloughs away over a period of days and must be protected from scratching or rubbing during the first several days after application.

Ace Wraps, Bandages, and Stretch Netting

Ace wraps are elastic stretch bandages used to provide light compression to an area or to secure dressings (Fig. 30-8). An Ace bandage should be applied in a distal to proximal direction when used on an extremity. Pressure should be snugger at the distal end to promote venous return. However, incorrectly applied, Ace wraps can result in impaired circulation, edema, and tissue injury. Gauze bandage rolls are also used to secure dressings, especially extremities. A gauze bandage roll does not apply compression. Tubular stretch netting is frequently used to secure dressings. It is easy to apply (slide over the dressing) and comes in multiple sizes for correct fit. Many bandages are routinely removed so that the area can be inspected and areas of pressure avoided.

> ## ❗ SAFETY ALERT
>
> Frequent assessment of body parts distal from the bandage site (e.g., fingers, toes) is necessary to detect impaired circulation promptly (see Fig. 30-9). Cyanosis, pallor, coolness, numbness, tingling, swelling, and absent or diminished pulse are signs that circulation may be decreased or that nerve function is impaired.

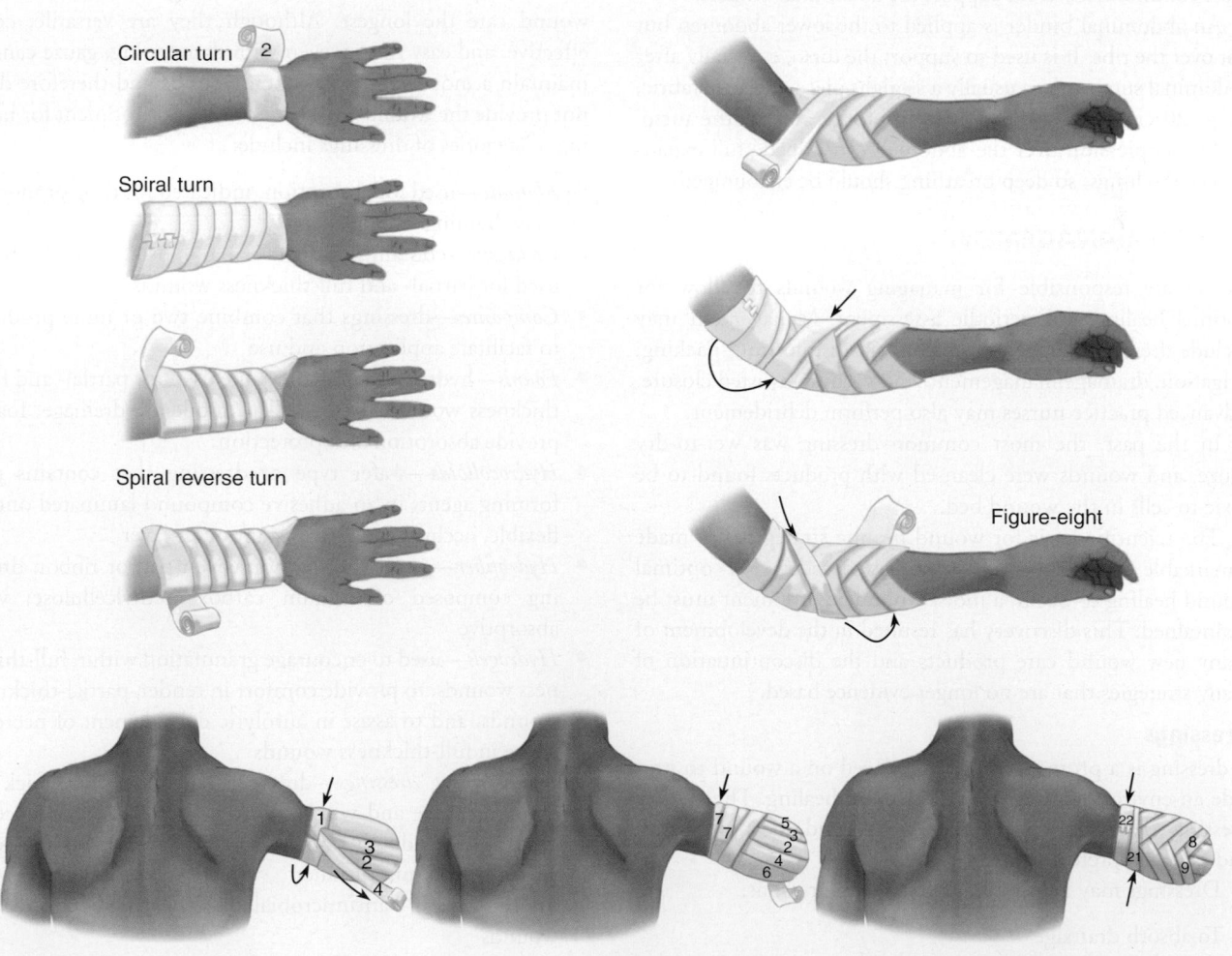

Circular turn

Spiral turn

Spiral reverse turn

Figure-eight

Recurrent-stump bandage

FIGURE 30-8 Techniques for bandage application.

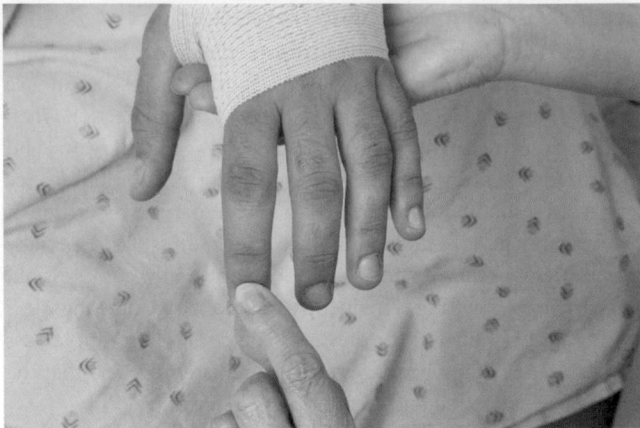

FIGURE 30-9 Assessing the body part distal to the bandage site for evidence of impaired circulation.

Binders

Binders are used to support a specific body part or to hold dressings in place. The use of Velcro in binders has increased their ease of application and comfort. Velcro fasteners permit individualized adjustments and securely fasten the binder in place while permitting quick and easy release. Binders come in different shapes and sizes depending on the area for use. The binders most commonly used for support are abdominal binders.

An abdominal binder is applied to the lower abdomen but not over the ribs. It is used to support the torso, especially after abdominal surgery. It is usually a straight piece of elastic fabric, 15 to 20 cm wide and long enough to go around the torso. Tight compression over the abdomen can impede full expansion of the lungs, so deep breathing should be encouraged.

WOUND MANAGEMENT

Nurses are responsible for managing wounds to allow for optimal healing and periodic assessment. Management may include dressing changes, cleansing and disinfection, packing, irrigation, drainage management, and vacuum-assisted closure. Advanced practice nurses may also perform debridement.

In the past, the most common dressing was wet-to-dry gauze, and wounds were cleansed with products found to be toxic to cells in the wound bed.

The scientific basis for wound healing strategies has made remarkable advances in the last few decades. For optimal wound healing to occur, a moist wound environment must be maintained. This discovery has resulted in the development of many new wound care products and the discontinuation of many strategies that are no longer evidence based.

Dressings

A dressing is a protective covering placed on a wound to provide an environment to promote wound healing. The type of dressing used depends on the type of wound, location, status, and personal preference.

Dressings may be used for the following reasons:

- To absorb drainage
- To prevent contamination
- To prevent mechanical injury to the wound
- To help maintain pressure so that excessive bleeding is avoided
- To provide a moist wound environment
- To provide comfort for the patient

Today, as the nurse participates in selection of the appropriate dressing, that selection must be based on an assessment of the wound and the principles of moist wound healing. If the wound bed is dry, the nurse will select products to add moisture to the wound bed. If the wound has copious exudates, the nurse will select a product to absorb the drainage without drying out the wound bed. Other factors affecting dressing selection are related to necrotic tissue, infection, tunneling, undermining, and location. The nurse must be aware that as the wound heals (or deteriorates), the appearance of the wound bed will likely change. Either an alternate type of dressing or the frequency of dressing changes may be indicated. The nurse continuously re-evaluates the wound for appropriate dressing type and frequency of dressing changes.

Types of Dressings

More than 2,000 products are available for the care of skin and wounds. These dressings can be broadly grouped into categories based on their characteristics and indications (Table 30-5). Of all the products listed, gauze dressings have been used in wound care the longest. Although they are versatile, cost-effective, and easy to use, even with dampening, gauze cannot maintain a moist surface on open wounds and therefore does not provide the wound with the optimal environment for healing. Categories of dressings include:

- *Alginate*—used for absorption; indicated for deep or moderately draining wounds
- *Collagens*—contain collagen, a major protein in the body used for partial- and full-thickness wounds
- *Composites*—dressings that combine two or more products to facilitate application and use
- *Foams*—hydrophilic polyurethane used for partial- and full-thickness wounds with small to moderate drainage; foams provide absorption and protection.
- *Hydrocolloids*—wafer type of dressing that contains gel-forming agents in an adhesive compound laminated onto a flexible, occlusive water-resistant outer layer
- *Hydrofiber*—a soft, sterile, nonwoven pad or ribbon dressing composed of sodium carboxymethylcellulose; very absorptive
- *Hydrogels*—used to encourage granulation within full-thickness wounds, to provide comfort in tender, partial-thickness wounds, and to assist in autolytic debridement of necrotic tissue in full-thickness wounds
- *Nonadherent dressings*—dressings that will not stick to wound surface and will minimize disruption of new cells; examples include silicone dressings or dressing impregnated with a petrolatum product.
- *Silver dressings*—antimicrobial dressings used for infected wounds
- *Transparent films*—adhesive semipermeable film dressings

TABLE 30-5 TYPES OF DRESSINGS, CHARACTERISTICS, AND INDICATIONS

Category	Characteristics	Indications
Alginate dressings	• Highly absorbent product designed to be placed inside the wound • Forms a gel as it absorbs wound exudate • Require a cover dressing • Available in sheet form or as packing strips	• Moderately draining wounds • Nontunneling wounds only
Gauzes	• Woven cotton material available in many sizes and thicknesses • Nonocclusive, allowing environmental oxygen to reach the wound surface • Absorbent • May be moistened with sterile saline to create a moist packing	• Newly created surgical incisions or wounds requiring pressure for hemostasis • Packing or filling of deep wounds
Hydrocolloid wafer dressing	• Adhesive-backed pad, often tan in color, made of hydroactive materials • Pad absorbs excess exudate into its matrix, maintaining a moist wound surface. • Most are occlusive, keeping environmental oxygen from reaching the wound. • Mild to moderate absorptive properties	• Partial-thickness wounds • Shallow full-thickness wounds • Minor autolytic debridement • Noninfected wounds only
Hydrogel	• Hydrophilic polymer product with a high percentage of water within the matrix • Available in transparent sheetlike wafer or as tube gel • Rehydrate a dry wound bed and maintain a moist wound environment • Mild absorption of drainage sheetlike wafer provides cooling sensation on the skin and reduces wound pain.	• Partial-thickness wound • Pressure ulcers, stages II–IV (with a cover dressing, such as gauze) • Minor autolytic debridement • Minor burns • Skin graft donor sites
Polyurethane foam	• Pads of compressed foam (vary in thickness according to brand; sometimes have an adhesive backing) • Moderate absorptive capacity, depending on thickness • Provide a moist wound surface	• Partial-thickness wounds • Shallow full-thickness wounds • Absorbent covering for deep wounds that have been packed or filled with a primary dressing
Transparent adhesive dressings	• Clear, polyurethane film with adhesive backing • Different brands allow varying levels of moisture vapor to evaporate through the dressing. • Maintain a moist wound surface • Multiple sizes and shapes • No absorptive properties	• May be used instead of tape over intact skin to secure a gauze pad or other type of absorbent dressing in place (e.g., intravenous sites)
Silver	• Contain ionic silver—either immediate or controlled release of silver into wound bed	• Infected or highly colonized wounds • Slow-release silver dressings may stay in place up to 7 d.
Hydrofiber dressings	• Consists of sodium carboxymethylcellulose fibers • Forms a gel as it absorbs wound exudates	• Moderately to heavily draining wounds • Available in sheets, ribbons, or composite dressing • Needs less frequent dressing changes r/t highly absorptive capacity while maintaining a moist wound bed

Advanced Wound Care Products

As our knowledge of microbiology of wound healing continues to grow, so does the number of new products available, including products derived from tissue-engineered skin, growth factors, extracellular matrix dressings, and porcine small intestinal submucosa.

Methods of Securing Dressings

"A medical adhesive is a product used to approximate wound edges or to affix an external device (i.e., tape, dressing, catheter, electrode, pouch, or patch) to the skin" (McNichol, Lund, Rosen & Gray, 2013). Tape is the most commonly used medical adhesive to secure dressings over wounds. However, many dressings are also packaged with the medical adhesive as an integral component of the outer layer of the dressing. **MARSI (Medical Adhesive-Related Skin Injury)** is now being recognized as a prevalent complication in healthcare settings. A consensus panel identified seven types of MARSI.

Prevention of MARSI is a basic nursing skill. Careful selection of tape and other medical adhesive products, along with proper application and removal, is key. See Box 30-6 for consensus panel recommendations for application and removal procedures.

Dressing Changes

The frequency of dressing changes is determined by wound status, type of dressing, amount of drainage, and frequency of wound assessment required. Sometimes, the provider orders the type of dressing and the frequency of dressing changes; other times, the nurse determines what type of dressing will best promote healing. Procedures for changing a dry sterile dressing and applying a saline-moistened dressing are given in **Procedures 30-1** and **30-2**, respectively.

Packing or Filling

Gauze or a hydrofiber dressing product placed into an open wound bed can prevent the wound surface from closing prematurely. A hydrofiber or nonadherent contact layer dressing is placed directly over the wound bed. Then, a gauze dressing is fluffed and shaped to fill in the contours of a wound bed so that dressing product is touching all surfaces of the wound bed. As the wound heals from the base to the surface, less dressing material will be needed to fill the wound bed.

Tunneling is a narrow passageway in the soft tissue of an open wound. Tunneling can extend in any direction from the wound bed or opening, and there may be more than one tunnel within a wound bed. In wounds with tunneling, filling the tunnel and wound bed with ¼ inch– or ½ inch–wide hydrofiber or gauze ribbon allows for healing from the base of the wound to the surface, helping to prevent abscess formation.

Undermining is an area of tissue destruction under the edge of the wound opening. Undermining is usually measured in centimeters and described in reference to the hours on a clock face, with the 12 o'clock position of the wound aligning with head of the patient. Filling the entire wound bed, including the undermined portions, also allows for healing from the base of the wound to the surface, helping to prevent abscess formation. Undermining may be present under the entire edge of the wound or only in specific sections of the wound edges. Gauze, or absorptive products such as calcium alginates, can be used to fill an undermined wound.

Packing also may be used after surgery on body areas that are hard to suture (e.g., vagina, nasal septum) to apply pressure and prevent blood loss from small capillaries. When packing has been inserted during surgery, it should be noted on the

---

BOX 30-6 | **Safe Application and Removal of Adhesive Products**

Application

- Clean periwound (around the wound) skin and allow to dry.
- Clip hair if necessary.
- Apply an alcohol-free skin barrier film to protect periwound skin.
- Allow the skin barrier film to dry.
- Then, apply the tape without tension, pulling, or stretching.
- Smooth the tape into place with firm, gentle pressure. Take care to avoid gaps and wrinkles.
- When securing a compression dressing, stretch the tape over the dressing only and then press remaining tape onto skin without tension.

Removal

- Use the fingers of one hand to push the skin down and away from the tape.
- Then, remove the tape low and slow back over itself in the direction of hair growth, keeping it horizontal and close to the skin surface.
- As the tape is removed, continue using the fingers of one hand as necessary to support newly exposed skin.
- Transparent film dressings may also be removed by loosening a corner of the dressing and stretching it horizontally in the direction opposite the wound (stretch and relax technique). Use one hand to stabilize the skin still adhered to the film dressing. Continue this method until dressing is completely removed.
- Use medical adhesive remover to loosen tightly adhered tape when above methods are not successful.
- Lotion, petrolatum, or mineral oil may be used to loosen tape if not reapplying another adhesive product to the same area.

Adapted with permission from McNichol et al. (2013, p. 372).

patient's record so that the packing is not accidentally removed when the dressing is changed. Pressure packing usually remains in place for 2 or 3 days and is removed by the surgeon or the nurse with a physician's order.

Cleansing and Disinfection

Intact skin is prepared for surgical incisions or invasive procedures by a process called *skin preparation*. Skin preparation often involves the use of antiseptic solutions, such as chlorhexidine, to scrub the skin's surface. Skin preparation decreases the possibility of the introduction of organisms breaking the intact skin barrier and is an appropriate use of disinfectants.

Open wound cleansing is performed to remove debris, contaminants, and excess exudate. The products used for intact skin cleansing and disinfection can be harmful to the cells involved in wound healing. Therefore, cleansers used on open wounds should not contain such agents. Many commercial wound cleansers are available that contain agents such as surfactant, which may facilitate the removal of wound debris. Sterile normal saline (0.9% NaCl) is the cleansing solution of choice for acute or chronic open wounds. **Procedure 30-3** describes how to irrigate a wound.

> ! **SAFETY ALERT**
> Using full-strength hydrogen peroxide, povidone-iodine, or other irritating solutions is caustic and damages new epithelial growth. This interferes with wound healing and is not appropriate for most open wounds.

DRAINAGE MANAGEMENT

A large amount of wound drainage can inhibit wound healing and impair skin integrity around the wound. Drainage devices are placed in the wound when the surgeon anticipates a large amount of fluid accumulation, which could inhibit wound healing. Closed drainage systems consist of a drain attached to a portable or external suction source. Open drainage systems, such as the Penrose drain, drain directly from the wound.

- The *Penrose* drain is a hollow, fat rubber tube placed directly into the incision or into a stab wound in the incisional area. It allows fluid to drain through capillary action into absorbent dressings. Penrose drains may be advanced or shortened to drain different areas.
- A *Hemovac* is placed into a vascular cavity where blood drainage is expected after surgery (Fig. 30-10). Suction is maintained by compressing a springlike device. When inspecting a Hemovac drain, expect bloody drainage and ensure that it remains in the compressed state. Suction can be interrupted if leaks are present in the system or if the Hemovac has filled with drainage.
- The *Jackson-Pratt* drain permits drainage to collect in a bulblike device that can be compressed to create gentle suction (see **Procedure 30-3**). Suction is lost when the bulb is expanded because of too much drainage or a leak in the system.

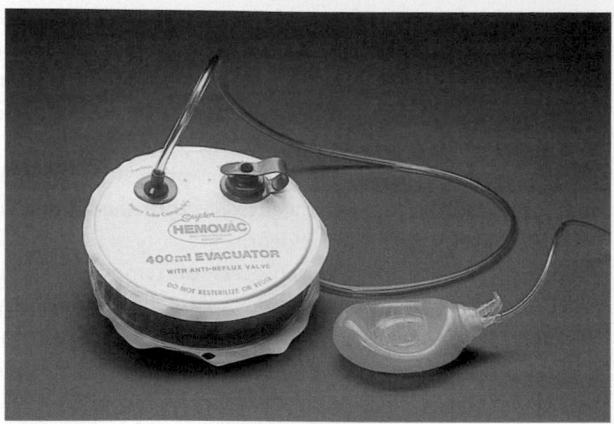

FIGURE 30-10 Closed drainage systems. *Left:* Hemovac. *Right:* Jackson-Pratt.

With any drainage system, inspect the system to ensure that it is patent and functioning. Drains may or may not be sutured in place, so take care not to inadvertently remove them during inspection. Nurses promote optimal wound healing by ensuring that closed drainage systems function properly and by selecting dressings that adequately absorb wound drainage. For large amounts of drainage, the nurse may utilize collection devices, wound drainage management systems, or pouching to contain the drainage and protect the skin. Nurses also protect skin from irritation from caustic drainage or constant moisture by applying a clear skin barrier/protectant to the surrounding or **periwound** skin. Skin barriers also help to prevent MARSI.

Negative-Pressure Wound Therapy

Use of **negative-pressure wound therapy (NPWT)**, sometimes referred to as vacuum-assisted closure, or VAC, has significantly changed the treatment for several types of wounds. NPWT is a method that uses specialized hydrophobic sponge dressings to fill a wound cavity, is covered by a transparent dressing, and then is connected to tubing and a machine that provides negative pressure to the wound. NPWT reduces excess moisture in the wound, reducing the bioburden (the number of microorganisms) and associated toxins. It also increases cell proliferation (including proliferation of granulation tissue) and perfusion in the wound bed. The negative-pressure system speeds tissue healing. NWPT is used on many types of open wounds, such as debrided pressure ulcers or abscesses, dehisced surgical wounds, vascular or diabetic lower extremity wounds, and acute trauma wounds.

When NPWT was first introduced, surgeons and wound care nurses applied and changed these dressings. While wound care specialists are available to provide consultation and assistance, nurses in various healthcare settings independently apply negative-pressure dressings. Refer to **Procedure 30-4** for instructional guidelines.

Debridement

Debridement is the removal of foreign material or dead tissue from a wound to discourage the growth of microorganisms and to promote wound healing. There are four main types of debridement: surgical, enzymatic, autolytic, and mechanical:

- *Surgical debridement* refers to the use of sharp instruments to debride the wound, as done during surgery or at the bedside. Physicians and other providers who specialize in wound care (e.g., WOCNs, nurse practitioners, physical therapists) perform sharp debridement.
- *Enzymatic debridement* refers to the process of placing chemical products (e.g., collagenase) within the wound to help break down the necrotic debris.
- *Autolytic debridement* is the process of removing debris and necrotic tissue using the body's own fluids and cells. Autolytic debridement occurs when an occlusive dressing or a hydrogel is applied over a wound and left in place while wound exudates, containing endogenous enzymes, build up. The wound exudate softens the nonviable tissue, making it easier to remove, and, in some cases, totally dissolves debris so that it can be irrigated from the wound during a subsequent dressing change.
- *Mechanical debridement* removes necrotic tissue using mechanical force. Although mechanical debridement is effective in removing necrotic tissue and debris, it is nonselective and likely will remove healthy granulating tissue as well. The simplest form of mechanical debridement is the wet-to-dry dressing. A wound bed is filled with saline-moistened gauze dressing, allowed to dry over several hours and then removed. Wound debris, including necrotic tissue, is trapped in the gauze dressing and removed along with the dressing. Removal of the dry dressing is often painful for the patient.

SAFETY ALERT

Because a wet-to-dry dressing harms new granulating tissue and is painful, it should never be used for clean granulating wounds (Bryant & Nix, 2012).

LOCAL APPLICATION OF HEAT AND COLD

Therapeutic uses of heat and cold to promote healing and patient comfort are summarized in Table 30-6. Cold therapies are usually used immediately after injury to control hemorrhage, edema, and pain. Cold is used to control local bleeding because it causes vasoconstriction, which decreases blood flow to the area and helps control swelling. Heat therapies are used to increase blood flow, resolve inflammation, improve healing of soft tissues, and relieve muscular pain and stiffness. Local heat causes vasodilation, increasing the supply of oxygen, nutrients, leukocytes, and antibodies to the tissues. The increased blood flow also promotes removal of metabolic wastes and dissipation of heat. Heat allows pus to consolidate in infected areas. Heat also promotes muscular relaxation and relieves muscle tension, spasms, and joint stiffness. A disadvantage of local heat is that increased capillary permeability can increase edema formation. **Procedure 30-5** gives the steps for heat application.

Patient safety is an important consideration when using heat or cold because these therapies can damage tissues or alter thermoregulation. Table 30-7 lists precautions for the safe use of heat and cold.

The duration of application is important. Maximum vasodilation or vasoconstriction usually occurs in 30 minutes, and prolonged application may result in burns or freezing. Very young patients and older patients have a decreased ability to tolerate heat and cold and are more likely to suffer adverse effects. Impairments to circulation, sensation, or cognitive abilities also increase the incidence of injury. Body areas where heat or cold therapy is used can be more or less sensitive, depending on the skin's sensitivity or thickness. Impaired skin integrity increases the chance that heat or cold application could damage tissues. Extensive exposure to heat or cold can have systemic and local effects. Unexpected adverse effects can occur, especially in high-risk patients, such as the very young and the elderly.

TABLE 30-6 USES FOR HEAT AND COLD

Effect	Physiologic Mechanism	Selected Uses
Heat Application		
Promotes healing and suppuration (consolidation of pus)	Results in vasodilation leading to increased blood flow, thus increasing oxygen and nutrients to the area and promoting removal of waste products	Surgical wounds, infected wounds, hemorrhoids, and episiotomies
Decreases inflammation by accelerating inflammatory process	Increases capillary wall permeability, increases leukocyte and antibody flow to area, and promotes action of phagocytes	Phlebitis and intravenous infiltration
Decreases musculoskeletal discomfort	Increases sensory nerve conduction, promotes muscle relaxation, and decreases viscosity of synovial fluid	Low back pain, menstrual cramps, contractures, arthritis, and muscle spasms
Cold Application		
Controls bleeding	Results in vasoconstriction, which decreases blood flow, and, in turn, decreases metabolic tissue demands and the supply of oxygen and nutrients	Fractures, trauma, superficial lacerations, and puncture wounds
Decreases edema	Decreases capillary permeability; causes vasoconstriction	Sprains, muscle strains, and sports injuries
Relieves pain	Decreases nerve conduction velocity; induces numbness or paresthesia	Arthritis, trauma, and musculoskeletal injuries

TABLE 30-7 PRECAUTIONS FOR THE SAFE USE OF HEAT AND COLD

Assessment Factor	Rationale
Acute sudden pain that may indicate abscessed tooth or appendicitis	Application of heat may cause rupture, with systemic spread of infection.
Broken skin or deep open wounds	Subcutaneous and visceral tissues are more sensitive to temperature extremes. Fewer pain and temperature receptors are available to warn of possible tissue damage.
Circulatory impairment (peripheral vascular disease, diabetes)	Cold application vasoconstricts, thus decreasing circulation to the already compromised area. Heat is not dissipated well from the area, making tissue damage more likely.
Sensory deficits (cerebrovascular) accident, paraplegia, and quadriplegia	Alterations in nerve conduction limit the sensation of temperature or pain, thus increasing the likelihood of tissue damage.
Mental status impairment (confusion, decreased level of consciousness)	Decreased reliability of reporting pain and altered sensation increases the possibility of tissue damage.
Age extremes	Very young children have immature thermoregulation, cannot communicate pain or discomfort specifically, and cannot alter their environment. Elderly may have reduced sensation to pain and often have another impairment (e.g., circulatory, sensory) that compounds the risk. Heat should not be applied to the abdomen of a pregnant woman because fetal growth could be affected.
Metallic implants (pacemakers, total joint replacements)	Metal is a good conductor of heat, thus increasing the potential for burns because the implant cannot be readily removed.

! SAFETY ALERT

During heating pad use, inspect the skin frequently, especially for patients with decreased sensation. Thermal burns may result. Never apply heat over a metal implant (joint replacement, pacemaker) because metal retains heat, causing serious thermal injury.

Cold Packs and Ice Bags

Cold packs and ice bags are used to deliver local dry cold. Some commercial cold packs contain a biochemical, non-toxic solution that is released inside the bag when it is squeezed or kneaded, creating a cold temperature. The outer covering is soft and pliable, so it can be molded to fit the body's contours and applied directly to the skin surface. These packs cannot be refrozen and are considered disposable. Reusable gel cold packs are also available; these packs are also flexible and can easily mold to a specific body area. The outer surface can be wiped/disinfected before being refrozen and reused.

Ice bags, which can be manually filled with crushed or cubed ice, come in various sizes and can be used to control localized bleeding, reduce swelling, and reduce pain. Most ice bags used at healthcare facilities come with a cloth or other protective covering attached. When administering cold therapy with children, marking a "face" on the bag may be helpful as a way of decreasing fear.

Cold Compresses

Cold compresses are used to relieve swelling and inflammation. Gauze pads or washcloths are moistened with chilled saline or water and applied to the appropriate area. Because cold compresses quickly warm to the temperature of the patient's skin, they need to be changed frequently.

Hot Packs

Dry local heat can be applied with commercially available packs or electric heating pads. Some commercial hot packs are squeezed or kneaded to activate the heat and then disposed of when cool. Some gel packs can be placed in a microwave to warm (follow manufacturer's instructions for timing). Some gel pads can be used for both heating and cooling—placed in a microwave for warming, a freezer for cooling. Local heat treatments are usually applied for 15 to 20 minutes at a time and may need a covering, such as a pillowcase, before application to the body. Use caution with local heat application to avoid burns.

Warm Compresses

Warm compresses may be applied to improve circulation and to promote suppuration. If commercially prepared compresses are unavailable, water can be warmed and applied to gauze pads or washcloths. Avoid using temperatures that might cause burns. The heat of a warm compress dissipates quickly. If a constant warm temperature is desired, apply a heating mechanism over the compress (e.g., an aquathermia pad). However, because moisture conducts heat, the temperature of the heating mechanism must be set at low.

Warm Soaks

Warm soaks involve immersing a body part in a warm liquid (usually water) to promote relaxation or improve circulation. They also can be used to apply a medicated solution. Warm soaks usually take about 20 minutes, and the solution may need to be changed because cooling commonly occurs.

Sitz Baths

A sitz bath provides moist heat to the pelvic and perineal areas. A sitz bath is used after rectal or perineal surgery or after vaginal delivery to decrease inflammation and discomfort. The patient sits in a special tub or in a basin that fits onto the toilet seat so that the legs and feet remain out of the water (See Fig. 24-5). Using a bathtub does not serve the same purpose because immersing the entire body in warm water nullifies the effect of local heat applied to the pelvic area. The patient's feet and upper torso should remain covered to prevent chilling. The sitz bath is filled with warm water (105°F to 110°F [40°C to 43°C]). A vinyl bag with attached tubing is filled with warm water and inserted into the portable sitz bath, where it slowly replenishes warm water during the procedure. Sitz baths usually last for about 20 minutes. Because heat is being applied to a large area, vasodilation can occur, causing the patient to feel light-headed and faint. If this occurs, assess the patient for a rapid pulse, pale facial color, or complaints of nausea. If these signs and symptoms are present, discontinue the sitz bath.

Aquathermia Pads

An aquathermia pad is a heating unit consisting of a waterproof pad through which water circulates. It is used to provide direct or indirect heat, treat muscle spasms, and reduce inflammation. The aquathermia pad is sometimes applied over a warm compress to apply continuous moist heat.

Home and Community Care

Skin disorders and wounds require regular care and assessment for complications. Some patients obtain their care at home or in outpatient wound care clinics, whereas others require hospitalization. Regardless of where the care is provided, the following principles apply:

- The environment should be clean.
- Wound care supplies must be accessible and available.
- The patient should receive adequate calories and nutrients to facilitate healing.
- The person providing wound or skin care should demonstrate the ability to perform the procedures and should know what symptoms to report to the healthcare provider.
- Provide information about methods to prevent pressure ulcers (frequent turning and proper positioning, hygiene, nutrition, and the use of pressure redistribution support surfaces) as indicated.
- Describe the topical wound care products and demonstrate the correct method of use.

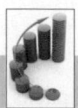

OUTCOME-BASED TEACHING PLANS

Sidney Smith, a 56-year-old engineer, is being seen in the clinic after a surgical procedure to repair a fracture in the foot. The site of the surgical incision has failed to heal. As a result, the incision site is open and requires daily dressing changes. He and his wife are here to learn the procedure.

OUTCOME

At the end of the teaching session, the patient/spouse can demonstrate the correct procedure for the dressing change.

STRATEGIES

- Describe the reasons for doing this dressing change with packing.
- Review the equipment necessary to perform the procedure.
- Demonstrate the correct way to remove the old dressing and cleanse the wound.
- Explain how to handle the new packing and dressing aseptically.
- Provide written steps of the procedure for their reference.
- Review both the procedure and plan to determine any questions.
- Have the patient, and spouse if indicated, return demonstrate the procedure before leaving the clinic.
- Arrange for follow-up with home care as necessary to evaluate performance and continue teaching.

OUTCOME

At the end of teaching session, the patient/spouse can verbalize the signs and symptoms to watch for in the wound.

STRATEGIES

- Discuss with Mr. and Mrs. Smith the changes in the wound site that might indicate infection or other aspects of poor healing.
- Provide a written list of warning signs that necessitate contacting their healthcare provider.
- Have Mr. and Mrs. Smith verbalize these factors back to you.
- Problem-solve with Mr. and Mrs. Smith how they will record the progress of the wound closure and healing and bring the record to the next clinic visit.

EVALUATION

2/17/17: 14:00— Signs of infection and poor wound healing discussed with the patient and wife and written instructions for dressing change provided. The patient is unable to look at the wound and deferred to wife saying she would take care of "it." Both the wife and patient were able to identify three signs of infection and the importance of notifying the provider if present in the wound. Wife performed dressing with cuing and support. She verbalized nervousness about doing it right. Home health referral submitted.

—Ben Eng, RN

Patients who need dressing changes must demonstrate the ability to perform wound care or receive assistance from a caregiver or healthcare worker in that process. Patients and involved caregivers should learn how to monitor the patient's wound, the signs and symptoms of infection, when and how to notify the healthcare provider, and recognition of adverse findings. Instructions (written and verbal) that include information on where to buy supplies should be provided. Patients who are unable to afford the needed products should receive assistance in making the treatment plan workable, which may include referral for assistance with healthcare expenses. Family members' acceptance of the skin impairment and their willingness to assist with care boost the patient's self-esteem.

Wound and skin problems can take an extended time to resolve. Therefore, many patients receive care at outpatient wound care clinics. Nursing staff in these clinics specialize in the care of chronic wounds. Adjunctive therapies such as peripheral compression wraps, electrical stimulation, sharp wound debridement, placement of tissue or skin grafts, or hyperbaric oxygen treatments are available. Nurses must instruct patients about the frequency of required follow-up medical appointments and symptoms of complications or recurrence. As indicated, teach about the disorder's etiology, control of risk factors, and the importance of maintaining healthy skin function.

EVALUATION

The evaluation of patient-centered goals determines whether the outcome criteria have been met for the prevention of tissue damage and promotion of optimal wound healing. Outcome criteria should be individualized for each patient and revised as necessary.

Goal

The patient's skin will remain intact without areas of local inflammation.

POSSIBLE OUTCOME CRITERIA

- The patient develops no skin lesions or pressure ulcers during hospitalization.
- The patient develops no redness or abrasions of the skin before next visit.
- The patient has intact skin without excessive drying or flaking.

Goal

The patient's wound will demonstrate evidence of healing.

PATIENT PLAN OF CARE
The Patient with Impaired Skin Integrity

NURSING DIAGNOSIS

Impaired Skin Integrity related to pressure, shear, and immobility as evidenced by 3- × 3- × 0.5-cm stage III sacral pressure ulcer

PATIENT GOAL

The patient/family will understand regimen to prevent and treat pressure ulcers.

PATIENT OUTCOME CRITERIA

- The patient discusses pressure ulcers in his or her own words.
- The patient describes five contributing factors to pressure ulcer development.
- The patient inspects skin daily.
- Before discharge, the patient demonstrates interventions to relieve pressure effectively.

NURSING INTERVENTION	SCIENTIFIC RATIONALE
1. Teach the patient and family what pressure ulcers are; use photographs.	**1.** Knowledge is important in developing values to maintain preventive health practices.
2. Discuss factors that can increase incidence of pressure ulcer formation.	**2.** Specific knowledge allows the patient to develop interventions that help prevent pressure ulcers.
3. Teach the patient or family to inspect all pressure points daily and to use a mirror for hard to visualize areas.	**3.** Daily inspection helps to detect any evidence of skin abnormality promptly.
4. Elicit the patient's preference for equipment (e.g., support surfaces), skin treatment, and turning schedules.	**4.** The patient's active involvement in individualizing prevention plan helps ensure compliance.

(Continued)

PATIENT GOAL

The patient's sacral pressure ulcer will heal without complications.

PATIENT OUTCOME CRITERIA

- The patient demonstrates increased granulation tissues in healing wound.
- The patient demonstrates absence of redness, swelling, and purulent drainage.
- The patient's sacral wound decreases in size.

NURSING INTERVENTION	SCIENTIFIC RATIONALE
1. Reposition every 2 hours, increasing frequency of positioning if redness or blanching does not disappear.	**1.** Repositioning relieves pressure, which can occlude capillary blood flow leading to tissue damage and ulcer formation.
2. Do not allow the patient to lie on healing pressure ulcer. Turn right to left and left to right.	**2.** Delicate healing tissues are more susceptible to trauma and impaired blood flow; pressure delays healing.
3. Use pillows to position and support pressure points.	**3.** Padding decreases pressure and shear, which can increase pressure sore development.
4. Instruct the patient to get up in chair at least 30 minutes twice a day.	**4.** Different body positions and movement improve overall circulation and relieve pressure from ulcer area.
5. Communicate turning schedule on wall at the patient's bedside.	**5.** Communication of specific times and positions helps promote compliance with turning schedule.
6. Avoid high Fowler's or semi-Fowler's position while the patient is in bed.	**6.** These positions increase shearing force, which impairs circulation as the patient slides down in bed.
7. Use turning sheet to lift, not drag, when moving the patient up in bed.	**7.** This action decreases shearing force from bed when moving the patient.
8. Inspect mattress; check for any areas of bottoming out. (Bottoming out can be checked by sliding one hand under the mattress directly under the patient; minimal contact of the body part should be felt.)	**8.** Pressure redistribution on the mattress is inadequate if bottoming out is felt. A powered, alternating pressure, low air loss redistribution mattress or mattress overlay may need to be obtained. These mattresses decrease the chance of occlusion of capillary blood flow, which can increase pressure sore development and delay healing.
9. Keep skin clean and dry, especially after episodes of incontinence.	**9.** Moisture promotes maceration of tissues and delays healing, which can lead to moisture-associated skin damage.
10. Apply a clear skin barrier/protectant to the periwound skin and cover with a foam dressing. Change the dressing every other day. Inspect daily.	**10.** A clear skin barrier protects the periwound skin from excess moisture and helps the dressing adhere to the skin while simultaneously preventing MARSI. Foam dressings will not dry out the wound bed, thereby maintaining a moist wound healing environment and protecting the ulcer to promote healing and prevent infection.
11. Encourage protein and vitamin-rich diet; assess dietary intake, and assist with menu choices.	**11.** Adequate nutrition is necessary for wound healing.

EVALUATION

8/1/17: 08:30—The patient's wife unable to attend teaching session. The patient listened to information re pressure ulcers but did not ask any questions. When asked what he could do to help heal his pressure ulcer, he said "move more." Pressure ulcer measures 3 cm × 4 cm × 1 cm deep. Will remeasure every Monday and contact WOCN re if powered pressure redistribution mattress can be ordered.

—S. Roberts, RN

POSSIBLE OUTCOME CRITERIA

- Within 24 hours, wound edges are well approximated.
- Within 48 hours, the wound shows evidence of increased granulation tissue.
- By discharge, the patient's wound is free from redness, swelling, and purulent drainage.

Goal

The patient will verbalize understanding of preventive skin care.

POSSIBLE OUTCOME CRITERIA

- After a teaching session, the patient verbalizes three interventions that can prevent pressure ulcer formation.
- After a teaching session, the patient identifies causes of mechanical or chemical tissue destruction.
- The patient demonstrates routine skin care measures to prevent excessive drying or abrasions at next visit.

Goal

The patient or family will demonstrate appropriate wound management technique.

POSSIBLE OUTCOME CRITERIA

- After a teaching session, the patient states important measures to promote skin integrity and wound healing.
- The patient maintains adequate nutritional intake as indicated on dietary journal.
- By discharge, the patient or family members demonstrate wound care and dressing change.
- The patient correctly verbalizes signs of wound infection and when to contact a healthcare provider.
- The patient or family members demonstrate proper use of special equipment needed to promote skin integrity.

KEY CONCEPTS

- The skin's physiologic functions are protection, thermoregulation, sensation, metabolism, and communication.
- The skin's health depends on sufficient blood flow, adequate nutrition, an intact epidermis, and proper hygiene.
- The very young and the very old are most susceptible to skin disruption.
- Altered skin integrity may be manifested by pruritus, rash, lesions, pain, and inadequate wound healing.
- Understanding the phases of wound healing is vital for proper wound assessment and management.
- Hemorrhage, infection, dehiscence, and fistula formation are potential complications of wounds.
- Factors affecting wound healing include oxygenation and nutrient supply, immune cellular function, age, obesity, smoking, drug intake, systemic disease, stress, nature of the injury, wound infection, and the environment.
- In the nursing assessment, data about normal skin status, risk for skin impairment, and identification of altered skin integrity are obtained.
- Planned nursing interventions are important to prevent pressure ulcer development and trauma to skin.
- Gauzes, transparent film, foam, hydrocolloids, hydrogels, alginates, hydrofibers, collagen, silver, and nonadherent are categories of dressings used in topical care.
- Sutures, staples, clips, Steri-Strips, cyanoacrylate glue, bandages, and binders can provide wound support.
- Effective management to promote optimal wound healing requires the use of moist wound healing.
- NPWT is a wound care treatment modality increasingly used for various acute and chronic wounds.
- Local application of heat and cold can decrease inflammation, improve healing, and reduce pain.
- Patient teaching is important for long-range promotion and maintenance of skin integrity.
- WOCNs are specialists in wound care and a valuable resource for patients, families, nurses, and other healthcare professionals.

PRACTICING FOR THE NCLEX

CHECK YOUR ANSWERS IN APPENDIX A.

1. Which of the following patients are at risk for altered integumentary function? Select all that apply:
    a. 23-year-old patient with anorexia nervosa
    b. 45-year-old obese patient with febrile sweats
    c. 61-year-old s/p renal transplant patient
    d. 72-year-old patient with congestive heart failure

2. A nurse is assessing a new colostomy stoma, finding it beefy, red, and moist though the surrounding skin appearing intact. What should be the nurse's conclusions?
    a. The patient is developing an infection.
    b. The patient is developing maceration at the site.
    c. The site is healing appropriately.
    d. The ostomy wafer and pouch have been too tight.

3. A patient is completely immobilized in spinal traction. Which type of mechanical force would put the patient at risk?
    a. Friction
    b. Shear
    c. Pressure
    d. All of the above

4. A patient is found to have a broken skin on his coccyx that has black eschar covering the base of the wound. How is this wound staged?
    a. Stage I
    b. Stage II
    c. Stage III
    d. Unstageable

5. A diabetic patient reports a nonhealing wound on his large toe. Which factors in this patient increase risk for this type of wound? Select all that apply:
   a. Decreased oxygenation
   b. Decreased blood flow
   c. Smoking
   d. Obesity

6. A nurse is assessing a patient's surgical wound. The wound shows beefy, red tissue at the base of the wound and the edges are gaping. Which words best describe this wound? Select all that apply:
   a. Fistula
   b. Hematoma
   c. Granulation
   d. Dehiscence

7. A patient with an existing pressure ulcer is scheduled for surgery. Which of the following interventions would be appropriate for this patient postoperatively? Select all that apply:
   a. Turn every 2 hours
   b. Pressure relief bed surface
   c. Silver dressings
   d. Debridement

8. A patient diagnosed with Risk for Impaired Skin Integrity is being assessed by the nurse. Which of the following would be priority areas to check? Select all that apply:
   a. Behind the ears
   b. Elbows
   c. Under TED hose on ankle and heels
   d. Skin under urinary catheter tubing on leg

9. A nurse is preparing to do wound care on several patients. Which patients would need sterile gloves?
   a. Emptying portable wound suction
   b. Irrigating an abdominal wound
   c. Applying a dry dressing to a surgical wound
   d. Applying hydrocolloid dressing to a coccygeal ulcer

10. A nurse is due to calculate intake and output, including the output from a Jackson-Pratt drain to the patient's flank. What should the nurse do as the last step?
   a. Clean the drainage spout with an antiseptic swab.
   b. Examine the tube and container.
   c. Compress the reservoir to establish suction.
   d. Pour the drainage in a calibrated container.

REFERENCES

Bryant, R., & Nix, D. (2012). *Acute and chronic wounds: Current management concepts* (4th ed.). St. Louis, MO: Mosby.

CDC. (2013). Necrotizing fasciitis: A rare disease, especially for the healthy. CDC.gov. Accessed July 7, 2014.

Edsberg, L. E., Langemo, D., Baharestani, M. M., Posthauer, M. E., & Goldberg, M. (2014). Unavoidable pressure injury: State of the science and consensus outcomes. *Journal of Wound, Ostomy, and Continence Nursing, 41*(4), 313–334.

European Pressure Ulcer Advisory Panel and National Pressure Ulcer Advisory Panel. (2009). *Prevention and treatment of pressure ulcers: Clinical practice guidelines.* Washington, DC: National Pressure Ulcer Advisory Panel.

Gray, M., Black, J. M., Baharestani, M. M., Bliss, D. Z., Colwell, J. C., Goldberg, M., et al. (2011). Moisture-associated skin damage: Overview and pathophysiology. *Journal of Wound, Ostomy, and Continence Nursing, 38*(3), 233–241.

Kaminski, M. V. Jr., & Drinane, J. J. (2014). Learning the oral and cutaneous signs of micronutrient deficiencies. *Journal of Wound, Ostomy, and Continence Nursing, 41*(2), 127–135.

Lie, P., He, W., & Chen, H.-L. (2012). Diabetes mellitus as a risk factor for surgery-related pressure ulcers: A meta-analysis. *Journal of Wound, Ostomy, and Continence Nursing, 39*(5), 495–499.

McNichol, L., Lund, C., Rosen, T., Gray, M. (2013). Medical adhesives and patient safety: State of the science: Consensus statements for the assessment, prevention, and treatment of adhesive-related skin injuries. *Journal of Wound, Ostomy, and Continence Nursing, 40*(4), 365–380.

Mudge, E. J., Meaume, S., Woo, K., Sibbald, R. G., & Price, P. E. (2008). Patients' experience of wound-related pain: An international perspective. *EWMA Journal, 8*(2), 19–20, 22, 24, 26, 28.

Herdman & Kamitsuru, S. (Ed.) (2014). *NANDA International. Nursing diagnoses: Definitions and classifications 2015–2017.* West Sussex, UK: Wiley-Blackwel.

Wound, Ostomy and Continence Nurses Society. (2010). Wound, ostomy and continence nurses: A smart addition to the healthcare team. Retrieved August 1, 2010, from www.wocn.org/resource/resmgr/smart_addition.pdf

Procedure 30-1 Changing a Dry Wound Dressing

Purpose

1. Protect wound from trauma and external contamination.
2. Provide opportunity to assess the wound.
3. Provide an absorbent covering over the wound.

Equipment

Clean gloves
Sterile, prepackaged foam dressing—with or without adhesive.
Syringe with normal saline flush (10 to 20 mL) (or dermal wound cleanser)
Clean, flat work surface
Silicone tape, if dressing does not include adhesive backing
Skin barrier wipe or spray
Plastic bag

Assessment

- Assess location and degree of pain. Medicate if necessary.
- Assess for generalized symptoms of infection (e.g., elevated temperature, leukocytosis, diaphoresis).
- Assess dressing for drainage.
- Review medical history and identify factors that may contribute to delayed wound healing (e.g., poor nutritional status, age, obesity, immunosuppressive therapy, disorders such as anemia or diabetes mellitus).
- Assess the patient's ability to cooperate during procedure. Arrange for assistance, if necessary, to ensure patient's safety during procedure.
- Note patient allergies to tape or dressing materials.

Procedure

1. **Perform hand hygiene and don gloves.**
   Rationale: Reduces microbe transmission.

2. **Identify the patient.**
   Rationale: Ensures correct patient receives proper assessment or treatment and reduces errors.

3. **Close door or bed curtains and explain the procedure to the patient and patient's family.**
   Rationale: Ensures patient privacy, increases patient compliance, reduces patient anxiety, and promotes learning.

4. **Position the patient comfortably. Expose only wound area.**
   Rationale: Keep the patient safe and comfortable.

5. **Ensure that an appropriate waste receptacle is within easy reach of work area.**
   Rationale: An easily accessible receptacle reduces the risk of contaminating the surrounding area and improves efficiency.

6. **Set up sterile supplies:**

   a. **Clear bedside table; wipe surface with paper towel and hand sanitizer, soap/water, or other disinfectant available.**
      Rationale: Provide a clean, organized work surface.

   b. **Open dressing package (or packages) by peeling paper down to expose dressing (Fig. 1). Smaller dressings may be carefully dropped onto inner package of larger dressings.**

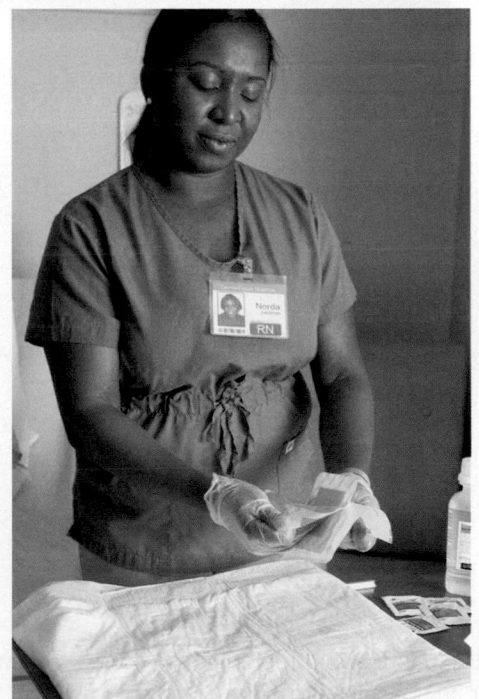

FIG. 1 Open dressing package, maintaining its sterility.

Rationale: The inside of the packaging is sterile and serves as a sterile field.

Procedure 30-1　*continued*

c. **Open normal saline flush syringe packaging, or place a dermal wound cleanser spray on the table next to the open dressing packages.**

   Rationale: Either normal saline or a commercially prepared wound cleanser is an appropriate cleanser to remove dried exudates on a closed wound or a shallow open wound.

7. **Change gloves.**

   Rationale: Gloves protect against contamination from wound drainage.

8. **Remove old dressing from the wound (Fig. 2). Remove the adhesive low and slow back over itself in the direction of hair growth, keeping it horizontal and close to the skin surface. Use fingers of the opposite hand to support newly exposed skin. (*Note*: If dressing adheres to wound, apply a small amount of sterile saline on the wound to loosen the dressing.) If dressing is small, hold the dressing in the palm of one gloved hand. Remove the glove holding the dressing first, then place the first glove into the palm of the second glove. Remove the second glove.**

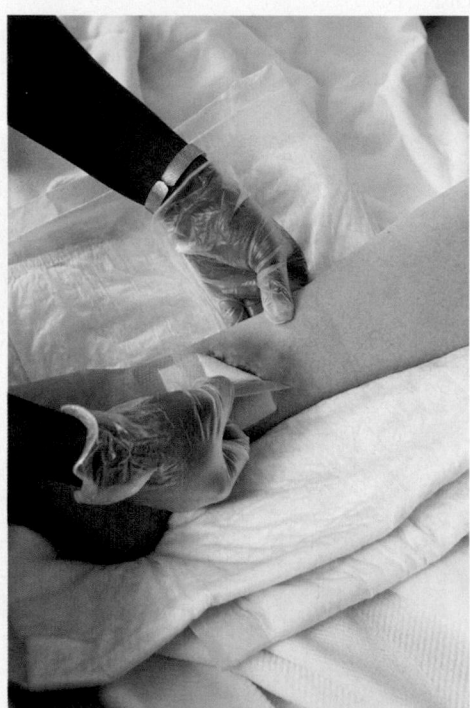

FIG. 2 Remove the old dressing from the wound.

Rationale: Avoid rapid vertical pulling to remove tape or an adhesive dressing to prevent MARSI.

   If the dressing is stuck, removing it without wetting will disrupt healing tissues and cause the patient pain.

9. **Dispose of gloves and old dressing in appropriate waste container. Perform hand hygiene if gloves are contaminated from wound drainage. Don clean gloves.**

   Rationale: Gloves are contaminated. Handwashing helps prevent spread of microorganisms.

10. **Apply normal saline or spray dermal wound cleanser to the wound. Use gauze to gently cleanse wound. Cleanse around a closed incisional wound with small circular strokes to gently remove adherent wound exudates (Fig. 3).**

    Rationale: Remove wound exudates to minimize environment for microorganism growth.

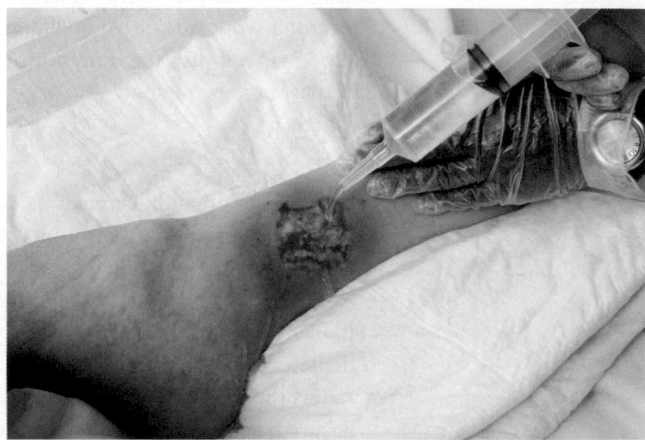

FIG. 3 Cleanse wound.

11. **Inspect the wound for bleeding, inflammation, drainage, and healing. Note any areas of dehiscence (opening or gaping of wound edges).**

    Rationale: Note and treat inadequate healing or complications immediately.

12. **Apply skin barrier to periwound skin and allow to dry (Fig. 4).**

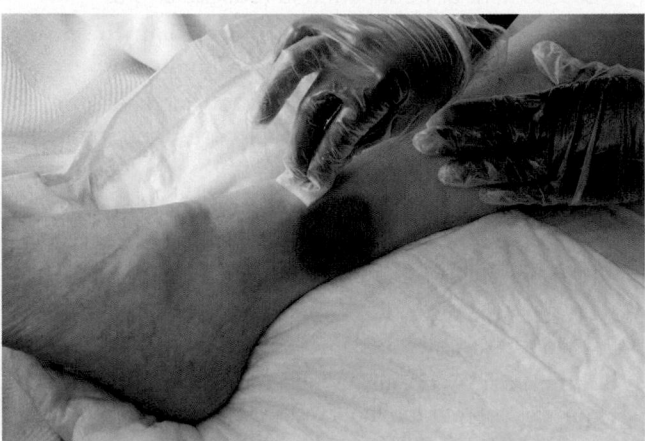

FIG. 4 Apply skin barrier.

Rationale: A skin barrier provides an interface between the skin and the adhesive to protect the skin from wound exudates and helps prevent MARSI.

Procedure 30-1   *continued*

13. Pick up the sterile foam dressing by touching only the outer center of the dressing or the outer edge of the adhesive layer, and apply over the wound (Fig. 5).

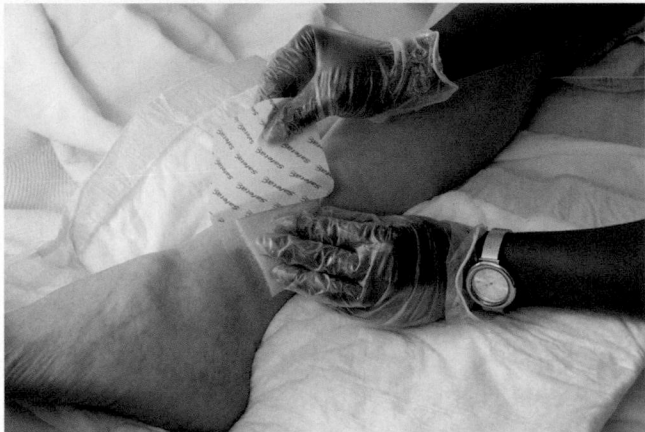

FIG. 5 Apply a sterile dressing over the wound.

Rationale: Careful application of dressings prevents introduction of microorganisms into the wound.

14. Secure the dressing to the skin. When using tape, place tape over center of dressing and evenly apply pressure to outward edges of dressings.

Rationale: Using even, gentle pressure without tension, pulling, or stretching when applying tape will prevent epidermal stripping of periwound skin or other type of MARSI when tape is removed.

15. Remove gloves. Perform hand hygiene.

Rationale: Handwashing helps prevent spread of microorganisms.

16. Document procedure.

Rationale: Maintains legal record and communicates with healthcare team.

Documentation

05/31/16: 16:15—PO day 3, dressing changed, wound edges approximating well, no drainage or signs of infection.

—S. Roberts, RN

Life Span Considerations

Child

- Remind young children not to touch the incision when their dressing is removed. Enlist the aid of assistants to prevent the child from moving and contaminating the wound or the sterile field.
- Preschool and young school-age children may think that the body part covered by a dressing is not there. Allow them to see their incision if they are interested. Seeing their body part will reassure them.
- Change the dressing immediately if a child is not toilet trained and the dressing becomes wet with urine or feces. Consider using wide plastic tape over the dressing to keep it dry.

Older Adult

- As skin ages, it loses its elasticity and becomes more sensitive, so adhesive tape may tear the skin. Apply a skin prep or skin sealant pad to periwound skin prior to applying tape to provide more protection to fragile skin. Apply and remove tape appropriately to prevent MARSI.

Home Care Modifications

- If a patient needs to change dressings at home, stress that handwashing before and after the dressing change is the most important aspect of maintaining asepsis. For some dressings, gloving is not required.
- Teach the patient where to buy and how to open and use dressings, how to clean the wound and which cleansing solution to use, and how to identify signs of infection that indicate the need to call the nurse or physician.

Collaboration and Delegation

- Instruct ancillary staff to observe for excessive drainage that may overwhelm the dressing and to report when dressings become soiled or loosened from the skin.

Procedure 30-2 Irrigating a Wound and Applying a Saline-Moistened Dressing

Purpose
1. Promote moist wound healing.
2. Cleanse the wound by removing debris and exudate.
3. Instill medication into the wound (if ordered).

Equipment

Clean disposable gloves
Sterile gloves
Sterile gauze dressings
Absorbent secondary dressing
ABD pad
Sterile saline—prefilled saline flushes or pour bottle of saline
Clean towel or absorbent drape
Tape or ties
Waterproof disposal bag
Sterile dressing instrument set with forceps and scissors (optional)
Sterile cotton-tipped applicators (optional)

Assessment

- Assess the wound's location and size to determine needed dressing supplies.
- Assess the patient's level of comfort. Give analgesics as needed before wound care.
- Review nursing notes for previous wound description and for generalized symptoms of infection (e.g., elevated temperature, leukocytosis).

Procedure

1. **Review the provider's orders for frequency of dressing changes.**
   Rationale: Prevents errors.

2. **Prepare the patient and remove dressing according to steps 1 through 6 of Procedure 30-1. (*Note*: Forceps may be used to remove a soiled dressing.) If dressing adheres to underlying tissues, moisten with saline to loosen. Gently remove the dressing while assessing the patient's comfort level.**
   Rationale: Moistening the dressing prevents disruption of healing tissue.

3. **Observe dressings for amount and characteristics of drainage. Note odor and color.**
   Rationale: Changes in the type or amount of drainage may be signs of wound infection.

4. **Observe wound for slough (a layer of dead cells and dried plasma, usually a yellow or yellow-brown color), granulation tissue (reddish capillary loops that bleed easily), or epithelial skin buds. Measure and record wound depth, diameter, and length.**
   Rationale: Assesses wound for healing.

5. **Place clean towel or absorbent drape pad on the patient's skin adjacent to wound area.**
   Rationale: Absorbs wound exudates and irrigant solution and keeps the patient's skin and bed linen clean.

6. **Don clean gloves for a chronic open wound (e.g., a pressure ulcer). Don sterile gloves for an acute full-thickness wound (e.g., dehisced surgical wound).**
   Rationale: Gloves prevent contamination of the wound or supplies. Chronic open wounds are considered colonized (microorganisms are present in wound but without signs and symptoms of infection). Clean gloves will prevent the introduction of pathogenic organisms into an already contaminated wound. Sterile gloves will reduce exposure to microorganisms and keep the wound as free from contamination as possible.

7. **Cleanse or irrigate wound as prescribed or with normal saline, moving from least to most contaminated areas. Use prefilled saline flush syringes to irrigate, or pour sterile saline from bottle into wound (Figs. 1 and 2). Use gauze pads to cleanse wound bed and absorb excess wound exudates and irrigant solution.**

Procedure 30-2   *continued*

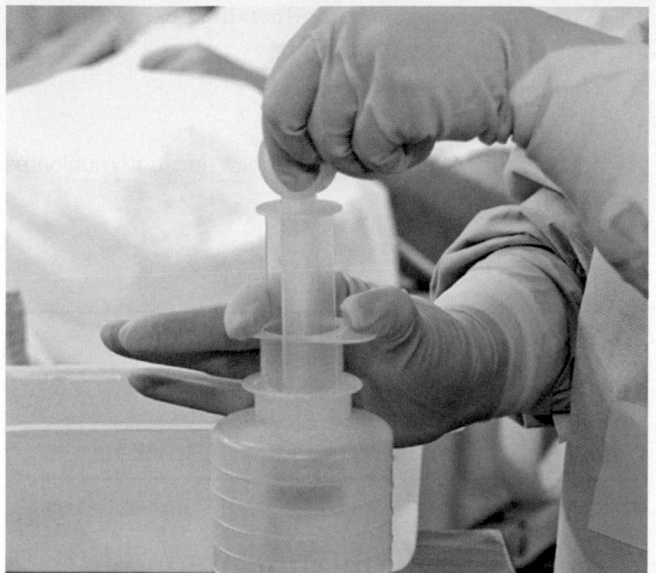

FIG. 1 Prepare syringe with irrigating solution.

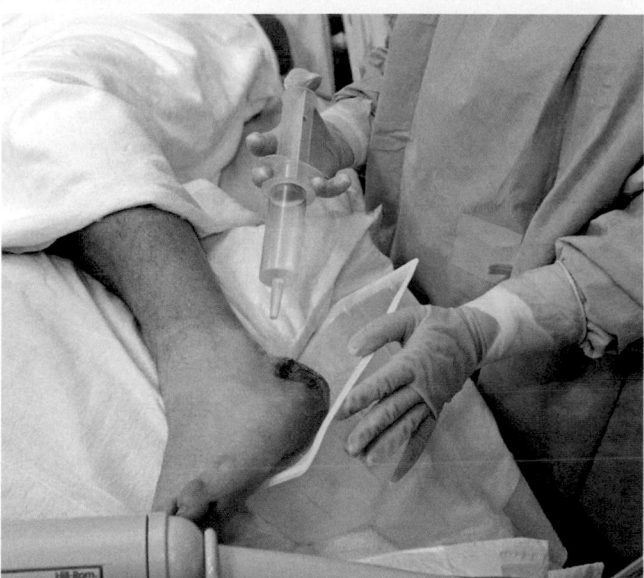

FIG. 2 Flush wound gently.

Rationale: When cleaning debris from wound, take steps to prevent spread of contamination.

8. Pick up dry gauze dressings in one hand, and pour or use syringe to apply a small amount of saline onto gauze dressings. Squeeze excess fluid from gauze dressing, then unfold and fluff out the dressings (Fig. 3).

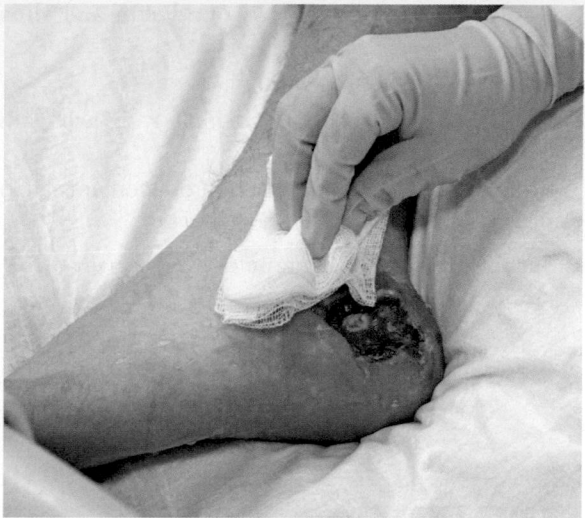

FIG. 3 Squeeze out excess fluid and fluff out dressing.

Rationale: Provides a thin, moist layer to contact all wound surfaces.

9. Check for tunneling so that all dead space can be filled. Gently fill moistened gauze into the wound cavity. If wound is deep, use forceps or cotton-tipped applicators to press gauze into all wound surfaces.

Rationale: Enhances healing from deepest part of wound first.

10. Apply several dry, sterile 4-inch × 4-inch pads over the wet gauze (Fig. 4).

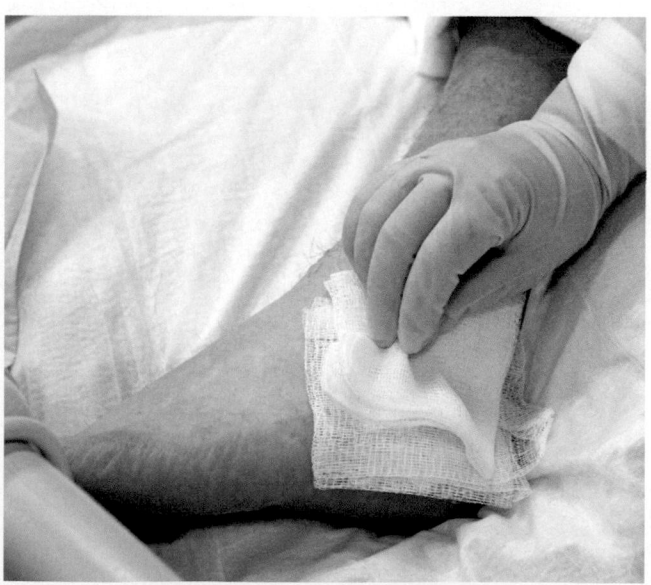

FIG. 4 Apply 4-inch × 4-inch pads.

Rationale: Extra pads help absorb excess moisture from under dressings.

Procedure 30-2   *continued*

11. Apply skin barrier to periwound skin and allow to dry.

    Rationale: Prevent MARSI.

12. Place ABD pad over dry 4-inch × 4-inch pads, if necessary.

    Rationale: Protects the wound from contamination.

13. Dispose of gloves.

14. Secure dressings with tape or Kerlix gauze (for circumferential dressings). .

15. Assist the patient to a comfortable position.

16. Perform hand hygiene.

    Rationale: Maintains asepsis.

17. Document procedure.

    Rationale: Maintains legal record and communicates with healthcare team.

Documentation

> 10/20/15: 10:00—Foot ulcer irrigated with NS and packed with moist gauze. 2-cm tunnel noted at 5 o'clock. Moderate amt of serous drainage noted.
>
> —S. Roberts, RN

Life Span Considerations, Home Care Modifications, and Collaboration and Delegation

- See **Procedure 30-1**.

Procedure 30-3 Maintaining a Portable Wound Suction

Purpose	1. Facilitate healing by removing drainage from the incisional area where granulation tissue is forming.
Equipment	Clean gloves Calibrated drainage receptacle Antiseptic swab
Assessment	• Assess the patient for generalized signs of infection (e.g., elevated temperature). • Assess type of surgery, postoperative day, and expected amount and type of drainage. • Assess drainage for amount, color, clarity, and odor. • Assess the patient for inflammation or discomfort around the drain.

Procedure

1. **Perform hand hygiene and don gloves.**
   Rationale: Reduces microbe transmission.

2. **Identify the patient.**
   Rationale: Ensures correct patient receives proper assessment or treatment and reduces errors.

3. **Close door or bed curtains and explain the procedure to the patient and patient's family.**
   Rationale: Ensures patient privacy, increases patient compliance, reduces patient anxiety, and promotes learning.

4. **Assist the patient to a comfortable position.**
   Rationale: Maintains the patient's comfort.

5. **Expose wound suction tubing and container while keeping patient draped (Fig. 1).**

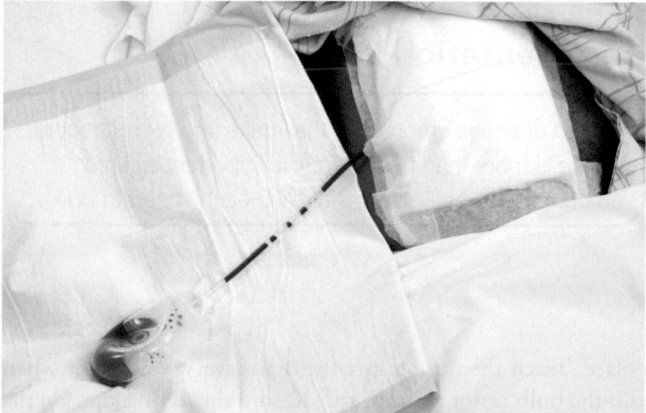

FIG. 1 Expose the portable wound suction device.

Rationale: Provides privacy and warmth for the patient.

6. **Examine tubing and container for patency and suction seal (Fig. 2). (*Note*: If the system's seal is broken, the bulb reservoir will be expanded and not compressed and suction will be lost.)**

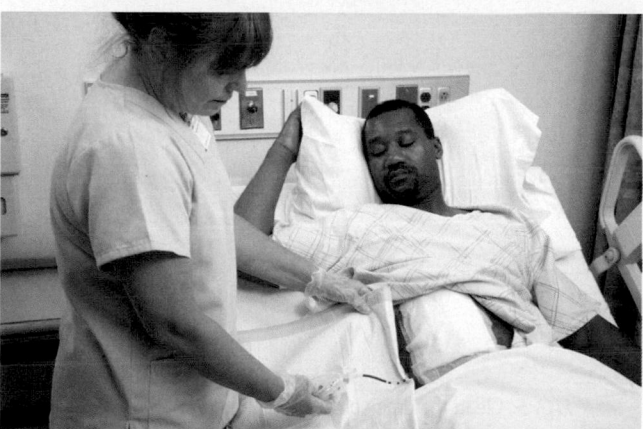

FIG. 2 Examine the tube and container.

7. **Open the drainage plug (Fig. 3).**

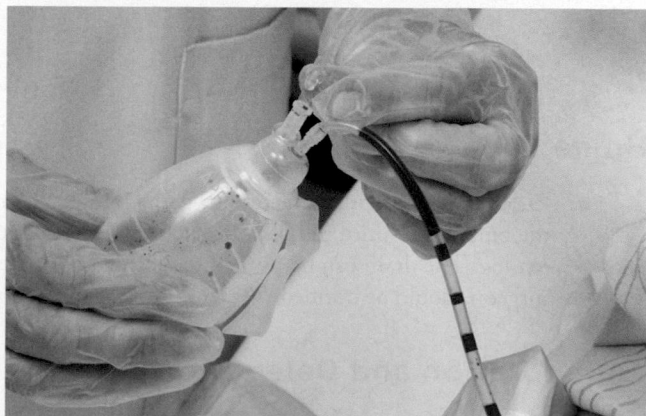

FIG. 3 Open the plug on the reservoir.

Rationale: Prepares the drain for emptying contents.

Procedure 30-3 *continued*

8. Pour drainage into a calibrated receptacle without contaminating the drainage spout (Fig. 4). Use an antiseptic swab to clean the drainage spout (Fig. 5).

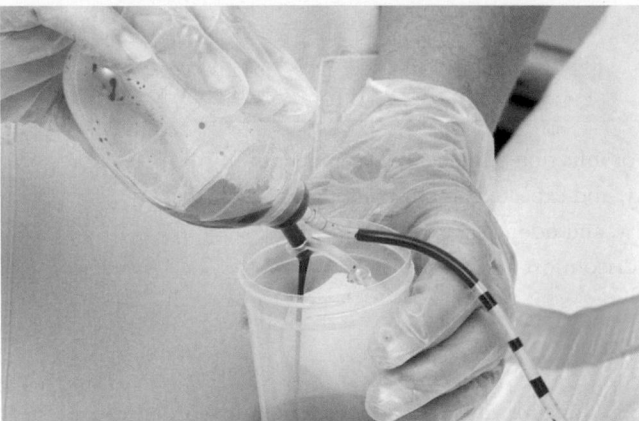

FIG. 4 Pour the drainage in a calibrated container.

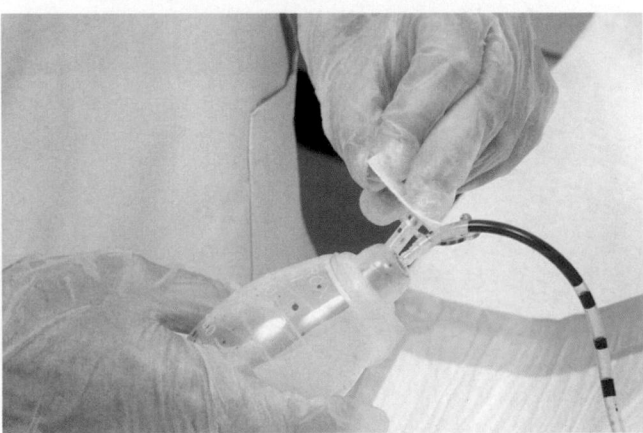

FIG. 5 Clean the drainage spout with an antiseptic swab.

Rationale: Prevents transfer of microorganisms to the wound.

9. Re-establish suction. With drainage plug open, compress the unit and reinsert drainage plug (Fig. 6).

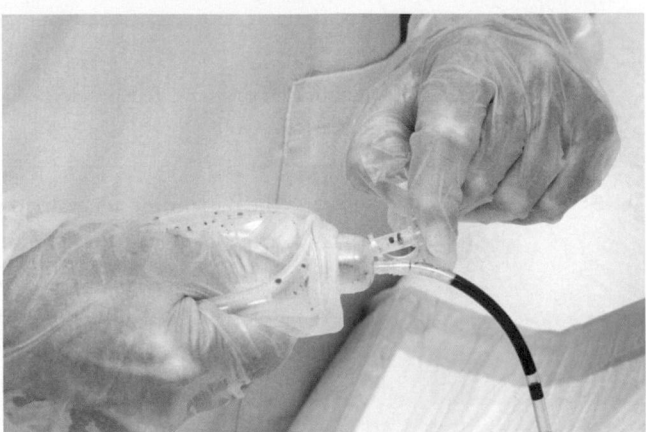

FIG. 6 Compress the reservoir to establish suction.

Rationale: A closed drainage system with gentle suction is established.

10. **Remove and discard gloves. Perform hand hygiene.**
    Rationale: Maintains asepsis.

11. **Return the patient to a comfortable position.**
    Rationale: Maintains patient's comfort.

12. **Measure drainage and record amount, color, and any other pertinent information.**
    Rationale: Obtains important information for the healthcare team to make clinical decisions.

13. **Document procedure.**
    Rationale: Maintains legal record and communicates with healthcare team.

Documentation

> Record drainage amounts in the intake and output record. If there is more than one drain, it is important to enter amounts separately, clearly labeling each separate drain.

Home Care Modifications

- Patients often are discharged with grenade (J-P) drains in place. Teach them to empty the drain every 8 hours or when the bulb is one-third full because suction is not maintained if the bulb is not compressed. Record the drainage in a written log. The drain can be pinned to clothing at waist height to avoid accidental dislodgement. If the drain falls out, the surgeon should be notified. When showering, a string can be looped around the patient's neck and the drain pinned to it.

Collaboration and Delegation

- Instruct unlicensed assistive personnel (UAP) to report if the suction device becomes filled with drainage or tubing appears dislodged. UAP often are responsible for emptying and recording drainage from drains. Be sure to label each drain (e.g., Rt & Lt, or A, B, C) if patients have multiple drains, and enter drainage totals separately.
- Surgeons use 24-hour drain totals to determine if the drain can be removed.

Procedure 30-4 Applying a Negative-Pressure Wound Therapy (NPWT) Dressing

Purpose

1. Promote wound healing by delivering negative pressure (a vacuum) at the wound site.
2. Vacuum-assisted wound therapy helps do the following:
   - Bring wound edges together
   - Remove wound exudates
   - Decrease edema at wound site
   - Develop granulation tissue

Equipment

Clean gloves
Sterile gloves for acute surgical wound
Negative-pressure therapy unit
Negative-pressure dressing kit (contains black foam dressing, transparent adhesive drape, connector tubing)
Negative-pressure drainage canister
Wound cleanser (normal saline or a dermal wound cleanser product)
4-inch × 4-inch pads (for cleansing wound bed)
Disposable measuring guide (centimeters)
Sterile cotton-tipped applicators
Skin barrier wipes
Scissors
Towel or other protective barrier
Plastic bag or other waste receptacle

Assessment

- Assess location and type of wound. Estimate wound size—decide on size of foam dressing kit to use.
- Assess degree of pain. Medicate if necessary.
- Assess the patient's ability to cooperate during procedure. Arrange for assistance, if necessary, to ensure the patient's safety.

Procedure

1. Follow steps 1 through 5 from Procedure 30-1.
2. Place towel or other protective barrier near wound and over bed linen.

   Rationale: Provides a barrier between the patient's skin and the bed linen to absorb debris and/or exudate from the wound.

3. Remove dressing from wound, and discard into appropriate waste container. When removing a negative-pressure dressing, close clamp on dressing pad tubing. Disconnect dressing tubing from canister tubing. Turn off negative-pressure therapy unit. Remove dressing. If dressing adheres to wound, pour a small amount of sterile saline on the dressing and wound. It may be necessary to allow the dressing to soak for up to 15 minutes.

   Rationale: Allows wound exudates to flow into the canister before turning the therapy unit off. Saline will safely loosen the dressing and prevent disruption of healing granulation tissue.

4. Dispose of gloves; apply new pair of clean gloves (sterile gloves for acute surgical wound).

   Rationale: Gloves are contaminated.

5. Cleanse wound using normal saline or dermal wound cleanser and 4-inch × 4-inch pads.

   Rationale: Prepares wound bed by removing exudates and wound debris.

6. Measure wound—length, width, and depth—and any undermined or tunneled areas using a disposable measuring guide and sterile cotton-tipped applicator.

   Rationale: Determines the amount and shape of foam dressing to place in the wound and evaluates the healing progress over time.

7. Dispose of gloves. Perform hand hygiene.

   Rationale: Gloves are contaminated.

8. Open sterile supplies (use the inside of packaging materials as sterile fields):

   a. Open black foam dressing kit.

   b. Open scissors or suture removal kit (containing scissors and forceps).

   c. Open skin prep wipes and place onto one of the sterile open packages.

      Rationale: All sterile supplies need to be open and ready before applying sterile gloves.

Procedure 30-4   *continued*

9. **Don sterile gloves when applying dressing to an acute surgical wound. Don clean gloves when applying dressing to a chronically contaminated wound such as a pressure ulcer.**

   Rationale: Gloves are standard infection control precautions for wound care.

10. **Apply skin barrier to 3 to 5 cm of periwound skin and allow to dry thoroughly.**

    Rationale: Skin prep protects intact skin and assists the transparent film dressing to adhere to the skin for a better vacuum seal.

11. **Cut or tear black foam to dimensions needed to fit gently into the wound bed without overlapping onto intact periwound skin; more than one piece of black foam may be used (Fig. 1). Do not cut or tear black foam over the wound.**

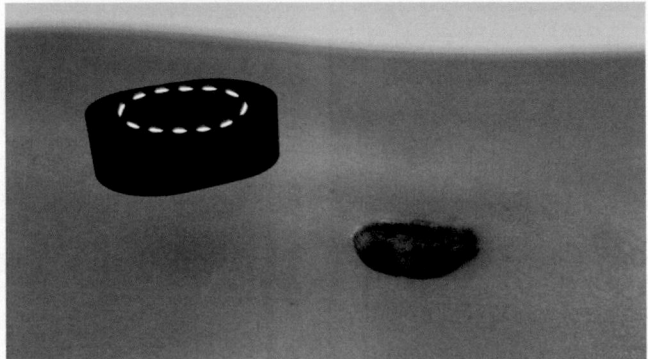

FIG. 1 Cut appropriate dressing to size. (From: V.A.C. Therapy, SENSA T.R.A.C. Pad. Courtesy of KCI Licensing, Inc.)

   Rationale: Black foam touching periwound skin will cause erythema to intact skin. No foam fragments should fall into the wound bed because small pieces can act as foreign bodies and disrupt healing.

12. **Place black foam dressing into wound bed to gently fill wound cavity (Fig. 2). If more than one piece of black foam is used, ensure foam to foam contact of adjacent pieces.**

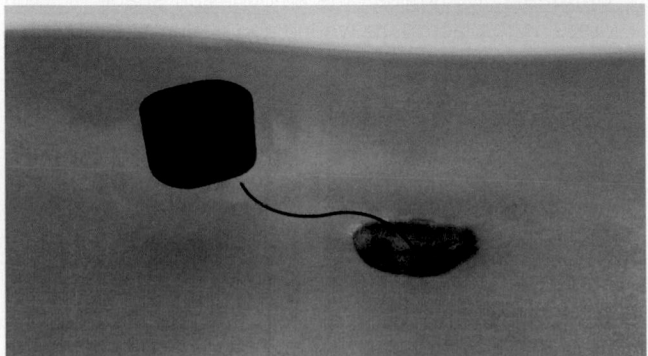

FIG. 2 Place dressing in wound. (From: V.A.C. Therapy, SENSA T.R.A.C. Pad. Courtesy of KCI Licensing, Inc.)

   Rationale: The black foam dressing must touch all the wound edges to allow for healing from the deepest part of the wound first (healing from inside to the outside). All foam pieces must be touching to assure effective negative pressure.

13. **Cover the foam pieces and 3 to 5 cm of periwound skin with the transparent film dressing. You may cut the drape into smaller pieces, as needed, to best fit over the wound and black foam sponge.**

    Rationale: The transparent film secures the dressing; extending the dressing beyond the wound edges is necessary for an effective vacuum seal.

14. **Select site for connector pad; pinch the drape and cut a 2-cm round hole. Remove the backing layers from connector pad and place directly over the 2-cm hole. Apply gentle pressure to pad and peel back stabilization layer on pad (Fig. 3).**

    Rationale: The hole needs to be large enough to allow wound exudates to flow out into the connector tubing. Pressing gently on the pad ensures complete adhesion.

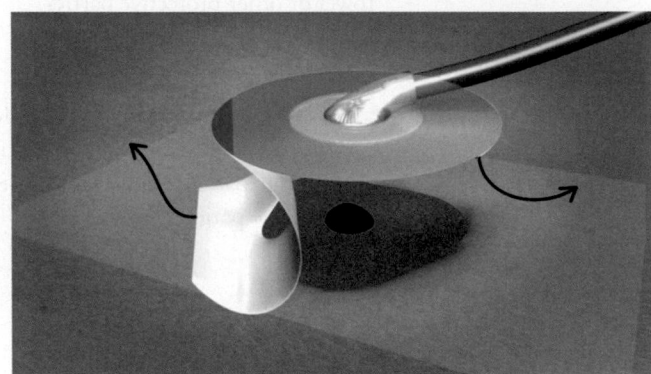

FIG. 3 Apply transparent film dressing over wound. (From: V.A.C. Therapy, SENSA T.R.A.C. Pad. Courtesy of KCI Licensing, Inc.)

15. **Insert drainage canister into negative-pressure therapy unit. Connect pad tubing to canister tubing and ensure both clamps are open (Fig. 4).**

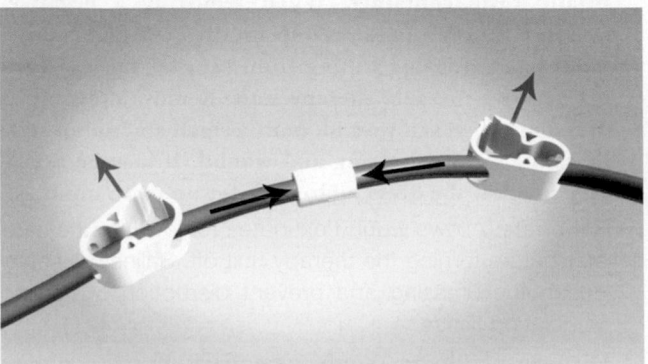

FIG. 4 Connect SENSA T.R.A.C. Pad tubing to canister tubing. (From: V.A.C. Therapy, SENSA T.R.A.C. Pad. Courtesy of KCI Licensing, Inc.)

Procedure 30-4   *continued*

Rationale: Wound exudates will flow from the foam dressing through the tubing and into the drainage canister.

16. **Turn on power to negative-pressure therapy unit; follow instructions to select prescribed therapy setting (Fig. 5). Assess for proper seal and functioning of the negative-pressure therapy.**

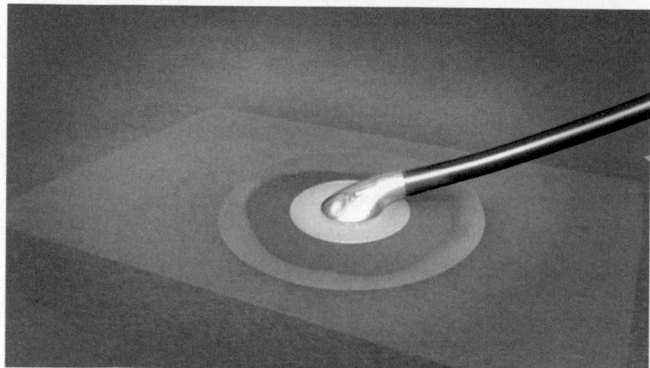

FIG. 5 Turn on power to V.A.C. Therapy unit. (From: V.A.C. Therapy, SENSA T.R.A.C. Pad. Courtesy of KCI Licensing, Inc.)

Rationale: The dressing will collapse and have a wrinkled appearance when negative pressure is functioning properly; exudate will begin to flow into the tubing and canister. The negative-pressure therapy unit will display the amount of negative pressure in mm Hg.

17. **Document procedure.**

Rationale: Maintains legal record and communicates with healthcare team.

Reference: *KCI. (2012). V.A.C. Therapy clinical guidelines: A reference source for clinicians. Retrieved April 19, 2014, from www.kci1.com/KCI1/vactherapyformsandbrochures*

Documentation

9/12/15: 16:00—Stage IV pressure ulcer 4 cm × 5 cm × 3 cm cleansed. Granulation tissue noted in wound bed. No undermining or tunneling. NPWT reapplied to wound.
—S. Roberts, RN

Life Span Considerations

Child

- NPWT is not approved by the Food and Drug Administration for use on children at this time.

Home Care Modifications

- A smaller, more portable negative-pressure therapy unit is used for patients at home. The unit has a longer battery life than hospital units but still is plugged into an electrical outlet for recharging.
- Home health nurses will assist patients and family members with application of NPWT dressings.

Collaboration and Delegation

- Consult a wound care specialist (WOCN) for advice regarding complex wounds and application of NPWT.
- Case managers can assist in obtaining insurance authorization for use of NPWT in the home setting.
- Request assistance from a second nurse or ancillary staff member when applying an NPWT dressing to a large wound.

Procedure 30-5 Application of Heat

Purpose

1. Increase blood flow, resolve inflammation, and improve healing of soft tissues.
or
2. Relieve muscular pain and stiffness.
3. Promote suppuration (discharge of purulent drainage) of indurated lesion.

Assessment

- Assess the wound's location and size to determine needed dressing supplies.
- Assess the patient's level of comfort. Give analgesics as needed.
- Assess for sensory deficits (e.g., diabetic neuropathy) that could increase the risk of thermal injury.

Procedure

1. **Review the physician's orders to determine the type and duration of heat treatment and the treatment area.**
   Rationale: Prevents errors.

2. **Perform hand hygiene.**
   Rationale: Reduces microbe transmission.

3. **Identify the patient.**
   Rationale: Ensures correct patient receives proper assessment or treatment and reduces errors.

4. **Close door or bed curtains and explain the procedure to the patient.**
   Rationale: Ensures patient privacy and increases patient compliance.

Commercial Heat Pack (Variations Depending on Source of Thermotherapy)

5. **Remove appropriate-size pack from wrapping paper. Note the directions for squeezing and rupturing a small vessel that releases the chemical into the larger bag.**
   Rationale: Breaking the vessel seal releases the chemical that produces the heat.

6. **Gently mix the bag, checking for leaks.**
   Rationale: Leaks could cause chemical reactions on the patient's skin.

7. **Apply the pack, checking back in 3 to 5 minutes to inspect the patient's skin for erythema.**
   Rationale: Excessive redness or swelling may indicate that the heat pack is too warm; tissue damage may result.

8. **Remove pack after 15 to 20 minutes or when it is no longer hot.**
   Rationale: Prevent thermal injury by restricting heat therapy to no more than 20 minutes per application. Leaving the pack in place when it is no longer hot serves no therapeutic purpose.

9. **Dispose of the heat pack. Do not reuse it.**
   Rationale: These units are designed for one-time use only.

Warm Moist Compress

Equipment

Aquathermia reservoir with pump and pad
Tape
Clean washcloth or towel

1. **Follow steps 1 through 4.**
2. **Check equipment to make sure connections are secure and cords are not frayed (Fig. 1).**

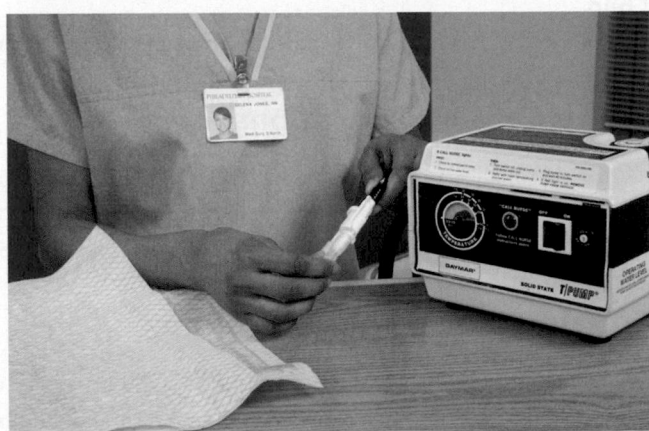

FIG. 1 Check the connections of the equipment.

Rationale: Prevents electric shock.

3. **Turn pump on and set the temperature with the pump key.**
   Rationale: Temperature should be about 35°C to 40°C. Remove key so that the temperature cannot be adjusted randomly.

Procedure 30-5 *continued*

4. **Apply warm water to washcloth or towel; wring out. Place cloth over lesion.**

   Rationale: Damp cloth provides moisture and will absorb any exudate that drains if the wound suppurates.

5. **Apply the pad with coiled surfaces on the warm moist cloth (Fig. 2).**

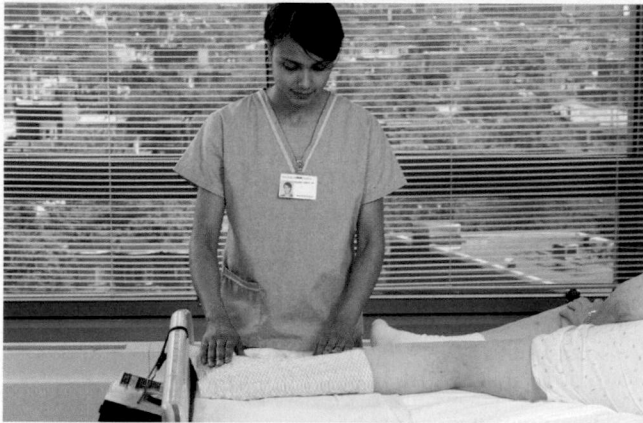

FIG. 2 Apply the aquathermia pad.

6. **Secure with tape, if needed.**

   Rationale: Sharp devices such as safety pins will puncture the pad and coils.

7. **Check the patient's skin and area of treatment every 10 minutes for the first 20 minutes to be sure the temperature is well tolerated. Discontinue compress after 30 minutes.**

   Rationale: Excessive redness or swelling may indicate that the heat pack is too warm; tissue damage could result.

8. **Check water level on aquathermia unit to make sure it is at the appropriate level.**

   Rationale: Lack of water in the unit can damage the unit and interfere with the supply of heat to the area.

9. **Document procedure.**

   Rationale: Maintains legal record and communicates with healthcare team.

Documentation

6/15/12: 15:00—Heat pack activated and applied to right forearm over the area of intravenous infiltration. Will recheck the arm in 20 minutes to assess for effectiveness.
—N. Blomquist, RN

Life Span Considerations

Child

- Children are at an increased risk of thermal injury; do not use a heating pack or pad on an infant.
- The use of warm compresses or heating pads needs to be closely observed because the child may change the heat setting or may change body position, making burns more likely.

Older Adult

- Older adults are more sensitive to heat therapy and require closer observation to avoid excess erythema or burns.

Home Care Modifications

- If warm compresses or a heating pad are ordered, be sure the patient and family know that the temperature should never be above the "low" setting and that the patient should not lie on it or use while sleeping.
- Teach the patient about signs of infection that indicate the need to call the nurse or other provider.

Collaboration and Delegation

- Instruct UAP to observe for edema or redness, which may indicate that the heat therapy may need to be adjusted.

Procedure 30-6 Application of Cold

Purpose	1. Relieve swelling and inflammation and decrease bleeding.
	2. Promote patient comfort in first 24 hours after an acute injury.

Equipment	Ice bag

Assessment	• Assess the injury's location and size.
	• Assess the patient's level of comfort. Give analgesics as needed.
	• Assess for sensory deficits (e.g., diabetic neuropathy) that could increase the risk of cold-related injury.

Procedure

1. **Review the provider's order to determine the duration of cold treatment and the treatment area.**

   Rationale: Damage to the skin can occur if cold therapy exceeds the prescribed duration.

2. **Perform hand hygiene and don gloves.**

   Rationale: Reduces microbe transmission.

3. **Identify the patient.**

   Rationale: Ensures correct patient receives proper assessment or treatment and reduces errors.

4. **Close door or bed curtains and explain the procedure to the patient and patient's family.**

   Rationale: Ensures patient privacy, increases patient compliance, and reduces patient anxiety.

5. **Fill ice bag with crushed/cubed ice to fill line; clamp bag closed. If not using commercially prepared bag, cover plastic bag with cloth.**

   Rationale: Protect the patient's skin from cold injury.

6. **Apply the pack, and use ties to keep cold application to desired location. Check back in 5 minutes to inspect the patient's skin for coldness or numbness (Fig. 1).**

Rationale: Excessive coolness may indicate that the heat pack is too cold; tissue damage may result.

7. **Remove bag after 15 to 20 minutes. Reapply fresh ice bag in 1 to 2 hours as needed.**

   Rationale: Prevent cold injury by restricting therapy to no more than 20 minutes per application.

8. **Document procedure.**

   Rationale: Maintains legal record and communicates with healthcare team.

Documentation

11/1/17: 11:45—Cold pack applied to right forearm. Encouraged rest and elevation of right extremity. Good circulation to extremity.

—S. Roberts, RN

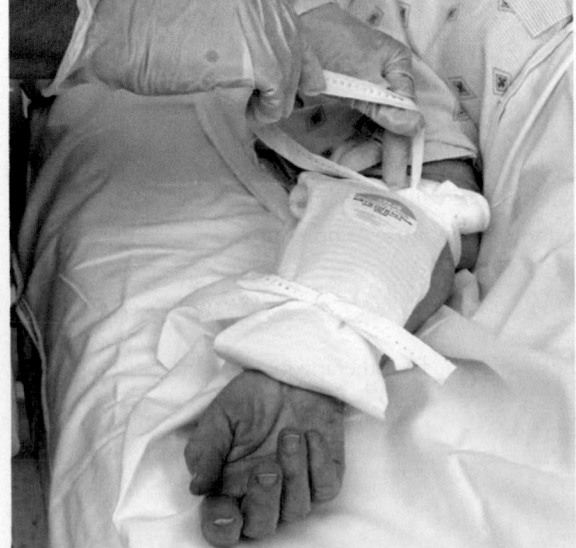

FIG. 1 Apply a cloth-wrapped ice bag to the wound site to promote healing and minimize pain.

Procedure 30-6   *continued*

Life Span Considerations

Child

- Infants cannot regulate body temperature and are very sensitive to thermal injury, so cold application is usually not indicated. Toddlers and older children often use cold packs to decrease pain and swelling for minor injuries.

Older Adult

- Cold therapies must be monitored more carefully in older adults, who are at risk for thermal injury due to poor sensation and circulation.

Home Care Modifications

- Cold packs often are kept in the freezer for use should an injury occur. Bags of frozen peas can be used if a commercial pack is not available.

Collaboration and Delegation

- UAP often fill ice bags or provide ice packs for patients. Stress the importance of frequent skin assessment and reporting any skin changes to the registered nurse.

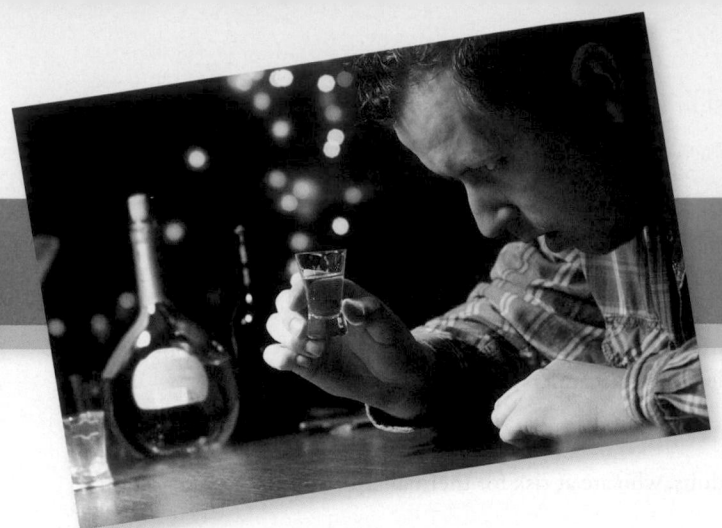

Infection Prevention and Management

Jeri Yoder

Case Scenario

You are a nurse doing tuberculosis (TB) surveillance for the public health department. A new patient is a 31-year-old man who had a positive purified protein derivative (PPD) test for TB last week when he was admitted to the hospital after a brawl in a local bar. Your patient left the hospital against medical advice (AMA) before a definitive diagnosis of TB could be made. When you find your patient, he is drinking in the same bar. After you introduce yourself, he swears at you, telling you to go away. He says he is not sick and does not need a nurse prying into his affairs.

Once you have completed this chapter and have incorporated information about infection prevention and management into your knowledge base, review the above scenario and reflect on the following areas of Critical Thinking:

1. Analyze how you would feel personally after this verbal attack.

2. Propose possible factors contributing to your patient's reluctance to talk to a nurse from the public health department.

3. Prioritize what is most important for your patient at this time, and explain how you can help your patient achieve his goals.

4. Weigh the rights of this patient to refuse treatment with the rights of the general public to live in a safe environment.

KEY TERMS

abscess
agranulocytes
anaerobes
antibodies
antigens
bacteremia
colonization
communicable disease
communicable period
complement system
endotoxins
extended-spectrum beta-lactamases (ESBLs)
granulocytes
healthcare-associated infections (HAIs)
interferon
leukocytosis
minimum inhibitory concentration (MIC)
multidrug-resistant organisms (MDROs)
neutropenia
normal flora
nosocomial infection
opportunistic
purulent
sepsis
shift to the left
superinfection
systemic inflammatory response syndrome (SIRS)
vaccination

LEARNING OBJECTIVES

Upon completion of this chapter, you will be able to do the following:

1. Name the major components of the body's normal resistance to infection and the role of each.

2. Differentiate between cellular and humoral immunity and between active and passive immunity.

3. Identify possible risk factors for infection or infectious diseases.

4. Discuss five common healthcare-associated infections (HAIs).

LEARNING OBJECTIVES *(cont.)*

5. Recognize common manifestations of infection.
6. Identify common diagnostic and laboratory tests used to identify or confirm an infectious process.
7. Describe major consequences of an infectious process.
8. Describe nursing measures that strengthen defense mechanisms against infection.

Infectious diseases have changed history by wiping out large numbers of people, stopping industrial growth, causing migrations, and altering social structures. They continue to significantly affect today's society. Infections consume billions of dollars in healthcare costs and are a major cause of absenteeism from work and school. They are a common cause of significant morbidity and mortality throughout the world. In the past several decades, changing sexual practices have led to a dramatic and rapid spread of disease to infection (STI), including herpes, gonorrhea, chlamydia, human papillomavirus (HPV), and acquired immunodeficiency syndrome (AIDS). All of these diseases have had enormous social consequences. Increasing numbers of **multidrug-resistant organisms (MDROs)**, including TB, methicillin-resistant *Staphylococcus aureus* (MRSA), **extended-spectrum beta-lactamases (ESBLs)**, resistant *Clostridium difficile* (*C. difficile*), and vancomycin-resistant enterococci (VRE) are posing a very serious challenge to healthcare providers.

For infection to occur, an uninterrupted chain of conditions must allow microorganisms to grow, reproduce, be passed from place to place, and enter a susceptible host. This "chain of infection" is described in detail in Chapter 19 and illustrated in Figure 19-1. Bodily defenses are relied on to combat pathogens when the chain of infection remains unbroken.

NORMAL RESISTANCE TO INFECTION

Microorganisms that live on the skin, in the nasopharynx, in the gastrointestinal (GI) tract, and on other body surfaces are referred to as **normal flora**. Normally, they pose no threat to the body. Sometimes, however, an agent can interact with a host that provides an environment for the agent's replication and growth. Infection results in such instances if the body's inflammatory and immune defenses fail.

Characteristics of Normal Resistance to Infection

The body's defenses against infection can be divided into two major groups: nonspecific natural defenses and specific acquired defenses. The types of human defenses against infection are outlined in Table 31-1.

NONSPECIFIC NATURAL DEFENSES

Nonspecific defenses that increase an individual's ability to resist infection include anatomic, mechanical, and chemical barriers; the inflammatory response; and fever.

Anatomic, Mechanical, and Chemical Barriers

The first line of defense against infection is intact skin and mucous membranes covering body cavities. They are the most important barriers to infection, and when they are intact, infection is rare. Chemical composition aids these physical barriers further. For example, the acidic nature of the skin and vagina helps to kill potential invaders before they enter the body. Some barriers, such as cells in the saliva, mucus, tears, and sweat, contain bactericidal enzymes.

Normal flora that grow on healthy tissues use local nutrients. Lack of nutrients and oxygen can inhibit the colonization and growth of pathogens. Mechanical forces, such as tears, saliva, and urine, wash bacteria from surfaces as they flow through the ducts and tracts. Peristalsis increases the mechanical cleansing of organ walls. Secretion of specific substances also defends against infection (Storey & Jordan, 2008). **Interferon** is a nonspecific chemical inhibitor that is secreted by body cells in response to viral invasion.

White Blood Cells

Leukocytes, also called white blood cells (WBCs), and the inflammatory response make up the second line of defense to microbial invasion. A normal WBC count is 5,000 to 10,000 cells/mm³. A count above this range is indicative of infection. Many leukocytes function as phagocytes, ingesting and thus destroying microbes. There are two categories of leukocytes:

- Granulocytes are polymorphonuclear cells that contain granules of digestive enzymes. Specific types of granulocytes include neutrophils, eosinophils, and basophils.
- Agranulocytes are mononuclear cells that lack digestive enzymes. Monocytes, which are immature macrophages, and lymphocytes are examples of agranulocytes.

Table 31-2 lists the actions of various WBCs.

Inflammatory Response

Inflammation is a nonspecific response to tissue injury that can be caused by microbial invasion or by mechanical, chemical, or heat injury. Inflammation attempts to limit an injury's extent. The blood vessels dilate, and plasma flows out of the capillaries into the irritated tissue. WBCs (typically neutrophils and then monocytes/macrophages) migrate into the area to attack and

TABLE 31-1 HUMAN DEFENSES AGAINST INFECTION

Defense	Examples
Nonspecific Natural Defenses Individual factors	Heredity Good hygiene practices Good nutritional status Immunization history
Anatomic barriers	Intact skin Intact mucous membranes
Mechanical removal of microorganisms	GI motility Ciliary action in the respiratory tract Cleansing effect of urine's flow Expulsive effect of coughing and sneezing Lavaging effects of tears and saliva Shedding of uterine lining in menstruation Flow of organ secretions through ducts (e.g., bile)
Chemical factors*	Acidity of gastric secretions, vaginal secretions, and fatty acids of the skin Lysozyme enzymes in tears, nasal secretions, urine, and saliva Hormones secreted by the adrenal cortex and pancreas Indigenous microflora (competition)
Local tissue factors	Tissue surface receptor (occupancy) Inflammation
WBC function	Fever Phagocytosis
Acquired specific defenses†	Cellular immunity (T lymphocytes elaborate killer cells and helper cells) Humoral immunity (B lymphocytes produce antibodies to specific microorganisms) Memory of the organisms produces lasting immunity.

*Factors that retard growth and provide less favorable media for growth.
†Person may acquire resistance naturally if he or she has had the infectious disease or has been immunized.

TABLE 31-2 WHITE BLOOD CELL FUNCTIONS IN INFECTION

Cells	Normal Values	Action
WBC count	4.1–10.0 × 10 million/mm³	
Granulocytes Neutrophils	50%–70%	Phagocytes. They ingest and break down foreign particles, particularly bacteria and parasites. They are also an important link in generating fever to combat the proliferation of microorganisms.
Eosinophils	0%–3%	Allergic reaction. They increase in response to allergic and parasitic conditions when an antigen–antibody response occurs.
Basophils	1%–3%	Unknown. They contain heparin and histamine in their granules, which may be important in preventing blood clotting during an inflammatory response.
Agranulocytes T lymphocytes		Synthesis of immunoglobulins. They produce cellular immunity and are effective in destroying bacteria, viruses, and cancer cells. They recognize antigens and stimulate B lymphocytes and macrophages. Three types have been identified: helper cells, which stimulate other leukocytes; killer T cells, which recognize and destroy virus-infected cells; and suppressor cells, which tell the other cells to stop fighting after the antigenic substance is cleared.
B lymphocytes		Synthesis of antibodies. They produce humoral immunity. They are important in the immune response. They are stimulated by the T cells to divide and produce the plasma cells, which then produce specific antibodies to antigens. The memory cells carry the memory of the antigen and produce lasting immunity to the specific microorganism.
Monocytes (macrophages)	2%–6%	Scavenger cells. They dispose of cellular debris. Their numbers increase in the late stage of acute infections and during chronic infections. Levels also rise in response to viral, bacterial, and parasitic infections. They are considered important in activating the lymphocytes and are found in the reticuloendothelial system.

ingest the invaders by the process of phagocytosis. This activity leads to the five signs of local inflammation at the injured area:

- Erythema (*redness*) from blood accumulation in the dilated capillaries
- *Warmth* from the heat of increased blood flow
- Edema (*swelling*) from fluid accumulation
- *Pain* from pressure or injury to the local nerves
- *Functional impairment* from edema and/or pain

The area becomes red, warm, swollen, and tender. It is inflamed but not necessarily infected.

Inflammation and phagocytosis work together to contain microorganisms. If these processes are successful, a collection of dead leukocytes, digested bacteria, dead tissue cells, and plasma may form into the material called pus.

Systemic responses due to inflammation may include increased WBC production, fever, fatigue, muscle aches, and loss of appetite. Due to the rise in body temperature and metabolic rate, the patient may also experience an increase in pulse and respiratory rate. Fatigue, muscle aches, and loss of appetite are a result of increased energy expenditures to support the inflammation process (Fig. 31-1).

Fever

Elevated body temperature also aids in the battle against infection. The hypothalamus raises the body's thermostat in response to pyrogens released by some phagocytic cells (macrophages)

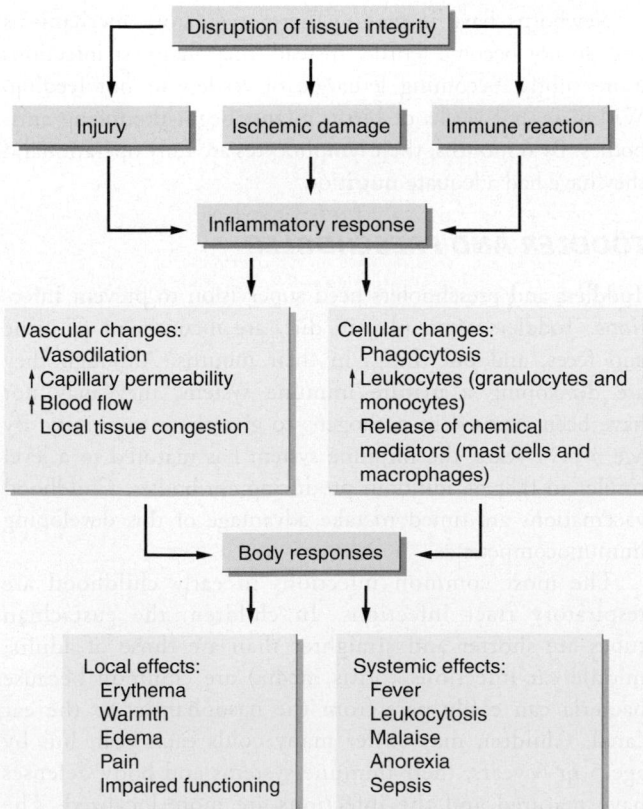

FIGURE 31-1 Inflammatory response.

after stimulation by microorganisms or endotoxins. The rise in temperature increases cell metabolism.

Fever (defined as body temperature greater than 38.2°C [101°F]) helps combat infection by interrupting viral replication and slowing the rate of bacterial growth. Fever also increases the mobility of leukocytes and enhances their ability to phagocytize microorganisms. In addition, the effects of endotoxins (toxins released by the immunogenic part of the bacterial cell wall of Gram-negative bacteria, which triggers an immune response) decrease with elevated temperatures.

SPECIFIC ACQUIRED DEFENSES: IMMUNITY

Another important defense against infection is immunity. **Antigens** are foreign particles, such as microbes, that enter a host. In some cases, such as in autoimmune diseases, the immune system senses or recognizes the person's own cells as antigens.

The immune system response is stimulated when antigens enter the lymphatic and circulatory systems. The antigens are phagocytosed by macrophages, monocytes, or neutrophils, and the microbes are digested. Portions of the microbe—antigenic particles—stay with the phagocyte and are carried to the lymphoid tissue in the lymph node or the spleen. The phagocyte, usually a macrophage, presents this processed antigen to the lymphocytes, which then stimulate immune responses.

The two types of lymphocytes are T lymphocytes and B lymphocytes. Both originate from stem cells in the bone marrow and differentiate to become the lymphopoietic cells. Some pass through the thymus gland and become modified to form the thymus-dependent or T lymphocytes (also known as T cells). Others are modified by unknown mechanisms to become B lymphocytes.

The immune system conveys lasting resistance to infection by forming a "memory" of the antigen by means of specialized T and B lymphocytes and memory cells. T and B lymphocytes, the building blocks of the immune system, accumulate in lymph nodes along lymphatic vessels and are exposed to all antigens except those that enter the bloodstream directly. These lymphocytes are heavily concentrated in the tonsils and spleen, which are important tissues in children and young adults.

The immune system, if properly functioning, can produce resistance to disease recurrence. After an active infection, which may or may not be symptomatic, immunity to a specific pathogen usually results.

Cellular Immunity

Cellular immunity, consisting principally of T-lymphocyte activity, is stimulated by fungi, protozoa, bacteria, and some viruses. After T lymphocytes are stimulated, they enter the circulation from the lymphoid tissues and seek the site of the microbe. At the site, the lymphocytes produce proteins called lymphokines that draw more phagocytes to the area, keeping them there to fight the invader and increasing their killing power. Lymphokines disappear after the antigen has been eliminated. Some T cells, however, remain in the tissues and keep a memory of the antigen. Memory T lymphocytes are reactivated rapidly if the same antigen reappears.

Humoral Immunity

Humoral immunity takes place in the bloodstream. B lymphocytes provide humoral immunity by producing **antibodies** that convey specific resistance to many bacterial and viral infections. B lymphocytes, stimulated by the antigenic particles contained within the macrophages, produce plasma cells. The plasma cells then produce antibodies that are released into the bloodstream from the lymphoid tissue. Antibodies, also called immunoglobulins, circulate in the bloodstream and interact with antigens they encounter.

Antibodies are formed in response to substances found in bacterial cell walls, toxins, microbial enzymes, viruses, and other individual allergens. Antibodies act to make bacteria more susceptible to phagocytosis or to help in bacterial cell lysis. Antibodies formed in response to a virus neutralize the virus, act as antitoxins, or cause microbes to clump together or precipitate. Other antibodies make it easier for phagocytes to ingest microbes. Memory B lymphocytes remain in lymphoid tissue, where they can become reactivated if the pathogen appears again.

The **complement system**, a series of proteins found in the bloodstream, also aids in the antigen–antibody reaction. The complement system enhances phagocytosis of microbes, helps in lysis of bacterial cell walls, and encourages the inflammatory response.

Active Immunity

Active immunity is produced when the immune system is stimulated, either naturally or artificially, to produce antibodies. Natural immunity occurs after an infection has run its course. The patient experiences a disease and produces an immune (antibody) response to the antigen. Active immunity can also be produced through **vaccination**. Vaccination is the process of injecting weakened or killed organisms into a person, stimulating antibody production. Vaccination produces an artificially acquired active immunity.

Passive Immunity

Passive immunity does not involve the host's immune response; rather, immunity is transferred to the recipient. This can be done in two ways. Antibodies can pass from a woman to her fetus by way of the placenta or to her newborn through breast milk. Also, antibodies from a person or animal that has had a disease can be taken from the blood and given to another person for temporary passive protection. Passive immunity, which provides only temporary protection, is given in the form of immune globulins when there is not enough time for the person to acquire active immunization or when a vaccine does not exist for the disease.

CULTURAL CONSIDERATIONS

Many ethnic groups have developed cultural habits that act as barriers to the spread of infection. Scientists are attempting to identify the roles of customs, genes, and religious rituals and practices in resisting infection.

A population can develop increased resistance to certain microorganisms over time or through other mechanisms. For example, Africans and African Americans living today who have inherited the genetic disease of sickle cell anemia do not contract malaria. This is because the sickled shape of the erythrocyte makes it impossible for the parasite causing malaria to grow and replicate. Malaria kills more than 1 million people each year, and although sickle cell anemia has its own serious consequences, this resistance provides a survival advantage for those living in areas where malaria is endemic, such as sub-Saharan Africa.

Life Span Considerations

NEWBORN AND INFANT

The immune system does not become fully operational until a baby reaches about 6 months of age. Before then, the infant's resistance to infection comes from the antibodies passed by way of the placenta and breast milk. Newborns have difficulty localizing infections (preventing the spread of organisms from the site of contact). Their phagocytes have difficulty trapping microbes, and they do not produce enough antibodies. At this time, viral diseases such as chickenpox or herpes simplex, acquired from the birth canal or from an infected sibling, can cause severe widespread disease (Storey & Jordan, 2008).

Newborns have immature thermoregulatory mechanisms and do not become febrile. Instead, they manifest infections more subtly, becoming lethargic or restless or not feeding. Within several weeks of birth, infants begin producing antibodies. By 6 months, their lymphocytes are fully operational if they have had adequate nutrition.

TODDLER AND PRESCHOOLER

Toddlers and preschoolers need supervision to prevent infections. Toddlers often play in dirt, are incontinent of urine and feces, and put things in their mouths. Although they are developing a mature immune system, they may not have been exposed to pathogens to give them immunity. By age 3 to 4 years, the immune system has matured to a level similar to that of adults in producing antibodies. Childhood vaccinations are timed to take advantage of this developing immunocompetence.

The most common infections in early childhood are respiratory tract infections. In children, the eustachian tubes are shorter and straighter than are those of adults; middle ear infections (otitis media) are common because bacteria can easily pass from the nasopharynx to the ear canal. Children may suffer many colds each year, but by age 5 or 6 years, their immune systems and body defenses have matured and the infections are more localized. The common communicable diseases are transmitted as children play with others.

Prevention of infections in early childhood requires the following:

- Good hygienic care of children and their food
- Adequate vaccinations
- Early infection treatment to prevent spread or complications
- Isolation from infected people

CHILD AND ADOLESCENT

Communicable diseases are most prevalent as children enter school and organized play activities. They are most common during the winter, when children stay indoors. Children are also exposed to skin diseases, such as impetigo (from staphylococcal infections), roundworm infestations, and lice (from sharing combs, clothes, and sports equipment). A high incidence of streptococcal infections occurs in children age 6 to 12 years, resulting in pharyngitis, tonsillitis, and scarlet fever.

The person's immune system should be fully mature by adolescence but may be compromised by malnutrition or acquired disorders such as chronic infections or illnesses. Adolescents are at high risk for STI. Those who contract STI run an increased risk of serious consequences. For example, pelvic inflammatory disease in young women is a major cause of ectopic pregnancy and infertility, and inflammation and infections of the urethra, epididymis, and testes can lead to sterility in men. Additionally, HPV has a causal relationship with virtually all cervical cancers. Two types of HPV (HPV 16 and HPV 18) are the cause of 70% of cervical cancers (CDC, 2014c). The CDC Advisory Committee on Immunization Practices (AICP) recommends routine vaccination at age 11 or 12 years of age. The vaccination series can be started as early as age 9 (CDC, 2014c).

ADULT AND OLDER ADULT

Immunity to many diseases is established by adulthood. Although adults have fewer respiratory tract infections, they have more chronic lung diseases, which can increase the risk of infection. Also, depending on the person's lifestyle, STI continue to be a major problem in this age group. ACIP also recommends routine HPV vaccination for females through 26 years and for males through 21 years who were not vaccinated previously. ACIP recommends vaccination of men who have sex with men, and immunocompromised persons (including those with HIV infection) through age 26 years if not previously vaccinated (CDC, 2014c). Infections during pregnancy can be transmitted across the placenta to the fetus. A minor or subclinical infection can be passed to the fetus, who may suffer minor consequences, major congenital anomalies, or death.

As people age, their lifestyle begins to affect their ability to resist infection. The thymus begins to shrink in late adolescence and continues to diminish into middle age, leading to a decline in cell-mediated and humoral immunity. Cardiovascular disease, cancer, diabetes, obesity or malnutrition, alcoholism, anxiety, depression, and stress have all been shown to decrease defense mechanisms against infection. Medications and treatments

used to combat these diseases may also impair immune system function. Adults with chronic diseases may require frequent hospitalizations and visits to outpatient clinics, putting them at risk for **healthcare-associated infections (HAIs)**.

With the increase in air travel and the development of global economic ties, people are traveling more and living in foreign countries, where they may be exposed to infectious diseases that are not indigenous to their native area. They may then bring these infectious organisms home, contributing to the spread of infection. Because the initial exposure occurs during adulthood, symptoms and complications of such diseases may be severe. The 2014 Ebola epidemic was the largest in history, affecting multiple countries in West Africa. Two imported cases, including one death, and two locally acquired cases in healthcare workers were reported in the United States (CDC, 2015a). Bedbug infestations have recently become a problem and can be contracted when sleeping in a hotel or motel and then brought back into the home environment.

As a person ages, the skin becomes thinner and drier. It loses elasticity and fat and receives less circulation, leading to an increased susceptibility to injury and subsequent infection. The body's pH secretions change, peristalsis slows, and endogenous flora also changes with age and use of medications. The cough and gag reflexes of older patients may be impaired after a stroke or from medications that cloud thinking. Loose-fitting dentures and impaired swallowing mechanisms may lead to aspiration, which can contribute to respiratory infection.

Older adults may have problems with urinary retention, possibly leading to bacterial growth in stagnant urine and decreased cleansing of the urethra by a brisk stream of urine. Adults who are incapacitated may be incontinent of urine and feces, leading to excoriation of the skin in the perineal and sacral regions and further contributing to infections. If confused or agitated, older patients may carry microorganisms from these areas to their nose or mouth if they are not given adequate help with hygiene.

The immune systems of older adults also may be impaired. Aging diminishes both nonspecific and specific defenses to microbial invasion. Metabolism, synthesis, and repair of body cells and tissues decrease. WBC counts do not always rise in response to infections, and phagocytosis is ineffective. There is a decreased inflammatory response, and body temperature may not be elevated in response to infection. The ability to wall off and limit the spread of infection is decreased. Cellular immune response is decreased, and old infections such as TB may be reactivated.

Respiratory diseases (including respiratory tract infections) as a cause of death in older adults are exceeded only by heart disease, cancer, and stroke (Healthy People 2020, 2010). Urinary tract infections (UTIs) and respiratory tract infections are the most common and most lethal. Infections consume energy that is necessary for other body processes. Older people have twice the incidence of influenza as young adults, and their mortality rate is higher. They are also vulnerable to HAIs, including surgical site infections (SSIs), particularly when the chest or abdomen is the operative site.

FACTORS AFFECTING NORMAL RESISTANCE TO INFECTION

Infectious Agents

In the past, only a few organisms were thought to be pathogenic. It is now recognized that almost any microorganism can cause disease, given the right conditions for entry and growth in the body. Even normal flora can cause disease under the right circumstances. Such organisms are **opportunistic**. Although normally not considered pathogens, they take advantage of being in the right place at the right time and cause infection, especially in patients with compromised immune systems. Bacteria, viruses, fungi, and parasites are pathogenic organisms.

BACTERIA

Bacteria contain thousands of species, but only a few hundred cause human disease. Bacteria are classified as Gram positive or Gram negative, referring to the differentiating process known as the Gram stain. This process, the initial process for bacterial identification, divides bacteria into one of two groups, depending on the characteristics of its cell wall. Gram-positive bacteria, such as staphylococci, are commonly found in wound infections and in food poisoning. Streptococci, also Gram positive, contribute to skin, wound, and respiratory infections. Gram-negative bacteria that reside in the GI tract (enteric) as normal flora are the source of many HAIs. Contamination of self and others by direct and indirect contact with Gram-negative pathogens, such as *Escherichia coli* and *Klebsiella pneumoniae*, is commonly the result of inadequate hygiene and handwashing practices.

Anaerobes, or organisms requiring reduced oxygen for growth, are often associated with serious infections. Anaerobic microorganisms are often seen with infections involving a combination of organisms (polymicrobial infections). These organisms are part of the normal flora of the mouth, intestines, and female genital tract.

Bacteria liberate toxins called exotoxins and endotoxins. **Endotoxins** are particularly potent poisons that can cause shock when large amounts are released into the blood. Exotoxins are liberated by the bacteria that cause tetanus, diphtheria, botulism, cholera, and staphylococcal food poisoning. Exotoxins of Gram-positive bacteria are able to move easily across cell membranes into healthy tissue and cause tissue injury.

VIRUSES

A virus invades a living cell many times its size, uses the cell's metabolism, and replicates itself while destroying the cell or changing the cell's genetic makeup. Viruses cause AIDS, chickenpox, colds, cold sores, encephalitis, hepatitis, herpes, HPV, influenza, measles, mononucleosis, mumps, polio, rabies, shingles, pneumonia, and many other diseases. They have been associated with some cancers and leukemias and with many autoimmune diseases, including multiple sclerosis, rheumatoid arthritis, and diabetes. For example, mononucleosis is caused by the Epstein-Barr virus, and cervical cancer is linked to certain types of HPV.

FUNGI

Only a few fungal infections cause disease in humans, but fungi can be deadly if they disseminate through the body tissues. Unicellular fungi, called yeasts, are often normal flora of the skin and mucous membranes. Yeasts do not injure the host until defenses are lowered, as with *Candida* in the mouth of infants (thrush) or in patients with cancer or AIDS. Antibiotics, which can destroy normal bacterial flora, can contribute to fungal infections. Infestations of yeast by inhalation of spores can cause coccidioidomycosis or histoplasmosis lung infections. The most common yeast infections affect the skin, hair, and nails (e.g., athlete's foot, ringworm, groin itch).

PARASITES

Parasites that infect humans are protozoa, helminths, or arthropods. Parasitic infections are associated with poor socioeconomic conditions, such as inadequate sanitation measures for water and sewage. When public health measures do not control these organisms, disease is prevalent.

Protozoal infections are common in underdeveloped countries and probably cause more suffering worldwide than does any other group of diseases. Trichomoniasis is considered the most common curable STI, affecting an estimated 3.7 million (CDC, 2012). Other diseases include African sleeping sickness, malaria, giardiasis, leishmaniasis, and toxoplasmosis. Pneumocystosis, a disease of the alveolar sacs, is increasing in frequency in patients with immunosuppression (e.g., cancer, AIDS).

Helminths include pinworms, flatworms, and roundworms. Some invade the tissues; others live in the GI tract or in the blood. Pinworms, found worldwide, are one of the most common parasites in humans. Roundworms, also passed among humans, are common. Flatworms are best known from reports of intestinal tapeworms.

Arthropods include mites, ticks, fleas, lice, and fly larvae, causing diseases such as plague, Lyme disease, and Rocky Mountain spotted fever. They irritate the skin because of the toxins introduced with human skin bites. Arthropods also serve as vectors for some protozoal infections and for dreaded bacterial infections.

Compromised Host

A few infections result directly from the virulence of the infectious agents or its by-products. Most infections result from decreased host defenses. Before an infectious process becomes a disease, a breakdown or impairment must occur in the physical and chemical barriers to bacterial colonization; the inflammatory and febrile response; and the response of the WBCs, including those involved in immunity.

Decreased resistance to infection may result from age, preexisting disease, medical therapy, malnutrition, or stress. Many conditions can compromise the body's anatomic barriers.

BREAKS IN SKIN AND MUCOUS MEMBRANES

Breaks in skin and mucous membranes predispose a person to infection. Both natural and therapeutic processes can alter intact epithelial surfaces. Skin in infants and older adults is thin and more easily broken or penetrated by microorganisms. Some medications, such as steroids, cause thinning of the skin and increase the potential for breakdown.

Surgical intervention and many diagnostic procedures break normal skin integrity, greatly increasing the possibility of infection. Therapeutic procedures invade every epithelial surface. Nasogastric tubes, urinary catheters, suction catheters, and rectal thermometers can cause surface abrasions and also obstruct the natural flow of cleansing fluids.

INVASIVE DEVICES

Any invasive device that enters the body provides a portal of entry for microorganisms, thus increasing the chance for infection. Invasive devices are often used to treat illnesses. Tubes through the skin and body orifices provide microorganisms with direct access to internal organs and the bloodstream. Intravascular lines are inserted to give medications and fluids or to serve as monitoring devices. Urinary catheters or tubes placed in the GI tract for decompression or feeding also increase infection risk. Surgical drains placed postoperatively to promote adequate wound drainage provide an access route for microorganisms into the wound.

STASIS OF BODY FLUIDS

Stagnant secretions in the body provide a warm, moist environment that fosters bacterial growth. Normal defense mechanisms prevent stasis of body fluids, but these can be altered. Tubes inserted into the trachea and drugs that cause sedation can bypass or suppress the normal cough and sneezing clearance of respiratory secretions. Smoking, with the associated inhalation of toxic chemicals, inhibits normal nasopharyngeal ciliary action. Tumors or other obstructions in ducts of exocrine glands hinder the flow of normal secretions, providing a rich medium for microbial growth. Decreased fluid intake, immobility, and urinary tract obstruction foster urinary stasis, increasing the risk of UTI.

INADEQUATE NUTRITION

Malnutrition depresses almost every normal defense to infection. Neutrophil and microphage function is defective, blood levels of complement are low, and both cellular and humoral immune reactions are diminished. When infection occurs, cellular metabolism increases as the body tries to fight it. Because increased metabolism requires increased calories and protein, inadequate protein stores decrease the body's ability to manufacture antibodies and WBCs. A vicious cycle occurs, with increased nutritional needs and decreased body reserves.

STRESS AND HYPERGLYCEMIA

Stress increases greatly when a patient is ill or hospitalized. Physical or emotional stress causes the body to release cortisol, which can increase the risk of infection by suppressing the immune response. Cortisol increases the level of serum glucose, providing a good medium for bacterial growth. The focus on tight glycemic control in the hospitalized patient can help prevent infection and promote postsurgical healing. The metabolic rate increases in periods of stress, depleting energy stores necessary for tissue healing and production of antibodies. Extreme continuous stress causes exhaustion, which limits a person's ability to resist infection.

IMMUNE SYSTEM DYSFUNCTION

The immune system's ability to produce memory cells and antibodies (humoral immunity) or to activate T lymphocytes (cell-mediated immunity) can be impaired in several ways. AIDS can compromise immune function by destroying helper T cells. Cancer can overwhelm the immune or inflammatory components.

COEXISTING MEDICAL PROBLEMS

Cancer, especially if it affects bone marrow production of leukocytes, increases the risk of infection. Cancers such as leukemia may accelerate the rate of leukocyte production, but the cells are immature and ineffective in fighting infection.

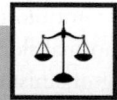

ETHICAL/LEGAL ISSUE

REACTION TO HIV/AIDS

Mabel is a nursing student who has just finished caring for her first HIV-infected patient. The patient is only 25 years old and very ill. When Mabel goes home, she relates to her family her sorrow concerning the patient's poor prognosis. Mabel's father gets very angry and states, "Under no circumstances are you to be taking care of those AIDS patients!" Mabel has always been very respectful, obeying her parents' wishes (especially those of her father). She believes he is being very unreasonable but is unsure how to proceed.

CRITICAL THINKING CHALLENGE

- What factors could have contributed to the father's outburst?
- Identify the conflicting emotions that Mabel may be experiencing.
- Does any healthcare worker have the right to refuse to care for patients with HIV?
- What supports might Mabel use to provide necessary information to her family regarding HIV?

Treatment for many forms of cancer by chemotherapy or radiation may suppress bone marrow and WBC production, affecting the body's ability to resist infection.

Some diseases affect the factors that attract neutrophils and circulating macrophages to the site of infection. This attraction, called chemotaxis, is decreased in diabetes mellitus, cirrhosis, and uremia. Patients with burns have impaired neutrophils that do not ingest and destroy microorganisms efficiently. Because neutrophils release chemical mediators of inflammation, impairment of their number and effectiveness profoundly affects host defenses.

Medical problems that affect blood circulation and nutrient transport can impair host defenses. Cardiovascular conditions, such as peripheral vascular disease or heart failure, can limit the body's ability to supply leukocytes and antibodies to the site of an infection, thus decreasing the infection-fighting potential.

Inflammatory disorders can also increase the risk of infection. The inflammatory response normally helps destroy and contain microbes to prevent systemic infection. Inflammation can be destructive, however, if it impairs vascular control and if the tissue exudate is extensive enough to provide a medium for microbial growth.

DRUG THERAPY

Drug therapy can cause defects in the host's response to infection. Steroids, chemotherapy, antimetabolites, and inappropriate or prolonged use of antibiotics can increase the risk of infection. Superinfection can and often does occur in these situations. For example, if the course of antibiotic administration is prolonged or prematurely stopped or an incorrect antibiotic is chosen, bacterial growth may be stimulated as normal flora in the gut, mouth, and skin is destroyed. Invading organisms can take advantage of the alteration in the normal flora, leading to serious infection in the host.

ALTERED RESISTANCE TO INFECTION

Type of Infection

Being infected and becoming ill are different. Illness results when the infectious agent overcomes the body's defenses and the normal state of health changes. When an obvious complex of symptoms occurs, the infection is called a clinical disease. When the body successfully resists being overwhelmed by the infection, the condition is called subclinical. There may be few symptoms, and the host may be unaware of the exposure, but antigens form that can be recovered from the person's blood.

Colonization is the introduction of microorganisms onto a body surface where they grow and multiply but do not invade the body or cause an immune response or symptoms. The host, if ill or in a vulnerable state, may develop an infection. Infection is described as primary when it occurs in an otherwise healthy person and secondary when it develops in a weakened patient.

LOCAL VERSUS SYSTEMIC

An infection may be localized to a single body area, or it may disseminate to other organs in the body. When it spreads to other body systems, the infection is called systemic. If bacteria spread through the bloodstream, the term **bacteremia** is used. Another term, *septicemia*, is often used as a synonym, but it more accurately refers to microorganisms (or their toxic products) in the bloodstream that are disrupting normal body functions. *Blood poisoning* is a common lay term for infectious agents such as *Staphylococcus* or *Streptococcus* in the blood.

ACUTE VERSUS CHRONIC

An infection may be acute or chronic, depending on the severity and duration of symptoms. An acute infection usually develops rapidly, causes symptoms, climaxes, and then fades fairly quickly. A chronic infection, on the other hand, can linger: Symptoms usually develop more slowly, and convalescence may take months. An acute infection can become chronic when the body cannot rid itself of the organism.

HEALTHCARE-ASSOCIATED INFECTIONS

The term **nosocomial infection**, which means hospital acquired, has been replaced by the more comprehensive term, *healthcare-associated infection*. An HAI is any infection associated with healthcare delivery. At times, symptoms are not apparent until after discharge. This change in terminology is due primarily to the transformation within the healthcare delivery arena to a more community- or outpatient-based approach. Today, many diseases and conditions once treated only in hospitals are now being treated in clinics, rehabilitation facilities, and surgery centers as well as in patient homes by home health nurses.

A person's defenses may be compromised when exposed to the healthcare system due to many reasons. HAIs often result from poor hand hygiene and invasive procedures occurring within the healthcare system. HAIs occur frequently in skilled nursing facilities (SNF), jails, and other residential facilities where auxiliary staff have varied levels of training to care for high-risk individuals.

Individuals in SNF and acute care facilities are often immunocompromised because of chronic diseases, such as diabetes or cancer and invasive procedures, which can predispose them to infection. Treatments such as antibiotic therapy also diminish the patient's ability to fight infection.

The impact of HAIs on healthcare and patients is astronomical. It is estimated the five most common HAIs (central line–associated bloodstream infections [CLABSI], catheter-associated urinary tract infections [CAUTI], ventilator-associated pneumonia [VAP], surgical site infection (SSI), and *Clostridium difficile* infection [CDI]) cost the US healthcare system $9.8 billion annually. HAIs are the fifth leading cause of death in acute care hospitals; up to 15% of patients will develop an HAI while hospitalized (Septimus et al., 2014). Risk factors for common infections, some of which may be healthcare associated, are presented in Box 31-1.

BOX 31-1	Factors Predisposing to Common Infections

Factors Predisposing to Urinary Tract Infection
Factors Increasing Contamination of Urethral Area
- Fecal incontinence
- Atrophic changes (senile vaginitis)
- Wiping back to front

Factors Facilitating Urethral Ascent of Organisms
- Catheterization
- Surgery
- Sexual intercourse
- Pelvic relaxation with aging
- Urethral incompetence (incontinence)
- Diapering incontinent patients

Factors Reducing Flow of Urine
- Outflow obstruction (urethral stricture, prostatic hypertrophy, fecal impaction)
- Neurogenic bladder
- Inadequate fluid intake (dehydration)

Factors Promoting Bacterial Colonization
- Foreign body (tumor, calculi)
- Aging (epithelial cell changes, reduced mucus production, waning immunity)
- Increased urinary glucose (diabetes)

Factors Predisposing to Wound Infection
Local Factors
- Degree of contamination of the wound
- Virulence of contaminating organisms
- Adequacy of local blood supply
- Amount of necrotic or injured tissue in the wound
- Degree of closure of the wound
- Dead spaces, hematomas, and seromas
- Presence and type of foreign bodies
- Location of the wound
- Mechanism of injury

Treatment Factors
- Length of stay in an acute care facility
- Time, type, and thoroughness of treatment
- Duration of operative procedure(s)
- Timeliness and appropriateness of antibiotic administration
- Appropriate surgical closure
- Surgical technique
- Appropriateness of wound dressing
- Nutritional support
- Adequacy of oxygenation and tissue perfusion
- Use of invasive devices for monitoring, drainage, and fluid or nutritional support
- Adequate treatment for coexisting infections

Host Factors
- Age
- General immunologic competence

- Chronic health problems
- Preoperative nutritional status
- Obesity
- Remote infections
- Extent of injury (multiple wounds or extensive surgery)
- Corticosteroid use

Factors Predisposing to Respiratory Infection
Factors Increasing Secretion Production
- Smoking
- Intubation
- Chemical irritation (air pollution, allergies, inhalation anesthetics, aspiration of gastric contents, impaired cough or swallowing mechanisms)

Factors Decreasing Chest Wall Movement
- Pain (chest or abdominal injuries or incisions)
- Obesity
- Abdominal distention
- Tight casts or bandages
- Age
- Skeletal deformities (traumatic or congenital [e.g., scoliosis])

Factors Inhibiting Secretion Clearance
- Weak cough
- Dry, tenacious secretions
- Dehydration
- Chronic lung disease
- Decreased diaphragmatic movement (neurologic deficits, paralysis, muscle weakness)

Factors Depressing the Respiratory Center (Hypoventilation)
- Sedatives
- Opioids
- Altered levels of consciousness (resulting from trauma or cerebrovascular events)
- Acid–base imbalance

Factors Increasing Risk of Microbial Colonization
- Extended hospital stay
- Residence in long-term care facility
- Endotracheal intubation
- Tracheostomy
- Superinfection after long-term use of antibiotics
- Malnutrition
- Primary or acquired immunodeficiency
- Contaminated respiratory equipment
- Steroids
- Immunosuppressive therapy
- Poor personal hygiene practices

SEPSIS

Sepsis is a severe systemic inflammatory response to a documented or suspected infection. Sepsis can progress to septic shock, with hypotension and a high mortality rate if not detected early. Severe sepsis cases in the United States exceed 750,000 cases per year and are reported to be rising. Often, the nurse is the person to identify and report sepsis even before an infection is confirmed. Early presenting symptoms of sepsis are referred to as **systemic inflammatory response syndrome (SIRS)** and include the following:

- Body temperature greater than 38°C or less than 36°C
- Heart rate greater than 90 beats per minute
- Respiratory rate greater than 20 per minute or $PaCO_2$ less than 32 mm Hg
- WBCs greater than 12,000, less than 4,000, or greater than 10% immature forms

Other symptoms to consider include chills, decreased urine output, poor capillary refill, skin mottling, and unexplained change in mental status. Early detection of sepsis saves lives.

Progress of an Infection

The course of an infection that results in a disease state is a dynamic series of events that express competition between the host and the invading organism. Disease usually results from the organism's growth and multiplication inside the host. The exception is when the disease is caused by the release of toxins, as in food poisoning or botulism. The pattern for most diseases follows a predictable course that includes four phases: the incubation period, the prodromal period, acute illness with symptoms, and the convalescent period. The time frame during which a disease can be passed from one person to another is known as the **communicable period**.

INCUBATION PERIOD

The incubation period is the time between the pathogen's entrance into the host and the appearance of symptoms. The length of this period varies depending on the number of organisms absorbed, the time they require to grow and multiply, their virulence, and the host's resistance. The point of entry may also be a factor.

PRODROMAL PERIOD

The prodromal period is characterized by nonspecific symptoms such as nausea, fever, general weakness, or aches and pains. Although prodromal symptoms are nonspecific, the cluster of symptoms and their order of appearance often help in the diagnosis of the disease.

ACUTE PHASE OF ILLNESS

The acute phase of an illness occurs when specific symptoms appear. Depending on the pathogen, there is a cluster of symptoms, and often, laboratory analysis can identify the disease.

The period during which the symptoms subside is included in this phase.

CONVALESCENT PERIOD

Convalescence completes the progress of an infection. The body systems return to normal, and appetite and energy return. Antibodies begin to appear in the person's blood.

Communicable Disease

If the causative agent of the disease is transmissible between one person and another, the disease is said to be a **communicable disease**. If the agent passes with ease from one host to the next, it may be called contagious. Childhood diseases (e.g., measles, mumps, chickenpox) are classic examples of communicable diseases. Not all diseases are contagious. For example, tetanus can be contracted in an isolated event when a person sustains a puncture wound. Infections among patients in healthcare facilities are not necessarily contagious, but because of the large number of patients with lowered host defenses, such infections are more easily transmitted in the facility than they would be in the community.

An infected person may be contagious during the incubation period, prodromal period, acute phase, or convalescent period, depending on whether organisms are being shed into the environment. When the agent is not present in body secretions but is hidden within the host's cells, the infection is called *latent*. The latent period refers to the time between exposure to the organism and the appearance of signs and symptoms. When the agent is being shed from the host's body in respiratory secretions, feces, blood, or urine or is cultured from body tissues, the infection is communicable. The period of communicability begins after the agent has multiplied sufficiently for shedding to begin and lasts as long as the level of shedding is sufficient for transmission. Diseases spread more rapidly if they have a short latent period. The latent period is almost always shorter than is the incubation period; therefore, the infected person usually is shedding microorganisms before any signs and symptoms appear.

Periods of communicability vary with each disease and with the control of microorganisms within the infected person's tissues. Because of the uncertainty of the period of communicability and the lack of identifiable infection in some people, all body secretions should be considered as potentially infectious, necessitating the use of gloves during contact and proper hand hygiene.

Use the concept map (Fig. 31-2) to help understand and manage the opening case scenario patient's situation and to plan for his care.

Manifestations of Infection

The human body has various internal sensors that signal when something is wrong. Often, this inner sense is the first warning of an impending infection. These early warnings include

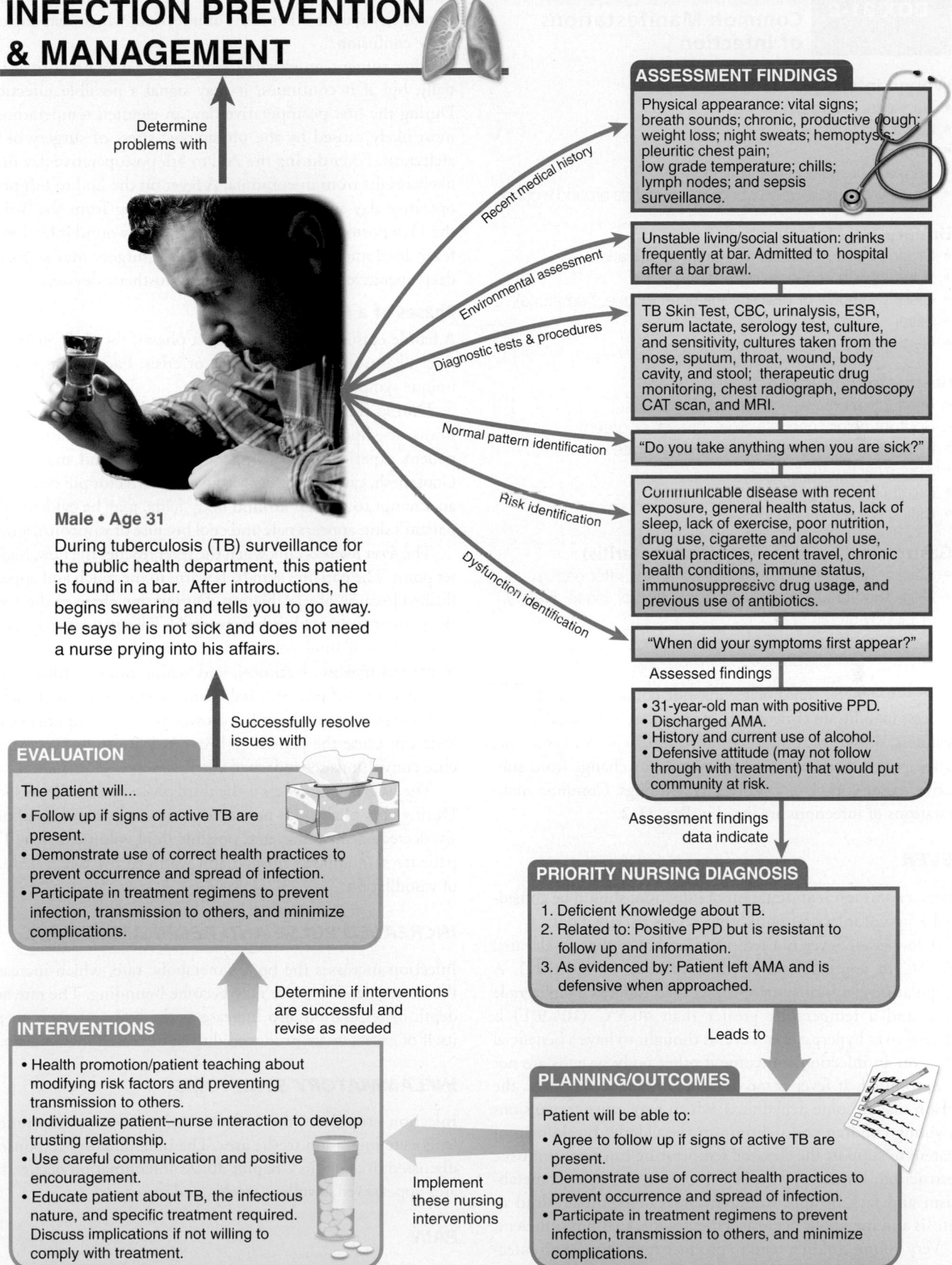

FIGURE 31-2 Concept map for infection prevention and management.

BOX 31-2 Common Manifestations of Infection

Wound Infection
- Redness, swelling, pain
- Localized heat
- Fever
- Purulent or malodorous drainage
- Bruising around incision or induration of area around wound

Urinary Tract Infection
- Urgency and increased frequency of urination
- Burning with urination (dysuria)
- Cloudy, bloody, or malodorous urine (pyuria, hematuria)
- Fever
- Flank pain

Respiratory Infection
- Productive cough
- Sputum color change (yellow, brown, or green)
- Fever, increased pulse and respiratory rate
- Abnormal breath sounds
- Painful breathing (pleuritic chest pain)
- Difficulty in breathing (dyspnea)

Gastrointestinal Infection (gastroenteritis)
- Severe abdominal cramping and nausea after eating
- More than usual number of stools and/or loose, watery, or bloody stools

malaise (a general sense of feeling not completely well), listlessness, inability to concentrate, uneasiness, light-headedness, weakness, muscle or joint discomfort, headache, and anorexia. As the person becomes more ill, symptoms change from subjective, vague complaints to objective findings. Common manifestations of infections are listed in Box 31-2.

FEVER

Fever, a common manifestation of infection, should be considered a sign of infection until other causes are ruled out.

A low-grade fever is a temperature that is slightly elevated (37.1°C to approximately 38.2°C [98.8°F to 100.6°F]). A temperature elevation above 38.2°C is considered a high-grade fever, and a temperature greater than 40.5°C (104.9°F) is referred to as hyperpyrexia. Fever is thought to have a beneficial effect on an infection's outcome if other body systems are not compromised. If fever is too high or prolonged, however, the person may become dehydrated, which may cause convulsions in young children and delirium in the elderly. Breakdown of protein to support the elevated temperature can result in tissue destruction. Protein and fat depletion due to increased metabolism and lack of appetite (anorexia) can eventually lead to ketosis and metabolic acidosis if dietary intake is not sufficient.

Very young children tend to produce high fevers with infection (up to 40°C [104°F]). Conversely, older people may not develop a fever or may produce only a low-grade fever when infection is present. Therefore, it is important with this population to observe for other signs of infection, which may include acute confusion.

After surgery, an elevated temperature may be normal initially, but if it continues, it may signal a possible infection. During the first postoperative day, an elevated temperature is most likely caused by the physiologic stress of surgery or by atelectasis. Fever during the 2nd to 5th postoperative day most likely results from pneumonia. A fever on the 2nd to 8th postoperative day suggests UTI. One occurring from the 3rd to the 11th postoperative day often suggests a wound infection. A fever developing weeks or months after surgery may suggest a deep operative infection or infected prosthetic device.

Phases of a Febrile Episode

A febrile episode has three distinct phases: the chill phase, the fever phase, and the flush phase or crisis. Each phase exhibits unique symptoms.

During the *chill phase*, the body's heat-producing mechanisms attempt to increase the core body temperature. The patient experiences a feeling of being cold and may shiver. Gooseflesh, caused by contraction of the arrector pili muscles in an attempt to trap air around body hairs, may be evident. The patient's skin appears pale and cool because of vasoconstriction.

The *fever phase* occurs when the fever reaches the new, higher set point. The patient's skin feels warm to the touch and appears flushed because of vasodilation. During this phase of the fever, the patient feels neither hot nor cold. The patient may experience thirst if fluid volume deficit has occurred. Complaints of general malaise, weakness, and aching muscles (due to the increased rate of protein catabolism) may be present. In addition, the patient may be either drowsy or restless. An unchecked fever can cause the patient to become delirious and to experience convulsions secondary to cerebral nerve cell irritation.

The *flush* or *crisis phase* is the third phase in a febrile episode. During this phase, the patient experiences profuse diaphoresis, decreased shivering, and possible fluid volume deficit. The patient's skin appears flushed and warm to the touch because of vasodilation.

INCREASED PULSE AND RESPIRATORY RATE

Infection increases the body's metabolic rate, which increases the heart rate. The pulse may become bounding. The rate and depth of respiration also increase as the body attempts to rid itself of excess waste produced during increased metabolism.

INFLAMMATORY SYMPTOMS

Infection stimulates the inflammatory response to promote leukocyte migration to the area. The inflammatory response is discussed in detail in Chapter 30. As inflammation occurs, the area appears red, swollen, tender, and warm.

PAIN

Most infections cause discomfort. Pain can occur when inflammation causes swelling within an enclosed area or when normal function is impeded. Examples of pain caused by infection include the following:

- Pleuritic pain when breathing with a respiratory infection
- Burning on voiding with a UTI
- Pain on swallowing with a streptococcal throat infection
- Pain at the incision site with a surgical site infection

PURULENT DRAINAGE

As WBCs migrate to the infection, **purulent** (containing pus) drainage may be observed. Because of the increased numbers of WBCs, body fluids such as urine or sputum may become cloudy or whitish-yellow. Purulent drainage is usually thicker than normal and is often foul smelling because it contains a great deal of cellular debris from the inflammatory response. An **abscess** occurs when the body attempts to localize infection by walling off the purulent drainage.

ENLARGED LYMPH NODES

During an infection, the lymph nodes that drain an infected area may become enlarged and easily palpable ("swollen glands"). As the swelling increases, the nodes may also become tender. During inflammation, the lymphatic capillaries dilate as excess interstitial fluid, proteins, and invading microorganisms enter the lymphatic system. The swelling indicates that lymphocytes and macrophages in the lymph node are fighting the infection and trying to limit its spread.

RASH

A rash may occur with primary infections of the skin (e.g., impetigo) but also may accompany some generalized infectious diseases. The diagnosis of many communicable childhood diseases is made on the specific characteristics of the rash. Many rashes cause pruritus (itching). Scratching may disrupt the skin's integrity, possibly resulting in secondary skin infections.

GASTROINTESTINAL SYMPTOMS

Viruses, bacteria, and toxins produced by certain bacteria and parasites may cause acute GI inflammation. Anorexia, nausea, and vomiting may occur when the stomach lining is inflamed; diarrhea is more common when the small or large intestine is inflamed.

"Traveler's diarrhea" may occur when tourists drink water or eat uncooked food that contains endemic bacteria or parasites. Travelers have little previous exposure to these microorganisms, so they have limited antibodies to fight the infectious agent.

ASSESSMENT

Normal Pattern Identification

Information about the patient's normal defense system against illness is important (Box 31-3). Ask the patient or caregiver about measures that are normally taken to avoid illness,

---

| BOX 31-3 | Health Interview Information |

- Immunization history, history of exposure to communicable diseases, and any recent acute infections
- Chronic diseases that have been complicated by infections and the usual method of treatment; signs and symptoms experienced and medications used
- Medications or medical therapy the patient is receiving (e.g., antibiotics, steroids, immunosuppression drugs, chemotherapy, or radiation therapy)
- Patient's usual diet and its nutritional adequacy
- Patient's patterns of sleep, exercise, and recreation to determine health beliefs and lifestyle factors that may contribute to the risk of infection
- History of nausea, vomiting, diarrhea, anorexia, general malaise, muscle aches, or headaches

---

including the patient's usual pattern of rest and exercise; nutrition; use of vitamins, herbs, and folk remedies; and understanding of germ exposure. Obtain a history of immunizations and determine whether it is complete and current. A description of the patient's usual experience of illness, including childhood diseases, provides valuable data to determine whether the pattern is normal.

Risk Identification

Closely screen the patient for infection risk, and document any recent exposure to infectious illness. Sometimes this means asking questions such as "Has anyone in your immediate family recently been infected with [specify disease]?" Consider school records and community documentation of infectious disease outbreaks in evaluating each patient for risk. Include questions about the patient's general health, such as normal sleep and exercise patterns; nutritional history; use of drugs, cigarettes, or alcohol; and sexual practices. Note any recent travel, especially to foreign counties. Explore any chronic health conditions, such as heart disease, lung disease, or diabetes, and their treatment. Determine whether the patient has received chemotherapy or radiation because such treatments often increase the risk of infection by suppressing the immune system. Also, obtain a medication history, focusing on immunosuppressive drugs (e.g., steroids) and current or previous use of antibiotics.

Dysfunction Identification

If infection was a reason the patient sought medical assistance, questions should elicit more specific information:

- How long has the infection been present?
- What symptoms first occurred?
- How does the infection affect your ability to perform activities of daily living?

If infection was not a reason the patient sought advice but the patient has symptoms of infection, address the following:

● Do you have any pain, redness, swelling, or abnormal drainage? When did it start? How long has it lasted? What is its intensity?
● Do you have a fever? If so, when did it start? Describe the pattern.
● Are you experiencing any nausea, vomiting, diarrhea, malaise, or general aches and pains (symptoms that accompany many viral infections)?
● Are you experiencing any wheezing or coughing? Is the cough dry or productive? Describe the color and consistency of the sputum.

The incidence of MRSA is increasing, both in the community and in healthcare settings. Many healthcare organizations have begun screening all patients for MRSA on admission to the facility in order to prevent the spread of MRSA to other patients. Determine if the patient has had a positive culture for MRSA in the past. If so, the patient may be placed in isolation until two separate negative cultures are obtained.

The nursing history and identifying infection promptly allow appropriate infection control practices to be instituted. The nursing history (as opposed to the medical history) also focuses on how the infection has affected the patient's ability to function normally and to perform usual activities and routines.

Physical Assessment

GENERAL INSPECTION

Determine whether the patient is comfortable or in obvious pain. Detect any signs of fatigue in the patient's posture and movement. Look for abnormal skin color, rashes or lesions, and any swelling and signs of inflammation.

VITAL SIGNS

Assess vital signs frequently to detect infection or to monitor its progress. The accuracy of such assessment is important in determining if infection is present. In a patient with an infection, look for elevations in temperature (above 38.4°C [101°F]), pulse rate, and respiratory rate.

Evaluate the significance of vital sign changes by comparing them to baseline values. If one vital sign is outside normal limits, make sure to check all vital signs. Consider other factors that could be responsible. Look at the pattern of changes in vital signs. A consistently elevated and rising temperature is significant. Usually, the physician obtains cultures and begins to look for the source of a possible infection when the temperature rises above 38.4°C (101°F). Older adults and immunosuppressed patients may not show a fever with infection.

AUSCULTATION OF BREATH SOUNDS

Auscultation of breath sounds can help detect respiratory infections. Pneumonia can alter normal breath sounds, producing crackles (rales), rhonchi, and wheezes. Atelectasis, which can predispose a patient to respiratory infection, is noted by crackles or diminished breath sounds.

 APPLY YOUR CRITICAL THINKING

Mr. Foscarelli, a 76-year-old patient with asthma, is recovering from abdominal surgery. He is having moderate incisional pain and is reluctant to move because of the pain. Your morning assessment reveals vital signs as follows: temperature 38°C, B/P 142/64, P 96, and R 26 and shallow. He appears slightly confused and has developed a productive cough of thick, tan sputum. Lung auscultation reveals diminished breath sounds with rhonchi in the right middle lobe. His urine is clear, and the output is good.

What risk factors does Mr. Foscarelli have for infection? What data support the presence of infection? What type of infection seems most likely? What laboratory tests would you expect the primary care provider to order?

Check your answers in Appendix B.

AUSCULTATION OF BOWEL SOUNDS

Auscultation of bowel sounds can help detect increased intestinal peristalsis. Increased peristalsis often accompanies microbial irritation of the gut, which can cause diarrhea and cramping.

PALPATION OF LYMPH NODES

Lymph nodes can enlarge and become tender because of localized or systemic infection. Gently palpate, using the tips of the middle three fingers, to detect any enlargement in lymph nodes. Normally, cervical lymph nodes are smaller than 1 cm in diameter, soft, and mobile. Note any tenderness during palpation.

SEPSIS SURVEILLANCE

The nurse is responsible for detecting possible sepsis by analyzing signs and symptoms present in the patient. Early recognition is essential to decrease morbidity and mortality. Screening for signs or symptoms of SIRS, detailed in the box titled Evidence-Based Bundles to Improve Patient Care: Recommendations Regarding Sepsis, is important to detect potential sepsis quickly so that interventions can save lives. Early detection and prompt intervention is the key. Often, the nurse is the health team member who first recognizes SIRS in patients and reports it to the physician so that the sepsis bundle can be started.

Diagnostic Tests and Procedures

Because clinical signs sometimes provide insufficient evidence to identify a pathogen, diagnostic procedures are used to detect and identify an infection's source. Laboratory analysis, culturing of body fluids, radiographic studies, and other imaging methods are used. Antibiotic sensitivities and therapeutic drug monitoring are used to identify optimal drug therapy. The following are common studies included in an initial workup for infection:

- Complete blood count (CBC) including hemoglobin, hematocrit, and WBC count

- Urinalysis
- Erythrocyte sedimentation rate (ESR or sed rate)

If infection is strongly suspected, the physician may also order a series of WBC counts with differentials and body fluid cultures and sensitivities. If sepsis is suspected, a lactate level is drawn.

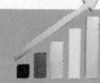

EVIDENCE-BASED BUNDLES TO IMPROVE PATIENT CARE
Recommendations Regarding Sepsis

BACKGROUND

The mortality associated with severe sepsis is approximately 30% to 50%. Severe sepsis is defined as sepsis plus sepsis-induced organ dysfunction or tissue hypoperfusion (Dellinger et al., 2012). Severe sepsis and septic shock affect millions around the world, killing one in four (Dellinger et al., 2012).

In 2003, critical care and infectious disease experts representing 11 international organizations developed management guidelines for severe sepsis and septic shock for the bedside clinician. The group published these guidelines in 2004 under the auspices of the Surviving Sepsis Campaign and teamed up with the Institute for Healthcare Improvement (IHI) to increase awareness and improve outcomes in severe sepsis. Updates to these guidelines were published in 2008 and 2012 (Dellinger et al., 2012).

Early Recognition of Sepsis

The presenting symptoms of sepsis have been termed the SIRS. Patients who manifest two of the four following criteria are considered to have SIRS and require intervention:

1. Body temperature greater than 38°C or less than 36°C
2. Heart rate greater than 90 beats per minute
3. Respiratory rate greater than 20 per minute or $PaCO_2$ less than 32 mm Hg
4. WBCs greater than 12,000, less than 4,000, or greater than 10% immature forms

Other symptoms to consider include chills, decreased urine output, poor capillary refill, skin mottling, and unexplained change in mental status.

NURSING IMPLICATIONS
- Early recognition of SIRS is critical.
- Alert the healthcare team if the patient exhibits two of the four criteria.
- Work diligently to reduce the patient's risk of sepsis—maintaining universal precautions, enforcing infection control measures, and vigilantly monitoring changes in physical assessment.
- Anticipate activation of the severe sepsis resuscitation bundle.

The severe sepsis resuscitation bundle describes seven tasks that should be accomplished within the first 6 hours of presentation for patients with severe sepsis or septic shock. A bundle is a group of interventions related to a disease process that, when executed together, result in better outcomes than when implemented individually.

KEY COMPONENTS OF THE SEVERE SEPSIS RESUSCITATION BUNDLE

1. Serum lactate measured.

Hyperlactemia is often present in patients with severe sepsis and may be secondary to anaerobic metabolism due to hypoperfusion. Obtaining serum lactate is essential to identifying tissue hypoperfusion in patients who are not yet hypotensive but who are at risk for septic shock.

NURSING IMPLICATIONS
- All patients with elevated lactate greater than 4 mmol per liter will enter the early goal-directed therapy for the severe sepsis resuscitation bundle, regardless of blood pressure.

2. Obtain blood cultures prior to antibiotic administration.

Collecting blood cultures prior to antibiotic therapy offers the best hope of identifying the organism causing severe sepsis.

NURSING IMPLICATIONS
- Two or more blood cultures are recommended.
- Patients with a central line in place should have one set of cultures from the central line and a second set drawn from a peripheral site.
- Blood cultures should be obtained as soon as possible after the onset of fever or chills.

(Continued)

EVIDENCE-BASED BUNDLES TO IMPROVE PATIENT CARE (*Continued*)
Recommendations Regarding Sepsis

3. From the time of presentation, broad-spectrum antibiotics should be *administered* within 3 hours for emergency department admissions and 1 hour for nonemergency department ICU admissions.

Evidence suggests that early administration of appropriate antibiotics reduces mortality in patients with Gram-positive and Gram-negative bacteremia.

NURSING	◆ Assure that antibiotic orders are sent to pharmacy noting first dose STAT (to be given immediately) in the patient with sepsis.
IMPLICATIONS	◆ Administer antibiotic as soon as it arrives on the unit.
	◆ Anticipate possible transfer of the patient to the ICU for increased monitoring.

4. **In the event of hypotension and/or lactate greater than 4 mmol per liter, deliver an IV fluid challenge.**

NURSING	◆ Fluid resuscitation should be started as early as possible in the septic patient, even prior to ICU admission.
IMPLICATIONS	◆ During a fluid challenge, large amounts of fluid may be administered intravenously over a short period under close monitoring to evaluate the patient's response.
	◆ A fluid challenge is not the equivalent to increasing the rate of maintenance fluid.
	◆ Fluid challenges require the following components:

   a. Type of fluid administered (crystalloids or colloids)
   b. Rate of infusion (500 to 1,000 mL over 30 minutes)
   c. End points (mean arterial pressure greater than 70 mm Hg, heart rate less than 110 beats per minute)
   d. Safety factor (development of pulmonary edema)

The following components must happen in the ICU:

5. **Apply vasopressors for hypotension not responding to initial fluid resuscitation to maintain mean arterial pressure greater than 65 mm Hg.**
6. **Achieve central venous pressure greater than 8 mm Hg.**
7. **Achieve central venous oxygen saturation (ScvO$_2$) of 70%.**

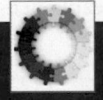

COLLABORATING WITH THE HEALTHCARE TEAM
Notifying a Physician of Signs of Possible Sepsis

Mrs. Chow, an 84-year-old widow, is 3 days post colon resection. The night nurse reported that her temperature was elevated (38.6°C), B/P 102/68, pulse 92, and RR 18 as compared with her baseline 130/80, 80, and 18. She still has no active bowel tones and received 1,000 mL of IV fluids during the night shift with urine output of 230 mL. Her blood glucose was 260 mg/dL, for which she received additional insulin. You note the vital signs that the nursing assistant took 30 minutes ago: 38.6°C, 96/62, 98, and 22. You decide to call the physician to report Mrs. Chow's status.

SITUATION: I am calling about Mrs. Chow in room 345 who had a colon resection 3 days ago.

BACKGROUND: Her temperature is 38.6°C for the last 6 hours. It was just taken and is up to 38.8°C. Her blood pressure is much lower than baseline, currently only 96/62 with minimal urine output of 230 mL over the last 8 hours. Her glucose was 260, for which she received 8 units of regular insulin.

ASSESSMENT: I am concerned that Mrs. Chow might have a serious infection or even may be becoming septic. She has symptoms of SIRS, including elevated temperature, elevated heart rate, and decreased urine output.

RECOMMENDATION: Could you please come evaluate Mrs. Chow right away? If you are not able to come soon, could you give me an order for an IV saline bolus to stabilize her blood pressure and see if that will increase her output? I could also draw labs (e.g., CBC and lactate) if you want.

CRITICAL THINKING CHALLENGE
- What risk factors does Mrs. Chow have for sepsis?
- Are there additional assessment data that would be helpful to have in this situation?
- What rationale would you use for asking the physician to come "right away" to evaluate Mrs. Chow?
- Why did the nurse request an IV fluid bolus for Mrs. Chow?

WHITE BLOOD CELL COUNT

The number of WBCs, or leukocytes, rises in response to infection, tissue necrosis, stress, or neoplastic changes in bone marrow. A rise in circulating WBCs above the normal adult range of 5,000 to 10,000 cells/mm³ is called **leukocytosis**. Infectious processes may be discovered by examining the WBCs and differentiating the cell types. Each type is based on a percentage of the total number.

Neutrophils normally comprise about 50% to 70% of all WBCs. Their numbers increase during infection. If the infection is severe or prolonged, the body cannot manufacture neutrophils quickly enough, resulting in the release of immature granulocytes (also called bands) into the blood. This increase in the number of immature cells is called a **shift to the left**, or leftward shift in the granulocytic differential count. A leftward shift is considered a strong indication of bacterial infection; the greater the leftward shift, the more worrisome the infection appears. When the proportion of neutrophils increases, the patient's resistance is good and the body is considered to be fighting the infection well.

Neutrophil counts below 2,000/mm³, often associated with cancer or chemotherapy, greatly increase infection risk. When the actual number of neutrophils, known as the absolute neutrophil count (ANC), is below 1,000/mm³, there is significant increase in the risk of infection. If the ANC falls below 500/mm³, the risk substantially increases.

Patients are instructed to institute measures to prevent possible lethal infections, including good personal hygiene and avoiding contact with infectious agents or individuals with infectious diseases. Common signs of infection are often caused by the actions by neutrophils, so when neutrophil counts are very low, symptoms of infection may be absent.

Some patients, such as those who are malnourished, elderly, immunosuppressed, or taking steroids, cannot produce more WBCs in response to an infection. In such cases, the absence of an increase in total WBCs or a lack of clarity on the differential count does not rule out infection.

ERYTHROCYTE SEDIMENTATION RATE

The erythrocyte sedimentation rate (ESR) measures, in millimeters per hour, the rate at which red blood cells (RBCs) settle in unclotted blood. The result is elevated in acute noninfectious inflammatory conditions and in infectious processes. Collagen disease, tissue necrosis, malignancy, or stress can also increase the rate of sedimentation. This test is most commonly used to provide a crude estimate of a disease process or of the response to therapy and is most helpful when used in conjunction with other lab tests, clinical findings, and the patient's health history. Because drugs and other factors affect the ESR, all medications the patient is taking should be brought to the laboratory's attention.

LACTATE LEVEL

Lactic acid, present in blood as lactate, is a by-product of metabolism that is usually metabolized in the liver. Normal levels are 0.3 to 2.6 mmol per liter. In sepsis, lactate levels increase secondary to anaerobic metabolism due to hypoperfusion. Obtaining a serum lactate level is essential to identify tissue hypoperfusion in patients who are not yet hypotensive but who are at risk for septic shock. All patients with lactate values of more than 4 mmol per liter should be treated with the severe sepsis resuscitation bundle (see the Evidence-Based Bundles to Improve Patient Care display in this chapter), regardless of blood pressure.

SEROLOGY TESTS

Serology tests that detect antigen–antibody reactions are sometimes done as part of a diagnostic workup for a fever. Early in an infection's course, an acute-phase blood specimen is collected. If the cause of the infection is not determined by the 3rd week, a convalescent-phase specimen is obtained, and both specimens are examined simultaneously for a change in antibody titer. The laboratory needs to know the patient's clinical signs and symptoms and immunization history. By comparing antigen–antibody reactions between the two specimens, a diagnosis can be made.

CULTURE, SENSITIVITY, AND MINIMUM INHIBITORY CONCENTRATION

Cultures are obtained from body fluids to isolate the source of unknown fevers and to identify the microorganism causing signs of clinical infection. Culture specimens are obtained from blood, sputum, stool, throat, wound exudate, urine or from spinal, joint, pleural, or other body cavity fluids.

Specimens are sent to the laboratory for Gram staining and culture and sensitivity results. Gram stains, when properly prepared, broadly classify the microorganisms. This information may be used to order antibiotic therapy while waiting for specific culture results. Results of Gram stains can be obtained from the laboratory in less than 30 minutes. Usually, 24 to 36 hours is required to grow good cultures, and 48 hours is needed to obtain growth and sensitivity results.

Sensitivity testing of microorganisms to antibiotics is a benefit of obtaining good culture specimens. After microorganisms are grown in culture media, various concentrations of antibiotics are used to test their ability to inhibit growth or to kill the organism. The laboratory reports the names of the organisms present and whether they are sensitive or resistant to specific antibiotics. A helpful way to report this information is the **minimum inhibitory concentration (MIC)**, which quantifies the minimal amount of the drug that is necessary to inhibit microbial growth in the laboratory. Use of the MIC permits primary healthcare providers to select antibiotics that can kill the organism with a concentration that will not be toxic to the patient. This approach is also beneficial for reducing the proliferation of MDROs because it narrows the therapeutic range and avoids prolonged use (CDC, 2006). The serum level of the drug is usually kept above the MIC value.

The accuracy of laboratory analysis for all cultures is only as good as the specimen provided. Factors affecting the results of the analysis include the following:

- Contamination of the specimen
- Delay in sending the specimen to the laboratory (which increases the growth of contaminating organisms and causes deterioration of the constituents to be examined)
- Use of inappropriate containers and/or culture media
- Failure to identify the source of the specimen
- Failure to tell the laboratory about current patient medications (e.g., antibiotics) that may affect the analysis

Always correctly identify the patient using two identifiers, and label the specimen container. Elicit the patient's cooperation by explaining why the specimen is being obtained. Obtain specimens before starting administration of antibiotics that could alter the results. Label the specimen with the patient's name, medical record number, time, date, and site of collection, and send it to the laboratory immediately.

SAFETY ALERT

When obtaining cultures, use aseptic techniques and wear gloves to avoid potential transmission of pathogens.

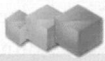

Concept Mastery Alert

It is unnecessary to wear sterile gloves when obtaining a wound culture since there is no intended contact between the nurse's hands and the wound bed or the swab. However, it is important to wear clean gloves because of the risk for contact with blood and body fluids.

Blood Cultures

Blood cultures are ordered when a high degree of suspicion exists that an infectious process is occurring in the bloodstream. Blood cultures are usually obtained from two separate venipuncture sites. Because indwelling intravascular lines may be contaminated with surface pathogens, blood is not usually drawn for culture from previously inserted lines. The ideal specimen is drawn just before or during the rise in temperature because the pathogens are usually circulating in high concentrations at that time.

Obtaining a blood culture requires use of a set of culture bottles, a sterile syringe, two sterile needles, skin preparation equipment, and a tourniquet. The skin is cleaned according to the institution's procedure. Usually, a combination preparation of chlorhexidine gluconate and alcohol or chlorhexidine gluconate alone is recommended. Clean the tops of the culture bottles, and allow them to dry. Apply gloves and then use the sterile needle and syringe to aspirate blood. Change the needle before inoculating the culture medium into special vacuum

bottles. After ensuring hemostasis at the puncture site, remove the gloves and wash your hands before transporting the specimen to the laboratory.

Nasal Swab Culture

Nasal swabs are commonly used to detect organisms such as *Staphylococcus aureus*, a common bacterium that lives on skin, in skinfolds, and in the nose. It usually survives in these areas without causing infection, a state known as colonization. Given the right environment and circumstances for bacteria multiplication, the colonized bacteria can multiply to a point that will cause a symptomatic infection.

Sputum Culture

Sputum cultures are obtained in a fever workup when the patient has a productive cough. Because infections may be located in either the upper or lower respiratory tract, a good culture specimen should not contain saliva (saliva and postnasal drip secretions contaminate the specimen). Sputum ideally should be obtained in the morning, before the patient eats. Collect the specimen in a sterile container with a lid, and transport it to the laboratory as soon as it is obtained (unless it is a 24-hour specimen, which usually is placed in a special fixative). Refer to Procedure 26-2 for guidelines on obtaining a sputum culture.

Occasionally, a patient cannot cooperate with sputum specimen collection or a specimen must be obtained from a patient who is endotracheally intubated. Obtain the specimen by suctioning with a sterile suction catheter by way of the nasotracheal or endotracheal route. The physician may also elect to perform a bronchoscopy or to insert a small catheter through a needle into the trachea to aspirate secretions transtracheally. Again, transport specimens to the laboratory immediately.

Throat Culture

Throat cultures are obtained with a sterile cotton swab that is touched to the back of the throat as the patient says "Aaahh." Perform this procedure as quickly as possible because it may trigger the gag reflex. Maintaining sterility, place the swab into a culture medium and transport it to the laboratory.

Wound Culture

Wound cultures are taken when signs of local inflammation or purulent drainage from the wound are noted (**Procedure 31-1**). Suitable culture media kits are used; they differ depending on whether the wound is being cultured for aerobic or anaerobic organisms.

Body Cavity and Fluid Culture

Body cavity and fluid cultures are obtained with the use of aseptic technique when inflammation in the area is indicated. Spinal, joint, and pleural cavity fluids are commonly cultured for microorganisms based on clinical observations and a high index of suspicion for an infectious process. Special kits are available, and sterile technique is always used. Assist the physician in obtaining these specimens by ordering supplies, positioning and draping the patient, and ensuring rapid transport of specimens to the laboratory.

Stool Culture

Stool cultures may be ordered to rule out infectious causes of diarrhea. Cultures are usually necessary to examine the stool for leukocytes and to identify enteric bacterial or fungal pathogens. Parasites, another common cause of diarrhea, lay eggs in the GI tract that can be detected on examination. Usually, when a patient is being screened for parasitic infection, stool specimens are collected daily for 3 days. Moving organisms can easily be detected in fresh specimens.

Collect stool specimens in a sterile bedpan, and transfer the specimens to a sterile container with a sterile tongue blade. On the laboratory form, identify the test required, the organism being screened, and whether the patient has been traveling or backpacking in remote areas. Urine, toilet paper, soap, disinfectants, antibiotics, antacids, barium, laxatives, enemas, and cool temperatures can affect stool specimens.

URINALYSIS

The urine is routinely examined to check for kidney and endocrine function and to identify UTI. Urinalysis provides information about the color, pH, specific gravity, and protein, glucose, and ketones in the urine. Microscopic examinations search for casts, RBCs and WBCs, epithelial cells, and bacteria. Changes in color, concentration, or odor of the urine may indicate an infectious process. Alkaline urine (pH > 8) may indicate bacteriuria. High levels of glucose and protein may indicate systemic infection or UTI. Erythrocytes (RBCs) or their cellular casts may indicate infection but also may be caused by noninfectious inflammatory conditions. Large numbers of WBCs in the urine usually indicate a UTI. A clean-catch or midstream urine specimen is requested if more than four WBCs are found or if bacteria are seen on the slide made from the urine sample. See Chapter 32 for more information on collecting urine samples.

THERAPEUTIC DRUG MONITORING

Drug monitoring is used to determine a drug's concentration in blood. Blood levels of antibiotics are tested to avoid possible toxic effects such as renal damage (nephrotoxicity) or eighth cranial nerve damage (ototoxicity). The timing of specimen collection is of critical importance. For the laboratory and physician to interpret the plasma drug level, they must know when the last dose of antibiotic was given and when the specimen was obtained. The highest level of drug concentration (*peak level*) should occur shortly after the drug is given, and the lowest level (*trough level*) should occur just before a dose is due to be administered. Specimens must be labeled as to whether they are being analyzed as a peak or a trough specimen. Depending on the test results, the amount of the antibiotic and the frequency of dosing may be adjusted to match the patient's rate of metabolism and drug clearance.

DIAGNOSTIC IMAGING

Medical advances have made possible the ability to visualize and scan internal organs and to evaluate them for infection. After these tests, monitor vital signs. When contrast material is used, observe for any signs of allergic reaction.

Chest radiographs are used to diagnose pneumonia, lung abscesses, and TB. Endoscopic procedures are used to visualize the respiratory and GI tracts and to obtain specimens for microbiologic testing. Computed axial tomography (CAT scan, or more commonly CT scan) is used to obtain multidimensional images of the body, which the computer interprets to construct images of internal structures. By visualizing the differences in density among organs and any organ deformities, the study can help locate abscesses or other areas of infection. The study can be done with the use of contrast medium, which enhances visualization of normal versus abnormal tissue.

Magnetic resonance imaging (MRI) is used with increasing frequency to detect infections of the nervous system. The procedure uses opaque contrast materials, injected intravenously, that have affinities for concentrations of WBCs in abscesses or other areas of infection.

 SAFETY ALERT

Because the MRI machine contains a very powerful magnet, metal objects must stay outside the room.

NURSING DIAGNOSES

Risk for Infection is the only nursing diagnosis related to infection that is accepted by NANDA-International (NANDA-I, 2014). Hyperthermia is a nursing diagnosis that may be used for patients with fever. If a patient has an actual infection, the problem is collaborative, necessitating intervention from nurses, physicians, pharmacists, and other members of the healthcare team. Nurses can independently develop individualized plans to help prevent infection for patients at risk by attempting to minimize introduction of organisms or to increase resistance, such as by improving nutritional status. Table 31-3 outlines these nursing diagnoses along with Nursing Outcomes Classification (NOC) and Nursing Interventions Classification (NIC).

Other nursing diagnoses are common in people with infection. Deficient Knowledge may occur, and inadequate knowledge of hygiene or infection control measures can contribute to increased incidence of infection. Many patients with infection are discharged with new treatments and protocols to master. Impaired Comfort and Fatigue are other common nursing diagnoses associated with infection. Depending on its location, infection can affect the function of various body systems.

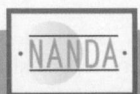

Table 31-3   SELECTED NANDA-I NURSING DIAGNOSES INVOLVING INFECTION

Nursing Dx	Risk/Related Factors	Dx Statement	NOC*	NIC†
Risk for Infection— Vulnerable to invasion and multiplication of pathogenic organisms that may compromise health	Chronic disease, inadequate vaccination, inadequate primary or secondary defenses, increased exposure to pathogens, immunosuppression, insufficient knowledge, malnutrition, trauma	Risk for Infection R/T malnutrition, chemotherapy, and the presence of invasive lines and catheters	Risk Control: infectious process and STI, Immune Status, Immunization Behavior, Knowledge: Infection Management, Infection Severity, Wound Healing; primary and secondary intention	Immunization/Vaccination Management, Infection Control, Infection Protection, Surveillance, Vital Signs Monitoring, Infection Control: Intraoperative, Health Education, Teaching: Safe Sex
Hyperthermia—Core body temperature elevated above normal range due to a failure of thermoregulation	Illness, trauma, medications, increased metabolic rate, anesthesia, dehydration	Hyperthermia R/T fever, increased metabolic rate, and wound infection AEB flushing and temperature above 39°C	Infection control, Thermoregulation, Vital Signs, Hydration, Comfort Status	Fever Treatment, hypothermia induction and Treatment, Temperature Regulation

Dx, diagnosis; AEB as evidenced by; R/T, related to; STI, disease to infection.
*From: Moorhead, S., Johnson, M., Maas, M., & Swanson, E. (2013). *Iowa Outcomes Project: Nursing Outcomes Classification (NOC)* (5th ed.). St. Louis, MO: C. V. Mosby.
†From: Bulecheck, G., Butcher, H., Dochterman, J., & Wagner, C. (2013). *Iowa Intervention Project: Nursing Interventions Classification (NIC)* (5th ed.). St. Louis, MO: Elsevier Mosby.
From: NANDA-International (NANDA-I). (2014). *Nursing diagnoses: Definitions and classification, 2015–2017.* West Sussex, UK: Wiley-Blackwell.

OUTCOME IDENTIFICATION AND PLANNING

Patient goals and outcome criteria focus on preventing infections, increasing knowledge about infection and the treatment, controlling fever and related discomforts, and minimizing potential complications. Examples of patient goals related to infection include the following:

- The patient or caregiver will demonstrate adequate knowledge to recognize and report signs of infection.
- The patient or caregiver will demonstrate use of good health practices to prevent occurrence and spread of infection.
- The patient will participate in treatment regimens to prevent or treat infection and minimize complications.

Planning for nursing interventions is directed at the following:

- Controlling the spread of infection
- Providing education to modify risk behaviors
- Supporting normal defense mechanisms and behaviors that prevent infection
- Reducing or eliminating the adverse effects of infection on functional abilities
- Detecting behaviors that increase the potential for infection
- Participating in community planning and activities for infection prevention

IMPLEMENTATION

Health Promotion

PERSONAL HYGIENE

Decreasing the number of microorganisms present on body surfaces can help prevent and fight infection. Encourage patients to wash their hands after using the toilet, before eating, and after coming in contact with articles likely to be contaminated. Regular bathing, shampooing, and general grooming help keep body surfaces clean. In some instances, such as before surgery, antimicrobial soap may be used to impede microbial growth.

SAFETY ALERT

Hand hygiene is the most significant measure to decrease the transient growth of microorganisms.

Daily brushing and flossing of teeth remove microorganisms that collect in the oral cavity. Regular dental checkups are important to remove plaque and tartar, which provide good foci for bacterial growth.

PROTECTION OF SKIN AND MUCOUS MEMBRANES

Intact skin and mucous membranes provide a physical barrier against invasion from possible pathogens. Encourage patients to prevent excessive drying of skin by ensuring adequate hydration and applying lubricants or cream. They should use a water-soluble lubricant applied to the nares or lips to prevent cracking. After bathing, be sure all areas are thoroughly dried, paying particular attention to skinfolds where maceration is likely to occur and fungal infections develop. Avoid trauma that could impair skin integrity. Remind patients to avoid harsh chemicals and excessive heat or friction that can abrade skin.

For bedridden patients, establish regular turning schedules to decrease the chance of skin breakdown and possible infection. Use specialized equipment such as low-air-loss beds or special mattresses for high-risk immobile patients.

REST AND RELAXATION

Adequate rest and freedom from stress are important in fighting and preventing infection. Sleep disturbances can occur when patients must be awakened at night. Keep the environment quiet and comfortable to induce sleep. Allow naps during the day as needed. Encourage activities that promote relaxation and reduce stress.

NUTRITION AND HYDRATION

A well-balanced diet and adequate hydration are important to maintain adequate host defenses against infection. The body's ability to synthesize antibodies, which are proteins, becomes ineffective if protein stores are depleted. Encourage foods that are rich in vitamins and minerals, such as fruits and vegetables. Consumption of eight glasses of water per day ensures adequate hydration, which helps maintain healthy skin and urine flow.

IMMUNIZATION PROGRAMS

Nurses participate in establishing programs for people to receive immunizations. They help to identify outbreaks of infectious disease in the community, give vaccinations, establish record-keeping mechanisms, and counsel people about precautions and possible complications of immunization. Many vaccination programs take place in clinics, schools, and industrial settings.

Immunizations may be given by injection, oral solution, or nasal spray. To avoid multiple injections, they are given in combination (when the compounds are stable and minimal danger exists of overwhelming the immune system). Booster injections of some vaccines are given throughout the life span to stimulate the memory cells. Guidelines for immunizations of a healthy infants, children, and adults are approved by the CDC's ACIP (CDC, 2014b). Because of frequent changes, new immunization guidelines must be obtained yearly. This information is available from the ACIP, the American Academy of Pediatrics, and the American Academy of Family Physicians. Similar committees exist in Canada and for the World Health Organization (WHO).

Encourage parents to maintain immunization records for their children and to give them to their children when they move away from home. Physicians need to record this information and make patients aware of any unusual reaction. Commonly, families maintain excellent vaccination records for children through their first years of school but then neglect to update records as children grow older. Children may need this information if questions arise about whether immunizations are current (especially for tetanus after an injury).

Vaccinations are contraindicated in patients with immunodeficiency states, an allergy to eggs, a history of previous allergic reactions, or who are currently febrile. Patients should not receive live vaccines during pregnancy, acute debilitating disease, or periods of severe malnutrition.

In addition to routine childhood immunizations, certain people who are at increased risk need additional immunizations. All healthcare workers and people exposed to blood and body fluids should receive immunizations for hepatitis B virus. Older adults, the chronically ill, and people with respiratory dysfunction should receive annual influenza shots and pneumococcal vaccines every 5 years. As noted in Chapter 19, annual influenza shots are also recommended for healthcare personnel as an essential patient safety measure. A person may require additional vaccinations when traveling to a foreign area, where different diseases are endemic.

In 1998, *The Lancet* published an article citing a possible link between the MMR vaccination and the appearance of autism. The article has since been retracted, its research discredited, and the author is no longer allowed to practice medicine (Jolley & Douglas, 2014). This idea has been propagated by various sources including media, the Internet, and Hollywood celebrities. Attributed at least partly as a result of this misinformation, healthcare workers have seen increasing number of parents over the last two decades refusing to vaccinate their children. In January of 2015, 100+ people from 11 states were reported to have measles, most of which are part of a large, ongoing outbreak linked to Disneyland in California (CDC, 2015b). It is of vital importance that healthcare workers are armed with up-to-date, accurate information regarding vaccinations and risks of both vaccinating and not vaccinating their children.

Nursing Interventions for Altered Function

When an infection becomes established, nursing measures focus at helping the patient combat the illness and preventing the infection from spreading to others. Because nothing is more important in controlling infection than maintaining natural barriers against it, nurses devote much time to supporting these defenses. Enhancing host defenses is both preventive and supportive therapy.

COMFORT MEASURES

Manifestations of infection (e.g., aches and pains, feelings of lethargy or malaise, fever, chills, nausea and vomiting, itching) cause generalized discomfort. This discomfort is most often managed by relieving the individual symptoms. Generally, comfort measures aim at relieving debilitating symptoms so as to conserve the patient's energy for healing and fighting infection.

Analgesics are used to relieve aches and pains and can positively affect rest, sleep, and ambulation. Warm broth, a cool cloth to the head, warm blankets, and rest may ease feelings of malaise. Prolonged or excessive fevers may be treated with tepid sponge baths, antipyretics, or cooling blankets. Warm blankets and warm fluids can relieve shaking chills. Removing objects with objectionable odors, offering carbonated beverages, and providing a darkened, quiet room may relieve nausea and vomiting. In more severe cases, oral intake may need to be restricted and antiemetics administered. Itching may be treated with moist, cool cloths; calamine lotion; pastes made from baking soda; or prescribed antihistamines (e.g., diphenhydramine).

AMBULATION AND POSITIONING

Encourage mobility unless a patient is severely debilitated from an infection. Regular periods of aerobic exercise, such as ambulating, help prevent respiratory infections that can occur in immobile patients. If mobility is limited, encourage as much activity as the patient can tolerate without excessive fatigue. Ambulation promotes circulation, facilitates chest wall excursion, promotes digestion, and decreases stasis of bodily fluids.

When ambulation is impossible, patients may require assistance with turning and positioning. Assist patients in turning every 2 hours while awake and every 2 to 4 hours while sleeping. Resume ambulation as soon as the patient's condition permits. When an infection is present in the extremities, elevation may be necessary to facilitate drainage and decrease edema.

RESPIRATORY INTERVENTIONS

Encouraging patients to cough, breathe deeply, blow the nose, and move promotes clearance of respiratory secretions, which may become infected if allowed to pool in the lower respiratory tract. Retained secretions prevent adequate gas exchange at the alveolar level and reduce oxygen available to the tissues to combat infection, heal injured tissues, and meet metabolic needs. Secondary infections are commonly associated with impaired respiratory tract function.

Teach patients to cough or sneeze into their sleeve and arm to prevent droplet transmission of microorganisms to others or their own hands. When blowing their noses, patients should always keep one nostril open to avoid forcing secretions into the ear canals. Caution youngsters not to pick their noses because they can easily transmit infected organisms to other body parts and other people. Instruct everyone to dispose of tissues and respiratory secretions properly. See Chapter 26 for detailed information on pulmonary hygiene and care.

FEVER MANAGEMENT

Because fever is thought to be an adaptive state that assists the body in fighting infection, interventions to reduce fever should be employed only when very high body temperatures exhaust body resources. Fever management focuses on comfort measures that differ for each fever phase (i.e., chill, fever, and flush). Appropriate nursing interventions are highlighted in Table 31-4.

Antipyretics

Drugs such as aspirin and acetaminophen are called antipyretics because they lower the setting of the hypothalamic thermostat so that body temperature falls. Antipyretics may be used to reduce temperature when fever threatens a patient's well-being. Most authorities agree that antipyretics are advisable for fever greater than 40°C (104°F).

Aspirin and acetaminophen are effective in lowering elevated temperature without reducing it to a lower-than-normal range. They promote heat loss by dilating blood vessels and fostering diaphoresis but do not affect the body's heat production. Usually, people take aspirin and acetaminophen mainly to reduce aches and discomforts associated with fever.

TABLE 31-4 CARING FOR THE FEBRILE PERSON

Phase	Signs/Symptoms	Nursing Interventions
Chill phase	Patient feels cold and shivers; skin is pale and cool to touch; "gooseflesh" appears; body temperature increases.	Apply extra blankets. Increase fluid intake. Restrict activity. Supply supplemental oxygen if patient has preexisting cardiac or respiratory problem.
Fever phase	Patient feels neither hot nor cold; oral mucosa is dry; patient is thirsty, possibly dehydrated; patient experiences feelings of general malaise, weakness, aching muscles, drowsiness, or restlessness.	Cover with light, warm clothing to avoid chilling patient. Encourage cool fluids. Promote rest. Apply lubricant to dry lips and nasal mucosa. Use tepid sponging if temperature becomes very high. Increase air circulation to encourage cooling. Implement safety precautions to protect patient if restless or delirious.
Flush phase	Patient sweats profusely, is possibly dehydrated. Shivering decreases. Skin is flushed and warm to touch.	Use tepid sponging. Avoid chilling patient. Encourage cool fluids. Restrict activity. Cover patient with light clothing or bed linens.

SAFETY ALERT

Do not give aspirin to children with flulike illnesses. The use of aspirin in such cases has been associated with Reye syndrome, a potentially fatal condition involving liver damage and encephalopathy.

When administering an antipyretic to a febrile patient, take the patient's temperature immediately before giving the medication and approximately 1 hour later to determine whether the medication has had the desired effect.

Tepid Baths

Tepid baths and sponging are used for febrile patients when their temperature reaches seriously elevated levels. Such baths should not be administered during a fever's chill phase. Use tepid, rather than cool, water to prevent chilling. Patients may find this procedure either soothing or uncomfortable, depending on skin temperature. Tepid baths or sponging is intended to artificially replace the body's sweating mechanism by cooling the skin's surface, thereby cooling the blood delivered to the body core. Also, this technique promotes cooling by the process of evaporation. Be careful to avoid chilling the patient, which will trigger the shivering mechanism. Measure the patient's temperature before and 30 minutes after the procedure to determine the intervention's effectiveness.

Hypothermia Blankets

These special blankets can be used to reduce the temperature of the hyperpyrexic patient. Such blankets consist of rubber or vinyl coils through which distilled water or alcohol is pumped. The fluid's temperature can be programmed by a control device similar to a thermostat. When cooling is desired, the blanket is usually set slightly lower than normal body temperature (e.g., 35°C [96°F]). A rectal probe is inserted to continuously monitor core body temperature so that excessive cooling does not occur. During use of the hypothermia blanket, medication may be necessary to block the shivering mechanism.

NEUTROPENIC PRECAUTIONS

Neutropenia poses a significant risk for infections when the ANC falls to fewer than 1,000 cells/mm³. This is considered stage 3 by the National Cancer Institute. Serious bacterial infection is almost certain if the ANC is less than 500 cells/mm³, which is considered stage 4 (National Cancer Institute, 2006). When neutropenic precautions are indicated, place the patient in a private room and limit visitors, especially children and people with any signs of infection. Hand hygiene is essential for all who enter the room. Hand hygiene and good hygiene are also important for the patient because endogenous flora causes many infections in the neutropenic patient. Keep the door closed to limit airborne exposure. When it is necessary for the patient to leave the hospital room, he or she should wear a mask. Take special care to prevent any breaks in mucous membranes. Provide gentle oral care, and avoid flossing. Avoid razors with blades and do not take rectal temperatures. Avoid injections whenever possible. Also, remove any sources of pathogens in the environment, such as stagnant water, fresh flowers, or potted plants. There is some controversy surrounding use of neutropenic diets, which eliminate fresh fruits or vegetables and undercooked, raw, or deli meat. The evidence to support such diets is limited and must be weighed with the patient's quality of life (Jubelirer, 2011).

Patients who are neutropenic after chemotherapy experience a predictable drop in neutrophils, which at its lowest point is referred to as nadir. Estimate when the patient will experience nadir based on the specific chemotherapeutic drug administered. Teach patients that this is when they will be most susceptible to infection and that preventive measures, such as avoiding crowds and other likely sources of infection, are essential during nadir. Febrile neutropenia is a complication of chemotherapy and can indicate serious infection or just delay treatment while a febrile workup is completed to rule out infection. Febrile neutropenia is generally defined as fever (single oral temperature 38.3°C or greater or 38.0°C or greater for more than 1 hour) with grade 3 out of 4 neutropenia (per the National Cancer Institute guidelines) and is associated with substantial morbidity, escalation of costs, and mortality risk (Aapro, Crawford, & Kamioner, 2010).

Granulocyte colony-stimulating factors (G-CSFs) have been developed with the use of DNA technology. These growth factors are administered to stimulate production of neutrophils in the bone marrow, thus decreasing the degree and duration of neutropenia.

ANTIMICROBIAL THERAPY

Antimicrobial agents are used to combat the growth and replication of microorganisms. Administration and monitoring of these drugs are collaborative functions of nurses, physicians, pharmacists, and laboratory technicians.

Prescribed antibiotics are based on the presumed antibiotic sensitivity of the infecting species. A culture and sensitivity analysis is obtained to determine appropriate antibiotic therapy. Antibiotics should not be used routinely for all infections. Studies indicate that 30% to 50% of antibiotics prescribed in hospitals are unnecessary or inappropriate (CDC, 2014a). Several species of organisms have mutated over the years since antibiotics were introduced and now are resistant to all but a few toxic drugs (see Chapter 19).

Remember what antibiotics can and cannot do. They cannot cure the patient; at best, they slow the growth of or kill the infecting organism, which is necessary for patients to recover from infection. They control the size of the microbial population against which the patient's immune system must contend. Antibiotics "buy time" during which the patient's own immune system can mobilize. Eliminating the microbes may prevent further injury, but a return to normal depends on the body's healing capacity.

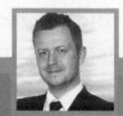

Infection Prevention and Management PICO

The patient who was treated for TB comes back to the clinic, 1 year later, with symptoms of rectal bleeding. He is diagnosed with colon cancer, which will require surgery. Danielle, the nurse, is prepping him for his surgery and tells him that he will be getting antibiotics prior to his surgery. The patient says to her, "I've had so many antibiotics in the past year, I really don't think it's going to make much of a difference." Seeing the exhausted look on her patient's face, Danielle decides to use evidence to help him understand. She uses the following PICO question to help with her search in the Cochrane Library. *In patients having colorectal surgeries, how does antibiotic therapy versus no antibiotic therapy prevent surgical site wound infections?*

P = patients having colorectal surgeries
I = antibiotic therapy
C = no antibiotic therapy
O = prevent surgical site wound infection

Danielle finds a systematic review that addresses many factors including how antibiotics prevent surgical wound infections. The study reviewed 260 studies with 43.451 patients and 68 different types of antibiotics. There was a positive statistical significance that indicated that surgical site wound infections were decreased in patients receiving prophylactic antibiotic.

Danielle shares her findings with the patient, who then seems a little more receptive to antibiotic treatment. She also notices from the patient's chart that he lives alone and inquires if he wants information about cancer support groups.

REFERENCE

Nelson, R. L., Gladman, E., & Barbateskovic, M. (2014). Antimicrobial prophylaxis for colorectal surgery. *Cochrane Database of Systematic Reviews, 5,* CD001181. doi: 10.1002/14651858.CD001181.pub4

As a group, antibiotics have a wide range of safety, but they can produce severe allergic reactions and toxic effects. Renal and hepatic failure, interactions with other drugs, underlying disease, and extremes of age predispose patients to adverse reactions. Both the very young and the very old have impaired renal clearance of drugs. Anticipate the need for dosage adjustments in these age groups. Monitor blood levels of antibiotics to ensure safety and optimal effectiveness.

! SAFETY ALERT

Always ask patients about allergies to foods or drugs and any drugs or herbs they currently use to prevent allergic reactions.

Antibiotics may eradicate the endogenous flora of the skin and mucous membranes of the mouth, GI tract, and vaginal tract. This flora normally protects the host's mucous membranes; when it is eliminated, opportunistic organisms may invade the tissues. A **superinfection** is a secondary infection that occurs when antibiotics, immunosuppression, or cancer treatment destroys normal flora. These infections are more common when antimicrobials are given in large doses, several antimicrobials are given concurrently, or broad-spectrum antibiotics are used. Usually, superinfection appears 4 to 5 days after antimicrobial therapy begins. Superinfections commonly are fungal infections of the mouth or vagina.

PREVENTION OF INFECTION SPREAD

Nurses perform interventions that prevent the spread of infection to others. Chapter 19 discusses aseptic practice: hand hygiene, disinfection and sterilization, use of barriers, isolation precautions, and surgical asepsis.

Hand hygiene and sterile technique are two significant measures to prevent the occurrence and transmission of infection in healthcare settings. Although healthcare professionals know the importance of handwashing in preventing the spread of infection, studies show that the rate of compliance continues to be less than 100%, sometimes as low as 50% to 60% (Ruef, 2009). Many reasons have been identified as the cause of noncompliance, such as time constraints, lack of available supplies (sinks with soap and water or hand sanitizer dispensers), a work climate that does not encourage staff to remind others of hand hygiene opportunities, lack of education, and a lack of workplace reminders. One study found a threefold increase in compliance when a hand hygiene auditor was visible on the unit. This is known as the Hawthorne effect: a behavioral change due to an awareness of being observed (Srigley, Furness, Baker, & Gardam, 2014).

Often, nurses are the first to identify symptoms indicating infection in patients and to institute precautions to prevent transmission. In addition to stressing the need for hand hygiene, instruct patients and their families about proper methods for disposal of body secretions such as sputum, feces, urine, and wound drainage. Also, provide patients with tissues to cover the noses and mouths while coughing and sneezing. Place disposal bags within convenient reach, and empty any bags that become full. Replace them as necessary.

Home and Community Care

Nurses work at various levels to plan, implement, and evaluate measures to prevent and control infection. Four levels are the person and family (household), the community, the nation, and the world.

HOME CARE MANAGEMENT

Many patients are discharged home with indwelling devices that increase the risk of infection. Whether such care is short or long term, avoiding infectious complications and supporting the family are important in helping patients maintain functional abilities. When discharging patients to home, education is the most important intervention for maintaining patient safety.

The trend is toward keeping all but the most seriously ill patients at home for the delivery of healthcare. Hospitalization, once thought to protect patients who are severely immunosuppressed, is now a matter of controversy. During hospitalization, patients are more likely to become infected with virulent, oftentimes MDROs.

Patients and their caregivers must learn how to evaluate vital signs, give medications, and observe for signs of infection. Stress the importance of basic hygiene measures such as bathing, toileting, and oral care as well as basic aseptic practices. Educate patients and caregivers about the importance of proper hand hygiene and proper disposal of contaminated supplies. Instruction in sterile technique is necessary for managing IV devices and IV medications.

Also, teach caregivers to wear gloves when caring for patients with known infections. If drug therapy is ordered, be sure to instruct patients and caregivers in the drug regimen, including taking the entire prescription, and symptoms of possible adverse effects or infection that they should report to the healthcare provider.

COMMUNITY, NATION, AND WORLD INFECTION CONTROL

Community regulations controlling the quality of drinking water, food served in public places, and disposal of sewage and solid waste are important aspects of community infection control. Community or regional health authorities gather statistics on the incidence of infectious diseases in their areas. They decide which diseases pose a hazard to the community's well-being and must be reported. Many communities and states have passed laws forbidding unimmunized children from attending school. Some bar children with active infections from classrooms.

Some countries have public health agencies that gather statistics from regional reports and compile them for yearly comparisons. These agencies govern quality of air, water, food, and wastes that cross state, regional, or international boundaries,

and they set standards for reduction of pollutants and microorganisms. They bar people with designated acute infections from immigrating into the country and prohibit the return of natives without proof of immunization against diseases endemic in the areas to which they have traveled.

Several international health organizations, such as the WHO, gather statistics from national groups and have formed commissions for the education of healthcare providers. These organizations establish priorities for infection control and make recommendations about immunizations for international travelers. International commissions also provide supplies and personnel for some immunization programs.

Community health nurses focus on health promotion, health maintenance, and disease prevention on both individual and population-based levels. Successfully planning, implementation, and evaluation of health-related education programs allow nurses to improve the health and well-being of many individuals. For people suffering from chronic diseases, such as diabetes, heart disease, or respiratory diseases, community health nurses focus on reducing comorbidities for these populations. Community health nurses often work for or in collaboration with health organizations to ensure safety within the community. Education and services that focus on communicable disease prevention are increasingly essential as infection rates continue to rise and infections once contained within the hospital setting are now emerging within the community.

EVALUATION

The success of a program to prevent or control infection requires cooperation from both the patient and the healthcare team. Excellent communication is necessary, and trust must be established. People must assume responsibility for their own behaviors and healthcare practices. The healthcare system must educate the public and scrutinize its own infection prevention methods. Healthcare workers must diligently practice infection control.

The optimal outcome of efforts to control infection (which is not always attainable) is freedom from signs and symptoms of infection. Some outcome criteria for goals involving infection are listed here.

Goal

The patient will demonstrate adequate knowledge to recognize and report signs of infection.

POSSIBLE OUTCOME CRITERIA

- After a teaching session, the patient or caregiver lists four signs of infection.
- After a teaching session, the patient or caregiver demonstrates accurate monitoring of body temperature.
- Before discharge, the patient or caregiver verbalizes indications that would require contacting a healthcare professional.

THERAPEUTIC DIALOGUE: FAMILY ILLNESS

SCENE FOR THOUGHT

The community health nurse is responsible for visiting 20 families per week. Today, she will see the Holden family, which consists of Ann, age 38 years; John, age 39 years; Maureen, age 11 years; and John Jr., age 9 years. As she drives up to the small, neat house, she notices that the family car is in the driveway, which is an unusual occurrence because John is usually at work when the nurse comes to see the family.

LESS EFFECTIVE

Nurse: *(Knocks on the door.)* Ann, it's Rosie Connors.

Ann: Hello, Rosie, come on in. *(Looks tired and pale.)*

Nurse: *(Settles on couch with Ann beside her.)* How are things?

Ann: Not wonderful. We're all sick with the stomach flu, and John and I have been up most of the night either with the kids or sick ourselves. It's just miserable.

Nurse: I know how that is! Especially when everyone gets it at once. No wonder you look tired. I'll bet a good night's sleep would feel just great! *(Smiles warmly and sympathetically.)*

Ann: That's the truth. *(Smiles wearily.)* I suppose you need to see Maureen now. I know you're busy.

Nurse: Okay. How's she doing, by the way? *(Goes with Ann to see Maureen, chatting as they go.)*

MORE EFFECTIVE

Nurse: *(Knocks on the door.)* Ann, it's Evelyn Mason.

Ann: Hello, Evelyn, come on in. *(Looks tired and pale.)*

Nurse: *(Settles on couch with Ann beside her.)* How are things?

Ann: Not wonderful. We're all sick with the stomach flu, and John and I have been up most of the night either with the kids or sick ourselves. It's just miserable.

Nurse: I noticed the car outside and wondered about John being home. What can I help you with while I'm here? *(Sits quietly and attentively.)*

Ann: Well, I know you usually come to check on Maureen's diabetes, and I don't want to trouble you with the rest of it.

Nurse: It's no trouble. Maureen's health and the family's health are connected. I'll be happy to do what I can.

Ann: *(Looks relieved.)* Well, could you maybe check us all over before you go, just to make sure it is the stomach flu and not something else? And then, I need some advice about what to eat. We're all thirsty, but some things don't really agree with me, and John Jr. won't drink juices. I'm not sure what to do.

Nurse: Sure, no problem. Shall I start with you since you're right here? *(Continues to sit with her without moving.)*

Ann: I'd rather you start with Maureen. You know, these things hit her harder than the rest of us. *(Face is somewhat anxious.)*

Nurse: Okay. Let's go see her.

CRITICAL THINKING CHALLENGE

• Detect what the first and second nurses did differently.
• Infer how likely Ann is to ask the first nurse questions about the family's health in the future.
• Compare this with Ann's inclinations in the future to ask the second nurse questions about the family's health.
• Analyze at what point the first nurse could have picked up cues from Ann that indicated she might like some help.

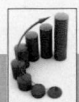

OUTCOME-BASED TEACHING PLANS

Mr. Petrenkov, a 76-year-old patient with asthma, developed pneumonia after abdominal surgery. He is being discharged with an antibiotic to take for the next 7 days. He will return to his primary care provider (PCP) in 1 week to have staples removed from his incision and to be evaluated.

OUTCOME

Mr. Petrenkov will verbalize signs and symptoms of any wound or respiratory infection and when to notify PCP.

STRATEGIES

- Review with Mr. Petrenkov a handout that lists the signs and symptoms of wound infection (elevated temperature, increased redness or pain in incision, drainage especially containing pus from the incision).
- Verbalize symptoms of respiratory infection (increased shortness of breath; increased sputum, change in tenacity or color of sputum) and add them to the list.
- Instruct Mr. Petrenkov to take his temperature daily and to notify PCP of any elevation over 100.8°F.
- Teach Mr. Petrenkov how to inspect incision every morning and evening for signs of infection.
- Have Mr. Petrenkov verbalize symptoms of infection that require calling PCP.

OUTCOME

Mr. Petrenkov will verbalize how to take antibiotic medication safely.

STRATEGIES

- Provide Mr. Petrenkov with written information about the prescribed antibiotic. Add the specific trade name, dose, and frequency.
- Review the handout with Mr. Petrenkov and reinforce plans and indications for antibiotic regimen.
- Have Mr. Petrenkov explain how he will take his medication after discharge. Provide positive reinforcement of an appropriate plan.
- Review common side effects such as diarrhea and rash, explaining the importance of contacting his PCP should they occur.
- Stress the importance of finishing the entire prescription to prevent recurrence of infection and possible drug resistance.

EVALUATION

5/12/16: 12:30—After the teaching session, Mr. Petrenkov was able to list four signs of infection and verbalized his intent to take his temperature daily and notify his provider of fever or signs of infection. He verbalized an appropriate plan for taking his antibiotic and promised to complete the prescription.

—B. Jones, RN

Goal

The patient will demonstrate use of good health practices to prevent the occurrence and spread of infection.

POSSIBLE OUTCOME CRITERIA

- After each teaching session, the patient or caregiver demonstrates correct hand hygiene technique.
- Before discharge, the patient or caregiver verbalizes proper methods of infection control to use at home.
- By the time of discharge, the patient verbalizes selected strategies to minimize the risk of infection.

Goal

The patient will participate in treatment regimens to prevent infection and minimize possible complications.

POSSIBLE OUTCOME CRITERIA

- The patient uses recommended aseptic practices for dressing changes or manipulation of invasive devices, as evidenced by a return demonstration at the next home visit.
- The patient takes prescribed medications to treat or prevent infections, as reported to the nurse at the next appointment.
- The patient keeps the next three appointments with healthcare providers.

PATIENT PLAN OF CARE
The Patient at Risk for Infection

NURSING DIAGNOSIS

Risk for infection related to delayed wound healing, immunosuppressive treatment for colon cancer, and age.

PATIENT GOAL

Patient/family will demonstrate knowledge about methods for preventing and detecting infection.

PATIENT OUTCOME CRITERIA

- Patient/family member describes methods to avoid infection after teaching session.
- Patient/family member verbalizes four signs and symptoms of infection after teaching session.
- Patient/family member demonstrates acceptable technique in applying a dressing after teaching session.
- Patient/family member describes food and fluid that will meet nutritional needs by next visit.

NURSING INTERVENTION	SCIENTIFIC RATIONALE
1. Begin instruction of wound care as early in the course of recovery as possible. Include family members.	**1.** Prepare the patient and involve family in wound management before discharge.
2. Review principles of good handwashing or the use of alcohol-based cleansers before wound care.	**2.** Hand hygiene is the single most important mechanism in stopping the transmission of pathogenic organisms.
3. Demonstrate the technique for dressing change. Allow time for practice and a return demonstration.	**3.** Patients can acquire technical skills better if they observe and practice them.
4. Demonstrate removal of old dressing, including how to discard in moisture-proof bag.	**4.** Proper waste disposal is important in preventing the spread of microorganisms.
5. Discuss activities that may cause trauma to the wound and how to avoid them.	**5.** Trauma can prevent wound healing and increase the chance of infection.
6. Review signs and symptoms of infection, encouraging the patient and family to ask questions.	**6.** Early detection of and treatment for infection decrease incidence of serious complications.
7. Instruct the patient in the importance of well-balanced diet high in protein and calories. Discuss sources of vitamin C and vitamin supplements.	**7.** Wound healing requires protein and calories for building new cells. The immune system depends on protein and calories to produce antibodies.
8. Provide the patient with written instructions concerning how to change the dressing, signs and symptoms of infection, and when to call the physician.	**8.** Providing more than one learning method optimizes retention. Written instructions provide a handy reference.

EVALUATION

> 4/12/16: 09:30—Wife and husband participated in teaching session; both stated that they didn't think they could do the dressing change and were unwilling to try. They have a neighbor who is a nurse, and their daughter may be able to help. Social work consult made. Will continue to follow up with additional teaching.
>
> —S. Roberts, RN

KEY CONCEPTS

- The body has an elaborate system of defenses to protect against infection.

- Most infections result from a breakdown of nonspecific and specific host defenses. Infections are responsible for most visits to healthcare facilities.

- Inflammation and fever are two nonspecific natural defenses. The five signs of inflammation are erythema, warmth, edema, pain, and functionality impairment. Fever is an important mechanism in fighting infection, but it consumes a great deal of metabolic energy.

- The immune response, a specific defense, involves two methods: humoral and cellular immunity. T lymphocytes and B lymphocytes form memory cells that can be reactivated on reexposure to an antigen.

- Infection progresses through four stages: incubation, the prodromal period, the acute phase, and convalescence.

- Very young and very old people have decreased resistance to infection. Age affects both nonspecific and specific barriers to infection.

- The inflammatory response helps control the spread of infection, but if it is prolonged, it can harm the patient.

- Fever supports host defense mechanisms and is treated with antipyretics, tepid baths, or hypothermia blankets only when very high (i.e., greater than 40°C [104°F]).

- A culture and sensitivity analysis is necessary to identify the specific organism causing an infection and antibiotics that may be useful for treatment. Proper antimicrobial therapy decreases the incidence of MDROs.

- Immunizations are given to children and adults to prevent some infectious diseases. Because communicable childhood diseases can result in severe complications, all children should be immunized.

- Preventing infection is an individual, community, national, and international responsibility.

- Increasing numbers of patients are being treated at home for chronic conditions or rehabilitation. Many of them have several risk factors for infection. Nurses must assume the responsibility for teaching these patients or their caregivers how to prevent and control infection.

PRACTICING FOR THE NCLEX

CHECK YOUR ANSWERS IN APPENDIX A.

1. A triage nurse receives a call from a mother worried about her formula-fed, 1-month-old infant. The infant is lethargic and not feeding regularly but is afebrile. The nurse tells the mother to bring the infant to the physician's office. Which of the following are relevant for this newborn's immunity and illness? Select all that apply:
   a. The immune system is not fully operational until 6 months of age.
   b. Formula does not provide the infant with antibodies.
   c. Newborns have immature thermoregulation and may not become febrile.
   d. Vaccinations will cover periods until the infant develops immunocompetence.

2. Elderly patients are at increased risk for infection related to which of the following? Select all that apply:
   a. Chronic disease (cardiovascular, cancer, diabetes, malnutrition, stress, etc.)
   b. Shrinking thyroid impairs cell immunity
   c. Medications and treatments
   d. Decreased efficacy of natural anatomic and chemical preventative factors

3. Healthcare associated infections are infections that are preventable with increased surveillance, proper hand hygiene, and judicial use of invasive procedures. Which of the following would be considered a healthcare associated infection? Select all that apply:
   a. Surgical site wound infection that develops 3 days following hospital discharge
   b. Ventilator-associated pneumonia in a skilled nursing facility
   c. Infection of a hemodialysis line in a person residing at home
   d. Gunshot wound in a jail prisoner

4. A nurse is assessing a college student with a severe headache and high fever. Which questions would be useful? Select all that apply:
   a. "Has someone in your immediate surroundings recently had similar symptoms or been diagnosed with meningitis?"
   b. "What are your normal sleep and eating patterns?"
   c. "Have you shared drinks or food with anyone recently?"
   d. "Have you traveled recently, especially to foreign countries?"

5. A coworker states that he is not feeling well but says that he is fine to work. Two days later, he is out of work due to illness. What phase of the communicable period was he in when at work earlier in the week?
   a. Incubation
   b. Prodromal
   c. Acute
   d. Convalescent

6. A patient is admitted with a diabetic foot ulcer. The nurse suspects that it is infected despite lack of pain at the site. Which of the following symptoms in this patient indicate infection? Select all that apply:
   a. Purulent drainage
   b. Increased WBC count
   c. Increased temperature
   d. Difficulty breathing

7. A patient admitted with pneumonia appears to be worsening. The patient is newly confused and has decreased blood pressure and increased heart and respiratory rate. Lab work also shows a very high WBC count. The nurse should be suspicious of what condition?
    a. Opportunistic infection
    b. Nosocomial infection
    c. Neutropenia
    d. Sepsis

8. A patient is experiencing new onset of diarrhea and abdominal pain following a course of chemotherapy. Which of the following best describes this illness?
    a. Opportunistic infection
    b. Colonization
    c. Neutropenia
    d. Immunodeficiency

9. A patient is receiving a third round of chemotherapy and has been determined to be neutropenic. Which precautions are appropriate in providing care for this patient?
    a. Place the patient in a semiprivate room.
    b. Encourage visitors to improve spirits.
    c. Avoid flowers and fresh fruit.
    d. Encourage comprehensive oral hygiene.

10. A nurse is performing a wound culture. Which order of steps is most appropriate?
    a. Apply clean dressing to arm, insert culture swab into wound, crush ampule of medium
    b. Remove soiled dressing, insert culture swab into wound, secure specimen in plastic bag
    c. Crush ampule of medium, insert culture swab into wound, secure specimen in plastic bag
    d. Insert culture swab into wound, crush ampule of medium, secure specimen in plastic bag

REFERENCES

Aapro, M., Crawford, J., & Kamioner, D. (2010). Prophylaxis of chemotherapy-induced febrile neutropenia with granulocyte colony-stimulating factors: Where are we now? *Support Care Cancer, 18,* 529–541.

Centers for Disease Control and Prevention. (2014a). *Get Smart for Healthcare.* Retrieved January 17, 2015, from http://www.cdc.gov/getsmart/healthcare/

Centers for Disease Control and Prevention. (2006). *Management of multi-drug-resistant organisms in healthcare settings, 2006.* Retrieved August 1, 2011, from www.cdc.gov/hicpac/mdro/mdro_0.html

Centers for Disease Control and Prevention. (2012). Trichomoniasis—CDC Fact Sheet. Retrieved January 17, 2015, from http://www.cdc.gov/std/trichomonas/stdfact-trichomoniasis.htm

Centers for Disease Control and Prevention. (2014b). *Immunization schedules.* Retrieved January 17, 2015, from http://www.cdc.gov/vaccines/schedules/

Centers for Disease Control and Prevention. (2014c). *Human Papillomavirus Vaccination: Recommendations of the Advisory Committee on Immunization Practices (ACIP).* Retrieved January 18, 2015, from http://www.cdc.gov/mmwr/preview/mmwrhtml/rr6305a1.htm

Centers for Disease Control and Prevention. (2015a). *Ebola (Ebola virus disease).* Retrieved January 17, 2015, from http://www.cdc.gov/vhf/ebola/index.html

Centers for Disease Control and Prevention. (2015b). Measles (Rubeola). Retrieved January 24, 2015, from http://www.cdc.gov/measles/index.html

Surviving Sepsis Campaign: International guidelines for management of severe sepsis and septic shock. (2013, February 1). Retrieved January 18, 2015, from http://link.springer.com/article/10.1007/s00134-012-2769-8

Dellinger, R. P., et al. (2012). Surviving Sepsis Campaign: International guidelines for management of severe sepsis and septic shock, 2012. *Intensive Care Medicine, 39*(2), 165–228.

Healthy People 2020. (2010). *A systematic approach to health improvement.* Retrieved October 23, 2010, from www.healthypeople.gov/document/html/uih/uih_2.htm

Jolley, D., & Douglas, K. M. (2014). The effects of anti-vaccine conspiracy theories on vaccination intentions. *PLoS one, 9*(2), e89177.

Jubelirer, S. J. (2011). The benefit of the neutropenic diet: Fact or fiction?. *The oncologist, 16*(5), 704–707.

NANDA-International (NANDA-I). (2014). *Nursing diagnoses: Definitions and classification, 2015–2017.* West Sussex, UK: Wiley-Blackwell.

National Cancer Institute. (2006). *Common terminology criteria for adverse events v3.0 (CTCAE).* Retrieved October 30, 2010, from http://ctep.cancer.gov/protocolDevelopment/electronic_applications/docs/ctcaev3.pdf

Ruef, C. (2009). Hand hygiene: Adherence influenced by knowledge and subjective norms. *Infection, 37,* 395.

Septimus, E., Yokoe, D. S., Weinstein, R. A., Perl, T. M., Maragakis, L. L., & Berenholtz, S. M. (2014). Maintaining the momentum of change: The role of the 2014 updates to the compendium in preventing healthcare-associated infections. *Infection Control and Hospital Epidemiology, 35*(5), 460–463.

Srigley, J. A., Furness, C. D., Baker, G. R., & Gardam, M. (2014). Quantification of the Hawthorne effect in hand hygiene compliance monitoring using an electronic monitoring system: A retrospective cohort study. *BMJ Quality & Safety, 23*(12), 974–980.

Storey, M., & Jordan S. (2008). An overview of the immune system. *Nursing Standard, 23,* 15–17.

Procedure 31-1 Obtaining a Wound Culture

Purpose	1. Identify organisms colonized within a wound so that antibiotics sensitive to the microorganisms can be prescribed, as needed.

Equipment	Sterile culture swab (anaerobic or aerobic) and transport container Normal saline to cleanse wound Clean gloves Sterile dressing and tape Name label and completed laboratory requisition

Assessment	• Frequently inspect surgical incisions and other wounds for signs of inflammation and infection (i.e., redness, swelling, warmth, drainage). • Monitor vital signs for evidence of infection (i.e., increased temperature, pulse). • Identify and document amount, color, and odor of any drainage from wounds. • Assess patient for level of discomfort associated with dressing changes and premedicate if necessary with analgesics. • Identify factors that contribute to potential development of wound infections.

Procedure

1. **Identify the patient using two separate identifiers**

   Rationale: Two separate identifiers are required for all specimen collection because incorrect identification or labeling of specimens could cause errors in treatment decisions.

2. **Close door or bed curtains and explain the procedure to the patient, if possible.**

   Rationale: Ensures patient privacy, increases patient compliance, reduces patient anxiety, and promotes learning.

3. **Verify order for culture noting site and type of culture. Label the specimen container and make sure the information includes the patient's name, medical record number, date and time specimen is obtained, and site of the culture.**

   Rationale: Prevents potential errors.

4. **Perform hand hygiene and don gloves.**

   Rationale: Prevents the transfer of microorganisms and protects hands from contact with drainage.

5. **Remove soiled dressing (Fig. 1). Observe drainage for amount, odor, and color.**

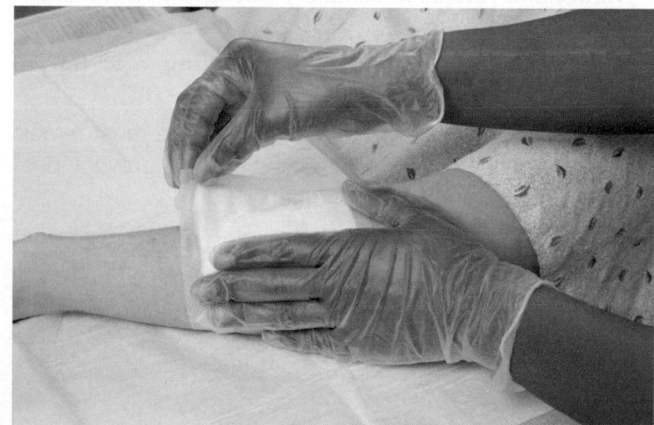

FIG. 1 Remove soiled dressing.

   Rationale: Assesses the wound for signs of infection.

6. **Clear and remove exudate from around wound and cleanse with normal saline.**

   Rationale: Old drainage and microorganisms from the wound could interfere with accurate culture and sensitivity report.

Procedure 31-1　*continued*

Obtaining Aerobic Culture

1. Perform steps 1 through 6 above.
2. Using sterile swab from culture tube, insert swab deep into area of active drainage (Fig. 2). Rotate swab to absorb as much drainage as possible.

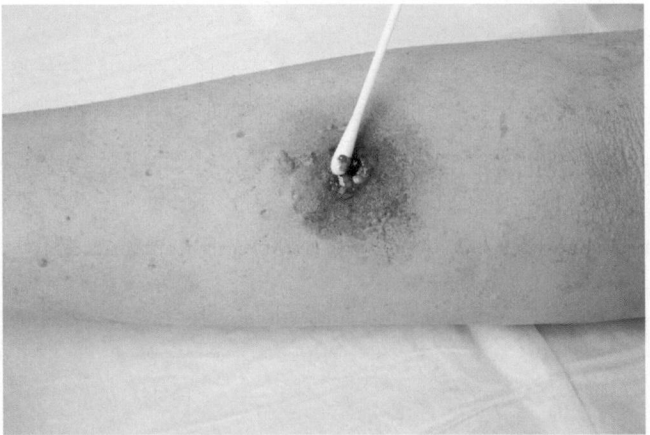

FIG. 2 Insert culture swab into wound to obtain sample.

Rationale: Adequate sample is necessary for culture of the organism.

3. Insert swab into culture tube, taking care not to touch the top or outside of the tube.

Rationale: The outside of the culture tube must remain free from pathogenic microorganisms to prevent possible spread of infection to others.

4. Crush ampule of medium and close container securely (Fig. 3).

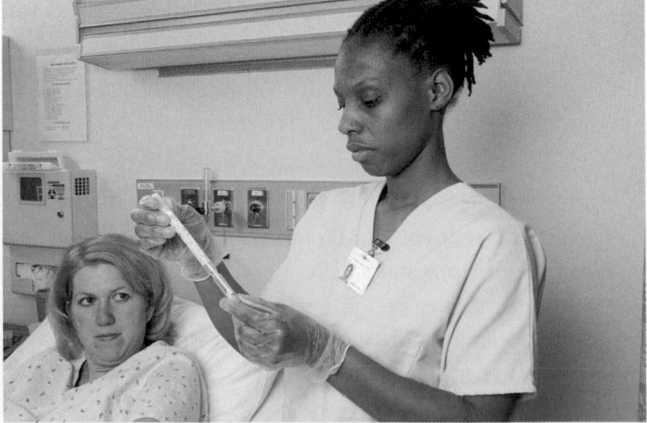

FIG. 3 Crush ampule of medium.

Rationale: Culture medium keeps bacteria alive until analysis is complete. Closing the container prevents transmission of microorganisms to other areas and also prevents introducing other microorganisms into the tube.

5. Continue with step 4 below.

Obtaining Anaerobic Culture

1. Perform steps 1 through 6 at the beginning of the procedure.
2. Using sterile swab from special anaerobic culture tube, insert swab deeply into draining body cavity.

Rationale: Take a drainage sample from a deep cavity to identify organisms that may grow where oxygen is not present.

3. a. Rotate swab gently and remove. Quickly place swab into inner tube of collection container.

   b. *Alternative method*: Insert tip of syringe with needle removed into wound and aspirate 1 to 5 mL of exudate. Attach 21-gauge needle to syringe, expel all air, and inject exudate into inner tube of the culture container.

Rationale: The inner tube of the culture container has either a carbon dioxide or a nitrogen environment to prevent potential contaminating organisms from growing until the laboratory analysis is complete. (*Note:* Drainage is sampled from only one drainage site per culture swab. If a specimen is required from another site, repeat the above steps to identify accurately microbes present at each drainage site.)

4. Send specimens in the prelabeled containers with appropriate requisition immediately to the laboratory. Some agencies require that specimens be transported in clean plastic bags to further prevent the transfer of microorganisms (Fig. 4).

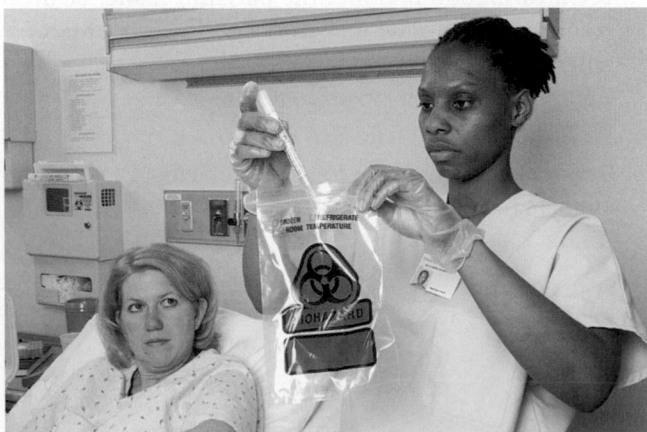

FIG. 4 Secure specimen in plastic bag.

Rationale: Bacteria grow rapidly within culture media of specimen tubes. Prepare cultures quickly for accurate results.

Procedure 31-1 *continued*

5. **Clean and apply sterile dressings to the wound, as ordered (Fig. 5).**

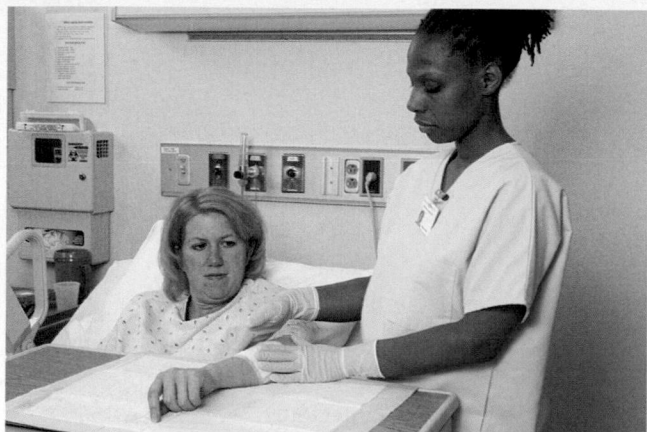

FIG. 5 Apply clean dressing.

Rationale: Protects the wound from environmental contamination; the dressing contains further drainage to prevent spread of infection.

6. **Remove and discard gloves. Perform hand hygiene.**

Rationale: Reduces the risk of transmission of microorganisms.

7. **Document all relevant information on the patient's chart. Include the location the specimen was taken from and the date and time. Record the wound's appearance and the color, odor, amount, and consistency of drainage. Record how the patient toler-** ated the procedure and any discomfort that he or she experienced.

Rationale: Documentation maintains accurate patient records and provides a means of communication with other health team members.

Documentation

4/22/16: 08:30— P: Risk for Infection: left arm ulcer
VS: T 38.6; BP 148/70; HR 110; RR 18
Pain: 7/10
Thick, foul-smelling green exudate in wound
I: Patient premedicated for pain (Percocet 2 tabs). Wound culture obtained using proper technique @ 0800. Crusted drainage removed and fluid culture obtained from deep within wound. Specimen placed in sterile culture tube with proper patient identification and wound location and transported to the lab @ 08:20.
E: Patient tolerated procedure well. Pain 2/10. Findings will be evaluated and MD will be notified ASAP.
—Jane Smith, RN
Addendum: MRSA in wound identified per lab findings. MD notified at 11:00. Patient moved to private room and contact precautions with appropriate barriers initiated. All necessary personnel notified. Two hour positioning schedule and heel protection continued.
—Jane Smith, RN 4/22/16 1231

Life Span Considerations

Infant and Child

- Perform procedures that are uncomfortable or potentially fear-inducing in areas other than the child's room so that the child continues to regard his or her room as a safe place.

Home Care Modifications

- Teach the patient the signs and symptoms of infection and what to report to the healthcare provider.
- When obtaining cultures from the patient at his or her home, transport the specimens as quickly as possible to the designated laboratory for analysis.

Collaboration and Delegation

- Notify the healthcare provider promptly of positive culture results, noting if prescribed antibiotics are indicated for the identified infectious agent.
- Supervise all personnel to ensure appropriate infection control measures to prevent the possible transmission of pathogens.

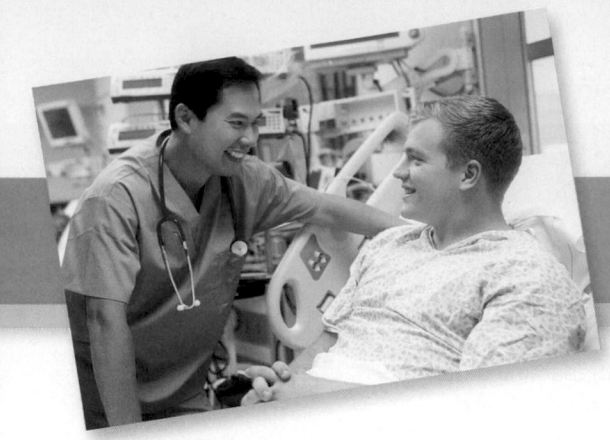

CHAPTER 32

Urinary Elimination

Shirley Kopf-Klakken

Case Scenario

You are a nurse working with John, a 17-year-old boy who has been recovering for 1 week after a motor vehicle accident on the night of his senior prom. John has had an indwelling (Foley) catheter in place for 3 days, draining large amounts of urine. Yesterday, you noted that John's urine was cloudy and he had a temperature of 37.8°C. When you reported these findings to the physician, he discontinued John's catheter and ordered a urine sample for culture and sensitivity.

Once you have completed this chapter and have incorporated urinary elimination into your knowledge base, review the above scenario and reflect on the following areas of Critical Thinking:

1. Identify risk factors that could alter John's urinary function.
2. Analyzing the information provided, determine what alteration in urinary function the data suggest.
3. Construct appropriate patient teaching for when an indwelling catheter is removed. Plan how you will individualize this teaching for John.
4. Consider which data are essential to identify whether John is voiding adequately after the catheter removal.

KEY TERMS

anuria
bladder ultrasound (BUS)
catheter-associated urinary tract infection (CAUTI)
cystectomy
cystocele
detrusor muscle
diuresis
diuretic
dysuria
enuresis
hematuria
hydronephrosis
ileal conduit
intermittent catheterization
micturition
nocturia
oliguria
overactive bladder
polyuria
pyuria
urgency
urinary incontinence
urinary retention

LEARNING OBJECTIVES

Upon completion of this chapter, you will be able to do the following:
1. Describe the structure and function of the urinary system.
2. Outline the process of micturition.
3. List and describe alterations in normal voiding patterns.
4. Recognize age-related differences in urinary elimination.
5. Describe factors that can alter urinary function.
6. Discuss nursing assessment of urinary function.
7. Identify nursing diagnoses related to urinary elimination.
8. Describe nursing interventions to promote normal urinary elimination.
9. Discuss interventions for altered urinary function.
10. Identify indications for proper indwelling catheter use.
11. Develop appropriate collaborative and community-based nursing interventions to manage problems with voiding.

The elimination of fluid waste is an essential function of the human body. Nurses are instrumental in promoting optimal urinary function and preventing urinary complications for all patients. Nurses individualize teaching and carry out specific interventions to help patients of all ages deal with problems of incontinence, **urinary retention**, and urinary tract infection (UTI). An understanding of the structure and function of the urinary system and factors that can affect normal urinary elimination is important for individualizing patient care.

NORMAL URINARY FUNCTION

Structures of the Urinary Tract

Structures within the urinary tract include the kidneys, where urine forms; the ureters, which connect the kidneys with the bladder; the bladder, which stores urine; and the urethra, which enables urine to leave the body (see Fig. 32-1).

KIDNEYS

The two kidneys are located on the posterior abdominal wall, in front of and on either side of the vertebral column between the 12th thoracic and 3rd lumbar vertebrae. Each kidney is enclosed by a fibrous capsule and supported by a mass of adipose tissue.

The functional unit of the kidney is called the nephron. Each kidney has more than 1,000,000 nephrons, and each nephron is capable of forming urine. The nephron consists of the glomerulus, Bowman capsule, proximal convoluted tubules, loop of Henle, distal tubule, and collecting duct. The glomerulus is a network of blood vessels, surrounded by Bowman capsule, where urine formation begins. The tubules, loop of Henle,

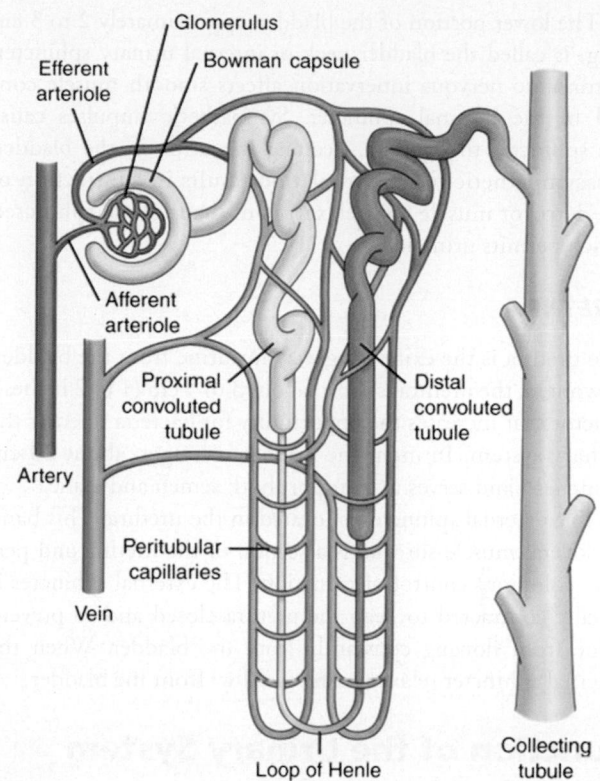

FIGURE 32-2 Representation of a nephron. Each kidney has about 1 million nephrons. (Reprinted with permission from Hinkle, J. L., & Cheever, K. H. (2014). *Brunner & Suddarth's textbook of medical-surgical nursing*. Philadelphia, PA: Wolters Kluwer.)

and collecting ducts are passageways that permit urine to flow to the renal pelvis and then to the ureters. More importantly, they selectively reabsorb or secrete substances from the urine to maintain fluid and electrolyte balance (see Fig. 32-2).

URETERS

The ureters are narrow (1.25 cm), smooth muscle tubes that serve as passageways for urine to flow from the kidneys to the bladder. Peristaltic movement in the ureters propels urine toward the bladder. A flap of mucous membrane, which acts as a valve, covers the juncture between the ureters and the bladder. Under normal conditions, this valve prevents reflux of urine up through the ureter into the kidney.

BLADDER

The bladder is the storage compartment for urine. It is a hollow, smooth muscle that lies behind the symphysis pubis when empty. In women, the bladder is located in front of the uterus and vagina. In men, the bladder is located in front of the rectum and above the prostate gland.

The body of the bladder is composed of three layers of smooth muscle. The inner and outer layers are longitudinal, whereas the middle layer is circular. Collectively, these three layers are called the **detrusor muscle**. The bladder is hollow when empty but is capable of expanding to hold a considerable amount of urine.

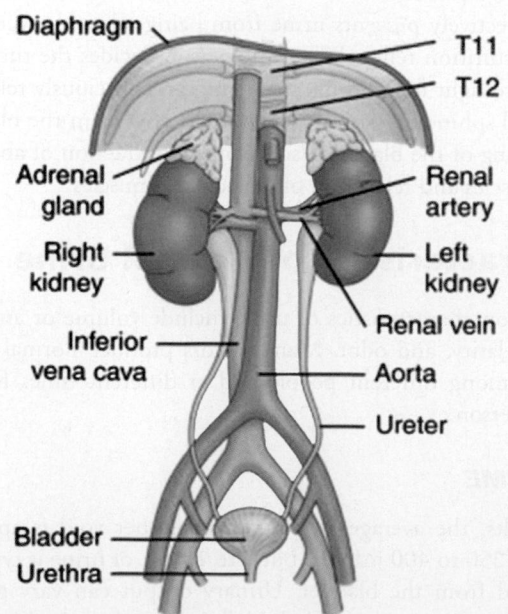

FIGURE 32-1 Kidneys, ureters, and bladder. (Reprinted with permission from Hinkle, J. L., & Cheever, K. H. (2014). *Brunner & Suddarth's textbook of medical-surgical nursing*. Philadelphia, PA: Wolters Kluwer.)

The lower portion of the bladder, approximately 2 to 3 cm long, is called the bladder neck or internal urinary sphincter. Autonomic nervous innervation affects smooth muscle control of the internal sphincter. Sympathetic impulses cause the sphincter to contract, keeping the urine in the bladder. Parasympathetic nerve stimulation results in contraction of the detrusor muscle and relaxation of the internal sphincter, which permits urination.

URETHRA

The urethra is the exit passageway for urine from the bladder. In women, the urethra is short, about 3 to 5 cm (1 to 2 inches), a factor that increases the opportunity for bacteria to enter the urinary system. In men, the urethra is longer, about 20 cm (8 inches), and serves to transport both semen and urine.

The external sphincter is located in the urethra. This band of skeletal muscle surrounds a section of the urethra and permits voluntary control of urination. The external sphincter is usually contracted to keep the urethra closed and to prevent urine from flowing constantly from the bladder. When the external sphincter relaxes, urine can flow from the bladder.

Function of the Urinary System

The elimination of fluid waste from the body is the function of the urinary system. This elimination process can be divided into two parts: urine formation and urine excretion.

URINE FORMATION

The kidney's major function is to regulate the volume and composition of the body's extracellular fluid (ECF). It performs this function by selectively retaining wanted water and other substances and excreting unwanted water and other substances in urine. Urine formation occurs by the processes of filtration, reabsorption, and secretion.

Filtration

The process of filtration begins at the glomerulus. The renal arteries bring blood to the kidneys; the smaller branches of these arteries bring blood to the glomerulus of each nephron. The capillaries of the glomerulus are porous, and as the blood passes through the glomerular capillaries, some constituents of the blood are actually filtered. The red blood cells and the proteins are too large to be filtered and remain in the capillary, but most remaining plasma constituents can be filtered. The fluid that is filtered from the glomerulus into Bowman capsule is called the glomerular filtrate.

Reabsorption

The glomerular filtrate then enters the second segment of the nephron—the tubule. The tubule actively and passively reabsorbs substances that the body wants to retain. These substances include varying amounts of water and electrolytes (Na^+, K^+, Cl^-, and HCO_3^-) as well as all glucose and amino acids. Reabsorption occurs mostly in the proximal convoluted tubule but also in the distal and collecting tubules. The tubules reabsorb almost 99% of the glomerular filtrate. The 1% that remains unabsorbed forms urine.

Secretion

In addition to reabsorbing substances, the tubules secrete some substances to rid them from the body. They secrete varying amounts of H^+ and K^+ ions as well as ammonia, creatinine, uric acid, and other metabolites.

URINE EXCRETION

Several words are used to describe the process of excreting urine from the body, including urination, voiding, and **micturition**. In adults, emptying of the bladder usually occurs when 250 to 400 mL of urine stretches or distends the bladder. Smaller amounts of urine trigger bladder emptying in children. When the volume of urine in the bladder reaches the range of 250 to 400 mL, the pressure of that amount stretches the detrusor sufficiently to begin to force the bladder neck to open. This sensation of stretch in the detrusor is transmitted to sacral segments of the spinal cord; reflex motor action is transmitted back to the detrusor muscle to cause it to contract. The detrusor contraction causes even more stretch and pressure; usually, at this point, the person perceives a full bladder and feels the need to urinate. This reaction of bladder stretch, leading to bladder contraction and perceived need to void, is called the micturition reflex, an involuntary spinal cord reflex.

In children younger than 3 years of age, the micturition reflex leads to spontaneous urination. Beyond 3 years of age, however, most people have learned to delay urination until the time and place are acceptable; this is because nerve centers in the brain ultimately control the act of urination. When the external sphincter, a skeletal muscle, is contracted in a closed position, a person can voluntarily delay voiding. This contraction effectively prevents urine from being released, even with the micturition reflex. When the person decides the time and place are right for voiding, he or she can consciously relax the external sphincter, permitting urine to flow from the bladder. Emptying of the bladder also involves contraction of abdominal muscles and relaxation of pelvic floor muscles.

Characteristics of Normal Urine

Common characteristics of urine include volume or amount, color, clarity, and odor. Many factors produce normal variations among different people and at different times for the same person.

VOLUME

In adults, the average amount of urine per void is approximately 250 to 400 mL. All but 5 to 10 mL of urine is typically emptied from the bladder. Urinary output can vary greatly, depending on intake and fluid losses. Catheterized patients should drain a minimum of 30 mL of urine per hour. Urine output of less than 30 mL per hour may indicate inadequate blood flow to the kidneys.

COLOR

The color of urine ranges from a light yellow, to a darker yellow, to a dark yellow-brown, called amber. The patient's state of hydration affects the color. Urine may be almost colorless if it is very dilute secondary to a high fluid intake. Urine may be dark amber or orange-brown if it is very concentrated secondary to a decreased fluid intake. Medications can also alter urine's color. Urine may appear cloudy, dark reddish brown, or streaked with blood when a woman is menstruating.

CLARITY

Urine is normally transparent. Freshly voided urine should appear clear, without sediment. Urine draining from an indwelling catheter should appear clear and without sediment in the tubing, but it may contain occasional mucus shreds. Urine that has been sitting unemptied in a urinal or collecting device for an hour or longer may normally appear cloudy secondary to separation or settling of urinary constituents.

ODOR

The odor of freshly voided urine is typically described as aromatic. Generally, the more dilute the urine, the fainter the odor; the more concentrated the urine, the stronger the odor. Collected urine that has been sitting unemptied for a long period may have a strong ammonia scent. Medications and certain foods can alter urine's odor. A strong, offensive odor is not normally present in urine that is free from infection.

Normal Pattern of Urinary Elimination

Many people have a routine pattern associated with urinary elimination. Most people void six to eight times a day. Typically, people void soon after getting out of bed in the morning. Many people tend to void within an hour after mealtime and once again before bedtime. Variations in patterns of fluid intake directly affect routine patterns of voiding.

The total amount of urine voided during a 24-hour period usually ranges between 1,200 and 1,500 mL. Each void should contain a minimum of approximately 200 mL and a maximum of 500 mL.

Lifespan Considerations

NEWBORN AND INFANT

From about the 3rd month after conception, the fetal kidneys begin functioning and the fetus voids urine in utero. Newborns, therefore, may have urine in their bladders at birth and should be able to void within the first 24 hours after birth. The first voiding may be of slightly pink-tinged urine, caused by an accumulation of uric acid crystals. Noting the first

TABLE 32-1 NORMAL RANGES FOR DAILY URINE OUTPUT DURING THE LIFESPAN	
Age (years)	Output (mL)
Newborn–2	500–600
2–5	500–800
5–8	600–1,200
8–14	1,000–1,500
14 and over	1,500

voiding after birth is important to verify that the infant's urine formation and excretion are adequate. At birth, the kidneys are still not fully developed; Bowman capsule and the tubules are still refining their respective filtering and reabsorption abilities. Newborns usually void small amounts (15 to 30 mL, up to 30 to 40 times a day) of dilute, light yellow urine.

As infants grow, they are able to void slightly larger amounts at less frequent intervals. The urine's color remains pale yellow throughout infancy. The total amount of urine that infants void in a 24-hour period depends on total fluid intake and fluid losses from other sources. The average urine output for newborns and infants is about 500 to 600 mL in 24 hours. Table 32-1 gives the normal ranges of daily urine output across the lifespan.

Infants lack voluntary control of urinary elimination. The sacral spinal cord segments innervating the bladder are still immature. The bladder empties in reflex fashion after a degree of bladder stretch occurs.

Congenital malformations of the urinary tract or the central nervous system may cause serious alterations in urinary elimination. UTIs, which are more common in female than in male infants, can also disrupt normal urinary function.

TODDLER AND PRESCHOOLER

During the toddler and preschool years, children usually achieve voluntary urinary continence because they become physiologically and psychologically capable of this task. Sometime between 12 and 18 months, the myelinization of the sacral spinal segments that control the bladder becomes complete, and children can then perceive bladder fullness. A good indicator of the maturation of the spinal cord is when a toddler begins to walk independently.

Beginning sometime between 2 and 3 years of age, parents watch for signs that a child may be ready for toilet training, such as staying dry for 2 hours at a time or dry after naps and the child can walk to the bathroom and is able to help undress. Most children will achieve daytime urinary control by 3 to 4 years of age. Sometimes, toddlers need to experience outdoor playtime without diapers to see what happens when they experience bladder fullness followed by urethral relaxation and bladder emptying. They begin to understand the relationship between bladder fullness and voluntary bladder emptying and are ready for toilet training. Children in North American cultures usually achieve daytime urinary continence by 3 years of age; boys may take longer than girls. Nighttime continence may not occur until 4 or 5 years of age.

SCHOOL-AGE CHILD AND ADOLESCENT

School-age children and adolescents have achieved both daytime and nighttime urinary continence. They are forming urinary elimination habits similar to those of adults, voiding straw-colored urine six or seven times a day. The amount of oral fluid intake greatly influences the amount of urine output; Table 32-1 lists average ranges of urine output in a 24-hour period for children of various ages.

Some healthy school-age children continue to experience involuntary **urinary incontinence**, which is termed *enuresis*. Many parents seek advice from healthcare providers when nocturnal **enuresis** occurs in their children older than 7 years of age. Specific nursing interventions for the management of nocturnal enuresis are discussed later in this chapter.

ADULT AND OLDER ADULT

Incontinence is not usually identified as a significant health problem in the early to middle adult years. For those affected with adverse urinary symptoms, a significant correlation exists between urinary incontinence symptoms and their negative impact on travel, social, physical, and emotional activities. In late middle age, men may experience altered urinary elimination related to prostatic hypertrophy, and women may experience altered urinary elimination related to weakened perineal muscles.

The ureters, bladder, and urethra lose some muscle tone with aging. The bladder becomes less able to hold large amounts of urine (decreased bladder capacity), and older persons may experience an **urgency** to empty the bladder more frequently of smaller amounts of urine. They may sense the urge to void only when the bladder is at the limit of its capacity, which diminishes the ability to delay voiding voluntarily. Uninhibited bladder contractions can further increase the sense of urgency. **Nocturia**, nighttime urination, is one of the most common reasons for interrupted sleep in the adult population, especially in older adults.

Symptoms of UTI are different in the older adult, especially if the immune system is depressed. Rather than experiencing painful urination and a high fever, the older adult will become acutely confused. UTI should be suspected for any older adult who develops sudden delirium.

As a result of cardiovascular changes that occur with aging, many older adults experience decreased perfusion to the kidneys. This decreased arterial flow to the renal arteries is a gradual change that results from decreased cardiac muscle strength, which reduces cardiac output to the periphery, and decreased elasticity of the peripheral blood vessels. Over time, owing to decreased arterial perfusion, kidney function progressively decreases; the kidneys become a less effective regulator of the body's ECF.

Women's risk of developing urinary incontinence during their lifetime is twice that of men's and is related to decreased

APPLY YOUR CRITICAL THINKING

You remove Mr. Phillips's Foley catheter, which had been in place for 5 days. You provide him with a urinal and ask him to let you know when he voids. Six hours later, he voids 100 mL of clear, light yellow urine. How would you assess his voiding after catheter removal?

Check your answer in Appendix B.

estrogen levels and weakened perineal muscles. Older men may experience urinary hesitancy and difficulty starting the urinary stream, related to prostatic hypertrophy. Nevertheless, although aging is a risk factor, urinary incontinence is not a normal or inevitable part of aging.

Older adults with incontinence may attempt to manage incontinence by restricting intake of fluids, using absorbent pads in clothing, and changing clothing and using powders and colognes to mask odors. They may also isolate themselves by restricting social interactions and activities.

Cultural Considerations

The privacy requirements for voiding can vary from culture to culture and among individuals within a culture. Many people cannot relax their perineal muscles without adequate privacy. Women, in particular, have been culturally trained to require more privacy for voiding: Women's public restrooms have private stalls for elimination, whereas men's public restrooms have open rows of urinals. In some third world countries, squatting over an in-ground receptacle rather than sitting on a commode is common. Hygiene practices after toileting can be culturally learned and dictated.

Parents in Western cultures usually begin toilet training their children by 24 months of age, although it is not uncommon to wait until age 3 years for some children. Training children prior to 24 months can lengthen the duration of training. Parents in non-Western countries often begin toilet training much earlier (Hockenberry & Wilson, 2013). In many cultures, the custom has always been toilet training from infancy. Parents become alert to infants' signals such as body language and sounds as well as patterns and timing after feeding or waking and simply place the infant over the toilet. Daytime urinary dryness is achieved much earlier (Palmer, Athanasopoulos, Lee, Takeda, & Wyndaele, 2012).

Urinary continence is a valued social behavior in all cultures. Urinary incontinence is a quality of life issue. Adults who experience urinary incontinence express shame and embarrassment. Patients in hospitals frequently attempt to get to bathrooms with or without assistance of healthcare personnel as they try to avoid embarrassment of wetting the bed. Incontinence is not a normal aspect of aging, yet many people, including some nurses and other healthcare professionals, accept incontinence as an inevitable aspect of aging. Older adults experiencing incontinence often attempt to maintain secrecy about their incontinence; urinary incontinence is not considered an appropriate topic for social conversation (Palmer et al., 2012). They also may not want to burden busy doctors and nurses regarding what they consider an inconvenience rather than an illness. Untreated urinary incontinence decreases satisfaction with life and is one of the major reasons for institutionalization of older adults in many countries and cultures (Barentsen et al., 2012; Siu & Lopez, 2012).

Factors Affecting Urinary Elimination

Fluid intake, loss of body fluid, nutrition, body position, cognition, and psychological issues can affect urinary patterns. Many other factors can predispose a person to disruption of normal patterns of urinary elimination (Box 32-1). Obstruction of urine flow, UTIs, hypotension, neurologic injury, decreased muscle tone, pregnancy, surgery, and medications are common causes.

FLUID INTAKE

The amount of fluid that a person ingests is the most influential factor in determining urine output. If a person increases his or her volume of fluid intake, an associated increase will occur in the volume of urine output. Conversely, a decrease in fluid intake will cause a corresponding decrease in urine output.

This relationship is hormonally controlled. Several hormones, the most important of which is antidiuretic hormone (ADH), play significant roles in the reabsorption of water in the tubules of the nephron. The name *antidiuretic* implies the function of ADH, which is to prevent **diuresis**, or water excretion.

BOX 32-1   Factors That Influence Urinary Patterns

- Fluid intake
- Loss of body fluid
- Nutrition
- Body position
- Psychological issues
- Cognition
- Obstruction of urine flow—renal calculi, prostatic enlargement, tumors, structural abnormalities
- Infection
- Hypotension
- Neurologic injury—spinal cord injury, cerebrovascular accident (stroke), brain tumor
- Decreased muscle tone—aging, multiple pregnancies, obesity
- Pregnancy
- Surgery—anesthesia, edema, immobility
- Medications
- Urinary diversions

ADH is secreted by the hypothalamus and released by the posterior pituitary in the brain. Increased plasma osmolarity stimulates the release of ADH (discussed in detail in Chapter 28). When ADH is present, the distal tubule of the nephron becomes more permeable to water. Release of ADH causes the kidney to reabsorb more water, thus producing more concentrated urine. When fluid intake increases, ADH release is suppressed. In the absence of ADH, the renal tubules become relatively impermeable to water, and little water is reabsorbed, producing an increased volume of dilute urine.

The amount of fluid intake not only affects the amount of urine produced but also influences the frequency of urination. If fluid intake is greatly increased, frequency of voiding increases because the bladder fills more quickly. Conversely, if fluid intake is low, voiding frequency decreases.

LOSS OF BODY FLUID

When a person loses a great deal of body fluid, the kidneys increase reabsorption of water from the glomerular filtrate to maintain the proper osmolarity of the ECF. This regulates the concentration of solutes in the ECF, resulting in decreased urine output. Increased loss of body fluids can occur with vomiting, diarrhea, excessive diaphoresis secondary to fever or exercise, excessive wound drainage, extensive burns, or blood loss from trauma or surgery.

DIET

Diet may affect urinary elimination. If the diet contains a high percentage of foods with high water content (e.g., soup, gelatin, fruits, vegetables), urine volume will be greater than if intake of such foods is limited. If a person ingests large quantities of salty foods without increasing water intake, urine output will decrease and the urine will be more concentrated. Alcohol and caffeine-containing fluids or food, such as coffee, tea, cola, or chocolate, irritate the bladder and contain a **diuretic** that can increase urine output when they are ingested in large amounts.

BODY POSITION

Body position plays an important role in the ability to empty the bladder completely with each voiding. The typical body position for urinary elimination in men is standing upright. Some men find it difficult to empty their bladder fully into a urinal while lying flat in bed. Commonly, this difficulty alters the voiding pattern, so voiding becomes more frequent but with less volume. The normal position for voiding in women is sitting. If a woman must use a bedpan while flat in bed, she also may be unable to empty her bladder completely.

COGNITION

Cognitive impairment interferes with a person's ability to maintain urinary continence. Neurologic conditions such as Alzheimer disease, brain tumor, or cerebrovascular accident (stroke) can reduce the person's ability to perceive bladder fullness or to delay voiding until he or she reaches the toilet. Medications or serious illness can cause temporary confusion called delirium, especially in older adults. People need to be alert, cognitively intact, and motivated to maintain urinary continence.

PSYCHOLOGICAL FACTORS

Because the release of urine from the bladder is ultimately under voluntary control, anything that causes a person to think about voiding can influence the process. Hearing another person talk about the need to void, reading a chapter about urinary elimination, or hearing running water may all produce the need for a bathroom break. Pouring warm water over a patient's inner thigh or perineal area may stimulate voiding; giving a patient a cold bedpan may temporarily delay voiding.

Stress and anxiety can affect urinary elimination. In stressful situations, a person can experience a strong urge to urinate. Stress can also cause the reverse problem of urinary retention: The person's muscles may become so tense that he or she cannot relax the perineal muscles, and voiding is inhibited.

OBSTRUCTION OF URINE FLOW

Obstruction of the normal flow of urine can lead to problems with urinary elimination and, when severe, can cause kidney damage. Structural abnormalities within the urinary tract, urinary tumors or other tumors that press against the urinary tract, renal stones, and prostatic enlargement are possible causes of urinary obstruction. Obstruction can also occur when patients have catheters or nephrostomy tubes in place that become plugged or kinked.

One of the complications of obstruction within the urinary system is **hydronephrosis**, which is distention of the kidney pelvis with urine secondary to the increased resistance caused by obstruction to normal urine flow. Unrelieved hydronephrosis can cause renal cell atrophy and necrosis, which can cause permanent kidney damage.

Urinary stasis also occurs secondary to urinary obstruction. The stagnant urine proximal to the obstruction provides a good growth medium for microorganisms, fostering the development of UTIs.

INFECTIONS OF THE URINARY TRACT

UTIs are usually caused by microorganisms normally found in the gastrointestinal tract. The species commonly responsible for UTIs are of the Enterobacteriaceae group and include *Escherichia coli, Klebsiella,* and *Proteus.* These microorganisms typically gain access to the urinary system by way of the urethral meatus. Thus, the most common UTIs are infections of the urethra (urethritis) or bladder (cystitis). Urethritis and cystitis are classified as lower UTIs, whereas infections of the ureters (ureteritis) and the kidney pelvis or tubule system are classified as upper UTIs. Upper UTIs are less common than lower UTIs, but they are more serious because kidney damage and renal failure may result.

Normally, the urinary tract is sterile, except at the urethral meatus. In the healthy person, the act of voiding tends to flush away bacteria. Infection occurs when microorganisms from the surrounding perineal skin or anal opening find their way to the urinary meatus and ascend the urethra. Women are more susceptible to lower UTIs because of the short length of their urethras and the proximity of the vagina and anus to the urinary meatus. Men are less susceptible to lower UTIs because of the longer length of the male urethra and also because of the antibacterial properties of prostatic secretions.

Other factors that can increase the incidence of UTIs include incorrect wiping of the anal area after bowel movements; sexual intercourse, which can bring perineal microorganisms into closer contact with the urinary meatus; and any procedure that places an object in the urethra or bladder for diagnostic or therapeutic reasons. Infections of the urinary tract can disrupt the normal pattern of urinary elimination in many ways. Voiding becomes painful and more frequent. The person with a UTI often experiences urgency, a subjective feeling of being unable to delay the urge to void voluntarily. Urine becomes abnormal, containing pus (**pyuria**) and blood (**hematuria**). Ultimately, if the infection ascends to the kidney, renal damage can occur, possibly resulting in renal failure.

Catheter-Associated Urinary Tract Infection

The Centers for Disease Control (CDC) defines **catheter-associated urinary tract infection (CAUTI)** as a UTI that develops when an indwelling urinary catheter is in place greater than 2 days prior to the onset of infection. UTI is responsible for 40% of all healthcare associated infections, and 80% of those infections are caused by indwelling urinary catheters. These infections can lead to gram-negative blood infections, which are sometimes fatal. CAUTI is caused by a biofilm that develops on the catheter surface and leads to multidrug resistant infections (CDC, 2014; Singhai, Malik, Shahid, Malik & Goyal, 2012).

Additionally, because CAUTI is considered preventable, the Centers for Medicare and Medicaid Services (CMS) will not provide additional reimbursement to hospitals for CAUTI if the UTI was not present upon admission (Bernard, Hunter, & Moore, 2012).

> **! SAFETY ALERT**
>
> Every day an indwelling catheter remains in the bladder, the chance of developing CAUTI increases 3% to 7% (Mori, 2014). The CDC recommends removal of indwelling catheters within 24 hours postoperatively whenever possible (CDC, 2014).

Use the concept map (Fig. 32-3) to help understand and manage the situation in the opening scenario of the patient who is at risk for CAUTI and to plan for his care.

URINARY ELIMINATION

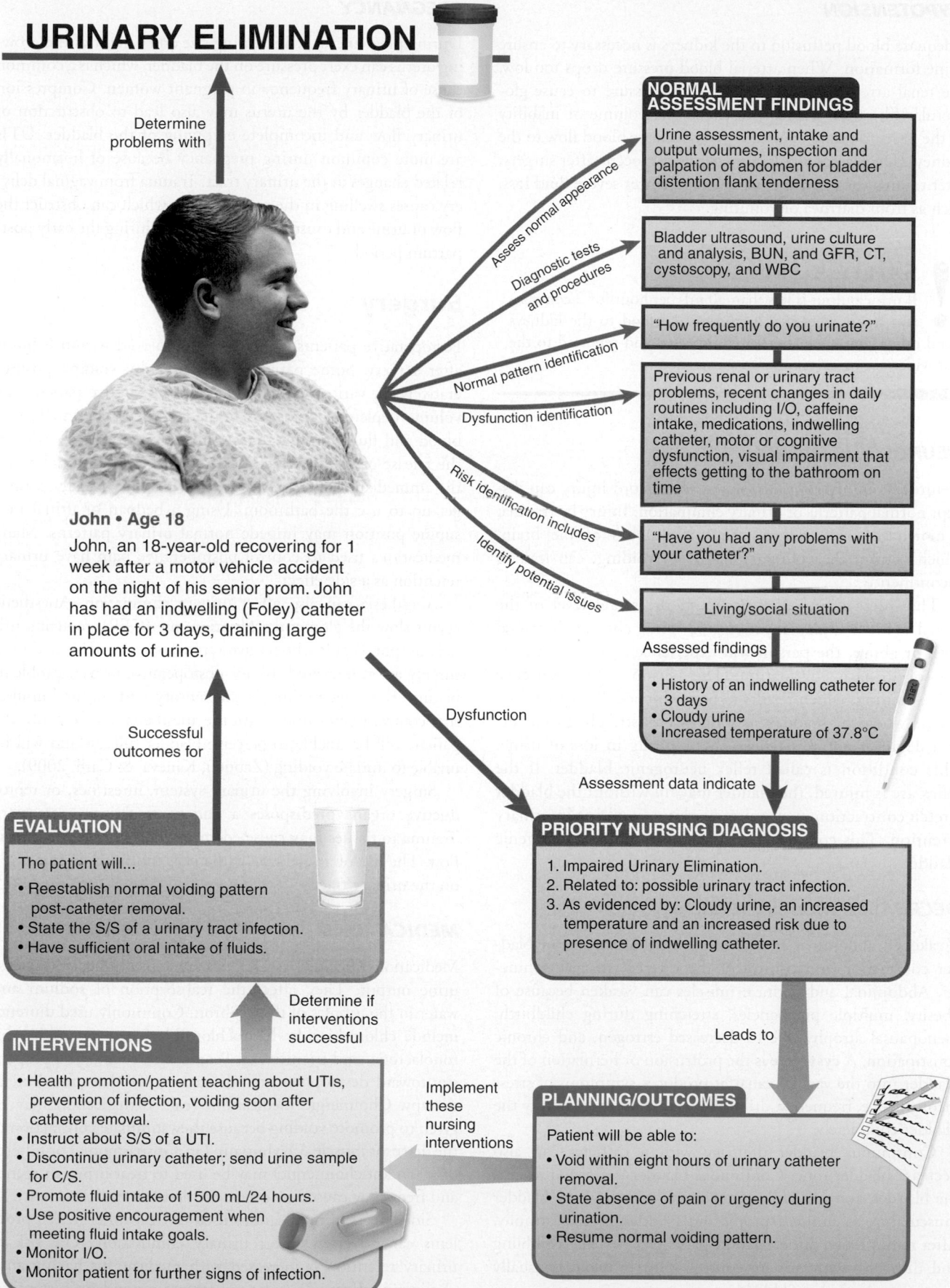

Determine problems with

Assess normal appearance

Diagnostic tests and procedures

Normal pattern identification

Dysfunction identification

Risk identification includes

Identify potential issues

John • Age 18

John, an 18-year-old recovering for 1 week after a motor vehicle accident on the night of his senior prom. John has had an indwelling (Foley) catheter in place for 3 days, draining large amounts of urine.

NORMAL ASSESSMENT FINDINGS

Urine assessment, intake and output volumes, inspection and palpation of abdomen for bladder distention flank tenderness

Bladder ultrasound, urine culture and analysis, BUN, and GFR, CT, cystoscopy, and WBC

"How frequently do you urinate?"

Previous renal or urinary tract problems, recent changes in daily routines including I/O, caffeine intake, medications, indwelling catheter, motor or cognitive dysfunction, visual impairment that effects getting to the bathroom on time

"Have you had any problems with your catheter?"

Living/social situation

Assessed findings

• History of an indwelling catheter for 3 days
• Cloudy urine
• Increased temperature of 37.8°C

Assessment data indicate

Dysfunction

Successful outcomes for

EVALUATION

The patient will...

• Reestablish normal voiding pattern post-catheter removal.
• State the S/S of a urinary tract infection.
• Have sufficient oral intake of fluids.

Determine if interventions successful

INTERVENTIONS

• Health promotion/patient teaching about UTIs, prevention of infection, voiding soon after catheter removal.
• Instruct about S/S of a UTI.
• Discontinue urinary catheter; send urine sample for C/S.
• Promote fluid intake of 1500 mL/24 hours.
• Use positive encouragement when meeting fluid intake goals.
• Monitor I/O.
• Monitor patient for further signs of infection.

Implement these nursing interventions

PRIORITY NURSING DIAGNOSIS

1. Impaired Urinary Elimination.
2. Related to: possible urinary tract infection.
3. As evidenced by: Cloudy urine, an increased temperature and an increased risk due to presence of indwelling catheter.

Leads to

PLANNING/OUTCOMES

Patient will be able to:

• Void within eight hours of urinary catheter removal.
• State absence of pain or urgency during urination.
• Resume normal voiding pattern.

FIGURE 32-3 Concept map for urinary elimination.

HYPOTENSION

Adequate blood perfusion to the kidneys is necessary to ensure urine formation. When arterial blood pressure drops too low, the renal arteries do not have enough pressure to cause glomerular filtration. Inadequate circulating volume or inability of the heart to pump adequately can decrease blood flow to the kidneys. Decreased circulating volume can occur after surgery, after trauma, or when the patient experiences severe fluid loss, such as from diarrhea or vomiting.

> **! SAFETY ALERT**
> If urine output is less than 30 mL per hour for 2 consecutive hours, decreased perfusion of blood to the kidneys and other vital organs must be suspected and reported to the provider.

NEUROLOGIC INJURY

Neurologic injury after a stroke or spinal cord injury can disrupt normal patterns of urinary elimination. Injury by trauma, hemorrhage, or tumor to the frontal lobes of the brain, which control the voluntary nature of voiding, can lead to incontinence.

The micturition reflex occurs at the sacral level of the spinal cord. If injury occurs to the spinal cord at the sacral level or above, the person will experience a change in control of urinary elimination. The person may experience reflex voiding, which results in incontinence. Reflex voiding occurs when the bladder, as soon as it is stretched to a certain degree, contracts reflexively, resulting in loss of urine. This condition is called reflex neurogenic bladder. If the reflex arc is injured, the bladder may fill without the bladder stretch contraction mechanism working, resulting in urinary retention. This condition is called autonomous neurogenic bladder.

DECREASED MUSCLE TONE

Weakened abdominal and perineal muscles can impair bladder contraction and control of the external urinary sphincter. Abdominal and perineal muscles can weaken because of obesity, multiple pregnancies, stretching during childbirth, menopausal atrophy due to decreased estrogen, and chronic constipation. A **cystocele** is the protrusion or herniation of the bladder into the vaginal canal; it produces symptoms of stress incontinence, frequency, dribbling, and inability to empty the bladder completely.

Continuous bladder drainage with a catheter can also decrease bladder tone. Continuous bladder drainage prevents the bladder from ever filling; therefore, stretch of the bladder musculature is limited, promoting bladder muscle atrophy. After removal of a catheter, some patients experience dribbling and difficulty with urinary control. This problem is usually temporary, lasting until bladder tone returns.

PREGNANCY

During pregnancy, the increasing size and weight of the growing uterus can exert pressure on the bladder, which is a common cause of urinary frequency in pregnant women. Compression of the bladder by the uterus may also lead to obstruction of urinary flow and incomplete emptying of the bladder. UTIs are more common during pregnancy because of hormonally related changes in the urinary tract. Trauma from vaginal delivery causes swelling in the perineal area, which can obstruct the flow of urine and cause urinary retention during the early postpartum period.

Surgery

Postoperative patients should be able to void within 8 hours after surgery. Some patients have difficulty voiding postoperatively for various reasons. Many postoperative patients are volume depleted because of limited fluid intake and loss of blood and fluid during surgery. The stress of surgery triggers the release of ADH, which decreases urinary output. During the immediate postoperative period, patients usually cannot get up to use the bathroom. Using a bedpan or urinal in a supine position may impede normal urinary patterns. Many medications used to control postoperative pain have urinary retention as a side effect.

Anesthesia can also affect urinary elimination. Anesthetic agents slow the glomerular filtration rate (GFR), reducing urinary output. People who receive a spinal or regional block during surgery are at increased risk for postoperative urinary problems because these agents impair the sensory and motor impulses that control micturition. Until the anesthesia has worn off, the patient will be unable to perceive bladder fullness and will be unable to initiate voiding (Zaouter, Kaneva, & Carli, 2009).

Surgery involving the urinary system, intestines, or reproductive organs predisposes a patient to urinary retention. Trauma to tissues may cause edema, which can obstruct urine flow. The use of a retention catheter is indicated after surgery on the urinary tract.

MEDICATIONS

Medications classified as diuretics are administered to increase urine output. They affect the reabsorption of sodium and water in the tubules of the nephron. Commonly used diuretics include chlorothiazide, hydrochlorothiazide, furosemide, spironolactone, and triamterene. People with edema or a propensity toward development of edema are candidates for diuretic therapy. Cholinergic medications (e.g., bethanechol) may be given to promote voiding because they stimulate contraction of the detrusor muscle. Oxybutynin (an antispasmodic) or tolterodine (an anticholinergic) may be used to treat urinary urgency and frequency caused by overactive detrusor muscle activity.

Side effects of medications used to treat other health problems can adversely affect urinary elimination. The risk of urinary retention is increased with medications having anticholinergic effects. Tricyclic antidepressants and antihistamines are examples of such drugs. Opioids can decrease the GFR and the sensation of bladder fullness.

Some medications change the color of urine. For example, phenazopyridine (Pyridium) causes urine to turn bright orange, and amitriptyline turns urine blue-green.

ALTERED URINARY FUNCTION

Altered urinary function manifests in many different ways including **dysuria**, **polyuria**, **oliguria**, urgency, frequency, nocturia, hematuria, pyuria, urinary retention, urinary incontinence, enuresis, and urinary diversion.

Dysuria

Dysuria means painful voiding. Pain is often associated with UTIs and is felt as a burning sensation during urination. Any bladder inflammation or trauma or inflammation of the urethra can cause dysuria. Painful voiding should be referred to a physician because dysuria has many causes.

Polyuria

Polyuria is the formation and excretion of excessive amounts of urine in the absence of a concurrent increase in fluid intake. Urine output of more than 2,500 to 3,000 mL in 24 hours is considered polyuria. Untreated diabetes insipidus and hyperglycemia can greatly increase urine output. Ingestion of diuretics, caffeine, and alcohol also results in polyuria.

Oliguria

Oliguria is the formation and excretion of decreased amounts of urine, or urinary output less than 500 mL in 24 hours. A severe decrease in fluid intake or any disease state or injury that leads to an excessive loss of body fluids can cause oliguria. For example, excessive vomiting, diarrhea, diaphoresis, burns, or bleeding can decrease urine output. People with renal disease may be oliguric. As the kidney approaches complete failure, the person may become anuric. **Anuria** is the formation and excretion of less than 100 mL of urine in 24 hours.

Urgency

Most adults can postpone emptying the bladder until it contains 250 to 400 mL of urine. **Urgency** is the subjective feeling of being unable to delay voiding voluntarily. Urgency implies a strong micturition reflex caused by inflammation or infection of the urethra or bladder, incompetent urethral sphincter, weak perineal muscle control, or psychological stress.

Frequency

Voiding at frequent intervals is known as frequency. Frequency occurs when a person voids more often than normal, without a significant increase in fluid intake. Each voiding usually contains less than 250 mL of urine. Frequency not associated with increased fluid intake can be related to other factors, such as UTI or pressure on the bladder from pregnancy. Frequency and urgency often occur together; the term **overactive bladder** is sometimes used in this situation.

Nocturia

Voiding during normal sleeping hours is called nocturia. If a person voids before going to bed, it should be possible to sleep for 7 to 8 hours without feeling a strong micturition reflex. Ingestion of large amounts of fluids before bed, especially those containing alcohol or caffeine, may promote nocturia. People with medical conditions such as congestive heart failure may also experience nocturia. When lying supine, edema decreases as fluid enters the circulation. Blood flow to the kidneys increases, increasing glomerular filtration and urine output.

Hematuria

Hematuria is blood in the urine; it can be gross (visible on visual examination) or occult (not visible on visual examination). Occult blood may change the color of urine from normal clear yellow or amber to a cloudy or hazy yellow or amber. As the number of red blood cells increases, the urine may become bright red. Pathologic causes of hematuria include UTIs, urinary tract tumors, renal calculi, poisoning, and trauma to the urinary mucosa. Hematuria is expected and temporary after urinary tract or prostate surgery.

Pyuria

Pyuria means that the urine contains pus, which is the accumulation of the end products of an inflammatory response. Pus-containing microorganisms and white blood cells give urine a cloudy color and, often, a strong, unpleasant odor. Pyuria occurs with UTI.

Urinary Retention

Urinary retention is the inability to empty the bladder of urine. In urinary retention, the person is either unable to perceive the feeling of bladder fullness or unable to relax the bladder neck and external urethral sphincter to allow urine to pass from the body. Because the kidneys continue to form urine, the volume within the bladder grows until, in extreme cases, the bladder holds up to 2,000 to 3,000 mL of urine. Bladder distention of more than 600 mL can often be palpated in the suprapubic area of the abdomen.

Urinary retention with overflow is the loss of small amounts of urine from an overdistended bladder. As the bladder becomes overdistended, it no longer responds to bladder stretch as a stimulus to initiate detrusor contraction and voiding. The bladder can maintain only a certain degree of overdistention before excess urine is eliminated in small amounts at frequent intervals. The small amounts of urine that are voided are known as "overflow."

Complications of urinary retention include the loss of bladder tone secondary to excessive stretch of the detrusor muscle fibers. Even after the primary retention is relieved, it may take weeks for the bladder stretch (i.e., bladder emptying response) to return to normal. Accumulation of urine in the bladder also leads to stasis of urine, which predisposes the person to UTIs and calculi development. Bladder distention also can lead to hydronephrosis, as the urine backs up into the ureters and renal pelvis. This pressure on the nephron can cause damage to the functional unit of the kidney and cause renal failure.

People at risk for development of urinary retention include those with neurologic impairment, such as spinal cord injury or brain lesions. Postoperative patients may experience temporary urinary retention until edema subsides and spinal anesthesia wears off. After vaginal delivery of a baby, swelling of the urinary meatus is common and may cause temporary obstruction to urine outflow.

Urinary Incontinence

Urinary incontinence is the involuntary loss of urine from the bladder. Five types of urinary incontinence are defined by patterns of uncontrolled voiding and related causative factors: stress, urge, reflex, functional, and total incontinence. Table 32-2 summarizes causes of and treatment for types of incontinence. Urinary incontinence can lead to social isolation and depressive symptoms because people fear that urinary incontinence will prove embarrassing in social situations. Incontinence in the older person often contributes to a family's decision to seek placement in a skilled nursing facility.

STRESS INCONTINENCE

The sudden, involuntary loss of small amounts (less than 50 mL) of urine that accompanies a sudden increase in intra-abdominal pressure is called *stress incontinence*. Examples of activities that increase intra-abdominal pressure are coughing, sneezing, laughing, lifting, and jumping.

Factors associated with stress incontinence include weakening of the pelvic floor muscles, high intra-abdominal pressure, damage to the bladder neck, and side effects of medications. Stretching that occurs during childbirth can weaken the pelvic floor muscles. Women who have experienced a long and difficult labor and delivery or who have borne several children are most likely to have weakened pelvic muscles. Estrogen is necessary to maintain the normal tone of reproductive organs and associated musculature; therefore, postmenopausal women who have decreased estrogen levels may experience stress incontinence. Obesity or pregnancy can cause high intra-abdominal pressure. Obese, postmenopausal women who have had multiple pregnancies are most likely to experience stress incontinence. Another cause of stress incontinence is direct trauma, which may result from a fractured pelvis or during genitourinary surgery.

URGE INCONTINENCE

The involuntary loss of urine after a strong feeling of the need to urinate is referred to as *urge incontinence*. The person with urge incontinence is unable simultaneously to perceive a full bladder and to hold urine until reaching the bathroom. The term *overactive bladder* is used to describe frequent strong urges to urinate; overactive bladder usually is eventually associated with incontinence. Frequency, dysuria, and nocturia

TABLE 32-2 CAUSES AND TREATMENT FOR INCONTINENCE

Type of Incontinence	Causes	Treatment
Stress Incontinence—increased abdominal pressure causes involuntary loss of small amounts of urine	High abdominal pressures from coughing, sneezing, jumping, or weak pelvic support from obesity, pregnancy Prostate surgery	Kegel exercises, weight loss if obese, vaginal pessary, estrogen vaginal creams, male external catheters, surgery
Urge Urinary Incontinence—random involuntary passage of urine after a strong urge to void	Overactivity of the detrusor muscle; decreased bladder capacity; irritation of the bladder; bladder infection; overdistension of the bladder; intake of diuretics, caffeine, or alcohol	Timed voiding schedule, anticholinergic drugs
Reflex Urinary Incontinence—involuntary loss of urine, occurring at somewhat predictable intervals when a specific bladder volume is reached overcoming sphincter control	Spinal cord impairment above the sacral reflex arc (spinal cord injury, stroke, brain tumor) or radical pelvic surgery; flaccid neurogenic bladder	In and out catheterization; alpha-adrenergic drugs to relax internal sphincter, baclofen to relax external sphincter
Functional Urinary Incontinence—inability of a normally continent person to reach the bathroom in time to avoid unintentional loss of urine	Altered environment treat and sensory, cognitive, psychological, neurovascular, or mobility deficits	Toileting routine, verbal cuing reminders with assistance to bathroom, alteration of environment for easy access to bathroom, clothing that is easy to remove
Total Urinary Incontinence—a person experiences continuous, unpredictable loss of urine	Neurologic lesion, trauma to or congenital malformation in the spinal cord or brain, severe cognitive deficits	Toileting routine and verbal reminders, external catheters for men, absorbent products, excellent skin care and hygiene

THERAPEUTIC DIALOGUE: URINARY INCONTINENCE

SCENE FOR THOUGHT

Mrs. Clements is a 55-year-old woman who has been referred for complaints of incontinence of urine for 3 months. The nurse is scheduled to perform a history and physical.

LESS EFFECTIVE

Nurse:	Good morning, Mrs. Clements. How are you today? Please sit down so I can ask you about your history. *(Asks about age, address, number of children, and other items on assessment sheet.)*
Mrs. Clements:	*(Answers all questions quietly.)*
Nurse:	I understand that you have an incontinence problem. Many women your age have that kind of difficulty, and I'm sure we can fix you up so you'll be just fine.
Mrs. Clements:	My mother's doctor told her that years ago, but she never got better. *(Looks down at her lap.)*
Nurse:	Well, we'll just see what we can do for you here. Could you undress and put on this gown? I'll be back in a minute to do your physical. *(Leaves room, closing the door quietly.)*

MORE EFFECTIVE

Nurse:	Good morning, Mrs. Clements. Please sit down so we can talk a while before I do your physical. *(Acknowledges Mrs. Clements, gives simple directions.)* What can I do for you this morning? *(Asks open-ended question.)*
Mrs. Clements:	You can help me stop wetting myself. *(Looks down at her lap.)*
Nurse:	You look worried about that. *(Observes behavior accurately.)*
Mrs. Clements:	Yes, I am. *(Looks relieved.)* Before my mother died last year, she had to wear adult diapers; she always smelled and had bladder infections, and it was awful for her and for everyone else. I don't want to get that way.
Nurse:	So what you would like is for me to help you figure out a way to deal with the wetting problem so you don't have to live the way your mother did. Is that right? *(States understanding of what Mrs. Clements wants and clarifies with her.)*
Mrs. Clements:	Yes! That would be great.
Nurse:	Okay. Why don't we start with some questions and then I'll do a physical and we can go from there. *(Gives Mrs. Clements some idea of planning.)*

CRITICAL THINKING CHALLENGE

- Critique what the nurse did that was effective in the second scene.
- Determine what was less effective about the first scene.
- Consider how you think Mrs. Clements felt in both scenes.
- Although each nurse spent the same amount of time with Mrs. Clements, analyze how the first nurse could have been more effective.

commonly accompany urge incontinence. Very few women who experience symptoms of urge incontinence seek medical help for their symptoms (Newman, 2009).

Factors associated with urge incontinence include UTIs, use of diuretics, consumption of fluids that contain caffeine or alcohol, smoking (nicotine), and increased fluid intake. An overdistended bladder can precipitate urge incontinence. Some patients experience urge incontinence for a short period after removal of an indwelling catheter: They have become accustomed to an empty bladder and need time to accommodate to the usual degree of bladder distention.

REFLEX INCONTINENCE

An involuntary loss of urine that occurs at somewhat predictable intervals when a specific bladder volume is reached is called *reflex incontinence*. The person is unable to sense bladder fullness because of neurologic impairment, and the bladder simply empties when a certain degree of bladder stretch occurs. Bladder emptying occurs at the sacral reflex level because of impairment of the connection to the cerebrum that allows voluntary inhibition of voiding. Reflex incontinence is seen in patients with neurologic impairment, such as a spinal cord lesion, cerebrovascular accident, or brain tumor.

FUNCTIONAL INCONTINENCE

Functional incontinence involves the inability or unwillingness of a person with normal bladder and sphincter control to reach the bathroom in time to void. Environmental barriers, disorientation, or physical limitations may contribute. The amount of urine that the person loses is typically large.

Many factors can interfere with the ability to reach the toilet in time. A poorly lit, cluttered room may obstruct easy access to the bathroom. Raised side rails or a call light that is out of reach can contribute to functional incontinence in a hospitalized patient. Sensory and cognitive factors are also associated with functional incontinence because confusion, disorientation, and sedatives or side effects of medications can impair cognitive functioning. Motor deficits, such as impaired gait and loss of the fine motor control needed to release necessary clothing, can also contribute.

TOTAL INCONTINENCE

The continuous, involuntary, unpredictable loss of urine from a nondistended bladder is called *total incontinence;* this term is sometimes used when the observed incontinence does not fit any other category and does not respond to usual treatment methods. Factors associated with total incontinence include a specific neurologic lesion in the brain or spinal cord, a traumatic or surgical injury to the genitourinary area or spinal cord, and a congenital malformation within the urinary tract or spinal cord.

Enuresis

Enuresis is involuntary voiding, with no underlying pathophysiologic origin, after the age at which bladder control is usually achieved. By the time most children are 4 or 5 years of age, they can control urinary elimination during both day and night. Enuresis beyond age 5 years is typically nocturnal and is commonly called *bed-wetting*. Involuntary voiding during sleep can also occur during daytime naps, but it is more common during longer periods of sleep at night. Factors associated with nocturnal enuresis include small bladder capacity, sound sleeping, bowel dysfunction, stress and anxiety at home or school, UTIs, and family history of nocturnal enuresis. Primary nocturnal enuresis can affect up to 20% of children between the ages of 5 and 7 years (Saldano, Chaviano, & Maizels, 2008). Enuresis can occur in older people too: In one study, 6% of the adults surveyed admitted to experiencing nocturnal enuresis (Buckley & Lapitan, 2009).

Urinary Diversion

A urinary diversion is a surgical procedure in which the normal pathway of urine elimination is altered. Muscle-invasive bladder cancer is the most common reason for a urinary diversion procedure in which the bladder is surgically removed (**cystectomy**) (Turner, 2009). Following cystectomy, the kidneys continue to produce urine. In an incontinent cutaneous urinary diversion, the ureters are implanted into the distal segment of the small intestine called the ileum. This section of ileum is then brought out to the abdomen to form a stoma. Urine is thus diverted to exit through the abdominal stoma. Urine (and small amounts of mucus produced by the ileum) is collected in a drainage bag applied over the stoma on the abdomen. This type of urinary diversion is called **ileal conduit**. A continent urinary diversion called neobladder is another type of urinary diversion. After removal of the urinary bladder, a pouch is surgically created from a portion of small bowel; the ureters are attached to the pouch and then the bottom of the pouch is attached to the urethra (Patel & Campbell, 2009). Since the urethral sphincter remains intact, urination occurs via the urethral meatus.

ASSESSMENT

Normal Pattern Identification

Patients may find it easier to describe alterations in urinary elimination than to describe normal urinary elimination. Many factors in daily living can affect normal elimination patterns, so some people have difficulty recognizing their own normal pattern within daily variations.

Specific questions regarding when the last voiding occurred, how many times per day urination usually occurs, whether each void contains a small, medium, or large amount of urine, and whether the patient often wakes during the night to void help identify normal patterns of urinary elimination. Ensure privacy, and be sensitive to feelings of embarrassment that patients may experience during discussion of urinary function. Clarify the term *urinating* by using other words that patients may be more familiar with, such as voiding, "peeing," passing water, or "going potty." Analyze data gathered from such questions to evaluate whether a patient's typical pattern falls within expected parameters.

Risk Identification

A nursing history identifies factors that could alter urinary elimination. Elicit information concerning previous renal or urinary tract problems, such as UTIs, renal calculi, or renal failure. If one of these conditions is present, obtain a history of the condition and how it was treated and resolved. Question the patient about any previous genitourinary surgery, such as prostate surgery or repair of a cystocele. Evaluate other acute or chronic medical problems, such as congestive heart failure or neurologic injury, in terms of their impact on urinary function.

Elicit data about recent changes in daily routines: exercise, diet, or fluid intake. Note any significant change in oral intake or consumption of beverages that contain alcohol or caffeine. Medications that can alter urinary output or function, such as diuretics or anticholinergics, should also be identified.

Assess any motor or cognitive dysfunctions that could impede getting to a bathroom. Visual impairment or communication difficulties could also affect the ability to reach the bathroom in time, especially in a new environment.

Dysfunction Identification

An open-ended question such as "Have you noticed any problems with voiding lately?" is a good way to begin. If the patient indicates no urinary difficulties, clarify the meaning of that answer by asking the following more specific questions:

- Do you have any pain or burning with urination?
- Have you noticed any pink or reddish color in your urine?
- Do you feel you are able to empty your bladder completely every time you urinate?
- Do you accidentally lose any urine when you sneeze or cough?
- Do you have any difficulty stopping or starting your urinary stream?

Such questions are useful because alterations in urinary function are usually gradual and patients may perceive them as normal. For example, an older man may have had difficulty starting his urinary stream for the past 10 years as a result of prostate enlargement, yet he may not view this as a urinary problem. When very specific details of urinary elimination are needed, request that the patient keep a voiding diary. A voiding diary can be as simple as recording on a piece of paper the times when the patient voids or logging the times on a computer on a programmed daily schedule. A voiding diary is most useful if it is kept for at least 3 days so that patterns can be established.

Abnormal patterns of voiding such as polyuria, oliguria, or anuria are important to document, as are hematuria, dysuria, frequency, or urgency. When one of these problems is present, question the patient about when it began and how long it has lasted.

If the patient has a chronic problem with urinary function, such as stress incontinence or a urinary diversion, ask how he or she manages the problem. When a problem in urinary elimination is identified, assess the patient's support systems. Because urinary elimination problems are stressful, support from family and friends is helpful for the patient.

Assessment of Urine

Assessment of urine is best done when the patient does not void directly into the toilet but instead voids into a collection device (urinal for men or bedpan or "hat" for women) or when an indwelling catheter is in place (see Fig. 28-9 in Chapter 28). If assessment of the urine is important, request that the patient void into one of these devices. A hat is a device that can be placed between the toilet and the toilet seat to catch urine. The use of the hat permits the patient to void normally in the toilet but still allows for visual inspection or measurement of urine.

Assessment of urine includes inspection for color, clarity, blood or mucus, and odor. Assess the amount of urine for each void and the total urine output over a 24-hour period.

Assessment of Intake and Output

When a patient's intake and output is being monitored on a flow sheet, urine output should be within approximately 200 to 300 mL of intake for any 24-hour period. Urine output that exceeds fluid intake may indicate diuresis. Urine output less than fluid intake may indicate decreased kidney perfusion, loss of body fluids from other sources (vomiting, diarrhea, bleeding, excessive perspiration), or physiologic conservation of body fluids. Trends of increasing or decreasing output require further evaluation.

The absence of voiding during any 8- to 12-hour period or frequent voiding of small amounts of urine (50 to 100 mL) per void suggests acute urinary retention or urinary retention with overflow voiding. Consider risk factors such as anticholinergic medications, surgery, vaginal delivery, and prostatic hypertrophy. If urinary retention is suspected, physical assessment of the lower abdomen is indicated. **Bladder ultrasound (BUS)** can also assist in determining the amount of urine in the bladder.

Physical Examination

Physical examination of the urinary tract includes inspection and palpation.

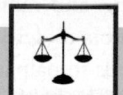

ETHICAL/LEGAL ISSUE

POSSIBLE NEGLECT OF A PATIENT
You are a home health nurse supervising nursing assistants who provide basic care for patients in their homes. A nursing assistant comes to you expressing concern regarding the care that the family is providing for one of her patients. She states, "I believe Mrs. James (an 86-year-old patient with dementia who is confined to bed because of medical problems) is being neglected and abused by her family. The last few times I arrived to bathe her, she was incontinent. She smelled strongly of urine, and it appeared that she had been sitting in urine for a long time. She even has a small area on her bottom that is beginning to break down."

CRITICAL THINKING CHALLENGE
- *Is there a difference between neglect and abuse? Outline what the nursing responsibility would be if neglect occurred and if abuse occurred.*
- How might Mrs. James's dementia and immobility contribute to this problem?
- Do you need to collect any additional information before drawing any conclusion concerning the neglect and/or abuse of this patient?
- Outline possible ways to collaborate with the family to improve the care that they provide for Mrs. James.

INSPECTION

Inspect the patient's lower abdomen. When the patient is lying in a supine position, a bulge in the central lower abdomen just above the symphysis pubis can be noted if the bladder is distended. If the bladder contains less than 500 mL, no bulge will be present. If the bladder holds more than 700 mL, the bulge may be observed extending in the direction of the umbilicus. It may not be easy to observe a distended bladder in an obese person.

It is not necessary to inspect the patient's perineal area routinely unless the patient reports severe dysuria and purulent drainage. When a patient has no specific complaints, examine the urinary meatus while performing perineal hygiene for the patient unable to meet his or her own hygiene needs. Always inspect the urinary meatus when inserting or removing a urinary catheter. If healthy, the skin surrounding the urinary meatus is not reddened, moist, and without discharge. Smegma, an accumulation of white, odorous secretions from sebaceous glands found under the labia minora in women and under the foreskin in men, is normal and does not represent discharge from the urinary meatus. Abnormal findings on inspection of the perineum are reddened, inflamed skin surrounding the urinary meatus and purulent discharge.

PALPATION

Palpation should start at the level of the umbilicus and move in a downward direction toward the symphysis pubis to detect bladder distention. Use the fingertips of both hands to palpate in an attempt to feel the top edge of the bladder. If the bladder contains more than 150 mL of urine, the edge of the bladder will feel smooth and rounded. Although palpation of the bladder must be deep to feel the edge of the bladder, be sure to perform it gently: Palpation can cause discomfort and stimulate voiding. Palpation of the bladder is often omitted because it is considered unnecessary when a bladder scanner is available to estimate bladder fullness.

BLADDER ULTRASOUND

Bladder ultrasound (BUS) is a noninvasive technology that can estimate the volume of urine in the bladder. This portable device consists of an ultrasound probe connected to a screen. Ultrasound gel is placed on the lower abdomen, and the probe is moved over the abdomen until a clear outline of the bladder is present on the screen. Two separate readings are taken, from which the machine computes the volume of urine.

Portable BUS allows the nurse to obtain measurements at the bedside, in the clinic, or in the home. It also can be used to measure post void residual (the amount of urine remaining in the bladder immediately after voiding, usually 50 mL or less). Provider orders or standard protocols can be used to guide interventions for postsurgical patients who have not voided or patients who have large post void residuals, thus avoiding unnecessary urinary catheterization. If acute urinary retention is present, catheterization to relieve bladder distention is necessary. **Procedure 32-1** details how to perform BUS.

Diagnostic Tests and Procedures

The physician can order many diagnostic urologic tests and procedures to understand the functioning of the patient's urinary system and to identify any abnormalities. Nurses are responsible for collecting or supervising the collection of urine specimens for laboratory examination. Nurses are also responsible for preparing the patient physically and psychologically for these tests, assisting with procedures, monitoring the patient during and after procedures, providing postprocedure care, and using information obtained to individualize the plan of care.

COLLECTION OF URINE SPECIMENS

Different tests require different collection procedures. Special considerations may be required during collection of urine from infants or small children. Guidelines are given in **Procedure 32-2**.

> ❗ **SAFETY ALERT**
> Because treatment decisions are made based upon tests results, it is important to identify the patient with two separate identifiers and properly label the specimen so that errors can be prevented.

Random Specimen

Random urine specimen collection is used when sterile urine is not required. The clean specimen may be collected in a urinal, bedpan, or hat or directly into a specimen cup. The urine should not be contaminated with feces or toilet paper. If a woman is menstruating, note this finding on the specimen. Properly label the specimen and promptly send it to the laboratory, or use it for tests to be done at the bedside.

Clean-Catch or Midstream Specimen

A clean-catch or midstream-voided specimen is used when a specimen relatively free of microorganisms is required. A sterile specimen cup or sterile bedpan or urinal is used to collect the urine specimen. Instructions for obtaining a clean-catch urine specimen are provided in **Procedure 32-2**.

Twenty-Four-Hour Specimen

A 24-hour urine specimen is required for accurate measurement of the kidney's excretion of substances (e.g., urine protein, creatinine, urobilinogen, uric acid, selected hormones) that the kidney does not excrete at the same rate throughout the day. Nurses are responsible for explaining the procedure to the patient and for ensuring the collection of all urine that the patient excretes during the 24-hour period. Inadvertently discarding even a small amount of urine invalidates the test results, and urine collection must start all over again. A sign over the patient's bed and on the bathroom door helps alert all healthcare personnel and family members to save all urine. The laboratory will usually provide a large container for urine collection. A preservative may be added to the container to prevent the breakdown of certain urinary constituents.

A 24-hour sample usually is started early in the morning, after the patient's first void. Instruct the patient to void until the bladder is completely empty. Discard this voided urine, and note the time as the beginning of the 24-hour period during which all urine will be saved. The patient may void into any clean urinary container (bedpan, hat, or urinal) but must take care to avoid contaminating the urine with stool or toilet paper. All voided urine is emptied into the 24-hour collection container, taking care not to splash, because the added preservative can be caustic. The large container should be refrigerated or placed in a bucket of ice during the 24 hours of collection. At the end of the 24 hours, ask the patient to empty his or her bladder, and add this urine to the collection container. Label the container and send it to the laboratory.

Specimen From a Catheter

Obtaining a specimen from a catheter may be necessary if a patient is unable to void or already has a catheter in place. Urine collected in this manner is sterile. When obtaining urine from a catheter, always maintain strict asepsis to prevent microorganisms from entering the bladder.

If catheterization is necessary to obtain urine, an in-and-out or straight catheterization is performed. This means the catheter remains in place just long enough to obtain the specimen (see later discussion and **Procedure 32-4**). The sterile urine is permitted to flow into the specimen container; the container is then properly labeled, placed in a plastic bag, and sent to the laboratory.

If the patient already has an indwelling catheter in place, the specimen is obtained by using a syringe to draw urine from a self-sealing port in the catheter, as outlined in **Procedure 32-2**. Some newer collection systems allow the urine to be collected directly into a vacuum tube specimen container that can be sent to the lab. Urine should never be collected from the catheter drainage bag. This urine is not considered sterile because the collection system has been opened to drain urine at various intervals. Also, as the urine sits for long periods in the drainage bag, growth of bacteria can occur.

Collecting Urine From Children

Collecting urine from an infant or a child may necessitate special attention if the child has not yet achieved control of voiding. Catheterization is often difficult and is not recommended because of the small meatal opening and the trauma to the young child. Plastic collection devices are a more acceptable method of collecting urine. Clear plastic bags with adhesive material can be attached over the child's urethral meatus (see **Procedure 32-2**).

Collecting specimens from children who have achieved bladder control can also be challenging. Many children find it difficult to start their stream on command. Giving the child a glass of water, running a faucet, and permitting the parent to help the child obtain the urine specimen may increase the chances of success.

URINE TESTS

The most common laboratory tests of urine include reagent strips, urinalysis, and culture and sensitivity for various urinary constituents.

Reagent Strips

Reagent strips (dipsticks) are available to measure the amount of certain substances such as glucose, protein, or ketones in the urine. Reagent strips can be used to determine urinary pH or detect occult blood. Leukocyte-esterase and nitrite assays by dipstick, to detect white blood cells in the urine as a screening indicator for UTI, are frequently used in the emergency room or outpatient clinics. The instructions for proper use of the various reagent strips are clearly printed on the container. Follow these instructions precisely to ensure accurate results. The procedure usually involves dipping the reagent strip into the urine sample and comparing any color changes to the color chart provided on the container. Timing is crucial for the accurate interpretation of results for some tests (e.g., glucose, ketones). Assessment of the urine by reagent strips is ordered by the physician when he or she wants to monitor closely certain parameters in high-risk patients (e.g., assessing a pregnant woman for protein in her urine). Nurses may independently decide to use reagent strips when necessary for comprehensive assessment of high-risk patients.

Urinalysis

Urinalysis is one of the most common screening tests performed on urine. A urinalysis provides data about the color, turbidity, pH, and specific gravity of the urine and detects protein, glucose, ketones, red blood cells, white blood cells, bacteria, or casts. Urinalysis can be performed on any random specimen of 20 to 30 mL of urine. Although the specimen can be collected at any time during the day, the first voided morning specimen is preferred. The first urine voided in the morning is ordinarily more concentrated because the patient usually consumes no fluids during the night and the effects of diet and activity are minimized. These factors make the first voided specimen most likely to reveal any abnormalities. Table 32-3 presents a summary of the parameters tested in a urinalysis, the range of normal values, and the clinical significance of abnormal values.

 **Concept Mastery Alert**

Urine collected for routine urinalysis must be clean and free of contaminants, but it does not need to be sterile. Urine collected for culture and sensitivity testing, however, must be sterile in order to avoid confounding the test results.

TABLE 32-3 URINALYSIS PARAMETERS

Parameter	Normal Values	Clinical Significance of Variations
Color	Light yellow-amber	Almost colorless: ↑ Fluid intake; dark color: ↓ fluid intake; pink, red, dark brown: red blood cells in urine; pink, orange, red, brown, blue-green: medications or foods
Turbidity	Clear	Hazy, cloudy, smoky: urine specimen allowed to stand at room temperature; red blood cells, white blood cells, bacteria, mucus threads: mucosal irritation secondary to indwelling catheter
pH	Normal: 6 Range: 4.6–8	<6: Diet high in meat or some fruits, metabolic acidosis (diabetes mellitus, starvation), respiratory acidosis (emphysema) >6: Diet high in vegetables and citrus fruits, UTIs, metabolic alkalosis (vomiting, prolonged diuretic therapy), respiratory alkalosis (hyperventilation)
Specific gravity	Range: 1.015–1.025	<1.015: ↑ Fluid intake, diuretic therapy, diabetes insipidus, renal diseases >1.025: ↓ Fluid intake, ↑ fluid loss (vomiting, diarrhea, fever), ADH secretion (trauma, stress)
Protein	None–trace	Present in severe stress, renal disease, preeclampsia of pregnancy
Glucose	None	Present in diabetes mellitus
Ketones	None	Present in diabetes mellitus, ketoacidosis, starvation
Microscopic examination: High-power field – Red blood cells – White blood cells – Bacteria/yeast – Casts (precipitation or clumping of protein substances)	 0–30 0–5 None–few None–occasional	 >3: Urinary tract infection, bleeding, urinary tract trauma, anticoagulant therapy >5: Urinary tract infection Few: Contamination from perineal skin Many: UTI Many: Possible renal diseases

Urine Culture and Sensitivity

Culture and sensitivity tests can be performed on urine to identify any microorganism causing a UTI and to determine which antibiotics can kill the organism. The culture allows bacteria to grow and multiply over a period of at least 48 hours. The laboratory is able to make a preliminary identification of the organism within 24 hours, but another 24 to 48 hours may be necessary to conduct the definitive analytic tests that identify the exact microorganism responsible for the infection. After identification of the organism, the laboratory can test to see which antibiotics will inhibit its growth. If an antibiotic inhibits bacterial growth, the bacteria is said to be sensitive to the antibiotic. If the antibiotic does not inhibit bacterial growth, the organism is considered resistant. The purpose of performing a culture and sensitivity test is to ensure effective antibiotic therapy in the treatment of UTIs.

BLOOD TESTS

Small samples of venous blood can be analyzed in the laboratory to screen for kidney disease. Two commonly performed tests are blood urea nitrogen (BUN) and serum creatinine. The BUN test measures the amount of urea nitrogen in the blood. Urea, the major nitrogenous end waste product of metabolism, is formed in the liver. The bloodstream carries urea from the liver to the kidneys for excretion. When the kidneys

are diseased, they are unable to excrete urea adequately and urea begins to accumulate in the blood, causing BUN to rise. Normal BUN is 8 to 25 mg per 100 mL. Because other factors, such as high dietary intake of protein, fluid deficit, infection, gout, or excessive breakdown of protein stores, can also elevate BUN, it is not a highly sensitive indicator of impaired renal function.

Serum creatinine is a more sensitive indicator of renal function. Creatinine is the waste product formed from the breakdown of skeletal muscle tissue; diet and other factors do not influence its formation. As creatinine forms, the bloodstream carries it to the kidneys for filtration and excretion. Damage to a large number of nephrons prevents efficient excretion of creatinine and causes it to accumulate in the blood. An elevated serum creatinine concentration is indicative of impaired renal function.

Creatinine clearance is a combination blood and urine test that measures the rate at which the kidneys clear creatinine from the blood. Creatinine is excreted in the urine by the process of glomerular filtration. Creatinine is not secreted by the kidney tubule, nor is it reabsorbed anywhere in the kidney tubule. Therefore, its excretion is an accurate measure of the kidney's glomerular filtration ability. To compute the creatinine clearance, measurements of the creatinine level in the blood, the creatinine level in the urine, and the amount of urine produced in a set period (usually 24 hours) are needed. A decreased creatinine clearance value indicates renal impairment.

The GFR is the amount of plasma filtered through glomeruli per unit of time and is the best indicator of kidney function. Many laboratories now calculate an estimated GRF for all patients who have a serum creatinine test. To calculate the GFR, you need the patient's age, race, gender, and serum creatinine. Laboratory reports usually only include GFR less than 60 mL per minute, indicating significant kidney disease that requires dosage adjustment for many medications.

IMAGING STUDIES

The most commonly performed imaging studies to visualize the urinary system are ultrasonography, computed tomography (CT), and the magnetic resonance imaging (MRI) scan.

Ultrasonography is a noninvasive scan used to estimate kidney size and position. It is also helpful to detect obstruction in the urinary tract, including kidney stones. Ultrasonography is not as useful in detecting masses or tumors of the kidney.

CT is a more reliable study for assessing for size and shape of the kidney and the presence of kidney tumors. A CT scan takes x-rays to make detailed pictures of parts of the kidneys and surrounding structures. CT can be performed with or without contrast dye. When contrast dye is used, the procedure is sometimes called a CT intravenous pyelogram (IVP). The CT IVP can detect kidney stones, blockage in the urinary tract, and detail of surrounding arteries and veins.

MRI can provide three dimensional images. The MRI uses a large magnet and radio waves to develop images of body structures. Patients who are allergic to contrast dye or who need a more detailed image of the kidneys and blood vessels would benefit from the MRI rather than the CT scan.

CYSTOSCOPY

Cystoscopy involves insertion of a tube into the bladder for the purpose of direct visualization. A cystoscope is a flexible tube that can be inserted into the urethra and guided into the bladder. A light at the end of the cystoscope allows the physician to look for abnormalities such as tumors, stones, or structural problems. Specialized instruments can be passed through the cystoscope to remove small stones or to take tissue biopsies. Radiopaque dye may be injected for subsequent kidney radiographic studies; this is known as a retrograde pyelogram. The patient needs to sign a consent form before the cystoscopy. After the procedure, assess for hematuria, urinary retention, dysuria, or bladder spasms, and any signs or symptoms of UTI. An indwelling catheter may remain in place for a short period after the cystoscopy.

URODYNAMIC STUDIES

Urodynamic studies are used to detect abnormalities in bladder function or voiding. These procedures (uroflowmetry, cystometrograms, and urethral pressure profile) measure pressure (in the bladder and urethra and within the abdomen), urinary flow, and striated muscle activity. The procedures require no special preparation before testing. Urodynamic studies usually are not painful, but the patient may experience some intermittent discomfort.

NURSING DIAGNOSES

Accepted NANDA-International (NANDA-I) nursing diagnoses involving alterations in urinary elimination include Urinary Incontinence: Stress, Urge, Reflex, Overflow, Functional, Total, and Urinary Retention (NANDA-I, 2014). See Table 32-4 for information on these nursing diagnoses as well as associated Nursing Outcomes Classification (NOC) and Nursing Interventions Classification (NIC).

OUTCOME IDENTIFICATION AND PLANNING

Outcomes for patients with urinary dysfunction should be individualized depending on assessment data. General patient goals might encompass the following:

- The patient will reestablish control over voiding.
- The patient will completely empty bladder with each void.
- The patient will strengthen or maintain adequate perineal muscle control.
- The patient will verbalize understanding of procedures necessary to promote optimal urinary function.

IMPLEMENTATION

Health Promotion

Health promotion interventions include patient teaching and measures to promote voiding. Teach all patients the importance of adequate fluid intake, ways to avoid UTIs, and measures to maintain adequate perineal muscle tone.

MEASURES TO PROMOTE VOIDING

Illness and hospitalization can disrupt a person's usual routines of urinary elimination. Unfamiliar and sometimes uncomfortable medical procedures, loss of privacy, strange surroundings, and anxiety concerning medical diagnosis or prognosis are just a few factors that can disrupt usual habits. In addition to promoting adequate fluid intake, the nurse can use a number of comfort measures to promote urinary elimination and assist patients in maintaining their usual patterns:

- Provide a private setting for voiding.
- Allow adequate, unhurried, and uninterrupted time for voiding.
- If nursing assistance is needed for voiding, assess the patient's usual voiding times (e.g., when awakening, before meals, at bedtime), offer assistance at those times in particular, and be available for assistance between those times.
- Encourage voiding every 4 hours.
- Promote relief of physical discomfort and anxiety-producing situations. Discomfort and anxiety may increase muscle tension and inhibit the relaxation needed for urination.

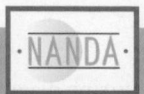

Table 32-4 SELECTED NANDA-I NURSING DIAGNOSES INVOLVING URINARY ELIMINATION

Nursing Dx	Related Factors	Dx Statement	NOC*	NIC†
Stress Incontinence— person experiences loss of urine with activities that increase intra-abdominal pressure	High abdominal pressures from obesity and multiple pregnancies; weak pelvic muscles and pelvic support	Stress Incontinence R/T five pregnancies causing weakened pelvic muscles AEB dribbling of urine when coughing or sneezing	Knowledge: Treatment Regimen, Urinary Continence, Symptom Control	Pelvic Muscle Exercise, pelvic muscle management, Urinary Incontinence Care
Urge Urinary Incontinence— person experiences involuntary passage of urine after a strong urge to void	Decreased bladder capacity; irritation of the bladder; bladder infection;overdistension of the bladder; intake of diuretics, caffeine or alcohol	Urge Urinary Incontinence R/T recent UTI and large intake of coffee AEB urgency and frequency and two episodes of incontinence before getting to the BR	Urinary Continence, Symptom Severity, Symptom Control, Urinary Elimination, Infection Severity	Infection management, Fluid Management, Urinary Bladder Training
Reflex Urinary Incontinence— person experiences involuntary loss of urine, occurring at somewhat predictable intervals when a specific bladder volume is reached	Spinal cord impairment above the sacral reflex arc (spinal cord injury, stroke, brain tumor) or radical pelvic surgery	Reflex Urinary Incontinence R/T recent stroke AEB inability to sense bladder fullness or initiate voiding after catheter D/C	Urinary Continence, Knowledge: Treatment Regimen, Neurological Status: Spinal Sensory/ Motor Function	Urinary Bladder Training, Urinary Habit Training, Fluid Management, Self-Care Assistance: Transfer, Self-Care Assistance: Toileting, Urinary Catheterization: Intermittent
Functional Urinary Incontinence— inability of a normally continent person to reach the toilet in time to avoid unintentional loss of urine	Altered environment and sensory, cognitive, psychological, neurovascular, or mobility deficits, weakened pelvic structures	Functional Urinary Incontinence R/T new long-term care facility environment and difficulty getting to the BR and managing clothing following hip replacement	Urinary Continence, Transfer Performance, Self-Care: Toileting, Knowledge: Treatment Regimen	Teaching: Toilet Training, Self-Care Assistance: Toileting, Self-Care Assistance: Transfer, Urinary Incontinence Care
Urinary Retention— state in which a person experiences incomplete emptying of the bladder	Weak detrusor muscles, inhibition of reflex arc, blockage, strong sphincter	Urinary Retention R/T postoperative swelling, weakened detrusor muscle AEB inability to void in an upright position	Urinary Elimination, Symptom Severity, Symptom Control	Urinary Retention Care, Urinary Catheterization: Intermittent, Prompted Voiding, FluidManagement

Dx, diagnosis; R/T, related to; AEB, as evidenced by; UTI, urinary tract infection; BR, bathroom; D/C, discontinued.
*From: Moorhead, S., Johnson, M., Maas, M., & Swanson, E. (2013). *Iowa Outcomes Project: Nursing Outcomes Classification (NOC)* (5th ed.). St. Louis, MO: C. V. Mosby.
†From: Bulecheck, G., Butcher, H., Dochterman, J., & Wagner, C. (2013). *Iowa Intervention Project: Nursing Interventions Classification (NIC)* (6th ed.). St. Louis, MO: C. V. Mosby.
From: NANDA-International (NANDA-I). (2014). *Nursing diagnoses: Definitions and classification, 2015–2017.* West Sussex, England: Wiley-Blackwell.

- Provide medications for pain as ordered, and give emotional support and reassurance.
- Aid patients in assuming a comfortable and, if possible, physiologic position for voiding (i.e., a sitting or squatting position for women and a standing position for men).
- If a patient has difficulty initiating urination, provide sensory stimuli that either promote relaxation or act as unconscious suggestions. Examples include pouring warm water over the perineum, running water from the faucet, having the patient relax in a warm bath, placing the patient's hands in warm water, stroking the inner thighs, providing music or reading material, and offering a beverage.

PROMOTING FLUID INTAKE

Educating people regarding the importance of adequate fluid intake is a significant nursing intervention. Normally, adults should drink between six and eight glasses (1,500 to 2,000 mL) of fluid, preferably water, each day. Water intake may have to be increased proportionally with any excessive loss of body fluid.

People should space their water intake throughout the waking hours to prevent transitory dehydration. They may need to restrict fluid intake before bed to avoid waking during the night. Water is the preferred fluid because excessive intake of caffeine (e.g., coffee, tea, cola), glucose (juices), or sodium (soda) can alter elimination patterns.

Explain why adequate fluid intake is important to the patient. First, adequate urine production flushes microorganisms out of the urinary system, thus decreasing the chance of infection or obstruction caused by stones. Second, production of large amounts of urine helps to distend and stretch the detrusor muscle, preventing atrophy. For these reasons, adequate fluid intake is helpful in preventing UTIs and maintaining bladder tone.

PREVENTING URINARY TRACT INFECTIONS

In addition to maintaining adequate fluid intake, other measures can prevent UTIs. Encourage people to void every 4 hours to avoid stagnant urine remaining in the bladder. Voiding immediately after engaging in sexual intercourse also helps prevent bacteria from entering the woman's urinary tract. Adequate perineal care is essential during menstruation and during the postpartum period. Instruct women to avoid tight-fitting pants, harsh soaps, bubble baths, and powders because they can irritate the urethra. Cranberry juice may be helpful in preventing chronic UTIs in women, but this has not been proven as a universal preventive measure (Moralejo, 2008); (Nowack & Schmitt, 2008). Remind men and women of the importance of washing their hands carefully with soap and water whenever they touch their perineal areas or body fluids.

Also, teach the signs and symptoms of UTIs, namely fever, flank pain, dysuria, frequency, urgency, pyuria, or hematuria. Teaching is especially important after any instrumentation of the bladder. These symptoms may be absent in older adults or the patient who is immune suppressed. Some people may be embarrassed to contact their physician about urinary problems, so stress the importance of prompt treatment.

SAFETY ALERT

Adequate perineal hygiene is important to prevent pathogens from the anus or vagina from entering the urethra. Instruct women always to wipe from front to back after urinary or fecal elimination.

PROMOTING OPTIMAL MUSCLE TONE

Loss of perineal and abdominal muscle tone can contribute to urinary retention and incontinence. Regular exercise of these structures can prevent loss of tone. Pelvic floor muscle exercises (or Kegel exercises) involve tightening of the perineal and anal muscles. Patients should perform this activity several times per hour, incorporating it into their daily life. Pelvic floor muscle exercises are discussed in Chapter 42.

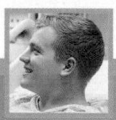

Urinary Elimination PICO

After reviewing the urine cultures, the physician orders Ciprofloxacin for the patient in the chapter-opening scenario. Jim, the nurse, goes in to talk to the patient about it. The patient is already frustrated with the situation of being in the hospital. He exclaims, "I don't understand how I got this infection!" "Why don't they have catheters that don't cause infection?" Jim is unclear of the answer and decides to look through the Cochrane library for help. He uses the following PICO to guide his search: *In adults, how do antimicrobial urinary catheters compared to standard urine catheters prevent urinary tract infections?*

P = opulation: adults
I = ntervention: antimicrobial urinary catheters
C = omparison: standard urinary catheters
O = utcome: prevent urinary tract infections

Jim's inquiry leads him to a systematic review article that compared various antiseptic and antimicrobial catheters to standard catheters. Even though Jim does not find a meta-analysis article, he knows that systematic reviews are one of the highest forms of evidence. The study included randomized controlled trials (RCT) and quasi-RCTs. Twenty-six trials with 12,422 adult patients in 25 parallel groups, and 27,878 patients in one large cluster-randomized crossover trial were reviewed (Lam, Omar, Fischer, Gillies, & MacLennan, 2014). The research showed that while the number of bacteria level reduced with the antiseptic catheters, it did *not* lower the incidence of UTIs. The evidence with using antimicrobial catheters also showed to be weak in preventing UTIs. In fact the expensive catheters proved to be more uncomfortable for patients.

Jim returns to his patient and shares his findings. Jim continues to encourage the patient by telling him that he is on the road to recovery because his catheter is out and he can start the antibiotics right away.

REFERENCE:

Lam, T. B. L., Omar, M. I., Fisher, E., Gillies, K., & MacLennan, S. (2014). Types of indwelling urethral catheters for short-term catheterisation in hospitalised adults. *Cochrane Database of Systematic Reviews*, 9, Art. No.: CD004013. DOI: 10.1002/14651858.CD004013.pub4

Another muscle-strengthening exercise involves voluntary stopping and starting of the stream of urine when voiding. Exercise instruction is especially important during the postpartum period. Patient teaching concerning weight reduction for obese persons is also helpful in improving muscle tone.

Nursing Interventions for Altered Function

In most patients, urinary incontinence can be managed with treatments that nurses can prescribe and implement independently (Newman, 2009). Lifestyle changes and behavioral interventions are recommended as first-line treatment of urinary incontinence. Medications, absorbent products, or external or indwelling catheters can be used for incontinent patients if behavioral interventions are unsuccessful.

BEHAVIORAL INTERVENTIONS

Behavioral interventions are the major independent nursing interventions used to treat urinary incontinence. Behavioral interventions include lifestyle modifications, scheduled voiding regimens, and pelvic floor muscle exercises.

Lifestyle Modifications

Regulating fluid intake, smoking cessation, losing weight, and establishing a good bowel regimen to prevent constipation are lifestyle modifications that promote bladder health and urinary continence.

Sufficient water intake is important for the success of a bladder-training program. The bladder requires at least 200 mL of volume to initiate the micturition reflex. A fluid intake of at least 2,000 mL daily is recommended to provide sufficient hydration to allow the normal bladder stretch–contraction reflex to occur. Help patients to decide on their daily fluid volume goal. Patients should ingest most fluids during daytime hours, decreasing fluid intake as bedtime approaches. Patients will find it best to avoid bladder irritants (e.g., coffee, tea, cola, alcohol) during bladder retraining. Nicotine is also a bladder irritant; thus, smoking cessation promotes urinary continence. In addition, the chronic cough often associated with smoking may predispose individuals to stress incontinence. Weight reduction is especially helpful for patients with stress incontinence. Interventions to prevent constipation are also important because the pressure of a full rectum can cause pressure against the bladder and bladder neck and impair bladder emptying.

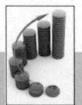

OUTCOME-BASED TEACHING PLANS

Jean Stedman, a young married woman, comes to the clinic with her third UTI since her wedding 18 months ago. Each time, she has received antibiotics as treatment. Today, you both decide to review methods to prevent recurrent UTIs.

OUTCOME

By the end of the teaching session, Jean will be able to identify personal factors that might contribute to her recurrent UTIs.

STRATEGIES

- Give Jean a list of factors that can contribute to UTIs (e.g., inadequate fluid intake; contamination from endogenous bacteria after sexual intercourse or defecation; delayed urination; tight, restrictive pants; urinary calculi).
- Ask Jean to select those factors that might apply to her situation, and develop a plan with Jean to reduce her risk. (She selects inadequate fluid intake, newly sexually active since wedding, and delaying urination.)

OUTCOME

On a return visit in 1 month, Jean's log will document compliance with prevention plan and no recurrent UTIs.

STRATEGIES

- Determine goal for daily fluid intake (3,000 mL per day).
- Brainstorm strategies for increasing fluid intake without caffeine (keep sports bottle at side, drink a full glass of water with meals, drink after every voiding).
- Increase intake during periods of increased fluid loss (e.g., exercise).
- Explain how contamination can occur after sexual activity. Encourage Jean to get up immediately after intercourse to void and to wash area from front to back.
- Explain the importance of frequent voiding to avoid stagnant urine in the bladder for long periods.
- Keep a log of fluid intake and voiding until next visit.
- Praise Jean for compliance with preventive measures.

EVALUATION

3/2/17: 08:30 — Jean identified low fluid intake and delaying voiding as factors that might increase her risk of UTIs. She verbalized that she would try to drink six glasses of water and void every 4 hours.

M. Klim, RN

Scheduled Voiding Regimens

Establishing and maintaining a voiding schedule is the most challenging aspect of behavioral therapy but is effective in decreasing urinary incontinence. Several options are available; if one is unsuccessful, another may be tried. These options include the following:

- *Timed voiding* is the continuous use of an unchanged, fixed voiding schedule (usually every 2 hours). This voiding regimen is used most often for patients with cognitive or physical impairments.
- *Prompted voiding* involves the use of regular checks (typically every 2 hours) to determine whether the patient perceives the urge to void. Sometimes just the reminder or suggestion of the need to void is sufficient stimulus to initiate the process. Prompted voiding can significantly reduce urinary incontinence in patients who have difficulty perceiving bladder fullness, including cognitively impaired older adults.
- *Habit retraining* schedules voiding times in an attempt to approximate the patient's usual voiding pattern. This voiding schedule can be used with patients who have predictable incontinent episodes—for instance, after a meal or taking medications (such as diuretics).
- *Bladder training* starts with scheduled voidings. Patients void at scheduled times (usually every 2 hours) and suppress the urge to void before scheduled times. The interval between voidings is gradually increased to 4 hours. This voiding schedule is more successful with cognitively intact patients with good mobility and motivation.

Patients and those responsible for their care must be aware of the method of bladder training and the voiding schedule. Posting the schedule at the bedside is a helpful measure. Success of bladder training depends on consistency over time because the bladder is being retrained to respond to a normal micturition reflex. Refer to the Patient Plan of Care near the end of this chapter for an example of a bladder retraining schedule.

Pelvic Floor Muscle Exercises

Muscle-strengthening exercises are the third part of an effective behavioral therapy program. Pelvic floor muscle exercises or Kegel exercises strengthen the pubococcygeal muscles and promote optimal urinary control. Pelvic floor muscle exercises are described in Chapter 42.

EXTERNAL CATHETERS AND ABSORBENT PRODUCTS

In addition to behavioral interventions, external catheters and absorbent products are often used, especially early in the treatment program before the patient attains continence. Alternative treatments are necessary when behavioral interventions are not successful.

COLLABORATING WITH THE HEALTH CARE TEAM
Discussing Urinary Incontinence With a Nursing Assistant

It is the beginning of an 8-hour shift, and your assignment on a geriatric unit includes providing care for five patients with the help of Sarah, a certified nursing assistant (CNA). You update Sarah on care requirements for Mrs. Wilson using the SBAR communication tool.

SITUATION: Sarah, let's take a few minutes to review Mrs. Wilson's plan of care before we get to work.

BACKGROUND: Mrs. Wilson, a 76-year-old widow with a history of dementia, was admitted with pneumonia yesterday. You will be responsible for taking her vital signs, providing hygiene, and getting her up to walk in the halls. Her history states she has been occasionally incontinent of urine during the last year, so I want to start her on a toileting program every 2 hours.

ASSESSMENT: Instituting a toileting program will help prevent incontinence and improve Mrs. Wilson's sense of dignity. Decreasing incontinence is important to prevent skin breakdown and possible falls.

RECOMMENDATION: Get her up to the commode or the bathroom so that she is likely to empty her bladder completely, and BUS her after she voids this morning so that we can assess her residual urine. Please let me know if you need help. If her residual is over 150, let me know, because that will increase her risk of UTI. Please be sure to document her voiding and BUS values in her record.

CRITICAL THINKING CHALLENGE

- Reflect on how clear communication with nursing assistants helps promote individualized patient care.
- Was delegation in this situation to the nursing assistant appropriate? If not, what tasks should not have been delegated?
- Is the SBAR communication respectful and given in a manner to encourage teamwork?
- Is there anything you would add to this report to the nursing assistant?

External Catheter

An external catheter is sometimes used for male patients who experience urinary incontinence. Patients who might benefit from the use of an external catheter include those who have sphincter damage following prostatectomy, spinal cord injury, or impaired skin integrity from incontinence. The external catheter is composed of a sheath that is placed on the penis and attached to tubing that inserts into a closed collection bag. The collection bag may be similar to the type used for indwelling catheters. Patients who are more mobile can use a collection bag that attaches securely to the leg. External catheters have a much lower risk of causing UTIs than do indwelling catheters. However, dislodgment and leaking are drawbacks of the external catheter. Ischemia or skin breakdown on the penis can be a complication if the sheath is applied incorrectly. When applying or removing an external catheter, follow clinical guidelines or the specific directions of the manufacturer. For general instructions on applying and removing an external catheter, see **Procedure 32-3**. Be sure to empty the patient's leg bag or larger urine collection bag at least every 8 hours or more frequently as needed.

 SAFETY ALERT

Remove the external catheter daily to cleanse the penis and surrounding tissues and to assess for any edema or areas of excoriation.

Absorbent Products

A satisfactory external catheter device for women has not been developed yet. As an alternative, some female patients (and some male patients) use absorbent products. These products (including pads, shields, or briefs) are typically disposable; waterproof; and lined with soft, absorbent material. Briefs open at the sides and have tape or Velcro closures that facilitate application for patients who have difficulty moving, turning, or pulling on clothes.

Patients need to change the protective pads or briefs frequently to avoid odor and to prevent skin irritation from prolonged exposure to moisture. Disposable briefs are not recommended for patients with total urinary incontinence because of the high risk of impaired perineal skin integrity known as incontinence-associated dermatitis (IAD). Patients wearing absorbent products should bathe at least daily. Each time the product is changed, the perineal area should be cleansed and examined for any areas of irritation.

Absorbent linen pads can be placed under patients to absorb urine and protect bed linen and mattresses. Most hospitals, long-term care facilities, and some home caregivers use thick cloth/washable linen underpads for incontinent patients. The fabric in the pad is designed to absorb urine and other fluid drainage and then wick the moisture throughout the pad rather than remaining in direct contact with perineal skin. Caregivers can also use clean bedpads to turn and move patients in bed. When bedpads become soiled with either urine or stool, the nurse cleans the patient's perineal skin and places a clean bedpad. Hospitalized patients should not use absorbent briefs and linen underpads simultaneously.

PERINEAL HYGIENE FOR THE INCONTINENT PATIENT

Good skin care and prevention of skin breakdown are very important for incontinent patients. Ammonia, a metabolite of urine, is a skin irritant. The process of skin softening caused by continuous moisture or soaking is called maceration. Incontinent patients are at high risk for impaired perineal skin integrity known as IAD. Gentle cleansing of the perineal skin after each episode of incontinence is standard incontinence care. Use either soap and water or a commercial perineal cleansing product. Skin needs to be dried after cleansing. If the perineal skin is reddened or fragile, apply a barrier cream or ointment or a nonsting barrier film (a quick-drying, liquid film-forming product that forms a waterproof barrier) as part of perineal hygiene.

URINARY CATHETERIZATION

Urinary catheterization involves inserting a small tube, called a catheter, through the urethra into the bladder to allow urine to drain. The most frequently used method is urethral catheterization. Urine can also be removed through a suprapubic catheter. When catheters remain in place to drain urine over an extended period, they are referred to as indwelling (or retention) catheters. When a urethral catheter is inserted temporarily to empty urine from the bladder and then is removed, it is referred to as straight catheterization. Straight catheterization performed on a routine, scheduled basis for a particular patient is called **intermittent catheterization**.

Indications for Catheterization

There is increased risk of UTI associated with urinary catheterization, especially when indwelling catheters are in place for more than 48 hours. Professional organizations, including the Wound Ostomy and Continence Nurses Society (2009), the Society for Healthcare Epidemiology of America, the Infectious Diseases Society of America, and the Healthcare Infection Control Practices Advisory Committee of the Centers for Disease Control and Prevention (CDC) (Lo et al., 2008) list the following as acceptable indications for the use of indwelling urinary catheters:

- Monitoring critically or acutely ill patients when accurate assessment of urinary output is necessary
- Management of terminally or severely ill patients
- Urinary retention not manageable by intermittent catheterization or other means
- Management of urinary incontinence in patients with stage III or stage IV pressure ulcers on the trunk

 SAFETY ALERT

Indwelling catheters should never be used solely for the convenience of either the staff or patients.

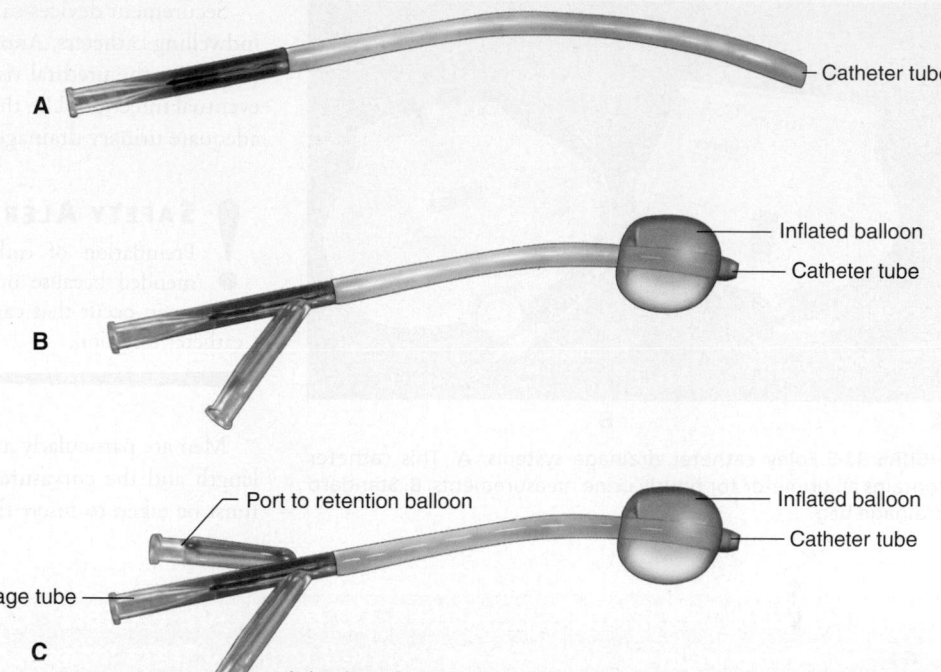

FIGURE 32-4 Types of urethral catheters. **A.** Intermittent (straight) catheter. **B.** Indwelling (Foley) catheter. **C.** Triple-lumen catheter.

Types of Catheters

Urinary catheters are usually made of latex, silicone, or rubber, and some are coated with silver hydrogel. Silver impregnated or coated catheters have been developed to discourage bacteriuria and prevent ureteral entry of microorganisms. A straight catheter with only one lumen is used for in-and-out or intermittent catheterization procedures (Fig. 32-4A). When an indwelling catheter is required, a double-lumen catheter known as a Foley is used. A Foley catheter contains one lumen to remove urine and a second, smaller lumen to inflate a balloon that keeps the catheter from falling out of the bladder. The balloon is located near the insertion tip of the catheter and can be inflated and deflated with a syringe (Fig. 32-4B). A third type of catheter, the triple-lumen indwelling catheter, is inserted when urine must be removed from the bladder and irrigation of the bladder with fluid or medications must also be performed. A triple-lumen catheter is normally used after urologic or prostatic surgery (Fig. 32-4C). A coudé catheter has a curved tip that permits easier insertion, especially as the catheter passes an area of urethral narrowing, such as that caused by prostatic hyperplasia.

Urinary catheters are available in various sizes. Catheters are sized on the French scale of numbers, according to the diameter of the lumen. According to this scale, the larger the lumen size the larger the French number. Available adult sizes range from 12 to 22 French, with sizes 14 to 18 French used most frequently.

❗ SAFETY ALERT

Selection of the proper size is important to help prevent trauma to urethral tissues. Use the smallest size catheter that will provide good urinary drainage (Gould, Umschied, Agarwal, Kuntz, & Pegues, 2009; Parker et al., 2009).

Catheterization

To avoid introducing microorganisms into the urinary system, which is sterile, hand washing before and after insertion of the catheter and the use of sterile aseptic technique is necessary for insertion of urinary catheters (Gould et al., 2009; Parker et al., 2009). Male patients can be positioned in a supine or semi-Fowler's position. Female patients usually are placed in a dorsal recumbent position (supine with knees flexed) for catheterization. An alternative, especially for female patients who have limited hip mobility, is the side-lying position. This position is more comfortable for weak female patients who may have difficulty keeping their legs flexed and spread apart to permit visualization. The side-lying position also permits excellent visualization of the urinary meatus.

Risks of Catheterization

Any break in sterile technique during catheter insertion carries the risk of infection to the bladder, the ureters, and, eventually, the kidneys. In addition, with an indwelling catheter, the risk of infection continues and increases as long as the catheter remains in place. The indwelling catheter must be connected to a closed drainage bag to prevent microorganisms from migrating up the inside of the catheter lumen to the bladder (Fig. 32-5). Even with the use of a closed drainage system, microorganisms can still migrate from the meatus up the outside of the catheter and drainage tubing toward the bladder.

❗ SAFETY ALERT

Manipulation of the catheter, especially advancing the catheter into the bladder after it has been originally placed, can increase the risk of infection.

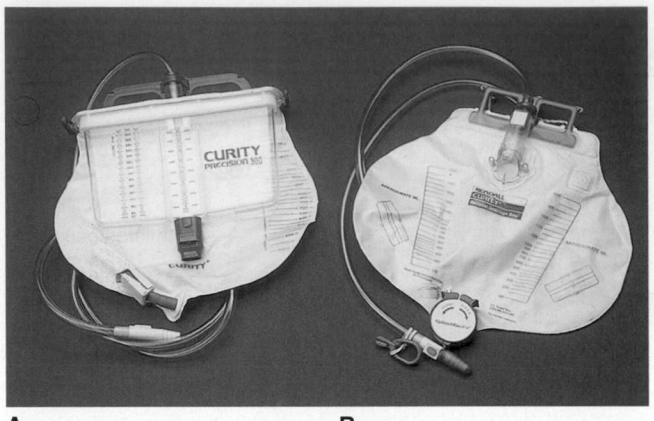

A **B**

FIGURE 32-5 Foley catheter drainage systems. **A.** This catheter contains an urimeter for hourly urine measurements. **B.** Standard drainage bag.

Securement devices can help minimize excess movement of indwelling catheters. Another risk of urethral catheterization is trauma to the urethral tissues, and this can also contribute to eventual infection. Use the smallest size catheter that will allow adequate urinary drainage.

 SAFETY ALERT

Preinflation of catheter balloon is no longer recommended because once the balloon is deflated, balloon ridges can occur that can increase the risk of trauma during catheter insertion.

Men are particularly at risk for tissue trauma because of the length and the curvature of the male urethra. Particular care must be taken to insert the catheter along the normal contour

EVIDENCE-BASED BUNDLES TO IMPROVE PATIENT CARE
Prevention of Catheter-Associated Urinary Tract Infections (CAUTI)

BACKGROUND

UTIs account for approximately 40% of all hospital-acquired infections annually, and fully 80% of these can be attributed to indwelling urethral catheters. In the United States, up to 5 million urinary catheters are placed annually. Between 12% and 25% of all hospitalized patients will receive a urinary catheter during their hospital stay, and up to half of these do not have an appropriate indication.

It is well established that the duration of catheterization is directly related to risk for developing a UTI. With a catheter in place, the daily risk of developing a UTI ranges from 3% to 7%. When a catheter remains in place for up to a week, the risk increases to 25%; at 1 month, this risk is nearly 100%.

RISK FACTORS

- Prolonged catheterization greater than 6 days
- Female gender
- Catheter insertion outside operating room
- Other active sites of infection
- Diabetes
- Malnutrition
- Azotemia (creatinine greater than 2.0 mg per deciliter)
- Ureteral stent
- Catheter in place solely for monitoring of urine output
- Drainage tube below level of bladder and above collection bag
- Antimicrobial drug therapy

KEY RECOMMENDATIONS

1. Avoid unnecessary urinary catheters.

NURSING IMPLICATIONS
- Catheters are appropriate in patients with acute urinary retention or bladder outlet obstruction or in patients undergoing prolonged surgeries or are anticipated to receive large-volume infusions or diuretics during surgery. Catheters are also indicated for patients with stage 3 to 4 decubitus ulcers with incontinence or for patients receiving palliative care if they request an indwelling catheter.
- Catheters are *inappropriate* if used as a substitute for nursing care of the patient with incontinence, as a means of collecting serial urine specimens, or for prolonged postoperative duration without appropriate indications (which include structural repair of urethra or other contiguous structures or prolonged effect of epidural anesthesia).

2. Insert necessary catheters using aseptic technique.

NURSING IMPLICATIONS
- Perform hand hygiene immediately before and after insertion or any manipulation of the catheter device or site.
- Ensure that only properly trained persons who know the correct technique of aseptic catheter insertion and

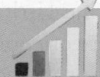

EVIDENCE-BASED BUNDLES FOR PATIENT SAFETY (*Continued*)
Prevention of Catheter-Associated Urinary Tract Infections

maintenance are given this responsibility. Consider using a portable ultrasound device to assess urine volume in patients undergoing intermittent catheterization to assess urine volume and reduce unnecessary catheter insertions. If ultrasound bladder scanners are used, ensure that indications for use are clearly stated, nursing staff are trained in their use, and equipment is adequately cleaned and disinfected in between patients.

◆ In the acute care hospital setting, insert urinary catheters using aseptic technique and sterile equipment. Properly secure indwelling catheters after insertion to prevent movement and urethral traction. Unless otherwise clinically indicated, consider using the smallest bore catheter possible, consistent with good drainage, to minimize bladder neck and urethral trauma.

◆ In the non-acute care setting, clean (i.e., nonsterile) technique for intermittent catheterization is an acceptable and more practical alternative to sterile technique for patients requiring chronic intermittent catheterization.

◆ Further research is needed on optimal cleaning and storage methods for catheters used for clean intermittent catheterization. If intermittent catheterization is used, perform it at regular intervals to prevent bladder overdistension. Further research is needed on the use of antiseptic solutions versus sterile water or saline for periurethral cleaning prior to catheter insertion.

3. Maintain catheters based on recommended guidelines.

NURSING
IMPLICATIONS

◆ Use Standard Precautions, including the use of gloves and gown as appropriate, during any manipulation of the catheter or collecting system. Maintain a closed drainage system. If breaks in aseptic technique, disconnection, or leakage occur, replace the catheter and collecting system using aseptic technique and sterile equipment. Maintain unobstructed urine flow (i.e., keep the collecting tube free from kinking, the collecting bag below the level of the bladder at all times). Do not rest the bag on the floor. Empty the collecting bag regularly using a separate, clean collecting container for each patient; avoid splashing, and prevent contact of the drainage spigot with the nonsterile collecting container.

◆ Changing indwelling catheters or drainage bags at routine, fixed intervals is not recommended. Rather, it is suggested to change catheters and drainage bags based on clinical indications such as infection, obstruction, or when the closed system is compromised. Unless clinical indications exist (e.g., in patients with bacteriuria upon catheter removal post urologic surgery), do not use systemic antimicrobials routinely to prevent CAUTI in patients requiring either short- or long-term catheterization. Routine hygiene (e.g., cleansing of the meatal surface during daily bathing or showering) is appropriate. Unless obstruction is anticipated (e.g., as might occur with bleeding after prostatic or bladder surgery), bladder irrigation is not recommended. Clamping of catheters prior to removal is not necessary (Gould et al., 2009).

4. Review the need for catheter daily and remove promptly.

NURSING
IMPLICATIONS

◆ If you believe a catheter has been inserted and is no longer needed or is being used when not appropriate, act as an advocate for getting it removed.

From: Gould, C. V., Umschied, C. A., Agarwal, R. K., Kuntz, G., Pegues, D. A., & Healthcare Infection Control Practices Advisory Committee (HICPAC). (2009). *Guidelines for prevention of catheter-associated urinary tract infections 2009*. Retrieved January 7, 2015, from www.cdc.gov/ncidod/dhqp/pdf/guidelines/CAUTI_Guideline2009final.pdf

of the urethra to avoid trauma to the tissues. The normal curve of the male urethra can be straightened somewhat by elevating the penis to a position perpendicular to the body. Coating the catheter with a small amount of 2% lidocaine gel or rubbing the gel over the urethral meatus (for women) or injecting it into the urethra (for men) is sometimes recommended to reduce the discomfort of catheter insertion. A coudé tip may facilitate catheter insertion in male patients with partial urethral obstruction.

Procedure 32-4 outlines the correct technique for catheterization.

Care of Indwelling Catheters

Indwelling urethral catheters increase the risk of acquiring CAUTI; thus, nursing personnel must take special care to minimize that risk. The CAUTI evidence-based prevention

bundle provides specific recommendations that when performed together are more effective in preventing CAUTI.

Standard precautions, including handwashing before and after handling an indwelling catheter, as well as use of clean gloves, are important. The catheter, drainage collection tubing, and bag represent a closed drainage system that should not be disconnected except to change to a new closed system. The system, including the catheter, should be replaced when the catheter becomes clogged, obstructed, or infected or is painful to the patient. Empty the drainage collection bag through the outlet port at the bottom of the bag at least every 8 hours, and more frequently if necessary, because pooled urine is an excellent growth medium for microorganisms.

To prevent the catheter from pulling or kinking, use either a nonadhesive leg strap or an adhesive-backed securement device to hold the catheter in place. The catheter should be affixed to the patient's body in a fashion that keeps the catheter securely in place but with enough slack to allow the patient to move freely. Nonadhesive straps are applied to the patient's thigh; the adhesive-backed devices can be applied to the inner aspect of the thigh for both men and women or to the lower abdomen for men. Affixing the securement device to a man's abdomen, rather than his leg, is thought to help prevent irritation at the penile–scrotal angle and minimize urethral trauma during spontaneous nocturnal erections; however, there is insufficient evidence to mandate this method (Gray, 2008).

The drainage collection bag and tubing should remain below the level of the bladder to maintain proper drainage and to prevent pooling or backflow. Most collection bags have a one-way valve at the insertion of the tubing into the collection bag that also prevents backflow. Attach the collection bag to the frame of the bed; do not attach it to the side rail or rest it on the floor. The collection bag and tubing come equipped with a way of attaching the collection bag to the bed frame and the tubing to the bed linens.

Cleanse the patient's perineal area and the catheter at least daily to remove normal secretions and after every bowel movement to help prevent infection. Most agencies suggest using soap and water or a commercially prepared perineal cleansing solution. It is not necessary to use an antimicrobial ointment or solution for catheter care. Cleanse the perineal area, wash the meatus carefully, and rinse and dry the area thoroughly. During catheter care, assess patients for any complaints of perineal irritation or burning, and inspect the area for redness or excoriation. Note the color of urine in the tubing and the presence or absence of mucus. When caring for patients with indwelling catheters, monitor intake and output to ensure a fluid intake adequate to produce 30 mL of urine per hour or 240 mL per every 8 hours.

 SAFETY ALERT
To avoid introducing microorganisms from the rectum forward toward the meatus, cleanse the woman's perineal area from front to back.

Bladder/Urinary Catheter Irrigation

The purpose of catheter irrigation is to cleanse the lumen of the catheter to promote patency of the tube. The purposes of irrigation of the urinary bladder include the instillation of solutions to help remove mucus, blood clots, or other tissue in the bladder (particularly after genitourinary surgery) and the application of medications to the bladder wall. For both types of irrigation, the closed method of irrigation is performed without disruption of the closed drainage system. In intermittent closed catheter irrigation, a specified amount of sterile irrigating solution is injected into a self-sealing port on the catheter tubing (Fig. 32-6).

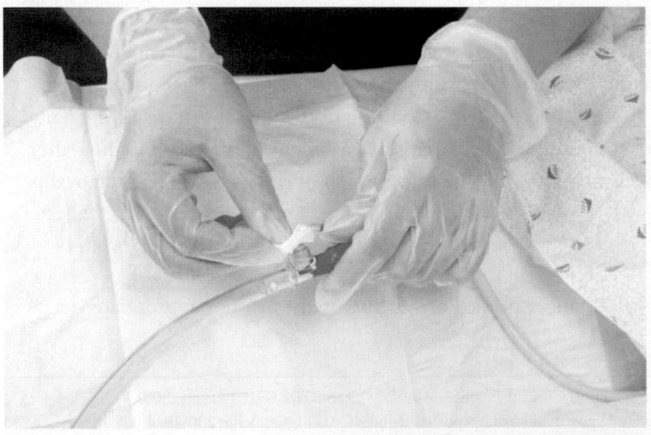

A

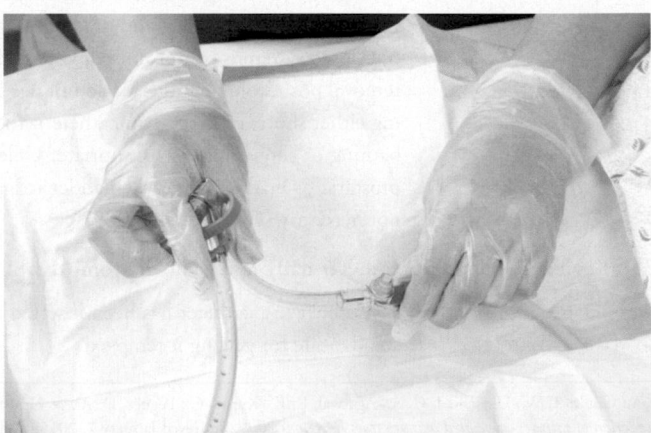

B

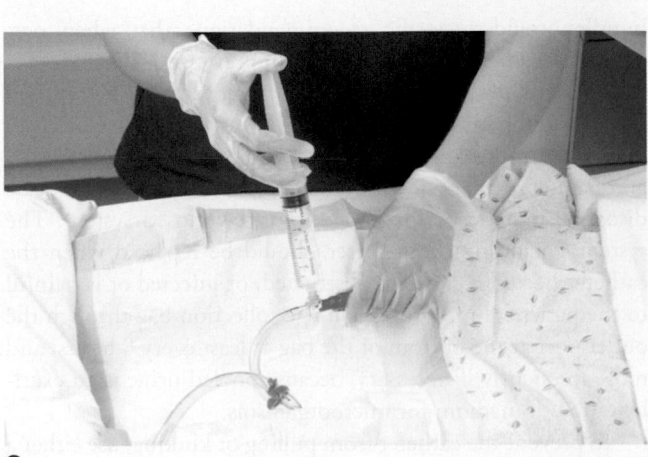

C

FIGURE 32-6 Intermittent closed catheter irrigation. **A.** Cleanse access port on catheter. **B.** Clamp the drainage tubing below the port. **C.** Irrigate the catheter.

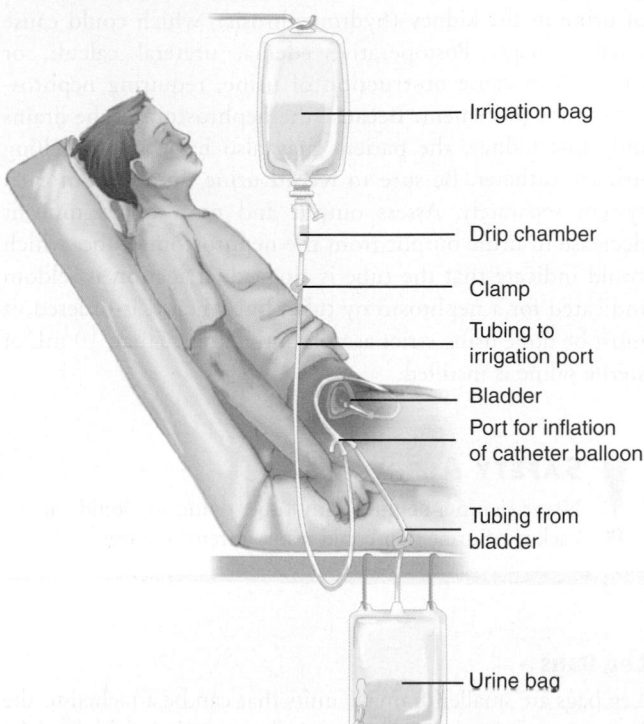

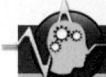

Irrigation bag

Drip chamber

Clamp

Tubing to
irrigation port

Bladder

Port for inflation
of catheter balloon

Tubing from
bladder

Urine bag

FIGURE 32-7 Irrigating an indwelling catheter using continuous bladder irrigation.

When performing continuous bladder irrigation, a triple-lumen indwelling urethral catheter must be in place. One lumen is used to inflate the balloon of the catheter to keep it securely inside the bladder, another lumen is used for the removal of urine into a closed drainage system, and the third lumen is connected to a container of sterile irrigating solution (Fig. 32-7). The specified type and amount of irrigating solution is administered by continuous drip at a rate prescribed by the physician or by written protocol. The catheter lumen used for removal of urine can be clamped until the prescribed solution has been instilled and then opened to allow drainage, or it can be left open to allow outflow of urine throughout the procedure. Throughout the closed method of irrigation, the catheter and drainage tube remain connected to decrease the risk of entry of microorganisms into the system, which could cause infection. If the catheter becomes encrusted or obstructed, change the entire system—the catheter and the drainage bag. Do not disconnect or open the system at the catheter–drainage tube junction.

Removal of Indwelling Catheter

Removal of the indwelling urethral catheter is a simple procedure performed with clean technique (see **Procedure 32-4**). Care is necessary to avoid trauma to the urethra and discomfort for the patient. Inform the patient about what to expect after catheter removal (delay in voiding for a few hours because the bladder is empty, the need to save first voided urine for measurement, the need to increase fluid intake).

After removal of the catheter, assess the patient's perineum and meatus for any signs of redness or irritation and then provide perineal care. Inform the patient that it is not uncommon to experience some dribbling of urine after catheter removal, particularly if the catheter was in place for several days.

Encourage the patient to drink plenty of liquids to distend the bladder. Voiding should be expected within the next 6 to 8 hours. Continue to assess the patient's intake and output. Note the time of catheter removal and also the time 8 hours later when the patient is due to void. If the patient has not voided in 8 hours, assess for urinary retention using a bladder scanner, if available. If the patient has difficulty reestablishing voluntary control of urination, notify the physician. It may become necessary to reinsert the catheter or to perform an intermittent catheterization.

APPLY YOUR CRITICAL THINKING

Mr. Sanchez, age 90 years, has been on the rehabilitation unit for 3 weeks. When you go to perform your morning assessment, Mr. Sanchez appears very confused and is mumbling incoherently (a significant change from the previous day when he was oriented to person, place, and time). His vital signs are T 37.5, B/P 142/86, P 92, R 18. He has a catheter in place with an output of 250 mL of dark amber urine with much cloudy sediment. What do you suspect is happening? How should you proceed?

Check your answers in Appendix B.

Suprapubic Catheter

A suprapubic catheter (Fig. 32-8) is a narrow-lumen tube with a curl at the distal end that helps prevent the bladder from expelling the catheter. A physician inserts the suprapubic catheter into the patient's urinary bladder from an abdominal entry point just above the symphysis pubis. Suprapubic catheterization can be performed under local anesthesia or in the operating room under general anesthesia and in conjunction with bladder or vaginal surgery.

The suprapubic catheter is kept in place by sutures at the abdominal entry point or by a form of body retention seal, which is a part of each catheter. The catheter tubing is then connected to a closed urinary drainage system. When the suprapubic catheter is to be removed, the sutures or body retention seal is removed and, as the catheter is guided out of the bladder, the bladder muscles contract over the entry site and seal off the opening made into the bladder. The abdominal entry point is then cleansed, and a sterile dressing is applied.

Complications that can occur with suprapubic catheters include obstruction of urine flow from the bladder due to accumulation of sediment or clots in the catheter as well as closing of the bladder wall over the catheter tip. The small lumen size of the suprapubic catheter also increases the incidence of tube

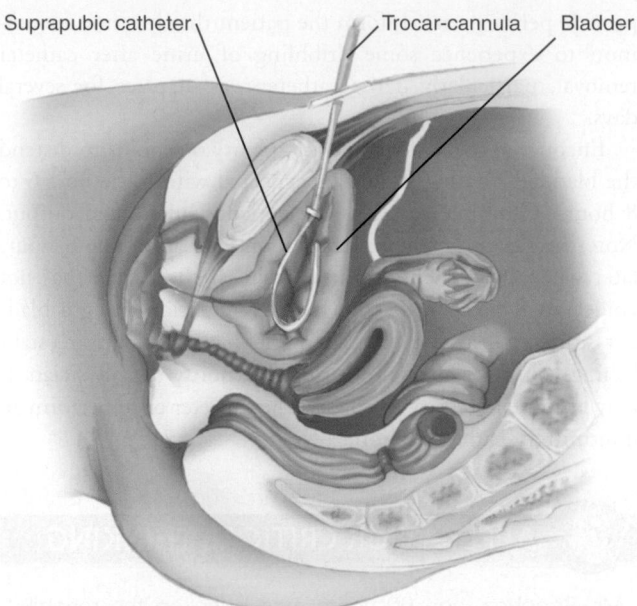

Suprapubic catheter   Trocar-cannula   Bladder

FIGURE 32-8 A suprapubic catheter is placed into the bladder through the abdomen to drain urine.

kinking and obstruction. The catheter can become dislodged, or trauma to the bladder wall can occur during suprapubic catheter insertion.

Nursing assessment of a patient with a suprapubic catheter includes frequent observations of the patient's urine for color, clarity, and quantity. In addition, assess the patient's fluid intake, temperature, and level of comfort and the condition of the abdominal insertion site.

Intermittent Catheterization

Intermittent catheterization involves the introduction and removal of a catheter into the bladder to permit drainage of urine at routine intervals, usually every 6 to 8 hours. Intermittent catheterization is used most commonly in patients with spinal cord injuries and those who are neurologically impaired and not able to void. The incidence of UTI is lower with intermittent catheterization than with an indwelling catheter but still remains a risk. Intermittent catheterization also permits the patient with chronic neurogenic bladder to have greater control and independence in self-care; emptying of the bladder occurs on a more physiologic schedule. Intermittent catheterization can be performed using clean or sterile technique; when done in the home setting, it is almost always performed using clean technique, which enables the patient to self-catheterize. A mirror helps the female patient visualize the meatal opening. To locate the meatus without a mirror, instruct the patient to place the index finger of her nondominant hand on the clitoris and the third and fourth fingers at the vagina, directing insertion of the catheter between these two landmarks. For the quadriplegic patient, a caregiver learns the procedure.

Nephrostomy Tubes

A nephrostomy tube is a tube placed in the renal pelvis of the kidney to permit outflow of urine and prevent backup

of urine in the kidney (hydronephrosis), which could cause renal damage. Postoperative edema, ureteral calculi, or tumors can cause obstruction of urine, requiring nephrostomy tube placement. Because the nephrostomy tube drains only one kidney, the patient may also have an indwelling urinary catheter. Be sure to record urine output from each system separately. Assess output and note any significant decrease in urine output from the nephrostomy tube, which could indicate that the tube is clogged. Irrigation is seldom indicated for a nephrostomy tube, but when it is ordered, it must be done using strict asepsis and no more than 10 mL of sterile saline is instilled.

> ❗ **SAFETY ALERT**
> Never clamp a nephrostomy tube; doing so would cause backup of urine that could result in renal damage.

Leg Bags

Leg bags are smaller drainage units that can be attached to the leg and worn under clothing. Leg bags are helpful when the patient must return home with a catheter or urinary drainage system (e.g., condom catheter, nephrostomy tube, suprapubic catheter) in place. Often, the leg bag is used during daytime hours, enabling the patient to participate in normal daily activities without having to carry a large urinary drainage bag. The leg bag contains a smaller volume of urine, so it must be emptied often. This is done by opening a clamp on the system and allowing urine to flow into the toilet or an appropriate container.

Teach patients how to change from one drainage system to another, as illustrated in Figure 32-9. First, have the patient gather equipment and wash his or her hands. If doing this for the patient, wear clean gloves. Wipe the connecting area with an alcohol wipe, using friction, before disconnecting the tubing from the collection system. Recap the old drainage system and connect the leg bag, keeping all ends sterile. Once connected, the bag can be attached to the leg using the rubber straps provided with the drainage unit. Leg bags should be cleaned daily, using a dilute (1:10) bleach solution.

RENAL DIALYSIS

In renal dialysis, a semipermeable membrane removes fluid, electrolytes, and other waste products from the body that healthy kidneys normally remove. It is used in patients with acute renal failure to allow the kidneys time to heal and to help prevent further complications of the disease process. In patients with irreversible chronic renal failure, dialysis is necessary to sustain life. Dialysis may be performed as a temporary or permanent measure, depending on the renal impairment. Hemodialysis (Fig. 32-10) and peritoneal dialysis are two types of renal dialysis.

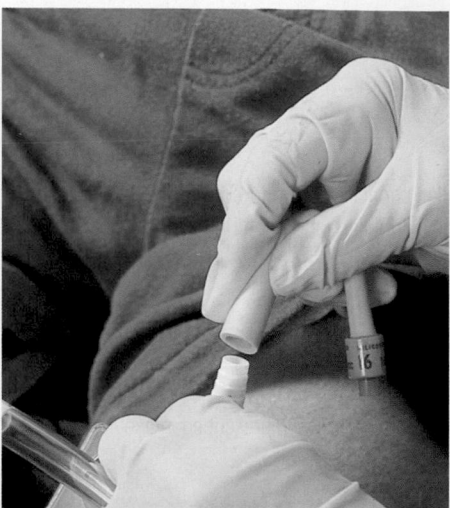
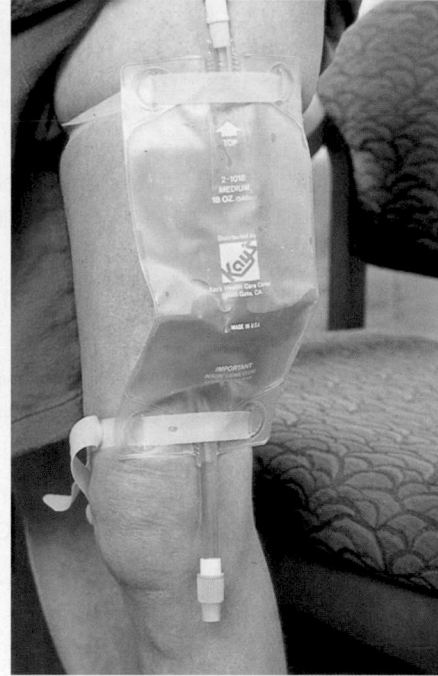

FIGURE 32-9 Changing from one drainage system to another when a leg bag is worn. **A.** Connect new drainage system, keeping ends sterile. **B.** Attach to leg with rubber straps.

A   B

Home and Community Care

Patients can manage urinary dysfunction, especially chronic conditions, in the home with assistance and support from their family. The nurse's role changes from that of direct care provider to teacher, enabling patients (or their care providers) to be successful in self-care and management. Teach all patients to recognize the symptoms of infection, and give clear guidelines regarding when to contact a healthcare provider.

Patients and their families may need to learn the correct methods to care for indwelling urethral or suprapubic catheters, to manage urinary diversion devices, or to perform intermittent straight catheterization. Standardized teaching

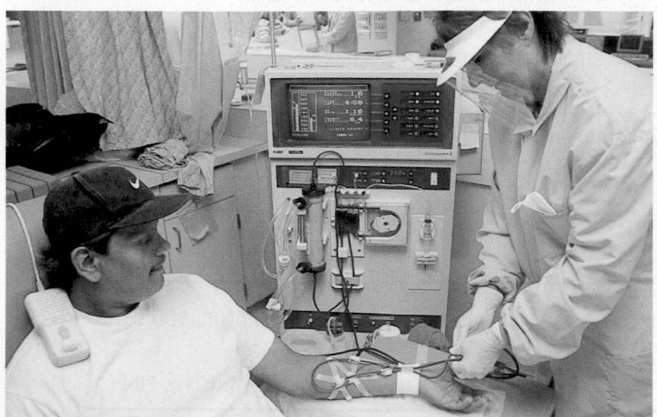

FIGURE 32-10 During hemodialysis, a machine filters the patient's blood because the kidney can no longer rid the body of waste products.

plans are often prepared for common procedures with appropriate audiovisual aids to assist in teaching the care of complex home care equipment. Urinary procedures in the home, such as self-catheterization, are performed with clean technique. When patients are sent home with an indwelling catheter, instruct them on how to use a leg bag for drainage, changing back to a drainage unit at night. Vinyl drainage bags and leg bags can be decontaminated with household bleach. A 10% bleach solution can be used for daily cleaning of the interior of the drainage bag. The drainage bag should be agitated twice with the bleach solution, rinsed well between cleanings, and then hung to air-dry.

Sometimes adjustments in the home environment may be necessary to promote optimal self-management. Patients can rent bedside commodes if ambulating or easy access to the bathroom is difficult, or the family may install a raised toilet seat for a patient with mobility limitations. Bathroom remodeling may be necessary in some situations (e.g., doorways too narrow to accommodate wheelchair entry).

Contacts with resource people in the community for follow-up and home management may be appropriate, especially if a patient is experiencing urinary incontinence, has recently learned self-catheterization, has a new urinary diversion, or will have dialysis in the home. Nurses can visit patients in their homes routinely to assess progress in the management of their healthcare needs. These nurses may be associated with the discharging hospital, but they are more likely to be associated with a city or county health agency or with an independent home healthcare agency. The hospital-based nurse should be involved in the decision to make referrals to community agencies.

PATIENT PLAN OF CARE
The Patient With Urge Incontinence

NURSING DIAGNOSIS

Urge Incontinence related to decreased bladder capacity and tone secondary to indwelling catheter postoperatively as manifested by strong urinary urge with incontinence, frequency, dribbling, and nocturia.

PATIENT GOAL

Patient will reestablish control over voiding.

PATIENT OUTCOME CRITERIA

- Patient remains continent for 2-hour intervals over next 48 hours.
- Patient verbalizes the importance of fluid intake and complies with prescribed intake.
- Patient will demonstrate Kegel exercises after teaching session.

NURSING INTERVENTION	SCIENTIFIC RATIONALE
1. Measure and record input and output.	**1.** Use data to assess for pattern of urinary output, relationship of intake to episodes of incontinence, relative overall fluid balance, success of bladder training.
2. Use bladder scan to assess for urinary retention after an incontinent episode.	**2.** Assessment is made to rule out urinary retention and overflow incontinence as the primary urinary alteration.
3. Teach the patient perineal muscle–strengthening exercises and tell him or her to perform them 10 times every 2 to 3 hours during the day.	**3.** These exercises strengthen the skeletal perineal muscles and increase voluntary contraction of urethral sphincter.
4. Work with the patient to develop acceptable regimen. Increase fluid intake to 1,500 to 2,000 mL per day, concentrating most fluid intake during day.	**4.** Adequate hydration is necessary to cause bladder filling and trigger the normal stretch/contraction response.
5. Post fluid intake schedule by the bedside.	**5.** Keeps a record and provides a visual cue for the patient. Schedule will allow tracking of intake.
6. *Begin bladder training routine:* **a.** Assist the patient, as necessary, to the bathroom to void every 2 hours during daytime, every 4 hours at night. Decrease between-voiding interval to 1.5 hours if the patient is initially unable to consistently remain continent for the longer intervals. **b.** Encourage the patient to "hold" his or her urine if he or she experiences the urge to void before the next scheduled voiding time. **c.** Increase between-voiding intervals by 0.5 hour after patient has successfully remained continent for 24 hours.	**6.** A consistent schedule for voiding helps to retrain the bladder and improves the chance for success. **a.** This regimen allows bladder to refill between voidings and gradually retrains the normal bladder stretch/contraction response. **b.** Suppressing the urge to void assists in retraining of voluntary contraction of external urethral muscles. **c.** Gradual retraining aims at achieving fewer voids with larger amounts, a more normal pattern.
7. Post voiding schedule in patient's room. Change prn. Include details of current voiding schedule at change of shift report.	**7.** Communication increases patient and staff compliance.

EVALUATION

5/1/17: 13:00—Bladder training begun and schedule posted on door. Voiding every 2 hours with prompting, 150 cc, 320 cc, and 75 cc. Incontinent × 1, Intake 620, Output 445 plus incontinence.

M. Klim, RN

EVALUATION

Some examples of goals and outcome criteria for patients with urinary dysfunction are listed in this section. Some criteria may be appropriate for more than one goal. Identify specific outcome criteria that will measure the attainment of the patient's goal.

Goal

The patient will reestablish control over voiding.

POSSIBLE OUTCOME CRITERIA

- The patient remains continent for 2-hour intervals over the next 48 hours.
- The patient voids four or five times a day, remaining continent for 48 hours, before discharge from rehabilitation.
- By the next home visit, the caregiver reports that the patient recognizes the urge to void in time to use the toilet or commode.

Goal

The patient will demonstrate understanding of procedures necessary to promote optimal urinary function.

POSSIBLE OUTCOME CRITERIA

- The patient verbalizes steps in intermittent self-catheterization by the end of the teaching session.
- The patient practices proper self-catheterization technique during teaching sessions and twice in the next 48 hours.
- The patient demonstrates proper application of the urinary stoma appliance before discharge.
- The patient demonstrates application of the leg bag before discharge.

KEY CONCEPTS

- The voluntary process of micturition is stimulated by stretch of the detrusor muscle as the bladder fills with urine.
- Between 250 and 400 mL of clear, yellow, aromatic urine per void is considered normal.
- As children approach 2 to 3 years of age, their kidneys mature and they achieve voluntary control over urinary elimination; kidney function declines in older adults because of normal age-related changes.
- Many factors, such as fluid intake, loss of body fluid, dietary intake, body position, psychological state, obstruction, infection, hypotension, neurologic injury, decreased muscle tone, pregnancy, surgery, and medications, can affect urinary elimination.
- Manifestations of altered urinary function include dysuria, polyuria, oliguria, urgency, frequency, nocturia, hematuria, pyuria, urinary retention, urinary incontinence, and enuresis.

- Physical assessment of urinary function includes inspection of urine and use of the bladder scanner to quantify residual urine in the bladder.
- Diagnostic tests and procedures that are helpful in identifying urinary dysfunction include urinalysis, urine culture and sensitivity, BUN, creatinine, cystoscopy, and urodynamic studies.
- Nursing measures to promote normal urinary function include ensuring adequate fluid intake, preventing UTIs, and promoting optimal perineal muscle tone.
- Independent nursing interventions for urinary incontinence include behavioral interventions such as timed voiding, prompted voiding, habit training, bladder training, use of external catheters and absorbent products, and perineal hygiene.
- Collaborative nursing interventions for management of altered urinary function include insertion of indwelling catheters and closed bladder irrigation.
- Self-management of many urologic problems occurs in the home setting with adequate support from the family, the community, and the healthcare provider.

PRACTICING FOR THE NCLEX

CHECK YOUR ANSWERS IN APPENDIX A.

1. Selective reabsorption of water and ions occurs in which part of the nephron?
   a. Bowman capsule
   b. Glomerulus
   c. Tubules
   d. Small intestine

2. Micturition occurs when:
   a. Glomerular filtration enters the tubule
   b. Increased pressure stretches the detrusor muscle
   c. Pelvic muscles relax and abdominal muscles contract
   d. Sympathetic impulses cause stimulation of the internal sphincter

3. Your patient is diagnosed with a UTI. Which urinary signs would best support this diagnosis?
   a. Cloudy urine
   b. Dark amber color
   c. No odor from urinal
   d. Sediment in the catheter tubing

4. Which patient condition would you expect to have decreased urinary output (volume)?
   a. A postoperative patient in recovery room
   b. An elderly patient with urinary frequency
   c. A pregnant patient with occasional nausea
   d. A patient following a cerebrovascular accident (CVA)
   e. All of the above

5. Which urinary output represents abnormal findings?
   a. Newborn voids 30 to 40 times per day
   b. Nighttime incontinence in a 6 year old
   c. Nocturia in elderly male patient
   d. Incontinence in an elderly female patient

6. Which of the following are expected findings?
   a. Polyuria in a patient with poorly managed diabetes
   b. Anuria in a patient with end-stage renal disease
   c. Hematuria in a patient with a UTI
   d. Urinary retention in patient with thoracic spinal cord injury
   e. All of the above

7. Your patient had a urinary catheter removed at 06:00, and it is now 14:00. What would you do first?
   a. Perform BUS
   b. Assess sensations of fullness, distention
   c. Encourage increased oral intake
   d. Assist patient to bathroom to void

8. Your assessment of an elderly female indicates the following: alert and oriented, ambulates independently, reports urinary frequency, and incontinence with coughing. Which nursing diagnosis best describes this patient's condition?
   a. Urge incontinence
   b. Functional urinary incontinence
   c. Reflex urinary incontinence
   d. Stress incontinence

9. You are working with an elderly patient with altered mental status and urinary incontinence. What nursing interventions would be most appropriate?
   a. Encourage patient to avoid smoking and drinking coffee
   b. Schedule toileting at least every 2 hours
   c. Provide medications to improve bowel function
   d. Request physician order to insert urinary catheter

10. Indwelling urinary catheters are not indicated in which of the following patient conditions?
    a. Recurrent urinary retention
    b. Surgical procedures with general anesthetic
    c. Incontinence with pressure ulcers
    d. Impaired mobility

REFERENCES

Bernard, M. S., Hunter, K. F., & Moore, K. N. (2012). A review of strategies to decrease the duration of indwelling urethral catheters and potentially reduce the incidence of catheter-associated urinary tract infections. *Urologic Nursing, 32*(1), 29–37.

Barentsen, J., Visser, E., Hofstetter, H., Maris, A., Dekker, J., & Bock, G. D. (2012). Severity, not type, is the main predictor of decreased quality of life in elderly women with urinary incontinence: A population-based study as part of a randomized controlled trial in primary care. *Health and Quality of Life Outcomes, 10*, 153. Retrieved August 2, 2014, from http://www.hqlo.com/content/pdf/1477-7525-10-153.pdf

Buckley, B. S., & Lapitan, M. C. M. (2009). Prevalence of urinary and faecal incontinence and nocturnal enuresis and attitudes to treatment and help-seeking amongst a community-based representative sample of adults in the United Kingdom. *International Journal of Clinical Practice, 63*(4), 568–573.

Centers for Disease Control and Prevention. (2014). *Catheter-associated urinary tract infection (cauti) event.* Retrieved from http://www.cdc.gov/nhsn/acute-care-hospital/CAUTI/

Gould, C. V., Umschied, C. A., Agarwal, R. K., Kuntz, G., Pegues, D. A., & Healthcare Infection Control Practices Advisory Committee (HICPAC). (2009). *Guidelines for prevention of catheter-associated urinary tract infections 2009.* Retrieved August 4, 2011, from www.cdc.gov/ncidod/dhqp/pdf/guidelines/CAUTI_Guideline2009final.pdf

Gray, M. (2008). Securing the indwelling catheter. *American Journal of Nursing, 108*(12), 44–50.

Hockenberry, M., & Wilson, D. (2013). *Wong's essentials of pediatric nursing* (9th ed.). St. Louis, MO: Elsevier.

Lo, E., et al. (2008). Strategies to prevent catheter-associated urinary tract infections in acute care hospitals. *Infection Control and Hospital Epidemiology, 29*(Suppl 1), s32–s50.

Moralejo, D. (2008). Review: Cranberry products may prevent urinary tract infection in women with recurrent infections. *Evidence-Based Nursing, 11*(3), 74.

Mori, C. (2014). A-voiding catastrophe: Implementing a nurse-driven protocol. *MEDSURG Nursing, 23*(1), 15–28.

Newman, D. K. (2009). Talking to patients about bladder control problems. *Nurse Practitioner, 34*(12), 33–45.

NANDA-International (NANDA-I) (2014). *Nursing diagnoses: Definitions and classification 2015–2017.* West Sussex, England: Wiley-Blackwell.

Nowack, R., & Schmitt, W. (2008). Cranberry juice for prophylaxis of urinary tract infections—conclusions from clinical experience and research. *Phytomedicine, 15*(9), 653–667.

Palmer, M., Athanasopoulos, A., Lee, K., Takeda, M., & Wyndaele, J. (2012). Sociocultural and environmental influences on bladder health. *International Journal Of Clinical Practice, 66*(12), 1132–1138. DOI: 10.1111/ijcp.12029

Parker, D., et al. (2009). WOCN fact sheet: Catheter-associated urinary tract infections: Fact sheet. *Journal of Wound, Ostomy, and Continence Nursing, 36*(2), 156–159.

Patel, A. R., & Campbell, S. C. (2009). Current trends in the management of bladder cancer. *Journal of Wound, Ostomy, and Continence Nursing, 36*(4), 323–421.

Saldano, D. D., Chaviano, A. H., & Maizels, M. (2008). Sustainability of remission of pediatric primary nocturnal enuresis—comparison of remission using try for dry vs. non-try for dry treatment plans. *Urologic Nursing, 28*(4), 263–266.

Singhai, M., Malik, A., Shahid, M., Malik, M. A., & Goyal, R. (2012). A study on device-related infections with special reference to biofilm production and antibiotic resistance. *Journal of Global Infectious Diseases, 4*(4), 193–198. Retrieved from http://www.jgid.org/article.asp?issn=0974-777X;year=2012;volume=4;issue=4;spage=193;epage

Siu, L., & Lopez, V. (2012). Chinese women's experiences of stress incontinence: a descriptive qualitative study. *International Journal of Urological Nursing, 6*(3), 125–136. DOI: 10.1111/j.1749-771X.2012.01155.x

Turner, B. (2009). Nursing care and treatment of patients with bladder cancer. *Nursing Standard, 23*(37), 47–56.

Zaouter, C., Kaneva, P., & Carli, F. (2009). Less urinary tract infection by earlier removal of bladder catheter in surgical patients receiving thoracic epidural analgesia. *Regional Anesthesia & Pain Medicine, 34*(6), 542–548. Retrieved from http://journals.lww.com/rapm/Abstract/2009/11000

Procedure 32-1 **Assessing Urine Volume Using a Bladder Ultrasonic Scanner**

Purpose
1. To noninvasively calculate the volume of urine in the bladder.
2. To determine the need for catheterization to relieve urinary retention.

Equipment
- Clean gloves
- Bladder scan device
- Ultrasound gel
- Isopropyl alcohol

Assessment
- Determine the patient's voiding pattern. Patients whose last void was more than 8 hours ago may be experiencing urinary retention. Patients who void small amounts (50 to 100 mL) frequently (every 1 to 2 hours) may be experiencing urinary retention with overflow voiding.
- Postoperative patients, patients taking anticholinergic medications, patients with urinary obstructive disease (e.g., enlarged prostate), and patients with neurologic impairments are at increased risk for urinary retention.

Procedure

1. **Perform hand hygiene and don gloves.**
   Rationale: Reduces microbe transmission.
2. **Identify the patient with two separate identifiers (name, medical record number, date of birth).**
   Rationale: Ensures correct patient receives proper assessment or treatment and reduces errors.
3. **Close door or bed curtains and explain procedure to the patient.**
   Rationale: Ensures patient privacy, increases patient compliance, reduces patient anxiety, and promotes learning.
4. **Raise the bed to a comfortable working height. Assist the patient to lie as flat as can be tolerated comfortably. Expose only the patient's lower abdomen and suprapubic area.**
   Rationale: Allows for better scanning of the bladder; prevents unnecessary patient chilling and provides privacy.
5. **Clean scan head probe (sound wave transducer) with isopropyl alcohol (Fig. 1).**

Rationale: Prevents transmission of microorganisms between patients.

6. **Turn the bladder scanner on and press "scan."**
   Rationale: Activates the ultrasonic scanner.
7. **Press "male" or "female" mode on scan device (Fig. 2). If a female patient has had a hysterectomy (removal of uterus), press "male."**

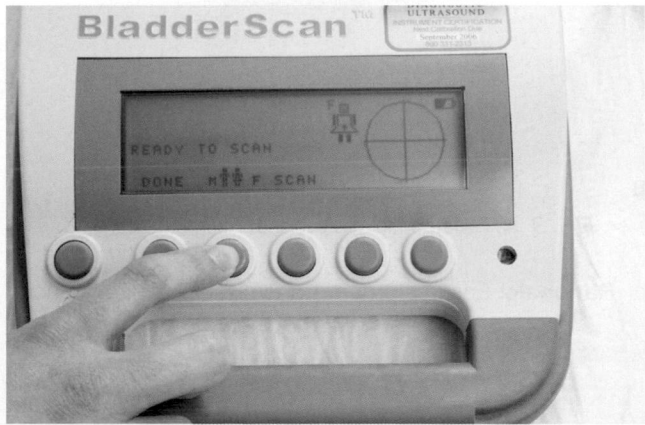

FIG. 2 Press "male" or "female" on scan device.

Rationale: The bladder scan machine is calibrated to adjust for uterus/bladder anatomy.

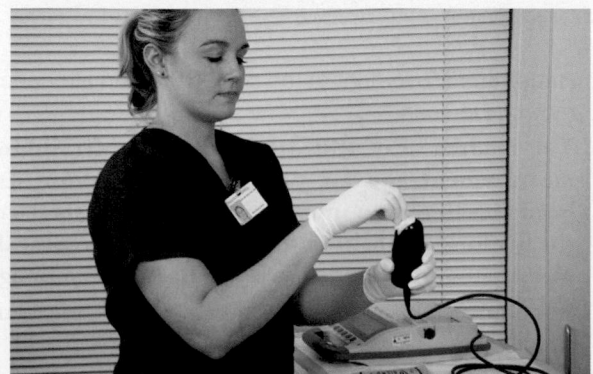

FIG. 1 Clean scan head probe.

Procedure 32-1   *continued*

8. Gently palpate the patient's symphysis pubis (Fig. 3A) and then apply ultrasound gel midline on the abdomen (about 1 to 1.5 inches above the symphysis pubis), or apply ultrasound gel directly to the scan head (Fig. 3B).

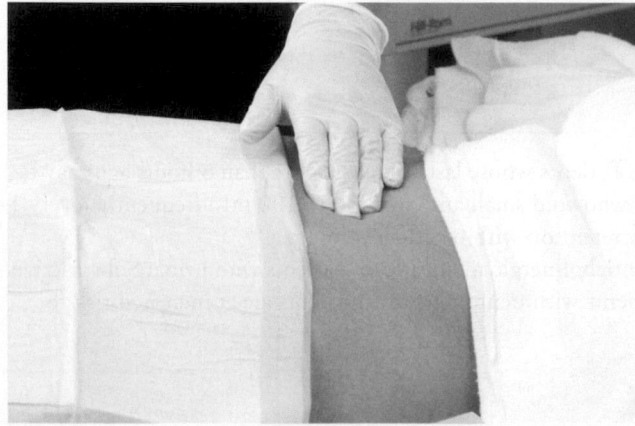

A

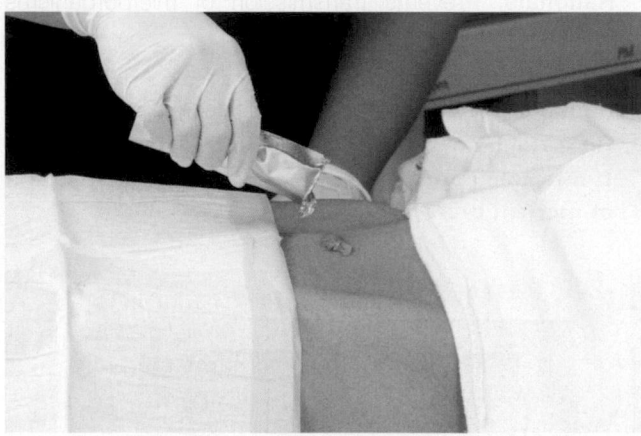

B

FIG. 3 A. Palpate symphysis pubis. **B.** Apply ultrasound gel.

Rationale: Ensures proper transmission of ultrasound.

9. Find the symphysis pubis (midline below the umbilicus) and place the scan head approximately 3 cm superior to the symphysis pubis, pointing toward the expected bladder location (Fig. 4). Locate the icon on the scan head and point the icon toward the patient's head.

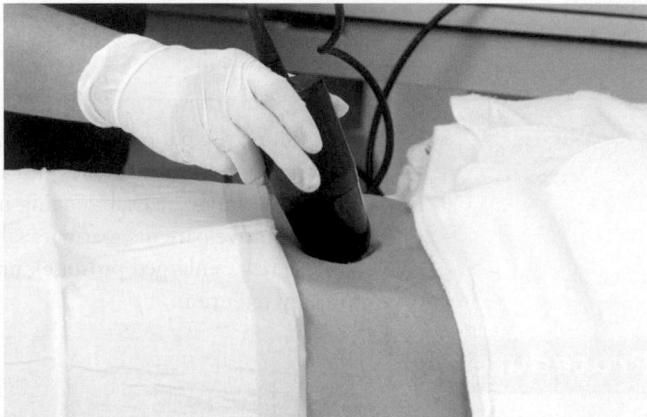

FIG. 4 Place the scan head.

Rationale: Correctly aligns the probe to scan the bladder.

10. Press the scan head button and hold the scan head steady until a beep is heard, then release (Fig. 5).

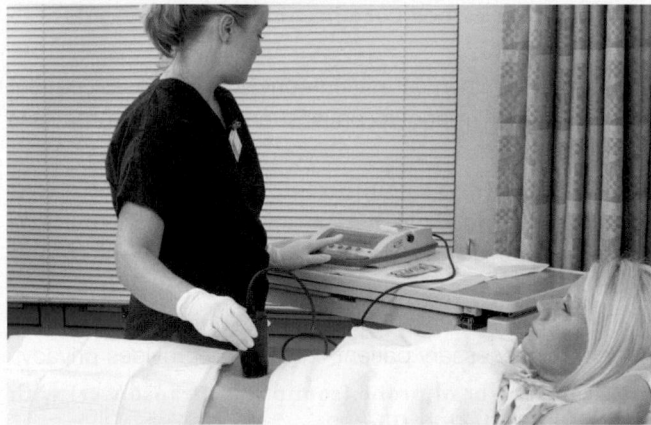

FIG. 5 Press the scan head button while holding the scan head steady to obtain reading.

Rationale: Movement of the scan head can alter accuracy of the scan.

11. The bladder scan will display the bladder volume measurement and an aiming display. Adjust scan head aim to obtain intersection of the crosshair and the bladder. Reposition the scan head and repeat the measurement as needed to obtain a centered image.

Rationale: Take several measurements for maximum accuracy.

Procedure 32-1   *continued*

12. **When finished, press "done" and print for a hard copy of results.**

    Rationale: Often, a printout of urine volume is placed in the patient's records as part of documentation.

13. **Wipe gel from patient's skin and reposition patient if needed (Fig. 6).**

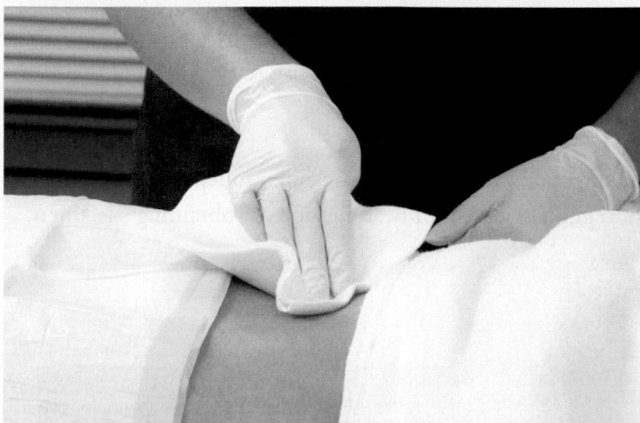

FIG. 6 Wipe gel from patient's skin.

Rationale: Maximizes patient comfort.

14. **Dispose of contaminated supplies. Clean scan head with isopropyl alcohol. Perform hand hygiene.**

    Rationale: Prevents transfer of microorganisms.

15. **Document urine volumes obtained via BUS.**

    Rationale: Communicates patient information to all members of the healthcare team.

Documentation

6/12/17: 04:30—

P: Risk for urinary retention—urinary catheter removed 8 hours ago.

I: Patient encouraged to increase fluid intake and save urine in hat placed in toilet, voided 150 mL of clear amber urine at 16:15, BUS at 16:30 for 375 mL. No abdominal distention or complaints of discomfort.

E: Urinary retention due to decreased bladder tone from Foley, MD notified, continue with plan and notify if BUS continues to be over 300 mL on subsequent voids.

—S. Roberts, RN

Collaboration and Delegation

- Assessing urine using a BUS is often delegated to unlicensed assistive personnel who have received training. Validate their technique and clarify residual urine volumes that should be reported to a registered nurse.

Procedure 32-2 Collecting Urine Specimens

Purpose	1. Obtain a noncontaminated urine specimen for routine analysis or culture and sensitivity.

Equipment

Disposable gloves
Container, label, and specimen biohazard bag
For collecting sterile urine specimen from indwelling catheter: Antimicrobial or alcohol swab and 10-mL syringe
For collecting midstream urine specimen: Cleansing solution, towel, and specimen container
For collecting a specimen from a child without urinary control: Cleansing solution, towel, pediatric urine collection bag, and diaper

Assessment

• Determine patient's ability to understand directions and to obtain specimen independently.
• Identify purpose for obtaining specimen to guide selection of best method for obtaining specimen.

Procedure

1. **Confirm the physician's order.**
   Rationale: Prevents errors.
2. **Perform hand hygiene and don gloves.**
   Rationale: Reduces microbe transmission.
3. **Identify the patient with two separate identifiers (name, medical record number, date of birth).**
   Rationale: Ensures correct patient receives proper assessment or treatment and reduces errors.
4. **Close door or bed curtains and explain procedure to the patient.**
   Rationale: Ensures patient privacy, increases patient compliance, reduces patient anxiety, and promotes learning.

Collecting Sterile Specimen From an Indwelling Catheter

5. **Position patient so that catheter is accessible.**
   Rationale: Proper positioning allows easy access during the procedure.
6. **Drain urine from tubing into collection bag. Allow fresh urine to collect in tubing by clamping or bending tubing (2 mL of urine is sufficient for a culture and sensitivity specimen, 30 mL for urinalysis) (Fig. 1).**

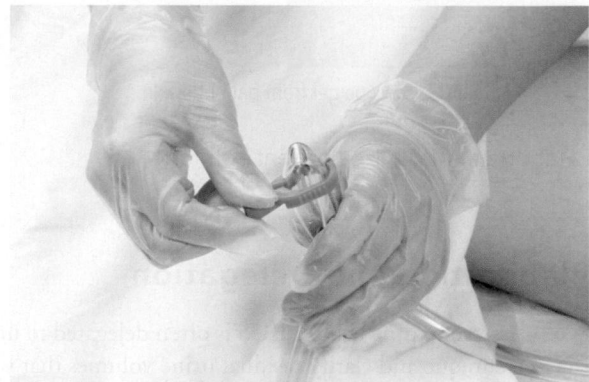

FIG. 1 Clamp tubing.

Rationale: Fresh urine is needed for accurate test results.

7. **Cleanse the aspiration port of the drainage tubing with alcohol or antimicrobial swab (Fig. 2).**

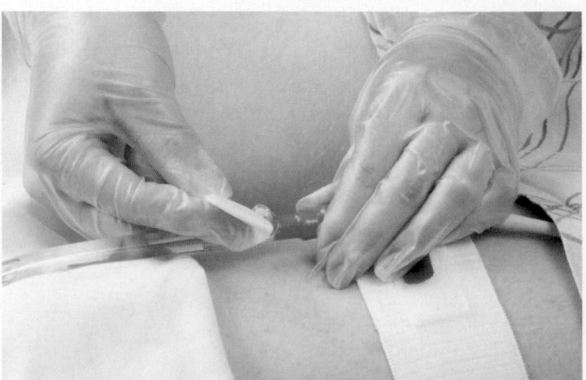

FIG. 2 Cleanse port.

Rationale: Prevents microorganisms from entering the drainage tubing.

Procedure 32-2   *continued*

8. Insert syringe into aspiration port (Fig. 3). Draw urine sample into syringe by gentle aspiration. Remove syringe from port and unclamp the drainage tubing.

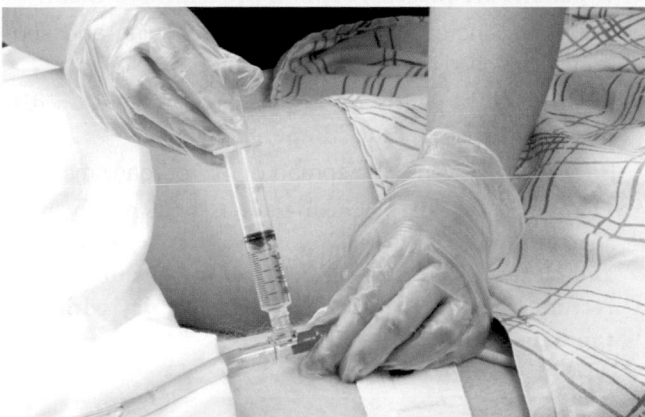

FIG. 3 Aspirate urine sample.

Rationale: Prevents contamination of the specimen.

9. Transfer urine from syringe into a sterile specimen container (Fig. 4).

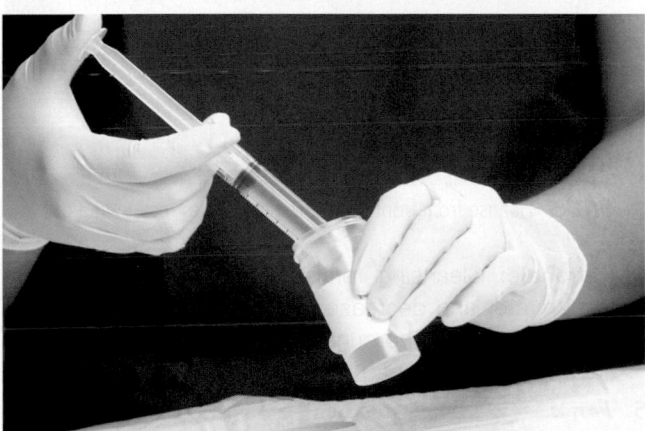

FIG. 4 Transfer urine from syringe into a sterile specimen container.

Rationale: Maintains sterility of the specimen.

10. Identify the patient with at least two identifiers (name, medical record number, birth date) and match this information to the label on the container. Note date and time on laboratory requisition form. Place in plastic biohazard bag for delivery to the laboratory.

Rationale: Prevents errors; bagging prevents spread of microorganisms.

11. Send specimen to laboratory within 15 minutes or place in specimen refrigerator. If specimen is for microbiology testing, it must be sent immediately and not refrigerated.

Rationale: Microorganisms grow quickly in urine, especially at room temperature. Refrigeration retards bacterial growth.

12. Dispose of all contaminated supplies. Perform hand hygiene.

Rationale: Prevents the transfer of microorganisms.

13. Document procedure and observations.

Rationale: Maintains accurate patient record.

Self-Collecting Midstream Urine Specimen for a Woman

1. Follow steps 1 through 4.
2. Give the patient the following instructions on how to cleanse urinary meatus and obtain a urine specimen:
   a. Perform hand hygiene.

   Rationale: Maintains asepsis.

   b. Separate labia minora and cleanse perineum with commercially prepared aseptic swabs, starting in front of the urethral meatus and moving swab toward the rectum.

   Rationale: Prevents spread of microorganisms from the rectum to the urinary meatus.

   c. Repeat this cleansing process three times with different cotton balls or swabs.

   d. Begin to urinate while continuing to hold labia apart. Allow first urine to flow into toilet.

   Rationale: First urine washes microorganisms and cellular debris out of the meatus.

   e. Hold specimen container under the urine stream.

   Rationale: Obtains specimen.

   f. Remove specimen container, release hand from labia, seal container tightly, and finish voiding; perform hand hygiene.

   Rationale: Maintains asepsis.

3. Put on disposable gloves to receive specimen container from the patient. Dry outside of container with a paper towel.

   Rationale: Prevents transfer of microorganisms to healthcare workers.

4. Date and time laboratory specimen. Verify the patient by two identifiers and make sure they match the label. Label the container and place specimen container in biohazard bag.

   Rationale: Prevents error; bagging prevents transfer of microorganisms to healthcare workers.

5. Send specimen to laboratory within 15 minutes or place in specimen refrigerator. If specimen is for microbiology testing, it must be sent immediately and not refrigerated.

   Rationale: Microorganisms grow quickly in urine, especially at room temperature. Refrigeration retards bacterial growth.

6. Dispose of all contaminated supplies. Wash hands.

   Rationale: Maintains good infection control practices.

Self-Collecting Midstream Urine Specimen for a Man

1. Follow steps 1 through 4.

2. Give the patient the following instructions on how to cleanse urinary meatus and obtain urine specimen:

   a. Perform hand hygiene.

      Rationale: Maintains asepsis.

   b. Starting at the top in a circular motion, cleanse end of penis with cotton balls and soap or commercially prepared antiseptic swabs. If the man is not circumcised, he should retract his foreskin to expose the urinary meatus before cleansing and throughout specimen collection.

      Rationale: Retraction of the foreskin is necessary to ensure adequate cleansing of the urethral opening. Circular cleansing from the meatus outward maintains asepsis.

   c. Repeat cleansing three times with three separate cotton balls or antiseptic swabs.

      Rationale: Adequate cleansing decreases the chance of infection.

   d. Begin to urinate, allowing first urine to flow into toilet.

      Rationale: The first urine washes microorganisms and secretions from the urethra before collecting the specimen.

   e. Pass specimen container into urine stream.

      Rationale: Allows collection of sample.

   f. Remove container, seal tightly, and finish voiding.

      Rationale: Promotes comfort and integrity of specimen.

3. Follow steps 3 through 6 above under the Self-Collecting Midstream Urine Specimen for a Woman section.

Collecting a Specimen From a Child Without Urinary Control

1. Follow steps 1 through 4.

2. If parents are present, explain procedure to them.

   Rationale: Increases parents' understanding and support of the child during the procedure.

3. Position child gently on his or her back. Put on disposable gloves. Remove diaper.

   Rationale: Prevents the spread of microorganisms.

4. *For a girl:* Clean perineal–genital area gently with soap and water, followed by antiseptic. Separate labia and cleanse from front of urethral meatus toward the rectum (Fig. 5). Rinse with water and dry with cotton balls.

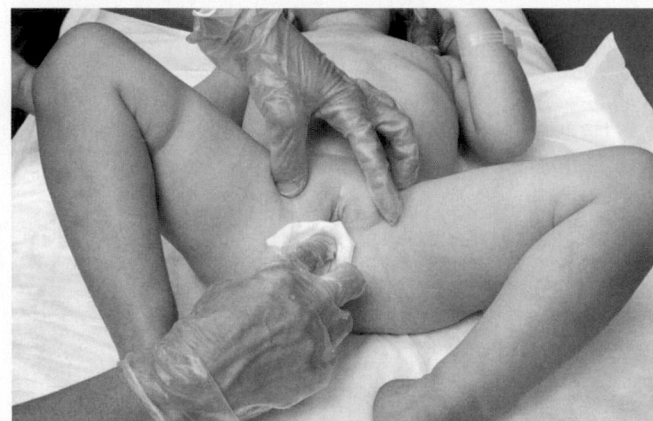

FIG. 5 Cleanse from front of urethral meatus to rectum in a girl.

Rationale: Cleansing removes lotions, powders, and fecal matter and decreases the number of microorganisms on the skin. Thorough drying facilitates adhesion of the urine collection bag.

5. *For a boy:* Clean perineal–genital area gently with soap and water, followed by antiseptic. Cleanse the penis and scrotum. If the boy is not circumcised, retract the foreskin and cleanse. Rinse with water and dry with gauze or cotton balls.

   Rationale: Same as for a girl.

6. Remove paper backing from adhesive of collection bag.

   Rationale: Prepares the bag for application.

7. Spread the child's legs widely apart.

   Rationale: Separates and flattens skinfolds to increase adhesion of the bag and decrease chances of leaking.

Procedure 32-2   *continued*

8. **Apply collection bag over child's perineum, covering penis and scrotum of a boy, urinary meatus and vagina of a girl (Fig. 6). Press adhesive to secure, starting at the perineum and working outward.**

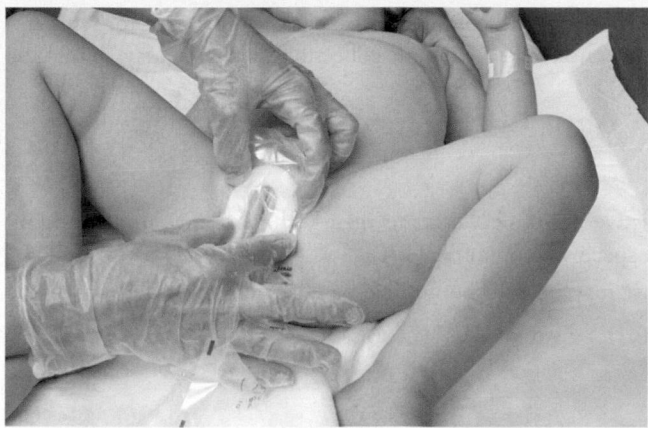

FIG. 6 Apply collection bag over urinary meatus and vagina in a girl.

Rationale: Securing adhesive from the center toward the outside decreases wrinkling and subsequent leaking of urine.

9. **Place a diaper on the child loosely.**

Rationale: A diaper helps hold the urine collection bag in place.

10. **Remove gloves and perform hand hygiene.**

Rationale: Maintains asepsis.

11. **Check the collector for urine every 15 minutes. Parents can check child for urine specimen.**

Rationale: Allows timely collection of specimen.

12. **When urine specimen is obtained, glove again, gently remove collection bag from the skin, and empty urine into specimen container (Fig. 7).**

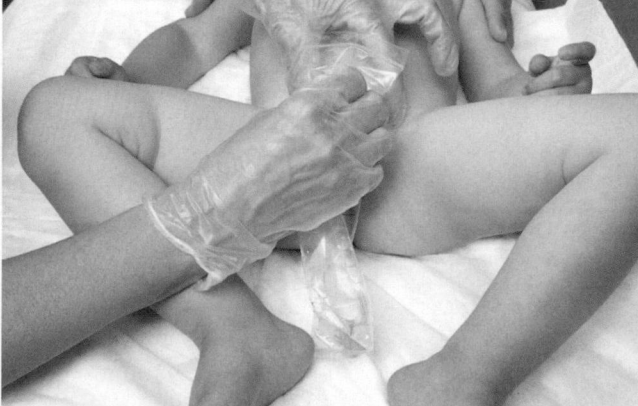

FIG. 7 Remove collection bag after obtaining urine specimen.

Rationale: Decreases skin irritation.

13. **Tighten lid, cleanse outside of container if contaminated with urine, and place in plastic biohazard bag for transfer to the laboratory.**

Rationale: Prevents spread of microorganisms.

14. **Label the container, making sure that patient information is correct. Record date and time on laboratory requisition form.**

Rationale: Prevents error.

15. **Send specimen to laboratory within 15 minutes or place in specimen refrigerator. If specimen is for microbiology testing, it must be sent immediately and not refrigerated.**

Rationale: Microorganisms grow quickly in urine, especially at room temperature. Refrigeration retards bacterial growth.

16. **Dispose of all contaminated supplies. Perform hand hygiene.**

Rationale: Maintains asepsis.

17. **Document that specimen was collected and sent.**

Rationale: Proper documentation is often necessary for reimbursement.

Documentation

7/1/17: 14:30—30 cc of clear, straw-colored urine obtained from collection bag, sent immediately to lab.
—S. Roberts, RN

Procedure 32-2   *continued*

Home Care Modifications

- Kits containing instructions, cleansing agents, specimen containers, and labels are often commercially available for patients who must collect urine specimens in their home.
- Remind patients to obtain a sample early in the morning for best results.
- When a 24-hour urine sample is collected in the home, an ice chest with commercial ice packs can be used for refrigeration of the sample; it should not be placed in the family refrigerator. End the sample collection during the day, so that the sample can be taken to the laboratory as quickly as possible.

Collaboration and Delegation

- Specimen collection is often delegated to unlicensed assistive personnel. Validate their technique and understanding because accurate collection methods are needed to prevent specimen contamination.
- Communicate clearly with laboratory personnel. Transport may need to be notified to ensure prompt delivery of the specimen to the laboratory.

Procedure 32-3 Applying an External Catheter

Purpose	1. Provide a means of collecting urine and controlling incontinence with less risk of infection that an indwelling urinary catheter imposes.

Equipment	Soap, warm water, washcloth, towel, prepackaged skin protector if not included in kit Commercially packaged external catheter Disposable gloves Urine collection bag with drainage tubing or leg bag with straps

Assessment	• Identify male patients who require control of incontinence. • Assess patient's mental status to determine ability to cooperate with procedure. • Inspect penis for irritation or areas of skin breakdown from previous incontinence. • Measure diameter of the penile shaft or use a measuring guide supplied by the manufacturer to determine appropriate catheter size. • Determine patient's activity level and need for leg bag or continuous drainage system for urine collection. • Assess for allergy or sensitivity to latex or cleansing solution.

Procedure

1. **Perform hand hygiene.**

   Rationale: Reduces microbe transmission.

2. **Identify the patient.**

   Rationale: Ensures correct patient receives proper assessment or treatment and reduces errors.

3. **Close door or bed curtains and explain procedure to the patient.**

   Rationale: Ensures patient privacy, increases patient compliance, reduces patient anxiety, and promotes learning.

4. **Raise the bed to a comfortable working height. Assist patient to supine position with thighs slightly apart. Drape patient so that only the area around the genitalia is exposed (Fig. 1).**

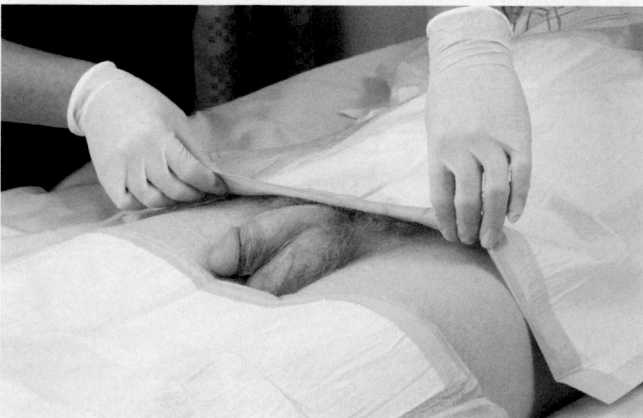

FIG. 1 Drape patient so that only the area of the genitalia is exposed.

Rationale: Provides the patient with comfort and privacy.

5. **Put on disposable gloves. Wash patient's genitals with plain soap and water. Clean the tip of the penis first using a circular motion from the meatus outward. Wash the shaft of the penis using downward strokes toward the pubic area (Fig. 2). Towel dry. For an uncircumcised male, retract the foreskin and clean the glans of the penis. Be sure to replace the foreskin after cleansing.**

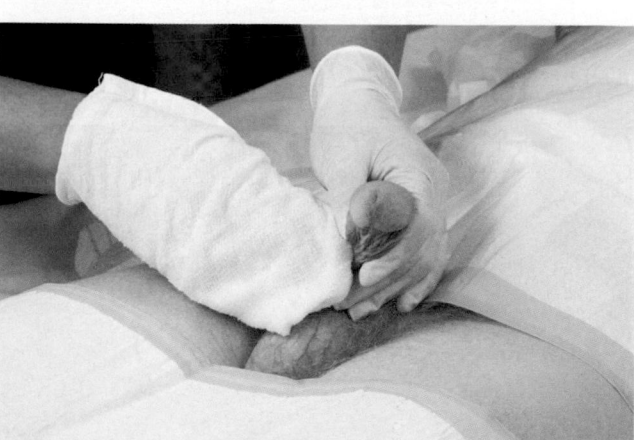

FIG. 2 Cleanse the shaft of the penis.

Rationale: Removes secretions to prevent skin breakdown. The catheter adheres best if the skin is thoroughly dry. Oils from lotions or emollients or soaps containing moisturizers or deodorants will interfere with the sheath adhesive. Replacing the foreskin prevents ischemia or necrosis to the penis from application of the catheter sheath to a retracted foreskin.

Procedure 32-3   *continued*

6. **Trim excess pubic hair from base of penis using blunt-end scissors, if necessary.**

   Rationale: Excess hair adheres to the condom adhesive, interfering with a good seal, and would cause removal to be uncomfortable.

7. **If not using a self-adhesive sheath, apply thin film of skin protector supplied in kit on penis shaft. Allow to dry for 30 seconds.**

   Rationale: Protects sensitive penile skin from irritation and provides better adherence to the external catheter.

8. **Grasp penis firmly with nondominant hand. Apply sheath by guiding opening over the glans of the penis and then unrolling the sheath the length of the penis using dominant hand (Fig. 3A,B). Leave only a small gap between the tip of the penis and the drainage port of the sheath. Gently press sheath to shaft of penis to secure adhesive inside the catheter to the skin.**

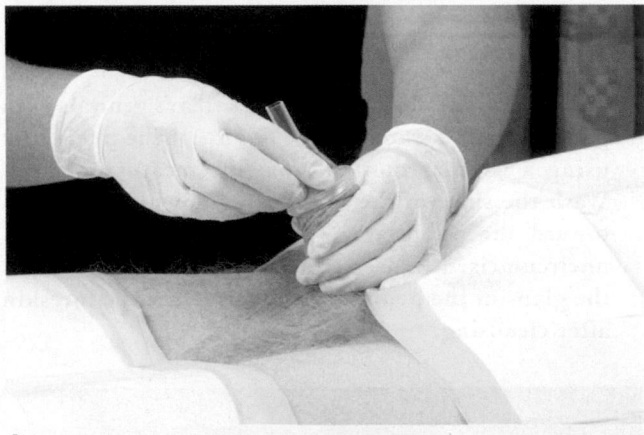

A

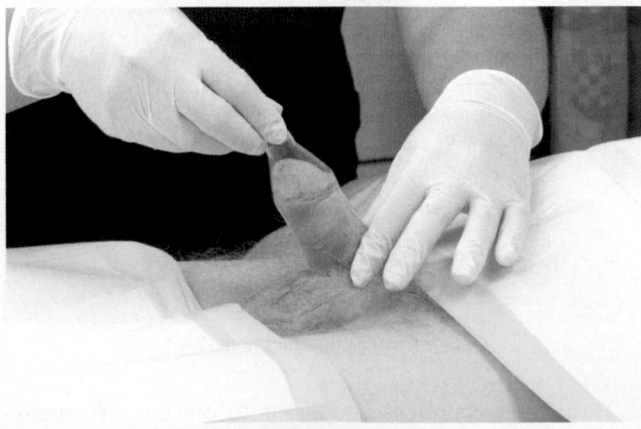

B

FIG. 3 **A.** Grasp the penis firmly with the nondominant hand. **B.** Unroll the sheath the length of the penis.

   Rationale: Proper placement of the condom sheath allows for urine collection and minimizes backflow that could interfere with the seal between the skin and the sheath.

9. **Attach drainage port of the sheath to collection system tubing (Fig. 4). Avoid kinks or loops in the tubing. Secure drainage tubing to patient's abdomen or inner thigh with securement device.**

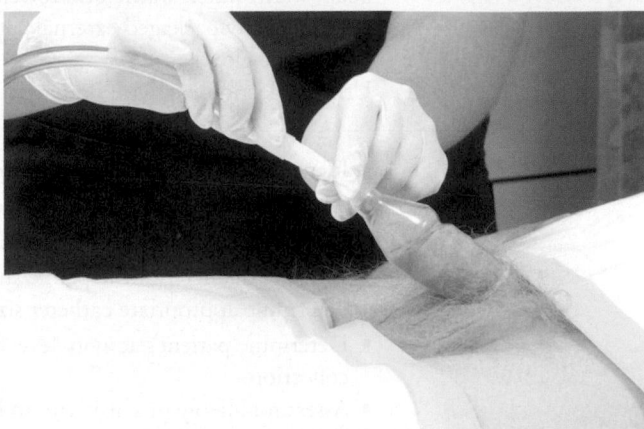

FIG. 4 Attach funnel end of condom to collection system tubing.

   Rationale: The collection system keeps the patient dry. Kink- and loop-free tubing allows free drainage and observation of color and quantity of urine. A securement device prevents disconnection of tubing as the patient turns and moves.

10. **Discard used supplies and perform hand hygiene.**

    Rationale: Maintains asepsis.

11. **Assist the patient to a comfortable position and cover him with bed linens. Place the bed in the lowest position.**

    Rationale: Provides warmth and promotes comfort.

12. **Secure collection system bag below the level of the bladder (Fig. 5). Check that the tubing is not kinked and that movement of bed rails does not interfere with the drainage system.**

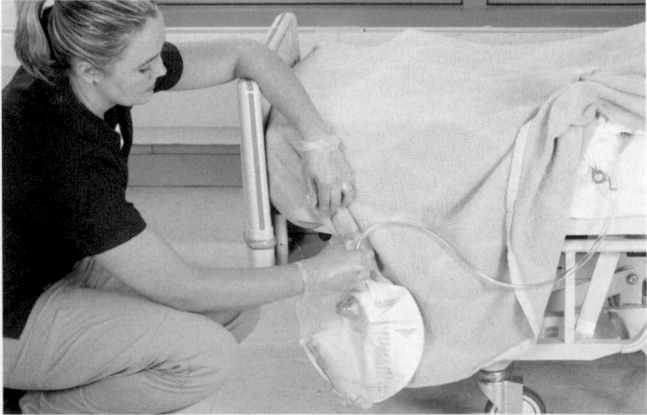

FIG. 5 Secure collection system bag below the level of the bladder.

   Rationale: Facilitates drainage of urine and prevents backflow of urine.

Procedure 32-3   *continued*

13. Observe penis 15 to 30 minutes after application of condom for swelling or changes in skin color. Routinely remove external catheter, examine the underlying skin, and reapply at least every 24 hours or if the patient complains of any discomfort.

    Rationale: Swelling or discoloration of the penis indicates that the condom is too tight and should be removed and reapplied in a larger size. Frequent monitoring and reapplication is necessary to promptly detect any areas of skin breakdown.

14. Document application and removal of external catheter and the condition of the skin.

    Rationale: Communicates information to all members of the healthcare team.

Documentation

07/18/17: 09:30—External catheter applied due to periods of incontinence over last 4 hours. Perineal skin abrasion free; external catheter intact and draining amber urine.

—S. Roberts, RN

Lifespan Considerations

- External catheters are not indicated for use in children.
- Young men might experience an erection as the penis is grasped for external catheter application.
- When the penis is grasped in older men, it may retract into lower abdominal skinfolds, making application difficult.

Home Care Modifications

- Teach patients using external catheters at home how to empty and care for their drainage collecting bag. In addition, instruct patients how to attach the external catheter to a leg bag to allow physical activity without fear of embarrassment from urine incontinence.
- Remind patients or caregivers to change external catheters daily to permit assessment of skin and to promptly detect skin breakdown. Extended-wear external catheters may be worn longer than 24 hours. Reevaluate wear time periodically and increase wear time based on individual needs; some patients may be able to tolerate an extended-use external catheter without complications for up to 72 hours.

Collaboration and Delegation

- Unlicensed assistive personnel frequently apply condom catheters. Make sure they apply catheters properly and check patients frequently for signs of constriction or skin breakdown.

Procedure 32-4 Inserting a Straight or Indwelling Urinary Catheter

Purpose

Indwelling Catheterization
1. Monitor urinary function.
2. Prevent or relieve bladder distention.
3. Provide continuous bladder drainage.
4. Provide a means for irrigating the bladder with fluids or medication.

Straight or Intermittent Catheterization
1. Obtain sterile urine specimens.
2. Routine emptying of the bladder in patients with neurogenic bladder.
3. Measure residual urine.

Equipment

A good light source
Prepackaged, sterile catheterization kit that usually includes:
- Sterile drapes
- Sterile gloves
- Sterile catheter (straight catheter or indwelling catheter, such as the Foley catheter, size 14 or 16 French with a 5-mL balloon)
- Antimicrobial cleansing solution with swabs or cotton balls
- Lubricant (in prefilled 10-mL syringe)
- Disposable forceps (optional)
- Sterile specimen cup (if specimen is required)

Sterile drainage bag and drainage tubing (included in some catheterization kits)
Catheter securement device
Disposable gloves
Washcloth and warm water to perform perineal hygiene before and after catheterization
Waterproof pad
2% lidocaine gel
Extra catheter

Assessment

- Assess why catheterization has been ordered.
- Assess the patient for bladder distention.
- Assess the patient's physical ability to tolerate positioning.
- Assess the patient for allergy to cleansing solution and latex.

Procedure

Initial Steps for Inserting Straight or Indwelling Catheters

1. **Confirm the physician's order.**
   Rationale: Prevents errors.

2. **Perform hand hygiene and don gloves.**
   Rationale: Reduces microbe transmission.

3. **Identify the patient with two separate identifiers (name, medical record number, date of birth).**
   Rationale: Ensures correct patient receives proper assessment or treatment and reduces errors.

4. **Determine if patient has any allergies (especially to iodine and latex).**
   Rationale: Prevents errors or allergic reactions.

Procedure 32-4   *continued*

5. **Close door or bed curtains and explain procedure to the patient.**

   Rationale: Patients who understand the procedure are more apt to relax, which facilitates the procedure and makes it more comfortable. Closing the curtain and door provides privacy.

6. **Set up good light source. Place trash receptacle within easy reach.**

   Rationale: Adequate lighting is crucial for clear visualization of the urinary meatus. Having a trash receptacle within easy reach allows for prompt disposal of used supplies and reduces the risk of contaminating the sterile field.

7. **Raise the bed to a comfortable working height. Stand on the patient's right side if you are right-handed, on the patient's left side if you are left-handed.**

   Rationale: Placing the bed at a comfortable working height reduces strain on the nurse's back while performing the procedure. Proper positioning allows for ease of use of the dominant hand for catheter insertion.

8. **Provide the patient with opportunity to perform personal perineal/penile hygiene. If the patient is unable or unwilling to perform personal hygiene, assist or perform hygiene as necessary. Slide waterproof pad under patient. For the female patient, wipe from front to back (Fig. 1A). For the male patient, clean the tip of the penis first, using circular motions from the meatus outward, and then cleanse the shaft of the penis using downward strokes toward the pubic area (Fig. 1B). Remove gloves and perform hand hygiene.**

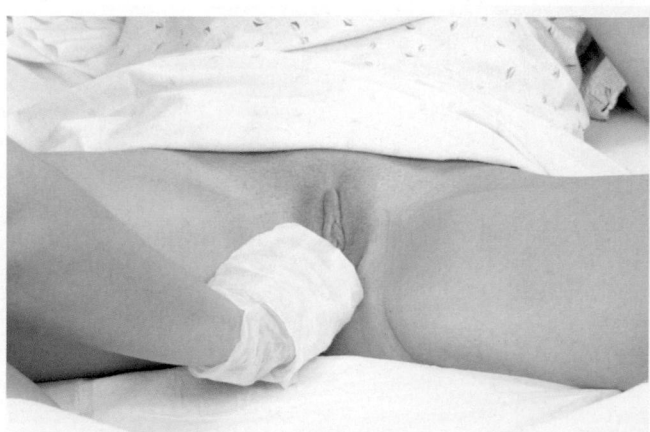

A

FIG. 1 **A.** Perform female perineal hygiene.

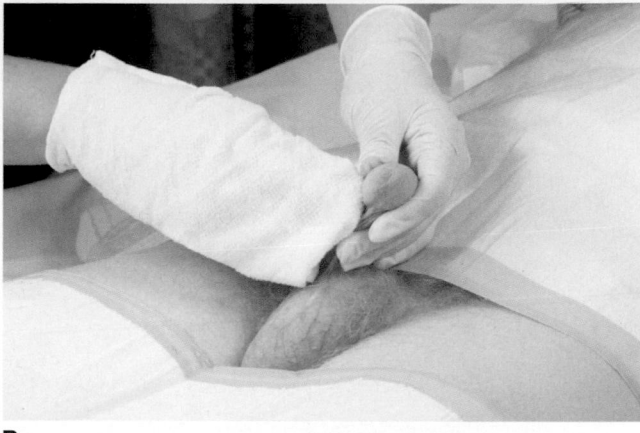

B

FIG. 1 (Continued) **B.** Perform male perineal hygiene.

Rationale: Strict asepsis must be maintained to reduce the possibility of introducing a UTI. Initial cleansing rids the body of gross contamination. Hand washing prevents transfer of microorganisms.

Inserting an Indwelling Catheter in a Female Patient

9. **Position patient in dorsal recumbent position (supine with knees flexed). Externally rotate thighs. Side-lying is an alternative position.**

   Rationale: Allows for visualization of the urinary meatus.

10. **Open the catheterization tray on clean bedside table while maintaining asepsis (Fig. 2). See Procedure 19-3 for preparing and maintaining a sterile field. If necessary, put on clean gloves. Pick up drape from the top of the catheterization kit, touching only the corners of the drape. Slide sterile drape under patient's buttocks; ask the patient to lift hips if possible so drape can be slid under easily (Fig. 3). Do not touch center of drape.**

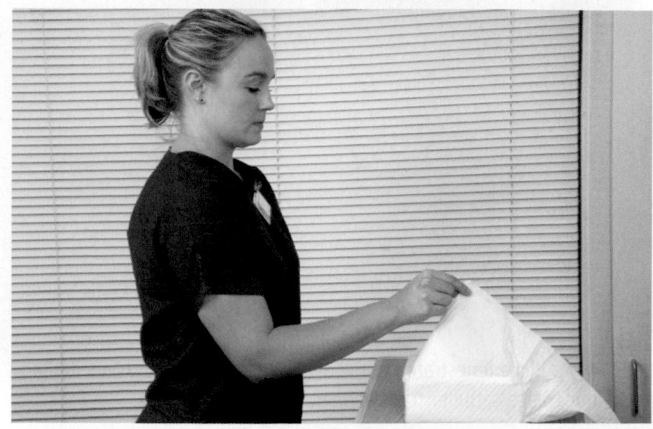

FIG. 2 Open catheter tray.

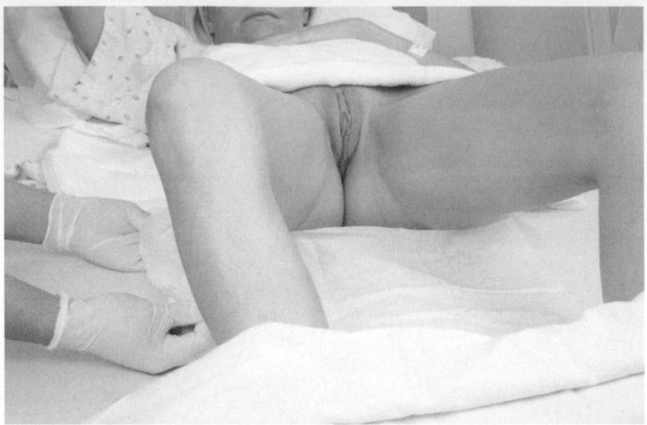

FIG. 3 Slide sterile drape under patient's buttocks.

Rationale: The drape provides a large sterile field.

11. **If used, remove clean gloves. Don sterile gloves. Place fenestrated sterile drape over the perineal area (Fig. 4A). Place sterile catheterization tray on sterile drape between patient's thighs (Fig. 4B).**

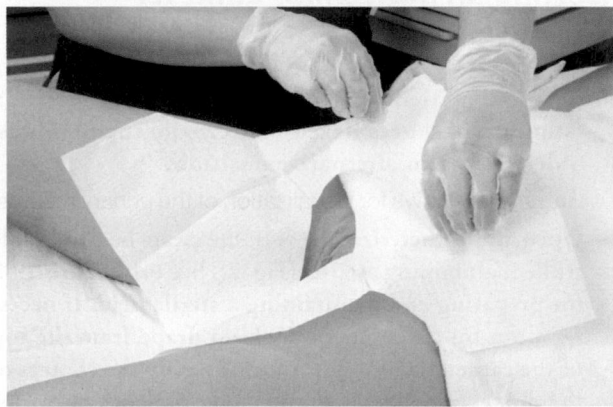

A

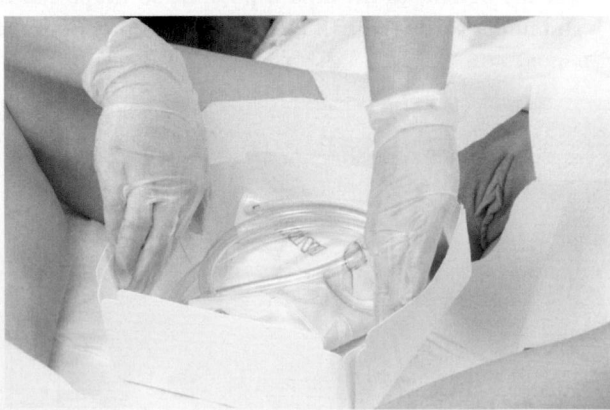

B

FIG. 4 A. Place fenestrated drape over perineal area. **B.** Using sterile technique, place catheter tray between the patient's thighs.

Rationale: This is a sterile procedure. Once gloves are on, all equipment in the kit can be touched yet remain sterile.

12. **Open sterile lubricant and lubricate the catheter tip. With a physician's order, 2% lidocaine gel can also be used for lubrication. Open cleansing solution and pour over half of the sterile balls or open antimicrobial cleansing swabs. Open the sterile specimen container. Do not test inflate the balloon.**

Rationale: Lubricant facilitates catheter insertion and reduces urethral trauma. Lidocaine decreases discomfort on insertion. Attention to preparation of the tray decreases chances of contaminating sterile hands or equipment before completing the procedure. Inflating the balloon before insertion can create balloon ridges that can traumatize the urethra upon insertion.

13. **Place nondominant hand on labia minora and gently spread to expose urinary meatus. (This hand is now considered contaminated.) Visualize exact location of meatus. During cleansing and catheter insertion, do not allow labia to close over meatus until after the catheter is inserted.**

Rationale: If the labia close over the meatus before catheter insertion, the meatus is considered contaminated and must be recleansed.

14. **Using sterile hand, pick up saturated cotton ball with sterile forceps or antimicrobial swabs.**

Rationale: Using forceps during cleaning protects the sterile hand from contamination. If the kit contains swabs, forceps are unnecessary.

15. **Cleanse the urinary meatus with a downward stroke (Fig. 5). Discard the cotton ball or antimicrobial swab. Repeat this step three or four times.**

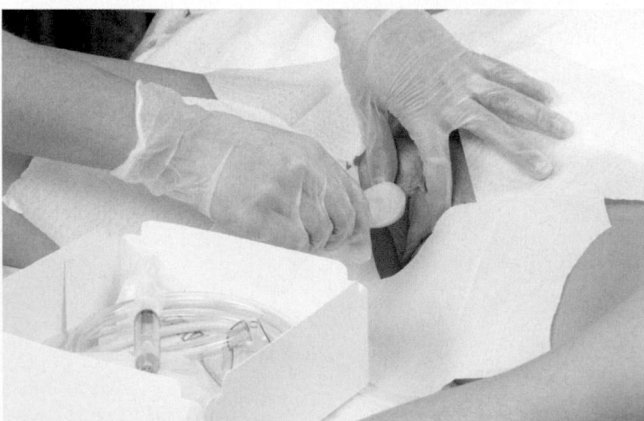

FIG. 5 Cleanse urinary meatus with a downward strokes.

Rationale: Cleansing from front to back avoids introducing microorganisms from the rectum to the urinary meatus.

16. **Use dry cotton balls to absorb excess antiseptic solution.**

Rationale: Absorbing excess antiseptic solution decreases slipperiness of tissues, aids in visualization of the meatus, and prevents introducing antiseptic into the urethra, which could cause discomfort.

Procedure 32-4   *continued*

17. **With sterile hand, pick up the catheter approximately 3 inches from the tip and place distal catheter end into sterile basin. If the catheter is attached to sterile tubing and drainage container (closed drainage system), position catheter and setup within easy reach on the sterile field. Make sure clamp on drainage bag is closed.**

    Rationale: Facilitates urine drainage and minimizes the risk of contaminating sterile equipment.

18. **Gently insert catheter into urethra (approximately 2 inches) until urine begins to drain (Fig. 6). If no urine appears, have patient cough or reposition catheter by rotating. Have patient take slow, deep breaths during catheter insertion.**

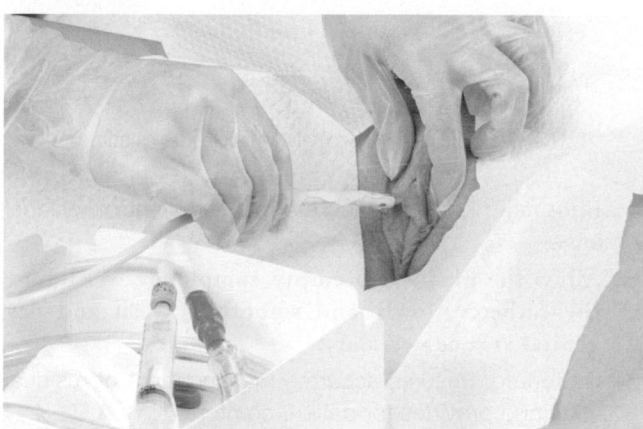

FIG. 6 Insert catheter into urethra.

Rationale: Coughing increases intra-abdominal pressure and may assist urine flow. When the patient takes slow, deep breaths, the external sphincter relaxes.

19. **Insert the catheter an additional 1 inch (2.5 cm).**

    Rationale: Ensures that the balloon inflates inside the bladder and not inside the urethra, where it would cause trauma. If the catheter enters the vagina by mistake, leave it there as a landmark and insert a second catheter into the meatus.

20. **Inflate the retention balloon with the prefilled syringe (Fig. 7). Check to ensure placement by gently pulling on catheter.**

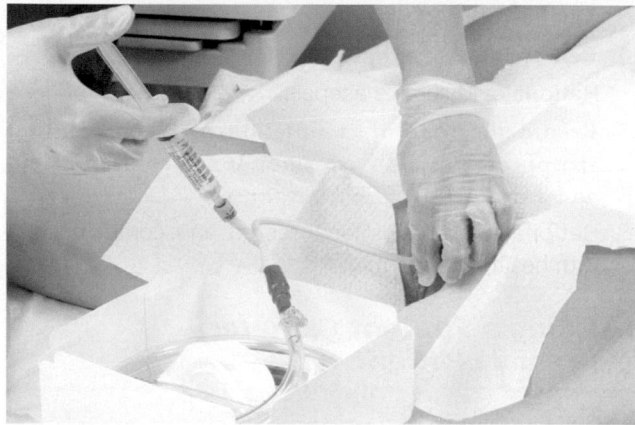

FIG. 7 Inflate retention balloon with prefilled syringe.

Rationale: If resistance is felt, the catheter balloon is properly inflated in the bladder.

21. **Connect distal end of catheter to drainage bag. In some kits, the catheter is already connected to the drainage unit. Some nurses prefer to connect equipment before catheter insertion.**

    Rationale: Maintains sterility of the system.

22. **Secure catheter tubing to the patient's inner thigh with Velcro leg strap or other securement device, with enough give, so that it will not pull when the legs move (Fig. 8).**

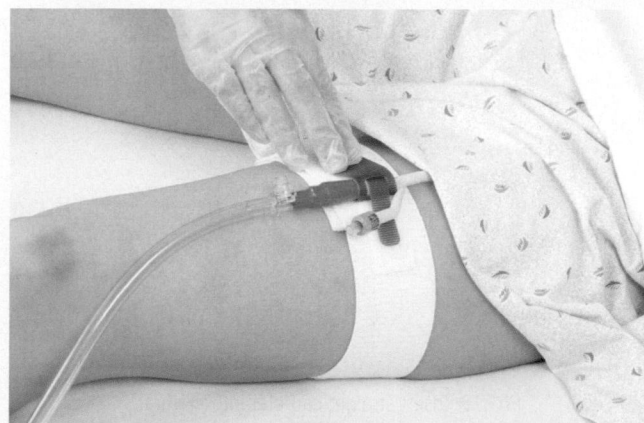

FIG. 8 Secure catheter tubing to patient's inner thigh.

Rationale: Securing the catheter tubing reduces urethral friction and irritation during patient movement.

Procedure 32-4   *continued*

23. Attach drainage bag to bed frame, ensuring that tubing does not fall into dependent loops and that side rails do not interfere with drainage system.

    Rationale: Dependent loops fill with urine and can prevent free drainage of urine.

24. Remove gloves and perform hand hygiene.

    Rationale: Maintains asepsis.

25. Record the time of completion of the procedure, size of catheter inserted, amount and color of urine, and any adverse patient responses.

    Rationale: Maintains legal record and communicates with healthcare team.

Inserting a Straight Catheter in a Female Patient

1. Follow steps 1 through 16.
2. With sterile hand, place the drainage end of the catheter in a receptacle. If a specimen is required, place the end into the specimen container in the receptacle.

    Rationale: Ensures accurate measurement of urine and proper specimen collection and prevents spillage of urine.

3. Gently insert catheter into urethra (approximately 2 inches) until urine begins to drain (Fig. 9). If no urine appears, have patient cough or reposition catheter by rotating. Have patient take slow, deep breaths during catheter insertion.

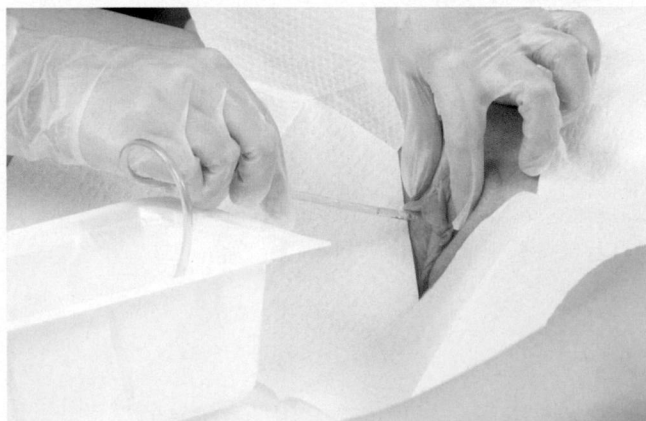

FIG. 9 Insert straight catheter into urethra.

Rationale: Promotes patient comfort and encourages urine flow.

4. Hold the catheter securely at the urinary meatus while the bladder empties (Fig. 10). If ordered, obtain urine specimen in sterile container, pinching catheter once specimen is obtained. Add volume of specimen to the residual volume obtained.

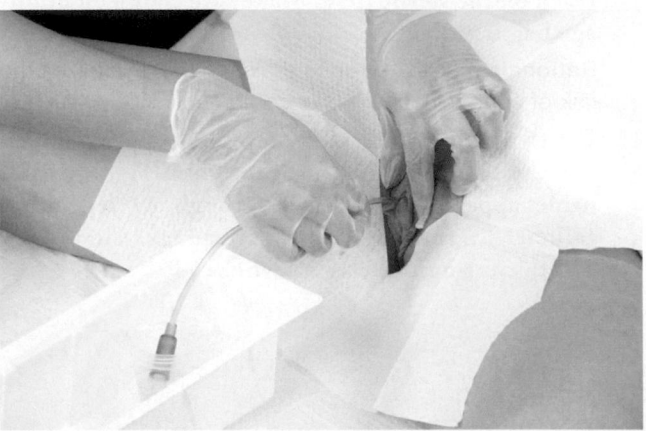

FIG. 10 Hold catheter securely while bladder empties.

Rationale: Ensures accurate measurement of residual urine.

5. Allow the bladder to empty completely. Withdraw the catheter slowly and smoothly. Wash and dry genital area as necessary.

    Rationale: Ensures accurate measurement of residual urine and provides for patient comfort.

6. Remove gloves and assist the patient to a comfortable position. Cover the patient with a gown and bed linens.

    Rationale: Provides patient comfort.

7. Put on clean gloves. Cover and label urine specimen if obtained and place in plastic bag with lab requisition form. Check patient identity with two separate identifiers. Send urine specimen to the laboratory immediately.

    Rationale: Properly labeling specimens prevents errors. Prompt transport prevents growth of microorganisms in the specimen.

8. Remove gloves and perform hand hygiene.

    Rationale: Maintains asepsis.

Inserting an Indwelling Catheter in a Male Patient

1. Confirm the physician's order.

    Rationale: Prevents errors.

2. Perform hand hygiene and don gloves.

    Rationale: Reduces microbe transmission.

Procedure 32-4 *continued*

3. **Identify the patient with two separate identifiers (name, medical record number, date of birth).**

Rationale: Ensures correct patient receives proper assessment or treatment and reduces errors.

4. **Determine if patient has any allergies (especially to iodine and latex).**

Rationale: Prevents errors or allergic reactions.

5. **Close door or bed curtains and explain procedure to the patient.**

Rationale: Patients who understand the procedure are more apt to relax, which facilitates the procedure and makes it more comfortable. Closing the curtain and door provides privacy.

6. **Set up good light source. Place trash receptacle within easy reach.**

Rationale: Adequate lighting is crucial for clear visualization of the urinary meatus. Having a trash receptacle within easy reach allows for prompt disposal of used supplies and reduces the risk of contaminating the sterile field.

7. **Raise the bed to a comfortable working height. Stand on the patient's right side if you are right-handed, on the patient's left side if you are left-handed.**

Rationale: Placing the bed at a comfortable working height reduces strain on the nurse's back while performing the procedure. Proper positioning allows for ease of use of the dominant hand for catheter insertion.

8. **Provide the patient with opportunity to perform personal perineal/penile hygiene. If the patient is unable or unwilling to perform personal hygiene, assist or perform hygiene as necessary. Slide waterproof pad under patient. For the female patient, wipe from front to back (Fig. 1A). For the male patient, clean the tip of the penis first, using circular motions from the meatus outward, and then cleanse the shaft of the penis using downward strokes toward the pubic area (Fig. 1B). Remove gloves and perform hand hygiene.**

Rationale: Strict asepsis must be maintained to reduce the possibility of introducing a UTI. Initial cleansing rids the body of gross contamination. Hand washing prevents transfer of microorganisms.

9. **Position the patient in supine position with only genitalia exposed.**

Rationale: Provides for comfort and privacy.

10. **Drape legs to midthigh with bath blanket or sheet.**

Rationale: Prevents chilling and increases comfort and aids patient relaxation.

11. **Open the sterile catheterization tray on a clean bedside table, maintaining asepsis (Fig. 11).**

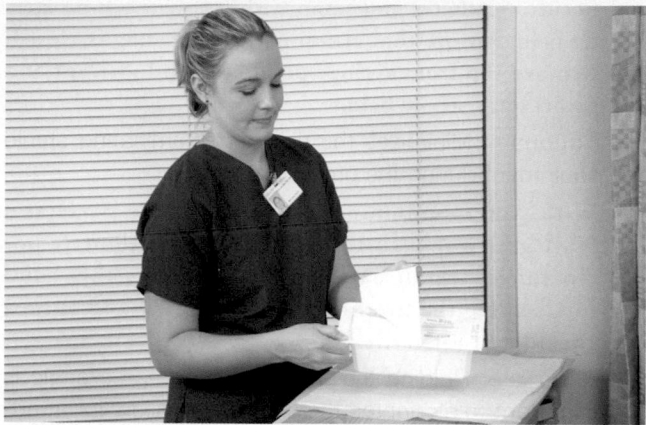

FIG. 11 Open catheter tray.

12. **Put on sterile gloves. Place the fenestrated drape over the patient's genitalia. Place sterile catheterization tray between patient's legs on the sterile drape (Fig. 12).**

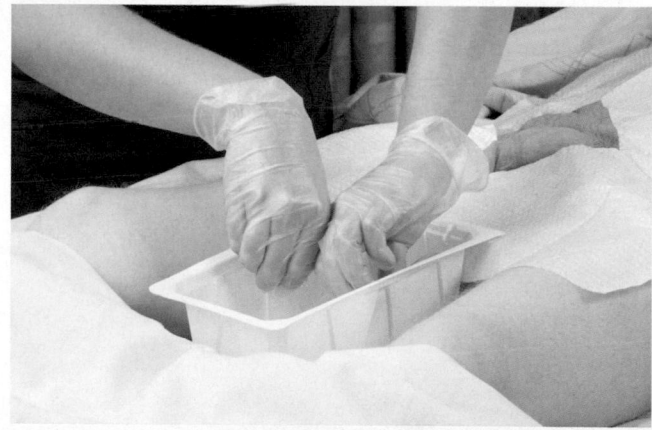

FIG. 12 Using sterile technique, place catheter tray between the patient's thighs.

Rationale: Maintains asepsis during sterile procedure.

13. **Open cleansing solution and pour over half of the sterile cotton balls, or open antimicrobial swabs. Open the sterile specimen container. Do not test inflate the balloon.**

Rationale: Attention to preparation of the tray decreases the chance of contaminating sterile hands or equipment before the procedure is completed. Inflating the balloon before insertion can create balloon ridges that can traumatize the urethra upon insertion especially with a male patient.

Procedure 32-4   *continued*

14. **Using sterile hand, place the distal catheter end into sterile basin. If catheter is preattached to sterile tubing and drainage container (closed drainage system), position catheter and setup within easy reach on sterile field. Ensure that clamp on drainage bag is closed. Remove cap from syringe prefilled with lubricant and squirt onto sterile field.**

    Rationale: Minimizes the risk of contaminating sterile equipment during the procedure.

15. **With your nondominant hand, hold the penis at a 90-degree angle to the body. If the patient is not circumcised, pull back the foreskin with this hand to visualize the urethral meatus. (This hand is now considered unsterile.)**

    Rationale: Holding the penis at a 90-degree angle is important to straighten the urethra and allow for atraumatic catheter insertion.

16. **Using the sterile hand, pick up the cleansing solution—either antimicrobial swabs or the soaked cotton ball (using sterile forceps).**

    Rationale: Using forceps during cleansing protects the sterile hand from contamination; if the kit provides swabs, no forceps are needed.

17. **Cleanse the urinary meatus with one downward stroke or use a circular motion from meatus to base of penis (Fig. 13). Discard the cotton ball or antimicrobial swabs. Repeat this step at least three or four times.**

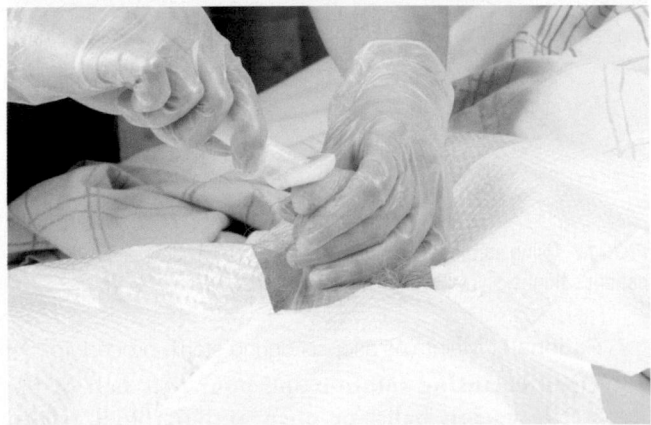

FIG. 13 Cleanse the urinary meatus.

Rationale: Cleaning from the meatus outward helps keep the insertion site as clean as possible.

18. **Use forceps to pick up one dry cotton ball to dry the meatus.**

    Rationale: Drying the meatus prevents introduction of cleansing solution into the meatus, which could cause discomfort.

19. **Hold penis with slight upward tension and perpendicular to the patient's body. Lubricate catheter well with lubricant or lidocaine. For a patient needing extra lubrication, the lubricant or lidocaine can be injected directly into the penis.**

    Rationale: Lubricant facilitates catheter insertion and reduces urethral trauma. Lidocaine gel reduces discomfort on insertion.

20. **Gently insert catheter into urethra (approximately 8 inches) until urine begins to drain (Fig. 14).**

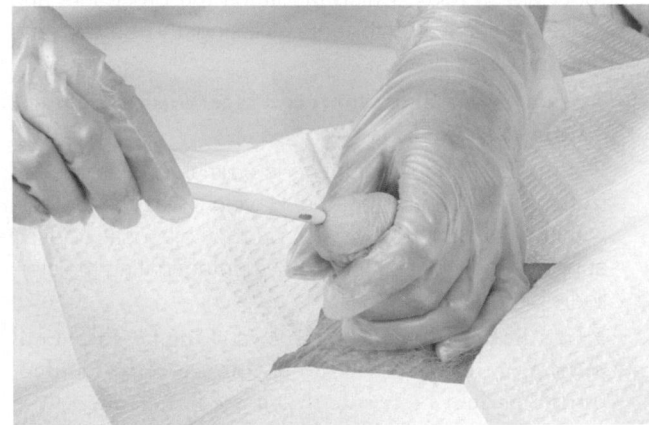

FIG. 14 Insert catheter into urethra.

Rationale: The urethra is much longer in the male than the female.

21. **Insert catheter an additional 1 inch (2.5 cm).**

    Rationale: Ensures that the balloon inflates inside the bladder and not inside the urethra, where it would cause trauma.

22. **Inflate the balloon with the prefilled syringe (Fig. 15).**

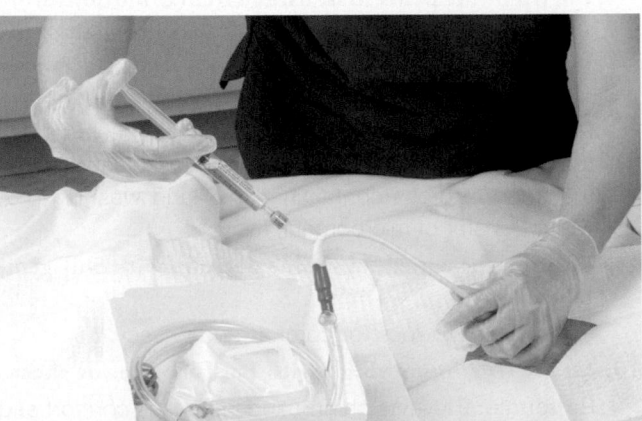

FIG. 15 Inflate balloon with prefilled syringe.

Rationale: Inflation prevents the catheter from slipping out of the bladder.

Procedure 32-4   *continued*

23. **Check for placement by gently pulling on catheter.**

    Rationale: If resistance is felt, the catheter balloon is properly inflated in the bladder.

24. **Connect distal end of catheter to drainage bag if necessary.**

    Rationale: Maintains asepsis of the system.

25. **Secure catheter tubing to the patient's thigh or abdomen using a Velcro leg strap or other securement device (Fig. 16). Leave some slack in catheter tubing to allow for movement.**

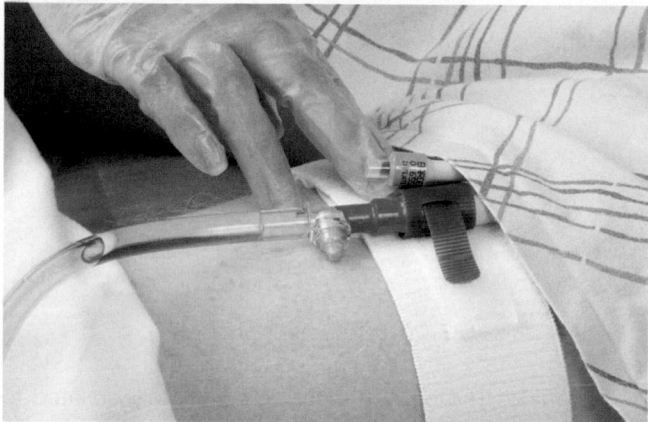

FIG. 16 Secure catheter to male patient's thigh using securement device.

    Rationale: Securely adhering the catheter reduces friction and irritation of the urethra from catheter movement.

26. **In the uncircumcised male, gently replace the foreskin over the glans.**

    Rationale: A foreskin left retracted can cause constricting edema and impair circulation to the penis.

27. **Attach drainage bag to bed frame, coiling tubing to ensure that tubing does not fall into dependent loops.**

    Rationale: Dependent loops fill with urine and can prevent free drainage of urine.

28. **Discard gloves and perform hand hygiene.**

    Rationale: Maintains asepsis.

29. **Record the time of completion of the procedure, size of catheter, amount and color of urine, and any adverse patient responses.**

    Rationale: Maintains a legal record and communicates with health team members.

Inserting a Straight Catheter in a Male Patient

1. **Follow steps 1 through 8 in the Initial Steps for Inserting Straight or Indwelling Catheters section.**

2. **Follow steps 9 through 19 in the Inserting an Indwelling Catheter in a Male Patient section.**

3. **Using your sterile hand, place the drainage end of the catheter in a receptacle. If a specimen is required, place the end into the specimen container in the receptacle.**

    Rationale: Maintains asepsis and proper collection of the sterile urine specimen.

4. **Gently insert catheter into urethra (approximately 8 inches) until urine begins to drain (Fig. 17).**

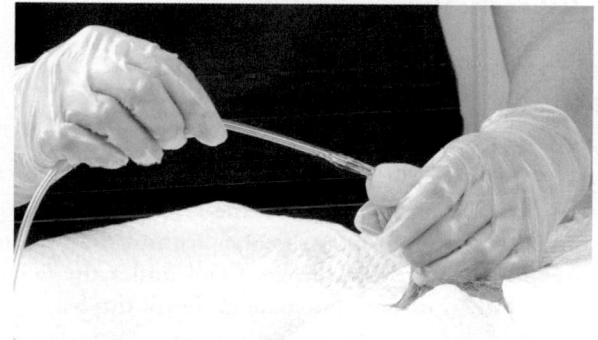

FIG. 17 Insert straight catheter into urethra.

    Rationale: The urethra is much longer in a male than a female.

5. **Hold the catheter securely at the meatus with your non-dominant hand while the bladder empties (Fig. 18). If a specimen is being collected, remove the drainage end of the tubing from the specimen container after the required amount is obtained and allow urine to flow into receptacle. Set specimen container aside.**

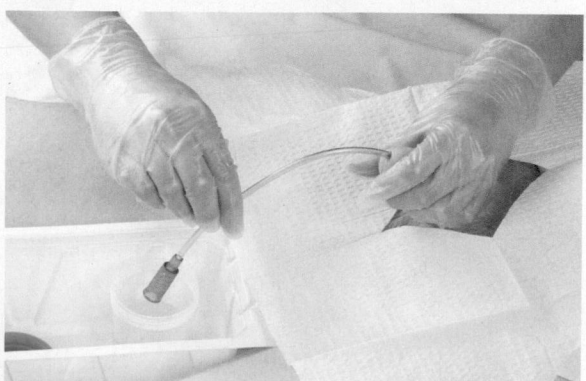

FIG. 18 Hold catheter securely at meatus while bladder empties.

    Rationale: Ensures accurate measurement of residual urine and proper specimen collection and prevents spillage of urine.

Procedure 32-4   *continued*

6. **Allow the bladder to empty completely. Withdraw the catheter slowly and smoothly. Wash and dry genital area as necessary. If necessary, replace foreskin.**
   Rationale: Promotes patient comfort.

7. **Remove gloves and assist the patient to a comfortable position. Cover the patient with a gown and bed linens.**
   Rationale: Promotes patient comfort.

8. **Put on clean gloves. Cover and label urine specimen and place in plastic bag with lab requisition form. Check the patient identity with two separate identifiers. Send urine specimen to the laboratory immediately.**
   Rationale: Proper identification prevents errors. Prompt transport prevents growth of microorganisms in the specimen.

9. **Remove gloves and perform hand hygiene.**
   Rationale: Maintains asepsis.

Removing an Indwelling Catheter

1. **Follow steps 1 through 4.**
2. **Position the patient as for catheter insertion. Drape the patient so that only the area around the catheter is exposed. Place a waterproof pad under the female patient's legs or over the male patient's thighs.**
   Rationale: Limits unnecessary exposure and promotes warmth. The waterproof pad will protect bed linens from moisture and will serve as a receptacle for the used catheter after removal.
3. **Clamp the catheter (optional).**
   Rationale: Clamping prevents urine collected in the catheter from leaking onto the bed after removal.
4. **Remove the securement device used to secure the catheter tubing to the patient's thigh or abdomen (Fig. 19).**

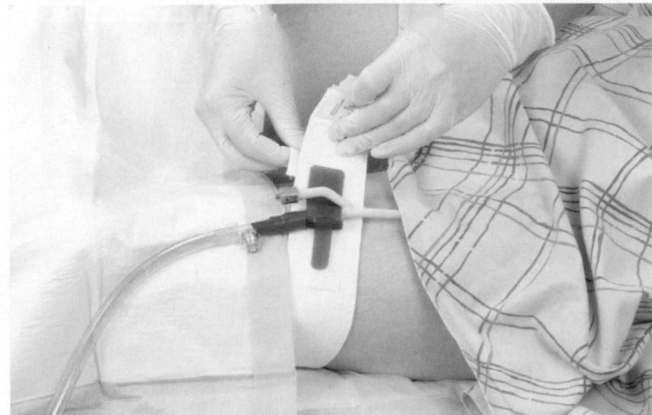
FIG. 19 Remove securement device from patient's thigh.

Rationale: Allows for removal of catheter.

5. **Insert hub of syringe into balloon inflation tube of catheter and allow syringe to fill with liquid from balloon. Do not pull on syringe to withdraw liquid (Fig. 20). Size of balloon is indicated on catheter; most commonly, sizes smaller than 10 mL are used. Larger balloons (30 mL) may be used after prostatic or urologic surgery.**

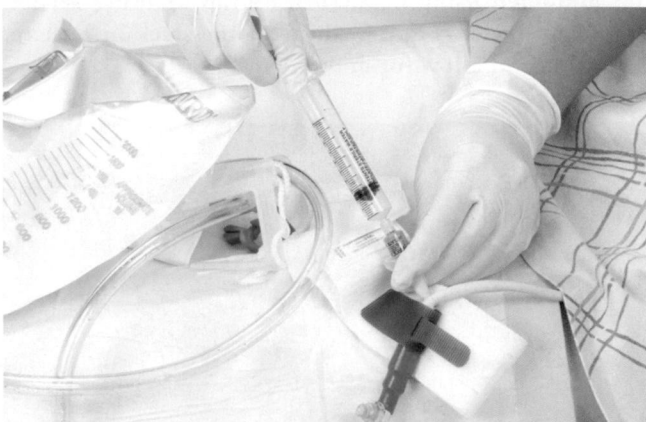
FIG. 20 Deflate catheter balloon.

Rationale: The balloon must be completely deflated to prevent trauma to the urethra as catheter is removed. Quick manual aspiration of fluid from the balloon with a syringe can cause ridges in the balloon that can cause trauma to the urethra when the catheter is withdrawn.

6. **Ask the patient to breathe in and out deeply. Pinch catheter and remove slowly and gently as patient exhales (Fig. 21).**

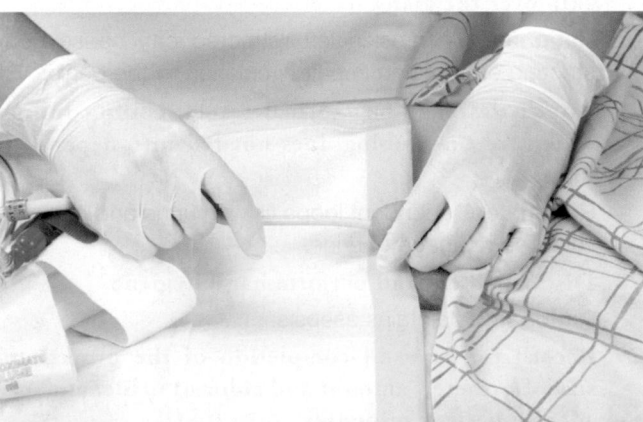
FIG. 21 Gently remove catheter as patient exhales.

Rationale: Breathing provides distraction, and exhalation prevents tightening of abdominal and perineal muscles as the catheter is withdrawn. Pinching the catheter prevents leakage of urine on the bed as the catheter exits the meatus.

Procedure 32-4   *continued*

7. Place catheter on waterproof pad and wrap in pad (Fig. 22).

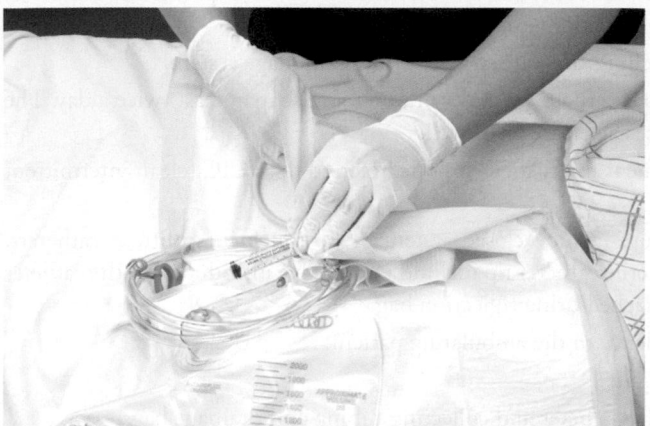

FIG. 22 Wrap used catheter in waterproof pad.

Rationale: Prevents contact with the catheter.

8. Assist the patient to cleanse and dry genitals. Remove gloves and assist the patient to a comfortable position. Place gown over the patient and cover the patient with bed linens.

Rationale: Provides for patient comfort.

9. Put on clean gloves. Remove and dispose of used equipment according to agency policy. Measure and document urine in drainage bag and time of catheter removal. Estimate when the patient should void (within 8 hours).

Rationale: Proper disposal prevents the spread of microorganisms. Maintains legal record and communicates with members of healthcare team.

10. Remove gloves and perform hand hygiene.

Rationale: Maintains asepsis.

11. Document the time of catheter removal, the time patient should void, and any adverse signs or symptoms.

Rationale: Maintains legal record and communicates information to all members of the healthcare team.

Documentation

07/13/17: 14:30—
P: Urinary retention, has not voided since 07:30, c/o of pressure, BUS 625 mL.
I: MD notified and order for I & O catheter obtained, 16 Fr Foley catheter inserted, 675 mL of straw-colored, aromatic urine obtained. Fluids encouraged.
E: Continue to assess for adequate output and urinary retention, BUS every 4 hours if not voiding or voiding in small amounts.
                                                            —S. Roberts, RN

Lifespan Considerations

Child

- Catheterization can be a frightening, painful procedure for a small child. It should be done in the treatment room so that the child's bed remains a "safe" area.
- An assistant may be necessary to help the child remain still during the procedure.
- Locating the urethral meatus on young girls takes extra care because the vaginal opening is more anterior than in women.
- Various sizes of catheters are available for use in children.

Older Woman

- The labia atrophies after menopause. The skinfolds can feel loose and slippery when they are being held before catheter insertion.
- Arthritis and other age-related musculoskeletal conditions may make it difficult for the older woman to maintain the position for insertion without an assistant. A side-lying position often is more comfortable.

Older Man

- The prostate gland often hypertrophies with aging, pressing in at the urethra–bladder junction. Always catheterize gently; if resistance is met, change the angle of the penis and advance the catheter again. If resistance continues, stop the procedure and notify the patient's physician.

Procedure 32-4　*continued*

Home Care Modifications

- Patients may return home with an indwelling or suprapubic catheter. Home health nurse follow-up is recommended.
- Instruct patients about UTI signs and symptoms, and give directions about whom to notify. Symptoms include fever; chills; cloudy, foul-smelling urine; and possibly a burning sensation around the catheter.
- Instruct patients to wash their hands before and after touching any part of their urinary drainage system.
- Patients or caregivers should cleanse the urinary meatus and catheter with warm water and soap at least twice a day. The uncircumcised man should retract the foreskin and cleanse the entire glans well.
- Intermittent self-catheterization in the home is usually done using clean technique, referred to as CIC (clean intermittent catheterization).
  - Products for intermittent catheterization for home use include closed system or no-touch intermittent catheters. Features to minimize even clean hands touching the sterile catheter tip include a protective introducer for the catheter tip, a self-contained gel/lubricant reservoir, and an attached urine collection bag.
- Leg bags (see Fig. 32-9) are available to increase independence in the ambulating patient.
- Bed-hanging, larger-volume collection bags are used at night.
- Check and follow home agency guidelines for changing the catheter and collecting tubing and drainage bags.

Collaboration and Delegation

- Nurses usually perform catheterization. Nursing assistants often help to maintain patient positioning.
- In rehabilitation units, where many patients are intermittently catheterized, a catheter team of technicians may be trained to perform catheterizations.
- If catheter insertion is very difficult or impossible, consult an urologist.

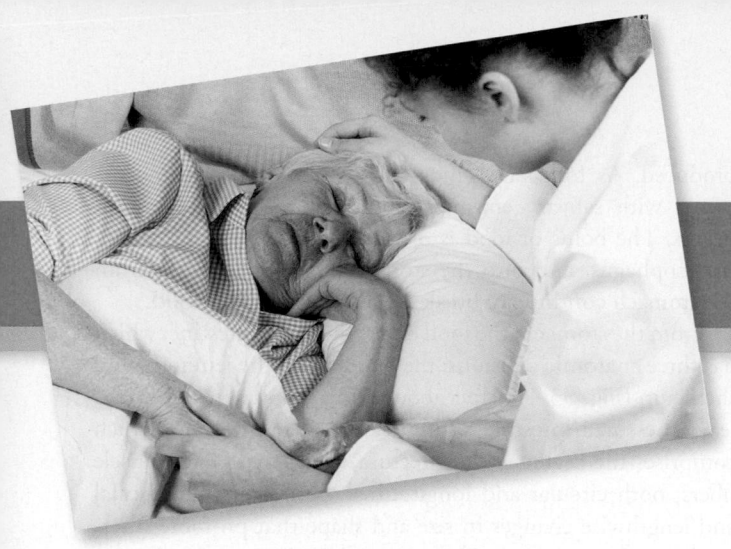

CHAPTER 33

Bowel Elimination

Susan A. Talbot

Case Scenario

You are working in a long-term care facility, caring for a 76-year-old woman with metastatic cancer. For the last few weeks, she has been receiving increasing doses of morphine to control her back pain. Her appetite is poor, and she spends most of the day in bed. At shift handoff, you learn that she has not had a bowel movement for 7 days and she has an order for an enema. When you go in to assess her and explain that she needs an enema, she replies, "Please leave me alone. Can't you see how tired I am and how much I hurt?"

Once you have completed this chapter and have incorporated bowel elimination into your knowledge base, review the above scenario and reflect on the following areas of Critical Thinking:

1. Examine factors that could contribute to the patient's constipation.
2. Reflect on how you feel when you must ask patients questions about elimination or perform procedures such as enemas.
3. Appraise possible factors that may have influenced the woman's refusal to have an enema.
4. Consider ethical and legal factors in determining how to respond to the patient.
5. Critique the use of therapeutic communication in responding to this patient.

KEY TERMS

borborygmi
Clostridium difficile (C-diff)
colonoscopy
colostomy
constipation
defecation reflex
diarrhea
distention
enema
fecal impaction
fecal occult blood test (FOBT)
flatus
gastric lavage
hemorrhoids
ileostomy
meconium
paralytic ileus
peristalsis
sigmoidoscopy
stoma
suppository
Valsalva's maneuver

LEARNING OBJECTIVES

Upon completion of this chapter, you will be able to do the following:

1. Identify factors that affect bowel elimination.
2. Describe the manifestations of altered bowel elimination.
3. Describe appropriate subjective and objective data to collect to assess bowel function.
4. Identify nursing diagnoses relating to altered bowel elimination.
5. Describe independent and collaborative nursing interventions to promote normal bowel function.

The elimination of waste from the bowel is an essential body function. Defecation is the process by which the solid waste products of digestion, known as feces or stool, are eliminated from the bowel. The major nursing responsibilities associated with bowel elimination include assessing bowel function, promoting normal bowel health, and intervening to manage alterations in bowel function.

Such responsibilities span many age groups and different health settings. For example, nurses might teach new parents about the color and consistency of stool to expect from their newborns, or they might help families cope with older parents in whom fecal incontinence has recently developed. Nurses who work in the community might develop an education program to alert workers to the symptoms of colorectal cancer. In acute care settings, nurses might assess the resumption of bowel motility during the postoperative period for patients who have had colon surgery, individualize bowel management programs for patients who have had strokes, and teach patients how to manage and adjust to a new colostomy.

NORMAL BOWEL FUNCTION

Structures of the Gastrointestinal Tract

Although the final formation of feces occurs in the large intestine, the type and amount of food and fluids ingested have a definite effect on the amount and consistency of the waste produced. As food and fluids enter the mouth, the food is mixed with salivary enzymes, and the process of digestion begins. The bolus of food is propelled to the pharynx, down the esophagus, and into the stomach, where secretions from the stomach continue to break down and digest the food.

From the stomach, the food enters the small intestine, which has three anatomic divisions: the duodenum, the jejunum, and the ileum (Fig. 33-1). After about 3 to 10 hours, the contents leave the small intestine and enter the large intestine, which comprises the cecum, colon, rectum, and anus. Here, muscle fibers, both circular and longitudinal, permit circumferential and lengthwise changes in size and shape that promote intestinal motility.

At the junction of the ileum and the cecum is the ileocecal valve, which serves to retard movement of semidigested food into the large intestine, allowing more time for the small intestine to absorb nutrients and to prevent the backflow of fecal contents from the large intestine into the small intestine.

The colon, the major portion of the large intestine, has four parts: the ascending, transverse, descending, and sigmoid colons (see Fig. 33-1). The rectum is the portion of the large intestine that immediately follows the sigmoid colon. The rectum, normally empty, is capable of considerable expansion to accommodate stool. The anus, the last portion of the large intestine, has two sphincters: the internal sphincter (smooth muscle that is under involuntary neural control) and the external sphincter (striated muscle under voluntary neural control). Both sphincters are normally in a contracted (closed) position.

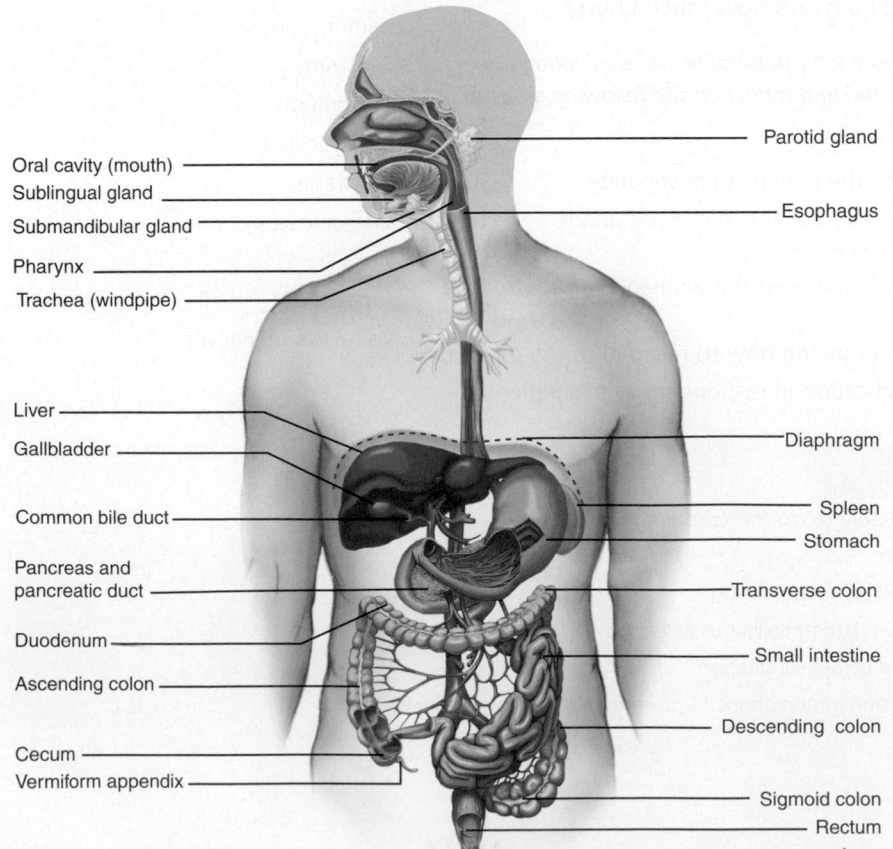

Oral cavity (mouth)
Sublingual gland
Submandibular gland
Pharynx
Trachea (windpipe)
Liver
Gallbladder
Common bile duct
Pancreas and pancreatic duct
Duodenum
Ascending colon
Cecum
Vermiform appendix

Parotid gland
Esophagus
Diaphragm
Spleen
Stomach
Transverse colon
Small intestine
Descending colon
Sigmoid colon
Rectum
Anus

FIGURE 33-1 Anatomic structures of the gastrointestinal tract.

Function of the Intestine

MOTILITY

Two types of movements—segmentation and peristalsis—occur within the intestine and are responsible for assisting with absorption and transportation of waste products over the full length of the intestines. During segmentation, alternating contraction and relaxation of the intestinal smooth muscle occur. This type of movement slows the passage of intestinal contents to permit more complete digestion and absorption of nutrients.

The second type of movement, **peristalsis**, propels the intestinal contents along the entire length of the small and large intestines. The walls of the intestine reflexively induce peristalsis, but peristalsis is particularly stimulated when partially digested food enters the duodenum from the stomach. This duodenocolic reflex is especially strong when food or fluids enter the duodenum after several hours of not eating.

Autonomic nervous system input affects the rate of intestinal motility. Sympathetic stimulation slows peristalsis and delays passage through the intestine, whereas parasympathetic stimulation increases bowel motility and emptying.

ABSORPTION

Partially digested food (also known as chyme) empties from the stomach into the small intestine, where the digestive process is completed and the absorption of nutrients and fluids begins. Most nutrient and electrolyte absorption occurs in the duodenum and jejunum. Some vitamins, iron, and fluid are absorbed in the ileum.

Final absorption of nutrients, especially the absorption of fluid and electrolytes, occurs in the large intestine. The amount of absorption that occurs depends on the speed at which the intestinal contents move through the colon: The longer that intestinal contents remain in the colon, the greater the absorption of fluid and electrolytes. The intestinal contents that enter the ascending colon are liquid. When the contents leave the transverse colon, they are semisolid and mushy and can be called feces. Although the distal colon's principal function is storage of feces, some sodium, chloride, and water continue to be absorbed during storage.

DEFECATION

The process of defecation begins when peristalsis propels feces into the rectum and causes rectal distention. This rectal distention begins a series of smooth muscle responses that can trigger bowel evacuation. When stool distends the rectum, parasympathetic afferent nerve fibers in the sacral segment of the spinal cord are stimulated, causing contraction of the descending and sigmoid colon, rectum, and anus and relaxation of the internal anal sphincter. This stimulus–response sequence is a sacral reflex, not under voluntary control. It is called the **defecation reflex**.

Defecation will automatically follow unless the external anal sphincter (a striated muscle under voluntary control) remains contracted. With the defecation reflex, the external anal sphincter can remain contracted until the person decides that the time and place for defecation are appropriate. At that time, the person can voluntarily relax the external anal sphincter. Defecation is assisted by taking a deep breath against a closed glottis (to move the diaphragm down), contracting the abdominal muscles (to increase intra-abdominal pressure), and contracting the pelvic floor muscles (to push the feces downward). These actions together are called **Valsalva's maneuver**.

Characteristics of Normal Feces

The feces consist of 75% water and 25% solids. The solids include bacteria, undigested fiber, fat, inorganic matter, and some protein. Cellulose is the major undigested fiber left in the feces after digestion and absorption have occurred. If dietary fiber intake is small, less stool is produced daily.

The normal color of feces is brown, resulting from the chemical conversion of bilirubin, an orange or dark yellow bile pigment, into urobilin and stercobilin (brown pigments) by intestinal bacteria and enzymes. The food ingested can affect the color (e.g., beets may give stool a reddish color). Ingestion of certain medications can also affect the stool's color and consistency.

The characteristic odor of feces comes from bacterial decomposition of proteins in the intestine. The feces normally have a soft consistency and a cylindrical form that approximates the shape of the rectum. Between 150 and 300 g of feces is produced daily. Table 33-1 compares normal and abnormal feces.

TABLE 33-1	CHARACTERISTICS OF NORMAL AND ABNORMAL FECES	
Characteristic	Normal	Abnormal
Frequency	Variable *Usual range*: 1–2/d to 1 every 2–3 d	Depends on usual pattern *Guideline*: >3/d; <1 every 3 d
Color	Brown	Black, tarry Reddish brown, maroon Clay colored Yellow green
Consistency	Soft, formed	Hard Loose, liquid High mucus content
Shape	Cylindrical	Narrow, pencil thin
Amount	100–300 g/d	<100 g/d >300 g/d
Odor	Aromatic, pungent	Foul, objectionable

Life Span Considerations

NEWBORN AND INFANT

Newborns usually evacuate stool within 24 to 48 hours after birth. This stool, which is softly formed and dark greenish, is called **meconium**. Meconium is the partially dried intestinal secretions that accumulated in the large intestine before birth.

By about the 3rd day after birth, the stool's characteristics begin to reflect the type of milk in the diet. If newborns are fed breast milk, the stools will be bright yellow, soft, and unformed with an unobjectionable odor. If newborns are fed formula, which is usually cow's milk, the stools will be dark yellow or tan, slightly more formed than the stools associated with breast milk, with a stronger, somewhat objectionable odor. Because the digestive and absorptive capacities of the gastrointestinal system are not mature at birth, intestinal contents pass through the system more quickly than in older children and adults, producing less firm stool. Stools become firmer as the gastrointestinal system matures and as the infant ingests more solid foods.

Frequency of bowel elimination varies among newborns and infants, as it does in adults. They may pass stool with every feeding, just once a day, or even only once every 3 days. As infants become older, they may seem to have bowel movements in more regular or identifiable patterns. Infants cannot control bowel elimination until their central nervous systems become more mature.

TODDLER AND PRESCHOOLER

The duodenocolic reflex is strong in toddlers and preschoolers. Any ingestion of food may stimulate a bowel movement, and toddlers and preschoolers may normally have more than one bowel movement per day. Toddlers are curious about the products their bodies produce. It is not unusual that, at some time during toddlerhood, smearing or playing with feces will occur. In a matter-of-fact manner that does not threaten the child's self-esteem, parents and caregivers should let the toddler know that smearing feces is unacceptable. They should encourage play with alternative substances, such as modeling clay or finger paints.

Privacy for bowel movements is a value learned early in one's culture. Young toddlers who are not yet toilet trained will sense the urge to defecate and then may hurry to another room or hide behind a piece of furniture to squat down for a bowel movement. Older preschoolers who have mastered the voluntary control of bowel movements usually prefer the privacy of their own bathrooms at home rather than public restrooms.

During toddlerhood, usually between 22 and 36 months, children are ready to learn voluntary control of bowel elimination. By this time, the central nervous system has matured enough to allow voluntary control. Myelinization of the sacral spinal cord segments, which control the anus, becomes complete between 12 and 18 months. When this occurs, toddlers can recognize that stool is present in the rectum. A good indicator of spinal cord maturation is the ability to walk independently.

Bowel training is easier when the number of daily bowel movements decreases to one or two. Successful bowel training usually does not occur before the age of 22 months. Until that age, a toddler's rectum and colon cannot hold large amounts of feces. Also, before that age, many toddlers do not have sufficient vocabulary to communicate the need to defecate and would not remember to do so before actually defecating. Children are seldom ready for bowel training until they can sense rectal distention, are able and willing momentarily to defer defecation, and can communicate the need to defecate. In the US culture, most parents believe that children are emotionally, socially, and physically mature enough to begin toilet training for bowel movements somewhere between the age of 22 and 36 months. Most children attain bowel control before 4 years of age. They usually achieve bowel control before bladder control.

SCHOOL-AGE CHILD AND ADOLESCENT

School-age children are approaching the bowel elimination habits of adults. Stools are brown and softly formed. Consistency and frequency of bowel movements depend on intake of sufficient fluids and dietary fiber and the amount of daily exercise. School-age children and adolescents may choose to defer defecation until they are in the privacy of their own bathrooms at home. Often, children delay elimination because they are enjoying an activity such as playing with friends. Continuous practice of this habit puts children at risk for decreased bowel responsiveness to rectal distention and may contribute to constipation.

ADULT AND OLDER ADULT

By the time individuals reach adulthood, they have developed bowel elimination patterns that are normal or typical. Because gastrointestinal motility slows with aging, frequency of bowel movements commonly decreases. Older adults need to increase the amount of fluids and high-fiber foods in the diet to prevent the formation of a harder stool. Weakened pelvic muscles and decreased activity level also contribute to constipation in older adults.

Normal physiologic changes within the lower intestinal tract that are associated with aging can contribute to factors that can lead to constipation. Although gut transit times and colonic motility are similar between adults and healthy older adults, older adults with chronic illness have prolonged gut transit times and delayed evacuation times. Long-term care facility residents can have delayed transit times, which can result in constipation and overflow fecal incontinence. Chronic health conditions, medication use, and mobility issues have more influence over constipation than does aging itself (Gardiner, 2013; McCrea, Miaskowski, Stotts, Macera, & Varma, 2008). Some people have a strong belief that a daily bowel movement is essential to health. Therefore, when normal age-related bowel changes occur, older persons may resort to a laxative to restore the "normal" daily pattern of bowel evacuation. Unfortunately, this type of laxative abuse is common among older adults. Educating older persons to recognize that decreased frequency of bowel movements is usually a normal result of aging, so encouraging a change in dietary habits and an increase in activity to prevent a change in stool consistency are important. With aging, the strength of the striated external sphincter muscles decreases, leading to decreased sphincter control, which increases the possibility of fecal incontinence.

Cultural Considerations

A patient's culture can affect issues related to bowel elimination and bowel-related problems. Cultural and generational influences can play a large part in infant and child care, especially in relation to toilet training. Additionally, folk remedies and old wives' tales can abound when bowel changes occur, especially in relation to babies and children. In all age groups, since bowel pattern changes are common and easily treated, home remedies or over-the-counter preparations are often employed first for relief of bowel pattern disruptions. Cultural beliefs are passed down from generation to generation, and when the desired outcome is achieved, there is reinforcement in that belief. For this reason, most cultures often may employ traditional therapies first and seek medical intervention only if those methods fail.

Cultural influence must also be considered when performing a health assessment. Many cultures would find it improper to discuss something as personal and intimate as bowel patterns. In addition, when English is not the primary language, there may be challenges in collecting subjective data concerning bowel patterns and elimination. Different cultures can use different terms to refer to bowel elimination patterns and stool. It would be important for the nurse to ascertain what typical terms the patient or family uses when discussing elimination patterns and stool. When performing patient teaching, some patients may answer yes to a suggestion for treatment, when in fact they are only acknowledging that something was said. It would be beneficial to ask the patient to restate in his or her own words what instructions were given in order to verify that understanding has taken place.

FACTORS AFFECTING BOWEL ELIMINATION

Nutrition

The 25% of feces that are solid comes chiefly from the intake of food that has a high cellulose or fiber content. Cellulose or fiber is contained in plant foods. Foods in the high-fiber category include fresh fruits and vegetables with the skins and intact outer coverings and cereal grains with the outer covering of bran in place. A person who consumes approximately 25 to 30 g of dietary fiber from fruits, vegetables, and grains will most likely have sufficient bulk in the stools to allow for easy defecation (Costilla & Foxx-Orenstein, 2014).

A person whose diet is deficient in fiber usually has less frequent bowel movements and stools with less bulk and may experience some difficulty in bowel elimination. Soluble fiber (found in foods such as oat bran, barley, and nuts) dissolves in water and increases intestinal transit time, whereas insoluble fiber (found in whole grains and fresh fruits and vegetables) decreases transit time in the colon, moving bulk through the bowels (O'Connor, 2013). Ingestion of large amounts of certain high-fiber foods, such as fresh fruits, may produce loose stools.

Food intolerances also may alter bowel function. Many people have difficulty digesting lactose (the sugar contained in milk products). The breakdown of lactose into its component sugars, glucose and galactose, requires a sufficient quantity of the enzyme lactase in the small intestine. If a person is lactase deficient, alterations of bowel elimination, including the formation of gas, abdominal cramping, and diarrhea, can occur after ingestion of milk products.

Some people cannot digest gluten, a protein found in wheat, rye, barley, and buckwheat. For these people, ingestion of gluten-containing food results in the retention of carbohydrates and fats, which cannot be digested and absorbed through the intestine. The person experiences abdominal distention and a bloated feeling, along with a diarrhea of bulky, greasy stools.

Fluid Intake

Because 75% of the feces is water, fluid intake also influences stool consistency. The need of body cells for water is a higher priority than is stool consistency. When the body needs to conserve fluid, it will absorb more water from the large intestine to meet its needs.

A fluid intake of approximately 2,000 mL per day is necessary to meet cellular needs and have enough left over to promote a soft stool consistency. When a person loses excessive water, such as from a high fever, profuse diaphoresis, or other abnormal drainage, the usual fluid intake may be insufficient. When fluid intake is inadequate, stools become harder and more difficult to pass.

Storage time in the large intestine also affects stool consistency. The longer feces remain in the large intestine, the more water will be absorbed; the result is a harder, drier stool. Conversely, feces that do not spend sufficient time in the large intestine will be watery and a source of fluid loss for the person.

Activity and Exercise

Physical activity and regular physical exercise promote muscle tone and facilitate peristalsis. Strong abdominal and perineal muscles are needed to increase intra-abdominal pressure during defecation. Muscle tone is lost when activity decreases or neurologic impairment results in loss of neurologic control. Any limitation of normal or usual physical activity can increase the risk of constipation. Most epidemiologic studies on constipation typically reveal a higher rate of constipation in long-term care facility residents, in whom physical inactivity is commonplace (Bouras & Tangalos, 2009).

Body Position

A sitting or a semisquatting position is the most advantageous position for defecation. This position allows gravity to assist the elimination of feces and also makes it easier for the patient to contract the abdominal and pelvic muscles, thereby applying external pressure to the large intestine and encouraging evacuation. Some people find it very difficult to defecate using a bedpan in a reclined position.

Ignoring the Urge to Defecate

Most people require a certain degree of privacy to feel psychologically comfortable defecating. Although part of the defecation reflex is involuntary, the external anal sphincter is under voluntary control, allowing one to ignore the urge to defecate until the time and place for defecation are appropriate.

The defecation reflex and the urge to defecate subside after a few minutes if the initial urge is ignored. The feces then remain in the rectum until another mass colonic movement propels more stool into the rectum, which may not be for several hours or longer. While the feces remain in the colon and rectum, the intestinal mucosa continues to absorb water from the feces, resulting in a harder and drier stool that may be more difficult to evacuate. Eventually, if the person continually denies the defecation reflex, recognition of the urge to defecate becomes more difficult and the defecation reflex weakens and subsides. Rather than relying on inherent body signals to initiate defecation, a person in this situation may have to depend on alternative methods, such as the persistent use of laxatives or enemas or manual disimpaction of stool.

People who experience pain during defecation may choose to deny the urge to defecate, which can lead to constipation. People at risk for delaying defecation because of pain include those with chronic constipation and those with rectal or anal abnormalities, such as hemorrhoids or fissures. **Hemorrhoids** are enlarged or varicose veins in the anal canal. Pain and rectal bleeding are sometimes associated with hemorrhoids and may lead to frequent denial of the defecation reflex to avoid pain. An anal fissure is an ulcerous crack or split in the anal mucosa. Bleeding and pain occur as the stool passes the fissure. In addition, patients may delay defecation after anal or perineal surgery because of the pain.

Lifestyle

Many people develop a pattern with respect to the timing of bowel elimination. For some people, ingestion of food or fluid first thing in the morning stimulates an urge to defecate. Over time, a pattern of bowel elimination every morning can be established and is considered a normal pattern for that person. Some people are ritualistic, using the same method to promote a regular pattern of bowel elimination, whereas others have no set pattern except to respond to the defecation urge whenever it occurs.

Alterations in a person's lifestyle or pattern of daily living can have an effect on bowel elimination. Vacations and travel often change daily routine enough to cause alterations. Lifestyle changes that cause either acute or chronic feelings of anxiety, anger, fear, depression, excitement, or other strong emotions can affect bowel function. Any acute stress or change in a person's lifestyle can increase bowel motility and mucus secretion. The result may be a sudden increase in frequency of bowel movements, with the stool containing large amounts of mucus. Hospitalization, a career change, a disruption in personal or family relationships, and anticipation of final examinations are just a few examples of situations that can stimulate acute stress. Chronic exposure to stress can slow bowel activity, resulting in decreased frequency of bowel movements. Long-term depression is an example of a chronic stressor that may slow bowel activity.

Pregnancy

Constipation frequently occurs during pregnancy because hormonal changes relax muscles of the gastrointestinal tract (Blackburn, 2013). Prolonged intestinal transit time and changes in water absorption increase risk of constipation in pregnancy (Jones & Gardiner, 2014). Also, the growing fetus puts pressure on the intestines, possibly affecting normal bowel function. Many pregnant women are instructed to take iron supplements, which are very constipating. Early in the postpartum phase, constipation can also occur from the fear of pain during a bowel movement, especially in the case of perineal repair.

Medications

Side effects of many medications can increase a person's risk for bowel elimination problems. For example, opioids and iron preparations can cause constipation, antibiotics can cause diarrhea, and antacids can lead to either constipation or diarrhea. Laxatives, stool softeners, and enemas are medications that are administered to promote stool evacuation. Antidiarrheal medications may be given to decrease stool frequency.

Diagnostic Procedures

Some radiologic and endoscopic procedures require cleansing fecal material from the large bowel before the procedure. The thorough cleansing of the large bowel alters the normal pattern of elimination for 2 or 3 days after the test. When the person resumes his or her usual diet, the normal bowel elimination pattern usually reemerges.

Bowel elimination also may be affected after a diagnostic test. For example, if barium is administered as a test agent, the stools after the procedure will appear chalky white or tan until all of the barium has been eliminated from the gastrointestinal tract. If barium remains in the colon, it hardens and can cause impaction of stool. Therefore, laxatives are commonly ordered after the diagnostic test to facilitate barium removal.

Surgery

Surgical intervention can place the patient at risk for altered patterns of bowel elimination. General anesthetics may slow gastrointestinal motility, causing the surgical patient to experience a period of decreased bowel functioning for 1 to 2 days after surgery.

Patients who have had abdominal surgery, especially surgery on a portion of the gastrointestinal tract, will require 3 or 4 days for bowel activity to return to normal. These patients are usually given preoperative laxatives or enemas to cleanse the large intestine of feces. During surgery, the bowel is exposed to air and manipulation, leading to further decreased bowel motility.

Postoperative use of opioid analgesics, reduced activity, and fear of pain further inhibit normal bowel motility. Until recently, postoperative patients were not allowed food and fluids orally until there was evidence of the return of active bowel motility. According to several evidence-based reviews of enteral nutrition following major gastrointestinal surgery, there was no increase in perioperative infection, anastomotic dehiscence, nitrogen imbalance, time for return of bowel function, or lengthening of hospital stay with early enteral nutrition (Osland, Yunus, Khan, & Memon, 2011; Shrikhande, Shetty, Singh, & Ingle, 2009). In fact, studies have demonstrated reductions in total complications during the postoperative recovery period (Osland et al., 2011). Although research over the past 30 years has demonstrated the safety and benefit of early postoperative feeding, clinical practice among surgeons has been slow to change.

Fecal Diversion

The presence of all or part of the large intestine is not necessary to maintain life. In some patients, cancer or other conditions, such as inflammatory bowel disease, necessitate surgical removal of all or part of the colon, rectum, and anus. In such cases, the proximal portion of the remaining bowel may be redirected through the abdominal wall to the abdominal skin surface. The portion of intestine brought through the abdominal wall is known as a **stoma**. When this surgery is performed, it is referred to as a fecal diversion because the normal route for feces is altered.

Fecal diversions can be permanent or temporary. The bowel segment used to form the stoma depends on the location of the bowel abnormality. For example, if the person has rectal cancer, the segment of bowel removed will be the cancerous rectum. The healthy, noncancerous sigmoid colon, which is the segment of the bowel just proximal to the rectum, can be used to form the stoma. A bowel diversion surgery that brings a segment of the large colon out to the abdominal skin is called a **colostomy**. It is also possible that the entire length of the large colon is so diseased that the next healthy proximal segment of intestine is the ileum. When a portion of the ileum is used to make the stoma on the abdomen, the procedure is called an **ileostomy**. Figure 33-2 illustrates fecal diversions.

People with colostomies or ileostomies evacuate feces through a stoma. The length of functioning intestine that remains after the surgery determines the consistency of the stool. When an ileostomy is created, the large intestine is no longer available to absorb water from the stool. Therefore, stool produced from an ileostomy is liquid and contains large quantities of electrolytes. In a person with a descending colostomy, in which only the rectum has been removed, stool is soft in consistency, and elimination may be controlled with daily colostomy irrigation. This may permit a pattern of bowel evacuation similar to that experienced before surgery.

Modern surgical methods aim for as little disruption of normal bowel patterns as possible despite fecal diversion. The ileoanal reservoir, sometimes referred to as a J pouch, involves construction of an internal pouch by removal of the colon and attachment of a segment of ileum to the anus. Fecal material goes directly from the small intestine out the anus. A Kock pouch or continent ileostomy is another development in fecal diversions. A pouch is made from 30 cm of ileum and an outlet valve is constructed. Although this procedure requires a stoma, feces can be drained at the patient's convenience rather than having it continually draining into an external pouch, as occurs in the traditional ileostomy. Figure 33-3 illustrates one type of continent ostomy.

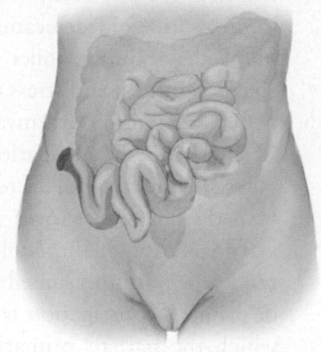 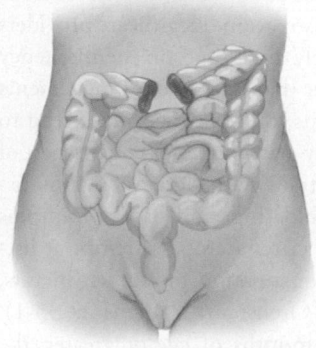 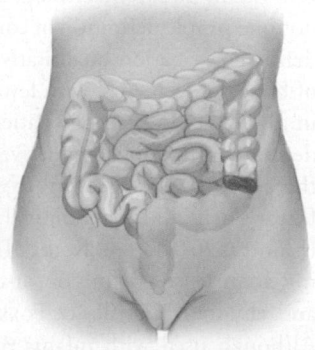

FIGURE 33-2 Intestinal diversions: ileostomy, transverse colostomy, and sigmoid colostomy.

Ileostomy   Transverse (loop) colostomy   Sigmoid colostomy

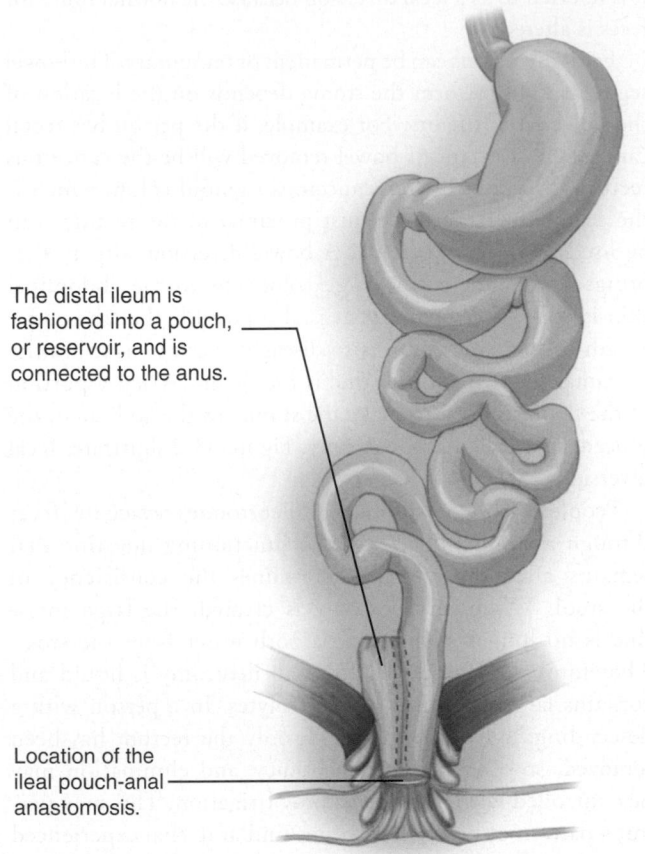

The distal ileum is fashioned into a pouch, or reservoir, and is connected to the anus.

Location of the ileal pouch-anal anastomosis.

FIGURE 33-3 Ileoanal reservoir. The distal ileum is fashioned into a pouch and connected to the anus to create a continent fecal diversion.

BOX 33-1   Rome III Criteria for Constipation

Adults

Must include two or more of the following for at least 12 weeks (not necessarily consecutive) in the preceding 12 months:

- Straining during more than 25% of bowel movements
- Lumpy or hard stools for more than 25% of bowel movements
- Sensation of incomplete evacuation for more than 25% of bowel movements
- Sensation of anorectal blockage for more than 25% of bowel movements
- Manual maneuvers to facilitate more than 25% of bowel movements (e.g., digital evacuation or support of the pelvic floor)
- Fewer than three bowel movements per week
- Loose stools not present and insufficient criteria for irritable bowel syndrome met

Infants and Children

- Pebblelike, hard stools for most bowel movements for at least 2 weeks
- Firm stools more than two times per week for at least 2 weeks
- No evidence of structural, endocrine, or metabolic disease

ALTERED BOWEL FUNCTION

Constipation

Constipation is a common condition, affecting an estimated 16% of Americans, with prevalence among older adults (over age 60) about 33% (Costilla & Foxx-Orenstein, 2014). In addition, it is more common in women, children under age 4, and lower socioeconomic populations (Costilla & Foxx-Orenstein, 2014; Greenwald, 2010; Mitchell, 2014). There is not one simple definition of constipation. Healthcare providers define constipation quantitatively and based on the frequency of bowel movements, with fewer than three bowel movements in a week as an example. Patients, on the other hand, tend to define constipation qualitatively based on the consistency of the stool (hard), necessity to strain with defecation, unsatisfactory defecation, abdominal bloating, and other symptoms (Hunter, 2014). The Rome III criteria are an attempt at listing a consensus definition of constipation for adults, infants, and children (Costilla & Foxx-Orenstein, 2014) (Box 33-1). Although used with infants 3 months of age or greater, the Rome III criteria also state that symptoms must be present for

at least 6 months. For infants younger than 3 months, 2 weeks of objective data are necessary. In general, constipation is the infrequent and sometimes painful passage of hard, dry stool. It occurs when stool moves through the large intestine too slowly or remains in the large intestine too long. Constipation is defined in relation to the person's normal defecation pattern and involves a change in stool consistency (harder and drier than usual) and a change in defecation frequency (less often than usual).

Chronic constipation is broadly categorized in one of three ways. Functional constipation occurs in patients with normal intestinal transit time. It is the most common type of constipation in adults as well as children. Some providers consider this a variant of functional bowel syndrome (Hunter, 2014). In children, it most often occurs when the child withholds feces in order to avoid defecation that may be unpleasant or painful. Toilet training, toilet availability, busy schedules, dietary changes, illness, and stress may contribute to fecal withholding and constipation (Greenwald, 2010).

Slow-transit constipation, sometimes referred to as colonoparesis, is the result of decreased peristalsis characterized by prolonged stool transit (over 3 days) (Costilla & Foxx-Orenstein, 2014). Although the etiology of this form of constipation is not known, it is presumed to be neurologic. The third category of primary constipation is outlet dysfunction constipation, in which the patient primarily experiences difficulty defecating or incomplete defecation. Pelvic floor dysfunction may result

SCENE FOR THOUGHT

Helen Palumbo is a 73-year-old woman who comes to the clinic for a checkup about every 6 months. She is busy, active, pleasant, and committed to staying healthy so that she can continue to enjoy life.

LESS EFFECTIVE

Nurse: Hi, Mrs. Palumbo. Glad to see you. How are you feeling?

Mrs. Palumbo: Hi, Barbara. I'm doing fine except I think I'm a little constipated. *(Whispers this last word.)*

Nurse: Tell me a little more. *(Listens attentively.)*

Mrs. Palumbo: Well, I usually go every morning, but over the last few months, I only go every 2 days and I'm worried. *(Looks worried.)*

Nurse: You certainly look worried. But, a woman your age is bound to slow down in some areas, even though you're still active and busy. Your bowel is slowing down, and so you don't need to evacuate every single day.

Mrs. Palumbo: *(Looks doubtful.)* Really?

Nurse: Absolutely. Many senior patients are perfectly fine even though they don't have a movement every day. They drink enough fluids, eat enough fruits and vegetables, exercise, and do just fine. I know from our last visit that you're doing all those things. Tell you what—if you have any questions, give me a call. But I think you're doing great, Mrs. Palumbo.

Mrs. Palumbo: Well, okay. I guess I'm just being silly. I'll call you if anything new comes up. *(Smiles and says good-bye.)*

Nurse: Great! I'll talk to you then. *(Smiles.)*

MORE EFFECTIVE

Nurse: Hi, Mrs. Palumbo. Glad to see you. How are you feeling?

Mrs. Palumbo: Hi, Mary Jo. I'm doing fine except I think I'm a little constipated. *(Whispers this last word.)*

Nurse: Tell me a little more. *(Listens attentively.)*

Mrs. Palumbo: Well, I usually go every morning, but over the last few months, I only go every 2 days and I'm worried. *(Looks worried.)*

Nurse: What worries you about that?

Mrs. Palumbo: Well, when I was in my 20s, I had a fistula. I put off having my first baby because of it. Then, 5 years ago, I had diverticulitis that put me in the hospital for a week with antibiotics. It wasn't fun, I'll tell you. If I get constipated, I'm worried about putting strain on my fistula scars or going back to the hospital. You see?

Nurse: I understand why you're concerned. Let me ask you a few questions about nutrition and fluids. I'll examine your abdomen, then we can talk more about some things you might do. Is that okay with you?

Mrs. Palumbo: Whatever you say. I always learn something new when I come here. *(Big smile.)*

Nurse: *(After the assessment.)* Well, you seem to be drinking lots of fluids, which is wonderful. You tell me you go every 2 days and have no gas or pain in the abdomen. I wonder if maybe our definitions of constipation are different.

Mrs. Palumbo: What do you mean?

Nurse: My definition of constipation is hard, dry stool that passes after 3 days or more and is accompanied by gas, bloating, and pain, maybe even nausea.

Mrs. Palumbo: *(Looks surprised.)* No, I don't get that!

Nurse: Lots of people believe that they're constipated if they don't go every day. They use laxatives and enemas, which can make it worse. From your description, it sounds as though your bowel function is fine for a healthy woman your age. You have none of the symptoms of constipation. *(Smiles.)*

Mrs. Palumbo: *(Smiles back.)* Good, I'm glad.

Nurse: Call me if you have any questions. You know I'm happy to talk to you anytime.

Mrs. Palumbo: Thank you so much. I will. *(Looks relieved and beams happily as she briskly leaves the office.)*

CRITICAL THINKING CHALLENGE

- Compare and contrast the different determinations made by Barbara and Mary Jo, as shown by their different responses to Mrs. Palumbo.
- Infer what Mrs. Palumbo needed from her nurse.
- If you were the nurse, what changes would you have made in Mary Jo's conversation with Mrs. Palumbo? In Barbara's conversation?

in impaired rectal relaxation, or paradoxical or impaired rectal and pelvic muscle contraction. Anatomical conditions such as anal–rectal fissures or strictures, rectocele, tumor, or conditions that impair rectal sensation may also contribute to outlet dysfunction constipation (Hunter, 2014). Factors previously discussed (such as nutrition, fluids, medications, activity, etc.) as well as other underlying medical disorders can be the cause of secondary constipation and can exacerbate any of the three primary conditions of chronic constipation.

Fecal Impaction

A **fecal impaction** is the accumulation of hardened feces in the rectum. The word *impaction* implies that the stool is lodged or stuck in the rectum; the person is unable to voluntarily evacuate the stool. A fecal impaction is usually the result of untreated and unrelieved constipation.

Suspect fecal impaction when there is a history or absence of a regular bowel movement for several days (3 to 5 days or more) followed by the passage of liquid or semiliquid stool. The person is typically incontinent of the liquid stool, complaining of an inability to perceive urge. The passage of liquid stool usually does not relieve the reported rectal and abdominal fullness. The passage of semiliquid stool results from seepage of unformed fecal contents around the impacted stool in the rectum; the pressure from the large volume of accumulated fecal contents forces liquid feces to the anus (Fig. 33-4). This liquid or semiliquid stool is not diarrhea but is sometimes confused with it. Fecal impaction is confirmed by the detection of hardened stool in the rectum on digital examination.

Symptoms similar to those experienced with constipation are also present—a subjective feeling of rectal and abdominal

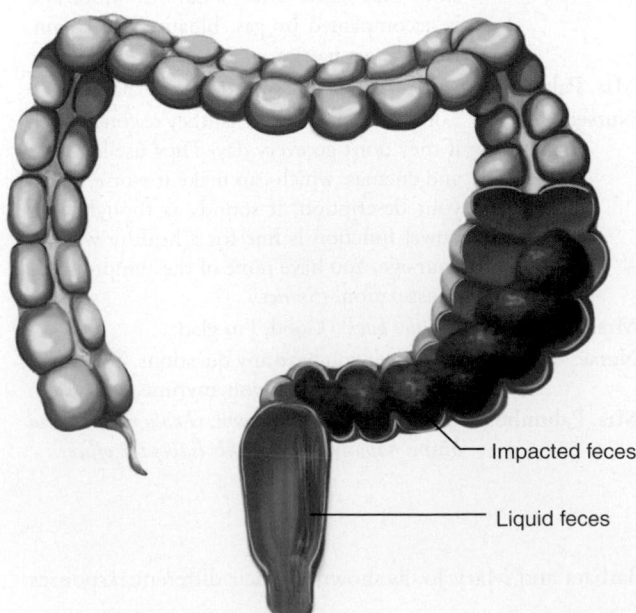

FIGURE 33-4 Fecal impaction in the sigmoid colon. Liquid stool may pass around the hard fecal plug.

fullness or bloating, an urge to defecate but an inability to pass stool, and a generalized feeling of malaise. Loss of appetite and nausea or vomiting also are typical. Abdominal distention is usually apparent.

Fecal impaction usually results from the same conditions as those associated with constipation. Fecal impaction also may result from the chronic use of opioid medication or the hardening of barium used in radiologic examination of the gastrointestinal tract. Patients who have swallowed barium or have received a barium enema should be monitored for complete evacuation of barium after the radiologic procedure. Some healthcare protocols require the use of laxatives for 1 or 2 days after the procedure to ensure complete evacuation of the barium.

Diarrhea

Diarrhea is manifested by frequent evacuation of watery stools. Diarrhea is usually associated with increased gastrointestinal motility and, therefore, a rapid passage of fecal contents through the lower gastrointestinal tract. It is the consistency of the stool (less formed and more watery than normal) that is more definitive of diarrhea than is the increased frequency of defecation. In addition to having a high water content, diarrheal stools may also have increased mucus; both of these factors contribute to increased volume. The extra volume and the rapidity with which it reaches the rectum cause rectal distention, resulting in an intense urge to defecate. Diarrheal stools may vary in color from light brown to yellow to green.

Abdominal cramping, nausea (with or without vomiting), and a painful burning sensation at the anus often accompany diarrhea. Diarrheal stool is usually highly acidic. Frequent passage of acidic stools can cause anal soreness and inflammation of the skin surrounding the anus, resulting in bleeding and breakdown of the perianal tissue.

The causes of diarrhea are many and varied. Any disease that inflames the intestinal tract can lead to diarrhea. Specific microorganisms or the toxins they produce can cause intestinal inflammation and diarrhea. The inflammation irritates the intestinal mucosa to increase its secretions and motility.

Medications, in addition to the inappropriate use of laxatives, can cause diarrhea. Antacids taken to decrease stomach acidity, especially those containing magnesium, also can lead to diarrhea. Antibiotics can promote diarrhea by irritating the gastrointestinal mucosa or by inhibiting the growth of normal intestinal flora. Normal intestinal flora inhibits the growth of ***Clostridium difficile*** (**C-diff**). C-diff is the most common cause of hospital-acquired diarrhea in the United States. Since the early 2000s, the incidence of C-diff infections has more than doubled, mostly among the elderly (Kee, 2012). However, C-diff is becoming more prevalent in populations previously unaffected, including young healthy persons without prior hospitalization and postpartum women (Dodin & Katz, 2014). Although numerous causes of *Clostridium difficile* infection (CDI) exist, 90% of the cases are caused by antimicrobial therapy either during or up to 8 weeks preceding the onset of diarrhea. Any antibiotic can cause CDI; however, clindamycin and cephalosporins have been implicated most often. When they are administered, normal flora is altered, thereby allowing ingested C-diff spores to proliferate and release toxins that cause antibiotic-associated diarrhea (Austin, Mellow, & Tierney, 2014).

Lifestyle changes causing acute stress and anxiety can result in episodes of diarrhea. Acute stress may increase stimulation of the large intestine, increasing the transit time of the feces through the intestines.

While traveling, some people experience diarrhea after ingesting food or water from an unfamiliar locale. Often, a waterborne foreign strain of *Escherichia coli* causes the intestinal inflammation and consequent symptoms known as traveler's diarrhea.

Additional diarrheal responses may be precipitated by lactase deficiency, gluten intolerance, or a specific food allergy. For example, apple juice can cause chronic diarrhea in some children. The hyperosmolality of parenteral tube feedings may precipitate a diarrheal response.

Fecal Incontinence

Fecal incontinence is the involuntary passing of bowel contents and is often associated with neurologic, mental, or emotional impairments. It is a stressful, embarrassing condition that can lead to withdrawal from social interactions and decreased quality of life. Patients with injury to the cerebral cortex may have difficulty perceiving a distended rectum or initiating the motor responses required to inhibit defecation voluntarily. People who have sustained sacral spinal cord injury or who have neurologic diseases that impair the nerve supply to the rectum and anal sphincters (e.g., multiple sclerosis) also may be unable to inhibit voluntary anal sphincters to postpone defecation.

Patients who are disoriented or confused may have lost the social inhibition that prevents immediate fecal evacuation. In the absence of voluntary contraction of the external anal sphincter, the immediate evacuation of the rectum follows rectal distention.

Diarrhea predisposes a person to fecal incontinence. Sometimes the volume of feces is so large and the defecation urge so intense that the person cannot maintain sphincter contraction long enough to access toilet facilities and remove the necessary clothing.

Flatulence

Flatus is the accumulation of gas in the gastrointestinal tract. Gas enters the gastrointestinal tract from three sources: swallowed air, bacterial action in the large intestine, and diffusion from the blood.

Excessive swallowing of air sometimes occurs with anxiety, rapid food or fluid ingestion, improper use of drinking straws, ingestion of large amounts of carbonated beverages, gum chewing, candy sucking, and smoking. Swallowed air is usually eliminated by burping or belching.

Gases produced by bacterial activity in the large intestine are eliminated through the anus. When larger than usual quantities of flatus are produced, they are most often a result of increased colonic motility secondary to intestinal irritation. The colonic activity propels the gases toward the anus before they have time to be absorbed by the intestinal mucosa.

Certain foods (e.g., broccoli, cabbage, onions, legumes) often increase the amount of flatus produced in the intestine. Many other high-fiber foods that are recommended to promote normal bowel elimination can cause excess flatus production when they are not introduced into the diet gradually.

Distention

An accumulation of excessive amounts of flatus or liquid or solid intestinal contents causes abdominal **distention**. Subjectively, the person complains of abdominal fullness and discomfort and the inability to pass flatus or stool. Visual inspection of the abdomen reveals a distended or a convexly stretched abdomen. Depending on the amount of flatus and feces in the intestines, the abdomen can appear only slightly distended or taut and stretched.

An obstruction that blocks the passage of flatus and intestinal chyme or feces is a primary cause of abdominal distention. Paralytic ileus and abdominal tumors are types of bowel obstruction that produce distention.

Long periods of bed rest or relative inactivity can slow peristalsis and lead to accumulated flatus in the large intestine. Peristalsis also slows after surgery with general anesthesia. In particular, surgery involving bowel manipulation, especially bowel surgery, causes decreased peristalsis postoperatively, with abdominal distention as a possible consequence. Constipation and fecal impaction also may lead to abdominal distention.

ASSESSMENT

Asking questions about a person's bowel habits is potentially an embarrassing situation for the patient and the beginning nursing student. Bowel elimination is considered a private function. For optimal care, obtain factual information both from the patient's perspective and through direct observation. The use of a matter-of-fact approach often eases the patient's embarrassment.

Think back to the patient with metastatic cancer in the case scenario. Recall that the patient has not had a bowel movement for 7 days. Use the concept map (Fig. 33-5) and assessment data to help understand the patient's situation and to plan for her care.

Normal Pattern Identification

The normal bowel elimination pattern is highly individualized. The frequency of defecation can normally range from one to two bowel movements per day to one bowel movement every 2 to 3 days.

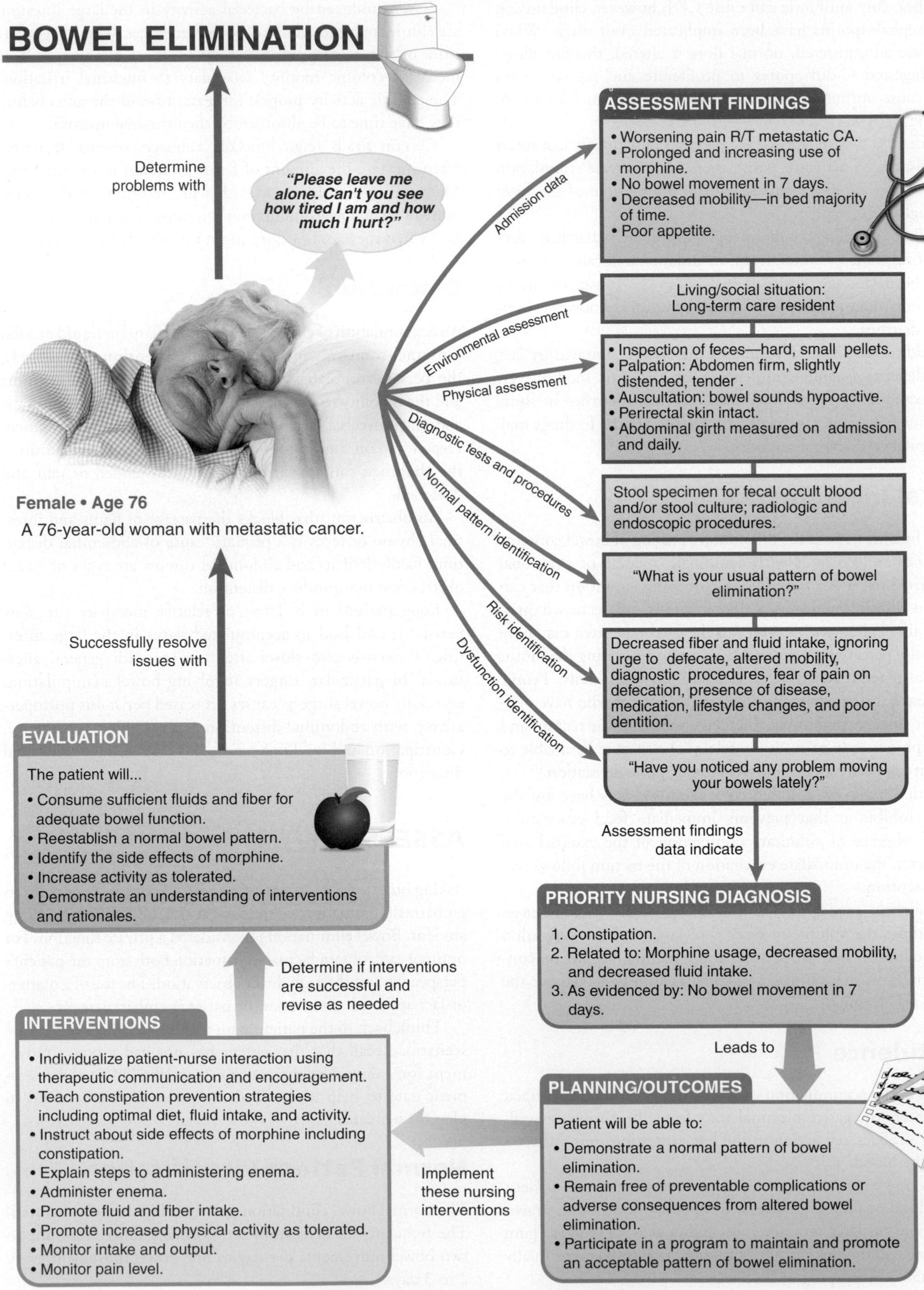

BOWEL ELIMINATION

Determine problems with

"Please leave me alone. Can't you see how tired I am and how much I hurt?"

Female • Age 76

A 76-year-old woman with metastatic cancer.

Successfully resolve issues with

EVALUATION

The patient will...

- Consume sufficient fluids and fiber for adequate bowel function.
- Reestablish a normal bowel pattern.
- Identify the side effects of morphine.
- Increase activity as tolerated.
- Demonstrate an understanding of interventions and rationales.

Determine if interventions are successful and revise as needed

INTERVENTIONS

- Individualize patient-nurse interaction using therapeutic communication and encouragement.
- Teach constipation prevention strategies including optimal diet, fluid intake, and activity.
- Instruct about side effects of morphine including constipation.
- Explain steps to administering enema.
- Administer enema.
- Promote fluid and fiber intake.
- Promote increased physical activity as tolerated.
- Monitor intake and output.
- Monitor pain level.

Admission data

Environmental assessment

Physical assessment

Diagnostic tests and procedures

Normal pattern identification

Risk identification

Dysfunction identification

ASSESSMENT FINDINGS

- Worsening pain R/T metastatic CA.
- Prolonged and increasing use of morphine.
- No bowel movement in 7 days.
- Decreased mobility—in bed majority of time.
- Poor appetite.

Living/social situation: Long-term care resident

- Inspection of feces—hard, small pellets.
- Palpation: Abdomen firm, slightly distended, tender .
- Auscultation: bowel sounds hypoactive.
- Perirectal skin intact.
- Abdominal girth measured on admission and daily.

Stool specimen for fecal occult blood and/or stool culture; radiologic and endoscopic procedures.

"What is your usual pattern of bowel elimination?"

Decreased fiber and fluid intake, ignoring urge to defecate, altered mobility, diagnostic procedures, fear of pain on defecation, presence of disease, medication, lifestyle changes, and poor dentition.

"Have you noticed any problem moving your bowels lately?"

Assessment findings data indicate

PRIORITY NURSING DIAGNOSIS

1. Constipation.
2. Related to: Morphine usage, decreased mobility, and decreased fluid intake.
3. As evidenced by: No bowel movement in 7 days.

Leads to

Implement these nursing interventions

PLANNING/OUTCOMES

Patient will be able to:

- Demonstrate a normal pattern of bowel elimination.
- Remain free of preventable complications or adverse consequences from altered bowel elimination.
- Participate in a program to maintain and promote an acceptable pattern of bowel elimination.

FIGURE 33-5 Concept map for bowel elimination.

To determine the patient's current bowel elimination pattern, obtain the following information from current medical records, the patient, or the caregiver:

- What is the patient's usual pattern of bowel elimination?
- What are the usual characteristics of the patient's stool?
- Which aids, if any, does the patient routinely use for defecation?
- When was the patient's last bowel movement?
- Are there any recent changes in the patient's normal bowel pattern?

Risk Identification

Areas of risk to assess include dietary factors, such as adequacy of fiber and fluid intake; ignoring the urge to defecate; factors or conditions that may alter the patient's mobility pattern; diagnostic procedures, especially those involving the use of radiographic contrast material such as barium; surgical procedures; fear of pain on defecation; physiologic alterations from disease; medications (especially opiates); and lifestyle changes.

A patient needs good teeth to chew high-fiber foods such as fresh fruits and vegetables. Poor dentition with concomitant chewing difficulty may lead to an insufficient intake of such foods and place the patient at risk for constipation.

Dysfunction Identification

Assessing a patient's beliefs about "normal" bowel function is necessary to determine the existence of a problem. Some people believe that a normal pattern is a bowel movement every day; they may further believe that a laxative or enema is necessary to correct any deviations from this pattern. People's concept of whether they have a bowel elimination problem usually depends on their beliefs about "normal" bowel elimination and whether their current pattern fits these beliefs. Many patients claim to be constipated despite having a daily bowel movement. Although a patient may believe that he or she has an altered bowel elimination pattern, analysis of the data may differ. Understanding the patient's beliefs about normal bowel patterns helps direct subsequent nursing interventions.

Bowel problems can be identified as significant deviations from the patient's normal pattern or a pattern that is outside the standards for bowel function. For instance, if a person usually has a bowel movement each day and states the absence of stool for the last 3 days, the nurse may identify constipation as a bowel problem. Also, a bowel problem may be identified if a patient states that he or she normally has a bowel movement every 3 weeks, because this does not fall within the range of normal bowel function.

Physical Assessment

Visual inspection of the feces and physical assessment of the abdomen and perirectal area provide objective data on the

TABLE 33-2	NORMAL AND ABNORMAL FINDINGS ON PHYSICAL EXAMINATION OF THE ABDOMEN AND PERIRECTAL AREA	
Examination	Normal	Abnormal
Abdomen		
Inspection		
Contour	Convex or flat	Hollow or scaphoid; distended
Symmetry	Symmetric	Asymmetric
Auscultation	Bowel sounds in all quadrants every 5–15s	Bowel sounds absent in all quadrants
Hypoactive bowel sounds—every 15–30s
Hyperactive bowel sounds—continuous or more than every 5s
Absent bowel sounds—no sounds in 1–2 min
Percussion	Hollow, tympany in LUQ (stomach)	Dull, tympany in quadrants other than LUQ
Palpation	Soft	Mass, firm distention
Perirectal		
Inspection	Intact, nonreddened skin	Excoriated, reddened skin, hemorrhoids, bleeding
Palpation	No stool or only soft, brown stool in rectum	Hard stool
Bleeding

LUQ, left upper quadrant.

patient's bowel elimination status. Inspection, auscultation, percussion, palpation, and measurement of abdominal girth are used. Table 33-2 compares normal and abnormal findings on physical examination of the abdomen and perirectal area.

INSPECTION

The abdominal examination begins with inspection. Observe the abdomen for contour and symmetry. Normally, the abdomen is convex (i.e., slightly rounded). It may be flat in a muscular or athletic person. An abdomen that appears hollow or scaphoid is not normal and may be associated with malnutrition. An abdomen that appears more than slightly rounded is called protuberant or distended; an abdomen may be protuberant because of excess subcutaneous fat, pregnancy, or accumulated fluid or gas. The umbilicus remains unchanged with gas distention but can be everted with abdominal distention related to ascites (O'Connor, 2013). The pannus is a thick abdominal fold that can be lifted from the abdomen in morbidly obese individuals. Note any signs of obvious asymmetry, comparing the contour of the right side of the abdomen with that of the left side and the upper quadrants with the lower quadrants. The normal abdomen shows no obvious asymmetry.

AUSCULTATION

Auscultation of the abdomen must be performed before percussion or palpation. Percussion or palpation of the abdomen may stimulate intestinal activity and therefore change the quality or frequency of bowel sounds. If the patient has a nasogastric or intestinal tube connected to suction, shut off the suction temporarily so that the sound of suction is not misinterpreted as bowel sounds. Bowel sounds, which are a result of peristalsis throughout the intestine, are heard through the stethoscope as a bubbling or gurgling noise. Everyone has heard his or her stomach "growl" without the benefit of a stethoscope. These loud bowel sounds are termed **borborygmi**. Bowel sounds heard through the stethoscope sound similar, only quieter.

Place the diaphragm of the stethoscope on the patient's abdomen, starting at the right lower quadrant, because bowel sounds are heard best at the ileocecal junction (Jarvis, 2012). If the patient complains of pain in the abdomen, auscultate that quadrant last. Normally, bowel sounds are heard in each of the quadrants within 5 to 15 seconds after the diaphragm is placed on the abdomen; infrequent bowel sounds suggest decreased gastrointestinal peristalsis and motility. Hypoactive bowel sounds in a patient previously without bowel sounds suggest the return of intestinal peristalsis.

An absence of bowel sounds means that the nurse has listened in each of the four quadrants for at least 1 to 2 minutes and heard no bowel sounds; it is the rare clinical nurse who has the time to listen to a patient's abdomen for 8 minutes. Clinically, most nurses define absent bowel sounds as no sounds heard within 30 seconds for each quadrant; this requires auscultation for only 2 minutes to document absent bowel sounds. A patient who has undergone abdominal surgery may have hypoactive or absent bowel sounds for 1 to 3 days postoperatively. Bowel sounds should gradually resume, indicating that normal peristalsis has begun. A continued absence of bowel sounds beyond 72 hours may signal **paralytic ileus**, a condition in which the bowel is temporarily paralyzed and distention occurs.

Abnormal bowel sounds also include hyperactive sounds. Continuous bowel sounds or sounds heard more frequently than every 5 seconds can be termed *hyperactive*. Patients with diarrhea usually have hyperactive, high-pitched bowel sounds, indicating hypermotility in the intestines. A patient with a bowel obstruction may have a combination of hypoactive and hyperactive bowel sounds, with hypoactive sounds below the level of the obstruction and hyperactive sounds above that level.

PERCUSSION

Percussion is used to identify air, fluid, or solid masses in the abdomen, usually when an abnormality has been identified during inspection or auscultation. Begin percussion in the quadrant that was first auscultated. It is normal to hear a high-pitched, hollow sound, called tympany, over the left upper quadrant (LUQ). The stomach is in the LUQ and contains more air than does the small or large intestine. The normal percussion sound heard in the other three quadrants is a hollow sound that is not quite as high-pitched as tympany, reflecting

a mixture of air and fluid in the intestines. When an abdomen is abnormally distended with air (or gas), tympanic percussion notes may be heard throughout the abdomen. When an abdomen contains an excess fluid accumulation, duller, lower-pitched sounds are heard over the fluid-filled areas. A mass or feces in the large intestine produces a dull sound.

PALPATION

Palpation is the last physical assessment technique used in examining the abdomen. If the history indicates problems in bowel elimination, or if abnormal findings have been observed during inspection, auscultation, or percussion, the nurse may wish to use light palpation. In light palpation, the examiner uses the warmed fingertips of one hand to press on the abdomen firmly yet gently enough to prevent causing discomfort. Palpate all quadrants of the abdomen in a systematic manner, saving the area that is thought to contain abnormalities for last (Jarvis, 2012). Instructing the patient to flex the knees during this part of the examination often helps the patient to relax abdominal muscles, resulting in less discomfort. From light palpation, the nurse can determine the firmness or softness of the abdominal muscles, the relative degree of abdominal distention, and possibly abdominal masses.

A special method called deep palpation is also part of the abdominal physical examination. During deep palpation, the examiner uses both hands and special techniques to assess deep abdominal masses and specific abdominal organs such as the liver and spleen. It is recommended that beginning nursing students not perform deep palpation independently. If possible, they should take the opportunity to observe the technique performed by a more experienced practitioner.

MEASUREMENT OF ABDOMINAL GIRTH

An assessment technique that nurses can perform independently is the measurement of abdominal girth. A plastic tape measure marked in inches or centimeters is wrapped around the patient's abdomen, and the measurement is taken. Comparison of abdominal girth measurements over time is an objective way of determining whether abdominal distention is increasing, decreasing, or unchanged. For the comparison of abdominal girth measurements to be valid, measure the same abdominal circumference each time. Mark an "X" with a marking pen on the patient's abdomen at the point of greatest distention, ensuring that any subsequent measurement will be made from the same location. Abdominal girth is especially helpful in assessing ascites, an accumulation of fluid in the peritoneum, usually from liver failure.

PERIRECTAL EXAMINATION

For selected patients, examination of the perirectal area completes the physical assessment. Place the patient in a side-lying position with one or both knees flexed forward. Gather disposable examination gloves and a packet of water-soluble lubricant. On inspection, perianal skin should appear intact.

Abnormal inspection findings include any of the following:

- Excoriation (red, bleeding, tender skin) often caused by the frequent evacuation of diarrheal stools
- Hemorrhoids, possibly resulting from the evacuation of hard, constipated stools over time
- Bleeding, such as from recent evacuation of a constipated stool past hemorrhoids

Palpation of the rectal area is next. To perform a digital examination of the rectum, separate the patient's buttocks and insert the lubricated index finger of a gloved hand into the patient's anus and rectum. Direct the finger toward the patient's umbilicus, feeling the sides of the rectal wall and for stool in the rectum at the tip of the finger. If any stool is felt, determine whether it is hard or soft. To help the patient relax the anal sphincter, ask the patient to bear down as if having a bowel movement as the examiner simultaneously inserts a lubricated finger. Then ask the patient to perform some slow deep breathing to aid in relaxation while the rectum is quickly assessed.

Sometimes, as the nurse's finger enters the rectum, the patient may exhibit a temporary loss of sphincter control and involuntarily release gas or stool from the rectum. This is especially true for weak patients, older patients, and infants and small children. Since this can be quite embarrassing for the patient, the nurse must not react if this occurs and must maintain a sense of professionalism. For these patients, place a disposable pad under the patient's buttocks before performing the digital examination. Normally, no hard stool is present in the rectum.

Diagnostic Tests and Procedures

Two laboratory tests are commonly performed on stool specimens for diagnostic purposes: the fecal occult blood test (FOBT), sometimes called the guaiac or Hemoccult test, and the stool culture. Other diagnostic procedures include radiologic examinations and endoscopic examinations.

STOOL SPECIMENS

Regardless of who tests a stool specimen, it is commonly the nurse's responsibility to collect it. First, explain to the patient the need for a stool sample. If the patient can walk to the bathroom, place a container (hat) used for obtaining specimens in the toilet. If the patient cannot ambulate to the bathroom, ensure that a bedpan or bedside commode is readily available in the patient's room. When obtaining a specimen for stool culture, inform the patient that it is best if urine is not mixed with the stool in the bedpan. The male patient can easily use a urinal to prevent this from occurring, but it is more difficult for the female patient. Having two bedpans ready in the room, one to be used for urine and the second to be used for the stool specimen, may be necessary.

FECAL OCCULT BLOOD TEST

The **fecal occult blood test (FOBT)** evaluates stool for blood that is not apparent upon visual examination. *Heme* refers to blood, and *occult* means "hidden." A small amount of stool is placed on a card or slide made especially for this purpose, and a few drops of a chemical developer are then placed on the slide. The nurse then observes the specimen for a color change. Blue is a positive diagnostic finding, indicating blood in the stool sample. No color change or any color other than blue is a negative diagnostic finding, indicating the absence of blood in the stool sample. Fecal occult blood testing is a simple procedure, as explained in **Procedure 33-1**, but the nurse should be sure to read the instructions that accompany the test slide and to follow them every time for accurate results.

Stool is tested for occult blood to check for pathologic sources of bleeding from the gastrointestinal tract. Gastrointestinal bleeding could be caused by ulcers or tumors in the stomach or intestines. If blood is on the surface of the stool, it is likely to be caused by bleeding from hemorrhoids and is not occult. If blood is mixed in the stool mass itself, its likely source is intestinal. When collecting a stool specimen for occult blood, a stool sample obviously contaminated by hemorrhoidal or menstrual blood should not be used.

An annual FOBT is recommended as a screening tool for colorectal cancer for all individuals beginning at age 50. Often, during a physical exam, a digital rectal examination (DRE) will be performed; however, it is not considered an adequate screening test for colorectal cancer (American Cancer Society, 2014b). Patients are often sent home from the doctor's office with an FOBT kit. It will be the nurse's responsibility to teach the patient the correct way to perform the test. Most tests require samples from more than one bowel movement. In order to obtain accurate results, the patient will be taught to avoid, 72 hours prior to testing, those foods and medicines that may give a false-positive result, such as red meat, iron preparations, aspirin, bismuth compounds, steroids, and nonsteroidal anti-inflammatory drugs (NSAIDs). Vitamin C in excess of 250 mg per day may cause a false-negative result (American Cancer Society, 2014a).

Another test for fecal blood, the fecal immunochemical test (FIT), is not affected by dietary intake, making the test easier for patients (American Cancer Society, 2014a). The frequency of screening for an FIT test is also annual. Most importantly, any positive test results or obvious blood in the stool should be evaluated, usually with a colonoscopy.

STOOL CULTURE

A culture for specific infectious organisms can be obtained from a stool specimen. The stool normally has a high bacteria count as a result of normal intestinal flora. A stool culture is performed to distinguish atypical intestinal organisms in the stool sample. Examples of atypical infectious organisms that might be cultured from a stool sample include *Salmonella* and *Shigella* species. When these organisms are in the intestine, they usually cause diarrhea. Specific antibiotics are necessary to kill the offending organism and stop the diarrhea. Stool is often cultured for C-diff, another potential cause of diarrhea.

A special kind of stool culture that is sometimes necessary is the testing of the stool for ova (eggs) and parasites. When collecting a stool specimen for specific parasitic organisms or their eggs, such as *Giardia lamblia* or *Entamoeba histolytica*, send the specimen to the laboratory soon after the patient defecates (i.e., while the stool is still warm).

RADIOLOGIC PROCEDURES

The small and large intestines can be visualized by x-ray imaging if a radiopaque substance, such as barium, is swallowed or instilled in the rectum. The small-bowel radiologic procedure is usually done in conjunction with a radiograph of the upper gastrointestinal (UGI) tract (commonly referred to as an UGI series with small-bowel follow-through). The patient must swallow barium, which aids visualization of the soft tissues of the gastrointestinal tract. The radiologist then monitors the progress of the barium from the esophagus through the ileum. The lower gastrointestinal tract can be radiologically visualized by instilling the barium through the rectum. The term *barium enema* is often used for this procedure.

The purpose of these two radiologic procedures is to visualize the segments of the small and large bowel to detect abnormalities in shape, motility, and functioning. Examples of abnormal findings include tumors, diverticula, obstructions, and filling defects.

For best results and maximum visualization, the bowel must be as free as possible from fecal contents. Patients need to take a combination of oral and rectal laxatives the day before and the morning of the procedure; tap water enemas can sometimes be substituted for the laxative regimen. The patient's oral intake is also restricted, usually beginning at midnight on the day of the test. The patient is NPO (allowed no food or fluids by mouth) until the procedure is finished; oral medications are also withheld until the procedure is completed if doing so will not pose an adverse risk to the patient. The nurse is responsible for informing the patient about the preparatory regimen and the purpose of the procedure, and the nurse may also be responsible for administering the laxatives or enemas and maintaining the patient's NPO status.

When the patient returns from the procedure, he or she may again eat and drink. Barium left in the bowel after the procedure can harden and become extremely difficult to eliminate. Therefore, orders to administer a laxative until the patient passes no more white-colored, barium-containing stool are followed.

ENDOSCOPIC EXAMINATION

Various endoscopic procedures permit visualization of internal structures of the gastrointestinal tract with the use of a flexible, fiber-optic instrument. Endoscopic procedures are helpful in diagnosing inflammation, ulceration, or tumors when less invasive tests, such as the barium enema, do not provide definitive results. Tissue can be extracted during endoscopic procedures and biopsied.

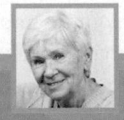

Bowel Elimination PICO

The patient in the chapter-opening scenario is going for an urgent endoscopy procedure because she has been vomiting blood. Sage, the endoscopy nurse on-call, will be assisting with the procedure. She notices a new drug that she is not familiar with, tranexamic acid, infusing through the patient's IV. She looks up the medication and finds out that it is an antifibrinolytic and reduces bleeding by preventing blood clots from breaking up quickly. After the procedure, Sage decides to look in the Cochrane library to understand how it compares to other antiulcer drugs. The PICO question she uses to guide her search is: *In patients with gastrointestinal bleeding, how does tranexamic acid compare to other antiulcer medications in the prevention of bleeding?*

P = Gastrointestinal (GI) bleeding patients

I = Tranexamic acid

C = Antiulcer medications

O = Prevention of bleeding

Sage finds a meta-analysis that compared tranexamic acid to no intervention, a placebo, cimetidine, and lansoprazole for GI bleeding. Eight randomized controlled trials involving 1,701 participants evaluated the effect of tranexamic acid on mortality, rebleed, and/or surgery. The evidence could not fully prove or disprove that tranexamic acid would be beneficial for GI bleeds. The study indicated that there was a large randomized controlled trial (8,000 participants) in progress that could shed more light in the future about the benefits and adverse effects of tranexamic acid for GI bleeds.

Sage reviews the patient's chart again and discovers that her patient is participating in the tranexamic acid study at her hospital. She decides to contact the person in charge of the study in hopes of gaining more information about it. Her plan is to present this case at the next staff meeting so that her peers will be informed about tranexamic acid and the study in progress.

REFERENCE

Bennett, C., Klingenberg, S. L., Langholz, E., & Gluud, L. L. (2014). Tranexamic acid for upper gastrointestinal bleeding. *Cochrane Database of Systematic Reviews*. (11), CD006640. DOI: 10.1002/14651858.CD006640.pub3

Sigmoidoscopy and Colonoscopy

Sigmoidoscopy examines the rectum and sigmoid colon. **Colonoscopy** can visualize the colon up to the ileocecal valve. During the sigmoidoscopy or colonoscopy, the endoscope is inserted into the rectum. The patient may be placed in a knee-to-chest position, which is an uncomfortable and somewhat embarrassing position for most people. For this reason, the left lateral position is the most often used position. Patients also feel the urge to defecate when the fiber-optic probe is inserted into the rectum, another embarrassing feeling for most people. For patients who are too weak to be examined in the knee-to-chest position, a side-lying position with the upper leg flexed (Sims position) can be used, although this position makes visualization of the sigmoid colon more difficult. Colonoscopy takes longer and produces more discomfort than does sigmoidoscopy or proctoscopy; therefore, the patient is given intravenous medications to control pain, reduce bowel spasm, and produce light anesthesia. General anesthesia is frequently used with pediatric patients (O'Connor, 2013).

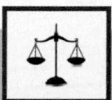

ETHICAL/LEGAL ISSUE

FAMILY CONFLICT OVER HEALTHCARE

Mrs. Diaz, age 79 years, is brought to the family practice clinic by her son because she has been complaining of feeling tired, is dizzy, and has fainted and fallen on at least one occasion. Mrs. Diaz has arthritis and has needed to take increasing doses of aspirin and ibuprofen (Motrin) to control the pain. The son also has some concerns because his mother is becoming increasingly forgetful. The physician decides to admit her to the hospital to complete a full gastrointestinal workup, including a colonoscopy, because he suspects gastrointestinal bleeding. You enter the examining room after the physician has discussed his plan with the patient and her son and find the mother very upset. She is saying to the son: "I don't want to go into the hospital and have all those horrible tests. I'm just fine the way I am, and I want to go home. My friend, Jenny, had that bowel test, and she told me she would rather be dead than have to go through something like that again."

CRITICAL THINKING CHALLENGE

- Refer to Chapter 7 to review informed consent. Identify those issues involving informed consent for Mrs. Diaz.
- What, if any, rights do you think Mrs. Diaz's son has if he wants his mother to consent to the tests for her own good?
- At this point, identify your responsibility to Mrs. Diaz, her son, and the physician.
- Role-play what you might say to Mrs. Diaz, her son, and the physician.

The esophagogastroduodenoscopy (EGD) is an endoscopic procedure that visualizes the esophagus, stomach, and duodenum. During the EGD, the endoscope is passed through the mouth while the patient is in a left lateral position with the head bent forward.

Informed consent must be obtained before an endoscopic procedure. A biopsy (retrieval of a small piece of mucosa or tumor for analysis) or polypectomy (complete surgical removal of a colonic lesion) can be done during endoscopy.

Before any endoscopic procedure (whether sigmoidoscopy, colonoscopy, or EGD), nursing responsibilities focus on educating the patient. Explain the purpose of the examination, the position necessary for the procedure, and sensations likely to be felt during the procedure. Also, discuss any dietary restrictions and test preparations. For example, the patient may be allowed only clear liquids the evening before and the morning of the test. Bowel preparation using laxatives, a rectal suppository, or enemas will also be required to cleanse the lower colon of stool before the procedure begins.

Afterward, the patient needs rest but must be closely monitored for signs of rectal bleeding or the onset of continuous, dull abdominal pain, possibly indicating colonic perforation. The patient will probably be tired and perhaps hungry and thirsty. Provide rest and offer food and fluids as allowed.

NURSING DIAGNOSES

NANDA-International (NANDA-I, 2014) nursing diagnoses concerning bowel elimination include Constipation, Perceived Constipation, Risk for Constipation, Chronic Functional Constipation, Dysfunctional Gastrointestinal Motility, Diarrhea, and Bowel Incontinence. Selected bowel elimination nursing diagnoses, along with Nursing Outcomes Classification (NOC) and Nursing Interventions Classification (NIC), are outlined in Table 33-3. Altered bowel status can contribute to or cause many potential or actual problems for the patient.

OUTCOME IDENTIFICATION AND PLANNING

After nursing diagnoses have been identified, a plan of care is developed. The overall goals for patients with bowel elimination pattern disturbances may include the following:

- The patient will demonstrate a normal pattern of bowel elimination without evidence of constipation, diarrhea, fecal incontinence, or distention.
- The patient will remain free from preventable complications or adverse consequences from altered bowel elimination.
- The patient will participate in a program to maintain and promote an acceptable pattern of bowel elimination.

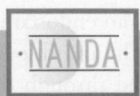

Table 33-3   SELECTED NURSING DIAGNOSES FOR BOWEL ELIMINATION

Nursing Dx	Related Factors	Dx Statement	NOC*	NIC†
Constipation—decrease in the normal frequency of defecation accompanied by difficult or incomplete passage of hard, dry stool	Insufficient fluids, insufficient fiber, decreased activity, abdominal muscle weakness, neurologic impairment	Constipation R/T inadequate activity, inadequate fluid and fiber intake AEB hard painful passage of stool every 3 d	Bowel Elimination Mobility Hydration Nutritional Status: Food and Fluid Intake	Constipation Management Fluid Management Teaching: Prescribed Diet
Diarrhea—passage of loose, unformed stool	Anxiety, stress, infectious processes, adverse effects of medications	Diarrhea R/T stress and antibiotics AEB cramping, urgency, and >6 liquid stools for last 24 h	Bowel Elimination Stress Level Medication Response Knowledge: Medications, Self-management: Acute Illness	Anxiety Reduction, Diarrhea Management
Perceived Constipation—state in which a person makes self-diagnosis of constipation and ensures a daily bowel movement through the use of laxatives, enemas, or suppositories	Faulty appraisal, impaired thought processes, family or cultural health beliefs	Perceived Constipation R/T belief that a daily BM is needed AEB abuse of laxatives and enemas	Knowledge: Health beliefs, Medication, Knowledge: Treatment Response, Bowel Elimination	Bowel Management, Nutrition Management, Fluid Management
Bowel Incontinence—a change in normal bowel habits characterized by involuntary passage of stool	Decreased muscle tone or sphincter control, impaction, chronic diarrhea, toileting self-care deficit	Incontinence R/T decreased sphincter control and decreased ability to self-toilet following a CVA AEB defecating prior to reaching toilet	Bowel Continence, Coping, Self-Care Toileting,	Bowel Incontinence Care, Bowel Training, Self-Care Assistance: Toileting
Dysfunctional gastrointestinal motility—Increase, decrease, ineffective, or lack of peristaltic activity within the gastrointestinal system	Immobility, treatment regimen, food intolerances, aging	Dysfunctional gastrointestinal motility R/T food intolerance, immobility, and treatment regimen AEB abdominal pain, cramping, and nausea	Bowel Elimination. Discomfort Level, Severity of Nausea	Nutritional Counseling and Monitoring, diet Staging, nausea Management, Flatulence Reduction

Dx, diagnosis; R/T, related to; AEB, as evidenced by; BM, bowel movement; CVA, cerebrovascular accident.
*From: Moorhead, S., Johnson, M., Maas, M., & Swanson, E. (2013). *Iowa Outcomes Project: Nursing Outcomes Classification (NOC)* (5th ed.). St. Louis, MO: C. V. Mosby.
†From: Bulecheck, G., Butcher, H., Dochterman, J., & Wagner, C. (2013). *Iowa Intervention Project: Nursing Interventions Classification (NIC)* (5th ed.). St. Louis, MO: Elsevier Mosby.
From: NANDA-International (NANDA-I. 2014). *Nursing diagnoses: Definitions and classification, 2015–2017.* West Sussex, England: Wiley-Blackwell.

The time frame for the patient to achieve a normal pattern of bowel elimination depends on the particular alteration involved. For example, constipation can usually be relieved in 1 or 2 days, whereas relief of diarrhea or incontinence is not always achievable in this time frame. The etiologic factors associated with the dysfunction also dictate the realistic time frame in which an outcome can be accomplished.

Promoting an acceptable bowel elimination pattern is, realistically, a long-term goal; in actual clinical practice, however, it is often subject to short-term management. Patient teaching is a major management tool for achieving this goal.

IMPLEMENTATION

Health Promotion

Nurses are responsible for teaching patients how to avoid bowel elimination problems and how to maintain normal bowel function. Such teaching often involves promoting optimal diet, fluid intake, and activity.

DIET

The nurse should assist the patient with planning a diet that contains sufficient daily intake of high-fiber foods because dietary fiber is necessary to provide bulk to the stool. High-fiber foods include fresh or cooked fruits and vegetables with their skins, whole-grain breads and cereals, and fruit and vegetable juices. The nurse can assist the patient in selecting foods from a list and identifying the foods the patient will most likely incorporate into his or her lifestyle. A dietitian can be consulted for a more extensive list of high-fiber foods and recipes using these ingredients. For example, unprocessed bran flakes can be added to cooked or processed cereals. The patient should start with small amounts (1 or 2 teaspoons) to determine whether bran causes any intestinal irritation or flatulence. Unprocessed bran can absorb eight times its weight in water. An acceptable amount of bran is added gradually to the diet to achieve an acceptable bowel elimination pattern. The daily intake of about 800 g of high-fiber foods (e.g., any combination of five or six servings of fruit or vegetables and whole-grain bread or cereal) is encouraged. A sandwich with two slices of whole-grain bread, served with a large fresh vegetable salad and two pieces of fruit, would provide about five servings of fiber.

FLUIDS

Fluid intake between 1,500 and 2,000 mL per day promotes a normal bowel elimination pattern. The nurse should discuss with the patient his or her fluid preferences and find a way to encourage the intake of 8 to 10 glasses of fluid per day.

Some fruit and vegetable juices provide not only fluid but bulk because of their high pulp or fiber content. A glass of prune juice is equivalent to more than one serving of the dried fruit, has high magnesium content, and is an excellent source of fluid to promote bowel elimination. Hot fluids, such as coffee, tea, or hot water with lemon juice, may also increase intestinal motility. A review of the literature of caffeine effects on fluid

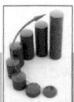

OUTCOME-BASED TEACHING PLANS

Mrs. Chin is being discharged from the acute care facility on Tylenol #3 for pain (an opioid analgesic), ferrous sulfate to improve her anemia, and Colace as a stool softener after hip replacement surgery. Mrs. Chin uses a walker, and her mobility is very restricted. After surgery, she required a suppository to have a bowel movement. Mrs. Chin states that she is very worried that she will be constipated after she is discharged home.

OUTCOME

At the end of the teaching session, Mrs. Chin can verbalize factors that could contribute to constipation during the surgical recovery period.

STRATEGIES

- Evaluate Mrs. Chin's normal bowel routine, including her knowledge of factors contributing to constipation, and her usual treatment for constipation.
- Discuss factors that slow bowel motility and increase risk of constipation (decreased mobility, altered diet and fluid intake, pain medication, iron supplements) during the postoperative period.
- Have Mrs. Chin verbalize factors back to you.
- Provide Mrs. Chin with a written list of factors for her reference.

OUTCOME

Before discharge, Mrs. Chin will verbalize a plan to decrease constipation risk and treat constipation if it should occur.

STRATEGIES

- Provide Mrs. Chin with a handout on promoting regular bowel function.
- From a list of foods high in fiber, have Mrs. Chin select those foods she likes and can easily incorporate into her diet.
- Problem solve together how to increase fluid intake (e.g., large sports bottle filled with water at side, fruit juices [e.g., prune] that are also high in fiber).
- Review prescribed medications and their effect on bowel function.
- Review medications (prescribed and over the counter) to prevent and treat constipation.
- Have Mrs. Chin verbalize how and when she will take laxative medications (e.g., Colace every day to keep my stool soft, milk of magnesia if no bowel movement for 3 days).

EVALUATION

Outcomes met. Mrs. Chin verbalized the impact of fluid intake, fiber, and activity level on bowel function. She also acknowledged that her pain medication and iron supplement can contribute to constipation. She verbalized her intent to drink at least 5 glasses of water daily, drink a glass of prune juice daily, and take her stool softener. She will take MOM if she goes without a bowel movement for 3 days and notify the MD if it is not effective.

balance by Maughan and Griffin (2003) shows that consuming moderate amounts of caffeine (250 mg) daily does not cause a diuretic effect. Caffeine intake greater than 300 mg may cause a diuretic response but depends on body mass and whether the person is habituated to drinking caffeine. Therefore, moderate amounts of caffeine taken as part of the various daily fluids poses no harm to total fluid balance in a healthy adult (Marcason, 2008).

ACTIVITY AND EXERCISE

A sufficient amount of daily exercise is necessary to promote general muscle tone. Exercise also encourages normal smooth muscle functioning, which is important for normal intestinal functioning. Walking is an excellent exercise in which most people can participate. Isotonic or isometric exercises also help to increase abdominal muscle tone. An example of these exercises is the alternate contraction and relaxation of the abdominal muscles for 8 to 10 repetitions. The many variations of sit-up exercises isometrically tone and strengthen the abdominal muscles. Assist the patient who is on bed rest to perform range-of-motion exercises until he or she can perform more independent activities.

BOWEL HABITS

Many people recognize that their bodies have a regular time for bowel elimination. Some people have a bowel movement at the same time of day or after a certain regular stimulus. The duodenocolic reflex is a strong reflex, especially when food or hot liquid is ingested after a period of fasting, such as after a night's sleep. For some people, ingestion of breakfast or a cup of coffee, tea, or any liquid is stimulus enough to activate the duodenocolic reflex. Teach patients to heed their body signals and stress that ignoring the urge to defecate can lead to constipation.

> ### ❗ SAFETY ALERT
>
> Teach patients to exhale slowly during defecation to avoid straining and Valsalva's maneuver, which for high-risk patients can lead to cardiac dysrhythmias, increased intracranial pressure, and syncope.

COLORECTAL SCREENING

Colorectal cancer is the third most common cause of cancer among men and women in the United States (American Cancer Society, 2014b). The risk of a person developing colorectal cancer in their lifetime is about 1 in 20 (5%). Risk for colorectal cancer increases significantly after 50 years of age and for people who have a positive family history; previous colorectal cancer, ulcerative colitis, or Crohn disease; or a history of benign adenoma (polyps). Teaching about annual screening beginning at age 50 years, including the FOBT, flexible endoscopic examination every 5 years, or colonoscopy every 10 years for normal-risk individuals, is an important nursing responsibility.

Nursing Interventions for Altered Bowel Function

Nursing interventions are individualized to reestablish optimal bowel function and treat common bowel alterations such as constipation, diarrhea, flatulence, abdominal distention, and related problems. Constipation is treated with laxatives, suppositories, enemas, and, if chronic, a bowel management program. Diarrhea is managed by treating the underlying cause, resting the bowel, and administering antidiarrheal medications. Fecal incontinence is managed by instituting a bowel-training program and using fecal collection devices. Problematic flatulence is treated by increasing activity, administering medications, using rectal tubes, and administering return-flow enemas. Persistent abdominal distention may require decompression by nasogastric intubation. Other nursing interventions may involve measures to relieve fecal impaction, to facilitate bowel training, and to care for the stoma and patient after fecal diversion surgery.

MEDICATION ADMINISTRATION

Almost all medications used to manage altered bowel function are available over the counter without prescription. People self-medicate to treat bowel problems, frequently seeking the advice of a healthcare professional only when symptoms become severe or extend over a long period. Teaching regarding normal bowel function and nonpharmacologic methods to regain normal bowel regularity is important to avoid overuse of laxatives. Also, inappropriate use of over-the-counter bowel medications can worsen some serious medical problems, such as bowel obstruction or appendicitis. Nurses are often in an ideal position to teach individuals or groups about appropriate use of bowel medications.

Laxatives

Usually, oral laxatives are the treatment of choice for constipation because these medications promote evacuation of hardened stool from the bowel. Table 33-4 presents some common agents, such as oral laxatives and stool softeners, that are used to relieve constipation. Oral laxatives take longer to evacuate stool than do laxatives given rectally. However, oral laxatives are preferred by most patients for their ease of administration and the more gradual effect on intestinal motility.

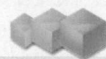 **Concept Mastery Alert**

Dependence is a significant risk among patients who use oral laxatives long term. It can develop over a relatively short period of time, posing a significant challenge to the resumption of normal bowel function.

Laxatives may be given in the form of a rectal suppository. A **suppository** is a medication prepared in a base (e.g., glycerin) that, when inserted into the rectum, melts and can be absorbed for systemic or local effects. Many suppositories are used to promote bowel evacuation, but other drugs that do

TABLE 33-4 COMMON AGENTS USED TO RELIEVE CONSTIPATION

Laxative Type	Examples	Mechanism of Action	Nursing Considerations
Bulk	Fibercon, Metamucil	Hydrophilic Nonabsorbable fibers attract water into large intestine	Usually well tolerated and used to regulate stool in constipation and diarrhea Additional fluid intake encouraged Concurrent administration with other medications avoided Contraindicated in bowel obstruction, fecal impaction, abdominal pain
Emollient (stool softeners)	Colace, Surfak, Dialose, Doss	Decrease surface tension of stool, allowing water to enter stool more readily	Short-term treatment when risk of constipation is high (e.g., when patient is less mobile or is taking opioids) Contraindicated in acute abdominal pain, nausea, vomiting, intestinal obstruction
Saline	Milk of magnesia (MOM), magnesium citrate, Fleet enema	Hyperosmolar Increase colon motility through release of cholecystokinin (a hormone)	Possible resultant electrolyte imbalances, especially hypermagnesemia Not for chronic use or use in renal failure Frequently used to prepare bowel for diagnostic testing
Stimulant	Castor oil, bisacodyl (Dulcolax), casanthranol (Peri-Colace), Ex-Lax, phenolphthalein (Correctol), senna (Senokot)	Direct stimulation of intestinal mucosa	Chronic use avoided Possible resultant electrolyte imbalances Use during pregnancy and lactation avoided

not affect bowel status (e.g., aspirin) can be administered in suppository form. A suppository is administered when a quick effect (15 to 60 minutes) is desired. For instructions for administering a rectal suppository, see Box 33-2.

BOX 33-2 Administering a Rectal Suppository

To administer a rectal suppository, gather the medication, a packet of water-soluble lubricant, and a pair of disposable gloves. If the patient cannot ambulate independently to the bathroom, place a bedside commode or bedpan nearby before administering the suppository. Placement of disposable underpads on the bed may be advisable if the patient's motor or mental abilities are compromised. Perform the following steps:
1. Ask the patient to assume a side-lying position.
2. With gloved hands, remove the outer wrapper from the suppository and cover the suppository with lubricant.
3. While separating the patient's buttocks, locate the anus and insert the suppository, pointed or rounded end first, past the internal sphincter. For the adult, the internal sphincter is at approximately 4 inches, or at the end of the nurse's index finger.
4. Guide the suppository with your index finger, aiming in a slightly upward direction toward the umbilicus. Typically, you will feel the patient's sphincter close around your finger. A suppository melts at body temperature and releases its medication as it rests against the rectal mucosa. Be sure that the suppository is not inadvertently deposited into stool that might be in the rectum, because this prevents absorption by the rectal mucosa.

Antidiarrheal Agents

Medications that act directly on the intestine to slow bowel motility or to absorb excess fluid in the bowel are called antidiarrheals. Table 33-5 lists the antidiarrheal agents that are most commonly administered. Absorbents and bulk-forming agents change the consistency of the stool to relieve diarrhea; they cause few adverse systemic effects and are considered safe for general use. Opiates and antispasmodics act systemically to decrease intestinal motility. Antidiarrheal agents are contraindicated when viral or bacterial infections cause diarrhea because diarrhea is a protective mechanism to shed the microorganisms from the body.

Medications may also be used to relieve the underlying problem causing diarrhea. For example, antibiotics are administered when an infectious microorganism causes diarrhea. Steroids may be given to decrease inflammation in the exacerbation of a chronic inflammatory bowel disease.

Fecal Microbiota Transplantation

Fecal microbiota transplantation (FMT), also referred to as stool transplant, is emerging as an effective treatment for recurrent CDI. Although treatment of CDI with antimicrobials such as metronidazole or vancomycin is usually initially successful, the recurrence rate of CDI can be as high as 35% (Austin et al., 2014; Burke & Lamont, 2013). This is thought to be the result of an imbalance of the intestinal microbiotic flora, due to antimicrobial suppression of normal intestinal bacteria in addition to the *C. difficile*. By replacing and normalizing the intestinal flora of the recipient, FMT helps to alleviate symptoms and eliminate infection. Reports from case studies and systematic reviews of the literature have shown success rates over 90% in curing of CDI (Pacheco & Johnson, 2013).

TABLE 33-5 MEDICATIONS USED TO RELIEVE DIARRHEA

Agent	Action	Nursing Considerations
Absorbents Kaolin/pectin (Donnagel) Attapulgite (Kaopectate) Bismuth subsalicylate (Pepto-Bismol)	Absorbs excess fluid and bowel irritants; provides soothing effect to irritated bowel	Do not use in suspected bowel obstruction.
Bulk-Forming Agents Psyllium (Metamucil, Effersyllium)	Attracts water to absorb excess fluid	Do not use in patients with swallowing difficulty or narrowing of the esophagus.
Opiates Paregoric	↓ Intestinal motility	Do not use in diarrhea caused by poisoning until toxin has been eliminated from the gastrointestinal tract.
Synthetic Opiates Loperamide (Imodium)	↓ Intestinal motility	Appropriate fluid and electrolyte replacement should be given; not for long-term use without monitoring electrolytes.
Diphenoxylate/atropine (Lomotil)	↑ Intestinal water and electrolyte absorption	Do not use in diarrhea associated with bacteria or colitis.
Antispasmodics Atropine	↓ Intestinal motility	Do not use in narrow-angle glaucoma or obstructive gastrointestinal diseases.

FMT is the infusion of human stool from a healthy donor into the gastrointestinal tract of the patient (Samuel, Crumb & Duba, 2014). It is considered an investigational biologic treatment by the Food and Drug Administration (FDA) (Samuel et al. 2014), and there is no standardized technique. Typically, the donor is a family member, though some studies have utilized unrelated healthy donors. All donors are screened according to guidelines of the FDA and the American Gastroenterological Association (AGA). Freshly donated, ideally within 6 to 24 hours, stool is mixed with saline or sterile water to create a suspension that can be injected through a tube. The most common delivery method is via a retention enema or a colonoscopy, although upper endoscopy or nasal–duodenal tubes have also been used. The procedural prep for the patient includes stopping the antibiotic regimen 2 to 3 days in advance and taking a cleansing colon prep. In the initial hours following procedure, many protocols involve using medications to diminish gut motility and bed rest, with rotating patient position in order to maximize contact of the infusion with intestinal mucosa. In addition to demonstrating safety and successful tolerance of the procedure, some studies have also indicated aesthetic acceptance of and even preference for this treatment, based on its success (Dodin & Katz, 2014). Continuing research will help define best practice in the treatment of CDI as well as possible applications in other intestinal diseases such as ulcerative colitis (Samuel et al., 2014).

Antiflatulence Agents

Antiflatulence agents, such as simethicone, are used to relieve gas. Simethicone coalesces gas bubbles in the intestine, allowing gas to pass from the gastrointestinal tract either by belching or by anal expulsion. It does not prevent the formation of gas. Antiflatulence medication is usually given in combination with an antacid. Suppositories that increase intestinal motility can also relieve accumulated intestinal flatus.

ENEMA ADMINISTRATION

An **enema** is the cleansing of a portion of the large bowel by insertion of fluid rectally. Enemas can be small volume, containing a laxative medication (approximately 150 mL), or large volume, containing only ordinary tap water or saline solution (up to 1,000 mL for the adult). A return-flow enema is administered to promote the expulsion of flatus. **Procedure 33-2** outlines the steps in administering an enema.

Small-Volume Enemas

Small-volume enemas are commercially prepared and usually are administered after an oral laxative fails to produce sufficient stool return or if a rapid evacuation is preferred. The laxative solution is hypertonic, osmotically drawing water from colonic mucosa to cause water retention in the lower colon. It also increases peristalsis. The volume of fluid itself distends the rectum to trigger a defecation reflex.

An oil retention enema is a small-volume enema containing a quantity of mineral oil. The mineral oil softens hardened stool, making the stool easier to pass. An oil retention enema usually is given only when a fecal impaction is suspected.

Small-volume enemas come from the manufacturer in disposable containers with prelubricated tips. The patient usually experiences the urge to defecate within 5 to 10 minutes after administration of the enema.

Large-Volume Enemas

Large-volume enemas cleanse the bowel of stool by distending the bowel with as much as 1,000 mL of fluid for the adult (15 to 60 mL is recommended for an infant, 240 to 360 mL for a child). Warm tap water or saline solution is used as the cleansing agent. However, saline solution is the only fluid recommended for infants and children. The large volume of fluid instilled into the bowel causes distention and stimulates the defecation reflex. The large-volume enema can be used as a treatment for constipation or as a method of cleansing the bowel before radiologic studies or surgery of the intestines.

After gathering the equipment, position the patient as for administration of a suppository or small-volume enema on the left side. Once the tubing has been flushed or primed, insert the lubricated tip of the tubing approximately 4 inches for an adult, aiming toward the umbilicus, and slowly instill the solution into the patient's rectum.

> ## ! SAFETY ALERT
> Care must be taken not to insert the tubing too far or to advance the tubing forcefully because doing so could injure mucosal tissue or, in extreme situations, perforate the intestine.

Control the amount and speed of the fluid instillation by opening and closing the tubing clamp and by adjusting the height of the solution container. Opening the clamp or raising the container increases the rate of flow of the solution into the rectum. Conversely, closing the clamp or lowering the enema bucket decreases the rate of flow. If the patient complains of abdominal discomfort or cramping, the nurse momentarily stops the flow of solution. To cleanse the bowel successfully of stool, the average adult needs to tolerate approximately 350 to 500 mL of solution instilled before expelling the enema. When the patient cannot tolerate any more solution per rectum, the nurse stops the enema and assists the patient to the bedpan, commode, or toilet.

A large-volume enema can be repeated up to three times in succession.

> ## ! SAFETY ALERT
> Never administer more than three large-volume tap water enemas in succession. Excess absorption of the hypotonic solution by colonic mucosa leads to fluid and electrolyte imbalances.

Guidelines for repeating an enema include the statement that the patient feels there is more stool in the bowel that needs to be evacuated, evidence of large pieces of stool in the enema returns, and heavily stool-colored water in the enema returns.

Return-Flow Enemas

The return-flow enema is used to relieve accumulated flatus. Use the same equipment and proceed in the same fashion as for the large-volume enema. However, only 300 to 500 mL of warm tap water is necessary. When the patient indicates that he or she feels abdominal discomfort or cramping, lower the enema solution container and allow the water to return through the tubing into the container. Flatus will also return, as evidenced by the bubbling of the water in the container.

Continue to repeat the procedure until there is no more evidence of expelled flatus or the patient reports relief. This procedure may take 15 to 20 minutes to be effective. The return-flow enema can be repeated as necessary.

FECAL IMPACTION REMOVAL

Removal of fecal impactions is a nursing responsibility. Manual removal of an impaction can be embarrassing for the patient. Explain the purpose and necessity of the procedure, telling the patient before beginning what will be done. Proceed in a matter-of-fact manner to reduce anxiety and embarrassment for the patient.

The equipment necessary for manual removal of fecal impaction includes plenty of disposable gloves, a gown, packets of water-soluble lubricant, several disposable underpads to protect the bed and floor, two bedpans, and a commode if the patient is capable of transferring to it. It is possible for the large intestine to distend to hold a large amount of stool. Because the nurse cannot accurately predict the volume before beginning the procedure, it is best to be prepared to remove a large quantity of stool. Also, wear an impermeable or disposable gown because some stool is likely to spill or splash during the procedure. The odor of the stool can be strong, and an open window or other form of ventilation should be provided.

Begin the procedure with the patient in the side-lying position. Then insert a double-gloved, lubricated index finger into the rectum. With a gentle hooking motion of the index finger, remove some of the stool from the rectum.

> ## ! SAFETY ALERT
> Be careful when using the hooking motion during normal disimpaction. Perforation of the rectum can occur.

The removal of stool begins slowly, but as the hardened stool that is blocking the lumen of the rectum is removed, the remaining stool may pass more quickly. The bedpan should be ready to place under the patient so that he or she can evacuate stool into it if possible; the stool may come so quickly that the patient is unable to control its evacuation. Weak patients with poor muscle tone may require assistance. Continue to remove stool manually until you can no longer feel stool at the fingertip and the patient is not voluntarily evacuating any more stool. Remove and dispose of collected stool and soiled linens, and provide hygiene care for the patient. Removal of a fecal impaction is a tiring procedure for the patient, so provide the patient with some uninterrupted time and a restful environment after the procedure. Reassessment and another disimpaction may be necessary for some patients.

Nursing interventions to prevent complications in the management of fecal impaction include effective yet gentle insertion of the gloved index finger into the patient's rectum when performing digital examination and manual removal of stool.

> ⚠ **SAFETY ALERT**
>
> Excess vagal stimulation during a digital rectal exam (DRE) and removal of stool can precipitate cardiac dysrhythmias in weak patients or those with cardiovascular disease. Forceful pressure against the rectal mucosa can damage the bowel tissue.

RECTAL TUBE INSERTION

A rectal tube, which is a short piece of plastic tubing similar to the tubing used for large-volume enemas, may be used if increased activity or medication does not relieve flatulence. The nurse inserts the lubricated tip of the tube about 4 inches into the patient's rectum and leaves it in place for 15 to 20 minutes or until the patient reports relief. The gas in the rectum can pass from the rectum through the tube and into a collecting device, such as a bag. Abdominal pain is the predominant adverse consequence of flatulence. It is wiser to relieve the cause of the pain by using antiflatulence agents or rectal tubes than to administer pain medications. Opioid analgesics, in particular, slow intestinal motility and compound the problem.

BOWEL TRAINING

A long-term approach to control bowel elimination may be necessary, especially for patients who are in the rehabilitation phase of a neurologic impairment (e.g., spinal cord injury, stroke, head injury). These patients are at high risk for constipation or fecal incontinence or both. Bowel training is not appropriate for patients with inflammatory bowel disease, infection, or lactose intolerance.

A standard bowel-training program aims to maintain a soft stool consistency and develop a routine method of stool evacuation. The routine is repeated at the same time each day with the same techniques to train and control the bowel's evacuation time. A common bowel-training program includes use of a stool softener twice a day, a bulking agent daily, and a suppository (glycerin or bisacodyl [Dulcolax]), usually given after breakfast, followed by toileting and digital stimulation. Bowel training may require weeks to months of persistence before success is attained. Reassurance and verbal expressions of confidence in the patient contribute to success of the program. Patient teaching about normal bowel function and factors to promote a soft stool is helpful.

For patients with anal sphincter control that is weak but not lost, a variation of the classic bowel-training program is implemented. Stool softeners and an increase in dietary fiber are used to maintain a soft stool, but instead of relying on the routine use of suppositories and digital stimulation, emphasis is placed on the patient's recognizing the body's own defecation signals. Careful assessment and documentation of incontinent episodes are performed for several days. From then on, the patient is assisted to the toilet at a time that has been identified as "routine." The time often coincides with a duodenocolic mass movement after eating. The intent is to establish a regular defecation time in synchrony with the patient's natural physiologic function.

Pelvic floor exercises, biofeedback, and abdominal massage have been used by some healthcare providers to promote regular stool evacuation. When performing pelvic floor exercises, the patient alternately contracts and relaxes the anal sphincter and puborectal muscles for a brief period (3 or 4 seconds) 25 to 30 times, repeating these exercises three times a day.

Biofeedback can be an effective adjunct to pelvic floor exercises because it has been demonstrated that verbally instructing someone on pelvic floor exercises is less than 50% effective. An anal probe provides visual feedback that helps the patient locate and therefore become more aware of the pelvic floor muscles needed to inhibit the passing of stool (Scott, 2014).

Abdominal massage stimulates peristalsis. The abdomen is massaged starting at the right iliac fossa, moving along the large colon and proceeding from the ascending to the transverse and descending colon.

Sensory retraining is a method to help patients achieve control over fecal incontinence. For any success, the patient must have some ability to perceive rectal sensations. This training, often done in an outpatient setting, involves three stages: increased recognition of the stimulus, exercises to increase maximal voluntary squeeze in the perianal area, and ability to coordinate external sphincter control (Gié & Christoforidis, 2011).

FECAL COLLECTION DURING INCONTINENCE

If bowel training is unsuccessful or fecal incontinence is considered intractable, a drainable fecal collector may be used. The drainable fecal collector is similar to an ostomy appliance. It consists of a collecting pouch and a skin-protective barrier designed to adhere firmly to the perineum, anal cleft, and inner surfaces of the buttocks. If a formed stool collects in the pouch, the drainage outlet can be cut off with scissors, the stool emptied, and the end of the pouch resealed with a plastic clamp.

Just as diapers are considered appropriate management for the infant or child who is not toilet trained, protective pants, called incontinence briefs, are sometimes used for intractable fecal incontinence in the adult. Such absorbent pads wick liquid stool away from the skin better than do plastic-coated underpads. Frequent assessment is important to promptly detect evacuation of stool so that skin irritation and patient embarrassment can be minimized. Shear force and trauma when cleansing the area should be avoided.

STOMA MANAGEMENT

Stoma management consists of a group of nursing interventions that may be necessary after fecal diversion surgery. Nursing responsibilities for patients with stomas include stoma assessment and management of feces collection by way of an ostomy appliance or through stoma irrigation. Many healthcare facilities have nurses with specialized training (wound ostomy continence nurses [WOCNs]) to assist patients and to support other nurses in the care of patients with fecal diversions.

Stoma Assessment

After surgery, the stoma and abdominal incision may be covered with a sterile dressing. When removing the dressing or when changing appliances over the stoma, the nurse should assess the stoma for color and position. Ideally, the stoma should be a healthy pink. A dusky pink or bluish tint (cyanosis) suggests inadequate circulation to the stoma. The stomal mucosa must remain on the abdominal surface. If the stoma retracts, feces may potentially enter the abdominal cavity and cause peritonitis. Prolapse (protrusion) of the stoma can also occur and should be reported to the surgeon. The stoma should also be inspected for bleeding and drainage. Some bleeding may occur because the stoma tissues are fragile.

Fecal Collection

Patients with ileostomies or colostomies that continuously drain liquid stool need an ostomy appliance (pouch or bag) over the stoma at all times. A large selection of ostomy appliances is commercially available; a common type of ostomy pouch is featured in Figure 33-6. Usually, when the WOCN visits a patient with a new ostomy, he or she inspects the condition of the stoma and discusses the methods for feces collection. The diameter of the stoma must be measured accurately for an appliance with the correctly sized opening to obtain proper fit.

> ### ! SAFETY ALERT
> An opening that is too small may constrict the stoma and restrict circulation, whereas an opening that is too large will allow stool to leak onto the abdominal skin.

The enzymatic juices contained in the liquid stool will cause irritation, maceration, and eventual skin breakdown. The back surface of the ostomy appliance contains a sticky substance that adheres to the abdominal skin. Also, the appliance is usually taped for extra security.

The ostomy pouch should be emptied of fecal contents when it is about one-fourth to one-third full. If the pouch becomes too full, the weight of fecal contents will disrupt the pouch seal, causing the stool to leak. The odor of the stool may be strong and offensive, especially to the patient with a new stoma. In such cases, the nurse can open the window or spray a deodorant in the room before emptying the pouch. The bottom of the pouch has an opening secured by a clip, which is removed to empty the pouch into the toilet. The appliance can also be emptied into a bedpan if the patient cannot get out of bed. As with all procedures in which the nurse handles feces or other bodily fluids, disposable gloves are worn and a gown used if splashing is likely.

Emptying an ostomy pouch is a clean, not a sterile, procedure. The pouch should be rinsed with clean, warm tap water after emptying. A large (60-mL) syringe works well for this purpose. Air is eliminated by compressing the pouch and reapplying the clip to close the pouch. Then, the pouch is checked for leaks from the stomal area, and the condition of the stoma is assessed. If the ostomy appliance leaks fecal contents where it is attached to the skin, the entire bag needs to be removed and replaced. The nurse or patient cleanses the abdominal skin surrounding the stoma, inspects the stoma's appearance, gently dries the abdominal skin, and applies a new ostomy pouch. The latter process is described in **Procedure 33-3**.

If the ostomy is continuously draining fecal material, the pouch change will need to be quick and well planned. A sterile or clean gauze 4″ × 4″ pad may be placed temporarily over the stoma to collect a small amount of fecal contents as the skin is dried and the new pouch is secured.

Stomal Irrigation

Bowel training to achieve a predictable evacuation of stool from a sigmoid colostomy can be assisted by stomal irrigation. Stomal irrigation is similar to giving a large-volume enema through the stomal opening instead of through the anus. More specialized equipment is necessary, but the principle of instilling fluid into the colon to cause distention and resultant elimination is the same. Because stomal irrigation is essentially an enema, it can also be administered to relieve constipation or to cleanse the bowel before diagnostic procedures or tests.

Figure 33-7 shows typical irrigation equipment, including an irrigating sleeve with belt and a water container

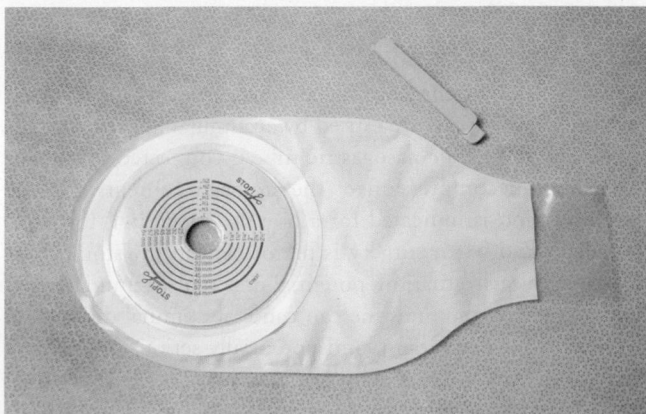

FIGURE 33-6 One-piece drainable ostomy pouch with clamp.

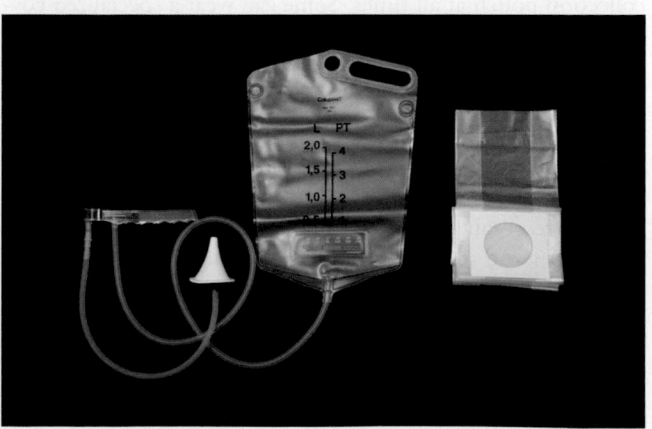

FIGURE 33-7 Colostomy irrigation equipment.

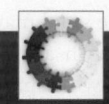

COLLABORATING WITH THE HEALTHCARE TEAM
Discussing Care for a Patient With a Colostomy

A WOCN who has consulted on Ellen White asks to discuss Mrs. White's care with you. Mrs. White is a 54-year-old obese patient who had a colostomy 3 days ago for colon cancer.

***S**ITUATION:* I am George Whynn, the WOCN. I received a consult to see Mrs. White and help her develop a plan for ostomy management. Do you have a few minutes to discuss this?

***B**ACKGROUND:* Mrs. White had her colon resection and colostomy 3 days ago. Her biopsy was positive for adenocarcinoma, and she will be followed up with chemotherapy. She and her family are quite overwhelmed with the diagnosis, and she was teary when I saw her. Her bowel tones are still hypoactive, and she is NPO. Her stoma is pink and moist, and she has serosanguineous drainage in the bag. Her stoma is located close to an abdominal fold, so I have fitted her with a new appliance. I will continue to see her daily, but I have written out the specific information on her plan of care.

***A**SSESSMENT:* Physically, Mrs. White's progress is on track. I'm concerned that once she starts producing stool, her bag will leak because of the challenges of getting a good seal around her abdominal folds. Also, Mrs. White and her family will need much ongoing support.

***R**ECOMMENDATION:* Could you make sure the nurses check her stoma bag for leakage every shift? Once her stoma starts producing stool, talk through how to empty her bag, and get her to participate as much as possible. I'm going to contact the Ostomy Association and see if an ostomate can visit her while she is still in the hospital. I have left my number on the plan of care, so call if any problems arise.

CRITICAL THINKING CHALLENGE

- Often, the nurse uses SBAR to communicate with others. How does it feel to receive a report from another team member using this framework?
- Why do you think the WOCN added certain information to the plan of care when he verbally discussed issues with the staff nurse?
- Was it clear from this communication what the two priority concerns were for this patient? Did the SBAR format affect clarity?
- Where might you find recommendations from consults if the WOCN did not seek you out to discuss his recommendations?

---

connected to an irrigating catheter with cone and lubricant. The evacuation of the colon at predictable times allows the patient a sense of control over his or her body and environment. Patients who have sigmoid ostomies and who have achieved reliable bowel training may not need to wear a fecal collection pouch at all times. Some can wear a specialized covering over the stoma between bowel evacuations. The covering protects the stoma from irritation by clothing.

Continent Fecal Diversion Management

The patient with an ileoanal reservoir is taught Kegel exercises before surgery to strengthen the perineal muscles. When the ileoanal reservoir begins to function, the patient may have 10 to 20 loose stools per day, but the number will decrease as the reservoir builds up capacity and the sphincter muscles strengthen.

The patient with a Kock pouch will need to learn how to drain the pouch of feces by passing a catheter through the surgically created one-way valve. Scheduled evacuation of the pouch should be planned to avoid overdistention.

NASOGASTRIC INTUBATION

A nasogastric tube is a thin, pliable plastic tube that can be inserted into a patient's nose and advanced into the stomach (Fig. 33-8). Nasogastric intubation may be ordered by the healthcare provider for gastric decompression, gastric lavage, or gastric feeding.

Gastric Decompression

Decompression drains stomach contents, relieving the stomach and intestines of pressure caused by accumulated gastrointestinal air and fluid. The nasogastric tube is connected to suction to facilitate decompression of the stomach contents. Gastric decompression is indicated for a bowel obstruction, for paralytic ileus, and when surgery is performed on the stomach or intestine. In each situation, potential or actual accumulation of fluid and gas in the intestine can cause abdominal distention, discomfort for the patient, and potentially serious physiologic alterations. The tube usually remains in place until normal bowel function resumes, as evidenced by active bowel sounds on auscultation.

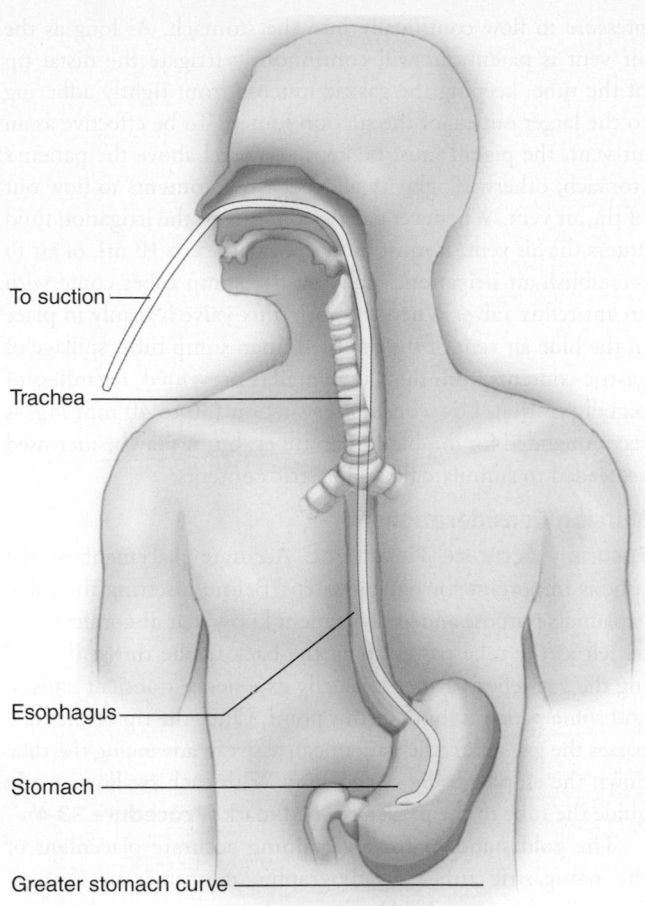

To suction

Trachea

Esophagus

Stomach

Greater stomach curve

FIGURE 33-8 Proper placement of the nasogastric tube.

Gastric Lavage

Gastric lavage is the irrigation of the stomach. In cases of accidental poisoning or accidental or intentional drug overdose, swift removal of stomach contents is required. If the patient cannot swallow an emetic medication, gastric lavage is necessary. In this situation, a nasogastric tube is inserted both to aspirate gastric contents and to instill a rinsing solution (usually normal saline) into the stomach to dilute the toxic substances. Patients with gastric bleeding are sometimes treated with an iced saline lavage, which involves instillation and aspiration of iced saline solution through the nasogastric tube to empty the stomach of blood and slow the bleeding at its source.

Gastric Feeding

For patients who cannot obtain adequate nourishment orally, liquid food can be instilled into the stomach through the nasogastric or nasointestinal tube. This type of feeding is also called enteral nutrition or gastric gavage. Nasogastric tubes for feeding are often used for a longer time than are nasogastric tubes used for decompression or lavage. They are narrower and are made of a more pliable material. Nasogastric feeding tubes and the nursing care associated with enteral nutrition are discussed in Chapter 29.

Equipment

Nasogastric Tubes. The most commonly used nasogastric tube for decompression is the double-lumen (two channels) gastric sump tube (Fig. 33-9). The double-lumen gastric sump tube is clear plastic and is sized according to the French method, which refers to circumference and is equal to three times the millimeter size (e.g., 2 mm is equal to 6 French) (O'Connor, 2013). Sizes 14 to 18 French are typical adult sizes, with a length of 120 cm (48 inches). The larger lumen is connected to suction and a drainage container to collect the aspirated gastric contents; the smaller second lumen terminates in a blue vent, often called the tube's "pigtail." The blue vent is always open to the air, providing continuous atmospheric air irrigation. Markings along the length of the tube serve as guides for depth of insertion. Both lumens have openings at the tip end to allow for fluid or air flow in and out of the tube.

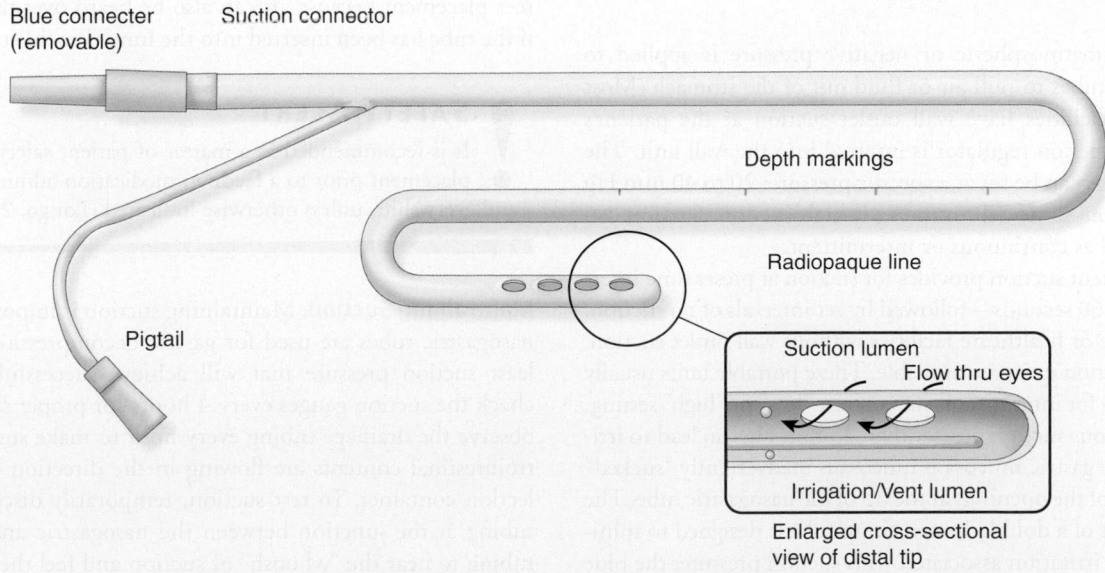

Blue connecter (removable)

Suction connector

Pigtail

Depth markings

Radiopaque line

Suction lumen

Flow thru eyes

Irrigation/Vent lumen

Enlarged cross-sectional view of distal tip

FIGURE 33-9 Double-lumen gastric sump tube.

Nasointestinal Tubes. When intestinal decompression for mechanical or nonmechanical bowel obstruction is the desired outcome, a longer tube capable of advancing the length of the intestine is used. These tubes may be single- or double-lumen. Some tubes permit stomach decompression as well as intestinal feedings.

The Harris tube (6 feet) and the Cantor tube (10 feet) are single-lumen tubes intended only for intestinal decompression. Both tubes have mercury-weighted bags attached to the tip of the tube. The weight of the mercury assists the tube in passing from the pylorus of the stomach into the duodenum. The weighted tip and the natural peristalsis of the intestine keep the tube advancing through the intestine.

The Miller-Abbot tube is a double-lumen, 10-foot tube. One lumen drains or decompresses the intestine; the second lumen is used to inflate the balloon at the tip of the tube with mercury. The double-lumen tube allows for insertion of the mercury after the tip of the tube has passed through the nose and into the stomach.

Nasointestinal tubes are inserted in the same manner as nasogastric tubes. When the tip of the tube has reached the stomach, the tubing is not taped to the patient's nose. The patient can be positioned on the right side, allowing gravity and the mercury bag to enhance passage of the tube into the duodenum. In a few hours, passage of the tube into the small intestine should be verified by radiography. If the tube has not advanced on its own, it can be advanced manually from the stomach into the duodenum under fluoroscopy by the healthcare provider or radiologist. Patient activity, position changes in bed, and ambulation encourage increased intestinal peristalsis and self-advancement of the tube along the length of the intestine. Markings along the length of the tube help to estimate progress of the tube through the intestine.

Nasointestinal tubes can be attached to a bag positioned below the patient's torso to achieve drainage of intestinal contents by gravity. Suction can also be applied, and contents can be emptied into a collecting device.

Suction. Subatmospheric or negative pressure is applied to nasogastric tubes to pull air or fluid out of the stomach. Most healthcare facilities have wall outlet suction at the patient's bedside. A suction regulator is inserted into the wall unit. The suction gauge can be set at a specific pressure: 20 to 40 mm Hg is low suction; 80 to 120 mm Hg is high suction. Suction can be regulated as continuous or intermittent.

Intermittent suction provides for suction at preset time intervals—up to 60 seconds—followed by set intervals of no suction. In the home or healthcare facilities without wall outlet suction, portable suction units are available. These portable units usually provide only for intermittent suction at a "low" or "high" setting.

Continuous suction greater than 25 mm Hg can lead to irritation of the gastric mucosa if mucosa is inadvertently "sucked" against one of the openings at the tip of the nasogastric tube. The blue air vent of a double-lumen sump tube is designed to minimize gastric irritation associated with suction pressure; the blue air vent is left open to the air, allowing air under atmospheric pressure to flow continually into the stomach. As long as the air vent is patent, air will continuously irrigate the distal tip of the tube, keeping the gastric mucosa from tightly adhering to the larger outlets of the suction lumen. To be effective as an air vent, the pigtail must be kept at a level above the patient's stomach; otherwise, gravity allows gastric contents to flow out of the air vent. Whenever gastric contents or the irrigation fluid enters the air vent, it must be cleared with 5 to 10 mL of air to reestablish air irrigation. Many gastric sump tubes come with an antireflux valve. When the antireflux valve is firmly in place in the blue air vent of the double-lumen sump tube, spillage of gastric contents from the blue pigtail is prevented, regardless of pigtail position. Low continuous suction (30 to 40 mm Hg) is recommended for double-lumen tubes, but it may be increased as needed to stimulate flow of gastric contents.

Nursing Considerations

Ensuring Accurate Placement. Accurate placement of the tube is important for patient safety. Before inserting the tube, explain its purpose and let the patient know that discomfort may be felt as the tube passes along the back of the throat (initiating the gag reflex). Patients usually experience transient nausea, and some patients vomit at this point. Once the tip of the tube passes the gag reflex, the patient can assist in advancing the tube down the esophagus by swallowing. With each swallow, gently guide the tube to the predetermined mark (**Procedure 33-4**).

The gold standard for ascertaining accurate placement of the nasogastric tube is radiographic confirmation (Longo, 2011; Proehl et al., 2011). Current best practice evidence for determining accurate placement includes measurement of tube length from nose–ear–midumbilicus (NIMU) and aspiration of fluid from the tube at the time of insertion to test the pH (Irving, Lyman, Northington, Barlett, & Kemper, 2014). If the pH is 5 or less, one can make the assumption that the tube is in the stomach. While some nurses still auscultate over the stomach while air is irrigated through the nasogastric tube with a syringe, it is not a safe or reliable method to use to assess correct placement because air can also be heard over the stomach if the tube has been inserted into the lung (Proehl et al., 2011).

> **! SAFETY ALERT**
> It is recommended as a matter of patient safety to verify placement prior to a feeding, medication administration, and every shift, unless otherwise indicated (Longo, 2011).

Maintaining Suction. Maintaining suction is important when nasogastric tubes are used for gastric decompression. Use the least suction pressure that will achieve successful drainage, check the suction gauges every 4 hours for proper setting, and observe the drainage tubing every hour to make sure that gastrointestinal contents are flowing in the direction of the collection container. To test suction, temporarily disconnect the tubing at the junction between the nasogastric and drainage tubing to hear the "whoosh" of suction and feel the suction at your fingertip. Replace any nonfunctioning suction units.

Maintaining Tube Patency. Tube patency is important to ensure proper functioning of the inserted tube. Occasionally, thick or solid particles of gastrointestinal contents plug the holes of a nasogastric or nasointestinal tube. The tube then ceases to drain gastrointestinal contents, even with properly functioning suction. When a tube clogs, minimal drainage appears in the tubing or collecting receptacle. The patient may begin to complain of nausea, which does not occur with a properly functioning system. The abdomen may appear distended.

 APPLY YOUR CRITICAL THINKING

You are caring for a postoperative patient who had colon surgery 2 days ago. During report, you are told that he has a nasogastric tube, which drained 350 mL of thick, green, mucus-filled liquid during the last shift. When you obtain your morning assessment, it reveals the following: vital signs stable, pain 6 on a 0 to 10 scale (patient frequently using patient-controlled analgesia), absent bowel sounds, no abdominal distortion, some complaint of nausea, NG to low suction, and no drainage in the suction container. What, if any, actions are indicated at this time, based on your assessment?

Check your answer in Appendix B.

The nurse can irrigate the tube with about 20 mL of water to dislodge particles or viscous gastrointestinal contents from the tip of the tube. When a large volume of irrigant is instilled, such as during gastric lavage, normal saline solution should be used to prevent fluid and electrolyte shifts that can occur when a hypotonic solution is used. Nasogastric irrigation is a clean, rather than a sterile, procedure because the gastrointestinal tract is not sterile.

When irrigating a double-lumen nasogastric tube, the nurse can instill irrigant in either lumen. If using the blue air vent, do not disconnect suction during irrigation, but always remember to clear the air vent with 10 mL of air after the procedure. Air clears the blue lumen of fluid and restores continuous air irrigation.

If a tube does not appear to be draining well even after irrigation, its placement may need to be checked. To do this, the nurse slightly advances or, alternatively, pulls back on the tube and assesses for any increase in drainage. Changing the patient's position sometimes improves nasogastric drainage.

A physician's order is required for irrigation after gastric or esophageal surgery.

❗ SAFETY ALERT

For gastric or esophageal surgeries, the tube has been placed in the operating room. To maintain patency and to avoid harm to the surgical site, the tube must not be advanced, pulled back, or manipulated in any way.

Monitoring Intake and Output

Intake and output (including the volume, color, and type of gastrointestinal drainage) are assessed and recorded every 8 hours. Gastrointestinal contents contain essential body fluids and electrolytes, including water, hydrogen (H^+), potassium (K^+), sodium (Na^+), chloride (Cl^-), bicarbonate (HCO_3^-), and magnesium (Mg^{++}). Losing too many fluids and electrolytes can lead to fluid volume deficit and metabolic acid–base imbalances. In addition, a patient with a nasogastric or nasointestinal tube for decompression is usually NPO. Any fluids swallowed would be immediately returned by way of the tube; any food swallowed would eventually clog the tube. Patients with nasogastric or nasointestinal tubes will receive intravenous therapy to supply needed fluids and electrolytes. It is the responsibility of the nurse to measure and record all intake and output and to monitor fluid and electrolyte status.

Some protocols require testing the pH of the stomach aspirate. An antacid or histamine blocker can be administered to make the stomach contents less acidic.

Providing Nasal and Oral Care

Nasal and oral care is an important nursing concern during a patient's intubation. Skin irritation and breakdown, and in severe cases pressure ulcers, at the nares (nostrils) develop. This can be prevented by appropriately taping the tube and providing frequent skin care. Applying a water-soluble lubricant to the nostrils provides moisturizing relief to dry skin.

To prevent constant tension and pulling on the tube, secure the tube to the patient's gown (channeling it through tape and securing with a safety pin). Ensure enough slack so that the patient can turn the head from side to side without pulling on the tubing.

Frequent oral hygiene can prevent the consequence of dry mouth associated with nasogastric intubation. Patients usually become mouth breathers with a tube in the nose. Sucking on ice chips or hard candies, if approved by the healthcare provider, can also provide some relief.

Encourage patients who can brush their teeth to do so frequently. An oral swab soaked in a solution of one-half water and one-half mouthwash is refreshing to many patients. The use of lemon–glycerin oral swabs or swabs soaked in full-strength mouthwash should be avoided. The immediate relief provided by the swab is sometimes followed by rebound dryness. Offer lubricant for the lips to prevent drying and cracking.

❗ SAFETY ALERT

The use of an oil-based lubricant (e.g., petroleum jelly) can inadvertently result in aspiration of oil particles into the lungs, leading to lipid pneumonia.

Administering Medication

Although usually patients with gastric decompression receive parenteral medications, medication intended for oral consumption may be administered through a nasogastric tube.

A liquid form of the medication is preferred, but many tablets can be crushed, mixed with water, and safely administered through the tube. Enteric-coated, extended-release, and sustained-release tablets are not suitable for administration through the tube, as they are designed specifically for protection of the GI tract or gradual drug release and therefore should not be crushed or opened (Guenter & Boullata, 2013). Each medication should be administered separately to avoid drug interaction that could occur when different tablets are ground into a powder, diluted in solution, and administered in the same syringe (Guenter & Boullata, 2013). All nasogastric tubes should be flushed before and after medication administration with at least 15 mL of sterile water to clear the tube and ensure that the medication has reached the stomach (Guenter & Boullata, 2013). This is especially important when small-bore feeding tubes are used, because they can clog easily. During gastric decompression, discontinue suction before administering the medication, and keep the tube clamped for 30 minutes afterward to permit absorption by way of the gastric mucosa.

Home and Community Care

To develop a teaching plan that meets the patient's unique needs, consider features of the patient's home environment that could affect optimal bowel management. For example:

- Does the patient have adequate access to toilet facilities?
- If the patient has to use a walker or wheelchair for mobility, will these devices fit through the bathroom doorway?
- Is there someone available to assist the person to the bathroom or with special interventions such as enema administration?
- Would the use of a bedside commode at home help a person with mobility or access problems prevent fecal incontinence?
- Does the patient have health insurance, and does it cover the necessary medications or special equipment?

If the assessment data disclose potential problems with financial or social support resources, a social worker should be consulted as soon as possible. The social worker is knowledgeable about the many community agencies available for assistance and can begin contacting the community agencies that will best meet the patient's unique needs.

Patients or their families may need assistance and advice in managing specialized equipment and techniques. The patients with a recent ostomy (known as an ostomate) and the patient at high risk for fecal incontinence particularly need assistance in home management of their bowel alterations. WOCNs are often responsible for patient education about ostomy care; however, the home health nurse must reinforce the concepts of stoma management and be available to answer questions.

The patient can be referred to ostomy organizations within the community. Usually, a member of an ostomy organization who also has an ostomy, and who has satisfactorily adjusted to the necessary lifestyle changes, visits with the new ostomate.

The first visit can be arranged before hospital discharge, or it can occur when the patient is at home. The "old" ostomate can be a source of support and advice for the "new" ostomate.

Diarrhea is still a leading cause (among the top ten) of death worldwide and in the top 5 causes of death among children younger than 5 years of age (World Health Organization, 2012). However, it and many other acute and chronic bowel problems can be managed in the home setting under the supervision of a healthcare provider. The viral and bacterial infections that cause severe diarrhea and that predispose the person to severe fluid volume deficit can be controlled as well. In such cases, adequate fluid replacement with rehydrating solutions containing electrolytes is important. Fortunately, various world relief organizations provide rehydrating solutions to decrease mortality from diarrhea. In developed countries, solutions such as Pedialyte or Gatorade can be purchased and used in the home during acute episodes of diarrhea. Hygiene teaching, especially good hand hygiene practice, is important in preventing transmission of microorganisms that cause diarrhea. Hand hygiene with soap and water rather than alcohol-based products is important for contact with anyone having diarrhea because C-diff is not controlled with alcohol-based cleansers.

EVALUATION

Evaluation includes assessing the patient and comparing the patient's current condition with established outcomes as a measure of attainment. Continuation, modification, or termination of problems in the plan of care is implemented based on the systematic evaluation of patient progress.

Examples of outcome criteria are listed here. Note that some are appropriate for more than one goal. It is important to identify specific outcomes that will most uniquely measure the attainment of the individual patient's goal.

Goal

The patient will demonstrate a normal pattern of bowel elimination without evidence of constipation, diarrhea, fecal incontinence, or abdominal distention.

POSSIBLE OUTCOME CRITERIA

- The patient experiences a bowel movement within 24 hours and then every other day during rehabilitation.
- The patient has a decrease in loose stools from four to five per day to one to two per day within 2 days.
- The patient demonstrates a stool consistency changing from liquid to semisoft within 24 hours.
- The patient experiences a bowel movement every morning after suppository and digital stimulation during rehabilitation.
- The patient has no evidence of hardened stool in the rectum on digital examination during each home visit.

PATIENT PLAN OF CARE
The Patient with Constipation

NURSING DIAGNOSIS
Constipation related to immobility manifested by straining and inability to pass stool for 3 days.

PATIENT GOAL
Patient will demonstrate a normal pattern of bowel elimination.

PATIENT OUTCOME CRITERIA
Patient has a formed brown stool within 24 hours and every 1 to 2 days during rehabilitation.

NURSING INTERVENTION	SCIENTIFIC RATIONALE
1. Notify dietitian to increase high-fiber foods in patient's meals.	**1.** High-fiber foods increase the amount of bulk in the lower gastrointestinal tract and result in softer, easier-to-eliminate stools.
2. Increase fluid intake to 2,000 mL per day.	**2.** A fluid intake of 2,000 mL in 24 hours is necessary to promote the formation of soft stools.
3. Assist patient to ambulate (within medically prescribed guidelines) at least three times daily.	**3.** Increased physical activity promotes increased gastrointestinal motility.
4. Assist patient to bedside commode or toilet. Fit commode or toilet with raised seat if needed.	**4.** The sitting position enlists gravity to promote bowel elimination. A raised seat may be necessary to increase patient comfort in sitting.
5. Provide privacy, but do not compromise patient safety.	**5.** Many people require a degree of privacy during bowel elimination, but do not leave the person alone if at risk for falling (wait outside the partially closed door).
6. Inspect patient's abdomen and auscultate for bowel sounds every shift.	**6.** Inspection and auscultation provide essential data about bowel elimination status.
7. Administer stool softeners and laxatives as necessary per bowel management program.	**7.** Daily administration of stool softeners can prevent constipation for patients in high-risk groups. Laxatives can stimulate the evacuation of bowel contents on an as-needed basis.
8. Record the patient's bowel movements in the patient's record.	**8.** Documentation provides essential data about patient's current bowel elimination pattern.

EVALUATION

6/13/17: Had medium, hard stool following Dulcolax suppository. Fluid intake only 900 mL during last 24 hours and ambulating only with encouragement. Senna added to daily meds. Will continue to assess bowel status daily and encourage plan.

—S. Roberts, RN

Goal

The patient will exhibit no preventable complications or adverse consequences from altered bowel elimination.

POSSIBLE OUTCOME CRITERIA

- The patient's perianal skin remains intact throughout the hospital stay.

- After a teaching session, the patient verbalizes the importance of exhaling during defecation.
- Throughout hospitalization, the patient washes his or her hands with soap and water after each bowel movement.

Goal

The patient will participate in a program to maintain and promote an acceptable pattern of bowel elimination.

POSSIBLE OUTCOME CRITERIA

- At the next appointment, the patient identifies methods to increase dietary fiber.
- The patient requests assistance to toilet at scheduled times during the day.
- The patient drinks 2,000 mL of fluid per day, as evidenced on a chart.
- The patient demonstrates correct ostomy bag application by the time of discharge.

KEY CONCEPTS

- Defecation, the process of eliminating feces from the body, is initiated by reflexes in response to intestinal distention.
- Many lifestyle habits affect stool consistency and the pattern of bowel elimination. Physiologic alterations of the intestines also can adversely affect bowel elimination.
- The characteristics of feces and bowel elimination patterns change during the life span.
- Altered bowel elimination can be a source of physiologic, psychological, and social distress.
- The manifestations of altered bowel elimination are constipation, fecal impaction, diarrhea, incontinence, flatulence, and abdominal distention.
- A focused nursing assessment of bowel elimination includes patient history, inspection of stool characteristics, and physical examination of the abdomen and perirectal area.
- The nurse has collaborative responsibilities in laboratory analysis of the feces and other diagnostic procedures.
- The nurse can diagnose and collaboratively treat altered bowel elimination. Treatment measures include medications, enemas, rectal tubes, nasogastric intubation, fecal impaction removal, bowel training, fecal collection during incontinence, and stoma care.
- Discharge planning considers the home environment, such as access to facilities, finances, and use of specialized equipment, and the unique learning needs of the patient and family.
- Continuation, modification, and termination of nursing strategies are based on systematic evaluation of patient response to therapy.

PRACTICING FOR THE NCLEX

CHECK YOUR ANSWERS IN APPENDIX A.

1. Which of the following bowel habits are abnormal?
   a. Breast-fed infant with stool once every 3 days
   b. Toddler smearing or playing with feces
   c. Preschooler with bowel control but not bladder control
   d. Elderly adult with fecal incontinence

2. You are assessing factors related to constipation in your postoperative patient. Which of the following could contribute to constipation? Select all that apply:
   a. Opioid analgesics
   b. Decreased mobility
   c. Fear of pain
   d. Supine position
   e. Lack of privacy

3. This morning, your adult patient reports new onset of frequent diarrhea with mucus and a foul odor. Which medication class would you suspect as being related?
   a. Antibiotic
   b. Dietary supplement
   c. Opioid analgesic
   d. Diuretic

4. Which of the following findings are abnormal?
   a. Borborygmi present
   b. Positive FOBT guaiac
   c. Tympany in LUQ
   d. Convex shape

5. You perform a FOBT guaiac test on a stool sample from a patient with a history of gastrointestinal bleeding. Which step would you do first after applying stool to the Hemoccult slide?
   a. Open flap on reverse side.
   b. Apply developing solution.
   c. Wait 3 to 5 minutes.
   d. Document.

6. You are caring for a female patient who is concerned that she has not had a bowel movement since yesterday and hasn't taken her laxative. You assess her abdomen and find bowel tones throughout all quadrants, reports of flatus, and abdomen is soft and not distended or tender. Which nursing diagnosis would be most appropriate for this patient?
   a. Constipation
   b. Perceived Constipation
   c. Deficient Fluid Volume
   d. Anxiety

7. You determine that your patient is at risk for constipation related to his postoperative status. What interventions can you provide to reduce this risk?
   a. Request high-protein foods to be included on the dietary tray.
   b. Encourage foods high in magnesium.
   c. Promote ambulation as tolerated.
   d. Promote intake of cold fluids.

8. You have just placed a nasogastric tube for gastric decompression secondary to a paralytic ileus. What is the first thing that you need to do?
   a. Connect tubing to intermittent suction.
   b. Ensure accurate placement.
   c. Provide liquid medications via tube.
   d. Irrigate tube to maintain patency.

9. You are providing discharge teaching to a patient with a colostomy. You include the following instructions about applying the colostomy wafer and bag. Select all that apply:

    a. Ensure that the opening in the wafer is tight to the stoma to prevent leakage.

    b. Leakage of colostomy contents to the surrounding area may lead to skin breakdown.

    c. Stoma coloring that is dusky or pale like the surrounding skin is normal.

    d. Some bleeding may occur because stoma tissues are fragile.

10. The wound nurse is visiting a patient with a new colostomy for a final appointment prior to discharge. Which patient statements would be most concerning?

    a. "I can't stand to even look at my stomach!"

    b. "I know that I have to empty the bag when it is one third full."

    c. "The stoma is beefy red, which is normal."

    d. "I have trouble securing the wafer because of abdominal discomfort."

REFERENCES

American Cancer Society. (2014a). *Colorectal cancer: Prevention and early detection.* Retrieved September 20, 2014, from www. cancer.org

American Cancer Society. (2014b). *Colorectal cancer: What are the key statistics about colorectal cancer?* Retrieved September 20, 2014, from www.cancer.org

Austin, M., Mellow, M., & Tierney, W. M. (2014). Fecal microbiota transplantation in the treatment of *Clostridium difficile* infections. *The American Journal of Medicine, 127*(6), 479–483.

Blackburn, S. (2013). *Maternal, fetal & neonatal physiology: A clinical perspective* (4th ed.). St. Louis, MO: Elsevier Saunders.

Bouras, E., & Tangalos, E. (2009). Chronic constipation in the elderly. *Gastroenterology Clinics of North America, 38*(3), 463–480.

Burke, K. E., & Lamont, J. T. (2013). Fecal transplantation for recurrent *Clostridium difficile* infection in older adults: A review. *Journal of the American Geriatrics Society, 61*(8), 1394–1398.

Costilla, V., & Foxx-Orenstein, A. (2014). Constipation: Understanding mechanisms and management. *Clinics in Geriatric Medicine, 30*(1), 107–115.

Dodin, M., & Katz, D. (2014). Facal microbiota transplantation for *Clostridium difficile* infection. *International Journal of Clinical Practice, 68*(3), 363–368.

Gardiner, A. B. (2013). The effects of ageing on the gastrointestinal system. *Nursing & Residential Care, 15*(1), 30–33.

Gié, O., & Christoforidis, D. (2011). Advances in the treatment of fecal incontinence. *Seminars in Colon & Rectal Surgery, 22*(1), 30–38.

Greenwald, B. J. (2010). Clinical practice guidelines for pediatric constipation. *Journal of the American Academy of Nurse Practitioners, 22*(7), 333–338.

Guenter, P., & Boullata, J. (2013). Drug administration by enteral feeding tube. *Nursing, 43*(12), 26–35.

Hunter, R. (2014). Nursing management of constipation in the medical-surgical setting. *MedSurg Matters, 23*(2), 4–9.

Irving, S. Y., Lyman, B., Northington, L., Bartlett, J. A., & Kemper, C. (2014). Nasogastric tube placement and verification in children: Review of the current literature. *Critical Care Nurse, 34*(3), 67–78.

Jarvis, C. (2012). *Physical examination and health assessment* (6th ed.). St. Louis, MO: Elsevier Saunders.

Jones, C., & Gardiner, A. (2014). Common gastrointestinal problems in pregnancy. *Gastrointestinal Nursing, 12*(6), 11–12.

Kee, V. (2012). *Clostridium difficile* infection in older adults: A review and update on its management. *The American Journal of Geriatric Pharmacotherapy, 10*(1), 14–24.

Longo, M. A. (2011). Best evidence: Nasogastric tube placement verification. *Journal of Pediatric Nursing, 26*, 373–376.

Marcason, W. (2008). Question of the month. Is caffeine considered a diuretic and should my clients increase their fluid intake to compensate for this effect? *Journal of the American Dietetic Association, 108*(5), 908.

Maughan, R. J., & Griffin, J. (2003). Caffeine ingestion and fluid balance: A review. *Journal of Human Nutrition and Dietetics, 16*, 411–420.

McCrea, G. L., Miaskowski, C., Stotts, N., Macera, L., & Varma, M. G. (2008). Pathophysiology of constipation in the older adult. *World Journal of Gastroenterology, 14*(17), 2633–2638.

Mitchell, G. (2014). Managing Constipation in primary care. *Primary Health Care, 24*(5), 18–22.

North American Nursing Diagnosis Association International (NANDA-I). (2014). *Nursing diagnoses: Definitions and classification, 2015–2017.* West Sussex, England: Wiley-Blackwell.

O'Connor, N, ed. (2013). *Gastroenterology Nursing: A Core Curriculum* (5th ed.). Chicago, IL: Society of Gastroenterology Nurses and Associates, Inc.

Osland, E., Yunus, R., Khan, S., & Memon, M. (2011). Early versus traditional postoperative feeding in patients undergoing resectional gastrointestinal surgery: A meta-analysis. *JPEN Journal of Parenteral & Enteral Nutrition, 35*(4), 473–487.

Pacheco, S., & Johnson, S. (2013). Important clinical advances in the understanding of *Clostridium difficile* infection. *Current Opinion in Gastroenterology, 29*(1), 42–48.

Proehl, J. A., Heaton, K., Naccarato, M. K., Crowley, M. A., Storer, A., Moretz, J.D., & Suling, L. (2011). Emergency nursing resource: Gastric tube placement verification. *Journal of Emergency Nursing, 37*, 357–362.

Samuel, B. P., Crumb, T. L., & Duba, M. M. (2014). What nurses need to know about fecal microbiota transplantation: Education, assessment, and care for children and young adults. *Journal of Pediatric Nursing, 29*(4), 354–361.

Scott, K. M. (2014). Pelvic floor rehabilitation in the treatment of fecal incontinence. *Clinics in Colon and Rectal Surgery, 27*(3), 99–105.

Shrikhande, S. V., Shetty, G. S., Singh, K., & Ingle, S. (2009). Is early feeding after major gastrointestinal surgery a fashion or an advance? *Journal of Cancer Research and Therapeutics, 5*(4), 232–239.

World Health Organization. (2012). Top 10 causes of death. Retrieved October 27, 2014, from www.who.org

Procedure 33-1 Assessing Stool for Occult Blood (FOBT)

Purpose
1. Screen patients who have or who are at risk for gastrointestinal bleeding.
2. Screen for early-stage colon cancer.

Equipment
Bedpan, bedside commode, or toilet hat to catch stool
Disposable examination gloves
Tongue blade or wooden applicator stick
Prepackaged Hemoccult cardboard slide, developing solution, and several drops of water

Assessment
- Review the patient's medical and drug history for risk factors for gastrointestinal bleeding.
- Assess the patient's understanding of need for the procedure and his or her ability to cooperate.
- Note the patient's dietary history and need for any modifications before the test. Red meat and iron preparations can cause false-positive test results for occult blood. Some physicians may restrict ingestion of these products for 72 hours before the test. Ingestion of large amounts of vitamin C can cause a false-negative result.
- Note use of medications such as aspirin, ibuprofen, or steroids, which can cause gastrointestinal irritation. These are often also restricted prior to testing.

Procedure

1. **Perform hand hygiene.**
   Rationale: Reduces microbe transmission.

2. **Identify the patient using two separate identifiers.**
   Rationale: Ensures correct patient receives proper assessment or treatment and reduces errors.

3. **Close door or bed curtains and explain procedure to the patient.**
   Rationale: Ensures patient privacy, increases patient compliance, reduces patient anxiety, and promotes learning.

4. **Ask the patient to void before collecting the stool specimen.**
   Rationale: Urine mixed with the stool sample could dilute the stool sample and prevent detection of occult blood. If urine has red blood cells, the test results might be positive but the source would be masked.

5. **Assist the patient onto bedpan or commode or to bathroom. Provide privacy; leave call bell handy.**
   Rationale: Provides for patient safety and dignity.

6. **Once the patient has passed stool and is clean and comfortable, don disposable gloves and obtain small amount of stool with a tongue blade or wooden applicator. Do not use any stool that has gross blood present.**
   Rationale: Prevents transmission of microorganisms to others. Observable blood probably originates from hemorrhoids and not from the intestines.

Hemoccult Slide Test

7. **Open flap of slide and apply a very thin smear of stool taken from the center of the specimen onto first window.**
   Rationale: Samples obtained from the edges are likely to be contaminated. The guaiac filter paper is very sensitive to blood content, so only a small sample is needed.

8. **Using second applicator, obtain a second sample from a different area of the stool. Smear thinly on second window of slide (Fig. 1).**

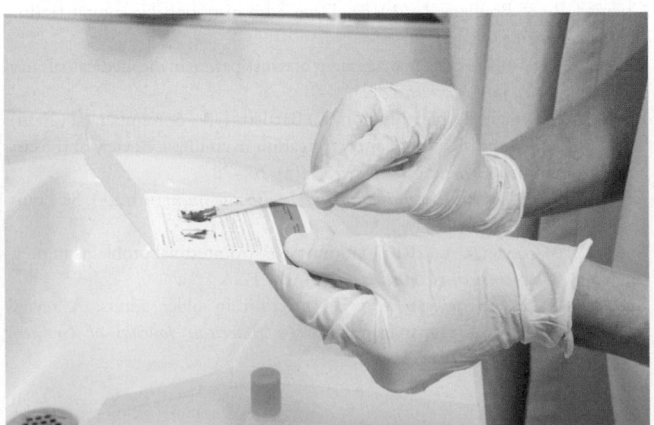

FIG. 1 Apply a thin smear of stool on Hemoccult slide.

Rationale: Blood may not be equally distributed throughout the stool sample. Testing findings from one area may not reveal blood in another area. In acute care agencies, physicians typically order samples to be tested on three different occasions.

Procedure 33-1   *continued*

9. **Wait 3 minutes.**

   Rationale: Fresh specimens require a minimum of 3 minutes of contact with the test paper to ensure validity of the test.

10. **Close slide cover and turn over. Then open the flap on the reverse side and apply two drops of the developing solution onto each window and one drop onto the control window (Figs. 2 and 3). Wait 30 to 60 seconds. Read test results (Fig. 4).**

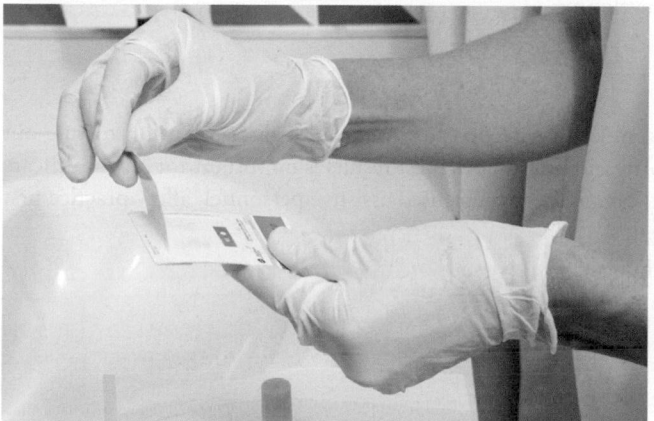

FIG. 2 Open flap on reverse side of slide.

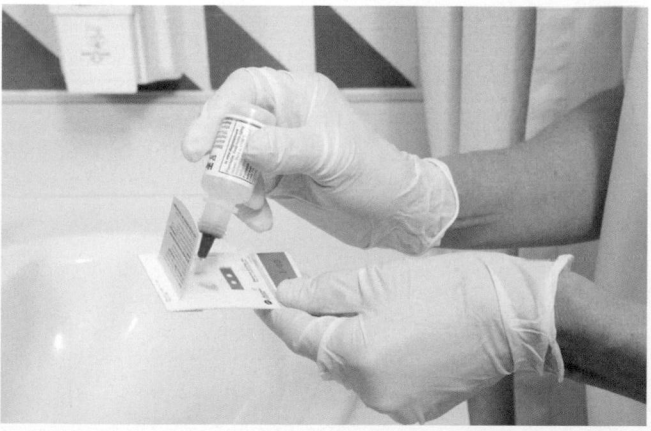

FIG. 3 Apply Hemoccult developing solution on slide window.

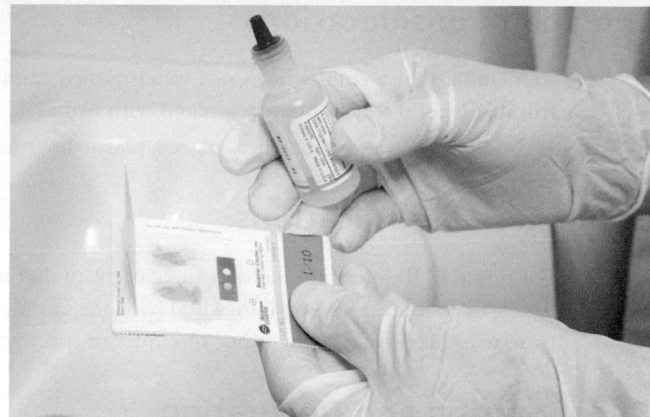

FIG. 4 Read test results. Blue discoloration indicates occult blood is present.

   Rationale: The developing solution penetrates the stool sample to react chemically with the blood. The positive control should turn blue, and the negative control should not change color. This indicates that the test paper will accurately detect occult blood. Stool test results are positive, indicating the presence of blood, if the filter paper has a bluish tint. Stool test findings are negative if there is no color change.

11. **Remove gloves, wash hands, and document findings.**

   Rationale: Maintains infection control and legal patient record.

Documentation

10/8/17: 14:00—Uncontaminated stool sample tested negative for occult blood; patient instructed that 2 more samples will be collected and tested to rule out GI bleeding.

—S. Roberts, RN

Procedure 33-1   *continued*

Life Span Considerations

- Remember that a child who is not toilet trained cannot cooperate with stool specimen collection. Obtain the specimen from a diaper if it is not contaminated with urine.
- If the child has watery diarrhea, place a plastic liner inside the diaper and use a cotton swab to obtain the specimen.

Home Care Modifications

- For home FOBT testing, instruct the patient in diet modifications that need to be made before collecting the specimen. Teach the patient to prepare the slide with the sample, close cardboard flap, write his or her name on the slide, and mail or return the sample to the office or clinic for specimen developing.

Collaboration and Delegation

- All personnel responsible for point of care FOBT testing must be screened for visual color discrimination to rule out color blindness. Validation of the ability to correctly perform and interpret the test results is important for any healthcare personnel performing the test. When teaching the patient, caregiver, or unlicensed assistive personnel, allow practice first with hamburger juice to see if technique has been mastered.
- Encourage validation of test results if color change is minimal.

Procedure 33-2 Administering an Enema

Purpose	1. Relieves gas, constipation, or fecal impaction 2. Cleanses the bowel in preparation for diagnostic tests or surgical procedures 3. Evacuates feces in patients with hemiplegia, quadriplegia, or paraplegia 4. Delivers medication
Equipment	Enema container with appropriately sized tubing (adult, size 22 to 32 French; child, size 14 to 18 French; infant—size 12 French or a bulb syringe) Possible solutions—normal saline, tap water, soap solution, medications, or commercially prepared small-volume enema Disposable gloves and water-soluble lubricant Personal hygiene items—disposable wipes or soap, towel, water Waterproof bed protector Clean bedpan or commode, and toilet paper. Children may use potty-chair or diaper.
Assessment	• Assess the patient's past and present elimination history: presence of hemorrhoids, external and internal. • Review the healthcare provider's order, and determine the purpose for the enema. • If constipation or impaction is suspected, palpate the abdomen for distention, and perform digital rectal examination. • Determine the patient's understanding of the purpose for the enema, what to expect during the procedure, and how he or she can help.

Procedure

Large-Volume Enema

1. **Assemble the needed equipment in one place.**
   Rationale: Increases efficiency and saves time.

2. **Prepare solution. Check temperature of solution by pouring some over your inner wrist. Fill enema bag with 750- to 1,000-mL lukewarm solution (105°F; for child, 500 mL or less, 100°F) (Fig. 1).**

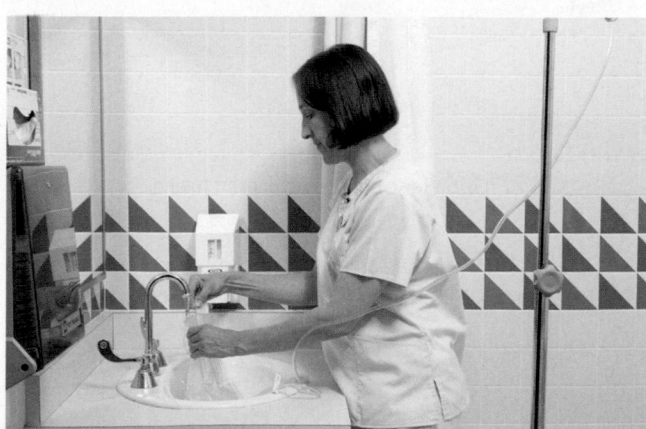

FIG. 1 Fill enema bag.

Rationale: Intestinal mucosa can be damaged if the solution is too warm. Cold solutions are difficult to retain and can cause abdominal cramping.

3. **Open clamp on tubing and allow solution to flow through tubing to remove the air (Fig. 2). Reclamp tubing.**

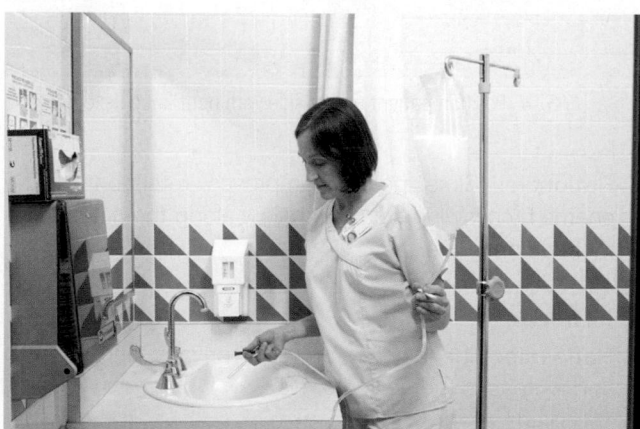

FIG. 2 Open clamp and allow solution to flow through tubing.

Rationale: Air in the rectum causes discomfort.

4. **Provide privacy by closing curtains or room door.**
   Rationale: Providing privacy reduces embarrassment for the patient and increases his or her ability to relax.

Procedure 33-2   *continued*

5. **Identify patient (Fig. 3). Position patient on left side (Sims position) with right knee flexed (Fig. 4).**

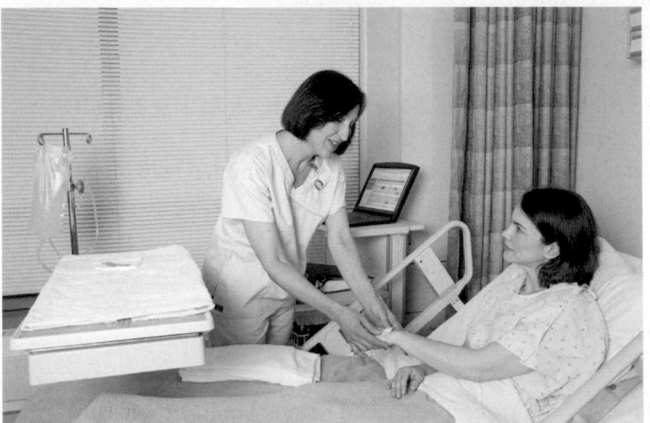

FIG. 3 Identify patient with 2 separate identifiers.

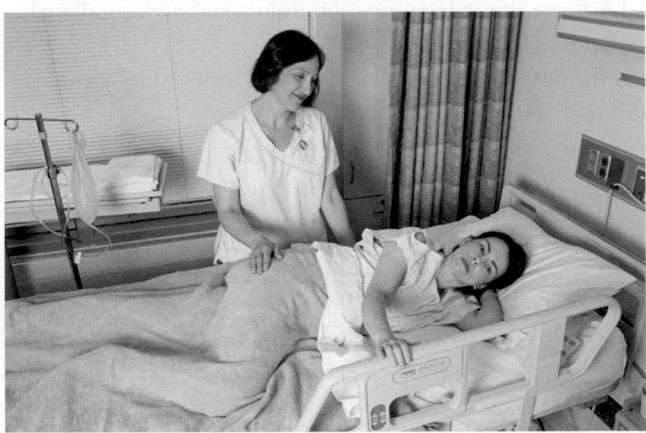

FIG. 4 Position patient on left side with right knee flexed.

Rationale: Sims position improves retention of the enema by allowing solution to flow along the natural sigmoid colon curve.

6. **Cover patient with bath blanket, exposing only the buttocks.**
   Rationale: The blanket provides privacy and warmth and increases the ability to relax.

7. **Put on disposable gloves. Place waterproof pad under patient's buttocks.**
   Rationale: Prevents soiling of linen and maintains infection control.

8. **Lubricate 2 to 3 inches of the tip of the rectal tube with water-soluble lubricant (Fig. 5).**

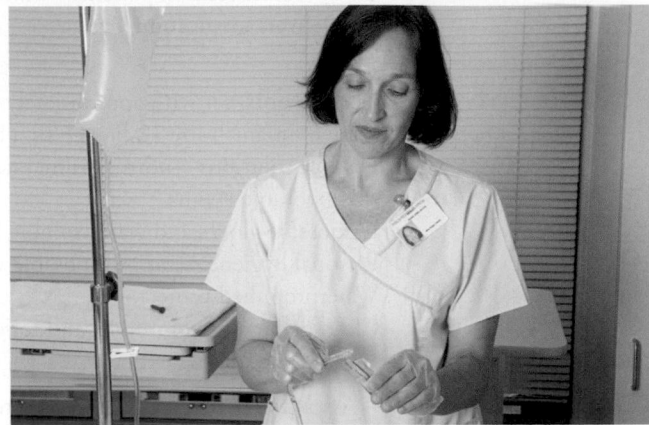

FIG. 5 Lubricate tube with water-soluble lubricant.

Rationale: Insertion is smoother, and trauma is minimized with lubrication.

9. **Separate the buttocks to visualize the anus. Observe for external hemorrhoids. Ask patient to take a slow, deep breath. Gently insert the tube, directing the tip toward the umbilicus (adult: 3 to 4 inches) (Fig. 6).**

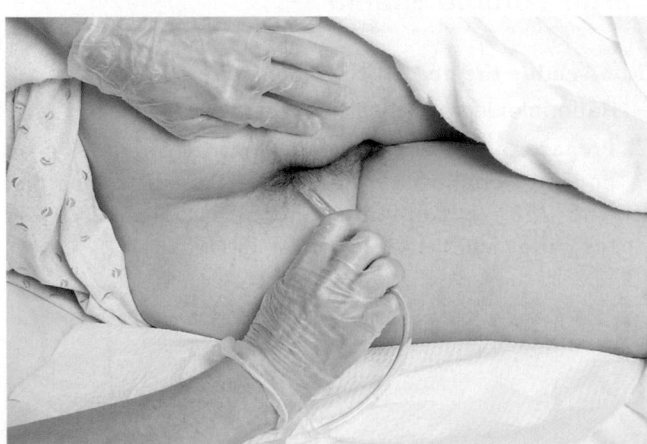

FIG. 6 Raise buttocks and insert tubing.

Rationale: Prevents injury to the intestinal mucosa by directing the tube along the natural bowel curve.

Procedure 33-2 *continued*

10. **Continue holding the tube in the rectum (Fig. 7). With other hand, open the clamp and allow solution to slowly enter the patient (Fig. 8). Raise container 18 inches above the anus, allowing solution to flow slowly over 5 to 10 minutes; if patient complains of cramping or pain, have patient breathe deeply and lower bag until the sensation stops.**

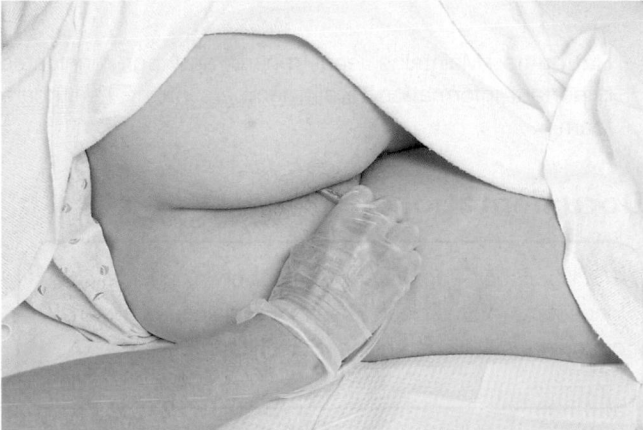

FIG. 7 Hold tube securely in place.

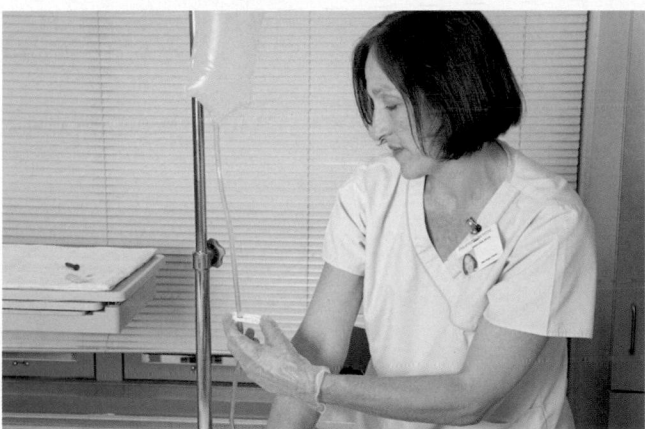

FIG. 8 Open clamp.

Rationale: Slow instillation reduces patient discomfort from bowel distention and cramping, thereby allowing a greater volume of solution to be retained.

11. **Reclamp tubing when desired amount of solution has infused.**

Rationale: Clamping prevents air from entering the rectum.

12. **Remove tube gently and have patient squeeze buttocks together firmly for several minutes.**

Rationale: The urge to defecate caused by tube removal will decrease if sphincters are contracted.

13. **Have patient retain solution as long as possible.**

Rationale: Longer retention enhances peristalsis and evacuation of bowel contents.

14. **Assist the patient to bathroom, commode, or bedpan. Place call bell within reach. Provide privacy until all of the solution has been expelled.**

Rationale: Increases patient comfort and safety.

15. **Visually inspect character of the feces and solution.**

Rationale: If enemas are ordered "until clear" as preparation for diagnostic testing, it is essential to assess expelled solution for fecal material. Allow the patient to rest, and then repeat as necessary.

16. **Assist the patient into comfortable position. Assist with cleansing as needed. Provide materials for the patient to wash hands. Open windows or provide air freshener if needed. Clean and dispose of equipment as necessary. Remove gloves and wash hands.**

Rationale: Spread of microorganisms is prevented, and patient comfort is increased.

Small-Volume Enema

1. **Follow steps 1 to 5 from the Large-Volume Enema procedure.**
2. **Remove protective cap from prelubricated catheter tip (Fig. 9). You may add more lubricant if necessary.**

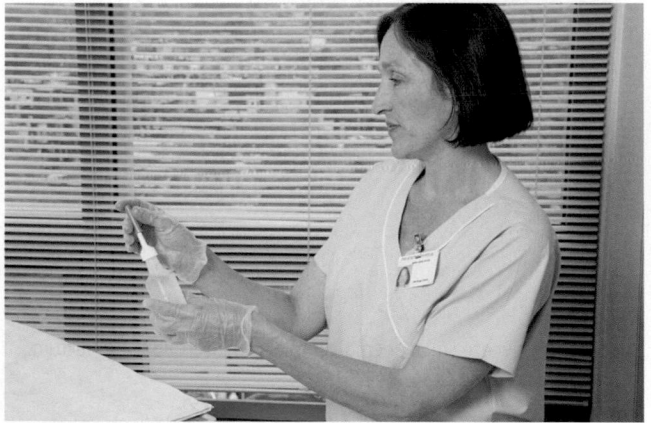

FIG. 9 Remove protective cap.

Rationale: Allows smooth insertion of the rectal tip and minimizes trauma to the rectal mucosa.

Procedure 33-2 *continued*

3. **Separate the buttocks to visualize the anus. Observe for hemorrhoids and gently insert rectal tip into rectum, directing the tip toward the umbilicus (Fig. 10).**

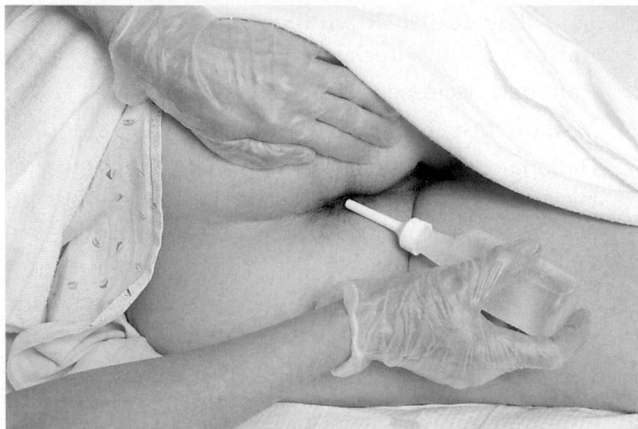

FIG. 10 Raise buttocks and insert rectal tip into rectum.

Rationale: Prevents injury to the rectal mucosa by following the natural curve of the bowel.

4. **Squeeze bottle to empty contents into the rectum and colon (approximately 240 mL of solution) (Fig. 11).**

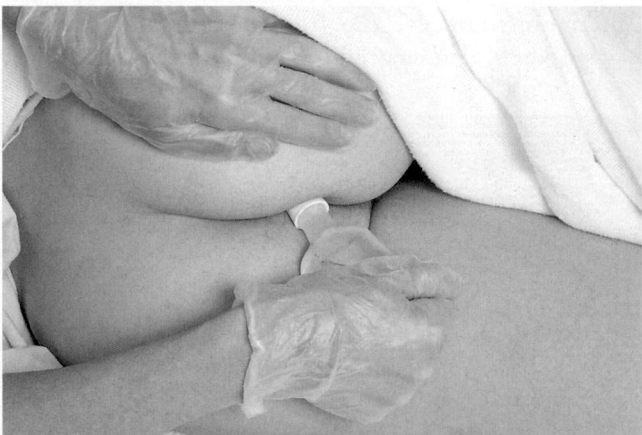

FIG. 11 Squeeze small enema container to insert fluid into rectum.

Rationale: Prepackaged solutions are usually hypertonic and require only small volumes to stimulate defecation. They are not to be used in children!

5. **Maintain pressure on the enema container until you withdraw it from the rectum.**

Rationale: Releasing the pressure while the container is still in the rectum will cause the liquid to be drawn back into the container.

6. **Continue with steps 13 through 16 above for a large-volume enema.**

7. **Document administration and the results from the enema.**

Rationale: Maintains legal record and communicates important information to all members of the healthcare team.

Documentation

4/3/17: 08:15—Tap water enema given X3 prior to colonoscopy, returns clear. Patient complained of minimal cramping. Awaiting transfer to GI unit for test.

—S. Roberts, RN

Life Span Considerations

Infants and Children

- Administer an enema with the child in the dorsal recumbent position. Children who are not toilet trained are incontinent, and other children may be unable to control their rectal sphincter sufficiently to retain enema solutions.
- Ensure that the healthcare provider orders the amount of solution to be administered for children under 2 years of age.
- Children and infants do not usually receive tap water or prepackaged hypertonic enemas because fatal water intoxication or circulatory depletion could occur.
- Insert the rectal tube 1 to 1.5 inches in an infant and 2 to 3 inches for a child.

Older Adults

- If an adult is incontinent, place clean, dry, waterproof linen under his or her buttocks until enema solution has been expelled and the buttocks are cleaned.
- Because the skin of older adults macerates easily from prolonged contact with moisture, check frequently for newly expelled stool and clean as necessary.
- If the older adult has poor sphincter control, administer the enema with the patient in the dorsal recumbent position on a bedpan.

Home Care Modifications

- Teach patients not to rely on enemas to maintain bowel regularity. Enemas do not treat the cause of irregularity and, if used frequently, can result in dependence on enemas for defecation because they can disrupt normal elimination reflexes.

Collaboration and Delegation

- Be sure to give clear instructions when delegating the enema procedure to patients, caregivers, or unlicensed assistive personnel.
- Reinforce the need to avoid inserting the enema tubing too far into the rectum, which could result in intestinal irritation or perforation.
- Mark the appropriate length on the tubing for the patient, caregiver, or personnel as necessary.
- When high colonic irrigations are ordered or in cases of severe impaction, consult a nurse who has extensive experience in gastroenterology.

Procedure 33-3 Applying a Fecal Ostomy Pouch

Purpose

1. Contains drainage and odors for the comfort of the ostomy patient
2. Protects the peristomal skin from excoriation
3. Allows accurate assessment of output, especially in the postoperative period
4. Provides visualization of the stoma and sutures during the postoperative period

Equipment

Clean, drainable pouch and clamp
Skin barrier and/or skin protectant
Disposable gloves
Disposable wipes or warm water, washcloth, mild soap, and towel
Toilet tissue
Gauze pad
Plastic disposal bag for old pouch

Assessment

- Observe color and amount of drainage from stoma.
- Assess existing pouch for leakage, and note appearance of stoma and incision to determine need to change pouch. A pouch does not have to be changed if it is not leaking and if the skin barrier is intact.
- Inspect condition of peristomal skin for erythema, excoriation, ulceration, or fistulas before selecting type of skin barrier to apply.
- Note presence of skinfolds, creases, scars, and abdominal softness or firmness before selecting pouch.

Procedure

1. **Perform hand hygiene and don gloves. The patient may perform the procedure without gloves.**
   Rationale: Reduces microbe transmission.

2. **Identify the patient.**
   Rationale: Ensures correct patient receives proper assessment or treatment and reduces errors.

3. **Close door or bed curtains and explain procedure to the patient.**
   Rationale: Ensures patient privacy, increases patient compliance, and reduces patient anxiety.

4. **Place a waterproof pad by stoma site (Fig. 1).**

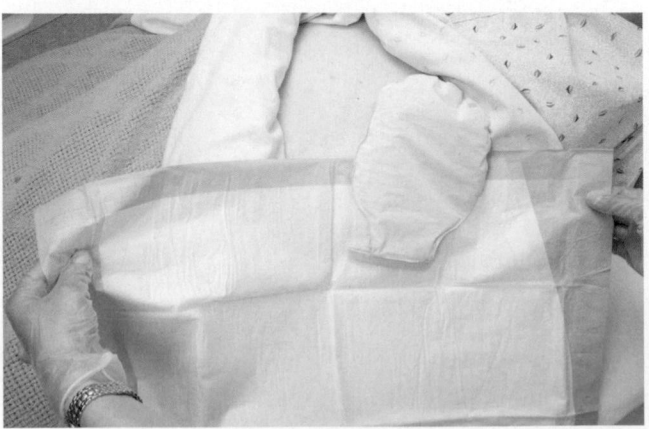

FIG. 1 Place a waterproof pad by stoma site.

Rationale: Prevents transmission of microorganisms to others.

5. **Start at the top of the appliance (Fig. 2); gently remove old appliance (and skin barrier if applicable) by pushing skin away from appliance (do not pull appliance from skin) (Fig. 3). If disposable, discard. If reusable, set aside for washing.**

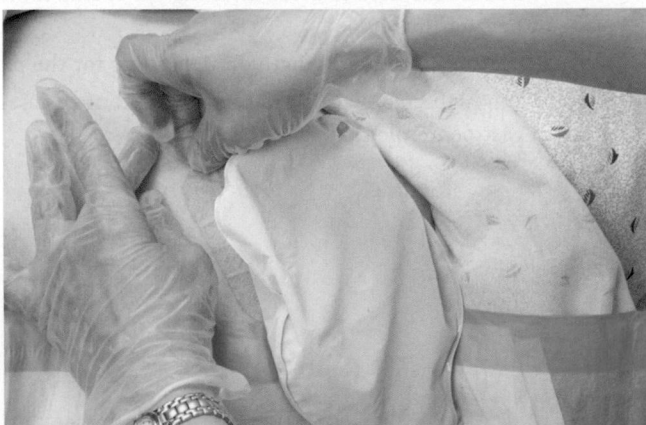

FIG. 2 Start at the top when removing the appliance.

Procedure 33-3 *continued*

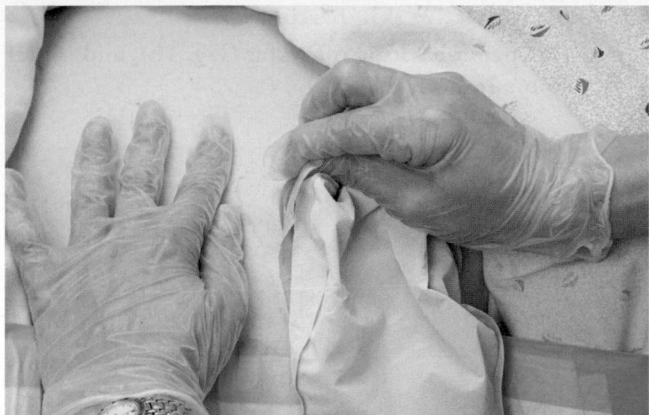

FIG. 3 Gently remove appliance by pushing skin away from the appliance.

> **Rationale:** Maintains skin integrity.

6. **Use toilet tissue to remove excess stool (Fig. 4). Wash skin thoroughly around stoma with skin cleanser or soap and water.**

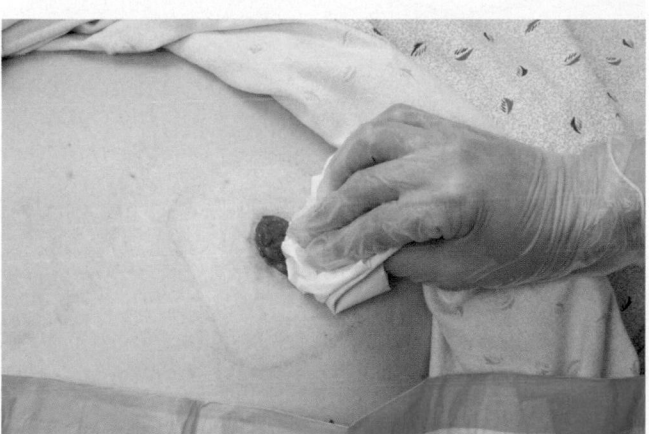

FIG. 4 Use toilet tissue to remove excess stool.

> **Rationale:** Bacteria in the fecal secretions can cause infection in the incisional area and irritate the skin.

7. **Rinse skin thoroughly and blot dry.**

> **Rationale:** Soap residue or dampness can interfere with pouch adhesion, resulting in leakage. Blotting the area dry minimizes trauma to the stoma.

8. **Observe condition of peristomal skin, the stoma, and the sutures. Teach the patient to make these observations daily.**

> **Rationale:** Observation allows monitoring for complications. The stoma is at risk for necrosis during the first postoperative week, as evidenced by dark color and lack of bleeding. The peristomal skin is at risk for breakdown from irritating fecal secretions. Infection is more easily corrected if detected early.

9. **Cover stoma with gauze while you prepare new appliance (Fig. 5). Prepare appliance and/or skin barrier: Measure stoma using a measurement guide (Fig. 6), and trace stoma measurement on the adhesive paper backing of appliance or barrier (Fig. 7). Cut the opening $\frac{1}{8}$ inch larger than tracing (Fig. 8).**

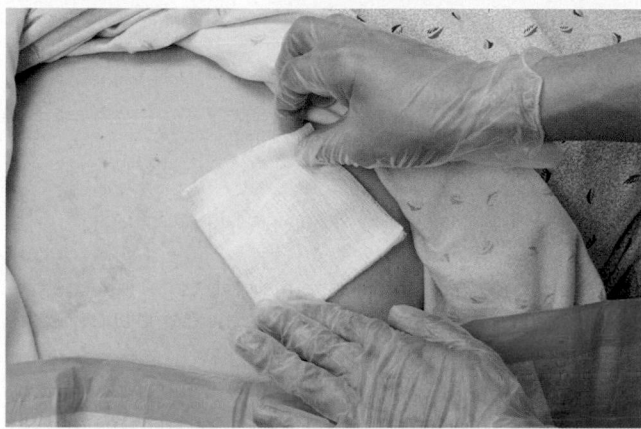

FIG. 5 Cover stoma with gauze.

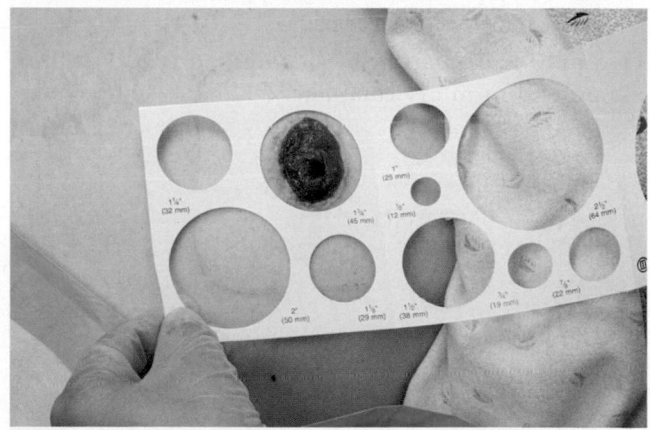

FIG. 6 Use measurement guide to measure stoma.

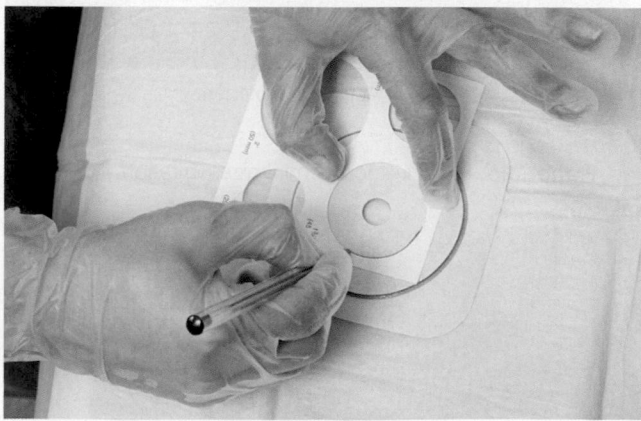

FIG. 7 Trace measurement on back of new appliance.

Procedure 33-3 *continued*

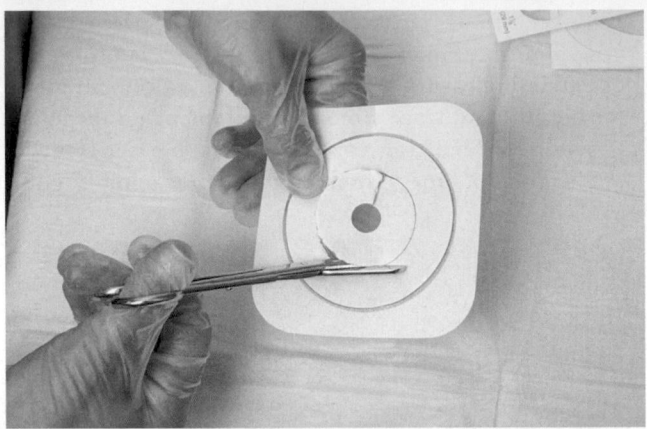

FIG. 8 Cut an opening ⅛ of an inch larger than tracing.

Rationale: Cutting the pattern slightly larger than the barrier avoids the risk of paper cuts to the stoma and ensures a tight seal with the barrier.

10. **If stoma is located in an abdominal crease or the skin is irregular, use a paste barrier to fill the irregularity.**

    Rationale: Minimizes leakage by providing a smooth surface for applying the skin barrier.

11. **Apply protectant as needed/desired (Fig. 9). Allow protectant to dry completely.**

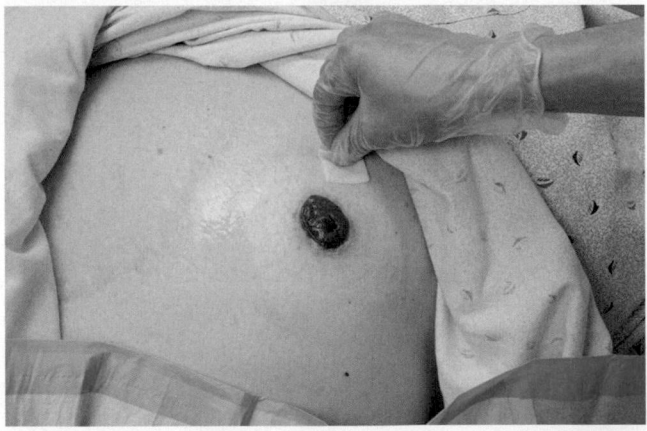

FIG. 9 Apply skin protectant.

Rationale: Skin protectant minimizes irritation.

12. **Apply protective skin barrier:**
    a. **Peel paper backing off wafer (Fig. 10), and center stoma in hole (Fig. 11).**

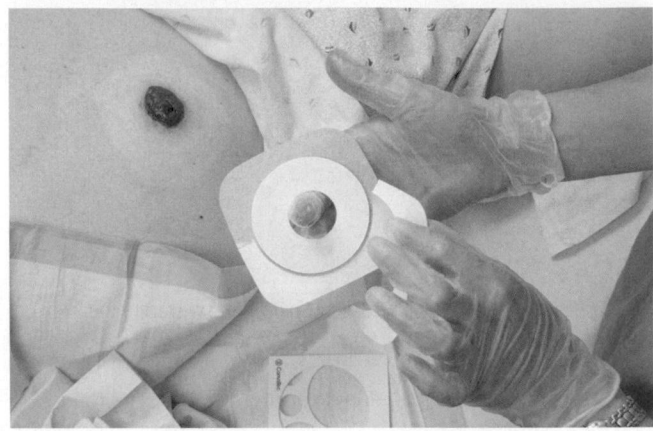

FIG. 10 Peel paper backing off barrier.

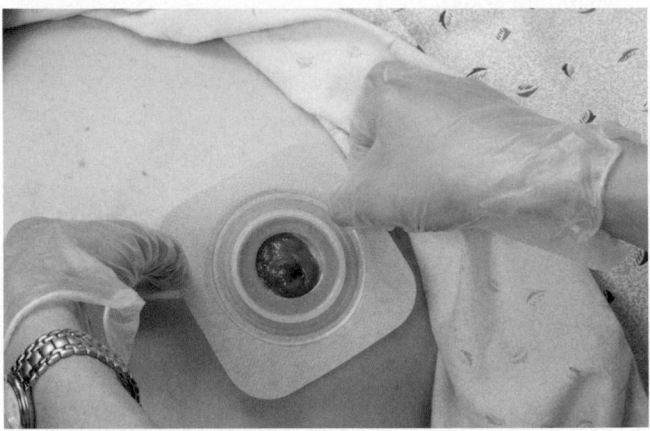

FIG. 11 Center barrier opening with stoma.

Rationale: Prepares the wafer for application.

Procedure 33-3 *continued*

b. Place on abdomen, pressing lightly over all areas of the barrier to promote adhesion with skin surfaces (Fig. 12).

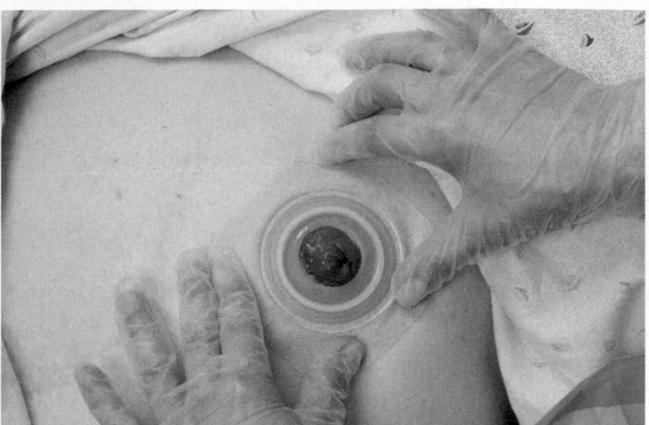

FIG. 12 Gently press to adhere barrier to skin.

Rationale: A tight fit will prevent leaking and protect the skin underlying the appliance.

13. Attach drainable pouch to skin barrier (Fig. 13). Some equipment attaches by means of a plastic flange that snaps in place; other models adhere through self-adherent tape that is exposed after protective paper backing is removed. Tug gently or inspect for secure fit.

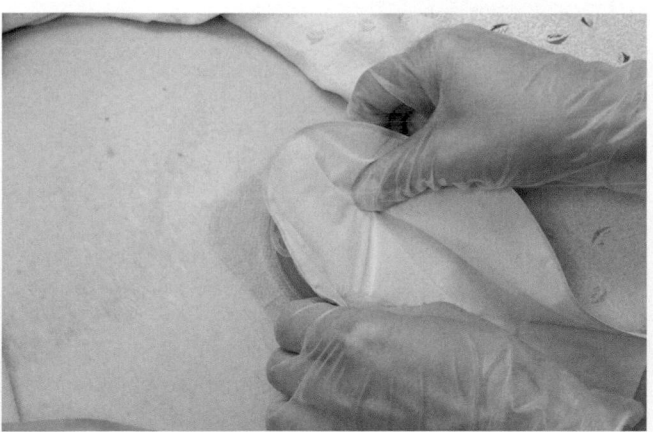

FIG. 13 Attach appliance to skin barrier.

Rationale: If the pouch is not securely attached to the protective barrier, leakage could occur, especially as weight from collected feces increases.

14. Fold over bottom edge of pouch and clamp (Fig. 14).

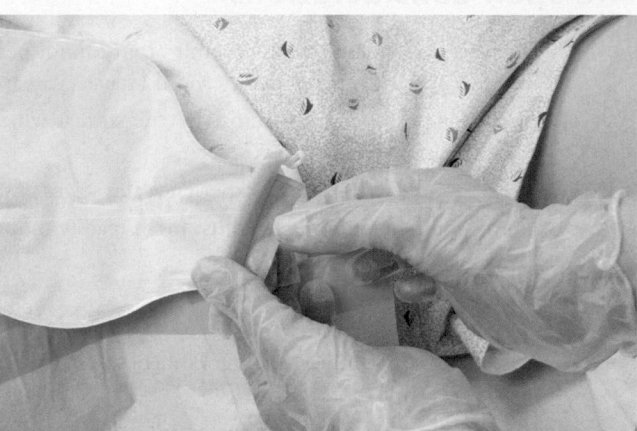

FIG. 14 Clamp edge of pouch.

Rationale: Prevents stool from leaking.

15. Dispose of old appliance. Clean and store any reusable supplies. Wash hands. Document observations.

Rationale: Maintains infection control standards and communicates with health team members.

Documentation

3/10/17: 07:30—
P: Risk for impaired skin integrity.
I: Colostomy bag changed with patient actively participating and asking questions. Stoma pink and moist, peristomal skin intact, draining moderate amount of liquid brown stool.
E: Current appliance working well and patient appears ready for discharge in 2 days. Will continue to work on independent emptying and flushing of bag and will complete WOCN referral for home care.

—L. Wren, RN

Procedure 33-3   *continued*

Life Span Considerations

- The very young and the older adult often cannot perform their own ostomy care. Any patient who is not able to change his or her pouch independently should have a caregiver instructed in this procedure.
- Assess for postoperative necrosis of the stoma, which occurs more commonly in obese patients. Notify the healthcare provider immediately if this is seen.
- New ostomy patients often experience the stages of grief as they try to adjust to their new body image.
- Young children and infants adjust more readily to lifestyle changes from ostomies than do adolescents and adults.

Home Care Modifications

- Teach spouses or other family members to assist with ostomy management, especially if the patient is impaired or weak or has poor fine motor skills.
- Provide good nurse–patient communication to help the patient develop a positive attitude about living with an ostomy.
- Provide the patient with the name and phone number of a WOCN therapist, community support groups, supply vendor, and other resource people to call if he or she has questions or problems after discharge.

Collaboration and Delegation

- Nurses who specialize in the management of ostomies (WOCNs) provide initial instruction and often follow the patient on an outpatient basis.
- Consult with this nurse so that you can reinforce teaching and coordinate the plan.

Procedure 33-4 Inserting a Nasogastric Tube

Purpose	1. Decompresses the stomach to relieve pressure and prevent vomiting 2. Provides a means for irrigating the stomach (lavage) 3. Provides access to gastric specimens for laboratory analysis 4. Provides a route for delivering liquid enteral feedings (gavage) in patients who can't swallow or ingest adequate calorie intake (see Chapter 29)
Equipment	Nasogastric tube of appropriate size (adult, 14 to 18 French; infant/child, 5 to 10 French) or small-bore feeding tube with guide wire if used for enteral feedings Water-soluble lubricant 20- to 50-mL syringe with catheter tip or adapter Glass of tap water with straw Towel, stethoscope, disposable gloves Hypoallergenic tape
Assessment	• Identify the patient's need for nasogastric intubation and type of tube to be placed. • Assess the patient's mental status and ability to understand and cooperate with procedure. • Ask the patient or review medical history for nosebleeds, deviated septum, or nasal surgery. • Assess nostrils for size, lesions, obstructions, or deformities. Have patient breathe through one nostril while occluding the other. The tube should be inserted through the most patent nostril.

Procedure

1. **Perform hand hygiene.**
   Rationale: Reduces microbe transmission.

2. **Identify the patient.**
   Rationale: Ensures correct patient receives proper assessment or treatment and reduces errors.

3. **Close door or bed curtains and explain procedure to the patient. Insertion is not painful, but it is uncomfortable because the gag reflex is usually stimulated.**
   Rationale: Ensures patient privacy, increases patient compliance, reduces patient anxiety, and promotes learning.

4. **Raise bed to high Fowler position, cover chest with towel or drape, and place emesis basin nearby (Fig. 1).**

5. **Determine length of tubing to be inserted by measuring nasogastric tube from tip of nose to tip of earlobe, then to tip of xiphoid process (Fig. 2). Mark tubing with adhesive tape or note striped markings already on the tube.**

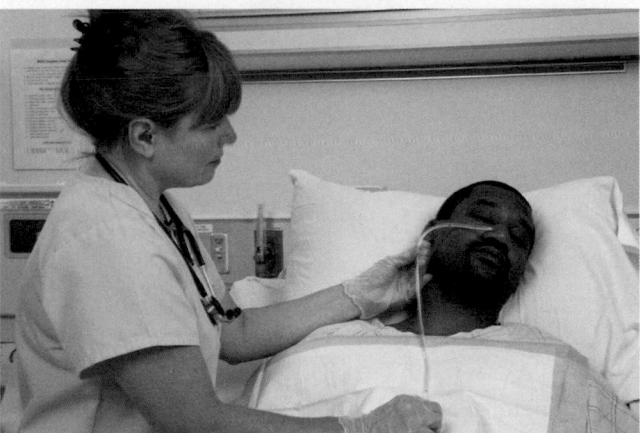

FIG. 2 Determine length of tubing.

Rationale: This measure determines the approximate length of the esophagus from the nares to the stomach, which varies among patients.

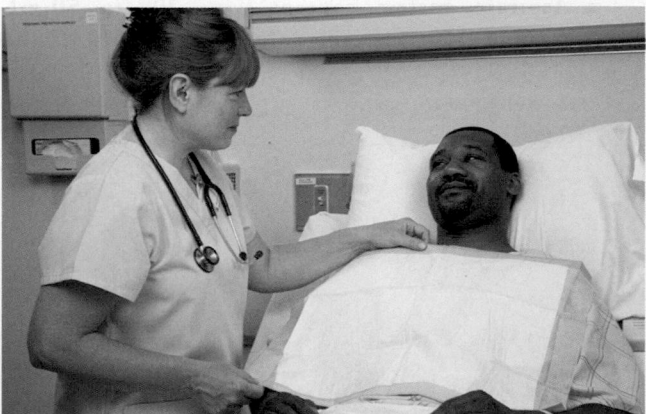

FIG. 1 Drape patient.

Rationale: Elevating the head protects against aspiration.

Procedure 33-4 *continued*

6. **Put on gloves. Lubricate tip of tube with water-soluble lubricant (Fig. 3).**

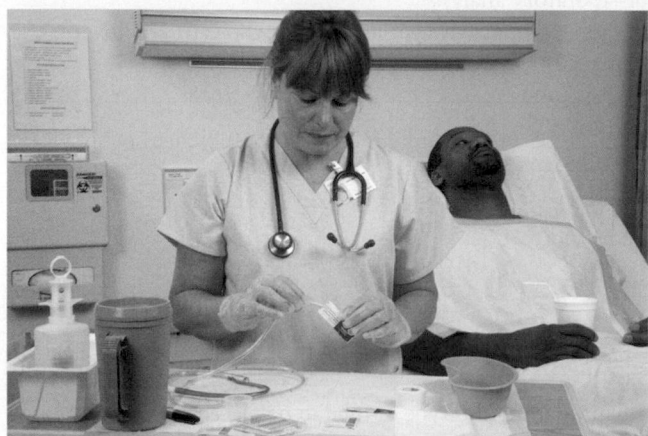

FIG. 3 Lubricate tip of tube.

Rationale: A water-soluble lubricant will be reabsorbed if the tube inadvertently enters the lung. Do not use an oil-based lubricant because respiratory complications may occur if aspirated.

7. **Gently insert tube into nostril (Fig. 4). Advance toward posterior pharynx.**

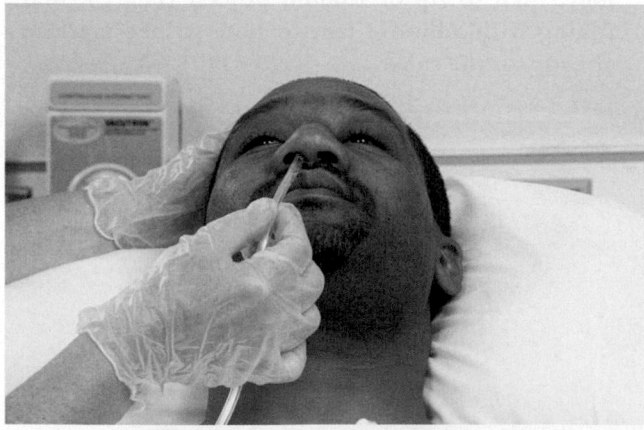

FIG. 4 Gently insert tube into nostril.

Rationale: Following the natural contour minimizes trauma to the nasal mucosa.

8. **Have patient tilt head forward and encourage patient to drink water slowly. Advance tube without using force as patient swallows (Fig. 5). Advance tube until desired insertion length is reached (Fig. 6).**

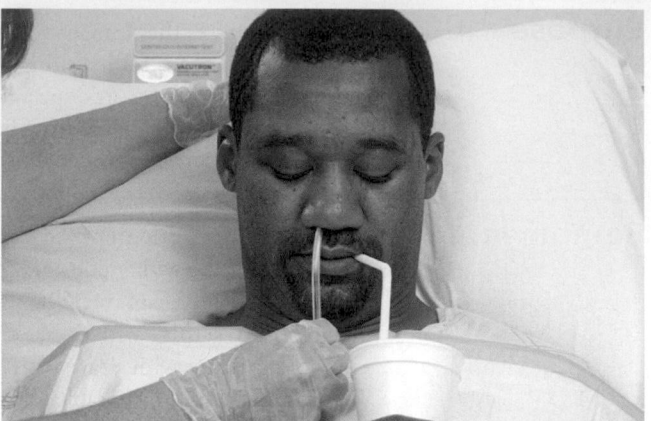

FIG. 5 Advance tube as patient swallows water.

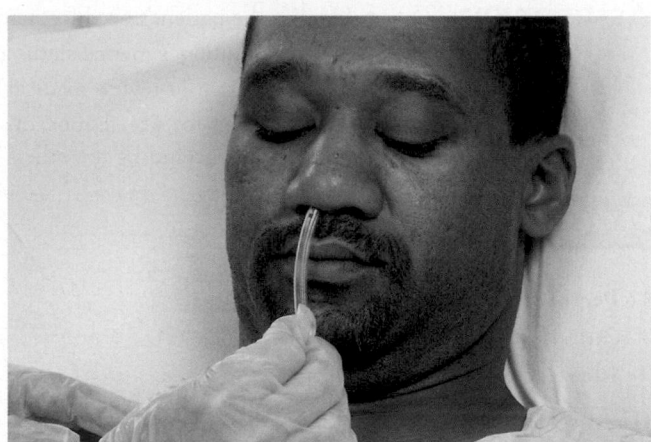

FIG. 6 Insert tube to premeasured mark.

Rationale: Forward tilt of the head facilitates passage of the tube into the esophagus and not the larynx. Swallowing moves the epiglottis over the larynx and facilitates tube passage.

9. **Temporarily tape the tube to the patient's nose, then assess placement of the tube:**

   a. **Aspirate gastric content with 20- to 50-mL syringe (Fig. 7); note color and test pH. If the**

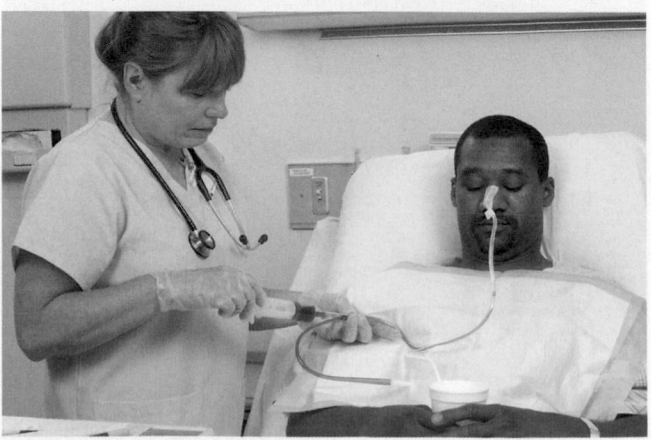

FIG. 7 Aspirate gastric content.

Procedure 33-4   *continued*

pH is 5 or less, it can be assumed that the tube is in the stomach (Fig. 8).

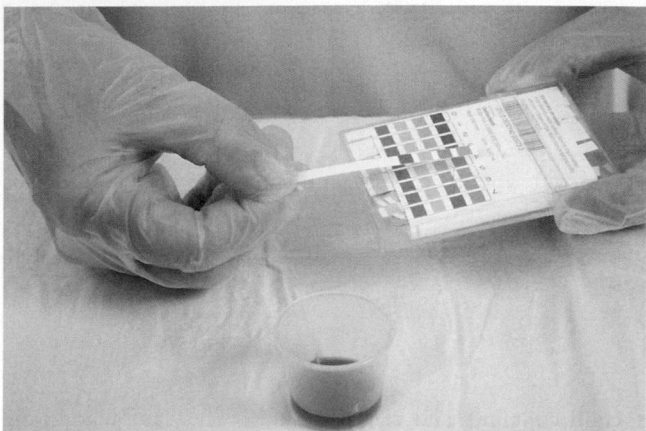

FIG. 8 Test pH of gastric content.

Rationale: Gastric content Is yellow to green and usually present in amounts greater than 10 mL; pH is acidic.

b. If feeding tube is placed, x-ray confirmation of placement is required before feeding is administered.

Rationale: Determining accurate placement is essential to prevent aspiration of feeding into the lungs once feedings are begun.

10. **If placement in stomach is not correct, untape tube, advance tube 5 cm, and repeat assessment in step 10.**

Rationale: Reassessment is required after any adjustments to ascertain whether the tube is correctly placed.

11. **Secure tube by taping to bridge of patient's nose (Fig. 9). Anchor tubing to patient's gown.**

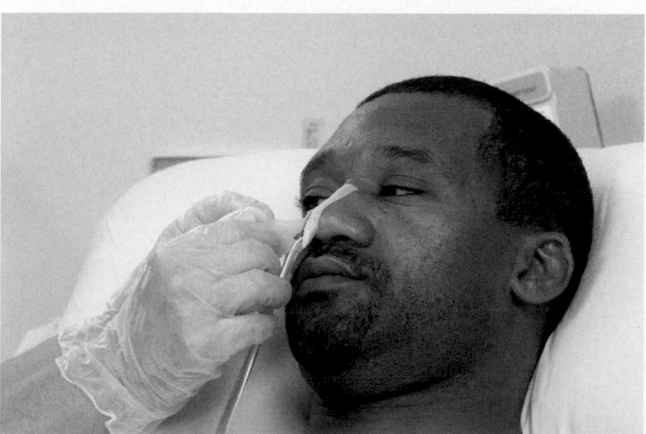

FIG. 9 Tape tubing to bridge of patient's nose.

Rationale: Correct taping prevents the tube from dislodging or pulling and traumatizing the nostril.

12. **Clamp end of tubing or attach to suction, as ordered by healthcare provider (Fig. 10).**

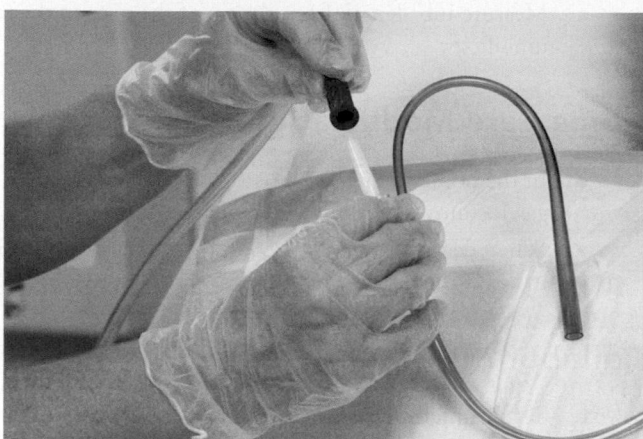

FIG. 10 Attach tubing to suction.

Rationale: Suction facilitates drainage.

13. **Wash hands, provide for patient's comfort, and remove equipment.**

Rationale: Reduces microbe transmission.

14. **Establish and document a plan for daily care of the nasogastric tube:**

a. **Inspect nostril for irritation.**

b. **Cleanse nostril frequently.**

c. **Change adhesive as required to prevent skin irritation or pressure sores on nostril from the tube.**

d. **Increase frequency of oral care because patients with nasogastric tubes often mouth breathe and may be NPO.**

Rationale: Provides for patient comfort and prevents nasal pressure ulcers.

Documentation

3/12/17: 17:00—

P: Abdominal distention, nausea and vomiting post abdominal surgery for 12 hours, absent bowel sounds.

I: 16 French NG tube placed, 500 mL of green bile drainage obtained, pH 2 confirming placement. Oral and nasal care provided.

E: Patient states nausea relieved and feels better. Continue to monitor NG output every shift and provide oral and nasal care.

Procedure 33-4 *continued*

Life Span Considerations

Infants
- Measure tube length from the tip of the nose to the ear lobe, then to the point halfway between the xiphoid process and umbilicus.

Home Care Modifications

- In the home setting, nasogastric intubation usually is done to provide enteral feedings, and a small-bore feeding tube or gastrostomy tube is used (see Chapter 29).
- When decompression is used in the home setting, a portable suction machine is used. Caregivers need to be taught how to assess the patient and monitor the equipment.

Collaboration and Delegation

- Teach unlicensed assistive personnel how to empty the suction container and clamp the tube when ambulating the patient. Encourage them to provide oral and nasal care frequently.

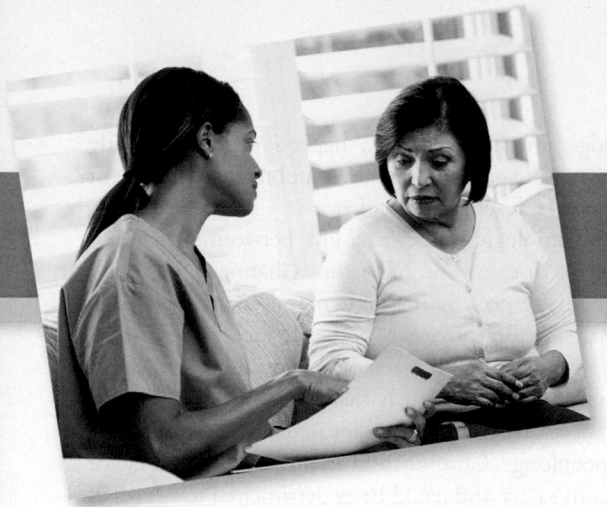

CHAPTER 34

Sleep and Rest

Carol Landis

Case Scenario

Ms. Song, a 57-year-old accountant, comes to see you in the clinic stating she is having significant problems with sleep that are impacting her quality of life. During your interview, you collect the following information:

- Work has been very stressful, especially during tax time when she has many deadlines
- Has trouble getting to sleep (average 45 minutes; some nights up to 2 hours)
- Wakes up two to three times a night to go to the bathroom or when her cat wakes her
- Drinks four to five cups of coffee a day but decaffeinated after 6 PM
- Usually has two glasses of wine at night to relax her
- Has trouble concentrating during the day and feels less productive
- Yawns frequently and at times has nodded off during boring meetings
- Has never used sleeping pills but now is willing if they will help her get a good night's sleep

Once you have completed this chapter and have incorporated sleep and rest into your knowledge base, review the above scenario and reflect on the following areas of Critical Thinking:

1. What poor sleep hygiene practices are influencing Ms. Song's sleep quality?
2. Script questions that could help her analyze factors that might have a negative impact on her sleep.
3. Identify nonpharmacologic interventions that could improve her sleep.
4. Discuss the advantages and disadvantages of pharmacologic use of hypnotics to treat Ms. Song.

KEY TERMS

circadian rhythms
enuresis
fatigue
hypnotics
hypopnea
insomnia
narcolepsy
parasomnias
polysomnography
rest
sleep
sleep deficiency
sleep-disordered breathing (SDB)
sleep health
sleepiness
sleep latency
sleep loss
somnambulism
sleep sufficiency

LEARNING OBJECTIVES

Upon completion of this chapter, you will be able to do the following:

1. Identify benefits of sleep sufficiency and consequences of sleep deficiency.
2. Describe normal patterns of sleep and of NREM and REM sleep stages throughout the life span.
3. Identify factors that affect quality sleep and rest.
4. Conduct an assessment interview regarding normal sleep patterns, risk for disturbance, and actual sleep problems.
5. Develop a daily schedule with a patient, incorporating his or her unique needs and patterns for sleep and rest.
6. Discuss interventions to promote sleep health.
7. Develop a nursing plan of care for a patient with sleep disturbance.

One third of human life is spent sleeping. **Sleep** is vital for survival, but its functions remain poorly understood. Lack of knowledge of sleep functions makes it difficult for somnologists (i.e., scientists who study sleep behavior, physiology, consequences of **sleep loss**, and sleep disorders) (Institute of Medicine, 2006) to answer questions such as "What is sleep good for?" "How much sleep do people absolutely need?" "Are there any good substitutes for sleep?" "Do daytime naps make up for less nighttime sleep?" "Do daily sleep requirements decline or stay the same as people age?" Ongoing research projects continue to address these questions. Sleep has long been assumed to have a restorative function, but somnologists still do not know what gets "restored" during sleep. Until recently, many people believed sleep to be a passive state of decreased stimulation, but active neurobiologic processes initiate and maintain states of sleep and waking.

Sleep, or the lack of it, has consequences at cellular, organ, and system levels of bodily function. Exciting new areas of research have discovered that brain synapses grow or shrink during sleep (Cirelli, 2013). Synapses become more efficient during waking and become either weaker or stronger during sleep in order to maintain a sustainable level of functioning. Structural and functional changes in brain synapses may underlie learning and memory processes and explain observations of reduced attention and task performance, memory lapses, and altered mood that occurs after acute sleep deprivation and chronic insufficient sleep (Porkka-Heiskanen, Zitting, & Wigren, 2013).

Adequate sleep and **rest** are essential for health and well-being. **Sleep health**, or **sleep sufficiency**, is multidimensional and includes sleep of adequate duration occurring at appropriate times of the day with sustained alertness during waking hours (Buysse, 2014). Poor sleep health or **sleep deficiency** is associated with an inadequate amount of or mistimed sleep and with specific primary and comorbid sleep disorders (Luyster, Strollo, Zee, & Walsh, 2012). Poor sleep and **sleepiness** influence a person's perceived levels of energy and **fatigue** and quality of life. People use phrases like "feeling well rested" and "energetic" to describe good sleep and health. The U.S. government recognized the importance of sleep health to public health, adding a new category "Sleep Health" to the objectives for Healthy People 2020 (www.healthypeople.gov/2020/topics objectives2020/overview.aspx?topicid=38, accessed 6-25-14). These objectives target obstructive sleep apnea (OSA), drowsy driving, and sufficient sleep both for teenagers and adults.

Chronic sleep deficiency from obtaining an inadequate amount of sleep increases disease risk and exacerbates health problems. Obtaining less than 6 to 7 hours a night of habitual sleep is associated with increased blood pressure; reduced blood levels of anabolic hormones (e.g., growth hormone and prolactin) required for tissue repair; and altered glucose metabolism and appetite regulation, higher blood levels of inflammatory cytokines, and the stress hormone cortisol during evening hours, when cortisol is usually low (Killick, Banks, & Liu, 2012; Porkka-Heiskanen et al., 2013). Many health problems affect sleep and are affected by sleep loss, either directly through shared pathophysiologic mechanisms (e.g., depression) or indirectly through symptoms (e.g., pain, impaired mobility) or treatment (e.g., medication side effects). Evidence is also accumulating from large epidemiologic studies of a link between sleep duration and chronic disease (Liu, Wheaton, Chapman, & Croft, 2013) and obesity, especially in children and adolescents (Liu, Zhang, & Li, 2012). Researchers hypothesize that chronic insufficient sleep is associated with metabolism, immune, and endocrine function abnormalities such that the risk of developing insulin resistance, diabetes, and cardiovascular disease increase, especially as people age. Chronic insufficient sleep is a risk factor for public health safety and could be as detrimental to health as lack of exercise and poor nutrition (Luyster et al., 2012).

NORMAL SLEEP AND REST

Sleep naturally occurs as a temporary perceptual disengagement from and unresponsiveness to environmental surroundings. Patients under the influence of sedating drugs or in a coma often display behaviors associated with sleep (e.g., closed eyes, little movement, recumbent posture, and reduced responsiveness to stimulation), but these states are not easily or naturally reversed and thus are not "sleep." With rest, one remains awake and aware of environmental surroundings. Whereas sleep involves the whole body, rest may involve total body relaxation or only a part of the body. The person relaxing in a hot tub during vacation may experience a generalized state of rest associated with decreased mental and physical activity, whereas a person with an injured arm in a sling rests only that body part and otherwise is active mentally and physically. It is important to distinguish sleep from rest. One can spend many hours at night "resting" in bed, as occurs in **insomnia**, but not obtain the benefits of a good night's sleep.

Sleep Physiology

POLYSOMNOGRAPHY

Sleep physiology involves electrophysiologic recordings of changes in brain waves (electroencephalogram [EEG]), eye movements (electrooculogram [EOG]), and muscles (electromyogram [EMG]), known as a **polysomnography**. From these recordings, two types of sleep are identified: non–rapid eye movement (NREM) sleep and rapid eye movement (REM) sleep. REM sleep is sometimes called paradoxical or active sleep because the EEG pattern resembles that of waking. During a typical sleep study, recordings also are made of a patient's heart rate (electrocardiogram), airflow through the nose and mouth, chest and abdominal movements, leg movements, and tracheal noise (snoring). Standards have been established for clinical polysomnography, including scoring sleep stages, and for events that are associated with sleep disturbance (e.g., arousals, periodic limb movements, apneas, **hypopneas**) (American Academy of Sleep Medicine [AASM], 2007). Physiologic waveforms associated with sleep stages are shown in Figure 34-1.

Awake:
low-voltage, fast

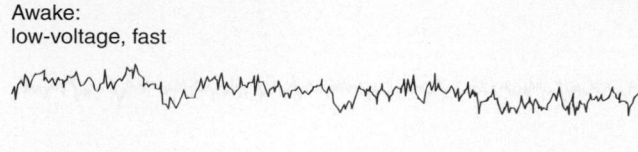

Awake, eyes closed:
alpha-waves, 8–12 cps

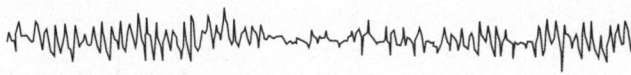

Stage 1:
theta-waves, 3–7 cps

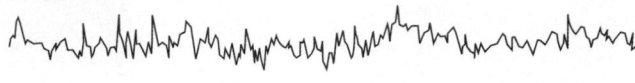

Stage 2:
sleep spindles, 12–14 cps;
K-complex

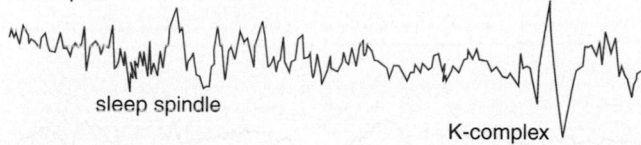

sleep spindle

K-complex

Stage 3 and 4:
delta-waves, 0.5–2 cps

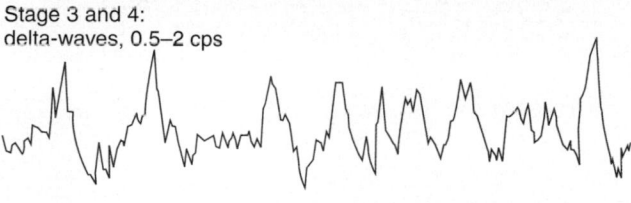

REM:
low-voltage mixed frequency
sawtoothed waves

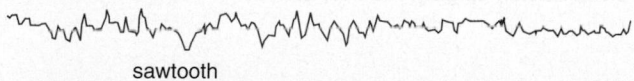

sawtooth

FIGURE 34-1 Characteristic EEG wave forms by sleep stage. (Courtesy of University of Washington School of Nursing, Sleep Laboratory, Seattle, WA.)

Non–Rapid Eye Movement Sleep

In healthy adults, NREM sleep comprises the largest percentage (75% to 80%) of a night's sleep time and is divided into three distinct stages, N1, N2, and N3 (AASM, 2007). Sleep usually begins with stage N1 and progresses to stages N2 and N3.

Stage N1. Stage N1 is the transitional stage between drowsiness and sleep, indicated by a shift from EEG alpha waves associated with relaxed wakefulness to low-voltage, theta, or vertex sharp waves and absence of other sleep stage signs. Muscles relax, respirations become even, and pulse rate decreases. In healthy adults, this stage usually lasts only a few minutes and, if awakened, the person may say he or she was not asleep.

Stage N2. Stage N2 constitutes 40% to 50% of a night's sleep time. Compared to N3 and REM, a person can be more easily wakened. Bursts of readily recognized sleep spindles and large slow waves, called K-complexes, appear on the EEG (Fig. 34-1). Rolling eye movements continue.

Stage N3. Stage N3 is called "deep" sleep, *slow-wave sleep* (SWS), or *delta sleep* after characteristic large amplitude EEG waves (see Fig. 34-1). N3 constitutes approximately 20% of a night's sleep in young adults, but by the 4th decade, SWS is reduced to as little as 5%. Slow waves need to comprise 50% of an epoch in order to be scored as N3. In the original scoring system for sleep stages (Rechtschaffen & Kales, 1968), SWS was differentiated into stages 3 and 4. However, when the scoring system was revised, these two stages were combined (AASM, 2007). During SWS, muscles are relaxed, but muscle tone is maintained; respirations are even; and blood pressure, pulse, temperature, urine formation, oxygen consumption, and swallowing are decreased. N3 is the stage during which sleepwalking (**somnambulism**) and bed-wetting (**enuresis**) are most likely to occur. During the early part of the sleep period, strong stimuli are necessary to awaken people during this stage. Dreams do occur and the content tends to be realistic. Examples are a dream of driving to work or phoning a friend that causes the patient to wonder, when awakening, whether it really happened!

Rapid Eye Movement Sleep

REM sleep closely resembles wakefulness in the EEG and is characterized by very low or absent EMG muscle tone (Fig. 34-2). REM sleep has been renamed as stage R (AASM, 2007). In healthy adults, REM sleep comprises about 20% to 25% of a night's sleep. The REMs from which REM sleep receives its name are documented through EOG recordings but may also be noted by careful observation of eye movements detectable through closed lids. Theta waves often have a sawtooth or notched appearance in stage R (see Fig. 34-1). Blood pressure and pulse rate show wide variations and may fluctuate rapidly. Respirations are irregular, and oxygen consumption increases. Thermoregulation is diminished or lost. Vaginal secretions increase in women, and erections may occur in men. Dreams occurring during REM sleep tend to be vivid, highly emotional, and implausible, often involving reports of movements (e.g., flying, running, being chased), but one is unable to actually move during this stage.

Sleep Cycles

Normal sleep architecture varies by age, gender, and individual characteristics but generally follows a regular pattern. For adults in industrial societies, 7 to 8 hours of sleep obtained in one period of time is considered optimal, sufficient sleep. After turning out the light and a brief period of waking (approximately 10 minutes) called **sleep latency**, electrophysiologic recordings of sleep show a rhythmic pattern of 90-minute NREM/REM cycles during which people progress in sequence through the sleep stages. The usual pattern is a fairly rapid progression through stages N1 to N3 and back through stage N2, from which the person enters REM sleep (Fig. 34-3).

EEG

C3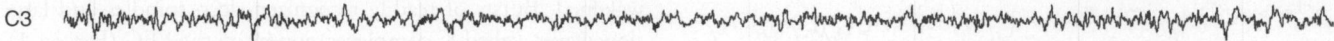

EEG

C4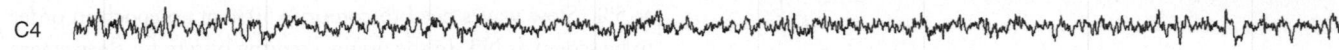

EMG

Chin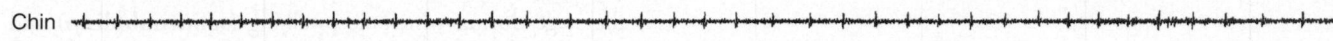

EOG

Left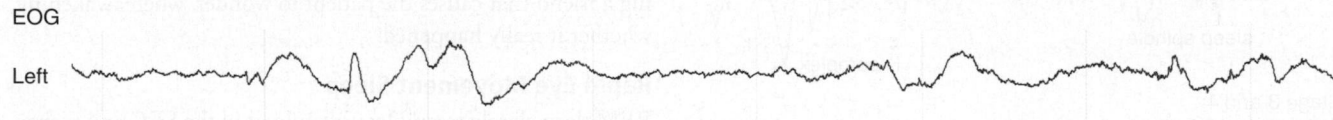

EOG

Right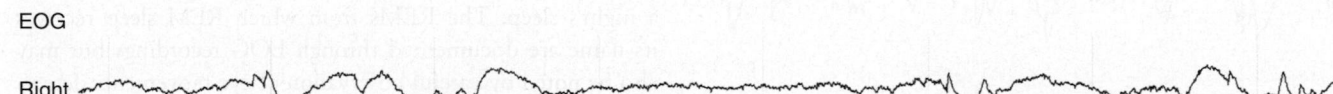

FIGURE 34-2 REM sleep on polygraph recording. Note the rapid, low-amplitude waves on the EEG, eye movements on EOG, and minimal muscle activity on EMG. (Courtesy of Alberta Lung Association Sleep Center, Calgary, Alberta, Canada.)

During the early part of the night, episodes of SWS are longer. In contrast, the time spent in REM sleep during the first sleep cycle may be very short (e.g., 3 to 4 minutes); toward morning, a REM episode may last as much as 45 minutes. If awakening occurs, the cycle begins again with stage N1. If the awakening was brief, the tendency is to re-enter the cycle from which the person was aroused. Thus, an early-morning awakening may be followed by return to one or more cycles in which a high percentage of REM sleep is present (Table 34-1).

Characteristics of Normal Sleep and Rest

Awareness of the need for sleep and rest is most commonly associated with the states of sleepiness and fatigue. Sleepiness refers to an urge of varying intensity to go to sleep. It may occur in response to too little or to lack of adequate sensory stimulation. Fatigue is a subjective state of weariness in which intense or rapid tiring accompanies physical activity. It is a common human response to illness, suggesting the need to conserve energy through rest. Women with disturbed sleep often complain of fatigue, and men often complain of daytime sleepiness, although these two symptoms overlap and are difficult to distinguish.

Typical Sleep and Rest Patterns

SLEEP DURATION

The range of "normal" sleep duration varies and changes across the life span from infancy to adulthood (see the "Life Span Considerations" section below). Optimum daytime performance with minimal sleepiness and no accumulation of sleep debt in adults is related to obtaining 8 hours of sleep each night.

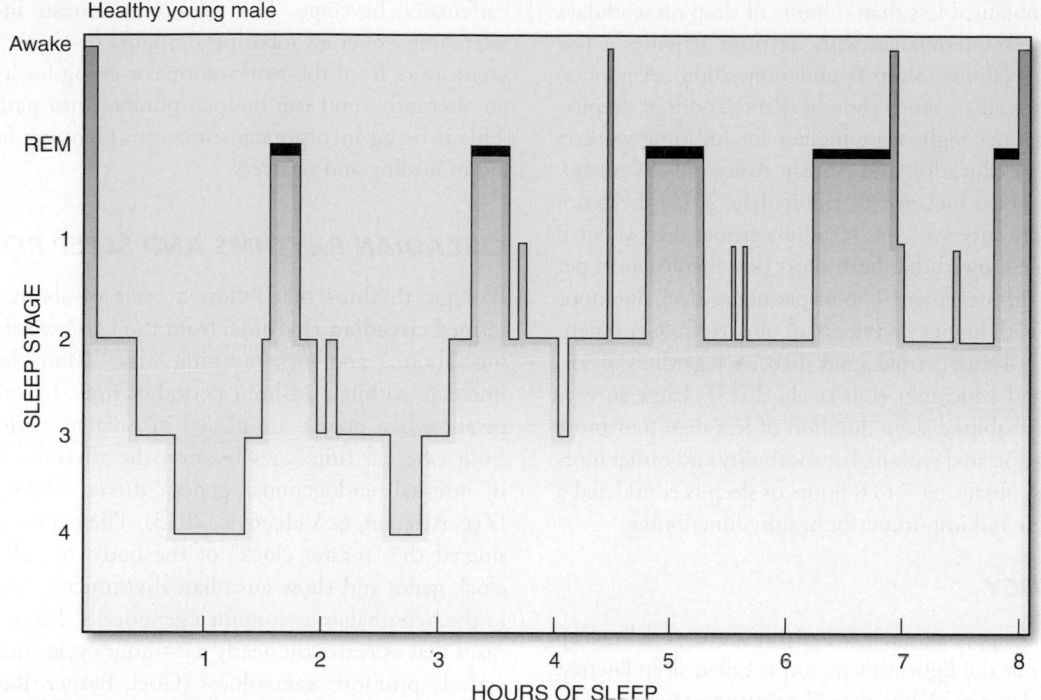

FIGURE 34-3 Typical sequence of sleep stages in a young, healthy man. Progression occurs through a sequence of 1–2–3–2 and into REM. Note increased amount of REM sleep and absence of SWS toward end of sleep period. (Courtesy of University of Washington School of Nursing, Sleep Laboratory, Seattle, WA.)

A well-rested person is mentally alert, energetic, and spontaneous. Daytime activity, even that of a monotonous nature, is maintained with a minimum of drowsiness and sleepiness.

Among adults, sleeping fewer than the recommended 8 hours has become quite common in modern society. In one population-based study, 28% of adults reported *less than 6* hours of habitual nightly sleep; Hispanic and African American adults

were more likely to report less than 5 hours compared to non-Hispanic White adults (Krueger & Friedman, 2009). Nearly half of the adults in the United States who work at least 30 hours each week report sleeping less than 7 hours per night on workdays and only sleep an average of 45 minutes longer on non-working days, which is not enough time to make up for the amount of lost sleep (National Sleep Foundation, 2008). Those

TABLE 34-1 PHYSIOLOGIC CHANGES DURING NREM AND REM SLEEP

Physiologic Variable	NREM	REM
Brain activity	Decreases from wakefulness	Increases in some areas compared to NREM
Heart rate and blood pressure	Decreases from wakefulness	Increases and highly variable compared to NREM
Sympathetic nerve activity	Decreases from wakefulness	Increases from both NREM and REM in some body areas
Muscle tone	Slightly lower from wakefulness	Absent
Blood flow to brain	Decreases from wakefulness	Increases from NREM, depending upon brain area
Respiration	Decreases from wakefulness	Increases and varies from NREM and may show brief stoppages; coughing suppressed
Airway resistance	Increases from wakefulness	Increases and varies from wakefulness
Body temperature	Regulated at lower level from wakefulness	Is not regulated, no shivering or sweating
Swallowing	Suppressed from wakefulness	Suppressed from wakefulness

Adapted with permission from Institute of Medicine. (2006). Sleep disorders and sleep deprivation: An unmet public health problem. Institute of Medicine of the National Academies. Washington, DC: National Academies Press.

who habitually obtained less than 6 hours of sleep on workdays reported sleepiness interference with daytime activities a few days each week (National Sleep Foundation, 2008). A population-based time-use diary study showed that the odds of sleeping less than 6 hours per night were highest for full-time workers with some college education and African Americans (Knutson, Van Couter, Rathouz, DeLeire, & Lauderdale, 2010). Evidence from a large health survey of 54,269 adults greater than or equal to 45 years of age showed that both short (less than 6 hours per night) and long (greater than 10 hours per night) sleep durations were associated with higher prevalence of obesity, frequent mental distress, heart disease, stroke, and diabetes regardless of sex, race/ethnicity, and education (Liu et al., 2013). Large surveys have shown that habitual sleep duration of less than 6 or more than 9 hours is associated with higher morbidity and earlier mortality. For adults, obtaining 7 to 8 hours of sleep is considered a sufficient amount and important for healthy functioning.

SLEEP LATENCY

Most people take approximately 7 to 10 minutes to fall asleep after they turn out the light; this period is called sleep latency. A regular sleep latency of less than 5 minutes suggests excessive sleepiness, which could be a sign of sleep deficiency. Sleep latency of longer than 30 minutes may be accompanied by some sense of frustration and is a symptom of sleep-onset insomnia.

BODY POSITION

Changes of position during sleep typically occur during the night. For people with impaired physical mobility, the normally unconscious act of changing positions during sleep may require awakening, conscious planning and effort, or the assistance of the bed partner or care provider.

NOCTURNAL AWAKENINGS

One to two brief awakenings per night are common for young adults; the frequency and duration of these awakenings increases with age. Waking up after a few hours of sleep and having difficulty falling back to sleep is quite common for women during the menopause transition (Kravitz & Joffe, 2011) and in older adults (Wennberg, Canham, Smith, & Spria, 2013). The final awakening is spontaneous for a well-rested person, who usually awakens feeling refreshed and energized. Reliance on an alarm clock to awaken can be a symptom of sleep deficiency.

NAPPING

Daytime naps and rest periods are infrequent among adults in some countries (see the "Cultural Considerations" section below), except when associated with illness, pregnancy, or "catching up" on a day off. Rest breaks in more industrialized nations are often associated with the use of stimulants such as caffeine in coffee or sodas and nicotine in cigarettes. However, a short 15- to 30-minute nap in the middle of the afternoon can be more energizing as a "rest break" than consuming a caffeinated beverage. The value of minirests in the form of stretching exercises, focusing thoughts or vision on a pleasant scene away from the workstation, or going for a short walk is an alternative and can be incorporated into patient teaching. This is being incorporated into care planning for patients to aid in healing and recovery.

CIRCADIAN RHYTHMS AND SLEEP REGULATION

Biologic rhythms that follow a cycle of about 24 hours are termed **circadian rhythms**, from the Latin words *circa*, meaning "about," and *dies*, meaning "day." Many bodily systems fluctuate within a 24-hour period of time. Circadian rhythms persist when people are placed in isolated environments free from external time cues because the rhythms are controlled by internal (endogenous), genetic-driven "clock" mechanisms (Zee, Attarian, & Videnovic, 2013). The hypothalamus is considered the "master clock" of the body, but all cells contain clock genes and show circadian rhythmicity. Specific neurons in the hypothalamus contain a genetically driven clock mechanism that operates on nearly a 24-hour cycle and is thought to actively promote wakefulness (Goel, Basner, Rao, & Dinges, 2013). This nearly 24-hour cycle is entrained to environmental light and dark periods primarily through specific light detectors in the retina (Zee et al., 2013). Physical activity and melatonin from the pineal gland also aid the entrainment of the endogenous clock to environmental time cues. This entrainment is considered important for both optimal functioning and health. Circadian rhythms are quite stable in an individual, but variations exist between people, called chronotypes. Some people are "morning" types, called larks, who get up early and function best in morning hours; others are "evening" types, called owls, who stay up late and function best in evening hours. There are probably multiple genes responsible for the biologic basis of one's chronotype (Goel et al., 2013).

The sleep–wake cycle is a prominent circadian rhythm in humans. The cycle is regulated by the interaction of two processes: a circadian rhythm process and a homeostatic process (Porkka-Heiskanen et al., 2013). The homeostatic process is responsible for the prolonged sleep that follows an episode of total sleep deprivation. In the previous years, the mechanisms underlying these processes have been considered separate, but the sleep–wake cycle is closely aligned with other circadian rhythms. Somnologists have discovered that some of the "clock" genes directly influence the homeostatic component (sleep intensity and duration) independent of regulating the timing of sleep (Franken, 2013).

Sleep and sleep loss affect certain blood hormone levels. Both growth hormone and prolactin secretion are closely tied to actual sleep time. Systemic blood levels of these hormones change in relation to variations in the sleep period, and levels of these hormones are greatly reduced when one stays up all night. Adrenocorticotropic hormone (ACTH) from the pituitary and cortisol from the adrenal gland follow a predominate circadian rhythm. ACTH levels begin to rise during the middle of the nocturnal sleep period, and levels of cortisol, its target hormone from the adrenal cortex, rise toward the end to reach a daily maximum in morning hours. This pattern remains stable in relation to endogenous "clock" time despite variations in actual sleep time (e.g., shift work), unless such changes are sustained for longer periods of time.

Life Span Considerations

Developmental variations in sleep patterns are quite prominent. Circadian rhythms develop in the first few months of life and persist throughout childhood and adulthood.

NEWBORN AND INFANT

Infants have three types of sleep: quiet (similar to NREM), active (analogous to REM), and indeterminate. Closed eyes, regular respirations, and absence of eye and body movements characterize quiet sleep. Eye movements observable through the closed lids, other body movements, and irregular respirations characterize active sleep. Of the three waking states—quiet awake, active awake, and crying—quiet awake would seem to correspond to a state of rest in adults. Based on a systematic review of the literature worldwide, infants up to 2 years of age sleep on average 12.8 hours (range 9.7 to 15.9 hours) with sleep episodes distributed throughout the day and night (Galland, Taylor, Elder, & Herbison, 2012). Newborns less than 2 months of age sleep up to 20 hours per day. Infant sleep patterns differ from those of adults in that the sleep often begins with active and not quiet sleep, sleep cycles are shorter, and the proportion of active or REM sleep is higher (approximately 50%).

One of the infant's major developmental tasks is to establish a circadian sleep–wake cycle (Fig. 34-4). By 2 to 3 months of age, circadian rhythms manifest and infants spend more time awake during the day and longer periods asleep at night. By 3 months of age, sleep onset begins with NREM sleep, REM sleep decreases, and sleep cycles become more regular. By 6 to 9 months of age, the number of sleep episodes drops, and infants begin "sleeping through the night" with one nighttime

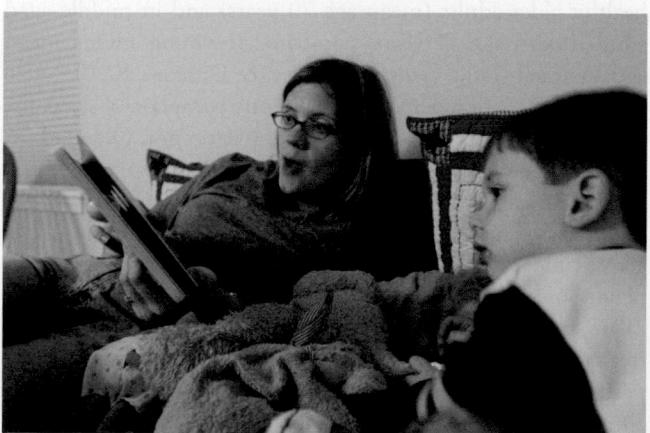

FIGURE 34-4 Bedtime rituals help minimize sleep issues by providing structure and a feeling of security.

episode of approximately 5 to 8 hours duration. By age 12 months, recommended total sleep time is 14 to 15 hours and napping usually has been reduced to once or twice a day, but many infants do not obtain the recommended hours of sleep (Galland et al., 2012).

TODDLER AND PRESCHOOLER

Few studies exist to describe sleep patterns in toddlers and preschool children compared to infants and school-age children (Galland et al., 2012). The number of hours of sleep drops from an average of 12.8 hours at 2 years of age to 11.9 hours (range 9.9 to 13.8 hours) by 5 years of age. REM sleep drops to about 30%, which is still higher than for adults. The percentage of SWS is also higher throughout childhood, whereas the amount of stage N1 sleep is lower. Getting the child to fall asleep is a common problem, but frequent awakenings and occasional night terrors may also occur.

SCHOOL-AGE CHILD

Developmental changes in sleep architecture have been documented by polysomnography for preschool children compared to early school-age children (Montgomery-Downs, O'Brien, Gulliver, & Gozal, 2006). In particular, the time to the onset of the first REM period occurs later in early school-age children compared to preschoolers, but both groups show similar amounts of slow-wave and of REM sleep. Sleep and rest needs fluctuate somewhat for school-age children in relation to activity patterns, but often, wake and sleep times are similar on weeknights and weekends and no differences in sleep between girls and boys are recognized. On average, school-age children sleep 9.2 hours per night (range 7.6 to 10.8 hours), but by 12 years of age, mean sleep duration has dropped to 8.9 hours (Galland et al., 2012). Clearly, some children are not getting a sufficient amount of sleep; beginning at 7 years of age, some children obtain less than 8 hours of sleep per day.

ADOLESCENT

During adolescence, major changes occur in sleep and in the sleep–wake cycle. SWS decreases, REM sleep reaches typical adult amounts, and daytime sleepiness manifests. There is a shift to a late evening bedtime and late morning rise time; an "owl-like" chronotype pattern develops. Adolescents still require about 9 hours of sleep for optimal functioning, but by 16 years of age, they often report sleeping less than 7 hours per night. Insufficient sleep has become an epidemic among adolescents in the United States and linked to greater risk of engaging in unhealthy behaviors (cigarette smoking, marijuana use, alcohol consumption, physical fighting) and thinking about suicide (McKnight-Eily et al., 2011). Adolescents have to get up early in the morning to go to school, so they end up being very sleepy, especially during the initial part of the day and again in the midafternoon. On weekends, they often sleep late in the morning attempting to catch up on lost sleep during school days. Work schedules, school-related or sports activities, homework, and other social pressures also interfere with time to obtain sufficient sleep and contribute to irregular sleep–wake schedules. Gender differences in sleep emerge with the onset of puberty; girls are at higher risk of developing and report more insomnia symptoms after puberty (Hysing, Pallesen, Stormark, Lundevold, & Sivertsen, 2013). The use of televisions, cell phones, computers, and video games and consumption of caffeinated beverages all contribute to sleep problems for adolescents.

Academic performance is negatively associated with shortened sleep time and irregular sleep–wake schedules for adolescents. Changing the time school starts to a later time in the morning increases the amount of sleep and reduces daytime sleepiness and caffeine intake among adolescents (Boergers, Gable, & Owens, 2014). The proportion of students obtaining greater than 8 hours of sleep increased from 18% at baseline to 44% after the school start time was shifted just 25 minutes later (Wahlstrom et al., 2014). Public high schools in Minnesota that have start times at 8:30 AM or later allow most students to obtain at least 8 hours of sleep on a school night. In these schools representing 9,000 students, academic performance and attendance rates were improved and tardiness was reduced. Perhaps most important, the number of car crashes for teen drivers was significantly reduced by 70% after a school shifted start times from 7:35 AM to 8:55 AM. Changing to later school start times is an important public health prevention strategy that provides adolescents more time for sleep, improves academic performance, reduces the risk of unhealthy behaviors, increases personal and public safety, and promotes better health practices that could impact a lifetime.

ADULT AND OLDER ADULT

Adults most often report a sleep duration of 7 hours, but the number of hours of sleep they obtain and in the preferred portion of the 24-hour period for sleep varies considerably. By middle age, the frequency of nocturnal awakenings increases, and satisfaction with sleep quality decreases. Situational variables such as lifestyle choice, work hours, computer-related stress, pregnancy, parenting and family caregiving responsibilities, and illness explain much of the variation in sleep among adults of all ages. Important findings from a meta-analysis of polysomnographic studies of approximately 3,577 healthy people showed percentages of nocturnal waking and N1 increased, while total sleep time and N3 decreased as people age (Ohayon, Carskadon, Guilleminault, & Vitiello, 2004). The intranight distribution in the duration of REM sleep episodes becomes more even, but the percentage of REM sleep in a night's sleep can remain stable until very old age (Fig. 34-5). Across the life span, women complain more of disturbed sleep and report more use of sleep medications compared to men, but age-related changes such as increased N1 and frequent awakenings occur earlier in men. Most age-related changes in sleep occur prior to, and reach a plateau after, age 60 years (Ohayon et al., 2004).

The amplitude of circadian rhythms becomes less prominent with increasing age. There is a tendency for a "phase

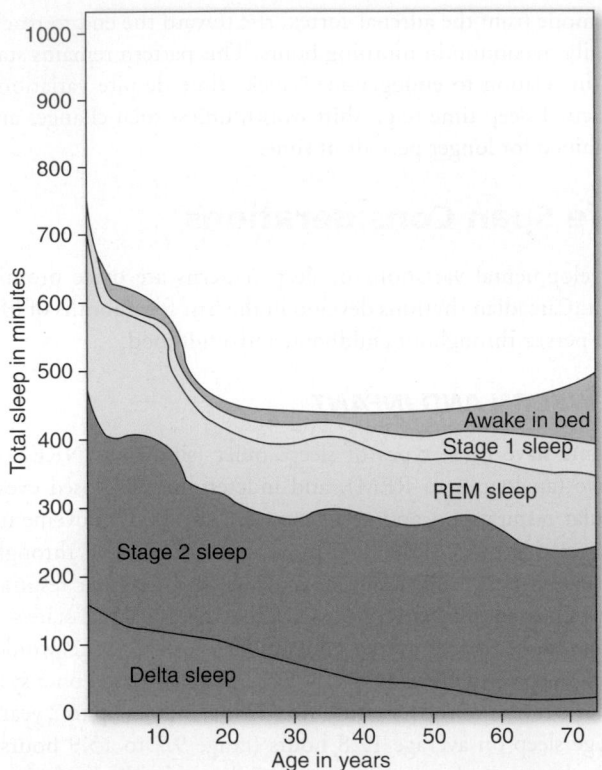

FIGURE 34-5 Schematic representation of the changes in sleep stages by age. Note that older adults spend more time in bed than younger adults but have less deep sleep. (Adapted with permission from Williams, R. L., Karacen, I., & Hursch, C. J. (1974). Electroencephalography (EEG) of human sleep: Clinical applications. New York, NY: Wiley.)

advance" to a "lark-like" chronotype pattern—that is, to go to bed earlier and awaken earlier. Sleeping patterns may become biphasic, with a shorter nocturnal period and daytime naps among retired individuals. Time spent in bed increases with advancing age such that sleep efficiency (time asleep/time in bed) decreases (Ohayon et al., 2004). Total time in bed gradually increases because of napping, longer sleep latency, increases in the number and length of awakenings, and general fatigue. However, physiologic propensity for daytime sleep is lower in healthy older adults (mean age 70 years) and in middle-aged adults (mean age 47 years) compared to young adults (mean age 25 years) (Dijk, Groeger, Stanley, & Deacon, 2010).

About 50% of older adults frequently complain of sleep disturbances, but of equal importance, 50% do not. Older adults express concerns about taking longer to fall asleep, awakening more frequently for long periods of time, and needing longer to adjust to changes in the sleep–wake schedule as they travel across time zones (Wennberg et al., 2013). Many of these complaints of poor quality sleep are related to episodes of medical or psychiatric illness, and if these problems are properly treated, sleep improves. However, symptoms of insomnia may persist, becoming a comorbid condition that requires therapy aimed at improving sleep (Wennberg et al., 2013). Important health promotion activities include helping healthy older adults to recognize that changes in sleep, such as more frequent awakenings or feeling sleepy earlier in the evening, are a natural part of aging and emphasizing the importance of keeping a regular sleep–wake schedule.

Cultural Considerations

A person's culture has profound effects on beliefs and many aspects of behavior, including sleep preferences and practices. However, very little research-based evidence has been published concerning cultural influences on sleep. Social scientists and anthropologists have begun to report findings from studies of sleep habits in various regions of the world. For example, daytime naps contribute to the total amount of sleep obtained in 24 hours in urban and rural families in Egypt (Worthman & Borwn, 2013). In this Egyptian study, when 8 hours of recommended nightly sleep was used as a marker of sufficient sleep, adults met this amount on only 20% of the days studied. However, when the amount of time spent napping was included in the total amount of daily sleep, sleep sufficiency more than doubled. Thus, in Egypt, naps are an important way to make up for shorter nighttime sleep, but one has to be able to take a nap, which is not always feasible given school and work schedules.

Cross-cultural aspects of children and parent sleep practices have been the most studied (Knutson & Orzech, 2013). Sharing the same bed or corooming among family members was the norm in both urban and rural families in Egypt, except for adolescents and unmarried young adults (Worthman & Borwn, 2013). Cosleeping was expected, valued, preferred, considered protective, and associated with better self-reported sleep quality, although it was associated with shorter episodes of nighttime sleep. Bed sharing between mothers and infants versus placing infants in a single bed in a separate room is heavily influenced by cultural practices (Knutson & Orzech, 2013). Pediatric authorities in Western industrialized countries recommend that infants should be placed supine in a separate bed in a separate room, but this practice is quite different from most other countries in the world. Anthropologists have documented that in most cultural groups studied, infants sleep in the same room as their parents, often sharing the same bed. Bed sharing, either in a separate bed in the same room or in the same bed, is increasing in the United States. Laboratory studies of mother–infant bed sharing have shown that both the mother and the infant have less stage N3, more N1 and N2, and more arousals from sleep yet overall obtain more sleep compared to mothers and infants who sleep in separate beds in separate rooms (Volpe, Ball, & McKenna, 2013). Cosleeping could have risks to the infant if the mother is smoking in bed, taking medications that cause sedation, or if using loose bedding and pillows.

Social and cultural determinants of sleep deficiency have been recognized. Among the most studied determinants in association with sleep include older age, female sex, depression, stress, loneliness, and African American race (Knutson, 2013), but this list is incomplete. These factors are not necessarily independent because many women are single mothers with less income and have longer life expectancies compared to men. Socioeconomic status, poverty, and place of residence both in urban and in rural locations also have been linked with sleep deficiency. Several studies have found that African American children and adults report shorter sleep duration (less than 6 hours nightly sleep) and more sleepiness during the day (Knutson, 2013). When the prevalence of short sleep duration (insufficient sleep) and symptoms of insomnia in a nationalized representative sample of men and women Mexican-born immigrants were compared to Mexican men and women born in the United States, the immigrant men and women, even though they were less educated, earned less income, and reported insufficient social support, had better health practices (lower rate of smoking, illegal drug use, lower body mass index) and were at lower odds of insufficient sleep and insomnia symptoms (Seicean, Neuhauser, Strohl, & Redline, 2011). However, even among Mexican-born immigrants, women had greater odds of reporting insufficient sleep compared to Mexican-born immigrants, which contrasted with U.S.-born Mexican men and women. The investigators attributed this difference to the possible influence of cultural norms and behaviors for household chores and care of children among immigrant men and women (Seicean et al., 2011).

FACTORS AFFECTING SLEEP AND REST

Need

Sleep is without question a biologic necessity because animals and humans deprived of sleep eventually die, but the functions of sleep remain a biologic mystery. Because infants and children obtain more sleep, many people believe that they need more sleep for normal growth and development. Similarly, because older adults obtain less sleep compared to young adults, many people believe that older adults require less sleep. Somnologists generally maintain that the need for sleep does not change with aging, but sleep drive is highest in children and adolescents and the ability or capacity to obtain good quality sleep declines as we age.

Environment

In general, people seek a safe and secure place for sleep, and environmental surroundings can promote or impede efforts to sleep. In a new environment, sleep latency increases, sleep is more fragmented, and total sleep time and the proportion of REM sleep decreases. This so-called first-night effect has long been recognized in sleep laboratory studies. Individuals who have insomnia may associate certain objects in the bedroom with poor sleep and may report sleeping better away from home, but most chronic sleep disorders manifest wherever an individual sleeps. If a sleeping room doubles as a work area, an individual may associate the room with work rather than sleep. Objects of play and electronic equipment in a child's room may disturb the child's sleep. Access to electronic devices such as computers and cell phones is a common cause of sleep disruption in adolescents.

Reduction of environmental light and noise facilitates sleep. People vary in their sensitivity to different stimuli and appear to vary in the intensity and degree of fluctuation of sensory input they require. Some people seem to require a slight elevation of sensory input and report sleeping better when surrounded by low-level noise such as a radio or television. However, a quiet environment is most conducive to sleep.

Awakenings, shifts to a lighter sleep stage, or brief arousals may occur when the bed partner changes position or snores. A habitual partner may provide a sense of security, and his or her absence may be disturbing. As discussed in the "Relationships" section, the nature, quality, and present state of the relationship are factors that contribute to the effect of the partner's presence or absence. For those who habitually sleep alone, the presence of another person may be disturbing.

NOISE

People who are chronically exposed to high noise levels have lighter sleep and more awakenings than their counterparts who live in quieter neighborhoods. Noise is more likely to awaken women and older people. The use of earplugs can be helpful if noises in the same room (e.g., partner snoring) or outside (e.g., traffic) are disturbing sleep.

Hospitals are busy, noisy places, and patients often complain of not being able to sleep, most often because of conversations among hospital staff. Noise levels recorded in critical care units are the equivalent of a noisy office. Nurses can modify the noise level in such settings by avoiding unnecessary conversations, keeping equipment noise to a minimum, and closing doors when possible. A designated "quiet time" for rest during the day has been shown to decrease noise levels and increase patient and staff satisfaction (Boehm & Morast, 2009).

LIGHT

Light levels in most homes can be readily controlled, but increasingly, individuals are exposed to the same level of dim indoor lighting during the day and night at home, at work, and during leisure activities. For people who live in northern latitudes during summer months and for night shift workers who try to sleep in the daytime, outdoor light brightness disrupts sleep. Control of lighting levels is important because exposure to even low levels of light at night can shut off melatonin secretion. Melatonin is the body's natural signal that it is dark outside. It is an important component of synchronizing endogenous circadian rhythms with the environment and has been shown to have anticancer properties (Rondanelli, Faliva, Perna, & Antoniello, 2013). Breast cancer risk is five times higher in industrialized societies where light exposure throughout a 24-hour day is higher compared to underdeveloped countries. It has been hypothesized that reduced melatonin may account, in part, for this increased cancer risk.

In acute care environments, especially in critical care units, control of light becomes a nursing responsibility often overlooked in the complexity of meeting other patient needs. Past studies have shown that some critically ill patients have very low levels of melatonin, but the significance of these findings in terms of recovery are difficult to assess because of the many factors that affect sleep in these patients (Drouot, Cabello, d'Ortho, & Brochard, 2008).

TEMPERATURE

Cool versus moderate room temperature is a matter of personal preference, but research has shown that either excessive hot or excessive cold increases restlessness and reduces sleep quality. Body temperature normally drops prior to sleep onset and drops further during sleep. The lowest point of the circadian rhythm of body temperature occurs in the early-morning hours when even shift workers find it difficult to remain awake regardless of the amount of sleep obtained the previous day. The use of an electric blanket to warm the bed before sleep may aid sleep onset, but if the blanket is left on during sleep, it will impair body heat dissipation and cause restless sleep or awakenings.

Relationships

Frequent awakenings associated with parenting of infants and young children may initiate and contribute to chronic insufficient sleep. It is not unusual to hear mothers speak of never getting more than an hour's sleep at a time over a period of 1 week or longer when caring for a sick child or colicky baby. The associated sleep loss may make coping even more difficult. Likewise, caregivers of people with advanced disease or Alzheimer disease may have disturbed sleep and experience chronic sleep loss.

Disruptions in primary relationships are commonly associated with sleep disturbance. Bereaved people often report nighttime as the most difficult time of the day and experience disturbed sleep. Children who are away from home are frequently homesick at bedtime. Marital discord may contribute to sleep disturbance in children as well as in the involved adults. Security needs are heightened at bedtime for people of all ages.

Healthcare providers are among the most frequent disturbers of sleep in institutional settings. In acute care environments, they must awaken patients frequently for various assessments and treatments. Where possible, nurses should strive to cluster activities to provide periods of 90 to 120 minutes of undisturbed time to permit rest and promote sleep. Nurses must assume an advocacy role by coordinating interruptions from the many disciplines involved in patient care.

Shift Work

Frequent changes in the sleep–wake schedule, such as those that occur with shift work, contribute to a misalignment between the internal circadian clock and the sleep–wake cycle. Individuals who work at night often are too sleepy to function well at work and too aroused to obtain sufficient sleep during the day. Trying to sleep at times when the body's circadian rhythm is set for wakefulness is thought to be the main reason for problems obtaining sufficient sleep in shift workers. Some people, particularly those who are younger and evening types, tend to adjust to shift work better, especially the swing shift, than do people who are predominantly morning types. Most shift workers get less sleep when doing night shift work than in a steady daytime or evening shift routine. The accumulated sleep debt of night shift workers compromises clinical judgment and decision making, an increasing concern in healthcare, and efforts to improve patient safety. Nurses are among the millions of people in industrialized countries who are involved in shift work. Consecutive night shift work is associated with reduced melatonin. Night shift workers have increased health risks, including higher risks for breast and prostate cancer, but whether reduced melatonin explains this risk is not clear (Rondanelli et al., 2013).

Research has shown that clockwise rotation of shifts (moving in the same direction of time, rather than counterclockwise) is preferable and that short naps during breaks enhance work performance. Attention to the sleeping environment is particularly important for nurses and others who work the night shift. Helpful simple strategies include blacking out windows with dark curtains or aluminum foil, shutting off or moving the telephone into another room, and allowing adequate time for sleep.

Nutrition and Metabolism

Hunger disturbs the sleep of some people, whereas others have difficulty sleeping after large meals. Individuals who suffer from gastrointestinal reflux should raise the head of the bed and not eat within three hours of bedtime. Ingestion of L-tryptophan, a precursor of serotonin found in foods such as milk, beef, eggs, wheat flour, turkey, and corn, has been found to decrease sleep latency and increase sleep propensity. Sleep tends to be disturbed during periods of either rapid weight loss or rapid gain. Consumption of foods and beverages high in caffeine and other stimulants (e.g., coffee, tea, cocoa, chocolate) in the late afternoon and evening should be avoided.

Elimination Patterns

The need to void during the night, called nocturia, is one of the most frequent events to disturb sleep, especially among middle-aged and older adults. Parents and other caregivers can assist children and encourage adults to establish a habit of voiding as part of preparing for bedtime. Limiting fluid intake after the evening meal and during the night may decrease nocturia. Using small nightlights rather than turning on bedside or overhead lights in the bedroom or bathroom are recommended to reduce the effects of light suppression of melatonin secretion. Frequent nocturia in middle age and older men could be a sign of an enlarged prostate.

Exercise, Passive Heating, and Thermoregulation

Habitual exercise is associated with self-reported better and longer sleep, but data from exercise intervention studies show only modest increased total sleep time. Passive heating, as in a sauna or tub of warm water, especially in the early evening and several hours before bedtime, has been shown to increase SWS similar to that of exercise. Given that sleep onset occurs most readily as body temperature is falling, it is preferable to schedule exercise or a hot bath several hours before bedtime. For a small group of older adults with sleep complaints, a warm footbath within an hour of sleep onset raised foot temperatures and core body temperature during sleep but was not associated with altered sleep architecture (Liao, Wang, Kuo, & Lo Chiu, 2013).

Vigilance

Another factor affecting sleep is the perceived need to maintain vigilance. Parents and others in protective roles apparently establish a variable arousal threshold in which they may respond to the faintest sound of a toddler changing position in the next room and yet sleep through a thunderstorm. Hospital patients, such as those recently disconnected from cardiac monitoring equipment, may deliberately prevent sleep for fear of succumbing to a complication that might go unnoticed by nursing staff.

Lifestyle and Habits

Habitual bedtime rituals are an effective way to decrease arousal and prepare for sleep. Participation in a routine such as putting out the dog, setting the alarm, teeth brushing, and changing into night attire becomes associated with the expectation of sleep.

Lifestyle patterns influencing sleep-wake schedules, such as time of rising, are closely linked with societal and occupational expectations. A habitual time of rising is one of the most effective means of improving sleep quality and in synchronizing endogenous circadian rhythms with clock time. Caregivers can help toddlers who are having difficulty settling into a bedtime routine by maintaining an early and consistent rising time and allowing them to stay up in the evening until they are sleepy enough to settle with quieting activities. Nurses can encourage adults who have difficulty getting to sleep to maintain a consistent rising time and to go to bed later if necessary rather than lying awake for long periods trying to sleep.

Illness

During acute and chronic illness, patients often have disturbed nighttime sleep and are sleepier in the daytime. The common cold, acute pain, and difficulty breathing are known to disturb sleep. Pain is often considered to cause poor sleep, and poor sleep to increase pain—a reciprocal relationship. However, findings from prospective and longitudinal studies of patients with chronic pain show disturbed sleep is more likely to increase pain the next day rather than pain to disturb sleep the next night (Finan, Goodin, & Smith, 2013). These findings are leading investigators to specifically target insomnia symptoms in addition to therapies for pain. For example, older adults with osteoarthritis classified as responders to an 8-week

SCENE FOR THOUGHT

Joanna and Paco Estevez are parents of two small children: Enrique, who is 3 weeks old, and Theresa, who is 3 years old. Paco works nights, and Joanna has recently returned to work at her day job as a nurse's aide in a large nursing home. Emily Arana, a community health nurse, is at their home for a follow-up visit.

LESS EFFECTIVE

Mrs. Estevez: I'm glad you came early, Ms. Arana. The kids are both asleep and so is Paco. We can talk in peace for a little while. (*Sits on sofa and motions Emily to sit down.*)

Nurse: Sounds like it's been busy around here lately. (*Settles onto sofa and sits attentively.*)

Mrs. Estevez: You got that right! Enrique isn't sleeping through the night yet, and Theresa wakes up, too. Plus, she has a cold, so she isn't feeling too good. And Paco isn't around to help much since he's working nights. It gets pretty hairy around here at 2 AM. (*Smiles tightly.*)

Nurse: And I understand you're working, too. Day shift?

Mrs. Estevez: Yes. (*Wearily.*) I had to go back or lose the job. I leave the kids with my mother all day until I get off at 3 PM. She lives close by. (*Yawns.*) Sorry! I didn't mean to yawn in your face!

Nurse: No problem. And is your husband able to help or is he too tired? (*Begins to open bag and take out assessment equipment.*)

Mrs. Estevez: He helps on his days off. He's really good with both of them. (*Sounds a little defensive.*)

Nurse: I'm sure he is, having had three brothers and sisters of his own to take care of. Maybe I could see the baby now and how he's doing. Do you think Theresa will be up soon? I can look at her, too, and see what we can do for her cold. What do you think?

Mrs. Estevez: Sure, you start on the baby, and I'll see if Theresa's about to wake up. (*Pauses to get a clean towel for the baby to lie on and goes in to the bedroom. Yawns again.*)

MORE EFFECTIVE

Mrs. Estevez: I'm glad you came early, Ms. Arana. The kids are both asleep and so is Paco. We can talk in peace for a little while. (*Sits on sofa and motions Emily to sit down.*)

Nurse: Sounds like it's been busy around here lately. (*Settles onto sofa and sits attentively.*)

Mrs. Estevez: You got that right! Enrique isn't sleeping through the night yet, and Theresa wakes up, too. Plus she has a cold, so she isn't feeling too good. And Paco isn't around to help much since he's working nights. It gets pretty hairy around here at 2 AM. (*Smiles tightly.*)

Nurse: How about you? (*Good eye contact.*)

Mrs. Estevez: I do what I can. (*Shrugs wearily.*) I had to return to work after the baby came home or lose my job. I get up at 5 to get the kids ready to take to my mother's while I work. So I don't get much sleep. Or much time with Paco. I really hate this night shift he's on. But it's extra money, and it won't be forever. He's put in for a shift change so we can have some sort of normal life, but it won't come through for a while. (*Yawns.*) Sorry! I didn't mean to yawn in your face!

Nurse: No problem. You have reason to be tired. What are you doing to try and get more sleep? (*Looks concerned, asking an open-ended question.*)

Mrs. Estevez: I try to nap here and there. Paco takes the night feedings on his nights off so I can sleep through at least two nights a week. Other than that, I wait for the baby to grow so he'll sleep through and for Theresa's cold to get better. (*Shrugs again with a resigned look.*)

Nurse: Have you thought about planning naps with Teresa and the baby at the same time? Would you be willing to discuss things that might help both kids move along faster?

Mrs. Estevez: (*Looks surprised.*) Sure! I didn't know there was anything else I could do for them. (*Baby begins to cry. Mrs. Estevez rushes to get him so Paco won't wake. She returns.*) Let me just change him and get a bottle and then we can talk! (*Looks eager.*)

CRITICAL THINKING CHALLENGE

- Determine the factors affecting this family's sleep and rest patterns.
- Explain how the nurse in the second dialogue elicited additional information from Mrs. Estevez.
- Explain what information the nurse in the first dialogue missed.
- Formulate your ideas of what consequences further sleep deficiency may have for this family.

trial of cognitive–behavioral therapy for insomnia (CBT-I) showed sustained improvements in sleep, pain, and fatigue for as long as 18 months following the trial (Vitiello et al., 2014).

Ventilatory responses to hypoxia and hypercapnia decrease during REM sleep, and although diaphragmatic function is essentially unchanged during REM sleep, the intercostals and other accessory muscles lose muscle tone. The pattern of frequent arousals seen in people with chronic obstructive lung disease may result from the body's need to maintain adequate oxygenation. **Hypnotics** should be used cautiously, if at all, in people experiencing ineffective breathing patterns or impaired gas exchange. Usually, these patients require low doses of oxygen at night.

Individuals with cardiovascular disease have heightened risk for heart attacks and strokes during the early-morning hours (Rimmele & Thomalla, 2014). Circadian variations in blood pressure, heart rate, and platelet aggregation around the time of wakening are associated with the observed frequency of myocardial infarction and stroke that occur in the latter part of the nighttime sleep period or within the first hours after wakening.

People with a history of seizure activity are at risk for increased occurrence of seizures with sleep loss or as the result of irregular sleep–wake schedules. Seizure activity may disturb sleep; some epileptic patients have seizures only at night. The recording of brain waves during sleep is an important method for diagnosing the site of abnormal electrical activity.

Hormonal changes associated with illness contribute to sleep pattern disturbances. Hyperthyroidism causes fragmented, short sleep with excessive SWS, whereas hypothyroidism seems to cause excessive sleepiness and a lack of SWS. The tremendous fatigue many women report after hysterectomy may be related to estrogen loss.

Medications

Hypnotics, or "sleeping pills," decrease sleep latency and improve sleep maintenance, but these drugs do not induce "natural" sleep. Benzodiazepine drugs (e.g., temazepam, lorazepam, triazolam) are well known to reduce SWS and REM sleep, have substantial side effects, often produce rebound insomnia when individuals abruptly stop taking them, and are not often prescribed any longer. Newer benzodiazepine receptor agonist drugs (e.g., zopiclone, zolpidem, eszopiclone) reduce sleep-onset latency and increase total sleep time, have fewer negative side effects, have less rebound insomnia, and are better tolerated even by older adults (Ancoli-Israel et al., 2010).

Alcohol is probably the oldest and most commonly used substance for promoting sleep, but its effects are of limited value. A moderate single dose causes early onset of sleep but increases wakefulness 3 to 4 hours later. With acute intoxication, REM sleep is suppressed; SWS may initially increase. Abrupt alcohol withdrawal in the heavy drinker will trigger sleep disturbance. Recovered alcoholics continue to have decreased SWS and gross cycle disturbance even after 1 or 2 years of abstinence.

Many medications affect sleep. Morphine, for example, increases the time spent awake during the sleep period and shortens total sleep time by decreasing both REM sleep and stage N3. Some antidepressants suppress REM sleep and may contribute to insomnia depending upon the dose and if central nervous system (CNS) arousal systems are up-regulated by the particular drug. Any drug that crosses the blood–brain barrier to reach the CNS has the potential to induce either sedation (e.g., antihistamines, adrenergic receptor blockers, anticholinergic agents) or insomnia (e.g., amphetamines or cholinergic receptor agonists). The effects of caffeine (adenosine receptor antagonist) on the CNS may last up to 6 hours, delaying sleep onset and affecting sleep patterns, even in those who believe that they are not affected. The half-life of caffeine in older adults is even longer, making them particularly vulnerable to its effects. Individuals with insomnia or difficulty sleeping should consume foods and beverages containing stimulants only in the morning hours. Nicotine, another mild CNS stimulant, accounts for the poorer sleep observed in heavy smokers compared with nonsmokers.

 *Concept Mastery Alert*

Hypnotics have the therapeutic benefit of inducing sleep, but they all have varying effects on the normal progression through the stages of sleep. This effect on the patient's sleep architecture must be considered when weighing the potential risks and benefits of hypnotics.

Mood States

Anxiety frequently delays sleep onset. Tension associated with psychological stress may also contribute to maintenance or early-awakening insomnia. Depression usually results in disturbed sleep. Poor sleep and depression are bidirectional and likely to further distress depressed people. Altered mood states are one the most frequent outcomes associated with sleep loss. Individuals with bipolar disorder need an adequate amount of sleep because insufficient sleep can trigger a mania.

ALTERED SLEEP AND REST

Insomnias

The most common sleep disorders in adults include insomnia, **sleep-disordered breathing (SDB)**, **narcolepsy**, and other hypersomnias, sleep-related movement disorders (restless legs syndrome [RLS], periodic limb movement disorder [PLMD]), and **parasomnias** (Box 34-1).

Insomnia is the most common sleep disorder. It is both a cluster of symptoms and a complex disorder of poor sleep quality, often associated with an insufficient amount of sleep. Insomnia has many causes and can be classified as onset insomnia (prolonged sleep latency), maintenance insomnia (prolonged

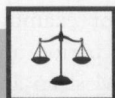

ETHICAL/LEGAL ISSUE

IMPACT OF NIGHT SHIFT ON HEALTHCARE WORKERS

Two months ago, you were hired for your first full-time position since graduating from your nursing program. You work the night shift permanently on a busy surgical unit. At first, you enjoyed the flexibility of having your days and evenings free and tended to sacrifice your sleep time. Lately, however, you have been having trouble sleeping during the day and staying alert during the night. Twice in the last week, you almost made medication errors. Tonight is the last night of this stretch, and you are experiencing difficulty concentrating on even the simplest procedures. You have asked your supervisor for a different shift rotation, but he says your schedule cannot be changed.

CRITICAL THINKING CHALLENGE

- What alternatives might you consider in the above situation?
- Is self-care an ethical issue? Explain why or why not.
- Reread the Code for Nurses in Chapter 7. List the statements in the code that apply to this situation. Give rationales for your choices.
- Identify the legal and ethical responsibilities of the supervisor in this context.

BOX 34-1 Common Sleep Disorders

Insomnias
- *Primary:* Difficulty falling and staying asleep or waking up too early
- *Comorbid:* Difficulty falling and staying asleep or waking up too early in conjunction with psychiatric or medical disorders

Sleep-Disordered Breathing
- *OSA:* Repetitive pauses in breathing with continued respiratory effort
- *UARS:* Increased ventilatory effort and snoring
- *CSA:* Decreased ventilatory effort and blood oxygen desaturation

Narcolepsy and Hypersomnias
- Repetitive, uncontrollable episodes of falling asleep, often associated with falling to the ground (cataplexy)
- Excessive sleepiness that interferes with daily function

Sleep-Related Movement Disorders
- *RLS:* Difficulty falling or staying asleep due to uncomfortable limb sensations
- *PLMD:* Frequent leg jerks that cause arousals from sleep
- *Parasomnias:* Sleepwalking, talking, night terrors, and enuresis

nocturnal awakenings), early-morning awakening insomnia, or complaints of nonrestorative sleep. About 5% to 10% of individuals who complain only of sleep-onset insomnia have delayed sleep phase disorder, a type of circadian rhythm sleep disorder (see the "Circadian Rhythm Sleep Disorders" section below). Polygraph recordings of people with insomnia are quite similar to those of self-defined good sleepers. However, people with insomnia consistently underestimate total sleep time and may overestimate the extent of their sleep problem compared to polysomnography. Insomnia with polysomnographic evidence of short sleep duration, for example, insufficient sleep of less than or equal to 6 hours, is a more severe type of insomnia associated with serious medical morbidity and mortality (Vgontzas, Fernandez-Mendoza, Liao, & Bixler, 2013). Insomnia associated with greater than or equal to 6 hours of sleep is associated with emotional arousal and cognitive rumination, but not with signs of serious medical morbidity.

Insomnia occurs when an individual has an adequate amount of time for sleep. This differentiates insomnia from *insufficient sleep syndrome*, which also is associated with an inadequate amount of sleep, but occurs because an individual *voluntarily restricts* the time available for sleep. Insomnia that occurs in individuals without any psychiatric or medical condition is called primary insomnia (Buysse, 2013). However,

insomnia symptoms and the disorder also commonly occur both with psychiatric and medical conditions. Once called secondary insomnia, the preferred term now is "comorbid insomnia" (Buysse, 2013). Insomnia is associated with the consumption of stimulants (e.g., caffeine, nicotine, methamphetamine, and other drugs of abuse) and as a side effect of many medications (e.g., antidepressants, antihypertensives, steroids, psychostimulants). Insomnia is common during and after hospitalization (Griffiths & Peerson, 2005). Pain, older age, preoperative medical status, pre-existing insomnia, anesthesia, analgesics, psychological and physiologic responses to surgery, and many aspects of the environment are likely contribute to insomnia symptoms in hospitalized patients.

As a chronic disorder, insomnia is diagnosed based on one or more symptoms of poor sleep quality, significant distress, and impairment of daytime function for at least 1 month duration (Buysse, 2013). The prevalence of insomnia disorder ranges from 10% to 20% (Buysse, 2013), but the prevalence of insomnia symptoms is much greater ranging from 35% to 50%. Chronic insomnia, lasting more than a month, is higher in women than men and higher in African Americans compared to Whites (Buysse, 2013). There is some evidence that insomnia is higher in divorced, widowed, and separated compared to married individuals and in individuals with low socioeconomic status and less education. Individuals prone to depressive symptoms and anxiety, but without evidence of a diagnosable psychiatric disorder, are more likely to complain of insomnia. Once chronic insomnia is manifested, symptoms are likely to persist over time. The prevalence of insomnia symptoms increases above 45 years of age and is nearly 50% in adults over 65 years as well as those who use healthcare services frequently. Insomnia symptoms in the elderly are frequently comorbid with depression, heart disease, bodily pain, and memory problems (Wennberg et al., 2013). Other sleep disorders (e.g., SDB, RLS, and PLMD) also increase with age and may manifest with insomnia symptoms. In the next few decades, it is likely that the number of individuals with a sleep disorder will increase as the population of older adults increases worldwide.

CBT-I is efficacious for the management of both primary and comorbid insomnia in adults (Buysse, 2013), including older adults (Wennberg et al., 2013). CBT for insomnia is typically delivered in 4 to 8 sessions and has shown long-lasting improvements in sleep quality. CBT-I is a safer alternative to the use of medications. Because of the increasing numbers of elders worldwide and the prevalence of sleep complaints, there is increased interest in making CBT-I available in primary care settings. Strategies to translate traditional CBT-I into self-management programs have shown efficacy (Morgan, Gregory, Tomeny, David, & Gascoigne, 2012) and are likely to become more popular.

Hypnotic and anxiolytic medications are efficacious and recommended at the lowest possible dose for the short-term management of insomnias, but their use in the management of chronic insomnia, particularly in the elderly, is controversial. Classes of medications most commonly used to treat insomnia in the United States are the benzodiazepine receptor agonists (eszopiclone, zolpidem, zaleplon) and the melatonin receptor agonist (ramelteon) (Table 34-2). Although many patients with insomnia use these agents for long periods of time, only for eszopiclone has efficacy been assessed for 6 months of daily use. Despite the lack of research evidence, trazodone is one of the most common agents prescribed "off label" in the United States to treat insomnia (National Institutes of Health State of the Science Conference Statement, 2005), although its anticholinergic properties make it an inappropriate drug to treat insomnia in the elderly.

TABLE 34-2 SELECTED HYPNOTICS: PROPERTIES AND IMPLICATIONS

Hypnotic	Properties	Nursing Implications
Zaleplon (Sonata)	Short acting *Half-life*: 1 h	Use for sleep-onset insomnia.
Zolpidem (Ambien)	Short acting *Half-life*: 2.5 h	Use for sleep-onset insomnia.
Ambien CR	Slow release	Use for maintenance insomnia.
Zopiclone (Imovane) Eszopiclone (Lunesta)	Short acting *Half-life*: 4–6.5 h	Use for sleep-onset and maintenance insomnia.
Ramelteon	Short acting *Half-life*: 0.5–1.5 h	Use only for sleep-onset insomnia.

Sleep-Disordered Breathing

SDB is a cluster of disorders associated with difficulty breathing and sleeping at the same time. SDB involves repeated interruptions of breathing during sleep that disrupt sleep and lead to hypoxemia. SDB includes OSA, upper airway resistance syndrome (UARS), and central sleep apnea (CSA). SDB essentially results in chronic sleep disturbance because of the frequency of miniarousals and often a lack of slow-wave and REM sleep.

SDB symptoms reported by patients referred to sleep disorders centers include excessive sleepiness, feeling tired (fatigue), depressed mood, difficulty concentrating, poor memory, and unrefreshing sleep. The problems of excessive daytime sleepiness and the large number of undiagnosed patients with SDB make this cluster of sleep disorders a major public health and safety issue.

 APPLY YOUR CRITICAL THINKING

Mrs. Wilson, a 45-year-old executive, comes in for a yearly physical examination. She reports that her only complaint is difficulty sleeping. She says that she wakes six to eight times each night from her husband's loud snoring. She is so tired some mornings that her productivity at work is beginning to suffer. She asks you if you think sleeping pills might help solve her problem. How will you respond to Mrs. Wilson?

Check your answer in Appendix B.

OBSTRUCTIVE SLEEP APNEA

OSA is the most common type of SDB. It refers to recurrent periods of absence of breathing for 10 seconds or longer (in adults), occurring at least five times per hour (AASM, 2007). OSA involves collapse of the upper airway despite respiratory effort. With sleep, the muscles of the upper airway relax, occluding an airway that may already be narrowed because of obesity, jaw structure, or enlarged soft tissue structures. With arousal or brief awakening, voluntary control of the upper airway muscles is restored, relieving the obstruction. Some people do not become completely apneic, but recurrent periods of very shallow breathing (hypopnea) have a similar effect.

OSA is a common condition, affecting about 3% to 7% of men and 2% to 5% of women with nearly equal prevalence in minority populations (Paiva & Attarian, 2014). Overweight and obese men and women of all ethnic groups are at increased risk for OSA. Weight gain increases the risk of developing OSA, and weight loss is an effective way to reduce disease severity in overweight patients. Abdominal obesity (high waist-to-hip circumference) is a core feature of metabolic syndrome and is associated with increased risk of OSA. With the increased numbers of overweight and obese children and adults in the United States and worldwide, the incidence of OSA is likely to increase in all age groups as well as cardiovascular and metabolic consequences of OSA (Drager, Togeiro, Polotsky, & Lorenzi-Filho, 2013).

An individual with OSA may be partially roused hundreds of times each night. Symptoms include excessive daytime sleepiness and reports from the bed partner of apneic periods, heavy snoring, and restless sleep. Common treatments include continuous positive airway pressure (CPAP) applied through a nose mask and surgical reconstruction of the upper airway with removal of most of the uvula, posterior portion of the soft palate, and tonsils. Current developments include laser-assisted pharyngoplasty and various dental splints. Weight control, relief of nasal congestion, and avoidance of sleeping on the back may be effective in milder cases. Despite the effectiveness of CPAP to relieve respiratory disturbances and reduce sleepiness, many patients fail to use the apparatus as prescribed or stop using it altogether; thus, adherence is a major problem in the treatment for OSA (Weaver, 2013).

OSA can be considered a chronic condition requiring ongoing participation in an evidenced-based clinical management program in order to improve patient outcomes (Heatley et al., 2013).

Independent of age, sex, and body mass, OSA has been linked to increased risk for cardiovascular disease (Paiva & Attarian, 2014). The prevalence of hypertension in patients with OSA is from 22% to 90% in different clinic populations. Reduced blood oxygen levels, increased sympathetic activity, and inflammatory processes that accompany apneic episodes are the main mechanisms linking OSA with increased risk for hypertension, ischemic heart disease, and stroke (Drager et al., 2013). Individuals who snore regularly are at higher risk for developing OSA and subsequent cardiometabolic consequences (Deary, Ellis, Wilson, Coulter, & Barclay, 2014).

OSA also has been linked in clinical studies to cognitive impairments (attention deficits, impaired concentration, and memory problems). Changes in cognitive function are present in patients with mild OSA, and impairments increase with the severity of the disease. A greater number of apneic episodes, sleep fragmentation, and greater hypoxemia correlate with worse neurocognitive and psychomotor performance deficits. Neural imaging studies have shown some improvement in cognitive function after the initiation of CPAP therapy in patients with OSA (Olaithe & Bucks, 2013).

Encourage people who have frequent apneas that exceed 20 seconds at a time and occur most nights (with or without snoring or excessive daytime sleepiness) to seek assessment for possible OSA. The use of hypnotics, alcohol, or antihistamines by patients with OSA can be dangerous.

Narcolepsy

Narcolepsy is a rare chronic disabling autoimmune neurologic disorder of excessive daytime sleepiness characterized by short, almost irresistible daytime sleep attacks, usually lasting

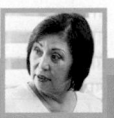

Sleep and Rest PICO

Ms. Song from the chapter-opening scenario discloses to you that one of her doctors had diagnosed her with OSA. She indicates that she is supposed to be using a CPAP machine at night. She states, "I hate that thing" "I can't sleep with it on …it's too big on my face." If I don't wear it, my husband tells me that I snore too loud and he ends up sleeping in another room. Ms. Song asks, "Isn't there any medication for sleep apnea?" Unsure about the answer, you turn to the Cochrane library for evidence. The PICO question you decide to use is: *In patients with obstructive sleep apnea, how does medication therapy versus no medication therapy improve breathing during sleep?*

P = patients with obstructive sleep apnea

I = medication therapy

C = no medication therapy

O = improve breathing at night

You find several studies in the Cochrane database. One systematic review catches your eye because it evaluates specific drug therapies to placebo and their effect on sleep apnea. The study analyzed 30 randomized controlled trials (RCTs) with 516 participants. Twenty-five drugs were studied with various time frames including acetazolamide (Diamox), eszopiclone (Lunesta), naltrexone (Revia), nasal lubricant (phosphocholinamine), physostigmine, donepezil (Aricept), fluticasone (Flonase), ondansetron (Zofran), fluoxetine (Prozac), and paroxetine (Paxil). Although some of the RTC seemed hopeful, the systematic review concluded that there is not enough strong evidence that proves that drug therapy benefited patients suffering from sleep apnea. More research is needed in this area. You share your findings with Ms. Song and provide her with teaching about modifying some of her habits to help improve sleep.

REFERENCE:

Mason, M., Welsh, E. J., & Smith, I. (2013). Drug therapy for obstructive sleep apnoea in adults. *Cochrane Database of Systematic Reviews.* Issue 5, Art. No.: CD003002. doi: 10.1002/14651858.CD003002.pub3

10 to 15 minutes, and abnormal manifestations of REM sleep (Partinen et al., 2014). Disease onset usually occurs in adolescence. People who have narcolepsy typically experience REM sleep within the first 20 minutes after falling asleep. Episodes of profound weakness in skeletal muscles during intense emotion (anger, laughter, or surprise), called cataplexy, are reported by 70% of narcoleptics. Other common signs related to disturbed REM mechanisms include episodes of feeling paralyzed (sleep paralysis) and vivid hallucinations when falling asleep or awakening. A deficiency of orexin (hypocretin), a neuropeptide linked to waking, in the hypothalamus is associated with narcolepsy, but the pathogenesis and pathophysiology are not well understood. Some patients with narcolepsy and cataplexy have low to undetectable levels of orexin in the cerebral spinal fluid. Examination of brain tissue after death has shown up to 95% loss of neurons that produce orexin in the posterior hypothalamus (Partinen et al., 2014). Orexin is a neuropeptide important for regulating waking behavior, physical activity, and hunger sensation. An autoimmune mechanism is hypothesized to lead to orexin cell loss in the hypothalamus in susceptible individuals.

The prevalence of narcolepsy is lower than other sleep disorders, estimated to affect 30 per 100,000 in various populations worldwide (Partinen et al., 2014). The genetics of narcolepsy are complex, but the relative risk for narcolepsy in first-degree relatives is estimated to be from 1% to 14% (Partinen et al., 2014).

Patients, regardless of ethnicity, complain of feeling drowsy, unable to remain awake while watching a movie, sitting in a classroom, reading, or doing other sedentary activities. As a result, they often show poor performance at work, have reduced quality of life, and are disabled with poor interpersonal relationships. Although excessive daytime sleepiness is a most troublesome symptom, people with narcolepsy also have disturbed nighttime sleep.

Pharmacologic management of narcolepsy includes amphetamine-like stimulants to relieve excessive daytime sleepiness and antidepressant drug therapy to control cataplexy. Drugs such as amphetamine, methamphetamine, methylphenidate, and modafinil are used in the pharmacologic management of daytime sleepiness. Tricyclic antidepressant drugs such as protriptyline, desipramine, and atomoxetine, as well as serotonin reuptake blocking drugs such as fluoxetine and venlafaxine, are used in the treatment for cataplexy. Side effects of stimulant and antidepressant medications hinder compliance with prescribed doses.

SAFETY ALERT

Encourage patients to seek assistance when getting up, especially at night, if they are at risk for dizziness (e.g., postoperatively, after sedation) or have impaired mobility.

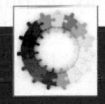

COLLABORATING WITH THE HEALTH CARE TEAM:
Requesting Consultation for Sleep Apnea

You are the assigned registered nurse for Mr. Matthews, a 48-year-old man who has just been admitted for an asthma exacerbation. While performing an initial nursing assessment, he tells you that he wakes multiple times per night and often awakes hyperventilating. He is often sleepy during the day and has frequent headaches. His wife reports that he "snores so loud, it sounds like a train is coming through the house." You are giving this information to the physician who arrives on the unit to continue admitting Mr. Matthews.

SITUATION: Mr. Matthews is reporting headaches and hyperventilation associated with poor sleep.

BACKGROUND: He is here for treatment for an asthma exacerbation, currently on 2 L of O_2 per nasal cannula with a saturation of 95%. When he was napping earlier, his oxygen levels dropped to 86%. He reports waking up multiple times per night hyperventilating, and he snores. He complains of persistent tiredness and frequent headaches when awake. He currently takes Advair daily and uses an albuterol MDI as needed.

ASSESSMENT: All of the symptoms Mr. Matthews reports are consistent with OSA.

RECOMMENDATION: I think we need to consider ordering a sleep study for Mr. Matthews, as he may need a CPAP device. Would you like to call the sleep lab or should I?

CRITICAL THINKING QUESTIONS
- Mr. Matthews's sleep study results show that he has OSA and is prescribed CPAP to use while he sleeps. At his follow-up appointment 1 week after discharge, he tells you (the clinic registered nurse) that he does not use the CPAP consistently. Can you think of at least three reasons people do not use a CPAP when they are recommended?
- What solutions could you and Mr. Matthews come up with to help him adjust to using CPAP?

Restless Legs Syndrome and Periodic Limb Movement Disorder

RLS and PLMD are neurologic disorders that commonly lead to insomnia and reduced quality of life (Rye & Trotti, 2012). An essential feature of RLS is unpleasant sensations (e.g., creepy, crawly, burning, twitching, aching) of the legs that lead to an irresistible urge to move them. Walking, pacing, or rubbing the legs temporarily provides relief. Symptoms of RLS occur during waking, but inactivity and lying down intensifies them such that individuals have difficulty falling and staying asleep. Many patients with RLS also have periodic limb movements, or sudden, brief jerks of the legs that occur repetitively during sleep. PLMD is characterized by repetitive dorsiflexion of the foot and flexion of the knee during sleep at a rate up to once every 15 to 20 seconds and occurs in association with insomnia symptoms and brief arousals from sleep.

There is some evidence that the prevalence of RLS is higher in individuals of European ancestry and in women compared to men (Rye & Trotti, 2012). RLS symptoms commonly occur in pregnancy and are associated with iron deficiency that resolves postpartum. The prevalence of RLS and PLMD increases with age. Gene studies have established multiple genetic links to RLS and PLMD.

Pharmacotherapy is the cornerstone of treatment to relieve RLS and PLMD symptoms. Drugs that enhance the activity of dopamine systems in the CNS are drugs of choice for severe RLS. Hypnotic medications, anticonvulsants, and analgesic (opioid) drugs are also used to treat RLS and PLMD. Because RLS and PLMD increase with age, patients need to be monitored carefully for side effects and drug interactions when taking these types of medications. Many of these drugs are contraindicated in pregnancy because they harm the developing fetus.

Circadian Rhythm Sleep Disorders

Circadian rhythm sleep disorders include transient disruptions, such as "jet lag" syndrome, shift work disorder (discussed previously), and more persistent problems of advanced or delayed sleep phase syndromes. Jet lag tends to be worst after west-to-east travel across time zones, and it affects poor sleepers and older adults most intensely. Effective treatments include exposure to bright light, taking exogenous melatonin or ramelteon, a melatonin receptor agonist with a longer half-life compared to melatonin, and appropriately timed so as to help advance or delay the endogenous circadian pacemaker depending upon whether one is traveling east or west across at least three time zones (Zee et al., 2013).

Delayed sleep phase disorder, a mismatch of circadian rhythm biology and societal expectations, is more common in adolescents and young adults (Zee et al., 2013). Adults who function best by going to bed in the early hours of the morning and sleeping into the afternoon find occupations and partners to match. Other people with this disorder find that the continued struggle with sleep-onset insomnia and to

awaken hours earlier than their internal clock dictates is not helped by simple treatments, such as establishing a consistent rising time. However, exposure to bright light therapy in the morning, combined with good sleep habits, such as consistent rising time and adequate total sleep time, can effectively alter circadian rhythms, but these behavioral routines must be maintained to be effective. Often, individuals with circadian rhythm disorders will revert to their preferred sleep–wake schedule during vacations and on days off and thus experience rebound symptoms.

Advanced sleep phase disorder is far less common than delayed sleep phase disorder. As noted earlier, with age, there is a tendency for the circadian timing of sleep onset to shift to an earlier hour in the evening and waking time to shift an earlier hour in the morning. Bright light therapy used in the evening is an effective treatment to offset sleepiness and delay bedtime (Zee et al., 2013).

Parasomnias

Parasomnias are activities that are normal during waking but abnormal during sleep, such as sleepwalking (somnambulism), talking, night terrors, and bed-wetting (enuresis). Parasomnias usually occur during SWS and are most common in children. Usually, a family history of similar behaviors is present. Occasional episodes of sleepwalking in children are fairly common, usually beginning before age 10 years and stopping by age 15 years (Carter, Hathaway, & Lettieri, 2014). Behavior during a sleepwalking episode may be purposeful, such as dressing or going to the bathroom, but lacking in coordination and appropriateness, such as voiding in the closet. Occurrence in adults is frequently associated with stress and anxiety. Parents and family members may need assistance in providing a safe environment to decrease the potential for injury.

Night terrors are repeated, sudden arousals accompanied by screaming, acute anxiety, and disorientation. They occur mainly among children and are associated with incomplete arousal from SWS early in the night. They are different from nightmares or bad dreams that occur during REM sleep.

Enuresis is not limited to SWS, although almost two thirds of all episodes occur in the first third of the night. The prevalence decreases from 30% at age 4 years to 10% at age 6 years and 3% at age 12 years. Enuresis is less common and tends to disappear earlier in girls than in boys.

Discourage attempts to awaken people from the parasomnias. Others should give help in the event of night terrors or somnambulism only to the extent that the person accepts, and they should encourage the person to return to sleep as the event subsides.

In addition to insufficient sleep, narcolepsy, and parasomnias, sleep apnea and insomnia are common in children and adolescents (Carter et al., 2014). Sleep apnea occurs in 1% to 5% of children, but this number may underestimate the actual prevalence. In a study of children with arthritis, 40% of the children snored, which is considered a mild form of sleep apnea (Ward et al., 2010), but physicians who care for children with arthritis rarely ask parents or children about sleep problems. Recognition of the potential prevalence of and the need for early detection of sleep apnea in children in primary care settings, clinical guidelines for the diagnosis and treatment were developed (Marcus et al., 2012). Habitual snoring, disturbed sleep, and daytime behavioral problems are the primary symptoms. Clinicians are encouraged as part of routine health maintenance to ask parents of children and adolescents about snoring, attention deficits, or learning problems. If the answers are positive, referral to a sleep specialist is warranted (Marcus et al., 2012). Treatment for sleep apnea in children and adolescents includes removal of the adenoids and tonsils (adenotonsillectomy), and if the problem persists, CPAP therapy is used. If the child or adolescent is overweight, weight loss improves apnea.

The risk of developing insomnia increases, especially in girls, after puberty (Hysing et al., 2013). However, "insomnia" in school-age children is not well documented. In a recent population-based polysomnographic study of 700 children 5 to 12 years old, the prevalence of insomnia symptoms was 19.3% and highest in girls 11 to 12 years old (Calhoun, Fernandez-Mendoza, Vgontzas, Liao, & Bixler, 2014). The girls, but not the boys, showed polysomnographic signs of sleep disturbance. A subsample from this study, children with insomnia and short sleep duration, but not "normal" sleep duration, had elevations in the stress hormone cortisol both in the evening before and in the morning after sleep (Fernandez-Mendoza et al., 2014). These findings suggest that signs of insomnia of short sleep duration begin early in life and some children may be more vulnerable to or hyperresponsive to environmental stressors. Unfortunately, to date, there is no research-based evidence of efficacious treatments for childhood or adolescent insomnia.

Recall Ms. Song in the case scenario. Use the concept map (Fig. 34-6) to help understand and manage Ms. Song's sleep problem to improve her function and quality of life.

ASSESSMENT

Sleep disturbances are frequent sources of concern to people sick or healthy. It is easy in hospital and outpatient settings for nurses to become preoccupied with assessments and treatments associated with the presenting illness. Likewise, in community practice, the diabetic's foot care or the new mother's ability to breast-feed may overshadow the concerns those people have regarding unsatisfactory sleep or inadequate rest. Regardless of the setting in which nurses' practice, sleep and questions about problems sleeping and obtaining adequate rest are important components of any routine clinical assessment. Professional nurses play a pivotal role in helping people to assess and to meet their needs for sleep and rest.

A useful framework for organizing an assessment about sleep and sleep disturbances is called the BEARS approach (Owens & Dalzell, 2005). *BEARS* is short for *B*edtime,

*E*xcessive daytime sleepiness, *A*wakenings, *R*egular Schedule, and *S*noring. The goal and questions to ask for each component of this assessment framework is summarized in Box 34-2. The questions assist in the identification of particular sleep problems. Spouses or other family members can provide additional information about the patient's sleep.

Normal Sleep–Wake Cycle Identification

An important criterion for adequacy of sleep and rest is the patient's report. The state of feeling rested is highly subjective. As discussed earlier, individual requirements and capacity for sleep vary. Besides the sense of feeling rested, people usually consider the congruency between their expectations and experience in relation to total sleep time, time in bed before sleep onset, number of awakenings, and time of final awakening. The history is the most important component of assessment of sleep and rest.

Determine the person's usual sleep–wake schedule through questions such as the following:

- How many hours of sleep do you usually get?
- What time do you usually go to bed? Get up?
- What helps you get to sleep?
- What makes it hard for you to sleep?
- How do you feel when you awaken?
- How much sleep do you believe you should be getting?
- What helps you relax?
- How often do you nap? Take rest periods?

Risk Identification

When assessing a person's risk for sleep problems, look for clues in the family history as well as developmental and situational changes (environmental, physical, social) that may increase the need for or interfere with sleep and rest. Assess caffeine, nicotine, and alcohol intake and involvement in shift work.

Sleep Problem Identification

Validate with the patient whether he or she perceives that getting adequate sleep and rest is a problem. If a problem is identified, determine whether it is chronic or situational, what has helped, and what has made it worse. In situations of chronic sleep disturbance, it may be useful to interview the sleep partner as well. Direct questions toward elaboration of the presenting concern; for example, if the person is concerned about daytime sleepiness, inquire about a history of snoring, awakenings accompanied by gasping, apneic periods that the sleeping partner may have observed, restlessness, and impact on activities associated with work, driving, and social interactions.

Having patients keep a sleep diary is part of a routine assessment and also as an intervention. Table 34-3 is an

SLEEP AND REST

Determine problems with

Resolution of problems with

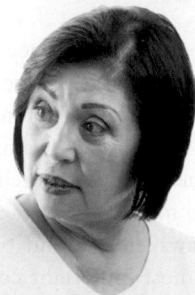

Ms. Song • Age 57

A 57-year-old accountant comes to the clinic with statements of significant sleep problems that are impacting her quality of life.

ASSESSMENT FINDINGS

Assess physical appearance

Normal assessment

Conduct assessment interview for sleep patterns

Poor sleep hygiene practices

- "How many hours of sleep do you usually get?"
- "What time do you go to bed and get up?"
- "What helps you get to sleep?"
- "What makes it hard to get to sleep?"
- "How do you feel when you awaken?"
- "What amount of sleep do you feel you should be getting?"
- "What helps you to relax?"
- "How often do you nap or rest?"

Patient verbalizes

- Work very stressful, especially during tax time with many deadlines.
- Trouble falling and staying sleep (average 45 minutes to fall asleep; some nights is awake 2 hours during the night).
- Gets up 2-3 times each night for the bathroom or when her cat wakes her.
- Drinks 4-5 cups of coffee/day; decaffeinated after 6 PM.
- Usually 2 glasses of wine at night to relax her.
- Trouble concentrating during the day and feels less productive.
- Yawns frequently and at times has nodded off during boring meetings.
- Has never used sleeping pills but now willing if they promote a good night's sleep.

Assessment findings data indicate

PRIORITY NURSING DIAGNOSIS

1. Disturbed Sleep Pattern.
2. Related to: job stress, caffeine and alcohol intake.
3. As evidenced by: difficulty getting to sleep, walking during night, daytime sleepiness, and decreased productivity.

Leads to

EVALUATION

The patient will...

- Be able to fall asleep more easily.
- Report feeling more rested.
- Demonstrate physical signs of being rested.
- Sleep less during the day and more at night.
- Demonstrate improved ability to cope.
- Demonstrate improved ability to participate in care/activities.
- On return visit, patient sleep log shows improvement in sleep - waking hours <2 per night and average of 20 minutes to fall asleep after switching to decaffeinated coffee and limiting alcohol to 1 drink per evening.

Determine if interventions successful

INTERVENTIONS

- Improve sleep hygiene (decrease activity, stimulants, adequate nutrition, exercise, sleep environment).
- Modify environment.
- Provide security (objects, backrub, anxiety reduction therapy, prayer, meditation).
- Maintain sleep ritual.
- Provide individual support (coping).

Implement these nursing interventions to promote sleep

PLANNING/OUTCOMES

Patient will be able to:

- Verbalize factors related to poor sleep.
- Verbalize psychological stress, facilitating ability to relax.
- Report decreased problems falling asleep.
- Feel rested.
- Demonstrate physical signs of being rested.
- Verbalize goals for sleep/rest.

FIGURE 34-6 Concept map for sleep and rest.

BEARS Approach To Sleep Assessment

Bedtime: Goal—find out what happens around bedtime.
- *Initial question:* Do you have any difficulty falling asleep?
- *Follow-up questions:* How long does it take you to fall asleep? What prevents you from falling asleep? How much coffee, tea, or cola do you drink each day?

Excessive Daytime Sleepiness, Fatigue: Goal—determine the extent of daytime sleepiness.
- *Initial question:* Do you find yourself falling asleep during the day when you don't want to?
- *Follow-up question:* How worn out or exhausted do you feel during the day?

Awakenings: Goal—characterize the extent of nocturnal and early-morning awakenings.
- *Initial question:* Are you having difficulty sleeping through the night or until the morning?
- *Follow-up questions:* What awakens you or keeps you from falling back to sleep? What is your mood in the morning? Has anyone else noticed that you jerk your legs during sleep?

Regularity and Sleep Duration: Goal—delineate sleep habits.
- *Initial question:* What time do you go to bed and get up in the morning?
- *Follow-up questions:* Do you feel that you get enough sleep? Do you need to use an alarm clock?

Snoring: Goal—screen for SDB.
- *Initial question:* Have you or anyone else noticed that you snore loudly?
- *Follow-up questions:* Does anyone complain about your snoring? Has anyone noticed that you stop breathing while you are asleep? Do you awaken from sleep with a feeling of being choked?

Reprinted with permission from Owens, J. A., & Dalzell, V. (2005). Use of the BEARS' sleep screening tool in a pediatric residents' continuity clinic: A pilot study. Sleep Medicine, 66, 63–69.

TABLE 34-3 SLEEP DIARY EXAMPLE

Name: Jane Doe

Complete in the AM (for previous night)	Day 1 (Example)	Day 2	Day 3	Day 4	Day 5	Day 6	Day 7
Day/date	Monday, 4/10						
Time you got into bed	10.00 PM						
Time you tried to sleep (turned out the light)	10:30 PM						
Time you finally awoke	6:30 AM						
Time you got up	7:00 AM						
Estimate time to fall asleep (previous night)	30 min						
Estimate number of awakenings during the night	5 times						
Estimate total time awake (previous night)	2 h						
Estimate amount of sleep obtained (previous night)	4 h						
Complete in the PM							
Naps (time)	3:30 PM						
Naps (duration)	45 min						
Alcoholic drinks (number and time)	1 drink @ 6 PM 2 drinks @ 9 PM						
Caffeine intake (number and time)	2 cups coffee @ 7:30 AM 1 cup @ noon 1 cup @ 7 PM						
List stresses today	Flat tire Argued with son						
How have you felt today? 1 = very tired/sleepy 2 = somewhat tired/sleepy 3 = fairly alert 4 = wide awake	2 = somewhat						
Irritability 1 = not at all/5 = very	5 = very						
Medications	2 Tylenol @ 10 PM						

Adapted from Informed Health Online. Relaxation techniques and sleep hygiene for insomnia. Sept. 24, 2013. Cited 12/3/14. http://www.ncbi.nlm.nih.gov/pubmedhealth/PMH0004995/.

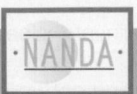

Table 34-4 SELECTED NANDA-I NURSING DIAGNOSES INVOLVING SLEEP

Nursing Dx	Related Factors	Dx Statement	NOC*	NIC†
Disturbed sleep pattern—time-limited disruption of sleep amount and quality	Sensory alterations may contribute to this change in functional health status, including illness or psychological stress that contributes to changing sleep stages.	Disturbed sleep pattern R/T difficulty falling asleep and awakening earlier than desired AEB decreased hours of nocturnal sleep	Anxiety Control Rest Sleep Well-being	Sleep enhancement
Sleep deprivation—prolonged periods of time without sleep	External sensory alterations from environmental changes or social cues may affect sleep patterns by modifying sensory input from changes in levels of light, noise, or social stimulation.	**Sleep deprivation** R/T daytime drowsiness and decreased ability to function AEB hallucinations, irritability, and disturbed perception	Anxiety Control Rest Sleep Well-being	Sleep enhancement

Dx, diagnosis; R/T, related to; AEB, as evidenced by.
*From: Moorhead, S., Johnson, M., Maas, M., & Swanson, E. (2013). Iowa Outcomes Project: Nursing Outcomes Classification (NOC) (5th ed.). St. Louis, MO: C. V. Mosby.
†From: Bulecheck, G., Butcher, H., Dochterman, J., & Wagner, C. (2013). Iowa Intervention Project: Nursing Interventions Classification (NIC) (6th ed.). St. Louis, MO: C. V. Mosby.
From: NANDA-Association International (NANDA-I). (2014). Nursing diagnoses: Definitions and classification, 2015–2017. West Sussex, England: Wiley-Blackwell.

example of a sleep diary. Giving patients responsibility for monitoring their own sleep will help them recognize factors that are related to their sleep. Young and middle-aged adults who are in the habit of sleeping late on days off sometimes express concern about sleep disturbances at the beginning of a workweek, which they may attribute to job stress, but are related to circadian sleep–wake cycle disturbances. Reviewing a sleep diary maintained for a couple of weeks will help them recognize erratic sleep–wake schedules, as well as good and bad sleep hygiene practices, and will assist them in an evaluation of their overall sleep quality and whether they are obtaining sufficient sleep.

Physical Assessment

In adults, observe for circles under the eyes, yawning, nodding, and slowness of response. Irritability, impaired concentration, and word-finding difficulties may indicate sleep disturbances but may also indicate other problems. Children often become hyperactive rather than sleepy.

Adequacy of rest after activity is often measured through return of heart rate and other physiologic parameters to baseline levels. Monitor vital signs after patient- or caregiver-initiated activity for return to baseline resting levels in severely compromised patients.

Diagnostic Tests

People with a suspected sleep disorder or excessive daytime sleepiness should be referred to a sleep center for a more thorough investigation. An overnight polysomnogram in a sleep center is the gold standard in diagnostic tests for OSA, PLMD, and narcolepsy. Home monitoring has the advantage of familiar surroundings and is being used more for screening but has not yet become the diagnostic standard.

NURSING DIAGNOSES

To formulate the nursing diagnosis, cluster the data, sifting out the incidental from the significant. A patient's seemingly casual comment regarding how the children at home are managing "without a disciplinarian around" may be a significant clue to sleep-disturbing anxiety. Diagnostic statements should be as specific as possible. Selected nursing diagnoses NANDA Association International (NANDA-I, 2014) are presented in Table 34-4 along with selected Nursing Outcomes Classification (NOC) and Nursing Interventions Classification (NIC).

OUTCOME IDENTIFICATION AND PLANNING

After the nursing diagnoses and related factors are identified, patient goals and interventions are planned. Patient goals for disturbed sleep pattern or sleep deprivation are specifically stated in terms such as minutes before sleep onset, hours of unbroken sleep, or verbal statement of feeling refreshed on wakening. Examples of specific patient goals are as follows:

- The patient will report fewer problems falling or staying asleep.
- The patient will report feeling more rested.
- The patient will demonstrate physical signs of being rested.

Involving people in setting their own goals for sleep and rest is a useful way of helping them explore what is realistic for their developmental stage, lifestyle, and state of health.

Counseling may be high on the priority list of nurses in helping patients establish periods of adequate sleep and rest. Nurses may need to meet with family members and caregivers to address environmental needs and to teach caregiving practices for enhancing sleep. Examples of nursing interventions commonly used in promoting sleep and rest are listed in Table 34-4 and discussed in the next section.

IMPLEMENTATION

Health Promotion

SLEEP HYGIENE RECOMMENDATIONS

Universal practices believed to enhance sleep quality include reduction of activity (e.g., work, strenuous exercise) and alcohol consumption several hours before bedtime; keeping the bedroom quiet, dark, and cool; eliminating caffeine intake within 6 to 9 hours of bedtime; engaging in relaxing activities before bedtime; and maintaining a consistent rising time.

ENVIRONMENT MODIFICATION

Encourage patients to reserve the sleeping room for sleep. Children should learn to play in other areas. Opportunities should be provided for home care, hospitalized, and residential patients to leave their rooms during the day when feasible. Objects associated with work, conflict, pain, or sleeplessness should be removed or disabled at bedtime.

Encourage patients to establish a quiet, darkened environment modified according to their preferred level (e.g., low light may be a source of comfort for children or those in a strange environment). Instruct parents to remind children to use the bathroom before going to bed. Patients may need to restrict fluids in the evening. Patients can learn simple relaxation exercises for use at bedtime. People with impaired physical mobility should be assisted with voiding before retiring and made comfortable in the bed. Some older male patients appreciate having a urinal within reach.

SAFETY ALERT

Caution patient with impaired gas exchange or sleep apnea to use hypnotics and alcohol cautiously, if at all.

PROVISION OF INTIMACY AND SECURITY

A bedtime hug for a child, the shared bed with a marriage partner, and an enjoyable evening with friends are some ways in which people enhance sleep quality for one another. If social isolation is suspected as a related factor in disturbed sleep pattern, assist the person to make or to improve social contacts. A favorite blanket or stuffed animal is a way of enhancing security for children.

In the hospital or extended care facility setting, arranging for family members to sit at a patient's bedside may be helpful. Assurance of frequent checks by nursing staff, prompt responses to call bells, and a caring manner can do much to allay the fears of anxious patients. For patients with particular religious beliefs, prayer and reading scripture may facilitate a sense of peacefulness and subsequent sleep. Other people find meditation helpful. A sensitive assessment of the person's values and beliefs (see Chapter 7) helps nurses to maximize the patient's strengths.

SLEEP RITUALS

Rituals can play an important role in facilitating sleep. Whether it is a bedtime story for the toddler or a cup of tea for the older couple, the regular association of certain activities with the end of the waking period is one of the most effective ways to create the expectation of sleep.

A routine of "settling" patients in institutional settings can provide a similar marking of the end of the day. Assisting with washing of hands and face, giving a gentle massage, plumping pillows, and providing extra blankets may be incorporated. Use this time as an opportunity to help patients focus on small goals they accomplished during the day, visits from loved ones, or whatever else is helpful to settle their minds as well as their bodies.

MANAGING INDIVIDUAL SLEEP NEEDS

Help patients to assess their individual sleep needs and to anticipate developmental changes. Remind middle-aged and older people that shorter unbroken sleep periods are normal. Likewise, people with insomnia may benefit from reassurance that they are probably getting more sleep than they realize. Parents and other caregivers may need anticipatory guidance regarding the wide variability in sleep needs of individual children.

Nursing Interventions for Altered Function

Despite major advances in medical therapeutics, rest remains one of the most common symptomatic treatments for various disease conditions. "Rest the affected part" is a common intervention for almost any condition.

REST

Patients who have suffered myocardial ischemia as a result of a blood clot are placed on a regimen of restricted activity with bed rest. Helping these patients maintain a resting state for the heart once the initial period of pain has subsided is a challenge to the nurse's creativity. Help these patients realize that although they may "feel great," the damaged heart needs further rest. Assist such patients to make lasting lifestyle changes that incorporate more rest and relaxation.

Maintaining traction to "rest" a patient's fractured femur and instilling eye drops temporarily to paralyze and thus rest the eye after surgery are ways in which nurses help patients meet situationally induced changes in rest requirements.

USE OF CONSISTENT ROUTINE

The single most important intervention for chronic insomnia is to establish a consistent rising time. Getting up is subject to voluntary control, whereas falling asleep usually is not. Decreasing the time in bed drives sleep need and tends to enhance sleep and, along with a consistent rising time, will finally lead to more regular times of sleep onset. Counseling regarding the maintenance of routines may be required for socially and occupationally isolated patients. For acutely ill patients, enhance cuing by turning lights down at night, keeping window drapes open during the day when possible, and providing verbal cuing regarding time of day.

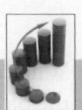

OUTCOME-BASED TEACHING PLANS

Ms. Song is an accountant with a heavy work schedule at the beginning of every calendar year. She finds that she has great difficulty getting to sleep and staying asleep at night. Yet she is drowsy during the day and worries that she may make accounting errors. She has come to the clinic to have her sleep problem assessed and to seek some advice.

OUTCOME

At the end of the teaching session, Ms. Song states factors that could contribute to her difficulty in falling asleep and maintaining sleep at night.

STRATEGIES

- Evaluate Ms. Song's normal sleep routine, her knowledge of factors that contribute to sleep disturbance, and her usual approach to managing her sleep problem.
- Discuss factors that interfere with sleep onset and maintenance, such as the use of alcohol or caffeine and lack of relaxation before bedtime.
- Have Ms. Song discuss these and related factors with you.

OUTCOME

Ms. Song will state a plan to decrease sleep disruption.

STRATEGIES

Suggest that Ms. Song employs the following approaches, and state how she will determine their effectiveness:

- Remind Ms. Song to get up at the same time each day and to avoid sleeping in on days off.
- Instruct Ms. Song to eat sensibly and regularly. If used to a bedtime snack, she should keep up the habit.
- Teach Ms. Song to avoid alcohol and caffeine. Their effects disturb sleep.
- Plan for Ms. Song to exercise daily but not too late in the day. Enjoyable activities will enhance the benefits for sleep and rest.
- Help Ms. Song determine ways to set her mind at rest before going to bed with relaxing music, a good book, or valued companionship. If she cannot sleep, Ms. Song will get up and do something relaxing until feeling sleepy.

EVALUATION

4/1/17: 08:30—Ms. Song's sleep routine is free from alcohol and caffeine, based on her report.

Ms. Song reports that she gets up at the same time each day on most days.

Ms. Song states she has started exercising 3 days a week in the early morning.

Ms. Song reports that she listens to relaxing music before going to bed, and it seems to have helped her fall asleep.

—J. Woodman, RN

COGNITIVE MEASURES

For many patients, racing thoughts and worries about the previous day's activity or anticipating activities the next day can be a major factor affecting the time it takes to fall asleep or to get back to sleep after a nighttime wakening. Nurses can assist by teaching relaxation exercises and stress management techniques such as thought stopping or writing down one's worries on paper and tossing the paper in the trash before sleep.

USE OF MEDICATIONS

Hypnotics may be useful as a short-term intervention for insomnia. CBT-I should be tried first. In making decisions and teaching patients regarding the use of hypnotics, the nurse should consider the following principles:

- Hypnotics require judicious use because they do not induce normal sleep and are not without side effects. Tapering withdrawal in long-term users can prevent rebound.
- Hypnotics can impair waking function as long as they are pharmacologically active. Perception of daytime drowsiness and impairment of psychomotor skills fades more rapidly

than do the actual effects, so individuals should avoid driving or handling machinery while the drug is in their system. Individuals should take safety precautions in the home or hospital when they have taken a hypnotic and need to get to the bathroom at night.

- Hypnotics are most appropriately used for insomnia of recent origin, such as after a situational crisis. Patients should take the smallest effective dose and then only for a few nights or intermittently as required.
- Certain people are at increased risk from the use of hypnotics. The time required for older adults to metabolize long-acting benzodiazepines is increased. Arousal because of decreased oxygen levels is depressed after the administration of hypnotics. Use particular caution in administering ordered hypnotics to older adults and those whose pulmonary function is compromised.

Table 34-2 shows how knowledge of the specific properties of each hypnotic can help nurses determine implications for assessment and teaching. The chart is not intended to be exhaustive but rather to highlight the need for nurses to be knowledgeable about the hypnotics that patients may take.

PATIENT PLAN OF CARE:
The Patient With Disturbed Sleep Pattern

NURSING DIAGNOSIS

Disturbed sleep pattern related to lack of cues for day–night schedule, manifested by erratic sleep schedule, frequent naps, nocturnal wandering, and asking for breakfast at 01:00 or 02:00.

PATIENT GOAL

Patient will sleep more at night and less during the day.

PATIENT OUTCOME CRITERIA

- Patient increases nocturnal sleep time by 10% to 20% over next 2 weeks.
- Patient verbalizes more appropriate orientation to time of day.

NURSING INTERVENTION	SCIENTIFIC RATIONALE
1. Offer meals at regular times, corresponding to patient's previous pattern.	**1.** Mealtimes are important social cues that reinforce circadian rhythms, which tend to weaken with advancing age.
2. Provide active, meaningful activities during daytime hours, with natural light exposure outdoors, when possible.	**2.** Light exposure is communicated through the retina to the hypothalamus, setting the circadian "clock."
3. Monitor frequency and duration of daytime naps and avoid napping in the early evening.	**3.** Napping is not contraindicated but is best at the time of day opposite to the midpoint of the nocturnal sleep period. Short, 15-minute naps are preferable.
4. Create an individualized bedtime ritual that includes a quieting activity, a light carbohydrate or protein snack, going to the bathroom, and a settling routine.	**4.** Reduced stimulation and rituals associated with sleep enhance sleep onset.
5. Do not waken even if incontinent. Change and assist the patient to the bathroom when he or she spontaneously awakens.	**5.** Older adults who can turn themselves generally do better to have their sleep undisturbed and tend to waken spontaneously if wet when their sleep cycle lightens.
6. If turning or other care is necessary, try to provide for periods of up to 2 hours of undisturbed sleep time whenever possible.	**6.** Sleep cycles average 90 minutes. A sleep latency of 20 to 30 minutes means that it would take about 2 hours to experience a full sleep cycle.

EVALUATION

4/3/17: 16:00—Patient reports increased nocturnal sleep time by about an hour over the last 2 weeks. Patient and family state that the patient has better appropriate orientation to time of day; will follow over the next 2 weeks.

—S. Roberts, RN

Home and Community Care

Patients often underestimate their need for rest when recovering from illness or surgery. Nurses may need to help them plan for periods of rest and for energy conservation. Assessment of and suggestions for correction or adaptation to environmental conditions may be necessary. Remember to consider the sleep and rest needs of home caregivers when ill or immobile patients need assistance during the night. Respite care may be an option, or caregivers may need counseling about their sleep and rest needs.

EVALUATION

Evaluate the degree to which disturbed sleep, sleep loss, or inadequate rest has been resolved according to the patient goals initially established. Particularly for this functional health pattern, validate findings with patients because of the subjectivity and individual variations in what people require for adequate rest and satisfying sleep. Examples of possible outcome criteria are listed below.

Goal

The patient will report fewer problems falling asleep.

POSSIBLE OUTCOME CRITERIA

The patient, within a designated time period:

- Reports decrease in sleep latency to 10 to 15 minutes
- Reports less anxiety regarding falling asleep

Goal

The patient will report feeling more rested.

POSSIBLE OUTCOME CRITERIA

The patient:

- Verbalizes feeling less fatigued within a designated period of time
- Nonverbally demonstrates increased restfulness (less dozing, greater animation in activity), as observed by the nurse

Goal

The patient will demonstrate physical signs of being rested.

POSSIBLE OUTCOME CRITERIA

The patient:

- Has decreases in circles under the eyes, excessive yawning, or slowness of response by the seventh day
- Reports to the nurse that he or she feels rested after activity within 10 days

KEY CONCEPTS

- Sleep is a naturally occurring behavioral state of decreased awareness and responsiveness to environmental surroundings.
- Rest is a physical and emotional state of decreased muscle and cognitive activity.
- Sleep and rest are important for health and recovery from illness.
- The two main types of sleep are NREM and REM sleep:
  - NREM sleep consists of three stages—stage N1, stage N2, and stage N3 or SWS.
  - REM sleep is similar to wakefulness in terms of brain activity, but muscle tone is absent and vital signs are highly variable.
- Young adults progress through stages 1–2–3–2–REM in cycles of approximately 90 minutes.
- Sleep duration and architecture change throughout the life span.
- Infants have frequent sleep cycles evenly distributed throughout the day and night.
- Adequate sleep is associated with waking up feeling alert and refreshed and with an absence of daytime sleepiness.

- Factors affecting sleep and rest include environmental stimuli, nutrition, exercise, illness, and hospitalization.
- Sleep disorders are common in both adults and children and include insomnia, SDB, narcolepsy, RLS, and PLMD, and the parasomnias.
- Anticipating changes in sleep and needs for rest can contribute to promotion of a healthy balance between rest and activity and a recognition that sleep changes are developmentally normal.

PRACTICING FOR THE NCLEX

CHECK YOUR ANSWERS IN APPENDIX A.

1. A patient seen at an annual physical is observed to be irritable and unable to concentrate. When questioned about his behavior, he attributes it to working two full-time jobs. What nursing diagnosis would be most appropriate?
   a. Disturbed sleep pattern
   b. Sleep deprivation
   c. Coping
   d. Activity intolerance

2. A postoperative patient with a history of OSA is admitted to your unit. With which assessment finding would you be most concerned?
   a. Apneic periods lasting more than 10 seconds
   b. Oxygen saturation of 94% when transferred to the room
   c. Oxygen desaturation to 90% when asleep
   d. Patient difficult to arouse
   e. Blood pressure 138/90

3. A patient complains about inability to sleep in the hospital. Which of the following nursing interventions would be most beneficial to do first?
   a. Providing warm milk like the patient has at home
   b. Transferring the patient to a room away from the nursing station
   c. Clustering nursing care to limit disturbances at night
   d. Complete a pain assessment

4. Which of the following factors influence sleep and rest needs? Select all that apply.
   a. Developmental stage
   b. Relationships
   c. Nutrition
   d. Alcohol
   e. Shift work

5. Normal circadian rhythms would be seen in which of the following individuals?
   a. A patient who is homebound without social contact
   b. Nurse who works in a hospital with variable night shifts
   c. Businesswoman traveling abroad
   d. A 1-year-old pediatric patient

REFERENCES

American Academy of Sleep Medicine. (2007). *Manual for the scoring of sleep and associated events: Rules, terminology and technical specifications.* Westchester, IL: Author.

Ancoli-Israel, S., Krystal, A. D., McCall, W. V., Schaefer, K., Wilson, A., Claus, R., et al. (2010). A 12-week, randomized, double-blind, placebo-controlled study evaluating the effect of eszopiclone 2 mg on sleep/wake function in older adults with primary and comorbid insomnia. *Sleep, 33*(2), 225–234.

Boehm, H., & Morast, S. (2009). Quiet time. *American Journal of Nursing, 109*(11 Suppl), 29–33.

Boergers, J., Gable, C. J., & Owens, J. A. (2014). Later school start times is associated with improved sleep and daytime functioning in adolescents. *Journal of Developmental & Behavioral Pediatrics, 35,* 11–17.

Buysse, D. J. (2013). Insomnia. *Journal of American Medical Association, 309*(7), 706–716.

Buysse, D. J. (2014). Sleep health: Can we define it? Does it matter? *Sleep, 37*(1), 9–17.

Calhoun, S. L., Fernandez-Mendoza, J., Vgontzas, A. N., Liao, D., & Bixler, E. O. (2014). Prevalence of insomnia symptoms in a general population sample of young children and preadolescents: gender effects. *Sleep Medicine, 15*(1), 91–95.

Carter, K. A., Hathaway, N. E., & Lettieri, C. F. (2014). Common sleep disorders in children. *American Family Physician, 89*(5), 368–377.

Cirelli, C. (2013). Sleep and synaptic changes. *Current Opinion in Neurobiology, 23,* 841–846.

Dijk, D.-J., Groeger, J. A., Stanley, N., & Deacon, S. (2010). Age-related reduction in daytime sleep propensity and nocturnal slow wave sleep. *Sleep, 33,* 211–233.

Deary, V., Ellis, J. G., Wilson, J. A., Coulter, C., & Barclay, N. L. (2014). Simple snoring: Not quite so simple after all? *Sleep Medicine Reviews,* May 9. pii: S1087-0792(14)00047-1. doi: 10.1016/j.smrv.2014.04.006. [Epub ahead of print]

Drager, L. F., Togeiro, S. M., Polotsky, V. Y., & Lorenzi-Filho, G. (2013). Obstructive sleep apnea: a cardiometabolic risk in obesity and the metabolic syndrome. *Journal of American College of Cardiology, 62*(7), 569–576.

Drouot, X., Cabello, B., d'Ortho, M.-P., & Brochard, L. (2008). Sleep in the intensive care unit. *Sleep Medicine Reviews, 12,* 391–403.

Fernandez-Mendoza, J., Vgontzas, A. N., Calhoun, S. L., Vgontzas, A., Tsaoussoglou, M., Gaines, J., et al. (2014). Insomnia symptoms, objective sleep duration and hypothalamic-pituitary-adrenal activity in children. *European Journal of Clinical Investigation, 44*(5), 493–500.

Finan, P. H., Goodin, B. R., & Smith, M. T. (2013). The association of sleep and pain: An update and a path forward. *The Journal of Pain, 14,* 1539–1552.

Franken, P. (2013). A role for clock genes in sleep homeostasis. *Current Opinion in Neurobiology, 23,* 864–872.

Galland, B. C., Taylor, B. J., Elder, D. E., & Herbison, P. (2012). Normal sleep patterns in infants and children: A systematic review of observational studies. *Sleep Medicine Reviews, 16,* 213–222.

Griffiths, M. F., & Peerson, A. (2005). Risk factors for chronic insomnia following hospitalization. *Journal of Advanced Nursing, 49*(3), 245–253.

Goel, N., Basner, M., Rao, H., & Dinges, D. F. (2013). Circadian rhythms, sleep deprivation, and human performance. *Progress Molecular Biology Translation Science, 119,* 155–190.

Heatley, E. M., Harris, M., Battesby, M., McEvoy, R. D., Chai-Coetzer, C. L., & Antic, N. A. (2013). Obstructive sleep apnoea in adults: A common chronic condition in need of a comprehensive chronic condition management approach. *Sleep Medicine Reviews, 17*(5), 349–355.

Hysing, M., Pallesen, S., Stormark, K. M., Lundervold, A. J., & Sivertsen, B. (2013). Sleep patterns and insomnia among adolescents: A population based study. *Journal or Sleep Research, 22*(5), 549–556.

Institute of Medicine. (2006). *Sleep disorders and sleep deprivation: An unmet public health problem. Institute of Medicine of the National Academies.* Washington, DC: National Academies Press.

Killick, R., Banks, S., & Liu, P. Y. (2012). Implications of sleep restriction and recovery on metabolic outcomes. *Journal of Clinical Metabolism, 97*(11), 3876–3890.

Knutson, K. L. (2013). Sociodemographic and cultural determinants of sleep deficiency: Implications for cardiometabolic disease risk. *Social Science & Medicine, 79,* 7–15.

Knutson K. L., & Orzech, K. M. (2013). Sleep, culture and health: Reflections on the other third of life. *Social Science & Medicine, 79,* 1–6.

Knutson, K. L., Van Couter, E., Rathouz, P. J., DeLeire, T., & Lauderdale, D. S. (2010). Trends in the prevalence of short sleepers in the USA: 1975–2006. *Sleep, 33,* 37–45.

Kravitz, H. M., & Joffe, H. (2011). Sleep during the perimenopause: A SWAN story. *Obstetrics Gynecology Clinics North America, 38,* 567–586

Krueger, P. M., & Friedman, E. M. (2009). Sleep duration in the United States: A cross-sectional population-based study. *American Journal of Epidemiology, 169,* 1052–1063.

Liao, W.-C., Wang, L., Kuo, C.-P., Lo, C., & Chiu, M.-J. (2013). Effect of a warm footbath before bedtime on body temperature and sleep in older adults with good and poor sleep: An experimental crossover trial. *International Journal of Nursing Studies, 50,* 1607–1616.

Liu, J., Zhang, A., & Li, L. (2012). Sleep duration and overweight/obesity in children: Review and implications for pediatric nursing. *Journal for Specialists in Pediatric Nursing, 17,* 193–204.

Liu, Y., Wheaton, A. G., Chapman, D. P., & Croft, J. B. (2013). Sleep duration and chronic diseases among US adults age 45 years and older: Evidence from 2010 Behavioral Risk Factor Surveillance System. *Sleep, 36*(10), 1421–1427.

Luyster, F. S., Strollo, P. J., Zee, P. C., & Walsh, J. K. (2012). Sleep: a health imperative. *Sleep, 35*(6), 727–734.

Marcus, C. L., Brooks, L. J., Draper, K. A., Gozal, D., Halbower, A. C., Jones, J., et al. (2012). Diagnosis and management of childhood obstructive sleep apnea syndrome. *Pediatrics, 130,* 576–584.

McKnight-Eily, L. R., Eaton, D. K., Lowry, R., Croft, J. B., Presley-Cantrell, L., & Perry, G. S. (2011). Relationships between hours of sleep and health risk behaviors in US adolescent students. *Preventive Medicine, 53,* 271–273.

Montgomery-Downs, H. E., O'Brien, L., Gulliver, T. E., & Gozal, D. (2006). Polysomnographic characteristics in normal preschool and early school-aged children. *Pediatrics, 117,* 741–753.

Morgan, K., Gregory, P., Tomeny, M., David, B. M., & Gascoigne, C. (2012). Self-help treatment for insomnia symptoms associated with chronic conditions in older adults: a randomized controlled trial. *Journal American Geriatric Society, 60*(10), 1803–1810.

National Sleep Foundation. (2008). *Sleep in America poll 2008.* Retrieved April 15, 2010, www.sleepfoundation.org/sites/default/files/2008%20POLL%20SOF.PDFblications/2008poll.html

National Institutes of Health State of the Science Conference Statement. (2005). Manifestations and management of chronic insomnia in adults, June 13–15, 2005. *Sleep, 28,* 1049–1057.

NANDA-Association International (NANDA). (2014). *Nursing diagnoses: Definitions and classification, 2015–2017.* West Sussex, England: Wiley-Blackwell.

Ohayon, M. M., Carskadon, M. A., Guilleminault, G., & Vitiello, M. V. (2004). Meta-analysis of quantitative sleep parameters from childhood to old age in healthy individuals. *Sleep, 27,* 1255–1273.

Olaithe, M., & Bucks, R. S. (2013). Executive dysfunction in OSA before and after treatment: a meta-analysis. *Sleep, 36*(9), 1297–1305.

Owens, J. A., & Dalzell, V. (2005). Use of the BEARS' sleep screening tool in a pediatric residents' continuity clinic: A pilot study. *Sleep Medicine, 6,* 63–69.

Paiva, T., & Attarian, H. (2014). Obstructive sleep apnea and other sleep-related syndromes. *Handbook of Clinical Neurology, 119,* 251–271.

Partinen, M., Kornum, B. R., Plazzi, G., Jennum, P., Julkunen, I., & Vaarala, O. (2014). Narcolepsy as an autoimmune disease: the role of H1NI infection and vaccination. *The Lancet Neurology, 13,* 600–613.

Porkka-Heiskanen, T., Zitting, K.-M., & Wigren, H.-K. (2013). Sleep, its regulation and possible mechanisms of sleep disturbances. *Acta Physiology, 208,* 311–328.

Rechtschaffen, A., & Kales, A. (1968). *A manual of standardized terminology, techniques, and scoring systems for sleep stages of human subjects.* Los Angeles, CA: Brain Information/Brain Research Institute UCLA.

Rimmele, D. L., & Thomalla, G. (2014). Wake-up stroke: clinical characteristics, imaging findings, and treatment – an update. *Frontiers in Neurology*, 5, 35.

Rondanelli, M., Faliva, M. A., Perna, S., & Antonicello, N. (2013). Update on the role of melatonin in the prevention of cancer tumorigenesis and in the management of cancer correlates, such as sleep-wake and mood disturbances: review and remarks. *Aging Clinical Experimental Research*, 25, 499–510.

Rye, D., & Trotti, L. M. (2012). Restless legs and periodic leg movements of sleep. *Neurology Clinics*, 30(4), 1137–1166.

Seicean, S., Newhauser, D., Strohl, K., & Redline, S. (2011). An exploration of differences in sleep characteristics between Mexico-born US immigrants and other Americans to address the Hispanic Paradox. *Sleep*, 34(8), 1021–1031.

Vitiello, M. V., McCurry, S. M., Shortreed, S. M., Baker, L. D., Rybarczyk, B. D., Keefe, F. J., et al. (2014). Short-term improvement in insomnia symptoms predicts long-term improvements in sleep, pain, and fatigue in older adults with co-morbid osteoarthritis and insomnia. *Pain*, doi: http://dx.doi.org/10.1016/j.pain.2014.04.032

Vgontzas, A. N., Fernandez-Mendoza, J., Liao, D., & Bixler, E. O. (2013). Insomnia with objective short sleep duration: the most biologically sever phenotype of the disorder. *Sleep Medicine Reviews*, 17(4), 241–254.

Volpe, L., Ball, H., & McKenna, J. (2013). Nighttime parenting strategies and sleep related risk to infants. *Social Science & Medicine*, 79, 92–100.

Wahlstrom, K., Dretzke, B., Gordon, M., Peterson, K., Edwards, K., & Gdula, J. (2014). *Examining the Impact of Later School Start Times on the Health and Academic Performance of High School Students: A Multi-Site Study.* St Paul, MN: Center for Applied Research and Educational Improvement, University of Minnesota.

Ward, T. E., Archbold, K. H., Lentz, M. J., Ringold, S., Wallace, C. A., & Landis, C. A. (2010). Daytime sleepiness and neurobehavioral performance in children with active and inactive Juvenile Rheumatoid Arthritis. *Sleep*, 33, 232–241.

Weaver, T. E. (2013). Don't start celebrating—CPAP adherence remains a problem. *Journal of Clinical Sleep Medicine*, 9(6), 551–552.

Wennberg, A. M., Canham, S. L., Smith, M. T., & Spria, A. P. (2013). Optimizing sleep in older adults: Treating insomnia. *Maturitas*, 76, 247–252.

Worthman, C. M., & Borwn, R. A. (2013). Sleep budgets in a globalizing world: biocultural interactions influence sleep sufficiency among Egyptian families. *Social Science & Medicine*, 79, 31–39.

Zee, P. C., Attarian, H., & Videnovic, A. (2013). Circadian rhythm abnormalities. *American Academy of Neurology*, 19(1):132–147.

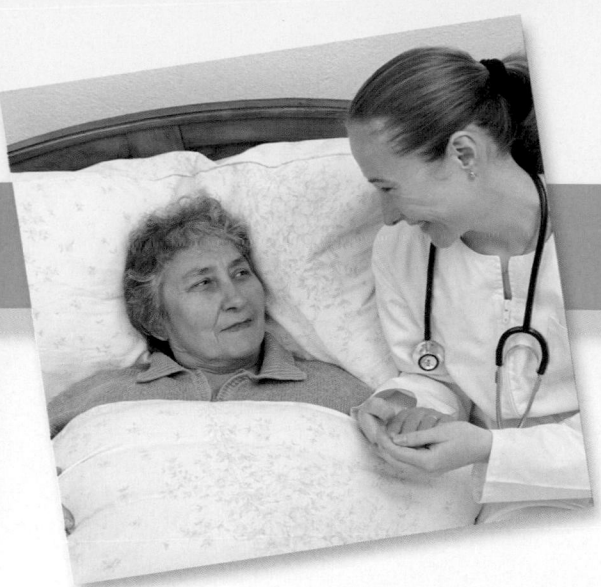

CHAPTER 35

Pain Management

Ellen Noel

Case Scenario

You are a home hospice nurse caring for an older patient who was diagnosed 3 months ago with lung cancer. The patient's history is positive for lung cancer (father died of it) and for smoking one to two packs of cigarettes per day for 50 years. Staging revealed metastases in the right lung, both kidneys, and the sixth cervical vertebra. Currently, the patient reports pain in the left shoulder, upper arm, and right upper thigh. The patient rates the pain as 6 on a scale of 0 to 10. The patient describes it as dull and aching but is unable to provide further description of its quality. She reports that the shoulder pain is constant and increases with particular movements. Her right leg pain is present only when ambulating and when turning onto her left side when in bed. The patient's ability to tolerate activity has diminished since radiation treatments began. Before treatment, the patient was out of bed 14 to 16 hours/day but now is out of bed 3 to 5 hours/day.

Once you have completed this chapter and have incorporated pain management into your knowledge base, review the above scenario and reflect on the following areas of Critical Thinking:

1. Give your interpretation of the patient's reports of pain and activity intolerance.
2. Reflect on your feelings about the patient's health history and present condition. Infer what the patient's thoughts and feelings may be.
3. Outline additional assessment data you need to develop a plan for relieving this person's pain.
4. Explain the rationale for using pharmacologic and nonpharmacologic methods of pain relief for this patient.
5. Plan at least two health promotion activities that may help this patient.

KEY TERMS

acute pain
addiction
adjuvant
allodynia
central sensitization
dermatome
endogenous opioids
exogenous opioids
hyperalgesia
multimodal therapy
neuropathic pain
nociception
nociceptive pain
persistent (chronic) pain
physical dependence
somatic pain
spinal dorsal horn
suffering
tolerance
transcutaneous electrical nerve stimulation
visceral pain

Upon completion of this chapter, you will be able to do the following:

1. Explain the basic process of normal pain transmission.
2. Outline how pain transmission is facilitated or inhibited.
3. Describe the four dimensions of pain.
4. Examine nonpharmacologic methods of pain relief based on individual needs.
5. Describe the types, actions, and adverse effects of analgesics.
6. List nursing implications for various classes of drugs used for pain management.
7. Develop a nursing plan of care for a patient experiencing pain.

PAIN PERCEPTION

Pain is a subjective and individual phenomenon that people encounter during their lives and is often the primary reason patients seek healthcare. Pain warns us of potential injury and alerts us when tissue damage has occurred. Although pain is a universal human experience, our unique genetic makeup and interpretations of pain make it extremely personal. The sensory and emotional complexities of pain contribute to the clinical challenges of pain management in multiple settings. Consequently, a strong pain management knowledge base that includes an understanding of the mechanisms of pain, evidence-based pain management standards, and a commitment to understanding the impact that pain has on patients' recovery, functioning, and quality of life is essential to professional nursing practice.

Structures and Pain Process

The International Association for the Study of Pain (IASP) defines *pain* as "an unpleasant sensory and emotional experience associated with actual or potential tissue damage or described in terms of such damage" (IASP, 1979, 1994). This definition reflects the adaptive characteristic of pain and its associated protective qualities. For instance, pain triggers sympathetic nervous system reflexes and makes a person pull his or her hand away from a hot stove. Pain from a surgical incision, angina, or pressure exerted on surrounding tissue from a pancreatic tumor alerts patients of actual or potential harm.

The subjective nature of pain is described simply in the groundbreaking definition of pain developed by nursing pain expert Margo McCaffery: "Pain is whatever the experiencing person says it is, existing whenever he says it does" (McCaffery & Pasero, 2011). This definition identifies the patient as the primary source of pain information and an expert in his or her pain experience. Integrating the patient experience into a pain management plan is essential to optimize outcomes and avoid additional physical and physiologic harm associated with suboptimal pain treatment.

PAIN PATHWAYS AND PROCESSES

Nociception involves the normal processing of painful stimuli and is described in terms of a four-step process that occurs when acute pain becomes a conscious event. As shown in Figure 35-1, the nociceptive system extends from the periphery through the spinal cord, brain stem, and thalamus to the cerebral cortex, where the sensation is perceived. The basic principles of nociception are outlined below.

Transduction

The first step in pain impulse transmission occurs in the periphery at the site of injury. Energy is converted from one form to another, and injured cells release substances that activate or sensitize nearby nociceptors. A nociceptor is a peripheral nervous system receptor that is sensitive to harmful stimuli. Nociceptors are sensitive to noxious stimuli from temperature (thermoreceptors), chemicals (chemoreceptors), pressure, or mechanical injury (mechanical receptors) and transmit a pain signal if the noxious stimuli are sufficiently strong.

Nociceptors that respond to noxious stimuli are found in the skin, blood vessels, subcutaneous tissue, muscle, fascia, periosteum, viscera, joints, and other structures. Nociceptors are located on two types of peripheral nerve cells (A-delta fibers and C-fibers) that are responsible for transmitting pain sensations from the tissues to the central nervous system (CNS). A-delta fibers give rise to bright, sharp, well-localized pain that is immediately associated with the injury. Slow-conducting C-fibers cause a second pain sensation that is dull, poorly localized, and persistent after injury.

The difference between pain from A-delta and C-fiber activation can best be described as first versus second pain. For example, if you hit your thumb with a hammer or puncture it with a needle, a fast, sharp pain alerts you to the injury. This pain is caused by stimulation of the A-delta fibers. Even though the hammer has stopped hitting your thumb, a burning, dull, aching sensation persists for minutes and is caused by stimulation of the C-fibers as the message travels through the periphery to the CNS for interpretation.

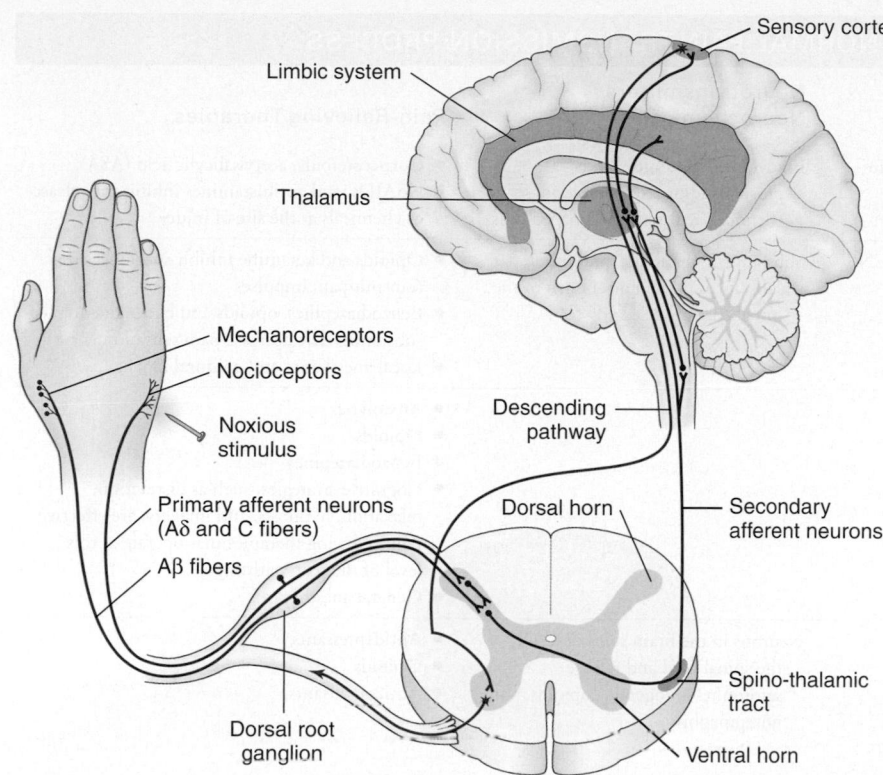

FIGURE 35-1 Transmission of pain stimuli starts at pain receptors and moves by way of sensory nerves into the dorsal root ganglia. The impulse enters the spinal cord, where it crosses the cord and ascends in the spinothalamic tract to areas of the brain where pain is perceived.

Transmission

Pain transmission from the peripheral nociceptive fibers to the brain is complex. Signals carried by A-delta fibers and C-fibers travel from peripheral tissues through the dorsal root of the spinal cord and terminate in the dorsal horn of the spinal cord. The **spinal dorsal horn**, where complex processing of messages occurs, is one of the most important areas for pain transmission. Signals communicate with excitatory or inhibitory interneurons that ascend to the brain by way of several crossed and uncrossed pathways. Input to dorsal horn excitatory interneurons releases substance P and glutamate, both of which have the potential to facilitate pain sensation. The spinothalamic tract transmits ascending impulses via secondary afferent neurons toward the brain and thalamus for interpretation. This crossed pathway is located in the white matter of the anterolateral quadrant of the spinal cord. The spinothalamic tract transmits sensations of pain and temperature and crudely localized touch. The spinothalamic tract enters the brain stem and terminates principally in the thalamus, where other neurons convey the information to the sensory cortex and limbic system (see Fig. 35-1).

Perception

Pain perception is the conscious awareness and personal interpretation of the painful experience as information is processed in the sensory cortex and limbic system. Sensation is combined with emotional, social, and behavioral components, and the individual meaning of pain is recognized. Current pain perceptions can be influenced by past experiences. For instance, a poorly managed past event can cause patients to anticipate that they will have uncontrolled pain. This can lead to feelings of anxiety and fear and ultimately heighten sensitivity to painful stimuli with decreased pain tolerance.

Modulation

Modulation is the inhibition of nociceptive impulses in the CNS. Neurons originating in the brain stem utilize the descending pathway in the spinal cord, releasing naturally occurring pain inhibitory substances that decrease pain sensation. Input to inhibitory interneurons and from descending neurons releases several neurochemicals that have inhibitory effects on pain sensations. These neurochemicals bind to several types of receptors. For example, the opioid receptors, important for the inhibition of pain perception, are sites where **endogenous opioids** (produced by the body) and **exogenous opioids** (administered to the person) bind. Endogenous opioids, serotonin, and norepinephrine are examples of substances that are released during the modulation step to inhibit pain impulse transmission.

Table 35-1 summarizes the four basic processes of normal pain impulse transmission and includes examples of pharmacologic and nonpharmacologic interventions for each process step.

Types of Pain

Understanding different types of pain helps nurses develop and execute an individualized pain management plan for their patients. Differences include the timing and duration of pain, causes, and objective signs. It is important to remember that some patients can experience both acute and persistent pain concurrently and that there are overlapping and unique pain management strategies for each.

TABLE 35-1 NOCICEPTION: THE NORMAL PAIN TRANSMISSION PROCESS

Process	Location	Neurotransmitters/ Neurochemicals	Pain-Relieving Therapies
Transduction	Peripheral nervous system at the site of injury	Bradykinin, histamine, and prostaglandins are examples of chemicals released by damaged cells	• Corticosteroids, acetylsalicylic acid (ASA), NSAIDs, and antihistamines inhibit the release of chemicals at the site of injury
Transmission	Peripheral nervous system to the CNS	Substance P, glutamate, and other substances in the dorsal horn of the spinal cord are released	• Opioids and ketamine inhibit substances that transmit pain impulses • Benzodiazepines, opioids and baclofen enhance substances that decrease pain sensation • Local anesthetics and epidural blocks
Perception	CNS		• Anxiolytics • Opioids • Benzodiazepines • Cognitive strategies, such as distraction, relaxation, hypnosis, and imagery, are effective pain-reducing therapies that operate at this level of the pain pathway • General anesthetics
Modulation	CNS	Neurons in the brain stem descend the spinal cord and release serotonin, endogenous opioids, and norepinephrine	• Antidepressants • Opioids • Anticonvulsants

ACUTE PAIN

Acute pain is the result of potential or actual tissue injury and includes activation of nociceptive nerve fibers at the site of localized injury. Acute pain is time limited and occurs after trauma, surgery, or a disease process. The cause of acute pain is usually known, and pain intensity usually decreases with healing. Acute pain may also have observable physical signs such as increased heart rate, increased respirations, or elevated blood pressure. Behavioral signs may also be present, such as facial grimacing or inability to cough and deep breathe after abdominal surgery. It is important to remember, however, that the absence of physical and behavioral signs does not mean that the patient is without pain since each patient will exhibit their own individual pain response.

PERSISTENT (CHRONIC) PAIN

Unlike acute pain, which follows the normal nociceptive pain process, persistent (chronic) pain serves no useful purpose. Healthcare providers are using the term *persistent pain* in place of *chronic pain* to help avoid the negative and often inaccurate assumptions associated with chronic pain patients. **Persistent pain** is an abnormal pain signaling process with origins that can occur both peripherally and centrally. Persistent pain is cyclical and irreversible and generally persists longer than 3 to 6 months. Untreated or undertreated acute pain may lead to a chronic pain syndrome that is difficult to treat (D'Arcy, 2014). Patients with severe persistent pain may not appear to be in pain and may exhibit a flat affect. Physical pain responses such as elevated blood pressure, tachycardia, or facial grimacing are usually not present, and stress, depression, or anxiety often heighten pain perception. Consequently, physiologic pain responses and

behaviors commonly seen during acute pain cannot be reliably used when assessing patients with prolonged persistent pain.

Several mechanisms can lead to persistent pain development. One proposed mechanism involves the process of **central sensitization**. During the process of central sensitization, nociceptive nerve signals (triggered by inflammation or nerve injury) bombard the CNS from the periphery. Prolonged and persistent bombardment leads to long-term changes in the CNS, resulting in persistent pain amplification with even mild noxious stimuli (Zacharoff, Pujol, & Corsini, 2010). Rheumatoid arthritis is an example of a chronic disease process that has persistent pain signal amplification due to prolonged autoimmune inflammation.

Central sensitization can lead to long-term changes in the CNS causing **hyperalgesia**, which is defined as an exaggerated response to normal painful stimuli. Hyperalgesia results in lower pain tolerance (threshold), spontaneous pain, and increased sensitivity. Patients with postherpetic neuralgia may experience hyperalgesia. **Allodynia** is another pain response phenomenon that occurs due to abnormal pain signaling and results in perceived pain with mild, nonpainful stimuli. Allodynia may be experienced by patients with diabetic neuropathy as even light touch, the weight of blankets, or rapid changes in temperature to the lower extremities can elicit a sudden, painful response.

CANCER PAIN

Patients with cancer at all stages of their disease and treatment require dedicated attention to pain management as part of their treatment continuum. Pain is often the first symptom that causes cancer patients to seek treatment. Early on, pain may be associated with diagnostic procedures, surgery, and cancer treatments. Cancer pain, like many pain types and syndromes, can have both acute and persistent pain qualities. Pain increases with the prevalence of cancer; however, it is important to remember that with appropriate interventions, pain does not have to be an inevitable outcome. Patients with cancer have been shown to be reluctant to report pain for fear that this is an indication that their cancer has progressed (Potter, Wiseman, Dunn, & Boyle, 2003).

NOCICEPTIVE PAIN

Prolonged, recurring pain that does not go away over time is a significant finding that differentiates persistent pain from acute pain. Pain is also classified in terms of its pathophysiology with two distinct categories. **Nociceptive pain** occurs in tissues other than the nervous system and is transmitted via intact nociceptors during normal pain transmission. Nociceptive pain can be acute, such as pain occurring from a laceration, or persistent, as seen in patients with ulcerative colitis. Nociceptive pain is divided into two unique pain types, each with its own specific characteristics. The first, **somatic pain**, originates in bone, skin, and soft tissue and is often well localized. Patients will describe somatic pain as aching or throbbing; when asked if they can point to the location of their pain, they are often able to specifically pinpoint where it hurts. Examples of somatic pain include a broken hip due to a femoral neck fracture or soft tissue injury such as a contusion from a sprained ankle. Somatic pain is also experienced by patients with a diagnosis of bone metastasis resulting from invasive cancer. The second type of nociceptive pain is **visceral pain**, which originates internally and is the result of stretching, distention, inflammation, or damage to the hollow and solid organs. Patients tend to describe visceral pain as aching, throbbing, cramping, pressure, deep, or radiating. This type of pain is often diffuse and difficult for patients to pinpoint. Chest pain from an acute myocardial infarct is an example of visceral pain; the patient describes chest pressure and heaviness with aching that radiates to the jaw or left arm. Inability to void resulting in significant bladder distention may also produce visceral pain.

NEUROPATHIC PAIN

Neuropathic pain arises from damage to the peripheral nerves or the CNS and unlike nociceptive pain is the result of abnormal sensory input. However, not all patients with nerve damage will experience neuropathic pain. Neuropathic pain may be evoked by stimulation or perceived spontaneously and often evolves over time with a great deal of variability in patient symptoms (Dahl, Gordon, Paice, Stevenson, & Brown, 2008). Neuropathic pain can occur in many syndromes, including diabetic neuropathy, central pain syndromes such as post stroke pain or phantom limb pain, impingement of tumors on nerves, and pain states associated with cancer. Some chemotherapy agents and radiation can damage the nervous system and contribute to the development of neuropathic pain. Postmastectomy and postthoracotomy patients may experience postneuropathic

pain syndromes due to nerve damage as a result of the surgical procedure. Patients describe neuropathic pain as tingling, itching, burning, cold, prickly, or "shocklike." Despite the variability in patient presentation, three symptoms are significant predictors of neuropathic pain: tingling, numbness, and pain with normal touch. Decreased strength and abnormal reflexes may also accompany neuropathic pain and should be taken into consideration during the systematic pain assessment.

Life Span Considerations

NEWBORN AND INFANT

Although a newborn or infant lacks the cognitive skills to verbally report pain, it is clear that painful stimuli is perceived from birth. Infants and newborns are considered one of the at-risk groups for the undertreatment of pain. Several studies have provided evidence that pain has both short- and long-term consequences in infants. Repetitive and prolonged pain in infants and newborns is associated with altered pain sensitivity and pain processing later in life. Studies have shown that infants circumcised without pain control exhibited increased pain response during their 4- and 6-month routine immunizations compared to the uncircumcised infants (Taddio & Katz, 2004). Objective signs of infant and newborn pain can be observed in the face, lower extremity positioning, activity level, crying, and level of consolation. Infants experiencing pain may exhibit brow bulge, eye squeeze, lip pursing, chin quiver, and tongue protrusion (Oaks, 2011).

TODDLER AND PRESCHOOLER

Young toddlers cannot identify the pain they are experiencing or its source. Older toddlers and preschoolers develop the ability to describe, identify, and locate sources of pain and can begin to use terms to define intensity and severity. Characteristics commonly associated with pain, such as lethargy, fatigue, anorexia, and regression, are important in these age groups.

During the toddler and preschool years, children are achieving a sense of autonomy. Because pain can be a source of fear and a threat to security, children respond with crying, anger, physical resistance, or withdrawal. Reasoning with these children about pain and its cause or management is difficult. Thus, children may withdraw from attachments for fear of being hurt again. Although parents are children's greatest source of comfort and support, children may appear ambivalent toward them, as though they blame them for the pain. Encourage and support parents in such instances, helping them understand children's response.

SCHOOL-AGE CHILD AND ADOLESCENT

School-age children develop a sense of competence and greater independence. They begin to rationalize in an attempt to explain what happens in their lives. Faced with a painful situation, children try to be "brave" and rationalize the pain. They are more responsive to explanations about pain than are younger children. School-age children can identify pain's specific location, intensity, quality, and frequency. If pain persists, school-age children may temporarily regress to an earlier stage of development in an attempt to handle the situation. For example, the young school-age child may temporarily lose bladder control and may revert to comfort measures such as thumb sucking, nail biting, and playing with favorite toys.

Because adolescents are developing an identity and personal independence, their physical appearance and abilities are important. When coupled with concern about peer relationships, adolescents demonstrate careful self-control and may be reluctant to acknowledge pain. To recognize or "give in" to pain may seem a sign of weakness. For example, a high school football player may know that his knee is injured but may prefer to deny the pain in an effort to be a "team player" and not let down his team or coach.

ADULT AND OLDER ADULT

Elders are the fastest-growing segment of our population, with the projected number of people older than 65 years by the year 2020 estimated at 52 million. The most frequent type of persistent pain in older adults is musculoskeletal (somatic) pain. Osteoarthritis of the lower back, knees, feet, and hips accounts for persistent pain in older adults and can greatly impact function and independence. The high incidence of postherpetic neuralgia and disease-related neuropathies (neuropathic pain) commonly seen in older adults can be disabling. Pain puts elders at increased risk for depression, social isolation, and cognitive dysfunction; interferes with the ability to care for self; and may impact their ability to remain in their home environment. An inadequate understanding of pain and self-management pain strategies in the older adult population is a barrier to helping the older patient remain active and enjoy healthy aging. Some older adults may incorrectly believe that pain is an unavoidable normal consequence of growing old. While the aging nervous system likely has decreased opioid receptors and increased inflammatory activity, and may be less sensitive to some types of mild pain, it is not desensitized to moderate or severe pain (Baumann, 2009). Older adults are more likely to become disabled due to pain than their younger counterparts and are at risk for poor pain control.

Nursing can assist the older adult in their awareness of human and environmental factors that contribute to pain and decreased functioning and help them appreciate those interventions that facilitate comfort and functionality. An example of an appropriate nursing intervention for an older patient experiencing pain due to lower back osteoarthritis would be for the nurse to suggest a physical therapy/occupational therapy consult and home health evaluation. Mobility aids, positioning and mobility awareness, and an evaluation of the home environment along with appropriate pain medications will likely increase function and decrease potential painful activities. Additionally, the nurse may explore the patient's awareness of cognitive interventions such as prayer or meditation as an effective nonpharmacologic pain management strategy. Application of heat or cold may also provide relief. Supplying information and resources that assist the older adult to choose, with awareness, the best holistic pain management strategies with the least side effects will positively impact mobility, coping, and well-being and improve overall quality of life (Baumann, 2009).

Cultural Considerations

Both culture and ethnicity affect how pain is interpreted and addressed on a personal, familial, and community level. Consequently, a culturally competent nursing approach to pain management for different ethnic groups is imperative, and acknowledgment and commitment to cultural sensitivity as part of the professional nursing framework is essential (Purnell & Paulanka, 2014).

Recent research has explored the cancer pain experience from a cultural and ethnic framework among White, Hispanic, African American, and Asian ethnic groups. Pain experience commonalities and differences among those ethnic groups have been identified.

Communication breakdown and pain as a gendered experience were two themes that surfaced as common patient experiences across ethnic groups. Patients expressed their difficulty communicating with healthcare providers regarding their pain, although the specific reasons for their communication difficulty differed. Ethnic minorities stated that it was hard to get someone to understand the severity of pain and how they were feeling and felt that they were sometimes perceived as having pain complaints that were unwarranted. Hispanic and Asian participants highlighted a lack of mastery of the English language as a barrier to expressing their pain experience to healthcare providers even if they came from a well-educated background (Im, Lee, Lim, Guevara, & Chee, 2009).

The gendered experience of cancer pain was also reported by female participants. The study cohort reported that their cancer pain was devalued compared to that of their male counterparts. Most of the women, especially mothers, reported having a higher tolerance to pain than men and attributed this to pain experienced in life through childbirth and menstruation. Additionally, the female cohort stated that they often were required to shoulder the burdens of household tasks and child-rearing despite disease progression (Im et al., 2009).

White patients exhibited stronger self-determination behaviors regarding cancer pain management and stated their strong desire to control their pain and pain management interventions. Agitation toward healthcare providers who neglected their pain or disregarded their pain was a common theme. White patients more often utilized their prerogative to change providers if they felt that they were not being cared for adequately or respectfully. Stoicism, concerns regarding addiction to opioid medications, and the development of tolerance to opioids were identified as factors influencing cancer pain management in African Americans (Im, 2008). Minority ethnic groups thought differently about their cancer pain, connecting malignancy with death and the belief that increased pain meant the cancer was getting worse. Consequently, many did not want to talk about their pain but instead minimized it. Asian patients wanted to hide their pain since they viewed their painful cancer experience as a result of "bad karma" and atonement for past sins. Most ethnic minorities minimized their pain by relying on religious faith and nonpharmacologic strategies such as meditation and prayer. Their belief in a divine healing power helped them to face cancer and make their pain tolerable (Im et al., 2009).

Most White participants wanted to treat their cancer and pain using diverse strategies of Western medicine. They searched for information on the Internet and through support groups, pain clinics, and other sources. They wanted an expert healthcare provider who was sensitive to their needs. It was not uncommon for the White cohort to continue to search for answers, try alternatives, ask questions, and network with others who had similar experiences.

In contrast, ethnic minorities focused on maintaining normal lives and more frequently used natural modalities for pain management. Ethnic participants wanted to reduce pain in natural, nonconventional ways instead of treating it aggressively through Western medicine (Im et al., 2009).

An individualized pain experience was more common in White patients experiencing cancer pain and contrasted a stronger familial focus in African American, Asian, and Hispanic ethnic groups. Whites tended to be more independent and autonomous. The ethnic minority viewpoint of the pain experience focused on fighting cancer and pain for their families. They received a high level of family support during treatments, and families involved to a greater extent in decision making, planning, and care delivery (Im et al., 2009).

FACTORS AFFECTING PAIN PERCEPTION AND PAIN RESPONSE

The multidimensional nature of pain includes cognitive and behavioral components that affect how pain is perceived. The multidimensional pain experience includes four domains: (i) affective, (ii) behavioral, (iii) cognitive, and (vi) physiological/sensory (Fig. 35-2). These factors are easily remembered using the ABC pain acronym (Cancer Pain Symposium Nursing Research Group, 2004). All four domains of the ABC pain acronym must be considered during assessment, planning, implementation, and evaluation to achieve a holistic and effective pain management plan.

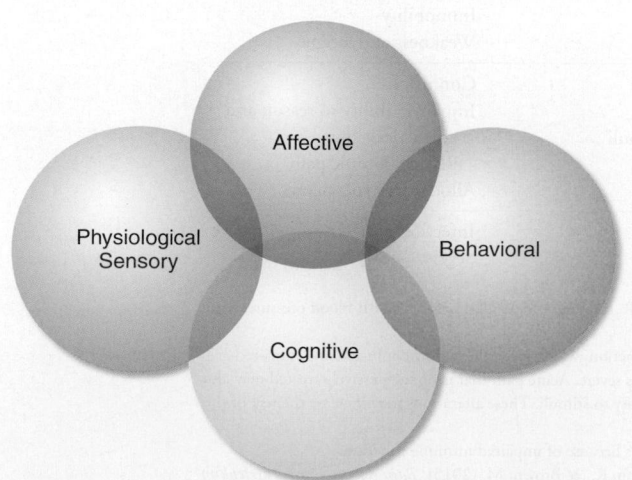

FIGURE 35-2 Affective, behavioral, cognitive, and physiological sensory factors all impact an individual's perception of pain.

Affective Factors

Suffering is an emotional response associated with increased pain, but pain and suffering are not synonymous. Suffering is associated with events that threaten the person's intactness, whereas pain is associated with events that threaten tissues. People can suffer without pain, have pain without suffering, or have pain and suffering simultaneously. Assessments and treatments for pain and suffering can be quite different.

Patients with unrelieved pain often have concurrent emotional responses, such as anger, fear, anxiety, sadness, or depression that can intensify pain perception. Emotions such as joy and pleasure may decrease the amount of pain perceived. Emotional factors can play a powerful role in pain perception. Helping patients understand the link between emotions and pain perception is an important role for nurses in all care settings.

Behavioral Factors

Many different behaviors are associated with pain; some aggravate it and others alleviate it. Patients with pain notice that certain activities can cause pain to be noticed or increased. Patients often avoid such activities, but this avoidance may not be in their best long-term interest. Pain may interfere with usual behaviors that bring joy and satisfaction. When pain prevents many activities, patients may experience increased emotional distress such as anxiety. Patients also engage in several behaviors to control their pain (reduce pain, prevent pain onset, reduce pain duration, and tolerate the pain). For example, watching television or talking with friends, staff, or family members helps to distract patients from their pain and can be effective in helping to control it. How patients comply with or adjust analgesic therapy plans also is an important aspect of pain behavior.

Emotional responses to pain, such as fear and anxiety, increase muscle tension, which increases perception of pain intensity. Fear of the unknown also may worsen pain because of tension and anxiety the patient brings to the situation. For instance, a toddler who fears an injection will cry and tense the muscles, thus intensifying pain. Aggressive behavior is not an uncommon way of "fighting back" against the pain. At the other extreme, the person in pain may withdraw from it by minimizing interaction with the environment and other people. Regression to earlier developmental stages may occur.

Pain can cause fatigue, possibly predisposing the patient to more pain. What might be tolerable to a well-rested person may be intolerable to one who is fatigued.

Cognitive Factors

Meanings associated with a disease (e.g., cancer) and pain, along with beliefs, attitudes, and expectations about them, can influence patient responses. Some cultures see pain tolerance as a virtue; often, men are expected to tolerate pain more stoically than are women. Healthcare providers need to recognize the patient's cultural beliefs and not impose their own judgments.

A sense of not knowing may increase a person's pain. The patient who does not understand treatments or does not know enough about decisions that need to be made may experience worse pain. A patient's goal for and expectations about pain relief and treatment outcomes are crucial in understanding pain. Treatment goals, however, must be realistic and attainable for the patient, healthcare providers, and environment. Identifying barriers to pain relief and determining realistic functional goals in partnership with the patient are necessary components of an optimal pain plan. Exhaustion and lack of sleep contribute to a chronically tired state, which may make it difficult to manage pain. Level of consciousness (sedation level), dementia, memory of past pain, source of motivation (internal vs. external locus of control), and cognitive resources to cope with the pain can dramatically influence the pain experienced.

Patients may use cognitive and behavioral activities to cope with pain. In general, when patients actively engage in behaviors to cope with the pain, they are less likely to be debilitated by it. Patients who focus on how terrible the pain is (coping by catastrophizing) are more likely to have functional and emotional problems related to the pain.

Manifestations of Pain

Physiologic and behavioral responses occur in the person in pain. Observers consider these responses indicators of pain, but for the person with pain, some responses represent dangerous effects of pain. Absence of these responses does not indicate that a patient has no pain or has less intense pain than he or she reports. Table 35-2 addresses the negative physiologic effects of untreated pain using a systems approach.

TABLE 35-2 CONSEQUENCES OF UNRELIEVED ACUTE PAIN

System	Physiologic Responses	Clinical Consequences
Endocrine/metabolic	↑ Stress hormones (ACTH, cortisol) ↑ ADH ↑ Epi, NE ↑ Renin, aldosterone Gluconeogenesis Glycogenolysis Protein catabolism	↑ RR, HR, BP Fluid overload Glucose intolerance Hyperglycemia Loss of lean body mass
Cardiovascular	↑ HR, cardiac output ↑ Peripheral vascular resistance ↑ O$_2$ consumption ↑ Coagulation	Hypertension Unstable angina MI Deep vein thrombosis
Respiratory	↓ Tidal volume ↓ Cough Hypoxemia	Atelectasis Pneumonia
Urinary	↓ Urinary output	Urinary retention Fluid overload Electrolyte imbalance
Gastrointestinal	↓ Gastric and bowel motility	Constipation Anorexia Ileus
Musculoskeletal	Muscle spasm Impaired muscle function	Immobility Weakness and fatigue
Neurologic	Impaired cognitive function Altered pain processing: ↑ sensitivity to noxious stimuli	Confusion Impaired ability to reason and make decisions ↑ Risk of chronic pain Allodynia, hyperalgesia
Immunologic	↓ Immune response	Infection Sepsis

ACTH, adrenocorticotropic hormone; ADH, antidiuretic hormone; RR, respiratory rate; HR, heart rate; BP, blood pressure; MI, myocardial infarction.

Note: Neurological consequences of pain include impaired cognitive function, which is manifested by confusion and impaired ability to reason and make decisions. This is especially true when pain is severe. Acute pain that is not aggressively treated may also cause persistent changes in pain processing, especially increased sensitivity to stimuli. These alterations may increase the risk of the development of chronic pain states with allodynia and hyperalgesia.

Patients with unrelieved pain are at increased risk of infection and sepsis because of impaired immune function.

Reprinted with permission from: Dahl, J., Gordon, D., Paice, J., Stevenson, K., & Brown, M. (2015). *Pain resource nurse curriculum & planning guide.* Madison, WI: Resource Center of the Alliance of State Pain Initiatives. Retrieved from http://trc.wisc.edu/items. asp?itemID=114

PHYSIOLOGIC RESPONSES

Observable physiologic signs of acute pain include changes in blood pressure, heart rate, respiratory rate, and metabolic responses. Commonly observed responses in acute pain are usually absent in persistent and chronic pain because adaptation occurs. It is unclear how long it takes for adaptation to occur. Therefore, lack of elevation in vital signs cannot be used as a reliable indicator of the presence or magnitude of persistent pain. Furthermore, other reasons for alterations in physiologic responses must be considered (e.g., effects of drug therapy lowering blood pressure in severe pain).

Increased Blood Pressure

The increase in blood pressure that may accompany acute pain is believed to be due to increased activity of the sympathetic nervous system. Peripheral vasoconstriction is an adaptive response as the blood shifts away from the periphery (skin, extremities) to the heart and lungs when the body perceives a threat. The increased blood pressure also increases the heart's work, possibly leading to myocardial ischemia. In addition, the decreased peripheral circulation can be dangerous to people undergoing vascular grafting procedures by diminishing blood flow needed to promote healing.

Increased Heart Rate

Increased heart rate reflects the body's attempt to increase available oxygen and circulating fluid volume to promote healing of damaged tissues. The shunting of blood from the periphery to the vital organs (brain, heart, liver, and kidney) is an effort to preserve the body's life-support systems.

Increased Respiratory Rate

An increase in the respiratory rate is an effort to increase the amount of oxygen available to the heart and circulation. Unrelieved pain classically includes rapid and shallow breathing that is inefficient to meet oxygen needs, which results in hypoxemia. The rapid, shallow breathing is corrected with effective pain relief.

Neuroendocrine and Metabolic Responses

Unrelieved pain produces a catabolic state. That is, stored energy is consumed to provide energy to vital organs and injured tissue. This response also is known as the stress response, which is capable of producing widespread metabolic effects. Some of these effects include generalized increase in metabolism, oxygen consumption, blood glucose, free fatty acids, blood lactate, and ketones. These effects related to the degree and duration of tissue damage can last for days.

BEHAVIORAL RESPONSES

Observable behavioral signs of acute and chronic pain include verbal, vocal, and nonverbal responses. As with physiologic signs, behavioral responses often adapt with time.

Verbal Responses

Verbal behavioral responses to pain, although subjective, are the most dependable indicators of pain in people who are able to communicate verbally. Therefore, healthcare providers should believe these reports and not dismiss them, even if they vary from other objective information. In people without verbal abilities (e.g., preverbal children, cognitively impaired patients), vocal responses (crying out) may provide important clues about pain's presence but do little to indicate where, what kind, or how much pain there is, or how it changes with time.

Nonverbal Responses

Nonverbal behaviors often give a clue about pain location, but verbal reports indicate more clearly its location, intensity, quality, and temporal pattern. Common nonverbal behavioral responses include rubbing painful areas, frowns and grimaces, and increased muscle tension that occurs with guarding and immobilization. Increased muscle tension shown by guarding, which is part of the body's fight-or-flight response, is a reaction to protect against further pain. Prolonged muscle tension, however, contributes to impaired muscle metabolism, muscle atrophy, and significantly delayed normal muscle function.

Think back to the patient in the case scenario who is undergoing radiation treatment for lung cancer. Use the concept map (Fig. 35-3) to help understand and manage the patient's pain to improve her function and quality of life.

ASSESSMENT

Inadequate and incomplete pain assessment is the most common reason for undertreatment of pain. The 2015 Joint Commission standards state that every patient has a right to have his or her pain assessed and treated in healthcare settings (hospital, ambulatory care, nursing care centers, home care, and office-based surgery programs). If assessment reveals the presence of pain, the organization is responsible for providing treatment or referring the patient for treatment (Joint Commission, 2015). A comprehensive, systematic pain assessment requires the nurse to use both subjective and objective data to inform care planning. Complete nursing pain assessment includes (i) physiologic characteristics and types of pain; (ii) patient's self-report of pain including how the pain impacts recovery, ability to function, and performance of normal activities and functions; and (iii) patient's response to current pharmacologic and nonpharmacologic treatments and interventions. Assessment is the critical first step to identify the patient's individual responses to the pain and enables the nurse to evaluate ongoing responses to the pain management plan.

Pain Assessment

Initial assessment should be at the first point of patient contact. Nurses in the ambulatory setting and home health nurses will assess pain at each visit. Routine screening for pain is a key component of a successful pain plan. Inpatient staff should assess pain no less than each shift and more often if pain is unrelieved and after the administration of pain medication to assess medication effectiveness. Pain assessment should occur on admission, when pain is reported, anticipated, or suspected. Assessment should also occur before, during, and after procedures known to cause pain and with each transition of care.

PAIN MANAGEMENT

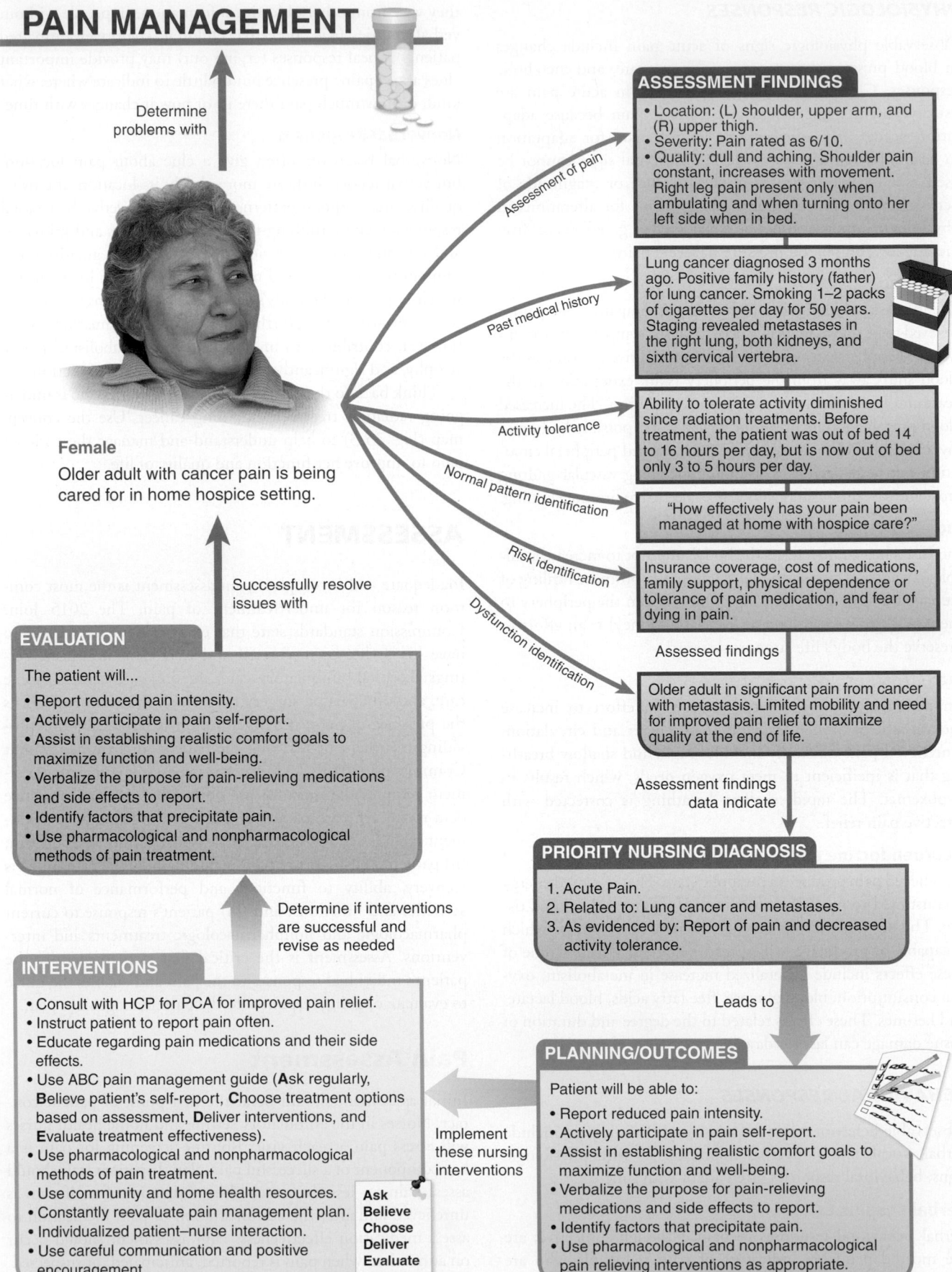

Determine problems with

Female

Older adult with cancer pain is being cared for in home hospice setting.

Assessment of pain

ASSESSMENT FINDINGS

- Location: (L) shoulder, upper arm, and (R) upper thigh.
- Severity: Pain rated as 6/10.
- Quality: dull and aching. Shoulder pain constant, increases with movement. Right leg pain present only when ambulating and when turning onto her left side when in bed.

Past medical history

Lung cancer diagnosed 3 months ago. Positive family history (father) for lung cancer. Smoking 1–2 packs of cigarettes per day for 50 years. Staging revealed metastases in the right lung, both kidneys, and sixth cervical vertebra.

Activity tolerance

Ability to tolerate activity diminished since radiation treatments. Before treatment, the patient was out of bed 14 to 16 hours per day, but is now out of bed only 3 to 5 hours per day.

Normal pattern identification

"How effectively has your pain been managed at home with hospice care?"

Risk identification

Insurance coverage, cost of medications, family support, physical dependence or tolerance of pain medication, and fear of dying in pain.

Dysfunction identification

Assessed findings

Older adult in significant pain from cancer with metastasis. Limited mobility and need for improved pain relief to maximize quality at the end of life.

Assessment findings data indicate

PRIORITY NURSING DIAGNOSIS

1. Acute Pain.
2. Related to: Lung cancer and metastases.
3. As evidenced by: Report of pain and decreased activity tolerance.

Leads to

PLANNING/OUTCOMES

Patient will be able to:

- Report reduced pain intensity.
- Actively participate in pain self-report.
- Assist in establishing realistic comfort goals to maximize function and well-being.
- Verbalize the purpose for pain-relieving medications and side effects to report.
- Identify factors that precipitate pain.
- Use pharmacological and nonpharmacological pain relieving interventions as appropriate.

Implement these nursing interventions

INTERVENTIONS

- Consult with HCP for PCA for improved pain relief.
- Instruct patient to report pain often.
- Educate regarding pain medications and their side effects.
- Use ABC pain management guide (**A**sk regularly, **B**elieve patient's self-report, **C**hoose treatment options based on assessment, **D**eliver interventions, and **E**valuate treatment effectiveness).
- Use pharmacological and nonpharmacological methods of pain treatment.
- Use community and home health resources.
- Constantly reevaluate pain management plan.
- Individualized patient–nurse interaction.
- Use careful communication and positive encouragement.

Ask
Believe
Choose
Deliver
Evaluate

Determine if interventions are successful and revise as needed

EVALUATION

The patient will...

- Report reduced pain intensity.
- Actively participate in pain self-report.
- Assist in establishing realistic comfort goals to maximize function and well-being.
- Verbalize the purpose for pain-relieving medications and side effects to report.
- Identify factors that precipitate pain.
- Use pharmacological and nonpharmacological methods of pain treatment.

Successfully resolve issues with

FIGURE 35-3 Concept map for pain management.

TABLE 35-3 ESSENTIALS OF PAIN ASSESSMENT: PATIENT SELF-REPORT

Pain Detail	Question	Considerations
Onset	When did the pain begin?	
Location	Can you point to where it hurts? Does your pain radiate?	*Somatic*: Localized *Visceral*: Vague or radiating
Duration	Is your pain constant? Is your pain intermittent?	Patients can have a combination of constant and intermittent pain.
Quality	How would you describe your pain?	*Nociceptive*: Aching, sharp, deep, gnawing *Neuropathic*: Shock-like, burning, tingling
Intensity	Can you rate your pain on a scale from 0 to 10? Zero is no pain, and 10 is the worst pain you could imagine.	Rating scales must be appropriate for age, culture, and cognitive ability.
Aggravating and alleviating factors	What makes your pain better? What makes your pain worse?	Include interventions that have helped or hindered pain management.

The impact pain has on ability to function and quality of life	How does pain affect your:
	   Sleep?
	   Activity level?
	   Appetite?
	   Relationships?
	   Ability to work?
	   Quality of life?
	 How would you describe your mood?
	 Is pain interfering with your ability to participate fully in your recovery?
		These exploratory questions are essential questions to ask patients with persistent pain.
		
		 In an acute care setting, pain often inhibits the ability to cough, deep breathe, and participate in activities.

Pain care goal	What level of pain, on the 0 to 10 scale, would let you participate fully in your life (recovery)?	Goals should be discussed with the intent that they are realistic and achievable. Track and measure progress toward goal.
Medications and treatments	What medication are you taking for your pain? What over-the-counter or herbal medications do you take for your pain? Do you use any nonmedication interventions to treat your pain?	A 24-hour recall total (mg) should be calculated for opioids and adjuvant medications.
Concerns or worries	Do you have any concerns or worries about your pain management plan?	Helps explore barriers to pain plan participation, such as fear of addiction, concerns about cost, or sociocultural influences that can influence patient response.

A comprehensive and systematic pain assessment including essential questions is found in Table 35-3.

PAIN SCALES

Reliable and valid pain intensity rating scales are used to measure and rank patients' pain levels and help monitor pain trends over time. The numeric rating scale (NRS), the verbal descriptor scale, and the faces pain scale (FPS) are the three most common pain rating tools used in adults. The Wong-Baker FACES Pain Rating Scale is useful for assessing children, although children as young as 8 years can use a 0 to 10 number scale. Teaching patients to use reliable tools to communicate pain intensity helps them to maintain a sense of control and actively participate in their care.

The pain intensity rating scale should be easy for the patient to use as well as age and culturally appropriate. It is important to remember that the intensity rating, based on the patient's self-report, is always important yet should never be considered a complete pain assessment. The nurse should assess pain intensity by asking the patient directly to rate his or her pain at rest, before and after pain medications or interventions, and after activity. Remember that patients may still have pain while asleep. Nurses should not assume comfort and rate pain as a zero but instead should document sleep instead of a pain rating.

Box 35-1 is an example of how a nurse might educate and support a patient on the use of the numeric pain scale.

ASSESSING NONVERBAL PATIENTS

Patients' self-report is the preferred method of pain assessment; however, there are situations where eliciting patients' self-report is not possible. Patients placed on a ventilator to support respiratory function or patients with severe dementia will not be able to self-report their pain levels. Cognitively impaired patients should always be given the opportunity to self-report first, and a validated nonverbal pain assessment tool should be used if this proves to be unsuccessful. Figure 35-4 is an example of a nonverbal assessment tool that assists the nurse in estimating the severity of pain for the nonverbal patient.

Risk Identification

Patients have the right to appropriate assessment and management of pain. Nevertheless, pain management is often suboptimal. Healthcare systems, the healthcare providers, and patient-related barriers to pain management contribute to the risk of poor pain control.

BOX 35-1   Assessing and Managing a Patient's Pain

Hello Mr. Jones, my name is Kim and I am the nurse caring for you today. The nursing assistant who answered your light a few moments ago told me that you are having some incisional pain. I would like you to rate your pain on a scale from 0 to 10. This will help ensure that you get the right dose of pain medication. Zero is no pain, and 10 is the worst pain you can imagine. On a scale from 0 to 10, what number would you call your pain?

Mr. Jones rates pain 6 out of 10.

Upon returning to the room with 2 mg of IV morphine, per the physician order, for a pain intensity rating of 6 out of 10, the following patient education is appropriate:

Mr. Jones, I have 2 mg of morphine to give you now. Take a couple slow breaths to relax as I give you the medication. Relaxing will actually help your body absorb the medication more quickly. The morphine will begin working in a few minutes, and you should feel less pain within the next 15 to

30 minutes. I will check back within the next half hour to see how you are feeling.

You return to Mr. Jones's bedside within 30 minutes. He is awake and resting quietly.

Mr. Jones, can you rate your pain now on a scale of 0 to 10? Zero is no pain, and 10 is the worst pain you can imagine.

Mr. Jones rates his pain 1 out of 10 at rest.

I am glad to hear you are more comfortable. You may notice a slight increase in your pain level with activity, deep breathing, and movement, but we want you to be comfortable enough to be able to rest and participate in your care. If your pain reaches a 3, please let your nurses know so they can help keep you comfortable. Keeping your pain level consistently at a mild level while you are recovering is the goal. Now that you are more comfortable, would you like to take a walk with me down the hallway before your lunch arrives?

HEALTHCARE SYSTEM

Lack of insurance coverage, high prescription costs, and limited access to healthcare resources are additional barriers that may impede a patient's ability to receive adequate pain management. Some institutions do not provide all types of pain management therapies that a person may need. For example,

a skilled nursing facility may not allow administration of continuous intravenous (IV) infusions of opioids, a treatment that a terminally ill person with pain might require. Nurses should take into consideration system issues, question barriers, and assess for alternative pain management options when planning care.

Checklist of Non-Verbal Indicators (CNVI)

	With Movement	At Rest
Vocal Complaints – nonverbal expression of pain demonstrated by moans, groans, grunts, cries, gasps, sighs)		
Facial Grimaces and Winces – furrowed brow, narrowed eyes, tightened lips, dropped jaw, clenched teeth, distorted expression		
Bracing – clutching or holding onto siderails, bed, tray table, or affected area during movement		
Restlessness – constant or intermittent shifting of position, rocking, intermittent or constant hand motions, inability to keep still		
Rubbing – massaging affected area		
Vocal complaints – verbal expression of pain using words, e.g., "ouch" or "that hurts"; cursing during movement, or exclamations of protest, e.g., "stop" or "that's enough."		
TOTAL SCORE		

FIGURE 35-4 Checklist of nonverbal indicators. (Reprinted with permission from Feldt, K. S. (2000). The checklist of nonverbal pain indicators (CNPI). *Pain Management Nursing, 1*(1), 13–21.)

Indications: Behavioral Health adults who are unable to validate the presence of or quantify the severity of pain using either the Numerical Rating Scale or the Wong-Baker Faces Pain Rating Scale.

Instructions:
1. Write a 0 if the behavior was not observed
2. Write a 1 if the behavior even briefly during activity or rest
3. Results in a total score between 0 and 5.
4. The interdisciplinary team in collaboration with the patient (if appropriate), can determine appropriate interventions in response to CNVI scores.

HEALTHCARE PROFESSIONALS

The healthcare professional's attitude toward pain may contribute to a poor assessment. For example, assuming that a patient will always report pain further interferes with the healthcare professional's awareness of the patient's actual discomfort level. Assuming that a patient with persistent pain is asking for pain medication because he or she is "drug seeking," when in fact there may be unrelieved pain due to a poor pain plan, can impede the nurse's ability to provide compassionate care. If the nurse fails to solicit the patient's self-report and complete a systematic objective assessment, there is risk that an inadequate pain plan will be developed and pain will go untreated.

Fear of addiction on the part of healthcare providers and patients can also lead to undertreatment of pain. Healthcare professionals and patients should be well informed of the differences between tolerance, physical dependence, and addiction so that incorrect assumptions regarding addiction are avoided when planning pain management strategies.

Tolerance occurs when a patient receives a drug, such as an opioid, continuously over an extended period time. A neuroadaptive

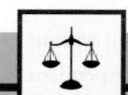

ETHICAL/LEGAL ISSUES

POSSIBLE DEPENDENCE ON PAIN MEDICATION

Mr. Stuart, 34 years old, has experienced first- and second-degree burns over 40% of his body. He was in good physical health before this accident but requires extensive treatment. Clearly, Mr. Stuart is going to survive his injuries, but the treatment process will be long-term and painful. He is anxious about the treatment. He requests you be sure that he experiences as little pain as possible and that you give him all the pain medication that he can have. You discuss this with the healthcare team, advocating for your patient regarding his concerns about pain relief. Another team member responds by saying that Mr. Stuart is exhibiting "drug-seeking" behavior, and the amount of pain medication has to be limited to prevent Mr. Stuart from becoming addicted.

CRITICAL THINKING CHALLENGE

- Identify your concerns about Mr. Stuart, his request for pain relief, and the other team member's response.
- For what reasons could the healthcare team member be responding as he is? What are your feelings in light of that opinion? What are ethical and legal consequences of complying with Mr. Stuart's request or withholding medication?
- Identify possible approaches to advocating for your patient in this situation.
- Recognizing the patient's injuries, his anxiety about pain, and the team member's opinion, define what you see as your ethically appropriate behavior.

response occurs, requiring a larger dose of the drug to produce the same effect (i.e., pain relief). Patients with a history of persistent pain will often have an elevated dose requirement compared to an opioid-naïve patient. Consequently, it is important to review home medication dosing carefully and communicate recent 24-hour opioid totals in milligrams to the physician so that medication dosing is adequate and pain is not left undertreated.

Physical dependence is a physiologic adaptation that is characterized by the development of withdrawal symptoms such as diaphoresis, anxiety, tachycardia, or nausea when the drug is stopped abruptly. Withdrawal symptoms are expected in patients receiving opioid analgesics for more than a few days and can be avoided by tapering (decreasing) the dose incrementally before discontinuation (Zacharoff et al., 2010). Patients using opioids to relieve pain will naturally self-taper their medication as their pain improves by extending the time between prn (as needed) opioid doses.

Addiction, on the other hand, is a chronic neurobiologic disease that has genetic, psychosocial, and environmental influences. Patients with addiction tendencies have impaired control over drug use, compulsive use, and continued use and craving despite harm (Zacharoff et al., 2010). Patients with true addiction will take opioids for other purposes such as mood alteration or to escape uncomfortable situations or feelings instead of using the medication for its intended pain-relieving properties. Patients with a history of substance abuse are entitled to pain relief, and because of tolerance require higher and even much higher doses to adequately manage pain (Jensen, 2015).

Physical Assessment

The physiologic response to pain results in autonomic nervous system activation. With acute pain, tachycardia, elevated blood pressure, increased respiratory rate, and diaphoresis may be objectively observed. With persistent or chronic pain, these responses may be modified or absent. Assessing the patient's vital sign trend is an important component of pain assessment. Baseline vital signs and pain levels should be obtained routinely during each outpatient or home visit. Inpatient vital signs and pain levels are obtained at least each shift and before and after potentially painful procedures or pain medication administration. For patients who have difficulty expressing pain or are unable to do so, vital signs along with the results of the nonverbal pain scale before and after pain relief measures will help evaluate pain management efficacy.

INSPECTION

Nursing inspection of the patient in pain can take numerous forms, and the results of objective observations will assist in planning pain management interventions and help to individualize a plan of care. For example, a nurse may inspect a painful incisional wound and find new erythema and purulent drainage, or notice that when the patient breathes deeply during auscultation of lung sounds that a painful productive cough produces greenish blood-tinged sputum. Consequently, pain is often an important associated symptom and should be reported along with other observations.

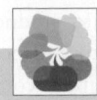

THERAPEUTIC DIALOGUE: PAIN MEDICATION

SCENE FOR THOUGHT

While walking down the hall, the nurse hears quiet moaning. She enters the room and sees Kathy Goodman looking toward the wall. Her body is restless, and she is breathing erratically. Her roommate says (a little irritably) that she's been that way for the last 10 minutes. The patient had abdominal surgery earlier today and is 42 years old.

LESS EFFECTIVE

Nurse: Ms. Goodman, I'm Liz Newman, the charge nurse. Can you tell me what's happening? *(Stands by the bed.)*

Kathy: My incision hurts. *(Grimaces and gasps as she moves.)*

Nurse: Has it gotten worse recently?

Kathy: No, it's just constant when I move. So I don't move.

Nurse: I'll just check your chart so I can see when you had your last pain medication. *(Does so.)* Okay, you're about due for more medication, but maybe we can get you an increase until your pain decreases and you start to heal a little.

Kathy: No! I don't want to take more.

Nurse: But you seem to be in such pain! Besides *(whispers)* I think your roommate is really concerned for you and may be a bit annoyed.

Kathy: *(Looks embarrassed.)* Oh, I didn't know I was bothering her. Are the pills safe to take? Someone told me I could become, you know, addicted. *(Body is tense.)*

Nurse: As long as you're in such pain, you won't become addicted. We're careful about that. I'll bet they'll help.

Kathy: *(Reluctantly.)* Okay.

Nurse: Great! I'll get them to you right away. *(Leaves in a hurry.)*

Kathy: *(Glances at roommate as if to speak but then remains silent. Roommate doesn't make eye contact. Kathy's body remains tense.)*

MORE EFFECTIVE

Nurse: Ms. Goodman, I'm Linda Norman, the charge nurse. Can you tell me what's happening? *(Stands by the bed.)*

Kathy: My incision hurts. *(Grimaces and gasps as she moves.)*

Nurse: Has it gotten worse recently?

Kathy: No, it's just constant when I move. So I don't move.

Nurse: I'll just check your chart so I can see when you had your last pain medication. *(Does so.)* Okay, you're about due for more medication, but maybe we can get you an increase until your pain decreases and you start to heal a little.

Kathy: No! I don't want to take more.

Nurse: I'm surprised to hear you say that. Could you explain?

Kathy: *(Looks down.)* I don't want to get too dependent on the pain pills.

Nurse: *(Pays silent attention.)*

Kathy: The last time I had my surgery, the nurses would give the pain pills only every 4 hours and no more. They said it wasn't allowed because I'd get addicted. So I don't want any more. *(Looks down.)* I'll just have to deal with it. *(Begins to close her eyes and settle her body stiffly into position.)*

Nurse: Can I help in any way?

Kathy: *(Opens her eyes wearily.)* How?

Nurse: Well, first, I need to examine your incision and ask you a few questions. Then we might be able to add a nonnarcotic pain pill to the ones you have to provide some overlap. When opioids are used for medical purposes, such as surgical pain, very few people become addicted—actually only 4 in 12,000 according to several studies. I also can teach you some relaxation techniques that might help relax you and reduce the pain. How do those options sound?

Kathy: *(Thinking about it.)* They might work. Worth a try, anyway.

Nurse: I thought you might be interested. Let's get started.

CRITICAL THINKING CHALLENGE

- Relate Kathy's body language to her pain.
- Explain the relationship between pain and stress.
- Detect what the first nurse taught Kathy. Compare and contrast what the second nurse taught her.
- Propose other ways to help Kathy handle her pain.
- Explain what happened by the end of the first dialogue to contribute to Kathy's tension.
- Describe each nurse's manner in talking to Kathy.

Visual inspection often includes how patients adapt their movements to decrease painful motion and activity. Observe the patient at rest and in motion noting altered gait, guarding parts of the body, limited range of motion, or avoiding certain activities altogether. These observations will provide clues to the source of pain and aggravating factors. Facial expressions and vocalization of pain can help gauge pain severity and is part of the inspection findings. All physical findings associated with the patient's pain should be described and documented clearly in the patient's chart.

PALPATION

Gentle palpation can be a useful addition to assess visceral pain involving the organs of the gastrointestinal and genitourinary systems. Gentle palpation can help provide information on the location, depth, and radiation of pain. Abdominal pain mediated along the visceral afferent pathways tends to be poorly localized and is often referred to the midline; however, the level of midline pain can prove helpful. *Rebound tenderness* is pain that is felt upon release of pressure over a part of the abdomen and is indicative of peritoneal inflammation. To test for rebound tenderness of the abdomen, have the patient lie flat in the supine relaxed position, and explain what you will do. Ask the patient to point to the general location and describe the pain. With three fingers of one hand, gently press down into the abdominal quadrant directly lateral from the painful location to a depth of approximately 2 inches, as patient comfort allows. Very quickly, release pressure. A positive rebound response is caused by the additional stimulation to the afferent visceral pathways and manifests as increased pain once pressure is released. The pain may be diffuse or sharp and localized. A new onset or change in pain should always be communicated directly to the physician, and complete pain assessment findings should be clearly documented in the patient's chart.

> **SAFETY ALERT**
>
> Do not palpate the abdomen of a patient complaining of sudden, severe abdominal pain, because doing so could rupture an inflamed appendix, causing peritonitis. Deep palpation is usually reserved for advanced practitioners.

OUTCOME PLANNING AND IDENTIFICATION

The overall goal in pain management is for the patient to participate in care, seeking culturally appropriate interventions that maximize comfort, function, and quality of life. General goals for the patient in pain may include the following:

- Active participation in pain self-report
- Assisting in establishing realistic comfort goals to maximize function

- Verbalizing the purpose for pain-relieving medications and side effects to report
- Utilizing nonpharmacologic pain-relieving interventions as appropriate

Persistent pain is present over time and difficult to manage; consequently, these attributes impact the patient's and provider's ability to set pain management goals. Often, the primary objective is to achieve a pain level that the patient considers manageable with interventions that address both short- and long-term pain management goals. With ongoing attention by members of the care team, patients with persistent pain can learn how to live with their pain over time, maximizing function, comfort, and their quality of life. Patients with persistent pain may benefit from the integration of behavioral and cognitive interventions into their care plan to improve their general well-being. If the patient is willing to keep a personal pain diary, doing so can help explore aggravating and alleviating factors including emotions, relationships, and environmental influences and can shed important insight into the patient's personal pain experience.

NURSING DIAGNOSES

Common NANDA-International (NANDA-I, 2014) nursing diagnoses that relate to pain include Impaired Comfort, Acute Pain, and Chronic Pain, Labor Pain, and Chronic Pain Syndrome. Selected pain diagnoses, along with appropriate Nursing Outcomes Classification (NOC) and Nursing Interventions Classification (NIC), are outlined in Table 35-4.

IMPLEMENTATION

To assist the patient in goal achievement, pain management nursing process essentials must be followed. Remember that timely and deliberate communication with all members of the care team (including patient and family) regarding treatment and goals is essential for success. The critical domains for successful execution of a pain management plan are outlined below using the ABC acronym (Dahl et al., 2008):

A. Ask regularly, assess systematically
B. Believe patients self-report
C. Choose treatment options based on comprehensive assessment
D. Deliver interventions in a coordinated way
E. Evaluate treatment effectiveness by reassessment

Complete elimination of acute pain during recovery may not always be possible. It is possible, however, to provide a level of comfort using pharmacologic and nonpharmacologic therapies that maximize the patient's ability to rest and heal, participate in activities, and engage in his or her environment. Persistent pain patients will need ongoing outpatient pain

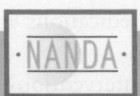

Table 35-4 SELECTED NANDA-I NURSING DIAGNOSES INVOLVING PAIN

Nursing Dx	Related Factors	Dx Statement	NOC*	NIC†
Acute Pain— unpleasant sensory and emotional experience associated with actual or potential tissue damage; sudden or slow onset of any intensity from mild-to-severe with an anticipated or predictable end	Injury agents either biological (e.g., infection, ischemia, neoplasm), chemical (e.g., burn), physical (e.g., trauma, surgery, overstraining)	Acute Pain R/T inflammation and trauma from surgical incision AEB verbalized 6 on a pain scale of 0–10, guarded movement, and inability to ambulate without pain medication	Pain Level, Stress Level, Patient Satisfaction: Pain Management, Knowledge: Pain Management	Active Listening, Acupressure, Analgesic Administration, Anxiety Reduction, Coping Enhancement, Distraction, Heat/Cold Application, PCA, Simple Massage, Guided Imagery
Chronic Pain— unpleasant sensory and emotional experience associated with actual or potential tissue damage; sudden or slow onset of any intensity from mild-to-severe constant or recurring without an anticipated or predictable end and a duration of >3 months	Chronic physical disability, chronic psychological disability, chronic musculoskeletal condition, history of abuse, nerve compression, tumor infiltration, crush injury	Chronic Pain R/T old back injury, multiple spinal surgeries, and anxiety AEB verbal report of pain, guarded movements, depression, and sleep disturbance	Pain Level, Stress Level, Client Satisfaction: Pain Management, Quality of Life, Patient Satisfaction: Symptom Control, Will to Live	Active Listening, Acupressure, Analgesic Administration, Anxiety Reduction, Coping Enhancement, Distraction, Heat/Cold Application, PCA, Simple Massage, Guided Imagery, Therapeutic Touch, TENS

Dx, diagnosis; R/T, related to; AEB, as evidenced by.
*From: Moorhead, S., Johnson, M., Maas, M., & Swanson, E. (2013). *Iowa outcomes project: Nursing outcomes classification (NOC)* (5th ed.). St. Louis, MO: C. V. Mosby.
†From: Bulecheck, G., Butcher, H., Dochterman, J., & Wagner, C. (2013). *Iowa intervention project: Nursing interventions classification (NIC)* (5th ed.). St. Louis, MO: Elsevier Mosby.
From: NANDA-International (NANDA-I, 2014). *Nursing diagnoses: Definitions and classification, 2015–2017.* West Sussex, England: Wiley-Blackwell.

management support and follow-up. For this unique patient population, a key nursing role is to assure that follow-up pain management resources are in place across transitions as part of seamless individualized plan of care.

Health Promotion

Teaching patients ways of anticipating and managing painful situations helps decrease the anxiety and fear associated with untreated or unexpected pain. Empowering patients with pain management information allows them to become active partners in their care experience. For instance, many routine procedures, such as peripheral blood draws and IV catheter insertions, can produce pain. The nurse's ability to anticipate painful events and then use appropriate pharmacologic and nonpharmacologic interventions ensures that untreated pain is avoided. For example, an order request for topical lidocaine jelly may be appropriate for a patient experiencing increased pain during an indwelling urethral catheter placement. If a patient is scheduled for a potentially painful procedure, such as a complex dressing change, demonstrating and practicing relaxation exercises and simple deep breathing techniques beforehand can add to the effectiveness of the prescribed preemptive analgesics.

Nursing Interventions for Pain Management

Nursing pain management interventions include physical, cognitive, behavioral, and pharmacologic therapies. Familiarity with pain management strategies is essential to nursing practice and includes an understanding of treatment options, strategies to maximize relief and minimize side effects, and competency in teaching the patient pain self-management.

Analgesics are the mainstay of a pain management plan, and these drugs can be classified based on their ability to treat different intensities and types of pain:

- *Nonopioids*: Acetaminophen (APAP) and nonsteroidal anti-inflammatory drugs (NSAIDs)
- *Opioids*: Morphine is the prototype
- *Adjuvant analgesics*: Drugs with primary indication other than pain (e.g., antidepressants and antiepileptics)
- *Adjuvants*: Drugs without analgesic properties that can be critical to pain management in certain populations and for treatment of related symptoms that may exacerbate pain (e.g., muscle relaxants, anxiolytics, sleep medications)

OUTCOME-BASED TEACHING PLANS

Dean Norman, 53 years old, has chronic back pain. He is in the clinic where he receives pain medication. He seems a little unsure how to best manage the medication and asks you to help him figure it out.

OUTCOME

The patient will verbalize a plan to monitor and report his pain.

STRATEGIES

- Discuss with Dean the way to describe his pain. Provide him with a body outline and a list of words that he can use as descriptors, and review the list periodically.
- Work with him to develop a plan about how to monitor his pain and record it in a journal, including the following points:
  - Where he has pain
  - How much pain he has at rest and with activity (using a 0 to 10 scale)
  - How his pain feels (descriptive terms)
  - How his pain changes with activity and time
- Ask him to practice reporting the information to you.
- Instruct Dean to write down any events that he thinks may be related to the occurrence of pain.
- Suggest that he anticipate possible painful events and alter his behavior to prevent or minimize pain.
- Advise Dean to take his journal with him to the healthcare provider, and encourage him to report this information to the provider.

EVALUATION

> 6/17/17: 11:00—Dean was able to verbalize how to use the pain scale and willingness to keep a journal recording pain symptoms, treatment, and relief.
>
> —G. Sloan, RN

OUTCOME

The patient will demonstrate appropriate measures to manage his pain.

STRATEGIES

- Discuss his plans to use nonpharmacologic methods for pain control. Provide written and verbal instructions for the methods chosen.
- Have him practice the methods to determine the most effective ones. Instruct him to use alternate methods if one seems ineffective.
- Review his medication prescription, including the following:
  - Drug name, dosage, and frequency
  - Analgesic action
  - Adverse effects and ways to minimize them, especially constipation
- Discuss the nature of his pain and prescribed time intervals for taking his medication, including:
  - Keeping the pain intensity level as close as possible to his goal for pain relief
  - Taking the medication regularly for constant pain and before pain begins for intermittent pain
  - Taking the medication before the pain becomes more intense than he would like to tolerate
- Discuss his plan to report inadequate pain relief to his healthcare provider.
- Urge him to obtain another prescription before the pain medications are all used.
- Discuss his concerns about using the pain medication, and provide clarification for any misconceptions that he may have.
- Review with Dean a plan of response in the event of a drug interaction.
- Give Dean the phone number of his healthcare provider and encourage him to keep it readily available.
- Advise him to always take a list of all medications with him to his healthcare provider appointments.

EVALUATION

> 6/17/17: 11:00—Dean accurately verbalized medication regimen and a willingness to try relaxation techniques for pain relief.
>
> —G. Sloan, RN

An overview of actions and nursing implications for the four pharmacologic categories are displayed in Table 35-5.

Without the knowledge of pain intensity or the type and location of pain, there is no basis for selecting a drug or drugs for pain relief. **Multimodal therapy** that uses two or more analgesics with different mechanisms of action to maximize pain relief and diminish side effects should always be considered as a pharmacologic strategy. For example, a patient with a mix of nociceptive and neuropathic pain will not get complete relief if prescribed NSAIDs alone since they

TABLE 35-5 DRUG ACTIONS AND NURSING IMPLICATIONS

Analgesic Classification	Nursing Implications
Nonopioids • Acetaminophen (APAP)—antipyretic, analgesic • NSAIDs—antipyretic, analgesic, anti-inflammatory	• Effective against nociceptive pain • Not effective for neuropathic pain • Analgesic ceiling (going beyond a maximum dose will not provide additional relief) • *APAP*: Metabolized in the liver; may cause toxicity. Do not go beyond 4 g in 24 h. Sometimes combined with opioids in pill format. Always check patient's 24-hour totals when APAP is an element in combination drugs not to exceed 4 g 24-hour maximum dose. • *NSAIDs*: Used effectively in multimodal therapy for the treatment of both acute and persistent pain. Use lowest effective dose over shortest period of time to decrease likelihood of side effects. • Inhibits prostaglandin production, which protects the stomach and kidneys. Also inhibits platelet aggregation. • Side effects include gastrointestinal irritation, renal toxicity, and bleeding. Use with caution in patients with gastrointestinal disorders, kidney disease, and patients with bleeding risk.
Opioids • Full agonist—morphine, hydromorphone, oxycodone, methadone, fentanyl • Antagonist—naloxone (Narcan)	• Drug of choice for moderate or severe pain • Used for treatment of persistent pain in select patients • Effective for both nociceptive and neuropathic pain • Versatile—works peripherally and centrally along the pain pathway and comes in many forms, routes, and doses • No analgesic ceiling, making these medications useful for upward dose titration if pain worsens • Constipation is the most common side effect. Other side effects are dose related and include sedation, nausea, vomiting, pruritis, respiratory depression, and delirium. Tolerance develops to many side effects over time except constipation. Always consider bowel management interventions with prescribed opioids. • Used to reverse oversedation and respiratory depression related to opioids in excess. Naloxone displaces the opioid at the receptor site and counteracts the opioid's effect. Naloxone has a much shorter duration than the opioids; consequently, repeat doses may be needed as soon as 30 minutes after initial dose. Monitor patient closely and frequently to avoid rebound sedation and respiratory depression and provide alternative pain relief as needed.
Adjuvant Analgesics • Antidepressants, anticonvulsants, local anesthetics, corticosteroids	• Primary use is for reasons other than pain management, but adjuvant analgesics have pain-relieving properties. • Many are helpful in treating neuropathic and persistent pain.
Other Adjuvants • Muscle relaxants, hypnotics, anxiolytics	• Do not have pain-relieving properties but are used to treat associated symptoms that can exacerbate pain (e.g., insomnia, anxiety, muscle spasm) • May compound sedative effects when used in combination with opioids; monitor sedation levels for safety

are not effective in treating neuropathic pain. A multimodal approach may be required that might include NSAIDs, opioids, and an antiepileptic medication such as gabapentin for neuropathic pain.

Finally, providers should consider five guiding principles for effective assessment, implementation, and evaluation of the pharmacologic pain management plan (Dahl et al., 2008):

• Base the initial drug choice on type and intensity of pain.
• Consider that patients may have more than one site and type of pain.
• Give adequate doses.
• Give drugs at appropriate intervals.
• When treating persistent pain, it is important to give drugs an adequate trial.

WORLD HEALTH ORGANIZATION ANALGESIC LADDER

The World Health Organization (WHO) pain relief ladder (Fig. 35-5) outlines a coordinated stepwise approach to

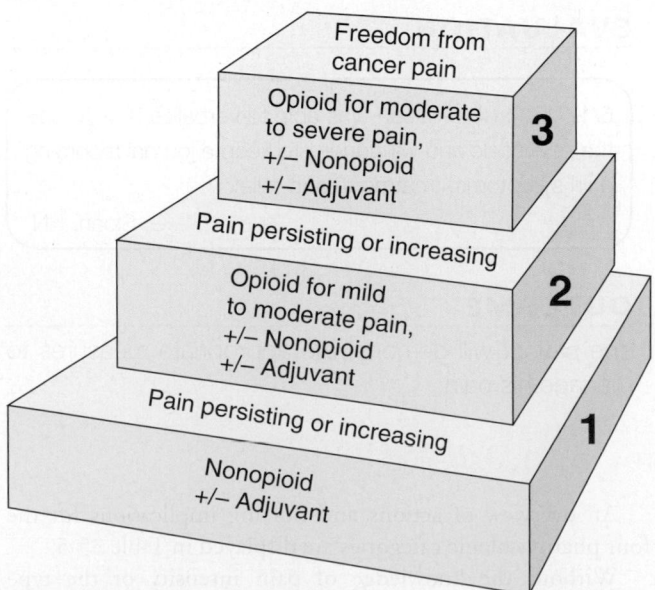

FIGURE 35-5 The WHO's pain relief ladder shows a stepwise approach to the pharmacologic management of pain. (Reprinted with permission from http://www.who.int/cancer/palliative/painladder/en/).

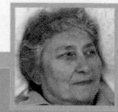

Pain Management PICO

Ruby is the hospice nurse visiting the patient in the chapter-opening scenario. She pulls out a fentanyl nasal spray to administer to the patient, who continues to experience uncontrolled pain. During the visit, the son approaches Ruby to ask her about the new pain medicine, fentanyl. He explains that he has never heard of it and wants to know if it is better than the other pain medications she is on. Ruby pulls evidence from the Cochrane Library to teach the son about efficacy of fentanyl. She uses the following question to guide her search: In cancer patients, how does oral fentanyl compare to other opioids or placebo to help with breakthrough pain?

P = cancer patients

I = oral fentanyl

C = opioids or placebo

O = help breakthrough pain

Ruby finds an updated systematic review that analyzed 15 studies with 1,699 participants. The studies looked at oral and nasal fentanyl administration and compared it to placebo and other opioids. The findings revealed that transmucosal (oral or nasal) fentanyl proved to be more effective in the treatment of breakthrough pain than placebo and oral morphine. Participants reported greater pain relief scores at all measured time intervals when compared to oral morphine or placebo. Using the evidence, Ruby is able to teach and reassure the son that oral fentanyl is a good treatment plan for his mother, and she assures him that she will carefully monitor his mother's response to the medication.

REFERENCE:

Zeppetella, G., & Davies, A. N. (2013). Opioids for the management of breakthrough pain in cancer patients. *Cochrane Database of Systematic Reviews* Issue 10. Art. No.: CD004311. DOI: 10.1002/14651858.CD004311.pub3

---

pharmacologic pain management and is widely used as a guideline for cancer and noncancer pain treatment. The ladder has three treatment levels or steps. Its effectiveness depends on patient pain intensity self-report and reflects a multimodal pain management approach.

Step 1 of the WHO ladder addresses patients with mild pain intensity, rating their pain between 1 and 3. Mild pain is often treated with around the clock administration of NSAIDs or acetaminophen. Pain that is unrelieved or progresses to a moderate level (step 2), with an intensity rating of 4 to 6 on the numeric pain scale, is treated with the addition of oral opioid analgesics. Low-dose IV opioid medications may also be used during step 2 if oral intake is restricted. Finally, step 3 of the WHO ladder addresses treatment options for severe pain, with a pain intensity rating of 7 to 10. Treatment includes the addition of higher-dose IV opioids and more frequent dosing as safety allows. Notice that each level of the WHO ladder includes the potential use of adjuvant medications. **Adjuvant** medications are drugs that have primary indications other than analgesia but act during the pain pathway phases of transmission, modulation, and perception to alter pain impulse transmission and perception. Examples of some common classes of adjuvant medication can be found in Table 35-5.

APPLY YOUR CRITICAL THINKING

You are assigned to care for Mr. Ward, a 69-year-old retired construction worker who had a total knee replacement 2 days ago. He is scheduled to be discharged later today after physical therapy. During handoff you were told that his PCA was discontinued at 06:00 and since his pain was 2/10 he did not receive any pain medication. He has the following medication orders for pain: Percocet 1 to 2 tablets every 4 to 6 hours PRN for moderate pain 4 to 7/10, morphine sulfate 1 to 2 mg IV every 4 hours for severe pain 8 to 10/10, Tylenol (acetaminophen) 650 mg every 6 hours. It is now 9 am and he is scheduled for PT at 10:00. He is rating his pain at 6/10 and states he would like the IV morphine the doctor ordered. How will you proceed to assist Mr. Ward in managing his pain?

Check your answer in Appendix B.

EQUIANALGESIC DOSING

The equianalgesic dosing table provides a comparison of various opioid agonists and is an important tool to use when

TABLE 35-6 APPOXIMATE EQUIANALGESIC DOSES

Drug	Oral (mg)	IV (mg)	Duration (h)
morphine	30	10	3–4
hydromorphone	7.5	1.5	3–4
oxymorphone	10	1	>4
Methadone*	2–5	2–5	6–8?
codeine	200	130	3–4
oxycodone	20–30	—	3–4
hydrocodone	30	—	3–4
meperidine	300	100	2–3

Note: This equianalgesic dosing table compares the potencies of various opioid agonists. It is traditional to compare opioids to a 10 mg dose of IV morphine. Note that hydromorphone and oxymorphone are more potent than morphine. That does not mean that they are more effective analgesics, but that a smaller dose of those drugs is required to get the same analgesic effect as with a dose of morphine. Note that morphine, hydromorphone, and oxymorphone are more potent when given intravenously than orally. This is because there is significant first-pass metabolism of oral drugs in the liver.

Tables of this sort provide **approximate**, not exact, equianalgesic doses, so exercise caution in their use. Many recommend that patients be given only 50% of the calculated dose of the "new" drug when they are being transitioned from one drug to another.

*Consult with a pain specialist before converting a patient to methadone from another opioid because the equianalgesic dose of methadone is dependent on the dose of that other opioid.

Reprinted with permission from: Dahl, J., Gordon, D., Paice, J., Stevenson, K., & Brown, M. (2015). *Pain resource nurse curriculum & planning guide.* Madison, WI: Resource Center of the Alliance of State Pain Initiatives. Retrieved from http://trc.wisc.edu/items.asp?itemID=114

patients convert from one opioid medication to another or from one route to another with the same drug. It is traditional to compare opioids to a 10-mg dose of IV morphine. Notice that hydromorphone and oxymorphone are more potent than morphine and therefore require a lower dose to achieve the same effect. Refer to Table 35-6 to have a better understanding of common opioid potencies.

ADVERSE EFFECTS OF OPIOIDS

Opioids are the drug of choice for the treatment of moderate-to-severe pain due to surgery, trauma, procedures, and cancer and are used to treat persistent noncancer pain in selected patients. If not delivered and monitored adequately, opioids have the potential to induce respiratory depression—a potentially serious and life-threatening side effect because of the drug's actions on the CNS. Consequently, it is important for nurses to understand their responsibility in monitoring patients receiving opioids so that patients remain safe and continue to receive the pain relief they deserve.

Sedation and Respiratory Depression

Patients at risk for sedation and respiratory depression related to opioid delivery include but are not limited to the following:

- Opioid-naïve patients
- Patients receiving other sedative medications
- Elders
- Patients with obstructive sleep apnea

BOX 35-2 Sedation Scale

S—Sleep, easy to arouse
1—Awake and alert
2—Slightly drowsy, easily aroused
3—Frequently drowsy, arousable, drifts off to sleep during conversation
4—Somnolent, minimal or no response to physical stimulation

From: McCaffery, M., & Pasero, C. (2011). Pain assessment and pharmacological management. St. Louis, MO: Mosby.

Most patients experience sedation at the beginning of therapy or when medications are changed or doses increased in response to increased pain levels. Assess the level of sedation when opioids are (i) initiated, (ii) before and after opioid administration, (iii) after a change in dose, and (iv) during opioid infusion monitoring. Box 35-2 outlines the four levels used to assess sedation in patients receiving opioids. Patients with a level of sedation greater than 2 should have their provider notified immediately, and the nurse should request a change in the pain plan and a provider visit to the bedside as warranted.

! SAFETY ALERT

An important safety rule of thumb is this—neurologically intact patients will *always* have an increased level of sedation before exhibiting signs and symptoms of respiratory depression. Paying attention to the level of sedation as an indicator of CNS depression will help avoid unwanted incidence of respiratory depression.

Monitoring Oxygenation Saturation with Pulse Oximetry. Oxygen saturation monitoring during intravenous opioid delivery is a common mechanical monitoring technique used to monitor patients for opioid induced respiratory depression. Pulse oximetry is the device used to measure the level of oxygenation in the blood. A noninvasive probe is clipped to the finger or the ear; then, with each pulsation of blood, the probe is able to calculate the difference between hemoglobin rich and hemoglobin poor blood and produce a percent saturation level. Despite widespread use of pulse oximetry to safeguard opioid delivery there are several drawbacks that nurses need to be aware of.

Pulse oximetry is a local measure of gas exchange in the circulatory system rather than a direct indicator of ventilator status. Pulse oximetry readings are influenced by changes in blood flow to the sensor area, which can alter the signal quality and produce inaccurate saturation levels. The most important disadvantage of pulse oximetry occurs when supplemental oxygen is delivered during pulse oximetry monitoring. Supplemental oxygen delivery saturates the circulatory system with oxygen rich blood, sending a signal to the pulse oximeter that blood oxygen levels are adequate. The device does not

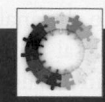

COLLABORATING WITH THE HEALTHCARE TEAM
Notifying Provider of Oversedation from Pain Medication

SITUATION: Hello Dr. Smith. My name is Luke, and I am the nurse caring for Mr. Young. I am concerned about Mr. Young's increasing sedation over the last 2 hours.

BACKGROUND: Mr. Young is a 62-year-old man, postoperative day 1 for a right colectomy, and he is opioid naïve. He is currently on a hydromorphone PCA for his incision pain. He had his dose increased from 0.2 mg every 8 minutes to 0.3 every 6 minutes during the night for pain out of control. He has used a total of 11.6 mg of hydromorphone over the last 4 hours.

ASSESSMENT: His sedation level is a 3. His respiratory rate is 10 to 12. His pupils are pinpoint. He is having trouble staying awake during conversation and nods off to sleep while using his incentive spirometer. He is too sleepy to sit at the edge of the bed this morning and rates his pain 2 out of 10 with movement.

RECOMMENDATION: I think he is receiving too much pain medication, and since he is comfortable, I would recommend that his PCA dose be decreased by 50%. I will continue to monitor him closely over the next 4 hours and will call you if his sedation level increases or his pain gets worse.

CRITICAL THINKING CHALLENGE
- What is the advantage of notifying the provider of an increased sedation level even though the patient's pain is well controlled and his respiratory rate is adequate?
- Is there any additional information you would add to this SBAR message?
- What assessment data would necessitate activating a medical emergency team?

---

assess the quality and efficacy of ventilation, which is the true measure for respiratory depression. See Pulse Oximetry guidelines in **Procedure 26-1**.

Monitoring Ventilation with End Tidal CO$_2$ (Capnography).
Ventilation is the process by which oxygen and CO$_2$ are transported to and from the lungs. End tidal CO$_2$ is the level of carbon dioxide released at the end of a breath. This level reflects cardiac output and pulmonary blood flow as gas is transported by the venous system to the heart and then pumped to the lungs. End tidal CO$_2$ is considered a highly reliable measure of the quality of ventilation and, unlike pulse oximetry, is an early indicator of impending respiratory depression (Kopra, Wallace, Reilly, & Binning, 2007).

End tidal CO$_2$ is measured using a device that measures expired CO$_2$. The nasal cannula probe is positioned under the nose. Adequate positioning of the probe is critical for accurate results. Cannula migration away from the nose, eating, and mouth breathing are a few of the factors that frequently trigger false readings and false alarms. The technology for monitoring End Tidal CO$_2$ is rapidly advancing and although further research and improved design are needed, end tidal CO$_2$ monitoring will most likely replace pulse oximetry monitoring in the future to detect respiratory depression (Kopra et al., 2007). See **Procedure 26-3**.

PATIENT-CONTROLLED ANALGESIA

Patient-controlled analgesia (PCA) is used to allow patients to self-administer drugs by various routes: subcutaneously, intravenously, and epidurally. IV administration is the most common PCA route for postoperative pain in the acute care setting. A major benefit of PCA is that the patient can control delivery of a predetermined dose and self-adjust the dosing frequency based upon individual pain management requirements (Fig. 35-6). Each PCA dose setting has safety parameters programmed into the infusion pump including (i) prescribed dose in milligrams or micrograms; (ii) minimum time interval between doses; and (iii) either a continuous infusion, on-demand setting, or a combination of both. PCA protocols help avoid delays in administration that can occur with nurse-administered analgesia. Routine self-administered PCA dosing decreases the likelihood of oversedation events because the patient will administer small doses of medication only when he or she is awake enough to do so.

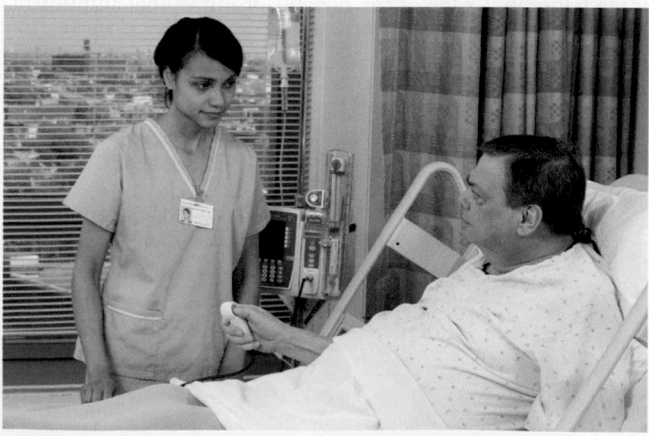

FIGURE 35-6 PCA allows the patient to self-administer only as much medication as needed to control pain.

❗ SAFETY ALERT

Patients should be instructed to push the delivery button when he or she feels pain, and family members are instructed to never deliver medication for their family member. Surrogate opioid delivery through the PCA can lead to oversedation and potential respiratory compromise or arrest and is not considered standard practice.

Patients must be cognitively and physically capable of using the PCA equipment safely. Educating patients and their families on the appropriate use of the PCA is a critical element of PCA nursing practice. In rare instances, such as a ventilator-dependent patient in the critical care unit, a nurse or designated family member who has been instructed on appropriate PCA delivery may be designated as a PCA surrogate and allowed to give opioids through the PCA route.

It is important to ensure that the patient is relatively comfortable before initiating PCA therapy. For example, clinician-administered IV boluses should be given to ensure a safe and reasonable level of pain relief prior to PCA initiation. Careful evaluation and response to clinician-delivered boluses includes documentation that addresses level of sedation, pain intensity, and respiratory status monitoring. The amount of medication that the patient received during the shift is required documentation since this information allows the physician and nurse to evaluate the effectiveness of the pain management plan. See **Procedure 35-1**, Pain Management: Patient-Controlled Analgesia.

Intraspinal Routes of Administration

Intraspinal routes of administration include intrathecal and epidural routes. Injecting opioids or combinations of opioids and local anesthetics directly into the epidural or intrathecal space has become a common technique used to control cancer pain, postoperative pain, and persistent nonmalignant pain. The intraspinal route is often referred to generally as "neuraxial analgesia." Figure 35-7 shows that the spinal cord is surrounded by the subarachnoid space, which contains cerebrospinal fluid (CSF). The subarachnoid space is called the intrathecal space, which is why "spinal" and "intrathecal" are often used interchangeably. One of the benefits of intraspinal administra-

tion of opioids is that the opioid is delivered close to the analgesic site of action—the opioid receptors in the dorsal horn. Because the site of delivery is so close to the action site, analgesia can be accomplished with much smaller amounts of opioid than by any other route of administration (Dahl et al., 2008).

Epidural catheters are placed in the epidural space, which is a potential space between the walls of the vertebral canal and the dura mater of the spinal cord. The epidural space is filled with fat, vasculature, and a network of nerve extensions. Epidural analgesia is extremely potent because distribution of the drug brings it very close to the action site (opioid receptor in the dorsal horn). Although the lumbar region is the most common site of placement, epidural catheters may be placed in the cervical, thoracic, lumbar, or caudal regions. Epidural analgesia may be delivered by bolus injection; however, in the inpatient setting, continuous infusion or a patient-controlled technique called patient-controlled epidural analgesia (PCEA) is the most common. Epidural medications are often a combination of opioids and dilute concentrations of local anesthetics (e.g., fentanyl 2 µg/mL/bupivacaine 0.05%). Epidural infusions require increased frequent monitoring of pain intensity, sedation levels, and vital signs.

❗ SAFETY ALERT

Hypotension is a fairly common side effect of epidural infusion therapy; consequently, sitting the patient upright at the bedside to acclimate him or her to an upright position, integrating calf pump exercises to increase blood flow prior to ambulation, and monitoring for hypotension and sensory/motor changes are important steps to ensure safe mobility and prevent falls.

Additional assessment is required for epidural infusions and includes monitoring the insertion site for exudate or inflammation, monitoring the patient for hematoma development, and sensory and motor function assessments (Table 35-7). Spinal dermatome maps, like the one in Figure 17-20 (Chapter 17, Health Assessment), help assess the level of sensation and the analgesic effects related to the infusion of dilute anesthetic agents. A **dermatome** is defined as the band of skin innervated by the sensory root of a single spinal nerve. To assess dermatomes, use an alcohol swab and touch the patient's skin gently just proximal to the site of injury. Compare sensation laterally on both sides of the body, moving down the torso in segments toward the feet. Ask the patient to tell you when he or she senses being touched; based on the dermatome map, record the level of analgesic effect. Typically, a patient with a well-placed and functioning PCEA for postoperative abdominal surgery will experience some decreased sensation and analgesia from the surgical site to T10, the location of the umbilicus. Refer to **Procedure 35-2**.

Intrathecal (into the CSF) administration and monitoring guidelines are similar to those for epidural administration. Doses administered, however, are much lower because the entire dose reaches the spinal cord (i.e., is not influenced by the dura and high vascularity of the epidural space).

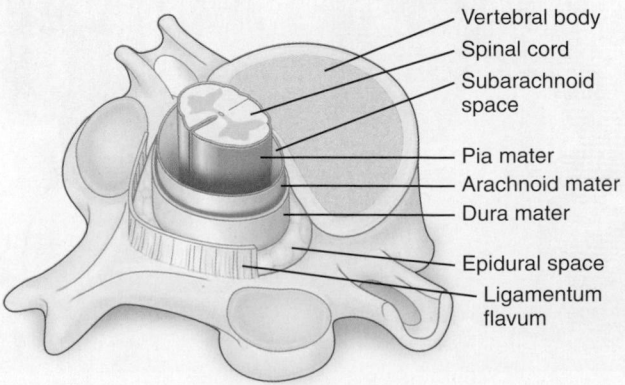

Vertebral body
Spinal cord
Subarachnoid space
Pia mater
Arachnoid mater
Dura mater
Epidural space
Ligamentum flavum

FIGURE 35-7 Anatomical location of the epidural space.

TABLE 35-7   EPIDURAL ANALGESIA

Assessment of motor function	• Ask the patient to move extremities with **dorsoplantarflexion** both feet (S1). • Supine leg lift against resistance (L2-4)	• Notify MD if abnormal. • Diagnosed by MRI
Assessment of sensory function	• Tingling, numbness, pain, burning, or feeling that an extremity is falling asleep. Instruct the patient to report this immediately. • Increased discomfort or back pain • Assess for bladder distention, inability to void, and incontinence. • Check dermatomes.	• Notify MD if abnormal. • Diagnosed by MRI
Exit site erythema or exudate	• Check site every shift, preferably at handoff. • Monitor for s/s infection • Check site for intact occlusive dressing.	• Notify MD if abnormal. • Consider *exit site culture*. • Use systemic antibiotics if culture is positive.
Swelling at insertion site	• Consider infection. • Consider catheter migration *(has dermatome or pain level changed?)*.	• Notify MD if abnormal. • Request *aspiration culture* (culture of the epidural space) if infection is suspected.
Epidural hematoma	• Back pain often first symptom • Sensory deficits (numbness, tingling, paresis) • Motor deficits • Bowel or bladder incontinence	• Notify MD if abnormal. • Heparin (LMWH), NSAIDs, platelet inhibitors, and anticoagulants put patients at risk. • *Catheter insertion*: For patients who have received preoperative LMWH, *delay insertion AT LEAST 12 h* after last SQ dose. • Indwelling catheters should be removed before beginning thromboprophylaxis.

MD, medical doctor; MRI, magnetic resonance imaging; s/s, signs and symptoms; LMWH, low-molecular-weight heparin; SQ, subcutaneous.
From: Pen, A. (2005). Care and management of epidural catheters. *Journal of Infusion Nursing, 28*(6), 377–381; Stillwell, S. (2000). When you suspect epidural hematoma. *American Journal of Nursing, 100*(9), 68–74.

NONPHARMACOLOGIC PAIN MANAGEMENT

Nonpharmacologic interventions are strategies other than medications that may be used to diminish pain and provide comfort. Comprehensive pain management plans that include both pharmacologic and nonpharmacologic strategies have been shown to improve pain control, decrease emotional distress, improve functional comfort, and in some cases reduce analgesic use. Nonpharmacologic interventions are used to enhance the effect, not replace analgesic medications. Three common nonpharmacologic intervention categories that are used frequently in mainstream healthcare are basic comfort measures, cutaneous stimulation techniques, and cognitive and behavioral strategies (Dahl et al., 2008).

Basic Comfort Measures

Basic comfort measures are simple fundamental actions that nurses can offer routinely to promote comfort and help diminish pain. Proper positioning to maintain body alignment, regular scheduled turning, and limb elevation to decrease edema are examples. Maintaining a therapeutic environment with appropriate lighting, low noise levels, a comfortable temperature, wrinkle-free sheets, nonconstrictive gowns or devises, and careful hygiene practices help release physical and emotional tension and will positively impact the patient's pain experience.

Cutaneous Stimulation

Cutaneous stimulation involves stimulation of the skin and underlying tissue, and this technique is thought to interrupt transmission of the pain signal. Examples of cutaneous stimulations include application of heat or cold, massage, and transcutaneous electrical nerve stimulation (TENS). Cutaneous stimulation requires little effort on the part of the nurse and can be used for all levels of pain intensity. Stimulation is commonly delivered directly over or near the painful site, but benefits can also be seen when stimulation is proximal to the pain, distal to the pain, or contralateral to the pain (on the opposite side of the body). Cutaneous stimulation should be moderate in frequency and duration, and its use should be determined by the extent of pain relief according to patient self-report. An important nursing function when using any cutaneous stimulation therapy is to frequently assess comfort level along with assessment of skin changes such as redness, blanching, irritation, blistering, or rash (Dahl et al., 2008).

Heat. Heat application decreases the sensitivity to pain and increases blood flow through local vasodilatation of vessels. Hot water bottles, electric heating pads, warm damp towels, and warm baths or showers are all options for delivering topical heating. Moist heat has been found to penetrate more deeply. The range for heat therapy should remain between 40°C and 45°C with duration between 5 and 30 minutes based on patient comfort and tolerance.

! SAFETY ALERT

Patients should be monitored frequently for signs of toler-ance and skin irritation, and special safety attention should be given to patients who are cognitively impaired. Heat applica-tion is contraindicated over areas of bleeding, over topical men-thol or other medication ointments, and over burned or irradiated skin. Heat should be used with caution in persons with impaired circulation, reduced sensation, or impaired communication that would prevent reporting of discomfort (Dahl et al., 2008).

Cold. Cold application decreases sensitivity to pain and is a use-ful therapy for muscle spasms, back pain, arthritis, headache, trauma, and surgical incisional pain (Fig. 35-8). Cold may act faster than heat and may provide a greater duration of relief. Cold can be delivered through ice packs, refrigerated gel packs, a frozen damp towel, or a towel dipped in ice water. Cold should be introduced gradually, and temperature should be based on patient comfort and skin tolerance. A temperature of 15°C and duration no longer than 20 minutes should be used.

! SAFETY ALERT

Cold application is contraindicated over areas of poor cir-culation, with peripheral vascular disease, with Raynaud's phenomenon, and over radiated skin.

Procedure 30-6, Application of Cold, in Chapter 30 pro-vides specific guidelines for safe application of cold therapy.

Massage. Massage is the scientific manipulation of soft tissue of the body. It is a healing art, an act of physical caring, and a way of communicating without words (Fontaine, 2014). Massage provides a tactile approach that has been found to decrease pain and symptom distress in individuals hospitalized with cancer. Backrubs lasting 3 to 5 minutes offer physiologic and mechani-cal benefits to patients in various settings. A backrub is usually given after a bath and if given in the evening may help with sleep. The massage is slow and rhythmical, stimulates circulation, and can ease stiffness and pain (Fontaine, 2014). It is important to

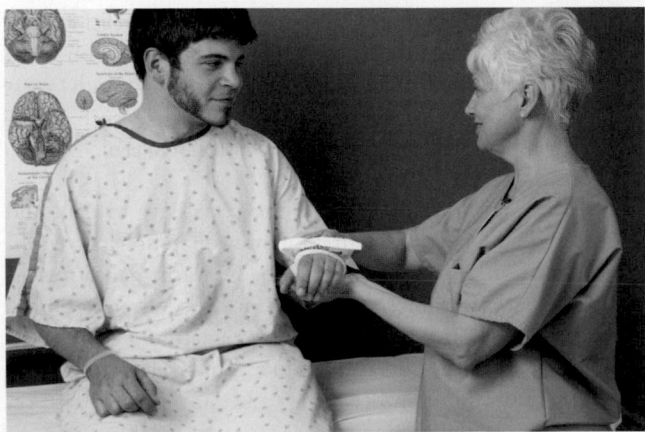

FIGURE 35-8 Application of a cold pack will decrease pain at the injury site.

1. Have the patient sit or lie in a comfortable position.
2. Sit comfortably so that the person's hands are easily accessible, facing the patient if possible.
3. Place a small amount of lotion in your hand and rub to warm it a bit or place lotion container in warm water.
4. Hold one hand palm down, and spread lotion on the skin.
5. Gently stretch skin over the hand outward on both sides from the wrist to the knuckles, pulling gently outward to the center.
6. Supporting the hand and using both thumbs, make cir-cular strokes over the top of the hand from the wrists to the knuckles.
7. Gently squeeze the webbing of one hand from the wrist to the knuckles and continue to gently squeeze the "pinky" finger to the fingertip. Repeat on each finger and the thumb. You may also do gentle range of motion with each finger.
8. Supporting the hand, gently turn the hand palm up:
   a. Stretch the palm gently outward from the wrist to knuckles.
   b. Massage the entire palm of the hand with small circu-lar strokes.

solicit patient preference and comfort with massage therapy. Some patients may prefer a hand or foot massage to a full back-rub. Box 35-3 outlines a simple hand massage that can easily be integrated into nursing practice as a pain-relieving measure.

Transcutaneous Electrical Nerve Stimulation. Transcutaneous electrical nerve stimulation (TENS) is used as an adjunct in the overall management of acute and chronic pain. The TENS unit consists of a palm-sized, lightweight, battery-operated stimulator that generates a mild electrical impulse. Two to four electrodes are taped to the skin near or over a pain zone, and the patient controls the electrode output to produce a tingling or tolerable muscle twitching (Fig. 35-9). TENS is thought to produce anal-gesia by interrupting pain impulse transmission.

The voltage intensity, frequency, and duration of the treat-ment are prescribed by the physician, and TENS is reserved for the treatment of moderate-to-severe pain since other less costly nonpharmacologic interventions are equally effective for mild pain intensity.

! SAFETY ALERT

TENS is contraindicated for patients with on-demand pace-makers and implanted electrical devices (Dahl et al., 2008).

Cognitive and Behavioral Strategies
Simple cognitive and behavioral strategies for the manage-ment of pain can be integrated into nursing practice as an additional therapy for patients with mild-to-moderate pain. Cognitive and behavioral strategies change the way that pain

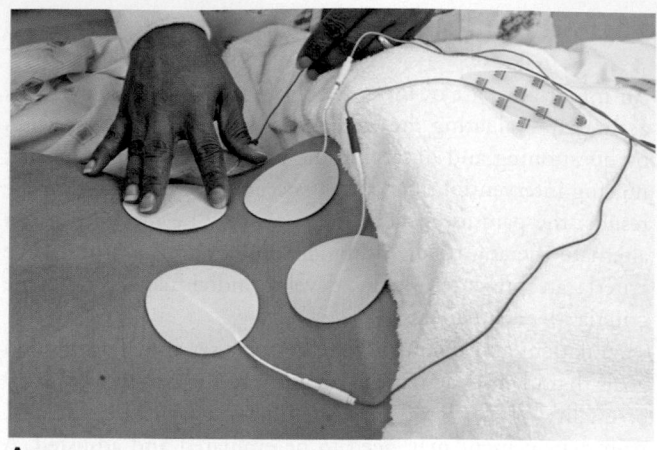

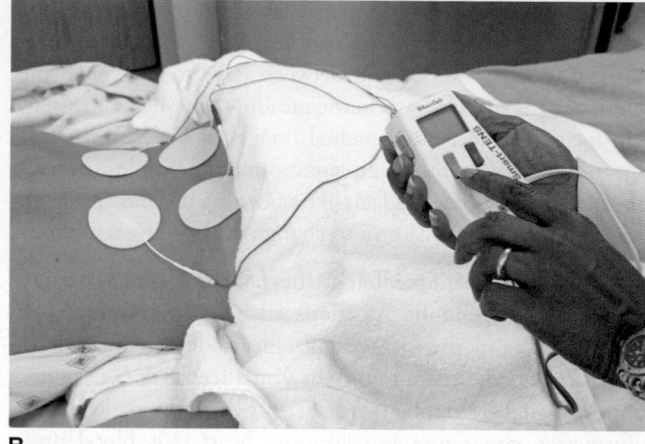

A   **B**

FIGURE 35-9 TENS. **A.** The nurse applies the TENS electrodes over the pain zone. **B.** The nurse adjusts the intensity setting on the unit so that it is comfortable for the patient.

is interpreted and experienced by modifying thoughts and behavior that exacerbate pain or interfere with coping efforts. Pain self-management that incorporates cognitive and behavioral strategies into the pain management plan provides the patient with a sense of control and self-determination and should be considered for patients who are able to put forth cognitive effort and mental focus. It is important to remember that the nurse must always assess the patient's interest and willingness to participate in cognitive and behavioral therapies, and the length and intensity should always be tailored to the patient's preferences.

Distraction. Distraction directs attention away from pain by directing mental focus onto other stimuli in the environment. Distraction is useful for brief pain periods, such as procedural pain, and pain relief tends to be temporary, lasting only through the distraction exercise (i.e., the Lamaze method for the woman in labor). Include multiple senses or high levels of concentration for mild-to-moderate pain. Distraction may be visual (reading—a complex stimulus; looking at pictures—a simple stimulus), auditory (playing an instrument—a complex stimulus; listening to music—a simple stimulus), or tactile (stroking a pet or rocking—a simple stimulus) (Fig. 35-10). The distraction is most effective if it is something the patient enjoys doing and is matched with the patient's energy level. Listening to music has been shown in many studies to be an effective way to reduce the intensity of many types of pain, including cancer pain.

Relaxation. Relaxation is a state of freedom from anxiety and muscle tension that results in a quiet and calm state of being. Relaxation decreases sympathetic nervous system activity, resulting in slowing of the heart rate, reduction in blood pressure, less oxygen use, and release of muscle tension. Relaxation techniques are useful for nearly all types of pain but are very effective in treating pain related to muscle tension (e.g., neck pain, back pain, headache) and helpful as a nonpharmacologic intervention for arthritis, procedural pain, postoperative pain, and cancer pain. Relaxation strategies are also helpful for pain associated with cognitive and affective components of the pain experience. There are various simple and short relaxation techniques—

rhythmic breathing, progressive muscle relaxation, meditation, and prayer are techniques commonly used in nursing practice across multiple settings. Rhythmic breathing involves focused attention on slow, deep respirations that originate from the stomach area. Progressive muscle relaxation combined with rhythmic breathing directs the patient to breathe deeply and relax specific parts of the body, starting from the head and progressing to the toes. A few minutes of coaching a patient through this technique not only provides comfort for the patient but also provides an avenue of relaxation for the nurse. Meditation and prayer can help clear the mind of bothersome thoughts. Focus on using a repeatable phrase, mantra, or prayer to reach a relaxed state.

Imagery. Imagery involves the use of one's own imagination to create sensory experiences to alter or change the pain experience itself. Imagery can be as simple as visualizing, with eyes closed, a favorite place or person and walking through the sensory experience in one's own mind. It is important that the image has significance to the person to be effective. As the nurse helps the patient imagine his or her favorite beach or mountain stream, she will walk the patient through the sensory experience: "As

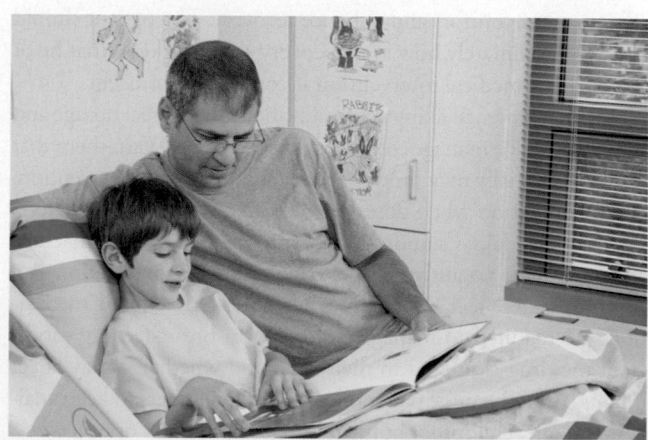

FIGURE 35-10 To promote comfort, the child is encouraged to participate in activities that provide distraction.

you walk into your favorite place, notice the beauty around you. Imagine the warm sun or cool breeze on your face." "Feel the cool water or warm sand between your toes." "Smell the wildflowers as you sit down in the meadow to rest." Conversely, pain-focused imagery uses mental images of the pain itself or objects that may alter the pain sensation. For example, a patient may imagine that the pain feels like a burning fire and creates an image of a dousing rainstorm to change the burning sensation.

Biofeedback. In **biofeedback**, the patient learns voluntary control over autonomic functions such as heart rate, hand temperature, and muscle tension. Electrodes are placed on the patient's body, and auditory or visual feedback (i.e., lights, sounds, digital or graphic readings) provides the patient with information about muscle relaxation, heart rate, blood pressure, and skin temperature. After baseline data are obtained, the patient learns relaxation and deep-breathing exercises. The relaxation decreases pain by decreasing anxiety and increasing the patient's sense of control over pain. With practice, the patient learns to call on the skills at will. This technique is helpful in patients with hypertension, muscle tension, tension headaches, migraines, temporomandibular joint syndrome, insomnia, chronic pain, and stress-related disorders. Motivation is an important component in its success because the technique requires extensive training.

Home and Community Care

Increasingly, pain management is occurring across various healthcare settings. Pain management in the home is critical to improve the quality of life of patients with persistent pain. Persistent pain may immobilize patients and hinder their daily activities, relationships, sleep, and appetite. Family members often provide complex symptom management. Ambulatory and home health nurses assess the interventions and test new interventions.

The nurse is responsible for anticipating the length of time pain will be experienced and, as early as possible in the course of care, teaching the patient and family about pain management and their roles and expectations. The postoperative patient needs information on the healing process with encouragement to maintain his or her pain at the lowest level possible, get adequate rest and nutrition, avoid fatigue, and increase mobility. These factors affect patient comfort and enhance recovery. The patient should know approximately how long recovery should take so that he or she can seek medical intervention if complications occur.

Instruct patients taking analgesics about the correct dosage and ways to avoid or manage common adverse effects. Warn them that analgesics initially may produce changes in judgment, perception, and coordination when doses are increased but that these effects clear in a few days. Caution them not to drive or operate machinery until these cognitive effects have cleared. Constipation is a common side effect, especially when long-term opioid medications are required to manage pain. Inform breast-feeding mothers if the drug is present in their milk and whether it may affect infants. At home, urge patients and family members to keep analgesics in safe, childproof bottles away from children or others.

EVALUATION

An important part of the nurse's role in pain management is accurately evaluating the effectiveness of pain relief measures by questioning and observing the patient. Never assume that nursing interventions have been successful. Depending on the results, the pain assessment measures may be modified or an alternate therapy tried. Although some examples of outcome criteria are presented below, develop individualized outcome criteria for each patient.

A patient and the nurse together may set comfort function goals that identify activities important to the patient's recovery or quality of life. If the comfort-function goals are not met, pain management may need to be evaluated and adjusted. A focus on comfort-function goals assists the nurse and team in maintaining accountability for patients' pain relief and should be included in documentation and discussed during nursing shift handoff and team rounds.

Goal

The patient will identify factors that precipitate pain.

POSSIBLE OUTCOME CRITERIA

- At the next appointment, the patient describes factors that precipitate pain.
- At the next appointment, the patient describes thoughts and feelings that aggravate pain.
- On the next home visit, the patient reports behaviors that aggravate the pain.

Goal

The patient will experience adequate pain relief to be able to participate in activities that will promote postoperative recovery.

POSSIBLE OUTCOME CRITERIA

- While in the hospital, the patient will use an incentive spirometer 10 times per hour and not develop postoperative respiratory complications.
- The patient will ambulate in the hall three times per day until discharge.
- During the first week at home, the patient will slowly resume normal activities within limitations outlined by the surgeon.

Goal

The patient will use techniques that decrease pain.

POSSIBLE OUTCOME CRITERIA

- Within 24 hours, the patient describes at least one behavioral intervention that helps to control pain.
- At the next appointment, the patient identifies the medication regimen that optimally controls pain.

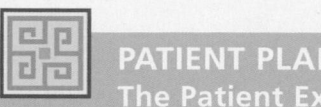

PATIENT PLAN OF CARE
The Patient Experiencing Pain

NURSING DIAGNOSIS
Acute pain related to abdominal surgical incision as evidenced by verbal report of pain (9 on a 0 to 10 scale) and nonverbal communication of pain.

PATIENT GOAL
The patient will experience pain level no greater than 2 (on a 0 to 10 scale) (number able to tolerate).

PATIENT OUTCOME CRITERIA
- The patient reports location, intensity, quality, and temporal pattern of pain and appropriate relief measures for pain.
- The patient reports pain immediately at each occurrence.
- The patient states pain is minimized at peak effect of analgesic therapy.

NURSING INTERVENTION	SCIENTIFIC RATIONALE
1. Evaluate preoperative comprehensive pain assessment.	**1.** The most important component of pain is an ongoing, accurate, thorough pain assessment.
2. Assess level of pain every 2 hours for first 24 hours using a self-rating scale of 0 to 10. Also assess location, quality, and temporal pattern if they have changed since initial assessment.	**2.** Frequent assessment provides data about how this person reports pain intensity and helps determine effectiveness of therapy.
3. Provide optimal pain relief with prescribed analgesics: **a.** Individualize medication regimen from assessment data. Collaborate with physician to prescribe opioid around the clock instead of prn in the first 36 hours to maintain opioid blood levels and provide good pain relief. **b.** Monitor for and minimize common adverse effects of medications (specify).	**3.** Optimal pain relief decreases anxiety and fear, both of which increase pain. Goal is to use a preventive approach to avoid severe pain: **a.** Ongoing assessment of severity of pain before and pain relief after medication is important. This identifies if the drug or dose is sufficient for the patient's pain. **b.** Opioids can cause sedation, respiratory depression, constipation, nausea, vomiting, and dry mouth.
4. Solicit techniques that have previously been helpful.	**4.** Individual techniques that a patient has used in the past enhance pain relief.
5. Establish a trusting relationship.	**5.** An effective nurse–patient relationship enhances all pain relief measures because it conveys caring and trust.
6. Instruct the patient to report pain promptly so relief measures can be instituted before severe pain occurs. Use therapeutic approaches for the prevention, not the relief, of severe pain.	**6.** Relief measures are instituted based on patient's verbal report of pain and regular patient assessments. This also informs patient of the expectation to communicate when in pain because many ethnic and cultural influences often discourage or prohibit expression of pain.
7. Allow rest periods during the day and periods of uninterrupted sleep at night when possible. Keep environment quiet.	**7.** Rest facilitates comfort and sleep, reduces stress, relieves muscle tension, and increases relaxation. Fatigue may enhance pain by lowering pain tolerance.
8. Collaborate with the patient to initiate the appropriate nonpharmacologic pain relief measure(s): **a.** Instruct in distraction technique (specify). *Example:* Engage in conversation or turn radio to favorite station during abdominal dressing change. **b.** Instruct in cutaneous stimulation (specify). *Example:* Give backrub after turning and before bedtime. **c.** Instruct in relaxation techniques (specify). *Example:* Relax muscles when turning.	**8.** Focus attention away from pain and increased pain tolerance results: **a.** Distraction may stimulate endorphins. **b.** Change of position and backrub increase circulation and decrease muscle tension. **c.** Relaxation reduces sympathetic nervous system effects.

EVALUATION

5/1/17: 09:30—Incisional pain 7/10, describes as stabbing, Vicodin 5 mg given, 40 minutes later rates pain as 3/10 and was able to ambulate in the hall.

—S. Roberts, RN

KEY CONCEPTS

- Pain is a subjective experience that occurs whenever the patient says it occurs.

- Initially, pain minimizes injury and warns of disease. Persistent pain has no purpose.

- Sedation does not always indicate pain relief.

- All pain relief measures are based on a thorough ongoing assessment. Because patients may not always report pain, the nurse must assess for pain regularly. Lack of pain expression does not mean a lack of pain.

- Pain may be expressed in physiologic, verbal, and nonverbal ways.

- Patients of all ages experience pain, but the way they express it differs with age, the type of pain, and their ability to cope with the pain.

- Cognitive and behavioral pain relief measures can augment the effectiveness of pharmacologic or invasive methods.

- All routes of opioid administration are effective for mild, moderate, and severe pain, but the IV route provides the fastest relief.

- Combining nonopioid, opioid, and adjuvant drugs with nonpharmacologic methods produces excellent analgesia because pain is relieved through different methods.

- Educating the patient and family about pain reduces anticipatory fear and anxiety, thereby decreasing the patient's pain.

- Using a preventive approach for pain relief is more beneficial than waiting until pain becomes severe.

PRACTICING FOR THE NCLEX

CHECK YOUR ANSWERS IN APPENDIX A.

1. A nurse is conducting a pain assessment on a patient with a spinal tumor and lower extremity pain. What questions would be important to characterize the pain? Select all that apply:
   a. "What is your current level of pain on a scale of 0 to 10?"
   b. "How would you describe your pain: sharp, shooting, radiating, stabbing, throbbing, etc.?"
   c. "How long have you had this pain, and is it constant?"
   d. "What do you usually take for pain at home?"

2. A patient with trigeminal nerve pain describes severe pain on her cheek when wind blows against her face or with the slightest touch of clothing. Which word best describes this phenomenon?
   a. Hyperalgesia
   b. Neural plasticity
   c. Nociception
   d. Allodynia

3. A nurse is caring for a nonverbal patient when she begins to suspect that the patient is in pain. Which nonverbal manifestations would indicate pain? Select all that apply:
   a. Decreased respiratory rate
   b. Increased blood pressure
   c. Facial grimacing
   d. Decreased urinary output

4. A nurse is working with a woman during the transition stage of labor. She asks the woman if should would like to change position and the woman retorts, "I didn't ask for any help, I'm fine where I am!" Which is the most appropriate reason for this behavior?
   a. Pain may evoke a wide range of responses, including anger.
   b. The patient may be disoriented or confused.
   c. There may be a psychiatric history involved with this patient.
   d. The patient's pain is well controlled.

5. A patient with chronic arthritic pain reports using several nonpharmacologic interventions. Which of the following would be examples of this type of intervention? Select all that apply:
   a. Cold compresses
   b. Massage
   c. Over-the-counter menthol ointment
   d. Lidocaine patches

6. A patient returns from the postanesthesia care unit following surgery with a PCA containing morphine. What assessment findings would be abnormal?
   a. Respiratory rate of 8 breaths per minute
   b. Pain scale rating of 3/10
   c. Blood pressure 106/76
   d. The patient is lethargic

7. A patient at the end of life is receiving comfort care. He is grimacing, and the family at the bedside are concerned that he is experiencing pain. They ask the nurse for pain medications. Which response by the nurse is most appropriate?
   a. "I am concerned about further depressing his respirations and cannot give him any opioid medications at this time."
   b. "It is important that he is comfortable. I will give him some oral morphine to help with his pain."
   c. "I am against euthanasia and will not be able to care for this patient any longer."
   d. "The patient has not verbalized his pain rating, and I am hesitant to give pain medication."

8. A postoperative patient is hesitant to receive opioid pain medication for fear of becoming addicted. Which nursing statement is most appropriate in encouraging correct use of opioid medications?
   a. "If you are taking opioids for pain relief and no other reason you will not become addicted."
   b. "You deserve to be pain free, and the medications will help this."

c. "It is important to take all of your medications as prescribed by the physician."

d. "You need to take the medications when you feel your pain level increasing, not once it is already at a high level."

9. A nurse is considering her options for pain relief for a patient with 10/10 pain in the lower extremities related to fibromyalgia. The physician has prescribed several pain interventions. Which would be the most immediately effective?

   a. Oxycodone 5- to 10-mg tablets
   b. Morphine 1- to 2-mg IV push

c. Acetaminophen 650-mg tablets

d. Extended-release oxycodone 20-mg tablet

10. A nurse is treating a Japanese man with cancer and spinal metastases resulting in severe back pain. She frequently asks him to state his pain level, and he responds with a 2/10. Which statement best explains this patient's response?

   a. The patient has a high pain tolerance.
   b. The patient's culture determines stoicism, particularly from men.
   c. The patient currently does not have pain.
   d. The patient does not understand the pain scale.

REFERENCES

Baumann, S. L. (2009). A nursing approach to pain in older adults. *Medsurg Nursing, 18*(2), 77–83.

Cancer Pain Symposium Nursing Research Group. (2004). In *Toolkit for nursing excellence at end of life transition: CD-ROM Version 1.0.* Funded by the Robert Woods Foundation and sponsored by the University of Washington School of Nursing.

D'Arcy, Y. (2014). *A compact clinical guide to woman's pain management.* New York: Springer Publishing.

Dahl, J., Gordon, D., Paice, J., Stevenson, K., & Brown, M. (2008). *Pain resource nurse curriculum & planning guide.* Madison, WI: Resource Center of the Alliance of State Pain Initiatives.

Fontaine, K. E. (2014). *Complimentary and alternative therapies for nursing practice* (4th ed.). Hammond, IN: Prentice Hall.

Im, E. (2008). The situation specific theory of pain experience for Asian American cancer patients. *ANS. Advances in Nursing Science, 31*(4), 319–331.

Im, E., Lee, S. H., Lim, H., Guevara, E., & Chee, W. (2009). A national online forum on ethic differences in cancer pain experience. *Nursing Research, 58*(2), 86–94.

International Association for the Study of Pain Subcommittee on Taxonomy. (1979). Pain terms: A list of definitions and notes and usage. *Pain, 6*(3), 249.

International Association for the Study of Pain Task Force on Taxonomy. (1994). Pain Terms: A current list with definitions and notes on usage. In H. Merskey & N. Bogduk (Eds.) *Classification of chronic pain* (2nd ed., pp. 209–214) Seattle: IASP Press.

Jensen, S. (2015). *Nursing Health assessment: A best practice approach* (2nd. Ed.). Philadelphia: Wolters Kluwer Health.

Joint Commission. (2015). Retrieved from http://www.jointcommission.org/assets/1/18/Clarification_of_the_Pain_Management__Standard.pdf

Kopra, A., Wallace, E., Reilly, G.,& Binning, A. (2007). Observational study of perioperative Ptc_{C0_2} and SpO2 in non-ventilated patients receiving epidural infusion or patient controlled analgesia using a single earlobe monitor. *British Journal of Anaesthesia, 99*(4), 567–571.

McCaffery, M., & Pasero, C. (2011). *Pain assessment and pharmacological management.* St. Louis, MO: Mosby.

NANDA-International (NANDA-I). (2014). *Nursing diagnoses: Definitions and classification, 2015–2017.* West Sussex, England: Wiley-Blackwell.

Oaks, L. (2011). *Compact clinical guide to infant and child pain management: An evidenced-based approach for nurses.* New York: Springer Publishing.

Potter, V. T., Wiseman, C. E., Dunn, S. M., & Boyle, F. M. (2003). Patient barriers to optimal cancer pain control. *Psychooncology, 12*(2), 153–160.

Purnell, L. D., & Paulanka, B. J. (2014). *Guide to culturally competent care* (3rd ed.). Philadelphia, PA: F. A. Davis.

Taddio, A., & Katz, J. (2004). Pain, opioid tolerance and sensitization to nociception in the neonate. *Best Practice & Research. Clinical Anaesthesiology, 18*(2), 291–302.

Zacharoff, K. L., Pujol, L. & Corsini, E. (2010). *The PainEdu.org manual: A pocket guide to pain management* (4th ed.). Newton, MA: Inflexxion.

Procedure 35-1 Pain Management: Patient-Controlled Analgesia

Purpose

1. Allow a patient to safely self-administer small preset doses of prescribed analgesic intravenously.
2. With continuous infusion, allow a patient to receive a baseline continuous IV infusion of analgesic and also to safely self-administer small preset doses of prescribed analgesic as needed for increased pain.

Equipment

Infusion pump for PCA

IV bag with correct medication and correct concentration of drug

(*Note:* To start PCA, an order must be written by the physician: Orders for PCA *medication* changes (e.g., changing from morphine to hydromorphone) or *medication concentration* changes (e.g., changing from 1 to 5 mg/mL) require that the entire order be rewritten.)

Assessment

- Assess if IV is patent without signs of infiltration or phlebitis. If a maintenance IV is no longer clinically required, standard protocols will often use D5½NS at a rate of 42 cc per hour to ensure line patency in between doses.
- Assess compliance, understanding, and acceptance on the part of the patient.
- Assess level of pain and sedation, respiratory rate and depth, and blood pressure.

Procedure

1. **Perform hand hygiene.**
   Rationale: Reduces microbe transmission.
2. **Identify the patient using two separate identifiers**
   Rationale: Ensures correct patient receives proper assessment or treatment and reduces errors.

Initiating PCA Therapy

3. **Close door or bed curtains and explain PCA to the patient:**
   a. **Explain to visitors/family that only the patient is to use the "pain button." Visitors/family may not push the pain button for the patient.**
   b. **Reinforce teaching throughout course of therapy.**
   c. **Document patient and family teaching.**
      Rationale: Ensures patient privacy. Appropriate teaching helps prepare the patient and family and reduces anxiety. Overdose is prevented since the patient will not use the PCA when sleepy or sedated.
4. **Check the prefilled syringe medication label against the medication order and the patient's identification (Fig. 1). Some agencies require two nurses to double check this step to ensure accuracy.**

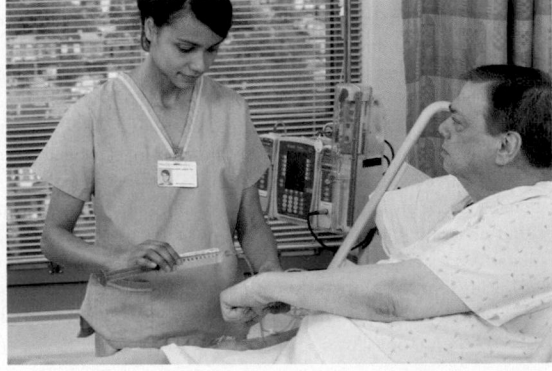

FIG. 1 Check the prefilled syringe with the patient identification.

Rationale: This ensures medication safety with a high-risk medication that could be dangerous to the patient.

5. **Connect prefilled syringe to the PCA device tubing. Load syringe into PCA device (Fig. 2).**

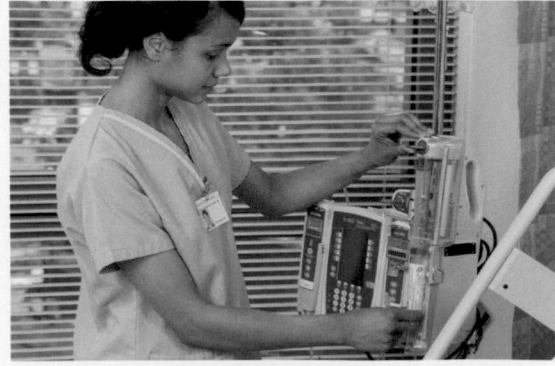

FIG. 2 Load prefilled syringe into PCA device.

Rationale: This prepares the device for medication administration.

Procedure 35-1   *continued*

6. **Prime PCA device tubing with the opioid medication. Program infusion dose and lockout interval according to the medication order (Fig. 3). If ordered, set up the EtCO$_2$ device according to manufacturer's instructions (see Procedure 26-3).**

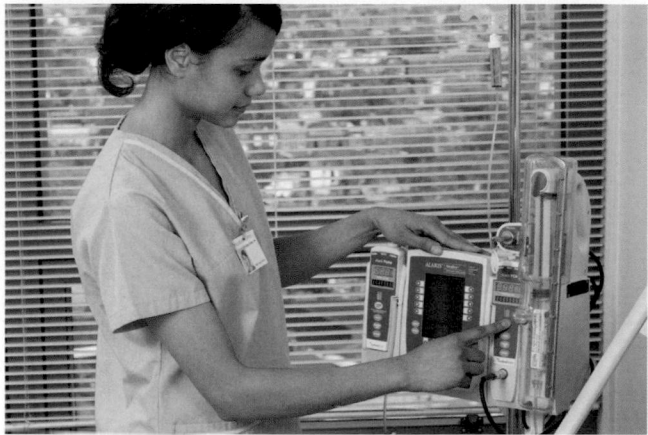

FIG. 3 Program dose and lockout interval.

Rationale: This purges air from the tubing and ensures that the ordered dose and lockout are programmed correctly. EtCO$_2$ device will detect respiratory depression quickly.

7. **Lock PCA device and remove key (Fig. 4).**

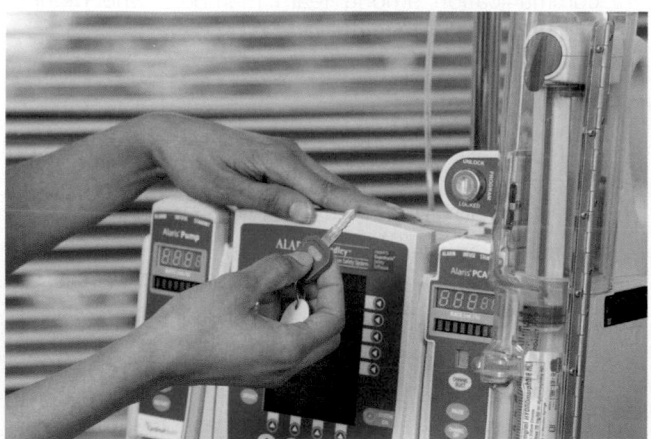

FIG. 4 Lock PCA device.

Rationale: This prevents tampering with dosage and infusion rate.

8. **Clean port with antimicrobial swab (Fig. 5A). Connect the PCA device tubing to the patient's primary IV tubing (Fig. 5B). Activate PCA device by pressing the start button.**

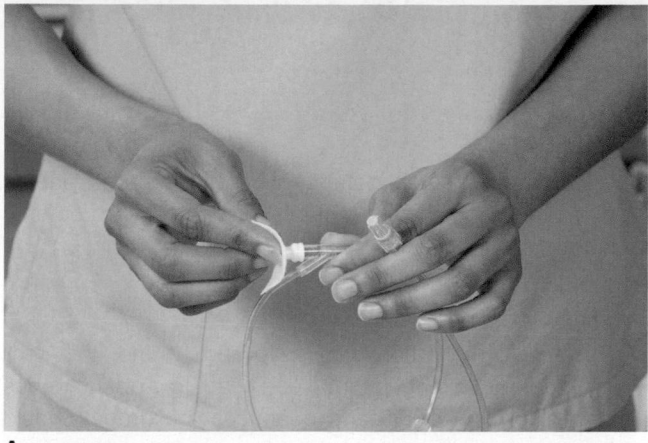

A

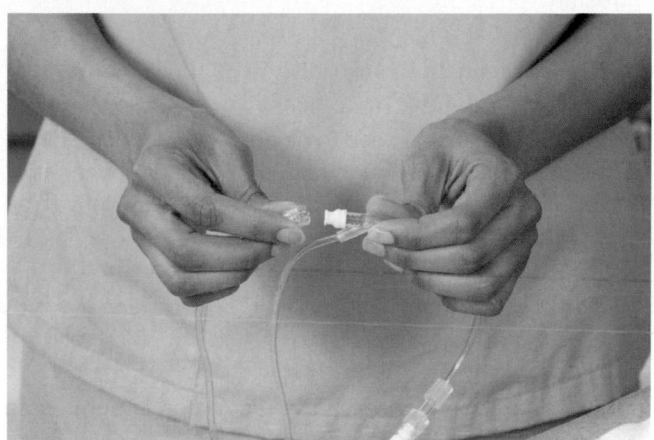

B

FIG. 5 **A.** Clean primary IV line. **B.** Connect PCA device tubing to primary IV line.

Rationale: Cleaning the port reduces the risk of infection. Connecting to the primary line allows for medication administration.

9. **Instruct patient to press button when experiencing pain. Reassure patient that lockout prevents possible overdose.**

Rationale: Patient teaching promotes compliance, understanding, and acceptance of therapy.

10. **Document administration of medication immediately, including date, time, dose, lockout interval, and any other observations of IV site and primary IV infusion.**

Rationale: Prompt documentation promotes safety of the patient.

Procedure 35-1   *continued*

Monitoring and Discontinuing PCA Therapy

3. **Close door or bed curtains and explain procedure to the patient.**

   Rationale: Ensures patient privacy, increases patient compliance, reduces patient anxiety, and promotes learning.

4. **Check the IV site frequently for signs of infiltration or occlusion.**

   Rationale: Infiltration with a flowing IV line, if unrecognized for a long period, can lead to subcutaneous deposition of significant quantities of drug. Should this happen, discontinue the IV and call the IV team to restart.

5. **If a patient is no longer capable of administering his or her medications, notify the physician so that another method of pain management can be used.**

   Rationale: Patients need to be able to understand directions and be alert enough to push the button when they are in pain. Appropriate communication with physician ensures adequate pain management.

6. **If problems occur with the PCA, refer to the troubleshooting guide on the pump. The pain management nurse specialist, the pain team, or the IV team also can help with problems related to PCA.**

   Rationale: **Using appropriate resources ensures safe administration.**

7. **Discuss with physician any problems with PCA or if transition to oral pain medication is appropriate.**

   Rationale: A physician's order is required for discontinuation of the PCA. Patients will often transition from IV medication to oral medication as they recover. An opioid transition order is required and will include directions that the registered nurse hold the PCA and deliver oral medications as prescribed. A "stop infusion" order is required once oral medications are evaluated for effectiveness and the infusion is discontinued.

8. **Discard all medication remaining in the opioid syringe in the presence of a second registered nurse. A second nurse witness is required for all wasted opioids. Record this information per individual hospital protocol.**

Rationale: Accurate wastage procedures and documentation prevents diversion of controlled medications and is required by law.

9. **Record total medication dose (mg/mcg), milliliters (mL) infused, and milliliters (mL) left in the patient's record *every shift* (Fig. 6).**

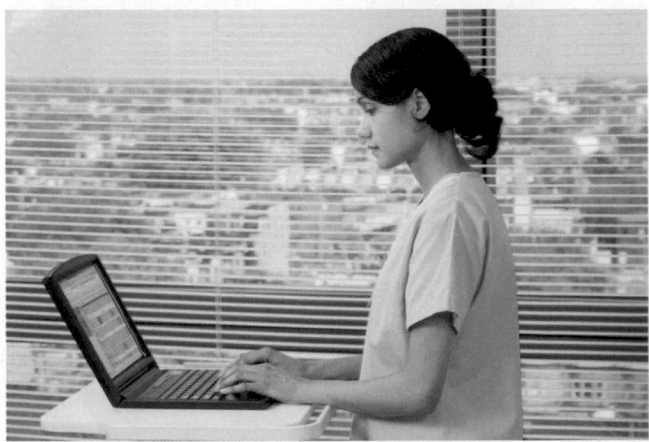

FIG. 6 Document medication administration on the medication administration record (MAR).

   Rationale: Appropriate documentation ensures safety and the tracking of the amount of medication used.

10. **Document times of syringe changes on the MAR.**

   Rationale: Appropriate documentation ensures clear communication among team members who monitor and care for the patient.

Documentation

6/15/17: 14:30—Patient received from PACU following total hip replacement. PCA intact.
Setting: 2 mg morphine/10-minute lockout. Total opioid delivered in PACU was 14 mg. Pain intensity is 4 on 0–10 scale. Level of sedation is 2, VS and rate and depth of respirations are within normal limits. PCA patient education reviewed and patient able to demonstrate appropriate PCA use. Family present and aware that PCA delivery is by patient only and that they should not prompt patient or push button.

—P. Day, RN

Procedure 35-1   *continued*

Collaboration and Delegation

- Discuss with the physician the efficacy of treatment based on functional comfort, level of sedation, and pain intensity and adjust treatment plan as needed. Request an acute pain service consult for inadequate pain management situations.
- Instruct nursing assistants to notify nurse if the patient demonstrates decreased level of consciousness, respiratory rate below 10, or unrelieved pain.

Life Span Considerations

Child

- PCA is generally not used in patients under the age of 18 years; however, there may be special exceptions, and these will require more vigilance by the nurse.

Older Adult

- Determine the cognitive alertness and abilities of the older adult to use PCA appropriately.
- Assess for handicaps that limit ability to use PCA as intended.
- Assess for obstructive sleep apnea (OSA), since respiratory depression is more likely with this condition. Patients with OSA will require continuous pulse oximetry monitoring and use of continuous positive airway pressure (CPAP) or bilevel positive airway pressure (BiPAP) to maintain airway patency.

Procedure 35-2 Pain Management: Epidural Analgesia

Purpose

1. Administer medications into the epidural or intrathecal space to control pain.

Equipment

Infusion pump for PCEA (*Note*: Pumps are color coded so that IV PCA pumps look different from epidural pumps.)
IV bag with correct medication and correct concentration of drug
One Betadine swab
One sterile 2″ × 2″ gauze pad
3-mL syringe
Sterile gloves

Assessment

- Assess compliance, understanding, and acceptance on the part of the patient.
- Assess pain intensity, sedation level, and vital signs.
- Assess sensory and motor function including dermatome levels.
- Assess epidural catheter site (Fig. 1).

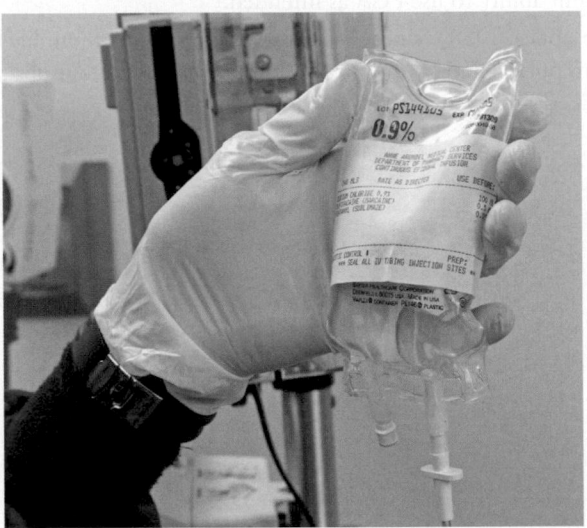

FIG. 1 Assess epidural catheter site.

Procedure

1. **Check physician order for current analgesia dose and complete six rights. The credentialed anesthesia provider who has placed the catheter has verified correct catheter placement and that the analgesia level of the patients is established and stabilized.**

   Rationale: Prevents potential errors and risk associated with medication delivery into a misplaced catheter (Fig. 2).

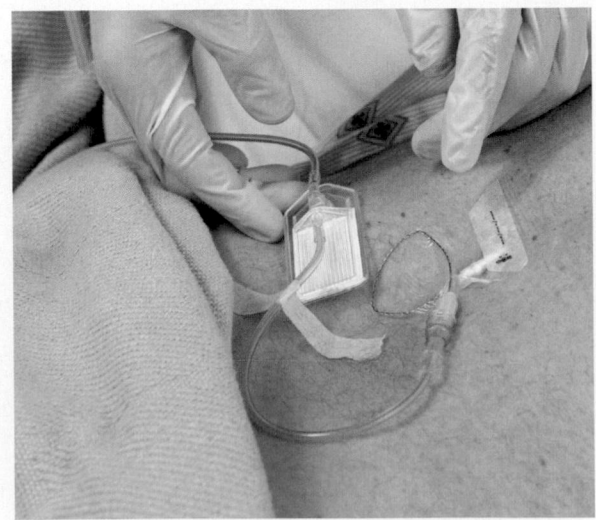

FIG. 2 Check epidural bag against physician order.

Procedure 35-2   *continued*

2. **Perform hand hygiene.**

   Rationale: Reduces microbe transmission.

3. **Check the prefilled medication bag against the medication order and the patient's identification using two separate identifiers.**

   Rationale: Ensures correct patient receives proper medication and reduces errors in high-risk medication administration.

4. **Close door or bed curtains and explain procedure to the patient.**

   Rationale: Ensures patient privacy, increases patient compliance, and promotes patient education.

5. **Insert tubing into medication bag; prime tubing and filter. Place tubing into color-coded pump with proper rate set to deliver ordered dose. Set limit to the amount of fluid in bag. Place epidural catheter label on tubing near pump.**

   Rationale: Ensures delivery of the correct dose and prevents potential errors.

   Flushes air from the tubing to prevent air entering the epidural space. Air in the tubing would cause the alarm to sound.

6. **If ordered, set up the EtCO$_2$ device according to manufacturer's instructions (see Procedure 26-3).**

   Rationale: EtCO$_2$ device will detect respiratory depression quickly.

7. **Cleanse connector of epidural catheter with Betadine swab. Wipe dry with sterile gauze.**

   Rationale: Alcohol swabs should never be used due to neurotoxic risk. Betadine cleansing decreases risk of infection and transmission of microorganisms.

8. **Recheck pump settings against physician's orders and turn on pump. Many agencies consider this a high-risk medication and require two nurses to double-check each other when the epidural infusion is started or changed.**

   Rationale: Double-checking is important in preventing potentially serious errors.

9. **Follow medical orders for ongoing monitoring of pain level, vital signs, and sensorimotor function.**

   Rationale: Promptly detects complications so that the dose can be adjusted.

10. **Document any change in PCEA protocol adjustments along with the patient's response as they occur. At the end of shift, retrieve the total doses administered from epidural pump and clear the totals for the next shift. Record amount administered and amount remaining on the eMAR.**

    Rationale: Prompt documentation promotes patient safety and allows the team to track the amount of medication used to help adjust the pain management plan as needed.

Life Span Considerations

Child

- Epidurals are now being used in some pediatric cases for postoperative pain management or for pain control related to cancer. Depending on the setting and acuity level, treatment may occur in an acute care unit or in a hospice setting. Generally, in-house application would occur in a high-level center.

Older Adult

- It is essential to assess dermatomes, especially in older adults. If sensorimotor function is impaired, falls might result.

Collaboration and Delegation

- Routine physician–nurse collaboration is necessary to ensure adequate pain plan evaluation. The nurse should communicate the 24-hour medication totals and trends in pain intensity. Abnormal vital signs and unexpected alterations in sensorimotor function should always be reported promptly. The patient's functional-comfort levels and patient goals should be discussed with the team as part of the evaluative process.

- Care of epidurals cannot be delegated to unlicensed assistive personnel, but they should be told to notify you if the patient complains of pain, if respirations fall below 10, if the level of sedation is 3 or greater, or if the patient is having difficulty ambulating because of motor or sensory deficits in lower extremities.

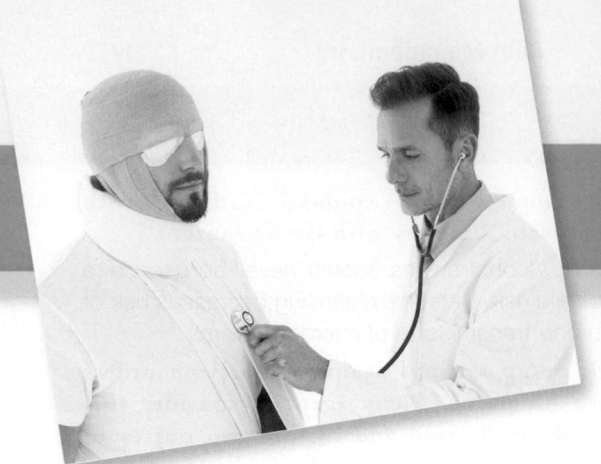

CHAPTER 36

Sensory Perception

Jean Yockey

KEY TERMS
delusions
hallucinations
perception
reticular activating system
sensation (sensory) information
sensoristasis
sensory deprivation
sensory overload
sensory perception

Case Scenario

Patrick Matthews, an active and popular college baseball star, was treated in your emergency department after being hit in the face with a baseball. He talked a great deal to the staff about his concerns, and the staff all commented on how likable he was. Patrick's eyes needed to be patched, and he received instructions to stay in an environment with minimal activity. His father has brought Patrick back to the hospital today. Patrick has refused to engage in conversation and has cut off contact with his friends. On the second night after the injury, Patrick showed signs of hallucinations that a roommate was talking to him and delusions that he was being poisoned through his meals. You have been assigned to give nursing care to Patrick the next morning.

Once you have completed this chapter and have incorporated sensory perception into your knowledge base, review the above scenario and reflect on the following areas of Critical Thinking:

1. Determine what additional information you might need.
2. Identify any specific concerns that you have about communicating with Patrick.
3. Considering the information and your concerns, describe how you feel about being assigned to Patrick.
4. Examine the possible sources for disturbances in sensory perception that you believe are critical for Patrick.
5. Prioritize the areas you need to address in determining your nursing care.

LEARNING OBJECTIVES

Upon completion of this chapter, you will be able to do the following:

1. Differentiate between sensation and perception.
2. Describe the five senses and their role across the life span in sensory perception.
3. Summarize factors affecting sensory perception.
4. Specify how sensory overload, deprivation, and deficit can occur, with interventions for each.
5. Relate manifestations of altered sensory function to their causes.
6. Identify patients who are at risk for altered sensory function in healthcare and community settings.
7. Discuss the relationship of safety to sensory dysfunction.

Sensory perception is needed for humans to interact with their environment. Sensation is the ability to perceive stimulation through the sensory organs that include the nose, eye, and mouth. The sensory stimulation can be from an internal source or from an external source such as temperature or light. **Perception** is the process by which we receive, organize, and interpret the internal and external sensations. The sensations must be converted into meaningful information. Therefore, sensory perception is the ability to receive sensory input and transform the inputs through various physiologic processes into meaningful information.

External stimuli are typically received through one of the five sensory pathways. The five senses of vision, taste, smell, touch, and hearing form the basis for communication, interpersonal interactions, and learning as well as provide a means of detecting and reacting to dangers in the environment. An alteration in any sensory pathway can potentially produce significant consequences. Persons with permanent sensory alterations, such as blindness, deafness, or paralysis, typically learn to make adaptations necessary to lead full and productive lives. However, when any new or temporary alteration in sensory function occurs, the person's risk for more serious mental and physical health deficits increases unless coping takes place.

Nurses encounter patients with preexisting sensory alterations and those with new alterations because of an illness process. The person's ability to adapt may also alter sensory perception. Assessment of sensory function and risk factors for sensory alterations is necessary for all patients, especially when the alteration is a new or temporary one. Older adults require close assessment because they experience age-related sensory changes and subsequent underlying visual and hearing impairments.

NORMAL SENSORY PERCEPTION

Sensory perception depends on the sensory receptors, reticular activating system (RAS), and functioning nervous pathways to the brain. The RAS influences awareness of stimuli, which are received through the five senses: sight, hearing, touch, smell, and taste. Kinesthetic (movement) and visceral (internal organ) senses are stimulated internally in the body.

Sensory Awareness

The **reticular activating system** is responsible for bringing together information from the cerebellum and other parts of the brain with that obtained from the sense organs. Awareness of the world depends on the RAS, which is located between the nerve centers of the medulla oblongata in the brain stem. Multiple sensory pathways, including visceral, kinesthetic, and cognitive input (Porth, 2015), stimulate the RAS. Multiple stimuli received by the senses reach the RAS. Here, certain selected impulses are conducted to the cerebral cortex of the brain to be perceived.

When the nervous system is oriented to a stimulus and receptive toward it, the neurons of the RAS arouse the brain, facilitating information reception (Widmaier, Raff, & Strang, 2013). The RAS is highly selective. For example, a parent may

be awakened in the middle of the night by the slightest murmur of an infant in a bedroom down the hall but may sleep through the sound of loud traffic noises outside the bedroom window. Destruction of the RAS produces coma and an electroencephalograph pattern characteristic of sleep (Widmaier, Raff, & Strang, 2013).

Input by Senses

Sensory function begins with reception of stimuli by the senses. Externally, stimuli are visual (sight), auditory (hearing), olfactory (smell), gustatory (taste), and tactile (touch). Their respective receptor organs are the eyes, ears, olfactory receptors in the nose, taste buds of the tongue, and nerve endings in the skin. Internally, the kinesthetic and visceral senses receive stimuli. Their receptors are nerve endings in the skin and body tissues. The kinesthetic sense influences awareness of the placement and action of body parts. The visceral sense receives stimuli that affect awareness related to the body's large interior organs. Vision, hearing, smell, and taste are termed *special senses*. Touch, kinesthetic (or proprioceptive) sensation, and visceral sensation are termed *somatic senses* (Widmaier, Raff, & Strang, 2013).

After stimuli are received, they are perceived with the help of the RAS. **Sensory perception** is a conscious process of selecting, organizing, and interpreting sensory stimuli that requires intact and functioning sense organs, nervous pathways, and the brain. (Chapter 37 provides more information on cognitive function.)

Characteristics of Normal Sensory Perception

Characteristics of normal sensory perception are the measures in quality and quantity of the special and somatic senses. Normal vision is associated with visual acuity at or near 20/20, full field of vision, and tricolor vision (red, green, blue). If you have 20/20 vision, you can see clearly at 20 feet what should normally be seen at that distance. Normal hearing is associated with auditory acuity of sounds at an intensity of 0 to 25 dB (decibels), at frequencies of 125 to 8,000 cycles per second. (For perspective, a whisper is approximately 30 dB.) Normal taste involves the ability to discriminate sour, salty, sweet, and bitter. Normal smell involves the discrimination of primary odors, such as camphoraceous, musky, floral, peppermint, ethereal, pungent, and putrid. The characteristics of somatic senses include discrimination of touch, pressure, vibration, position, tickling, temperature, and pain (Widmaier, Raff, & Strang, 2013).

Normal Sensory Pattern

SENSORISTASIS

Each person has his or her own comfort zone or zone of optimum arousal (Hasson, Brown, & Hasson, 2010). This comfort zone varies from person to person and is the range at which a person performs at his or her peak. **Sensoristasis** is a state of optimum arousal—not too much and not too little. Some theorists view the RAS as a monitor for sensoristatic balance.

ADAPTATION

Beyond the point of sensoristasis, sensory adaptation occurs. Sensory receptors adapt to repeated stimulation by responding less and less. Eventually, the brain will not perceive constant stimulation, such as background traffic noise. Varied and irregular stimuli will still be perceived, however.

Lead time and afterburn are two necessary time periods crucial to helping a person deal with new stimuli (Hasson et al., 2010). *Lead time* is the time each person needs to prepare for an event emotionally and physically. *Afterburn* is the time needed to think about, evaluate, and come to terms with the activity after it happens. The necessary amount of lead time and afterburn is different for each person. Lead time and afterburn help a person process stimuli so that he or she can respond appropriately without becoming overwhelmed.

Life Span Considerations

NEWBORN AND INFANT

At birth, sensory perception is rudimentary. External experiences and stimulation of sensory systems are needed for development of the brain. Newborns and infants receive most stimulation by touch, needing to feel objects in the environment and learning to feel comfortable with their own bodies in space. They respond to holding, cuddling, soothing, rocking, and changing position. Newborns see only gross patterns of light and dark or bright colors. As newborns grow, vision becomes more discriminating; at 2 weeks of age, infants can distinguish patterns with stripes 3 mm apart, and by 6 months, their vision is as acute as that of an adult.

TODDLER AND PRESCHOOLER

Children's growth, development, and attachment are directly linked with sensory stimulation (Fig. 36-1). Full acquaintance

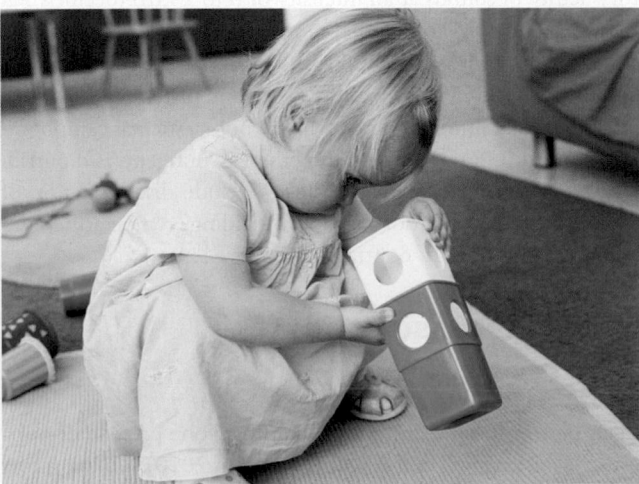

FIGURE 36-1 Young children explore using the senses, including sight and touch. Such exploration facilitates learning and knowledge of the world.

with the world includes exploration with the senses. As children grow, they react to a world of people and things. Lack of meaningful stimulation can lead to developmental and motor delays (Gesell & Ilg, 1949). Successful adaptation to change occurs when stimulation is not too much or too little.

Toddlers are explorers; they investigate and learn about the environment by seeing, hearing, touching, tasting, and smelling. Preschoolers seek out information using more organized play, such as singing and storytelling, to perceive and respond to stimuli through the senses.

CHILD AND ADOLESCENT

Children and adolescents experience rapid changes in their world, and learning occurs at an accelerated pace. Reading and listening to school lessons dominate a child's day. School-age children and adolescents are learning to make independent responses based on what is perceived through the senses, such as crossing the street when the light turns green or reporting a fire when smelling smoke.

ADULT AND OLDER ADULT

An adult's sensory perception function is at its peak. However, as people reach middle age, they begin to notice certain changes in their sensory system. Eyesight diminishes, sounds become more muffled, and the other sensory systems deteriorate. As the average life span increases, the number of people with sensory changes will increase. Early identification of problems can help older persons be more healthy and active (Lewis, Dirksen, Bucher & Camera, 2013).

Cultural Considerations

A person's culture may determine the amount and type of stimulation that he or she considers normal. For example, a child reared in a single-family dwelling may be accustomed to a different level of stimulation than a child raised in a setting where extended family is responsible for the children. The amount of sensory input associated with a person's religious affiliation also affects the amount of stimulation he or she believes to be meaningful. A sudden change in cultural surroundings, especially if there are differences in language, foods, behaviors, and health expectations, may also result in sensory perception problems.

FACTORS AFFECTING SENSORY PERCEPTION

Environment

Sensory stimuli in the environment affect sensory perception. For example, a teacher may not notice the noise in a consistently noisy environment, such as the school cafeteria. But the same teacher may perceive a loud television set very differently in his or her own home, which is usually quiet.

Previous Experience

Previous experience affects sensory perception in that people become more alert to stimuli that evoke a strong response. For example, a person may drive to work by the same route each day, noticing little along the way. A person may listen to the radio inattentively until a favorite song is played and then listen to every word. A new experience, such as hospitalization, may cause a patient to perceive a barrage of threatening new stimuli.

Lifestyle and Habits

Lifestyle affects sensory perception. One person may enjoy a lifestyle of abundant stimulation, surrounded by many people, frequent changes, bright lights, and noise. Another person may prefer less contact with crowds, less noise, and a slow-paced routine. People with different lifestyles perceive stimuli differently.

Cigarette smoking causes atrophy of the taste buds, decreasing the sensory perception of taste. Chronic alcohol abuse may lead to peripheral neuropathy, a functional disorder of the peripheral nervous system that results in sensory impairment. Intranasal drug abuse with cocaine or amphetamines can alter the sense of smell.

Illness

Certain illnesses affect sensory perception. Diabetes and hypertension cause changes in tiny blood vessels and nerves, leading to visual deficits and decreased sensation of touch in the extremities. Cerebrovascular disorders impair blood flow to the brain, possibly blocking sensory perception. Pain, fatigue, and stress caused by illness also affect perception of stimuli. For example, a person dealing with hospitalization and the associated illness, diagnostic tests, pain, and new information may request that only selected support persons visit.

Medications

Some antibiotics, including streptomycin and gentamicin, can damage the auditory nerve, impairing hearing. Central nervous system (CNS) depressants, such as opioid analgesics, decrease awareness and impair perception of stimuli.

Age

Among older adults, 30% of those 65 to 74 years and 50% of those older than 75 years have some form of hearing loss, making hearing impairment one of the most chronic ailments in this age group. Negative effects of hearing impairment include higher rates of depression, social dysfunction, functional disability, decreased cognitive functioning, and reduced quality of life (Ignatavicius & Workman, 2013). Reduced skin innervation is associated with nerve degeneration and ultimately results in decreased perception of thermal and nociceptive (pain) stimuli (Farrell & Gibson, 2007). According to the Eye Disease Prevalence Group, the projected increase will be approximately 72% by 2030, when the last of the baby boomers turn 65,

because most people with low vision are 65 years old or older. (National Eye Institute, 2013). Consequences of vision impairment include greater disability in activities of daily living (ADL), depression, loss of valued activities (reading and driving), and increased risk of falls; it also predicts a person's overall disability (Ignatavicius & Workman, 2013).

Variations in Stimulation

If a person experiences more sensory stimulation than he or she is used to, or can make sense of, then distress and **sensory overload** may occur. On the other hand, if a person experiences less than the usual stimulation, that person is below his or her optimum state of arousal and may be at risk for **sensory deprivation**.

Reactions to sensory overload or sensory deprivation are special challenges that nurses frequently encounter in themselves and patients. Sensory overload or sensory deprivation can lead to perceptual, cognitive, and decisional problems. Separating where one area begins and another ends is often difficult. For example, when a person's senses are bombarded with seeing, feeling, and hearing too much information at one time, it may be difficult to perceive accurately, think clearly, or make a good decision.

When the RAS is overwhelmed with input, a person may experience *sensory overload* and feel confused, anxious, and unable to take constructive action. When the RAS fails to recognize a stimulus because it is below the threshold level or lacks relevant meaning to the person, *sensory deprivation* may occur, and the person experiences boredom, depression, restlessness, and vivid sensual imagery, including hallucinations. These two conditions may be referred to as hyperactive or hypoactive delirium, respectively, and should resolve within 3 weeks (Mistraletti, Pelosi, Mantovani, Berardino, & Gregoretti, 2012; Solberg, Plummer, & May, 2013).

SENSORY OVERLOAD (HYPERACTIVE DELIRIUM)

Sensory overload occurs when a person is unable to process or manage the intensity or quantity of incoming sensory stimuli. The person feels out of control and overwhelmed by the excessive input from the environment. Clinical signs of sensory overload include anxiety, irritability, and inability to concentrate (Box 36-1). Routine activity in the healthcare setting can contribute to sensory overload in patients.

These activities fall into three main categories: internal factors, information, and environment.

Internal Factors

Internal factors, such as thinking about impending surgery or the meaning of a medical diagnosis, can contribute to anxiety and cognitive overload so that the person cannot process additional stimuli. Pain, medication, lack of sleep, worry, hypoxemia, electrolyte disturbances, and brain injury also can contribute to a person's vulnerability to sensory overload.

Information

Imparting information to a patient may lead to sensory overload. Some examples include teaching a patient about a procedure, informing a patient about a diagnosis, making requests of a patient, or helping the patient solve a problem.

BOX 36-1   Clinical signs of Sensory Overload and Sensory Deprivation

Sensory Overload
Irritability
Confusion
Decreased problem-solving ability
Insomnia
Anxiety
Decreased ability to concentrate
Restlessness

Sensory Deprivation
Irritability
Confusion
Decreased problem-solving ability
Depression
Delusions (misinterpretation of stimuli)
Hallucinations (seeing, hearing, smelling something that is not real)

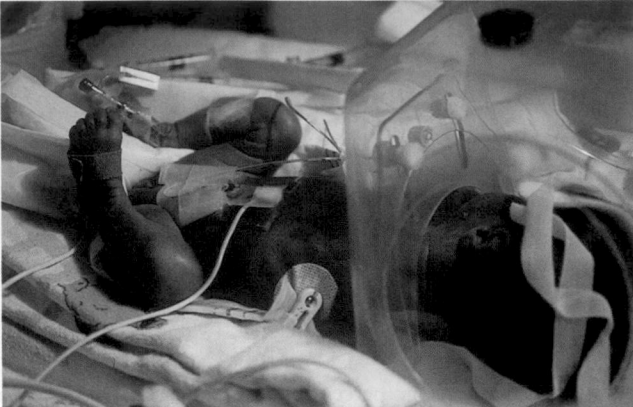

FIGURE 36-2 Lights and frequent activity can cause sensory overload in a premature newborn in the neonatal intensive care unit.

Environment

The environment of the healthcare agency provides a higher than usual amount of sensory stimulation. A patient newly admitted, for example, may have to cope with adjusting to a new roommate, having the television on more than usual, bright lights, paging systems, unexpected intrusions, meeting many staff members, having the bed move up and down at someone else's bidding, waiting for someone to answer the call light, uncontrolled pain, and having strangers touch and probe private body areas. Patients in intensive care units often exhibit symptoms of sensory overload because of the high degree of light, noise, and activity around the clock (Fig. 36-2). Disorientation can occur when expected day/night differences in levels of general activity are lost. To reduce such disorientation, provide a clock displaying a clear distinction of AM/PM time, day, and date (Bell, 2011; Mistraletti et al., 2012; Van den Boogaard, Schoonhoven, vander Hoeven, van Achterberg, & Pickkers, 2012).

SENSORY DEPRIVATION (HYPOACTIVE DELIRIUM)

Although sensory deprivation can be thought of as the opposite of sensory overload, they share many elements. Think about the paradoxical statement "the silence was deafening." **Sensory deprivation** generally means a lessening or lack of meaningful sensory stimuli, monotonous sensory input, or an interference with the processing of information (Mistraletti et al., 2012).

Sensory deprivation (understimulation) can be just as disruptive as sensory overload. Cognitive and emotional deterioration can occur when stimuli are reduced below a person's optimum level of stimulation (Hasson et al., 2010). Some clinical signs of sensory deprivation are similar to those of sensory overload (Box 36-1). One common source of sensory deprivation is a sudden decrease in stimuli when a person moves from a fast- to a slow-paced environment. Any time a patient experiences an

interference with or a decrease in sensory input, that person may be at risk for sensory deprivation. In a healthcare agency, such occurrences fall into two general categories: altered sensory reception and deprived environments.

Altered Sensory Reception

Altered sensory reception occurs in such conditions as spinal cord injury, brain damage, changes in receptor organs, sleep deprivation, and chronic illness. The person does not receive adequate sensory input because of an interference with the nervous system's ability to receive and process stimuli. This inability also can lead to secondary problems, as in the following example: A patient who suffered a spinal cord injury in an automobile accident was left paraplegic with loss of motion and sensation in the lower extremities. One day, he decided to sneak a cigarette while no one was looking. He accidentally dropped the lighted match on his knitted slipper and burned his foot because he could not feel the heat when his slipper began to smolder.

Older people are especially susceptible to sensory deficit, as shown in the following example: An elderly patient stopped attending her senior citizen group. She began to spend most of her time sitting alone. She became more depressed, ate less, and began to show signs of confusion. Nurses who observed these actions were able to intervene to assist her to increase her socialization and communication with others.

Deprived Environments

Deprived environments can have negative effects on a person's sensoristasis. A person who is immobilized or isolated for any reason is deprived of the usual amount of stimulation and may show manifestations of sensory deprivation (Fig. 36-3). Consider the circumstances of Patrick Matthews as presented in the Case Scenario at the beginning of the chapter. His verbal communication diminished dramatically after his injury. Because Patrick could not see, he did not have visual senses and therefore experienced perceptual distortions. He misinterpreted sounds outside his room. He changed from being a likable, open person to being angry and suspicious.

Patrick was showing signs of sensory deprivation. Used to being active, Patrick suddenly needed to change his environment to nonstimulating and quiet. To compensate for temporary loss of sight, his senses of hearing and taste became more

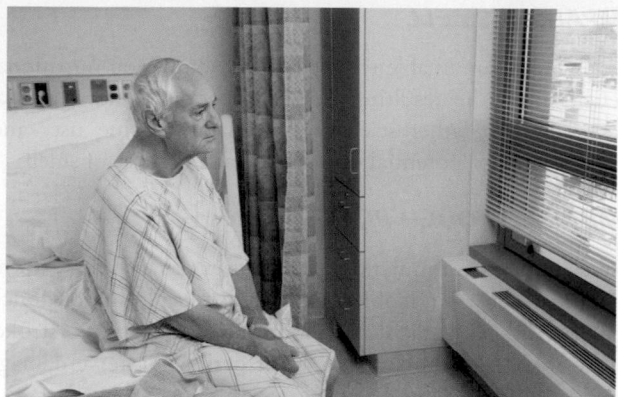

FIGURE 36-3 Isolation from routine environments may contribute to sensory deprivation.

acute, leading to misinterpretations of sounds and taste of food. His personality changed drastically.

As another example, consider a patient who is in isolation due to having a methicillin-resistant *Staphylococcus aureus* infection. Due to the protective measures needed, touch is altered due to the need for protective gowns and gloves worn by staff. Visitors are limited. The patient does not leave her room. Staff interaction is decreased due to the extra time needed to don protective wear to enter the room. Nurses notice that the patient starts spending long periods of time lying in her darkened room without having the radio or television on, and they begin developing a plan to increase interactions with the patient.

ALTERED SENSORY PERCEPTION FUNCTION

Anxiety

Altered sensory perception frequently leads to anxiety, and anxiety can further compound altered sensory perception. For example, an older woman with poor hearing who lives alone may be anxious about going to bed at night because she believes that she might not hear a smoke alarm, the telephone ringing, or someone trying to break into the house. Anxiety stems from not being able to interact fully with the environment due to sensory deficit, fear of embarrassment when trying to communicate with others, or misinterpretation of information perceived through the senses.

Cognitive Dysfunction

Disturbances in remembering, reasoning, and problem solving can occur with sensory overload. Decision making may be irrational or dysfunctional. Other common behaviors indicative of cognitive dysfunction include disorientation; verbalizing disconnected thoughts; complaining of too much going on, sleeplessness, and fatigue; inability to think; and poor work performance (Gordon, 1994). Sensory deprivation also reduces mental capabilities. Mind wandering occurs, along with fantasy activity. The person may have difficulty concentrating and thinking logically.

Hallucinations and Delusions

Hallucinations, sensory impressions that are based on internal stimulations, have no basis in reality. Hearing voices when no one is there is a typical auditory hallucination. **Delusions**, beliefs not based in reality, reflect an unconscious need or fear (e.g., believing that the hospital food is poisoned). Both hallucinations and delusions have been documented in cases of sensory deprivation, sensory overload, and sensory deficits, such as hearing or vision loss. For example, an older woman with glasses and a hearing aid is suddenly hospitalized. Her glasses are misplaced, and the battery is weak in her hearing aid. She may not understand why strange people come into her room at night. She has difficulty ambulating and locating the call light to ask for assistance with toileting, so she soils her bed. Her sensory deficits cause her to misinterpret stimuli and distort reality. She has delusions that she is in a prison, the nurses are guards, and other prisoners are trying to take advantage of her. She hallucinates that her dead sister is telling her to join her in heaven.

Sensory Deficits

A sensory deficit is impaired function in sensory reception or perception. The deficit may be blindness due to disease of the eyes, such as glaucoma. In this case, reception is affected. Spinal cord injuries and strokes that cause loss of tactile sensation affect perception because of disruption in nerve pathways or the brain.

A sudden loss of sensory perception through a sensory deficit can cause total disorientation because compensation does not occur immediately. Compensation for a deficit usually occurs when loss of function is gradual. The patient may change his or her behavior to adapt to the sensory deficit, such as turning a functioning ear toward a speaker to hear or measuring the temperature of bath water with a thermometer (if there is decreased sensation of the extremities). Physiologic compensation also occurs, with the remaining senses becoming more acute. For example, a blind person may develop a more acute sense of smell or hearing.

A sensory deficit may occur due to either a temporary or permanent treatment or illness condition. Temporary bandaging after eye surgery may render a patient totally unable to care for himself or herself. Nasal packing that temporarily eliminates the sense of smell affects taste, possibly leading to anorexia. The patient with sudden loss of lower extremity sensation from a spinal cord injury is at risk for injury to the lower extremities. Specific sensory deficits are discussed in the following sections.

IMPAIRED VISION

Visual deficits may occur due to CNS disorders, microvascular changes such as those that occur in diabetes and hypertension, diseases of the eye such as an infection, or damage to the eye such as from infection or a stroke. Age-related changes may include cataracts (a clouding of the lens resulting in blurred vision), glaucoma (vision loss caused by increased pressure in the eye that can lead to blindness), and macular degeneration (a progressive loss of central and near vision due to damage of the central portion of the retina). Changes in vision can affect all aspects of daily life, including interactions with others and activity levels.

IMPAIRED HEARING

Hearing deficits may occur after an injury or disease in any of the structures of the ear or the neural pathways needed for the conduction of sound waves. An infection or arthritis may decrease the ability to transmit sound vibrations. Damage to cranial nerve VIII or receptors in the cochlea may be a result of medications toxic to the ear (e.g., gentamicin), viral infections, or chronic exposure to loud noise. Impacted cerumen, where tightly packed earwax blocks the ear canal, can decrease hearing. Otitis media, an infection of the middle ear, may be caused by a virus or bacteria. Impaired hearing can negatively impact communication and create safety hazards due to an inability to hear warnings such as a smoke detector or the sounds of traffic.

IMPAIRED TASTE

Impaired taste commonly results from xerostomia, or excessively dry mouth. This condition may be caused by medications, poor fluid intake, poor nutrition, or poor oral hygiene. Other causes include infections of the nose, mouth, or sinuses, the common cold, smoking, or injury to the mouth or nose.

IMPAIRED SMELL

Patients who are unable to smell may also develop nutritional deficits from the resulting loss of appetite. Tumors, cranial nerve damage, atherosclerosis, intranasal cocaine use, and sinusitis are also potential causes of impaired sense of smell.

IMPAIRED TOUCH PERCEPTION

Touch, or tactile stimulation, transmits external stimuli, warns of injury (such as a hot object), and transmits pleasurable touch sensations. Loss of tactile sensation may result from a stroke, brain or spinal tumors or injury, or peripheral nerve damage from an illness such as diabetes.

Depression and Withdrawal

Depression may result from sensory deficits or sensory deprivation. Helplessness and loss of self-esteem lead to depression and withdrawal. The patient who is placed on isolation precautions may show signs of poor appetite, sleeplessness, and loss of interest in activities or interaction with others as he or she becomes depressed, leading to further sensory deprivation.

Think back to Patrick in the Case Scenario. Recall that after 2 days, Patrick began to show signs of sleep deprivation. Use the concept map (Fig. 36-4) to help understand and manage Patrick's situation and to plan for his care.

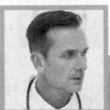

Sensory Perception PICO

As the student nurse from the chapter-opening scenario finishes helping the patient from that scenario cope with his situation, the charge nurse asks the student nurse to admit another patient. The new patient is being admitted for dehydration, loss of appetite, and malnutrition. The student nurse, upon reviewing the patient's home meds, notices that the patient is on zinc supplements. When the student nurse inquires about it, a family member replies, "They have her on it to improve her taste buds." Having never heard of this, the student nurse decides to look it up, using the following PICO question to search the Cochrane library: *In adults, how does zinc supplements versus no supplements improve taste alterations?*

P = In adults
I = Zinc supplements
C = No supplements
O = Improve taste alterations

The student nurse finds a current meta-analysis that reviews several interventions for taste disorders. The study examined nine trials with 566 participants, which included children, adolescents, and adults. There were a group of studies within the meta-analysis that showed moderate evidence in favoring zinc supplements in idiopathic/zinc-deficient disorders. However, the *overall* quality of evidence proved to be low to consider that zinc supplements would improve taste perception. Also, the following adverse effects were reported with zinc supplements: "eczema, nausea, abdominal pain, diarrhea, constipation, decrease in blood iron, increase in blood alkaline phosphatase, and minor increase in blood triglycerides." The researchers concluded that more studies are needed to fully determine if zinc supplements would be a treatment plan.

The student informs the charge nurse about the patient's inquiry and his findings. After reviewing the study, the charge nurse agrees with the student that Zinc supplements might not be the best recommendation for the patient. The charge nurse agrees to consult with the care provider as to appropriateness.

REFERENCE

Kumbargere, N.S., Naresh, S., Srinivas, K., Renjith, G. P., Shrestha, A., Levenson, D., et al. (2014). Interventions for the management of taste disturbances. *Cochrane Database of Systematic Reviews, 11*, CD010470. doi: 10.1002/14651858.CD010470.pub2.

SENSORY PERCEPTION

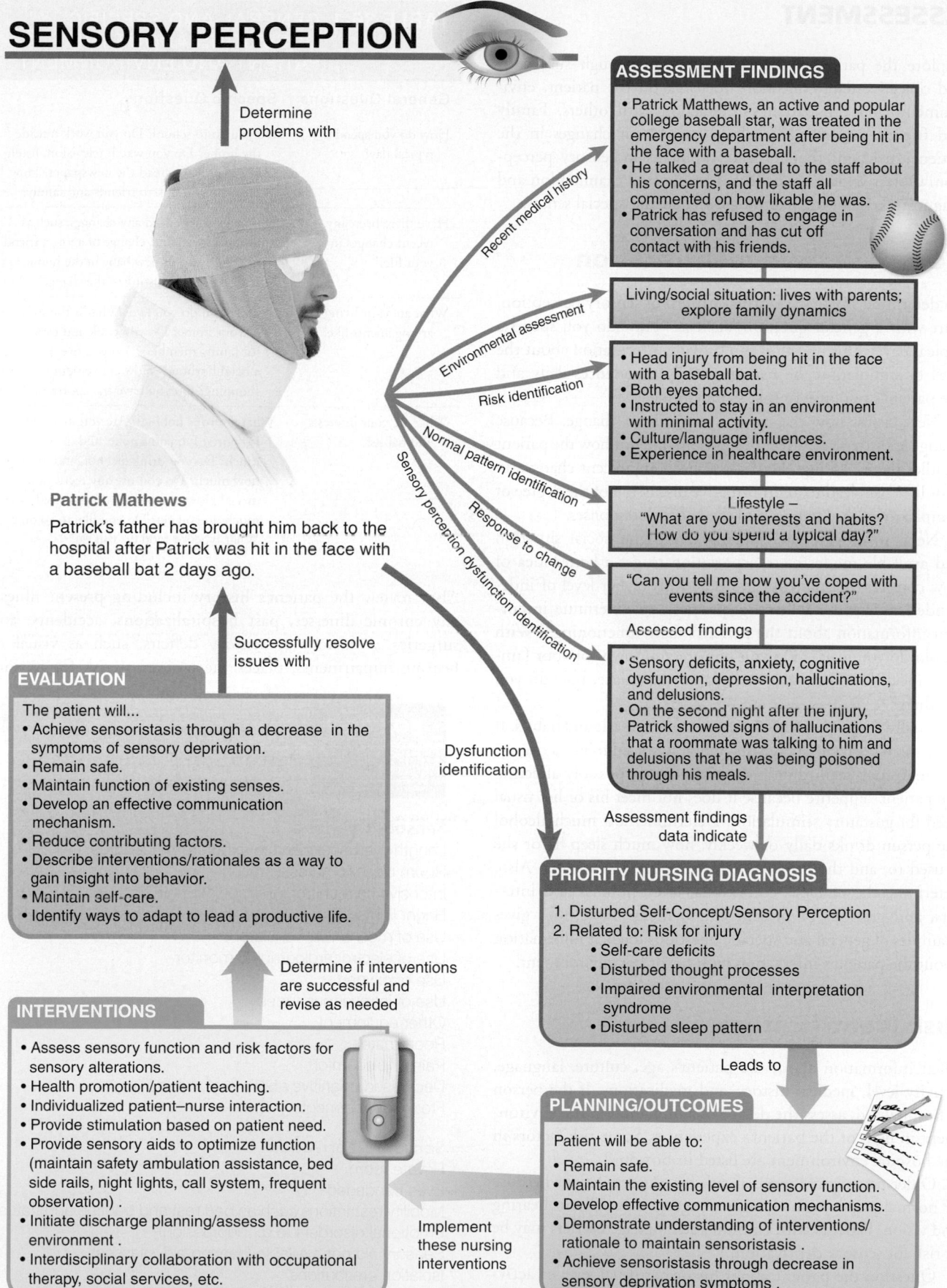

Determine problems with

ASSESSMENT FINDINGS

- Patrick Matthews, an active and popular college baseball star, was treated in the emergency department after being hit in the face with a baseball.
- He talked a great deal to the staff about his concerns, and the staff all commented on how likable he was.
- Patrick has refused to engage in conversation and has cut off contact with his friends.

Recent medical history

Patrick Mathews

Patrick's father has brought him back to the hospital after Patrick was hit in the face with a baseball bat 2 days ago.

Environmental assessment

Living/social situation: lives with parents; explore family dynamics

Risk identification

- Head injury from being hit in the face with a baseball bat.
- Both eyes patched.
- Instructed to stay in an environment with minimal activity.
- Culture/language influences.
- Experience in healthcare environment.

Normal pattern identification

Lifestyle –
"What are you interests and habits? How do you spend a typical day?"

Response to change

"Can you tell me how you've coped with events since the accident?"

Sensory perception dysfunction identification

Assessed findings

- Sensory deficits, anxiety, cognitive dysfunction, depression, hallucinations, and delusions.
- On the second night after the injury, Patrick showed signs of hallucinations that a roommate was talking to him and delusions that he was being poisoned through his meals.

Successfully resolve issues with

EVALUATION

The patient will...
- Achieve sensoristasis through a decrease in the symptoms of sensory deprivation.
- Remain safe.
- Maintain function of existing senses.
- Develop an effective communication mechanism.
- Reduce contributing factors.
- Describe interventions/rationales as a way to gain insight into behavior.
- Maintain self-care.
- Identify ways to adapt to lead a productive life.

Dysfunction identification

Assessment findings data indicate

PRIORITY NURSING DIAGNOSIS

1. Disturbed Self-Concept/Sensory Perception
2. Related to: Risk for injury
   - Self-care deficits
   - Disturbed thought processes
   - Impaired environmental interpretation syndrome
   - Disturbed sleep pattern

Determine if interventions are successful and revise as needed

Leads to

INTERVENTIONS

- Assess sensory function and risk factors for sensory alterations.
- Health promotion/patient teaching.
- Individualized patient–nurse interaction.
- Provide stimulation based on patient need.
- Provide sensory aids to optimize function (maintain safety ambulation assistance, bed side rails, night lights, call system, frequent observation).
- Initiate discharge planning/assess home environment.
- Interdisciplinary collaboration with occupational therapy, social services, etc.

Implement these nursing interventions

PLANNING/OUTCOMES

Patient will be able to:

- Remain safe.
- Maintain the existing level of sensory function.
- Develop effective communication mechanisms.
- Demonstrate understanding of interventions/ rationale to maintain sensoristasis.
- Achieve sensoristasis through decrease in sensory deprivation symptoms.

FIGURE 36-4 Sensory perception concept map.

ASSESSMENT

Explore the patient's sensory perception through subjective and objective data collection, focusing on the patient, environment, and the patient's interaction with others. Family and friends may provide helpful data about changes in the patient's behavior that indicate problems in sensory perception. Objective data are collected by physical examination and diagnostic tests of the neurologic system and special senses.

Normal Pattern Identification

To determine a patient's normal pattern of sensory perception, start with a general question, such as "How do you spend a typical day?" This question can provide information about the level of stimulation the patient usually experiences daily and the patient's response to that stimulation.

Next, assess how the patient responds to change. Because change and stress can affect perception, find out how the patient handles them. Asking "Have there been any recent changes in your life?" can lead to an informative discussion of the degree of complexity of the changes and the patient's responses.

Next, investigate the patient's living and social situation and available modes of transportation to get a better idea of how complex the patient's life is and his or her level of independence. Use the following questions to determine important information about the patient's daily functioning: "With whom do you live?" "Do you prepare your own (or your family's) meals?" "When you want to go someplace, how do you get there?"

Finally, focus questions on the person's lifestyle and habits. If the patient's usual diet consists of highly spiced foods, a change in menu may seem dull and uninteresting, possibly affecting the patient's appetite because it does not meet his or her usual need for gustatory stimulation. Determine how much alcohol the person drinks daily or weekly, how much sleep he or she is used to, and the usual time for sleeping and waking. Also, determine the patient's educational level, hobbies and interests, and previous or present employment. Table 36-1 gives examples of general and specific questions to elicit information about the patient's interaction with his or her environment.

Risk Identification

Elicit information about the patient's age, culture, language, activity level, medical history, and medications. If the person is hospitalized, assess the degree of stimulation in the environment in light of the patient's experiences. Some risk factors in the hospital environment are listed in Box 36-2.

Older patients are more at risk for sensory deficits because of normal physiologic changes of aging, especially in hearing and vision. Patients with cultural and language barriers may be at risk for sensory deprivation.

Question the patient about his or her usual level of activity. For example, immobilization due to physical disability restricts patients from their usual amount of stimulation.

TABLE 36-1 GENERAL AND SPECIFIC QUESTIONS ABOUT THE PATIENT AND ENVIRONMENT

General Questions	Specific Questions
How do you spend a typical day?	Do you go to school? Do you work outside the home? Do you watch television, listen to the radio, or read the newspaper? How often do you talk to friends and family?
Have there been any recent changes in your life?	Have you experienced any changes, such as loss of a loved one, change of a job, a friend moving away, or new baby in the house? How are you adjusting to the change?
What are your living arrangements like?	With whom do you live? What is the size of your home? Do you cook and care for family members? Do you live in a neighborhood? How convenient is shopping? Do you have transportation?
What are your interests and habits?	What are your hobbies? Are you involved in sports? Do you smoke, and, if so, how much? Do you drink alcohol, and, if so, how much? Do you use any recreational drugs? How much sleep do you need; how much do you get? Do you like to go out? What types of food do you eat?

Also, review the patient's history including present illness, any chronic illnesses, past hospitalizations, accidents, and surgeries. A history of sensory deficits, such as visual or hearing impairments, places the patient at risk for sensory

BOX 36-2   Risk Factors for Sensory Perception Dysfunction in the Healthcare Environment

Sensory Overload
Lengthy verbal explanations before procedures
Room close to nurse's station
Intensive care unit or intermediate unit
Bright lights
Use of mechanical ventilator
Use of electrocardiographic monitor
Use of oxygen
Use of intravenous tubes
Other equipment
Roommate
Pain or discomfort
Decreased cognitive ability (e.g., head injury)
Frequent treatments

Sensory Deprivation
Private room
Eyes bandaged
Mobility restrictions such as bed rest and traction apparatus
Emotional disorders (e.g., depression)
Sensory aid not available (hearing aid, glasses)
Isolation precautions
Few visitors, especially if from a different culture

THERAPEUTIC DIALOGUE: SENSORY DYSFUNCTION

SCENE FOR THOUGHT

Charlie Brisco is 62 years old and in the intensive care unit (ICU) after a car accident. He sustained internal injuries and many lacerations on his face and arms. He has an IV, urinary catheter, heart monitor, and nasogastric (NG) tube. The pumps and monitors give off soft beeps. The ICU has been busy and noisy since Charlie was admitted.

LESS EFFECTIVE		MORE EFFECTIVE	
Nurse:	Hi, Charlie. How're you doing? *(Checks the IV and NG tube pumps.)*	**Nurse:**	Hi, Charlie. How're you doing? *(Checks the IV and NG tube pumps.)*
Charlie:	Who are you?! What are you doing with those machines?! *(Sits up in bed abruptly, wincing with pain, looking frightened.)*	**Charlie:**	Who are you?! What are you doing with those machines?! *(Sits up in bed abruptly, wincing with pain, looking frightened.)*
Nurse:	*(Turns to look at him, then continues to check the equipment.)* I'm Gigi, Charlie, your nurse.	**Nurse:**	*(Turns to look at him, stands still with arms at side and hands open.)* I'm Georgia. I'm your nurse.
Charlie:	Gigi? I don't know you! Where's my wife? What did you do with her? *(Looks frightened.)*	**Charlie:**	Georgia? I don't know you! Where's my wife? What did you do with her? *(Looks frightened.)*
Nurse:	She's right over there, Charlie, at the desk. See her? Sounds like you need a little sedative to calm you down. I'll go get it right now.	**Nurse:**	She's right there, Charlie. Do you see her standing at the desk?
Charlie:	Betty! Betty! Where are you?! *(Struggles to sit up in bed.)*	**Charlie:**	Oh. Yeah. *(Focuses on his wife. Slumps back on the pillows.)* Sorry. *(Starts to cry but tries to hide it.)* I get confused.
Nurse:	*(Gets sedative and calls for help to restrain Charlie so he won't dislodge his tubes.)*	**Nurse:**	I can see that.
		Charlie:	Yeah. *(Closes his eyes wearily.)* And I can't sleep too good.
		Nurse:	I know. I was wondering if you had a personal music player at home.
		Charlie:	Yeah. Why?
		Nurse:	Well, how about using it to shut out noise with some music. Not loud music, something mellow.
		Charlie:	Yeah, that would be good. *(Shifts and winces.)*
		Nurse:	You look uncomfortable.
		Charlie:	I am.
		Nurse:	I'll get you some more pain pills, and I'll talk to your wife about the music player, too. You can tell her what tapes to bring later.
		Charlie:	Okay. Thanks. *(Closes his eyes and lies still.)*

CRITICAL THINKING CHALLENGE

- Name and explain some factors that contributed to Charlie's sensory dysfunction.
- Decide whether this dysfunction was sensory overload or deprivation. Give your reasons.
- Describe the relationship between traumatic events and pain and sensory dysfunction.
- Appraise how each nurse related to Charlie, and summarize the outcomes.

deprivation. A history of illnesses such as diabetes, hypertension, stroke, or spinal cord injury also increases the patient's risk for sensory deficits.

The patient's experience with the healthcare environment determines the effect of stimulation on the patient. Needed treatments such as admission to an intensive care unit or isolation precautions increase the risk of sensory overload or deprivation. An evaluation of the patient's medication history, including CNS depressants such as opioid analgesics and sedatives, can reveal factors that affect sensory perception. Large doses of antibiotics may affect the patient's hearing.

PATIENT DECISION MAKING

Jane Nelson, 24 years old, was admitted to intensive care after a motor vehicle accident. She had multiple injuries to the chest and abdomen, leg fractures, and facial lacerations. She has improved sufficiently now to be transferred to a hospital unit. Her face is still bandaged, and the damage to her eyes is unknown at this time. Although she is expected to fully recover from her other injuries, a strong possibility exists that she may lose her sight in one or both eyes. She has said that if she is going to lose her vision, she doesn't want to know. You have heard her say, "I don't know what I might do to myself if I thought I was going to be blind the rest of my life." You have overheard the physicians say that Jane will, in all likelihood, be blind. One of the other nurses believes that Jane should know and start preparing for the possibility.

CRITICAL THINKING CHALLENGE

- Explore your own feelings about these interactions.
- Identify your personal values and beliefs in this situation.
- Think about ways in which you can respond to Jane about her situation.
- Think about ways in which you can respond to the other nurse about her beliefs.
- Identify possible approaches that might be needed in this situation.

Dysfunction Identification

During the nursing assessment, collect data about any actual sensory perception problems, determining whether the patient has difficulty with vision, hearing, smell, taste, and touch. If problems are identified, find out when the problem started, its severity, what actions the patient has taken, and the effectiveness of those actions. This information is useful in helping the patient adapt to his or her environment.

Also, determine whether the patient is anxious, depressed, withdrawing from social contact, or having difficulty concentrating, making decisions, or remembering. Has the patient ever experienced hallucinations or delusions? This information will uncover any manifestations the sensory dysfunction may have caused.

Physical Assessment

The focus of the physical assessment is to determine whether the senses are impaired. The following must be assessed: hearing, vision, taste, smell, touch, somatic senses, and mental status. Mental status data, including level of consciousness, orientation, attention span, memory, and cognitive skills, can

TABLE 36-2 PHYSICAL ASSESSMENT OF SENSORY FUNCTION

Sense	Technique for Assessment
Vision	Use Snellen chart to measure visual acuity (or have patient read newspaper, menu, or whatever is available). Test visual fields.
Hearing	Whisper numbers in each ear while occluding the other; ask the patient to repeat. Perform Weber and Rinne tuning fork tests. Observe the patient's conversation with others.
Smell	With eyes closed, have the patient identify three odors, such as coffee, tobacco, and cloves, one nostril at a time while occluding the other nostril.
Taste	With eyes closed, have the patient identify three tastes, such as lemon, salt, and sugar, waiting 1 min and giving sips of water in between. Have the patient close the eyes for all tests.
Somatic sensation	Test light touch of extremities with a wisp of cotton. Test sharp and dull sensation using the point and blunt end of a pin. Test two-point discrimination using two pins held close together. Test hot and cold sensation using test tubes filled with warm and cold water. Test vibration sense using a tuning fork over joints. Test position sense by moving the patient's fingers or toes. Test stereognosis by giving the patient a common object (quarter, paper clip) to identify by feel.

be collected during the patient history. See Chapter 17 for more information on assessment.

To collect objective data about the sensory system systematically, first inspect and then perform simple tests. Inspect the head for any abnormalities of the eyes, ears, nose, or mouth and the extremities for any burns or injuries. Table 36-2 lists tests used to assess sensation.

Diagnostic Tests and Procedures

Electrolyte imbalances, alterations in blood chemistry (e.g., elevated ammonia, elevated blood urea nitrogen), and toxic levels of drugs that affect the CNS can alter sensoristasis (Mistraletti et al., 2012). Special visual and auditory acuity tests also may be ordered. Neurologic tests, such as nerve conduction studies, computed tomographic scanning of the brain, and cerebral angiography, may be performed to determine the cause of sensory deficits.

NURSING DIAGNOSES

The accepted NANDA-International (NANDA-I, 2014) for Domain 5 Perception/Cognition related to the human information processing system includes attention, orientation, sensation, perception, cognition, and communication. The selected nursing diagnosis is Unilateral Neglect, which is

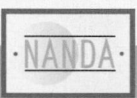

Table 36-3 SELECTED NANDA-I NURSING DIAGNOSES INVOLVING SENSORY PERCEPTION/COGNITION

Nursing Dx	Related Factors	Dx Statement	NOC*	NIC†
Unilateral Neglect— impairment in sensory and motor response, mental representation, and spatial attention of the body, and the corresponding environment, characterized by inattention to one side and overattention to the opposite side. Left-side neglect is more severe and persistent than is right-side neglect.	Altered sensory integration, reception, and transmission, unaware of positioning of the neglected limb, failure of hygiene tasks on affected side, and impaired mobility performance	**Unilateral Neglect** R/T altered decrease in sensory awareness of one side of the body manifested by neglected hygiene on that side, balance problems, and misinterpretation of sensory stimuli	Adaptation to physical disability; heedfulness of affected side; Cognitive Orientation to affected side; Improved Balance and Fall Prevention Behavior. Self-Care: Activities of Daily Living	Monitor for abnormal responses to three primary types of stimuli: sensory, visual, and auditory; ensure that affected extremities are properly and safely positioned; encourage patient to touch and use affected body part; assist patient to bathe and groom affected side first; focus tactile and verbal stimuli on affected side; and assist patient in ambulating and preventing falls.

Dx, diagnosis; R/T, related to.

*From: Moorhead, S., Johnson, M., Maas, M., & Swanson, E. (2013). *Iowa Outcomes Project: Nursing Outcomes Classification (NOC)* (5th ed.). St. Louis, MO: C. V. Mosby.

†From: Bulecheck, G., Butcher, H., Dochterman, J., & Wagner, C. (2013). *Iowa Intervention Project: Nursing Interventions Classification (NIC)* (6th ed.). St. Louis, MO: C. V. Mosby.

From: NANDA Association International (NANDA-I. 2014) *Nursing diagnoses: Definitions and classification, 2015–2017*. West Sussex, UK: Wiley-Blackwell.

impairment in sensory and motor response, mental representation, and spatial attention of the body, and the corresponding environment, characterized by inattention to one side and overattention to the opposite side. Left-side neglect is more severe and persistent than right-side neglect.

This selected nursing diagnosis is presented in Table 36-3 along with selected Nursing Outcomes Classification (NOC) and Nursing Interventions Classification (NIC).

OUTCOME IDENTIFICATION AND PLANNING

Patient goals are individualized but focus on achieving optimal sensory function. The patient goals for Disturbed Sensory Perception may include the following:

- The patient will remain safe.
- The patient will demonstrate an understanding of contributing factors to disturbed sensory perceptions by reducing or eliminating them.
- The patient will maintain the functioning of existing senses.
- The patient will develop an effective communication mechanism.
- The patient will demonstrate an understanding of interventions and rationales by using this information as foresight in maintaining sensoristasis.
- The patient will achieve sensoristasis through a decrease in the symptoms of sensory overload or deprivation.
- The patient will demonstrate achievement or maintenance of self-care.

Planning centers on the patient's ability to function on a perceptual level. Patient teaching, procedure preparation, provision of stimulation or stimulation reduction, and safety are major issues. Examples of nursing interventions commonly used in problems with sensory overload and deprivations are listed in Table 36-3 and discussed in the following section.

IMPLEMENTATION

Health Promotion

PATIENT TEACHING

Patient teaching to promote sensory health and function focuses on ways to prevent sensory loss and to maintain general health. Teaching topics include the importance of frequent eye examinations and close control of chronic illnesses such as diabetes.

Teaching healthcare consumers the importance of sensory function and the roles of sensory receptors and the CNS in receiving and perceiving stimuli is important. Preventing sensory dysfunction enables patients to interact with the environment optimally. Yearly eye examinations (or more frequently if problems arise) help promote optimal visual function. Other measures to prevent visual dysfunction include avoiding eye strain, infection, and injury. Prompt recognition and treatment for ear infections and childhood immunization against illnesses such as rubella may prevent hearing loss.

People should wear protective eyewear whenever there is a risk of injury or contamination to the eyes. Plain glasses without side shields are not effective protection. Protective ear-wear is essential to avoiding hearing loss, particularly related to occupational noises.

Teach older adults who are at risk for sensory loss due to physiologic changes of aging about the need for routine checkups. Education regarding the prevention of falls related to sensory deficits is imperative. Encourage these patients to seek attention for any developing problems. They may delay medical attention, fearing that hearing loss is inevitable, when simple ear irrigation might dislodge impacted cerumen and restore hearing. Instruct patients with chronic illnesses such as diabetes or hypertension about the importance of closely controlling blood sugar and blood pressure, respectively. Control can help prevent pathophysiologic changes that might lead to tactile and visual dysfunction. Self-monitoring of blood sugar or blood pressure, compliance with medications, diet control, and medical follow-up are essential.

PROCEDURE PREPARATION

A primary nursing concern is to prevent symptoms of sensory overload for patients. Risk for sensory overload greatly increases when unfamiliar procedures are taking place. Overstimulation can be prevented by preparing patients before procedures, using a technique called **sensation (sensory) information**. The purpose of this intervention is to alleviate a patient's distress responses to threatening stimuli and to improve the patient's coping through stimulation of the cognitive processes. The technique involves objectively and specifically describing to the patient, in serial order, what he or she typically will see, hear, smell, taste, or feel (tactile) in a particular situation (rare or atypical events are not to be included). This preparation must be from the patient's point of view, not from that of the observer.

A solid understanding of this technique is necessary before it can be used. In general, sensation information is useful when a patient feels threatened by a procedure. The patient, not the nurse, must make that appraisal. Patients who indicate a high level of anxiety before a procedure seem to benefit from sensation information more than those with low levels of anxiety. Finally, determine what patient outcomes are desired. Sensation information does not help patients achieve new coping skills, but it may enhance their current coping mechanisms.

Other interventions to help prevent sensory overload include educating patients about why a procedure will be done, who will do it, and how long it will take. Helping patients gain a sense of control through interventions, such as establishing a schedule for routine care, providing a calendar and clock, and allowing choices whenever possible, also can reduce the risk of sensory overload.

NURSE–PATIENT INTERACTION

Individualized nurse–patient interaction promotes sensory health function. Patients at risk for sensory deprivation may need frequent interaction initiated by the nurse, whereas others may not. In any case, provide appropriate stimuli, such as

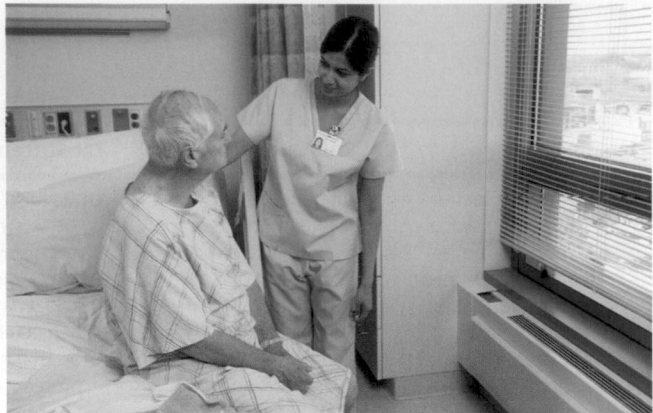

FIGURE 36-5 The simple act of touching a patient, talking, or listening may provide sensory stimulation.

addressing the patient by name, introducing and reintroducing yourself as necessary, explaining all activities, and when leaving, acknowledging when you will return. Length, frequency, and content of interactions should be based on individual needs. Talking to the patient, showing the patient equipment or articles used in care, encouraging the patient to smell and taste food that is served, and touching the patient are appropriate stimuli during interactions (Fig. 36-5).

> ### ! SAFETY ALERT
> When assisting a visually impaired patient with ambulation, stand on the patient's nondominant side, about 1 foot in front of him or her. Have the patient grasp your arm with the nondominant hand and use the dominant hand to feel around for barriers or landmarks. Always maintain an uncluttered environment.

Nursing Interventions for Altered Sensory Perception Function

STIMULATION PROVISION

Providing meaningful external stimuli can help a patient overcome sensory deprivation or sensory deficit. Measures to provide stimulation include playing the television or the radio occasionally, playing music for brief periods, encouraging use of a clock and calendar, encouraging the patient to dress for the day's activities, putting up colorful pictures, encouraging visitors, encouraging family to bring in personal items such as photographs, opening the drapes, and turning on lights. Place the bed or chair so the patient can see or hear activities in the area and when someone enters the room. Diets that include various flavors and textures can stimulate the taste buds.

Frequent interaction with the patient also may help. Discussing scheduling of care and placement of equipment, encouraging self-care activities, providing tactile stimulation through backrubs, combing and brushing the patient's hair

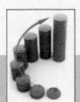

OUTCOME-BASED TEACHING PLANS

When Nicole Travis, mother of an 11-month-old child named Jessie, comes to the clinic for a routine well-child visit, you learn that Jessie is not paying attention when spoken to. Her mother reports that Jessie frequently ignores her when she tries to get her attention. Nicole states, "I'm not sure what kind of discipline or punishment I should use."

OUTCOME

Nicole Travis will verbalize a realistic plan to determine whether Jessie is ignoring her on purpose or is truly not hearing her.

STRATEGIES

- Discuss with Nicole the common methods of determining adequate hearing in an infant.
- Suggest a referral to an audiologist.
- Have Nicole observe Jessie's response to sounds that are out of her vision.

- Instruct Nicole to record Jessie's reactions to sounds and her facial expressions.
- Encourage Nicole to record and describe the verbal sounds and words that Jessie says, including listening for inflections in Jessie's voice.
- Urge Nicole to bring these observations to the next appointment and to the audiologist for a more detailed discussion.
- Encourage Nicole to avoid discipline about not responding until Jessie's hearing is thoroughly evaluated.

EVALUATION

- 3/29/17: 13:00—Nicole Travis is able to identify resources to evaluate Jessie's hearing levels.
- Nicole Travis has utilized strategies appropriately to determine if Jessie has a hearing deficit.

—J. Woodman, RN

(or encouraging the patient to do so), reading to the patient, speaking slowly and clearly, and identifying yourself verbally and with a name tag are meaningful interactions. Encouraging the use of crossword puzzles or games stimulates mental functioning. Reorienting the patient frequently to person, place, and time may be necessary. Because the patient may be having difficulties concentrating, he or she may need repeated direction to accomplish even simple tasks.

Orienting the patient to the environment can help avoid misinterpretations. Visiting the patient often and letting him or her know when to expect another visit helps the patient overcome a feeling of isolation. Providing a calendar and a clock to assist in keeping track of time helps keep the patient in touch with activities in the environment. A roommate for a patient experiencing sensory deprivation can help a great deal. Preparation for any procedure that may add to the sensory deprivation, such as being restricted to bed rest postprocedure, gives time to develop an intervention plan to prevent problems.

Also, encourage patients to provide self-stimulation, such as singing, reading, and talking into a tape recorder and playing it back. Self-care activities also are forms of self-stimulation. Provide various different types of stimulation to encourage maximum use of the patient's available senses. Doing so also helps the person adapt to any changes.

A patient can use up restless energy and prevent symptoms of sensory deprivation by using physical movement. Encourage the patient to move around in the bed or walk around the room, sit in a chair, do ADLs as independently as possible, and do exercises in the room or in bed to provide stimulation to the patient's senses.

SAFETY ALERT

Add stimulation slowly so that patients are not overwhelmed. Include various stimuli, and keep the amount of sensory input at a moderate level.

STIMULATION REDUCTION

If the patient is experiencing sensory overload, interventions should focus on reducing stimulation involving information, the environment, and internal factors. Limiting extraneous noise, lights, room clutter, interruptions, pain, and stress reduces stimulation.

Patients with sensory overload may neglect their ADLs to the point that they need assistance. Such assistance can be problematic because it can add to sensory overload. With this in mind, assist the patient only with the immediately essential ADLs (moving, eating, toileting, and resting). Additional tasks may be added as the patient is able to cope. If the overload leads to unilateral neglect of one side of the body, the patient stops responding to the affected side, which can lead to problems with self-care, balance, and sensory awareness of the side that needs the most rehabilitation attention.

BOX 36-3   Sensory Aids

Vision
- Eyeglasses with the proper prescription, clean, and in good repair
- Adequate room lighting, drapes open
- Sunglasses or window shades to reduce glare
- Literature with large print
- Uncluttered environment, no furniture rearranging
- Clock with large numbers
- Telephone dial with large numbers
- Magnifying glass
- Bright, contrasting colors in environment
- Color-coded dials on appliances, medication bottles, and so forth
- Braille, recorded books, seeing-eye dog, and so forth, as necessary

Hearing
- Hearing aid in good repair with working battery
- Speaking slowly and distinctly in patient's full view, no mouth covering or gum chewing
- Avoidance of background noise
- Amplified phone ringer, doorbell, smoke alarm, and so forth
- Headset for telephone communication
- Closed-caption television

Smell
- Fresh food served for meals
- Fresh flowers or fragrance in the room
- Others wearing light perfume or fragrance
- Notice of environmental smells

Taste
- Fresh food, seasoned appropriately, not overcooked or overprocessed (to preserve texture)
- Foods served at appropriate temperature and time of day
- Note smell and taste of food
- Sips of water between foods
- No mixing of foods

Touch
- Therapeutic touch
- Massage (self or nurse)
- Turning and repositioning
- Hairbrushing and grooming (self or nurse)
- Activity around environment
- Amount of pressure individualized to patient's comfort level
- Clothing of various textures

SENSORY AIDS

If a patient is experiencing a sensory deficit, sensory aids help promote optimal function of that sense and other available senses (e.g., hearing aids in good working order, use of cochlear implant devices, clean eyeglasses, good oral hygiene). In addition to providing actual physical and situational sensory aids, enlist significant others whenever possible to assist the patient in dealing with the deficit. Suggestions for sensory aids are listed in Box 36-3.

Sensory aids can be used in the healthcare environment and taught to patients for use at home. When one sense is lost, sensory aids can be used for other senses to enhance general stimulation. For example, a blind patient should be encouraged to savor the aroma, taste, and texture of food.

At times, the nurse may be called upon to assist patients with sensory aids such as contact lenses and hearing aids. See **Procedures 36-1** and **36-2**.

SAFETY

Implementation of safety precautions is essential for patients with sensory perception dysfunction. Sensory deficits and the cognitive effects of sensory deprivation or sensory overload place the patient at risk for injury from the environment. Implement actions such as assisting patients with ambulation; use of bed side rails, night-lights, and a call system; and frequent or continuous observation as necessary.

Teach patients with sensory deficits how to ensure safety at home. For example, advise patients with decreased sensation to temperature in the extremities to adjust their hot water heater to a lower temperature and to test water temperature with a thermometer before bathing. If the patient is unable to check the temperature, encourage a family member to help. Also, instruct patients to inspect their legs and feet for any injuries or pressure sores that they cannot feel.

Teach patients with a decreased sense of smell about the dangers of using gas and chemicals. For example, cleaning with ammonia in a confined space such as a bathroom may cause the patient to be overcome by fumes before he or she can smell them. A patient may not smell a gas leak in the home, so if a stove or gas heater is not working properly, it should be reported promptly. Urge the patient to inspect food for freshness, looking for color and texture and checking the expiration date as the patient may not smell spoiled meat or dairy products. Patients with hearing and visual deficits need to take additional safety precautions as well. See Chapter 23 for more information on safety.

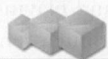 **Concept Mastery Alert**

When assisting a visually impaired patient with ambulation, the patient should be encouraged to hold on to the nurse's arm rather than the nurse grasping the patient's arm. This allows the patient more control during ambulation, better preventing falls.

Home and Community Care

With rising costs and shorter hospital stays, a patient may be discharged while still adjusting to his or her condition. This can be a new or worsening sensory deficit or an illness or treatment that causes sensory deprivation or sensory overload. Initiate planning as soon as possible to help the patient adjust to sensory dysfunction. Include patient teaching, enlisting the help and cooperation of family and friends, assembling sensory aids and equipment, contacting home health services, and locating additional support groups as needed.

Assess the patient's home environment as necessary to determine what will be needed to help the patient adapt to his or her sensory dysfunction. Teach the patient and family how to interact in the home environment, using other senses and sensory aids to adapt and remain safe. The patient may need much help during the adaptation process, but eventually he or she may become independent. At first, the patient may need help with basic care and hygiene; ongoing nursing assessment will determine the need for further interventions.

Because family roles can be changed suddenly (e.g., if the breadwinner becomes the care receiver), family members may need as much help and support as the patient for their own issues and concerns. Enlist the aid of social services to help with financial problems related to the patient's sensory dysfunction. Occupational therapy may be appropriate for helping the patient with assistive devices and modifications in the home. Nurses are in a unique position to assess the patient's needs before discharge and to organize services that can continue the patient's care after discharge.

EVALUATION

Evaluation of the care of a patient with sensory/perceptual dysfunction is based on the answers to the following questions developed from the patient goals:

 APPLY YOUR CRITICAL THINKING

Stan Myer, 76 years old, lives in an assisted living facility and occasionally has some confusion. He has been telling you that his new glasses are worthless. The glasses seemed to work at first, but now, he says he sees something wavy or distorted in the center of his vision. He keeps asking you to clean the glasses and get rid of whatever is making it difficult for him to see. You have cleaned his glasses several times and they look clear to you, yet you have noticed that Mr. Myer no longer reads the paper and his signature has changed.

What assessment data do you need to collect at this point? Discuss how you will help to clarify Mr. Myer's sensory perception.

Check your answers in Appendix B.

- Was safety maintained?
- Was sensoristasis achieved?
- Were contributing factors to sensory dysfunction reduced or eliminated?
- Can the patient describe the interventions and rationale so that this information can be used in the future to deal with sensory dysfunction?
- Was self-care maintained?

Examples of positive outcome criteria for a patient at risk for sensory overload are described below.

Goal

The patient will remain safe.

POSSIBLE OUTCOME CRITERIA

The patient:

- Accurately and consistently uses safety devices such as side rails, night-lights, and a call system
- Reports absence of injuries

Goal

The patient will maintain the functioning of existing senses.

POSSIBLE OUTCOME CRITERIA

The patient:

- Receives appropriate sensory input
- Will control chronic diseases to protect sensory function
- Will receive regular eye and hearing examinations

Goal

The patient will develop an effective communication mechanism.

POSSIBLE OUTCOME CRITERIA

The patient:

- Will maintain eyewear and hearing aid in working order
- Will use paper, pencil, or computer communication when necessary
- Will use large-button phone, large-print text, or speaker phones as needed
- Will maintain social interactions

Goal

The patient will demonstrate an understanding of contributing factors to disturbed sensory perceptions by reducing or eliminating them.

POSSIBLE OUTCOME CRITERIA

The patient:

- Uses earplugs and eyeshades during sleep for the next three nights
- Limits television and radio use to 1 to 3 hours per 8-hour period for next 48 hours
- Asks appropriate questions about care before and during treatment during next 24 hours

Goal

The patient will demonstrate an understanding of interventions and rationales by using this information as foresight.

POSSIBLE OUTCOME CRITERIA

The patient:

- During next 24 hours, describes procedures to the nurse before they are done, including what he or she might see, hear, feel, smell, or taste
- Gives the rationale for a procedure and asks questions

Goal

The patient will achieve sensoristasis through a decrease in the symptoms of sensory overload or deprivation.

POSSIBLE OUTCOME CRITERIA

The patient:

- Demonstrates the ability to concentrate by listening to an explanation of medications, asking appropriate questions, and repeating the medication schedule every time medication is given during next 24 hours
- Sleeps 5 to 7 hours each night without awakening every night
- Is oriented to person, place, and time during visiting hours for the remainder of the day as reported by the nurse
- Listens to a relaxation tape with earphones when housekeeping personnel are cleaning the patient's room

Goal

The patient will maintain self-care.

POSSIBLE OUTCOME CRITERIA

The patient:

- Bathes and performs adequate oral care daily
- Performs toileting independently and safely
- Ambulates in the hall three times a day
- Feeds himself or herself food and liquid for next three meals

---

COLLABORATING WITH THE HEALTHCARE TEAM
Calling the Physician Concerning a Patient's Change in Mental Status

Mr. Knaack, age 77 years, has had cognitive changes over the 3 hours that you have been caring for him. He has gone from being oriented to time, place, and person to confusion about where he is or why he is here.

SITUATION: Mr. Knaack has demonstrated cognitive changes over a short period of time. His speech is slightly slurred, he is lethargic, and he has some left-sided weakness. His blood pressure is 155/96 and pulse is 82.

BACKGROUND: Mr. Knaack, age 77 years, was admitted last night following a home repair accident in which he fell from a ladder. He was admitted for observation with a moderate headache and numerous bruises.

ASSESSMENT: The family is staying with the patient, but they are concerned about his changing mentation and stability. I am also concerned that his change in mental status might indicate increasing intracranial pressure, possibly a subdural hematoma or possibly a stroke.

RECOMMENDATION: Could you come and evaluate Mr. Knaack within the next hour and provide orders for how to proceed?

CRITICAL THINKING CHALLENGE

- Consider advantages and disadvantages of providing this information to the physician over the phone or via a text message.
- Discuss the rationale for requesting that the physician come and evaluate Mr. Knaack rather than just providing orders over the phone.
- Are there other data you could collect to support your assessment that Mr. Knaack may have increased intracranial pressure or a stroke?
- What could you do if the physician does not agree to see the patient and you are still worried about his declining neurologic status?
- Is there any time when a change in mental status would not require contacting the physician?

PATIENT PLAN OF CARE
The Patient with Disturbed Sensory Perception

NURSING DIAGNOSIS

Disturbed Visual Sensory/Perception related to temporary decrease in visual sensory input manifested by fear of body image alteration, irritability, withdrawal, and misinterpretation of sensory stimuli

PATIENT GOAL

Patient will demonstrate an understanding of the sensory deprivation experience.

PATIENT OUTCOME CRITERIA

- Within 8 hours, patient accurately describes this eye injury and expected medical outcome (i.e., full visual recovery).
- During hospitalization, patient freely discusses problems with the staff, asking appropriate questions.
- Before discharge, patient describes his or her behavioral changes and relates them to temporary deficit. Before discharge, patient explains his or her behavioral changes to the family.

NURSING INTERVENTION	SCIENTIFIC RATIONALE
1. Introduce self from doorway before entering room and explain reason for being there.	*1.* Avoid startling the patient and prevent misperceptions.
2. Post schedule for day on wall for all staff, visitors, and family to follow. Review schedule with patient for input.	*2.* A schedule assists others to know and to inform the patient about what is going to happen, reducing anxiety.
3. As rapport and trust build, invite the patient to share his or her concerns about recovery; answer questions and correct misconceptions.	*3.* By focusing on concerns, the nurse can help the patient separate fears from reality.
4. Encourage patient to identify his or her frustrations and feelings related to being temporarily "blind" and to ask questions about his or her environment.	*4.* Expression of feelings helps to allay anxiety while also providing reassurance and various sensory stimulation.
5. Hold a conference with the patient's family to promote mutual discussion of the experience. Encourage patient to teach the family what he or she understands about sensory deprivation.	*5.* Mutual discussion and sharing provide outlets for the patient and family, aid in understanding of sensory deprivation, and provide opportunities for additional teaching related to the family's concerns about home management.

PATIENT GOAL

Patient will demonstrate achievement of sensoristasis through a decrease in the symptoms of sensory deprivation.

PATIENT OUTCOME CRITERIA

- Before discharge, patient uses various sensory pathways to increase sensory variation.
- Before discharge, patient reports no difficulty related to misperceiving sensory stimuli.
- During hospitalization, patient visits with family and friends for a minimum of 15 minutes per visit.

NURSING INTERVENTION	SCIENTIFIC RATIONALE
1. Schedule 5-minute conversations every hour on the hour while patient is awake for the first 24 hours.	*1.* Regular conversations provide gradual cognitive and sensory stimulation at a time the patient can count on, so he or she is not overwhelmed.
2. Orient patient to any noises that can be misinterpreted (e.g., air-conditioner thermostat on the wall, chimes indicating a fire drill, sound of the food cart being wheeled in at mealtimes).	*2.* Awareness of specific sounds helps the patient stay focused in reality.

(Continued)

PATIENT PLAN OF CARE (Continued)
The Patient with Disturbed Sensory Perception

NURSING INTERVENTION	SCIENTIFIC RATIONALE
3. After the first 24 hours, on day and evening shifts, provide a minimum of two and maximum of four staff per shift, other than assigned caretakers, to talk with the patient for a minimum of 10 minutes. Post a schedule in front of the patient's chart to sign up for these social visits.	**3.** Help build trust, reduce anxiety, and provide cognitive stimulation and sensory variation.
4. Teach the patient the importance of gradually increasing input from other sensory pathways when vision is temporarily unavailable; include teaching about self-stimulation, such as counting, singing, and using a tape recorder to talk into; isometric exercises; tactile stimulation; auditory variation; and gustatory and olfactory stimulation.	**4.** The patient needs information about management of sensory deficit, how to increase stimulation gradually, and prevention of further sensory deprivation or overload.

EVALUATION

5/11/17: 09:30—Patient demonstrates the use of multiple sensory pathways to increase stimulation, both in the hospital and at home.
- Prior to discharge, patient correctly interprets sensory stimuli.
- Documentation of 15-minute or longer visitation sessions with family and friends present while patient is oriented to accurate interpretation of sensory stimuli.

—A. Ferran, RN

KEY CONCEPTS

- The senses are vision, hearing, taste, smell, and touch. Senses related to touch are the somatic senses of kinesthesia, or position sense, and visceral, or deep sensation.
- The RAS controls arousal and awareness to stimuli.
- Sensoristasis refers to a person's optimum state of arousal through stimulation. When stimulation is constant, adaptation occurs.
- Sensory perception generally decreases as a person approaches 60 to 70 years of age.
- Sensory overload occurs when a person is unable to process the intensity or quantity of incoming stimuli. Sensory deprivation is a lack of meaningful stimuli.
- Sensory deficits, impaired function in sensory reception or perception that occurs gradually, may bring about behavior changes and sharpening of other senses to help the person adapt.
- Anxiety, cognitive dysfunction, depression, hallucinations, and delusions are manifestations of sensory perception dysfunction.
- Nursing assessment of sensory perception function includes subjective information about the patient and his or her usual environment and physical examination for vision, hearing, taste, smell, and the somatic senses of touch, pressure, position, vibration, pain, and temperature.
- Goals for the patient with altered sensory perception function include achieving sensoristasis, reducing contributing factors, describing intervention and rationales, achieving self-care, and maintaining safety.
- Patient teaching about the importance of regular eye examinations and prompt treatment for ear infections may help promote sensory function. Preparing patients for procedures and their associated sensory experiences is another crucial nursing intervention.
- Nurses must provide appropriate stimulation for patients with sensory deprivation while reducing excess stimulation for those with sensory overload.
- Sensory aids may be physical (e.g., glasses, hearing aids, large-print books, sound amplifiers) or situational (e.g., speaking directly in front of a hearing-impaired patient, encouraging a patient to smell and taste food).
- Safety precautions, crucial for patients with altered sensory perception function, include assisting with ambulation and care; encouraging use of side rails, night-lights, and call systems; and frequently observing the patient.

PRACTICING FOR THE NCLEX

CHECK YOUR ANSWERS IN APPENDIX A.

1. A patient with a history of cerebrovascular accident with residual left hemiparesis and dysphagia is hospitalized for malnutrition. Which of the following could contribute to his altered sensory perception? Select all that apply:
   a. Overstimulation caused by IV pump and bed alarms
   b. Nutrition imbalance caused by poor oral intake at home
   c. Loss of peripheral vision on the left
   d. Loss of self-esteem related to chronic health condition

2. An elderly patient is experiencing signs of sensory perception dysfunction related to the hospital environment. What nursing interventions could reduce her risk factors?
   a. Lengthy verbal explanations of procedures
   b. Controlling the patient's pain
   c. Use of bright lights to minimize visual problems
   d. Placing the patient in a shared room for companionship

3. A patient is identified as having Disturbed Sensory Perception. Nursing goals for this patient include the ability to do which of the following? Select all that apply:
   a. Demonstrate understanding of contributing factors
   b. Remain free from falls during the hospitalization
   c. Minimize sensoristasis by altering the level of sensory intake
   d. Demonstrate need for assistance in ADLs

4. A patient is admitted to your skilled nursing facility with moderate confusion following a hospitalization. Which of the following should be done first?
   a. Clean patient's glasses and confirm that they are hers.
   b. Assess current pain level.
   c. Secure a bed alarm to prevent falls.
   d. Administer Haldol 0.5 mg IV to decrease agitation.

5. You are assigned a patient who is impulsive and unsteady on her feet. Which of the following would be appropriate to delegate to the nursing assistant that you are working with?
   a. Encourage the patient to ambulate.
   b. Provide bedside commode to maximize independence.
   c. Turn out all lights to decrease sensory stimulation.
   d. Assist with bathing and oral hygiene.
   e. It is not appropriate to delegate care of this patient to a nursing assistant.

REFERENCES

Bell, L. (2011). *Delirium Assessment and Management Practice Alert (with AACN Levels of Evidence and Complete Reference List)* [PDF: 11/2011] Retrieved February 1, 2015 at http://www.aacn.org/WD/practice/docs/practicealerts/delirium-practice-alert-2011.pdf

Gesell, A., & Ilg, F. (1949). Child development. New York, NY: Harper Brothers.

Gordon, M. (1994). Nursing diagnosis: Process and application (3rd ed.). St. Louis, MO: C. V. Mosby.

Hasson, H., Brown, C., & Hasson, D. (2010). Factors associated with high use of a workplace web-based stress management program in a randomized controlled intervention study. *Health Education Research, 25*(4), 596–607.

Ignatavicius, D. D., & Workman, M. L. (2013). Medical-surgical nursing: Patient-centered collaborative care. St. Louis, MO: Saunders.

Lewis, S. L., Dirksen, S. R., Heitkemper, M. M., Bucher, L., & Camera, I. M. (2013). Medical-surgical nursing: Assessment and management of clinical problems. St. Louis, MO: Mosby.

Mistraletti, G., Pelosi, P., Mantovani, E. S., Berardino, M., & Gregoretti, C. (2012). Delirium: Clinical approach and prevention. *Best Practice and Research in Clinical Anaesthesiology, 26*(3), 311–326. doi: 10.1016/j.bpa.2012.07.001

National Eye Institute. (February 1, 2013). New NIH resources help growing number of Americans with vision loss. National Institutes of Health. Retrieved January 29, 2015 from https://www.nei.nih.gov/news/pressreleases/020113

North American Nursing Diagnosis Association International (NANDA-I). (2014). *Nursing Diagnoses: Definitions and Classification, 2015–2017.* West Sussex, UK: Wiley-Blackwell.

Porth, C. M. (2011). Essentials of pathophysiology: Concepts of altered health states. Philadelphia, PA: Lippincott Williams & Wilkins.

Solberg, L.M., Plummer, C.E., May, K.N., & Mion, L.C. (2013). A quality improvement program to increase nurses' detection of delirium on an acute medical unit. *Geriatric Nursing, 34,* 75–79.

Van den Boogaard, M., Schoonhoven, L., vander Hoeven, J. G., van Achterberg, T., & Pickkers, P. (2012). Incidence and short-term consequences of delirium in critically ill patients: A prospective observational cohort study. *International Journal of Nursing Studies, 49,* 775–783.

Procedure 36-1 Removing Contact Lenses

Purpose   1. Remove contact lenses in the event that the patient is unable to do so.

Equipment   Wetting/cleaning and soaking solution for hard contact lenses
                     Sterile lens disinfecting and/or enzyme solution for soft contact lenses
                     Contact lens storage container
                     Lens suction cup
                     Clean disposable gloves

Assessment   • Review the physician's order to determine the need for contact lens removal.
                     • Assess the patient's medical history to determine risk for complications from contact lens removal.
                     • Assess the eye area for open lesions or ecchymosis.
                     • Assess the patient's understanding of the purpose of the procedure and his or her physical and
                       emotional ability to learn and perform the procedure independently, if possible.

Procedure

1. **Perform hand hygiene and identify the patient.**
   Rationale: Reduces microbe transmission and ensures safety.

2. **Close door or bed curtains and explain the procedure to the patient, if possible.**
   Rationale: Ensures patient privacy, increases patient compliance, reduces patient anxiety, and promotes learning.

Removing Hard Contact Lenses

3. **Position patient comfortably in a sitting position, if possible.**

4. **Pull the patient's upper and lower lid apart and pull tautly toward the lateral side.**

5. **Ask the patient to blink, and the lens should pop out into your hand.**

6. **An alternative method for removing hard contact lenses is the use of a lens suction cup. This is particularly useful for a patient who cannot consciously assist with the removal.**

Removing Soft Contact Lenses

3. **Position the patient comfortably in a sitting position, if possible.**

4. **Ask the patient to look upward. Pull down on the lower lid and place your index finger on the lower edge of the lens, moving it onto the white part of the eye (Fig. 1).**

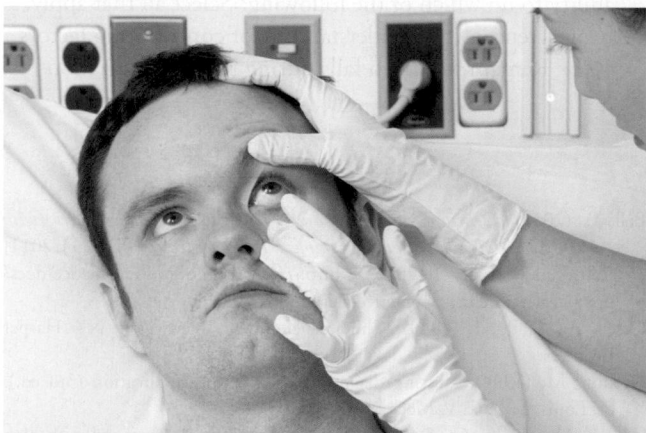

FIG. 1 As the patient looks upward, pull down on the lower lid.

5. **Gently grasp lens between your thumb and index finger to release the suction of the lens. The lens will fold over and can easily be removed. Gently roll the lens, using normal saline as needed, to separate it and return it to its normal form.**

Procedure 36-1   *continued*

Storing Lenses

3. Rinse lenses thoroughly with recommended rinsing solution (Fig. 2).

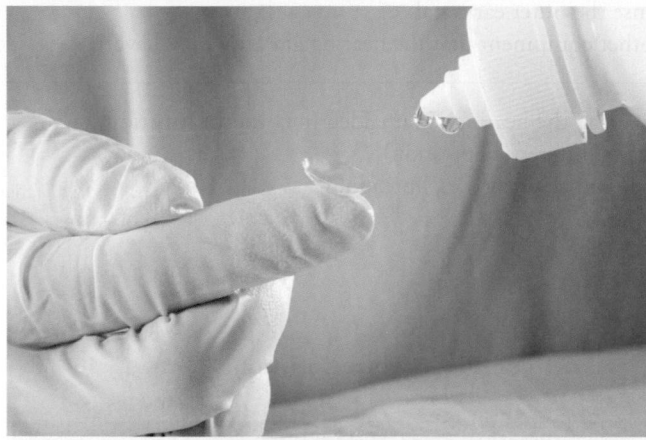

FIG. 2 Rinse lens thoroughly.

4. Identify the left and right cups marked on the storage case.
5. Place the first lens in its designated cup in the storage case before removing the second lens (Fig. 3).

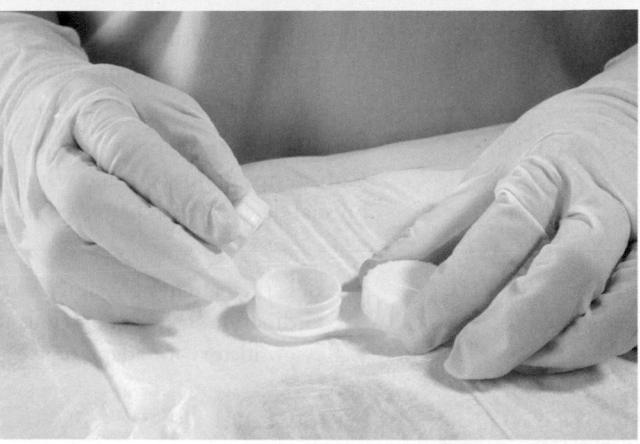

FIG. 3 Store lens in designated cup.

Rationale: Lenses might be different prescriptions for each eye. Placing them in the proper cup avoids mixing them up.

Documentation

4/15/17; 15:00—Patient responsive to teaching about correct insertion and removal of contact lenses. Demonstrated proper hygiene in care of eyes and in care of lenses within the lens case.

—M. Klim, RN

Life Span Considerations

Infant and Child

For babies or small children who may be required to wear contact lenses, more assistance is needed for both insertion and removal of the lenses. Closer observation of the child is necessary to be sure that the lenses are staying in place, because the child may not be able to tell you.

Older Child and Adolescent

Older children and adolescents need to be reminded to follow all cleanliness precautions and not to share their lenses with each other because they are uniquely fitted for the individual.

Older Adult

Depending on their cognitive and physical capabilities, older adults can generally handle contact lenses with no problem. If they need assistance, the preceding procedure can be used.

Home Care Modifications

The primary concern in managing contact lenses at home is the attention to cleanliness, not wearing contacts longer than recommended, and safe cleaning and storage.

Collaboration and Delegation

With small children and babies, special teaching may be done to assist parents in managing contact lenses for children. Referral to an eye care specialist can assist parents in deciding if it is appropriate for young children to have contacts and any special care needed.

Procedure 36-2 Assisting an Adult with Inserting a Hearing Aid

Purpose

1. Maintain hearing status.
2. Provide assistance with insertion.

Equipment

Personal hygiene supplies for cleaning the ear mold as recommended by the manufacturer
Cotton tips, mild soap, and water to cleanse the outer ear canal
Special devices (fresh battery, if needed; other equipment that the hearing aid style may have)

Assessment

- Assess the patient's physical ability to manage the hearing aid unaided (i.e., motor function, coordination, level of consciousness, vision, interest, depression).
- Review history for adaptations to hearing impairment (i.e., lipreading).

Procedure

1. **Perform hand hygiene and identify the patient.**
   Rationale: Reduces microbe transmission and ensures safety.

2. **Close door or bed curtains and explain the procedure to the patient, if possible.**
   Rationale: Ensures patient privacy and increases patient compliance.

3. **Check to be sure the battery is functional. Hold hearing aid in your hand and turn up the volume until you hear a "feedback" whistle. The feedback results from sound leaking around and back into the microphone and being amplified.**

4. **Inspect the hearing aid to be sure that tubing and ear mold are intact and not cracked or broken (Fig. 1). The opening in the ear mold should be free from cerumen.**

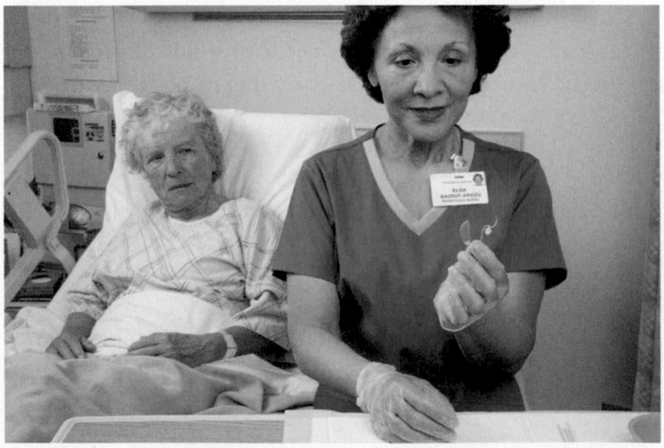

5. **Clean the hearing aid according to manufacturer's guidelines (Fig. 2). Place in storage unit.**

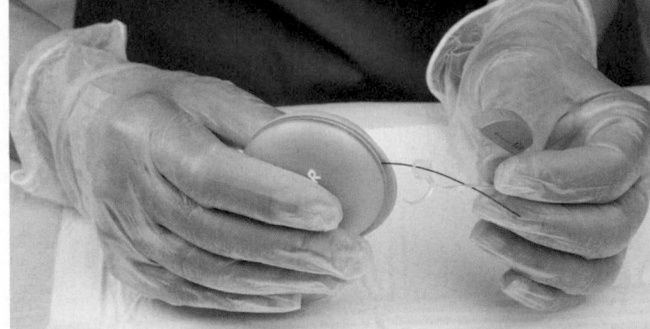

FIG. 2 Clean the sound tube as directed.

6. **Assess the patient's ear for redness, irritation, drainage, and excessive cerumen. Moisten swab and clean the ear as necessary (Figs. 3 and 4).**

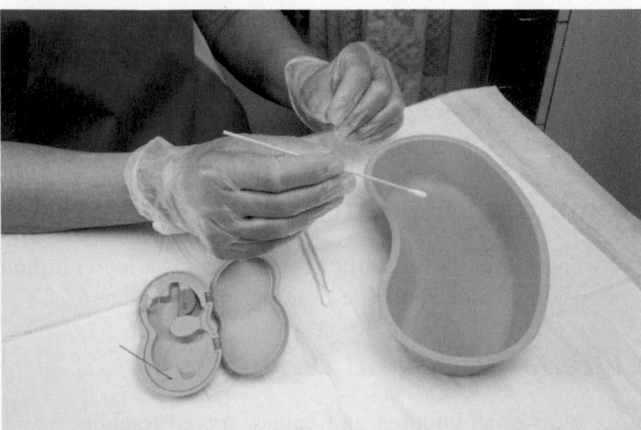

FIG. 3 Moisten a swab with warm water or normal saline.

FIG. 1 Inspect the hearing aid.

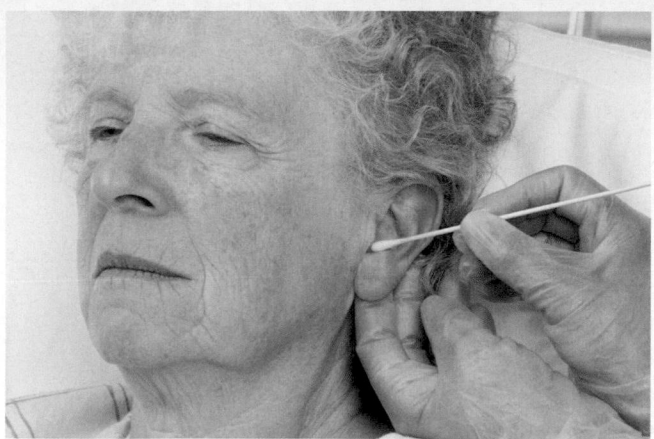

FIG. 4 Clean the patient's ear with the moistened swab.

7. With the volume turned down, insert the ear mold into the ear canal, twisting slightly for a snug fit.
8. Secure the battery behind the ear, if of that type (Fig. 5). There are other styles of hearing aids that may fit in other ways.

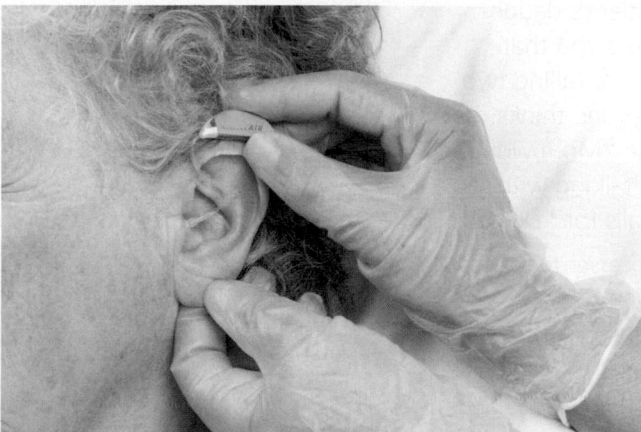

FIG. 5 Secure the hearing aid behind the patient's ear.

9. **Turn the volume up slowly while speaking to the patient in a normal voice tone. Ask the patient to let you know when the sound level is comfortable.**
   Rationale: Helping the patient to participate in the environment through improved hearing assists in the sensory function of communication.

Documentation

4/15/17: 15:30—Patient successfully demonstrated insertion, removal, and cleaning of hearing aid. Stated understanding of care of hearing aid when not in use.

—M. Klim, RN

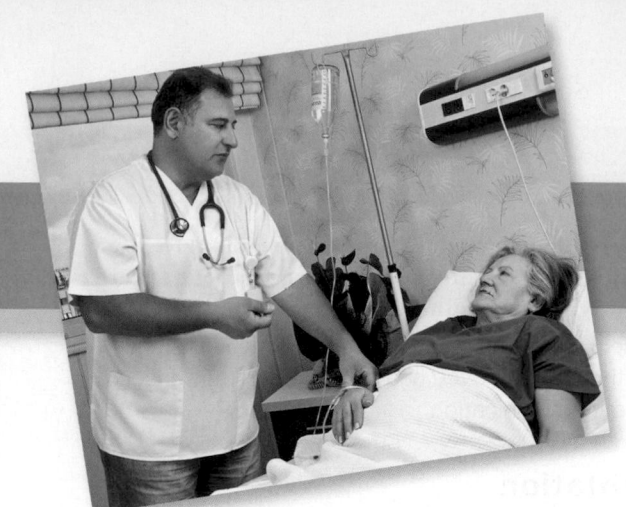

CHAPTER 37

Cognitive Processes

Heather A. Martin

Case Scenario

You are a nurse working on a general surgical unit of a hospital. A patient returns to the unit after repair of a broken hip. She appears agitated and confused despite a pain control regimen of morphine. The patient's daughter, Donna, comes to visit and looks acutely anxious. Donna tells you that her mother lived in a long-term care facility for 16 months before falling two nights ago after getting up to go to the bathroom. Donna says she thinks that the nurses at the home ignored her mother's call light because "Mom would never get up at night without calling a nurse." While you are talking with Donna, the patient moans, pulls at intravenous tubing, and calls for "Dorothy."

Once you have completed this chapter and have added cognitive processes to your knowledge base, return to the above scenario and reflect on the following areas of Critical Thinking:

1. Describe your immediate impressions of this situation.
2. Determine how the information in the scenario and your own knowledge and values contributed to these impressions.
3. Given the situation as presented, formulate and prioritize your plans for nursing interventions.
4. Organize your plans for assessing the patient's cognitive function.

KEY TERMS

anomia
aphasia
articulation
attention
cognition
coma
communication
comprehension
consciousness
delirium
dementia
dysarthria
judgment
learning
memory
orientation
perceiving
phonation
reality orientation
schizophrenia

LEARNING OBJECTIVES

Upon completion of this chapter, you will be able to do the following:

1. Identify key components of cognition and communication.
2. Describe characteristics of normal cognition.
3. Describe influences on cognitive function related to the lifespan.
4. Explain factors that can affect cognitive processes.
5. Identify manifestations of altered cognitive processes.
6. Apply the nursing process to the care of persons experiencing altered cognitive processes.
7. Discuss socialization needs of people with altered cognition and their families.
8. List resources available to families of people with altered cognitive processes.

In all practice settings, nurses work with people experiencing temporary or irreversible impairment of cognitive function. Nurses play a central role in identifying people at risk for and experiencing cognitive impairment and in the ongoing assessment of the impairment's impact on self-care and safety. Nursing interventions focus on promoting optimal function by preventing, minimizing, or restoring factors affecting function and by compensating for deficits. Planning and evaluating nursing care require an understanding of normal **cognition**, factors that place a person at risk for cognitive impairment, and effective interventions to be individualized as appropriate.

NORMAL COGNITIVE PROCESSES

Cognition is the systematic way in which a person thinks, reasons, and uses language. Each instant of awareness can be defined as a thought, and awareness itself can be defined as **consciousness**. **Attention** is the ability to concentrate on and take in specific sensory stimuli. **Memory** is the ability to recall a thought at least once and usually again. **Learning** is the capability of the nervous system to store memories. **Communication** is the exchange of information between at least two people and involves the use of language to store, process, and transmit thought content. The cerebral cortex coordinates consciousness, thought, memory, learning, and communication.

Anatomic Structures Involved in Cognition

For information to be processed, the person must be able to perceive it. Perception of information begins when the information enters the person's awareness through the senses; consciousness, thought, memory, learning, and language all play roles in further processing that information. Intact structure and functioning of the sensory receptors, the afferent nervous pathways, and the cerebral cortex are necessary for a person to take in information through the senses and to assimilate and interpret that information in the cerebral cortex. Additionally, the efferent nervous pathways, major reflexes, and muscles are needed to communicate information to others. Detailed information on the senses and sensory perception is presented in Chapter 36.

Normal Cognitive Function

PERCEPTION OF INFORMATION

Perception of information includes sensing and interpreting stimuli from the external and internal environments. Perception depends on functioning sensory receptors, neurotransmission, and central processing.

Sensory receptors can be classified into three groups: exteroceptors (external sensors), proprioceptors (position sensors), and interoceptors (internal sensors). Neurotransmission occurs when the stimuli to the sensory receptors are converted to neural impulses and transmitted to the appropriate area of the brain for central processing and interpretation.

Exteroceptors

The exteroceptors respond to stimuli from the external environment. They include the receptors for vision (rods and cones) and hearing (hair cells in the organ of Corti) and the somatic receptors for pain, touch, and pressure in the skin. Vision permits people to link abstract concepts with concrete objects, thus contributing to learning and memory. Hearing, also present from birth, links concepts with the frequency, intensity, and duration of sounds. Both vision and hearing enhance environmental awareness and facilitate experiences that amplify cognitive development.

Touch, pressure, heat, cold, or chemicals in the tissue activate somatic sensors in the skin. Resulting nerve impulses enter the spinal cord through the posterior roots. From the spinal cord, sensory information is transmitted through the thalamus to the somatosensory cortex in the brain's parietal lobes.

Taste is a function of the taste buds of the tongue and includes sweet, sour, salty, and bitter components. The sensation of taste is transmitted to the brain stem. Ascending fibers carry the impulses to the taste center of the sensory area. Smell is a function of the olfactory cells located in the upper nose and is the least understood of the special senses. Taste and smell seem to be closely related because diminished function in one usually affects the function of the other (McCance & Heuther, 2013).

Proprioceptors

Proprioceptors are located in the inner ear, muscles, tendons, and joints. Proprioceptive sensations relate to the body's physical state, including the relative position of different body parts and the sensation of movement. The proprioceptive function of the inner ear is discussed in Chapter 36.

Interoceptors

Interoceptors are located in and respond to stimuli from the body's viscera and deeper tissues such as bone. Sensations relate to changes in the internal environment. With the exception of visceral pain receptors, the interoceptors operate at a reflex level (Koeppen & Stanton, 2010).

CONSCIOUSNESS

Consciousness, a state of awareness and full responsiveness to stimuli, relies on an intact reticular activating system (RAS) and cerebral cortex. The RAS influences awareness of stimuli, which are received through the five senses: sight, hearing, touch, smell, and taste. The RAS mediates level of arousal, and the cerebral cortex mediates perception and interpretation of stimuli, as discussed in Chapter 36. When the facilitatory and inhibitory areas are balanced, the person is conscious but neither excited nor inhibited.

THOUGHTS

Each thought results from a momentary pattern of stimulation of many parts of the nervous system at the same time. The stimulated area of the cortex determines discrete characteristics of thought (what is seen in the visual field), discrete patterns of sensation (texture of objects), and other specific characteristics (Guyton & Hall, 2011).

MEMORY

Memory is the process by which information and experiences are stored and retrieved. Physiologically, changes in nerve transmission from one neuron to the next due to previous neural activity (learning) result in memories. Plasticity, the tendency of synapses and neural circuits to change as a result of activity, allows new synaptic pathways to form. These new pathways are called memory traces and, once established, can be activated to reproduce the memories (Guyton & Hall, 2011).

Memory is subdivided into three basic types based on the time span between stimulus presentation and memory retrieval. Immediate memories last for a few seconds to a few minutes and may be caused by local reverberating neural impulses. Intermediate memories may last for minutes or weeks but will be lost unless converted to long-term memories. Physiologically, intermediate memories involve changes in the strength of the synaptic connections, which may be attributed to changes in neurotransmitter or intracellular chemicals. Long-term memories, those that can be recalled indefinitely, are stored at the same site as intermediate memories but require the activation of previously inactive genes and the expression of new proteins (e.g., the number of cell membrane channels may increase).

The hippocampi, part of the limbic system located within both temporal lobes, play a role in determining which memories are committed long term. The ability to retain some things and forget others is essential to intelligent behavior. Assimilating experiences and new information is a process involving memory. The hippocampi play a vital role in retaining new knowledge and preventing dissipation of the information.

Memory impairment is a concern for old and young alike. Situational and emotional stress usually has few effects on long-term memory. Significant impairment of long-term memory usually indicates a central nervous system (CNS) disorder or a severe confusional state. Short-term memory is much more sensitive to stress. For example, hospitalized patients may have little recall of conversations with healthcare professionals because the stress of illness interferes with usual memory functioning.

Characteristics of Normal Cognition

INTELLIGENCE

Intelligence is the measurable product of intellectual functioning, which consists of memory (discussed earlier), **comprehension**, and concentration. Comprehension, a part of learning, involves grasping the meaning of stimuli (see below discussion on learning). Concentration is the ability to filter extraneous stimuli to focus on a task. People depend on intellectual functioning to learn in school settings, vocational surroundings, and living environments.

REALITY PERCEPTION

Perception of reality, or **reality orientation**, includes awareness of time, place, situation, and self. It is the knowledge of how self and environment interact over time and transform sensory information into meaning. Reality perception is complex and depends on functioning sensory receptors, neurotransmission, and intact central processing. People with affective disorders, such as depression, experience alterations in reality perception.

ORIENTATION

Orientation is the basic process by which people know their location in the dimensions of time and place. Orientation also includes the ability to know who one is as a person and in relation to others. People tend to take orientation for granted until they experience confusion. On a simple level, one can experience disorientation upon awakening in a new setting (e.g., on vacation) and momentarily forgetting where one is.

JUDGMENT

Judgment, or insight, is the process of reasoning. It is the ability to process incoming stimuli and to determine the complex meanings associated with many aspects of a situation. For example, a person driving down the street may see a truck blocking the road ahead. The person determines that the truck is an obstacle and that evasive action is required to prevent a crash. The term *insight* is often used to express perceptions that people make about behavior or feelings. For example, recognizing that a craving for chocolate while studying for exams is an indicator of stress is an insight.

RECALL AND RECOGNITION

Recall and recognition are abilities used to retrieve information from long- and short-term memory. Recall involves the ability to retrieve information directly or by relating it to other information (e.g., seeing a person and "recalling" his or her name accurately). Recognition is the ability to relate accurately something in the current environment with what is stored in memory (e.g., seeing a rose and "recognizing" it as a type of flower). People depend on these abilities to perform in school, on the job, and in everyday life. Recall and recognition are cognitive characteristics that can be developed and need practice to remain actively useful.

LANGUAGE

Language is the ability to convey needs, ideas, and feelings through the systematic use of symbols. Humans are unique in being able to use symbolic codes to communicate abstract ideas through a highly refined verbal language. The biophysical interaction and integration of the brain, neural system, and organs of speech permit humans not only to produce sounds but also to remember what they said in the past and to speak about the future.

Language enables people to relate to others in their families and communities. It helps people identify and express their roles in relationships. For instance, a father may discipline a child, an instructor may give an assignment, or a student may ask questions for clarification. In each example, people use language to communicate a relationship.

NORMAL COGNITIVE PATTERNS

Cognition is the sum of the various thinking processes through which a person gains, stores, manipulates, and expresses knowledge. Cognition enables the person to interact with the environment meaningfully and purposefully. Normal cognitive patterns integrate the processes of attending, **perceiving**, thinking, learning, remembering, and communicating.

Attending

Attending is the process of concentrating on a specific stimulus without being distracted by other, irrelevant stimuli. Ability to concentrate is a cortical function of the brain's frontal lobe. Attending is different from alertness; an alert but inattentive person will be attracted to any environmental stimulus.

Perceiving

Perceiving is the process of receiving and interpreting sensory stimuli that function as a basis for understanding, knowing, or learning. In perceiving, a person integrates information obtained through vision, hearing, touching, taste, and/or smell with past experiences to understand or make sense of the environment. An example of perceiving is hearing a phone ring, seeing the phone, touching and holding the receiver, listening to the person speaking, interpreting the meaning, and responding appropriately. The integration of motor activities involved in handling the phone, sensory activities of seeing and hearing, and central perceptual activities of interpretation results in a meaningful interaction.

Thinking

Thinking is the process of sorting, organizing, and categorizing information to form mental concepts or perceptions. "Thinking" is forming ideas or arriving at conclusions; "reasoning" is following a logical thought sequence, starting with what is known and proceeding to a conclusion. A person is capable of different types of thinking. Concrete thinking involves objects that can be perceived by the senses. An example of concrete thinking is proving the arithmetic proposition that $1 + 1 = 2$ by attaching the numbers to objects such as apples. Abstract thinking is a higher-level process that involves a thought or idea apart from any material object. For example, the idea of beauty is a value. Beauty can be attributed to a flower but is not a concrete object in itself. Abstract thinking is required for people to interpret a veiled or abstract truth from the use of concrete objects and terms. Creativity is an innate human attribute that enables us to bring something new into existence.

Learning

Learning is the multidimensional process of acquiring knowledge that depends on abstract functions such as symbols, language, classifications, and concepts as well as concrete operations. Comprehension is the capacity for understanding and reasoning. For learning to be useful, the person needs to develop strategies for organizing information in memory so that he or she can recall it as needed (for more discussion on learning, see Chapter 36).

Remembering

Memory is a complex biochemical storage system that is not yet completely understood. Experiences, ideas, and images are chemically coded and integrated for later retrieval (Koeppen & Stanton, 2010). The content of long-term memory, which is the storehouse of a person's knowledge, depends on the perceived value and significance of the past event. Specific significant life events, such as weddings or the birth of a child, hold great value and memory potential. The reason some items move from short- to long-term memory is not clear but is probably related to the perceived value of the information and its relation to other memories.

Communicating

Communication brings people together while differentiating them from one another. Communication allows people to be unique. People may communicate thoughts and ideas verbally through spoken or written language or nonverbally through facial expressions, body posture, movements, gestures, and touch (see Chapters 6 and 36). Touch, a very effective means of nonverbal communication, has many different meanings; understanding the true meaning may be difficult because of its personal nature. Familial, regional, class, and cultural influences shape tactile expressions. Age and gender also shape meanings that are associated with touch.

Life Span Considerations

Physiologic health and the quality of the social and physical environments affect the complex process of cognitive development. Environment can strongly influence the rate at which a person proceeds through the usual stages of cognitive development. Each developmental phase has unique aspects related to language and communication. People need emotional security, human interaction, and various sensory experiences to develop optimally. Jean Piaget (1969) is the most widely recognized theorist in cognitive development, although the work of other theorists, such as Erikson (1963) and Havighurst (1972), contributes to the understanding of cognitive development throughout the life span.

NEWBORN AND INFANT

Newborns and infants are in the "sensorimotor period" in which sensory experience is the major developmental task (Piaget, 1969). Infants interact with the environment through the five senses and learn to modify behavior in response to stimuli. Language skills are not developed, and infants express thoughts or needs through behavior. Bonding is essential to the development of basic trust. Primary caregivers are lifelines for infants. Through consistent relationships, infants learn to differentiate self from others, to communicate, and to relate to others.

Babies perform the cognitive developmental work of infancy by exploring the environment and playing. Infants learn to connect some behaviors with expected responses. For example, moving a toy in a certain way may cause a pleasing sound; that process is play. With repetition and maturity though, infants may begin to remember and repeat the action at will. Similarly, infants begin to assimilate language, linking specific words and sounds with objects of meaning such as "Mama" or "bottle." Providing stimulation through varied objects, different sounds, and face-to-face communication and interaction enhances cognitive development (Santrock, 2012).

Crying, smiling, pointing, and tugging are kinds of nonverbal communication that babies use. Language skills begin with cooing and progress to vocalizations that express various emotional states (Santrock, 2012). During the babbling period, infants produce sounds that form the basis of language. As they mature, babies begin to understand language and use words to communicate. Most babies speak their first words by the end of the first year.

TODDLER AND PRESCHOOLER

During these stages, young children develop the concept of object permanence and begin to label familiar items. Object permanence means that children learn that objects have constancy; they give objects names and use those names to communicate with others (Piaget, 1969). Vision and hearing are necessary to understand the environment as a basis of thinking. Language and thinking develop side by side. Preschoolers have concrete thinking patterns and demonstrate pronounced egocentrism, or self-concern. These children view the world only from their point of view.

By the time infants become toddlers, they have transformed vocalizations and gestures into words to express themselves. At 2 years of age, most children understand more than 300 words and can speak about 200 words (Santrock, 2012). Although children vary in their rate of language acquisition, uniformity exists in the way all children acquire language. Language is acquired not only in terms of learning principles but also through biologic, environmental, and cognitive factors. Any serious change or interruption in these factors can affect a child's acquisition of language. Children who are abandoned, abused, or not exposed to language rarely learn to speak normally.

The process of reasoning begins as young children try to make sense of the world. When two events occur simultaneously, children think one caused the other (transductive reasoning). Thus, preschoolers believe their thoughts to be all powerful. For example, if a child spilled her milk and later fell and scraped a knee, she might interpret the pain associated with the abrasion as punishment for spilling the milk. More

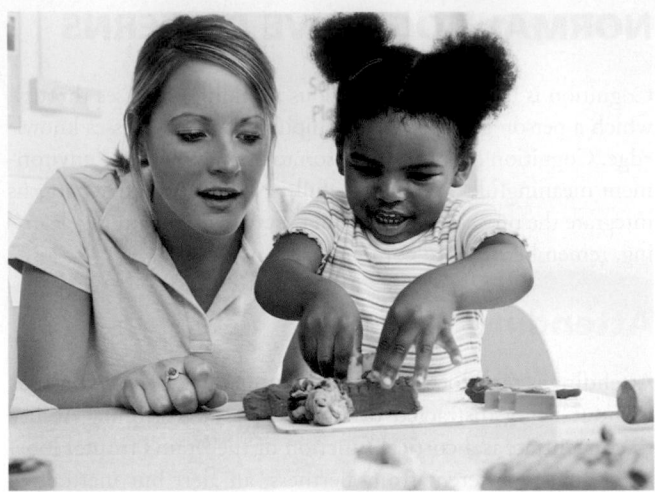

FIGURE 37-1 Play activities that incorporate imagination and creativity help to develop cognitive abilities in preschoolers.

significantly, a child may interpret parental divorce as punishment for "bad" thoughts or behavior. Because adults find this thinking so absurd, they may underestimate its seriousness to children.

As part of cognitive development, young children develop confidence in abilities and gain independence through encouragement in each new area of learning (Erikson, 1963). Positive, nurturing environments that encourage imaginative play, interaction, questioning, and use of language and symbols, while reinforcing earlier knowledge, will foster the preschooler's cognitive development (Fig. 37-1).

SCHOOL-AGE CHILD AND ADOLESCENT

School-age children can carry out complex mental operations such as addition, subtraction, grouping, classifying, and ordering (Piaget, 1969). They understand and can mentally represent multiple dimensions of objects and symbols and can encode stimuli for later retrieval. School-age children understand conservation, which is the idea that the properties of an object stay the same even if the object is altered in certain ways. For example, if an equal volume of fluid is poured into two differently shaped containers, a preschooler will perceive that the volume of water has changed, whereas the school-age child will recognize that there's a change in shape but the water volume is constant. This shift in comprehension indicates the ability to incorporate abstract thinking with concrete processes. At this stage, children derive great pleasure in accomplishments resulting from new learning and thinking skills (Erikson, 1963) (Fig. 37-2). Learning and play environments that reward children's achievements contribute positively.

Adolescence is a particularly difficult time for the development of thinking processes because of enormous emotional stress from many sources, including the struggle for separateness from family and a strong need to identify with the peer group (Erikson, 1963). Fluctuating hormonal levels add to the emotional stress. Abstract reasoning and logical judgment are two functions that emerge with increasing maturity.

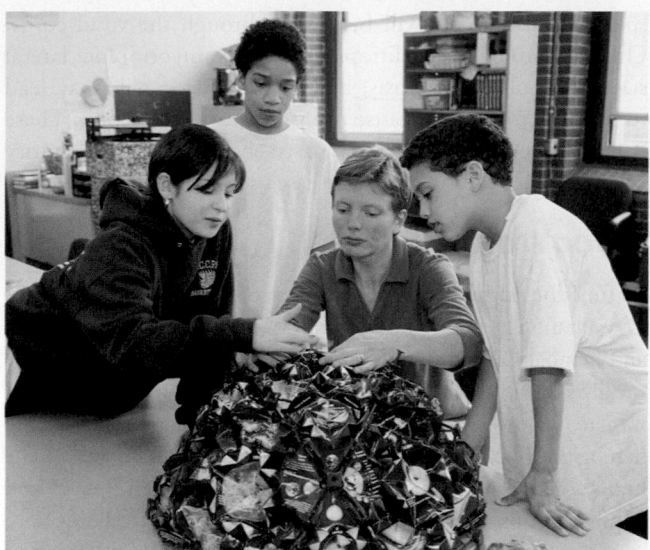

FIGURE 37-2 School-age children delight in learning and show an intense interest in every experience.

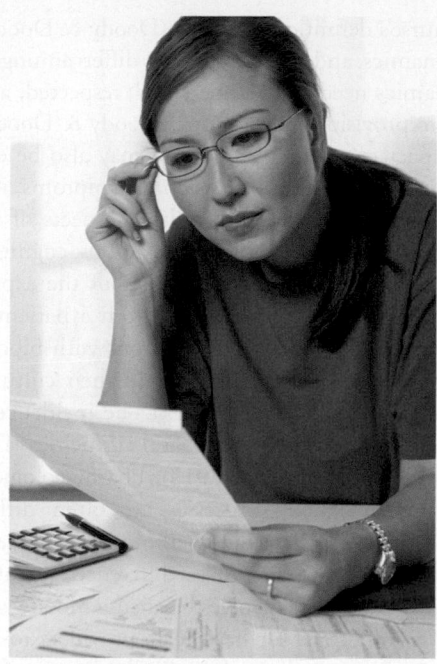

FIGURE 37-3 Cognitive development is an ongoing process as adults encounter educational, career, and life experiences.

During adolescence, teenagers become able to think abstractly and to perform complex mental processes. They are able to hypothesize situations and solutions as well as to conceptualize abstract ideas (Piaget, 1969). Teenagers develop the cognitive capacities of classification, serialization, spatial abilities, verbal skills, and abstract relationships. Communication with peers takes priority over communication with adults. At the same time, adolescents need adult guidance and protection. During illness, peer relationships provide support and companionship. Providing opportunities for independent thinking and decision making encourages increased maturity.

ADULT AND OLDER ADULT

Throughout young and middle adulthood, people make steady progress in rational thinking abilities, formal and informal educational opportunities, career development, and life experiences. As adults feel progressively more competent, they become less rigid and more flexible. Making decisions and adjusting to changes usually creates less disruption during adulthood than in teenage years. Creativity and productivity in work contribute to continual cognitive development and to innovative use of integrated abstract and concrete thinking (Fig. 37-3). Adults depend on communication for dealing instrumentally with the world, managing careers and vocations, maintaining relationships, and carrying out various roles. Communication conveys thoughts, feelings, and the innermost aspects of the human experience.

As aging progresses in the adult years, cognitive function remains relatively unchanged, although processing information may require more time. Problems with thought processes and communication are more common among older adults than younger groups, but they usually relate to a decrease in coping reserves, trauma, or a specific condition. They are not a normal part of aging. Age-associated memory impairment is a mild memory impairment that does not significantly interfere

with activities of daily living (ADLs). Items forgotten are usually unimportant. People can use memory enhancement techniques to compensate for benign forgetfulness. Although the brain undergoes some degenerative changes as the ventricles enlarge slightly and brain weight decreases, significant cognitive impairment in older persons is never normal but is indicative of a disorder.

Diminished vision and hearing are common among older adults and can interfere with effective communication. Because these senses usually diminish gradually, older adults develop compensatory mechanisms for adapting to the changes and their effects on communication.

Cultural Considerations

Comprehension and meaning vary among cultures, and communication is often inhibited or blocked as a result. Words and their meanings carry different nuances and significance depending on a person's culture, values, beliefs, language, and customs. Ability to interact with others and to express one's self develop from each aspect of one's personal cultural framework.

Language barriers, which may exist with different cultures, can result in anxiety, fear, and frustration for people who are unable to communicate effectively. It is equally frustrating trying to understand and to be understood. Because communication involves nonverbal and verbal language, the meaning of body position and expression can further facilitate or impede communication.

Values regarding thoughts and feelings about an individual's customs, healthcare, or way of life may be difficult to understand for the healthcare providers and difficult to explain for patients. Health as defined by one ethnogroup may be different from the nurse's definition of health (Doody & Doody, 2012). Family dynamics and roles may also differ among cultures. These dynamics need to be understood, respected, and incorporated into provision of healthcare (Doody & Doody, 2012).

The impact of cultural framework may also be evident in other ways. These include expression of symptoms, incidence/types of disease processes, and multiple aspects of treatment methodologies. Symptomatology of various cognitive disorders is the same across cultural groups, but the expression of symptoms and the treatment evolve from a patient's unique cultural framework. For example, persons with bipolar disorders experience symptoms based within their cultural beliefs and values (Doody & Doody, 2012). The incidence of some diseases is greater for certain races and ethnicities (Dillworth-Anderson, Pierre, & Hilliard, 2012). Pharmacologic research indicates that metabolic processes are often different for individuals from racially and ethnically diverse groups. Ethnopharmacology studies these differences. Treatment for some cognitive disorders involves balancing moods with medications. It is important for healthcare providers to know the differences in how racially and ethnically diverse groups react to medication. Adherence to the treatment plan also improves when cultural frameworks are integrated into the patient teaching plan (Doody & Doody, 2012).

FACTORS AFFECTING COGNITIVE FUNCTION

The interaction of personal (physiologic and emotional) and environmental factors can affect cognitive processes. Culture, values, and beliefs are contextual factors that influence meaning and understanding.

Physiologic Factors

Any physiologic abnormality that affects the body's cellular environment can interfere with brain function and affect cognition. Disturbances range from mild mental clouding to disorientation and acute confusion to **coma** and death (Tabloski, 2013). Physiologic abnormalities contribute to **schizophrenia**, depression, and some kinds of **dementia**. Similarly, physiologic abnormalities that cloud the senses or interfere with usual cortical functioning may alter communication.

Communication may be altered by the functional impairment of the speech apparatus of the larynx, the ability to move air, the use of the tongue and the oral pharynx, and/or innervation to each of these structures. Cancer of the throat is the major risk for impaired **phonation**. Neurologic impairment and muscular dysfunction also have the potential for affecting communication.

Muscular dysfunction can be related to cortical, cerebellar, or cranial neurologic impairment or from effects of drugs (e.g., alcohol, sedatives, or other medications). People who have a high cervical (C2, C3 quadriplegia) injury also have a permanent tracheostomy (and ventilatory support). They cannot speak because no air will be forced through the vocal cords. Other neurologic conditions, such as amyotrophic lateral sclerosis, multiple sclerosis, and myasthenia gravis, may lead to inability to speak because of loss of muscle function. These conditions may also necessitate a tracheostomy or ventilatory assistance, depending on the disease's severity.

BLOOD FLOW

To function optimally, all cells need a continuous oxygen supply. Oxygenation depends on respiratory and circulatory function and hemoglobin production. During respiration, oxygen enters the alveoli, diffuses across capillary membranes to enter the pulmonary venous system, and binds with hemoglobin. Then, the hemoglobin-bound oxygen is transported to brain cells. The brain accounts for 20% of the body's total oxygen uptake and requires a constant oxygen supply to support brain cell life.

Any interruption in blood flow to the brain cells causes cellular hypoxia, resulting in changes in function. A chronically inadequate blood supply causes cellular dysfunction and deterioration of mental processes (Porth & Matfin, 2013). Any disease process that interferes with alveolar ventilation, pulmonary circulation, cardiac function, cerebral blood flow, or production of normal hemoglobin can result in hypoxia and altered cognition. A cerebrovascular accident (CVA) or stroke usually occurs because a thrombus occludes a cerebral blood vessel, resulting in inadequate blood flow. Approximately 20% of all stroke survivors require the specialized services of a speech pathologist to help them regain communication skills. The other 80% have only minor or temporary damage to the brain's language centers (Baxter & Wilson, 2012). The location of the insult and the extent of damage affect the pattern and severity of speech impairment.

NUTRITION AND METABOLISM

The brain cells need glucose for metabolic energy and other nutrients for optimal functioning. The brain consumes 25% of the glucose the body uses. The efficiency with which oxygen is delivered to the cells is related to hemoglobin production, which requires an adequate dietary intake of iron. Vitamins and minerals are essential for effective neurologic functioning and neurotransmitter activity.

People with inadequate nutrition usually have low hemoglobin levels (anemia). Abnormal hemoglobin can be produced in people with specific genetic disorders such as sickle cell anemia. Disorders that impair metabolic processes and oxygen use, such as hypothermia and hypothyroidism, can also alter cognition (Porth & Matfin, 2013). The body's inadequate intake or impaired use of glucose will limit the quantity available for the brain's metabolic demands.

FLUID AND ELECTROLYTE BALANCE

The brain cells require a constant extracellular environment of fluid and electrolytes for optimal function. The brain's cellular processes depend on the active and passive movement of water and charged particles across cell membranes (see Chapter 28). The brain is protected by the blood–brain barrier, a shield that prevents or delays the entry of certain substances from the blood into the cerebrospinal fluid or interstitial spaces. The blood–brain barrier protects the brain cells from substances (other than normal fluid and electrolytes) that could damage sensitive nerve cells. Maintenance of a dynamic state of fluid balance and electrolyte levels provides the ideal internal environment for neurologic function.

Disturbance in the concentration and balance of intracellular and extracellular fluid and electrolytes can cause cellular dysfunction and accompanying cognitive changes. Such disturbances have various causes, including abnormal loss of body fluids, dietary deficiencies, acute and chronic disease, and effects of medications. Although any disturbance in fluid or electrolyte balance can impair cognitive processes, a few common disturbances are hyponatremia and hypernatremia (variations in the serum sodium level), hypokalemia (reduced serum potassium level), hypercalcemia (elevated serum calcium level), and hypoglycemia and hyperglycemia (abnormal serum glucose levels) (Porth & Matfin, 2013).

Accumulated metabolic by-products (metabolic end products) that are not eliminated from the body can be toxic to CNS function. Impaired function of the kidney, liver, or both can impair the ability to break down and excrete such potential toxins. The liver converts ammonia, a by-product of protein metabolism, into urea that the kidneys excrete. Liver or kidney dysfunction can interfere with this process, resulting in elevated ammonia levels and a **delirium** known as hepatic encephalopathy.

SLEEP AND REST

Sleep's restorative function allows people to regain energy for cognitive functions (see Chapter 34). Sleep is necessary for consolidating learning and moving information from short-term to long-term memory. Rapid eye movement (REM) sleep seems to be particularly important to efficient cognitive functioning. Lack of sleep (sleep deprivation) can cause irritability, decreased calculation and problem-solving skills, poor concentration, and/or impaired memory. Everyone has experienced feeling dull and slow after a sleepless night or staying up too late. Rotating shifts can cause similar problems, particularly if a person changes shifts frequently with inadequate time to adjust to new sleep patterns. Inadequate REM sleep may impair both learning and memory and decrease the subjective feeling of being rested.

SELF-CONCEPT

The way a person feels about himself or herself is called self-concept (see Chapter 38). Communication conveys the way a person feels about him- or herself in relation to the world. If a person feels competent, successful, and in control, the quality of his or her communication will reflect that confidence and security.

People who feel disadvantaged or less competent are likely to believe they have little control over their lives. Their self-concept is apt to be correspondingly less confident. If a person sees the self as unable to compete in a given arena (e.g., school, work, or play), the person's communication reflects that lack of confidence.

Others usually reflect the manner in which a person communicates. If a person communicates confidence and security, he or she will usually receive that response from others. Conversely, if the person communicates insecurity, lack of control, or inadequacy, responses from others will mirror this communication.

The relationship between self-concept and communication is susceptible to change. People vary in personal skills, and one can compensate for weaknesses in some areas with strengths in others. This adaptation and adjustment help create a balanced self-concept and more confident communication.

INFECTIOUS PROCESSES

Infectious processes of the CNS, including encephalitis and brain abscesses, and the subsequent inflammatory response of nerve cells, are obvious causes of altered cognition. HIV can invade the CNS, causing acute infection or progressing to AIDS. Infections elsewhere in the body can also cause changes in mental status. Any person with a severe infection in the circulation (e.g., bacteremia, septicemia) may experience CNS effects, including lethargy and confusion. Common sources for bacteremia or septicemia include the urinary tract, respiratory system, and any open wounds (Dunne, 2013). Altered cognitive function in an older adult may be the earliest indication of an infectious process anywhere in the body.

DEGENERATIVE PROCESSES

Any process contributing to degeneration of the brain cells may ultimately affect cognitive function. Causes of degeneration may be related to an organism (viral or bacterial infection), aging, or unknown sources. Degeneration can impair judgment, insight, planning, memory, problem solving, and communication. Potential impairments range from mild disability to severe dysfunction that may be incompatible with normal cognition.

Clarifying the terms used to describe degenerative processes related to cognition is important. *Senility*, which literally means the process of aging, is a term used to describe cognitive impairments that are mistakenly thought to be a normal part of aging. Actually, significant memory and problem-solving impairment is never normal but rather indicates a pathologic process (Cummings, Arsland, & Jarvik, 2013). The terms *senile dementia* and *organic brain syndrome* have no place in current nursing practice.

PHARMACOLOGIC AGENTS

Medications that primarily act on the CNS (e.g., anticonvulsants, antidepressants, antianxiety agents, antipsychotics, opioids, and hypnotics) can impair thinking and cause confusion. In the early stages of use or with moderate to heavy dosages, the person may experience impairment in speech motor control (slowness and slurring) and in comprehension and expression (inability to think of the correct word or response). Discontinuing or decreasing the dosage of these medications will often improve cognitive function within a few days. Medications commonly prescribed to manage agitated or confused behavior, such as haloperidol and the benzodiazepines, may cause a paradoxical increase in confusion in some people, especially older adults.

Medications that do not have primary pharmacologic effects on the CNS can also cause confusion, either alone or in combination (Tabloski, 2013). The mechanism varies and is not well understood. In some cases, such as with strong diuretics, the drug predisposes the person to another physiologic cause of confusion—hyponatremia. In practice, it is wise to consider almost any medication as a possible contributing factor to altered cognition.

Toxicity states can occur with overdose of a medication or alcohol and can cause confusion. Overdosage of drugs that normally have no CNS effects can potentially cause significant mental status changes. Overuse of drugs affecting the CNS alone or combined with alcohol will also impair thinking.

HEAD TRAUMA

People of all ages sustain head trauma. The leading causes are falls and motor vehicles crashes. In many cases, alcohol and drugs are contributing factors. Head trauma is a common cause of childhood hospitalization. The elderly are prone to falls and traffic accidents resulting in head trauma. Young men have a high incidence related to motor vehicle and work-related accidents and physical violence (Baxter & Wilson, 2012). Most seriously injured patients have prolonged hospital, long-term care, and rehabilitation stays for major disabilities. Because specific injury sites vary, classification of brain injury and prediction of outcome are difficult. The more severe the head injury, the more likely communication will be interrupted. Communication problems in head-injured patients are usually compounded by impairments in cognitive function, such as behavior, memory, orientation, and attention.

Environmental Factors

The basic cognitive processes of perceiving, thinking, learning, and remembering depend on the ability to receive and organize stimuli. The amount of stimuli in the environment, either increased or decreased, can influence cognition. For example, one student preparing for exams in an environment of noisy students, television, and loud music may find it difficult to study effectively. Another student may find that some background noise, depending on the level of distraction, assists with concentration.

As people age, perceptual ability, which contributes to cognitive functioning, declines as sense organ functions diminish. For example, older adults need more light to see objects, have more problems with light glare, and experience loss of accommodation for near objects (presbyopia). Hearing diminishes, especially in the high-frequency range, and acuity of sense of touch declines. These normal changes affect the ability to organize incoming stimuli.

Emotional stress or physical discomfort can lead to disorganized thinking, memory impairment, and poor judgment. A person learning of an injury to a loved one, finding out about a failed exam, or planning a wedding may have difficulty maintaining the usual level of cognitive performance. Concentration and problem solving are also difficult when a person is in pain, has a full bladder, or experiences other discomfort. Sometimes, such everyday problems combine and accumulate, creating enough stress to impair thinking.

Psychological disorders, such as depression, interfere with cognitive function and can contribute to altered thought processes. Psychological and emotional disorders can interfere with sleep, rest, and nutrition and can affect cognitive functions directly.

The stress of an unfamiliar environment can affect the basic cognitive processes of orientation and arousal, which depend on the ability of the cerebral cortex to receive and organize incoming stimuli. Numerous stimuli are found in any environment, some of which are attended to and some ignored. Through a complex perceptual process, habituation or familiarization occurs to routine background stimuli, such as the feel of clothing and the tick of a clock. As a result, the person is not "overloaded" with meaningless input. The brain can also conjure up input when none is available. People experiencing inadequate sensory input are at risk for cognitive dysfunction as the brain attempts to stimulate itself (see Chapter 36).

Hospitalization removes people from familiar surroundings and daily activities that provide orienting cues and places them in an environment of strange noises, sights, feelings, and procedures (Fig. 37-4). All of these unfamiliar stimuli demand attention because the person has not had time to habituate to the new surroundings. This state of sensory overload can overwhelm the person's ability to find meaning, and a state of perceptual dysfunction may occur.

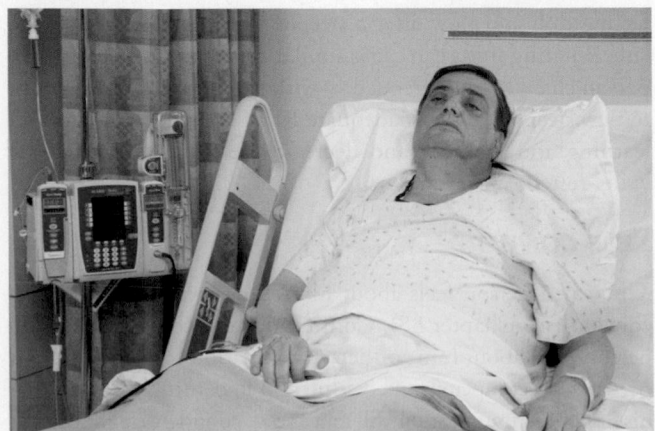

FIGURE 37-4 Patients might be at risk for cognitive dysfunction related to unfamiliar environments and procedures.

ALTERED COGNITIVE FUNCTION

Cognition is a complex process; the normal outcome is an appropriate, adaptive behavioral or emotional response. Anything that interrupts this complex process can result in impaired thinking and abnormal behavioral or emotional responses.

Disorganized Thinking

Clinical manifestations of altered cognitive function include delirium (acute confusion), dementia (chronic irreversible confusion), sensory perceptual alterations, and impaired language skills. Dysfunctions can be either temporary or permanent, depending on the cause.

A person experiencing disturbed thought processes or disorganized thinking interacts inappropriately with others or the environment and may have an altered perception of reality. Thinking, learning, reasoning, and remembering occur in a disorderly fashion. Manifestations of disorganized thinking may include inappropriately interacting and conversing with others, talking or gesturing to one's self, performing inappropriate activities, or exhibiting bizarre behavior. Withdrawal from others, hallucinations, and delusions are other common manifestations, especially in schizophrenia and affective disorders. They may also occur in acute confusion and, less commonly, in Alzheimer.

Cognitive impairment frequently interferes with perception of reality, which is based on life experience, personal relationships, and environment. When thought processes become altered, the person may find it difficult to separate accurately altered perceptions from reality. **Delusions** (fixed false beliefs) and **hallucinations** (perceptions arising from the person's own thoughts) are examples of altered perceptions of reality. Both responses are attempts to cope with or to manage stress or physiologic dysfunctions that impair cognition.

In disorganized thinking, the content of the person's speech may make no sense in the context of the conversation or a sentence may contain multiple unrelated ideas. Interactions with people with disorganized thinking are difficult because they are unable to follow a logical sequence or to respond rationally or predictably. The patient who ignores the meal tray but tries to eat the tissue box with a spoon or who asks to go to the bathroom but resists assistance to get out of bed displays impaired reasoning processes.

Impaired Thought Processes

Abnormal levels of arousal, attention span deficits, and memory impairments can affect judgment, insight, planning, and problem solving. Most people with impaired thought processes have aspects of all three elements, and severity can fluctuate.

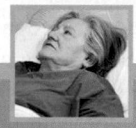

Cognitive Processes PICO

The patient in the chapter-opening scenario is going to be discharged back to the long-term care facility. Rose has also been taking care of the patient for the past week and has noticed that the patient seems sad and quieter. The patient has been diagnosed with some mild dementia; however, she has been interactive with the staff and family during the hospital stay. The patient tells Rose that even though "everyone at the home is nice," she still feels "anxious and sad" about going back. This is Rose's first time preparing a patient for discharge. Rose wonders if a psych consult might be beneficial for patients suffering from dementia. She looks for evidence in the Cochrane Library and uses the following PICO question: *In patients with mild dementia, how do psychological interventions compare to standard care (or no intervention) in helping with feelings of anxiety and depression?*

P = Patients with mild dementia
I = Psychological interventions
C = Standard care or no psychological interventions
O = Help feelings of anxiety and depression

Rose finds a meta-analysis involving 439 participants from six randomized controlled trials. The studies evaluated if cognitive–behavioral therapy (CBT), interpersonal therapy, relaxation therapy, and counseling interventions improved anxiety and depression. These treatments were modified and geared toward people suffering from dementia or cognitive impairment. The CBT combined social support and Tai Chi exercises as well as strategies to combat challenging and negative thoughts. Counseling session included education and therapeutic conversations. The interpersonal therapies focused on identifying and resolving conflicts that caused distress. The overall evidence seems to indicate that these interventions helped decrease anxiety and depression in patients with mild dementia. After reading the study, Rose decides to ask the doctor about a possible outpatient psychiatry referral as part of the discharge plan for her patient.

REFERENCE:

Orgeta, V., Qazi, A., Spector, A. E., & Orrell, M. (2014). Psychological treatments for depression and anxiety in dementia and mild cognitive impairment. *Cochrane Database of Systematic Reviews*, Issue 1, Art. No.: CD009125. doi: 10.1002/14651858.CD009125.pub2

Delirium, depression, and dementia are the three primary mental impairments that affect cognition throughout the life span.

DELIRIUM

Delirium is an acute change in mentation and represents a high risk to patients. Delirium, which is considered a medical emergency, is defined per the DSM-IV as "acute and fluctuating brain organ dysfunction, presenting with a disturbance of consciousness with reduced ability to focus, sustain, or shift attention" (APA, 2000). Delirium is quite common among hospitalized patients; as many as 80% of patients in intensive care units and up to 30% of patients in acute medical surgical units will experience delirium (Kostas, Zimmerman, & Rudolph, 2013). Multiple studies have shown that delirium poses a risk to patients both while they are in the hospital and when they are discharged. Patients have a higher incidence of mortality, longer time spent in the hospital, increased costs of care, and greater long-term cognitive dysfunction (Ely et al., 2004).

There are three types of delirium: hypoactive, hyperactive, and mixed. Patients are agitated in hyperactive delirium and often disruptive within the unit (Kostas et al., 2013). Hypoactive delirium is often termed "quiet delirium" because patients are withdrawn and lethargic and appear sedated. Hypoactive delirium, the most common subset, is underdiagnosed and carries a higher risk for mortality (Kostas et al., 2013). In the mixed form, which is a combination of hypoactive and hyperactive delirium, the patient's behavior waxes and wanes over a 24-hour period.

Nurses must identify delirium early and ensure interventions are in place that will hasten delirium and mitigate potential complications associated with undiagnosed delirium. The first step in delirium identification is to know the patient's baseline cognitive status. Institutions need an organized baseline tool that will allow healthcare givers to identify early changes that indicate delirium. Multiple tools are available that have proven successful in the identification of delirium. A commonly used and validated tool is the Confusion Assessment Method (CAM), first established in the 1990s (Inouye et al., 1990). (See http://www.healthcare.uiowa.edu/igec/tools/cognitive/CAM.pdf.) In addition, the CAM-ICU is a version of the CAM for the specialized assessment needs for intensive care unit patients. Essentially, both scales assist caregivers in identifying the key features of delirium: acute onset/fluctuating course and inattention, in combination with either disorganized thinking or altered level of consciousness (Inouye et al., 1990).

An essential caregiver role is identifying potential causes of delirium. Nurses spend the largest amount of time with patients and are well posed to identify factors contributing to delirium. Nurses also should work with providers and pharmacists to review patients' medication and identify common medications that exacerbate delirium. A multidisciplinary approach to delirium prevention and management facilitates resolution of delirium symptomatology. It is essential that nurses and providers are able to recognize an acute neurologic emergency in a delirious patient (see Table 37-1). Physicians may order

TABLE 37-1 RED FLAGS OF NEUROLOGIC EMERGENCY	
Neurologic Emergency	Red Flags
Stroke	Facial droop
	Motor weakness
	Pronator drift
	Ataxia
	Speech dysfunction
Seizure	Staring spells
	Eye deviation and unresponsiveness
	Periods of loss of consciousness
	Muscle twitching
	Periods of stuttering

medications to manage behavior; effort should be taken to not use medications that may exacerbate delirium including benzodiazepines.

Multiple nursing interventions facilitate improvement in delirium. Many of the interventions directly relate to the patient's environment and include managing the patient's sensory needs, early mobilization, minimizing use of restraints, promoting sleep/wake schedule, and frequent reorientation to the patient care environment (Fong, Tulebaev, & Inouye, 2009). Sensory strategies include ensuring use of glasses/hearing aids and eliminating nuisance environmental noise.

Another protective strategy is for nurses to recognize patients at high risk of developing delirium. Several populations of patients have been identified as having an increase likelihood of delirium development and include those who have experienced stroke, history of alcohol/drug abuse, dementia, sepsis, and respiratory failure, those patients who have received anesthesia, and those in isolation (Desai, Chau, & George, 2013). Acute stroke patients have a 13% to 48% incidence of delirium, and strokes in certain areas in the brain pose a higher risk (Kostalova et al., 2012). Intensive care unit patients are at the top of the risk category, and risk increases with length of time spent on a ventilator (Kostas et al., 2013).

Delirium has been a diagnosis dating back to 500 BC when Hippocrates described a syndrome with "acute onset of behavioral change, sleep disturbance, and cognitive deficit most commonly associated with the onset of fever. A second syndrome, lethargus, described inertia and dulling of the senses" (Field & Wall, 2013, p. 170). Some advancements that have been made in the care of delirious patients focus on early identification and management of symptoms, yet delirium remains a significant cause of morbidity and mortality in the hospitalized patient. Nurses continue to play a strong role in decreasing mortality associated with delirium.

DEMENTIA

Dementia is a clinical syndrome involving progressive impairment of intellectual function and memory. It is not associated with disturbance in level of consciousness, but it does interfere with social or occupational functioning. People with dementia experience a gradual decline in all cognitive processes,

TABLE 37-2 CHARACTERISTICS OF DEPRESSION, DELIRIUM, AND DEMENTIA

	Depression	Delirium	Dementia
Onset	Weeks to months	Hours to days	Months to years
Mood	Low/apathetic	Fluctuates	Fluctuates
Course	Chronic; responds to treatment	Acute; responds to treatment	Chronic, with deterioration over time
Self-Awareness	Likely to be concerned about memory impairment	May be aware of changes in cognition; fluctuates	Likely to hide or be unaware of cognitive deficits
ADLs	May neglect basic self-care	May be intact or impaired	May be intact early, impaired as disease progresses
Instrumental Activities of Daily Living (IADLs)	May be intact or impaired	May be intact or impaired	May be intact early, impaired before ADLs as disease progresses

Reprinted with permission from: Gagliardi, J. P. (2008, June). Differentiating among depression, delirium, and dementia in elderly patients. *Virtual Mentor, 10*(6), 383–388. http://virtualmentor.ama-assn.org/2008/06/cprl1-0806.html

as contrasted to delirium, in which dysfunctions may be reversible (Table 37-2). Potential causes for dementia include trauma, circulatory interferences, genetic predisposition, alterations in neurotransmitters, and infectious agents.

Twenty-five million people worldwide have dementia including 7% of the patients over the age of 65 (Gealogo, 2013, p. 347). Dementia differs from delirium in that in dementia, the cognitive changes occur over time and are permanent versus the acute onset of delirium. The five main subsets of dementia include Alzheimer dementia (AD), vascular dementia (VAD), frontotemporal dementia (FTD), Lewy body dementia (LBD), and Parkinson disease dementia (PDD) (Jablonski, 2013).

Alzheimer Dementia

Alzheimer is a progressive disease in which there is cerebral atrophy or shrinking of the cortex. Approximately 5 million people in the United States have Alzheimer, and it is expected that as many as 16 million will have AD by 2050 (Uriri-Glover, McCarthy, & Cesarotti, 2012). Common characteristics of AD are memory loss, behavioral issues, and sleep problems. Typically, patients will have symptoms that worsen over many years. Early diagnosis allows the patient and family to plan for the future including preference for advanced life directives. Diagnosis is mainly dependent on the progressiveness of the symptoms, family history, and, ultimately, on pathology found on autopsy.

Vascular Dementia

One of the early theories of origin of Alzheimer disease revolved around the idea that lack of adequate blood flow to the brain caused formation of plaques. With the advancement of neurovascular imaging, vascular changes can be diagnosed. VAD is a term that refers to cognitive impairment caused by arterial brain lesions. VAD is heterogeneous in its presentation as symptoms will revolve around areas of brain affected. Examples of symptoms can include **aphasia**, motor weakness, vision changes, and seizures. Patients with previous stroke are at high risk for developing VAD with or without onset of new ischemic injuries (Korczyn, Vakhapova, & Grinberg, 2012).

Frontotemporal Dementia

FTD refers to the clinical manifestation of nerve cell loss and impairment of the frontal and anterior temporal lobes.

Diagnosis can be challenging as the presenting symptoms are often either behavioral or language difficulties versus cognitive in nature. Age of onset is typically in patients less than 65 years old, and patients have an average survival of 6 to 11 years once symptoms begin (Kurz, Kurz, Ellis, & Lautenschlager, 2014). No current medications are available to treat the progression of FTD.

Lewy Body Dementia/Parkinson Disease Dementia

LBD refers to a specific type of dementia with clumps of protein aggregating that cause neurodegeneration over time. Core features of LBD include fluctuating cognition, REM sleep disorder, falls, orthostatic hypotension, and urinary incontinence (Gealogo, 2013). Diagnosis is made when dementia onset occurs less than one year after diagnosis with Parkinson disease. If dementia occurs greater than 1 year after Parkinson disease occurs, then the dementia is considered Parkinson dementia.

Some forms of dementia have medications that are available to treat symptoms and to attempt to slow the progression of the disease. However, the most effective interventions remain those focused on environmental management, therapeutic reorientation, safety promotion, and maintaining quality of life. Nurses play a key role in not only providing direct care to patients but also identifying caregiver stress.

DEPRESSION

As patients age, they experience multiple losses that can include loss of spouse or friends, physical limitations, changes in living situations, and financial strain. Changes in mood might happen quickly and not be recognized by the patient or their family as depression. Caregivers and providers need to screen patients when interacting with them because depression is not a consequence of the normal aging process. In addition, depression is a largely treatable disease (Downing, Caprio, & Lyness, 2013).

Common symptoms of depression in the elderly include forgetfulness, increased fatigue, and a definite change in mood or behavior. Unlike dementia symptoms, cognitive impairment related to depression is typically connected to a specific issue and is not widespread. Patients might describe feelings of being overwhelmed and that their memory worsens when they are stressed.

Suicide risk is a realistic concern for older patients as "5% to 10% of older adults experience suicidal ideation but that rate rises to 30 % when we only consider older adults with a diagnosis of major depression" (Downing et al., 2013, p. 7). Therefore, nurses need to screen patients routinely for potential suicide risk. Suicidal ideation is directly correlated to suicide in the older adult as compared to younger individuals where suicide is typically associated with drugs and alcohol. Some providers may be reluctant to start antidepressants in the elderly due to the presence of polypharmacy, but antidepressants have shown to be effective in the elderly population.

ALTERED LEVEL OF AROUSAL

Arousal is a person's level of reactivity to incoming stimuli. Levels of arousal may be categorized as hypervigilant, alert, lethargic, obtunded, and comatose. Hypervigilant means the person is acutely aware of environmental stimuli and may startle at unexpected noise; hypervigilance is often accompanied by a decreased ability to concentrate. Alert means the person is awake and fully aware of incoming stimuli. Lethargic describes the patient who is not fully awake and tends to drift off to sleep when not actively stimulated. Obtunded describes the patient who is difficult to arouse and when aroused is confused. Coma describes the patient who is completely unresponsive to incoming stimuli. Arousal does not imply the ability to focus attention.

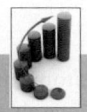

OUTCOME-BASED TEACHING PLANS

Mrs. Harold has come to the clinic with concerns about her husband. Mr. Harold has had increasing problems with memory as evidenced by repeatedly asking the same questions, telling his wife the same things repeatedly, and forgetting where he puts things. Mrs. Harold thinks that he is beginning to realize this too. She wants some guidance on how to help him.

OUTCOME

Mrs. Harold will assist Mr. Harold to maintain orientation as to time and place.

STRATEGIES

- Explore with Mr. Harold his concerns about his memory.
- If Mr. Harold is motivated to improve his memory, use cues for reality data such as clocks, calendars, and verbal reminders.
- Encourage Mrs. Harold to speak clearly and in short, simple statements.
- Discuss the need to maintain a predictable routine or schedule for Mr. Harold.
- Promote the use of lists and of stability of familiar objects in the home so that he can develop habits of always placing things in the same location.
- Encourage activities, visits, and meaningful interaction with family and friends.
- Positively reinforce small changes in behavior that indicate increasing orientation to reality.
- Encourage Mrs. Harold to focus Mr. Harold's attention deliberately (with little stress and distractions) on information that he needs to remember.
- Suggest the use of both vision and hearing to provide input from two perceptual sources.
- Discuss the usefulness of making lists and using other association techniques to help Mr. Harold remember tasks and information.

- Encourage the regular practice or rehearsal of retrieving information from memory, such as doing crossword puzzles.

EVALUATION

8/19/17: 15:30—The patient
- Maintains orientation to time and place during the daytime
- Discusses his concerns about his memory with family and health providers
- Utilizes clocks, calendars, and verbal reminders as evidenced by verbal responses
- Speaks clearly and in short, simple statements and responds appropriately to a predictable routine/schedule
- Develops habits of placing things in the same location as a result of the use of lists and familiar objects being in the same place in the home with a moderate degree of regularity
- Participates appropriately in activities, visits, and meaningful interaction with family and friends
- Receives positive reinforcement for small changes in behavior that indicate increasing orientation reality and responds favorably
- Receives encouragement to focus attention on information that is necessary to remember
- Receives both visual and auditory input to improve communication
- Participates in creating lists to help remember tasks and information
- Practices retrieving information from memory such as doing crossword puzzles until he becomes frustrated

—M. Klim, RN

Impaired Communication

Aphasia is the complete or partial loss of language abilities including understanding speech (auditory comprehension), reading, speaking, writing, arithmetic, and expression through pantomime. This acquired communication dysfunction results from brain damage but does not affect intelligence. Aphasias are produced mostly through damage to the cortical language areas of the dominant left hemisphere. Rarely, an injury affects one isolated area of speech, but injury usually affects all speech and language functions. The most common cause of aphasia is related to an interruption in circulation as a result of a cerebrovascular incident. Significant improvement in speech and communication may occur in the first 6 months and can continue up to 18 months after the onset of aphasia. The prognosis of poststroke aphasia depends on the type of language impairment. According to a research study by Bakheit, Shaw, Carrington, and Griffiths (2007), the rate of improvement in language function is highest in the first 4 weeks after a stroke. Recovery from aphasia may be influenced by the intensity and duration of the language therapy.

The manifestation of speech impairment depends on location and extent of damage. It can range from slight slurring of speech to total loss of communication. Aphasia has been described and categorized based on lesion location and linguistic deficit ("Merck Manual," 2014). The four most common types of aphasia are expressive (Broca's), receptive (Wernicke's), anomic, and global.

EXPRESSIVE APHASIA

Expressive aphasia (also called Broca, motor, or nonfluent aphasia) is characterized by limited speech that is slow and halting with great effort, reduced grammar, and poor **articulation**. Because intellect is not necessarily impaired, the person knows what he or she wants to say but cannot find the needed words. **Anomia** refers to problems with word retrieval. In expressive aphasia, the person's speech often sounds like a telegraph message consisting of isolated or small groups of words and lacking tone or inflection. Writing is also affected and can be as severely or more severely impaired than speech.

Expressive aphasia can cause extreme frustration and anger. Sometimes, the anger shows in physical behaviors such as pushing objects or people away and shouting. Often, patients direct anger at people who care the most about them. Such behavior makes it difficult for spouses or significant others to understand what is happening.

RECEPTIVE APHASIA

Receptive aphasia (also called Wernicke, sensory, or fluent aphasia) is characterized by speech that is well articulated and has good melody and normal or slightly faster rate. The major manifestations are impaired auditory comprehension and feedback. People with receptive aphasia have difficulty understanding spoken and written words. They talk a great deal but may not make sense. Their speech lacks specific content. Their ability to read, write, listen, concentrate, or follow instructions is impaired; the severity level is usually consistent with or worse than the speech impairment. The affected person is unaware of the language impairment and appears euphoric in relation to his or her language problems.

A person with receptive aphasia also has a pattern of symptoms referred to as right hemisphere syndrome. He or she neglects the paralyzed side of the body, even to the point of not knowing that the left arm or leg is really his or hers. Behaviorally, these patients are impulsive, lack insight into their deficits, and have poor judgment. They are said to display inappropriate behavior when actually their behavior is a result of their injury. The combination of these symptoms and behaviors makes rehabilitation difficult.

GLOBAL APHASIA

Global aphasia results from severe and extensive damage to all language areas (Broca and Wernicke). These patients have no consistent functional skills in any language modality. They cannot speak or understand speech, nor can they read or write. Some patients' speech consists of meaningless, recurrent sounds.

DYSARTHRIA

Dysarthria refers to a group of speech disorders that result from a disturbance of motor control, weakness, paralysis, or incoordination of the oral musculature. It results from damage to the central or peripheral nervous system. Patients with dysarthria usually have normal auditory comprehension and can select and order words correctly. They have a motor speech disorder that causes them difficulty in saying words and sounds precisely, using appropriate stress, loudness, pitch, and control. The result is speech described as "slurred," "heavy," or unclear. There are numerous types of dysarthria. The specific type depends on the site of the neurologic lesion.

Recall the older patient from the case scenario who has just returned to the unit after repair for a fractured hip. Recall that she is more agitated and confused than she was before surgery. Use the concept map (Fig. 37-5) to help understand and manage the patient's confusion and agitation.

ASSESSMENT

Assessment is essential to nursing care for patients with actual or potential alterations in cognitive function. Assessment identifies patients with alterations in cognitive processes and describes the patient's ability to function safely within his or her environment. Determining how a person functions and the quality of the social and physical environment guides the establishment of patient goals and nursing interventions. When assessing a patient with communication difficulties, remain attentive and be patient when the person is attempting to communicate. Doing so places the person at ease and encourages him or her to initiate communication. Taking time to ask appropriate questions, pausing, listening, and being genuinely interested in what is being communicated are patient centered. Patient-centered interviewing can enhance effectiveness and efficiency of care (Boscart, 2009; Lein & Wills, 2007).

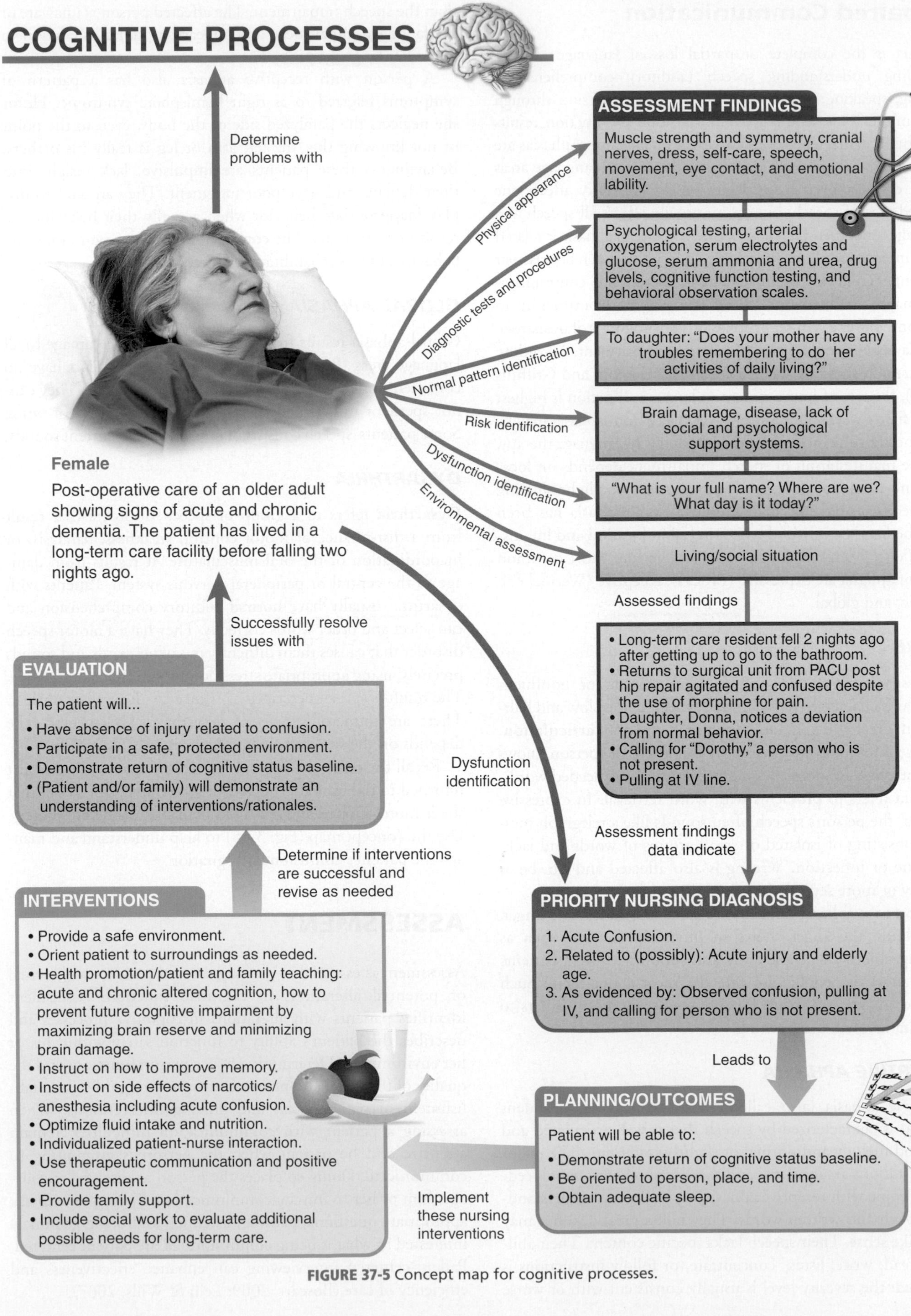

COGNITIVE PROCESSES

Determine problems with

Female

Post-operative care of an older adult showing signs of acute and chronic dementia. The patient has lived in a long-term care facility before falling two nights ago.

Physical appearance

Diagnostic tests and procedures

Normal pattern identification

Risk identification

Dysfunction identification

Environmental assessment

ASSESSMENT FINDINGS

Muscle strength and symmetry, cranial nerves, dress, self-care, speech, movement, eye contact, and emotional lability.

Psychological testing, arterial oxygenation, serum electrolytes and glucose, serum ammonia and urea, drug levels, cognitive function testing, and behavioral observation scales.

To daughter: "Does your mother have any troubles remembering to do her activities of daily living?"

Brain damage, disease, lack of social and psychological support systems.

"What is your full name? Where are we? What day is it today?"

Living/social situation

Assessed findings

- Long-term care resident fell 2 nights ago after getting up to go to the bathroom.
- Returns to surgical unit from PACU post hip repair agitated and confused despite the use of morphine for pain.
- Daughter, Donna, notices a deviation from normal behavior.
- Calling for "Dorothy," a person who is not present.
- Pulling at IV line.

Successfully resolve issues with

EVALUATION

The patient will...

- Have absence of injury related to confusion.
- Participate in a safe, protected environment.
- Demonstrate return of cognitive status baseline.
- (Patient and/or family) will demonstrate an understanding of interventions/rationales.

Dysfunction identification

Determine if interventions are successful and revise as needed

INTERVENTIONS

- Provide a safe environment.
- Orient patient to surroundings as needed.
- Health promotion/patient and family teaching: acute and chronic altered cognition, how to prevent future cognitive impairment by maximizing brain reserve and minimizing brain damage.
- Instruct on how to improve memory.
- Instruct on side effects of narcotics/anesthesia including acute confusion.
- Optimize fluid intake and nutrition.
- Individualized patient-nurse interaction.
- Use therapeutic communication and positive encouragement.
- Provide family support.
- Include social work to evaluate additional possible needs for long-term care.

Assessment findings data indicate

PRIORITY NURSING DIAGNOSIS

1. Acute Confusion.
2. Related to (possibly): Acute injury and elderly age.
3. As evidenced by: Observed confusion, pulling at IV, and calling for person who is not present.

Leads to

PLANNING/OUTCOMES

Patient will be able to:

- Demonstrate return of cognitive status baseline.
- Be oriented to person, place, and time.
- Obtain adequate sleep.

Implement these nursing interventions

FIGURE 37-5 Concept map for cognitive processes.

Normal Pattern Identification

Collection of subjective information helps to identify patterns of cognitive function; risk factors that may predispose patients to alterations in roles, relationships, or functional patterns; and actual cognitive or communication dysfunction. Gathering subjective data about cognitive abilities is a time-consuming process that usually involves multiple, brief, planned interactions with many people. Keep a general assessment framework in mind to remember all key areas (Box 37-1). The situation can be especially complex when the patient is hospitalized and unknown to the staff. Nurses, physicians, and social workers may individually gather then collaboratively share information from many sources. Nurses are in the best position to gather data related to the patient's normal pattern of function, areas of risk, and areas of actual dysfunction. All healthcare team members must document essential subjective data for consistency and collaboration.

BOX 37-1   **Nursing Assessment: Cognition**

Current Cognitive Function
A. Objective tool—Mini-Mental Status or Pfeiffer
B. Subjective evaluation
  1. Attention
  2. Ability to answer questions
  3. Appropriateness of affect

History and Time Course of Cognitive Impairment
A. Previous difficulties with thinking, perception, or communication
B. Previous head trauma—details of accidents or periods of unconsciousness
C. Previous stroke, hypertension, and elevated blood cholesterol
D. When current symptoms began and how they evolved; include information from family and friends

Contributing Factors
A. Chronic or acute illness
  1. Laboratory abnormalities
  2. CNS disorders
  3. Multisystem disease
B. Use/abuse of medications
  1. Drugs with CNS effects
  2. Drugs with CNS side effects
  3. Drugs with potential for toxicity
  4. Use of recreational drugs or alcohol
C. Sensory impairment
  1. Vision
  2. Hearing
D. Quality of environment
  1. Family support
  2. Frequency and number of social contacts
  3. Availability of transportation
  4. Adequacy of financial resources
  5. Nutritional status
  6. Living situation
E. Psychological stressors
  1. Bereavement
  2. Major life change
  3. Lack of financial resources
  4. Family crisis
  5. Loss of independence
  6. Serious illness
F. Family history of dementia, schizophrenia, or affective disorders

Current Functional Status
A. Ability to communicate verbally or nonverbally
B. Ability to understand spoken and written word
C. Literacy
D. Ability to perform ADLs
E. Amount of assistance currently available in the home
F. Ability to exercise good judgment
G. Safety of home environment
H. Nutritional adequacy
  1. Protein, iron, sodium, and calcium intake
  2. Adequacy of fluid intake
  3. Previously identified nutritional disorder
I. Sleep and rest
  1. Restfulness after a night's sleep
  2. Changes in life events, patterns, or current environment
J. Motor activity
  1. Agitation or withdrawal from activity
  2. Recent patterns of increased or decreased mobility
K. ADLs
  1. Level of independence in hygiene and home maintenance
  2. Problem-solving abilities, such as money management, use of telephone, and interactions with needed services

Physical Assessment
A. Respiratory function
  1. Rate, rhythm, and depth of normal respirations
  2. Lung and breath sounds
B. Cardiovascular function
  1. Rate, rhythm, and quality of heartbeat
  2. Carotid pulses and bruits
C. Nutrition and metabolism
D. Height, weight, and skin turgor
E. Musculoskeletal function
  1. Muscle tone and strength
  2. Gait
F. Sensory function
  1. Vision
  2. Hearing
G. Neurologic function
  1. Cranial nerves
  2. Involuntary movements
  3. Deep tendon reflexes

TABLE 37-3 EXPRESSION AND COMPREHENSION WITH MAJOR TYPES OF APHASIA

Types of Aphasia	Oral Expression	Written Expression	Comprehension
Expressive (Broca or motor)	Nonfluent, telegraphic	Limited	Usually good
Receptive (Wernicke or sensory)	Fluent, speech well articulated, disorganized content	Impaired	Impaired
Anomic	Speech fluent, talks around the subject	Variable, mild to severe impairment	Variable, mild to severe impairment
Global	Speech very poor, meaningless recurrent sounds	Severely impaired	Severely impaired

When assessing thought processes, gather information about the patient's usual cognitive function and its impact on daily living. The patient's ability to communicate usually will be apparent in the assessment interview. Systematic assessment can determine the nature and extent of the impairment and its effects on the patient and family. Changes in other cognitive functions are often nonspecific and most obvious to those who know the affected person well. For this reason, elicit information from family and friends as well as from the patient.

To determine the type of communication disorder the patient is experiencing, assess verbal expression, written expression, comprehension, and nonverbal expression. Table 37-3 defines the expected comprehension and verbal and written expression for the four major types of aphasia. Box 37-2 also delineates communication abilities to assess for in the major types of aphasia. Answers to these questions assist in determining the degree of the patient's communication dysfunction.

Information about other cognitive functions is best obtained systematically. Assess consciousness, the most basic cognitive process, first. Describe it in terms of the intensity of the stimulus used and the nature of the patient's response. Next, evaluate ability to pay attention. Then, assess abilities to use language and memory because they are basic to reasoning and problem solving.

The significance of any cognitive impairment lies in its relationship to function in daily living, not in the impairment itself. For example, an older woman may tell the nurse that she does not remember the names, dosages, and purposes of her medications. On the surface, it seems that she has a problem with medication management. Upon further questioning, the nurse learns that the patient identifies her pills by color and uses a medication management system that groups pills in daily dosage units. The patient's granddaughter, a registered nurse, oversees the medication management. This woman and her family have developed an effective system to compensate for a mild cognitive deficit.

BOX 37-2 | **Initial Assessment Concerns About Communication**

Is the Person Able to Speak at All?
If so, is the speech intelligible and appropriate to the situation?
Does the person use gestures or point in an effort to communicate?
Is the person literate?
How much formal education does the person have?
Is the person able to speak another language?
Can the person understand and follow simple one-step commands?
Did the person have a speech difficulty before this most recent difficulty?
Was the person previously an active conversationalist, or did he or she prefer to listen?

Assessment for Major Types of Aphasia Verbal Expression
Does the person speak easily, fluently?
Is the content appropriate in context?
Does the person initiate speech on his or her own?
Is the speech telegraphic (short, choppy)?
Is the speech organized?
Does the verbal output contain recurrent sounds?
Does the person name objects correctly?
Does the person repeat words and phrases easily?

Written Expression
Can the person write his or her own name and address correctly?
Can the person produce a short narrative written paragraph?
Does the written product have appropriate meaning?

Comprehension
Does the person give any indication of hearing impairment?
Does the person answer simple, open-ended questions appropriately?
Does the person answer yes/no questions in appropriate context?
Can the person correctly point to an object that has been named?
Does the person respond appropriately to simple commands?

Nonverbal Expression
Observe for the type of affect (sign of emotion):
- Flat—no sign of emotion
- Labile—wide fluctuation in emotions
Observe gestures for appropriateness to the situation.
Observe for the integrated context of voice tone, emotional expression, and body movement.

Detecting mild to moderate cognitive impairment during an interview or casual conversation can be difficult. People who are aware of and embarrassed by their poor memory can become experts at giving vague answers and steering conversations into "safe" territory. Using a formalized approach to cognitive testing (such as the Folstein or Pfeiffer mental status examinations) is advisable if cognitive impairment is suspected. A nonjudgmental, warm, and friendly demeanor is important to put the person at ease.

Assessing perception of reality includes determining the person's orientation to time, place, and person (sometimes referred to as "orientation times 3"). Determine orientation to time by asking questions pertaining to time: year, day, date, and approximate time of day. Determine orientation to place by asking questions related to city or location. Assess orientation to person by asking the patient his or her name. Orientation to time will usually show deficits first, with deficits in orientation as to identity being the last and most severe form of dysfunction.

Levels of consciousness and orientation are not by themselves adequate assessments of cognitive function. Comprehensive assessment includes the use of a mental status questionnaire (such as Folstein's Mini-Mental State Examination) and a behavioral rating scale (such as the classic Clinical Assessment of Confusion–A or the NEECHAM Confusion Scale) (Hattori et al., 2009). In assessing reality, clarify how the environment may be contributing to disorganized thinking. For example, an older woman in a long-term care facility calls for her son and does not understand why he will not stop to see her when she saw him pass by her door. In exploring the environment, the nurse realizes that the woman is not wearing her glasses and that the man who walked by had a build and clothes similar to that of her son. As a result, the patient misperceived the information. Failure to be thorough in assessment might lead to a wrong conclusion that results in attaching a label of "confused" to a patient who is actually having difficulty with perception. Do not allow personal perceptions of reality to overshadow the ability to monitor another person's perception of reality.

Risk Identification

Risk identification assesses for physiologic, psychological, and environmental factors that increase the likelihood of impaired cognitive processes. The degree of risk from each category will depend on the individual patient and setting.

Patients with brain damage from stroke or head injury, impaired speech apparatus (e.g., laryngectomy or tracheotomy), and other temporary dysfunctions are at greatest risk for communication impairment. Pathophysiologic factors, such as cerebral, neurologic, respiratory, or auditory impairments, and laryngeal infection or edema place the person at high risk for altered communication. A community health nurse making a home visit to an older patient will include a detailed assessment of social and psychological support systems as well as physiologic assessment.

Medications can be a primary risk factor for altered thought processes, either alone or in combination with other substances. Patients and families need to know the expected actions of medications, potential side effects, potential interactions, and indications of toxicity. Many instances of altered cognitive function can be traced directly to the addition of a new medication, toxic levels of a usual medication, or unexpected interactions with other substances. Patients and families need to be alert to subtle changes in cognition and mental status in relation to their pharmacologic therapies. As part of the assessment process, obtain a detailed medication history from primary or secondary sources. Include all medications (prescribed, over-the-counter preparations, herbal remedies, and others) that the patient takes. Note medications recently added and stopped. Be sure to obtain information about the amount of alcohol the patient consumes.

Having multiple risk factors does not always lead to dysfunction. Individual strengths and resources can enable a person to withstand multiple stressors. An important part of a nursing assessment is identifying existing and potential coping resources. Interventions can then be designed to support and develop these resources.

Dysfunction Identification

Analyze information to determine if dysfunction is present for a specific patient. When identifying dysfunction, document assessed data in clear terms that others can easily understand. Instead of using vague terms like "slightly confused" or "poor attention span," describe the behaviors associated with the deficits precisely, using anecdotes when appropriate. Phrases like "oriented to self only," "needs verbal cuing to wash face," and "when given toothbrush, combed hair with it" provide clear information for identifying dysfunction.

Physical Assessment

Assessment of physiologic function provides clues as to the source of altered cognitive processes. Because the earliest clinical signs of changes in the levels of oxygen, electrolytes, and metabolic by-products are lethargy, mild confusion, and impaired thinking, assess those components. Assessing these functions requires skill in the physical examination and laboratory evaluation. Physical functions to be assessed are listed in Box 37-1. The mouth, tongue, and facial muscles must be intact to form and articulate words correctly. Patients with altered communication related to impaired motor functioning or brain damage need a thorough examination of the muscles and organs of speech. Chapter 16 discusses assessment methods for cranial nerves.

Observation is useful for identifying clues to impaired thinking and to defining possible causes of impaired communication. Disheveled appearance, disorganized speech, and abnormal movements are obvious indicators of dysfunction, especially when they represent a change in status. Difficulty maintaining eye contact, a tendency to repeat the same story, inappropriate responses to stress or stimuli, and emotional lability can also indicate difficulty with thought processes. At times, these behavioral changes are subtle; repeated observation of behaviors is necessary.

The tongue receives its motor innervation from the 12th cranial nerve (hypoglossal). Assess motor control of the tongue by instructing the patient to protrude the tongue. If there is damage to the hypoglossal nerve, the tongue will deviate to the side of the weakness as the strong side pushes it forward unopposed.

The facial muscles are innervated by the fifth (trigeminal) and seventh (facial) cranial nerves. Assess the motor function of these nerves by noting the symmetry of facial movement when asking the patient to show teeth, purse lips, and frown. When the patient's face is at rest, note any asymmetry of the forehead or cheeks along with facial drooping or drooling.

The muscles of swallowing and the gag reflex are supplied by the 9th (glossopharyngeal), 10th (vagus), and 11th (accessory) cranial nerves. The larynx is supplied by the 10th cranial nerve alone. Motor weakness of the soft palate contributes to difficulty swallowing (dysphagia). To test swallowing, ask the patient to swallow chips of ice. The ice gives some substance for the patient to manipulate in the mouth yet introduces only water if he or she is unable to swallow successfully.

Impairment in the use of the larynx is immediately obvious with an endotracheal tube or tracheostomy or a ventilator. Because the movement of air bypasses the laryngeal function, the patient is unable to communicate verbally. Assess if the patient is able to use other modes of communication such as gestures, codes using eye blinks or hands, or written notes.

Many factors complicate the assessment of cognitive function in infants and young children. Because their language skills are not fully developed and they have difficulty expressing thoughts, observation of behavior becomes the primary data source.

Diagnostic Tests and Procedures

Patients with altered communication are evaluated by speech pathologists, who perform detailed assessments of speech, expression, comprehension, and swallowing. Results from this assessment contribute to the plan of care and help to establish communication with patients. Patients with altered thought processes may require extensive testing to determine contributing (and possibly reversible) factors.

PHYSIOLOGIC TESTS

Physiologic causes of confusion can result from disorders of multiple systems. Their diagnoses and management require multiple tests and procedures, from simple urinalysis to highly technical scans. Nurses use tests such as weight, vital signs, serum electrolytes, complete blood count, cultures, and measures of oxygen saturation to identify potential contributors. Monitoring these parameters helps to identify imbalances and to target early interventions to prevent complications.

Arterial Oxygen

Arterial oxygen level is best determined by measuring arterial blood gases. An oxygen partial pressure greater than 60 mm Hg reflects adequate oxygenation. A noninvasive technique for assessing oxygenation is pulse oximetry, which measures oxygen saturation (percentage of hemoglobin that is bound to oxygen). A saturation of 90% correlates with a partial pressure of 60 mm Hg, given a normal level of hemoglobin. If a low (less than 90%) value is determined, oxygen therapy and further evaluation may be indicated.

Electrolytes

A serum sodium level less than 135 mEq/L or greater than 145 mEq/L may result in cognitive impairment. Mild confusion can progress to agitation or severe confusion, with hallucinations or delusions followed by stupor and coma if the condition is untreated. Because brain cells can adapt to slow changes, severity of symptoms is related to how rapidly the sodium level drops.

Calcium

An elevated level of serum calcium can cause severe defects in neuromuscular activity with cognitive manifestations of lethargy or decreased level of consciousness. When the total serum calcium exceeds 14 mg/dL (normal level is 8.5 to 10.5 mg/dL), confusion is common, and further increases in calcium concentration may result in coma or death.

Serum Glucose

Serum glucose levels below 70 mg/dL typically cause shakiness or nervousness but can progress to cause altered cognition. Although the determination of serum glucose from venipuncture is the most accurate method of measurement, the widespread availability of capillary blood glucose monitoring has promoted reliable self-assessment for patients at home and rapid assessment of patients in a clinical setting.

Ammonia and Urea

Ammonia and urea are potentially toxic by-products of protein metabolism. Liver failure can cause elevated ammonia levels; high blood ammonia levels are toxic to the brain cells. Kidney failure can cause an elevated blood urea nitrogen level and produce confusion.

Toxic Levels of Drugs

Toxic levels of drugs can result from impaired ability to metabolize or excrete them. Serum concentration of many drugs can be measured to determine therapeutic and toxic levels. People with impaired hepatic or renal function are at risk for drug toxicity and require dosage reduction and regular monitoring. Drug and toxicologic screening is indicated for drug overdose or toxic exposure.

TESTS OF COGNITIVE FUNCTION

Intellectual function consists of short- and long-term memory, comprehension, and concentration. These straightforward abilities are easily tested and converted to objective measurements with standardized tools. IQ tests attempt to measure intellectual function. These tests rely on measuring verbal ability and vocabulary within a structured questioning format. They are standardized to the vocabulary and cultural experience of white, middle-class Americans and have questionable validity when administered to other ethnic and socioeconomic groups. Remember that standardized tests of verbal ability are not sensitive to sociocultural differences and so should not be used to assess "normality" for all groups. The primary usefulness of standardized tests is that each person using them encounters the same information, thus providing a common base of information and quantification for comparison.

Because of their limited attention span, children find it difficult to cooperate with tedious assessment procedures. Assessment tools for children focus on the observation of behavior, especially behavior elicited by a standard set of stimuli.

Standardized tools are available for the objective assessment of mental status. Two examples are the Pfeiffer Short Portable Mental Status Questionnaire (Pfeiffer, 1975) (Box 37-3) and the Mini-Mental State Examination (Folstein, Folstein, & McHugh, 1975). A score of 7 or less on the Pfeiffer or 20 or less on the Mini-Mental State Examination indicates significant cognitive impairment. These tools are most useful when given to healthy people repeatedly, which allows identification of changes from baseline. Administering these tools during an acute confusional state can help quantify daily changes. Without a premorbid baseline and with physiologic imbalance though, little can be determined about the patient's change from baseline function. There is a specific battery of tests used to diagnose dementia.

BEHAVIORAL OBSERVATION SCALES

Several instruments have been designed to measure behavioral aspects of acute confusion/delirium in hospitalized patients. The NEECHAM Confusion Scale is an observational scale designed to unobtrusively detect cues to the onset of acute confusion and to monitor recovery (Hattori et al., 2009). The Delirium Index (DI) is intended to measure the severity of delirium based on patient observation of seven domains including attention, thought, consciousness, orientation, memory, perception, and psychomotor activity. The total score ranges from 0 to 21, with the higher scores indicating greater severity. The Mini-Cog is a screening tool recommended for use with older people admitted to the hospital. It measures high to low likelihood of cognitive impairment and predicts that patients with abnormal results are five times more likely to develop delirium (Sendelbach & Guthrie, 2009).

APPLY YOUR CRITICAL THINKING

Joe Moran, age 52 years, is admitted to the neurologic unit after a brawl in a bar where he fell and hit his head. When you enter his room to do the morning assessment, he is very agitated and starts yelling, "I don't belong here!" He has an intravenous infusion and is trying to get out of bed.

What additional assessment data do you need to collect at this time? How can you help maintain safety for Mr. Moran?

Check your answer in Appendix B.

NURSING DIAGNOSES

The accepted NANDA-International (North American Nursing Diagnosis Association International, [NANDA-I], 2014) nursing diagnoses for patients with cognitive/perceptual impairment are Acute Confusion, Chronic Confusion, Impaired Memory, Impaired Environmental Interpretation Syndrome, Wandering, Unilateral Neglect, and Impaired Verbal Communication. Each diagnosis describes alterations in cognitive function that interfere with daily living. Selected nursing diagnoses are presented in Table 37-4 along with selected Nursing Outcomes Classification (NOC) and Nursing Interventions Classifications (NICs).

OUTCOME IDENTIFICATION AND PLANNING

After nursing diagnoses and related factors are identified, nurses plan outcomes and interventions with patients and/or family. The goals of nursing intervention for patients with

---

BOX 37-3   Pfeiffer Mental Status Questionnaire

1. What is today's date? _____
2. What day of the week is it? _____
3. What is the name of this place? _____
4. What is your telephone number? _____
   If none, what is your address? _____
5. How old are you? _____
6. When were you born? _____
7. Who is the President of the United States now? _____
8. Who was the President before him? _____
9. What is your mother's maiden name? _____
10. Subtract 3 from 20 and keep going down to 0. _____

Total numbers of errors _____

Reprinted from Pfeiffer, E. (1975). A short portable mental status questionnaire for the assessment of organic brain deficit in elderly patients. Journal of the American Geriatrics Society, 23, 433–441.

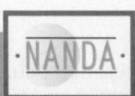

Table 37-4 SELECTED NANDA-I NURSING DIAGNOSES INVOLVING COGNITION

Nursing Dx	Related Factors	Dx Statement	NOC*	NIC†
Acute Confusion—abrupt onset of a cluster of global, transient changes and disturbances in attention, cognition, psychomotor activity, level of consciousness, and/or sleep–wake cycle	Age older than 70 y, alcohol abuse, abuse, cognitive impairment, uncontrolled pain, multiple comorbidities, medications, dehydration, infection, sensory deficit, and compromised ADLs	**Acute Confusion** R/T medications, dehydration, infection AEB fluctuation in cognition, sleep–wake cycle, level of consciousness, and in agitation or restlessness	Cognitive Orientation Distorted Thought Self-Control Electrolyte and Acid/Base Balance Fall Prevention Behavior Fluid Balance Neurologic Status: Consciousness	Cognitive Restructuring Neurologic Status: Consciousness Delirium Management Fall Prevention Memory Training Neurologic Monitoring Reality Orientation
Chronic Confusion—irreversible, long-standing, and/or progressive deterioration of intellect and personality characterized by decreased ability to interpret environmental stimuli and decreased capacity for intellectual thought processes, and manifested by disturbances of memory, orientation, and behavior	Multi-infarct dementia; Korsakoff psychosis; and brain injury, Alzheimer disease, and related dementias	**Chronic Confusion** R/T Alzheimer disease AEB altered interpretation and/or response to stimuli, altered personality, impaired memory (short and long term), impaired socialization, and decreased ability to participate in self-care	Patient Satisfaction: Safety Cognitive Orientation Distorted Thought Self-Control Fall Prevention Behavior Identity Safe Home Environment Sleep	Neurologic Status: Consciousness Dementia Management Fall Prevention Memory Training Reality Orientation

Dx, diagnosis; R/T, related to; AEB, as evidenced by.
*From: Moorhead, S., Johnson, M., Maas, M., & Swanson, E. (2013). *Iowa Outcomes Project: Nursing Outcomes Classification (NOC)* (5th ed.). St. Louis, MO: C. V. Mosby.
†From: Bulecheck, G., Butcher, H., Dochterman, J., & Wagner, C. (2013). *Iowa Intervention Project: Nursing Interventions Classification (NIC)* (6th ed.). St. Louis, MO: C. V. Mosby.
From: North American Nursing Diagnosis Association International (NANDA-I). (2014). *Nursing diagnoses: Definitions and classification, 2015–2017.* West Sussex, England: Wiley-Blackwell.

impaired cognition focus on the prevention and early recognition of the disturbance, reversal of contributing factors, and provision of an environment that compensates for existing impairments, does not predispose to new impairments, and protects patients from harm. For patients with impaired verbal communication, the goals of nursing intervention focus on establishing alternate communication methods and preventing sequelae such as loneliness and role alterations. Goals need to be individualized and take into consideration each patient's history, areas of risk, evidence of dysfunction, and related objective data. Examples of goals for the patient with Acute Confusion include the following:

- The patient will demonstrate return of cognitive status to baseline.
- The patient will obtain adequate sleep.

Examples of goals for the patient with Chronic Confusion include the following:

- The patient will function at maximal cognitive level.
- The patient will participate in ADLs at a maximum level of functioning.

Examples of goals for the patient with Impaired Memory include the following:

- The patient will report decreased forgetfulness.
- The patient will discuss methods to help with memory loss.

Examples of goals for the patient with Impaired Verbal Communication include the following:

- The patient will use effective communication techniques.
- The patient will demonstrate ability to understand what was communicated.

Examples of some nursing interventions useful in planning are outlined in Table 37-4 and discussed in the next section of the chapter.

IMPLEMENTATION

Appropriate nursing interventions vary with the specific nursing diagnosis. Preventing, reversing, and slowing the progression of dysfunction along with providing for safety and dignity are central goals of nursing care. For patients with impaired cognition, preventing alterations in roles and relationships and supporting effective relationships are central focuses of nursing intervention. Relationships are affected by the ability to communicate thoughts, feelings, needs, and other intimate aspects. Nursing interventions need to recognize those relationships and their importance.

Health Promotion

ENCOURAGING HEALTHY LIFESTYLES

Primary prevention of cognitive impairment involves maximizing brain reserve and minimizing brain damage across the life span. Maximizing brain reserve begins with adequate prenatal and early childhood nutrition and educational experiences. Preventing brain damage means preventing unintentional injuries and toxic exposures. Prevention of cardiovascular disease by controlling risk factors such as blood pressure, cholesterol, diabetes, and obesity, which can lead to cerebrovascular disease and stroke, will prevent the major cause of impaired verbal communication (Day, McGuire, & Anderson, 2009).

Maintaining a lifestyle that includes adequate nutrition, rest, regular exercise, stress management, and social activity is essential to promote cognitive function. A balanced diet with sufficient protein, iron, and other nutrients is required for cells to function optimally. A lower risk of mental decline has been noted among people who follow a Mediterranean diet, which is rich in fruits, vegetables, whole grains, and healthy fats. Serum imbalances of water, sodium, calcium, and glucose can be prevented through adequate fluid intake throughout the day in conjunction with a balanced diet. For people with known dysfunctions that place them at risk for some serum imbalances (e.g., diabetes mellitus), teach the importance of regulating the dysfunction, recognizing early indications of imbalances, and initiating preventive dietary or fluid therapy. Chapters 27 and 28 present complete discussions of ways to promote fluid and electrolyte balance and good nutrition.

Oxygen perfusion to brain cells is enhanced through the practice of regular exercise. Regular exercise also enhances cardiovascular conditioning, improves circulation throughout the body, contributes to a sense of well-being, and improves cognitive functioning. Encourage patients to develop the habit of regular, vigorous exercise. Depending on the patient, exercise may range from energetic walking to active sports. Studies have revealed that aerobic activity has an effect on cognitive functioning compared to nonaerobic activity, and participation in moderate intensity activity (approximately 1 hour a day, at least three times a week) appears to have an effect on cognitive function (Clarke, Shaw, Villalba, Alli, & Sink, 2013).

Consult a dietitian to help patients plan menus, change recipes, and learn to read food labels. Patients should monitor their serum cholesterol regularly to determine the effects of a low-fat diet and an exercise program. Encourage patients who have high blood pressure to maintain their prescribed medication regimen, check their blood pressure routinely, and follow up with their physicians.

Smoking increases the risk of cardiovascular disease and throat cancer. Encourage patients to quit. Early warning signs of throat cancer are nagging cough and chronic hoarseness. Awareness of the warning signals can be helpful for early detection or prevention.

Equally important as sufficient exercise are adequate sleep and rest. Inadequate or interrupted sleep cycles usually result in loss of REM sleep. Manifestations are fatigue and, if prolonged, forgetfulness, confusion, and disorientation. Encourage people to maintain regular sleep patterns so that they obtain sufficient sleep and feel rested when awake. Counsel patients to create an environment that is conducive to rest and sleep.

Stress management can contribute to healthy cognition by minimizing distractions, improving rest, and enhancing concentration. Effective coping skills allow patients to channel stress productively and to dissipate resulting tension. Exercise, as discussed previously, is one type of coping skill to encourage. Alcohol intake is not an appropriate coping mechanism to handle stress. Alcohol intake should be limited.

Cognitive skills developed throughout life need to be practiced regularly to be maintained. Social interaction is one such skill in which patients need to participate regularly for enjoyment of human contact, stimulation of conversation, and confirmation of personhood. Use social interaction on a one-on-one basis with patients, and encourage opportunities for interaction with others in informal groups. These interactions can provide patient feedback related to reality orientation, self-concept, and sensory perception.

For people with sensory impairments, several assistive devices can help maintain and promote cognitive function. People who have hearing difficulties can often be fitted with hearing aids. Telephone/cell phone companies can provide equipment to assist with communication, and television offers programs with printed captions that permit hearing-impaired people access to cognitive stimulation. Talking books, voice-activated computer technology, and other services from public libraries help supplement cognitive input for the visually impaired.

IMPROVING MEMORY

Fatigue, stress, and illness may temporarily reduce the efficiency with which patients are able to store information or retrieve it from memory. Reassure patients that, in most situations, no organic basis exists for simple, occasional forgetfulness. Reducing stress, relieving fatigue, or recovering from illness should eliminate the temporary difficulty.

For people with minimal memory problems, memory training programs and devices may be beneficial. Memory training programs focus on personal and compensatory capabilities to stimulate cognitive function. Encourage such patients to participate in memory training or to use principles of memory enhancement. Focusing attention deliberately on the information to be remembered helps to reduce stress and to minimize distractions. Using visual, auditory, and olfactory senses provides important sources of perceptual input for cognition. The olfactory sense has been found to have an important role in the process of memory. The more senses used in learning, the more your brain will be involved in retaining the memory. Making lists, using mnemonic devices (formulas or patterns of letters to aid in remembering), putting things on a calendar/planner, repeating what you want to remember, and developing other association techniques can assist with remembering tasks or information. The regular practice or rehearsal of retrieving information from the memory helps maintain the skill. For example, doing crossword puzzles regularly helps many people rehearse the skill of knowledge and information retrieval from the long-term memory. Challenging your brain promotes cognitive functioning. Mental exercise is thought to activate processes that help maintain brain cells and stimulate communication between them. This might be accomplished by learning a skill such as a language, pursuing a hobby, reading, taking a class, attempting music or art, or volunteering for something you haven't done before (President and Fellows of Harvard, 2010).

MAINTAINING LEARNING SKILLS

Developing learning skills is nearly as important as the actual knowledge gained. These learning skills, developed in childhood, need to be practiced, reinforced, and used throughout life. The goal is always to keep learning and making lifelong learning a priority. Identify the type of learner and strengthen learning skills when teaching. People learn better when the relevance of the information is apparent; for example, if a person has experienced side effects of a medication, the learning related to potential effects of other medications has increased relevance because of the desire to prevent problems in the future.

Learning improves when it is meaningful and linked with previous learning. To illustrate, if the nurse wants to teach an automobile mechanic about the importance of exercise, associating various body parts with analogous parts of an automobile may increase meaningfulness. As another example, for a person needing to learn about medications, the classifications and generic names of drugs will be less meaningful than the color, shape, size, and frequency of the medication.

Nursing Interventions for Impaired Cognitive Function

When a diagnosis of impaired cognitive function is made, nurses can intervene to help identify causative factors, restore or improve cognitive function, protect the patient from injury, and help the family cope. Nurses have both an independent and a collaborative role in identifying patients at risk for acute confusion, modifying or structuring the environment, and initiating appropriate teaching. Nurses, as the healthcare professionals with the most patient contact, are in the best position to monitor changes in cognitive function, communicate these to the healthcare team, and intervene as appropriate.

Cognitive deficits may be acute and reversible or chronic and irreversible, or an acute insult may exacerbate a chronic deficit. Nursing interventions designed to improve function include similar measures and activities for patients with each of these deficits. The major focus of nursing care is restoring physiologic balance while creating an environment that provides appropriate sensory stimulation, adequate assistance with ADLs, and protection from physical injury.

THERAPEUTIC COMMUNICATION

Therapeutic communication means that nurses respect the patients' individuality and use modes of communication to convey that respect. Therapeutic communication is used in assessment to obtain accurate information but is equally important in ongoing interactions between nurses and patients. Communication techniques are presented in detail in Chapter 6.

Therapeutic communication enables nurses to re-evaluate and intervene consistently by using information that is as accurate as possible. Regular use of these communication techniques allows nurses to detect cognitive changes whenever they occur, so the interventions are free from personal bias.

Understanding verbal and nonverbal responses is important in caring for people with chronic confusion. For example, patients who repeatedly call for "Mama" may be expressing needs for nurturing and affection. Patients who take food from the plates of others may be communicating that they are still hungry (Skinner, 2009; Smith, Fortin, Dwamena, & Frankel, 2013). Nonverbal communication can express positive regard through touch, facial expression, and eye contact. Finally, patients without other means of communication may express distress or dislike through behaviors such as spitting, turning away, or striking out. The importance of nonverbal communication may increase as other cognitive abilities decline.

Therapeutic communication with patients who have chronic confusion may be enhanced by assuming a nonthreatening posture (e.g., sitting at eye level with the patient). Explain what you are going to do in a calm, friendly tone of voice. Avoid using commands or asking "why" questions. Do not try logically to persuade a resistive patient to comply with your requests. Do not try to argue or change the patient's beliefs; instead, deal with the patient's reactions to the beliefs. Accept that the patient may have a distortion of reality and focus on the feelings that are related.

ORIENTATION TO SURROUNDINGS

Patients who have difficulty with understanding require special considerations. Patients who are experiencing receptive (Wernicke) aphasia may also be suffering from confusion related to this unfamiliar state. Maintaining a structured environment assists patients in adapting to cognitive alteration and in re-establishing communication. Structured routines minimize the factors on which patients must focus. Sequenced events, consistent daily schedules and care providers, calendars, and frequent reminders contribute to structure. To assist with orientation, ask patients why they are in the healthcare facility or where they are; gently correct false answers and ask the orientation questions again later. Supportive environmental cues, such as a current calendar and a large, visible clock, assist patients with orientation to time.

SAFETY ALERT
Provide structure and predictable routines whenever possible to minimize distractions and potential injuries.

ALTERNATIVE COMMUNICATION METHODS

A plan of care that provides patients with Broca or nonfluent aphasia with an effective, efficient means to communicate is essential. Encourage patients to use any means available to express themselves. Methods of communication that may be helpful include offering patients pictures at which to point, having patients use gestures, or letting them show what they want. Writing and reading skills may be impaired along with speech; therefore, these skills may not be useful alternatives.

Adjust the communication style to the patient, including speed, length of content, and written versus spoken method. If it is difficult to understand what a patient has said, be honest and let the patient know. Ask the patient to try again and perhaps use gestures to assist with understanding. If the patient tries again and you still do not understand, take a rest and come back in a few minutes. Do not pressure the patient; some symptoms worsen if patients are fatigued, upset, or anxious. Be alert to the patient's daily schedule, and allow for adequate rest at night and naps during the day.

For patients who have lost the ability to produce sound because of a laryngectomy, communication may be restored through the use of sophisticated electronic or computer communication devices or an electronic larynx. In these cases, nurses should know how to use these devices. Patients with disabilities, such as visual, mobility, hearing, learning, and communication disorders, may benefit from computer adaptations.

The Patient with Dysarthria

To facilitate communication with a dysarthric patient, face the patient to read his or her lips. Augment communication by gestures, written messages, a communication board, or flash cards. Encourage the patient to use slow speech, to speak loudly, and to take breaths between sentences. Ask the patient to repeat unclear words. If the patient appears tired, ask questions that require short answers. Establish a specific care plan and a routine for delivering care to reduce the time the patient would otherwise need to explain his or her care to others.

ENVIRONMENTAL RESTRICTIONS

The number of visitors with whom patients have to communicate may increase frustration for patients with impaired verbal communication. Many people and noises in the environment can interfere with cognitive functioning and understanding. Quiet environments allow patients to focus on understanding, speaking, or communicating.

Nurses may find that environmental restrictions are advantageous in assisting communication with patients. Be aware of excessive noise levels caused by equipment, loudspeaker systems, and/or other people. Limit the number of visitors present at any given time. Teach visitors how to communicate effectively with patients by using thoughtful methods, such as one person speaking at a time and not carrying on simultaneous conversations.

FLUID INTAKE AND NUTRITION

Because shifts in nutrients, electrolytes, and fluids contribute to cognitive changes, monitor the food and fluid intake of patients. People who are ill may not feel like eating or may not find food appealing. Allow patients to choose foods they particularly like. Give supportive encouragement and monitoring so that diets are reasonably balanced.

Similarly, patients may not experience thirst even when increased fluid intake is needed. Keep fluids within easy reach of patients, and give reminders to drink. Fluid intake and output records are useful to observe for patterns of fluid intake. The most accurate guideline for the adequacy of food and fluid intake is regular measurement of body weight. For patients at risk for fluid imbalances, a regular schedule of weighing will need to be established.

Patients and families will need health teaching regarding the factors that place them at risk for food and fluid imbalances. Diabetic patients who may have fluctuations in serum glucose must understand appropriate diet and medication management. Persons taking diuretics must understand the effects and side effects and know not to withhold water unless specifically prescribed by the physician or nurse practitioner. Patients who have any identified risk factors for the development of cognitive dysfunction should receive health teaching related to the problem, along with supportive nursing care.

Patients with chronic confusion need particularly close monitoring of food and fluid intake. With loss of judgment, some patients fail to respond to normal signals of appetite, thirst, or satiety. They may not eat or drink unless reminded, may overeat, may eat inappropriate things, or forget how to eat. Sitting with these patients while they eat, reminding them to eat, and assisting them with the mechanics of eating may be useful. For some patients, socialization opportunities when eating at a table with others may help to reinforce desired behaviors and activities. For others, a quiet environment free from distractions is best.

Patients with dysarthria need to be evaluated and treated by a speech therapist to ensure safe swallowing. Their intake should be monitored to ensure adequate caloric intake. Patients with difficulty swallowing should be placed in a full upright position when eating. They will usually tolerate foods with texture and consistency and thickened liquids better than thin, clear fluids. If patients are unable to consume an adequate number of calories safely, tube feeding may be required.

MOBILITY

Encourage isolated or withdrawn patients to move around. Physical activity improves ventilation, cardiovascular function, and oxygenation of the brain. It also helps people feel better physically and personally. Improved socialization is an important aspect of increased mobility. As patients move around more, even on hospital units, they increase contact with other people. Contact with others and exposure to more environments provide increased stimulation and reinforcement of reality.

Selectively providing sensory stimulation for all of the senses is an important consideration, particularly for patients with chronic confusion. In addition to hearing and seeing, make use of touch through personal contact and varied fabric textures, taste through varieties of food and beverages, and smell through food and flowers. While providing stimulation, be sure to avoid overstimulating patients who have chronic confusion. Overstimulation can result in apparently purposeless behaviors, such as wandering, agitation, and aggression. Recognize signs of overstimulation (i.e., inability to maintain eye contact, increased or decreased verbalizations, or attempts to avoid or retreat from the situation), and reduce the level of stimulation to prevent these behaviors.

❗ SAFETY ALERT

Supervise patients with confusion during ambulation and other activities. They may have altered judgment as to where they are. To prevent potential falls, be sure the environment is free from unnecessary obstructions. Provide adequate lighting.

SAFETY

Persons with altered cognitive function are at risk for injury and require nursing interventions to ensure safety. For example, when patients are hospitalized or ill, in an unfamiliar location, and/or subject to strange routines, they may temporarily lose orientation. Elderly patients are at particularly high risk for confusion and cognitive decline when hospitalized because of stress, illness, unfamiliar surroundings, and loss of routine (Kostas et al., 2013). More specifically, the illness/hospitalization and cognitive decline may be related to oxygenation, blood glucose, inflammation, or side effects of medications (Kostas et al., 2013). Patients may be at risk for falling while trying to get out of bed or while going to the bathroom. Safety measures, such as orienting patients to the room and the nurse call system, using lights at night to help orient patients to their environment, keeping beds in the lowest possible position, and placing patients in rooms closest to the nursing station for closer observation, help to prevent accidents and injuries.

Safety becomes a primary concern for patients with progressively impaired judgment. In institutional settings, safety measures for patients with chronic confusion involve frequently checking on patients, providing company, and interacting with them; keeping the bed at the lowest level; frequently assisting patients to get in and out of bed to meet elimination needs; supervising wandering behavior; gently redirecting lost or wandering patients; providing secured locks or alerting systems for elevators and door; providing motion detection devices that can be applied to the patient or to the bed to signal nursing staff when movement occurs; staying with patients who are agitated; and removing items that may be potentially harmful from the area.

Physical restraints are sometimes used to reduce patient interference with their treatment and to protect patient safety. Types of restraints include side rails, vest/chest/jacket restraints, wrist or ankle ties, belts, hand mitts, sheet ties, lap tables, or locked Geri chairs/recliner chairs. Patient safety with the use of restraints is related to preventing falls. Falls can occur with patients getting out of bed or chairs, being unstable sitting in chairs, and experiencing emotional disturbance (Burock & Naqvi, 2014). Persons most likely to be restrained are older adults. The use of physical restraints has actually not been shown to reduce or prevent falls and injury and has been associated with poor patient outcomes. Facilities have been cited for both not using and using restraints. Court cases related to restraint use include inappropriate ordering, incorrect application, failure to monitor the patient, and failure to correct the negative effects of the restraint (De Bellis et al., 2011). Some nurses hold misconceptions about the use of restraints in acute care and would improve knowledge, attitude, and skills related to use of restraints if in-service education were provided (De Bellis et al., 2011). Nurses should determine the reason for patient behavior and recognize those at risk for restraint use through appropriate assessment. Determine if patient behavior is related to physical factors such as alterations in senses, elimination, pain, or impaired mobility; physiologic factors such as altered cognitive level related to the patient's cardiac, respiratory, neurologic status, or medication; psychological factors such as anxiety or fear; or environmental factors such as noise, lighting, or unfamiliarity. Nursing interventions should then be focused on treating or eliminating the cause for behavioral changes, meeting the patient needs, and collaborating with team members. Restraint-free care is the current standard. Facilities and staff should move toward restraint-free care while maintaining safety and use restraints only when nonrestricting procedures have failed (De Bellis et al., 2011).

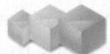 ***Concept Mastery Alert***

Supervise patients with confusion during ambulation and other activities. They may have altered judgment as to where they are. To prevent potential falls, be sure the environment is free from unnecessary obstructions. Provide adequate lighting.

When caring for a confused patient, the potential risks and benefits of side rails must be weighed carefully. The nurse must consider the patient's recent behavior and overall level of consciousness. For some patients, raising all of the side rails may have a protective effect; for others, they may heighten the risk for falls. It is rarely necessary to keep all of a patient's side rails raised at all times.

Consider also that changes in routine and environment may upset and distress patients with chronic confusion. For this reason, the care environment should be as predictable and consistent as possible. Meals, baths, treatments, and other activities should be at regular times with familiar staff people. Objects in the room should be kept in the same place. If changes are

SCENE FOR THOUGHT

Carmen Morales has come in for a regular blood pressure check and has brought her grandmother, Rosa Gomez, to be checked too. Mrs. Gomez, age 84 years, smiles and affectionately pats the nurse's hand as they meet. Carmen tells the nurse that "Abuelita" is having some trouble with her memory, and the family is worried that she might be unsafe at home. She forgot to turn off the stove, has trouble with the household appliances, and is getting irritable when the children make noise after school. This problem has been occurring over the last 2 months. Mrs. Gomez has no physical problems except controlled high blood pressure and occasional constipation.

LESS EFFECTIVE

Nurse: Mrs. Gomez, you've heard what Carmen and I have been talking about? (*Mrs. Gomez nods, smiling brightly.*) What do you think?

Mrs. Gomez: I lose my memory sometimes, but it's nothing to worry about. I'm old, I'm supposed to lose my memory sometimes. (*Continues to smile.*)

Nurse: It's true that as we get older our memories get a little worn out (*pats her hand*), but Carmen is worried about your safety while you're taking care of the cooking, cleaning, and so on. I think that it would be a good idea for you to see one of the geriatric nurse specialists here in the clinic. He could talk with you, maybe run some tests, work with you on your memory. He's very good, caring, and has lots of experience with people your age. What do you think?

Mrs. Gomez: Am I sick or something? Why do I need a specialist? (*Looks at Carmen anxiously.*)

Carmen: It's okay, Abuelita, we'll go see what this other nurse has to say. I'm sure he can help us with your memory. (*Rises to leave.*) Come on Abuelita, let's go and make the appointment.

Mrs. Gomez: Okay, querida, if you say so. But I don't understand all this fuss over a little memory loss. (*Grumbles on her way out.*)

MORE EFFECTIVE

Nurse: Mrs. Gomez, you've heard what Carmen and I have been talking about? (*Mrs. Gomez nods, smiling brightly.*) What do you think about that?

Mrs. Gomez: I lose my memory sometimes, but it's nothing to worry about. I'm old. I'm supposed to lose my memory sometimes. (*Continues to smile.*)

Nurse: You expect that you will lose your memory as you grow older?

Carmen: Sure. My parents didn't live to be very old, but I remember my grandmother not remembering things very well by the time she was 70! So I'm doing fine. (*Gives a little laugh.*)

Nurse: I'm wondering if you can think of times that you have more trouble remembering than others.

Mrs. Gomez: (*Concentrates for a minute.*) I think it's when there's too much commotion in the house or when I don't get enough sleep. Then I can't remember things very well. (*Turns to Carmen.*) That's when I forgot to turn off the stove, querida mia, and it was only once. Yes, it's when there's a lot to distract me from my work.

Nurse: I understand. You said you don't get enough sleep sometimes? Tell me a little more, please.

Mrs. Gomez: Certainly. I sometimes have to go to the bathroom in the middle of the night. Then it's hard for me to get back to sleep all alone in that big bed. My husband died 2 years ago, and it's still hard for me to sleep in that big bed. (*She doesn't smile now.*)

Nurse: You're still missing him, I can see that. I guess it helps to take care of the family the way you do.

Mrs. Gomez: Yes, it does help. And I want to do the best I can for them. I don't want them to worry about me or send me away. (*Looks at Carmen with tears in her eyes.*)

Carmen: No, Abuelita, we don't want to send you away; we just want you to be safe and comfortable. Don't cry, don't cry. (*Puts her arm around her grandmother.*)

Nurse: I think if we three talk together we can come up with some ways to help you get better sleep, Mrs. Gomez. And there are some tricks I can think of to help you remember things better. Let's work together on this. What do you say?

Mrs. Gomez: I would be happy to! Thank you very much! (*Squeezes the nurse's hand and smiles.*)

CRITICAL THINKING CHALLENGE

- Although Mrs. Gomez ultimately received effective care in both dialogues, detect what made the second dialogue "more effective" from the patient's point of view.
- Explain what factors the first nurse never found out about.
- Describe the relationship between anxiety and cognitive processes.

necessary, remember that patients with chronic confusion will need additional support and reassurance.

REALITY ORIENTATION

Reality orientation is a nursing technique used to assist patients in restoring awareness of reality (Fig. 37-6). A hallmark in reinforcing reality for hospitalized patients is to provide those environmental cues on which people depend for orientation to time and place. Having the change in lighting match the usual day and night cuing is helpful. Patients who are in specialized units with few windows and lights have greater difficulty relying on environmental cues.

Clocks and calendars that allow patients to know the date, day of the week, and time of day are important sources of input for reality orientation. Additional interventions include allowing uninterrupted sleep periods when possible and encouraging visits from family and friends. Contact with familiar objects, such as photographs, favorite chairs, or special books, is also useful.

Allowing patients the maximal advantage in relation to sensory–perceptual data is equally important in reinforcing reality. If patients normally wear glasses or hearing aids, ensure that these are available. Glasses must be clean and hearing aids adjusted correctly. If information that patients take in is as accurate as possible, interpreting and responding to reality are easier.

Although patients with irreversible changes such as dementia will not return to previous levels of cognitive functioning, nurses need to assist them in maintaining existing levels of function for as long as possible. Nonconfrontational reality orientation is an appropriate intervention, and various modalities can be used, such as clocks, calendars, lighting cycles, or personal contact. However, verbal attempts to orient a patient with dementia to time, place, or person are often futile and may exacerbate behavioral problems. For this type of patient, avoid reorienting and redirect his or her thoughts. Assist the family in understanding how to work with the patient.

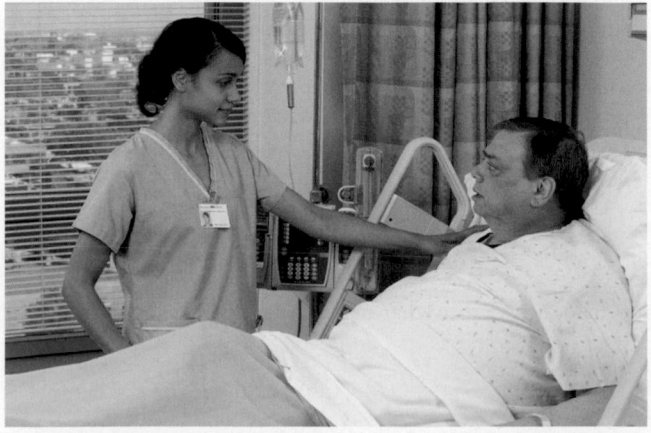

FIGURE 37-6 Stimulation of the senses through touch and other environmental cues helps the patient maintain touch with reality.

ETHICAL/LEGAL ISSUE

MISTREATMENT OF PATIENT BY STAFF

Mr. Schooner, 80 years old, has entered a long-term care facility because of his forgetfulness, wandering behavior, and inability to care for himself. He is in good physical health but has a history of progressive dementia. Although his family members were reluctant to admit him, they were exhausted from the constant care that Mr. Schooner required.

At the long-term care facility, Mr. Schooner becomes agitated, has increased wandering, and talks loudly, which disturbs the staff and the other residents. You overhear a staff member saying to him, "If you don't sit still and be quiet, I'm going to tie you to your bed and put tape on your mouth!" You are aware that such behavior on the part of healthcare staff is not reflective of nursing philosophy, but you have to work closely with this staff member.

CRITICAL THINKING CHALLENGE

- Identify your concerns about Mr. Schooner. How could the move to this facility and his cognitive dysfunction be contributing to his behavior?
- Describe your feelings about the staff member. What ethical concerns do you face in this situation?
- Identify possible approaches to this state of affairs.
- Recognizing the patient's dependence and the staff member's behavior, define what you feel is your ethically appropriate behavior.

SOCIALIZATION THERAPIES

Socialization therapies can take many forms such as pets, music, recreation, and reminiscence. The purpose of these therapies is to encourage patients to expand contact with others in social settings in an effort to increase cognitive and sensory stimuli. For some people, contact within usual social groups, such as senior citizen centers, volunteer groups, church groups, or recreation groups, may provide beneficial stimulation. Interaction with pets may provide cognitive and sensory stimuli as the patients observe, hold, stroke, and communicate with an animal.

For patients who are at risk for being isolated or who require more protected environments, reality orientation groups or day care centers provide the same type of human contact and stimulation. Developing an ongoing relationship with people who staff these groups or centers provides continuity of care and consistent support for cognitive function.

In reminiscence therapy, patients use recall of the past to assist in clarifying meaning in the present or reconciling conflict. This therapy is particularly useful for older patients because it contributes to successful aging by maintaining self-esteem and reinforcing cognitive function. It requires facilitation by a nurse or other health professional skilled in group process and in reminiscence therapy.

Recreation therapy involves using recreation or hobbies to increase meaningful experiences and contact with others. It is another way of using familiar objects or past abilities to help patients ascribe meaning. Although recreation therapy may be prescribed and directed by another health professional, nurses also may use recreation or hobbies appropriate to the individual patient to stimulate cognitive function. Activities that elicit pleasant memories may be used to engage chronically confused or withdrawn patients. Examples are the review of a personal scrapbook or photograph album.

Music therapy enhances cognitive contact through the familiarity of music. The music may be in the background or used for exercise or in group sings. Both the music and the socialization and recreation inherent in musical group opportunities are stimulating. Some therapists may use music in a specific, prescriptive fashion; however, nurses can use music as a part of nursing care, as deemed appropriate. Although selected music may provide therapeutic cognitive stimulation, it must be individualized to the patient's preferences, and the risk of overstimulation must be kept in mind.

FAMILY SUPPORT

Families of patients with acute confusion are often anxious and fear a progression to chronic confusion. Reassure patients and families that, in most cases, cognitive function will improve with time. Encourage families to participate actively in the planning and care of patients; the collaborative intervention goal will be to prevent or minimize patients' altered thought processes.

Many patients with chronic confusion live at home and receive care from family members. Family caregivers usually receive inadequate training for this difficult task (Clarke et al., 2013). Teaching family caregivers about the nature and progression of chronic confusion, along with techniques for managing the behavioral manifestations, may reduce exhaustion and delay institutionalization. Nurses should assess evidence of abuse by the caregiver or abuse and violence by the patient. At the appropriate time, nurses should advise family members to determine the patient's competence and ability to make decisions regarding healthcare. Legal counsel may need to establish guardianship or power of attorney.

Nurses may also provide direct care and support to family members. Families have a difficult time adjusting to the fact that their loved ones are losing or have lost all memory of them and their lives together. The grief process begins before the death of patients with dementia. In essence, the person whom the family members once knew and interacted with is no longer present mentally but is still present physically. Use nursing interventions that aid the family in its grief, as discussed in Chapter 38 or 39.

Home and Community Care

Because of shorter hospital stays, patients may be discharged before cognitive function has returned to normal. Careful discharge planning is imperative. Planning may need to include teaching family caregivers effective techniques in communicating with and caring for patients. Community self-help groups, such as stroke clubs, the Alzheimer's Disease and Related Disorders

Association, the Multiple Sclerosis Society, the National Spinal Cord Injury Society, and the International Association of Laryngectomies, can be beneficial. These groups offer support and provide patients and families with tips to make role adjustment easier and to improve the quality of relationships.

HOME CARE

Home care services, which include nurses; occupational, physical, and speech therapists; and home health aides, should be arranged as necessary before patients are discharged. Going home may help reverse the dysfunction of mildly cognitively impaired patients as they return to a familiar environment and routines. Patients who have more severe impairments may need frequent home visits for nursing care and homemaking.

If impaired cognitive function interferes with the ability to perform higher-level skills (e.g., managing medications and maintaining the home), support systems usually can be created to promote safety and independence. For people with minor memory impairment, ways to support and compensate include making lists of medications to take, things to do, or appliances to turn off. Maintaining organization in the home and in routines creates a predictable environment with few distractions so that memory functions more effectively. Resources like chore service, volunteers, subsidized van service, Meals on Wheels, and grocery delivery can be arranged.

DAY AND RESPITE CARE

Day care and respite care are two useful support services for irreversibly cognitively impaired people and their family caregivers. Fatigue is constant for caregivers of progressively impaired family members. One means of managing fatigue is access to services that allow some time away from caregiving while providing impaired persons with health and rehabilitative services. Caregivers are assured that impaired family members are benefiting from the alternative care and simultaneously having much-needed rest and personal time.

LONG-TERM CARE

Many times, people with progressive cognitive impairment or dementia need consistent support from long-term care settings with 24-hour supervision, structured environments, and extended health services. Caregivers need the support and reinforcement from healthcare providers as they make the decision to admit loved ones to long-term care. They need assurance that they have made the right decision, whatever that decision ultimately is.

Admission to long-term care can be very positive for patients, who will have contact with people, objects, and situations that provide increased stimulation. Full-time care allows the environment to be structured and predictable, which may actually increase a patient's level of cognitive functioning even temporarily. The actual process of relocation can be stressful, but patients can be helped to cope through diligent orientation and unhurried repetition. A caring attitude on the part of healthcare professionals is essential.

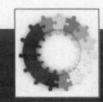

COLLABORATING WITH THE HEALTH CARE TEAM
Calling the Physician Concerning a Patient's Increased Agitation

Mrs. Latapie, age 67 years, has had cognitive changes over the 3 hours that you have been caring for her. She has gone from being oriented to time, place, and person to being acutely agitated and hallucinating.

SITUATION: Mrs. Latapie has demonstrated rapid cognitive changes over a short period of time. She is acutely agitated about the "bugs" she thinks she sees in her bed and on the walls.

BACKGROUND: Mrs. Latapie, age 67 years, was admitted yesterday following an accident in which she tripped over an electric cord in her home. She was admitted for repair of a fractured hip, which is scheduled for tomorrow morning.

ASSESSMENT: The family were here briefly but have now gone. They think that maybe Mrs. Latapie may have been drinking more over the past month and that may be why she tripped. I am concerned that her change in agitation and hallucinations might indicate alcohol withdrawal.

RECOMMENDATION: Could you come and evaluate Mrs. Latapie within the next hour and provide orders for controlling the agitation and the hallucinating and determining whether she should go to surgery tomorrow?

CRITICAL THINKING CHALLENGE

- Discuss the rationale for requesting that the physician come and evaluate Mrs. Latapie rather than just provide orders over the phone.
- Are there other data you could collect to support your assessment that Mrs. Latapie may be experiencing alcohol withdrawal?
- Would you try to contact the family for more data about Mrs. Latapie and their comment about her increased alcohol consumption?
- Would you want to consider using restraints? What would be your decision-making process?

EVALUATION

Evaluation of the effect of nursing interventions toward patient goals includes a patient assessment related to the outcome criteria. Continuation, modification, or termination of nursing interventions depends on the assessment. This process may be ongoing. Some examples of the relationship between goals and outcome criteria for patients with alterations in thinking and communicating are listed below.

Goal

The patient will have absence of injury related to confusion.

POSSIBLE OUTCOME CRITERIA

- At discharge, there are no reports of injury (e.g., falls, abrasions, burns) related to cognitive dysfunction.

Goal

The patient will experience adequate support to compensate for deficits.

POSSIBLE OUTCOME CRITERIA

- Before discharge, patient demonstrates adequate nutrition, safety, and mobility.
- Before discharge, patient receives support services as needed to offset needs presented by cognitive deficits.

Goal

The patient will participate in a safe, protected environment.

POSSIBLE OUTCOME CRITERIA

- Patient demonstrates the absence of injury from environmental hazards.
- Patient demonstrates relaxed behavior and other indications of comfort with the environment.

Goal

The patient will communicate basic needs.

POSSIBLE OUTCOME CRITERIA

- By discharge, patient demonstrates ability to express needs using a new method (gestures, writing, blinking, or electronic device) with the nurse.

Goal

The patient will verbalize experiencing less frustration with communication.

POSSIBLE OUTCOME CRITERIA

- Patient verbalizes to the nurse a decrease in frustration with communication problems.
- Patient expresses a decrease in feelings of isolation and depression.

PATIENT PLAN OF CARE
The Patient Experiencing Chronic Confusion

NURSING DIAGNOSIS

Chronic Confusion related to Alzheimer's disease, cerebrovascular attack, Korsakoff psychosis, head injury, or multi-infarct dementia manifested by impaired short- or long-term memory, impaired socialization, altered response to stimuli, and progressive cognitive impairment

PATIENT GOAL

Patient will function at maximal cognitive level.
Patient will be free from harm.

PATIENT OUTCOME CRITERIA

- Patient will participate in ADLs at the maximum level of functional ability.
- Patient will be free from harm in a safe environment.

NURSING INTERVENTION	SCIENTIFIC RATIONALE
1. Determine patient's cognitive level using a screening tool such as the Mini-Mental State Examination.	**1.** Using a standard evaluation tool can help determine the patient's abilities and assist in planning care.
2. Obtain patient information about underlying cause for chronic confusion and predementia social, physical, and psychological level of functioning.	**2.** Knowing possible cause will influence treatments and provide information about possibility of improvement. Knowing prior functioning will help with understanding of patient reminiscence, delusions, or hallucinations.
3. Ensure the patient is in a safe environment. Remove clutter or obstacles that may contribute to falls. Remove items that may cause harm or injury, such as chemicals or cleaning solutions.	**3.** Patients with confusion/dementia are prone to falls and are not able to use good judgment, which may result in harm to self or others.
4. Avoid unfamiliar situations. Assign consistent caregivers when possible. Maintain a routine for meals, bathing, and sleeping.	**4.** Minimizing the number of caregivers allows the patient to recognize staff and feel comfortable with their care. Maintaining consistency of ADLs minimizes situational anxiety that may prevent escalation of agitated behavior.
5. Assess patient's ability to perform and encourage patient to participate in ADLs as much as possible.	**5.** Performing ADLs helps the patient regain a sense of control and gives the nurse an opportunity to assess functional ability.
6. Give one simple direction at a time and repeat as necessary. Use verbal and physical prompts.	**6.** Patients with dementia/confusion need extra time to comprehend communication. They can't understand complex commands and may not remember the steps to complete their ADLs.
7. Keep the environment quiet and reduce stimuli immediately with signs of patient anxiety.	**7.** Sensory overload can result in agitated behavior in patients with dementia/confusion.
8. Provide quiet activities such as listening to music and simple activities such as folding or sorting washcloths.	**8.** Quiet activities provide a calming environment. Repetitive activities provide a positive outlet for energy and behavior for the dementia patient.
9. Encourage family and friends to visit; put cards and flowers where patient can see them.	**9.** The ability to recognize family and friends persists even in a state of severe confusion. Loved ones can be reassuring and can minimize the negative effects of the dementia experience.

(Continued)

PATIENT PLAN OF CARE (Continued)

EVALUATION

10/30/17: 10:00—The patient:

- Participates in completing the Mini-Mental State Examination with a score of 7 at 2 weeks.
- Family relates that prior to the diagnosis of Alzheimer disease, the patient was physically active and involved at the senior citizen center several times a week.
- Is cooperative with staff but provides minimal assistance in ADLs such as bathing and dressing.
- Is able to feed self.
- Is free from injury and has no history of falling.
- Responds appropriately to simple verbal commands.
- Participates in simple games, reminiscing, and craft activities.
- Recognizes and visits with family members.

—M. Klim, RN

KEY CONCEPTS

- Cognition is the process of knowing, thinking, learning, and communicating; it is the complex processing of information by which sensory input, past experiences, awareness, and emotions are integrated and made meaningful, thereby enabling the person to interact with the environment in a purposeful way.

- To provide comprehensive nursing care, nurses need to be aware of factors affecting cognitive function, such as physiologic state, infectious processes, medications, personal and environmental stressors, and affective states.

- Manifestations of impaired cognition include disorganized thinking, attention deficits, memory impairment, impaired thought processes, and impaired communication.

- For the person with disturbed thought processes, ADLs are disrupted, and the amount of support in the living situation must be assessed.

- Disorders in cognition can markedly disrupt the quality of life for the person affected and the person's family.

- To guide the development of the nursing process, the nurse needs to determine how a person functions along with assessing the quality of the social and physical environment.

- Identifying risk factors for disturbed thought processes will assist the nurse in defining the actual dysfunction and the appropriate interventions.

- Thorough assessment of physiologic and psychosocial function is essential in identifying causes of impaired cognitive processes.

- In adults, the main cause of impaired communication is brain damage. Other major causes are cancer and neurologic disorders.

- The plan of care involves collaboration of nursing, speech therapy, and other disciplines, as needed.

- Nursing goals should focus on restoring physiologic balance while providing an environment that supports function, does not cause new impairments, and protects the patient from harm.

- If the nurse is aware of potential risk for dysfunction, preventive interventions will concentrate on minimizing those factors and supporting the patient and caregivers.

- Among many supportive interventions for the impaired patient is reality orientation, which is used to reinforce and restore awareness of reality.

- People with altered cognitive processes require careful discharge planning and home care along with referral for families to long-term care, day care, or respite care, as appropriate.

PRACTICING FOR THE NCLEX

CHECK YOUR ANSWERS IN APPENDIX A.

1. A nurse is caring for an elderly patient with altered mental status. Which of the following are potentially related to impaired cognition? Select all that apply:
   a. Stroke
   b. Hypoglycemia (low blood sugar)
   c. Hyponatremia (low sodium level)
   d. Inadequate sleep
   e. Urinary tract infection

2. In assessing an elderly patient diagnosed with delirium, which of the following data would support this diagnosis? Select all that apply:
   a. Patient mental status changes began yesterday.
   b. Patient believes that the year is 1990.
   c. Patient is lethargic.
   d. Patient has no history of drug/alcohol use.

3. A nurse is caring for a patient following a head trauma. He is able to understand well, but when he talks, he is unable to speak fluently or find the correct words. How would the nurse best characterize his speech?

    a. Expressive aphasia

    b. Dysarthria

    c. Receptive aphasia

    d. Global aphasia

4. A nurse is setting up the room for a patient with cognitive impairments related to a brain lesion. Which intervention would best create a supportive environment for this patient?

    a. Posting a sign to remind the patient to call for assistance before rising

    b. Placing a large clock next to the bed

    c. Leaving the bed in a locked, low position

    d. Limiting visitors and loud stimuli

5. The nurse is discharging a patient with impaired cognition to home. Which of the following elements would be important? Select all that apply:

    a. Teaching family caregivers effective communication techniques

    b. Delaying discharge until cognition improves

    c. Discussing options for occupational and speech therapists

    d. Providing resources for respite care for family members

REFERENCES

American Psychiatric Association. (2013). Diagnostic and Statistical Manual of Mental Disorders. In *Diagnostic and statistical manual of mental disorders* (5th ed.). Arlington, VA: American Psychiatric Publishing.

American Psychiatric Association. (2013). *Diagnostic Criteria from DSM V TR.* Washington, DC: Author.

Aphasia. (2014). Retrieved from http://www.merckmanuals.com/professional/neurologic_disorders/function_and_dysfunction_of_the_cerebral_lobes/aphasia.html

Bakheit, A. M., Shaw, S., Carrington, S., & Griffiths, S. (2007). The rate and extent of improvement with therapy from the different types of aphasia in the first year after stroke. *Clinical Rehabilitation, 21*(10), 941–949.

Baxter, D., & Wilson, M. (2012). The fundamentals of head injury. *Neurosurgery, 30*(3), 116–121.

Boscart, V. M. (2009). A communication intervention for nursing staff in chronic care. *Journal of Advanced Nursing, 65,* 1823–1832.

Burock, J., & Naqvi, L. (2014, June). Practical management of Alzheimer's dementia. *Rhode Island Medical Journal, 97,* 36–40.

Clarke, P., Shaw, E., Villalba, J., Alli, R., & Sink, K. (2013). Therapeutic interactions to enhance the mental health and wellness of dementia caregivers and patients. *Journal of Gerontological Nursing, 39*(11), 7–10.

Cummings, J. L., Arsland, D., & Jarvik, L. (2013). Dementia. In C. K. Cassel, R. Leipzig, H. J. Cohen, E. B. Larson, & D. Meier (Eds.), *Geriatric Medicine: An evidence based approach* (4th ed.). New York, NY: Springer.

Day, K., McGuire, L., & Anderson, L. (2009). The CDC healthy brain initiative: Public health and cognitive impairment. *Journal of the American Society on Aging, 22*(1), 11–17.

De Bellis, A., Mosel, K., Curren, D., Predergast, J., Harrington, A., & Muir-Cochrane, E. (2011). Education on physical restraint reduction in dementia care: A review of the literature. *Dementia, 12,* 93–110.

Desai, S., Chau, T., & George, L. (2013). Intensive care unit delirium. *Critical Care Nurse Quarterly, 36,* 370–389.

Dillworth-Anderson, P., Pierre, G., & Hilliard, T. (2012, spring). Social justice, health disparities, and culture in the care of the elderly. *Journal of Law Medicine & Ethics, 40*(1), 26–32.

Doody, O., & Doody, C. (2012). Intellectual disability and transcultural care. *British Journal of Nursing, 21*(3), 174–180.

Downing, L. J., Caprio, T. V., & Lyness, J. M. (2013, May 2). Geriatric psychiatry review: Differential diagnosis and treatment of the 3 D's—delirium, dementia, and depression. *Current Psychiatry Report, 15*(365), 1–10. http://dx.doi.org/10.1007/s11920-013-0365-4

Dunne, W. M. (2013). Mechanisms of infectious disease. In C. M. Porth, & G. Matfin (Eds.), *Pathophysiology: concepts of altered health states* (9th ed.). Philadelphia, PA: Lippincott Williams & Wilkins.

Ely, E. W., Shitani, A., Truman, B., Speroff, T., Gordan, S. M., Harrell, F. E., et al. (2004). Delirium as a predictor of mortality in mechanically ventilated patients in the intensive care unit. *Journal of American Medical Association, 29*(14), 1753–1762.

Erikson, E. H. (1963). *Childhood and Society* (2nd ed.). New York, NY: Norton.

Field, R. R., & Wall, M. H. (2013). Delirium: Past, present, and future. *Seminars in Cardiothoracic and Vascular Anesthesia, 17,* 170–179. http://dx.doi.org/10.1177/1089253213476957

Folstein, M. F., Folstein, S. E., & McHugh, P. R. (1975). Mini-mental state: A practical method of grading the cognitive state of patients for the clinician. *Journal of Psychiatric Research, 12,* 189–198.

Fong, T. G., Tulebaev, S. R., & Inouye, S. K. (2009). Delirium in elderly adults: diagnosis, prevention and treatment. *Nature Reviews Neurology, 4,* 210–220. http://dx.doi.org/10.1038/nrneurol.2009.24

Gealogo, G. (2013, December). Dementia with Lewy bodies: A comprehensive review for nurses. *Journal of Neuroscience Nursing, 45*(6), 347–359.

Guyton, A. C., & Hall, J. E. (2011). *Textbook of medical physiology* (12th ed.). Philadelphia, PA: W.B. Saunders.

Hattori, H., et al. (2009). Assessment of the risk of postoperative delirium in elderly patients using E-PASS and the NEECHAM Confusion Scale. *International Journal of Geriatric Psychiatry, 24*(11), 1304–1310.

Havighurst, R. J. (1972). *Developmental tasks and education* (3rd ed.). New York, NY: David McKay.

Inouye, S. K., Van Dyck, C. H., Alessi, C. A., Balkin, S., Siegal, A. P., & Horwitz, R. I. (1990). Clarifying confusion: The confusion assessment method. A new method for detection of delirium. *American College of Physicians, 113*(12), 941–948.

Jablonski, R. (2013). Dementia is not dementia is not dementia. *Journal of Gerontological Nursing, 39*(1), 3–5.

Koeppen, B. M., & Stanton, B. S. (2010). *Berne & Levy physiology* (6th ed.). St. Louis, MO: Mosby.

Korczyn, A., Vakhapova, V., & Grinberg, L. (2012). Vascular dementia. *Journal of Neurological Sciences, 322,* 2–10.

Kostalova, M., Bednarik, J., Mitasova, A., Dusek, L., Michalcakova, R., Kerkovsky, M., et al. (2012). Towards a predictive model for post-stroke delirium. *Brain Injury, 26,* 962–971.

Kostas, T. R., Zimmerman, K. M., & Rudolph, J. L. (2013). Improving delirium care: Prevention, monitoring, and assessment. *Neurohospitalist, 3,* 194–202. http://dx.doi.org/10.1177/1941874413493185

Kurz, A., Kurz, C., Ellis, K., & Lautenschlager, N. (2014). What is frontotemporal dementia? *Maturitas, 79,* 216–219.

McCance, K. L., & Heuther, S. E. (2013). *Pathophysiology: The biologic basis for disease in adults and children* (7th ed.). St. Louis, MO: Mosby.

North American Nursing Diagnosis Association International. (2014). *Nursing diagnoses: Definitions and classification, 2012–2014.* West Sussex, England: Wiley-Blackwell.

Pfeiffer, E. (1975). A short portable mental status questionnaire for the assessment of organic brain deficit in elderly patients. *Journal of the American Geriatrics Society, 23,* 433–441.

Piaget, J. (1969). *The Psychology of the child.* New York, NY: Basic Books.

Porth, C., & Matfin, G. (2013). *Pathophysiology: Concepts of altered health states* (9th ed.). Philadelphia, PA: Lippincott Williams & Wilkins.

President and Fellows of Harvard. (2010). Preserving and improving memory as we age. *Harvard's Women's Health Watch, 17*(6), 1–3.

Santrock, J. W. (2012). *Life-span development* (14th ed.). Madison, WI: Brown & Benchmark.

Sendelbach, S., & Guthrie, P. F. (2009). Acute confusion/delirium: Identification, assessment, treatment and prevention. *Journal of Gerontological Nursing, 35*(11), 11–18.

Skinner, K. (2009). Nursing interventions to assist in decreasing stress in caregivers of Alzheimer's patients. *ABNF (Association of Black Nursing FacultyJournal), 20*(1), 22–24.

Smith, R., Fortin, A., Dwamena, F., & Frankel, R. (2013). An evidenced-based patient-centered method makes the biopsychosocial model scientific. *Patient Education and Counseling, 91*, 265–270.

Tabloski, P. A. (2013). *Gerontological nursing* (3rd ed.). Upper Saddle River, NJ: Prentice Hall.

Uriri-Glover, J., McCarthy, M., & Cesarotti, E. (2012, November). Alzheimer's disease: What new evidence shows. *Nursing Management, 26–31.*

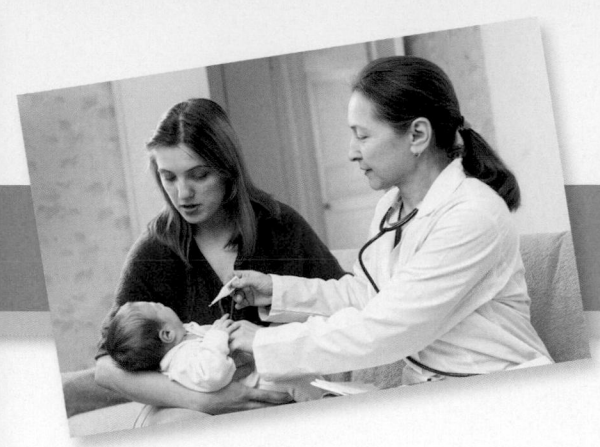

CHAPTER 38

Self-Concept

Anne P. Poppe

Case Scenario

You are a nurse working in a well-baby clinic. A 31-year-old woman brings in her 3-month-old child for a scheduled appointment. While you are weighing the baby, the mother talks about feeling tired and makes comments about her body such as "These breasts are so big and heavy" and "I don't think I'll ever wear normal-sized clothes again." She tells you that she misses the baby when she goes to her parttime job and wonders if she really wants to be away from the baby at all, but she feels better now that she is back to aerobics class. When you ask about the baby, she smiles and tells you how happy she and her significant partner are to have him. She describes how much more rewarding it is to care for her own child than to babysit her nieces and nephews. She then looks at the baby and says, "I wonder if I'll ever feel rested again."

Once you have completed this chapter and have incorporated self-concept into your knowledge base, review the above scenario and reflect on the following areas of Critical Thinking:

1. Describe your immediate impressions of the woman and her situation.
2. Reflect on the information provided as well as your own experience, knowledge, and beliefs. Consider how these might influence your impressions.
3. Analyze how the mother and infant may feel.
4. Consider additional assessment data that you might need to collect; develop appropriate questions to ask to obtain this data.
5. State possible nursing diagnoses for this family and identify some desired outcomes.
6. Given your assessment, nursing diagnoses, and outcome identification, plan interventions that may be appropriate.

Upon completion of this chapter, you will be able to do the following:

1. Describe the functions of self and self-concept.
2. Define self-concept, self-perception, self-knowledge, self-expectation, social self, and self-evaluation.
3. Identify the four patterns of self-concept.
4. Discuss how self-concept develops throughout the life span.
5. Discuss factors that can affect self-concept.
6. Identify possible manifestations of altered self-concept.
7. Apply theory to assess for self-concept functioning.
8. Plan care for a person with an altered self-concept.

As people adapt to changes in life, body image, role performance, self-esteem, and personal identity evolve. Self-concept is dynamic, influenced by experiences and expectations. A sound self-concept is a prerequisite for mental health. Nursing responsibilities associated with self-concept include self-knowledge, assessment of self-concept, promotion of adequate self-concept functioning, and interventions when self-concept is at risk or altered. The nurse who possesses a healthy self-concept will be better equipped to deal with the unique and varied needs of patients. Conversely, if a nurse's self-concept is dysfunctional, he or she will be unable to meet the needs of patients. In fact, coping with such a nurse may actually add to a patient's work.

NORMAL FUNCTION OF SELF

Because of its importance in understanding human behavior, the concept of self has been examined by many disciplines and defined in various ways. Self may be defined as a person's unique dimensions, potentials, and purposes (Rogers, 1961). Self-concept is the mental image a person has of oneself. It is the person's meaning when stated as "I" or "me." Self-concept is the frame of reference that influences how a person handles situations and relationships. It is crucial to esteem and self-actualization, the highest needs in Abraham Maslow's hierarchy of needs.

Characteristics of Self-Concept and Self-Perception

People who have a healthy self-concept exhibit a clear sense of self and others. They understand who they are in the world. They can and do distinguish themselves as separate individuals with strengths and weaknesses. These people acknowledge their emotions and find constructive ways to bring meaning into life. The person with a healthy self-concept views others realistically and is able to relate to them in a satisfying manner, which includes the capacity for intimacy and love. The person

with a healthy self-concept handles life's realities and problems with appropriate coping behaviors.

According to Brown (2007), self-concept is the way a person thinks about himself or herself, whereas self-perception is how a person explains behavior based on self-observation. How one perceives oneself has several dimensions: self-knowledge, self-expectations, social self, and self-evaluation.

SELF-KNOWLEDGE

Self-knowledge or self-awareness involves a basic understanding of oneself, a cognitive perception. It is consciousness of one's abilities: cognitive, affective, and physical. Self-knowledge involves basic facts (age, weight, sex) and qualities (sincere, athletic, intelligent) related to oneself.

SELF-EXPECTATION

Self-expectation involves the "ideal" self—the self a person wants to be. It is the setting of present and future goals. If goals are realistic, the person may attain them. Unrealistic goals, however, can be defeating. Self-expectation is based on the limits of a person's awareness. For instance, the goals of the person who watches glamorous shows on television may be to be thin, beautiful, popular with the opposite sex, and wealthy. The person who spends time reading may have increased knowledge as a goal. Significant others influence a person's self-expectation. If a mother pushes her son to be a physician, the son may share this goal or may feel like a failure if he lacks interest.

SOCIAL SELF

Social self is how a person sees himself or herself in relation to social situations, including behavior and interaction with others. One never fully knows how others see him or her. One can only guess, and the guess may be far from reality. Conversely, people may tend to wear masks in their social obligations, trying to hide their true selves. The "religious" self that a person displays in church may differ from the self shown at parties. A person may hide aggressive feelings when being interviewed but display aggression later on the job.

SELF-EVALUATION

Self-evaluation is the conscious assessment of the self, leading to self-respect or self-worth. "Have I met my expectations? Do I like who I see in the mirror? Do I like how I behave?" Self-evaluation involves the aforementioned dimensions plus self-esteem (discussed below).

Normal Self-Concept Patterns

Body image, self-esteem, personal identity, and role performance comprise the mental image of the self. The whole of self represents more than the sum of these four components. To clarify the dynamics of these components, consider the mother and 3-month-old child described in the case scenario. The woman's body image and role performance have clearly changed with pregnancy and motherhood. These components then influence her self-esteem and identity into which motherhood must be incorporated. If her self-concept is healthy, she will be able to make the necessary changes to cope with and adapt to the dynamics of self.

POSITIVE BODY IMAGE

The human body is the self's physical manifestation. How a person pictures and feels about his or her body describes body image. Body image includes the total conscious and unconscious disposition toward one's body. It is the unifying concept behind feelings about one's size, sex, and sexuality; the way one looks; the way one's body functions; and whether one's body can help one accomplish goals.

Culture and social experience influence body image. Western cultures are influenced by the media, value beauty, health, and youth. Other cultures may value weight or old age. Most people have a picture of how they hope they look, an *idealized body image*. In addition, people have an awareness of how they really look, a *mirrored image*. When the real image is close to the ideal image, the person experiences positive regard for self. These positive feelings about body image are part of self-esteem.

A nursing research study found that African American women had positive body images regardless of their weight, and they considered physical exercise as a luxury they could not afford in their busy everyday life (Im et al., 2012). Such ethnic-specific attitudes are important to consider when planning dietary and exercise counseling.

SELF-ESTEEM

Whereas self-concept refers to the way people think about themselves, self-esteem refers to how people feel about themselves (Brown, 2007). Two sources for esteem are self and others (Fig. 38-1). Self-esteem develops throughout childhood and adolescence and becomes more stable in adulthood. People who receive more positive comments than negative comments about their body size and physical appearance tend to have higher self-esteem, less body

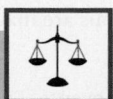

ETHICAL/LEGAL ISSUE

ANOREXIA

Angela Jackson, age 14 years, comes to the clinic with her mother. Angela is reluctant, but her mother is insistent and worried. Mrs. Jackson states that Angela has lost weight regularly over the past 6 months and seems to just pick at her food. She wants you to "do something" and make Angela eat, even if it means force-feeding her. Angela, who is 5 feet, 6 inches and weighs 98 lb, says she just isn't hungry. She doesn't understand her mother's worry. Angela states that she thinks she is "fat" and has to watch her weight. You recognize that Angela may have an eating disorder that may be a source of conflict between mother and daughter.

CLINICAL THINKING CHALLENGE
- Identify additional information that you may want to obtain.
- Examine the relationship between mother and daughter and the potential ethical dilemmas that may involve you.
- Consider additional resources that you need to manage this situation.
- Determine your ethical and legal responsibilities in this situation.

dissatisfaction, and more positive body image (Herbozo, Menzel, & Thompson, 2013).

Early in life, children accept their parents' evaluations as their own. Then children incorporate others' appraisals and expectations to form a self-ideal. They then slowly begin self-evaluation, emerging into adulthood with a basic or core self-esteem. Coopersmith (1967) identified antecedents of high self-esteem: parental acceptance, clear expectations, limitations, and freedom to express opinions. From these four antecedents,

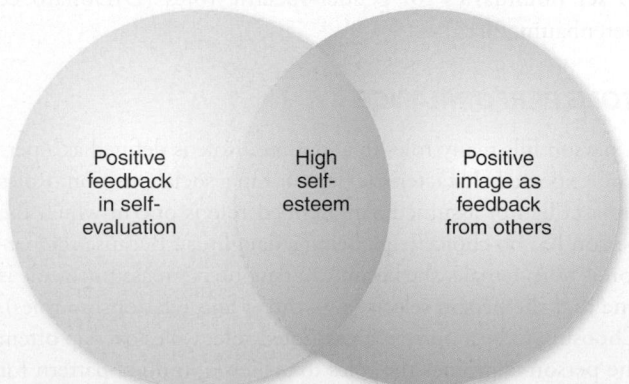

FIGURE 38-1 A person develops high self-esteem when he or she receives positive feedback from both self and others.

fundamental criteria by which people's self-appraisals are made have been proposed:

- *Power*: The ability to influence people and events—the sense that one's opinion counts and will be heard
- *Meaning*: The sense of being valued and worthwhile—one's existence matters to others
- *Competence*: The ability to achieve personal goals—personal success
- *Virtue*: Behaving in a manner consistent with personal values—adherence to a moral or ethical standard

Core self-esteem is the person's consistent, overall appraisal of self. The person acts or perceives events in ways that tend to support his or her level of self-esteem. Although core self-esteem is relatively stable, people do change their perceptions of self based on current experience (Rosenberg, 1979). Such an example is the woman described in the case scenario at the beginning of this chapter.

The person with adequate self-esteem has learned to cope with personal deficiencies and to maximize strengths. This person is self-accepting. The person with high self-esteem accepts others, experiences less anxiety, and functions effectively in social situations.

STRONG PERSONAL IDENTITY

Identity is an organizing principle of the self, the awareness that one is a distinct individual separate from others. The person with a strong sense of personal identity has integrated self-esteem, body image, and various roles into a whole self-concept. This whole or "I" is not associated with any one aspect. Identity provides the person with a sense of continuity through time. "I am not the person I was yesterday, but similarities and consistency provide links for today and the future."

The concept of boundaries is central to identity. Actual body boundaries (this is my hand; that is your hand) and ego boundaries (this is my thought or feeling, not your thought or feeling) must be intact for a person to maintain identity. To maintain mental health, the person must be able to differentiate self from others. Gender gives meaning to identity, but it is more than sexual function. A person's gender helps to set boundaries for gender-specific roles (DiDonato & Berenbaum, 2013).

ROLE PERFORMANCE

A person fills many roles in a lifetime. Role is defined as a person's expected characteristic behavior in a social position. Roles are ascribed or assumed. An ascribed role is one in which the person has no choice (e.g., being a daughter). Because the person is born female, she becomes a daughter. An assumed role is one that the person selects (e.g., career and relationship roles). Choosing to be a nurse is an assumed role. Roles overlap often; the person combines the roles to achieve a unified pattern for functioning. When the person perceives self as adequate in various roles, self-esteem is enhanced.

Life Span Considerations

Each developmental stage requires the completion of specific tasks that foster the development of positive self-concept. Prominent theories regarding development of self-concept are those of Erikson (1963), Freud (1920/1966), Havighurst (1972), Kohlberg (1969), and Piaget (1969). Sullivan (1953) discussed an interpersonal theory of life span development. Freud's, Sullivan's, Erikson's, and Havighurst's theories related to development of self-concept are listed in Table 38-1.

NEWBORN AND INFANT

Newborns have undifferentiated selves; they do not experience a separate existence from others. Parents and other caregivers transmit their self-concepts, sense of competence in new roles, and amount and intensity of anxiety they feel to newborns. When parents are reasonably calm and communicate warmth and acceptance to newborns, they help their babies establish the basis for positive self-concept.

Both family and newborn experience dramatic changes that can potentially affect the baby's self-concept. The mother shifts from being pregnant with a pregnant body to not being pregnant. If the mother chooses to breast-feed, she experiences further body-image changes and has concerns about milk production, sexuality, and competence. If she chooses not to breast-feed, she may experience guilt or doubt concerning the mothering role. During this same time, the mother is shifting in existing roles and developing new roles. The father also experiences shifts in and development of new roles. He must integrate new relationships into his identity. The family's relationships with others change during this time. Extended family may either help or confuse role transition. Friends may treat the couple differently after a child is born. Any siblings of the newborn experience shifts in roles also. Healthy acceptance and working through changes during this period set the stage for positive self-concept development.

Infants begin to understand self as separate and that feelings (e.g., hunger) are their own. As an infant begins to distinguish self from others, self-concept starts to develop. As an infant interacts with meaningful others, he or she begins to read the wants of others.

For example, when mom smiles and plays pat-a-cake, mom smiles even more when the infant smiles and makes noises. Thus, the infant begins to learn social role expectations. During infancy, children learn to sit, stand, and possibly walk. This managing of the body allows infants to experience the world in different ways and teaches children body boundaries. Bodily control helps to establish a beginning sense of separateness from others. Through play, infants learn to control aspects of the environment. For instance, early during this stage, infants bat objects such as colorful items on a mobile. Later, they grasp items and, toward the end of infancy, may be able to stack two blocks. This play helps children during the earliest stages of acquiring identity, just as social control (e.g., smiles) helps children with beginning roles.

In addition, infants begin to communicate through symbols. For example, smiles mean good, cries mean bad, "ma-ma"

TABLE 38-1 THEORIES OF SELF-CONCEPT DEVELOPMENT

	Freud: Psychodynamic (1920/1966)	Sullivan: Interpersonal (1953)	Erikson: Ego (1963)	Havighurst: Tasks (1972)
Newborn/infant	Oral stage, 0–3 mo; child is undifferentiated from mother.	*Infancy*: beginning self-concept formed; security = good me; anxiety = bad me; overwhelming anxiety or deprivation = not me	Trust vs. mistrust; adequate mothering helps infant establish trust in self and others.	*Task*: establishes physiologic stability
Infant	3 mo to 1.5 y; child begins to distinguish his or her body from objects (people and things) in the environment.	Infant has no separateness from caretaker.		
Toddler	Anal stage; personal identity pronounced "I"; role performance learned in family.	*Early childhood*: beginning differentiation; if relationship is adequate, child begins to integrate good me, bad me, and not me into self-concept.	Autonomy vs. shame; personal identity—body image and self-esteem develop as child experiences self-control through exploration in the world.	*Tasks*: learns body image through walking, talking, control of waste
Preschooler	Phallic stage; sex role, body image, and personal identity become more clearly differentiated.		Initiative vs. guilt; beginning role established through sexual identity development and family relationships.	Learns own sex role and identity through above tasks
School-age child	Latency; role performance is primary work of this stage; body-image problems may manifest if previous stages not resolved successfully.	*Juvenile*: process of individuation occurs as peer relationships develop; individual learns competition, compromise, and collaboration.	Industry vs. inferiority; socialization and competence are developing, helping continued growth of self-concept.	*Tasks*: learns physical skills for games; roles (i.e., sex, student, and friend); values
Adolescent	Genital stage; body image is altered as the individual establishes self as sexual being; separation from parents leads to enhanced sense of identity; role choices are made.	Identity, body image, and role continue to develop or be redefined as individuation progresses.	Identity vs. role confusion; search for self	*Tasks*: acceptance of body and sex role; independence from parents; occupational preparation and other roles learned (i.e., marriage, citizen)
Adult	Individual works on conflicts/deficits from previous developmental stages.		Intimacy vs. isolation; primary task role related—acquisition of love, sexual fulfillment, and closeness Generativity vs. self-absorption; as person concerns self with next generation(s), new sense of identity develops, increasing self-comfort and integration of varied roles.	*Tasks*: marriage, parenting, occupation *Tasks*: adjusting to physiologic changes; role with aging parents
Older adult			Integrity vs. despair; individual accepts personal accomplishments or feels decreased worth; body image changes as the person experiences physical alterations associated with old age (e.g., decreased sensory acuity).	*Tasks*: adjusts to decreased physical strength, retirement, possible death of self or spouse, decreased income

is associated with mothering persons, and infants begin to respond to their names. Infants accomplish these developmental tasks by interacting with caregivers and exploring.

TODDLER AND PRESCHOOLER

Toddlers have a rudimentary body image. Although they know the self as separate from others, they have no clear definition of where the body ends. For example, some toddlers may not want to flush the toilet after defecating because they see the stools as part of them. Toddlers are not aware of specific influences, only general feelings or thoughts. They do, however, understand others' responses to behavior. Thus, excessive punishment leads to bad feelings, and praise leads to good feelings. Gradually, toddlers incorporate these feelings into self-concept.

Self-concept continues to develop actively during preschool years. Preschoolers' sense of self becomes more defined as they realize that they are separate and unique. During this stage of development, children exhibit great sexual curiosity. They are aware that they are different from others. In addition to this sense of sexual self, preschoolers are incorporating both spatial relationships and increased coordination into their body image.

Sense of how one relates to others is more defined in the preschool stage than in previous stages. Children's roles in the family and the world are beginning to take shape. Preschoolers often imitate adult roles (Fig. 38-2). During this stage, children may share in older siblings' accomplishments or perceive themselves as not as good because they cannot achieve the same things. If a new baby is added to the family, preschoolers may respond with anger, jealousy, or regression. The family's response to the child's reaction influences his or her role performance and self-esteem.

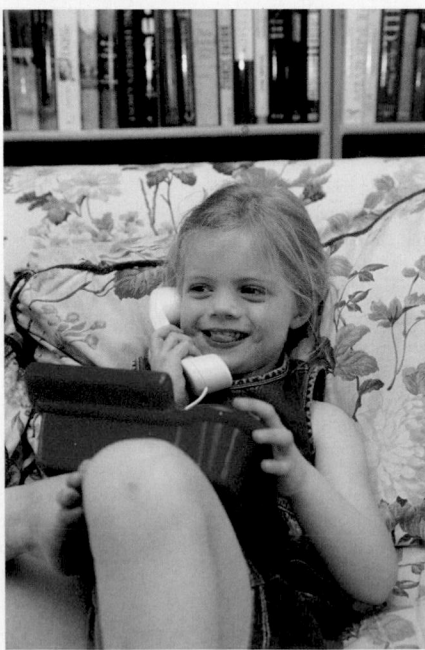

FIGURE 38-2 Preschoolers like to imitate adult roles as they learn about the world around them.

Because of curiosity, preschoolers learn body parts and names as well as attitudes about body and self. If questions are discounted, met with great anxiety, or answered with misinformation, children may develop a negative self-concept or poor body image.

SCHOOL-AGE CHILD AND ADOLESCENT

The school experience can strongly reinforce or alter a child's body image, sense of self, and identity. Teachers and peers become important influences on self-concept. Basically, children compare self to peers and measure looks, abilities, and social self against them. Because of rapid change and growth during school-age years, self-concept remains quite flexible, and changes are very individual. Figure 38-3 illustrates the flow of a child's self-concept development from 6 to 12 years of age.

Through life experiences, children "place values on feelings and on themselves as individuals, they make decisions about how to behave. When significant others accept a person's expression of feelings, the self grows and thrives, and the individual feels valued and loved simply for existing. This acceptance is particularly important to the adolescent who is concerned with self-understanding of inner emotions and psychological characteristics" (Brown, 2007).

Adolescents experience remarkable changes. Their bodies grow rapidly, secondary sex characteristics appear, and hormone secretion increases—all of which necessitate rapid changes in view of self. Adolescents must incorporate these changes to establish a coherent body image. Peers and role models, such as sports or media stars, strongly influence self-concept. Clothes, hairstyles, and movement are extensions of body image influenced by peers. Sexual changes and peer group expectations regarding sexual behavior may lead to a sexually active role.

As adolescents seek added responsibility, parents need to learn new methods of parenting. All family members can perceive an adolescent's striving for independence as a conflict. Adolescents may act in ways that seem to directly oppose the family's values and expectations. This behavior occurs because the chief developmental task of adolescence is to develop and to define personal identity.

 APPLY YOUR CRITICAL THINKING

Boden V., age 10 years, comes to the well-child clinic with his mother. Her concern is that Boden is always "sick" on gym days, yet he does not have systemic symptoms. While discussing this with Mrs. V., you notice how uncomfortable and embarrassed Boden is. He reluctantly tells you that because he is overweight he gets some teasing in gym activities, so he tries to get out of attending school on those days. How would you seek to understand the self-esteem issues that pertain to this visit? How would you suggest that the mother and son approach this challenge?

Check your answer in Appendix B.

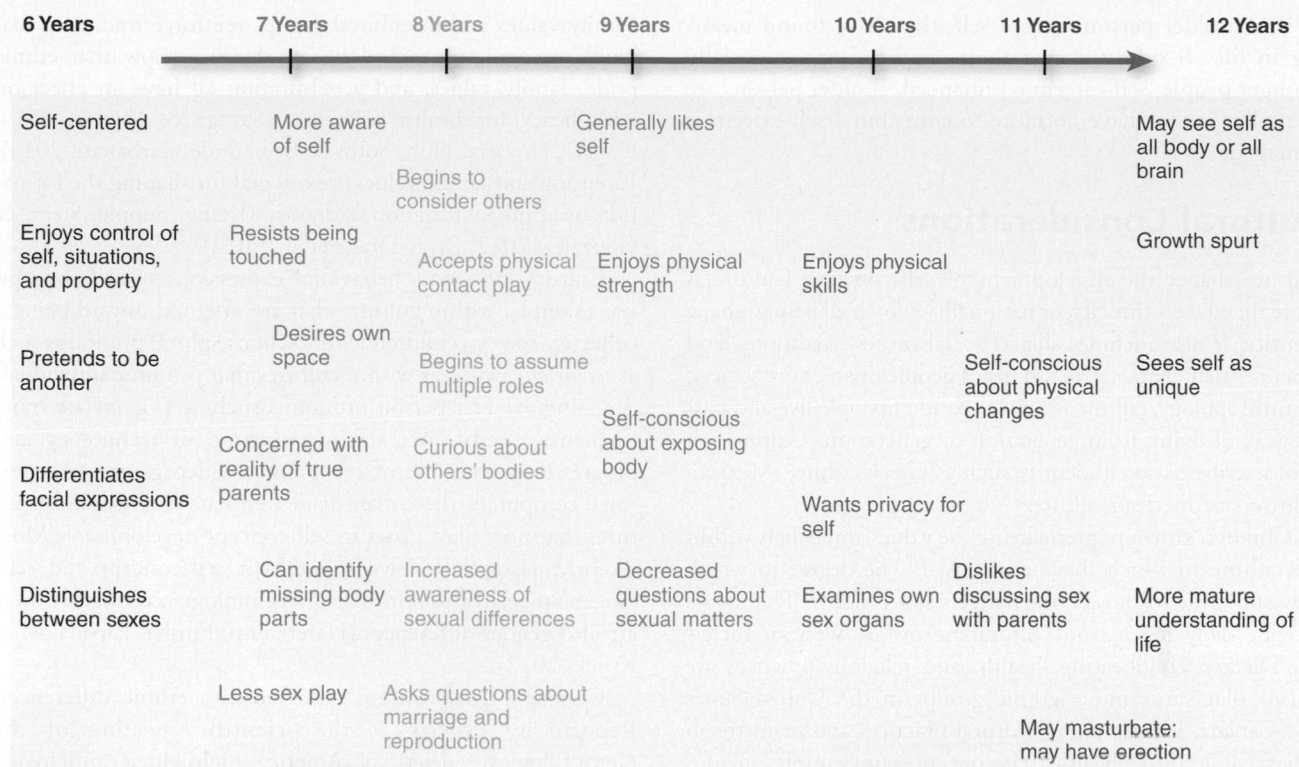

6 Years	7 Years	8 Years	9 Years	10 Years	11 Years	12 Years
Self-centered	More aware of self		Generally likes self			May see self as all body or all brain
		Begins to consider others				
Enjoys control of self, situations, and property	Resists being touched	Accepts physical contact play	Enjoys physical strength	Enjoys physical skills		Growth spurt
Pretends to be another	Desires own space	Begins to assume multiple roles			Self-conscious about physical changes	Sees self as unique
Differentiates facial expressions	Concerned with reality of true parents	Curious about others' bodies	Self-conscious about exposing body			
				Wants privacy for self		
Distinguishes between sexes	Can identify missing body parts	Increased awareness of sexual differences	Decreased questions about sexual matters	Examines own sex organs	Dislikes discussing sex with parents	More mature understanding of life
	Less sex play	Asks questions about marriage and reproduction				May masturbate; may have erection

FIGURE 38-3 Self-concept development as shown on a continuum from age 6 to 12 years. Attributes are approximate. Although there is general consistency in development, each child is unique.

ADULT AND OLDER ADULT

Adults continue to modify self-concept. Young adults move away from the conforming peer group with a struggle for personal identity modified through life experiences. Much of assumed role formation happens early in the adult stage. Common life experiences for early adulthood include forming intimate relationships, choosing a career, establishing a home base, and starting a family.

During the fourth and into the fifth decade, adults may question the fit of their chosen identity and experiences. They may examine the meaning of self and contemplate the parts of self not previously explored. They examine roles and options taken and discarded as they look for more meaning in life. Sheehy (1974), in her classic book *Passages*, has called this process an "authenticity crisis." The outcome of this authenticity crisis is renewal or resignation. With renewal, the person emerges with an expanded sense of self. With resignation, the person's self remains defined by the narrow constraints of his or her roles.

Retirement requires extraordinary changes in role performance and self-esteem. Because career roles have much to say about whom a person is, retired persons are often described by who they were, which implies that they no longer have value; this greatly affects self-esteem.

Most older Americans live independently in their own homes. Independence and self-care are related to higher self-esteem and life satisfaction (Fig. 38-4). Those who have the ability to manage stress and adapt to new situations are better

able to function independently, and physiologically, the brain continues to regulate the ability to withstand life challenges (Karatsoreos & McEwen, 2013).

Physical changes such as decreased strength, skin turgor, and sensory acuity affect body image in later life. Because of the valuation of youth in the media and popular culture, some older adults experience lowered self-esteem with the changed body image. Sensory changes also affect personal identity. If the environment does not provide feedback, a person may have difficulty determining what is part of self.

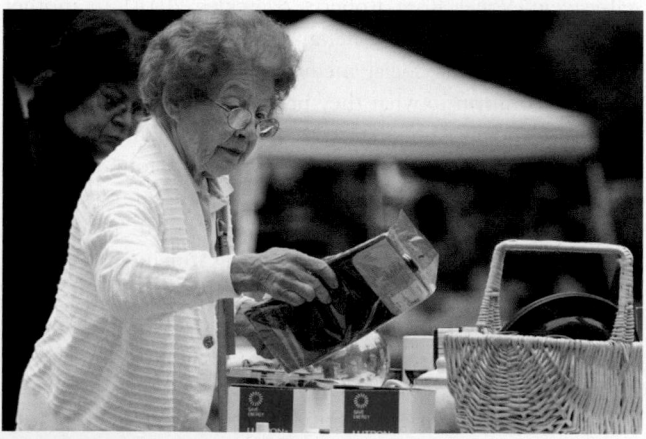

FIGURE 38-4 Independence is an important aspect of self-concept or personal identity.

When older persons accept self, they have found meaning in life. If others accept their contributions, especially younger people, self-esteem is enhanced. If older persons are treated as if they have no more to contribute, self-esteem is damaged.

Cultural Considerations

Culture shapes the development of self-concept. Culture is more than race, ethnicity, or nationality, which all help to shape identity. It also includes shared social mores, traditions, and practices that characterize groups of people or an entire society. In anthropology, culture is how a group of people live and pass the way of living from generation to generation. Culture can also describe national identity such as Greek culture, Mexican culture, or American culture.

Children grow up internalizing the values and beliefs within the culture to which they are exposed. The degree to which they subscribe to those norms affects self-concept. The media provide daily lessons on cultural norms in Western societies. Dietary, childbearing, health, and religious practices are norms that vary among ethnic groups in the United States and Canada. Integration of cultural practices and mainstream beliefs can lead to a healthy self-concept. For example, an adolescent who cultivates an interest in ethnic music and dance but still shares a love of rock music with his peers will have a strong identity and high self-esteem.

Social settings are common places for experiencing culture. Starting in the 1950s, the corner drug store and later fast-food restaurants that served inexpensive burgers and milkshakes became the social setting for developing teenagers. With the advent of computers, handheld technology devices, and social media such as Facebook, Twitter, and Instagram, there are new factors in modern culture that affect many aspects of individuals, especially self-esteem. Increasing social interaction via social media could improve self-esteem. However, many studies have shown that social media has the potential to impact individuals in unexpected ways. For example, one study found that frequent use of social media such as Facebook and seeing profiles of successful individuals led to a temporary decrease in self-esteem (Vogel, Rose, Roberts, & Eckles, 2014). In another study conducted in the Netherlands, preteens interacting with another preteen via social media altered their food (candy) intake to conform to what they perceived their peer to be eating (Bevelander, Anschütz, Creemers, Kleinjan, & Engels, 2013). In young adults of college age, a study found that frequent social media usage was associated with communication overload and reduced self-esteem, which led to psychological distress (Chen & Lee, 2013). During nursing assessment, it becomes important to discover whether a patient's social engagement is through in-person interactions or via social media because these factors have the potential to impact the individual's self-esteem differently.

Ethnic pride is an expression of a person's affiliation with their ethnic and or cultural group. This is also a display of ethnic identity, particularly among minority cultural groups.

Family values within cultural groups reinforce traditions that build personal values and beliefs. Studies show that ethnic pride, family values, and acculturation all have an effect on self-efficacy for health behaviors (Savage & Mezuk, 2014; Unger, Schwartz, Huh, Soto, & Baezconde-Garbanati, 2014). Parenting and family values are integral for shaping the formation of ethnic and national identity (Kiang, Supple, Stein, & Gonzalez, 2012; Rivas-Drake et al., 2014).

Culture influences behavioral expressions of self-concept. For example, within cultures that are oriented toward being a collective society, children tend to choose plural pronouns such as *we* or *our*, whereas within cultures that promote individualism, singular first person pronouns such as *I* or *my* are more frequently used. Since the introduction of technology and progressively wide use of cell phones, video games, and personal computers, these man-made items are factors within cultures that now play a part in self-concept development. More recently, researchers have found that self-concept and self-esteem are related to information technology use and that there are also gender differences (Haferkamp, Eimler, Papadakis, & Kruck, 2012).

Genetic predispositions contribute to ethnic differences. Reports by experts at the scientific meeting of the Gerontological Society of America highlighted anticipated increases in our ethnically diverse elderly population and the importance of providing ethnic-specific culturally appropriate healthcare. For example, elders with the same diagnosis and treatments who come from varied ethnic groups rate their pain differently (Laguna, Goldstein, Braun, & Enguidanos, 2014). Programs based on cultural beliefs of the patient can improve adherence to health-promoting behaviors (Eschiti et al., 2014).

Acculturation occurs when people move from the culture where they grew up to an unfamiliar culture, either in a different country or in another area within the same country, and must learn a new set of cultural values, beliefs, and traditions. Acculturation can help minority groups be successful within the greater adopted society, but the process of acculturation affects self-concept development and self-efficacy. For example, there are differences within cultures as seen in studies that explored development of ethnic and national identity among Dutch ethnic minority adolescents (Eichelsheim et al., 2010). Integrating identified cultural values and practices of specific cultural groups into tailored health promotion programs will make them more acceptable to those communities of people (Pan et al., 2013).

FACTORS AFFECTING SELF-CONCEPT

Biologic Makeup

Biologic makeup comprises many characteristics that affect self-concept. Sex, height, weight, skin color, and appearance are characteristics that self and others perceive to help form

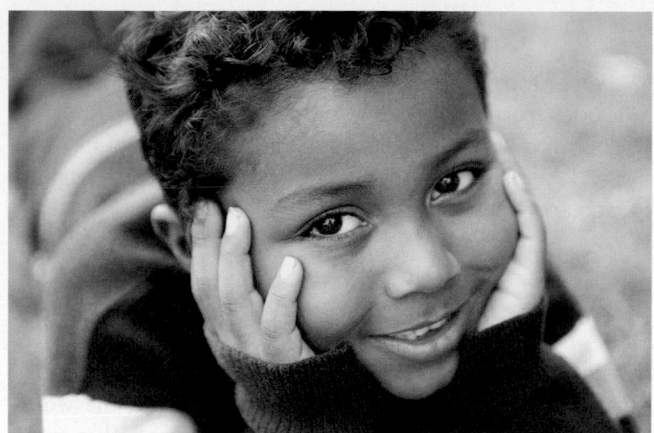

FIGURE 38-5 Sex, skin color, hair color, and eye color affect self-perception.

self-concept (Fig. 38-5). These factors also influence what a person experiences. For example, men often have more opportunities to play competitive sports, which may enhance self-concept, whereas in some cases, women are more limited in playing certain sports. Women who are athletically inclined may perceive their abilities as inferior, a perception damaging to self-concept. Recently, opportunities for athletics and competitive sports for women have increased, thus helping to promote positive self-concepts. Likewise, someone who is black in a predominantly white society may have difficulty securing a positive self-concept if others' perceptions are discriminatory. People who are tall, slender, and attractive may easily develop positive self-concepts because these qualities are favorably perceived.

The continuing debate over nature (biology) versus nurture (environment) indicates that biology plays a significant role because of the results of studies of twins (Polderman, Hoekstra, Posthuma, & Larsson, 2014). Many attributes such as assertiveness, happiness, and even vulnerability to stress have been found to have a heritable component (Zhao et al., 2013; Cole et al., 2014). Although genes are not exclusive causes of such attributes, they are increasingly important to understanding nature's power and influence on nurture. Knowledge of biology offers hope for clearer understanding of therapeutic nursing interventions that build on inherent traits while simultaneously shaping environmental conditions to promote self-esteem and self-concept.

Coping and Stress Tolerance

Coping and stress tolerance influence self-concept. People who are able to adapt to stress and resolve conflicts through coping tend to develop healthy self-concepts. Internal resources, such as a sense of humor and productivity under pressure, and external resources, such as strong support groups, enhance coping. A single mother who has strong family support may master the roles of parenthood, financial provider, and activist for women's rights while enhancing self-esteem and likewise strengthening performance in these roles. Poor stress tolerance may lead to crisis, however, and a damaged self-concept.

Older adults with a strong self-concept are better able to maintain a positive attitude when dealing with adverse conditions. For example, mental attitude with the ability to cope and staying engaged in one's own continuity of care can improve recovery from joint replacement surgery (Tay Swee Cheng, Klainin-Yobas, Hegney, & Mackey, 2014).

STRESSFUL LIFE EVENTS

Most people face numerous daily stressors, many of which occur simultaneously. Common stressors include financial difficulties, job problems, change or loss of employment, relationship concerns, sexuality concerns, divorce, moving, making new friends, loss of loved ones, parenting, competition, and making important decisions. Stressful events often challenge the person's identity and self-esteem. One stressor may be so intense that it paralyzes the person and damages self-concept. More often, however, cumulative stress wears away at self-concept (see Chapter 41). For example, a young couple marries and must move to another city where the husband found a job. They have difficulty buying a house because of the high cost of living in the new area and immediately have financial difficulties. The wife would like to start a family but must take a job for which she feels overqualified. They have difficulty making new friends and are overwhelmed by the numerous decisions that have to be made while starting their life together. The husband begins to feel that he is not a good provider and cannot afford the lifestyle he would like. The couple experiences stress in their relationship, and both may feel that self-esteem and identity are damaged.

INADEQUATE COPING

Inadequate coping can lead to problems with self-concept. In the previous example, the young couple needs strong coping skills to maintain intact self-concepts. Lack of support systems and inability to prioritize and problem solve, however, contribute to further problems. Some people with inadequate coping develop defensive self-esteem. Defensive self-esteem is a protective mechanism in which the person reports high self-esteem to deny negative personal information. The person has a high need for social approval while defending the self against hurt, failure, or anxiety through denial, grandiosity, or projection.

For example, an adolescent heart transplant recipient who accepts this body change is able to develop a new sense of self. However, if he or she is not able to accept this experience, the adolescent continues to worry about being normal and idealizes about relationships rather than discusses the problem. One research study found that self-accepting, positive body talk was related to satisfaction with body image and self-esteem (Rudiger & Winstead, 2013).

In teenagers, suicide is the third leading cause of mortality Centers for Disease Control and Prevention, 2013. Many teenagers that are at risk for suicide have not learned adequate coping skills for daily stresses, which can lead to depression and self-concept issues. A study in Brazil assessed factors leading to increased suicide risk for pregnant teenagers and found that factors related to poor development of coping skills such as low education, prior abortion, previous major depressive episode, and physical abuse all were significant contributing factors (Vitriol et al., 2014). Additionally, social and cultural factors such as the growth of social media can influence teenage suicide risk. For example, bullying, including cyberbullying, has been linked to increased risk for suicide by teenagers (Bazelon, 2013). However, technology can also be used positively to deliver suicide prevention interventions. In a research study, Whittaker et al. (2012) used text messaging to deliver two depression prevention messages each day to a group of teenagers. They found that the teenagers preferred reading the messages over talking to a friend, and the teens stated that these messages led to increased positive thinking and to decreased negative thinking.

Self-Efficacy

Self-efficacy theory (Bandura, 1977) suggests a link between perceived self and coping behaviors. Self-efficacy is the degree of confidence a person has about the ability to perform specific activities (Bandura, 1994). Stated another way, self-efficacy is related to how much a person believes that his or her efforts can effect a desired outcome. In Bandura's self-efficacy model, individuals with high self-efficacy believe they can perform well and are thus more likely to perceive difficult tasks as within their abilities and something to be mastered. Conversely, those with low self-efficacy believe they are unable to do well and frequently won't even attempt a difficult task. Four factors influence self-efficacy: experience, modeling by others, social persuasion, and physiologic factors. Experience refers to a person's actual successful or unsuccessful attempts to master a skill such as trying to quit smoking. Modeling can come from many sources, including family, friends, and media. Social persuasion involves trying to convince the individual of the merits of changing. Finally, physiologic factors are the physical responses to new situations. For example, a person who experiences a high heart rate or sweaty palms when asking someone out on a date may interpret that physiologic information as being incompetent, even though it is simply physical responses to a stressful new event. Each of these factors is influential though may be subtle depending on the situation.

Self-efficacy offers nurses a tool for use in health promotion, patient teaching for smoking cessation, dietary modification, and compliance with many therapeutic regimens. For example, individuals with high self-efficacy were far more likely to successfully quit smoking after participating in a web-based smoking cessation intervention study (Smit, Hoving, Schelleman-Offermans, West, de Vries, 2014). In working with adults with diabetes, self-efficacy level was an important factor in predicting improved diabetes self-care and overall quality of life (Walker, Gebregziabher, Martin-Harris, & Egede, 2014). In a study of Taiwan patients who experienced heart failure symptoms, those who were taught self-management skills via modeling and social persuasion techniques improved in their self-efficacy and experienced lower symptoms (Shao, Chang, Edwards, Shyu, & Chen, 2013).

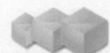

Concept Mastery Alert

When providing care for a patient whose self-concept includes feeling dependent and a burden, avoid performing all of the patient's ADLs. It is important to provide assistance where necessary while still promoting a sense of achievement and self-efficacy.

Previous Experience

Self-concept is the individual's complex, ever-changing personal perspective on his or her relationship with the world. It is affected by one's previous experiences with the world. Experiences include opportunities for success and failure. If the person meets with success, he or she builds self-esteem and role satisfaction and begins to expect success. The person also learns what and whom he or she can influence.

An *expectancy* is a belief that one's behavior will lead to a given response. Two expectancies incorporated into the self are expectancy for success and locus of control, which can be external or internal. Expectancy for success means the person has a belief that personal behavior will lead to something desired. A person with *external locus of control* perceives that outcomes happen because of luck, chance, or the influence of powerful others. A person with *internal locus of control* believes that personal behavior influences outcome and that he or she can achieve desired results. These expectancies develop from life experiences and influence the self. For instance, if a person believes that luck brought about an outcome, that person would not feel increased esteem because of the outcome, whereas a person with internal locus of control would have increased esteem. Illness may threaten a person with strong internal locus of control; however, self-concept can be preserved by the person's belief that subsequent health-seeking behavior will bring about wellness.

Experience also allows the person to develop and use coping strategies. As the person experiences stress in life, he or she uses the coping skills that fit with his or her views of self and the world. The person who is able to use healthy-coping mechanisms that worked in the past will reinforce self-esteem with future successful coping.

Bullying is an unwanted, aggressive behavior among school-aged children that involves a real or perceived power differential (stopbullying.gov, 2014). For most individuals, bullying occurs only a few times, but some children experience pervasive episodes of bullying. Unfortunately, bullying can continue into adult life and be experienced at home or at work. Bullying may alter an individual's self-concept and be part of a number of psychological factors leading to many negative physical, emotional, relational, and other outcomes. For example, bullying, including "cyberbullying," was associated with lowered self-efficacy along with other psychological issues in a study of Hong Kong middle school-aged students (Wong et al., 2014). In a study conducted in Greece, Kokkinos and Kipritsi (2012) found that bullying was more common among boys than girls and that being a bully and

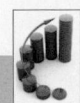

OUTCOME-BASED TEACHING PLANS

Maria Benet, age 16 years, comes to the high school clinic for a "sore throat." Assessment reveals that her throat is not inflamed, and she does not have a fever. As you explore the situation, Maria states, "I'm too sick to go to class today. Besides, I'm no good at math and never will be. I think I'll just drop out of school." You realize that Maria may have some self-concept problems. You decide to try to help her overcome them.

OUTCOME

Maria will express more confidence in her ability to learn new things.

STRATEGIES

- Explore Maria's feelings about her performance in math class.
- If Maria is motivated to try to change:
  - Have Maria discuss her performance privately with her teacher and/or counselor.

- Discuss possible support mechanisms (e.g., peer tutors, special study sessions).
- Discuss ways she uses math every day (e.g., memorizing phone numbers, figuring "percent off" at sales, making change when she shops).
- Suggest she practice math activities and realize that she can handle them.
- Problem solve with Maria a plan that she feels motivated to follow.
- Provide regular opportunities for follow-up to assess and provide encouragement from you and others.

EVALUATION

4/15/17: 09:00—After discussion with Maria, she has decided to talk with her teacher privately, explaining her math fears and asking for tutoring assistance. Maria has agreed to talk with her counselor on a biweekly basis about her progress in managing her math class.

—M. Klim, RN

being a victim of bullying were both related to lower overall self-efficacy in academic achievement and empathy. Other studies have demonstrated a relationship between level of self-efficacy and whether or how an individual responds to witnessing episodes of bullying (Thornberg & Jungert, 2013). It is important for nurses to assess level of self-efficacy in areas of coping and empathy to design effective interventions to promote safety and wellness.

Developmental Level

Developmental level influences self-concept from birth through older adulthood. Whereas newborns have no separate sense of self and young children are learning that their identities are separate from others, adolescents must deal with body-image changes. Each developmental level brings unique experiences that can reinforce or alter self-concept. If developmental tasks are not completed, problems with self-concept occur, possibly leading to uncompleted tasks at a later developmental level. Accomplishment of key tasks at each level enhances self-concept.

Incomplete developmental tasks can lead to problems with self-concept. Adolescence is a particularly difficult time because many physical, emotional, and sexual changes occur during this period. Adolescents make decisions about the future, seek independence from their parents, and feel pressure from peer groups. Body image and identity are not secure but depend on others' perceptions. Self-esteem is fragile.

Changes in role or body image can affect personal identity during developmental transitions. If personal identity is disturbed, the person has difficulty stating who he or she is.

This person may be unable to differentiate personal thoughts and feelings from those of others. Decreases in amount or quality of social interaction may affect relationships.

For example, regardless of ethnicity, girls with higher body mass index and percentage body fat experienced more social anxiety, depression, victimization from their peers, and decreased self-worth (Lanza et al., 2013). Also, women with eating disorders may have low or lack self-esteem. Being sensitive and giving positive feedback can improve their self-esteem (Vancampfort et al., 2014).

Role Transition

People make multiple role transitions in a lifetime. Two types of role transition are developmental and situational. *Developmental* role transitions are commonly associated with aging and growth, such as the transition from student to wage earner. *Situational* transitions are associated with change in relationships, such as the death of a spouse leading to changing one's status from married to being widowed. Either type of role transition can prompt role problems, including role ambiguity, role strain, and role conflicts.

Role ambiguity occurs when the person lacks knowledge of role expectations, which fosters anxiety and confusion. For example, a person assumes a new job without receiving an orientation to his or her expected job performance and responsibilities. As a result, this person may feel uncertain about how to be successful in this new role.

Role strain occurs when the person perceives himself or herself as inadequate or unsuited for a role. This can occur in any role or because of numerous roles. One example is a

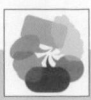

THERAPEUTIC DIALOGUE: SELF-CONCEPT

SCENE FOR THOUGHT

Gwen Jacobs is 12 years old. She comes to the clinic for her school sports physical, accompanied by her mother.

LESS EFFECTIVE

Nurse: Hi, Gwen, I'm Barbara Thompson, the nurse practitioner who will do your physical today. What sport are you trying out for this year?

Gwen: All of them. *(Looks at the nurse curiously.)* I thought only doctors did physicals.

Nurse: Actually, nurses do physicals, too. What sports do you particularly like? *(Checks head, eyes, ears, nose, and throat [HEENT].)*

Gwen: I like soccer and softball best. I want to play them in high school too.

Nurse: Good for you. *(Asks mom a question and continues to do exam, taking out stethoscope.)*

Gwen: Are you going to listen to my heart with that? *(Looks at stethoscope.)*

Nurse: Sure am. *(Opens patient's gown and listens to heart sounds.)*

Gwen: *(Hunches shoulders as if to hide chest from view.)*

Nurse: Okay, now I'll listen to your lungs from the back. Breathe in for me. *(Completes exam. Gwen is silent.)* I can see you look pretty healthy, Gwen. All the normal milestones are being reached, Mrs. Jacobs, including some breast development. If you need any information about menstruation or anything like that, the clinic has some terrific pamphlets I could give you. Otherwise, we'll see her for her next exam next year. Hope you have a good year, Gwen. Win a lot of games! *(Smiles and leaves the room.)*

Gwen: *(Blushing.)* I hope we don't get her again! Let's go, Mom, I'm going to be late for practice.

MORE EFFECTIVE

Nurse: Hi, Gwen, I'm Becky Thomas, the nurse practitioner who will do your physical today. What sport are you trying out for this year?

Gwen: All of them. *(Looks at the nurse curiously.)* I thought only doctors did physicals.

Nurse: Actually, nurses do physicals, too. What sports do you particularly like? *(Checks HEENT.)*

Gwen: I like soccer and softball best. I want to play them in high school too.

Nurse: Good for you. You really look strong, especially your leg muscles. Been playing sports a long time? *(Warms up the stethoscope for heart and lung assessment.)*

Gwen: Yes, since I was little. *(Looks at the stethoscope.)* Are you going to listen to my heart with that?

Nurse: *(Stops to look at her.)* Yes. And your lungs too. Any problems?

Gwen: *(Looks down at the floor.)* Do I have to take my gown off?

Nurse: No. I can examine your heart this way *(shows her how the drape will continue to cover her chest)* and listen to your lungs through your back. Does something worry you about being examined?

Gwen: No. *(Blushes.)*

Nurse: I wonder if you're a little embarrassed about being examined. *(Listens to heart sounds under the gown.)*

Gwen: Yeah. *(Looks guilty.)*

Nurse: I understand. I have a daughter your age. She's also pretty shy about people seeing her body. She says it's because it's changing so fast, and she doesn't understand it all. *(Listens to lung sounds.)*

Gwen: Yeah. *(Looks interested.)* Does she play sports too? The hardest part is taking a shower after gym. Everybody always looks. I hate it.

Nurse: Not an easy time, I imagine. Could you lie down, please? *(Examines abdomen.)*

Gwen: *(Big sigh.)* Yeah. Are you almost done? *(Giggles.)* That tickles!

Nurse: Almost. *(Finishes exam.)* I'm going to leave the room so you can get dressed, then you, your mom, and I can sit and talk for a bit. If you or your mom have any questions you want to ask, I can answer them then. Okay?

CRITICAL THINKING CHALLENGE

- Explain the relationship between body image and self-concept.
- Interpret how you think Gwen would describe herself.
- Compare and contrast how each nurse talked to Gwen and her response to each.
- Describe how Becky used self-disclosure to help Gwen.
- Identify to whom Barbara was primarily talking and why she was less effective.

contemporary woman trying to fulfill the roles of wife, lover, mother, employee, and professional. As she tries to meet the demands of all of these roles, she may experience the feeling that she is not fulfilling any role the way she believes that she should.

Role conflict is related to expectations concerning the role. Role conflict can be described as intrapersonal, interpersonal, or inter-role. *Intrapersonal* role conflict exists when role expectations conflict with the person's values, such as a nurse being asked to assist with an abortion when she believes it is immoral. *Interpersonal* role conflict exists when the person's expectations differ from that of some significant other. For example, an adolescent might want to play in a rock band, but his or her parents value intellectual pursuits rather than artistic pursuits. *Interrole* conflict exists when a person is expected to fulfill two or more roles simultaneously. In the case of a spouse's death, the surviving spouse may become sole wage earner for the family, single parent, and caretaker of the house. He or she may be unsure what is expected in a new job. The role as wage earner may conflict with parenting responsibilities, and the combination of roles may be overwhelming. Self-concept can be damaged by such role transitions.

Illness, Trauma, and Surgery

Positive self-concept is usually based on a healthy self. Acute and chronic illness, trauma, or surgery can adversely affect self-esteem and body image, thereby producing stress and role strain, reducing self-esteem, and altering body image. Even physical changes associated with normal aging may alter self-concept. Successful coping during illness, however, may enhance self-esteem. For example, a person with cancer who tolerates chemotherapy, can hold down a job, and becomes closer to the family may emerge feeling emotionally stronger and more resourceful and with a more positive self-concept than before the illness.

Altered body image occurs when the person experiences a disruption in the perception of the body image. Obviously, if the person has an actual loss of a body part or function, he or she will have a disrupted body image until the change is incorporated. Feelings associated with disturbed body image include helplessness, hopelessness, powerlessness, fear of others' reactions, and anger.

People who experience trauma during their childhood are more likely to develop depression and self-concept changes. Interventions focused on these childhood traumas can help patients understand the cause of their psychological difficulties. Women in Chile who had depression after suffering childhood traumas showed improvement in their social role functioning after receiving these treatments (Vitriol et al., 2014).

Amputation, mastectomy, burns, and facial trauma cause significant change in body structure and appearance. Cardiac disease that limits activities, renal disease requiring dialysis, and a colostomy all impact the body's function. The ability to retain an intact self-concept in the face of illness, trauma, and surgery varies among people. The person's perception of the alteration and the importance that he or she places on the body part or function affected influences body image dysfunction. For example, an athlete who places great importance on his or her long, strong legs for running would be devastated by

a neurologic illness that produces weakness, placing him or her in a wheelchair. The athlete experiences decreased self-esteem and change in body image.

ALTERED SELF-CONCEPT

Self-Care Deficit

Manifestations of self-concept dysfunction range from subtle emotional and behavioral changes to full-blown, self-destructive behaviors. These manifestations also may reflect other problems, such as anxiety, depression, or substance abuse. Accurate identification of the underlying problem is essential. People with dysfunctional self-concept may exhibit self-care deficit. For example, people with chronic disease may disregard special diet instructions, not take medications, and miss follow-up appointments. Hospitalized patients may avoid participation in medical and nursing treatment. Self-care deficit may also be characterized by poor personal hygiene, disregard for health maintenance activities, inappropriate exposure or concealment of body parts affected by disease, and lack of health-seeking behaviors. The person may refuse to acknowledge health concerns or express feelings of not being worth special care or concern. For example, a middle-aged diabetic woman with an amputated leg keeps her lower body covered by a blanket, even in warm weather. She rarely combs her hair or puts on makeup, frequently misses appointments, and eats sweets because she feels she is "not worth it."

Emotional and Behavioral Changes

Emotional changes with self-concept dysfunction include feelings of depersonalization, hopelessness, helplessness, alienation, fear of rejection, anger, sadness, shame, guilt, inadequacy, worthlessness, and suspicion of others. Emotional responses may be blunted or inappropriately intense.

Behavioral changes indicating self-concept dysfunction include lack of interest in activities, inability to make decisions, withdrawal from social situations, isolation, refusal to look in the mirror, refusal to look at an affected body part or discuss a limitation, avoidance of responsibility, show of hostility toward others, refusal to make eye contact, and negative verbalizations about self.

Behavior may become more dependent on or independent of others, including healthcare providers. A woman who has undergone cancer chemotherapy, lost her hair, and undergone significant weight loss may show emotional and behavioral manifestations of self-concept dysfunction. She may refuse to look in the mirror, assume independence in bathing and dressing to prevent others from seeing her body, avoid eye contact with the staff, refuse visitors by saying she is tired, and seem emotionally apathetic.

Anxiety and Depression

Anxiety and depression are two common psychological disturbances that are manifestations of self-concept dysfunction. Whenever there is a change in body image, problems with roles or identity, and low self-esteem, the person is threatened.

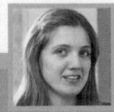

Self-Concept PICO

After hearing the comments of the mother in the chapter-opening scenario, you wonder if parenting programs might be helpful in providing some psychosocial support for the array of feelings she has been experiencing since giving birth. You look around the clinic and see several brochures describing different types of parenting classes and notice one for group-based therapy, but you are unsure of how it might help. You decide to look for evidence in the Cochrane Library and use the following PICO for your search: *With parents, how does group-based parenting programs compare to no programs improve psychosocial well-being?*

P = parents

I = group-based parenting programs

C = no programs

O = improve psychological well-being

You find a meta-analysis that reviewed 48 randomized controlled trials with 4,937 participants. Some studies included fathers. Three types of group-based programs were evaluated in the review: behavioral, cognitive–behavioral, and multimodal. Some of the interventions in these programs focused on empowering parents, strategies to deal with the child's behaviors, and tactics to decrease parenting stress between the two parents and improve marital relations. The studies did show a statistical difference in psychosocial well-being of parents who participated in these programs, although short term. Feelings such as depression, anxiety, stress, anger, guilt, and partner relationship satisfaction had shown improvement with these programs. The research showed in particular that stress and confidence of participating individuals continued to improve for up to six months. You decide to offer the brochure to the mother since you know that psychosocial well-being of parents can impact the child's development.

REFERENCE:

Barlow, J., Smailagic, N., Huband, N., Roloff, V., & Bennett, C. (2014). Group-based parent training programmes for improving parental psychosocial health. *Cochrane Database of Systematic Reviews*, (5), CD002020. doi: 10.1002/14651858.CD002020.pub4

This threat is often the cause of great anxiety and is frequently followed by the grieving process. As an example, an older man who has recently experienced loss of a job, loss of a wife, and loss of good health may very likely show signs of depression. A person may experience brief episodes of sadness in response to temporary self-concept dysfunction. However, if they lack adequate coping or self-efficacy, they may exhibit signs of clinical depression that is characterized by symptoms that last longer than 2 weeks such as persistent sadness, difficulty sleeping, difficulty concentrating, and social withdrawal.

The percentage of adults that is considered elderly, age 65 years and older, has dramatically increased over the past few decades. As in other age groups, geriatric populations are susceptible to depression. About 1 in 7 of those over age 65 experience depression, and suicide rates are highest in the United States for those over age 85 (Geriatric Mental Health Foundation, 2014). Additionally, approximately 25 percent of those experiencing a chronic medical condition such as heart disease, lung disease, cancer, arthritis, and Alzheimer disease are likely to suffer from depression. Given the higher rate of chronic medical conditions, social isolation, and decreased activity level of many elderly individuals, it is important to help identify the source of their self-concept disturbance and apply nursing interventions that build coping skills and increase situational self-efficacy.

When parents have anxiety or depression, they tend to perceive lower self-efficacy in their adolescent children who have diabetes. This then may lead to the adolescents having less confidence in their own abilities to manage their diabetic symptoms. Therefore, interventions with a family approach that focus on the self-concept of each family member and how they affect each other may be more effective than focusing on the adolescent alone (Berg et al., 2013).

Self-Destructive Behavior

Substance abuse (drugs, alcohol), sexual promiscuity, gambling, and overeating can be manifestations of self-concept dysfunction. Brown (2007) described the intoxicated person's progression from becoming less self-aware to failing to use good judgment and subsequently behaving atypically. These self-destructive behaviors are addictive, giving immediate gratification only. Persons with low self-esteem and negative self-image find it difficult to change self-destructive behaviors because they have difficulty seeing themselves more positively. For example, a 40-year-old male alcoholic attributes loss of a job, financial insecurity, and injuries in an alcohol-related car accident to bad luck. This person is exhibiting self-destructive behavior and self-concept dysfunction.

Recall the new mother in the case scenario. While she is very happy to be a mother, she is experiencing some body image issues. Use the concept map (Fig. 38-6) to help understand and manage the mother's concern about body image.

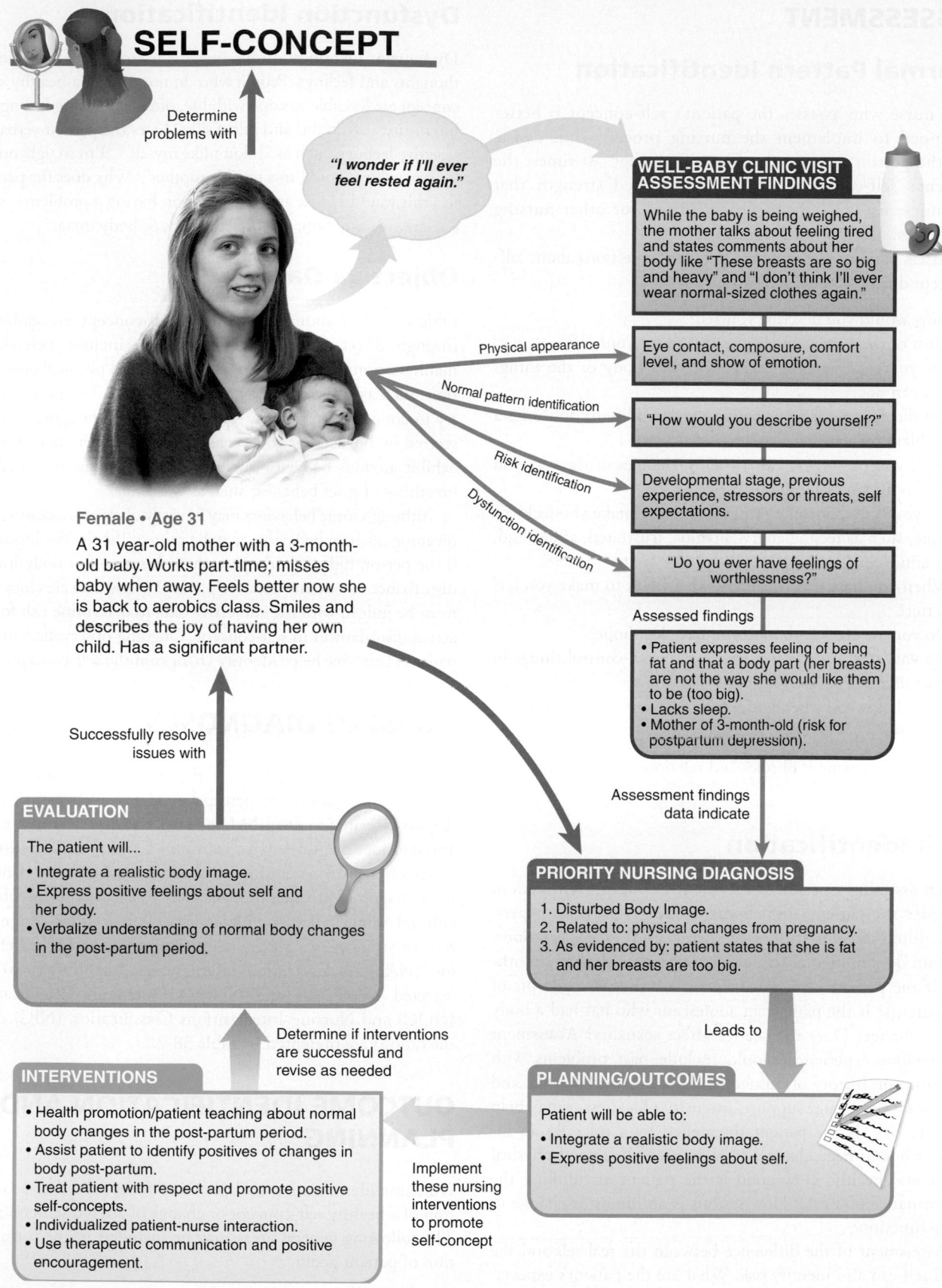

SELF-CONCEPT

Determine problems with

"I wonder if I'll ever feel rested again."

Female • Age 31

A 31 year-old mother with a 3-month-old baby. Works part-time; misses baby when away. Feels better now she is back to aerobics class. Smiles and describes the joy of having her own child. Has a significant partner.

Physical appearance

Normal pattern identification

Risk identification

Dysfunction identification

WELL-BABY CLINIC VISIT ASSESSMENT FINDINGS

While the baby is being weighed, the mother talks about feeling tired and states comments about her body like "These breasts are so big and heavy" and "I don't think I'll ever wear normal-sized clothes again."

Eye contact, composure, comfort level, and show of emotion.

"How would you describe yourself?"

Developmental stage, previous experience, stressors or threats, self expectations.

"Do you ever have feelings of worthlessness?"

Assessed findings

- Patient expresses feeling of being fat and that a body part (her breasts) are not the way she would like them to be (too big).
- Lacks sleep.
- Mother of 3-month-old (risk for postpartum depression).

Assessment findings data indicate

Successfully resolve issues with

EVALUATION

The patient will...

- Integrate a realistic body image.
- Express positive feelings about self and her body.
- Verbalize understanding of normal body changes in the post-partum period.

Determine if interventions are successful and revise as needed

INTERVENTIONS

- Health promotion/patient teaching about normal body changes in the post-partum period.
- Assist patient to identify positives of changes in body post-partum.
- Treat patient with respect and promote positive self-concepts.
- Individualized patient-nurse interaction.
- Use therapeutic communication and positive encouragement.

Implement these nursing interventions to promote self-concept

PRIORITY NURSING DIAGNOSIS

1. Disturbed Body Image.
2. Related to: physical changes from pregnancy.
3. As evidenced by: patient states that she is fat and her breasts are too big.

Leads to

PLANNING/OUTCOMES

Patient will be able to:

- Integrate a realistic body image.
- Express positive feelings about self.

FIGURE 38-6 Self-concept concept map.

ASSESSMENT

Normal Pattern Identification

The nurse who assesses the patient's self-concept is better equipped to implement the nursing process, thus assisting the person in strengthening self-concept. At times, the patient's self-concept will be an identified strength that the nurse uses to enhance interventions for other nursing diagnoses.

Assess patients by asking the following questions about self-concept during a nursing history:

- How would you describe yourself?
- Most of the time, how do you feel about yourself?
- Are you experiencing changes in your body or the things you can do?
- Are the changes in your body or your ability to do things a problem for you?
- Have you or are you experiencing changes in the way you feel about yourself or your body?
- Do you find that some things frequently make you feel irritable, such as feeling angry, anxious, frustrated, afraid, sad, or annoyed?
- When you have those feelings, what helps to make you feel better?
- Do you ever feel as though you have lost hope?
- Do you ever feel that you are not able to control things in your life?
- What helps you when you feel hopeless or out of control of your life?

Further assessment of roles and relationships is discussed in Chapter 39.

Risk Identification

When assessing a person at risk for self-concept dysfunction, consider the patient's developmental stage, previous experience, intensity of a stressor or threat, and self-expectations. Certain developmental stages pose a greater risk than do others. If the patient is an infant, what are the self-concepts of the parents? Is the patient an adolescent who has had a body image change? Does the change affect sexuality? Assessment of previous experience should include past problems with self-concept, history of unsuccessful coping mechanisms, and lack of resources and support. Intensity of a stressor may help identify risk. Is the patient threatened by a role? By an illness or body image change? How important is good physical or mental health? How good is the patient at fulfilling the performance of a role? How serious is an illness or change in body function?

Assessment of the difference between the real self and the ideal self can also identify risk. What are the patient's expectations? How far is he or she from meeting these expectations? Are expectations unrealistic?

Dysfunction Identification

Dysfunction identification also involves assessment of the patient's thoughts and feelings. People who do not possess a healthy self-concept are less able to cope with life, often expressing feelings of inferiority, self-doubt, and self-dislike. Does the patient verbalize negative feelings, such as "I don't like myself," "I'm so ugly now," "I'm worthless," or "I'm a terrible mother"? Why does the person feel this way? In what area is the person having a problem—self-esteem, role function, personal identity, or body image?

Objective Data

Objective data about the patient's self-concept are gathered through direct observation. These data include behavioral manifestations such as lack of eye contact and physical observations such as a missing body part or function. The person may try to conceal a body part, for example, by bandaging an arm scarred by burns after the burns have healed. The person may exhibit anxious behavior such as hand wringing and shallow breathing or grief behavior such as weeping.

Although some behaviors may be easily observed, assessing the meaning of these behaviors may be more difficult. For instance, if the person hides a body part, does this manifest body image disturbance or extreme need for privacy? These data are clues and must be judged with the subjective data to determine risk for or actual disturbances in self-concept. Ongoing observation of the patient's behavior helps identify changes in the self-concept.

NURSING DIAGNOSES

Disturbed personal identity is the inability to maintain an integrated and complete perception of self. When making a diagnosis related to disturbed personal identity, the nurse must also consider diagnoses with common defining characteristics. These often are inherent in disturbed personal identity. Among these diagnoses are alteration in body image; confusion about cultural values, goals, or ideologic values; feelings of emptiness or strangeness; gender confusion; or inconsistent behaviors (NANDA-Association International [NANDA-I] 2014). Selected NANDA-I and Nursing Outcomes Classification (NOC) and Nursing Interventions Classification (NIC) considerations are presented in Table 38-2.

OUTCOME IDENTIFICATION AND PLANNING

Outcome identification and planning focus on either promotion of a healthy self-concept or change of altered self-concept. The following general areas may be included in the formulation of patient goals:

- Patient will integrate a realistic body image.
- Patient will express positive feelings about self or self-capabilities.

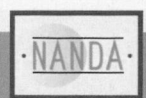

Table 38-2 SELECTED NANDA NURSING DIAGNOSES INVOLVING SELF-PERCEPTION

Nursing Dx	Related Factors	Dx Statement	NOC*	NIC†
Disturbed body image—confusion in the mental picture of one's physical self	Effect of altered body perception, surgery, colostomy, urinary diversion, congenital deformity, eating disorders, morbid obesity, trauma with altered body part—structure or function, chronic illness resulting in structural or functional change, body scheme/perceptual disorders, lifestyle change, depression, trauma (e.g., rape), cultural or spiritual differences, developmental or age-related factors	**Disturbed body image** R/T lack of acceptance of amputation of the lower leg AEB verbalization of perceptions that reflect an altered view of one's body in appearance, structure, or function. Behaviors of avoidance, monitoring, or acknowledgment of one's body	Acceptance: health status; adaptation to physical disability; body image; coping; decision making; grief resolution; health beliefs: perceived ability to perform; personal well-being; role performance; self-esteem	Active listening; anxiety reduction; body image enhancement; self-awareness; enhancement self-esteem; enhancement self-modification assistance
Chronic low self-esteem—state in which a person has long-standing negative self-evaluation/feeling about self or self-capabilities	Long-standing or chronic self-negating verbalizations (the person discounts, minimizes, or criticizes self, personal ideas, or accomplishments), expressions of shame or guilt, evaluation of self as unable to deal with events, rejection of positive feedback or exaggeration of negative feedback, or hesitancy to try new things or situations (the person says "I can't" in relation to new experiences)	**Chronic low self-esteem** R/T statements of shame and excessive food intake AEB exaggerated negative self-feedback and statements of "I can't" or "I'm no good"	Acceptance: health status; body image; coping; decision making; personal well-being; self-esteem	Active listening; anticipatory guidance; anxiety reduction; body image enhancement; decision-making support; self-esteem enhancement; self-modification assistance; socialization enhancement

Dx, diagnosis; R/T, related to; AEB, as evidenced by.

*From: Moorhead, S., Johnson, M., Maas, M., & Swanson, E. (2013). *Iowa Outcomes Project: Nursing Outcomes Classification (NOC)* (5th ed.). St. Louis, MO: C.V. Mosby.
†From: Bulecheck, G., Butcher, H., Dochterman, J., & Wagner, C. (2013). *Iowa Intervention Project: Nursing Interventions Classification (NIC)* (6th ed.). St. Louis, MO: C.V. Mosby.
From: NANDA-Association International (NANDA-I). (2014). *Nursing diagnoses: Definitions and classification, 2015–2017*. West Sussex, England: Wiley-Blackwell.

- Patient will distinguish between self and nonself.
- Patient will perform capably.

Patient goals will differ according to the defining characteristics that apply to each patient. The patient and nurse plan together to identify goals and interventions. Some interventions used in planning are listed in Table 38-2 and discussed in the following section.

IMPLEMENTATION

Health Promotion

IDENTIFICATION OF STRENGTHS

Nurses can promote positive self-concept in their patients by assisting them in identifying strengths. The continued use of internal and external resources helps strengthen identity, role

performance, self-esteem, and body image. Various personal strengths include good sense of humor, good communication skills, good problem-solving ability, a nice smile, strong health maintenance patterns, strong values, hobbies, strong social support systems (e.g., family relationships), a stable marriage, enjoyment in work, and a good education (Fig. 38-7). When presented with stressors such as illness or loss of a loved one, point out these strengths to patients to reinforce a positive self-concept. Encourage patients to cultivate these strengths and use them in the coping process whenever the self is threatened.

SENSE OF SELF

Always treat patients respectfully and personally to help them maintain a sense of self. By respecting each patient's individuality, nurses promote positive self-concepts. Pay special attention to verbal and nonverbal interactions with all patients. Introduce yourself to patients, address patients by name, speak

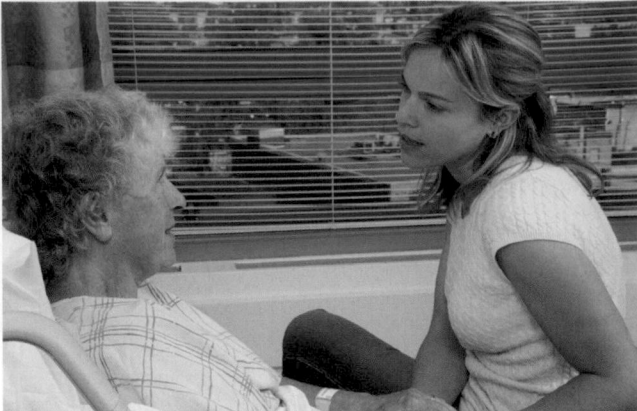

FIGURE 38-7 Families can provide stability and strength during changes. Strength may come from intergenerational relationships.

respectfully, and maintain the privacy of patients at all times. Explain all procedures and nursing activities, and pay attention to emotional responses of patients.

DEVELOPMENT OF SELF-CONCEPT

Helping patients to develop self-concept is related to developmental periods. Table 38-3 lists nursing interventions for development of self-concept as specific to age group.

Newborn

During the neonatal period, anticipatory guidance assists family members to adapt to their new roles and the self-concept related to these roles. Most often, this is accomplished through a therapeutic relationship that allows for exploration of expectations and provides support to deal with anxiety. Educate the family about parental roles, body changes, emotional changes, and family role expectations. When done early, care provided minimizes disturbances in self-concept for all family members, including the newborn.

Infant

Teach parents about the infant's need for movement, stimulation, and safety. If a child has an acute or chronic illness during this period, an environment that facilitates continued development is crucial. Activities should be age and health appropriate, providing safety and security. Parents need to provide as much care as possible for hospitalized infants. Assist parents to decrease their anxiety (to cope with the hospitalization). Doing so helps infants to feel more secure, fosters trust, and promotes continued self-concept development.

Toddler

Toddlers need an environment that allows practice of newly developing skills, especially movement-related skills, for body image and esteem to develop positively. Educate families that repetitive positive input and allowing toddlers to explore support the development of a favorable self-concept.

TABLE 38-3	DEVELOPMENTAL INTERVENTIONS TO PROMOTE SELF-CONCEPT AND PERSONAL IDENTITY
Developmental Level	Interventions
Newborn	Assist family in adapting to new roles by establishing therapeutic relationship and educating members.
Infant	Teach family about infant's need for movement, stimulation, and safety. Encourage parents to help provide physical care and security for hospitalized infants.
Toddler	Allow toddler to develop skills through exploration. Support family and help toddler maintain self-control.
Preschooler	Teach preschooler and family health maintenance behaviors. Encourage family to stay with the child if hospitalized, and let the child make some decisions about care.
School-age child	Allow privacy. Teach parents of need for socialization and belonging. Allow liberal visitation and age-appropriate activities if hospitalized.
Adolescent	Educate adolescent about sexual health and drug and alcohol use. Educate family about identity and body-image changes. If adolescent is hospitalized, offer choices in care to maintain autonomy.
Adult	Use therapeutic relationship to support adult and significant other. Support decisions adult makes in relationships and work roles.
Older adult	Treat older adult with respect and allow independence and individuality. Help older adult integrate loss of spouse, job, social support network, health, and the like.

Hospitalization or illness during toddlerhood affects the development of self-concept. Support toddler and family by helping the toddler maintain self-control.

Preschooler

During the preschool years, educate the family about normal development and support the family's establishment of an effective environment that facilitates growth. Because children have increased sexual feelings, preschoolers fear damage to their bodies. Therefore, they need support and education concerning health maintenance behaviors such as personal hygiene and healthcare visits. This can be accomplished through visits to healthcare providers with other family members or through supportive treatment during routine examinations. Hospitalization or serious illness in preschoolers is especially difficult. Preschoolers have many fantasies about punishment, abandonment, or physical harm. Combat these fantasies by including preschoolers in decisions as much as possible.

In addition, encourage families of hospitalized preschoolers to stay with their children as much as possible. Remember that a family may respond to a child's hospitalization with guilt, helplessness, and anxiety. To aid the child, assist the family in dealing with these feelings.

School-Age Child

Continue to teach and help parents understand their children's need for socialization and belonging. Frequently school nurses teach reproduction and health in school settings. If a child is hospitalized during this period, be cognizant of changing needs for privacy and the child's need to know that he or she still belongs to the family and peer group. In addition, school-age children need information about their illnesses and treatments. Parents again need support and help dealing with their fear and anxiety.

Adolescent

Support adolescents and families through the process of assuming roles and establishing independence. The need for privacy is a major concern of teenagers. Teach the family about the developmental process and why individual family members may have intense feelings during this period. Adolescents experiment as they make choices to establish identity. Provide health teaching including information concerning birth control, AIDS, and sexually transmitted diseases. A further concern is drug use and alcohol abuse. Adolescents need to know the ramifications of choosing drugs or alcohol as a coping style. They may need assistance to learn and practice alternate coping behaviors.

Many adolescents are hospitalized on pediatric units, which may contradict a teen's view of himself or herself as an independent, grown-up person. Offering adolescents choices regarding care helps them maintain some autonomy. Provide feedback about the adolescent's strengths and weaknesses to help him or her establish a realistic self-concept.

Adult

Assist adults with role satisfaction primarily in intimate relationships and occupation through use of a therapeutic relationship. Structure the environment to provide for successes and allow adults time and support while exploring the meaning of life. A feeling of generativity enhances self-concept. Continue to offer support to significant others.

Older Adult

Older people do not seek care as "old" people but as people with needs. Loss of independence associated with aging may bring loss of self-esteem. Support appropriate independence and self-care for older adults, which enhances self-concept. In working with older people, assist them in integrating changes, most often loss, into their self-concept. Also, enhance their self-concept by using respect and allowing individuality. Interventions aimed at older adults include allowing them to keep personal belongings in their settings for healthcare, listening to their stories, respecting privacy, explaining procedures, and allowing them extra time to accomplish tasks (Fig. 38-8).

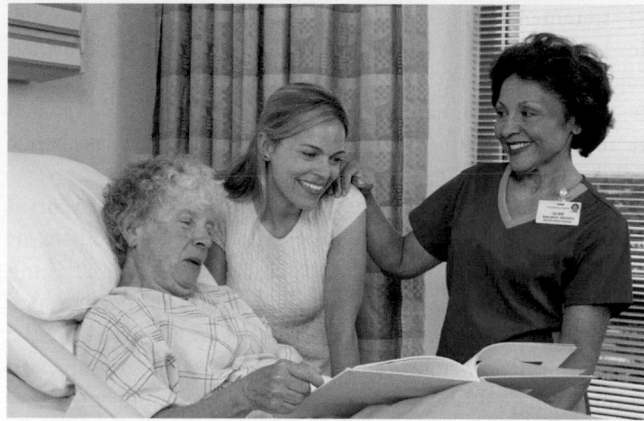

FIGURE 38-8 An older patient tells her story through family pictures and mementos.

Nursing Interventions for Disturbed Personal Identity

THERAPEUTIC RELATIONSHIP

Nurses intervene with patients with disturbed personal identity through therapeutic relationships. To develop therapeutic relationships, nurses must demonstrate great self-awareness and effective communication. Conveying a sense of friendship and trust helps establish rapport with patients. When empathy is shown, patients believe that nurses understand their feelings and will care for their needs. Once the relationship is established, use therapeutic communication techniques such as active listening, reflection, and reality-based feedback. Therapeutic communication assists patients with defining self-concept problems and attempting to problem solve.

SELF-EVALUATION

Nursing interventions that assist patients with positive self-evaluation can help change poor self-concept or disturbed personal identity. People with low self-esteem frequently put themselves down and act in ways that perpetuate negative self-evaluation. To break this cycle, patients need help in realistically evaluating the self and developing more positive thoughts and feelings about the self. Emphasize positive attributes rather than negative behaviors. Assist patients to point out tasks or accomplishments that deserve positive feedback. Offer praise honestly and encourage patients to make positive self-statements. Also, be a model for patients by acting confident, making positive statements, and accepting compliments.

BEHAVIORAL CHANGE

Nursing interventions aimed at changing behavior also assist patients with personal identity problems. General measures that bring about behavioral changes include accepting responsibility for self, defining realistic goals, using resources to enact change, and rewarding positive outcomes. Help patients accept responsibility for self by suggesting they make

"I" statements that reflect thoughts and feelings. For example, for a patient with role performance problems, instead of saying, "nothing ever goes right," a more active statement might be "I can't get the hang of my new job." This is the first step in realizing that the patient may have the power to change behavior.

In helping patients define realistic goals, assist them in evaluating expectations. If expectations are unrealistic or the discrepancy between the real self and the ideal self is too great, behavior will not change. Goals should be specific, such as "I will ask my boss for a 2-week training period on the new computer system." Help patients identify resources to accomplish goals including, for example, a computer training department at the office, night school courses, or someone to help around the house so the patient can temporarily devote more time to work.

Patients will be more likely to change behavior if they believe they will be rewarded for more positive behavior. Point out rewards such as a feeling of greater competence, less time spent at the office, greater productivity, and praise by others. By assisting patients with problem solving, role performance should improve, which strengthens self-concept.

Home and Community Care

Patients with disturbed personal identity usually require psychosocial assistance beyond the scope of routine nursing. Assist such patients to recognize difficulties and to accept additional therapy. Afterward, work with these patients to initiate plans for additional care. The goals of discharge planning are effective teaching and referral.

The teaching plan may include where and how to use community resources such as support groups or individual teaching concerning stages of loss. Referral may be to a specialized support group, such as for mastectomy patients, or may be for therapy through a psychiatric nurse specialist, psychologist, or psychiatrist. Consult the healthcare provider about ambulatory referrals. If the patient is to receive home health services, communicate with the home care nurse about the plan of care. For example, home care for the patient after mastectomy should include interventions to help incorporate a change in body image and to strengthen self-esteem, if those problem areas were identified while the patient was hospitalized. Describe interventions that have worked for continuity of care.

EVALUATION

Specific outcome criteria are used to measure the attainment of goals in self-concept. If the nurse asks what the patient hopes to see or hear if the interventions chosen are effective, goals will be behavioral in nature. The nurse then asks under what circumstances the patient will exhibit that behavior and by when. Such goals are measurable. Because the nurse and patient (in most cases) establish goals and outcome criteria, they can discuss whether or not these criteria have been met. Outcome criteria for patient goals discussed earlier in the chapter may include the following.

Goal

Patient will integrate a realistic body image.

POSSIBLE OUTCOME CRITERIA

- Patient speaks about his or her body within 2 days after surgery.
- Patient views self in mirror within 3 days after surgery.
- Patient assists with dressing changes within 4 days after surgery.

Goal

Patient will express positive feelings about self or self-capabilities.

POSSIBLE OUTCOME CRITERIA

- Patient establishes eye contact with nurse during conversation within 2 days.
- Patient lists negative and positive attitudes and their effects on self by discharge.
- Patient verbalizes feelings of success with self-care activities by discharge.
- Patient verbalizes strategies to support self-care and positive feelings related to self at home.

Goal

Patient will distinguish between self and nonself.

POSSIBLE OUTCOME CRITERIA

- Patient identifies feelings of depersonalization as related to illness within 2 days.
- Patient states realistic expectations for discharge within 5 days.
- Patient expresses feelings of hope and power over own life within 7 days.

Goal

Patient will perform capably.

POSSIBLE OUTCOME CRITERIA

- Patient expresses interest in caring for newborn within 1 day.
- Patient identifies three coping strategies to help assume new role within 2 weeks.
- Patient performs basic care of newborn successfully within 24 hours and more complex care within 2 weeks.
- Before discharge, patient verbalizes whom the patient will contact for social support when home.

PATIENT PLAN OF CARE
The Patient With Disturbed Personal Identity

NURSING DIAGNOSIS
Disturbed body image in related to confusion in mental picture of one's physical self.

PATIENT GOAL
Patient will express improved perception of physical appearance.

PATIENT OUTCOME CRITERIA
- Patient discusses his or her physical changes within 2 days of surgery.
- Patient demonstrates participation in ADLs within 3 days.
- Patient uses coping skills to prepare for changes in physical appearance within 3 days.
- Patient views affected body part within 1 week of surgery.

NURSING INTERVENTION	SCIENTIFIC RATIONALE
1. Assess patient's strengths that will positively affect body image, such as family relationships.	**1.** Assessment of factors that can contribute to improved body image builds on patient's strengths.
2. Provide opportunities to discuss altered appearance and self-worth.	**2.** Stating feelings verbally often helps patient to clarify and achieve perspective.
3. Assist with grooming.	**3.** When patient is unable physically or emotionally to groom self, the nurse's care activities indicate concern for the patient's welfare and help to establish rapport.
4. Encourage the patient to participate in self grooming and to strive for independence.	**4.** Encouraging participation in self-care provides patient with a sense of control.
5. Encourage identification and use of positive coping strategies.	**5.** Use of coping strategies that have worked effectively for the patient aids in successful coping with body image.
6. Encourage patient to cultivate positive coping strategies.	**6.** Use of internal and external resources helps strengthen self-esteem and body image.
7. Provide a mirror for the patient to view self. The patient may want to do so in privacy.	**7.** Patient must view physical changes before integrating them into a realistic body image.
8. Provide information and education regarding altered appearance, support groups, and other resources.	**8.** Individualized education and information meet the patient's unique needs.

EVALUATION

11/15/17: 09:30—Patient discussed physical changes caused by the surgery the second day after surgery.
- During participation in ADLs, the patient demonstrated using coping skills on the third day after surgery and was able to view affected body part.

—M. Klim, RN

KEY CONCEPTS

- Self-concept is the mental image a person holds of the self.
- Characteristics of normal self-concept include the dimensions of self-perception: self-knowledge, self-expectation, social self, and self-evaluation.
- Positive body image, self-esteem, strong personal identity, and role performance are normal patterns of self-concept.
- Factors that affect self-concept include biologic makeup; culture, values, and beliefs; coping and stress tolerance; self-efficacy; previous experience; developmental level and completion of developmental tasks; and illness, including trauma and surgery.

- Manifestations of altered self-concept or disturbed personal identity include self-care deficit, emotional and behavioral changes, anxiety and depression, and self-destructive behavior (e.g., alcoholism, drug abuse, acting out, and sexual promiscuity).

- Personal strengths that nurses can encourage patients to cultivate to promote positive self-concept include sense of humor, communication skills, strong health maintenance patterns, hobbies, social support systems, enjoyment in work, and education.

- Nurses help patients with low self-esteem by assisting them with realistic self-evaluation and development of more positive thoughts and feelings about themselves, including emphasizing positive attributes rather than negative ones.

- Nurses can also help bring about behavioral change in patients with altered self-concept by assisting them to accept responsibility for themselves, define realistic goals, use resources to enact change, and reward positive outcomes.

PRACTICING FOR THE NCLEX

CHECK YOUR ANSWERS IN APPENDIX A.

1. Self-perception or personal identity is how a person explains behavior based on self-observation. Which of the following are dimensions of self-perception?
   a. Self-knowledge, self-expectation, self-esteem, and role performance
   b. Self-knowledge, self-esteem, social self, and self-evaluation
   c. Self-esteem, self-expectation, social self, and self-evaluation
   d. Self-knowledge, self-expectation, social self, and self-evaluation

2. You are caring for a patient following bilateral mastectomy surgery. The patient refuses to look at her chest and states "I'm hardly even a woman now." What nursing diagnosis would be most applicable to this situation?
   a. Impaired coping
   b. Anticipatory grieving
   c. Disturbed body image
   d. Powerlessness

3. A teenage girl seen for her annual physical remarks that she is "so ugly." What should the nurse do first?
   a. Recommend counseling to the parent and physician.
   b. Ask the patient to explain why she feels this way.
   c. Recognize this as a developmentally appropriate statement for teenagers.
   d. Evaluate physiologic changes since the last appointment.

4. A nurse is performing patient education related to a new therapeutic regimen. Incorporating which of the following factors would be most applicable in promoting adherence? Select all that apply:
   a. Social support and coping
   b. Self-efficacy
   c. Education about evaluation
   d. Role ambiguity

5. The nurse is discussing home care of a patient with a below-the-knee amputation 1 month ago. She suspects a self-care deficit because the patient reported that he "sits in his chair and watches television all day" and does not shower or eat regularly. What intervention would be most appropriate to address this altered self-concept?
   a. Risk identification
   b. Classification of developmental level
   c. Self-evaluation
   d. Assess stressors

REFERENCES

Bazelon, E. (2013). *Sticks and stones: Defeating the culture of bullying and rediscovering the power of character and empathy*. New York, NY: Random House.

Berg, C. A., Butner, J. E., Butler, J. M., King, P. S., Hughes, A. E., & Wiebe, D. J. (2013). Parental persuasive strategies in the face of daily problems in adolescent type 1 diabetes management. *Health Psychology, 32*(7), 719–728.

Bevelander, K. E., Anschütz, D. J., Creemers, D. H. M., Kleinjan, M., & Engels, R. C. M. E. (2013). The role of explicit and implicit self-esteem in peer modeling of palatable food intake: A study on social media interaction among youngsters. *PLoS ONE, 8*(8), e72481. doi: 10.1371/journal.pone.0072481

Bandura, A. (1977). Self-efficacy: Toward a unifying theory of behavior change. *Psychological Review, 84*, 191–215.

Bandura, A. (1994). Self-efficacy. In V. S. Ramachaudran (Ed.), *Encyclopedia of human behavior* (Vol. 4, pp. 71–81). New York, NY: Academic Press. (Reprinted in H. Friedman [Ed.], *Encyclopedia of mental health*. San Diego, CA: Academic Press, 1998). Retrieved April 25, 2010, from http://www.des.emory.edu/mfp/BanEncy.html

Brown, J. (2007). *The self*. London, England: Psychology Press.

Bulecheck, G., Butcher, H., Dochterman, J., & Wagner, C. (2013). *Iowa Intervention Project: Nursing Interventions Classification (NIC)* (6th ed.). St. Louis, MO: C.V. Mosby.

Centers for Disease Control and Prevention, National Center for Injury Prevention and Control. 10 Leading Causes of Death by Age Group, United States, 2013. Available from http://www.cdc.gov/injury/wisqars/leadingcauses.html

Chen, W., & Lee, K. (2013). Sharing, liking, commenting, and distressed? The pathway between Facebook interaction and psychological distress. *Cyberpsychology, Behavior and Social Networking, 16*(10), 728–734. doi: 10.1089/cyber.2012.0272

Cole, D. A., Dukewich, T. L., Roeder, K., Sinclair, K. R., McMillan, J., Will, E., et al. (2014). Linking peer victimization to the development of depressive self-schemas in children and adolescents. *Journal of Abnormal Child Psychology, 42*(1), 149–160.

Coopersmith, S. (1967). *Antecedents of self esteem*. San Francisco, CA: Freeman.

DiDonato, M. D., & Berenbaum, S. A. (2013). Predictors and consequences of gender typicality: The mediating role of communality. *Archives of Sexual Behavior, 42*(3), 429–436.

Eschiti, V., Lauderdale, J., Burhansstipanov, L., Weryackwe-Sanford, S., Weryackwe, L., & Flores, Y. (2014). Developing cancer-related educational content and goals tailored to the Comanche Nation. *Clinical Journal of Oncology Nursing, 18*(2), E26–E31.

Eichelsheim, V., Buist, K., Deković, M., Wissink, I., Frijns, T., van Lier, P. A., et al. (2010). Associations among the parent–adolescent relationship, aggression and delinquency in different ethnic groups: A replication across two Dutch samples. *Social Psychiatry and Psychiatric Epidemiology, 45*(3), 293–300.

Erikson, E. (1963). *Childhood and society* (2nd ed.). New York, NY: W. W. Norton.

Freud, S. (1920/1966). *Lectures on psychoanalysis* (J. Strachey, Ed. and Trans.). New York, NY: W.W. Norton.

Herbozo, S., Menzel, J. E., & Thompson, J. K. (2013). Differences in appearance-related commentary, body dissatisfaction, and eating disturbance among college women of varying weight groups. *Eating Behaviours, 14*(2), 204–206.

Geriatric Mental Health Foundation (2014). Consumer patient information sheet: Late life depression. Retrieved September 10, 2014 from http://www.gmhfonline.org/gmhf/consumer/factsheets/depression_factsheet.html

Haferkamp, N., Eimler, S. C., Papadakis, A. M., & Kruck, J. V. (2012). Men are from Mars, women are from Venus? Examining gender differences in self-presentation on social networking sites. *Cyberpsychology, Behaviour, and Social Networking, 15*(2), 91–98.

Havighurst, R. (1972). *Developmental tasks and education* (3rd ed.). New York, NY: David McKay.

Im, E. O., Ko, Y., Hwang, H., Yoo, K. H., Chee, W., Stuifbergen, A., et al. (2012). "Physical Activity as a Luxury": African American Women's Attitudes Toward Physical Activity. *Western Journal of Nursing Research, 34*(3), 317–339. First published on March 14, 2011. doi: 10.1177/0193945911400637

Karatsoreos, I. N., & McEwen, B. S. (2013). Annual Research Review: The neurobiology and physiology of resilience and adaptation across the life course. *Journal of Child Psychology and Psychiatry, 54*(4), 337–347.

Kiang, L., Supple, A. J., Stein, G. L., & Gonzalez, L. M. (2012). Gendered academic adjustment among Asian American adolescents in an emerging immigrant community. *Journal of Youth and Adolescence, 41*(3), 283–294.

Kohlberg, L. (1969). Stage and sequence: The cognitive developmental approach to socialization. In D. A. Goslin (Ed.), *Handbook of socialization: Theory and research*. Chicago, IL: Rand McNally.

Kokkinos, C. M., & Kipritsi, E. (2012). The relationship between bullying, victimization, trait emotional intelligence, self-efficacy and empathy among preadolescents. *Social Psychology of Education, 15*(1), 41–58. doi: 10.1007/s11218-011-9168-9

Laguna, J., Goldstein, R., Braun, W., & Enguidanos, S. (2014). Racial and ethnic variation in pain following inpatient palliative care consultations. *Journal of the American Geriatrics Society, 62*(3), 546–552.

Lanza, H., Echols, L., & Graham, S. (2013). Deviating from the norm: Body mass index (BMI) differences and psychosocial adjustment among early adolescent girls. *Journal of Pediatric Psychology, 38*(4), 376–386. doi: 10.1093/jpepsy/jss130

Moorhead, S., Johnson, M., Maas, M., & Swanson, E. (2013). *Iowa Outcomes Project. Nursing Outcomes Classification (NOC)* (5th ed.). St. Louis, MO: C.V. Mosby.

NANDA-Association International (NANDA-I). (2014). *Nursing diagnoses: Definitions and classification, 2015–2017*. West Sussex, England: Wiley-Blackwell.

O'Connor, R. C., Rasmussen, S., & Hawton, K. (2014). Adolescent self-harm: A school-based study in Northern Ireland. *Journal of Affective Disorders, 159*, 46–52. doi: 10.1016/j.jad.2014.02.015

Pan, S. C., Tien, K. L., Hung, I. C., Lin, Y. J., Yang, Y. L., Yang, M. C., et al. (2013). Patient empowerment in a hand hygiene program: Differing points of view between patients/family members and health care workers in Asian culture. *American Journal of Infection Control, 41*(11), 979–983.

Pavlickova, H., Turnbull, O. H., & Bentall, R. P. (2014). Discrepancies between explicit and implicit self-esteem and their relationship to symptoms of depression and mania. *Psychology and Psychotherapy: Theory, Research and Practice, 87*(3), 311–323. doi: 10.1111/papt.12015

Piaget, J. (1969). *The psychology of the child*. New York, NY: Basic Books.

Polderman, T. J., Hoekstra, R. A., Posthuma, D., & Larsson, H. (2014). The co-occurrence of autistic and ADHD dimensions in adults: An etiological study in 17,770 twins. *Translational Psychiatry, 4*, e435.

Rivas-Drake, D., Syed, M., Umana-Taylor, A., Markstrom, C., French, S., Schwartz, S. J., et al. (2014). Feeling good, happy, and proud: A meta-analysis of positive ethnic-racial affect and adjustment. *Child Development, 85*(1), 77–102.

Rogers, C. R. (1961). *On becoming a person*. Boston, MA: Houghton Mifflin.

Rosenberg, M. (1979). *Conceiving the self*. New York, NY: Basic Books.

Rudiger, J. A., & Winstead, B. A. (2013). Body talk and body-related co-rumination: Associations with body image, eating attitudes, and psychological adjustment. *Body Image, 10*(4), 462–471.

Savage, J. E., & Mezuk, B. (2014). Psychosocial and contextual determinants of alcohol and drug use disorders in the National Latino and Asian American Study. *Drug and Alcohol Dependence, 139*, 71–78.

Shao, J., Chang, A. M., Edwards, H., Shyu, Y., & Chen, S. (2013). A randomized controlled trial of self-management programme improves health-related outcomes of older people with heart failure. *Journal of Advanced Nursing, 69*(11), 2458–2469.

Sheehy, G. (1974). *Passages*. New York, NY: E. P. Dutton.

Slovinec D'Angelo, M. E., Pelletier, L. G., Reid, R. D., & Huta, V. (2014). The roles of self-efficacy and motivation in the prediction of short- and long-term adherence to exercise among patients with coronary heart disease. *Health Psychology, 33*(11), 1344–1353. doi: 10.1037/hea0000094

Smit, E., Hoving, C., Schelleman-Offermans, K., West, R., & de Vries, H. (2014). Predictors of successful and unsuccessful quit attempts among smokers motivated to quit. *Addictive Behaviors, 39*(9), 1318–1324. doi: 10.1016/j.addbeh.2014.04.017

Sullivan, H. (1953). *The interpersonal theory of psychiatry*. New York, NY: W.W. Norton.

Tay Swee Cheng, R., Klainin-Yobas, P., Hegney, D., & Mackey, S. (2015). Factors relating to perioperative experience of older persons undergoing joint replacement surgery: An integrative literature review. *Disability and Rehabilitation, 37*(1), 9–24..

Thornberg, R., & Jungert, T. (2013). Bystander behavior in bullying situations: Basic moral sensitivity, moral disengagement and defender self-efficacy. *Journal of Adolescence, 36*(3), 475–483. doi: 10.1016/j.adolescence.2013.02.003

Unger, J. B., Schwartz, S. J., Huh, J., Soto, D. W., & Baezconde-Garbanati, L. (2014). Acculturation and perceived discrimination: Predictors of substance use trajectories from adolescence to emerging adulthood among Hispanics. *Addictive Behaviours, 39*(9), 1293–1296.

Vancampfort, D., De Herdt, A., Vanderlinden, J., Lannoo, M., Soundy, A., Pieters, G., et al. (2014). Health related quality of life, physical fitness and physical activity participation in treatment-seeking obese persons with and without binge eating disorder. *Psychiatry Research, 216*(1), 97–102.

Vitriol, V., Cancino, A., Weil, K., Salgado, C., Asenjo, M. A., & Potthoff, S. (2014). Depression and psychological trauma: An overview integrating current research and specific evidence of studies in the treatment of depression in public mental health services in Chile. *Depression Research and Treatment, 2014*(2014), 608671.

Vogel, E. A., Rose, J. P., Roberts, L. R., & Eckles, K. (2014). Social comparison, social media, and self-esteem. *Psychology of Popular Media Culture, 3*(4), 206–222. doi: 10.1037/ppm0000047

Walker, R. J., Gebregziabher, M., Martin-Harris, B., & Egede, L. E. (2014). Independent effects of socioeconomic and psychological social determinants of health on self-care and outcomes in type 2 diabetes. *General Hospital Psychiatry, 36*(6), 662–668. doi: 10.1016/j.genhosppsych.2014.06.011

Whittaker, R., Merry, S., Stasiak, K., McDowell, H., Doherty, I., Shepherd, M., et al. (2012). MEMO—A mobile phone depression prevention intervention for adolescents: Development process and postprogram findings on acceptability from a randomized controlled trial. *Journal of Medical Internet Research, 14*(1), 169–179. doi: 10.2196/jmir.1857

Wong, D. W., Chan, H., & Cheng, C. K. (2014). Cyberbullying perpetration and victimization among adolescents in Hong Kong. *Children and Youth Services Review, 36*, 133–140. doi: 10.1016/j.childyouth.2013.11.006

Zhao, X., Li, J., Huang, Y., Jin, Q., Ma, H., Wang, Y., et al. (2013). Genetic variation of FYN contributes to the molecular mechanisms of coping styles in healthy Chinese-Han participants. *Psychiatric Genetics, 23*(5), 214–216.

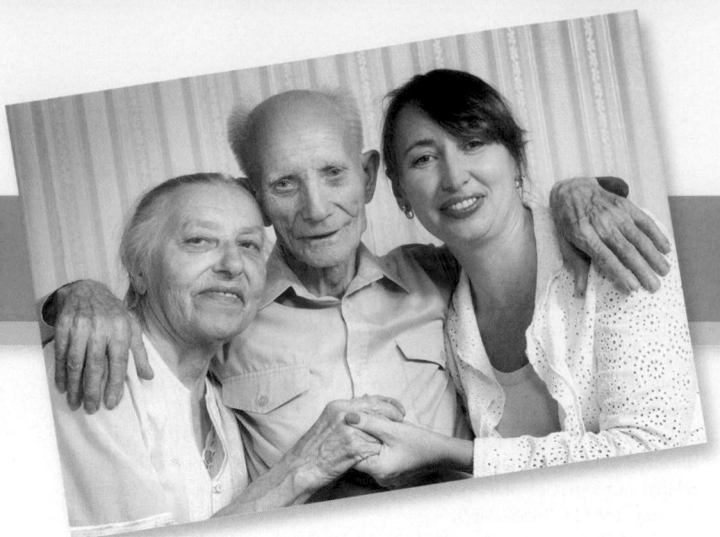

CHAPTER 39

Families and Their Relationships

Georgia L. Narsavage

Case Scenario

You are the home care nurse coordinator meeting with Jeffery and Sarah Jones and their 23-year-old granddaughter, Marissa, for the first time. Their family nurse practitioner has obtained an order for home care after consultation with a neurologist. Mrs. Jones, 78 years old, has noted that her husband, 82 years old, has become increasingly forgetful, "getting lost" if he walks even a block away from home. Mr. Jones has recently begun several inappropriate behaviors such as "using the flowerpot as a toilet." She suspects that he is "getting senile" just like his father was before he died. She has asked Marissa to live with them for a while to help her handle Mr. Jones, especially during the nights when he is restless and wanders. Marissa sits quietly and does not look at her grandmother. When you ask if she has been able to stay full-time, the grandmother immediately replies that she has. "But," she continues, "I don't think she can do it much longer—it really interferes with her sleeping and makes it hard for her to keep her job. Besides she should get married before it's too late!" You find out that Marissa's mother, a 56-year-old social worker, is struggling to maintain her own career while caring for Marissa's younger brother, who has limited functioning due to a heart condition. Marissa does not know her father. The family members seem very concerned about each other, but they don't know how they can continue to cope if things get any worse.

Once you have completed this chapter and have incorporated families and their relationships into your knowledge base, review the above scenario and reflect on the following areas of Critical Thinking:

1. Analyze your initial feelings about this family's ability to care for the older male (Mr. Jones).

2. Plan how you will elicit the family's perception of needs, goals, and outcomes.

3. Describe what you think are the perceptions of the wife, daughter, and granddaughter in this situation. Compare and contrast them with your own feelings.

4. Summarize key areas to assess when you visit the family within 48 hours after referral.

5. Differentiate the potential impact of stress on each family member.

6. Recommend ways to facilitate family-centered care, particularly if disagreements arise about the home care plan.

Upon completion of this chapter, you will be able to do the following:

1. Describe variations in family structure and function.
2. Identify demographic, sociocultural, and economic factors that affect family relationships.
3. Describe manifestations of altered family function.
4. Evaluate the possible impact of altered family function on activities of daily living.
5. Differentiate subjective and objective data needed to assess family function.
6. Identify nursing diagnoses and related factors associated with altered family function.
7. Discuss evidence-based nursing interventions to promote family health and function.
8. Discuss evidence-based nursing interventions for altered family function.
9. List family-centered healthcare services in the community.

Two hundred years ago, children were raised in extended families that consisted of several generations of family members living in close proximity to one another. Large families were desired, members were interdependent, and socialization was accomplished by passing traditions from one generation to the next. Dynamic public policy and social changes, together with demographic trends, including expanded opportunities for higher education, diverse avenues of employment, women's economic independence, and electronic/social media have changed family life (Cruz, 2013). In the 21st century, family structures are much more varied than in the past. The small, traditional family unit, known as the nuclear family, has decreased to 20% in 2012; 9% of family units consist of children who live with a single parent and an additional 9% of children live with unmarried individuals (U.S. Census Bureau, 2013). Blended families, extended families, cohabitated families, and communal families are among the many other variations in family units. Married couples without children increased to 29%, likely related to delayed childbearing and an aging population. One-person households overall increased from 17% to 27% between 1970 and 2012 (U.S. Census Bureau, 2013). Increased lifestyle options have established new family norms with a concurrent need for nurses to focus on helping individuals and families to adapt to these changes.

Although nurses deal with individuals, those individuals are not isolates but are integral parts of families. They influence and are influenced by other people and the environment. Individuals can meet some basic needs independently, but they require interaction with family and community to meet other needs.

Consider the older couple, their career-focused daughter, and their granddaughter in the Case Scenario. You can see from this example how the entire family influences the health perceptions and practices of its members. Nurses must understand the importance of family functioning to affect positively each person's health status. Nurses who practice family-centered care, which means caring for the patient and family as a unit, recognize the positive aspects of diversity and facilitate patient/caregiver/professional collaboration in multiple settings (Kuo et al., 2012; Donahue et al., 2013).

FAMILY RELATIONSHIPS

Traditionally, the family has been considered the basic unit of human society and has played a central role in the organization of social relations. A family is a social group whose members share common values, occupy specific roles in relation to one another, interact over time, and have diverse strengths and needs. The family provides for the following needs: sexual, reproductive, economic, nurturing, educational, socialization, caring, status, and political. Several, if not all, of these seem to be necessary to designate a group as a family. Family members may bear and rear children, cooperate economically and politically, and care for the ill and infirm of all ages.

Family Structure

Family structure means who the members are and what their relationships are to one another. Structure varies among families as well as within each family over time. Although the traditional structure of the family in the United States is no longer the nuclear family, many family structures are common today. Family members do not always live together in one household but remain connected by their relationships. Persons themselves define who is in their family.

NUCLEAR FAMILY

The **nuclear family** traditionally includes a married man and woman and their children (Fig. 39-1). Members live in the same house, usually until the children leave home to support themselves or to attend college. In 2011, 20.1% of the nation's 115 million households were composed of a married couple with children younger than 18 years (Vespa et al., 2013). Variations in the nuclear family include couples who remain childless or whose older children return home after a period of independence (e.g., after college). As of 2012, 36% of adult children (older than 18 years) lived with their parent(s), an increase from 11% in 2007 (Fry, 2013).

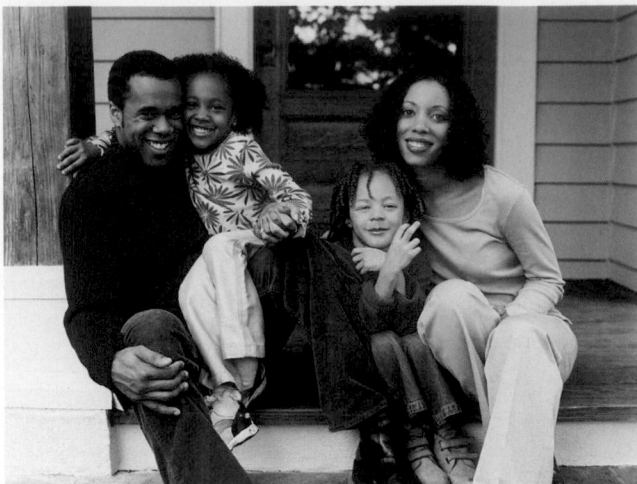

FIGURE 39-1 The traditional nuclear family consists of a married man and woman with one or more children living together in one household.

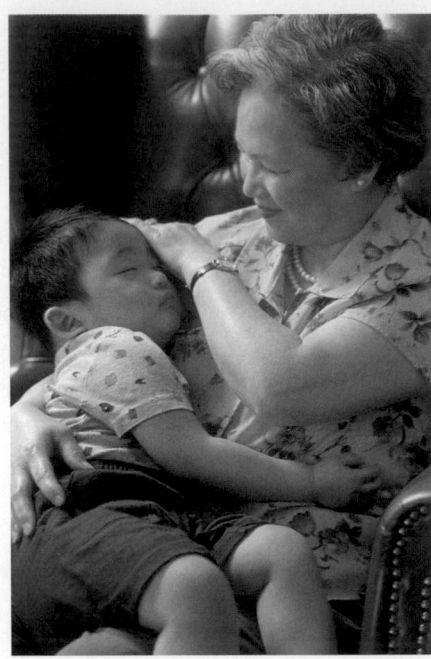

FIGURE 39-2 As part of the extended family, grandparents contribute to nurturing young children.

In the 1970s, traditional roles in the nuclear family were the man as breadwinner outside the home and the woman as responsible for physical provision of the home and children. The average of nuclear family households with their own children declined from 40% of all households in 1970 to 20% in 2012 (Vespa et al., 2013). However, there was a dramatic increase from 1975 (47%) to 2012 (70%) of mothers with children younger than 18 years who worked outside the home (Bureau of Labor Statistics, 2014). In addition, growing numbers of men are leaving the workforce to take care of children, while their partners assume the breadwinner role.

SINGLE-PARENT FAMILIES

Single-parent families, composed of one parent and one or more children, have more than doubled in the last 50 years. One third of American children—a total of 15 million—are being raised without a father. Nearly five million more children live without a mother according to the 2010 census. Women head more single-parent families than do men by a margin of 3:1 (Vespa et al., 2013). Death of a spouse or desertion can be the basis for single-parent families. These families may experience increased financial strain and parenting stress because of inadequate support systems and unemployment, with 7.7 million families having at least one member unemployed in 2013 (Bureau of Labor Statistics, 2014).

BLENDED FAMILY

Members of a **blended family** (stepfamily) include children who live with one birth parent and one parent as well as any offspring of the non–birth parent. Each member faces the challenge of forming relationships with the new members while possibly maintaining ties and loyalties to biologic family members who are not part of the new unit. In 2000, 43% of all marriages involved a remarriage for one or both spouses; in 2010, the remarriages accounted for 30% of all

marriages (Cruz, 2012). Blended families that form are also at risk for altered family function as members maintain or break ties to previous marriages and question extended family relationships.

COHABITATED FAMILY

Cohabitated family structure means people living together without the formal or legal bond of marriage. Such couples include men and women who live together as a trial or an alternative to marriage as well as gay and lesbian couples. Cohabitated families may include children.

EXTENDED FAMILY/MULTIGENERATIONAL FAMILY

The **extended family** structure expands the previously listed family types by adding grandparents, aunts, uncles, and cousins (Fig. 39-2). Members may or may not live under the same roof and exert varying influence on each person. Extended families may also be categorized as **multigenerational families**, with several generations living together in one residence. Multigenerational family units made up 5% of households in 2012 (Vespa et al., 2013; U.S. Census Bureau, 2013).

COMMUNAL FAMILY

A **communal family** includes a number of members who share a common bond, such as religious affiliation, ideology, or economic need. Another example is when young adults share living quarters while attending college. Membership in this type of situation may be short term, with instability in the unit, or long term, such as farming cooperatives.

NONTRADITIONAL AND OTHER FAMILIES

Nontraditional families do not fit the description of the other families. Same-sex parents (two adults of the same gender) who have established a functioning household may have children from other relationships, or children may have been adopted or conceived through medical procedures. Increasingly, same-sex parents have been seeking legitimization of their relationship through same-sex marriage.

Still other variations in family structure exist, including commuter marriages, in which one member lives away from the rest of the family part-time to work or to attend school. Caring for foster or adopted children is another way to include children in a family. Many families have adopted children of a race different from their own, including orphans from Southeast Asia, South America, and Eastern Europe. A single adult living alone who has never married or has been widowed, separated, or divorced is described in census data as a "nonfamily household" but may still belong to a larger extended family. In Census 2012, 32 million people (27%) lived alone (Vespa et al., 2013; U.S. Census Bureau, 2013). Information on the changing demographics of the U.S. population can be found through the website of the U.S. Census Bureau (www.census.gov).

FAMILY FUNCTION

Although family functions differ in each family, all families exist to meet some common goals. Family assessment includes six historical support functions of the family and social groups (Kaakinen et al., 2015). The usual functions of families involve physical and economic provisions of care, sexual intimacy, reproduction, education, socialization (including communication), and nurturing and support for problem solving and goal setting. Besides the physical bonds of family relationships, members experience emotional bonds that provide support and security for members, thereby fostering growth and development. Like family structures, family functions evolve over time within individual families.

Physical Provision

Providing physical care is a common need for all family members but is greater for those who are dependent because of age or illness. Physical care includes food, clothing, shelter, and healthcare. In most families, some members provide comfort and safety for others. Members cook, clean, shop for food and clothing, and possibly feed and bathe other members. Those cared for and those providing the care may change in situations such as illness or with new family structures.

ECONOMIC PROVISION

One or more family members contribute money to provide basic necessities such as food and clothing, as well as luxuries and provisions for the future such as college tuition. Families usually share the funds that some members earn. Dual-career families are common because of today's economic climate and standard of living. Almost 60% of U.S. women are in the labor force, constituting nearly 50% of today's total workforce (U.S. Department of Labor, 2014). Policy and legislation in the past 20 years, particularly the Family Medical Leave Act that guarantees up to 12 weeks of job-protected leave annually, have advanced the issues of workforce equality (Workplace Flexibility, 2010).

SEXUAL INTIMACY

Most couples in families need sexual intimacy. This basic human need and developmental concern can be met within a family. In a supportive family, partners play an active role in meeting each other's sexual needs. Human sexuality is discussed in Chapter 42. The development of dependable methods of family planning has influenced the couple's ability to express sexuality with less concern over unplanned pregnancies.

REPRODUCTION

Reproduction is not a function of all families; it is more often a choice rather than a given in family life. Couples may postpone or be unable to accomplish childbearing or may choose to eliminate it as an option. Alternative methods of having children, such as adoption, foster parenthood, use of donor sperm, and surrogate mother/donor programs, exist to fulfill a family's desire for children.

EDUCATION

Education, whether formal or informal, is a function of all families. Parents and other adults correct children, teach them how to care for themselves, help them mature, and send them to school for formal learning. Older members share with younger family members information that they have learned through experience; younger members, in turn, teach older members about the changing world. Education not only involves communicating information but also techniques for problem solving, coping, attitudes, and values. Education is ongoing and lifelong in most families.

SOCIALIZATION

Socialization is a function in all families, especially in close extended families. Gathering together at the dinner table and converging for holiday celebrations are prime opportunities for socialization. Through such events, family members learn to get along, to behave appropriately in various situations, and to express culture, tradition, and religious beliefs.

NURTURING AND SUPPORT

Families provide nurturing and support to their members from initial bonding at birth through old age and death. Nurturing and support may be provided through the emotional tasks of love, belonging, and affection as well as safety and security for growth.

FUNCTIONAL FAMILY PATTERN

A functional family meets its developmental tasks and guides members to accomplish individual tasks appropriate for age and developmental level. There are many forms for assessment and planning to develop supportive families. For example, an ecomap, a genogram, the 15-minute interview, and a social history with developmental stages and tasks are all forms that may be used to guide families (Holtslander et al., 2013). Any formal assessment should be very flexible in order to address strengths, needs, and particular concerns of each family member and the family as a whole (Wright, & Leahey, 2013).

Life Span Considerations

An understanding of life span developmental transitions helps us understand families. Critical transitions can be grouped into three types of events: changes in the number of family members, changes in the ages and relationships of members, and changes in status such as retirement (Kail & Cavanaugh, 2013). A classic useful resource for understanding these life span transitions can be found in Erik Erikson's theory of development from infancy through adulthood; this theory was selected to organize life span considerations because it integrates historical, biologic, psychological, and sociocultural dimensions (Kail & Cavanaugh, 2013). Erikson's Psychosocial Stages Summary Chart can be viewed online at http://psychology.about.com/od/psychosocialtheories/fl/Psychosocial-Stages-Summary-Chart.htm (Cherry, 2015).

NEWBORN AND INFANT

The process of infant–parent attachment or bonding after birth is critical to family development. Factors that affect bonding include availability of both parents after birth, flexibility of schedules, feelings about the birth, comfort in parenting roles, emotional responsiveness of baby and parents, financial security, other demands such as care of another child, and supportive others.

By 8 months of age, most infants have become attached to their primary caregivers and are developing *trust*. An interactive family environment can support the socialization process. Changes in the infant's environment that involve separation (such as hospitalization of a primary caregiver or of the infant) may slow down the infant's development. Studies of nurses, mothers, and preterm infants hospitalized in the neonatal intensive care unit reinforced the need for family-centered care and supported the important role nurses play in family growth and positive development during this stressful experience (Faber, 2013; Lee, Carter, Stevenson, & Harrison, 2014).

TODDLER AND PRESCHOOLER

In toddlerhood, learning to walk imparts mobility, and increasing cognitive ability stimulates curiosity. Protection from harm is an important focus for caregivers of toddlers and preschoolers.

At the same time, the child's need to develop self-control can strain family interactions as power struggles, frequently accompanied by temper tantrums, become the norm. Encourage caregivers to promote children's independence within established limits for children to develop *autonomy*. Sibling rivalry may escalate as self-centered toddlers resent the dominance of older children and the attention given to younger children. Despite power struggles, toddlers remain attached to their caregivers, and severe separation anxiety may be noted when primary caregivers leave these children, who are from 18 to 24 months of age. Hospitalization or other types of separation at this time may be especially traumatic. Role changes required by the need to care for a disabled family member in the home may decrease a parent's contact time with the toddler, who may then regress into an earlier developmental stage.

Psychosocial development escalates during the preschool years. Preschoolers identify with the role of boy or girl as they interact differently with parents or primary caregivers. The caregiver of the opposite sex becomes the focus of the child's love, whereas the child may direct aggression toward adults of the same sex. Consistent involvement with people of both genders enhances preschoolers' development.

Playing together with interaction but little organization evolves into cooperative play as children approach school age. Cooperative play and generally increasing social skills help preschoolers to develop mutually supportive roles with siblings, although rivalry continues (Fig. 39-3).

The preschool years are crucial for the development of *initiative*, which is the ability to begin actions independently. Stable family relationships can enhance the development of creativity. Adults can prepare preschoolers for changes such as surgery by playing out feelings and focusing attention on the event one part at a time. Family members should assure children that changes such as death are not their fault.

Significant others can expand the socialization process as preschoolers develop an ability to separate from home and family. Preschoolers need independence and security. Fear of separation remains, and parental anxiety may reinforce it. Types of interactions with preschoolers can develop different

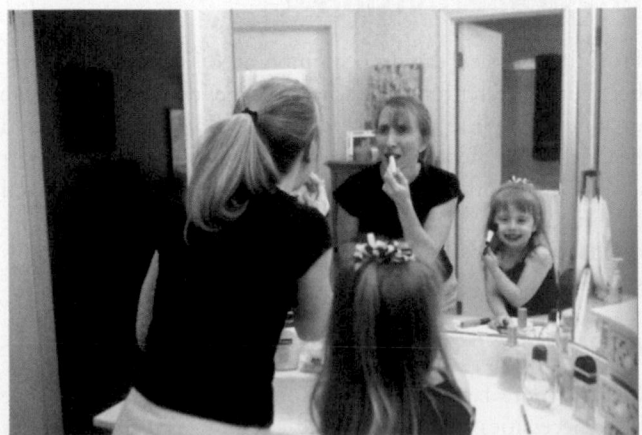

FIGURE 39-3 The preschool-age child learns to identify with the parent of the same sex.

skills, including moral behaviors (Hetherington, Hendrickson, & Koenig, 2014) Research has also shown that book reading helps children develop language skills, and modeling and shaping with clay helps them develop independence and control of conversation (Wasik, 2012).

SCHOOL-AGE CHILD AND ADOLESCENT

The school years are a time of change for both children and their adult caregivers. A need for relationships with peers, usually of the same sex, is enhanced. The role of "best friend" assumes importance. Family atmosphere continues to provide a sense of security as children move away from obvious signs of dependence on parents. Sibling rivalry is still present but continues to resolve unless adults compare children (e.g., for differing levels of ability).

Children's perceptions of their own abilities are significant as they seek to accomplish the task of being productive and to avoid feeling inferior. Fears of illness, injury, punishment, and death of self or significant others are evidenced during this developmental stage. Children may use phobias and ritualistic "good luck" behaviors as adaptive mechanisms. Understanding of such behaviors, rather than denial, is important on the part of significant adults (Browning, 2011; Peterson, Wellman, & Slaughter, 2012). Dying children are helped by open communication about death, based on research findings and clinical experience (Smith, 2014).

In some cultures, puberty, after the completion of identifiable "rites of passage," signals the assumption of adult roles. The family plays an important role in preventing emotional and behavioral problems and promoting resilience in adolescents (Melnyk et al., 2013). Western culture is less clear in defining the steps for transition into adulthood. To the extent that independence is desirable, alterations in family and social relationships are normal and inevitable in adolescence. Psychosocial development is closely related to changes in physical development. Peer group identity is strongly desired; adolescents strive to look and act like each other. Shame and stigma of not being accepted by their peers can lead to increased risk for substance **abuse**, anxiety, and depression among both adolescents and parents. Stability in the home and supportive relationships with others can help adolescents avoid "role confusion" in developing a sense of self and identity. A relational approach by clinicians can show respect for the role that adolescents can play in making decisions (Walter & Ross, 2014).

ADULT AND OLDER ADULT

Chief developmental tasks of the adult period are *intimacy*, which involves commitment to others, and *generativity*, which focuses on productivity. Both social and job-related concerns strongly influence development in adulthood. Critical life junctures (e.g., cohabitation, marriage, childbirth, career advancement, and mobility) influence development of intimacy and generativity (Wright, Pincus, & Lenzenweger, 2012).

A decision to remain single does not exclude the development of intimate relationships. Many young adults leave their families of origin, usually to form families of procreation. Social relationships with peers remain important for feelings of identity. The need for peer group support may be intertwined with such serious problems as substance abuse, sexually transmitted diseases such as HIV/AIDS, unplanned pregnancies, and abortion. Family support can have a positive impact on outcomes when facing these serious health problems (Wellings et al., 2013; Wouters, Masquillier, Ponnet, & le Roux Booysen, 2014).

In the middle years, adults' relationships with children gradually change as children gain independence, and relationships with partners change as each person matures. Menopause in the woman and climacteric in the man can precipitate family crises that require role adjustments but also present opportunities for positive changes in lifestyle (McCloskey, 2012; Magon, Chauhan, Malik, & Shah, 2012). Relationships with aging parents may result in conflict, frustration, and/or anger as older adults become more dependent. Healthcare support workers can be integral to successfully caring for parents who are dying at home as the family deals with the challenging legal and ethical issues that can affect the individual/family/nurse relationships (Herber & Johnston, 2013).

Demographic trends document the increased numbers of adults over age 65 years; the group over age 85 years is growing fastest. Nearly all families are concerned about at least one older adult member. Formidable tasks face the family with aging adults as members try to balance personal and work obligations. Support from family is essential to help older adults achieve "ego integrity" and to avoid despair. Changes in family structure occur as children leave home (and sometimes return), as family members die, and as new relationships develop. Another substantial change has been noted in the increasing role that grandparents today play in raising and providing care for grandchildren. From 1970 to 2011, the number of children living with or in a home maintained by their grandparent(s) increased from 2.2 million to 7.7 million (Livingston, 2013). Changes related to caring for grandchildren and spouses, retirement, death, and decreasing social contacts alter family and social structure because members must redefine their usual roles. Nurses can play a significant role in helping aging adults cope with changes (Zauszniewski, Au, & Musil, 2012).

Cultural Considerations

Cultural considerations for developmental assessment include ethnic patterns, language, food customs, patterns of communication, role expectations, healthcare beliefs, childrearing practices, availability of extended family support, and religious beliefs and practices. Nurses may encounter many variations in family structure and function among different cultures; each variation can relate to the patient's health status. For example, the extended family that is basic to Native American society values children and older adults, and childrearing is a group endeavor (Karanja et al., 2012). Other research has helped to define the role of family members in adopting healthy eating patterns within a different ethnic group (Rawlins, Baker, Maynard, & Harding, 2013). The extended family acts as an essential support system to help families cope when stressors such as illness occur and should be included within a cultural context as well.

Cultural traditions impact the family as it functions in Western society. Variations occur even within cultures, as seen among Asians and Asian Americans, where caregivers' relationships with their care recipients have been shown to affect caregiver burden and depression, emphasizing the importance of family relationships to depression among Asian Americans (Chae, Lee, Lincoln, & Ihara, 2012).

When extended family support is unavailable, parents employed outside the home may express concerns over the amount of time they spend separated from their children. Research has shown that children of employed mothers are able to develop well and have their needs met as long as the parent is comfortable with the child's care arrangements (Bianchi, 2012; Coley, McPherran, & Lombardi, 2013). Inadequate child care remains a concern for dominant as well as minority cultures in the United States due to public policy's limited response to social change and the existence of quality differences that could be addressed by stricter requirements and financial support (Hillemeier, Morgan, Farkas, & Maczuga, 2013).

Religious customs and expressions of spirituality also influence how children grow up in families. The Jewish religion considers the bar or bat mitzvah as the "rite of passage" (Hilton, 2014) (Fig. 39-4). Mormons emphasize self-discipline and strong family ties that find positives in parenting of special-needs children, and Seventh-Day Adventists strictly observe their holy day of rest and worship with the family, even in hospital settings (Koenig, King, & Carson, 2012). End-of-life decision making for a Muslim patient should involve the family and a religious scholar, as hastening death by withdrawing nutrition and hydration is forbidden in Islamic law (Alsolamy, 2014). However, spirituality—behaviors that give life meaning and purpose—may or may not be connected to a specific religious group. In some Latino cultures, the belief that death extends life can provide a positive aspect to grieving, and the nurse's role in allowing Latino patients to respond in their own culturally appropriate way can enhance the family relationship (Adames et al., 2014).

In addition to spiritual influences, families pass down attitudes about male and female roles and childrearing through the generations; they also pass on beliefs and practices about health, illness, and healthcare. Even those people born and raised in traditional "American" culture may exhibit behavior arising from various cultural beliefs (Spector, 2012).

FACTORS AFFECTING FAMILY FUNCTION

In addition to age, factors that may affect family relationships include community, cultural beliefs, economic status, lifestyle, and previous life experience. Acute and chronic illness, traumatic experiences, and substance abuse are other factors that influence family function related to the impact of stress on families (Sieh, Dikkers, Visser-Meily, & Meijer, 2012). Evidence has shown that a family's lower socioeconomic status and parental negativity, mediated by genetic factors, are predictors of behavior problems in children (Alemany, Rijsdijk, Haworth, Fañanás, & Plomin, 2013). Such influences may be mild, affecting only some members or lasting only briefly, or they may be stressors that propel the entire family through a prolonged crisis. Crises may actually strengthen family bonds, however, if members become more committed to the family's common goals and strong support systems are in place (Schappin, Wijnroks, Uniken Venema, & Jongmans, 2013). Table 39-1 lists common family stressors.

Community

Nurses in every setting must be aware of their patients' interactions with and within the community and view patients as individuals within a family within a community. Appropriate nursing care incorporates the interaction of patients with family members with community institutions (e.g., employer, religious institution, school, other social group) on any level of need (individual, family, or community) while not losing sight of the relationships among all three levels.

DEFINITION OF COMMUNITY

For the purposes of this discussion, **community** is defined as a social group whose members may or may not share common geographic boundaries yet who interact because of common interests or shared values to meet their needs within a larger society.

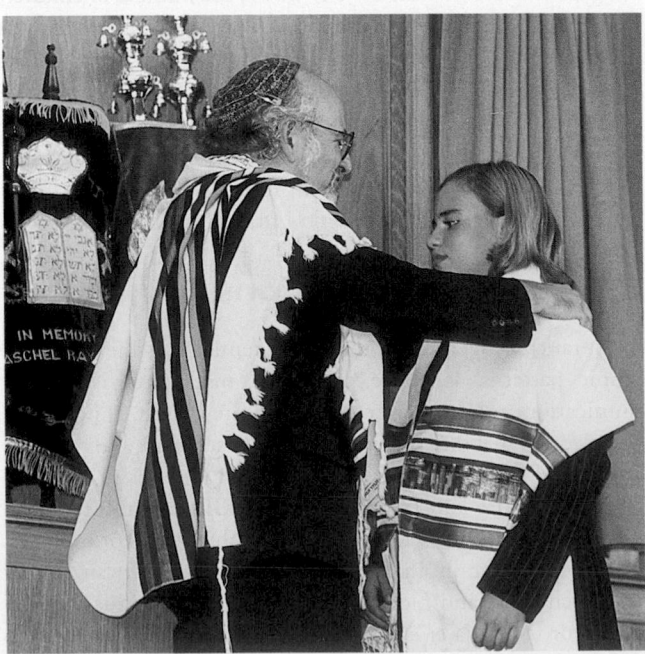

FIGURE 39-4 Cultural and religious traditions like the bat mitzvah can serve as "rites of passage" for members and can promote further family bonding.

TABLE 39-1	SOURCES OF FAMILY CONFLICT
Source	Problem Areas
Finances	Lower socioeconomic status; income inadequate to meet needs; disagreement on money management
Occupation	Unemployment; semiskilled status, task sharing when both adults working
Culture/religion	Mixed religious or cultural background; in-laws; disagreement on childrearing practices
Education	Incongruent levels of education, especially if school dropout
Residence	Mixed rural/urban background; relocation for benefit of only one family member; isolation
Sexual	Dissatisfaction with intimacy level; disagreement on family planning
Substance abuse	Difference in values; physical/psychological changes due to chemical addiction
Social ties	Dissimilar selection of friends; single vs. couple focus in friendships
Situational	Fatigue; loss; illness; separation, trauma, disaster
Developmental	Change in number, age composition, or status of family members

Economic Resources

A clear economic influence on family and social relationships can be observed as people with marginal incomes struggle to survive. Economic constraints often create problems in maintaining a family's lifestyle after a divorce or change in employment or with a change from two wage earners to one (Lavelle & Smock, 2012). Resentment toward society or other family members for forcing a below-standard lifestyle may arise. Functioning in single-parent families is difficult given chronic problems of limited economic support and role stress but can be balanced by positive aspects, such as decreased psychological stress, increased family cohesiveness, family resilience, and use of creative coping strategies (Luhmann, Hofmann, Eid, & Lucas, 2012).

Lifestyle

The mobility of families can affect relationships as adults change jobs or retire and children change schools. Support people and friendships also change. The family's lifestyle in terms of rest and relaxation, nutrition, smoking, drug and alcohol use, and exercise influences the health status of all members. Lack of support from extended family due to geographic distance can increase the effect of stress on individuals and families after relocation. The health and development of family members when a child or an adult with a chronic condition is in the family depends on adequate communication and support

(Rosland, Heisler, & Piette, 2012). The need for employment and challenges in finding affordable childcare have created the "latchkey" practice in childrearing in which children are responsible for their own care and supervision after school. The difficulty families may have in providing care to infirm older adults has also created a need for more long-term care facilities, assisted living, and community-based services.

Previous Life Experience

Previous life experience greatly affects a family's functioning. Children learn about relationships almost exclusively from their families of origin. They carry beliefs to their families of procreation about forming relationships, making decisions and solving problems, carrying out roles, raising children, using resources, and showing affection. Some coping strategies, such as using alcoholic beverages to numb mental pain and stress, may have been accepted in a person's previous life experience and yet destroy present relationships. Active or problem-focused coping behaviors have been associated with positive, although mixed, outcomes and passive emotion-focused approaches with problematic adjustment to chronic illness; accommodative coping or efforts to adapt to sources of stress have been most useful, even when situations are unchangeable (Compas, Jaser, Dunn, & Rodriguez, 2012).

Coping and Stress Tolerance

Any stress on an individual can affect the entire family's functioning. For example, the term **sandwich generation** has been used to describe adult children facing the dilemma of meeting their own generativity needs while assisting the older generation (their parents) and the younger generation (their children) (Fingerman, Pillemer, Silverstein, & Jill Suitor, 2012). Even with variations in baseline psychological distress, caregivers of the sandwich generation have been shown to cope with increasing needs of other family members (Hoffman, Lee, & Mendez-Luck, 2012). Other stresses, such as the loss of a family member, involvement in a natural or man-made disaster, or loss of employment, can also alter a family's relationships.

Social Isolation

Social isolation may result when family members are separated, communication within families is poor, or others do not accept a family or its members. Isolation can be physical or psychological. Separation may result from hospitalization, job commitments, or going away to college. Today, many nuclear families, single adults, and older adults are separated from their extended families because the young have sought employment elsewhere. People without the usual family support may feel isolated in a new town. Daily demands of a job, parenting, home maintenance, college studies, finances, and illness may overburden the persons involved. They may not know where to turn for support if they have depended on family in the past. The nurse–family relationship becomes extremely important

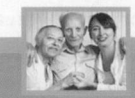

Families and Their Relationships PICO

Brenna, a home health nurse, has been working with the Jones case for 3 months. She is noticing that the family members are struggling to deal with Mr. Jones' situation. They are attending support groups and giving each other respite time. However, Brenna notices that Mrs. Jones is becoming a little more withdrawn with each visit. Brenna recently heard that the community offers telephone counseling for family caretakers. She wonders if this will be a good option to offer Mrs. Jones. She turns to the Cochrane library for evidence. Brenna uses the following PICO statement to lead her search: *For caregivers of dementia patients, how does telephone counseling versus no telephone counseling provide support?*

P = caregivers of dementia patients
I = telephone counseling
C = no telephone counseling
O = support

Brenna finds a meta-analysis that reviewed telephone counseling services to family members who are taking care of patients with dementia. The study evaluated nine randomized control trials and two qualitative studies. The studies were considered moderate quality and needed further research. However, there was some evidence that indicated that telephone counseling did provide an immediate form of support to families who served as a caretaker. Brenna decides to offer the information to Mrs. Jones on the next visit.

REFERENCE

Lin, S., Hayder-Beichel, D., Rücker, G., Motschall, E., Antes, G., Meyer, G., et al. (2014). Efficacy and experiences of telephone counselling for informal carers of people with dementia. *Cochrane Database of Systematic Reviews*, (9), CD009126. doi: 10.1002/14651858.CD009126.pub2

in helping families adjust to stress and illness in both hospital and home settings (Gottlieb, 2013). Older adults are facing their final years away from their children and grandchildren and may be living alone after their spouses die. They may feel isolated by a society that values youth.

Poor communication within a family can isolate individual members. Another form of isolation occurs when a family is not accepted socially or fears such rejection. Members may be discriminated against because of race, color, religion, ethnic origin, or stigma associated with illnesses such as AIDS (Betancourt, Meyers-Ohki, Charrow, & Hansen, 2013). Fear of isolation by the community, in the workplace, or from others adds to tension within the family.

Role Strain

Role strain is a manifestation of family function when events and family developments force changes in roles. For example, when a husband becomes chronically ill and unable to work, the wife may become the family's primary economic provider. She may experience role strain because she must combine the role of caregiver with the roles of wife, mother, and employee. The husband may experience stress as he gives up his role as economic provider and spends more time at home. Children may be assigned additional tasks including some physical care for the father.

Giving up familiar roles and assuming new ones may be by choice, as in the case of a two-career family that decides to suspend or temporarily give up one parent's career for childrearing. Family developmental stages call for changing roles

periodically; however, role strain develops when family members cannot adapt and meet their needs (Scott, Whitehead, Bergeman, & Pitzer, 2013). Inherent decision-making power may either increase or decrease role strain (Lawn, Delany, Sweet, Battersby, & Skinner, 2013).

Acute Illness

Acute illness may place sudden demands on a family. The ill member often looks to the others for validation that he or she is sick; with such validation, the ill member can seek healthcare. Roles may change as the ill member depends on others for physical care, nurturing, and economic security. The ill member's self-esteem may decrease if he or she feels less valued.

Other members may temporarily sacrifice their own needs to provide for the ill person's needs. In a family with a seriously ill older female, the older male may become her primary caregiver and neglect his own health. Needs such as sexual intimacy may go unmet. Problems may arise when members cannot adjust to new roles or as needs remain unmet. Stressors rarely occur in isolation, and the caregiver role adds an unprecedented and unequally distributed burden of care (Bradley & Dahman, 2013). One member in particular may feel overburdened. For example, when a construction worker is unemployed while receiving treatment for fractured vertebrae, his spouse may work additional hours to provide for the family economically. Children may have to assume more responsibility for meeting their own needs, and housework may be left undone. The family tries to fit in support of the ill member, meal preparation, and chauffeuring the children around varied work schedules. Anxiety increases about the illness as well as about how the children are managing with decreased support. Consequently, the caregiver's own physical needs for sleep and nutrition, as well as the family's need for nurturing, may go unmet. Depending on the severity of the illness and how suddenly it occurred, the family might need increased attention at this time. Stability of the family structure is essential when one or more members are absent or incapacitated. Some flexibility is necessary to share roles and still meet needs such as economic provision and physical care.

> ### ! SAFETY ALERT
> Assist families with finding resources for child care, finances, and other basic needs while a parent or primary caregiver is hospitalized.

Chronic Illness

Because chronic illness lasts longer than does acute illness, it can influence the family to a greater extent. The course of chronic illness may require both individual and family adaptation to changes in lifestyle and roles and may result in the ill person's increased dependence on others. In caring for children with chronic illness, family functioning can be influenced by both the caregiver's role adaptation and support provided by healthcare professionals (Lawn et al., 2013). Actions by family or significant others can be supportive, but behaviors such as overprotection are problematic.

Because of the inherent dependency of children and frail older adults, their illnesses provoke yet other family adjustments. A newborn who has a congenital defect or the diagnosis of a chronic illness such as dementia or an older adult with a traumatic disability may result in severe stressors to family relationships. The ability of a family to function will influence the affected person's ability to develop and to cope and will affect the course of the illness or disability (Tschanz et al., 2013). A congenital birth defect that is initially stressful but ultimately correctable is likely to have less impact on family function than would a chronic illness or developmental disability that requires lengthy treatment (Lemacks, Fowles, Mateus, & Thomas, 2013).

Common stressors in chronic illness include exhaustion, anxiety, needing help from relatives and friends, alterations in social contacts or travel abilities, concern about sibling needs, and financial concerns, especially for single-parent families (Granek et al., 2014). Family roles, responsibilities, and social relationships change to meet the needs of the family system as well as the ill child or adult.

People with chronically ill children, parents, or other family members may express negative feelings about themselves, such as guilt, inadequacy, failure, rejection, and helplessness (Whittemore, Sarah, Chao, Jang, & Grey, 2012). The family may be in denial initially as members struggle with the shock of the illness, but after acknowledging the problem, the family will strive toward the goal of simply functioning as close to "normal" as possible (Toly, Musil, & Carl, 2012).

Traumatic Experiences

Trauma, because it entails stress and disruption of usual interactions, can alter family relationships. Traumatic experiences can be physical (e.g., a gunshot wound) or emotional (e.g., robbery). They can involve one person or many and can be caused by humans (e.g., surgery) or nature (e.g., flood). Personal involvement or involvement of a family member or significant other in a disaster or mass trauma (e.g., school shooting, severe fire; flood; hurricane; or car, train, or plane accident) is associated with loss of control and role change (Pfefferbaum, Noffsinger, & Wind, 2012). The role of "survivor" is fraught with conflicts. A family member may experience guilt that she or he was responsible or should have been the victim. One family member may blame another for contributing to the event. The victim may experience difficulty concentrating as he or she relives the event or may move from numbness to awareness. Coping within these contexts is a complex process, requiring multiple approaches to care.

Separation or divorce may be a trauma or a positive solution to **altered family function** in which the family unit is chronically disorganized, leading to family conflicts. Intervention may be needed if a family is unable to create and maintain a system to nurture and support its members. A major family transition occurs when separation or divorce breaks the family unit. Each member's confidence and self-esteem must be strengthened through careful handling of the transition (Fig. 39-5). An increasing number of families are being thus affected. Most commonly, the mother and children form a new unit while the father moves into a separate environment. A problem that can lead to further altered family function is role overload for the custodial parent. Shared custody may help to reduce the strain on a single parent, but no single solution is best for all families.

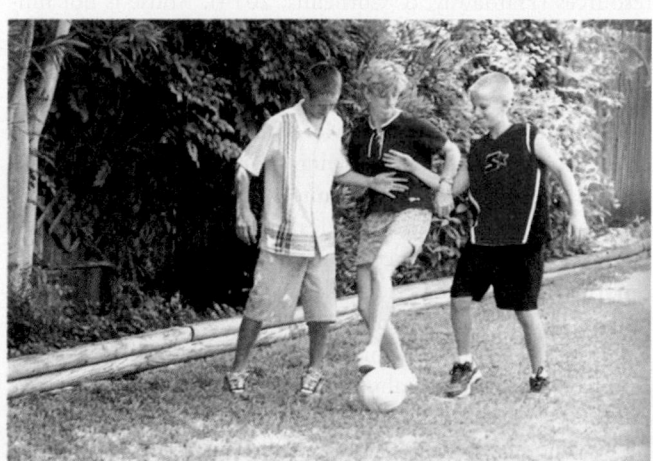

FIGURE 39-5 These children adjust to the transition in their lives, gaining security and confidence as they enjoy time together with their newly divorced mother.

EMOTIONAL PROBLEMS

Parenting may suffer whenever family emotional and developmental function is altered. Problems with bonding and attachment may arise, and children may have difficulty with emotional development. When family conflict arises, psychosocial development may be arrested. Family relationship patterns are associated with optimal and problematic adolescent adjustment (Jager, Yuen, Bornstein, Putnick, & Hendricks, 2014). For example, if tension arises while a person is in adolescence and the family responds poorly, the adolescent may be left confused, indecisive, and unable to plan for the future.

The family's ability to teach, nurture, educate, and socialize offspring is important, according to many developmental models (Wasik, 2012; Gottlieb, 2013). Children usually display emotional problems by behaving inappropriately for age or situation. Acting out may occur in the form of temper tantrums, poor school performance, or sexual promiscuity.

As older adults face retirement, depression may become evident, especially if the family has not actively planned for this change. Without communication of worth from other family members, maladaptation in retirees has been found (Tanabe, Suzukamo, Tsuji, & Izumi, 2012). Depression leading to suicide in older adults is an increasing societal problem (Lapierre et al., 2011; Bekhet, & Zauszniewsk, 2012).

ABUSE

Family abuse and violence are social problems of increasing significance. Abusive behaviors may cause physical harm, arouse fear, force people to do something against their will, or prevent them from doing what they wish. Abuse may be physical, sexual, or emotional or involve threats or intimidation or economic deprivation. It may be aimed at the spouse or partner, children, older parents, or grandparents. Factors that contribute to abuse in families include unemployment, economic hardship, substance abuse, chronic illness, inadequate housing, and lack of education and other resources (Hardaway, & Cornelius, 2014). Abuse is not limited to any one socioeconomic level and frequently is passed down through the generations. Many abused children grow up to abuse family members (Nunes, Hermann, Renee Malcom, & Lavoie, 2013). More than 3 million reports of child abuse and neglect involving more than 6 million children were reported in the United States in 2012 (Moyer, 2013; US Department of Health and Human Services, 2013). Domestic violence or intimate partner violence was reported by more than 12 million women and men in 2010 (Walters, Chen, & Breiding, 2013). The abuser is usually a family member in a long-standing relationship (Walters et al., 2013). Changing abusive patterns of behavior is difficult (Sanders-McDonagh, 2013). The nurse's ability to detect subtle behavioral cues is crucial when abuse is suspected because victims frequently attempt to hide their suffering. Violence increases during pregnancy and with the birth of children as relationships change (Kramer, Nosbusch, & Rice, 2012).

Abuse in families is often manifested in parenting behaviors (Lereya, Samara, & Wolke, 2013). A lack of attachment (bonding) may be evidenced by an adult's failure to care for the child's physical or emotional needs or by verbalized resentment or indifference toward the parenting role. Evidence of neglect or physical abuse may be noted as well as *failure to thrive*. Rigidity in role expectations may be present in either or both parents; the consequence may be inhibited flexibility in meeting children's needs.

Sexual abuse, especially of children, is another area of concern (Walthen et al., 2012; Trindade et al., 2014). Emotional turmoil escalates when family members fail to report such abuse or ignore it to avoid shaming the family. The child is often confused about the appropriateness of the abuser's behavior and may feel that he or she is to blame.

It is estimated that 1 in 10 older adults are victims or elder abuse; abuse of older adults is a growing problem (Dong, 2013; National Center on Elder Abuse, 2014). As they become physically dependent, in addition to physical abuse, older adults may be neglected or verbally and financially abused by their own children or other caregivers. Depression, loneliness, and psychosocial distress are risk factors for elder abuse. Immobility or sensory disabilities may prevent them from seeking help. They may also be reluctant to prosecute because of family loyalty. Signs of elder abuse may be missed by professionals working with older Americans because of lack of training on detecting abuse, and only a small percentage of cases are reported, even though almost all states have legislated mandatory reporting requirements. Additionally, with an increasingly diverse population, nurses need to better understand the ethical and cultural issues related to elder abuse (Dong, 2013). The National Center for Elder Abuse (NCEE; www.ncea.aoa.gov) has resources to use in detecting and addressing the problem.

Substance Abuse

The consequences of coping with substance abuse in a family are many (Bröning et al., 2012). For each person afflicted with alcoholism, there are family members who also suffer social and emotional problems. Alcoholics and possibly family members will deny that alcoholism is a problem. A spouse or child usually becomes the alcoholic's *enabler*, the person who keeps the family functioning even at an altered level. The enabler assumes tasks that the alcoholic cannot accomplish and cares and makes excuses for the alcoholic. These behaviors enable the alcoholic to continue drinking, which contributes to the deterioration of the family unit.

> **❗ SAFETY ALERT**
> Discuss the deleterious effects of alcohol or drug abuse with the abuser and his or her family, and refer the person to a substance abuse treatment program.

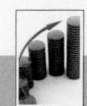

OUTCOME-BASED TEACHING PLANS

Janet Williams, age 46 years, comes to the primary care clinic for a "headache." Assessment reveals that her body has bruises on her arms and shoulders, which are not visible unless her clothing is removed. She does not have any marks of trauma on her head or elsewhere on her body. As you explore the situation, Janet states, "I'm really concerned that my husband has lost his job and is drinking more than he used to. He's not really an alcoholic you know—but he does get upset more often these days—if only he didn't drink so much at one time." You realize that Janet may be a victim of alcoholism and might be having trouble coping. You decide to try to help her recognize the problem and identify possible resources to help her and her husband.

OUTCOME

Janet will state the difference between alcohol use, abuse, and alcoholism and make a list of resources that can be used to help her and her husband.

STRATEGIES

- Explore Janet's knowledge about alcohol use, abuse, and alcoholism.

- If Janet wants to get help for her and her husband:
  – Have Janet describe her distress when her husband is drinking and gets upset.
  – Discuss possible support mechanisms (e.g., AA, Al-Anon, other family members).
  – Discuss ways that she can prevent further injury to herself (e.g., have phone numbers to call family or friends with "code words" for help, leave the house when her husband starts drinking, obtain legal restraining orders if problem gets worse).
- Suggest she find the nearest group of Al-Anon and attend a meeting.
- Problem-solve with Janet a plan that she can use if her husband denies the problem and refuses to work with her to get help.

EVALUATION

- At 1 week, Janet can state the difference between alcohol use, abuse, and alcoholism.
- At 2 weeks, Janet has a list of resources that can be used to help her and her husband.
- At 1 month, Janet reports which resources have been used by her and/or her husband within the past month.

Drug abuse also alters family function (Norman et al., 2012). Economic destruction may play a greater role in the family of a drug abuser than in that of an alcoholic, owing to the higher cost of illegal drugs. Because drug use is less socially acceptable than is alcohol use, the drug abuser and family may be isolated from the community. The threat of drug testing in the workplace may prevent the drug abuser from holding a job, which further compromises the family's economic security. Arrest and incarceration may completely disrupt the family unit. Legal drugs can also be abused, especially by those who suffer from chronic illness or use multiple medications. Both alcohol and drug abuse may lead to physical problems from the effects of the substance as well as injury incurred while intoxicated. Chronic liver disease, poor nutrition, and eventual heart failure are common in alcoholics. Intravenous drug abusers experience frequent infections, hepatitis, and possibly AIDS. These illnesses further alter family dynamics.

Recall the Jones family in the case scenario at the beginning of the chapter. They are exploring how their daughter and granddaughter can support them and what other options are available. A concept map diagramming the relationships between the nursing concepts you have learned can help you organize your knowledge about family relationships. Use the concept map (Fig. 39-6) to help you understand and manage Mrs. Jones's concern about caring for her husband and the family's role in his care.

ASSESSMENT

Family functional assessment can be accomplished in terms of structure, function, development, communication, and support. Subjective and objective data are both important. Gather subjective data by interviewing patients and family members to explore their strengths and needs; gather objective data by observing family interactions and performing the physical examination. Nursing assessment helps to identify functional patterns, risks, and dysfunction. Assessment findings serve as a basis for making nursing diagnoses and formulating interventions.

 APPLY YOUR CRITICAL THINKING

You are working in a medical walk-in clinic when a woman, accompanied by her boyfriend, brings in her 3-year-old child who has fallen and injured his arm. The boy appears very stoic and emotionless: although he is in obvious pain, he does not cry. When you try to talk with him, he avoids eye contact. When you undress him to examine his injury, you notice old and new bruises on his arm, which he is unable to move. What might your assessment findings reveal? How should you proceed?

Check your answers in Appendix B.

THERAPEUTIC DIALOGUE: FAMILIES

SCENE FOR THOUGHT

The Loeman family (Ronald and Marilyn, both age 50 years; Jeff, age 18 years; and Stefanie, age 14 years) are in the hospital visiting Mr. Loeman, Ronald's father, who lives with them. Mr. Loeman, otherwise healthy, was admitted for replacement of his pacemaker and is doing well at this time, 2 days postoperatively. He, his family, and his nurse are chatting in the unit's solarium.

LESS EFFECTIVE

Ronald: Dad looks great, doesn't he, Mr. Boren? *(Beams at his father and pats his shoulder.)*

Nurse: He does seem to be recovering well after the surgery. How do you feel today, Mr. Loeman? *(Sits next to the wheelchair.)*

Mr. L: Wonderful, wonderful! Why do all of you keep treating me like I'm a baby? *(Grumpily.)*

Nurse: Now, now, Mr. Loeman, your family are all here to see you because they love you. You were looking forward to seeing them this morning, remember? *(Gives his hand a reassuring pat.)*

Jeff: Mom, Stef and I are going to the cafeteria for a soda. *(Starts to leave with his sister.)*

Ronald: Not now, Jeff. Stay and visit with Opa for a little while. We've only been here 5 minutes. *(Sternly.)*

Mr. L: Never mind, Ronald. Let them go. I'll see them later. Here, Jeff, have a soda on me. *(Hands Jeff a few dollars. The children quickly leave.)*

Nurse: That's sweet, Mr. Loeman. I'll bet they really appreciate you. *(Smiles at Ronald and Marilyn. They smile back weakly.)*

Mr. L: Mr. Boren, wheel me back to my room. I'm tired.

Nurse: Sure, Mr. Loeman. *(To Ronald and Marilyn.)* I'll be right back. I'll just get him settled.

Mr. L: What are you going to talk to them about? *(Suspiciously.)*

Nurse: Just about how to help you recover when you go home tomorrow. Don't worry, we'll take good care of you. *(Wheels Mr. Loeman into his room. Marilyn and Ronald silently watch them go.)*

MORE EFFECTIVE

Ronald: Dad looks great, doesn't he, Mr. Ballard? *(Beams at his father and pats his shoulder.)*

Nurse: He does seem to be recovering well after the surgery. How do you feel today, Mr. Loeman? *(Sits next to the wheelchair.)*

Mr. L: Wonderful, wonderful! Why do all of you keep treating me like I'm a baby? *(Grumpily.)*

Marilyn: Now, Dad, don't start that. We're just concerned about you. *(Smiles tightly and throws a significant look at Ronald.)*

Jeff: Mom, Stef and I are going to the cafeteria for a soda. *(Starts to leave with his sister.)*

Ronald: Not now, Jeff. Visit with Opa for a little while. We've only been here 5 minutes. *(Sternly.)*

Mr. L: Never mind, Ronald. Let them go. I'll see them later. Here, Jeff, have a soda on me. *(Hands him a few dollars. The children quickly leave.)*

Ronald: You spoil them, Dad. *(Exasperated.)*

Mr. L: Why not? They're my only grandchildren. When I go, they won't get much but they'll think of me fondly. *(Looks sad, defiant, and angry.)* Mr. Ballard, wheel me back to my room. I'm tired.

Nurse: Sure, Mr. Loeman. Is it okay with you if I talk to Ronald and Marilyn while you rest? *(Continues to sit next to him.)*

Mr. L: What are you going to talk to them about? *(Suspiciously.)*

Nurse: What they need to do to help you recover when you're discharged tomorrow. Would you rather stay and participate? Or would you like to rest in bed and participate there?

Mr. L: *(Thinks about it.)* I'd rather rest in bed and listen to you in my room. I'm tired.

Nurse: Good idea. Let's go. I'll get us all some juice on the way. *(Wheels Mr. Loeman to his room; he looks tired but more relaxed. Ronald and Marilyn are surprised at how easily the decision was accomplished. They make a mental note to try it at home with Mr. Loeman.)*

CRITICAL THINKING CHALLENGE

- Analyze the effect that Mr. Loeman's illness has had on his family (individually and collectively).
- Detect and examine how the stress appeared in the dialogues.
- Construct what the family must be like at home together.
- Evaluate indications of dysfunctional patterns in this family.
- Compare and contrast how the two nurses hindered or facilitated family coping.

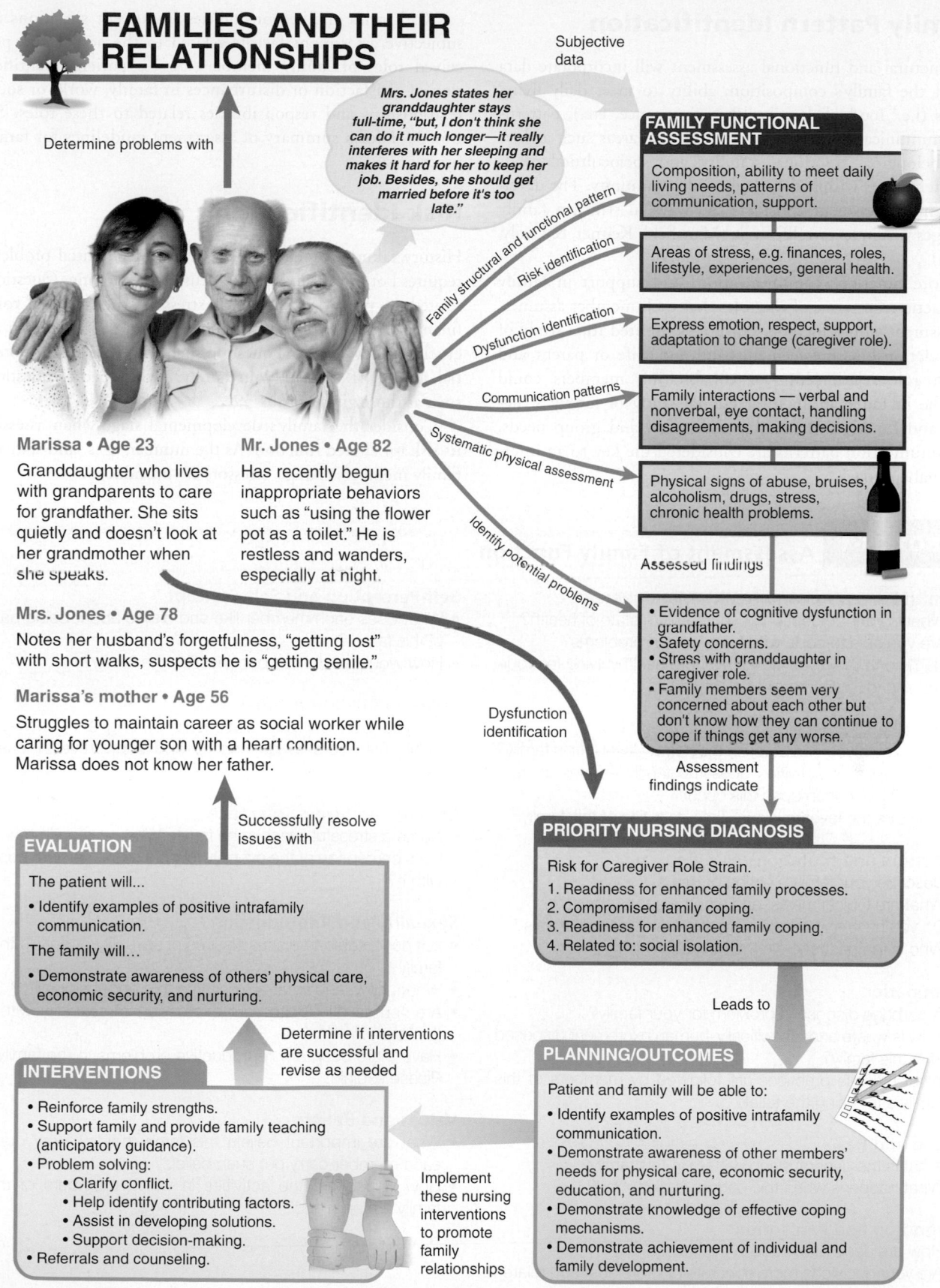

FAMILIES AND THEIR RELATIONSHIPS

Determine problems with

Subjective data

Mrs. Jones states her granddaughter stays full-time, "but, I don't think she can do it much longer—it really interferes with her sleeping and makes it hard for her to keep her job. Besides, she should get married before it's too late."

Marissa • Age 23

Granddaughter who lives with grandparents to care for grandfather. She sits quietly and doesn't look at her grandmother when she speaks.

Mr. Jones • Age 82

Has recently begun inappropriate behaviors such as "using the flower pot as a toilet." He is restless and wanders, especially at night.

Mrs. Jones • Age 78

Notes her husband's forgetfulness, "getting lost" with short walks, suspects he is "getting senile."

Marissa's mother • Age 56

Struggles to maintain career as social worker while caring for younger son with a heart condition. Marissa does not know her father.

Family structural and functional pattern
Risk identification
Dysfunction identification
Communication patterns
Systematic physical assessment
Identify potential problems

FAMILY FUNCTIONAL ASSESSMENT

Composition, ability to meet daily living needs, patterns of communication, support.

Areas of stress, e.g. finances, roles, lifestyle, experiences, general health.

Express emotion, respect, support, adaptation to change (caregiver role).

Family interactions — verbal and nonverbal, eye contact, handling disagreements, making decisions.

Physical signs of abuse, bruises, alcoholism, drugs, stress, chronic health problems.

Assessed findings

- Evidence of cognitive dysfunction in grandfather.
- Safety concerns.
- Stress with granddaughter in caregiver role.
- Family members seem very concerned about each other but don't know how they can continue to cope if things get any worse.

Dysfunction identification

Assessment findings indicate

PRIORITY NURSING DIAGNOSIS

Risk for Caregiver Role Strain.
1. Readiness for enhanced family processes.
2. Compromised family coping.
3. Readiness for enhanced family coping.
4. Related to: social isolation.

Leads to

EVALUATION

The patient will...
- Identify examples of positive intrafamily communication.

The family will...
- Demonstrate awareness of others' physical care, economic security, and nurturing.

Successfully resolve issues with

Determine if interventions are successful and revise as needed

INTERVENTIONS

- Reinforce family strengths.
- Support family and provide family teaching (anticipatory guidance).
- Problem solving:
  - Clarify conflict.
  - Help identify contributing factors.
  - Assist in developing solutions.
  - Support decision-making.
- Referrals and counseling.

Implement these nursing interventions to promote family relationships

PLANNING/OUTCOMES

Patient and family will be able to:
- Identify examples of positive intrafamily communication.
- Demonstrate awareness of other members' needs for physical care, economic security, education, and nurturing.
- Demonstrate knowledge of effective coping mechanisms.
- Demonstrate achievement of individual and family development.

FIGURE 39-6 Families and their relationships concept map.

Family Pattern Identification

A structural and functional assessment will incorporate data about the family's composition, ability to meet daily living needs (i.e., food, shelter, health maintenance, etc.), patterns of communication, and support. Examine areas such as love and belonging, emotional stability, and sociocultural needs or interactions within the family and community. The developmental assessment considers the ways in which a family changes within its own life cycle (Mansfield, Keitner, & Dealy, 2014).

Note function, communication, and support in family interactions in terms of the roles that each member assumes. Assessment would include, but not be limited to, a study of the relationships between husband and wife or parent and child; role relationships of cohabiting members could also be included in an interactional study of family structure and function in meeting individual and group needs. Communication patterns are considered the key to an interactional approach.

Work roles and responsibilities in current situations are subjective assessment factors related to the actual and perceived roles of family members. Assess patient identification of satisfaction or disturbances in family, work, or social relationships and responsibilities related to these roles. See Box 39-1 for a summary of assessment guidelines for family function.

Risk Identification

History taking to identify areas of risk or potential problems requires both open-ended and focused questioning. Questions related to potential sources of stress in the areas of roles, finances, lifestyle, previous experience, and general health are crucial. Follow a general question such as "What are the potential sources of stress in your family?" with specific questions such as those given in Box 39-2.

Consider the family's developmental stage when assessing its risk for altered function. As the number, ages, and status of family members change, stressors are introduced.

BOX 39-1   Assessment of Family Function

Health Perception and Health Management
- What is your perception of your family's state of health?
- Are you able to cope with family health problems?
- Name one thing you do to promote healthy living for yourself and for each member of the family.

Activity and Exercise
- How would you characterize the activity level in this family?
- What types of activities does the family engage in as a group? How often does this occur?
- What are the favorite leisure-time activities of this family?

Nutrition and Metabolism
- Describe your family's eating patterns.
- What are typical meals, and when are they served?
- Do you have any special way of preparing family meals?
- Who is the best cook in the house? Why?

Elimination
- Is garbage disposal a problem for your family?
- How is waste and, specifically, human excrement disposed of in this family?
- What hygiene practices are followed by members of this family after using the toilet?

Sleep and Rest
- What is the general sleep pattern in this family?
- What happens when this pattern is disturbed?

Cognition and Perception
- How are decisions made in this family?
- Are your decisions more concrete or more abstract, related to the past, present, or future?

Self-Perception and Self-Concept
- What does each member like and dislike about being part of this family?
- How would each member describe the family?

Roles and Relationships
- Do you consider the relationship among and between family members to be healthy and supportive? Please explain.

Coping and Stress Tolerance
- Name a stressful event in the family. What was each member's perception of the event? How did each member cope with it?

Sexuality and Reproduction
- Is it acceptable to discuss issues of sexuality openly in this family?
- When, how, and what are children told about sexuality?
- Are you satisfied with your expression of sexuality within the family?
- Have there been any reproductive problems in the family? Please explain.

Values and Beliefs
- What are important beliefs this family holds? How does each member carry out such beliefs?
- How valued are the activities in which members of the family are engaged?

BOX 39-2   Assessment of Family Social Relationships

Family Structure and Function

- Description of patient's family unit—age, sex, and so forth
- Patient's responsibilities in the household
- Persons responsible for decision within patient's household
- Management of finances
- Ways in which family responsibilities are distributed
- Pattern of eating, sleeping, and health practices

Family/Social Interaction

- Most significant person in patient's life
- Availability of significant others to patient
- Any other people whom patient can turn to if necessary
- Number of friends
- Patient's socialization with friends, neighbors, and relatives
- Description of patient's neighborhood and neighbors

Indicators of Change

- Any major change in patient's role(s) or responsibilities (explain)
- Patient's anticipated future changes in the coming years
- Preparations made for these changes
- Any family stressors—how are they being handled

Parental Role Function (If Person Is a Parent)

- Patient's relationship with his or her children? Parents? Friends?
- Any plans to expand his or her family?
- Comparison of parenting patterns to those of patient's parents (e.g., discipline). Explain.

Occupational Role Factors

- Patient's occupation (include work role and responsibilities)
- Hours worked per week; work interfering with other aspects of patient's lifestyle?
- Ability of patient's income to maintain patient's lifestyle

Leisure-Time Management

- Usual activity pattern? Joint activities?
- Vacations taken and frequency
- Patient's plans for retirement; if retired, is patient enjoying it?

Cultural Factors

- Ethnic/religious background
- Similarity of family values
- Family childrearing practices

Source: University of Scranton, Department of Nursing. (1994). *University of Scranton guide to care plan assessment.* Scranton, PA: Author.

Characteristic risk factors for potential alterations in family processes include unrealistic expectations of self or others, lack of appropriate role models, history of abuse, inability to bond with others, inadequate support systems, stress, skill or knowledge deficit, acute or chronic illness, and unmet psychosocial needs of children or adults (Dever, Schulenberg, Dworkin, O'Malley, Kloska, et al., 2012; Kuo et al., 2012; Gottlieb, 2013).

Dysfunction Identification

Altered family functioning can be identified when there is a significant difference from an effective pattern of functioning. Inability to express or accept emotions, lack of respect or support for other family members, and inability to adapt to change are contributing factors (Nanni, Biancosino, Grassi, et al., 2014).

As an ill family member experiences change, the caregiver's role changes as well. This may be evidenced by verbalization of feelings of inadequacy, guilt, anxiety, failure, helplessness, and powerlessness. Parents may express concerns about the effects of a child's illness on siblings and finances. Noncompliance with treatment may be a manifestation of denial or refusal to acknowledge a problem's existence. Denial may serve as a mechanism to maintain or to restore "normality" in family life, but it can indicate dysfunction if it

prevents a family from dealing with the situation (Dennis & Halberstadt, 2013).

Objective Data

Objective data for assessing family function include observation of family interactions and the behavior of members as well as physical examination. Behavioral signs of family dysfunction include labile emotions, withdrawal, irritability, poor sleeping and eating, inability to concentrate, and dependency (Dever et al., 2012; Keeton, Ginsburg, Drake, Sakolsky, Kendall, et al., 2013). Observe family communication patterns. How do members relate to one another, and how effectively do they communicate? Observe who does the talking, who remains silent, whether members listen to one another, how they handle disagreements, how they make decisions, and what they communicate nonverbally. Observation of which family members visit the ill person, how often, and how the patient responds can also provide clues in family assessment.

Physical assessment includes inspection, palpation, auscultation, and percussion performed systematically. While assessing physical health, look for clues of family dysfunction. Pay special attention to injuries or bruises that may indicate physical abuse, enlarged liver and other signs of chronic alcoholism, track marks indicating intravenous drug injection, nasal inflammatory symptoms of cocaine abuse, signs of stress (e.g., weight loss, fatigue, and impaired cognitive function), and multiple acute and chronic physical problems (Dong, 2013; Trindade et al., 2014; Dinis-Oliveira, Carvalho, Duarte, Proença, Santos, et al., 2012).

NURSING DIAGNOSES

Careful assessment of individual members and the family as a whole is needed to identify actual or potential problems. As suggested in the Case Scenario, nurses work with families to formulate a diagnosis by eliciting each member's perceptions of needs, goals, and expectations. NANDA International (NANDA-I, 2014) has identified the following accepted nursing diagnoses in family problems: Class 1, Caregiver Role Strain, Impaired Parenting, and Readiness for Enhanced Parenting; Class 2, Risk for Impaired Attachment, Dysfunctional Family Processes, Interrupted Family Processes, and Readiness for Enhanced Family Processes; and Class 3, Ineffective Relationship, Parental Role Conflict, and Impaired Social Interaction selected nursing diagnoses are presented in Table 39-2 along with

selected Nursing Outcomes Classification (NOC) and Nursing Interventions Classification (NIC).

OUTCOME IDENTIFICATION AND PLANNING

After the nursing diagnoses and related factors are identified, patient goals and nursing interventions are planned. Goals are designed to identify the general and specific changes that the patient and family think will demonstrate that the situation has improved. Patient- and family-centered care goals are often derived from identifying the contributing factors and are designed to indicate specific, discernible behaviors. General goals can be identified for family functioning and then individualized for each situation. Common patient- and family-centered goals for families experiencing problems include the following:

- The patient and family will identify instances in which they have achieved intrafamily communication (Wittenberg-Lyles, Washington, Demiris, Shaunfield, 2014).

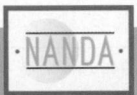

Table 39-2 SELECTED NANDA-I NURSING DIAGNOSES INVOLVING FAMILIES

Nursing Dx	Related Factors	Dx Statement	NOC*	NIC†
Caregiver Role Strain—a caregiver's felt or exhibited difficulty in performing the caregiver role	Illness severity, addiction or codependency, or other instability in health Psychosocial or cognitive problems Situational factors	Caregiver role strain R/T difficulty in doing specific caregiving activities AEB-specific dysfunctions in family relationships	Caregiver Home Care Readiness Caregiver Stressors Caregiver Well-Being Caregiver–Patient Relationship Knowledge: Parenting	Caregiver Role Strain Complex Relationship Building Conflict Mediation Family Involvement Promotion Family Therapy
Dysfunctional Family Processes—behavior which often results in conflict, denial, resistance to changing behavior, ineffective problem solving, and ongoing crises	Anxiety, stress, depression, job loss, grief	Dysfunctional family processes R/T alcoholism AEB denial, reluctance to change, ongoing crises	Abuse Cessation Abuse Protection Support: Domestic Partner Abuse Protection Support: Elder Caregiver Stressors Caregiver Well-Being Caregiver–Patient Relationship	Abuse Protection Support: Child Abuse Protection Support: Domestic Partner Abuse Protection Support: Elder
Impaired Parenting—a state in which a nurturing figure experiences a change or modification in ability to create, continue, or regain an environment that promotes the optimum growth and development of another human being	Abuse of the parent, lack of support between significant others, unmet needs, lack of knowledge, unrealistic expectations	Impaired parenting R/T inability to parent effectively AEB inappropriate parental behaviors, neglect or inattention to child needs, observed role inadequacy	Parent–Infant Attachment Parenting Parenting Performance Role Performance Child Adaptation to Hospitalization Child Development Knowledge: Child Physical Safety	Childbirth Preparation Development Enhancement: Child Family Involvement Promotion Family Therapy Teaching: Infant Safety Teaching: Infant Stimulation Teaching: Toddler Nutrition Teaching: Toddler Safety

Dx, diagnosis; R/T, related to; AEB, as evidenced by.
*From: Moorhead, S., Johnson, M., Maas, M., & Swanson, E. (2013). *Iowa Outcomes Project: Nursing Outcomes Classification (NOC)* (5th ed.). St. Louis, MO: C. V. Mosby.
†From: Bulecheck, G., Butcher, H., Dochterman, J., & Wagner, C. (2013). *Iowa Intervention Project: Nursing Interventions Classification (NIC)* (6th ed.). St. Louis, MO: C. V. Mosby.
From: NANDA-Association International (NANDA-I). (2014). *Nursing diagnoses: Definitions and classification, 2015–2017.* West Sussex, England: Wiley-Blackwell.

- The patient and family will demonstrate awareness of other members' needs for physical care, economic security, education, and nurturing (Williams, 2014).
- The patient and family will demonstrate knowledge of effective coping mechanisms (Stamataki, Ellis, Costello, Fielding, Burns, et al., 2014).
- The patient and family will demonstrate achievement of individual and family development (Williams & Bakitas, 2012).

When using family-centered care, the nurse in the case scenario at the beginning of the chapter will need to review and to clarify expectations with both the caregivers and extended family before proceeding to interventions. Implementation is most effective when the patient, family, and nurse have collaboratively set goals and developed interventions (Kuo et al., 2012).

Nurses plan with the patient, the family, or both to promote healthy family patterns and function or to assist directly in meeting the needs of the family with altered function. Motivation and educational needs will influence planning. Examples of nursing interventions commonly used in family care are listed in Table 39-2 and discussed in the following section.

IMPLEMENTATION

To promote family function, nurses support, reinforce, and teach. Interventions for altered family functioning include referral, counseling, and assistance with problem solving. The more family members the nurses can involve, the more family centered the care will be and the greater its potential impact (Kuo et al., 2012) (Fig. 39-7).

Health Promotion

Identifying strengths, reinforcing positive behaviors, and providing anticipatory guidance and resources can support the family (Toly et al., 2012). These strengths and resources are key areas to assess that you can include in your first visit with the family.

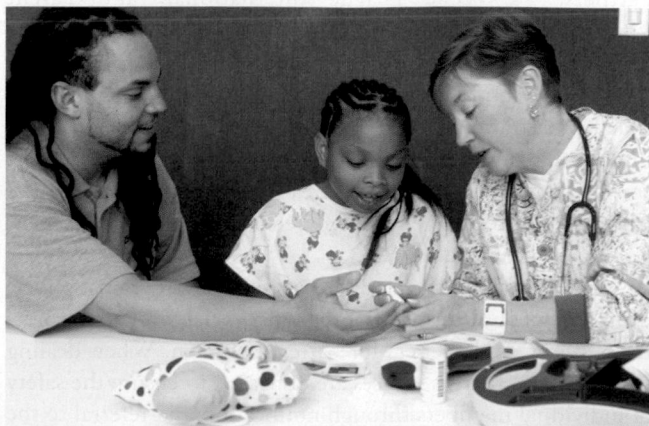

FIGURE 39-7 Involving family members in the care of an ill member helps them cope with the illness and understand their role in the healing process.

REINFORCEMENT OF FAMILY STRENGTHS

From information obtained during assessment, help the patient and family to identify their own areas of strength (Fig. 39-8). Strengths may include effective communication, mutual support of members, flexible roles, general stability, healthy coping mechanisms, and good support systems. Identification of strengths will help the family target resources to draw from for daily functioning as well as when crises develop. Focus on the family's strengths rather than weaknesses (Wright & Leahey, 2013). Point out examples of strengths, such as a family member's ability to take a leave of absence to care for the ill person to relieve the primary caregiver or the spiritual support that the family's clergy or spiritual consultant provides. Encourage the patient and family to think of examples of strengths that they have used when faced with problems in the past and how they can draw on these strengths if needed. Identify both individual and family strengths.

SUPPORT AND TEACHING

Support the patient and family in actions that promote family functioning by listening to and educating them. During serious or chronic illnesses, many nurses form close bonds with patients and their families. Families come to look to nurses for emotional support. Help families identify other sources of support as well, such as extended family, religious affiliations, work groups, peers, and community groups (Kuo et al., 2012; Magon et al., et al., 2012; Wright & Leahey, 2013). Then the family can strengthen contact with support groups. Assure the family that using support systems is a strength, not a weakness. **Anticipatory guidance** is a technique combining teaching and support. Instead of focusing on what has happened during the course of an illness, using anticipatory guidance prepares the patient and family for what will happen next and why (Garfield, Lee, Kim, et al., 2014).

Nursing Interventions for Altered Family Function

If altered family functioning has been identified, interventions focus on behaviors that will return the family to positive outcomes, improve the problem, and support family relationships (Kuo et al., 2012; Donahue, Kazer, Smith, & Fitzpatrick, 2013). Assist with problem solving, offer referrals, and facilitate family counseling if necessary.

PROBLEM SOLVING

Families who are experiencing altered family function attain goals with assistance in problem solving. Aim interventions at resolving family conflicts by first identifying the participants' willingness to acknowledge a problem and to work on their ability to communicate. Stress effective communication practices. Allow each member to speak, listen, and

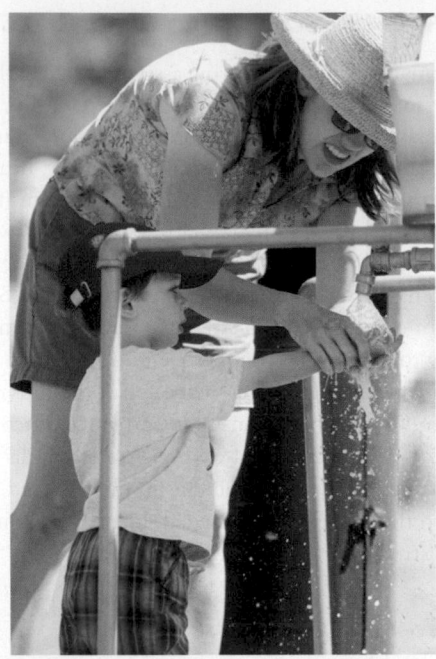

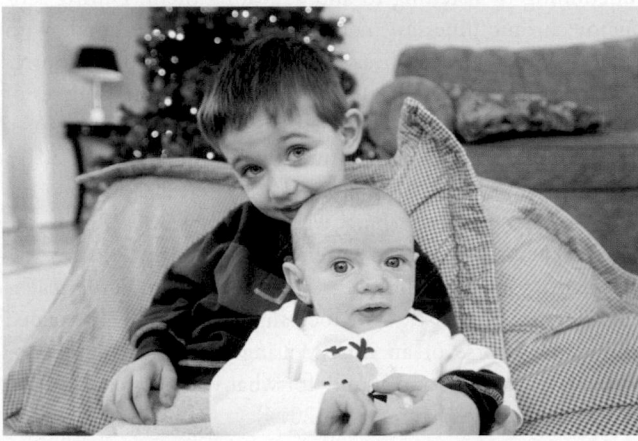

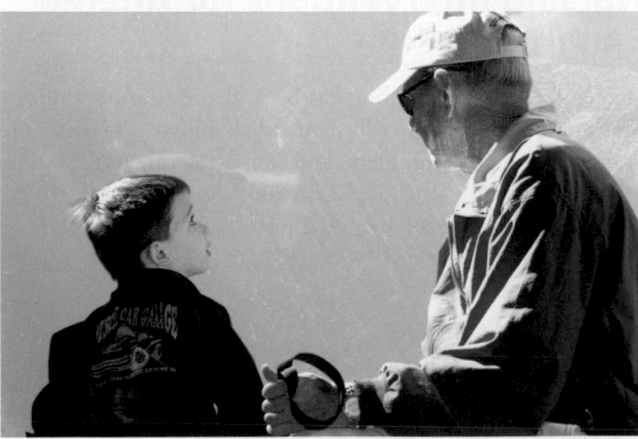

FIGURE 39-8 Sources of strength and support are found in various family relationships such as between mother and son **(A)**, siblings **(B)**, and grandparent and grandchild **(C)**.

express feelings as well as facts (White, Cua, Walk, Pollice, Weissfeld, et al., 2012; Holtslander et al., 2013; Haslam et al., 2015); nursing interventions to foster problem solving include the following:

- Clarify the conflict with participants.
- Help participants identify contributing factors.
- Correct misconceptions.
- Provide concrete feedback based on nursing observations.
- Assist participants to develop solutions.
- Support decision making among participants.

Focus on helping the participants develop self-awareness, and identify a working method to solve problems (Law, Fisher, Fales, Noel, Eccleston, 2014). Lead the family through problem solving while teaching them how to conduct the process themselves. Guide the family in solving a small problem first, providing reassurance that they can deal with larger problems as well.

Along with improving communication and problem solving, nurses must help the family strengthen its coping mechanisms (see Chapter 41). Assist the family in identifying what coping mechanisms worked in the past and what coping mechanisms were detrimental.

REFERRAL AND FAMILY COUNSELING

Nurses may be able to refer families with altered function to other resources (Kevern, 2012; Polivka, Chaudry, Mac Crawford, et al., 2012). Members of the social service department or spiritual ministry may assist families with unmet financial or spiritual needs. Clinical nurse specialists, nutritionists, and physical and occupational therapists may provide information and training for patients and family members who have physical care needs.

Professional referrals and peer support groups may be sources of help to those experiencing difficulty with parenting roles (Sarrami-Foroushani, Travaglia, Debono, & Braithwaite, 2014). Self-help groups for parents include Parents Without Partners, La Leche League International, and Parent Effectiveness Training. Numerous support groups listed in the blue pages of phone books are valuable resources for referrals. The Association for the Care of Children's Health, an international organization located in Bethesda, Maryland, can provide information and a comprehensive list of support groups, their activities, and resources. The Area Agency on Aging and the American Association of Retired Persons (AARP) are excellent resources for older adults.

Other possible referrals are to psychiatric programs, police, drug and alcohol treatment programs, social workers, protective services, and shelters for battered women. When dealing with families in crisis, nurses are obligated to ensure the safety of individual members through notification and referral to the appropriate groups (Schappin et al., 2013). Evidence of suspected child abuse necessitates notification of the police and referral to appropriate agencies.

Ongoing counseling may be necessary for families with chronic stressors such as chronic illness, substance abuse, loss of a family member, role strain, separation, or divorce (Schappin et al., 2013). Family or marital counseling focuses on the interaction of the members, not on counseling any one person. Roles and relationships are examined, communication and problem solving are fostered, and bonds are strengthened. Nurses can be instrumental in leading families to counseling if members are unable to overcome altered function without outside help.

> ! **SAFETY ALERT**
>
> If you suspect child or elder abuse, notify the police and local child protective services or area center for elder abuse. Tell the family that you are acting as an advocate for the child or adult and are legally responsible to report your suspicions.

Healthcare Planning and Home or Community-Based Nursing

Altered family relationships usually must be dealt with in the home environment, placing stress and additional responsibility on family members. When illness is the causative factor of alteration, assess the home for supports and barriers to providing appropriate care and quality of life (Mansfield et al., 2014). Family members can differ in their willingness to assume new or additional responsibilities. Referral to social agencies, such as home healthcare providers, may be necessary to ensure adequate support.

Healthcare planning should address specific needs, types of assistance and equipment needed, learning needs, and availability of alternative support (Toly et al., 2012). Teach family members techniques of care to meet the patient's physical needs to assist in their adaptation to the caregiver's role. Teach signs of risk factors for complications to promote confidence in caring for the patient at home. Provide the family with the name and phone number of someone to contact with questions to ease anxiety. An interdisciplinary approach should include referrals to social workers, counselors, spiritual advisors, community resource centers, and self-help support groups as needed.

Examples of self-help and support groups that are often community-based include Alcoholics Anonymous (AA), Al-Anon, Alateen, Opioids Anonymous, cancer support groups, Compassionate Friends, stroke support groups, and Alzheimer support groups. These groups can help the family solve problems by providing information and emotional support (Herber, & Johnston, 2013). Peer adherence programs and social media have also been used to provide support for families (Wouters et al., 2014).

Case management, a means of coordination and ongoing evaluation of care, is used to help the patient and family deal with the complex healthcare system. Case management

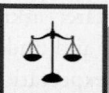

ETHICAL/LEGAL ISSUE

PLACEMENT OF AN ELDER IN A LONG-TERM CARE FACILITY

Janine Sanders was an independent 75-year-old woman despite multiple illnesses including chronic lung disease, osteoporosis, and diabetes. She had been able to remain in her own apartment with visits and help from home care nurses and neighbors. Her family lives over 300 miles away and visits only occasionally. Recently, Janine was hospitalized for a fractured hip. Her doctor cannot recommend discharge to the home; he says the most reasonable option is to admit her to a long-term care facility because no one is available to care for her on a 24-hour basis. Janine wants to move in with her daughter, although her daughter is not home during the day. Janine and her family ask you what you think about placement in a long-term care facility and if you can suggest any other options. The hospital will discharge Janine within a week.

CRITICAL THINKING CHALLENGE

- Reflect on your feelings as the family asks you to help them consider moving the previously independent woman to a long-term care facility. Try to identify any areas that you are uncomfortable discussing.
- Identify your underlying assumptions about the ethics of hospital discharge into facilities such as long-term care facilities.
- Reflect on how the Patient Bill of Rights in Chapter 7 applies to this situation. What information does the family need to make an informed decision?
- Think of at least three different ways to respond to the family's request for help. Identify a possible approach that could help Janine's family feel that they have supported Janine's right to independence along with her need for continuous support. How could her quality of life be maintained?

includes identifying, coordinating, and evaluating the provision of services, including cost, quality, and continuity (Kramer et al., 2012; Jensen, 2014). People must be connected to outside resources and support systems and assisted to maximize their own strengths in caring for patients at home. Family members, neighbors, and community organizations can form a "family-centered" network of care (Kuo et al., 2012). Their goal is to provide as "normal" a lifestyle as possible with the patient and family acting in partnership with the nurse case manager and other professional healthcare providers. If the caregivers, patient, and family members disagree, the case manager needs to remain nonjudgmental and show acceptance of the differences. Encouraging everyone's active involvement facilitates family-centered care; asking questions about each family member's knowledge and understanding of past and present situations, as well as expectations for the future, should help to define problems and suggest solutions (Donahue et al., 2013; Garfield et al., 2014). In the Case Scenario, questions addressed to the spouse, daughter, and granddaughter could facilitate optimal home care for the patient.

EVALUATION

Evaluation is an ongoing process of determining progress toward the stated goals in the outcome identification phase. For alterations in family function, expected outcome criteria focus on patient and family communication, family needs, use of coping mechanisms, and family development. The following are examples of possible outcome criteria for general goals.

Goal

Patient will identify instances in which intrafamily communication has been achieved (Toly et al., 2012).

POSSIBLE OUTCOME CRITERIA

• By home care discharge, each family member engages in conversation during visit, as observed by the nurse.
• By home care discharge, other members listen while family member is talking, as observed by the nurse.

• Family member relates that content of conversations includes feelings within 48 hours.
• Caregiver expresses use of alternatives such as telephone and letter writing when personal visits are impossible due to distance or other time constraints.

Goal

Family members will demonstrate awareness of other members' physical care, economic security, educational needs, and nurturing (Schappin et al., 2013).

POSSIBLE OUTCOME CRITERIA

Within 48 hours, family states that bills are being paid and family members are attending social functions.

Within 48 hours, family members display affection toward one another, as observed by nurse.

Goal

Patient will demonstrate knowledge of effective coping mechanisms (Wright & Leahey, 2013).

POSSIBLE OUTCOME CRITERIA

During first counseling sessions, caregiver discusses family coping mechanisms that worked in the past.

During first counseling session, caregiver states coping mechanisms that were detrimental in the past.

By discharge, the patient verbalizes coping mechanisms that he or she will use in future.

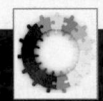

COLLABORATING WITH THE HEALTHCARE TEAM
Calling the Home Health Nurse Concerning Care Issues in the Home

Mr. House, age 78 years, has advanced Alzheimer disease with occasional wandering at night.

SITUATION: Mrs. House needs her sleep in order to do all the things she needs to do, so she ties Mr. House in bed at night so that he'll stay put.

BACKGROUND: Mrs. House, age 74 years, provides care for her husband, holds a part-time child day care job because their income is limited, and she is getting increasingly fatigued but is adamant about not finding another care situation for her husband. Mrs. House has no other family close by.

ASSESSMENT: Mrs. House needs the home health nurse to spend time with her, assess her situation, and help her to understand what other options she may have to assist her with Mr. House's care as well as her own well-being.

RECOMMENDATION: Could you go as soon as possible and talk with Mrs. House and support her in her caregiving responsibilities? I am quite concerned about her mental and physical state.

CRITICAL THINKING CHALLENGE
• Discuss the rationale for requesting that the home health nurse be called instead of another professional colleague.
• Which other members of the collaborative team could be called on to help provide some advice?
• What support does Mrs. House need in this situation? Mr. House?

PATIENT PLAN OF CARE
The Family with Caregiver Role Strain

NURSING DIAGNOSIS
Caregiver Role Strain related to anxiety, lack of knowledge, money, and emotional support manifested by altered sleep patterns; frequent crying; verbalized inadequacy of knowledge, finances, and husband

FAMILY GOAL
Caregiver will develop a realistic care plan that includes support from the family and community.

FAMILY OUTCOME CRITERIA
- Caregiver demonstrates decreased anxiety with increased confidence in caretaking behaviors within 1 month.
- Caregiver receives and accepts support from family and community within 1 month.
- Family seeks external resources within 2 weeks.

NURSING INTERVENTION	SCIENTIFIC RATIONALE
1. Assess caregiver's knowledge of dementia disease characteristics by questioning and observation. Be nonjudgmental. Encourage expression of feelings.	**1.** Objective data can validate verbal responses. Need to identify knowledge without provoking resentment.
2. Reinforce positive caregiving, accept expressions of negative emotions, and focus on positive behaviors.	**2.** Reinforcement encourages caregiver and decreases anxiety.
3. Role-model effective communication techniques: talk directly to older adult and maintain eye contact.	**3.** Communication is important for developing coping techniques.
4. Explore with caregiver ways to involve all family members in meeting the older adult's needs consistently and securely.	**4.** By decreasing denial, realistic planning can occur. Likelihood of compliance increases if all members are involved.
5. Initiate a plan to develop caregiving skills by providing information and opportunities for wife–family interaction with feedback.	**5.** Information about realistic expectations and solutions can promote effective coping. Practice reinforces these measures.
6. Explore possible sources of support. Offer to make initial contacts. Fear of authorities may inhibit initiating action.	**6.** Support needs to be ongoing for change to be maintained.
7. Refer to Area Agency on Aging for caregiver relief assistance; refer to Alzheimer support groups for respite care planning.	**7.** Continuity of care includes assessment and support.

EVALUATION

- At 1 month, caretaking behaviors demonstrate decreased anxiety with increasing confidence.
- Caregiver reports increased support from family and community over the last 4 weeks.
- Family identifies community and healthcare resources that have been used within the past 2 weeks.

KEY CONCEPTS

- Many family structures exist, including nuclear families, single-parent families, blended families, cohabitated families, extended/intergenerational families, communal families, and nontraditional families.

- Each family functions uniquely, but all families share some common goals. Needs that families address for their members include physical and economic provision of care, sexual intimacy, reproduction, education, socialization, and nurturing and support.

- Factors that affect family function include culture, values and beliefs, economic resources, lifestyle, previous life experience, stress, social isolation, role strain, illness, and traumatic experiences.

- Families and their relationships change in reaction to daily and situational stress as well as acute and chronic illness. Roles may be redefined to meet individual and family needs.

- Common manifestations of altered family function include separation or divorce, emotional problems, role overload, abuse/violence, substance abuse social isolation, and emotional problems.

- Both subjective and objective data are useful for assessment of altered family function. Assessment seeks to identify usual patterns, families at risk, and family dysfunction.

- Outcome identification and planning focus on the patient and family members and the family as a whole. Goals, which involve applying family-centered care, include improved communication and coping mechanisms, fulfilled family needs, and accomplished development.

- A multidisciplinary approach is useful in interventions for altered family function. Interventions to promote health and family functioning include reinforcement of family strengths, support, and use of anticipatory guidance. Interventions for families with altered function include problem solving, referral, and family counseling.

- Evaluation of nursing care is an ongoing process of determining progress toward goals established during the outcome identification stage.

PRACTICING FOR THE NCLEX

CHECK YOUR ANSWERS IN APPENDIX A.

1. A 58-year-old patient, a Boeing employee, is hospitalized with a myocardial infarction. The wife, a homemaker, is present at the bedside along with their two teenage children but seems unable to make decisions related to the patient's care and discharge plan. The wife is also terse with nursing staff and questions all prescribed interventions. The nurse suspects that this behavior may be attributed to which of the following nursing diagnoses?
   a. Caregiver Role Strain
   b. Interrupted Family Processes
   c. Impaired Parenting
   d. Ineffective Family Therapeutic Regimen Management
   e. Parental Role Conflict

2. A patient is admitted with congestive heart failure exacerbation and an ejection fraction of 40% with her husband at the bedside. The nurse suspects Caregiver Role Strain as a pertinent nursing diagnosis. Which of the following husband's comments best indicate this diagnosis? Select all that apply:
   a. "I hardly sleep because I'm so worried about my wife's breathing."
   b. "I make sure that she has her inhalers and medications exactly as scheduled."
   c. "I recently stopped working to help my wife full-time at home."
   d. "My wife was just admitted last month for the same breathing problems."

3. Family function is an aspect of all family structures and evolves over time within each individual family. Which of the following are elements of family function?
   a. Sexual Intimacy
   b. Culture
   c. Chronic/Acute Illness
   d. Role Strain
   e. Parental Role

4. A patient is seen in the clinic for a diabetic foot ulcer and states that she is socially isolated related to her limited mobility. Which of the following problem-solving strategies should be done first by the nurse in addressing Altered Family Function? Select all that apply:
   a. Help the patient identify contributing factors.
   b. Assist the patient to develop solutions.
   c. Refer to counseling for social isolation.
   d. Refer to resource agencies for assistance.

5. Which of the following would NOT be an example of a *family*?
   a. One birth parent, one non–birth parent, and children
   b. Same-sex partnerships without children
   c. Homeless group raising a child
   d. Parent who lives across the country for most of the year
   e. Widowed parent with adult children, living alone

REFERENCES

Adames, H.Y., Chavez-Dueñas, N. Y., Fuentes, M. A., Salas, S. P., & Perez-Chavez, J. G. (2014). Integration of Latino/a cultural values into palliative health care: A culture centered model. *Palliative & Supportive Care, 12*(2), 149–157. doi: 10.1017/S147895151300028X

Wright, A. G., Pincus, A. L., & Lenzenweger, M. F. (2012). Interpersonal development, stability, and change in early adulthood. *Journal of Personality, 80*(5), 1339–1372. doi: 10.1111/j.1467-6494.2012.00761.x

Alemany, S., Rijsdijk, F. V., Haworth, C. M. A., Fañanás, L., & Plomin, R. (2013). Genetic origin of the relationship between parental negativity and behavior problems from early childhood to adolescence: A longitudinal genetically sensitive study. *Development and Psychopathology, 25*(2), doi: 10.1017/S0954579412001198

Alsolamy, S. (2014). Islamic views on artificial nutrition and hydration in terminally ill patients. *Bioethics, 28*(2), 96–99. doi: 10.1111/j.1467-8519.2012.01996.x

Bekhet, A. K., & Zauszniewski, J. A. (2012). Mental health of elders in retirement communities: Is loneliness a key factor? *Archives of Psychiatric Nursing, 26*(3), 214–224. doi: 10.1016/j.apnu.2011.09.007

Betancourt, B. S., Meyers-Ohki, S. E., Charrow, A., & Hansen, N. (2013). Mental health and resilience in HIV/AIDS-affected children: A review of the literature and recommendations for future research. *Journal of Child Psychology and Psychiatry, 54*(4), 423–444. doi: 10.1111/j.1469-7610.2012.02613.x

Bianchi, S. M. (2012). Family change and time allocation in American families. *Work and Family Commons (WFC): Alfred P. Sloan Foundation.* pp. 1–29. https://workfamily.sas.upenn.edu/wfrn-repo/object/1tu90df23ih550x4

Bradley, C. J., & Bassam Dahman. (2013). Time away from work: Employed husbands of women treated for breast cancer.. *Journal of Cancer Survivorship, 7*(2), 227–236. doi: 10.1007/s11764-012-0263-5

Bröning, S., Kumpfer, K., Kruse, K., Sack, P.-M., Schaunig-Busch, I., Ruths, S., et al. (2012). Selective prevention programs for children from substance-affected families: A comprehensive systematic review. *Substance Abuse Treatment, Prevention, and Policy, 7*, 23. doi: 10.1186/1747-597X-7-23

Browning, D. L. (2011). Testing reality during adolescence: The contribution of Erikson's concepts of fidelity and developmental actuality. *The Psychoanalytic Quarterly, 80*(3), 555–593.

Bureau of Labor Statistics, US Department of Labor. (2014). *Employment Characteristics of Families —2013*. Washington, DC. http://www.bls.gov/news.release/famee.nr0.htm

Chae, D. H., Lee, S., Lincoln, K. D., & Ihara, E. S. (2012). Discrimination, family relationships, and major depression among Asian Americans. *Journal of Immigrant and Minority Health, 14*(3), 361–370. doi: 10.1007/s10903-011-9548-4

Cherry, K. (2015). Erikson's psychosocial stages summary chart. *Erikson's Stages of Psychosocial Development*. Retrieved September 11, 2015. http://psychology.about.com/od/psychosocialtheories/fl/Psychosocial-Stages-Summary-Chart.htm

Coley, R. L., McPherran, C., & Lombardi, B. (2013). Does maternal employment following childbirth support or inhibit low-income children's long-term development? *Child Development, 84*(1), 178–197. doi: 10.1111/j.1467-8624.2012.01840.x

Compas, B. E., Jaser, S. S., Dunn, M. J., & Rodriguez, E. M. (2012). Coping with chronic illness in childhood and adolescence. *Annual Review of Clinical Psychology, 8*, 455–480. doi: 10.1146/annurev-clinpsy-032511-143108

Cruz, J. (2012). Remarriage Rate in the U.S., 2010. (FP-12-14). National Center for Family & Marriage Research. Retrieved from http://ncfmr.bgsu.edu/pdf/family_profiles/file114853.pdf

Cruz, J. (2013). *Marriage: More than a Century of Change (FP-13-13)*. National Center for Family & Marriage Research. Retrieved from http://www.bgsu.edu/content/dam/BGSU/college-of-arts-and-sciences/NCFMR/documents/FP/FP-13-13.pdf

Dennis, P. A., & Halberstadt, A. G. (2013). Is believing seeing? The role of emotion-related beliefs in selective attention to affective cues. *Cognition & Emotion, 27*(1), 3–20. doi: 10.1080/02699931.2012.680578

Kuo, D. Z., Houtrow, A. J., Arango, P., Kuhlthau, K. A., Simmons, J. M., & Neff, J. M. (2012). Family-centered care: Current applications and future directions in pediatric healthcare. *Maternal and Child Health Journal, 16*(2), 297–305. http://www.ncbi.nlm.nih.gov/pmc/articles/PMC3262132/

Dever, B. V., Schulenberg, J. E., Dworkin, J. B., O'Malley, P. M., Kloska, D. D., & Bachman, J. G. (2012). Predicting risk-taking with and without substance use: The effects of parental monitoring, school bonding, and sports participation. *Prevention Science, 13*(6), 605–615. doi: 10.1007/s11121-012-0288-z

Dinis-Oliveira, R. J., Carvalho, F., Duarte, J. A., Proença, J. B., Santos, A., & Magalhães, T. (2012). Clinical and forensic signs related to cocaine abuse. *Current Drug Abuse Reviews, 5*(1), 64–83.

Donahue, M., Kazer, M. W., Smith, L., & Fitzpatrick, J. J. (2013). A geriatric family-centered care model for hospitalized elders. *American Nurse Today, 8*(4), 3 pages. Retrieved September 11, 2015. http://www.americannursetoday.com/a-geriatric-family-centered-care-model-for-hospitalized-elders/

Dong, X. (2013). Elder abuse: Research, practice, and health policy. *Gerontologist.* doi:10.1093/geront/gnt139, 1–10. http://gerontologist.oxfordjournals.org/content/early/2013/11/18/geront.gnt139.full.pdf+html

Faber, K. (2013). Relationship-based care in the neonatal intensive care unit. *Creative Nursing, 19*(4), 214–218.

Fingerman, K. L., Pillemer, K. A., Silverstein, M., & Jill Suitor, J. (2012). The baby boomers' intergenerational relationships. *Gerontologist, 52*(2), 199–209. doi: 10.1093/geront/gnr139

Fry, D. (2013). *A rising share of young adults live in their parents' home*. Washington, DC: Pew Research Center Social & Demographic Trends Project, March. http://www.pewsocialtrends.org/files/2013/07/SDT-millennials-living-with-parents-07-2013.pdf

Garfield, C. F., Lee, Y., & Kim, H. N. (2014). Paternal and maternal concerns for their very low-birth-weight infants transitioning from the NICU to home. *The Journal of Perinatal & Neonatal Nursing, 28*(4), 305–312.

Gottlieb, L. N. (2013). *Strengths-based nursing care: Health and healing for person and family*. New York, NY: Springer Publishing Co.

Granek, L., Rosenberg-Yunger, Z. R., Dix, D., Klaassen, R. J., Sung, L., Cairney, J., et al. (2014). Caregiving, single parents and cumulative stresses when caring for a child with cancer. *Child: Care, Health and Development 40*(2), 184–194. doi: 10.1111/cch.12008. Epub 2012 Nov 2.

Haslam, D., Filus, A., Morawska, A., Sanders, M. R., & Fletcher, R. (2015). The Work-Family Conflict Scale (WAFCS): Development and initial validation of a self-report measure of work-family conflict for use with parents.

Child Psychiatry & Human Development, 46(3), 346–357. doi: 10.1007/s10578-014-0476-0.

Hardaway, C. R., & Cornelius, M. D. (2014). Economic hardship and adolescent problem drinking: Family processes as mediating influences. *Journal of Youth and Adolescence, 43*(7), 1191–1202. doi: 10.1007/s10964-013-0063-x

Herber, O. R., & Johnston, B. M. (2013). The role of healthcare support workers in providing palliative and end-of-life care in the community: A systematic literature review. *Health & Social Care in the Community, 21*(3), 225–235. doi: 10.1111/j.1365-2524.2012.01092.x

Hetherington, C., Hendrickson, C., & Koenig, M. (2014). Reducing an in-group bias in preschool children: The impact of moral behavior. *Developmental Science, 17*(6), 1042–1049. doi: 10.1111/desc.12192

Hillemeier, M. M., Morgan, P. L., Farkas, G., & Maczuga, S. A. (2013). Quality disparities in child care for at-risk children: Comparing head start and non-head start settings. *Maternal and Child Health Journal, 17*(1), 180–188. doi: 10.1007/s10995-012-0961-7

Hilton, M. (2014). *Bar Mitzvah: A history*, Lincoln, NE: University of Nebraska Press

Hoffman, G. J., Lee, J., & Mendez-Luck, C. A. (2012). Health behaviors among baby boomer informal caregivers. *Gerontologist, 52*(2), 219–230. doi: 10.1093/geront/gns003

Holtslander, L., Sola, J., & Smith, N. R. (2013). The 15-minute family interview as a learning strategy for senior undergraduate nursing students. *Journal of Family Nursing, 19*(2), 230–248. doi: 10.1177/1074840712472554.

Jager, J., Yuen, C. X., Bornstein, M. H., Putnick, D. L., & Hendricks, C. (2014). The relations of family members' unique and shared perspectives of family dysfunction to dyad adjustment. *Journal of Family Psychology, 28*(3), 407–414. doi: 10.1037/a0036809.

Jensen, S. L. (2014). A valuable education: Teaching case management to tomorrow's clinicians. *Professional Case Management, 19*(4), 194–195. doi: 10.1097/NCM.0000000000000046

Kaakinen, J. R., Coehlo, D. P., Steele, R., Tabacco, A., & Hanson, S. M. (2015). *Family health care nursing: Theory, practice, and research* (5th ed.). Philadelphia, PA: F. A. Davis. ISBN-13: 978-0803639218.

Karanja, N., Aickin, M., Lutz, T., Mist, S., Jobe, J. B., Maupomé, G., et al. (2012). A community-based intervention to prevent obesity beginning at birth among American Indian Children. Study design and Rationale for the PTOTS study. *Journal of Primary Prevention, 33*(4), 161–174. doi: 10.1007/s10935-012-0278-8.

Kail, R. V., & Cavanaugh, J. C. (2013). *Human development: A life-span view* (6th ed.). Belmont, CA: Cengage Learning.

Keeton, C. P., Ginsburg, G. S., Drake, K. L., Sakolsky, D., Kendall, P. C., Birmaher, B., et al. (2013). Benefits of child-focused anxiety treatments for parents and family functioning. *Depression and Anxiety, 30*(9), 865–872. doi: 10.1002/da.22055

Kevern, P. (2012). Who can give 'spiritual care'? The management of spiritually sensitive interactions between nurses and patients. *Journal of Nursing Management, 20*(8), 981–989. doi: 10.1111/j.1365-2834.2012.01428.x

Koenig, H., King, D., & Carson, V. B. (2012). *Handbook of religion and health*. New York, NY: Oxford University Press.

Kramer, A., Nosbusch, J. M., & Rice, J. (2012). Safe mom, safe baby: A collaborative model of care for pregnant women experiencing intimate partner violence. *The Journal of Perinatal & Neonatal Nursing, 26*(4), 307–316; quiz p. 317–318. doi: 10.1097/JPN.0b013e31824356dd

Krista Lynn, M. (2012). Family structure, gender, and the work–family interface: Work-to-family conflict among single and partnered parents. *Journal of Family and Economic, 33*(1), 95–107.

Lapierre, S., Erlangsen, A., Waern, M., De Leo, D., Oyama, H., Scocco, P., et al.; International Research Group for Suicide among the Elderly. (2011). A systematic review of elderly suicide prevention programs. *Crisis, 32*(2), 88–98. doi: 10.1027/0227-5910/a000076

Lavelle, B., & Smock, P. J. (2012). Divorce and women's risk of health insurance loss. *Journal of Health and Social Behavior, 53*(4), 413–431. doi: 10.1177/0022146512465758

Law, E. F., Fisher, E., Fales, J., Noel, M., & Eccleston, C. (2014). Systematic review and meta-analysis: Parent and family-based interventions for children and adolescents with chronic medical conditions. *Journal of Pediatric Psychology, 39*(8), 866–886.

Lawn, S., Delany, T., Sweet, L., Battersby, M. C., & Skinner, T. (2013). Control in chronic condition self-care management: How it occurs in the health worker-client relationship and implications for client empowerment. *Journal of Advanced Nursing, 70*(2), 383–394.

Lee, L. A., Carter, M., Stevenson, S. B., & Harrison, H. A. (2014). Improving family-centered care practices in the NICU. *Neonatal Network, 33*(3), 125–132. doi: 10.1891/0730-0832.33.3.125.

Lemacks, J., Fowles, K., Mateus, A., and Thomas, K. (2013). Insights from parents about caring for a child with birth defects. *International Journal of Environmental Research and Public Health, 10*(8), 3465–3482. doi: 10.3390/ijerph10083465

Lereya, S. T., Samara, M., & Wolke, D. (2013). Parenting behavior and the risk of becoming a victim and a bully/victim: A meta-analysis study. *Child Abuse & Neglect, 37*(12), 1091–1108. doi: 10.1016/j.chiabu.2013.03.001

Livingston, G. (2013). *At grandmother's house we stay: One-in-ten children are living with a grandparent*. Washington, DC: PEW Research Center. http://www.pewsocialtrends.org/files/2013/09/grandparents_report_final_2013.pdf

Luhmann, M., Hofmann, W., Eid, M., & Lucas, R. E. (2012). Subjective well-being and adaptation to life events: A meta-analysis on differences between cognitive and affective well-being. *Journal of Personality and Social Psychology, 102*(3), 592–615. doi: 10.1037/a0025948

Magon, N., Chauhan, M., Malik, S., & Shah, D. (2012). Sexuality in midlife: Where the passion goes? *Journal of Midlife Health, 3*(2), 61–65. doi: 10.4103/0976-7800.104452

Mansfield, A. K., Keitner, G. I., & Dealy, J. (2014). The family assessment device: An update. *Family Process, 54*(1), 82–93. doi: 10.1111/famp.12080

McCloskey, C. R. (2012). Changing focus: women's perimenopausal journey. *Health Care for Women International, 33*(6), 540–559. doi: 10.1080/07399332.2011.610542

Melnyk, B. M., Jacobson, D., Kelly, S., Belyea, M., Shaibi, G., Small, L., et al. (2013). Promoting healthy lifestyles in high school adolescents: A randomized controlled trial. *American Journal of Preventive Medicine, 45*(4), 407–415. doi: 10.1016/j.amepre.2013.05.013

Donahue, M., Kazer, M. W., Smith, L., & Fitzpatrick, J. J. (2013). A geriatric family-centered care model for hospitalized elders. *American Nurse Today, 8*(4) http://www.americannursetoday.com/article.aspx?id=10152&fid=10122

Moyer VA; U.S. Preventive Services Task Force. (2013). Primary care interventions to prevent child maltreatment: U.S. Preventive Services Task Force recommendation statement. *Annals of Internal Medicine, 159*(4), 289–295. doi: 10.7326/0003-4819-159-4-201308200-00667

Nanni, M. G., Biancosino, B., & Grassi, L. (2014). Pre-loss symptoms related to risk of complicated grief in caregivers of terminally ill cancer patients. *Journal of Affective Disorders, 160*, 87–91. doi: 10.1016/j.jad.2013.12.023.

National Center for Elder Abuse. (2014). *The elder justice roadmap*. Washington, DC: National Center on Elder Abuse. Retrieved September 11, 2015. http://www.ncea.acl.gov/Library/Gov_Report/docs/EJRP_Roadmap_and_Appendices.pdf

Norman, R. E., Byambaa, M., De, R., Butchart, A., Scott, J., and Vos, T. (2012). The long-term health consequences of child physical abuse, emotional abuse, and neglect: A systematic review and meta-analysis. *Public Library of Science Medicine, 9*(11), e1001349. doi: 10.1371/journal.pmed.1001349

NANDA-Association International (NANDA-I). (2014). *Nursing diagnoses: Definitions and classification, 2015–2017*. West Sussex, England: Wiley-Blackwell.

Nunes, K. L., Hermann, C. A., Renee Malcom, J., & Lavoie, K. (2013). Childhood sexual victimization, pedophilic interest, and sexual recidivism. *Child Abuse & Neglect, 37*(9), 703–711. doi: 10.1016/j.chiabu.2013.01.008.

Peterson, C. C., Wellman, H. M., & Slaughter, V. (2012). The mind behind the message: Advancing theory-of-mind scales for typically developing children, and those with deafness, autism, or Asperger syndrome. *Child Development, 83*(2), 469–485. doi: 10.1111/j.1467-8624.2011.01728.x

Pfefferbaum, B, Noffsinger, M. A., & Wind, L. H. (2012). Issues in the assessment of children's coping in the context of mass trauma. *Prehospital and Disaster Medicine, 27*(3), 272–279. doi: 10.1017/S1049023X12000702

Polivka, B. J., Chaudry, R. V., & Mac Crawford, J. (2012). Home environmental hazard education for undergraduate and prelicensure nursing students. *Journal of Nursing Education, 51*(10), 577–581. doi: 10.3928/01484834-20120820-07

Rawlins, E., Baker, G., Maynard, M., & Harding, S. (2013). Perceptions of healthy eating and physical activity in an ethnically diverse sample of young children and their parents: The DEAL prevention of obesity study. *Journal of Human Nutrition and Dietetics, 26*(2), 132–144. doi: 10.1111/j.1365-277X.2012.01280.x

Rosland, A. M., Heisler, M., & Piette, J. D. (2012). The impact of family behaviors and communication patterns on chronic illness outcomes: A systematic review. *Journal of Behavioral Medicine, 35*(2), 221–239. doi: 10.1007/s10865-011-9354-4

Sanders-McDonagh. (2013). Rebuilding lives after domestic violence: Understanding long-term outcomes A Book Review of Abraham – women back into society Community, *Work & Family, 16*, Number 4, 1, 435-436(2).

Sanders-McDonagh. (2013). A book review: Rebuilding lives after domestic violence: Understanding long-term outcomes by H. Abrahams (2010). *Community, Work & Family, 16*(4), 435–436.

Sarrami-Foroushani, P., Travaglia, J., Debono, D., & Braithwaite, J. (2014). Key concepts in consumer and community engagement: A scoping meta-review. *BMC Health Services Research, 14*(1), 250.

Schappin, R., Wijnroks, L., Uniken Venema, M. M., & Jongmans, M. J. (2013). Rethinking stress in parents of preterm infants: A meta-analysis. *PLoS One, 8*(2), e54992. doi: 10.1371/journal.pone.0054992

Scott, S. B., Whitehead, B. R., Bergeman, C. S., & Pitzer, L. (2013). Combinations of stressors in midlife: Examining role and domain sressors using regression trees and random forests. *Journals of Gerontology. Series B, Psychological Sciences and Social Sciences, 68*(3), 464–475. doi: 10.1093/geronb/gbs166

Sieh, D. S., Dikkers, A. L. C., Visser-Meily, J. M. A., and Meijer, A. M. (2012). Stress in adolescents with a chronically Ill parent: Inspiration from Rolland's Family Systems-Illness Model. *Journal of Developmental and Physical Disabilities, 24*(6), 591–606. doi: 10.1007/s10882-012-9291-3

Smith, H. (2014). Giving hope to families in palliative care and implications for practice. *Nursing Children and Young People, 26*(5), 21–25. doi: 10.7748/ncyp.26.5.21.e412

Spector, R. E. (2012). *Cultural Diversity in Health and Illness* (8th ed.). Upper Saddle River, NJ: Prentice-Hall.

Stamataki, Z., Ellis, J. E., Costello, J., Fielding, J., Burns, M., & Molassiotis, A. (2014). Chronicles of informal caregiving in cancer: Using 'The Cancer Family Caregiving Experience' model as an explanatory framework. *Support Care Cancer, 22*(2), 435–444. doi: 10.1007/s00520-013-1994-1

Tanabe, M., Suzukamo, Y., Tsuji, I., & Izumi, S.-I. (2012). Communication training improves sense of performance expectancy of public health nurses engaged in long-term elderly prevention care program. *International Scholarly Research Notices Nursing, 2012*, 430560. doi: 10.5402/2012/430560

Toly, V. B., Musil, C. M., & Carl, J. C. (2012). Families with children who are technology-dependent: Normalization and family functioning. *Western Journal of Nursing Research, 34*(1), 52–71. doi: 10.1177/0193945910389623

Trindade, L. C., Linhares, S. M., Vanrell, J., Godoy, D., Martins, J. C., & Barbas, S. M. (2014). Sexual violence against children and vulnerability. *Revista Da Associacao Medica Brasileira, 60*(1), 70–74.

Tschanz, J. A. T., Piercy, K., Corcoran, C. D., Fauth, E., Norton, M. C., Rabins, P. V., et al. (2013). Caregiver coping strategies predict cognitive and functional decline in dementia: The Cache County Dementia Progression Study. *The American Journal of Geriatric Psychiatry, 21*(1), 57–66. doi: 10.1016/j.jagp.2012.10.005

U.S. Department of Health and Human Services, Administration for Children and Families, Administration on Children, Youth and Families, Children's Bureau. (2013). *Child Maltreatment 2012*. Available from http://www.acf.hhs.gov/programs/cb/research-data-technology/statistics-research/child-maltreatment and http://www.childhelp.org/pages/statistics

Vespa, J., Lewis, J. M., & Kreider, R. M. (2013). America's families and living arrangements: 2012. *Current Population Reports*, P20-570, U.S. Census Bureau, Washington, DC.

Walter, J. K., & Ross, L. F. (2014). Relational autonomy: Moving beyond the limits of isolated individualism. *Pediatrics, 133*(Suppl 1):S16–S23. doi: 10.1542/peds.2013-3608D.

Walters, M. L., Chen, J., & Breiding, M. J. (2013). *The National Intimate Partner and Sexual Violence Survey (NISVS): 2010 Findings on Victimization by Sexual Orientation.* Atlanta, GA: National Center for Injury Prevention and Control, Centers for Disease Control and Prevention.

Wasik, B. H. (2012). *Handbook of Family Literacy.* 2nd ed. New York, NY: Routledge.

Wathen, C. N., MacGregor, J. C., Hammerton, J., Coben, J. H., Herrman, H., Stewart, D. E., et al.; PreVAiL Research Network. (2012). Priorities for research in child maltreatment, intimate partner violence and resilience to violence exposures: Results of an international Delphi consensus development process. *BMC Public Health, 12,* 684, 1–12. http://www.ncbi.nlm.nih.gov/pmc/articles/PMC3490760/pdf/1471-2458-12-684.pdf

Wellings, K., Jones, K. G., Mercer, C. H., Tanton, C., Clifton, S., Datta, J., et al. (2013). The prevalence of unplanned pregnancy and associated factors in Britain: Findings from the third National Survey of Sexual Attitudes and Lifestyles (Natsal-3). *Lancet, 382*(9907), 1807–1816. doi: 10.1016/S0140-6736(13)62071-1

White, D. B., Cua, S. M., Walk, R., Pollice, L., Weissfeld, L., Hong, S., et al. (2012). Nurse-led intervention to improve surrogate decision making for patients with advanced critical illness. *American Journal of Critical Care, 21*(6), 396–409. doi: 10.4037/ajcc2012223

Whittemore, R., Sarah, J., Chao, A., Jang, M., & Grey, M. (2012). Psychological experience of parents of children with type 1 diabetes: A systematic mixed-studies review. *The Diabetes Educator, 38*(4), 562–579. doi: 10.1177/0145721712445216

Williams, A. L. (2014). Psychosocial burden of family caregivers to adults with cancer. *Recent Results in Cancer Research, 197,* 73–85. doi: 10.1007/978-3-642-40187-9_6

Williams, A. L., & Bakitas, M. (2012). Cancer family caregivers: A new direction for interventions. *Journal of Palliative Medicine, 15*(7), 775–783. doi: 10.1089/jpm.2012.0046.

Wittenberg-Lyles, E., Washington, K., Demiris, G., Oliver, D. P., & Shaunfield, S. (2014). Understanding social support burden among family caregivers. *Health Communication, 29*(9), 901–910. doi: 10.1080/10410236.2013.815111.

Workplace Flexibility 2010, Georgetown University Law Center, "Different Types of FMLA Leave". (2007). *Memos and Fact Sheets.* Paper 38. Retrieved September 11, 2015. http://scholarship.law.georgetown.edu/legal/38

Wouters, E., Masquillier, C., Ponnet, K., & le Roux Booysen, F. (2014). A peer adherence support intervention to improve the antiretroviral treatment outcomes of HIV patients in South Africa: The moderating role of family dynamics. *Social Science & Medicine, 113,* 145–153. doi: 10.1016/j.socscimed.2014.05.020

Wright, A. G., Pincus, A. L., & Lenzenweger, M. F. (2012). Interpersonal development, stability, and change in early adulthood. *Journal of Personality, 80*(5), 1339–1372. doi: 10.1111/j.1467-6494.2012.00761.x.

Wright, L. M., & Leahey, M. (2013). *Nurses and families: A guide to family assessment and intervention* (6th ed.). Philadelphia, PA: F.A. Davis.

Zauszniewski, J. A., Au, T.-Y., & Musil, C. M. (2012). Resourcefulness training for grandmothers raising grandchildren: Is there a need? *Issues in Mental Health Nursing, 33*(10), 680–686. doi: 10.3109/01612840.2012.684424

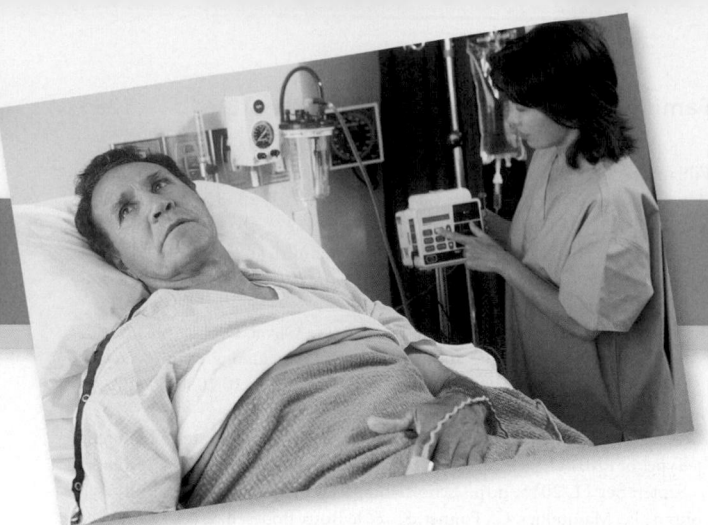

Loss and Grieving

Craig R. Sellers

Case Scenario

You are a nurse in an inpatient medical surgical unit. The patient, a middle-aged man, is admitted to your unit for evaluation, monitoring, and management following an episode of coffee-ground emesis. As you complete your admission assessment, you obtain the following data: (1) Mr. Brown, who asks you to call him "Jim," has been HIV positive for 14 years and (2) his partner, John, with whom he lived for 15 years, died of AIDS 6 months ago after numerous hospitalizations. Jim complains of abdominal pain that is "like the pain" his partner had just before his death. Jim is retired, lives by himself, has few close friends, and is estranged from his family. During the examination, he becomes tearful and states, "I don't know what is wrong with me. I just can't get myself together and do things like I used to."

Once you have completed this chapter and have incorporated loss and grieving into your knowledge base, review the above scenario and reflect on the following areas of Critical Thinking:

1. From the information provided, consider possible nursing diagnoses for this patient.
2. Identify additional information you need to make a thorough assessment of this patient and his social support system.
3. Plan actions you should take to assist this patient.
4. Examine other resources (professional and nonprofessional) that you think could be mobilized to assist this patient.
5. Propose how the patient could best use such professional and nonprofessional resources.

LEARNING OBJECTIVES

Upon completion of this chapter, you will be able to do the following:

1. Define selected terms related to loss, dying, death, and grief.
2. Identify the normal functions of grief.
3. Compare models of grief related to dying and grief related to bereavement.
4. Identify the common signs and symptoms of grief.
5. Evaluate grief reactions across the life span.
6. Identify variables that influence normal grieving.

7. Discuss the effects of multiple losses on the grief process.
8. Apply the nursing process to grieving patients.
9. Differentiate between normal and dysfunctional grieving.
10. Identify the principles of hospice and palliative care.
11. Recognize physical and emotional signs and symptoms of dying.
12. Identify nursing interventions to assist dying patients and their families.

Loss and **grief** are universal experiences that each person experiences from birth until **death**. Losses vary in importance, from insignificant losses that cause minor and brief sadness to major losses that cause intense and long-lasting distress.

Some losses are the result of normal development, whereas other losses are the result of unexpected events. Regardless of the source of the loss, grief is a necessary and normal reaction to loss: Grief is the price we pay for becoming attached to people, objects, and beliefs. Through the grief process, the person is able to change the attachment to the lost person or object and become attached to other people or objects.

NORMAL GRIEVING

Grief is the characteristic pattern of psychological and physiologic responses a person experiences after the loss of a significant person, object, belief, or relationship. Grief has several important functions:

- To make the outer reality of the loss into an internally accepted reality
- To alter the emotional attachment to the lost person or object
- To make it possible for the bereaved person to become attached to other people or objects

Characteristics of Normal Loss and Grieving

TYPES OF LOSS

Loss is defined as the experience of parting with an object, person, belief, or relationship that one values; the loss requires a reorganization of one or more aspects of the person's life. Losses range from minor ones, which necessitate only minor adjustments, to major ones, which necessitate major adaptations.

Losses are part of the normal developmental cycle. At birth, the newborn loses the warmth and security of the mother's womb. Later, the infant loses the comfort and gratification of the mother's breast. When a sibling is born, the child loses his or her place as the youngest in the family. Each loss has both negative and positive aspects. For example, by no longer being the youngest in the family, the child gains certain rights

and responsibilities, but the child also loses the family's undivided attention and the special benefits attached to being the youngest.

A material loss is a loss of some tangible object or possession; a psychological loss is a loss of something that has no physical form but has some important symbolic meaning. Many losses have both material and psychological components. For example, loss of a job results in the material loss of income, but it also may result in numerous psychological losses, such as loss of status, self-esteem, relationships with coworkers, and meaning for living.

An *expected* loss occurs with forewarning, whereas an *unexpected* loss occurs without warning. When a loss is expected, as in the case of terminal illness, survivors have time to prepare for it; thus, the distress associated with the loss may, but not always, be decreased. In contrast, when a loss is unexpected, individuals have no time to prepare and are at risk to experience greater distress. When a family member has a terminal illness, the survivors may have time to express their love, make amends, and make legal and financial arrangements. This is impossible when an unexpected loss occurs, such as a sudden death from an accident or acute myocardial infarction.

TERMS RELATED TO GRIEVING

Grief is person centered and encompasses the entire range of physical, psychological, cognitive, and behavioral responses to a loss. Grief comes from the Middle English and French words for *heavy* or *grave*.

Bereavement, which comes from the old English word for *bereft*, meaning "to take away or be deprived of," is a state of desolation that occurs as the result of a loss, particularly the death of a significant other. Bereavement manifestations are the person's total response to a loss and include emotional, physical, social, and cognitive responses.

Mourning encompasses the socially prescribed behaviors after the death of a significant other. Such behaviors may vary significantly from culture to culture. Mourning behaviors are socially conventional bereavement behaviors and do not necessarily indicate the presence or absence of grief. The word *mourning* comes from a Greek word meaning "to care," which aptly describes mourning, as it encompasses the outward and social expressions of loss.

TABLE 40-1 MODELS OF GRIEF

Engel's Model	Parkes's Model	Demi's Grief Cycle Model	Kübler-Ross's Stages of Dying
1. Shock and disbelief	1. Numbness	1. Shock	1. Denial
2. Developing awareness	2. Yearning	2. Protest	2. Anger
3. Restitution	3. Disorganization	3. Disorganization	3. Bargaining
4. Resolving the loss	4. Reorganization	4. Reorganization	4. Depression
5. Idealization			5. Acceptance
6. Outcome			

Anticipatory grief is the characteristic pattern of psychological and physiologic responses a person makes to the impending loss (real or imagined) of a significant person, object, belief, or relationship (Potter & Wynne, 2015). It is generally believed that anticipatory grief facilitates coping with loss when the loss actually occurs.

MODELS OF GRIEVING

Many researchers and theorists have attempted to describe the characteristics of the normal grief process. Some have proposed stage models of grief, others task models, and still others models including subconcepts, such as bereavement guilt. Although these models and concepts are useful in guiding nursing care of patients who are experiencing loss, remember that there are no clear-cut stages of grief, nor are there any exact timetables. Expecting all patients to conform to a specific model is both inappropriate and unrealistic. Table 40-1 outlines several models of grief, which are discussed in the following paragraphs. In addition, Kübler-Ross's (1969) theory of the stages of grief is discussed in more depth later in this chapter.

Two popular stage models of grief are those proposed by Engel (1964) and by Parkes (1986). A third model (Fig. 40-1) is the Grief Cycle Model (Demi, 1981), which was derived from Parkes's theory of grief. It can be used to guide practice with bereaved patients and (with minor modifications) with people who have experienced other types of loss. Hogan (2002) proposed a fourth model, the Grief to Personal Growth Model.

Engel's Model

Engel (1964), one of the first to study grief, proposed six phases of grief: (a) shock and disbelief, (b) developing awareness, (c) restitution, (d) resolving the loss, (e) idealization, and (f) outcome. In the shock and disbelief stage, the survivor either refuses to accept the loss or shows intellectual acceptance of the loss but denies the emotional impact. Developing awareness occurs as the reality and meaning of the loss penetrate the person's consciousness. The numbness of the first phase is replaced with feelings of intense psychological pain, often expressed through crying and anger. The next phase, restitution, consists of the work of mourning and includes the various funeral and religious rituals. The fourth phase, resolving the loss, occurs intrapsychically as the grieving person focuses energy on thoughts of the deceased. In the phase of idealization, first, all negative feelings toward the deceased are repressed; then, through identification, the survivor incorporates certain

characteristics of the deceased into his or her own personality. Gradually, the grieving person's psychological dependence on the deceased diminishes, and his or her interest in new relationships returns. This is the final phase. According to Engel, the resolution of grief takes 1 year or longer.

Parkes's Model

Parkes (1986) proposed four stages of grief: (a) numbness, (b) yearning, (c) disorganization, and (d) reorganization. In the numbness stage, which is usually brief, trauma so overwhelms the bereaved survivor that he or she must use denial as a psychological defense. The next stage, yearning, usually lasts several months and is characterized by intense psychological distress, with thoughts focusing on the deceased. The disorganization stage is characterized by severe depression, social withdrawal, and lack of interest in people and activities. The last stage, reorganization, usually begins 6 to 9 months after

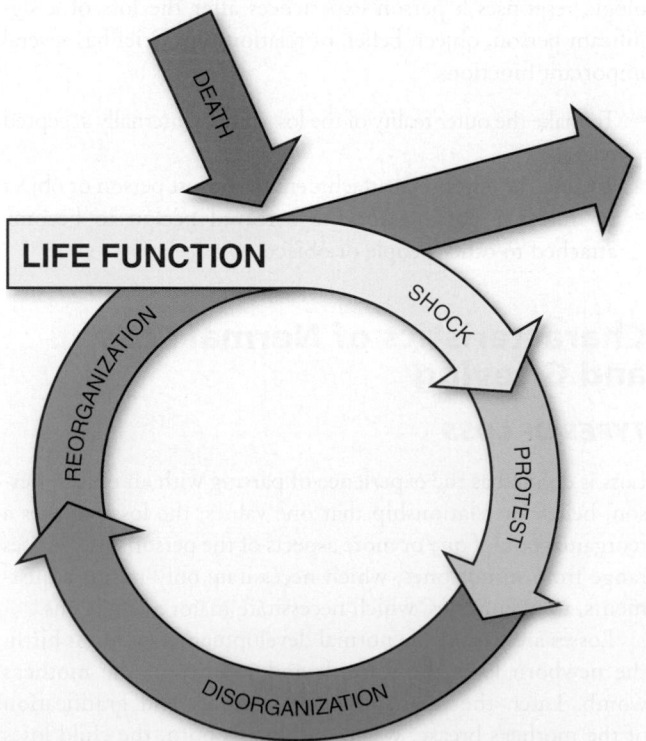

FIGURE 40-1 Grief wheel. (*From:* Demi, A. (1981). *Bereavement support group: Leadership manual.* Littleton, CO: Grief Education Institute.)

TABLE 40-2 MAJOR FUNCTIONAL MANIFESTATIONS DURING GRIEF

| | Stages/Phases of Grief | | | |
Realm	Shock	Protest	Disorganization	Reorganization
Cognitive	Slowed and disorganized thinking Blocking of thoughts Wish to join deceased Thoughts of suicide Denial of the loss and its significance	Preoccupation with thoughts of deceased Searching for deceased Dreams/nightmares Hallucinations Concerns about others' health and safety Continued death wishes	Difficulty making decisions Aimlessness Loss of interest in people, work, usual activities Perception of life as meaningless Focus on memories and reminders of deceased	Realistic memory of deceased Comfortable when remembering deceased Return to previous level of ability
Emotional	Blocking of emotions Emotional outbursts May appear unaffected Emotionally numb Feeling of unreality	Sadness Anger Guilt Relief Anxiety Yearning for deceased Feel deceased's presence	Depression Loneliness Meaninglessness Decreased self-esteem Apathy	Feels life has meaning Able to experience pleasure
Physical	Feels physically numb Hyperactive/underactive, immobile	Pain in heart Sleep or appetite problems Weight loss Neglect of appearance Fatigue Lethargy Poor hygiene	Continued sleep and appetite problems Restlessness Decreased sexual interest/satisfaction Aimless activity Decreased resistance to illness Accident prone Increased alcohol intake Increased drug use Increased tobacco use	Renewed vigor Restoration to previous level of health Improved health habits Sexual drive renewed
Social	Passive Unaware of others	Depends on others Seeks help and advice of others	Loss of interest in people and work	New or renewed social relationships New or renewed activities Development of close relationship with at least one person

the loss and is characterized by a gradual renewal of interest in people and activities and return of a sense of meaning in life. Parkes proposed that progression through the stages of grief normally takes 2 years or longer.

Grief Cycle Model

The grief cycle model (Demi, 1981) assumes that before a major loss, the person is functioning on a relatively unchanging level. Table 40-2 describes the manifestations of each stage of the grief cycle model: shock, protest, disorganization, and reorganization.

When a loss occurs, the first reaction is shock and a drop to a lower level of functioning. This stage may last several hours to several days. The second stage of grief, protest, usually starts during the first week after the loss and continues through the 3rd month. The person continues to drop in his or her level of functioning. Intense physical and psychological distress marks this period. The disorganization stage starts around the 3rd month and continues for 3 to 6 months. The person sinks to the lowest level of functioning. Feelings of depression and social withdrawal characterize this stage. The reorganization

stage starts at approximately the 6th month and usually continues for at least 1 year, but it may continue for a much longer period. People who have sufficient resources during this period are likely to continue to improve their level of functioning and often emerge from the grief cycle at a higher level of functioning than before the loss. Others with more stressors and fewer resources may be unable to recover fully from the grief experience and therefore function at a lower level than before the loss.

In reality, these stages are not as discrete as the grief cycle model indicates. However, it is helpful to use the model as a general guide, while keeping in mind that people may vary greatly in their responses to loss and still fall within the normal response range. Grieving persons may go through the stages at varying rates, go back and forth between stages, or skip stages.

Grief to Personal Growth Model

Hogan (2002), in the grief to personal growth model, proposes that there are two pathways of grief: the *grief to growth* pathway and the *mired in grief* pathway. She further proposes that social support can help the bereaved person move out of his or her distress into personal growth.

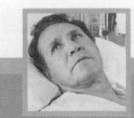

Loss and Grieving PICO

The patient in the chapter-opening scenario returns to his primary care clinic. All the diagnostic tests and blood work have come back negative. The nurse practitioner (NP) tells the patient that his symptoms are somatic and may be related to his depression. The patient is not interested in taking prescribed antidepressants and wants to know if something like St. John's wort will work better. The NP looks for evidence in the Cochrane library. He uses the following PICO question for his search: In adults, how does St. John's wort compare to antidepressants to help relieve somatoform disorders?"

P = Adults
I = St. John's Wort
C = Antidepressants
O = Relieve somatoform disorders

The NP finds a recent meta-analysis that looked at natural products and antidepressants for somatoform disorder. The authors reviewed 26 randomized control trials involving 2,159 participants. The studies included various tricyclic antidepressants, new-generation antidepressants such as serotonin reuptake inhibitors, serotonin and noradrenaline reuptake inhibitors, antipsychotics, and natural products (e.g., *St. John's wort*). The natural products were only compared to placebos (not to antidepressants). The evidence seems to indicate that the severity and intensity of medically unexplained physical symptoms that manifest from somatoform disorders can decrease with St. John's wort. However, the authors do note these are low-quality studies with high risk to bias. The NP shared his finding with his patient who decided to give St. John's wort a try. The provider also gave names of counselors and therapists to help the patient work through his grief.

REFERENCE

Kleinstäuber, M., Witthöft, M., Steffanowski, A., van Marwijk, H., Hiller, W., & Lambert, M. J. (2014). Pharmacological interventions for somatoform disorders in adults. *Cochrane Database of Systematic Reviews*, Issue 11. Art. No.: CD010628. doi: 10.1002/14651858.CD010628.pub2.

Life Span Considerations

The person's developmental stage must be considered when assessing reactions to loss and planning interventions. The impact of a traumatic event and the person's reaction to it depend on the individual's developmental stage at the time the traumatic event occurs. For example, Blank and Werner-Lin (2011) discuss how loss of a parent in early childhood often cannot be resolved until the child reaches adulthood. Shapiro's (1994) classic work on grief as a "family process" is an excellent resource.

NEWBORN AND INFANT

Newborns have no concept of life and death (Favazza & Munson, 2010). Growing infants have the ability to sense alterations in existence during cycles of wakefulness and sleep, which can be likened to a beginning understanding of the states of "being" and "nonbeing." The infant's concept of death or loss is related to feelings of separation anxiety when the parent or other caregiver is out of sight. The game of "peekaboo" introduces children to the death-related concepts of absence and presence. The child's delighted reaction to the other person's reappearance in the peekaboo game is the result of relief from the terror of separation.

TODDLER AND PRESCHOOLER

Cognitive powers are evidenced by 18 to 24 months and intensify the toddler's experience of separation anxiety. The developmental task of toddlers is to gain a sense of autonomy. Achievement of this task helps toddlers break the tie with their mother or other primary caregiver, who can now be out of sight for some time without the toddler being overly anxious. However, because toddlers vacillate between independence and attachment, such separations still cause them to fear abandonment by the primary caregiver (Favazza & Munson, 2010).

Preschoolers perceive death as reversible, avoidable, and occurring in degrees. They develop an increasing awareness of themselves as separate physical and emotional beings. With this deepening awareness of self comes the vague realization that one may cease to exist. Although preschoolers sense their own vulnerability and begin to make the distinction between being alive and being dead, they still cannot grasp death's universality, inevitability, and finality. Preschoolers develop their concept of death from their experiences in real life and the depictions of death in books and the media. On television, animals and people die only to pop up again live in the same program, or on another program, reinforcing the perception that death is reversible. Preschoolers think of death as a long sleep. The death of a pet or a family member plays an important part in a child's development of a concept of death, although the preschooler's cognitive ability does not yet allow a clear understanding.

SCHOOL-AGE CHILD AND ADOLESCENT

In the early school years, the child perceives death as unnatural, reversible, and avoidable; the child may also personify death (e.g., perceive *death* to be a person or an animal). At about 9 years of age, the child's concept of death matures, and the child perceives death realistically as irreversible, universal, inevitable, and natural.

Society reinforces concepts of life and death. By school age, children usually have been touched by death in some way (e.g., family member, classmate, friend's family member, pet, news story). Some children live in violent neighborhoods where death is common. The modern school curriculum includes discussions about deaths and traumatic events that are prominent in the news or that occur locally. Religious institutions teach diverse beliefs about death and about life after death. The school-age child gradually realizes that death is an event no one escapes.

As age increases, the child's understanding of death becomes more realistic. A high level of cognitive development allows the adolescent to view life and death with an adult understanding. Adolescents begin to develop a philosophy of life and death. Nevertheless, the thought of one's own death is overwhelming and consequently is suppressed. Adolescents are already in the midst of a developmental crisis during which they experience constant change. Adolescents generally have the capacity to mourn fully, but they are at greater risk for poorer outcomes than are adults because of the numerous other stressors and developmental changes they are experiencing during this stage of the life cycle.

ADULT AND OLDER ADULT

In contrast to children, adults tend to grieve more intensely and more continuously but for a relatively shorter period of time. Furthermore, adults usually do not seek an immediate replacement for the lost loved person but rather may move toward this after achieving some resolution of their grief.

Young adults often experience many losses within a short period of time, which places them particularly at risk for poor outcomes. They may experience the death of a family member, the ending of their schooling and consequent separation from peers, broken relationships, or failure in their attempt to achieve a satisfying job. These multiple losses, coupled with their inexperience with loss and grief, make them particularly at risk.

Middle-aged adults who have a relatively stable lifestyle and adequate support systems usually cope well with loss; however, an untimely loss, such as the death of a child or the death of a spouse, may be extremely stressful because it is perceived as out of the normal sequence of events. When children move away from home (the "empty nest syndrome"), middle-aged adults may also face challenges in coping.

Older adults are also at risk for challenges associated with loss. They may be faced with retirement, loss of regular income, death of a spouse and also of peers and other relatives, and moving into more manageable living arrangements versus remaining in the home where they raised their family. As some older adults age, they may grieve the losses associated with functional and cognitive decline. In addition, many may be forced by circumstances to move into assisted living or long-term care situations, due to loss of their ability to remain independent. Older adults with dementia may also have altered coping with loss due to their cognitive dysfunction and warrant individualized intervention from caregivers (Johansson & Grimby, 2013).

Older adults often experience numerous losses, sequentially or simultaneously; therefore, they are at higher risk than other adults for poor outcomes after major losses. At a time when their stressors are highest, their resources are often the most meager. Deaths of relatives and friends, retirement, impaired health of self or family members, and decreased economic resources are all common stressors for the older adult. Fewer support networks are available to older adults because of deaths and illnesses of family and friends. Therefore, they may need to rely more heavily on healthcare providers to assist them in coping with their losses.

Cultural Considerations

It is critical for the nurse to understand that *how* individuals who are **dying** and their families react to their losses and grieving is largely impacted by cultural beliefs and traditions. Recall that *mourning* is mostly a cultural phenomenon. Nurses are encouraged to develop an understanding of the typical cultures and religious practices with whom they often come in contact. Before they can do that, however, they must thoughtfully reflect on their own beliefs and traditions in order to avoid imposing their personal beliefs and practices on patients and families who may not want them.

Matzo and colleagues (2002) identified three primary themes related to culturally sensitive care of people experiencing loss and grief: (a) various factors including, but not limited to, race and ethnicity, gender, sexual orientation, differing abilities, religious and spiritual beliefs, and social class are relevant; (b) communicating with patients and their families is strongly affected by culture; and (c) the best care is provided by working with an interdisciplinary team. Many resources for learning about other cultures and how they impact the grief process are available both in print as well as via the Internet. In addition, an excellent source for developing enhanced cultural awareness and understanding can be found by simply being inquisitive and showing patients and their families that the nurse is interested in understanding them more fully. An important caveat, however, is to not fall into the trap of confusing cultural stereotypes with expected, anticipated, or actual behavior of individuals who are all unique, despite any cultural heritage they may claim. Additional information is widely available (D'Avanzo, 2008; Dayer-Berenson, 2011; National Cancer Institute, 2014).

THERAPEUTIC DIALOGUE: LOSS AND GRIEVING

SCENE FOR THOUGHT

Maureen O'Hagan, 48 years old, had a simple mastectomy 2 months ago. She is married with two grown children and runs her own business. She is returning to the clinic for a check of her operative site. The nurse notes that she looks pale and tired, although she is dressed well and is wearing makeup.

LESS EFFECTIVE

Nurse: Hi, Ms. O'Hagan, I'm Natalie, one of the office nurses. How are you doing?

Maureen: Okay, I guess.

Nurse: Good! Any pain in the incision or in the muscles underneath? (*Patient shakes head no.*) How about your general health? Any problems there? (*Looks at patient and chart.*)

Maureen: Well, I haven't been eating or sleeping too well since the operation. (*Looks down at her hands.*)

Nurse: Really? Your lab work looks good. I wonder what the problem is. Do you have any ideas?

Maureen: Not really.

Nurse: Well, let me see about getting you some sleep medication to relax you. Getting enough sleep usually makes people feel better right away. Okay? (*Writes in chart and leaves the room. Ms. O'Hagan sighs.*)

MORE EFFECTIVE

Nurse: Hi, Ms. O'Hagan. I'm Rosalie Smith, your Registered Nurse. I'm going to check your mastectomy site today and see how you're doing in general.

Maureen: Fine. (*Gives a small smile to be polite.*)

Nurse: So, how are you doing? (*Shows concern; uses good eye contact.*)

Maureen: I … I'm not too sure, actually. I have no pain, the arm feels fine, the scar is okay, but I don't seem to be back to normal yet. My husband is beginning to complain about our not having sex like we used to. I don't get it. (*Looks confused, annoyed, and depressed.*)

Nurse: I'm checking your chart and all your blood work is fine. How have you been eating and sleeping? (*Assessment of the physical signs of grief.*)

Maureen: Not too well. I can't get to sleep very easily and then I wake up in the middle of the night with dreams I can't remember. And I have no appetite.

Nurse: It sounds like you've been going through a difficult time. You're having trouble with sleep, disturbing dreams, fatigue, appetite loss, decreased sex drive, and not feeling like yourself. Is there anything else you want to add? (*Summarizes, asks open-ended question.*)

Maureen: Uh, well, yes, but it's stupid. (*Looks embarrassed.*)

Nurse: Oh? (*Continues with good eye contact and interested posture.*)

Maureen: I, ah, thought about driving into a wall one day last week. Quickly. I would never do it, but I got worried when I thought about that. Besides, what does it have to do with feeling tired and everything else?

Nurse: I think you haven't finished grieving for the loss of your breast. (*Says gently.*)

Maureen: (*After a short silence.*) Oh. So, you think I'm depressed? And that I haven't accepted that the breast is gone?

Nurse: Let's talk some more about it. I know some ways to help you feel better. Would that be okay?

Maureen: Well, maybe. I'm willing to try.

CRITICAL THINKING CHALLENGE

- Compare and contrast the signs that Natalie missed to which Rosalie paid attention.
- Propose the stage of grief Maureen might be in. Give your reason.
- Analyze Maureen's potential support systems.
- Specify other assessment factors to consider.
- Select interventions you would use if you were Rosalie.

FACTORS AFFECTING GRIEVING

Many factors influence the grieving process, including the meaning of the loss to the individual, the circumstances of the loss, personal resources and stressors, and sociocultural resources and stressors (Field & Filanosky, 2010).

Meaning of the Loss

People have a tendency to ascribe their own values to others and therefore incorrectly assume that a specific loss is or is not traumatic to a specific person without first assessing the meaning of the loss to that person. Loss of a finger would have very different meanings to a classical guitarist and a manual laborer. Divorce may be extremely undesired and cause intense grief in one person, whereas it may be welcomed and a cause for rejoicing in another. The age at which a loss occurs has a major impact: The loss of a parent has different meanings to an infant, a child, and an adult (see the "Life Span Considerations" section).

Circumstances of the Loss

Whether a loss is expected or unexpected, violent or peaceful, timely or untimely, natural or unnatural, it affects the grief process. A loss that occurs under violent or frightening conditions is much more difficult to cope with than is a loss that occurs under more peaceful conditions. A death that occurs as a result of homicide or suicide is usually more stressful than is a death from natural causes. The perception that one in some way caused or contributed to the loss increases the grieving person's distress, such as when loss of function in an auto accident is caused by one's own carelessness. Loss of the ability to conceive a child may be stressful if it is untimely (occurs at a young age), but in middle age, it is timely and therefore may not be stressful.

Religious or Spiritual Beliefs and Loss

An individual's faith (religious) or spiritual beliefs may affect the grief process. Some people find strength in dealing with loss through their faith, whereas others experience greater distress due to their beliefs. Some people believe that death is the end; others believe that death is the beginning of a life in heaven or hell, and still others believe in reincarnation in another form. Some may think that their loss is a punishment for past sins. Other individuals may declare no specific religious or spiritual beliefs. Nurses should gain knowledge of the specific religious or spiritual beliefs of the patients they are serving and help their patients deal with loss in a manner that is congruent with those beliefs and practices of theirs. Nurses must hold a nonjudgmental stance with regard to others' faith or spiritual beliefs, as well as lack of such beliefs.

Personal Resources and Stressors

Each person enters a loss situation with a unique combination of personal resources and stressors. What is a resource for one person may be a stressor for another. For example, health status may be either a resource or a stressor: The person who has good health habits, various coping strategies, and a generally high level of wellness has a major advantage over the person who has poor health habits, limited coping skills, a chronic or acute illness, and a history of emotional instability.

Personal resources and stressors that influence response to a loss include coping skills, previous experiences with loss, emotional stability, spiritual beliefs, physical health, individual developmental stage, family developmental stage, other concurrent stressors, and socioeconomic status (Choi & Jun, 2009). Research indicates that socioeconomic status is one of the major factors related to ability to cope with loss. People with higher levels of education, higher income, and higher job status tend to have better outcomes after a major loss.

Sociocultural Resources and Stressors

Sociocultural resources include the social support (Lin, Simeone, Ensel, & Kuo, 1979) that is available from family, friends, coworkers, and formal institutions. Absence of these social supports creates additional stressors for the grieving person. Sometimes these supports can also be stressors, particularly if the resource people are not able to empathize with the grieving person. Further, if a community is able to deal with loss and has reasonable expectations of the survivors, this reduces stress; however, if the community tends to blame the survivors for their plight (as sometimes happens in the case of AIDS), or if the community has unrealistic expectations, the grieving person will have much more difficulty coping with the loss.

ALTERED GRIEVING

Dysfunctional grief is grief that falls outside the normal response range and may be manifested as exaggerated grief, prolonged grief, or absence of grief (Maccallum & Bryant, 2013; Stroebe, Hansson, Schut, & Stroebe, 2008). In dysfunctional grief, the grieving person often becomes stuck in one stage of the grief process and is unable to progress to the next stage or stages. Furthermore, the grieving person expends so much energy either repressing the grief or dealing ineffectively with the grief that little time or energy is left to invest in normal growth and development.

Manifestations of Altered Grieving

In a classic study of bereavement experts' perceptions of "grief that falls outside normal parameters," Demi and Miles (1987) found that more than 30 different terms were commonly used to label dysfunctional grief. The most commonly accepted

BOX 40-1   **Normal and Abnormal Grief Manifestations**

May Be Normal at 1 Year after Bereavement

- Excessive or persistent expression of affect
- Inability to experience joy
- Clinical symptoms of depression
- Inability to form new relationships
- Inability to speak of the deceased without intense emotion
- Hearing or seeing the deceased
- Feelings of emptiness or meaninglessness

Abnormal if Present beyond 3 Years

- Leaving the deceased's room and belongings intact
- Reporting physical symptoms similar to those the deceased had before death
- Talking about the loss as if it had just happened
- Inability to remember or talk about the deceased
- Being preoccupied with thoughts of the deceased
- Talking or acting as if the deceased were still alive
- Experiencing physical illness that seems to be related to the loss

terms were *pathologic grief, unresolved grief, dysfunctional grief,* and *prolonged grief.* Many symptoms that had been considered abnormal or dysfunctional were identified as components of the normal grief process. At 1 year after bereavement, most experts believed that the grief manifestations listed in Box 40-1 were within normal parameters.

Bereavement experts reported that they considered almost all bereavement manifestations to be normal during the early stages of grief but considered most of the manifestations to be abnormal if they continued beyond 3 years after bereavement (Demi & Miles, 1987). Symptoms considered abnormal if present beyond 3 years are also listed in Box 40-1.

Recall the patient from the case scenario at the beginning of the chapter. Use the concept map (Fig. 40-2) to help manage and understand the patient's grief.

ASSESSMENT

Questions about losses (actual and anticipated) need to be incorporated into the assessment of every patient. Frank physical illness may be the result of a loss, actual or anticipated; often, the patient does not connect the presenting symptom with the loss. On the other hand, physical illness or accident may result in loss, both actual and anticipated. The skillful nurse recognizes the relationship of loss to health status and helps the patient recognize and acknowledge this connection.

Normal Pattern Identification

Many behaviors previously thought to be dysfunctional are being recognized as normal components of grief. Observation

and assessment of a grieving person at a single point in time is not a good way to assess the normality of the grief response. To distinguish between normal and altered grief reactions, one must assess the severity of the symptoms and the pattern of change over time. *Establishing rapport is an essential communication activity.*

It is helpful to start the interview with the patient with broad, general, nonthreatening questions before asking specific, potentially emotion-laden questions about the loss; this is known as the laddered interviewing technique (Price, 2002). A major factor in understanding the patient's loss reaction is assessing the relationship to the lost person or object and the particular circumstances surrounding the loss. Important considerations include the following:

- What was the physical and psychological significance of the lost person or object?
- Was the loss unexpected or expected?
- Did the survivor contribute, or perceive that he or she contributed, to the loss?

Assessment of the patient's personal resources and personal stressors is essential. Personal resources are strengths within the person that contribute to a healthy pattern of grieving. Personal stressors are limitations within the person that may inhibit healthy grieving. Personal stressors and resources include personality characteristics, coping skills, communication skills, physical health status, spirituality, and previous experiences with loss. To assess personal stressors and resources, ask the following:

- How do you usually cope with stress?
- How well do you communicate with others?
- What previous losses have you experienced?
- How did you cope with the previous losses?
- Are any of those previous losses still unresolved?
- Do you have any physical health problems?
- Do you have a history of emotional illness or mental health concerns?
- Do you have spiritual beliefs? If so, what are they?
- Do you follow a particular faith (religious) tradition?
- Are your spiritual/faith beliefs helpful or unhelpful to you in coping with your loss?
- What other personal stressors are you experiencing?

Also assess sociocultural resources and stressors. Sociocultural resources are the assets that are available to the patient from the interpersonal environment; they include social support, material support (financial assistance, assistance with tasks), and cultural traditions and customs. Sociocultural stressors are strains and tensions that the social and cultural systems exert on the patient. Family members, peers, friends, coworkers, and employers can function as either resources or stressors. Cultural traditions also may be either resources or stressors. For example, if the cultural tradition dictates a long mourning period and the bereaved person is ready to move into the reorganization stage of grief, this may create feelings of conflict. However, it is more likely that sociocultural

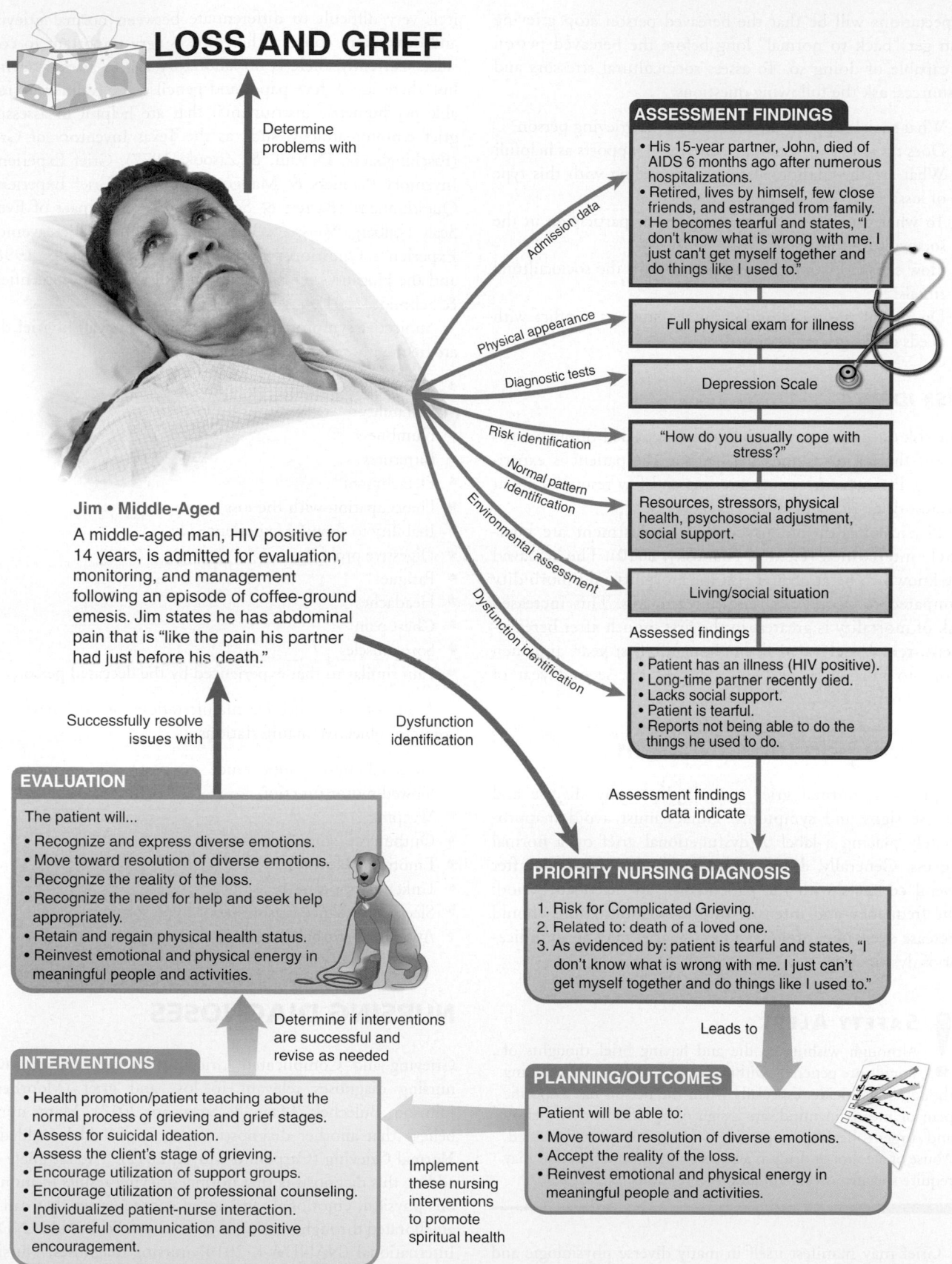

LOSS AND GRIEF

Determine problems with

Jim • Middle-Aged

A middle-aged man, HIV positive for 14 years, is admitted for evaluation, monitoring, and management following an episode of coffee-ground emesis. Jim states he has abdominal pain that is "like the pain his partner had just before his death."

Admission data

Physical appearance

Diagnostic tests

Risk identification

Normal pattern identification

Environmental assessment

Dysfunction identification

ASSESSMENT FINDINGS

• His 15-year partner, John, died of AIDS 6 months ago after numerous hospitalizations.
• Retired, lives by himself, few close friends, and estranged from family.
• He becomes tearful and states, "I don't know what is wrong with me. I just can't get myself together and do things like I used to."

Full physical exam for illness

Depression Scale

"How do you usually cope with stress?"

Resources, stressors, physical health, psychosocial adjustment, social support.

Living/social situation

Assessed findings

• Patient has an illness (HIV positive).
• Long-time partner recently died.
• Lacks social support.
• Patient is tearful.
• Reports not being able to do the things he used to do.

Assessment findings data indicate

Dysfunction identification

PRIORITY NURSING DIAGNOSIS

1. Risk for Complicated Grieving.
2. Related to: death of a loved one.
3. As evidenced by: patient is tearful and states, "I don't know what is wrong with me. I just can't get myself together and do things like I used to."

Leads to

Successfully resolve issues with

EVALUATION

The patient will...

• Recognize and express diverse emotions.
• Move toward resolution of diverse emotions.
• Recognize the reality of the loss.
• Recognize the need for help and seek help appropriately.
• Retain and regain physical health status.
• Reinvest emotional and physical energy in meaningful people and activities.

Determine if interventions are successful and revise as needed

INTERVENTIONS

• Health promotion/patient teaching about the normal process of grieving and grief stages.
• Assess for suicidal ideation.
• Assess the client's stage of grieving.
• Encourage utilization of support groups.
• Encourage utilization of professional counseling.
• Individualized patient-nurse interaction.
• Use careful communication and positive encouragement.

Implement these nursing interventions to promote spiritual health

PLANNING/OUTCOMES

Patient will be able to:

• Move toward resolution of diverse emotions.
• Accept the reality of the loss.
• Reinvest emotional and physical energy in meaningful people and activities.

FIGURE 40-2 Loss and grieving concept map.

expectations will be that the bereaved person stop grieving and get "back to normal" long before the bereaved person is capable of doing so. To assess sociocultural stressors and resources, ask the following questions:

- What social supports are available to the grieving person?
- Does the grieving person perceive these supports as helpful?
- What are the traditional rituals for dealing with this type of loss?
- To what extent did the grieving person participate in the sociocultural rituals?
- How satisfied is the grieving person with the sociocultural rituals?
- Do any of the social and cultural traditions conflict with needs of the grieving person?

RISK IDENTIFICATION

The risk of dysfunctional grief can be identified through analysis of the resources and stressors that the patient is experiencing. Patients with many stressors and few resources are at greatest risk.

Physical health and psychosocial adjustment are intricately intertwined (Field & Filanosky, 2010). The bereaved are known to be at greater risk for mortality and morbidity compared to people who are not grieving. This increased risk of mortality is greatest in the first month after bereavement, remains elevated throughout the first year, and then drops to normal range by the end of the second year of bereavement.

Dysfunction Identification

People with normal grief may display many diverse and intense signs and symptoms. Nurses must avoid inappropriately placing a label of dysfunctional grief on a normal process. Generally, dysfunction can be identified only after several contacts with the patient over an extended period. The frequency and intensity of grief manifestations should decrease over time; prolonged intense grief may be an indicator of dysfunction.

> ### ❗ SAFETY ALERT
> Although wishing to die and having brief thoughts of suicide are generally within the normal range, continuing thoughts of suicide, especially when the person has a specific plan or means in mind, are a sign of significant dysfunction and urgent healthcare provider intervention is warranted. Abuse of alcohol or drugs is also a sign of dysfunction that may require specific assessment and intervention.

Grief may manifest itself in many diverse physiologic and psychological signs that are directly observable. Many of these signs are identical to the signs of depression; consequently,

it is very difficult to differentiate between normal grieving and depression; context, therefore, is very important to consider. Currently, there is no laboratory test to assess grieving, but there are a few paper-and-pencil tests (valid and reliable psychometric instruments) that are helpful in assessing grief symptomatology, such as the Texas Inventory of Grief (Faschingbauer, DeVaul, & Zisook, 1977), Grief Experience Inventory (Sanders & Mauger, 1979), the Grief Experience Questionnaire (Barrett & Scott, 1989), the Impact of Event Scale (Zilberg, Weiss, & Horowitz, 1982), the Bereavement Experience Questionnaire (Guarnaccia & Hayslip, 1998), and the Hogan Grief Reaction Checklist (Hogan, Greenfield, & Schmidt, 2001).

Subjective symptoms (emotional and physical) of grief that are frequently reported include:

- Sadness
- Irritability
- Numbness
- Bitterness
- Detachment
- Preoccupation with the loss
- Inability to show or experience joy
- Digestive problems
- Fatigue
- Headaches
- Chest pain
- Sore muscles
- Pain similar to that experienced by the deceased person

Many of the subjective manifestations of grief have concomitant objective manifestations:

- Dejected physical appearance
- Slowed motor function
- Weeping
- Outbursts of anger
- Emotional blunting
- Unkempt appearance
- Sleep disturbance (insomnia or hypersomnia)
- Appetite disturbance (excessive weight loss or gain)

NURSING DIAGNOSES

Grieving and Complicated Grieving are the two approved nursing diagnoses relevant to loss and grief (Moorhead, Johnson, Bulechek, Maas, & Swanson, 2013). Many nurses believe that another diagnostic category should be added—Normal Grieving (Carpenito-Moyet, 2012). The rationale for adding this diagnosis is that normal grieving results in numerous physical, emotional, and social consequences that can be ameliorated through nursing interventions. Selected NANDA-International (NANDA-I, 2014) nursing diagnoses, Nursing Outcomes Classification (NOC), and Nursing Interventions Classifications (NIC) are presented in Table 40-3.

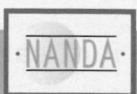

Table 40-3 SELECTED NANDA-I NURSING DIAGNOSES INVOLVING GRIEF AND LOSS				
Nursing Dx	Related Factors	Dx Statement	NOC*	NIC†
Grieving—a normal complex process that includes emotional, physical, spiritual, social, and intellectual responses and behaviors by which individuals, families, and communities incorporate an actual, anticipated, or perceived loss into their daily lives.	Anticipatory loss of significant object; expression of distress at potential loss; denial of potential loss; guilt, anger, or sorrow; changes in eating habits; alterations in sleep patterns or in activity level; despair; and disorganization	Grieving R/T loss of significant person AEB denial of loss; expression of guilt or expression of unresolved issues; anger, sadness, or crying; difficulty in expressing loss; alterations in eating habits and sleep patterns	Acceptance: Health Status Coping Family Coping Psychosocial Adjustment: Life Change	Identify the loss and the nature of attachment Active Listening Anxiety Reduction Coping Enhancement Counseling Crisis Interaction Emotional Support Family Involvement Promotion Family Support Grief Work Facilitation Spiritual Growth Facilitation
Complicated Grieving—a disorder that occurs after the death of a significant other in which the experience of distress accompanying bereavement fails to follow normative expectations and manifests in functional impairment.	Differentiating grieving from complicated grieving requires consideration of the interval between the time of loss and the time of assessment. To be considered complicated, the grief must be unusually prolonged and turbulent. The major etiologic factors include perceived object loss ("object loss" is used in the broadest sense). Objects may include people, possessions, a job, status, home, ideals, or parts and processes of the body.	Dysfunctional Grieving R/T stress and inability to move forward with life AEB dysfunction in daily activities	Coping with Depression; Self-Control; Family Coping; Grief Resolution; Spiritual Support	Active Listening; Anxiety Reduction; Coping Enhancement; Counseling; Family Support; Grief Work Facilitation

Dx, diagnosis; R/T, related to; AEB, as evidenced by.

*From: Moorhead, S., Johnson, M., Maas, M., & Swanson, E. (2013). *Iowa Outcomes Project: Nursing Outcomes Classification (NOC)* (5th ed.). St. Louis, MO: C. V. Mosby.
†From: Bulecheck, G., Butcher, H., Dochterman, J., & Wagner, C. (2013). *Iowa Intervention Project: Nursing Interventions Classification (NIC)* (6th ed.). St. Louis, MO: C. V. Mosby.
From: NANDA-Association International (NANDA-I). (2014). *Nursing diagnoses: Definitions and classification, 2015–2017*. West Sussex, England: Wiley-Blackwell.

OUTCOME IDENTIFICATION AND PLANNING

After the nursing diagnoses and related factors have been identified, patient goals and nursing interventions are planned. Development of patient goals centers on the stage of grief the patient is in and whether the grief is normal, anticipatory, or dysfunctional. The patient should have input in deciding what his or her personal needs are at the moment. Short- and long-term goals are needed. The following patient goals are samples of what may need to be addressed with such a patient:

- The patient will move toward resolution of diverse emotions.
- The patient will accept the reality of the loss.
- The patient will reinvest emotional and physical energy in meaningful people and activities.

Planning evolves around the phase or stage the patient is in. It may vary from emotional support to counseling to finding a support group.

IMPLEMENTATION

Nurses frequently have contact with people who are anticipating or experiencing a major loss; therefore, they have many opportunities to provide care for grieving people. Because grief can be both devastating and long lasting, opportunities for intervention occur throughout the grief process.

Health Promotion

In addition to the diagnoses of Grieving and Complicated Grieving, patients who have experienced a major loss may

TABLE 40-4 SAMPLE NURSING DIAGNOSES RELATED TO GRIEF AND BASED ON FUNCTIONAL HEALTH

Functional Health Area	Nursing Diagnosis
Health perception and health management	Ineffective Health Maintenance Risk for Injury Delayed Development Noncompliance
Activity and exercise	Activity Intolerance Deficient Diversional Activity Impaired Home Maintenance/ Management
Nutrition and metabolism	Imbalanced Nutrition: Less Than Body Requirements
Sleep and rest	Disturbed Sleep Pattern
Cognition and perception	Deficient Knowledge Acute Confusion Decisional Conflict
Self-perception	Anxiety Fear Hopelessness Powerlessness Disturbed Body Image Situational Low Self-Esteem
Roles and relationships	Impaired Family Processes Risk for Loneliness Impaired Parenting Social Isolation
Coping and stress tolerance	Ineffective Individual Coping Impaired Adjustment Ineffective Family Coping Risk for Suicide
Sexuality and reproduction	Sexual Dysfunction
Values and beliefs	Spiritual Distress

BOX 40-2 Preparing Children for Death

Instruct the parent as follows:

DOs
- Know your own feelings and beliefs.
- Be honest.
- Begin at the child's developmental level.
- Offer to include the child in family rituals related to death and mourning.
- Encourage expression of feelings.
- Provide security and stability.
- Encourage remembrance of the deceased.
- Recognize that children grieve differently than do adults.
- Expect the child to alternate between grieving and normal functioning.
- Talk openly about death and the feelings it generates.
- Introduce death concepts into conversation naturally.

DON'Ts
- Praise stoicism.
- Encourage forgetting of the deceased.
- Force the child to participate in grief and mourning rituals.
- Emphasize the likeness of the child to the deceased.
- Compare the child to the deceased.
- Use euphemisms ("Grandpa went to sleep"; "your brother went on a long journey").
- Protect the child from exposure to experiences with death.

also be found to have nursing diagnoses based on functional health given in Table 40-4. Whenever feasible, nursing interventions to promote normal grieving should occur before the loss occurs.

PATIENT TEACHING

Loss education should begin in early childhood. Preschoolers should learn about the normality of loss and grief through exposure to naturally occurring events. A visit to a long-term care facility, the death of a distant relative, the death of a pet, or the loss of a friend all provide opportunities to discuss the natural life cycle and loss in nonthreatening ways. The parent, other caregiver, or healthcare professional who can talk about loss honestly and openly, in terms that the child can understand, will help the child establish a healthy attitude toward loss and will serve as a role model (Favazza & Munson, 2010).

Loss education should continue throughout childhood and adolescence. Encourage parents to include children in

mourning rituals; however, family members should never force children to participate in such rituals. Also, encourage parents to allow children to express their diverse feelings about various losses (Box 40-2 contains helpful instructions for intervening with parents). Gradual exposure to loss and death situations concurrent with appropriate preparation and support will prepare the child to cope with losses later in life.

Nurses should also be directly involved in education of children about grief and loss. Incorporate grief education naturally into your contacts with children in various healthcare settings, such as schools, hospitals, physicians' offices, and clinics.

WORKING THROUGH GRIEF STAGES

The following is a discussion of nursing interventions based on the patient's present stage of grief. Box 40-3 provides additional information.

During the shock phase, nursing interventions should focus on protecting the patient from physical harm and on assisting the patient to accept the reality of the loss. During this phase, help the patient mobilize normal support systems; for example, help the patient contact family members and tell them about the loss. Patients may act out impulsively or may have decreased reaction time; therefore, make an effort to protect the patient from self-harm (suicide attempts) and from accidents. It usually is helpful to have a family member present

BOX 40-3   Examples of Nursing Interventions Used in Helping Patients Move through Grief

Interventions During Shock Phase
- Help the patient mobilize a support system.
- Protect the patient from physical harm.
- Have a family member present when notifying the patient of a loss.
- Have someone drive the patient home.
- Help the patient establish coping behaviors used in past.
- Encourage the patient to participate in mourning rituals.

Interventions During Protest Phase
- Encourage expression of diverse feelings (e.g., sadness, loneliness, anger, guilt, resentment, relief).
- Encourage remembering and talking about that which was lost.
- Provide anticipatory guidance regarding the normal grief process.
- Provide role models who have successfully coped with similar loss.
- Encourage the patient to use existing support systems.

- Identify new support systems.
- Discourage use of alcohol, drugs, and caffeine.
- Promote appropriate sleep habits.
- Promote good nutrition.
- Refer for complete physical examination.
- Encourage participation in religious rituals.
- Encourage use of previous healthy coping behaviors.
- Introduce new coping behaviors.

Interventions During Disorganization Phase
- Continue interventions begun in shock phase.
- Refer the patient to self-help groups.
- Refer the patient for individual or group counseling.

Interventions During Reorganization Phase
- Refer the patient for career counseling.
- Refer the patient to educational programs.
- Refer the patient to social activity programs.

when the patient is notified of a loss or an anticipated loss and to have this person drive the patient home; this is particularly important if the loss was unanticipated. Encourage patients to use coping behaviors that have been helpful to them in the past, such as participation in religious/spiritual activities or talking with a friend or relative, or perhaps a pastoral care professional. If the loss was a death, encourage patients to participate in funeral and mourning rituals.

During the protest phase, nursing interventions should focus on getting the patient to express thoughts and feelings about the loss and maintaining the patient's normal health status.

During the disorganization phase, place emphasis on getting the patient to accept the reality of the loss and to begin reorganization of his or her life. Continue interventions instituted during the shock phase.

During the reorganization phase, place emphasis on helping the patient to continue changing patterns of behavior so that he or she can find new or renewed meaning in life. Some losses, such as the death of a spouse, a spinal cord injury, or sudden deafness or blindness, require a major reorganization of many life activities, whereas other losses, such as reproductive sterility or amputation of a finger, may require reorganization in only a few areas. Patients who experience a greater degree of life reorganization may need additional interventions.

ENCOURAGING SUPPORT GROUPS

To prevent or ameliorate intense emotional distress or lack of social support or prolonged grief, encourage patients to participate in support groups for bereaved persons (Fig. 40-3).

Programs such as GriefShare, Widow-to-Widow, Reach-to-Recovery for mastectomy patients, Survivors of Suicide, and Compassionate Friends for bereaved parents provide support by nonprofessionals who have experienced a similar loss and have made a satisfactory recovery from the loss. These programs provide role modeling, education, and emotional support.

Recently, Internet-based support programs such as GriefNet have flourished; however, the effectiveness of these programs has not been evaluated (Oliveri, 2003).

Some bereaved people need more specialized help than self-help groups can provide. For such people, professionally led support groups or individual counseling may be more helpful. **Hospice** and other formal bereavement programs may be of assistance.

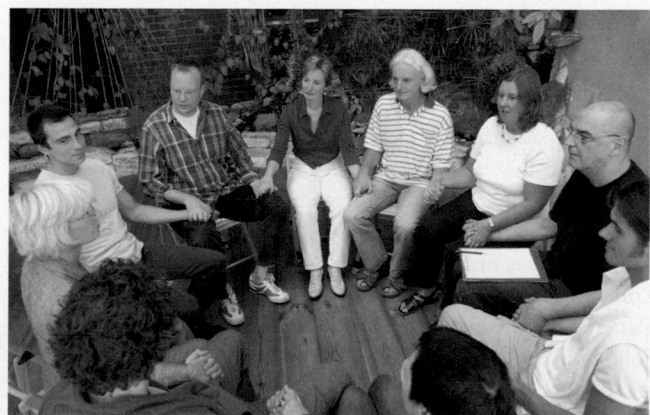

FIGURE 40-3 Support groups can help people work through their feelings with others who share similar experiences.

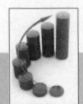

OUTCOME-BASED TEACHING PLANS

Henry Jones, 88 years old, recently died after a long illness. His daughter, Angela, has two young grandchildren, Aisha (age 9 years) and Kayla (age 6 years). Tanya, the mother of Aisha and Kayla, wants her children to attend the memorial service for their great-grandfather. Angela, the grandmother, thinks it would be better to not discuss the death with the children and to just tell them that Henry has "gone away." Tanya turns to you, the nurse in the pediatric clinic, for advice.

OUTCOME

Family can verbalize feelings about the death and the memorial service with respect to the children's feelings and understanding.

STRATEGIES

- Encourage Tanya to explore her own feelings and beliefs.
- With Tanya, evaluate each child's level of understanding of the event.
- Encourage expression of the children's feelings about the event.
- Help the family recognize that children grieve differently than adults.

- Talk openly about death and feelings it generates, expecting children to alternate between grieving and normal functioning.
- Encourage the children and family to discuss their desires about remembrance of the deceased and convey those inclinations to other family members as the basis of their decision making about the upcoming memorial service.

EVALUATION

Tanya effectively explored and verbalized her feelings about death and realized that she was fearful of her children's reactions, was already grieving the loss herself of her grandfather, and was having difficulty focusing on her children's needs.

- Aisha and Kayla were given the opportunity to attend calling hours for Henry; Aisha decided to attend with her parents, and Kayla chose to stay at home with neighbors.
- After the funeral, Aisha and Kayla recalled stories from their childhoods about their great-grandfather.

Nursing Interventions for Altered Grieving

Patients experiencing dysfunctional grief need professional help to resolve their problems. This help generally takes one of two forms: individual therapy or professionally led support groups. This type of help may be prescribed in addition to self-help. Professional support is particularly important if the patient has inadequate support systems. Many nurse therapists specialize in grief therapy; psychotherapists and professional grief counselors also provide these services.

Home and Community Care

When a patient has experienced a major loss, or is anticipating such a loss, adequate discharge planning and follow-up are essential. Because the grief process extends over a long period, the severity of the patient's grief may not be obvious during hospitalization. Nurses may misperceive the patient's shock and denial and conclude that the patient is "unaffected by the loss." Actually, the patient who appears unaffected by a loss is particularly in need of follow-up care because he or she may have a delayed grief reaction.

Referral

Discharge planning should include referral to social support programs, self-help groups, professionally led support groups,

public health nurses, or hospice/**palliative care** programs, depending on the patient's specific needs and the resources available in the community. Widow and widower groups may help when the patient is ready for such a program. Pastoral counselors and other clergy are helpful resources for many people. Be aware, however, that some grieving individuals may not feel empowered to participate in the more common referrals due to their unique circumstances, such as being an ex-spouse or partner, persons in same-sex relationships, parents of murdered children; these people may need more individualized and specialized attention. Encourage patients to continue contact with their primary healthcare provider (physician or nurse) as well, because the grief process often decreases resistance to disease and exacerbates existing illnesses.

EVALUATION

This section lists some general goals and outcome criteria for a grieving patient that can be used as a guide for evaluation. Remember, however, that evaluation must be individualized based on the patient's specific needs and goals. The items presented here are suggestions, to be amended based on knowledge about the specific patient.

Evaluation is an ongoing process that includes assessing the patient and comparing the patient's status to the outcome criteria. During this process, recall the long-term nature of grief

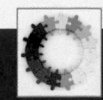

COLLABORATING WITH THE HEALTHCARE TEAM
Calling the Hospital Chaplain Concerning a Child's Death

Baby Barry, 3 months old, died unexpectedly an hour ago in the pediatric ward.

SITUATION: Mrs. Barry sits in the rocking chair, rocking her baby, and crooning to him. When approached, she just keeps saying, "Shhh, my baby's sleeping. We don't want to waken him." Her husband is out of town, and Mrs. Barry has no other family close by. She belongs to a faith community, but her clergy person has not yet been reached.

BACKGROUND: Baby Barry was in the hospital for an intestinal procedure that was expected to go smoothly; however, he apparently had a pulmonary embolus and could not be resuscitated.

ASSESSMENT: Mrs. Barry needs the chaplain to spend time with her and help her to understand what has happened and what decisions she needs to make.

RECOMMENDATION: Could you come immediately and talk with Mrs. Barry and support her in her grief? I am quite concerned about her mental state.

CRITICAL THINKING CHALLENGE
- Discuss the rationale for requesting that the chaplain come to speak with and stay with the mother.
- Which other members of the collaborative team could be called on to help provide some comfort?
- What support do you, as the nurse, need in this situation?

---

and that progress toward these outcomes may be very slow but nevertheless within the normal range. Use astute clinical judgment to determine whether the patient is making satisfactory progress and revise the nursing care plan as appropriate.

APPLY YOUR CRITICAL THINKING

You are working in an emergency department when Carlos, 18 years old, is brought in after a terrible accident. His parents, Juan and Maria Sanchez, are called and arrive less than 1 hour before Carlos dies. They are able to say good-bye, but Carlos never regains consciousness. After Carlos's death, his mother sits crying, saying over and over, "How could this happen? How could this happen?" In which phase of grieving is Maria? What interventions would be most helpful? For all of the Possible Outcome Criteria, remember that the time frames noted may not be appropriate for all persons and must be individualized by the nurse for each patient.

Check your answer in Appendix B.

Goal

The patient will recognize and express diverse emotions.

POSSIBLE OUTCOME CRITERIA

- Within 7 days, the patient expresses diverse emotions, such as sadness, anger, guilt, loneliness, or relief.
- Within 14 days, the patient states that experienced emotions are normal components of the grief process.

Goal

The patient will move toward resolution of diverse emotions.

POSSIBLE OUTCOME CRITERIA

- Within 6 months, the patient reports decreased frequency and intensity of painful emotions.
- Within 9 months, the patient expresses decreased frequency of preoccupation with thoughts of the lost loved one or object.

Goal

The patient will recognize the reality of the loss.

POSSIBLE OUTCOME CRITERIA

- Within 4 weeks, the patient discusses the loss and its meaning.
- Within 4 weeks, the patient discusses potential life changes necessary because of the loss.
- Within 6 months, the patient disposes of articles no longer needed (e.g., paraplegic gives away skis, widow gives away deceased spouse's clothing).
- Within 12 months, the patient plans for major life changes to accommodate the loss (e.g., selling home, taking new job).

Goal

The patient will recognize the need for help and seek help appropriately.

POSSIBLE OUTCOME CRITERIA

- Within 24 hours, the patient reaches out to family and friends for emotional and practical help.
- Within 2 months, the patient uses family and friends for social support.
- Within 6 months, the patient uses community resources for support.
- Within 12 months, the patient assumes major responsibility for self.

Goal

The patient will retain or regain physical health status.

POSSIBLE OUTCOME CRITERIA

- The patient does not use sleeping pills, alcohol, caffeine, tobacco, or tranquilizers as crutches to ease the pain.
- Within 3 months, the patient follows his or her prescribed medical regimen and adheres to healthful behaviors.
- Within 12 months, the patient states that he or she has returned to normal eating, sleeping, and exercise habits.

Goal

The patient will reinvest emotional and physical energy in meaningful people and activities.

POSSIBLE OUTCOME CRITERIA

- Within 9 months, the patient participates in new activities.
- Within 12 months, the patient reports making necessary changes in social, recreational, and occupational spheres.
- Within 12 months, the patient identifies renewal of old friendships and development of new friendships.
- Within 24 months, the patient expresses a sense of satisfaction with life and a sense of meaning in life.

CARING FOR THE DYING PATIENT

Definition of Death

Death is defined in three ways: as irreversible cessation of heart–lung function, or of whole-brain function, or of higher-brain function. The classic heart–lung definition (cessation of heartbeat and respirations) is widely used to define clinical death. Higher-brain death results in a vegetative state in which the patient has no consciousness, speech, or feelings but is able to independently maintain respirations. Lower-brain death results in inability to maintain circulation and respiration; such patients depend on a ventilator for breathing and circulation. The President's Commission for the Study of Ethical Problems in Medicine and Biomedical and Behavioral Research (1983)

ETHICAL/LEGAL ISSUE

DURABLE POWER OF ATTORNEY FOR HEALTHCARE AND ADVANCE DIRECTIVES

You are a registered nurse working in a neurosurgeon's office. Two weeks ago, a 45-year-old physician, Dr. Smithson, had a complete neurologic workup because she was having headaches that were increasing in severity and some short-term memory loss. At that time, she was told that she had an operable brain tumor. She was given the choice of (i) having a type of surgery with minimal risk of death, but with the likelihood that she would lose some cortical brain function, or (ii) having a type of surgery that had a high risk of death but would not affect her cortical brain function. She chose the latter. Today, she and her husband have come to the office for preoperative preparation and teaching. Mr. Smithson tells you that she is extremely worried about his wife's prognosis and potential for full recovery.

CRITICAL THINKING CHALLENGE

- Consider your own feelings as you encounter this situation. Which type of surgery would you have chosen?
- Think about three different ways you could respond to this situation and the consequences of responding in these different ways.
- What additional information would you need to help the couple prepare for the impending surgery?
- What do you need to know about advance directives? What information should you provide to Dr. and Mr. Smithson about a durable power of attorney/healthcare proxy for healthcare and a living will? Which laws apply in your state? How would you go about discussing these topics?

defined death as either (i) irreversible cessation of circulatory and respiratory functions or (ii) irreversible cessation of all functions of the entire brain (whole brain), including the brain stem. A determination of death must be made in accordance with accepted medical standards. An organ donor may have an organ harvested while he or she is clinically alive if either higher- or lower-brain death occurs (i.e., only when respiration is completely controlled by use of mechanical ventilation). Given an important societal need for organ donation, new standards for the determination of death while, at the same time, providing for quality of care at the end of life, are under debate (President's Council on Bioethics, 2008). State laws determine who can pronounce and certify a death. In many states, the nurse may pronounce death (note the date and time that the patient was found without a pulse or respirations), and the death will be certified by other designated providers (e.g., physician, NP, physician assistant, medical examiner, coroner). Certification of death is reported on a death certificate, a legal document.

Response to Dying and Death

Kübler-Ross's (1969) theory of the stages of grief when an individual is dying has gained wide acceptance in nursing and other disciplines as well as with the general public. Kübler-Ross, a Swiss psychiatrist, was an early pioneer in developing sensitive, compassionate care for the dying. Her work provided the impetus for increased attention to the needs of the dying and the bereaved and had an influence on the later development of hospice programs. She proposed five stages of grief: (i) denial, (ii) anger, (iii) bargaining, (iv) depression, and (v) acceptance. Denial may range from complete denial of the illness and impending death to denial of the effect that dying will have on self and others. In the second stage, anger may be directed toward fate, God, family members, healthcare providers, or others. Bargaining occurs as the patient seeks to delay the dreaded event; the patient bargains with God for more time and, in return, promises to do something to repay God for this favor. Depression occurs when the patient acknowledges the reality and inevitability of the impending death. In the final stage, acceptance, the patient comes to terms with the loss, begins to detach from supportive people, and loses interest in worldly activities.

Although Kübler-Ross's theory provides a general guideline for understanding responses to dying, many patients do not follow this progression through stages. Many go back and forth from one stage to another; others remain in one stage until their death. Nurses must be aware that there is no one right way for a patient to respond to dying. Nurses must adapt their care based on patients' current responses and needs and not expect them to always progress through defined stages. Review the other models of grieving provided earlier in this chapter.

Physical Signs of Dying

When a patient is dying, the lungs become less efficient for gas diffusion and oxygenation. As blood pressure and heart rate decrease, the body becomes increasingly unable to maintain circulation and to perfuse tissues, and the brain ceases to regulate vital centers (Norlander, 2008). The following physical signs (Hui et al., 2014; Matzo & Hill, 2015) often occur:

- Skin may become extremely pale, cyanotic, jaundiced, mottled, or cool
- Heart rate is irregular and the pulse is weak, rapid, and irregular

- Respirations are changed, shallow, labored, faster or slower, or irregular (e.g., Cheyne–Stokes respirations, death rattle, apnea)
- Urine output is decreased due to worsening renal function and limited fluid intake
- Fecal retention or impaction occurs due to reduced gastrointestinal motility
- Incontinence occurs due to relaxation of the sphincter tone
- Difficulty swallowing, loss of appetite
- Generalized weakness
- Increased fatigue or somnolence or restlessness and increased anxiousness
- Decreased responsiveness to external stimuli.

Hui et al. (2014) reported that apnea periods, Cheyne–Stokes breathing, death rattle, peripheral cyanosis, pulselessness of radial artery, respiration with mandibular movement, and decreased urine output occurred most frequently in the last 3 days of life in the group of cancer patients they studied, although most of the patients had only one or two of the symptoms.

Unfortunately, decreased pain does not always occur with people who are dying. When patients cannot tell us about their pain, closer observation for nonverbal signs of pain is essential. As death approaches, the signs of impending death increase and become more pronounced.

Hospice and Palliative Care

Hospice and palliative care are two terms that many people, including some healthcare providers, confuse with one another. *Hospice care* is a viable alternative for dying patients and their families. Hospice programs, which, in effect, are a type of insurance benefit, focus on relieving symptoms and supporting patients with a life expectancy of 6 months or less, rather than years, and their families. *Palliative care*, on the other hand, may be given at any time during a patient's illness, from diagnosis to end of life. The World Health Organization (WHO, 2015) offers the following definition of palliative care:

> An approach that improves the quality of life of patients and their families facing the problems associated with life-threatening illness, through the prevention and relief of suffering by means of early identification and impeccable assessment and treatment of pain and other problems, physical, psychosocial, and spiritual.

Specifically, palliative care (WHO, 2015):

- Provides relief from pain and other distressing symptoms
- Affirms life and regards dying as a normal process
- Intends neither to hasten or postpone death
- Integrates the psychological and spiritual aspects of patient care
- Offers a support system to help patients live as actively as possible until death

- Offers a support system to help the family cope during the patient's illness and in their own bereavement
- Uses a team approach to address the needs of patients and their families, including bereavement counseling, if indicated
- Will enhance quality of life and may also positively influence the course of illness
- Is applicable early in the course of illness, in conjunction with other therapies that are intended to prolong life, such as chemotherapy or radiation therapy, and includes those investigations needed to better understand and manage distressing clinical complications

The first home hospice in the United States was founded in 1974; these care homes for the dying have since become a routine component of the U.S. healthcare system (Matzo & Sherman, 2015). Since the mid-1990s, palliative care has become an increasingly important specialty within the U.S. healthcare system as well (National Hospice and Palliative Care Organization, n.d.).

Hospice and palliative care programs provide care that focuses on quality rather than length of life. Both hospice and palliative care share a similar foundation. The philosophy of hospice is that patients and families are empowered to achieve as much control over their lives as possible (Sherman, Bookbinder, & McHugh, 2015). Hospice-type care can be provided in hospitals, extended care facilities, freestanding hospices, and patients' homes. Palliative care extends the principles of hospice care to a broader population to benefit those who need this type of care at an earlier stage of their illness. Under a palliative care approach, patients may focus on managing symptoms at the same time they are seeking curative therapies. Hospice focuses on treatments and care aimed only at relieving symptoms in the last few months of life. The philosophy of hospice focuses on caring at the end of life and seeks to neither hasten nor delay death. Hospice and palliative care programs provide comfort care such as control of pain and nausea; they also help patients and families to attain a degree of mental and spiritual preparation for death in accordance with their wishes. Hospice and palliative care provide physical, social, psychological, and spiritual support through a team of healthcare professionals and lay volunteers (Holley, Gorawara-Bhat, Dale, Hemmerich, & Cox-Hayley, 2009). Researchers have shown that psychological distress is lower among bereaved spouses whose partners received hospice care than among those who did not (McCorkle, 2006). Temel et al. (2010) studied the effects of palliative care with a group of lung cancer patients and found that patients who received early palliative care survived longer (by almost 3 months) and had less aggressive care at the end of life compared to patients who did not receive the intervention.

Nursing Diagnoses and Nursing Implementation

The ultimate outcome for dying patients is to achieve good end-of-life care and a good death. A death is defined as "good" if there is an awareness, acceptance, and preparation for death by all those concerned and there is control of physical and emotional pain and distress. Patients often define a "good death" as being pain free, dying with dignity, and dying in their sleep (DeJong & Clark, 2009; Matzo & Sherman, 2015). A good death may be defined differently based on patients' cultural and health beliefs (Pattison, 2008). DeJong and Clark described a "bad death" as one where there was poor pain management along with loss of independence and control. The nursing care needs of patients may vary based on their cultural belief systems (D'Avanzo, 2008).

Nurses need to address the physical, emotional, social, spiritual, and cultural needs of dying patients and their families, and they need to recognize that these needs vary across the stages of dying. Three core competencies are necessary: ability to talk to patients and families about dying, pain and other symptom control techniques, and comfort care nursing interventions (Ferrell & Coyle, 2010). An interdisciplinary healthcare team is necessary to best meet the complex needs of dying patients and their families. Nurses alone cannot meet these needs. Caring for dying patients can be very stressful to caregivers. Working as a team often provides the support necessary to help the caregivers cope with these stressors. Nurses should always be attentive to their own self-care needs.

The following are some of the common nursing diagnoses for dying patients: Pain; Fatigue; Deficient Fluid Volume; Imbalanced Nutrition (Less than Body Requirements); Impaired Gas Exchange; and Interrupted Family Process. These nursing diagnoses are explored in more depth in previous chapters. Selected nursing diagnoses related to grieving are presented in Table 40-3.

Caring for the Deceased

Nursing care continues after the death of the patient. Concern for dignity in the care of the body and sensitivity to the needs of the deceased patient's family are nurses' responsibilities. Immediately after the patient's death has been pronounced, family members may wish to spend some time alone with the patient's body. In an effort to limit exposure to the disturbing sight of equipment and medical supplies, the nurse should, if possible, remove unneeded items and clean, position, and cover the patient. Under some circumstances (such as an unexpected death), intravenous and other lines and tubes should not be removed because the body may need to be examined by a med-

PATIENT PLAN OF CARE
The Patient Who is Grieving

NURSING DIAGNOSIS
Grieving (normal) related to actual loss of significant person manifested by expression of unresolved issues

SHOCK STAGE
PATIENT GOAL
The patient will move toward resolution of diverse emotions.

PATIENT OUTCOME CRITERIA
- The patient cognitively accepts the reality of death within 1 week.
- The patient participates in funeral and mourning rituals within 1 week.
- The patient expresses emotional affect in discussion, facial expressions, and reactions within 72 hours.
- The patient uses family and friends for social support in resolving emotional responses within 1 week.

NURSING INTERVENTION	SCIENTIFIC RATIONALE
1. Encourage mourner to see the deceased and allow mourner to touch or hold the deceased, if desired.	**1.** Cognitive recognition of the reality of death is necessary before beginning to work on acceptance of the emotional significance of the death.
2. a. Provide anticipatory guidance regarding physical appearance of the deceased. **b.** Encourage mourner to participate in grief and mourning activities that are congruent with his or her sociocultural and spiritual/religious beliefs.	**2.** Cognitive acceptance of the death is facilitated by participating in funeral and mourning rituals.
3. Notify family members of the death in person in a private setting whenever possible.	**3.** Trauma of notification of the death can be eased by sensitive attention to family members' needs.
4. Encourage mourner to express diverse feelings (e.g., guilt, sadness, relief, numbness, anger).	**4.** Open expression of feelings facilitates gradual resolution of these feelings; some feelings may be perceived as socially unacceptable.
5. Encourage mourner to talk about the deceased and to ask questions about the death.	**5.** Preoccupation with thoughts of the deceased is a normal part of the grief process.
6. Provide anticipatory guidance on the grief process, including common thoughts, feelings, and behaviors; emphasize that there is no one right way to grieve.	**6.** Most people have little knowledge about the normal grief process, and it is reassuring for them to know that what they are experiencing is normal.
7. Assist mourner with making decisions regarding urgent postdeath responsibilities; help mourner contact family members and other support persons, clergy, funeral director.	**7.** The bereaved person is often in crisis and needs the emotional and practical support from family and other support systems.
8. Protect mourner from deliberate or unintentional harm (e.g., inquire about suicidal thoughts, encourage mourner not to drive own car immediately after learning of the death).	**8.** Bereaved are at greater risk of mortality and morbidity, particularly from accidents and suicide.

(Continued)

PATIENT PLAN OF CARE (*Continued*)
The Patient Who is Grieving

PROTEST STAGE
PATIENT GOAL
The patient will begin acceptable transition to life without the deceased.

PATIENT OUTCOME CRITERIA
- The patient recognizes and accepts emotional feelings as acceptable within 2 months.
- The patient begins transition to new roles within 2 months.
- The patient experiences minimal deterioration of physical health during first 3 months after death of loved one.

NURSING INTERVENTION	SCIENTIFIC RATIONALE
1. Encourage mourner to remember and talk about both negative and positive memories of the deceased. Use counseling skills of empathy, warmth, and positive regard. Facilitate reality testing. Assess need for individual or family who have numerous stressors.	**1.** The process of altering bonds with the deceased continues over an extended period of time. Counseling skills can be used to elicit unrecognized thoughts and feelings. Bereaved people who have numerous stressors and few resources benefit from professional therapy.
2. Teach support people about the emotional needs of the bereaved.	**2.** Adequately prepared support people can augment professional services or may be the only intervention needed.
3. Provide appropriate reading materials on the grief process.	**3.** Identification with other bereaved people can be therapeutic.
4. Reinforce use of healthy coping skills.	**4.** During a crisis, people may be too overwhelmed to use their usual coping skills; therefore, the nurse must help them remember these skills.
5. Assess for suicidal ideation.	**5.** Transition to new roles is a major stressor for the bereaved; role models and education on the new roles facilitates ease in role transition.
6. Encourage the patient to assume some new roles, relinquish other roles, and allow support people to fill some of the deceased's roles. Provide role models for new roles (e.g., Widow-to-Widow befriender). Recommend participation in self-help or mutual help support groups.	**6.** The death of a significant other precipitates role changes. Patients often do not know how to function in new roles; role models can show them how to function.
7. Teach problem-solving skills related to new roles.	**7.** New roles require diverse problem-solving skills.
8. Provide appropriate reading materials on practical aspects of role transition (e.g., financial management, automobile maintenance, child care, home maintenance).	**8.** Seeing things in written form helps to reinforce ideas and knowledge; books become references.
9. Encourage complete physical assessment.	**9.** The risk of increased mortality and morbidity is highest during the early bereavement period but continues throughout the first year of bereavement.
10. Promote good health habits (e.g., nutrition, rest, avoidance of alcohol and tobacco).	**10.** Good health habits and early identification of health problems may prevent serious illness.

DISORGANIZATION STAGE

PATIENT GOAL

The patient will reinvest emotional and physical energy in meaningful people and activities.

POSSIBLE OUTCOME CRITERIA

- The patient emotionally accepts the loss within 9 months, as disclosed by the patient.
- The patient experiences improved functioning in new roles within 9 months.
- The patient discusses with nurse a search for new meaning in life within 9 months.
- The patient/family verbalizes experiencing increased family cohesiveness within 9 months.

NURSING INTERVENTION	SCIENTIFIC RATIONALE
1. Assist the patient in decision making regarding disposal of deceased's belongings.	1. During the disorganization state, the patient recognizes the emotional significance of the loss and begins to accept the meaning of the loss.
2. Support the patient's expression of grief (e.g., cemetery visits, memorial services, visiting places of special meaning to the deceased).	2. Activities focusing on grief can facilitate resolution of the loss.
3. Normalize thoughts and feelings.	3. Same as above.
4. Use role-play to work through unresolved issues.	4. Same as above.
5. Encourage the patient to express thoughts and feelings through writing.	5. Same as above.
6. Enhance previous coping skills.	6. New roles continue to cause stress; effort must be directed toward strengthening the bereaved person's intrapersonal and interpersonal competence.
7. Introduce additional coping techniques.	7. Same as above.
8. Support independent problem-solving skills.	8. Same as above.
9. Keep support systems mobilized.	9. Same as above.
10. Encourage the patient to delay major decisions until out of acute grief.	10. Same as above.
11. Support the patient's reevaluation of the meaning of his or her life.	11. The death of a loved one leads the bereaved to question the meaning of life.
12. Encourage participation in spiritual/religious activities.	12. Same as above.
13. Encourage the patient to participate in social and recreational activities.	13 Same as above.
14. Teach family members that each person expresses grief differently and resolves his or her grief at a different speed.	14 The family functions as a system; death of a family member affects all parts of the system.
15. Encourage open family communication about the loss and the feelings engendered.	15. Each subsystem affects other subsystems and the system as a whole.
16. Identify and reinforce the strengths of each family member.	16. Strengthening any part of the system has a positive effect on the other subsystems and on the system as a whole.
17. Encourage family members to provide support to each other.	17. Same as above.
18. Mobilize extra family support systems.	18. Friends, coworkers, and others can supplement support received from family members.

(*Continued*)

PATIENT PLAN OF CARE (Continued)
The Patient Who is Grieving

REORGANIZATION STAGE

PATIENT GOAL

The patient will increase level of physical, emotional, social, and spiritual functioning (previous level or higher level of functioning)

POSSIBLE OUTCOME CRITERIA

- The patient resolves emotional reactions to the loss within 2 years.
- The patient reports satisfaction with new roles within 2 years.
- The patient reports finding new meaning in life within 2 years.
- The patient reports achievement of personal growth within 2 years.
- The patient reports improved coping skills within 2 years.

NURSING INTERVENTION	SCIENTIFIC RATIONALE
1. Avoid unrealistic expectations for mourner to recover quickly.	**1.** Resolution of grief after the death of a significant other often takes 2 to 5 years. By the end of the first year, the bereaved should have resolved the major portion of his or her grief but may continue to experience a resurgence of grief on anniversaries and holidays.
2. Remind the patient that it is normal for grief feelings to be rekindled by trigger events such as holidays and anniversaries.	**2.** Same as above.
3. Support renewal of old friendships/interests and development of new friendships/interests.	**3.** Meeting with friends and finding new activities eases the emotional loss and gives new meaning to life.
4. Use gentle confrontation to deal with unresolved feelings toward the deceased.	**4.** It is important to deal with all feelings before the grief period can end.
5. Facilitate recognition of patient's own strengths and limitations.	**5.** Knowing oneself aids in acceptable functioning.
6. Encourage continued participation in support group.	**6.** Support is still needed from people with similar problems.
7. Support continued involvement in religious, social, and recreational activities.	**7.** By the end of the second year, bereaved should have found a satisfactory level of health and functioning.
8. Encourage reevaluation of diverse meanings in life.	**8.** By the end of the second year, bereaved should be functioning satisfactorily in roles.
9. Praise the patient for satisfactory achievement of roles.	**9.** The search for meaning continues for a long time after resolution of other aspects of grief.
10. Support changes in patient's behavior and lifestyle.	**10.** The crisis of bereavement often produces profound personal growth.
11. Reinforce use of various coping skills.	**11.** Bereaved people often report greatly increased coping skills after resolution of grief and also report a sense of confidence that because they managed to handle their grief satisfactorily, they will be able to handle any other stressor satisfactorily.

EVALUATION

10/1/17: 09:30—The patient has met the goal and outcome criteria for the shock, protest, and disorganization stages of grief.

- The patient reports that now, 12 months following the death, she is beginning to shape a life that accepts the reality of death and that she has some comfort in moving on.

—S. Roberts, RN

ical examiner. Having time alone with the patient is important for some families, whereas others appreciate the presence of a nurse, a spiritual leader, or friends. Religious/spiritual and cultural beliefs and customs should be observed as much as possible.

KEY CONCEPTS

■ Loss is a universal experience, and grieving is a normal response to loss.

■ Models of the grief process provide direction for nursing assessment.

■ The grief process is similar regardless of the type of loss experienced.

■ A major loss results in a long-term life transition.

■ Response to loss is influenced by the person's stage of development.

■ The characteristics of the loss, personal resources and stressors, and sociocultural resources and stressors affect the grief process.

■ The outcome of a loss experience is not predetermined but rather is determined by the balance of stressors and resources present during the grief period.

■ Risk of dysfunctional grieving can be identified through analysis of the stressors and resources that the patient is experiencing.

■ Physical health and psychosocial adjustment during the grief process are intricately intertwined.

■ Nursing interventions should be based on knowledge of the long-term nature of the grief process.

■ Many grief manifestations, identified in previous literature as dysfunctional, are considered to be components of the normal grief process.

■ Caution should be used in labeling a patient as having dysfunctional grieving.

■ Discharge planning must consider the long-term nature of the grief process.

■ End-of-life care should promote quality of life through comfort care measures and open communication.

■ Palliative care should be offered to all patients experiencing a serious or life-threatening illness.

■ Hospice care is a viable option for dying patients and their families.

PRACTICING FOR THE NCLEX

CHECK YOUR ANSWERS IN APPENDIX A.

1. In admitting a patient with confusion and labile affect, the nurse discovers that the patient recently lost his son in a motor vehicle accident. Which nursing diagnosis best describes this patient?
    a. Anticipatory Grieving

    b. Ineffective Health Maintenance
    c. Dysfunctional Grieving
    d. Impaired Family Processes

2. The nurse is caring for an East African family that has just experienced a fetal demise at full term. The family initially refuses to see the stillborn infant. What should the nurse do first?
    a. Assist family members to see the infant in order to gain closure
    b. Ask the family about their expectations for mourning
    c. Evaluate the need for emotional and practical help
    d. Provide educational materials about loss of an infant

3. A nurse is talking with a wife whose husband just expired. What would appropriate nursing interventions be for someone in the Shock Phase of the Grief Cycle Model? Select all that apply:
    a. Help mobilize a support system
    b. Encourage expression of diverse feelings
    c. Help to establish coping behaviors used in past
    d. Provide role models who have coped with similar loss

4. The nurse is caring for a patient newly diagnosed with metastatic lung cancer. What would be the most appropriate statement for the nurse to make regarding palliative care resources?
    a. "Palliative care is for when you have a prognosis of less than 6 months."
    b. "Once you decide that you don't want to receive further treatment, palliative care will help keep you comfortable."
    c. "Palliative care can only be done once you discharge from the hospital."
    d. "Palliative care focuses on quality of life and may be used from the time of diagnosis."

5. The nurse is caring for an actively dying, unresponsive patient while the family sits at the bedside. The husband asks "Isn't she hungry? She hasn't had anything to eat in 24 hours." Which response by the nurse would be most appropriate?
    a. "The body doesn't need food at this stage."
    b. "We should talk to the physician about placing a feeding tube to help with intake."
    c. "Here is a menu—we can order some foods that she enjoys eating."
    d. "Motility of the stomach and intestines are decreased, so eating could make her nauseous."

REFERENCES

Barrett, T. W., & Scott, T. B. (1989). Development of the grief experience questionnaire. *Suicide & Life Threatening Behavior, 19*(2), 201–215.

Blank, N. M., & Werner-Lin, A. (2011). Growing up with grief: Revisiting the death of a parent over the life course. *Omega: Journal of Death and Dying, 63*(3), 271–290.

Bulecheck, G., Butcher, H., Dochterman, J., & Wagner, C. (2013). *Iowa intervention project: Nursing Interventions Classification* (6th ed.). St. Louis, MO: Mosby.

Carpenito-Moyet, L. (2012). *Nursing diagnosis: Application to clinical practice* (14th ed.). Philadelphia, PA: Lippincott Williams & Wilkins.

D'Avanzo,, C. E. (2008). *Pocket guide to cultural health assessment* (4th ed.). St. Louis, MO: Mosby/Elsevier.

Dayer-Berenson, L. (2011). *Cultural competencies for nurses: Impact on health and illness.* Sudbury, MA: Jones & Bartlett.

De Jong, J. D., & Clarke, L. E. (2009). What is a good death? Stories from palliative care. *Journal of Palliative Care, 25*(1), 61–67.

Demi, A. (1981). *Bereavement support group: Leadership manual.* Littleton, CO: Grief Education Institute.

Demi, A., & Miles, M. (1987). Parameters of normal grief: A Delphi study. *Death Studies, 11*, 397–412.

Engel, G. (1964). Grief and grieving. *American Journal of Nursing, 64*(9), 88–100.

Faschingbauer, T., DeVaul, R., & Zisook, S. (1977). Development of the Texas Inventory of Grief. *American Journal of Psychiatry, 134*, 696–698.

Favazza, P. C., & Munson, L. J. (2010). Loss and grief in young children. *Young Exceptional Children, 13*(2), 86–99.

Ferrell, B. R., & Coyle, N. (Eds.). (2010). *Oxford textbook of palliative nursing* (3rd ed.). New York, NY: Oxford University Press.

Field, N. P., & Filanosky, C. (2010). Continuing bonds, risk factors for complicated grief, and adjustment to bereavement. *Death Studies, 34*(1), 1–29.

Guarnaccia, C. A., & Hayslip, B. (1998). Factor structure of the bereavement experience questionnaire: The BEQ-24, a revised short-form. *Omega: Journal of Death and Dying, 37*(4), 303–316.

Hogan, N. S. (2002). Testing the grief to growth model using structural equation modeling. *Death Studies, 26*(8), 615–634.

Hogan, N. S., Greenfield, D. B., & Schmidt, L. A. (2001). Development and validation of the Hogan Grief Reaction Checklist. *Death Studies, 25*(1), 1–32.

Hui, D., dos Santos, R., Chisholm, G., Bansal, S., Silva, T. B., Kilgore, K., et al. (2014). Clinical signs of impending death in cancer patients. *Oncologist, 19*(6), 681–687.

Johansson, A. K., & Grimby, A. (2013). Grief among demented elderly individuals: A pilot study. *American Journal of Hospice and Palliative Care, 30*(5), 445–449.

Johnson, M., Bulechek, G., McCloskey-Dochterman, J., Maas, M., & Moorhead, S. (2013). *Nursing diagnoses, outcomes and interventions.* St. Louis, MO: Mosby.

Kübler-Ross, E. (1969). *On death and dying.* New York, NY: Macmillan.

Levetown, M. (2008). Communicating with children and families: From everyday interactions to skill in conveying distressing information. *Pediatrics, 121*, 1441–1460.

Lin, N., Simeone, R. S., Ensel, W. M., & Kuo, W. (1979). Social support, stressful life events, and illness: A model and an empirical test. *Journal of Health & Social Behavior, 20*, 108–119.

Maccallum, F., & Bryant, R. A. (2013). A Cognitive Attachment Model of prolonged grief: Integrating attachments, memory, and identity. *Clinical Psychology Review, 33*(6), 713–727.

Matzo, M., & Hill, J. A. (2015). Peri-death nursing care. In M. Matzo & D. W. Sherman (Eds.), *Palliative care nursing: Quality care to the end of life* (4th ed.; pp. 649–674). New York, NY: Springer.

Matzo, M., & Sherman, D. W. (Eds.). (2015). *Palliative care nursing: Quality care to the end of life* (4th ed.). New York, NY: Springer.

McCorkle, R. (2006). A program of research on patient and family caregiver outcomes: Three phases of evolution. *Oncology Nursing Forum, 33*(1), 25–31.

NANDA-Association International (NANDA-I). (2014). *Nursing diagnoses: Definitions and classification, 2015–2017.* West Sussex, England: Wiley-Blackwell.

National Cancer Institute. (2014). Grief, bereavement, and coping with loss-for health professionals. Retrieved from http://www.cancer.gov/about-cancer/advanced-cancer/caregivers/planning/bereavement-hp-pdq#section/all

National Hospice and Palliative Care Organization. (n.d.). Retrieved from http://www.nhpco.org/

Norlander, L. (2008). *To comfort always: A nurse's guide to end-of-life care.* Indianapolis, IN: Sigma Theta Tau International.

North American Nursing Diagnosis Association International (NANDA-I). (2014). *Nursing diagnoses: Definitions and classification, 2015–2017.* West Sussex, England: Wiley-Blackwell.

Oliveri, T. (2003). Grief groups on the Internet. *Bereavement Care, 22*(3), 39–40.

Parkes, C. M. (1986). *Bereavement: Studies of grief in adult life* (2nd ed.). New York, NY: International Universities Press.

Pattison, N. (2008). Caring of patients after death. *Nursing Standard, 22*(1), 48–58.

Potter, M. L., & Wynne, B. P. (2015). Loss, suffering, bereavement, and grief. In M. Matzo & D. W. Sherman (Eds.), *Palliative care nursing: Quality care to the end of life* (4th ed.; pp. 205–234). New York, NY: Springer.

President's Commission for the Study of Ethical Problems in Medicine and Biomedical and Behavioral Research. (1983). *Deciding to forego life-sustaining treatment: A report on the ethical, medical, and legal issues in treatment decisions.* Washington, DC: U.S. Government Printing Office.

President's Council on Bioethics. (2008, December). *Controversies in the determination of death: A white paper by the President's Council on Bioethics.* Washington, DC: White House. Retrieved from http://bioethics.georgetown.edu/pcbe/reports/death/index.html

Price, B. (2002). Laddered questions and qualitative data research interviews. *Journal of Advanced Nursing, 37*(3), 273–281.

Sanders, C., & Mauger, P. (1979). *A manual for the Grief Experience Inventory.* Tampa, FL: University of Florida.

Shapiro, E. R. (1994). *Grief as a family process: A developmental approach to clinical practice.* New York, NY: Guilford Press.

Sherman, D. W., Bookbinder, M., & McHugh, M. (2015). Palliative care: Responsive to the need for health care reform in the United States. In M. Matzo & D. W. Sherman (Eds.), *Palliative care nursing: Quality care to the end of life* (4th ed.; pp. 21–31. New York, NY: Springer.

Stroebe, M. S., Hansson, R. O., Schut, H., & Stroebe, W. (Eds.). (2008). *Handbook of bereavement research and practice: Advances in theory and intervention.* Washington, DC: American Psychological Association.

Temel, J. S., Greer, J. A., Muzikansky, A., Gallagher, E. R., Adamane, S., Jackson, V. A., … Lynch, T. J. (2010). Early palliative care for patients with metastatic non–small-cell lung cancer. *New England Journal of Medicine, 363*, 733–742.

World Health Organization. (2015). *WHO definition of palliative care.* Retrieved from www.who.int/cancer/palliative/definition/en/

Zalenski, R., Gillum, R. F., Quest, T. E., & Griffith, J. L. (2006). Care for the adult family members of victims of unexpected cardiac death. *Academy Emergency Medicine, 13*, 1333–1338.

Zilberg, N., Weiss, D., & Horowitz, M. (1982). Impact of event scale: A cross validational study and some empirical evidence supporting a conceptual model of stress response syndromes. *Journal of Consulting and Clinical Psychology, 50*(3), 407–414.

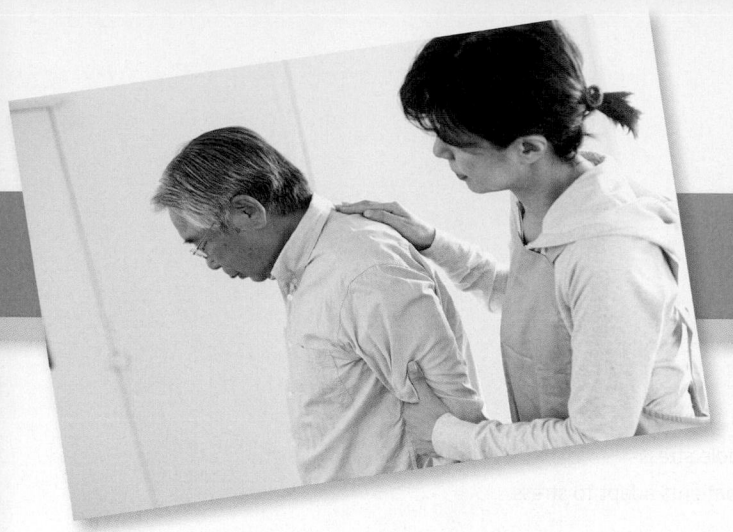

CHAPTER 41

Stress, Coping, and Adaptation

Marilyn J. Hammer

Case Scenario

An 82-year-old male patient with a 20+ year history of type 2 diabetes (T2D) was diagnosed with Alzheimer disease 2 years ago and has just been admitted to the hospital for pneumonia. The patient's oldest daughter is with him and expresses her concern to you that her father will have to move in with her family so she can take care of him. Her mother passed away 5 years ago, and her father has been living on his own since that time; however, his Alzheimer disease is progressing, he is neglecting to carefully monitor his blood sugar, and he needs assistance. It is financially and emotionally difficult for the daughter to place him in an assisted living type of facility. She also promised her mother before her death that she would take care of him. The daughter is feeling terribly stressed at the thought of how this will disrupt her family's home life in addition to her father having to move from his home of 54 years.

Major nursing responsibilities associated with assisting patients to manage stress include assessing a patient's ability to cope with stressors, identifying personal factors that could interfere with coping, promoting effective coping and stress management, and implementing nursing interventions to modify coping as the situation warrants. Once you have completed this chapter and have incorporated stress, coping, and adaptation into your knowledge base, review the above scenario and reflect on the following areas of Critical Thinking:

1. Illustrate how you will proceed with this assessment.
2. Identify potential stressors to the people in the situation.
3. Identify factors that may affect the daughter's coping behaviors.
4. Explore factors that place this family at risk for dysfunctional coping.
5. Describe possible manifestations of altered coping in this scenario.
6. Based on the information, plan appropriate nursing interventions.

KEY TERMS

adaptation
allostasis/allostatic load
appraisal
coping
coping mechanisms
homeostasis
hypothalamic-pituitary-adrenal axis
inflammation
plasticity
resistance
resilience
stress
vulnerability

Upon completion of this chapter, you will be able to do the following:

1. Identify physiologic signs and symptoms of stress.
2. Identify psychological responses to stress.
3. Discuss pathophysiologic processes of stress.
4. List examples of biophysical and psychosocial stressors.
5. Give examples of variables that affect a person's ability to cope with stress.
6. Describe various types of coping patterns people typically use to handle stress.
7. Identify stress management techniques that nurses can use to help patients adapt to stress.

What is stress? Defined by Hans Selye in 1936 as "the non-specific response of the body to any demand for change" (American Institute of Stress, 2010), **stress** is a complex process that solicits our psychological and physiologic systems. Stress has been further described as an actual or potential threat to homeostasis (Chrousos, 2009), the body's maintenance of physiologic balance within a certain range or "set point" (McEwen & Wingfield, 2010). In essence, stress is part of our lives from conception through death, an everpresent component of our physical and social environments. Whether changes occur as a natural progression of life (e.g., starting a new school or job, beginning or ending relationships, relocating, etc.) or a sudden unexpected event (e.g., a trauma), stress is psychologically processed and physiologically manifested.

The perception of stress is an individual experience that can express itself in various ways. Although stress predominately has a negative overtone, it can be a positive experience as well. Good stress, or eustress, is when a sense of accomplishment or even exhilaration is felt with overcoming a challenge or obstacle with limited duration (McEwen, 2007). For example, these types of positive challenges can include good athletic and academic performances. On the negative end of the spectrum, with prolonged challenges that are not easy to resolve, stress can lead to illness, disease, and even death (Chrousos, 2009).

The initial reaction to a potentially stressful situation is appraisal. **Appraisal** is the process of interpreting a situation and determining if it is a stress (Bacon, Milne, Sheikh, & Freeston, 2009). Once a real or perceived stress is actualized, physical and/or emotional action is engaged. Managing stress can be accomplished through the mechanism of coping. Coping can be problem focused through actions that directly mitigate the stressor (the event or situation causing the stress) or emotion focused through finding ways to lessen the feelings of anxiety and angst triggered by the stressful event (Bacon et al., 2009). The ability to cope well can lead to a sense of well-being. The outcome of coping is **adaptation**, or the adjustments made in response to the stressful event. Adaptation is the successful adjustment to stress, ensuring continued health and well-being. Failure to adapt can lead to pathologic manifestations.

NORMAL COPING AND ADAPTATION TO STRESS

Life is a dynamic process. Through constantly changing environments, from the smallest cellular components to the largest global levels, stress is encountered. Successful adaptation to these ever-changing environments perpetuates survival.

Stress can be acute or chronic. Historically, acute stress was described as daily life encounters that led to the "fight-or-flight" response, such as coming in close proximity to a large wild animal. The stress response was described as an emotional and physiologic reaction to either fight off the animal or run away from it, ensuring survival. In this context, stress was periodic short-term events. We experience these types of acute stress reactions frequently—for example, swerving to avoid another vehicle. Chronic stress, however, is a sustained response or repeated event that impedes coping (Sierra, Beccari, Diaz-Aparicio, Encinas, & Comeau, 2014) Indeed, stress occurs on many levels in many situations and is a constant element throughout life. Changes and adjustments to these changes are ongoing and range from subtle to extremely overt. The process of appraisal, stress, coping, and adaptation are the elements of managing these changes.

Physiologic Function Related to Stress, Coping, and Adaptation

HOMEOSTASIS

Based on work by Claude Bernard in the late 1800s, the Harvard physiologist Walter B. Cannon in 1932 described the term **homeostasis** as the physiologic parameters that must be maintained for the human body to survive under emergency circumstances (McEwen & Wingfield, 2010). According to Cannon, these events were sympathetically driven and included the secretion of epinephrine to increase heart rate, blood coagulation, and blood glucose levels, while also decreasing digestion and removing cellular fatigue waste products from muscle.

The contemporary understanding of homeostasis encompasses complex regulatory processes necessitating the coordination of various systems, such as regulation of pH, oxygen levels, blood pressure, heart rate, blood glucose levels, fluid and electrolytes, and body temperature within narrow therapeutic ranges to maintain the body's dynamic equilibrium (McEwen & Wingfield, 2010). Overall, the process of maintaining homeostasis is constant and not just engaged in during emergent situations as Cannon presumed (McEwen & Wingfield, 2010).

Homeostasis involves sensors in various tissues and organs that are responsible for detecting imbalances and responding by producing or inhibiting specific molecules and/or sending out small signaling molecules to trigger other cells, organs, and tissues to respond (Chovatiya & Medzhitov, 2014). In essence, homeostasis maintains the biologic system of an entire organism. The components of homeostasis and the interplay of the numerous biologic factors involved in maintaining this balance are complex.

The 82-year-old patient in the case study, for example, has been living with T2D for more than 20 years—a chronic stress. The normal homeostatic process of endogenously regulating blood sugar became impaired. Although diagnosed 20 years prior, the decline in cellular regulatory function began many years earlier. Due to multiple factors, likely including a genetic predisposition coupled with a lifestyle void of physical activity and a diet high in fat and sugar, the patient's cellular functions of insulin production, gluconeogenesis, glycolysis, and cellular uptake and utilization of glucose ultimately became imbalanced to a point of chronic impairment. The patient is able to continue living his life through the exogenous help of medications that now regulate his blood sugar. Without them, he would not have survived long enough to have encountered the Alzheimer disease. In fact, the history of T2D is a risk factor for Alzheimer disease and other forms of cognitive impairment and dementia (Bornstein, Brainin, Guekht, Skoog, & Korczyn, 2014; Cheng, Huang, Deng, & Wang, 2012). The snowballing effect created when the body can no longer maintain homeostasis is tremendous.

ALLOSTASIS

Allostasis is the process of maintaining or reestablishing homeostasis in response to stress (Chrousos, 2009; McEwen & Wingfield, 2010). This process of physiologic adjustments ensures survival when environmental changes or stressors are encountered (Bellar, Kunkler, & Burkett, 2009). In the late 1980s, Sterling and Eyer described allostasis as (a) ongoing assessments between internal resources and external demands, (b) physiologic adjustments in anticipation of oncoming events, and (c) adaptation occurring over time.

Allostasis also takes into account the larger schema of life, including circadian (daily internal physiologic) and circannual (annual external, e.g., seasonal) alterations (McEwen & Wingfield, 2010). For example, the body temperature has a circadian rhythm, meaning the set point during the day (higher temperature) is different from the set point during the night (lower temperature). The allostatic response is managed through physiologic mediators including the hypothalamus, anterior pituitary, adrenal glands, and nervous and immune systems (Bellar et al., 2009; Bilkei-Gorzo, Racz, et al., 2008; McEwen, 2007).

The ability to effectively respond to an environmental change or stressor varies with each individual. Both genetic and epigenetic factors, particularly early environmental predisposition, influence an individual's response. Whereas effective responses restore stability, ineffective responses result in lack of recovery with sustained states of allostasis. Sustained allostatic states lead to **allostatic load**, which, in turn, can lead to disease (Bellar et al., 2009; McEwen, 2007).

PHYSIOLOGIC MEDIATORS OF ALLOSTASIS

The physiologic mediators of allostasis include an orchestration of various systems working in harmony to reestablish or maintain homeostasis. Higher cognitive areas of brain function assimilate the stress information and interface with other parts of the brain such as the hypothalamus and brain stem. In turn, brain activity regulates autonomic, neuroendocrine, and immune responses (McEwen, 2007).

The Central Nervous System

The central nervous system (CNS) consists of the brain and spinal cord and controls behaviors in the body. The brain has the overarching control over neuroendocrine, autonomic, and immune function (McEwen, 2007). The CNS regulates sensory and motor functions and their integration. With stress, the brain is integral in processing stress perception and initiating physiologic responses (Bilkei-Gorzo, Racz, et al., 2008; McEwen, 2009). More specifically, the limbic system receives and integrates information about the stressor and sets off the neurologic cascade of responding events (Bilkei-Gorzo, Racz, et al., 2008). The hippocampus, amygdala, thalamus, and limbic cortex are major components of the limbic system responsible for reactions to perceived sensory stimuli. The amygdala, for example, regulates alterations in respiratory function when a stressor is perceived (Bondarenko, Hodgson, & Nalivaiko, 2014). With an anxiety-provoking situation, the respiratory rate may increase rapidly, then decrease once the stimulus is removed (Bondarenko et al., 2014).

Information about olfaction (smell), emotions, behavior, and long-term memory is processed through this system. Olfactory pathways are highly plastic in that structure and function in neurons can be altered through the experiences from different odors or scents (Claudianos et al., 2014). This **plasticity** can be appreciated through the example of how a certain scent can sometimes trigger a memory along with an emotion attached to that memory.

The response initiated from limbic assimilation of the information depends on how the individual interprets the information. This can be variable because it depends on each individual's genetic and early environmental experiences.

A repeated negatively interpreted stressor can turn into a chronic stress, leading to neuronal maladaptive plasticity. On the positive side, the aberrant adaptation can be reversible, especially once the stressor is removed (McEwen, 2009). In essence, the brain bridges the psychological and physiologic aspects of stress (McEwen, 2009).

Neuroendocrine Regulation

Endocrine glands synthesize and secrete hormones, chemical messengers that cause changes in other cells of the body. The pituitary, pineal, thymus, thyroid, and adrenal glands, and pancreas are major endocrine glands. Additionally, hormones are secreted from the testes in men and ovaries in women. The action of hormones is often a cascade event. Hormones released from one gland travel through the bloodstream to another gland, and trigger the secondary gland to release certain hormones. Eventually, the final hormones released from the cascade will act on cells for a specific purpose such as the regulation of growth and development, metabolism, and stress. Increased levels of hormones act as a negative feedback loop to the original glands, causing them to decrease or completely stop secreting the triggering hormones (Holsboer & Ising, 2010).

Neuroendocrine regulation of stress is a complex process involving the hypothalamus, pituitary, and adrenal glands known as the **hypothalamic–pituitary–adrenal** (HPA) axis.

The primary triggering of this system stems from the CNS. Once stress is perceived by the limbic system, signals will be sent to the hypothalamus. The basic functioning consists of secretion of corticotropin-releasing hormone (CRH) from the hypothalamus, which in turn triggers the secretion of adrenocorticotropic hormone (ACTH) from the anterior pituitary (Timmermans, Xiong, Hoogenraad, & Krugers, 2013). ACTH then stimulates the secretion of corticosteroids from the adrenal cortex (Holsboer & Ising, 2010) (Fig. 41-1). The corticosteroids include glucocorticoids, which increase glucose levels, and mineralocorticoids, such as aldosterone, which regulate electrolytes (Holsboer & Ising, 2010).

Under normal daily activity, glucocorticoids are released in a circadian pattern, peaking in humans in the early morning hours (Di, Maxson, Franco, & Tasker, 2009). Under the duress of stress, glucocorticoid levels can elevate at any time (Di et al., 2009). Cortisol is the primary glucocorticoid released from the adrenal cortex. It is involved in numerous functions, including glucose, lipid, and protein metabolism; immune activity (anti-inflammatory and immunosuppressive actions); and regulatory activity in the nervous, muscular, gastrointestinal, cardiovascular, and genitourinary systems. Additionally, cortisol influences behavior, mood, and cognitive function. Under acute stress, cortisol is protective of mood whereas under chronic stress, it is associated with depression and anxiety.

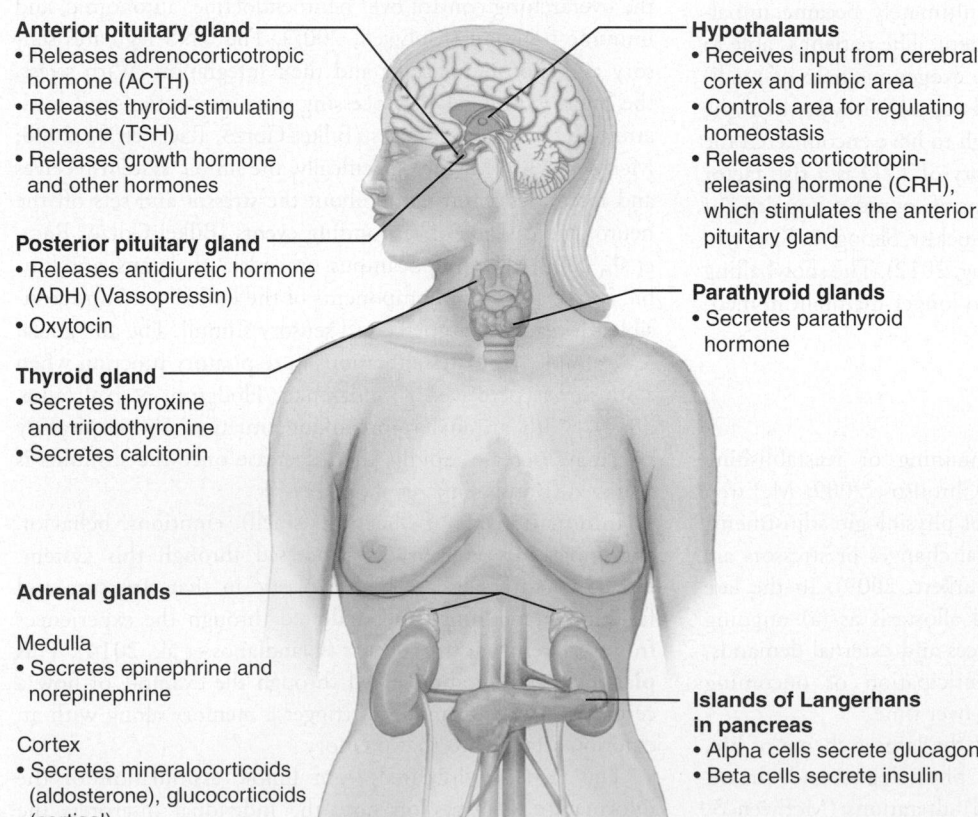

Anterior pituitary gland
• Releases adrenocorticotropic hormone (ACTH)
• Releases thyroid-stimulating hormone (TSH)
• Releases growth hormone and other hormones

Posterior pituitary gland
• Releases antidiuretic hormone (ADH) (Vassopressin)
• Oxytocin

Thyroid gland
• Secretes thyroxine and triiodothyronine
• Secretes calcitonin

Adrenal glands

Medulla
• Secretes epinephrine and norepinephrine

Cortex
• Secretes mineralocorticoids (aldosterone), glucocorticoids (cortisol)

Hypothalamus
• Receives input from cerebral cortex and limbic area
• Controls area for regulating homeostasis
• Releases corticotropin-releasing hormone (CRH), which stimulates the anterior pituitary gland

Parathyroid glands
• Secretes parathyroid hormone

Islands of Langerhans in pancreas
• Alpha cells secrete glucagon
• Beta cells secrete insulin

FIGURE 41-1 Location of specific endocrine glands that affect the body's adaptation to stress.

Autonomic Regulation

The autonomic nervous system (ANS) is integral in responding to actual or potential stress. The ANS response involves several systems throughout the body by inducing contraction of both smooth and cardiac muscles to regulate cardiovascular, respiratory, gastrointestinal, renal, and endocrine function. Starting at the CNS level in response to stress or other emotional events, noradrenergic nerve fibers from the locus caeruleus act on β-adrenergic receptors in the limbic region, including the amygdala, hippocampus, and prefrontal cortex (Timmermans et al., 2013). Assimilation and response to the perceived event is further processed through the two main divisions of the ANS. The sympathetic and parasympathetic divisions of the ANS each have specific target tissues and functions. The sympathetic nervous system (SNS) has nerves that exit the spinal column from the thoracic and lumbar regions and secrete the neurotransmitter norepinephrine (also known as noradrenaline). Activation of the SNS also causes the secretion of the neurohormone epinephrine (also known as adrenaline) from the adrenal medulla into the bloodstream, causing sympathetic stimulation to all organs of the body, not just the ones directly innervated by the sympathetic nerves releasing the norepinephrine. Depending on the targeted tissue or organ, epinephrine and norepinephrine will be excitatory or inhibitory. During a stressful situation, the excitatory actions will cause pupil dilation, increased heart rate and force of contraction, bronchial dilation, and stimulation of converting glycogen to glucose. The sympathetic inhibitory responses decrease activity in certain organs that would interfere with other activities needed at that time. These inhibitory effects include decreasing digestive function, inhibiting insulin secretion from the pancreas, and preventing urination. The nerves of the parasympathetic nervous system (PNS) exit the spinal column from the brain stem along with fewer branches leaving from the sacral region. The major neurotransmitter secreted is acetylcholine. Following the resolution of a stressful event, PNS activation ensues, causing pupil constriction, watery secretions of salivary glands, decreased heart rate, constriction of the bronchioles, increased digestive function, increased insulin secretion, and promotion of the release of urine, thus helping the body return to a state of dynamic equilibrium. In all of its actions, the ANS is a key physiologic regulator of the stress response (Holsboer & Ising, 2010).

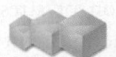 **Concept Mastery Alert**

In times of stress, norepinephrine and epinephrine have similar, not opposing, physiologic functions. These include increased heart rate and contractility, bronchial dilation, heightened awareness, and pupil dilation. Norepinephrine and epinephrine are not counterpoints in the manner of the SNS and the parasympathetic nervous.

Immune Regulation

The immune system is a complex network of protective mechanisms that has key roles in maintaining homeostasis. From mechanical barriers such as skin and mucous membranes that keep harmful microorganisms from entering body's internal environment to specialized cells produced by the bone marrow, immune function prevents and fights infections and the formation of abnormal cells. As a stress responder, the immune system is activated to maintain homeostasis with acute stress onset, such as when trauma, infections, and autoimmune responses occur. In particular, interleukin-6 (IL-6), one of the proinflammatory cytokines expressed when the immune system is activated, stimulates activation of the HPA axis.

Sustained **inflammation** can occur with chronic stress, referred to as neuroinflammation (Sierra et al., 2014). With neuroinflammation, the HPA axis triggers an oversecretion of glucocorticoids, leading to maladaptive plasticity with resultant cognitive impairment (Sierra et al., 2014). For the patient in our case study, this pathway is prominent with his T2D, an indicator of uncontrolled hyperglycemia. Hyperglycemia triggers oxidative stress that, in turn, impairs normal immune cell functioning (Buchholz & Stephens, 2008). Additionally, mitochondria (the cell's energy source) in muscle tissue can become impaired (Iqbal & Hood, 2014), potentially interfering with the ability to appropriately respond to future acute stresses. In the case of this patient, the physiologic stress of the T2D appears highly associated with the Alzheimer disease, both with linkages to impaired immune system functioning.

In general, immune system inhibition from chronic stress can increase the risk of infections, allergies, autoimmune disorders, and cardiovascular disease. Stress at the immune level, therefore, can lead to a cascade of multiple health-related challenges.

Characteristics of Stress, Coping, and Adaptation

The word *stress* can have different meanings as well as mean different things to different people at different times. The mechanical definition of stress describes a load or force placed on a structure. It is the psychoemotional definition that can be elusive. Mostly thought of in terms of an event or situation (the stressor or stimulus) causing feelings of anxiety, discomfort, fear, or similar, stress is predominately perceived as negative. Stress is also unavoidable. Stress interpreted as angst and grief is sometimes labeled *distress*. The ability to appraise and cope with stress, and the subsequent physiologic responses, are an integral part of the experience of life.

STRESS AS A STIMULUS

The classical transactional stress model created by Lazarus and Folkman in 1984 describes the process of stress from the point of appraisal through **coping mechanisms** (Bacon et al., 2009). The triggering event or stressor initiates the cascade of events. A stressor can be any number of triggering events, including environmental changes, alterations in routine activities, or unexpected traumas or tragedies (Bellar et al., 2009). The stressor, therefore, is the stimulus initiating the stress response.

In the middle of the last century, Selye and Fortier (1950) described how a stressor triggers the physiologic response through a model they termed the *general adaptation syndrome* (GAS). The GAS explains how the initiating stressor triggers an alarm reaction (initial physiologic response) by the body followed by a stage of resistance (reestablishment of homeostasis) and finally a stage of exhaustion (resolution and full recovery or disease) (Selye & Fortier, 1950). In this model, the stressor was presented as the onset of a physical injury to the body and the associated emotional and physiologic responses. Current studies and discussions include psychosocial events such as work and relationship issues as well as unexpected events, which can be physical (natural disasters, trauma, injuries) or emotional (death of a loved one) stressors. Social stress, for example, can alter neural function and lead to adverse experiences. An epidemiologic study examined the impact of social marginalization among ethnic minorities and found correlations between perceived discrimination and alterations in brain activity (Akdeniz et al., 2014). These researchers believe there may be a linkage between such social stress and mental illness (Akdeniz et al., 2014).

In this context, stressors create an overt adverse outcome. Stress, however, can also be favorable. Selye coined the term *eustress* (Greek; with *eu* meaning "well" or "good") to describe positive stress (American Institute of Stress, 2010). Eustress also activates the physiologic stress pathways but in this context includes pleasurable stimuli such as participating in fun sports activities or enjoying treatments at a spa. Because stress is reliant upon individual interpretation and experiences, measuring stress can be challenging.

The Everyday Hassles Scale (Box 41-1) was created by Lazarus, a renowned stress researcher, to evaluate and quantify stressors in life, both negative and positive (Lazarus, 1981). This model was tested in comparison to a major life events model for its effectiveness. The Hassles scale, which includes "hassles" or stressors that create undesirable stress and "uplifts" that create the positive feelings of exhilaration and well-being, was found to perform more accurately than did the standard life events model (Kanner, Coyne, Schaefer, & Lazarus, 1981). The Everyday Hassles measurement tool of stress continues to be the basis for current stress studies. Since stress is so variable and an individual experience, using such measurement tools of stress can help define the stressors and degree of emotional and related physiologic response for each individual. In essence, it quantifies the allostatic load and risk for disease.

Both genetic predisposition and life events (or epigenetic factors) shape how an individual assimilates to stress and the risk of the outcome of disease. Numerous factors including age at each event, gender, cultural beliefs, and values can contribute to the outcome. Gillespie and colleagues (2009)

BOX 41-1 Lazarus's Everyday Hassles Scale

The following scale rank-orders "hassles," which contribute to stress, and "uplifts," which contribute positively to stress management, as evaluated by several middle-aged patient groups. Nurses may determine the patient's hassles and uplifts for purposes of providing anticipatory guidance. Individual patients may perceive hassles and uplifts differently from the groups studied by Lazarus.

Hassles (Rank Ordered)
1. Feeling concerned about weight
2. Worrying about health of a family member
3. Worrying about rising cost of living
4. Dealing with home maintenance
5. Having too many things to do
6. Misplacing or losing things
7. Doing yard work or outside home maintenance
8. Worrying about property, investment, or taxes
9. Worrying about crime
10. Feeling concern about physical appearance

Uplifts (Rank Ordered)
1. Relating well to spouse or lover
2. Relating well with friends
3. Completing a task
4. Feeling healthy
5. Getting enough sleep
6. Eating out
7. Meeting responsibilities
8. Visiting, telephoning, or writing someone
9. Spending time with family
10. Taking pleasure in one's home

Source: Lazarus, R. S. (1981). Little hazards can be hazardous to your health. *Psychology Today, 15*(7), 58–62.

explored genetic and environmental influences on the development of the stress response in relation to depression and posttraumatic stress syndrome. The HPA axis was found to be a central component in early exposures related to long-term outcomes such as anxiety and depression (Gillespie et al., 2009).

STRESS AS A RESPONSE

Early research based on Cannon's 1932 definition of stress described the stress response in terms of sympathetic activity triggered from the causative agent or stressor (Selye, 1950). The fight-or-flight scenario (discussed above) explained the physiologic reactions of needing an increased heart rate, dilation of the bronchi, and increased synthesis and release of glucose for the individual to best respond to the situation at hand. The response choices were to stay and physically fight or run away to escape harm. This is the classic example of encountering a large animal in the wild.

Over time, research has refined these definitions and models to incorporate all of the complexities involved. The newest model, termed the Reactive Scope Model, expands on the allostatic load model and incorporates homeostasis, stress, and allostasis (Romero, Dickens, & Cyr, 2009). Within the reactive scope model, the integration of each physiologic system involved, along with their corresponding mediators and outcomes are used to describe the process of the sequence of events and predict outcomes. Furthermore, the model allows for predictions, such as who is more likely to recover under the duress of a prolonged response versus who is more likely to develop a pathology under the same parameters of the prolonged response (Romero et al., 2009).

Studies also show stress response differences between men and women. In addition to structural differences of the brain (e.g., men have more brain volume and white matter, while women have more gray matter and a more complex cortical structure), studies have shown that women have greater verbal skills, while men have greater spatial ability (although these findings warrant further investigation) (Darnall & Suarez, 2009). Women have higher levels of estrogen, which are associated with greater sensitivity to stress and a tendency towards being emotionally supportive and building meaningful relationships. The higher testosterone levels in men are associated with more aggressive reactions (Darnall & Suarez, 2009). The sympathetic fight or flight is therefore more masculine in context, while the feminine role is sometimes termed *tend and befriend.*

The interpretations of stress are as individual as the responses to stress. The physiologic pathway triggered, however, is predominately the same. The genetic predisposition coupled with the various experiences or environmental challenges throughout each stage of life shape how stress is assimilated at subsequent stages of life. Individuals who adapt effective coping skills tend to do well and experience the positive sense of accomplishments. These individuals are often good "problem solvers" and can even enjoy the process of overcoming life's challenges. Each challenge with a successful outcome reinforces the skills and confidence.

Physiologic Stress Response

The physiologic response to stress begins with processing of the stressor by the brain. The emotional regions of the brain (limbic system) assimilate the stimulus and have neural communication with various areas of the brain, including the hippocampus, basal ganglia, amygdala, hypothalamus, parts of the prefrontal cortex, insula, and various medullary and brainstem nuclei (McEwen, 2009). Many neural connections exist between the limbic system regions and the hypothalamus. Ultimately, it is the hippocampus that regulates the emotional information processes in the various areas and serves as the coordinator of activity in the HPA axis.

Although activation of the HPA axis is critical to the stress response, the first responder is actually the ANS. In particular, immediate stimulation of the SNS division of the ANS causes release of the catecholamines epinephrine and norepinephrine. The catecholamines trigger initial responses of increased heart rate and dilation of the pupils, bronchi, and blood vessels. Feelings of nervousness, excitement, and heightened awareness are associated with these physiologic responses.

Following ANS stimulation, the HPA axis is activated with the hypothalamus being at the forefront of the stress response. The parvocellular CRH and arginine-vasopressin (AVP) neurons of the hypothalamus coordinate activity with central catecholaminergic neurons of the brain stem (Holsboer & Ising, 2010). CRH, in particular, is the key hypothalamic stimulator of the pituitary and, in turn, adrenal glands. Signals from the hypothalamus from CRH stimulate release of ACTH from the anterior pituitary, and concurrent AVP stimulation enhances the action of CRH (Holsboer & Ising, 2010). ACTH is released into circulation, where it ultimately stimulates the adrenal cortex to synthesize and release glucocorticoids (Holsboer & Ising, 2010). The glucocorticoids, particularly cortisol, activate several systemic activities. Glucocorticoids provide energy to the CNS, muscles, and other systems throughout the body. These steroids have anti-inflammatory effects, suppress immune activity, increase blood glucose levels, and increase arousal and cognition.

The activated HPA axis depends on signal feedback for regulation. A negative feedback mechanism occurs with increased levels of glucocorticoids. Glucocorticoids regulate HPA activity and terminate the stress response through engaging receptors on cells within the hypothalamus. Under conditions of excessive stress, the feedback mechanisms may fail to function optimally and offset the normal process. Since glucocorticoids are extensively involved in the functioning and regulations of tissues, organs, and systems throughout the body, interferences in the system can lead to numerous problems.

Regulation of this stress perception/stress response system can be influenced by psychobiologic allostasis, or the degree to which an individual has resistance and resilience. **Resilience** can be described as being able to recover from an adverse event, whereas **resistance** is adaptability to adversity (Karatsoreos & McEwen, 2011). The opposite is vulnerability or the inability to adapt to adversity (Karatsoreos & McEwen, 2011). **Vulnerability** is suspected to evolve following a major adverse event or multiple adversities, leading to decreased resistance and resilience in future adverse situations. Many molecules are involved in the adaptive plasticity of the brain that will shift towards greater resistance and resilience or vulnerability. Brain-derived neurotrophic factor (BDNF), in particular, is greatly involved in brain remodeling with stress (Gray, Milner, & McEwen, 2013). With chronic stress, BDNF levels are diminished, resulting in cognitive alterations and increased anxiety (Karatsoreos & McEwen, 2011). Once again, the case study patient is reflective of these pathophysiologic processes.

Further, under chronic stress conditions, allostatic load is progressive, leading to any number of disease processes.

The overexpression of the stress response mediators (e.g., sympathetic activity, glucocorticoid release, etc.) leads to cellular damage, which, in turn, can evolve into pathologies (McEwen, 2007). In fact, several specific disease processes have been found to have strong associations with psychological stress, including depression, cardiovascular disease, and HIV/AIDS. Furthermore, studies show evidence for stress-associated respiratory problems, infections, autoimmune disorders, and poor wound healing, with less evidence for some cancers. Physiologically, it would appear that stress is a contributor to cancer. Cortisol released during the stress response impairs immune activity. Immunosuppression is associated with several malignancies. Further studies are needed to assess the extent to which stress is associated with cancer, response to treatment, and survival.

Cognitive and Psychological Response to Stress

Psychological stress, as implied, begins at the cognitive level. The challenge, threat, or obstacle encountered, be it real or not, is *perceived* as real and the physiologic responders engage accordingly. As the various parts of the limbic system assimilate the information, the ANS initiates the start of the physiologic response, followed by HPA activation, as described above. The physiologic component, however, is also part of the cognitive reaction. Normal basal levels of glucocorticoids (small doses that are released throughout the day and night as part of normal physiologic functioning without the influence of stress or other events) are part of normal cognitive function. With stress, glucocorticoid levels increase, creating heightened awareness of the impending situation while also temporarily dampening long-term memory. The acute stress response enhances mood. Under chronic stress, however, depression and anxiety can manifest.

Appraisal precedes stress, and once the situation is accepted as stress, appraisal continues as an assessment of how to deal with the situation (Bacon et al., 2009). This is called secondary appraisal and is associated with engaging in coping mechanisms to deal with the stress. Buffering as a mechanism for coping can be helpful or harmful depending on the activity. Social buffering or the act of soliciting other individuals to help resolve or provide comfort during a stressful event can be quite effective.

Defense mechanisms such as daydreaming, fantasizing, or sleeping may be used as a form of temporary removal from the stressor. Table 41-1 is a comprehensive list of defense mechanisms. Other buffers or defense mechanisms can also help an individual to escape but might be more harmful, such as the use of alcohol or drugs. These temporary mechanisms, called avoidance coping, may alleviate the feelings of anxiety brought on by the stress for a short period of time, but the stressor still needs to be addressed. Prolonged avoidance of the situation can lead to allostatic load with possible disease manifestations as well as decreasing the ability to cope and adapt during future stressful events.

TABLE 41-1 COMMON DEFENSE MECHANISMS

Compensation	The attempt to achieve respect or recognition in one activity as a substitute for inability to achieve in another endeavor
Denial	Refusing to believe or accept something as it is but rather as one wishes it to be
Displacement	Transferring emotion away from the person or situation that incited the emotion to an inappropriate person or object
Introjection	Taking into one's personality the characteristics of another
Projection	Attributing one's own thoughts, emotions, characteristics, or motives to another
Rationalization	Concealing the motive for behavior by giving some socially acceptable reason for the action
Regression	Return to behaviors more appropriate to an earlier stage of development
Repression	Immersing something in the subconscious or unconscious level of thought
Sublimation	Release of libido in socially acceptable behavior rather than using it to obtain sexual gratification
Suppression	Consciously dismissing something from the mind and thoughts

Normal Coping Patterns

Coping is the process of applying thoughts and actions to deal with stressful events. There are various mechanisms to coping. The two major types of coping strategies are problem focused and emotion focused (Box 41-2). Coping strategies can also be long-term or short-term and may include actions that are beneficial or detrimental. Problem-focused coping directly deals with the challenge, and the successful outcome can lead to psychosocial well-being. Emotion-focused coping is directed at controlling emotions during a stressful event that is perceived as unchangeable (Bacon et al., 2009). Coping and appraisal are constant during the stressful period, especially in chronic stress situations. As different aspects of the event unfold, appraising the moment and engaging in coping strategies may shift as needed. For example, dealing with a hospitalized loved one can be quite stressful. There may be a period of time with an unknown outcome. As information about the patient's status evolves, appraisal of the new information along with coping strategies will be implemented. Each new piece of information may also reignite the physiologic stress response. The technique known as *cognitive reappraisal* may be valuable in such a situation. Cognitive reappraisal uses "reality checking" to reduce future negative emotions and behaviors. In the above example, cognitive reappraisal would help the loved one to put the situation into perspective. Instead of assuming the worst and becoming fully anxious about the thought of the patient dying, the information known would become

> ### BOX 41-2 Examples of Coping Strategies

Examples of Problem-Oriented Coping Mechanisms
- Making a time schedule for studying and sticking to it
- Applying for a job at another company because your current position is not supporting your professional growth
- Trying to find out more about an illness, such as diabetes, to manage it better

Examples of Emotion-Focused Coping Mechanisms
- Accepting sympathy and understanding from a friend in the loss of a family member
- Releasing tension after a hard day at work by meditating, crying, or taking a walk
- Blaming someone else—for example, a spouse or teacher—for the situation you are in

Examples of Long-Term Coping Mechanisms
- Working out stress through physical exercise
- Talking with others about problems (friend, counselor)
- Relying on belief in a higher power
- Seeking additional information about a situation
- Drawing on past experience
- Developing alternative plans for handling the situation

Examples of Short-Term Coping Mechanisms
- Smoking
- Alcohol use
- Overeating
- "Pill-popping"
- Excessive caffeine intake

The case study patient, therefore, is at increased risk for poor coping skills by virtue of his physiologic conditions. The patient's daughter and other family members affected by his comorbid conditions on a psychosocial level are also at increased risk for coping deficiencies, decreased resistance and resilience, and increased vulnerability. Even in the absence of disease, chronic stress impairs healthy neuronal adaptation (Wosiski-Kuhn et al., 2014). These family members, however, are at a potential increased risk for T2D themselves, as genetic linkages have been found (Verhoog et al., 2013). The added stress of a dependent family member can only exacerbate this, triggering his or her own aberrant HPA responses.

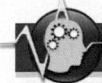 **APPLY YOUR CRITICAL THINKING**

You are a nursing student about to take your second pathophysiology test of the quarter. You received a poor grade on the first exam, so you stayed up all night studying hard to do better on this test. You left the house in a hurry this morning without eating breakfast because your stomach felt upset. Now as you sit down to take the exam, your heart is racing, your hands are sweaty and cold, and you are having trouble concentrating. What do you think is the physiologic cause of your symptoms? In what positive ways could you cope with the stress of the situation?

Check your answers in Appendix B.

Life Span Considerations

Genetic predisposition, the environment, and the ability to deal with each stressful event throughout life set the tone for each successive stressful event. In effect, the response to stress and adaptability has a cumulative effect throughout the lifespan (McEwen, 2007). Additionally, evidence is emerging how stressful events to a woman during pregnancy influence how her children handle stress in their lives. There is also evidence that HPA alterations occur in preterm infants whose mothers received glucocorticoids during pregnancy, also leading to problems with the stress response for these offspring. From conception through old age, each stage of life has an impact on stress and conversely, stress at all ages impacts current and future life (Wagner et al., 2014). Some parental stress, however, may benefit the offspring. A large historical study found greater survival among children who were conceived during disease epidemics in the 1700s (Willfuhr & Myrskyla, 2014). This idea of epigenetic transgenerational phenotypic expression of stronger survivability (Willfuhr & Myrskyla, 2014) would be in alignment with the notion of eustress (Selye, 1950). It is important to evaluate the numerous influences at each stage of life.

the focus instead of dwelling on the information unknown. If the situation were such that is was most likely the patient would not survive, starting to deal with that impending loss would be appropriate. In both scenarios, the use of social buffering in having a support system close at hand would be most beneficial.

Coping mechanisms in a current situation are dependent on the individual's level of resistance, resilience, and vulnerability acquired through prior adverse events. The HPA axis is greatly involved in the stress resilience/vulnerability response (Franklin, Saab, & Mansuy, 2012). Integral to HPA activation is the hippocampus, a major regulator of corticosteroids. Stimulation of the hippocampus decreases glucocorticoid levels; conversely, with stress, these levels are inhibited, causing increase activation of the HPA axis resulting in higher levels of glucocorticoids (Franklin et al., 2012). Glucocorticoids, in turn, can regulate hippocampal function (Franklin et al., 2012). Chronic stress-induced glucocorticoid exposure suppresses BDNF, causing decreased synaptic plasticity (Wosiski-Kuhn, Erion, Gomez-Sanchez, Gomez-Sanchez, & Stranahan, 2014). Diabetic stress contributes to this impaired system (Wosiski-Kuhn et al., 2014).

NEWBORN AND INFANT

Newborns and infants depend on the care of others for survival. Innate reflex responses are their initial strategies for coping with stress. Under normal healthy circumstances, the stressors of feeling hungry or the need for touch are quickly relieved with the mother's or other adult's attentive response to the crying baby. The need for touch, bonding, and attachment are essential for the development of the infant. A study by Figueiredo and Costa (2009) evaluated newborn/infant attachment in mothers and infants 3 months before and 3 months after birth. From pregnancy to the postpartum period, several measurements, including cortisol levels, were evaluated. Findings suggested that with the mother's increased cortisol and anxiety levels, emotional involvement toward the child decreased. Stress and poor emotional involvement during pregnancy predicted poor emotional involvement after birth. Human outcomes such as failure to thrive in infants are associated with lack of maternal or similar nurturing contact and emotional involvement.

Newborns who spend the first days, weeks, or even months in the neonatal intensive care units are exposed to stressful stimuli of light, sounds, unpleasant and unnatural handling for diagnostic procedures and treatments, and even painful procedures.

Healthy newborns may also be vulnerable to health issues later in life if their essential needs are not met. Infant brain development depends on parents or caregivers providing protection, the process of healthy attachment, responsive care, and breast milk/breast-feeding (Bryanton & Beck, 2010). Although many newborns/infants cannot be breast-fed and develop without problems, attention to nutrition in this area is important for optimal brain development and how well the individual can respond to and adapt to stressful events throughout life.

TODDLER AND PRESCHOOLER

Coping strategies become more evolved as a child develops. Learning behaviors and how to handle stressors, such as not getting something that is wanted right away or at all, depend on how parents, siblings, and others who are an integral part of the child's early life respond to the child's needs and desires. Children who are used to immediate gratification may grow up to always have such expectations.

Stressful events such as getting injured can have a significant impact later in life. Protection and safety of the child is the responsibility of adults. Minor stressors can feel major to this age group as well. Family members set boundaries and help the toddler/preschooler in handling stressful events (Fig. 41-2).

SCHOOL-AGE CHILD AND ADOLESCENT

School-age children and adolescents are in the expanded environment of school and related social activities in addition to their family environments. Stress from various events can occur. In these age groups, stress is most commonly due to new, unfamiliar/uncomfortable and/or unpredictable situations, uncertain expectations, and/or fear of unpleasant events or failure

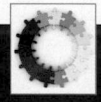

COLLABORATING WITH THE HEALTHCARE TEAM
Contacting the Social Worker Concerning a Patient's Relocation Anxiety

Mrs. Ella Roe, age 85 years, has severe vision and hearing problems along with lack of stability in gait and movement.

SITUATION: Mrs. Roe's children have decided that for her own safety and their peace of mind, their mother must relocate to an adult living facility where she can have more assistance if needed.

BACKGROUND: Mrs. Roe has always prided herself on being independent and overcoming all odds, so she sees this relocation from her home as a defeat and a denial of everything she has accomplished.

ASSESSMENT: The family needs the social worker to spend time with Mrs. Roe and the children to help them clarify the problem from both viewpoints and reach an agreeable decision.

RECOMMENDATION: Could you work with this family in finding some accommodation in the concerns of both Mrs. Roe and her children?

CRITICAL THINKING CHALLENGE
- Discuss the rationale for requesting that the social worker be the health team member to work with Mrs. Roe and her family.
- Are there other members of the collaborative team who could be called on to help if you do not have access to a social worker?
- If you needed to start the negotiating among all parties, what would be the concerns that you would want brought to the forefront for consideration?

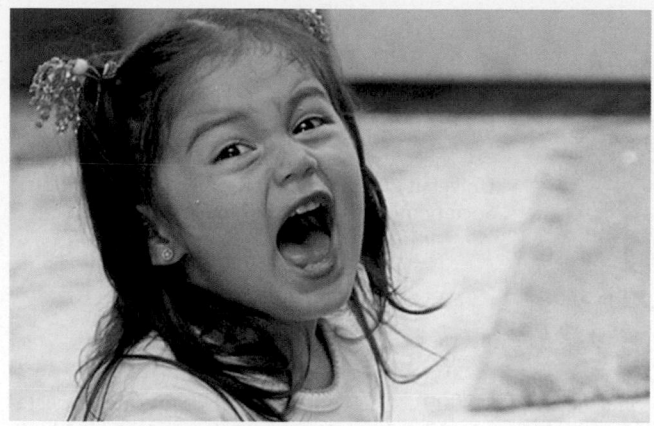

FIGURE 41-2 Temper tantrums are a natural result of the frustration that toddlers experience when attempting to assert their independence. During a tantrum, a trusted adult needs to remain nearby to reassure the child and provide security.

(Washington, 2009). At this stage, there is great pressure to perform well in school and fit in with peers and friends. Added stress may come from parental and sibling expectations.

Several factors influence stress and coping in children and adolescents. Age, gender roles, the onset of menarche in girls, developmental maturation, family dynamics, temperament, and parental models can lead to good or maladaptive coping strategies (Washington, 2009). Younger children use their cognitive abilities, motor skills, emotional states, social abilities, and feelings of self-worth (or lack of) in coping with stressful situations. They can incorporate reason into the experience but may not be able to rationalize. Magical thinking can cloud the truth. An example is a child thinking that his or her sibling became sick because the child had done something "bad." Coping may manifest as assertive behavior, engaging in symbolic play, and going to parents for comfort (Washington, 2009).

During adolescence, the ability to cope with stress becomes more evolved and complex. Adolescents' level of reasoning matures, and they can begin to rationalize events. They are also better at using emotion-focused coping mechanisms and problem solving. Furthermore, adolescents can use cognitive reframing and self-talk to better handle stressful events (Washington, 2009). They will continue to use other family members as models. For some adolescents, development of coping skills can be difficult. Events perceived as traumatic disruptions to their lives such as moving/changing schools can have an enormous negative impact until they adapt to their new environment and establish new friends and peer groups. The adjustment phase can be quite difficult. The need to fit in is enormous in this phase of life, and negative behaviors such as smoking and using alcohol and drugs to fit in is not uncommon. Adolescents having problems adjusting may also withdraw or overeat to feel comforted. Further, loneliness has been found to be associated with engaging in risky behaviors such as alcohol and illegal drug use in adolescents—a type of coping mechanism that can be carried forward in life (Stickley, Koyanagi,

Koposov, Schwab-Stone, & Ruchkin, 2014). Congruent with this, another study found that adolescents with high physiologic stress reactivity were able to mitigate such effects when they had effective coping skills (Paysnick & Burt, 2014).

It is important to note that coping strategies vary within different age groups. Early adolescent years may rely on metacognitive (awareness of one's own knowledge and abilities) coping, middle adolescents may tend toward using personal values, and late adolescents may use coping mechanisms with a focus on long-term goals.

Gender differences are also prominent. Girls may be more focused on family, personal appearance/body image, personal health, peer acceptance, and family issues compared to their male counterparts, who may be more focused on sports and game-related activities (Washington, 2009). Distraction coping techniques such as exercise or daydreaming are common for both genders. Family security continues to be of high importance.

ADULT AND OLDER ADULT

Exposure to stress from conception through adolescence contributes to adaptability to stress during the adult and older adult years. The responsibilities of adulthood add a new dimension of stress. Even under the happy occasions of new relationships, marriage, having children, career developments, and even moves that are a reflection of these happy events, stress can be part of the process. Successful coping strategies in younger years will add to the success of coping with these new life changes (Fig. 41-3).

Being in the adult/parental role of the family can compound stress. The adults are now the model for how their children will, in part, learn to cope with stress. Moving and starting a new job can add direct stress on the parents while they also have to help their children cope with the move and

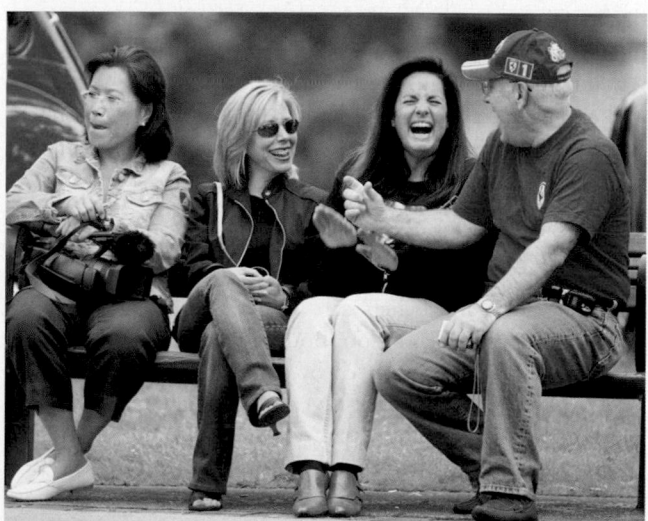

FIGURE 41-3 After retirement, the older adult can adapt to life changes by finding avenues for new relationships and social interaction.

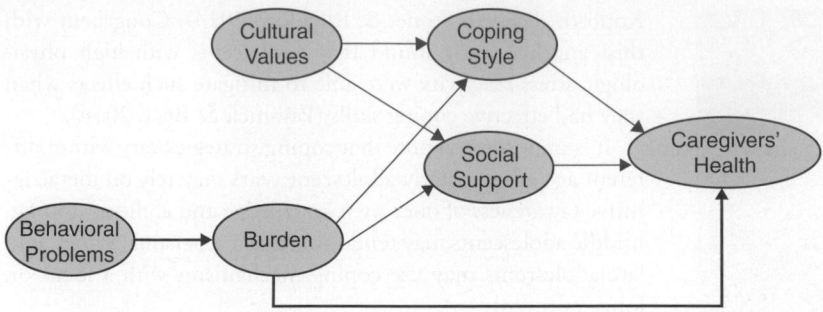

adjustment phase. In situations of divorce or death of a parent, stress levels can be significantly greater. Adults may also be in a position of having to take care of their aging parents. Balancing the demands of work and family along with caring for an aging parent can compound stress and may require advanced coping strategies.

Physiologic changes in adulthood add to this dynamic process. Adult brains go through a process of neurogenesis (development of new neurons), which further contributes to coping strategies and stress adaptability. In older age, this process of neurogenesis declines significantly. Cortical synapses, however, can undergo bidirectional modifications in adulthood (Verhoog et al., 2013), which can strengthen coping strategies. Stress, though, actually inhibits adult neurogenesis contributing to depression. More so, stress in early life can alter HPA axis function, leading to depression later in life (Juruena, 2013).

Additionally, declining neurogenesis may compound new stressful events in older age. Children are now adults and have established their own families, peers may die, their physical and cognitive abilities may decline, and with retirement their sense of self-worth may be diminished. Further, those who used alcohol as a coping mechanism in adolescence are at increased risk for encountering chronic mild stress in adulthood (Raineki et al., 2014). For women, the process of menopause with the decline of estrogen and associated physiologic symptoms (e.g., hot flashes, night sweats, mood alterations, dizziness, and the inability to concentrate) alters the HPA axis. Responses to stress and coping mechanisms may not be as fruitful as in younger years. For both men and women, the biomarkers related to the stress response are altered.

Cultural Considerations

Cultural values and beliefs can have a significant impact on stress, coping, and adaptation. Both psychological and biologic aspects of stress are influenced by culture. Cultures tend to be either individualistic or collectivistic. The main culture within the United States is individualistic, in which the self is seen as an independent entity with self-defining attributes and personal beliefs and goals (Sherman, Kim, & Taylor, 2009). Those who are individualistic also engage in self-chosen, limited-obligation relationships and tend to be more cognitively analytic. Cultures that are collectivistic, such as those seen in Asian countries, view the self as an interdependent part of others

(Sherman et al., 2009). The expression of emotions, expectations, and roles within the culture can shape an individual's response to stress. Some cultural beliefs, for example, discourage admitting feeling pain, as it may be thought of as a sign of weakness. A patient experiencing pain may hesitate to ask for pain medication so as not to break the cultural norm.

The Revised Sociocultural Stress and Coping Model (Fig. 41-4) considers such cultural differences. Based on evaluating how various cultures deal with caring for an older family member with chronic health issues, this model describes several major premises of sociocultural influences on stress and coping. In terms of caregiving, these include a common core model of caregiver stress, the cultural identity within a family (*familism*), and the resources used (such as social support) (Knight & Sayegh, 2010). In Asian cultures, there tends to be a strong sense of filial piety (high respect for parents and ancestors) compared to White, African American, and Hispanic Americans. The sense of filial piety in Asian cultures under the circumstance of an elder ill family member may have younger family members naturally assuming the caregiver role. In individualistic cultures, who will assume this role and the burden it will place on that individual's life may be perceived as a more stressful situation.

Coping strategies also vary by culture. One study evaluated the self-healing techniques used in Indo-Tibetan culture in terms of stress and allostasis. These techniques (e.g., interventions that integrated mindfulness with techniques of cognitive analysis, affect modulation, motivational imagery, and reinforcing breathing) appeared to minimize stress and promote healing. Furthermore, the various techniques allowed for individual differences and temperaments, all leading to similar outcomes.

FACTORS AFFECTING COPING PATTERNS

Many factors that can influence coping patterns can be as various as each individual is unique. Genetic predisposition, family and cultural environments, and prior exposures to stress and related outcomes all contribute to coping patterns. As stressors are initially perceived events, they will be interpreted differently by different people. The level of stress in one individual may be very different from the level of stress in another, given the same stressor. For example, one student in a class might feel a little bit of stress, but also excitement, over having to stand up in front of the class and give an oral presentation. This type of event may be a eustress for this student, with a feeling of accomplishment and exhilaration after the presentation. Another student in that same class may feel completely petrified at the thought of presenting in front of others, causing days of anxiety, lack of sleep, and an inability to concentrate leading up to the event. The event itself might feel terrifying. The aftermath could leave that student feeling exhausted and just relieved that it is over without reaping any benefits of a sense of accomplishment. Unexpected events can further influence subsequent stress responses. Natural disasters, terrorism, unexpected hospitalizations, or death of a loved one can greatly impact the interpretation and coping of future stressors, large or small.

Underlying these different experiences by individuals is self-efficacy. Described in the 1970s by Albert Bandura (1977), self-efficacy was hypothesized to determine the initiation and level of coping behaviors. In effect, various influences in life reinforce responses to stimuli and shape the behavior response (Bandura, 1977). Positive experiences can build self-confidence, which can lead to better coping skills with similar or increasing levels of stress. The converse is also true; for some, continued ineffective behavioral responses to stress remain after the stressor has been removed or diminished, leading to maladaptation to future stressors (McEwen, Eiland, Hunter, & Miller, 2012).

Lifestyle Considerations

Lifestyle is another contributor to stress, coping, and adaptation. Nutritional choices, exercise/fitness level, sleep, career choices, and socialization each influence the psychoemotional and physiologic processing of stress. Allostatic load may be greater in an individual with poor nutritional selections, a sedentary lifestyle, and self-destructive behaviors. A stressor to this individual may be perceived as significantly greater compared to an individual with a relatively healthy lifestyle of good nutrition, exercise, rest, and all around sense of well-being. The individual with the unhealthy lifestyle is at increased risk for a host of diseases, not just from the lifestyle habits but also as compounded by allostatic load due to ineffective coping with stress.

DIET

Good nutrition is essential for optimal functioning of cells throughout every tissue and organ in the body. Ideally, all of the nutrients needed are obtained from food. If certain vitamins or minerals are lacking, supplements may be beneficial. Overnutrition can be as detrimental as being undernourished. T2D, for example, is a condition of overnutrition that can lead to multiple morbidities, including impairing the ability to effectively cope and, as seen with the case study patient, contribute to cognitive impairment. Conversely, undernutrition or

malnutrition can be equally if not more detrimental. Cancer-related cachexia, for example, can cause severe physiologic and psychological stress (Vaughan, Martin, & Lewandowski, 2013). Such an extreme aside, having the right nutrients and balance will ready the body for action under stress.

ACTIVITY AND EXERCISE

Physical activity and exercise can greatly enhance an individual's ability to cope. Combined with good nutrition and other healthy lifestyle choices (not smoking, not drinking excessive amounts of alcohol, not using drugs, etc.), physical and psychological fitness can be achieved. Exercise not only improves cardiovascular function, helps with weight control, improves muscle tone, and enhances bone integrity but can greatly benefit psychological well-being. Additionally, exercise can be used as a coping mechanism in helping to decrease feelings of anxiety (emotion-focused coping) and help with processing of the situation to take action (problem-focused coping). Conversely, lack of exercise can contribute to poor health and a decreased ability to effectively cope.

SLEEP

Glucocorticoids, essential components of the stress response, regulate several actions in the body, including sleep. The basal release of cortisol also varies between day and night, and disturbances in sleep can shift this balance. Sleep is an important part of health and well-being. It becomes increasingly difficult to function optimally when there is a sleep deficit. With extreme sleep deficit in cases of chronic insomnia, the stress response system may not function adequately. Subsequently, sleep deprivation can increase allostatic load and lead to pathologic processes. People who do not get enough sleep tend to be irritable and have a lower threshold for minor disturbances throughout the day. Adults tend to sleep 1½ hours less than a century ago, but today life expectancy is about 30 years longer, mostly attributable to advances in science and medicine.

SAFETY AND SECURITY

Security depends on the perception of safety. The level of safety perceived may vary with each situation stimulating the stress. For example, stress caused by a mugger in a dark alley would be quite high with a very low sense of security. Stress induced by wanting to perform well in an athletic event while being surrounded by loving family and friends cheering the athlete on would have a considerably higher sense of security. The degree of safety and security will influence the effectiveness of coping mechanisms.

Previous Experience

The way each stressor is handled and the outcome of the event will influence subsequent stressful situations (McEwen & Wingfield, 2010). Successful outcomes will build confidence and aid in a subsequent similar stressful situation. In fact, repeated stressors that affect coping may stimulate less heightened perceptions of stress with each encounter. An example would be an actor in a play. On opening night, the actor may feel extreme levels of stress. A good performance will lead to slightly less feelings of stress at the start of the next performance. Continued good performances will build confidence, and eventually the start of a performance will have minimal stress. The feelings of accomplishment and achievement would be classified as a eustress.

The perception of stress can also be learned from other's experiences. A child whose parents display stress over finances may grow up and act similarly as an adult.

Involuntary Relocation

Moving to a new place is stressful even when the event is exciting and fully supported by all who are going. The transition part, however, of leaving behind the safety of familiarity, community, and comforts of an established home, along with setting up the new home, new routines, and building new relationships, can be quite stressful. For families with a parent in the military, multiple moves might be necessary. Children and adolescents in school may experience extreme stress with having to adjust to new schools and establish new friends and peer groups.

Older adults may also face involuntary relocation from an established home to an assistive living facility. This can be extremely stressful because the individual must leave the comforts and familiar surroundings of a long-established home. The individual may have also lost his or her spouse, compounding the sense of loss. In some instances, such a move can ultimately be positive as the individual gains a new sense of safety with on-hand caregivers, social activities, and less responsibility with activities of living such as preparing meals. Whether such a move is perceived as favorable or not, coping mechanisms are needed while adjusting to the new environment.

People at any age who become hospitalized for illnesses also face the stress not just of the illness but of adjusting to the new environment, people, and unfamiliar stimuli. A sense of security can also be established in this environment with constant care. Patients can sometimes feel stressed when it's time to be discharged back home.

The case study patient will endure another level of stress by his forced relocation to his daughter's house following hospitalization. Compounding this is his progressive Alzheimer disease, which will further inhibit his adaptation and coping mechanisms. This, in turn, will likely be disruptive to the dynamics of his daughter and her family in their home life. How well each of the family members adapts and copes with the changing life situation will depend on both their shared and personal genetic and epigenetic factors (McEwen et al., 2012).

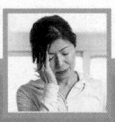

Stress, Coping, and Adaptation PICO

David is the triage nurse working in an Alzheimer clinic. The daughter from the chapter-opening scenario calls because she is concerned that her father is more depressed with all the changes. She tells David that her dad has been diagnosed with depression for years. Now with the onset of his Alzheimer disease and changes to his lifestyle, he seems to be really struggling. The daughter is not interested in putting her father on more medications. She is inquiring about other therapies to help his depression. David is familiar with some psychological therapies for depression and anxiety, but he is not quite comfortable discussing the success rates on it with the daughter. He turns to the Cochrane Library for help. David uses the following PICO question to start his search: *In Alzheimer patients, how do psychological treatments compared to no psychological treatments effect depression?*

P = Alzheimer patients
I = psychological treatments
C = no psychological treatments
O = effect depression

David finds a meta-analysis study involving patients with dementia. The research examined six randomized control trials involving 439 patients that compared psychological treatments with their usual care (i.e., social contact). Psychological treatments included cognitive behavioral therapy, counseling, and interpersonal psychodynamic therapy. The overall results concluded that psychological treatments used in addition to just social contact did improve depression in patients with dementia. Unfortunately, the studies did not reflect if one type of psychological therapy was better than the other, nor did it discuss success rates. David calls the daughter back to help her find options for her father.

REFERENCE

Orgeta, V., Qazi, A., Spector, A. E., & Orrell, M. (2014). Psychological treatments for depression and anxiety in dementia and mild cognitive impairment. *Cochrane Database of Systematic Reviews*, Issue 1, Art. No.: CD009125. DOI: 10.1002/14651858.CD009125.pub2.

Social Interaction

Stress is encountered under the best home circumstances. When there is separation, divorce, a death, a newborn with disabilities, the addition of an older adult moving in (as with the case study scenario), or any disruption to the established household, stress is encountered and adaptations must be made. Divorce can be particularly stressful on children as they enter a new routine of living part-time at each parent's home in addition to the loss of the family dynamic they once knew. Difficulty adjusting can lead to distress and impaired coping skills. Children may adapt new unfavorable behaviors and even join new peer groups with negative influence.

Dysfunctional home situations, especially those that entail abuse, can lead to ineffective coping techniques that can last a lifetime. Adults with poor coping skills may become abusers. Abuse can take many forms, including physical, sexual, and neglect. Children in an abusive home may find ways to protect themselves through forms of escape such as talking to imaginary friends or learning to shut off feelings. Increased neuroendocrine and ANS stress response with increased allostatic load has been shown in those on the receiving end of abuse, particularly in the young (McEwen, 2008). There are many agencies and support groups in the United States to protect against abuse at all levels (children, adults, and older adults).

Sensory Deficits

Sensory deficits such as loss of vision or hearing can impair the stress response, coping, and adaptation. Under stress, it is increasingly difficult for the person with an impaired sense to judge the situation, interpret the environment, and effectively cope. Misinterpretations can heighten the feelings of anxiety and enhance the physiologic stress response while being unable to adequately cope. Maladaptive coping skills can develop for future events.

ALTERED COPING PATTERNS

Addictive Behaviors

Maladaptive behaviors or altered coping mechanisms can manifest in numerous ways. Substance abuse, beginning or increasing smoking, oversleeping, over- or undereating, oversleeping, overexercising, excessive daydreaming, and fantasizing are various way individuals with the inability to cope with stress successfully deal with stress. Illness is another outcome that can be a result of stress. Additional examples are presented in Box 41-3.

The use of drugs and alcohol as a means of emotional escape is common among individuals with poor coping skills. Phrases such as "I just can't cope" and "I need to numb the pain" are not uncommon. Alcohol is legal, readily accessible, and a frequently used and abused substance. Alcohol, nicotine, and caffeine all cross the blood–brain barrier. Alcohol interferes with cognition, memory, and even motor movement; hence, it can interfere with the stress response, including blocking or clouding the emotional response from areas of the limbic system. Similarly, excessive use of both legal and illegal drugs alter brain function and help the individual to feel better and avoid dealing with the situation in the short term. These behaviors become addictive from repeated use to continue the escape in addition to the substances themselves, creating an addiction or "craving" of the substances. Dependency, psychological problems, and ultimately physiologic damage can ensue. The capacity to cope will decline the more the individual escapes coping. Adolescents are at particular risk for substance abuse due to their need for acceptance and the peer pressure related to this stage of development.

Smoking and caffeine also cross the blood–brain barrier, and can both be addictive. Increased caffeine intake is sometimes used to help counter feelings of exhaustion if the stress is also interfering with sleep. As opposed to alcohol, caffeine is a stimulant and will not mask the emotions.

Smoking often begins at the adolescent stage, also with peer pressure and the enormous need to fit in. Although smoking is considerably less promoted through marketing efforts than it once was, the habit can still be viewed as macho, cool, or sophisticated. Once the addiction is formed, it is difficult to quit. Additionally, smoking then becomes

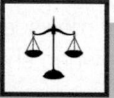

BOX 41-3   Psychosocial and Physiologic Expressions of Stress

Psychosocial Expressions

BEHAVIORS

Crying
Decreased motivation
Decreased self-esteem
Decreased intellectual processes
Forgetfulness
Impulsive behavior
Inability to make decisions
Learning disabilities
Poor concentration
Insomnia

EMOTIONS

Anger, anxiety
Nervousness
Moodiness, depression
Emotional instability
Irritability
Fears, phobias

Feeling out of control
Frustration
Feelings of worthlessness

Physiologic Expressions

Back, neck, or shoulder pain
Breathing irregularities
Elevated blood pressure
Change in appetite
Stuttering, trembling
Jaw tension
Sexual dysfunction
Constipation or diarrhea
Irregular heartbeat
Muscle cramps, spasms
Stomach, digestive disorders
Sweating, skin problems
Tension headaches
Fatigue

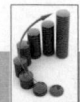

OUTCOME-BASED TEACHING PLANS

While caring for an older woman suffering from manic depression, you interview her 46-year-old daughter, Sophia. Sophia tells you that her mother has been married for 51 years to a man who has had quadruple cardiac bypass surgery, recurrent kidney and bladder cancer, and a long history of alcoholism, although he is not drinking currently. Sophia cooks and takes meals to them, drives them to their many healthcare appointments, handles their finances, and provides most of their support. Sophia is married, has three children, and works full-time. She states that she frequently is torn between her responsibilities to her parents and to her husband and children. You realize that Sophia, as the caregiver, may have some problems with stress and needs your attention. You decide to try to help her cope with them.

OUTCOME

Sophia will express more confidence in her ability to cope with competing responsibilities.

STRATEGIES

- Explore Sophia's feelings about the competition for her time.
- If Sophia is motivated to try to change:
  - Have Sophia discuss her specific concerns privately with a counselor.

- Discuss possible support mechanisms for the parents (e.g., Meals on Wheels, faith-based volunteers).
- Discuss ways she can maximize her time and efforts every day (e.g., making food for multiple meals at once to limit kitchen time, making changes when she shops).
- Suggest that she make specific time for herself and learn some coping techniques (e.g., relaxation techniques).
- Problem solve with Sophia to create a plan that she feels motivated to follow.
- Provide regular opportunities for follow-up to assess and provide encouragement from yourself and others.

EVALUATION

10/16/17: 08:00—Sophia has begun to discuss her feelings of stress.

- Sophia has met with her counselor to discuss these issues.
- Relaxation training sessions have been arranged by Sophia.
- Sophia meets with you and her counselor for follow-up sessions.

—J. Woodman, RN

THERAPEUTIC DIALOGUE: STRESS

SCENE FOR THOUGHT

Kathleen O'Brien, a registered nurse and staff member at a clinic, is sitting in the break room alone one morning, looking sad and preoccupied. Jean enters to get a cup of coffee.

LESS EFFECTIVE	
Jean:	Hi, Kathleen, how are you?
Kathleen:	Okay, I guess. *(No eye contact. Looks at the floor.)*
Jean:	*(Sits down next to her.)* You don't seem okay. Anything wrong?
Kathleen:	*(Smiles embarrassedly.)* I just don't seem to have my usual energy, that's all.
Jean:	I've noticed. It's been pretty hectic around here lately. We're all tired, including me! Are you getting enough rest with your busy schedule? *(Concerned tone of voice.)*
Kathleen:	Not really. Finals are coming up at school, and I've been working on those. *(No eye contact.)*
Jean:	Well, if I can do anything to help, let me know. I've got to get back to my meeting. See you later.
Kathleen:	Okay. Thanks. *(Gets up and walks back to her desk to prepare for her next patient.)*

MORE EFFECTIVE	
Jean:	Hi, Kathleen, how are you?
Kathleen:	Okay, I guess. *(No eye contact. Looks at the floor.)*
Jean:	*(Sits down next to her.)* You don't seem okay. Anything wrong?
Kathleen:	*(Smiles embarrassedly.)* I just don't seem to have my usual energy, that's all.
Jean:	I noticed you've seemed a little tired. What's going on?
Kathleen:	Just stressed out, I guess. *(Looks down again.)*
Jean:	You mean more stressed than usual? Are the kids and George okay?
Kathleen:	Yes, thank goodness.
Jean:	How about school? Are you still taking two courses at night?
Kathleen:	Yes, I'm doing alright.
Jean:	*(Silence.)*
Kathleen:	*(Takes a deep breath.)* The only thing that's changed is my brother Tom. He was diagnosed with a malignant brain tumor last week. The cancer is already in his bowel and liver. *(Tears well in her eyes.)* I feel so helpless. My other brothers expect me to help them and Tom and his family to handle the shock and sorrow. I guess I'm feeling a little overwhelmed.
Jean:	I guess so! Who's supporting you? *(Puts her hand on Kathleen's.)*
Kathleen:	George has been wonderful and helps all he can. *(Squeezes Jean's hand and sighs.)* It's a matter of finding enough time to keep up my schoolwork and talk on the phone to all the people calling about Tom. I haven't been for a run in weeks. *(Sighs again.)*
Jean:	Can I do anything to help?
Kathleen:	No, but thanks. Just talking about it to someone who'll listen is comforting.
Jean:	Let me know if you need a change in your schedule for anything, including a chance to exercise. Come talk to me anytime.
Kathleen:	Thanks. I appreciate that.

CRITICAL THINKING CHALLENGE

- Examine psychosocial expressions of stress that Kathleen exhibited.
- Suggest what you think prevented Kathleen from being able to cope with all the stressors at this time.
- List who and what her resources are, and give reasons.
- Propose what you would do to reduce your stress level if you were Kathleen.

a comfort tool around stress. During stressful situations, an individual may considerably increase the amount that he or she smokes. Smokers may say that they feel more relaxed when smoking. The consequences to their lungs, cardiovascular structures, and other organs can be tremendous. The ultimate illnesses from smoking can create significantly more stress than the prior stressors that were dealt with through smoking.

Overeating can also become addictive, although not as a substance that crosses the blood–brain barrier to alter cognitive function and emotions. Eating does increase glucose levels, which play a significant role in the stress response, but the physiology is not clear. Stress has been shown to induce the maladaptive behavior of overeating in people who are obese. Speculations have been made about how eating "stuffs" the negative emotions, elicits feelings of comfort, and can give temporary pleasure. Overeating also leads to several physiologic health issues systemically. Think about the impact the T2D has on the patient in the case study. Aside from Alzheimer's disease, he is also at risk for multiple other co-morbidities. The rate of T2D, commonly associated with a high body mass index due to overeating, continues to increase with 8.3% of the U.S. population, over 11% of adults ages 20 and older, and more than 23% of older adults ages 65 and older, living with diabetes (National Institute of Diabetes and Digestive and Kidney Diseases, 2014). The prevalence of T2D is expected to double worldwide by the year 2030 (WHO, 2014).

Undereating can also be associated with stress. Some individuals lose their appetite during stressful situations. This is actually part of the normal sympathetic stress response that diminishes appetite and digestive function (Holsboer & Ising, 2010). SNS activity, however, should be short term, and a person's appetite should return. Undereating is sometimes associated with those who overuse or abuse substances, preferring alcohol and/or drugs over food. Lack of nutrition can be as dangerous, if not more dangerous physiologically, than overeating.

People exhibiting stress and altered coping through substance abuse or overeating require a comprehensive treatment program to address their coping and adaptation problems.

Physical Illness

Prolonged stress increases allostatic load and can lead to physiologic dysfunction and, ultimately, pathologic processes. Chronic stress impairs immune function, leaving the individual more susceptible to colds, infections, poor wound healing, autoimmune disorders, and other ailments. Studies in psychoneuroimmunology (PNI) have shown the link between alterations in psychological well-being interfering with the HPA axis and ultimately impairing immune function. The brain not only interprets stimuli that can be perceived as emotional stress, but is itself an organ that endures physiologic stress (McEwen & Getz, 2013). The biophysiologic responses can lead to disease at the immune level and

virtually all systems of the physical body. Some techniques that help with coping strategies and promote relaxation and a sense of well-being target these pathways, with a primary focus on strengthening immune function.

Anxiety and Depression

Stress can cause anxiety, a subjective reaction to a real or imagined threat. Anxiety related to stress starts at the neuronal level, particularly in fetal life with a stressed mother. The offspring can develop anxiety in response to stress during life (Bilkei-Gorzo, Otto, & Zimmer, 2008). The sense of uneasiness or dread may range from mild to severe. Anxiety may be further exacerbated by lack of sleep, poor nutrition, excessive caffeine intake or smoking, or physical illness.

The extreme response to prolonged stress may be depression and suicide. People with poor coping mechanisms or inadequate support may see suicide as a desirable way to end stress and depression. Adolescents experiencing various kinds of stress have a high rate of suicidal behaviors.

Violent Behavior

Violent behaviors are another maladaptive approach to dealing with stress. Individuals with poor impulse control or inadequate coping mechanisms may respond to stress by acting out violently or abusively. For example, a man experiencing difficulties at work may come home and behave violently with his wife or children as an outlet for stress.

Recall the patient's daughter in the Case Scenario at the beginning of the chapter. She is struggling with the stress of caring for her father who suffers from both T2D and Alzheimer disease and will be moving him into her home. Use the concept map (Fig. 41-5) to help understand and manage the daughter's stress.

ASSESSMENT

Patients with health problems face many stressors and have various ways of coping with them. Nurses must understand the methods or strategies that patients use to deal with stress in order to best individualize care.

Normal Pattern Identification

The focused functional assessment of coping patterns includes obtaining subjective data from patients through a series of purposeful questions and interviews and through observation and mental notation of nonverbal communication, such as body position, facial expressions, gestures, voice, and speech. The nursing history is one of the earliest sources of these data, and in continued interactions, nurses may become increasingly focused on specific considerations.

Subjective data help identify normal coping patterns and strategies, determine factors that place patients at risk for

STRESS, COPING, AND ADAPTATION

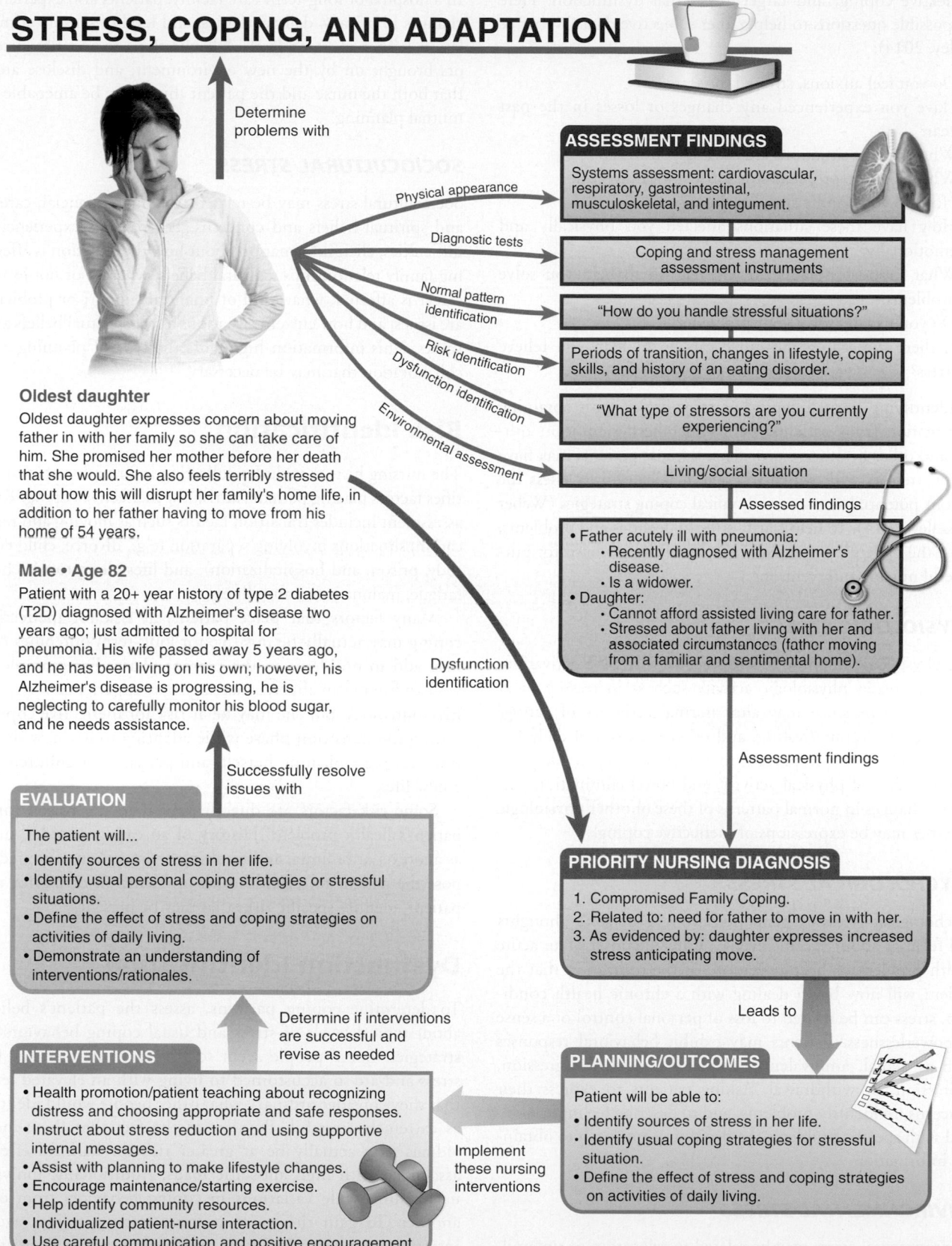

Determine
problems with

Oldest daughter

Oldest daughter expresses concern about moving
father in with her family so she can take care of
him. She promised her mother before her death
that she would. She also feels terribly stressed
about how this will disrupt her family's home life, in
addition to her father having to move from his
home of 54 years.

Male • Age 82

Patient with a 20+ year history of type 2 diabetes
(T2D) diagnosed with Alzheimer's disease two
years ago; just admitted to hospital for
pneumonia. His wife passed away 5 years ago,
and he has been living on his own; however, his
Alzheimer's disease is progressing, he is
neglecting to carefully monitor his blood sugar,
and he needs assistance.

Physical appearance

Diagnostic tests

Normal pattern
identification

Risk identification

Dysfunction identification

Environmental assessment

ASSESSMENT FINDINGS

Systems assessment: cardiovascular,
respiratory, gastrointestinal,
musculoskeletal, and integument.

Coping and stress management
assessment instruments

"How do you handle stressful situations?"

Periods of transition, changes in lifestyle, coping
skills, and history of an eating disorder.

"What type of stressors are you currently
experiencing?"

Living/social situation

Assessed findings

• Father acutely ill with pneumonia:
   • Recently diagnosed with Alzheimer's
     disease.
   • Is a widower.
• Daughter:
   • Cannot afford assisted living care for father.
   • Stressed about father living with her and
     associated circumstances (father moving
     from a familiar and sentimental home).

Dysfunction
identification

Assessment findings

Successfully resolve
issues with

EVALUATION

The patient will...

• Identify sources of stress in her life.
• Identify usual personal coping strategies or stressful
  situations.
• Define the effect of stress and coping strategies on
  activities of daily living.
• Demonstrate an understanding of
  interventions/rationales.

PRIORITY NURSING DIAGNOSIS

1. Compromised Family Coping.
2. Related to: need for father to move in with her.
3. As evidenced by: daughter expresses increased
   stress anticipating move.

Leads to

Determine if interventions
are successful and
revise as needed

INTERVENTIONS

• Health promotion/patient teaching about recognizing
  distress and choosing appropriate and safe responses.
• Instruct about stress reduction and using supportive
  internal messages.
• Assist with planning to make lifestyle changes.
• Encourage maintenance/starting exercise.
• Help identify community resources.
• Individualized patient-nurse interaction.
• Use careful communication and positive encouragement.

Implement
these nursing
interventions

PLANNING/OUTCOMES

Patient will be able to:

• Identify sources of stress in her life.
• Identify usual coping strategies for stressful
  situation.
• Define the effect of stress and coping strategies
  on activities of daily living.

FIGURE 41-5 Stress, coping, and adaptation concept map.

ineffective coping, and target any actual dysfunction. Here are possible questions to help gather subjective data (Weber & Kelley, 2014):

- Do you feel anxious, stressed, or scared?
- Have you experienced any changes or losses in the past year?
- What present situations are causing you stress?
- What does the problem/stressor/loss mean to you?
- How do you handle stressful situations?
- How have these situations affected you physically and emotionally?
- What support systems do you rely on to help you solve problems?
- Do you usually solve your problems?
- Is there something the nurse can do to help you relieve stress?

Identifying normal coping patterns begins with obtaining information from patients, family members, significant others, and other healthcare providers. Because patients may have many stressors with which to cope, it is helpful to assess the various potential stressors and typical coping strategies (Weber & Kelley, 2014). To help clarify stressful feelings and problems, enlist the patient's participation in establishing a basis for purposeful nursing interventions.

PHYSIOLOGIC STRESS

The physiologic response to stress begins with SNS activation, which increases physiologic activity such as increasing heart rate. This experience may alter normal activities of eating/eliminating, sleeping/resting, and other activities of daily living. Therefore, it is important to ask about fatigue, adequacy of sleep, level of physical activity, and bowel elimination patterns. Changes in normal patterns of these or other physiologic activities may be expressions of ineffective coping.

PSYCHOLOGICAL STRESS

Psychological stress is generated from a person's thoughts and feelings about specific events. With the onset of an acute health problem or hospitalization, or the realization that the patient will now begin dealing with a chronic health condition, stress can be related to loss of personal control or a sense of powerlessness. Patients may exhibit behavioral responses such as denial, ambivalence, suspicion, hostility, regression, depression, or withdrawal. Asking patients to express their concerns, to identify problems, and to describe feelings associated with specific problems is a beginning approach to obtaining information.

ENVIRONMENTAL STRESS

Environmental stress may be related to relocation or unfamiliarity with the setting. A change in surroundings with unfamiliar sounds, odors, and sights may induce stress for patients.

In a hospital or long-term care facility, patients also experience changes in privacy, daily activities, and level of sensory stimulation (either more or less). Ask questions to identify stressors brought on by the new environment, and disclose areas that both the nurse and the patient think may be amenable to mutual planning.

SOCIOCULTURAL STRESS

Sociocultural stress may be related to family, financial, career, and spiritual beliefs and concerns. For patients experiencing difficulties, elicit information about how the situation is affecting family relationships, cultural beliefs, whether or not job or career is affected, what kind of financial support or problems are issues, and how current situations affect spiritual beliefs and values. This information highlights the type of planning and collaboration that may be necessary.

Risk Identification

The nursing history includes collecting information that identifies factors placing patients at risk for ineffective coping. Risk assessment includes transition factors such as moving and relocation; situations involving separation (e.g., divorce, child custody, prison, and hospitalization); and lifestyle factors such as fatigue, malnutrition, and illness.

Many factors that place patients at risk for ineffective coping may actually be positive for long-term outcomes but may add to problems in the current phase. For example, a woman leaving an abusive marriage may experience very positive outcomes, but she may be at risk for ineffective coping during the transition phase while adapting to her new situation and reestablishing herself, and perhaps her children, in a new life.

Some risk factors are directly related to the reason for a patient's health problem. History of an eating disorder, such as anorexia or bulimia, and resulting malnutrition may predispose the patient to related health problems. In caring for the patient, identify specific risks that may be present.

Dysfunction Identification

To determine coping patterns, assess the patient's beliefs about typical levels of stress and usual coping behaviors or strategies. Some people seem to have a high tolerance for stress and are so accustomed to living with an elevated level that they consider ordinary what other people would identify as extremely stressful. Be alert to the fact that these individuals may actually be at greater risk for harmful effects associated with high allostatic loads. Additionally, individuals exhibit wide variations in coping behaviors from one another. To gain the most accurate understanding, avoid inserting your personal biases and coping expectations into the assessment. Stay open to learning how patients identify situations.

Altered coping patterns can be identified as significant differences in a patient's need to use typical coping behaviors and/or as coping and adaptation patterns outside the range of typical behaviors for that patient. For example, the person who usually handles job stress by exercising but reports a current response of fatigue and excessive sleep has identified an altered coping pattern.

Physical Assessment

With activation of the ANS and the HPA axis, physiologic responses occur and can be observed in the physical assessment. Because physiologic arousal responses involve general and nonspecific responses, there may be many other causes for some of these same responses. Do *not* assume that the only cause of some physical findings is stress.

CARDIOVASCULAR SYSTEM

The cardiovascular system is the target system for the effects of epinephrine and norepinephrine, which include increased heart rate, vasoconstriction of peripheral organs, and increased oxygen consumption by the heart. The manifestations of prolonged stimulation by these hormones may include the following:

- An increase in the resting heart rate related to direct stimulation of the myocardium; the patient may describe a "pounding in the chest" or palpitations
- An increase in systolic or diastolic blood pressure related to peripheral vasoconstriction
- Dysrhythmias related to ischemia (tissue oxygen deprivation in the face of increased energy demand), noted in an irregular heartbeat or rhythm changes
- Angina, or chest pain, and ischemia-related changes in the electrocardiogram
- Headaches related to vasoconstriction

RESPIRATORY SYSTEM

Norepinephrine affects the respiratory system, which leads to an increased breathing rate and to bronchiolar dilation. Hyperventilation, a feeling of "air hunger," dizziness, and tingling in the hands and feet are the most common physical manifestations.

GASTROINTESTINAL SYSTEM

The gastrointestinal system is a common target system in stressful situations. Whereas epinephrine and norepinephrine usually slow gastric motility, people experiencing stress often report loss of appetite, nausea, vomiting, and increased peristaltic activity. Increased peristalsis is manifested by increases in bowel sounds, secretion of hydrochloric acid in the stomach, and number of bowel movements. The increase in hydrochloric acid secretion may also contribute to nausea and vomiting,

and, in combination with cortisol, to gastrointestinal ulcerations or gastritis.

MUSCULOSKELETAL SYSTEM

The musculoskeletal system responds to stress by exhibiting increased tension in larger muscles and shakiness and tremor in smaller muscles. The muscle tension is related to the fight-or-flight response. Prolonged tension can lead to muscle spasm, particularly in the back, shoulders, and neck.

INTEGUMENTARY SYSTEM

The skin, or integumentary system, manifests the peripheral effects of norepinephrine and epinephrine by being diaphoretic (sweating) and cool and by exhibiting smooth muscle tension caused by contraction of the arrector pili muscles ("making the hairs stand on end").

Diagnostic Tests and Procedures

Although there are many physiologic responses to stress, they are difficult to measure clinically. Stress-related hormones (epinephrine, norepinephrine, and cortisol) can be detected through laboratory tests, and a stress state can be inferred from their existence; these hormones are most often measured in research studies rather than in clinical situations. Furthermore, these hormones may be expressed for numerous reasons and cannot be exclusively labeled as due to stress.

Gathering objective data about coping and adaptation incorporates the structured interview and the use of coping and stress management assessment instruments, such as the Everyday Hassles Scale (Lazarus, 1981) and the Coping Self-Efficacy Scale (Chesney, Neilands, Chambers, Taylor, & Folkman, 2006) (Fig. 41-6). These measurement tools attempt to identify and quantify stressors and levels of stress to predict outcomes. Using such instruments helps identify behaviors and feelings that may relate to the amount of stress and the corresponding vulnerability to illness and dysfunction. Nurses may use the scales, which turn subjective factors into objective measures. Other healthcare team members who may use such scales include psychosocial clinical nurse specialists, psychologists, or other mental healthcare providers.

NURSING DIAGNOSES

NANDA-International (NANDA-I, 2015–2017) has approved several categories of nursing diagnoses related to coping and stress tolerance. Currently, the diagnoses include Posttrauma responses; Coping responses; and Neurobehavioral stress. A selected nursing diagnosis, Ineffective Coping, is presented in Table 41-2 along with selected Nursing Outcomes Classification (NOC) and Nursing Interventions Classification (NIC).

When things aren't going well for you, or when you're having problems, how confident or certain are you that you can do the following:

Cannot do at all				Moderately certain can do				Certain can do

0   1   2   3   4   5   6   7   8   9   10

For each of the following items, write a number from 0–10, using the scale above.

When things aren't going well for you, how confident are you that you can:

1. Keep from getting down in the dumps.   _____   99
2. Talk positively to yourself.   _____   99
3. Sort out what can be changed, and what can not be changed.   _____   99
4. Get emotional support from friends and family.   _____   99
5. Find solutions to your most difficult problems.   _____   99

6. Break an upsetting problem down into smaller parts.   _____   99
7. Leave options open when things get stressful.   _____   99
8. Make a plan of action and follow it when confronted with a problem.   _____   99
9. Develop new hobbies or recreations.   _____   99
10. Take your mind off unpleasant thoughts.   _____   99

11. Look for something good in a negative situation.   _____   99
12. Keep from feeling sad.   _____   99
13. See things from the other person's point of view during a heated argument.   _____   99
14. Try other solutions to your problems if your first solutions don't work.   _____   99
15. Stop yourself from being upset by unpleasant thoughts.   _____   99
16. Make new friends.   _____   99

17. Get friends to help you with the things you need.   _____   99
18. Do something positive for yourself when yon are feeling discouraged.   _____   99
19. Make unpleasant thoughts go away.   _____   99
20. Think about one part of the problem at a time.   _____   99

21. Visualize a pleasant activity or place.   _____   99
22. Keep yourself from feeling lonely.   _____   99
23. Pray or meditate.   _____   99
24. Get emotional support from community organizations or resources.   _____   99
25. Stand your ground and fight for what you want.   _____   99
26. Resist the impulse to act hastily when under pressure.   _____   99

FIGURE 41-6 Coping self-efficacy scale. (Reprinted from Chesney, M. A., Neilands, T. B., Chambers, D. B., Taylor, J. M., & Folkman, S. (2006). A validity and reliability study of the coping self-efficacy scale. *British Journal of Health Psychology, 11*(Pt 3), 421–437. Retrieved August 18, 2011, from www.ncbi.nlm.nih.gov/pubmed/16870053).

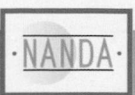

	Table 41-2 SELECTED NANDA-I NURSING DIAGNOSIS RELATED TO COPING				
Nursing Dx	Related Factors	Dx Statement	NOC*	NIC†
---	---	---	---	---
Ineffective Coping — inability to form a valid appraisal of the stressors, inadequate choices of practiced responses, and/or inability to use available resources	Gender differences in coping strategies, inadequate level of confidence in ability to cope, uncertainty, inadequate opportunity to prepare for stressor, inability to conserve adaptive energies, and disturbance in pattern of appraisal of threat	**Ineffective Coping** R/T inadequate level of perception of control AEB use of forms of coping that impede adaptive behavior, poor concentration, fatigue, inadequate problem solving	Acceptance Health Status Adaptation to Physical Disability Coping Risk Control: Drug Use Self-Esteem Social Interaction Skills Social Support	Coping Enhancement Counseling Decision-Making Support Family Support Risk Identification Self-Awareness Enhancement Self-Esteem Enhancement Sleep Enhancement Support Group

Dx, diagnosis; R/T, related to; AEB, as evidenced by.

*From: Moorhead, S., Johnson, M., Maas, M., & Swanson, E. (2013). *Iowa Outcomes Project: Nursing Outcomes Classification (NOC)* (5th ed.). St. Louis, MO: C. V. Mosby.

†From: Bulecheck, G., Butcher, H., Dochterman, J., & Wagner, C. (2013). *Iowa Intervention Project: Nursing Interventions Classification (NIC)* (6th ed.). St. Louis, MO: C. V. Mosby.

From: NANDA-Association International (NANDA-I). (2014). *Nursing diagnoses: Definitions and classification, 2015–2017*. West Sussex, England: Wiley-Blackwell.

OUTCOME IDENTIFICATION AND PLANNING

After establishing nursing diagnoses and related factors, nurses work with patients to identify goals and interventions. Goals for patients with ineffective coping need to be individualized by considering each patient's history, areas of risk, evidence of dysfunction, and related objective data. Examples of patient goals include the following:

- The patient will identify sources of stress in his or her life.
- The patient will identify usual personal coping strategies for stressful situations.
- The patient will define the effect of stress and coping strategies on ADLs.

For patients who have related nursing diagnoses or more complex problems with stress, coping, and adaptation, the goals need to be adjusted accordingly along with the time frame in which they can be realized. Examples of some interventions useful in planning are listed in Table 41-2 and discussed in the following section.

IMPLEMENTATION

Nurses can intervene independently or collaboratively to help restore function. When working with patients, assist them to recognize signs and symptoms of stress, to identify sources of distress, and to choose appropriate and safe responses. Patients may not recognize that muscle tension or feelings of depression and anxiety are stress related. Because the stress response is highly complex and individualized, management of that response must also be individualized. Stress management techniques that are effective for one person may not help another. People may use the same type of intervention differently.

For example, there are various methods for the Indo-Tibetan self-healing strategy that take into consideration different patient dispositions and needs. Assist patients to find techniques that are most effective for them.

Health Promotion

Helping patients to recognize and manage stress is an important aspect of health promotion and disease prevention. Learning to cope effectively with stress requires self-awareness and recognition of personal manifestations of stress; this is true for nurses as well as patients (Box 41-4).

REDUCING STRESSORS

Assist patients to recognize stress, its sources, and meanings through careful observations. Nurses and patients can partner together to formulate approaches to either reduce stressors or remove them entirely. Through health education, which leads to learning the causes of stress, patients can develop strategies for coping and adapting. They can continually appraise their symptoms with respect to significance for well-being and survival and can cope accordingly. For example, the working mother who is tired from putting in overtime and is struggling to spend time with her family may find herself feeling angry, fatigued, and short tempered with her children. Help her to realize that the mood changes she is experiencing are stress induced and that coping strategies may include changing jobs to accommodate her own and her family's needs, asking her spouse for help, or hiring part-time help.

ADDRESSING PERFECTION

Striving for perfection can enhance stress. Feelings of having to perform without error or making sure certain things are completed at all costs can be detrimental. Feelings that

BOX 41-4   Stress Management for Nurses

Nursing practice often involves working in stressful environments, caring for patients in noisy or overcrowded spaces, visiting homes or situations that are depressing, adjusting to various work shifts, and being understaffed. Nursing literature describes two conditions that commonly affect nurses: burnout and tedium.

Burnout results from working with people who are demanding and needy, which can produce conflict within the nurse and can lead to depleted energy and low morale. Tedium results from environmental factors that create conflicts or place demands on the nurse. Physical and emotional depletion, negative self-concept, negative attitudes, and feelings of helplessness and hopelessness characterize both burnout and tedium.

Be aware of your own stress levels. Recognize your personal stress and its manifestations. One step is realizing that increased fatigue, anger, disorganization, or other behavior changes may be related to an increased level of stress. Noting changes in lifestyle factors, such as smoking, eating behaviors, or alcohol or other substance use, may provide further evidence of personal stress.

Once you recognize the ways in which you respond to stress, attend to the times when stress is most pronounced and to situations that stimulate a stress response. As you do so, take positive action to institute effective coping strategies by preventing, managing, and alleviating stress.

Suggestions for Stress Management

- Establish a regular program of exercise and activity to focus energy expenditure.
- Eliminate or restrict the amount of alcohol, caffeine, and other mood-altering substances as a means of managing stress.
- Learn to accept failure (your own and others) and turn it into a constructive experience.
- Develop techniques for assertiveness to have more feelings of personal control.
- Develop support systems with colleagues and friends to bolster personal resources.
- Have an optimistic view of the world and believe that most people are doing the best they can.

---

one "should, ought, or must" do something may compound a negative response to stress. An example is the person who tells him- or herself "I must never make a mistake" or "I should always clean the house before going to work." Help such patients realize that a desire for perfection and unrealistic self-expectations are stress inducing. Encourage patients to be realistic about how much they can and need to accomplish and to remember that relationships are more important than things or tasks. If an individual suffers from obsessive–compulsive disorder (OCD), accomplishing certain tasks before moving on to something else might feel essential. Dealing directly with the OCD may help alleviate the associated stress.

USING SUPPORTIVE INTERNAL MESSAGES

Self-support through positive self-talk is an important part of stress management strategies (Esch & Stefano, 2010). An internal dialogue, whereby the person describes and interprets his or her environment, is referred to as "self-talk" or internal messages. Internal messages are constant and influence daily functioning and self-concept. A constant stream of negative self-messages can lead to generalized feelings of inferiority and self-doubt. Patients can learn to replace defeating negative internal messages with supportive messages to help cope with difficulties. Changing internal messages involves these three steps:

- Identify what one says when the situation occurs (self-talk).
- Evaluate how rational or irrational these messages are.
- Replace the negative messages with supportive coping statements and integrate supportive statements into daily life.

For example, a person interviews for a job but is not hired. Instead of saying "I blew it, I'm a failure; I'll never get the job I want," the person learns to restructure the negative thoughts into supportive self-statements such as "I feel disappointed that I didn't get this job. I know I presented myself well. I have the ability to get the job I want." Encourage patients to examine internal messages and to practice rephrasing those that are negative or irrational.

Another useful behavioral strategy for gaining control over self-defeating thoughts is called "thought stopping." Thought stopping can be accomplished by using the following technique:

- When a negative or self-defeating thought crosses the mind (e.g., "I'll never be able to find a job"), say "stop" inwardly or out loud.
- Substitute a positive, assertive statement for the negative thought (e.g., "I have the skills needed to get the job I want").
- If using the word *stop* is ineffective, place a rubber band around the wrist and snap it whenever negative, unwanted thoughts occur.

USING ASSERTIVENESS

Another useful technique for changing behavior in response to stressful encounters is assertiveness. Assertive behavior enables people to act in their best interests, to stand up for themselves, to express their feelings openly and honestly, and to exercise their rights without infringing on the rights of others. Assertiveness is a learned skill that requires practice. When working with patients who have difficulty expressing feelings or meeting their needs, suggest that the patient enroll in a class or workshop in assertiveness training.

MAKING LIFESTYLE CHANGES

Adequate rest and nutrition are important components to managing stress and coping effectively. Any person will be more capable of handling daily stressors if the body is well nourished and rested. Encourage patients to get adequate sleep and nutrition; limit or eliminate smoking; reduce caffeine consumption; and avoid dependence on using substances to mask pain or ill feelings, such as "pill popping" (e.g., taking aspirin or tranquilizers). All such measures will promote healthier management of stress.

EXERCISING

Physical activity or exercise is a technique that helps counter the effects of the stress response. Physical exertion helps to release tension from the muscles and is a natural outlet when the body is in a fight-or-flight state of arousal. Exercise also triggers the release of endorphins and enkephalins (natural opioids), promoting a better sense of well-being. Of the broad categories of exercise, aerobic exercise and moderate, low-intensity exercise is recommended. Aerobic exercise involves sustained activity of the large muscle groups and places an increased demand on the cardiopulmonary system. Examples of aerobic exercise include running, bicycling, swimming, cross-country skiing, brisk walking, and rowing. Moderate and low-intensity exercise is less vigorous than aerobic exercise; however, it can increase muscle strength and flexibility. Researchers have recognized that walking programs such as the First Step Program, which uses pedometers to count out steps taken per day, significantly improve health and well-being (Tudor-Locke, 2009). Low-intensity exercise is particularly a good preparation for sedentary persons before they progress to more vigorous aerobic exercise. Additional examples of low-intensity exercise include calisthenics, gardening, and housecleaning.

Regular, moderate-intensity exercise and physical activity have substantial health benefits. Such exercise may take the form of active or passive range of motion either encouraged or performed by nurses. Box 41-5 gives examples of the benefits of exercise.

RELAXATION TECHNIQUES

Various relaxation techniques can be effective in decreasing physiologic stimulation. The physiologic arousal response can affect all body systems. During this state, muscle tension and heightened awareness begin to compete with a state of relaxation. The body has the ability to elicit the "relaxation response" that directly opposes the physiologic arousal response through countering the physiologic and biochemical actions during the acute stress response. Techniques such as meditation can lead to decreased oxygen consumption, respiratory rate, heart rate, and metabolic shifts, which all lead to success in countering the stress response (Dusek & Benson, 2009).

Dr. Herbert Benson established the relaxation response in the 1970s and is the director emeritus of the Benson-Henry Institute for Mind Body Medicine at Massachusetts General Hospital. This organization's website (www.massgeneral.org/bhi/) contains an overview of stress, stress warning signals, and links to how to carry out the relaxation response. Several techniques have been shown to elicit the relaxation response, including deep breathing, progressive relaxation, autogenics, visualization, meditation, yoga, and biofeedback. Table 41-3 presents some selected advanced stress management techniques.

BOX 41-5   Health Benefits of Exercise

- Improves muscular strength, endurance, and flexibility
- Improves cardiovascular efficiency
- Lowers resting heart rate
- Reduces blood cholesterol levels
- Reduces general anxiety and depression
- Reduces chronic fatigue and insomnia
- Lowers body weight by burning calories and suppressing appetite
- Increases absorption and use of food
- Improves appearance and self-image

TABLE 41-3   SELECTED ADVANCED STRESS MANAGEMENT AND RELAXATION TECHNIQUES

Autogenic training	A systematic technique teaching the body and mind to respond to verbal commands, allowing the person to achieve a deep state of relaxation through self-suggestion (or self-hypnosis).
Visualization and imagery	An attempt to affect an unconscious process by using a conscious suggestion or a mental picture of the desired change.
Affirmations	Strong, positive, feeling-rich statements about a desired change to reinforce and increase the effectiveness of visualization; can be done silently, out loud, in writing. For example, a person with a strong sense of time urgency might use this affirmation: "I am relaxed and centered. I have plenty of time for everything."
Meditation	A traditional Eastern religious technique to achieve mental and physical relaxation. Four elements include a quiet place, a comfortable position, an object to dwell on such as a word or symbol, and a passive attitude.
Biofeedback	A specialized relaxation technique in which the person learns to monitor physiologic processes, feedback a measure of that function, and exert control over autonomic functions. Information, such as heart rate, muscle tension, and finger temperature, is translated into an auditory or visual signal that the person senses, and through these signals the person learns to discriminate between tension and relaxation.
Therapeutic touch	The use of touch to reduce anxiety and stress, relieve pain, and provide comfort.
Massage	The manipulation of soft tissue, generally with the hands, to provide stimulation and relaxation and to reduce stress and anxiety.
Yoga	A form of exercise (usually combined with meditation) to foster relaxation, mental alacrity, and good health.

Deep Breathing

Breathing is an important element of the relaxation response. As stress and tension mount during the day, breathing becomes shallow and irregular and the heart rate accelerates. Poorly oxygenated blood contributes to lethargy, tension, and depression. When a person is relaxed, breathing slows and deepens and the heart rate returns to normal. Because breathing is the easiest physiologic system to control, a person can use slow, deep breathing to trigger the relaxation response. In fact, many relaxation techniques begin by having the person slowly inhale and exhale for a few minutes.

As a method to get into the practice of deep breathing, an individual can train him/herself by deep breathing during daily routine tasks such as answering the phone or looking at the clock. Frequently, the act of taking a few deep breaths before a stressful situation can decrease fear and anxiety, allowing for a more relaxed frame of mind.

Meditation

Meditation is a technique that can be used to help individuals enhance positive emotions, termed *psychological thriving* (Epel, Daubenmier, Moskowitz, Folkman, & Blackburn, 2009). This can be quite useful for the process of shifting thoughts from threats to challenges and decreasing stress arousal (Epel et al., 2009). Mindfulness meditation, in particular, brings an individual to a state of awareness in which he or she can better adapt to stressful life events (Garland, Gaylord, & Park, 2009). Box 41-6 describes the elements of meditation.

BOX 41-6   Elements of Meditation

A quiet location: Meditation is usually practiced in a quiet place with as few distractions as possible. This can be particularly helpful for beginners.

A specific, comfortable posture: Depending on the type of meditation being practiced, meditation can be done while sitting, lying down, walking, or in other positions.

A focus of attention: Focusing one's attention is usually a part of meditation. For example, the meditator may focus on a mantra (a specially chosen word or set of words), an object, or the sensations of the breath. Some forms of meditation involve paying attention to whatever is the dominant content of consciousness.

An open attitude: Having an open attitude during meditation means letting distractions come and go naturally without judging them. When the attention goes to distracting or wandering thoughts, they are not suppressed; instead, the meditator gently brings attention back to the focus. In some types of meditation, the meditator learns to "observe" thoughts and emotions while meditating.

Adapted from: National Institutes of Health, National Center for Complementary and Alternative Medicine. *Meditation.* Retrieved August 18, 2011, from http://nccam.nih.gov/health/meditation/

Nursing Interventions for Altered Function

Nurses have a significant role in identifying people at risk for ineffective coping and in initiating appropriate teaching to promote optimal health. Many techniques that promote healthy coping can also be used for altered coping. An advantage of using stress control techniques and promoting effective coping when patients are well is that they then have the skill to use these techniques when altered function exists.

RELAXATION TRAINING

Nurses may encounter many stressful situations in all healthcare settings where it is appropriate to teach or remind patients to use relaxation techniques. Such situations include the following:

- Before and after diagnostic tests or treatments
- During childbirth
- After surgery to help manage postoperative pain
- During recovery from myocardial infarction
- During chemotherapy and radiation treatments for cancer
- While calming an anxious or agitated person
- Before a painful procedure such as an intramuscular injection or inserting an intravenous line

Having relaxation tapes available for patients to use is becoming a common practice in institutional and community settings. Patients may purchase relaxation tapes or may want to make their own personal recordings. Telling the patient to take a few deep breaths before a procedure can decrease anxiety. For example, before a painful procedure or intramuscular injection, ask the patient to take two or three slow, deep breaths. Usually, patients experience less discomfort physically and emotionally if they are relaxed and calm.

MODIFYING THE ENVIRONMENT

Nurses should be aware of environmental stressors and make adjustments whenever possible to reduce sensory overload and to assist patients with coping and adaptation. For hospitalized patients, that environment, which affords little privacy and is unfamiliar, may be the source of stress. Increased noise levels, constant lights, and unfamiliar procedures all contribute to stress.

Nurses may be instrumental in making modifications in the environment that assist patients to manage the stress of the situation and to cope with the environment. Organizing nursing care to decrease patient disturbance, having as few extra lights on as possible, and keeping down the conversational noise in the hallways are a few examples. In the home, encourage families to create a room or space where patients can control the noise level and stimuli (Boehm & Morast, 2009).

CRISIS INTERVENTION AND DE-ESCALATION

Acute health problems, illness, loss, or trauma may precipitate a crisis in a person's life. A crisis suggests a situation in which usual coping strategies are ineffective and the person is disorganized or unable to problem solve appropriately. During crisis, social buffering is essential. Patients need assistance from family, friends, clergy, and healthcare providers, including nurses. Adequate support during a crisis and its resolution can help patients realistically perceive the problem or stress and relearn or reinstitute coping strategies.

A person under stress without good coping mechanisms can reach a state of becoming dysfunctional or even nonfunctional. An otherwise benign situation can escalate into a dangerous one for the patient and those around him/her. It is important to recognize a developing situation that can become unsafe. One effective mechanism to de-escalating a difficult situation is the Listen, Empathize, Affirm, and Partner (L.E.A.P.) approach (Amador, 2001; NAMI, 2014). The key to the L.E.A.P. approach is building trust with the individual and following the steps to diffuse or de-escalate the situation. It is important to remember that emotional stress triggers physiologic responses (Bilkei-Gorzo, Racz, et al., 2008; McEwen, 2009). In an escalated situation, not only is the noncoping individual experiencing emotional and physiologic responses, but so are those directly involved in dealing with the individual. As a healthcare provider, it is imperative to understand one's own reactions to situations to ensure the most effective care can be provided.

The following is an example of L.E.A.P. in action pertaining to the case study at the beginning of this chapter:

You are a nurse on an in-patient medical/surgical unit assigned to an 82-year-old gentleman being admitted for pneumonia. The patient's oldest daughter is with him, and through the history intake you learn of his T2D and new diagnosis of Alzheimer disease. He is started on treatments for the pneumonia and has a peaceful first night in the hospital. In the middle of your second day assigned to the patient, you find him wandering down the hall, dripping blood from his arm where you had placed an intravenous line that is no longer intact. You approach him in a friendly manner and he looks at you as if he's never seen you before. He starts yelling for you to get away from him. He starts repeating, "They are trying to harm me."

Your heart begins to race, and you are unsure what to do first. You take a deep breath and remember the steps of L.E.A.P.

The first step is *listen*. Listening includes providing full attention to the patient, calmly asking him why he is upset, and nodding in an understanding manner. Your nonverbal cues are open and nonthreatening. The patient repeats that he feels threatened, but this time you notice his tone is softer, with less conviction. You reassure him that you only want to help him. You also *empathize* with him. You label his emotion by noting that he feels uncomfortable and unsafe. You repeat back the words he uses, emphasizing that you understand what he is experiencing. You ask him if he would be more comfortable sitting, and you provide a chair. You ask others in the area to leave so that he feels safer. As the patient sits, you *affirm* his feelings. You restate that he feels "they" are trying to harm him. You offer support by telling him that you will ensure no one will harm him. You pull up another chair and sit across from him so that you are at the same level and not looking down on him.

You ask him if you can take care of his arm that now has dried blood around the area where the IV catheter was pulled out. He holds out his arm and, wearing gloves, you gently apply sterile gauze to the area with a reassuring touch. You now begin to *partner* with him. You engage him in planning the next steps—problem-solving together. After he correctly answers your questions about who he is and where he is, you ask him if he'd like to go back to his room. You discuss with him the steps to his recovery and the goal of being discharged home. The patient has gained trust in you.

Situations such as this one, where medical and mental health issues collide, are not uncommon. Particularly with a disease such as Alzheimer's (Stone, Johnstone, Mitrofanis, & O'Rourke, 2014), declining mental status is part of the process. Healthcare providers must be aware of and prepared for such encounters. Using the L.E.A.P. method to de-escalate a potentially dangerous situation is ideal.

Home and Community Care

People who are convalescing from stress-producing situations are increasingly vulnerable to other stresses and to ineffective coping. Continued support for coping and adaptation is particularly important. Support groups can be especially effective (Fig. 41-7). These groups may be informal, such as family, friends, and spiritual sources, or they can be formal. An example of a formal support group is the Alzheimer Association, which is composed of people who have family members with Alzheimer disease. Similarly, cancer support groups can benefit patients and loved ones enormously. A list of cancer support groups can be accessed through the American Cancer Society. Groups such as these can be particularly helpful for those experiencing the stress associated with caring for others and can offer many useful ideas for coping strategies and effective adaptation.

Many support groups offer assistance for specialized problems and needs. Be aware of these groups, and develop networks with other healthcare professionals to link patients with them appropriately.

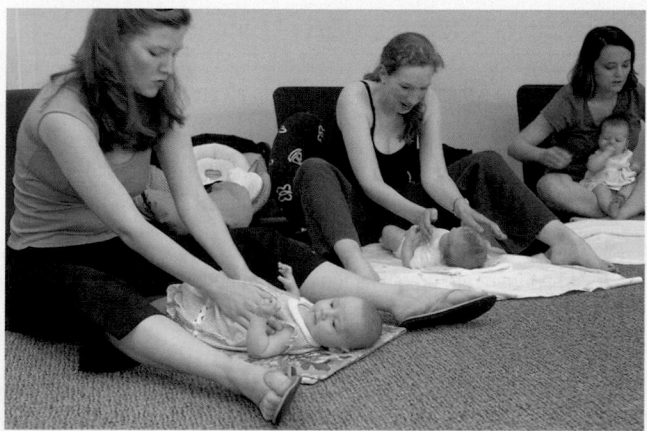

FIGURE 41-7 Many support groups, like this group for new parents, offer valuable outlets for people with similar needs.

PATIENT PLAN OF CARE
The Patient With Ineffective Coping

NURSING DIAGNOSIS
Ineffective Coping related to situational crises manifested by inability to manage stressors

PATIENT GOAL
Patient will identify cause of current problems and usual personal coping strategies for stressful situations.

PATIENT OUTCOME CRITERIA
- Patient verbalizes feelings related to present emotional state within 24 to 48 hours.
- Patient identifies recent stressful life events or sources of stress during first week.
- Patient identifies signs and symptoms of current stress.
- Within 1 week, patient identifies current coping patterns and consequences of such behavior.

NURSING INTERVENTION	SCIENTIFIC RATIONALE
1. Assess causative and contributive factors by discussing with patient (i.e., loss, grieving, inadequate support, recent life changes).	**1.** Assessment of causative factors provides information from which to develop a treatment plan.
2. Assess the person's present coping status: – Determine onset of symptoms and correlation with recent life changes. – Assess for risk of self-harm.	**2.** Identification of current coping skills helps to assess adequacy/inadequacy of coping.
3. Encourage the patient to evaluate the effectiveness of current coping skills.	**3.** Personal understanding of coping skills and outcomes reinforces use of acceptable coping or encourages the patient to look for alternatives in coping.

PATIENT GOAL
Patient will demonstrate appropriate coping strategies.

PATIENT OUTCOME CRITERIA
- Patient makes environmental changes to reduce stress within 1 to 3 months.
- Patient practices several new coping skills (i.e., relaxation techniques, assertiveness, exercise, talking about feelings, thought stopping, affirmations) and chooses at least one skill to practice consistently.
- Patient assesses effectiveness of social support network.

NURSING INTERVENTION	SCIENTIFIC RATIONALE
1. Assist the patient to problem solve in a constructive manner.	**1.** Development of healthy coping strategies helps to eliminate or reduce stress and decrease possibility of chronic illness.
2. Help the patient identify problems in the environment that are stressful. Discuss how to change them, if this is possible.	**2.** The patient may need help in knowing how to make necessary changes.
3. When there are problems the patient cannot control directly, help him or her identify stress-reducing techniques to use.	**3.** In addition to identifying techniques, the patient needs to understand them and learn proper skills for their usefulness.

PATIENT PLAN OF CARE (*Continued*)
The Patient With Ineffective Coping

NURSING INTERVENTION	SCIENTIFIC RATIONALE

4. Assist the patient in identifying a social support network.
  a. Encourage the patient to develop this support if it is helpful.
  b. If desired, assist the patient in finding support groups to meet his or her needs.
	4. People need external as well as internal resources for coping.

EVALUATION

10/17/17: 15:00—Patient begins to verbalize feelings related to current stress within first week.
- Patient identifies signs and symptoms of current stress and effective coping patterns during the first week.
- Patient states what environmental changes need to be made to reduce stress within 1 month.
- Patient starts practicing coping skills of relaxation techniques and affirmations.
- Patient evaluated the effectiveness of social and family support network within the month.

—J. Woodman, RN

EVALUATION

Specific outcome criteria are the tools for measuring the attainment of patient goals. Nursing interventions are the means for achieving those goals. Outcome criteria need to be specifically tailored to the individual patient so that they will uniquely measure the attainment of a patient's goals.

Goal

The patient will identify sources of stress in his or her life.

POSSIBLE OUTCOME CRITERIA

- The patient defines events that create personal stress by listing them before the next meeting with the nurse.
- The patient demonstrates anticipation of stressful situations by discussing them with the nurse before they occur.
- The patient identifies the difference between positive and negative sources of stress in the next discussion with the nurse.

Goal

The patient will identify usual personal coping strategies for stressful situations.

POSSIBLE OUTCOME CRITERIA

- The patient names at least 10 personal coping patterns.
- The patient describes techniques that he or she uses to reinforce previous responses or to establish new responses in the next teaching session with the nurse.

- The patient consciously initiates effective stress management techniques during a stressful period, as observed by the nurse.

Goal

The patient will define the effect of stress and coping strategies on ADLs.

POSSIBLE OUTCOME CRITERIA

- At the first home visit, the patient describes to the nurse specific ADLs that elicit stress effects.
- After the next teaching session with the nurse, the patient describes how specific coping strategies interfere with or promote ADLs.
- At the next home visit, the patient demonstrates new coping skills effective in managing stress and assisting ADLs to the visiting nurse.

KEY CONCEPTS

- Stress, an inherent part of life, may have positive or negative effects.
- Coping with stress successfully requires ongoing adaptation or change in response to stress.
- Homeostasis consists of coordinated physiologic processes that maintain steady functioning.
- Allostasis reflects the body's capacity to maintain stability in the face of constant change and to adjust to new levels of functioning.
- Allostatic load is the cumulative effect of chronic stressors and can lead to pathologic processes.

- The HPA axis and the SNS mediate the physiologic response to stress.

- Coping is a process the person uses to manage stresses or events that he or she encounters.

- Altered coping may be manifested by use of alcohol and drugs, excessive smoking, increased sleeping, withdrawal, and illness.

- Manifestations of altered coping can interfere with the person's effective management of ADLs.

- A focused nursing assessment of coping and adaptation includes the history of the patient's previous coping methods, areas of risk for ineffective coping, and identification of coping and adaptation dysfunction.

- Nursing interventions include assisting the patient to develop effective coping strategies to promote healthy adaptation to stress and supporting the patient in using those strategies in unusually stressful situations.

- Community-based care encompasses the use of support people or groups to maintain effective coping strategies.

PRACTICING FOR THE NCLEX

CHECK YOUR ANSWERS IN APPENDIX A.

1. The capacity of physiologic systems to maintain stability yet alter the set point required for optimum system functioning is known as which of the following?
   a. Homeostasis
   b. Allostasis
   c. Coping
   d. Adaptation

2. An unemployed, single woman is seen at a prenatal visit. Which of the following assessment findings would indicate the effects of chronic stress?
   a. Elevated blood glucose
   b. Decreased immune response
   c. Dilated pupils
   d. Rapid breathing pattern

3. A new mother seen in a postpartum visit reports high levels of stress associated with her new role as a mother. Which of the following nursing interventions would be most appropriate?
   a. Recognizing stressors
   b. Using assertiveness to express feelings
   c. Encouraging adequate exercise and diet
   d. Offering crisis intervention resources

4. A patient is admitted with malnutrition and bilateral pneumonia. During the admission process, it is discovered that the patient's significant other recently died. Which nursing diagnosis is most appropriate?
   a. Defensive Coping
   b. Caregiver Role Strain
   c. Chronic Sorrow
   d. Ineffective Coping

5. A nurse is conducting a patient assessment of coping and adaptation. Which of the following questions would be appropriate? Select all that apply:
   a. "How have you coped with difficult situations in the past?"
   b. "What type of stressors do you find most difficult?"
   c. "Are you able to discuss your feelings when you are stressed?"
   d. "Whom do you rely on for social support?"

REFERENCES

Akdeniz, C., Tost, H., Streit, F., Haddad, L., Wust, S., Schafer, A., et al. (2014). Neuroimaging evidence for a role of neural social stress processing in ethnic minority-associated environmental risk. *JAMA Psychiatry.* DOI: 10.1001/jamapsychiatry.2014.35.

American Institute of Stress. (2010). *Stress, definition of stress, stressor, what is stress? eustress?* Retrieved February 17, 2010, from www.stress.org/topic-definition-stress.htm

Amador, X. (2001). *I am not sick I don't need help - How to help someone with mental illness accept treatment.* New York: Vida Press.

Bacon, E., Milne, D. L., Sheikh, A. I., & Freeston, M. H. (2009). Positive experiences in caregivers: An exploratory case series. *Behavioural and Cognitive Psychotherapy, 37*(1), 95–114.

Bandura, A. (1977). Self-efficacy: Toward a unifying theory of behavioral change. *Psychological Review, 84*(2), 191–215.

Bellar, A., Kunkler, K., & Burkett, M. (2009). Understanding, recognizing, and managing chronic critical illness syndrome. *Journal of the American Academy of Nurse Practitioners, 21*(11), 571–578.

Bilkei-Gorzo, A., Otto, M., & Zimmer, A. (2008). Environmental modulation of anxiety-related neuronal activity and behaviors. *Behavioural Brain Research, 186*(2), 289–292.

Bilkei-Gorzo, A., Racz, I., Michel, K., Mauer, D., Zimmer, A., & Klingmuller, D. (2008). Control of hormonal stress reactivity by the endogenous opioid system. *Psychoneuroendocrinology, 33*(4), 425–436.

Boehm, H., & Morast, S. (2009). Quiet time: A daily period without distractions benefits both patients and nurses. *American Journal of Nursing, 109*(11 Suppl), 29–32.

Bondarenko, E., Hodgson, D. M., & Nalivaiko, E. (2014). Amygdala mediates respiratory responses to sudden arousing stimuli and to restraint stress in rats. *American Journal of Physiology Regulatory, Integrative and Comparative Physiology.* DOI: 10.1152/ajpregu.00528.2013.

Bornstein, N. M., Brainin, M., Guekht, A., Skoog, I., & Korczyn, A. D. (2014). Diabetes and the brain: Issues and unmet needs. *Neurological Science.* DOI: 10.1007/s10072-014-1797-2.

Bryanton, J., & Beck, C. T. (2010). Postnatal parental education for optimizing infant general health and parent-infant relationships. *Cochrane Database of Systematic Reviews, Issue 1,* Art No. CD00468. DOI: 10.1002/14651858.CD004068.pub3.

Buchholz, K. R., & Stephens, R. S. (2008). The cytosolic pattern recognition receptor NOD1 induces inflammatory interleukin-8 during *Chlamydia trachomatis* infection. *Infection & Immunity, 76*(7), 3150–3155. DOI: 10.1128/iai.00104-08.

Cheng, G., Huang, C., Deng, H., & Wang, H. (2012). Diabetes as a risk factor for dementia and mild cognitive impairment: A meta-analysis of longitudinal studies. *Internal Medicine Journal, 42*(5), 484–491. DOI: 10.1111/j.1445-5994.2012.02758.x.

Chesney, M. A., Neilands, T. B., Chambers, D. B., Taylor, J. M., & Folkman, S. (2006). A validity and reliability study of the coping self-efficacy scale. *British Journal of Health Psychology, 11*(Part 3), 421–437.

Chovatiya, R., & Medzhitov, R. (2014). Stress, inflammation, and defense of homeostasis. *Molecular Cell, 54*(2), 281–288. DOI: 10.1016/j.molcel.2014.03.030.

Chrousos, G. P. (2009). Stress and disorders of the stress system. *Nature Reviews Endocrinology, 5*(7), 374–381.

Claudianos, C., Lim, J., Young, M., Yan, S., Cristino, A. S., Newcomb, R. D., et al. (2014). Odor memories regulate olfactory receptor expression in the sensory periphery. *European Journal of Neuroscience.* DOI: 10.1111/ejn.12539.

Darnall, B. D., & Suarez, E. C. (2009). Sex and gender in psychoneuroimmunology research: Past, present and future. *Brain, Behavior, and Immunity, 23*(5), 595–604.

Di, S., Maxson, M. M., Franco, A., & Tasker, J. G. (2009). Glucocorticoids regulate glutamate and GABA synapse-specific retrograde transmission via divergent nongenomic signaling pathways. *Journal of Neuroscience, 29*(2), 393–401.

Dusek, J. A., & Benson, H. (2009). Mind-body medicine: A model of the comparative clinical impact of the acute stress and relaxation responses. *Minnesota Medicine, 92*(5), 47–50.

Epel, E., Daubenmier, J., Moskowitz, J. T., Folkman, S., & Blackburn, E. (2009). Can meditation slow rate of cellular aging? Cognitive stress, mindfulness, and telomeres. *Annals of the New York Academy of Sciences, 1172,* 34–53.

Esch, T., & Stefano, G. B. (2010). The neurobiology of stress management. *Neuro Endocrinology Letters, 31*(1), 30.

Franklin, T. B., Saab, B. J., & Mansuy, I. M. (2012). Neural mechanisms of stress resilience and vulnerability. *Neuron, 75*(5), 747–761. DOI: 10.1016/j.neuron.2012.08.016.

Garland, E., Gaylord, S., & Park, J. (2009). *The role of mindfulness in positive reappraisal.* Explore (New York, N.Y.), 5(1), 37–44.

Gillespie, C. F., Phifer, J., Bradley, B., & Ressler, K. J. (2009). Risk and resilience: Genetic and environmental influences on development of the stress response. *Depression and Anxiety, 26*(11), 984–992.

Gray, J. D., Milner, T. A., & McEwen, B. S. (2013). Dynamic plasticity: The role of glucocorticoids, brain-derived neurotrophic factor and other trophic factors. *Neuroscience, 239,* 214–227. DOI: 10.1016/j.neuroscience.2012.08.034.

Holsboer, F., & Ising, M. (2010). Stress hormone regulation: Biological role and translation into therapy. *Annual Review of Psychology, 61,* 81–109, C101–111.

Iqbal, S., & Hood, D. A. (2014). Oxidative stress-induced mitochondrial fragmentation and movement in skeletal muscle cells. *American Journal of Physiology: Cell Physiology.* DOI: 10.1152/ajpcell.00017.2014.

Juruena, M. F. (2013). Early-life stress and HPA axis trigger recurrent adulthood depression. *Epilepsy and Behavior.* DOI: 10.1016/j.yebeh.2013.10.020.

Kanner, A. D., Coyne, J. C., Schaefer, C., & Lazarus, R. S. (1981). Comparison of two modes of stress measurement: Daily hassles and uplifts versus major life events. *Journal of Behavioral Medicine, 4*(1), 1–39.

Karatsoreos, I. N., & McEwen, B. S. (2011). Psychobiological allostasis: Resistance, resilience and vulnerability. *Trends in Cognitive Sciences, 15*(12), 576–584. DOI: 10.1016/j.tics.2011.10.005.

Knight, B. G., & Sayegh, P. (2010). Cultural values and caregiving: The updated sociocultural stress and coping model. *Journals of Gerontology. Series B, Psychological Sciences and Social Sciences, 65B*(1), 5–13.

Lazarus, R. S. (1981). Little hazards can be hazardous to your health. *Psychology Today, 15*(7), 11–31.

McEwen, B. S. (2008). Central effects of stress hormones in health and disease: Understanding the protective and damaging effects of stress and stress mediators. *European Journal of Pharmacology, 583,* 174–185.

McEwen, B. S. (2007). Physiology and neurobiology of stress and adaptation: Central role of the brain. *Physiological Reviews, 87*(3), 873–904.

McEwen, B. S. (2009). The brain is the central organ of stress and adaptation. *NeuroImage, 47*(3), 911–913.

McEwen, B. S., Eiland, L., Hunter, R. G., & Miller, M. M. (2012). Stress and anxiety: Structural plasticity and epigenetic regulation as a consequence of stress. *Neuropharmacology, 62*(1), 3–12. DOI: 10.1016/j.neuropharm.2011.07.014.

McEwen, B. S., & Getz, L. (2013). Lifetime experiences, the brain and personalized medicine: An integrative perspective. *Metabolism, 62*(Suppl 1), S20–S26. DOI: 10.1016/j.metabol.2012.08.020.

McEwen, B. S., & Wingfield, J. C. (2010). What is in a name? Integrating homeostasis, allostasis and stress. *Hormones and Behavior, 57*(2), 105–111.

NAMI. (2014). *National Alliance on Mental Illness.* Retrieved October 26, 2014, from http://www.nami.org/

NANDA-Association International (NANDA-I). (2014). *Nursing diagnoses: Definitions and classification, 2015–2017.* West Sussex, England: Wiley-Blackwell.

National Institute of Diabetes and Digestive and Kidney Diseases. (2014). *National Institute of Health Statistics.* Retrieved September 7, 2011, from http://diabetes.niddk.nih.gov/DM/PUBS/statistics/#i_people

Paysnick, A. A., & Burt, K. B. (2014). Moderating effects of coping on associations between autonomic arousal and adolescent internalizing and externalizing problems. *Journal of Clinical Child and Adolescent Psychology, 34*(10), 1–13. DOI: 10.1080/15374416.2014.891224.

Raineki, C., Hellemans, K. G., Bodnar, T., Lavigne, K. M., Ellis, L., Woodward, T. S., et al. (2014). Neurocircuitry underlying stress and emotional regulation in animals prenatally exposed to alcohol and subjected to chronic mild stress in adulthood. *Front Endocrinol (Lausanne), 5,* 5. DOI: 10.3389/fendo.2014.00005.

Romero, L. M., Dickens, M. J., & Cyr, N. E. (2009). The Reactive Scope Model—a new model integrating homeostasis, allostasis, and stress. *Hormones and Behavior, 55*(3), 375–389.

Selye, H. (1950). Stress and the general adaptation syndrome. *British Medical Journal, 1*(4667), 1383–1392.

Selye, H., & Fortier, C. (1950). Adaptive reaction to stress. *Psychosomatic Medicine, 12*(3), 149–157.

Sherman, D. K., Kim, H. S., & Taylor, S. E. (2009). Culture and social support: Neural bases and biological impact. *Progress in Brain Research, 178,* 227–237.

Sierra, A., Beccari, S., Diaz-Aparicio, I., Encinas, J. M., Comeau, S., & Tremblay, M. E. (2014). Surveillance, phagocytosis, and inflammation: How never-resting microglia influence adult hippocampal neurogenesis. *Neural Plasticity, 2014,* Article No. 610343. DOI: 10.1155/2014/610343.

Stickley, A., Koyanagi, A., Koposov, R., Schwab-Stone, M., & Ruchkin, V. (2014). Loneliness and health risk behaviours among Russian and U.S. adolescents: A cross-sectional study. *BMC Public Health, 14*(1), 366. DOI: 10.1186/1471-2458-14-366.

Stone, J., Johnstone, D. M., Mitrofanis, J., & O'Rourke, M. (2014). The mechanical cause of age-related dementia (Alzheimer's Disease): The brain is destroyed by the pulse. *Journal of Alzheimers Disease.* DOI: 10.3233/jad-141884.

Timmermans, W., Xiong, H., Hoogenraad, C. C., & Krugers, H. J. (2013). Stress and excitatory synapses: From health to disease. *Neuroscience, 248,* 626–636. DOI: 10.1016/j.neuroscience.2013.05.043.

Tudor-Locke, C. (2009). Promoting lifestyle physical activity: Experiences with the First Step Program. *American Journal of Lifestyle Medicine, 3*(1 Suppl), 508–548.

Vaughan, V. C., Martin, P., & Lewandowski, P. A. (2013). Cancer cachexia: Impact, mechanisms and emerging treatments. *J Cachexia Sarcopenia Muscle, 4*(2), 95–109. DOI: 10.1007/s13539-012-0087-1.

Verhoog, M. B., Goriounova, N. A., Obermayer, J., Stroeder, J., Hjorth, J. J., Testa-Silva, G., et al. (2013). Mechanisms underlying the rules for associative plasticity at adult human neocortical synapses. *Journal of Neuroscience, 33*(43), 17197–17208. DOI: 10.1523/jneurosci.3158-13.2013.

Wagner, R., Staiger, H., Ullrich, S., Stefan, N., Fritsche, A., & Haring, H. U. (2014). Untangling the interplay of genetic and metabolic influences on beta-cell function: Examples of potential therapeutic implications involving TCF7L2 and FFAR1. *Molecular Metabolism, 3*(3), 261–267. DOI: 10.1016/j.molmet.2014.01.001.

Washington, T. D. (2009). Psychological stress and anxiety in middle to late childhood and early adolescence: Manifestations and management. *Journal of Pediatric Nursing, 24*(4), 302–313.

Weber, J., & Kelley, J. (2014). *Health assessment in nursing* (5th ed.). Philadelphia, PA: Lippincott Williams & Wilkins.

Willfuhr, K., & Myrskyla, M. (2014). Disease load at conception predicts survival in later epidemics in a historical French-canadian cohort, suggesting functional trans-generational effects in humans. *PLoS One, 9*(4), e93868. DOI: 10.1371/journal.pone.0093868.

World Health Organization. (2014). *Diabetes Facts.* Retrieved April 25, 2014, from http://www.who.int/diabetes/facts/world_figures/en/

Wosiski-Kuhn, M., Erion, J. R., Gomez-Sanchez, E. P., Gomez-Sanchez, C. E., & Stranahan, A. M. (2014). Glucocorticoid receptor activation impairs hippocampal plasticity by suppressing BDNF expression in obese mice. *Psychoneuroendocrinology, 42,* 165–177. DOI: 10.1016/j.psyneuen.2014.01.020.

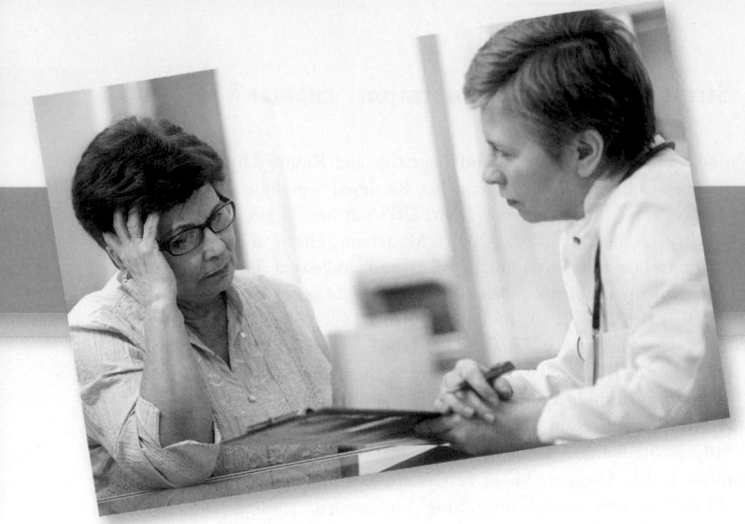

CHAPTER 42

Human Sexuality

Nancy Westvang

Case Scenario

You are a nurse working in a women's health clinic. A divorced woman comes in for an examination because she has not menstruated for 2 months. She tells you that she is sexually active and has a new male partner who refuses to use condoms. She is not using anything for contraception herself.

Once you have completed this chapter and have incorporated human sexuality into your knowledge base, review the above scenario and reflect on the following areas of Critical Thinking:

1. Reflect on your feelings and impression about this situation. Distill possible explanations for your reactions.
2. Propose additional information that you would need to elicit from this woman, including your rationale for needing such information.
3. Describe how you would best approach this woman to get as detailed a history as possible.
4. Describe a plan for follow-up for this patient.

KEY TERMS

bisexual
celibacy
climacteric
clitoris
dyspareunia
erectile dysfunction (ED)
foreplay
foreskin
heterosexual
homosexual
impotence
intersex
masturbation
menarche
menopause
menstruation
orgasm
premature ejaculation
prepuce
sexuality
sexually transmitted infection (STI)
transgendered
transsexual
vaginismus

LEARNING OBJECTIVES

Upon completion of this chapter, you will be able to do the following:

1. Describe the structures of the male and female reproductive systems.
2. Discuss sexual expression, menstruation, and reproduction as functions of human sexuality.
3. Compare the male and female sexual response cycles.
4. Relate sexuality to all stages of the life cycle.
5. Identify factors that affect sexual functioning.
6. Describe common risks and alterations in sexuality.
7. Understand the nursing process as it relates to sexual functioning.
8. Teach patients to perform breast self-examination or testicular self-examination.

Despite the marked openness of today's media regarding sexual matters, many people are hesitant to discuss their own **sexuality** and sexual issues, especially with strangers. But nurses need to overcome patient hesitance so that they can accurately gather important health information related to this core human function.

Most nurses work with patients in settings that are not directly related to sexuality. Patients in any setting, however, may approach nurses with concerns regarding sexuality. Or sexual issues may exist for the patient, but he or she is hesitant to acknowledge them to the nurse or to other healthcare providers. Thus, sexual issues should be part of the patient history. Although some common problems can be dealt with in the healthcare facility (by healthcare providers with general knowledge of human sexuality), more advanced problems require attention from specially trained personnel. Each nurse must be aware of his or her personal attitudes, expertise, and limitations. These should not, however, interfere with care given.

The 2001 *Surgeon General's Call to Action to Promote Sexual Health and Responsible Sexual Behavior* emphasized the importance of encouraging responsible sexual behavior to the public with the goal of promoting general health and wellness in our society (U.S. Office of the Surgeon General, 2001). Responsible sexual behavior has been one of the top 10 health indicators of the nation since 2000 and will continue to be in Healthy People 2020 (HealthyPeople.Gov). The importance of addressing issues of human sexuality in routine healthcare practices cannot be overemphasized. According to the World Health Organization (WHO), readily available access to sexual and reproductive health promotes the realization of basic human rights (WHO, 2014).

NORMAL HUMAN SEXUALITY

Sexuality includes function of the sexual organs, gender identity, reproduction, eroticism, intimacy, the person's perceptions of his or her own functioning, sexual expression, and sexual preferences. All throughout a person's life, sexuality is an essential facet of being human (WHO, 2011). Human sexual response varies and is influenced by many factors. Such factors include psychological, emotional, and cultural issues; values and moral views; and comfort with one's body and the quality of any sexual relationships (National Institutes of Health, 2009). Patients may experience various emotions related to sexual dysfunction such as embarrassment, guilt, anger, sadness, or frustration (Latif & Diamond, 2013). A person not involved in a sexual relationship is still a sexual being with a sexual identity.

Structure of the Reproductive Systems

Although sexuality is not synonymous with reproduction, the reproductive organs are involved in human sexual response. For purposes of clarity, the male and female reproductive systems are discussed separately.

MALE REPRODUCTIVE SYSTEM

The male reproductive system (Fig. 42-1) is composed of both external and internal organs. The external organs include the penis and scrotum. The penis is a pendulous organ composed of two sections, the shaft and the glans. Inside the penis are cylindrically shaped areas of spongy tissue filled with tiny blood vessels. Normally flaccid, the penis becomes erect in

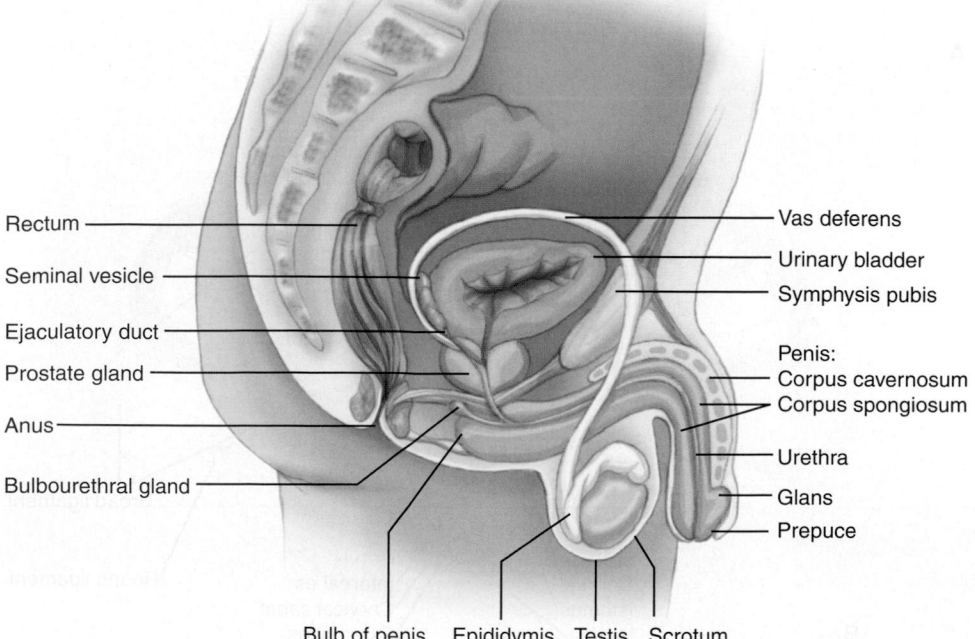

FIGURE 42-1 Internal and external organs of the male reproductive system.

Rectum

Seminal vesicle

Ejaculatory duct

Prostate gland

Anus

Bulbourethral gland

Vas deferens

Urinary bladder

Symphysis pubis

Penis:
Corpus cavernosum
Corpus spongiosum

Urethra

Glans

Prepuce

Bulb of penis   Epididymis   Testis   Scrotum

response to arousal or other stimuli. Blood is pumped into the tiny vessels and the spongy areas fill, causing the penis to become hard. The shaft also contains the urethra, the outlet for urine from the urinary bladder. The glans is the cone-shaped head of the penis; it is covered with loose skin called the **prepuce** or **foreskin**. Uncircumcised men can retract the glans for intercourse and cleaning. In circumcised men, the glans is exposed because the foreskin has been removed surgically. The scrotum is the loose, pouchlike sac containing the testes. The testes are the male gonads, which are the reproductive glands that produce male cells (spermatozoa) and testosterone (male hormone).

The internal organs include the prostate gland and seminal vesicles. These glands produce and store most of the seminal fluid. The combination of seminal fluid and spermatozoa forms semen, the secretion discharged from the urethra during **orgasm**.

FEMALE REPRODUCTIVE SYSTEM

The female reproductive system also includes external and internal organs.

External Genitalia

The major structures composing the external genitalia include the mons pubis, labia majora, labia minora, **clitoris**, urethral meatus, Skene and Bartholin glands, and vaginal orifice (Fig. 42-2A). Collectively, these external parts are referred to as the vulva.

The mons pubis is a pad of fatty tissue over the bony prominence called the symphysis pubis. The labia are the fleshy borders of the external genitalia. The labia majora lie on either side of the vaginal opening, forming the lateral borders. The labia minora are thinner folds that lie just inside the labia majora.

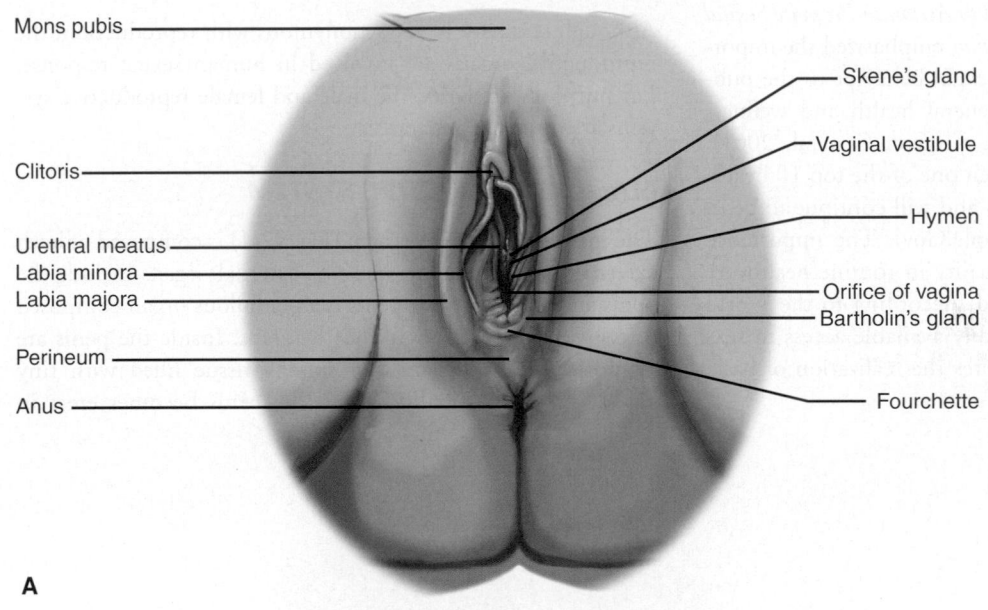

Mons pubis

Clitoris

Urethral meatus
Labia minora
Labia majora

Perineum

Anus

Skene's gland

Vaginal vestibule

Hymen

Orifice of vagina
Bartholin's gland

Fourchette

A

FIGURE 42-2 Female reproductive system. **A.** External genitalia. **B.** Internal genitalia.

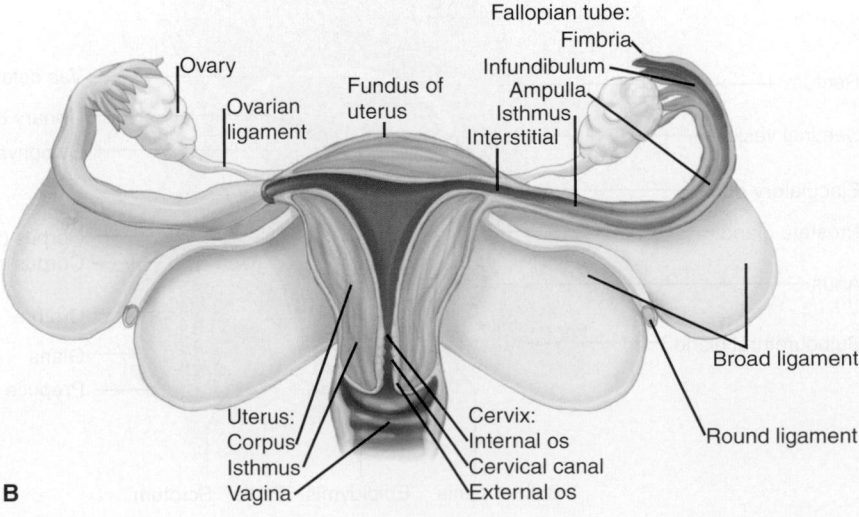

Ovary

Ovarian
ligament

Fundus of
uterus

Fallopian tube:
Fimbria
Infundibulum
Ampulla
Isthmus
Interstitial

Broad ligament

Round ligament

Uterus:
Corpus
Isthmus
Vagina

Cervix:
Internal os
Cervical canal
External os

B

The clitoris sits just above the point where the labia minora come together. It corresponds to the penis in the male in that both organs contain erectile tissue and respond to stimulation that can result in orgasm. Skene or paraurethral glands lie inside of and on the posterior of the urethra, and Bartholin glands are small mucous glands on the lateral wall of the vestibule of the vagina. The Skene and the Bartholin glands produce a small amount of lubricant. Although it was once believed that these glands were responsible for producing enough vaginal lubricant during sexual arousal, in actuality, they produce only a very small amount.

Internal Genitalia

The internal genitalia include the ovaries, fallopian tubes, uterus, and vagina (Fig. 42-2B). The ovaries are two almond-shaped bodies lying on either side of the pelvic cavity. They contain the ova (female sex cells) and female hormones, specifically estrogen and progesterone. Fallopian tubes are narrow ducts about 4.5 inches (11.4 cm) in length. They extend laterally on either side of the uterus and terminate in fingerlike projections near, but not touching, the ovaries.

The uterus is a muscular, pear-shaped organ that lies between the sacrum and the symphysis pubis. It consists of three areas: the fundus or upper portion; the cavity, which is hollow; and the cervix at the lower end, which connects the uterus to the vagina. The uterus is expandable.

The vagina is a musculomembranous tube that forms a passageway from the uterus to the vulva. It lies between the urinary bladder and the rectum. The vagina represents a potential space—the walls of the vagina, which are normally in contact, stretch for sexual intercourse or delivery of a baby.

Breasts

The female breasts (also called "mammary glands") are considered organs of reproduction because the reproductive hormones—estrogen and progesterone—directly influence them and because they are organs of lactation. Each breast is composed of fatty and glandular tissue and consists of 15 to 20 lobes (Fig. 42-3). Each lobe drains through a lactiferous duct that opens on the tip of the nipple. A circular pigmented area called the areola surrounds the nipple; the color of the areola is a pale to deep pink in light-skinned women and a light to darker brown in dark-skinned women. Breast size varies among women and throughout each woman's life span.

Function of Sexuality and the Reproductive Systems

Reproduction is only one component of sexuality. Human beings can be sexual—engage in sexual relationships and find sexual expression—without reproducing. When reproduction occurs, the male reproductive system is responsible for the generation, maturation, and ejaculation of spermatozoa. The female reproductive system is responsible for cyclic maturation and release of ova and, should fertilization occur, preparation of the uterus for implantation of a fertilized ovum. The experiences of **menstruation**, ovulation, and lactation are related to the woman's reproductive process.

SEXUAL EXPRESSION

Human beings are sexual beings. Their sexual expression varies. People may present themselves outwardly in terms of their own views of their sexuality. Sexual behaviors also vary. When engaging in coitus or stimulation, people use many different body positions without any particular one being considered "normal." Typical **heterosexual** sexual expression involves penile penetration of the vagina. Other expressions among both heterosexual couples and same-sex couples may include oral–genital stimulation or penile–anal penetration. The frequency of sexual expression also varies, with no determined "normal." Additionally, the amount and kind of **foreplay** (activity before sexual intercourse) may vary greatly. Some people engage in **masturbation** (self-stimulation) with a partner or alone. Others choose **celibacy** (abstention from sexual intercourse), although they still consider themselves sexual beings.

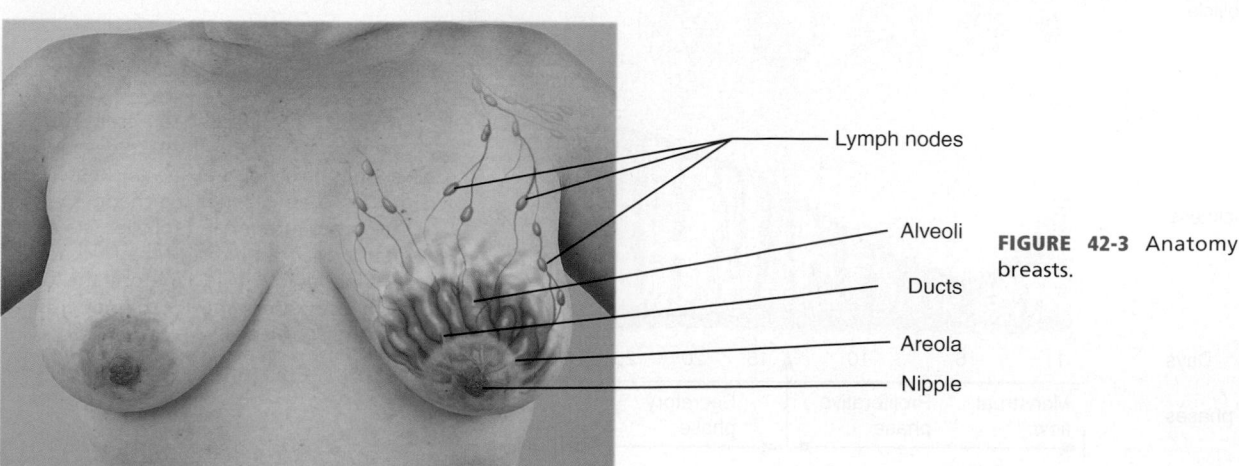

Lymph nodes

Alveoli

Ducts

Areola

Nipple

FIGURE 42-3 Anatomy of the breasts.

MENSTRUATION AND OVULATION

Menstruation is an external sign of complex physiologic processes essential to the reproductive function of women. Sexual expression can occur in the absence of menstruation (e.g., a woman who has gone through **menopause** or a woman with Turner syndrome, a genetic condition in which a woman is born without ovaries and does not menstruate). Because of its direct connection with reproduction, however, menstruation is appropriate to discuss in this chapter. Menstruation is a cyclic, periodic discharge of bloody fluid from the uterus through the vagina during the woman's reproductive years. The length of a menstrual cycle varies among women and during each woman's life span. The cycle repeats itself approximately every 28 days, although a normal range can be every 21 to 35 days.

Menstruation depends on the interplay of various hormones (Fig. 42-4). The hypothalamus secretes gonadotropin-releasing hormone, which stimulates the pituitary gland to secrete follicle-stimulating hormone and luteinizing hormone. These hormones stimulate the ovaries to produce estrogen and progesterone, which are necessary for stimulation of the target organs (vagina, breast, uterus) in preparing the body for possible pregnancy. If pregnancy does not occur, levels of estrogen and progesterone fall, menses ensues, and the feedback mechanism begins again with a new menstrual cycle.

The menstrual cycle is discussed in terms of the ovarian cycle and the endometrial or uterine cycle. The ovarian cycle consists of the follicular phase, the ovulatory phase, and the luteal phase. The follicular phase is estrogen dominant; during this phase, the follicles mature, with usually only one follicle reaching full maturity. This follicle, or oocyte, ruptures from the ovary at the time of the ovulatory phase. Progesterone then becomes the dominant hormone during the luteal phase, preparing the uterus for possible implantation and maintenance of a fertilized ovum.

The endometrial or uterine cycle is divided into the proliferative and secretory phases. The proliferative phase refers to the proliferation of the endometrium, or uterine lining.

Estrogen is the dominant hormone during the proliferative phase. During the secretory phase, which is progesterone dominant, the endometrial glands continue to grow, becoming edematous and dense, in preparation for implantation and maintenance of a fertilized ovum.

Hormones also affect the uterus at the cervical level. Under the influence of estrogen, the cervical mucus becomes more watery, alkaline, and stretchy, resembling the quality of egg whites. These qualities are conducive to sperm's survival, thus preparing for the possibility of conception.

CONCEPTION, PREGNANCY, AND BIRTH

For conception and reproduction to occur, several complicated factors must fully operate. First, the man must produce fully mature spermatozoa in sufficient numbers and with enough motility to penetrate the woman's cervix and to ascend the uterus and fallopian tubes. This transportation occurs by way of cervical mucus, which becomes alkaline and thus receptive to sperm. When the spermatozoa reach the fallopian tubes, they undergo capacitation, a process in which the sperm's surface characteristics change, releasing enzymes that enhance their ability to penetrate the ovum.

The occurrence of ovulation must correspond to the process described earlier because the time period in which the woman can be impregnated is only a few days. In ovulation, the ovary releases a mature follicle into one of the fallopian tubes. The fimbriae (fingerlike projections at the end of each fallopian tube) assist in extracting the ovum from the ovary and bringing it into the fallopian tube.

Fertilization of one ovum with one spermatozoon normally occurs in the outer third of the fallopian tube (see Fig. 42-2). After fertilization, the fertilized ovum undergoes several cell divisions and moves toward the uterus, where it implants in the uterine wall. The first 2 weeks after fertilization are critical; many pregnancies do not continue beyond this point because of a defective ovum or spermatozoon or because of hormone imbalances. If a pregnancy continues despite these

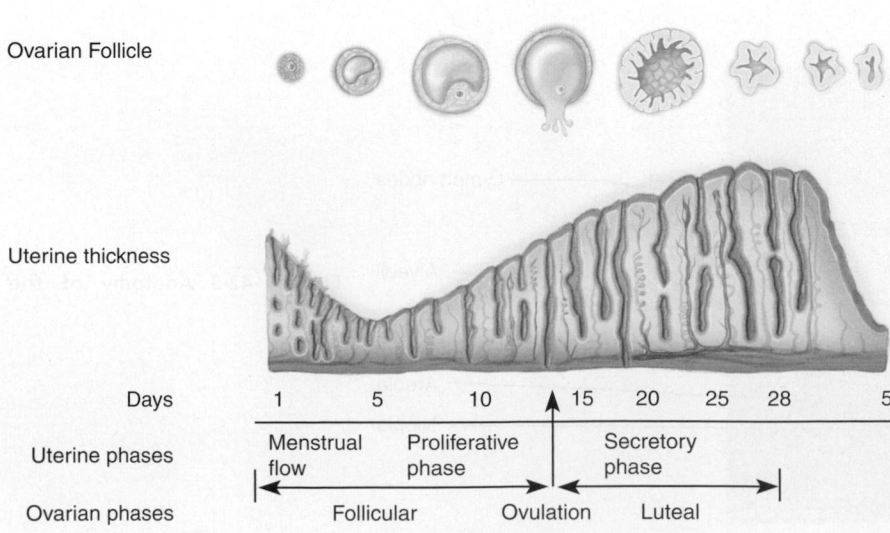

FIGURE 42-4 Schematic representation of one ovarian cycle and the corresponding changes in endometrial thickness. The ovarian cycle includes the changes within the corpus luteum and follicle. The endometrial changes indicate the thickness of the endometrium just before the onset of menstruation and its thinness just as menstruation ends.

complex factors and potential risks, the fertilized ovum, now called an embryo, develops rapidly. The average length of pregnancy, counted from the time of conception, is approximately 267 days, or 38 weeks, but may vary by about 2 weeks in either direction.

Birth is a normal process that occurs in three stages of labor. Although how labor begins is not entirely understood, stimulation by hormones causes the uterus to contract, ultimately pushing the fetus through the birth canal after several hours.

MILK PRODUCTION

With pregnancy and lactation, the woman's breasts undergo anatomic and physiologic changes (Fig. 42-5). They enlarge and become more sensitive. The nipples expand and darken, and the sebaceous glands in the areola hypertrophy. During the second half of pregnancy, the alveolar cells may begin to secrete colostrum. This yellowish fluid, considered a precursor to actual milk, contains important nutrients for the newborn.

Milk production occurs under the influence of prolactin, glucocorticoids, insulin, and parathyroid hormone. Estrogen and progesterone actually inhibit milk production; thus, with the delivery of the placenta, estrogen and progesterone levels fall dramatically.

Characteristics of Normal Sexuality

SEXUAL ORIENTATION

Sexual orientation is the core inner physical, romantic, or emotional attraction toward people of a specific gender (Fenway Institute, 2010). Various forms of sexual orientation exist. As mentioned earlier, no one way is "normal" in terms of sexuality and sexual orientation. Some people are heterosexual, attracted sexually to members of the opposite gender. Others are **bisexual**, attracted to both men and women sexually. Still others are **homosexual**, attracted sexually to members of the same gender. In an effort to address healthcare disparities among lesbian, gay, bisexual, and transgender (LGBT) individuals, questions regarding sexual orientation were included for the first time in the 2013 National Health Interview Survey (NHIS). Among US adults, nearly 97% of adults identified themselves as being heterosexual, while 1.6% identified as gay/lesbian and 0.7% identified as being bisexual (Centers for Disease Control and Prevention [CDC, 2014a]). Although the United States is becoming more open, there are many areas of this country and worldwide where those who view themselves as homosexual or bisexual are victims of family rejection, reproach, and verbal and physical abuse. This can impede the patient–provider relationship. Sexual orientation is not always consistent with sexual behavior or choice of partner. Some people choose to abstain totally from sexual relations either permanently or temporarily.

GENDER IDENTITY AND ROLES

Gender identity is a person's psychological identification as a man, a woman, or something else (Fenway Institute, 2010). Gender expression refers to the way in which a person chooses to demonstrate which gender he or she identifies with by way of outward appearance and voice. Individuals who identify with the opposite gender may still be heterosexual, bisexual, or homosexual in their expression of sexual orientation (APA, 2011). Gender role is the normative behavior a culture expects based on gender. Gender identity and corresponding roles influence sexuality, and it is important to understand the complexities of various gender identities and roles (Green, 2009). Nurses must understand each patient's perception of his or her gender and the meaning of that gender in terms of identity and roles. The CDC has many excellent online resources available to healthcare providers addressing the specific issues of LGBT health issues (CDC Resources for Serving LGBT Patients).

Sometimes a person's biologic gender does not coincide with his or her gender identity, as in the case of people who are **transsexual**. A **transgendered** person is someone who appears as, may have had surgery for, or desires to be a member of the opposite sex. The word transsexual is often used. A transsexual man views himself as a woman trapped in a man's body; the reverse is true for a female transsexual. Social roles

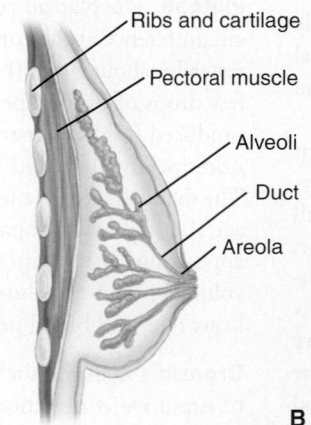
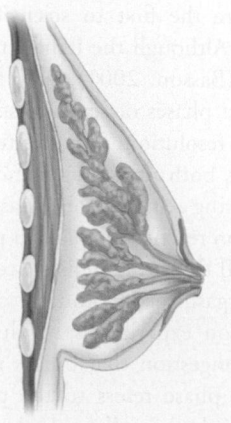
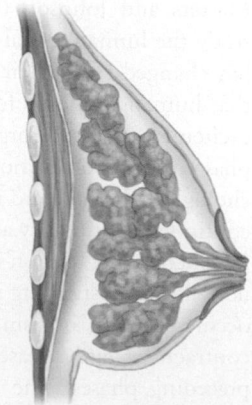

Ribs and cartilage

Pectoral muscle

Alveoli

Duct

Areola

FIGURE 42-5 The structure of the breast varies among women and during a woman's lifetime. The illustration shows the breast in the nonpregnant woman **(A)**, pregnant woman **(B)**, and lactating woman **(C)**.

A   B   C

are usually confusing for transsexuals. Some marry and have families; others do not. Some seek medical intervention in the form of hormones and surgery to change their physical gender. Sometimes the terms *transsexual* and *transvestite* are used interchangeably, although incorrectly. Transsexuals may maintain an appearance consistent with their biologic gender. *Transvestite* is an outdated term used to describe a person who dresses like someone of the opposite sex but views himself or herself according to his or her biologic gender. The term is now considered pejorative. Cross-dressing can range from wearing only one article of clothing to entire ensembles. People who cross-dress do not always do so for erotic pleasure, but rather simply feel more comfortable in opposite gender clothing. The cross-dresser has no desire to change sexual orientation (APA, 2011). Some people are **intersexed**, meaning they were born with what is referred to as "ambiguous genitalia," in which it is difficult to determine sex. These people may eventually undergo surgery to differentiate and determine their gender. The literature, although growing, remains sparse in regard to gender identity issues, but these matters are of great importance to nurses and other healthcare providers. It is critical that healthcare providers develop sensitivity and understanding of these issues to provide optimum care for these people if they become patients for any reason. It is important to recognize the humanness in all people (Denny, 2004). The University of Pittsburgh has established the Center for Research on Health and Sexual Orientation (www.crhso.publichealth.pitt.edu/index.htm), which promotes research to better understand the experience of sexual minorities.

Normal Sexual Patterns

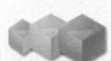

Concept Mastery Alert

Biologic sex is an outcome of genetic factors, while gender identity is a more complex and varied psychosocial construct. However, it is simplistic to claim that gender identity is something that is consciously "chosen" at a particular time of development.

SEXUAL RESPONSE

Masters and Johnson (1966) were the first to scientifically study the human sexual response. Although the female model has changed since their research (Basson, 2001), they found that humans undergo four distinct phases of sexual response: excitement, plateau, orgasm, and resolution. The excitement phase results from various stimuli, both physiologic and psychological. If there are no distracting stimuli, this phase will continue and intensify as the person reaches the plateau phase, in which sexual tension increases. If this sexual tension continues without distracting stimuli, orgasm or involuntary climax occurs. During orgasm, the person experiences involuntary contractions and release of vasocongestion that builds in the preceding phases. The resolution phase refers to the period after orgasm in which physiologic changes allow the body to

return to its preexcitement state. These phases will be discussed more specifically as experienced by men and women. Other researchers revised the definition (Lauver & Welch, 1990). Kaplan (1979), for example, believed that desire was an important part of the cycle and redefined the sexual response cycle according to three phases: desire, excitement, and orgasm. The American Psychiatric Association (APA) (1994) developed a slightly different description of the sexual response, consisting of four phases: appetitive, excitement, orgasm, and resolution. More recently, Basson described a different sexual response cycle that focuses on the importance of the interaction and interpersonal relationship with the sexual partner in eliciting the sexual response. In Basson's nonlinear model of female sexual response, women are in a state of sexual neutrality, receptive to sexual activity, with arousal seen before desire. This differs from men, where desire always precedes arousal (Neuroscience Education Institute, 2010).

Because Masters and Johnson's work is considered "classic" and much subsequent research is based on their work, this chapter presents detailed descriptions based on their model.

Male Sexual Response

Masters and Johnson (1966) found one pattern of sexual response in men, although it is unlikely that male sexual response occurs without variation. In fact, for both men and women, many factors affect sexual response, which is a psychophysiologic response (Sadock, 2009). The predominant pattern identified by Masters and Johnson (1966) includes a rapid excitement phase, a short plateau phase with orgasm occurring immediately, and a resolution phase that includes an obligatory refractory period.

Excitement. The excitement phase is characterized by rapid erection of the penis with tensing and thickening of the scrotal skin and elevation of the scrotal sac. The spermatic cords shorten, causing partial elevation of both testes toward the perineum. Vasocongestion during this phase is responsible for penile erection, thickening of the scrotal skin, and elevation of the scrotal sac. The testes increase in size. The man may experience nipple erection during the excitement phase. It is not unusual for the man partially to lose his penile erection and regain it. Distractions may interfere with excitement.

Plateau. The plateau phase involves a thickening of the penis circumference at the coronal ridge and an increase in size of the testes by about 50% (Hacker, Gambone, & Hobel, 2010). A few drops of fluid appear at the urethral meatus. This fluid is produced from Cowper glands and contributes to lubrication. Additionally, this fluid may contain some active spermatozoa. The man may experience nipple erection, and a sex flush, characterized by a maculopapular rash over the epigastric area, may appear during the latter part of this phase. Increases occur in voluntary and involuntary muscle contraction, ventilation, heart rate, and blood pressure.

Orgasm. Orgasm is the climax of the plateau phase and consists of expulsive contractions of the entire length of the urethra. The initial three or four contractions are strongest and then they subsequently decrease. Concurrently, the force of ejaculation is greatest with the first several contractions and decreases thereafter. Ejaculation can be viewed as composed of two stages. The first stage consists of expulsion of seminal fluid substrate from the seminal vesicles into the prostatic urethra. The second stage consists of expulsion of the seminal fluid from the prostatic urethra to the urethral meatus.

Resolution. Resolution, the fourth and final phase, occurs immediately after orgasm and consists of an initial rapid loss of vasocongestion with an accompanying decrease in penis size. The scrotum becomes less congested, and the testes descend back into the scrotum, decreasing to their preexcitement size. Sex flush and nipple erection, if they occurred, disappear. Men experience an obligatory refractory period during which they are unable to be restimulated to erection. The length of this period varies individually.

Female Sexual Response

Although they found only one response pattern in men, Masters and Johnson (1966) found variability in the patterns of sexual response among women. Their classic model was linear, starting with excitement, progressing to plateau, then orgasm, and ending with resolution. Kaplan (1979) modified this classic model by emphasizing desire as the first stage instead of physiologic excitement. Basson published her model of female sexual response in 2001. This intimacy-based circular model emphasized the multifactorial nature of the female sexual response, which encompasses emotional intimacy, sexual stimuli, psychological factors, and relationship satisfaction (Kingsberg & Rezaee, 2013). Some women experience a plateau phase with several peaks without actually experiencing orgasm. Others experience a definite orgasm; still others experience multiple orgasms.

Excitement/Arousal. The excitement phase or arousal stage in women consists of clitoral enlargement and vulvar swelling. Vaginal lubrication occurs in response to vasocongestion from increased pressure in the capillaries as well as fluid escape from the vaginal wall. The vaginal space expands in the inner one-third portion, and the uterus becomes elevated. The vaginal orifice opens as the labia majora and minora either separate or move away slightly. The woman may also experience nipple erection and breast enlargement. She may experience a sex flush similar to that described earlier for men.

Plateau. The plateau phase involves retraction of the clitoris under the clitoral hood. The labia minora increase, and the vagina expands in width and depth. Full elevation of the uterus with concurrent rising of the cervix occurs. Nipple erection may continue, and the sex flush may spread. Both voluntary and involuntary muscle contractions increase, as do ventilation, heart rate, and blood pressure.

Orgasm. The orgasmic platform, or the outer third of the vagina and the labia minora, is the location of primary response during the orgasmic phase. Contractions occur very quickly and strongly in this area. After the initial three to six

contractions, intensity and frequency decrease. The woman experiences increased respiratory rate, heart rate, and blood pressure. Controversy exists as to whether women experience fluid expulsion during orgasm. Some research reports that women have described feeling a gushing of fluid along with orgasm. More recently, attention has focused on the differences in women's subjective experiences of orgasm.

Resolution. The resolution phase includes a return of the clitoris to normal size and position. Vasocongestion dissipates with resulting decrease in size of the orgasmic platform and vaginal relaxation. The woman does not have an obligatory refractory period and may experience multiple orgasms in a short period.

Life Span Considerations

Sexuality continues throughout a person's life. This section examines sexuality at each developmental stage, emphasizing physiologic, emotional, and social aspects. Figure 42-6 shows couples at two ends of the spectrum of male–female relationships.

INTRAUTERINE

The new organism's chromosomal formation is determined when the ovum and spermatozoon unite during fertilization. The sperm carries either an X or a Y chromosome to combine with the X chromosome that the ovum supplies. An XX combination becomes a female and an XY combination becomes a male at about the fifth or sixth week of prenatal life. Hormonal influences also play an important part in determining gonadal sex. In addition to an XY zygote, androgens must be present and cells must be sensitive to androgens for male genitalia to form. Lack of sensitivity to androgens, even with an XY genotype, will lead to development of female genitalia.

If genetic errors occur that lead to ambiguous genitalia, parents will have difficulty assigning gender to their newborn. Under normal circumstances, parents automatically interact with their child according to the child's gender. Problems such as ambiguous genitalia or lack of particular sex hormones may create serious problems in relating to a child as male or female and may create serious problems for the child as he or she matures.

NEWBORN AND INFANT

All beings are sexual. Male fetuses have been observed with erections on ultrasound, and it is known that sexuality is present from birth, with newborns of both genders having sexual responses of erection and vaginal lubrication (Gray, 2013). Healthy and normal psychosexual development is derived from parents and caregivers who cuddle, soothe, and touch their infants. Development of trust should occur during these stages, paving the way for future healthy interpersonal relationships. Parents normally relate to their infants as either male or female, which has consequences for later development. Because infants are very sensitive to touch, they commonly explore their own

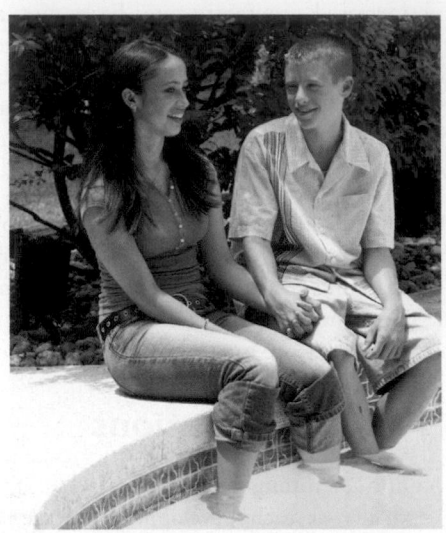

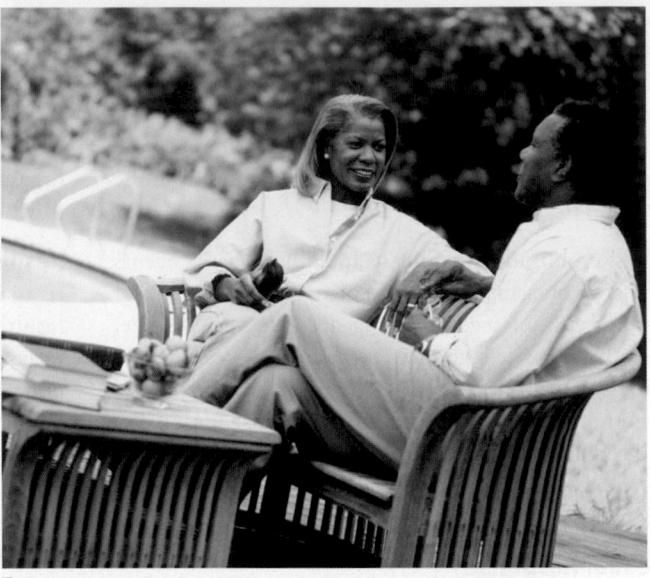

A   B

FIGURE 42-6 Expressions of sexuality from two aspects of the life span. **A.** A key aspect of adolescent development is learning to develop relationships. **B.** In older adulthood, warmth, intimacy, and companionship are comfortable aspects of sexuality.

bodies, including genitalia. Parents and other caregivers should recognize this developmental process as normal.

TODDLER AND PRESCHOOLER

As children become toddlers, they learn to walk and gain independence. They begin to explore their bodies even more while developing a body image that includes sexual identity. Toddlers may engage in masturbation, and parents should be reassured that this behavior is normal and healthy for development.

As toddlers become preschoolers, they begin to engage in further exploration of the body. Playing with friends and exploring their own bodies are normal. Children at this stage are curious about body parts and may often ask questions related to such things as where babies come from, breast-feeding, and physical differences between men and women and boys and girls.

SCHOOL-AGE CHILD AND ADOLESCENT

During elementary school, children establish their gender identity, continue to adopt certain sex role behaviors, and usually maintain friendships with those of the same sex. Children learn about anatomy, are curious about the opposite gender, and are interested in sexual jokes or stories. Masturbation in private situations remains normal as school-age children learn that public masturbation is not acceptable social behavior (APA, 2013). Experimentation in both heterosexual and homosexual roles is a normal part of childhood and adolescence, although homosexual youth may delay acting out sexual behaviors due to negative views held by family and society.

Adolescence is a turbulent time of psychosexual development. Adolescents not only cope with development of identity and independence from parents but also concurrently

experience a surge of hormonal changes leading to the physiologic changes of puberty. Adolescents of both sexes masturbate regularly and find it a pleasing outlet for sexual expression (APA, 2013). It is important to address in an open manner issues of sexuality with adolescents, with the understanding that adolescents are sexual beings by virtue of curiosity regarding sex, even if they are not yet sexually active A social phenomenon that has been gaining in popularity among adolescents is that of "sexting" or sending pornographic messages and images via cellular phones. Although this behavior is seen as an extension of sexual expression, in certain jurisdictions, it is seen as child pornography, and participants have been prosecuted to the full extent of the law (Fortenberry, 2013).

Outward physical changes in sexual maturity occur primarily from age 9 to 10 years through age 18 years and can be described using the five Tanner stages. Stage 1 is predevelopment, and stages 2 through 5 involve early development of pubic hair, breast budding, and then breast development in girls and maturing of the testes and scrotum and enlargement of the penis in boys (Slough, Hennrikus, & Chang, 2013). A key point in the development of adolescent girls is the onset of menstruation. The first menstrual period is termed **menarche**. The average age of menarche in the United States is 12.5 years (CDC, 2006–2010). Tanner stages of development of breasts and pubic hair and an emerging adult female shape and proportions coincide with puberty. Adolescent girls become concerned with these physical changes, some equating them with acceptance, confidence, and popularity, as well as sexual identity, while others find the changes disturbing.

Adolescent boys begin to experience nocturnal emissions. They assume a masculine sexual identity and behaviors based on role models and personal expectations. Teen boys are usually competitive in all areas of life, particularly sexual activity. In the

United States, the typical adolescent engages in sexual behavior that is unrelated to marriage. A growing practice among adolescents is termed "hooking up" in which they engage in sexual activity outside of a meaningful relationship (Garcia et al., 2012).

Sexual experimentation during adolescence is not without consequences. According to the CDC's *2013 Youth Risk Behavior Surveillance Report*, 46.8% of high school students have had sexual intercourse; 5.6% reported having had their first intercourse under the age of 13, and 15% have had four or more lifetime partners. Thirty-four percent were currently sexually active, and almost 40% of those who were sexually active did not use a condom during their last sexual intercourse (CDC MMWR, 2013). US birth certificate data from 2009 demonstrated that teen pregnancy rates for ages 15 to 19 were at the historic low of 39.1 births per 1,000 and down from their historic high of 61.8 births per 1,000 seen in 1991. However, the rate of 39.1 births per 1,000 is three times the rate of that seen in Canada and nearly four times the rate of teen pregnancy seen in Germany. The rate of teen pregnancy in Italy for the same period was 7 per 1,000 (Vital and Health Statistics, 2011). Interpersonal relationship conflicts, **sexually transmitted infections (STIs)**, and pregnancy are common problems during adolescence.

Awareness of sexual orientation usually begins during the early teen years. During 2006 to 2008, 8% of females and 3% of males ages 18 to 19 reported homosexual or bisexual orientation (Guttmacher Institute, 2014c). Adolescents who recognize homosexual feelings but are unable to express these feelings due to societal pressures tend to suffer higher incidence of depression, low self-esteem, alcohol and drug abuse, and violence. Studies have indicated that homosexual teens may be at a higher risk for suicide. Understanding this phenomenon is of critical importance for nurses caring for teenagers.

ADULT AND OLDER ADULT

The period between the tumultuous changes of adolescence and the **climacteric** spans about 35 years. Many changes may occur during this time, such as becoming involved in adult intimate relationships, raising children, letting children go, and beginning to experience aging. A review of adult sexuality found that men masturbate more often than women across the adult age span, with both sexes engaging in less frequent masturbation with declining age. Similarly, while 54% of men report thinking about sex at least once per day, only 19% of women do (Gray, 2013). Adults are responsible for educating their children about sexuality and have much influence in shaping their children's attitudes. Adults will continue to grapple with their own issues about sexuality and sexual behavior if they have not developed a high enough comfort level in the past. Many myths and stereotypes persist surrounding sexuality and sexual behavior, and some people fear certain aspects, such as homosexual feelings or behaviors. Adults, therefore, also need guidance from healthcare professionals.

During adulthood, many women experience pregnancy, which poses developmental issues related to sexuality. Additionally, physical and contextual changes that accompany pregnancy may lead to increased or decreased sexual activity. Some people may fear intercourse during pregnancy, or there may be contraindications to sexual intercourse due to high-risk conditions. People who limited the time engaged in sexual intercourse to prevent pregnancy no longer have that deterrent. Couples who desire pregnancy but encounter fertility problems may face other issues caused by the need to engage in sexual intercourse according to a rigid schedule.

The climacteric, or perimenopause, refers to the period during which significant sexual changes occur in the transition from middle to old age. This term more commonly refers to the transition that women experience as they begin to lose their reproductive function and approach cessation of their menstrual cycles. Menopause occurs exactly 1 year after the woman's last menstrual period. Essentially, it is a single point in time that marks the permanent cessation of menstrual activity. It normally occurs between the ages of 51 and 56 but may be surgically induced earlier. Postmenopause is the time after menopause. The most common symptom of menopause, experienced by as many as 75% of women, is hot flushes (ACOG, 2013). A decrease in sexual desire, termed loss of libido, may be reported in nearly half of all postmenopausal women. This is attributed to a decrease in hormones, especially when abrupt, as in the case of surgical menopause (Kingsberg & Rezaee, 2013). However, those women who do not experience a loss of libido may be engaging in less sexual activity with a partner as they age, not because they are unwilling, but because many women outlive their partners. Masturbation may be undertaken as an outlet for sexual desire.

Certain physiologic changes result from decreasing amounts of estrogen and testosterone during peri- and postmenopause. Women may experience thinning of vaginal and vulvar tissues, resulting in genitourinary atrophy with vaginal dryness, irritation, itching, and **dyspareunia** (Pinkerton & Stanczyk, 2013). Often, a lubricant is useful to counteract vaginal dryness. Either local or systemic estrogen may also be employed for vaginal dryness. The use of long-term systemic estrogen replacement therapy has been controversial because there is concern that regular systemic estrogen may promote or support malignancies. Vasomotor symptoms that may disrupt daytime activities and sleep can result in heightened fatigue. There are also cognitive changes associated with menopause, including decreased verbal fluency/memory and increased depressive symptoms and diagnosis of major depression (Weber, Maki, & McDermott, 2014). Osteoporosis is also common among some postmenopausal women, especially those with slight body types and those who are sedentary. Symptoms are typically absent until a fall, when a broken bone results. Physiologic changes also occur in older men. Specific effects can be noted in relation to the sexual response cycle, as described by Masters, Johnson, and Kolodny (1988). During the excitement phase, women experience slower onset of and decreased amounts of lubrication, whereas men experience slower and decreased firmness of erection. In women, the clitoris becomes smaller. Men may need more direct genital stimulation during the excitement phase. During the plateau phase, the vaginal canal does not increase as much as it did earlier, and the uterus does not become as elevated as it did previously. Men experience a decrease in the amount of Cowper gland secretion, are less able to maintain an erection, and have decreased testicular elevation. The orgasmic phase may become shortened for women and may not occur for men as their need to ejaculate is decreased. Men also experience a decreased force and volume of ejaculate and may experience less pleasure from ejaculation (Wylie & Kenney, 2010). Men experience longer refractory periods. Both men and women experience more rapid return to nonengorgement of the genitals. Cultural assumptions in the United States that sex is for the young is gradually being replaced by an understanding that many people are sexually active throughout their lives After divorce or death of a partner, many older adults are returning to the dating scene, often without considering the ramifications of unprotected intercourse. Additionally, with newer drugs and devices available for **erectile dysfunction (ED)** and vaginal atrophy, older adults are often remaining sexually active well into their 80s (Stewart & Graham, 2013). However, many people are comfortable with little or no sexual activity. Despite this, they may feel worried or pressured by a growing social belief created by the media and pharmaceutical influences that continued sexual activity is the norm. Older adults are as reluctant as are younger patients to bring up sexual issues with their healthcare providers; however, they will open up if the provider asks questions about sexual issues (Corona et al., 2013). Older women and men may wish to ask about and should be given the opportunity to discuss sexual concerns based on their individual desires.

CULTURAL CONSIDERATIONS

The practice of showing affection and sexuality has extensive cultural variation. Most Americans kiss and embrace in public. Some nationalities kiss only in private; others kiss publicly, often two times (once on each cheek); and, finally, some may kiss three times starting with one cheek. Some cultures show affection by rubbing noses, and other cultures choose not to show any demonstrative affection in public. All of these variations are valid for members of that culture.

A growing cultural phenomenon is the use of the Internet for sexual gratification, expression, and human sexuality. The number of online dating websites has increased dramatically, and many men and women seek to build relationships with the use of the Internet. Internet searches conducted by persons living in the United States were analyzed and reported on in the study titled "A Billion Wicked Thoughts." It was found that whereas men prefer to look at sexual images of a graphic nature, women desire romance and relationship-based stories (Ogas & Gaddam, 2011). In assessing beliefs that people hold in regard to sexuality, it becomes clear that we are all prejudiced by our family influences, religious beliefs, and personal experiences. These influences are embedded in our cultural understanding and knowledge. As a nurse, our personal perspective may be quite different from the viewpoints of those we encounter. It is important to keep an open, nonjudgmental attitude with respect for the beliefs and values of others.

FACTORS AFFECTING SEXUALITY

All people have a basic human need to be loved. Sexuality involves much more. The WHO (2006, 2010) defines *sexual health* as "a state of physical, emotional, mental and social well-being in relation to sexuality and not merely the absence of disease, dysfunction or infirmity."

Sexuality is a core part of human existence throughout a person's life (WHO, 2010):

- It encompasses sex of the physical body and the inner sense of gender identity and role as well as sexual orientation, eroticism, pleasure, intimacy, and reproduction.
- It is experienced and expressed through thoughts, behaviors, roles, relationships, and many other ways.
- It is influenced by "biological, psychological, social, economic, political, cultural, ethical, legal, historical, religious and spiritual factors" (p. 10).

As described previously, not all people are involved in sexual relationships, but they still regard themselves as and are sexual beings. Sexuality or experiences with sex can influence other areas. Addressing sexual health is an important part of any comprehensive approach to healthcare.

Relationships

The quality of a person's relationships can strongly influence the quality of his or her sexual experiences. Love and trust may be key factors in facilitating comfort with sexuality and sexual relations. Again, referring to the Case Scenario at the beginning of the chapter, the quality of the woman's relationships, particularly sexual relationships, may be important in allowing her to voice any fears or concerns (even perfectly normal concerns).

Cognition and Perception

Psychological factors include aspects leading to sexual arousal, such as certain mental images being triggered in the mind. Emotional state may greatly influence sexual response. For example, a person who is depressed may be less concerned with sex than a person who is happy or content. In addition, the degree of knowledge or misperceptions about sexuality will influence sexual functioning.

Culture, Values, and Beliefs

Cultural factors include society's predominant views of sexuality and the social context within which people experience it. Values and morals are additional influences. Religious beliefs and/or personal values may shape views concerning contraception, abortion, sex education, and sex outside marriage. The woman in the Case Scenario may be from a culture or ethnic group whose values influence her feelings about a pelvic examination, particularly one done by a male healthcare provider.

Self-Concept

People who are comfortable with themselves as sexual beings are likely to experience pleasure and comfort with sexual relations. A person who feels decreased self-esteem and self-confidence may experience negative effects in sexual functioning. The person may have a decreased sexual drive or conversely may attempt to compensate for this negative self-concept by over-emphasizing involvement in sexual relations.

Previous Experience

Previous experience with sexuality or ideas about sexuality influence current sexual functioning. For example, a person who was sexually abused in the past is likely to experience repercussions that will negatively affect current sexual functioning. A more subtle example is that of a man or woman who has grown up with many cultural taboos related to sexuality and finds it difficult later on to engage in a healthy sexual relationship. Fearing another unwanted pregnancy, a woman who has experienced an unwanted pregnancy or possibly an abortion may feel apprehensive about having sexual intercourse.

Pregnancy

Pregnancy clearly influences sexual functioning. Although sexual intercourse is not contraindicated during a normal, low-risk pregnancy, pregnancy may affect sexual drive. Many women find their sexual drive decreased during the first trimester, when they are tired and may feel nauseated. They may worry about miscarriage during the first trimester and thus fear having sexual intercourse. Problems with sexual desire, arousal, lubrication, and orgasm are reported in 63% to 90% of pregnancies. Dyspareunia is common as gestational age increases (Ribeiro et al., 2014). Decreased sexual function continues for some women for as long as 3 to 6 months after birth. Men also may vary in their sexual desires regarding pregnancy. Some men find pregnant women sexually attractive, whereas others are apprehensive about sexual relations during pregnancy for fear of harming the woman or fetus.

Infertility can place profound stress on a couple's sexual relationship. Couples who are trying to conceive must have sex according to when the woman ovulates. Sex becomes programmed and loses its spontaneity. In addition, couples may feel that they are having sex for a specific purpose rather than for enjoyment and mutual satisfaction. The sharing of their most private and intimate parts of their relationship can cause psychological distress. They may believe that they are being judged for how well they have sex in that pregnancy symbolizes "success" and lack of pregnancy symbolizes "failure." Mourning a child that has never been conceived can contribute to sexual problems. Many couples report that normal sexual relations resume after time elapses or they discontinue fertility treatments.

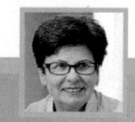

Human Sexuality PICO

Angie is a nurse working in the women's clinic. She receives a call from the patient in the chapter-opening scenario. The patient tells Angie that she recently found out that she is pregnant and is worried about miscarrying. The patient states that she has a history of miscarriages and has been researching this topic on the Internet. She learned that progestogen therapy prevents miscarriages and is requesting that the gynecologist put her on this treatment. Angie tells the patient that she will need to talk to the doctor and will call her back. Angie looks for evidence in the Cochrane Library before talking to the gynecologist. She uses the following PICO statement for the search: *In women of childbearing age, how does progestogen therapy compared to no progestogen therapy prevent miscarriages?*

P = women of childbearing age
I = progestogen therapy
C = no progestogen therapy
O = prevent miscarriage

Angie finds a meta-analysis study that reviewed 14 studies with 2,158 participants. The review showed no statistical evidence that progestogen therapy would prevent miscarriages. However, there was some evidence within the subgroups that seemed to indicate that women who suffered from three to four consecutive miscarriages found progestogen therapy to be beneficial. The authors noted that these findings were of low quality due to small trial groups and methodologic factors.

Angie takes these findings along with the patient's request to the gynecologist. The doctor asks Angie to bring in the patient's medical records and schedule lab work for progesterone levels with the patient's next office visit.

REFERENCE

Haas, D. M., & Ramsey, P. S. (2013). Progestogen for preventing miscarriage. *Cochrane Database of Systematic Reviews*, Issue 10. Art. No.: CD003511. doi: 10.1002/14651858.CD003511.pub3.

Environment

Environment can greatly affect sexual functioning. Hospitalized patients, particularly those undergoing long-term treatments, may find it inhibiting to have sexual relations with a partner or to masturbate within the confines of a hospital room. Lack of privacy becomes a major issue. The same is true for people in long-term care facilities. Environment is also a factor for people who are not hospitalized. Living in crowded conditions may preclude privacy. Fears about environmental pollutants affecting fertility may also influence sexuality.

ILLNESS AND DISABILITY

Illness poses a threat to normal sexual functioning. A person with cardiac problems may fear overexertion from engaging in sexual relations. Although this fear may not be based on physiologic principles, it can still be inhibiting. A person with an STI may fear transmitting the disease to a partner, or conversely, a person may fear contracting an STI from a partner. Although the individual may follow safer sex guidelines, this fear can inhibit sexual relations. Pain and joint disorders may make normal sexual intercourse uncomfortable. Motor vehicle accidents have created a sizable population of people with spinal cord injuries (paraplegia and quadriplegia); those affected must develop alternate methods of sexual functioning.

Medication

Some medications affect sexual desire and the ability to perform sexually. These include prescription drugs, over-the-counter drugs, and social/recreational drugs. Many conventional therapeutic drugs may adversely affect sexual functioning; those drugs include antihypertensives, antipsychotic tranquilizers, antidepressants, neurotransmitters, and hormones. Social drugs that can affect sexuality and sexual response include alcohol, opiates, marijuana, cocaine, sedative–hypnotics, amphetamines, amyl nitrite, LSD, cantharides, and yohimbine. Specific drugs have been developed to enhance male sexual functioning, particularly for erectile dysfunction (e.g., Viagra, Cialis).

Surgery

Cesarean births, hysterectomy, and mastectomy are examples of surgical procedures that affect a woman's sexuality. Women who undergo cesarean deliveries may experience longer recovery periods than do women who deliver vaginally and thus may feel less desire to resume sexual relations. Women who do not deliver vaginally may believe that they "failed" the labor and birth process, even though this thought is irrational. Such thoughts may affect subsequent sexual functioning.

Women who have had hysterectomies may believe that their femininity has been adversely affected. Again, this belief is irrational because women with hysterectomies are certainly able to engage in sexual intercourse and have orgasms. The meaning of the hysterectomy may be so negative to some women, however, that it adversely affects sexual functioning.

Women who have had mastectomies may also believe that femininity has been adversely affected, particularly in a society that highly emphasizes breasts as sexual objects. A mastectomy may negatively affect a woman's view of herself, which, in turn, may negatively affect her sexual functioning.

Men's sexuality may be profoundly affected by prostate cancer surgery as this can often result in problems related to maintaining an erection or difficulties with incontinence.

ALTERED HUMAN SEXUALITY

Certain conditions directly related to sexuality influence a person's ability to engage in mutually satisfying sexual relations. Conditions other than those mentioned in this section also may affect sexuality. Responsive sexual desire is increased desire following sexual arousal. One of the most important changes of the DSM-5 has been the merging of desire and arousal diagnoses into one, which is now referred to as female sexual interest and arousal disorder (FSIAD). This single diagnosis now takes into account both hypoactive sexual desire disorder (HSDD) as well as women without responsive desire, originally defined by Basson (Sungur & Gunduz, 2014).

Manifestations of Altered Sexuality

Alterations in normal patterns of sexuality can be seen in the following manifestations: sexual abuse, hypoactive sexual desire, **impotence**, ejaculatory dysfunctions, orgasmic dysfunction, and genitopelvic pain/penetration disorder (GPPD) (commonly known as dyspareunia and vaginismus; please see section on GPPD later in this chapter). The prevalence of sexual dysfunction is difficult to accurately ascertain. A survey conducted in the United States in 1999 demonstrated that 43% of women and 13% of men reported altered sexuality. Difficulty with desire is most prevalent in women reporting sexual dysfunction, followed by problems with orgasm, problems with arousal, and, finally, sexual pain (Latif & Diamond, 2013). Nurses can play a key role by assessing alterations in sexuality, assisting in prevention of problems, and helping patients cope with existing problems.

SEXUAL ABUSE

Some people manifest altered sexual functioning by being sexually abusive to others, such as children, spouses, acquaintances, or strangers. Regarding childhood sexual abuse, girls are victims more often than boys; however, the exact incidence of child sexual abuse is impossible to know. Psychiatric issues such as depression, anxiety, sleep and eating disorders, posttraumatic stress disorder, and attempted suicide are all attributed to child sexual abuse (Martin & Silverstone, 2013). Sexual abuse results in sexual problems for abused people as well.

HYPOACTIVE SEXUAL DESIRE

Lack of or hypoactive sexual desire is subjective. Because there is no "normal" frequency of sexual relations, determining the frequency that reflects hypoactive sexual desire is difficult. A key feature may be the partner's dissatisfaction with frequency of sexual relations. Thus, relationships play an important role in this issue. Sometimes, inhibited sexual desire in one partner accompanies inhibited desire in the other partner. More commonly, though, each partner's desires are incongruent and thus become a problem. Many factors contribute to inhibited sexual desire. Physical factors include use of certain medications, neurologic problems, and hormonal imbalances. Psychological factors may be depression and interpersonal difficulties. It may be difficult to determine if depression has resulted from inhibited sexual desire or if it is a cause of inhibited sexual desire and consequent marital problems. Other possible causes are history of sexual abuse and GPPD.

ERECTILE DYSFUNCTION

Also known as impotence, ED is the inability to attain or maintain an erection long enough for satisfactory sexual intercourse. It is a common occurrence in men over 40, and in men over age 70, the prevalence can be as high as 50% to 100%. As populations are aging worldwide, the predicted incidence of ED by the year 2025 is estimated to reach 322 million. Most cultures highly value a man's "virility" and view ED as a manifestation of his "failure to perform." ED can be primary or secondary. Primary ED refers to a man who has never been able to achieve an erection necessary for intercourse; secondary ED refers to a man who was once successful in attaining and maintaining erections but who has subsequently experienced difficulty.

ED is caused by physiologic conditions such as diabetes, hypertension, hyperlipidemia, depression, and lower urinary tract conditions. It is also closely associated with coronary artery disease, and it is suggested that men presenting with ED be worked up for cardiac problems if not previously done. Lifestyle factors may also lead to ED, including obesity, smoking, and little to no exercise (Shamloul & Ghanem, 2013). A study of over 500 men without ED that were followed for 8 years demonstrated that above all, regular physical exercise resulted in a 30% decrease in the development of ED, regardless of BMI. Those at most risk for ED were those men that remained sedentary. Various neurogenic conditions may also be associated with ED. These include Parkinson disease, multiple sclerosis, temporal lobe epilepsy, and spinal cord injury. Nerve damage from radical prostatectomy frequently results in ED. Certain manifestations may indicate the probability that the problem is secondary to a psychological factor such as fear of performance failure. For example, if a man is able to attain an erection in certain situations but not others, has erections during sleep, or has experienced periods with no erection difficulties, the problem is probably psychological. However, if erection is impossible in any of these situations, the problem is probably physiologic.

First-line treatment for ED includes modifying medications that may be interfering with function and lifestyle changes such as weight loss, exercise, and smoking cessation (Glina, Sharlip, & Hellstrom, 2013). Phosphodiesterase type 5 (PDE5) inhibitors such as Viagra, Cialis, and Levitra are oral drugs effective in treating ED by producing an erection caused by physical problems such as spinal cord injury, diabetes, and antidepressant therapy (Heidelbaugh, 2010). The drugs do not work to improve libido.

EJACULATORY DYSFUNCTION

Premature Ejaculation

Premature ejaculation (PE) is the most commonly reported male sexual dysfunction. Until recently, it was poorly understood and had no clear definition. As a result of marketing of PDE5 inhibitors and ED research, new interest and opportunity to better understand PE has arisen. It is now seen primarily as a neurophysiologic disorder (Keel et al., 2010), and the International Society of Sexual Medicine recently agreed on one common definition, where PE is diagnosed when ejaculation nearly always happens prior to penetration or occurs within 1 minute of vaginal penetration, there is an inability to delay ejaculation nearly all the time, and the man experiences negative personal consequences (Althof et al., 2014). Because there are few studies addressing PE with regard to homosexual activity, this definition is solely based on heterosexual intercourse with vaginal penetration. PE can be classified as lifelong (primary) or acquired. All men who present with a complaint of PE should have a thorough history and physical exam, including a prostate examination if over 40. A careful assessment of sexual history is obligatory because some men may incorrectly label normal sexual function as PE (McMahon et al., 2013). Treatments have included psychotherapy using both behavioral methods and cognitive interventions. Medications include topical medications to decrease sensation as well as the use of short-acting selective serotonin reuptake inhibitors (SSRIs), which are known to delay ejaculation. Dapoxetine, a potent SSRI, is the first medication that has been marketed specifically for the treatment of PE. This is taken several hours prior to intercourse and has been shown to be efficacious in delaying ejaculation (McMahon et al., 2013).

Inability to Ejaculate

Most men ejaculate within 4 to 10 minutes after entering the vagina. Delayed ejaculation ranges from a limited ability to ejaculate in the vagina to a complete inability to ejaculate under any condition (Corona et al., 2013). Delayed ejaculation occurs when sexual activity is longer than 20 to 30 minutes or has to be stopped due to tissue irritation or exhaustion. Inability to ejaculate actually refers to inability to ejaculate in the vagina. This condition is less common than PE. The cause of ejaculatory incompetence may be primary or secondary. Primary causes include psychological disturbances; secondary causes may be related to interpersonal problems with one's sexual partner or organic causes such as lumbar sympathectomy or antiadrenergic drugs such as guanethidine or methyldopa.

ORGASMIC DYSFUNCTION

There are multiple neural pathways that can produce a female orgasm. Some originate in the clitoris, while others exist independently deep in the vagina. Female orgasms vary by intensity, frequency, and pleasure produced. Even the ability to have an orgasm varies. Women often take four times as long to experience an orgasm than men do. Some women have never had an orgasm, while others have regular orgasms. Some women can have an orgasm without direct genital stimulation by using fantasy thoughts or nipple stimulation (Albaugh, 2014). Difficulty achieving orgasm has been reported by as many as 20% to 30% of women, and many causes have been identified. Lack of information, lack of adequate stimulation, or problems in an intimate relationship may cause difficulty attaining orgasm. Sometimes women feel pressured to have an orgasm to please their partners, and some partners feel pressure to "bring" the woman to orgasm so that they will have been "successful" at sex. This kind of pressure may inhibit the woman's ability to attain an orgasm. Physical problems such as illnesses that decrease quality of life or impact cardiovascular, neurologic, hormonal, or musculoskeletal systems may interfere with orgasm, as may conditions that cause chronic worry, pain, or mental illnesses including depression. As with men, certain pharmacologic agents or treatments may interfere with orgasm, such as SSRIs, chemotherapy, or radiation. Developmental and physiologic changes such as pregnancy, menopause, and gynecologic surgeries may lead to decreased ability to have an orgasm.

GENITOPELVIC PAIN/PENETRATION DISORDER

In the DSM-IV-TR, two separate diagnoses of dyspareunia and **vaginismus** appear. With the new DSM-V diagnostic criteria, they have made the determination to group these disorders into one known as GPPD. Both disorders singly addressed painful intercourse along a continuum from superficial vaginal pain to pain with deep penetration. It also now considers fear of pain with penetration to be a key emotional element necessary for diagnosis (Sungur & Gunduz, 2014). Dyspareunia, or painful intercourse, is thought to be the direct result of physical or structural problems or the result of psychological traumas or problems (Van Lankveld et al., 2010). It is reported to occur at some time in 14% to 34% of younger women and up to 45% of older women. Dyspareunia may occur with insertion, suggesting pain at the vaginal opening or with deep thrusting (Schorge et al., 2008). There may be coexisting problems, such as vulvodynia, which produce similar symptoms of burning and pain in areas of the vulva. Common causes of dyspareunia are organic problems, including lack of adequate lubrication at the vaginal opening or within the vaginal walls. Inadequate sexual arousal, drugs (antihistamines, certain tranquilizers, marijuana, alcohol), or estrogen deficiency may inhibit lubrication. Vaginal infections may lead to painful penetration on intercourse. Barrier methods of contraception may irritate the vagina, causing painful intercourse. Pelvic diseases may also cause pain. It used to be believed that vaginismus was the involuntary contraction of the muscles surrounding the vaginal orifice so that penetration may be impossible and very painful. It is now known that very little vaginal muscle contraction occurs (Sungur & Gunduz, 2014). Women with vaginismus have higher rates of anxiety disorders and report less self-stimulation and sexual desire (Van Lankveld et al., 2010). There usually is no concurrent anatomic abnormality, and rarely is there a physiologic abnormality, although these must be ruled out. Vaginismus is believed to result from psychological problems, namely, fear of penetration due to a negative association such as rape, sexual abuse, or fear of sexual intercourse (Lahaie et al., 2010). The new definition pays particular attention to the fear and extreme anxiety of anticipated pain associated with penetration (Sungur & Gunduz, 2014).

Recall the patient in the case scenario at the beginning of the chapter. Use the concept map (Fig. 42-7) to help manage and understand the patient's situation.

ASSESSMENT

Although many patients are willing to discuss sexual problems with their healthcare provider, most are only willing to discuss problems if the provider starts the conversation. Just as with any other body system, inquiring about sexuality issues should be included in a thorough assessment (Jensen, 2012; Lamont, 2012). Assessment involves collecting subjective and objective data regarding normal sexual function, risk factors for sexual dysfunction, and any present sexual dysfunction(s). Assessments are made by asking direct questions, observing nonverbal behavior, and evaluating information obtained through physical assessment and diagnostic and laboratory tests.

The historical content is important, although the assessment technique and approach influence the content obtained. Narrigan (2006) and the Association of Reproductive Health Professionals (2008) suggest specific types of questions for a sexual history. These include questions about current sexual relationships (i.e., Does the person partner with men, women, or both? Is the person satisfied with the current sexual relationship and function?). An outline of important content to elicit in the context of a sexual history is presented in Box 42-1; however, not all patients need to be questioned on all areas. Assess which areas are appropriate for each patient.

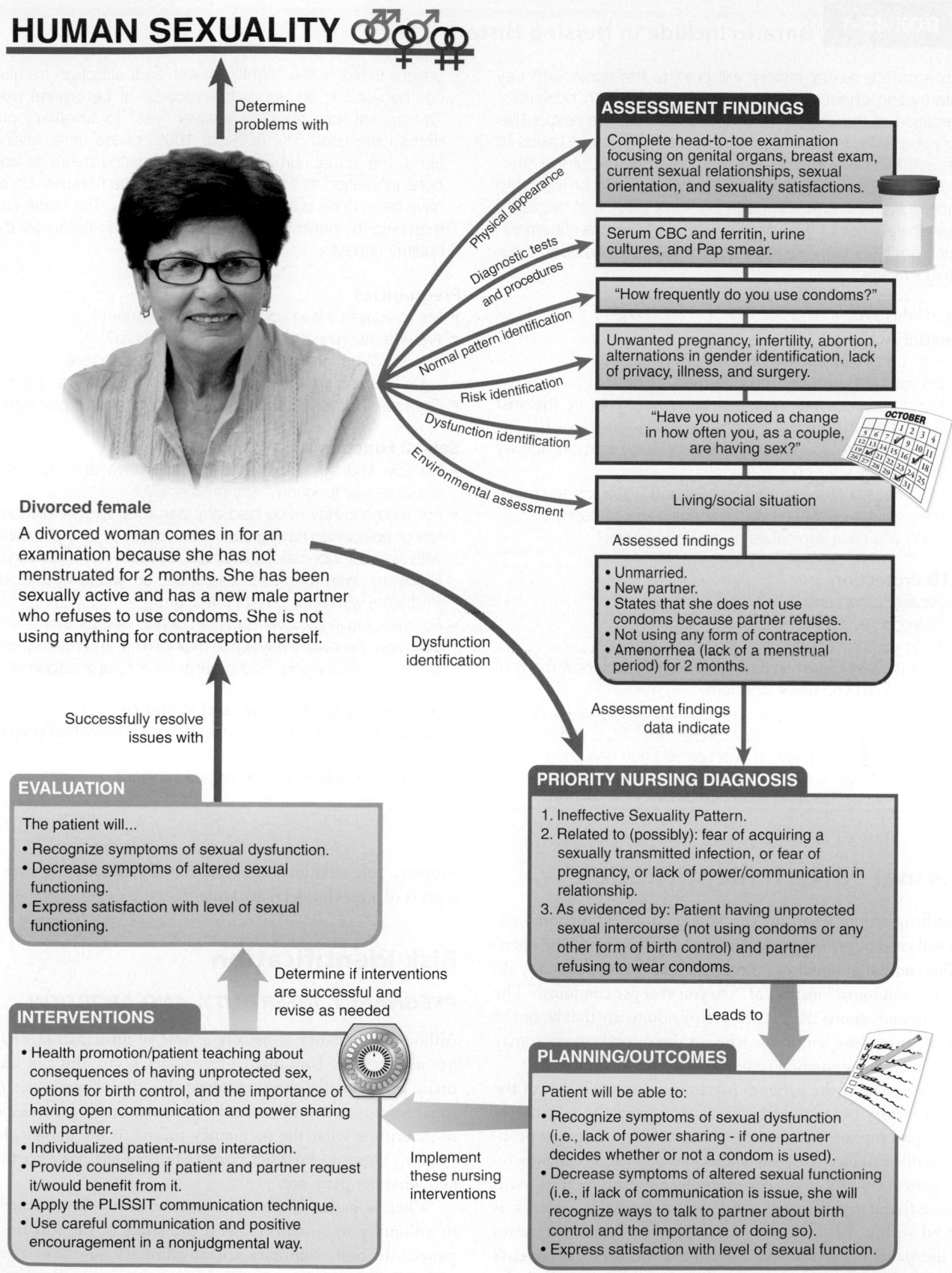

FIGURE 42-7 Human sexuality concept map.

BOX 42-1   Data to Include in Nursing History

An accurate sexual history will provide the nurse with key information about a person's health and health behaviors. Because of the sensitivity of the questions, the sexual history is usually asked later in an interview. The nurse needs to be comfortable with the questions, the content of the interview, and possible responses. Questions should be limited to those pertinent to the specific person's care. It is helpful to start this section of the interview with a transitional statement, such as "Now I am going to ask some questions about your sexual health."

Sexual History

Sexual Activity
- Are you sexually active?
- Do you have sex with men, women, or both?
- How many sexual partners have you had in the last 6 months? In your lifetime?
- How old were you when you first became sexually active? Was this by your choice?
- In settings such as family planning or STD clinics, the nurse may include questions about specific sexual behaviors:
  - Do you have vaginal, anal, and/or oral sex?

STD Protection
- Have you had any STIs? If so, which ones?
- How do you protect yourself against STIs?
  - Do you use condoms when you have sex?
  - Of the last five times that you have had sex, how many of those did you use a condom?*
- Have you had any abnormal Pap tests? If yes, what was the outcome of that?
- Asking a global question such as "do you use condoms?" tends to elicit a "yes" or "no" response, often what the

patient thinks is the "right" answer and, although truthful, not necessarily an accurate indicator of behavioral risk. The patient may honestly answer "yes" to whether condoms were used 5%, 50%, or 100% of the time. Asking about the actual number of times a healthy behavior was done in relation to the number of times the behavior could have been done is a useful indicator of risk. The nurse can then help the patient explore barriers and facilitators for the healthy behavior.

Pregnancies
- *For a woman:* Have you ever been pregnant?
- Are you planning a pregnancy in the future?
  - *If not:* What are you doing to prevent pregnancy?
  - Do you use contraception? What kind of contraception?
- *For a man:* Have you ever caused someone to be pregnant?

Sexual Function
- Do you find sex satisfying? Do you have any concerns about sexual function? Any problems?
- *For women:* Have you had any pelvic or vaginal discomfort or pain when having sexual intercourse? Any problems with vaginal lubrication, dryness, irritation, or discharge? Problems with bacterial vaginosis or yeast infections? Problems with urinary tract infections?
- *For men:* Have you ever had pain during sex, problems with urination, problems having or maintaining an erection, any lesions on your penis, or discharge or scrotal enlargement?

Potential Exposure to Sexual Violence
- Has anyone ever done anything to you sexually that you did not want the person to?
- Do you feel safe with your sexual partner?

Normal Pattern Identification

Specific questions regarding the patient's normal functional status will yield information. Approach the patient by asking open-ended, nonjudgmental questions, such as "How frequently do you use condoms?" instead of "Do you ever use condoms?" The first question grants the patient permission to say that he or she doesn't always use condoms, whereas the second question may imply a more judgmental response to a "no" answer.

Assessment of the patient's psychosocial status is part of the sexual history but should be discussed separately to reinforce the importance of such an assessment. Often, assessing a problem with sexuality is highly subjective because it depends on the patient's perspective. For example, an assessment of inadequate frequency of sexual relations is meaningless unless it is placed within the context of what adequate frequency means to the patient. Psychosocial assessment includes the patient's perception(s) of his or her sexuality. In addition, it includes the healthcare provider's assessment, based on data elicited, of the patient's psychosocial functioning. Outlook on life, social

support, role relationships, and family functioning are all aspects of a psychosocial assessment.

Risk Identification

PREGNANCY, INFERTILITY, AND ABORTION

Although pregnancy is usually a time of anticipation, that is not always true. Unwanted pregnancies occur and can create many problems for those involved. Be careful not to let personal assumptions influence the assessment. Phrase questions to determine what the pregnancy means to the patient, how she feels about it, how her partner feels (if she has a partner), and what her plans are.

When a patient loses a pregnancy, either by miscarriage or voluntary termination, assess the effect of the loss on the patient. In both voluntary and involuntary abortion, a sense of loss is usually present. Sensitive assessment will assist the patient and nurse in planning the type of support from which the patient can derive the greatest benefit.

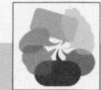

SCENE FOR THOUGHT

Richard Meyers and his wife Aileen are both in their 60s and had been healthy and active until Richard's car accident 3 months ago. At that time, he sustained a comminuted fracture of his right femur that had to be reduced surgically. He still needs crutches to help him ambulate and sometimes has pain in his right leg. Maddie Hines, his clinic health nurse, has been visiting the family since Richard was discharged from the hospital.

LESS EFFECTIVE

Nurse: Hi, Mr. Meyers. How are you today? (*Sits next to him at the kitchen table.*)

Richard: Glad to see you, Maddie. Who would have thought a broken leg would give a body such trouble! (*Laughs a little.*)

Nurse: Well, it wasn't just a broken leg, you know. It was pretty severe. What's giving you trouble? (*Good eye contact. Smiles.*)

Richard: I'm still having trouble negotiating around the house. The furniture and rugs are still in my way even though you helped us move them. (*Sighs.*) I'm just having trouble with those crutches.

Nurse: (*After assessing Mr. Meyer's ability to maneuver and making some suggestions.*) There, that should work better, don't you think?

Richard: Yes, that's fine. Could I ask you about something else? (*Looks embarrassed but determined.*)

Nurse: Sure. (*Sits quietly.*)

Richard: Um, I seem to be having some trouble in the bedroom.

Nurse: What kind of trouble? (*Looks skeptical about this subject.*)

Richard: It's the positioning of this darned leg. It hurts when Aileen and I try to, uh, get close, and then she gets worried and I get annoyed and it all goes to heck! (*Sounds frustrated.*)

Nurse: Oh, I see. Let me tell you about a few things you might try to alleviate the pain that would work for you. (*Settles in for a teaching session.*)

Richard: I don't know about trying anything new. We're pretty happy with the way we do it. (*His turn to look skeptical.*)

Nurse: Don't worry, these will work just fine. Other orthopedic patients have told me they were happy with the way things worked out. (*Talks to him about some ways to alleviate pain and pressure on his leg during sex. Says she'll bring pamphlets on the subject next time.*) What do you think? (*Smiles brightly at him.*)

Richard: Well, I suppose they're worth a try. I'll let you know. Now, I wonder if you could take my pressure. I've felt it was a little high lately. (*They go on to other subjects, both feeling vaguely unfinished.*)

MORE EFFECTIVE

Nurse: Good afternoon, Mr. Meyers. How are you this week? (*Sits down at the kitchen table with him.*)

Richard: Glad to see you, Maddie. Who would've thought a broken leg would cause a body such trouble! (*Laughs a little.*)

Nurse: Are you having trouble? (*Good eye contact. Smiles but does not laugh so as to pay attention.*)

Richard: Well, I'm still having trouble negotiating around the house. The furniture and rugs and all are still in my way, even though you helped us move them. (*Sighs.*) I'm just having trouble with those crutches.

Nurse: (*After assessing Mr. Meyer's ability to maneuver and making some suggestions.*) Is there something else that's causing you trouble?

Richard: Uh (*looks to see where his wife is*), I am having some trouble in the bedroom. (*Looks embarrassed but determined.*)

Nurse: Okay, tell me a little more. (*Sits quietly.*)

Richard: It's the positioning of this darned leg. It hurts when Aileen and I try to, uh, get close, and then she gets worried and I get annoyed and it all goes to heck! (*Sounds frustrated.*)

Nurse: Frustrating, huh? (*Mr. Meyers nods.*) Let me ask you a few questions so I can find out what you're used to and then we can talk about modifications you might want to try. (*Assesses usual sexual habits and practices, including willingness to experiment with positions and effective use of analgesics. Then suggests two different positions that would afford pleasure without undue pain on the affected leg.*)

Richard: That sounds doable, Maddie. I think we'll start out with some dinner and flowers. I'm going to call my son and see if he can help me arrange a dinner here tomorrow night. Aileen's worked hard these last weeks. She deserves it. Then we'll see what we can manage after that. (*Said with a wink. Looks eager to start planning.*)

Nurse: How romantic! Sounds like you two are going to have a great evening. I'm glad we were able to talk about this.

Richard: Me too, me too. (*Big smile.*)

CRITICAL THINKING CHALLENGE

- The patient in both dialogues received the same information. Discern what was more effective about the second dialogue.
- Distinguish what Maddie did the second time that made it effective for the patient's sexual needs.
- Analyze your thoughts about a couple in their 60s, 70s, or 80s having sex.
- List effects that pain has on a person's desire to have sex.

ETHICAL/LEGAL ISSUE

ABORTION

You are caring for a 35-year-old woman who has come to the primary care clinic for a routine annual examination. You ask her if she has any concerns. She tells you that she has experienced a significant decrease in sexual desire since having a therapeutic abortion 3 years ago. She says her previous healthcare provider told her that if she gets pregnant and has another abortion, her pelvic organs will be damaged. She does not want to take birth control pills and does not trust any other form of contraception.

CRITICAL THINKING CHALLENGE

- Identify your concerns related to what the woman's previous healthcare provider told her.
- Consider your own feelings about this situation. How might your views influence your assessment?
- Explain how you would approach this woman's concerns.
- Is there any way to address the information given by the previous healthcare provider?

Be particularly sensitive to the stress placed on infertile couples. Assessing the feelings of both partners is essential; there may be guilt, self-blame, or other feelings affecting the situation and the relationship. Inquiring about past illnesses, infections of the reproductive system, and previous nonterm pregnancies may provide useful assessment and counseling information.

SEXUALLY TRANSMITTED INFECTIONS

Unless condoms are used, both heterosexual and homosexual encounters result in the transmission of potentially infected bodily fluids. However, condoms are not foolproof, and the term "safer sex" has replaced the absolute term of "safe sex" in patient education. Chlamydia, gonorrhea, syphilis, herpes, and HPV will be briefly discussed here.

Chlamydia

Chlamydia is the most frequently reported STI in the United States, with the highest prevalence among females between the ages of 15 and 24. The cases of chlamydia are highest in the south and lowest in the northeast (CDC, 2014b). There are no symptoms of chlamydia and, if left untreated, can result in pelvic inflammatory disease (PID), which can lead to tubal scarring, chronic pelvic pain, and infertility. Local inflammation caused by chlamydia and other STIs can promote the spread of human immunodeficiency virus (HIV). Once recognized, it is easily treated with antibiotics. Both partners must be treated to prevent reinfection.

Gonorrhea

The second most frequently reported STI in the United States is gonorrhea. The incidence of gonorrhea had decreased since 1975 to an all-time low in 2009; however, since 2009, it has been increasing again. Its prevalence is highest in blacks and higher in males than females. There have been increasing instances of drug-resistant gonorrhea. Currently, the treatment regimen recommended is dual therapy with ceftriaxone and either azithromycin or doxycycline (CDC, 2014b). Like chlamydia, gonorrhea can cause PID and lead to infertility.

Syphilis

A third STI of concern is syphilis. Although it starts as a genital ulcer, if left untreated, it can lead to complications such as perinatal infection and stillbirth during pregnancy as well as neurologic complications in the adult. The prevalence is growing among men who have sex with men (MSM) (CDC, 2014b). The diagnosis of syphilis is divided into primary and secondary. Primary syphilis is the presence of a sore that is not painful and can often go unnoticed. If left untreated, progression to secondary syphilis occurs. This is manifested by a generalized rash, swollen lymph nodes, and malaise. Untreated syphilis past the secondary stage is termed latent syphilis and is further classified into early latent, late, and late latent. Late syphilis can result in paralysis, dementia, and death 10 to 30 years after the initial infection. Syphilis passed from mother to fetus is known as congenital syphilis. As with chlamydia and gonorrhea, treatment is successful with antibiotic therapy, and partners must be treated to prevent reinfection.

HSV

The herpes simplex virus (HSV) type I and type II are responsible for genital herpes. Unlike bacterial infections, HSV does not go away with treatment. It can lie dormant for long periods of time but is always present in the body. In the first year of infection, numerous outbreaks of herpes are common. Antiviral medications may be prescribed to lessen the frequency of outbreaks. Many people with genital herpes are asymptomatic. Transmission of HSV by shedding of the virus is via oral, genital, or anal sex. Because HSV is not a reportable condition, the incidence in the United States is not fully known. It is estimated that the prevalence is nearly as high as one in five (CDC, 2014b). Condoms may reduce the risk of transmission; however, because the area of the body with active HSV may not be on the penis, condoms do not reliably prevent the spread of HSV. Initial outbreaks may be more symptomatic with pain, lymphadenopathy, fever, and malaise. Active HSV outbreaks during labor increase the risk of transmission to the neonate during childbirth and are an indication for an elective C-section.

HPV

Human papillomavirus (HPV) is the most commonly transmitted sexual infection. It is estimated that up to half of all sexually active individuals will contract HPV. Some cases of HPV will be automatically cleared by the body, whereas others will proceed to more serious conditions. A vaccine to prevent HPV was approved for use in females between the ages of 9 and 26 in 2006 and was further approved for males of the same age group in 2009. It is recommended that the vaccine, which is a series of three injections, begins at age 11 to 12 to provide immunity prior to the adolescent becoming sexually active. The vaccine offers protection against four subtypes: Subtypes 6 and 11 account for 90% of genital warts, and subtypes 16 and 18 are responsible for 70% of cervical cancers. Female vaccination rates are low, with only 25% of women ages 18 to 26 being vaccinated. For boys, the rates for the full first year that it was available were dismally low, with only 2% starting the series of vaccinations and only 0.5% completing the three shot series (Printz, 2013). HPV infections are also contributing to the increasing rates of oropharyngeal cancers in young people, possibly transmitted via oral sex.

ALTERATIONS IN GENDER IDENTIFICATION

For patients experiencing alterations in gender identification, be tactful and discerning. Although the beginning nurse will not have many opportunities to work with these patients, it is useful to be aware of assessment needs, including the patient's feelings about self, how others regard the patient, treatments and medications, and other underlying feelings.

ENVIRONMENT

Lack of privacy, especially in acute and long-term care settings, is a concern related to sexuality. Sensitive assessment of the patient's response to the environment is essential. Because acute care settings involve relatively short stays, long-term care settings are where the nurse will particularly encounter and need to assess the effect of the environment on sexuality. Assessing the patient's need for privacy is necessary in long-term care facilities and other similar settings.

ILLNESS

Assessment of present illness, past illnesses, chronic conditions, and medications is integral. Illness may have placed some constraints on sexual relations or sexual performance. Attentive assessment may reveal areas of previously unspoken. Careful assessment may reveal misconceptions that some patients (e.g., those with cardiac problems or cancer) have about the advisability of sexual relations. Obtaining this information may assist in planning further assessment or counseling.

If the illness a patient is concerned about is an STI, diligently assess the person's feelings regarding the diagnosis, fears related to the consequences, and anxiety about future sexual relations. A nonjudgmental approach will support the patient in clarifying and focusing on the aspects of greatest concern.

SURGERY

Surgical procedures that relate to the reproductive organs create sexual concerns. Procedures such as prostate resection, mastectomy, and hysterectomy may initiate apprehension regarding sexuality, desire, disfigurement, and future sexual relations. Thoughtful questioning and listening as part of assessment may target areas of anxiety and clarify misunderstandings.

Dysfunction Identification

Dysfunctional patterns can be identified as those that differ significantly from the patient's or couple's normal patterns—such as a difference in desire for frequency of sexual intercourse, lack of interest, or anger—which may indicate an underlying problem. Annon (1976) suggests an approach to discovering important data regarding any problem. This technique includes eliciting information in several areas: description of the current problem; onset and course of the problem; patient's perception of what has caused the problem and what prevents the problem from being alleviated; any past treatment and treatment outcome; whether treatment was medical, professional, or self-treatment; and the patient's current expectations and treatment goals.

Physical Assessment

A thorough physical examination includes a complete, systematic, head-to-toe examination with specific focus on the genital organs or any infectious process that might be the result of or might impair sexual activity. Provide privacy, and use careful draping. Instruments should be warm. Be sure to wear gloves during physical examination of a patient's genitals.

Physical examination includes inspection and palpation, as described in Chapter 26. The nurse's role in examination of the genitals varies according to nursing preparation and type of healthcare facility. Nurses may perform the assessment directly or assist other clinicians.

EXAMINATION OF MALE GENITALIA

Help the male patient into a position for examination of the penis, scrotum, and testicles. Having the man stand or lie on his back with the knees bent exposes the genitals for examination. Inspect and palpate the genitals. Observe the distribution of hair in the area.

Pay careful attention to any skin masses, skin lesions, discharge from the penis, or anal/rectal abnormalities. Note the absence or atrophy of the testicles and the presence of the foreskin or of circumcision. The urethra's location will indicate whether hypospadias exists. Hypospadias is an abnormal congenital opening of the urethra on the undersurface of the penis rather than at the center of the glans penis. Observe male breasts for deviations from normal. Although rare, breast cancer can occur in men.

EXAMINATION OF FEMALE GENITALIA

Help the female patient into the lithotomy position. Ensure that she is comfortable. Inspect her external genitalia for normal and abnormal characteristics, including hair distribution and genital development.

A complete pelvic examination is necessary and includes checking for pelvic masses, pelvic tenderness, vaginal discharge, other signs of infection, and vaginal or vulvar lesions. The pelvic examination is conducted in two parts: a speculum examination and bimanual palpation. The speculum examination allows visualization of the vagina and cervix. The speculum is a two-bladed instrument that, after insertion in the vagina, is expanded for viewing. To minimize discomfort, it is helpful if the patient relaxes. The speculum should be warm before insertion. Samples and smears for culture are taken while the speculum is in place. As the speculum is withdrawn, the clinician views the vaginal walls.

In bimanual palpation, the clinician places the gloved index and middle fingers of one hand into the vagina while placing the other hand on the lower abdomen. The cervix, ovaries, and uterus are palpated by this method.

SAFETY ALERT

Use sterile equipment for gynecologic examinations to avoid introducing organisms into the vagina.

SAFETY ALERT

Always wash your hands and wear gloves when assessing or performing hygiene in the perineal area. Handle equipment or dressings used in the perineal region appropriately. Limit the spread of contact with body substances.

EXAMINATION OF THE BREASTS

A breast examination is included with the assessment of the reproductive organs. The breast examination is discussed in Chapter 26. The clinician checks for size, symmetry, contour, color, lesions, and nipple discharge. This is also a good time to teach the woman how to do a breast self-examination (BSE), which is discussed later in this chapter.

Diagnostic Tests and Procedures

Certain diagnostic tests may be performed in conjunction with the physical examination. Blood work to detect anemia or infection is routinely ordered. Vaginal, rectal, urethral, or urine tests to detect STIs such as gonorrhea or chlamydia may be indicated. For women, a Papanicolaou (Pap) smear to screen for cervical cancer may be appropriate depending on age and previous Pap history. Pap tests are no longer recommended for

TABLE 42-1	DIAGNOSTIC TESTS AND PROCEDURES OF THE REPRODUCTIVE SYSTEMS
Test/Procedure	Description
VDRL (Venereal Disease Research Laboratories)	Blood test to detect syphilis (for both men and women)
Chlamydia testing (nucleic acid amplification techniques [NAAT]) or cell culture	Clinician or patient obtained vaginal NAAT swab for women or urine tests for males (optimal tests); also cervical culture, rectal swab, or as part of ThinPrep Pap to detect *Chlamydia*
Gonorrhea testing (NAAT) or cell culture	Clinician or patient obtained vaginal NAAT swab for women, urethral swab for men or urine tests; endocervical culture or as part of ThinPrep Pap test to detect gonorrhea
HPV	Reflex HPV may be done on already collected ThinPrep specimen for certain Pap abnormalities.
Wet preparation (KOH, potassium hydroxide; NS, normal saline)	Slide preparation from vaginal secretions to detect *Candida (monilia), Gardnerella, Trichomonas!*
Pap smear	Endocervical cells from the squamocolumnar junction of cervix placed in a vial of ThinPrep liquid to detect cellular changes in cervix, cervical cancer!

women until age 21 years, regardless of sexual history. Liquid-based cytology Pap tests or conventional Pap smears should be done every 3 years from ages 21 through 29 years. For women between the ages of 30 and 65 with normal Pap smear results, the recommendations are for either a liquid-based cytology Pap test every 3 years or cytology plus HPV testing every 5 years. For women over 65 with normal Pap smear history on three consecutive tests, the recommendation is for Pap smear testing to be discontinued (Burd, 2014). If an actual or potential problem is found, certain other tests, such as HPV typing, may be performed. A summary of various diagnostic tests and procedures is given in Table 42-1.

NURSING DIAGNOSES

The NANDA-International (NANDA-I, 2014)–approved nursing diagnoses in the area of sexuality are Sexual Dysfunction and Ineffective Sexuality Patterns. Also included in this pattern is Rape-Trauma Syndrome, although this diagnosis will not be discussed here because it is beyond the scope of information presented in this chapter. The nursing diagnoses for sexuality and the related Nursing Outcomes Classification (NOC) and Nursing Interventions Classification (NIC) considerations are shown in Table 42-2.

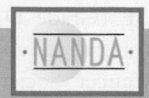

Table 42-2 SELECTED NANDA-I NURSING DIAGNOSES INVOLVING SEXUALITY

Nursing Dx	Related Factors	Dx Statement	NOC*	NIC†
Sexual Dysfunction— state in which a person experiences a change in sexual function that is viewed as unsatisfying, unrewarding, or inadequate	Any change in sexuality, whether biologic, psychological, or sociologic, may lead to sexual dysfunction. Any abuse indicates the presence of harmful relationships, which can lead to vulnerability, values conflict, lack of privacy, and lack of a reliable significant other. Misinformation or lack of knowledge also contributes to sexual dysfunction.	**Sexual Dysfunction** R/T modified radical mastectomy AEB verbalization of perceived limitations imposed by disease or therapy, conflicts involving values, alteration in achieving sexual satisfaction, inability to achieve desired satisfaction, or alteration in relationship with significant other	Body Image Self-Esteem Sexual Identity	Behavior Management: Sexual Body Image Enhancement Self-Esteem Enhancement Sexual Counseling
Ineffective Sexuality Patterns—state in which a person expresses concern regarding his or her sexuality	Lack of knowledge or skills regarding alternative responses to health-related transition. Changes in body function or structure, illness, or certain medical diagnoses can bring on these health-related transitions.	**Ineffective Sexuality Patterns** R/T removal of breast AEB "reported" difficulties in achieving sexual satisfaction	Body Image Self-Esteem Sexual Identity Knowledge: Sexual Functioning	Body Image Enhancement Self-Esteem Enhancement Self-Responsibility Facilitation Sexual Counseling

Dx, diagnosis; R/T, related to; AEB, as evidenced by.
*From: Moorhead, S., Johnson, M., Maas, M., & Swanson, E. (2013). *Iowa outcomes project. Nursing Outcomes Classification (NOC)* (5th ed.). St. Louis, MO: C. V. Mosby.
†From: Bulecheck, G., Butcher, H., Dochterman, J., & Wagner, C. (2013). *Iowa intervention project: Nursing Interventions Classification (NIC)* (6th ed.). St. Louis, MO: C. V. Mosby.
From: NANDA-Association International (NANDA-I). (2014). *Nursing diagnoses: Definitions and classification, 2015–2017.* West Sussex, England: Wiley-Blackwell.

OUTCOME IDENTIFICATION AND PLANNING

After the nursing diagnoses and related factors are identified, patient goals and nursing interventions are planned. Common goals for the patient or couple with sexual dysfunction should be individualized, depending on assessment findings. General goals for most patients include the following:

- The patient/couple will recognize symptoms of sexual dysfunction.
- The patient/couple will decrease symptoms of altered sexual functioning.
- The patient/couple will express satisfaction with level of sexual functioning.

Planning revolves around the patient's motivation to be healthy. Use educational interventions to teach patients about self-care and responsible sex. Examples of nursing interventions commonly used in caring for patients with sexuality needs are listed in Table 42-2 and discussed in the next section of this chapter.

IMPLEMENTATION

Nurses play a key role in assisting patients with any of the diagnoses listed previously. At times, however, they must refer patients to other healthcare providers—for example, if a major sexual dysfunction is noted.

Health Promotion

Concerns about sexual issues may or may not be obvious. Patients may enter the healthcare system for a primary problem unrelated to sexuality. Put patients at ease, develop rapport, and allow them to discuss any issues of concern.

PATIENT TEACHING

Anticipatory guidance is a major nursing role. Assist patients in anticipating outcomes and consequences; help them to devise plans to cope with or to manage such outcomes and consequences.

Self-Awareness

Assist patients to become more aware of their bodies and body functions. Exploring and understanding the body are essential in assisting men and women to achieve healthy sexual relationships. Women need assistance in understanding their anatomy. The use of a mirror during a pelvic examination is one way to begin this process; a second way is to encourage women to examine themselves with a mirror. Understanding the anatomy of their genitals may help women understand how their bodies respond to sexual stimulation and what helps them achieve orgasm. Women need to understand what happens to their bodies during menstruation, pregnancy, and menopause.

Men also need assistance in becoming more aware of their bodies. Understanding their anatomy and particularly what kind of stimulation causes them to have an erection will help men to develop healthy sexual relationships.

Self-Examination

As part of developing awareness of their own bodies, men and women may need assistance in learning techniques of self-examination. Men should learn to perform testicular self-examination (see Box 42-2). BSE is controversial. Although promoted since the 1950s, BSE was only recently studied scientifically. Beginning in 2002, several large studies demonstrated that breast cancer mortality was unaffected by BSE. In addition, in one large study, it was shown that women who did perform BSE had twice the number of breast biopsies performed without any difference in the number of cancers diagnosed. The impact, both financially and emotionally, of negative biopsies is considerable. In 2009, the U.S. Preventive Task Force recommended against teaching BSE (Grade D). Despite this, both the American College of Obstetricians and Gynecologists (ACOG) and the American Cancer Society (ACS) have thus far not recommended *against* SBE. The ACS lists it as "an optional" screening method. ACOG has changed the terminology, using the term breast self-awareness. Both entities continue to have information on BSE available to the public (Mark, Tempkin, & Terplan, 2014). Women who are interested and want to continue BSE can be shown how to perform the examination (ACS, 2014).

Exercises

Self-awareness for women also involves control of the muscle of the pelvic floor. Provide needed instruction in the simple steps necessary during assessment or in a teaching situation. Kegel exercises involve contraction and release of the pubococcygeus muscle, which contracts to prevent urine flow or a bowel movement (Neilson, 2009). Muscle tone can be restored in about 6 weeks of regular practice of Kegel exercises. Benefits of Kegel exercises are increased vaginal lubrication during sexual arousal, enhanced sexual excitement, stronger gripping of the base of the penis, more rapid postpartum recovery of the pelvic floor muscles, increased flexibility of episiotomy scars, and relief of constipation (May & Mahlmeister, 1994). Kegel exercises are also used in bladder training for both men and women (Dumoulin & Hay-Smith, 2010). Box 42-3 lists steps of the Kegel exercises.

Sex Education

Parents and caregivers of preschool children need guidance in becoming comfortable answering questions as well as in volunteering information their children may not directly request. They also need education in the normalcy of masturbation and self-exploration in this age group. During adolescence, both teens and their families need guidance. The focus of sex education in the United States tends to be aimed at abstinence,

---

BOX 42-2   Testicular Self-Examination

What Can I Do?
Your best hope for early detection of testicular cancer is a simple 3-minute monthly self-examination. The best time is after a warm bath or shower, when the scrotal skin is most relaxed.

Roll each testicle gently between the thumb and fingers of both hands. If you find any hard lumps or nodules, you should see your doctor promptly. They may not be malignant, but only your doctor can make the diagnosis.

After a thorough physical examination, your doctor may perform certain x-ray studies to make the most accurate diagnosis possible.

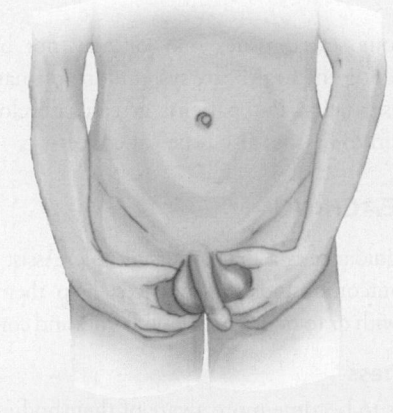

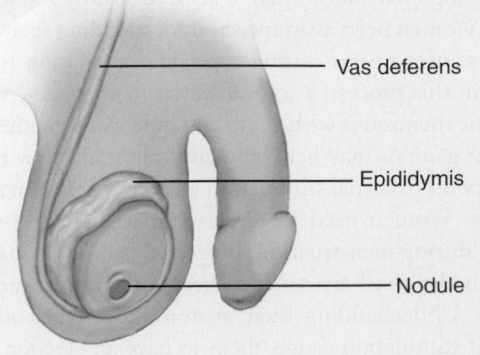

Vas deferens

Epididymis

Nodule

BOX 42-3   Kegel Exercises

1. Locate the muscles surrounding the vagina by sitting on the toilet and starting and stopping the flow of urine.
2. Test the baseline strength of the muscles by inserting a finger in the opening of the vagina and contracting the muscles.
3. *Exercise A:* Squeeze the muscles together, and hold the squeeze for 3 seconds. Relax the muscles. Repeat.
4. *Exercise B:* Contract and relax the muscles as rapidly as possible 10 to 25 times. Repeat.
5. *Exercise C:* Imagine sitting in a pan of water and sucking water into the vagina. Hold for 3 seconds.
6. *Exercise D:* Push out as during a bowel movement, only with the vagina. Hold for 3 seconds.
7. Repeat exercises A, C, and D 10 times each and exercise B once. Repeat the entire series three times a day.

From: May, K. A., & Mahlmeister, L. R. (1994). *Comprehensive maternity nursing: Nursing process and the childbearing family* (3rd ed.). Philadelphia, PA: J. B. Lippincott.

prevention of pregnancy, and the avoidance of STIs while leaving out instruction about orgasm, sexual expression, and masturbation (Fortenberry, 2013). Adolescents need reassurance that their confusing and conflicting feelings are normal, and adults need to treat teens with patience as they vacillate between wanting to be taken care of and wanting to assert their independence. Assist parents in dealing with adolescent mood swings and unpredictability. Give reassurance and support regarding the parents' approach to their children. In addition, parents need help maintaining their own intimate relationships during this turbulent time that often calls attention to their own aging as their children are growing older.

Responsible Sex

Teaching men and women to participate in responsible sex is important. Specifically, limiting the number of sexual partners and using condoms in nonmonogamous relationships are very important. In a nonjudgmental manner, present the importance of limiting sexual contacts. However, if such a discussion might defeat the purpose of the counseling or teaching session, stress the importance of hygiene and condom use. Condoms should always be used in nonmonogamous heterosexual and same-sex partner relationships and in other relationships with the potential for STIs. Much has been said in the media about "safer sex," and nurses should build on this groundwork. Encourage potential sexual partners to talk openly with one another about how to have safer sex and to be honest with one another about any history of STIs.

As part of responsible sex education, teach patients about the prevention of STIs. Some STIs are easily treatable, whereas others are not (e.g., herpes). Currently, AIDS is considered incurable and ultimately fatal. The importance of teaching about prevention of STIs cannot be overemphasized.

CONTRACEPTIVE USE

Statistics demonstrate that the typical woman in the United States wants to limit her family to two children. This means that she must use some form of birth control for almost three decades (Guttmacher Institute, 2014a). Decisions regarding family size and spacing are possible largely because of the various birth control methods available to meet specific needs. There are 62 million women in the United States of childbearing age, and 7 out of 10 of those women who are sexually active do not want to become pregnant (Guttmacher Institute, 2014a). Child spacing, limiting family size, and timing the first birth are preventive health measures that will be met with limited success unless contraceptives are available and used. Almost 90% of women who do not want to become pregnant are using some form of contraception. Less than 2% of adolescents under the age of 12 report having had sexual intercourse and only 16% report intercourse by the age of 15. Sex becomes more common in middle and later teen years, with more than half reporting first intercourse by age 17. Among teens, engaging in sexual behavior is equally reported among both genders (Guttmacher Institute, 2014c). Most teens have been using contraceptives

during sexual encounters, with the condom being the most common method (Guttmacher Institute, 2011). This consistent contraceptive use among teens led to a decline in teen pregnancy rates from 1991 to 2012. Still, 700,000 teens in the United States become pregnant each year, and over 300,000 teens ages 15 to 19 give birth, which is one of the highest rates among developed countries (MMWR, 2014).

Men, women, and teens need information on available contraceptive methods. Nurses are responsible for being familiar with the various contraceptive methods: their advantages and disadvantages, contraindications, effectiveness, safety, cost convenience of use, and directions for use. Methods are grouped into highly effective, moderately effective, and slightly effective methods. The most highly effective reversible methods are subdermal implants (Implanon) and two forms of intrauterine devices (IUDs; copper IUD and levonorgestrel IUD). These methods allow for quick reversal should the woman desire to conceive. Although reversal surgery exists, the methods considered irreversible are sterilization methods (tubal ligation for women and vasectomy for men). The most common contraception method worldwide is surgical sterilization (Cleland et al., 2012). All of these methods are responsible for less than one pregnancy per 100 women in a year. Another highly effective but temporary method of contraception is that of lactation amenorrhea method (LAM) when strict criteria are met (exclusively breast-feeding, no onset of menses, and less than 6 months postpartum). The next effective methods are those that result in 6 to 12 pregnancies per 100 women in a year. They are all hormonal methods with the exception of diaphragm use. Injectable contraceptives, oral contraceptives, transdermal patches, and vaginal ring that contains hormones are in this group. Finally, those methods considered least effective with 18 or more pregnancies per 100 women in a year are all nonhormonal methods of contraception. These include female and male condoms, fertility awareness methods (FAMs), spermicides, contraceptive sponge, and withdrawal method (MMWR, 2014). However, even these least effective methods are still more effective than no method being used at all. The most effective method for any one patient or couple is the one that they decide will work for them. The couple needs to be comfortable with the method and know how to be able to use it correctly and consistently (Fig. 42-8).

 APPLY YOUR CRITICAL THINKING

You are a school nurse, and two junior high school students drop by the health office to have you settle an argument that they have been having. One student thinks that you cannot get pregnant if you have sex during your period; the other student thinks that it might be possible. How can you answer this question in a way that allows the opening for further discussion about sex?

Check your answer in Appendix B.

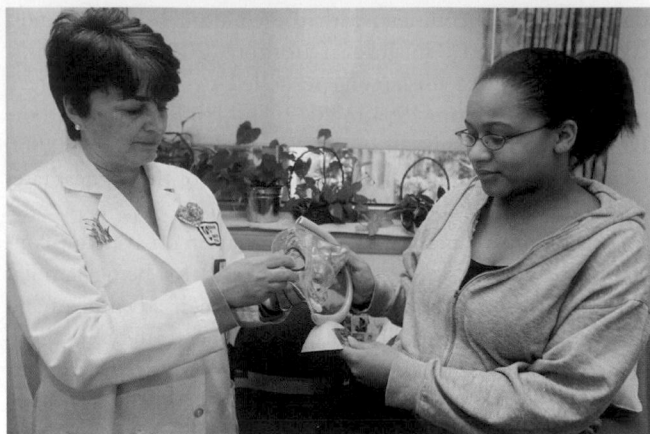

FIGURE 42-8 Providing information about contraceptive methods is an important component of reproductive health for patients.

Nurses and patients need to be continually aware of the growing, and often changing, body of evidence to support the safety and effectiveness of various contraceptive methods. As yet, there is no perfect contraceptive method—all have

advantages and disadvantages. Although it is beyond the scope of this text to discuss them in detail, they are summarized in Table 42-3 and in the following sections.

Natural Family Planning

FAMs help couples understand the biologic markers to determine when a woman's fertile period occurs. Therefore, it is used in natural family planning to avoid or achieve pregnancy. For those couples wishing to avoid pregnancy, FAMs require motivation and a willingness to abstain from sexual intercourse during the fertile period. There are three phases to the menstrual cycle: before ovulation (infertile), 5 to 7 potentially fertile days in the middle of the cycle, and after the fertile phase. FAM requires the woman to have regular periods and relies on estimating the day of ovulation/fertility. Natural family planning methods rely on one of five methods.

Calendar calculations rely on regular menstrual cycles to predict fertility by means of menstrual cycle dating. The *calendar method* uses calculations of menstrual cycles by first recording cycles for 6 months and then using a formula to calculate a window of probable fertility for future periods. In the *standard days method*, women with regular cycles

TABLE 42-3 METHODS OF FERTILITY CONTROL IN INCREASING ORDER OF EFFECTIVENESS*

Percentage of women experiencing an unintended pregnancy during the first year of typical use* and the first year of perfect use† of contraception and the percentage continuing use at the end of the first year—United States

Method	% of Women Experiencing an Unintended Pregnancy Within the First Year of Use		% of Women Continuing Use at 1 y‡
	Typical Use	Perfect Use	
No method§	85.0	85.0	
Spermicides∥	28.0	18.0	42.0
Fertility awareness-based methods	24.0		47.0
Standard days method¶		5.0	
2-d method¶		4.0	
Ovulation method¶		3.0	
Symptothermal method		0.4	
Withdrawal	22.0	4.0	46.0
Sponge			36.0
Parous women	24.0	20.0	
Nulliparous women	12.0	9.0	
Condom**			
Female	21.0	5.0	41.0
Male	18.0	2.0	43.0
Diaphragm††	12.0	6.0	57.0
Combined pill and progestin-only pill	9.0	0.3	67.0
Evra patch	9.0	0.3	67.0
NuvaRing	9.0	0.3	67.0
Depo-Provera	6.0	0.2	56.0

TABLE 42-3   METHODS OF FERTILITY CONTROL IN INCREASING ORDER OF EFFECTIVENESS *(Continued)*

Percentage of women experiencing an unintended pregnancy during the first year of typical use* and the first year of perfect use† of contraception and the percentage continuing use at the end of the first year—United States

Method	% of Women Experiencing an Unintended Pregnancy Within the First Year of Use		% of Women Continuing Use at 1 y‡
	Typical Use	Perfect Use	
Intrauterine contraceptives			
ParaGard (copper T)	0.8	0.6	78.0
Mirena (LNG)	0.2	0.2	80.0
Implanon	0.05	0.05	84.0
Female sterilization	0.5	0.5	100.0
Male sterilization	0.15	0.1	100.0

Emergency Contraceptives: Emergency contraceptive pills or insertion of a copper intrauterine contraceptive after unprotected intercourse substantially reduces the risk of pregnancy.‡‡

Lactational Amenorrhea Method: LAM is a highly effective, temporary method of contraception.§§

Source: Adapted from Trussell, J. (2011). Contraceptive efficacy. In R. A. Hatcher, J. Trussell, A. L. Nelson, W. Cates, D. Kowal, & M. Policar (Eds.), *Contraceptive technology* (20th revised ed.). New York, NY: Ardent Media.

*Among typical couples who initiate use of a method (not necessarily for the first time), the percentage of couples who experience an accidental pregnancy during the first year if they do not stop use for any other reason. Estimates of the probability of pregnancy during the first year of typical use for spermicides and the diaphragm are taken from the 1995 National Survey of Family Growth corrected for underreporting of abortion; estimates for fertility awareness-based methods, withdrawal, the male condom, the pill, and Depo-Provera are taken from the 1995 and 2002 National Survey of Family Growth corrected for underreporting of abortion. See the text for the derivation of estimates for the other methods.

†Among couples who initiate use of a method (not necessarily for the first time) and who use it perfectly (both consistently and correctly), the percentage of couples who experience an accidental pregnancy during the first year if they do not stop use for any other reason. See the text for the derivation of the estimate for each method.

‡Among couples attempting to avoid pregnancy, the percentage of couples who continue to use a method for 1 year.

§The percentages becoming pregnant in columns labeled "typical use" and "perfect use" are based on data from populations in which contraception is not used and from women who cease using contraception to become pregnant. Among such populations, approximately 89% become pregnant within 1 year. This estimate was lowered slightly (to 85%) to represent the percentage of women who would become pregnant within 1 year among women now relying on reversible methods of contraception if they abandoned contraception altogether.

‖Foams, creams, gels, vaginal suppositories, and vaginal film.

¶The Ovulation and 2-day methods are based on evaluation of cervical mucus. The Standard Days method avoids intercourse on cycle days 8 through 19. The Symptothermal method is a double-check method based on evaluation of cervical mucus to determine the first fertile day and evaluation of cervical mucus and temperature to determine the last fertile day.

**Without spermicides.

††With spermicidal cream or jelly.

‡‡Ella, Plan B One-Step, and Next Choice are the only dedicated products specifically marketed for emergency contraception. The label for Plan B One-Step (1 dose is 1 white pill) says to take the pill within 72 hours after unprotected intercourse. Research has indicated that all of the brands listed here are effective when used within 120 hours after unprotected intercourse. The label for Next Choice (1 dose is 1 peach pill) says to take one pill within 72 hours after unprotected intercourse and another pill 12 hours later. Research has indicated that both pills can be taken at the same time with no decrease in efficacy or increase in side effects and that they are effective when used within 120 hours after unprotected intercourse. The Food and Drug Administration has in addition declared the following 19 brands of oral contraceptives to be safe and effective for emergency contraception: Ogestrel (1 dose is 2 white pills), Nordette (1 dose is 4 light orange pills), Cryselle, Levora, Low-Ogestrel, Lo/Ovral, or Quasense (1 dose is 4 white pills), Jolessa, Portia, Seasonale, or Trivora (1 dose is 4 pink pills), Seasonique (1 dose is 4 light blue–green pills), Enpresse (1 dose is 4 orange pills), Lessina (1 dose is 5 pink pills), Aviane or LoSeasonique (one dose is 5 orange pills), Lutera or Sronyx (1 dose is 5 white pills), and Lybrel (1 dose is 6 yellow pills).

§§However, for effective protection against pregnancy to be maintained, another method of contraception must be used as soon as menstruation resumes, the frequency or duration of breast-feeds is reduced, bottle feeds are introduced, or the baby reaches age 6 months.

Reprinted from Centers for Disease Control and Prevention. MMWR April 2014. Appendix D: Contraceptive Effectiveness: http://www.cdc.gov/MMWR/preview/mmwrhtml/rr6304a5.htm#Tab

---

between 26 and 32 days long can match color-coded beads (CycleBeads) to their menstrual cycle to indicate probable fertile days (Institute for Reproductive Health, 2010). They do not have to record 6 months of cycles before beginning. A third method (cervical mucus ovulation detection or Billings method) takes into account the quality of cervical mucus as an indicator of fertility. Fertile mucus indicating ovulation is clear, wet, and stretchy, similar to raw egg white. It facilitates movement of sperm into the uterus. Mucus at other times is scant, cloudy, or thick. The *2-day method* also uses cervical secretions but is simpler because it is based only on the presence or absence of secretions and not on their characteristics. If there are no secretions on the present day or the previous day, pregnancy is unlikely and it is safe to have intercourse. Finally, symptothermal methods involve a combination of either BBT or calendar calculations in addition to cervical mucus monitoring (Smoley & Robinson, 2012). All of these methods are useful for couples who are highly motivated, those willing to commit to abstinence, women who want to avoid using hormones or devices, or those following the tenets of certain religions. Fertility awareness is useful information for women to better understand their bodies. Disadvantages are that the methods require motivation, time, consistent daily records, and abstinence for long periods. Miscalculations can occur in any of the methods, and these methods do not allow for spontaneous sex.

Hormonal Methods

Hormonal contraceptives may be combined contraceptives (estrogen and some form of progestin) that come in pill, patch, or vaginal ring form. Some hormonal contraceptives do not contain estrogen and rely instead on a progestin-only (or progestinlike) hormone. Nonestrogen hormonal contraceptives include progestin-only pills (POPs), injectables (Depo-Provera), subdermals (Implanon), and the Mirena IUD. In addition to preventing pregnancy, hormonal contraceptives have many health benefits, including reduction in risk of ovarian cancer, endometrial cancer, reducing symptoms of premenstrual discomforts, decreasing blood loss and anemia, reducing symptoms of endometriosis, and many other benefits (Cleland et al., 2012).

Hormonal contraceptives also have disadvantages. They do not protect against STIs. Oral contraceptives need to be taken on a daily basis to prevent breakthrough ovulation. Historically, higher doses of estrogen were used in combined oral contraceptives (COCs), and some women on higher doses subsequently developed cardiovascular events such as myocardial infarction and blood clots. Current lower-dose estrogen has decreased that risk. Estrogen has been implicated in a slightly increased risk of deep vein thrombosis and increased clotting, particularly in women with risk factors. The CDC adapted the WHO's medical eligibility criteria for contraceptive use (Curtis, 2010). The CDC report emphasizes that the risks of pregnancy and associated complications are greater than the risks of various contraceptive methods. However, they do state that women with significant hypertension, migraines with aura, a history of deep vein thrombosis, known clotting disorder such as factor V Leiden, diabetes with vascular disease, smokers over age 35 years, or prolonged immobilization not use COCs or other forms of combined estrogen-containing hormones. Breast-feeding mothers are also discouraged from using COCs, but POPs are safe. See Curtis (2010) for a full discussion surrounding medical eligibility.

Oral contraceptives fall into two main categories: COCs (combined estrogen and progestin) and POPs or minipills that contain only progestin. COCs and POPs suppress ovulation; thicken cervical mucus; slow tubal motility, making it difficult for sperm to reach an egg; and cause temporary uterine atrophy, leading to decreased monthly blood loss. Forgetting to take a pill results in a sudden drop in hormone. Today's very low-dose pills are less forgiving than pills of the past, and a missed pill can lead to ovulation and a potential pregnancy. Detailed contraceptive specific explanations accompany pills and other forms of contraception and should be referred to when troubleshooting contraceptive problems. The only transdermal formulation of combined estrogen and progestin currently available is the Evra® patch. The advantage is that it is worn for 7 days, thereby eliminating the risk of forgetting a daily pill. The patch is worn for three consecutive weeks followed by a week off, when withdrawal bleeding occurs. A disadvantage of the patch is that the risk of VTE is increased due to the higher circulating estrogen blood levels. Many additional transdermal contraceptive patches are in the testing phases and several

are soon to be released. One is a progestin-only patch, which would be approved for breast-feeding women or those women with contraindications to estrogens. Testing of transdermal contraceptive gel or spray is also being done (Bahamondes & Bahamondes, 2014). Oral contraceptives ("the pill") are most commonly used despite years of controversy about them. The vaginal ring is another alternative method of delivering hormonal contraception without having to remember a daily pill.

Emergency postcoital contraception (EC) has been available for nearly 40 years and is a highly effective method of pregnancy prevention if used correctly. Although the mechanism of action is not completely understood, it is thought to prevent pregnancy through inhibiting or delaying ovulation long enough for the 5 days that sperm remain viable. In addition, with copper IUDs, there is toxicity from the copper to the ovum and sperm, inhibiting fertilization. The ethical ramifications of EC continue to raise controversy among proponents of the prolife movement who may view EC as abortifacients. Three oral medications are currently approved for use within the United States. The most effective method of EC is insertion of the copper IUD within the first 120 hours following intercourse. The pregnancy rate with this method of EC is 0.14% (Koyama, Hagopian, & Linden, 2013). An added benefit of the copper IUD is that it may be left in place and used up to 12 years as a reversible contraception method in women without contraindications. Available providers who are competent with IUD insertion may not be available in all geographic areas, limiting access. In addition, cost may be a factor. The oldest form of EC, the Yuzpe method, involves ingestion of combination estrogen/progesterone pills taken in higher than usual doses. This is only available by prescription, and it would be accompanied by precise doctor or pharmacist directions and/or counseling. Alternately, a woman can look up the EC dosing for her combination pills at www.not-2-late.com. This method is not as effective as is the progestin-only method (ACOG, 2013).

The most commonly used method of EC in the United States is a progestin-only pill that is available without a prescription. Currently on the market are two formulations; Plan B One-Step is available to all women who are at least 17 years of age, and Next Choice One Dose is available without a prescription to those over age 16. Adolescents under age 17 may obtain a prescription for this EC by calling 888-NOT-2-LATE to locate a provider. EC prescriptions may also be written to have available as needed. Efficacy of all oral preparations of EC is best soon after unprotected intercourse. Although off-label use is described for up to 120 hours postcoitus, the efficacy of progestin-only EC decreases after 72 hours. It is also less effective in women who are morbidly obese. Another oral preparation, ulipristal acetate, which is a progesterone receptor modulator, was approved by the FDA in 2010. The efficacy of this method remains constant for 120 hours following unprotected intercourse. This is only available by prescription. An additional method, mifepristone, which is an abortifacient when taken in high doses, is currently available only in China, Russia, Vietnam, and Armenia for use as EC (Koyama et al., 2013).

Regardless of the method of EC chosen, all women should be counseled to use a barrier method of contraception until their next menses and to report to their healthcare provider if they do not resume menses 1 week after their next expected cycle. Women should also be counseled on future contraception options that they may employ.

For women who cannot use estrogen or prefer a longer-term contraceptive, depot medroxyprogesterone acetate (DMPA) is an injectable form of progesterone that is given approximately every 3 months. A progestin implant, Norplant, was introduced to the United States in 1991. It required five small rods to be inserted under the skin. It proved to be not successful and was taken off the market. It has now been replaced by a single capsule subdermal implant called Implanon, which is effective for at least 3 years.

There are side effects to these methods, and they can become expensive if used for a lengthy period. Health insurance coverage for contraception is also controversial. Some insurance companies cover such expenses, but much debate and discussion continue regarding the advantages and disadvantages about providing such coverage. The Affordable Care Act (ACA) or as it is more commonly known, "ObamaCare" after President Barack Obama, was signed into law in 2010 and upheld by the Supreme Court on June 28, 2012. The ACA is a law that reformed the American health insurance system. It requires all Americans to have healthcare coverage and mandates coverage for preexisting conditions. It also mandated for contraception coverage (Obamacarefacts, 2014). However, in 2014, the Supreme Court sided with Hobby Lobby, which states that it should be able to bow out of providing birth control coverage based upon religious views. There is still much controversy regarding ObamaCare, and numerous attempts to repeal this law have continued to make this a political hotbed issue.

Intrauterine Devices

IUDs were the subject of much controversy when older models produced untoward effects (specifically PID); consequently, some IUDs were taken off the market in the 1970s and 1980s. Newer IUDs do not have those problems; they are safe and growing in popularity in the United States. Worldwide, IUDs are the most common reversible contraception method being used (Cleland et al., 2012) Three IUDs are currently available in the United States: the nonhormonal copper T-380A (ParaGard), which is approved for 10 years, and two hormonal IUDs containing the progestin levonorgestrel (Mirena, approved for 5 years, and Skyla, approved for 3 years) (Yoost, 2014). Efficacy rates are high. In this contraceptive method, a small soft "T"-shaped device, approximately 1 inch long and 1 mm in diameter, is inserted through the cervix into the uterine cavity, where it remains until removed by a healthcare worker. The copper "T" is useful for women who want to or need to avoid hormones and need an extremely reliable form of reversible contraception. Women do experience heavier periods with the copper T, which acts as a spermicide. Mirena continuously releases small amounts of levonorgestrel into the uterus.

This causes cervical mucus to thicken and block the cervix, preventing sperm from entering the uterus. This prevents sperm from fertilizing an ovum. One side effect is that Mirena gradually decreases menstrual flow to scant or none. This effect is being put to use in older women with heavy menstrual bleeding, decreasing the need for hysterectomy until menopause provides a permanent resolution.

Barrier Methods

Chemical and mechanical barriers are popular with women who cannot or prefer not to use hormonal contraception. Barrier methods are readily available, and some can be purchased over the counter. Mechanical barriers include diaphragms, cervical caps, and condoms. Diaphragms and cervical caps are washable and reusable. They need to be initially fitted by a healthcare provider such as a certified nurse–midwife, nurse practitioner, or physician and can then be purchased with a prescription. The diaphragm and FemCap (the only cervical cap currently approved for use in the United States) are used with spermicide. The diaphragm stays in for 8 hours after intercourse; the FemCap can stay for 48 hours. In both cases, the woman needs to learn correct insertion methods and must plan ahead for sexual encounters because the devices must be inserted before intercourse. Both are effective. Their use may result in discomfort to one or both partners.

The major form of male birth control is the condom. Male condoms can be made of latex, polyurethane, or natural membranes. Male latex condoms, when used correctly, are an effective means of contraceptive and very effective at preventing transmission of STIs. Nonlatex, natural membrane condoms are not as effective in preventing STIs, including transmission of HIV. Female condoms came on the market in the early 1990s. They are made of nonlatex polyurethane and more recently nitrile, an inexpensive alternative to polyurethane. Female condoms provide women with the ability to use a condom when a male condom is not being used. Male and female condoms cannot be used together. Female condoms can be inserted up to 8 hours before intercourse to avoid interrupting sexual activity. They also protect against STIs.

Foams, creams, jellies, and suppositories are chemical barriers. These vaginal spermicides act in two ways: blocking and killing sperm. They have a high failure rate. Chemical barriers are purchased without a prescription. Nonoxynol-9 (N-9), the spermicide available in the United States, does not prevent against HIV, and frequent use can cause irritation to the vaginal mucous membranes, increasing the risk of infection.

Elective Abortion

Nearly half of all pregnancies in the United States each year are unplanned, and 4 out of 10 end by elective induced abortion. In 2011, there were 1.06 million abortions performed. This was the lowest rate of abortions since the Roe v. Wade Supreme Court decision allowed for legal abortions performed by healthcare providers prior to the age of viability. Each year, approximately 1.7% of reproductive-age women have an elective abortion, and half of those women have had at least one previous abortion. Sixty-one percent of women who have abortions have had at least one child. Women who are age 20 to 24 have the most abortions, followed by those ages 25 to 29. Teenagers account for 18% of all abortions. Abortion rates are highest among non-Hispanic White women, followed by non-Hispanic Black women and Hispanic women. Of the women who had an abortion, more than half were using some form of birth control when they got pregnant (Guttmacher Institute, 2014b). Nurses who are familiar with family planning resources and contraceptive options are in the position to improve access to effective user-friendly contraception, patient education, and patient-centered family planning. There are several methods for performing an abortion. The rate of complications, such as infection, bleeding, and uterine or cervical trauma, may be extremely high in illegal abortions that are not regulated. However, risk of complication in legal induced abortion is extremely low, especially when performed during the first trimester. Less than 0.05% of abortions end in complications that require hospital care.

Withdrawal (Coitus Interruptus)

People have used coitus interruptus, or withdrawal of the penis just before ejaculation, for centuries. Although no expense is involved in its use and there are no medical side effects, the effectiveness is limited because of difficulty using the method.

Surgical Sterilization

Surgical sterilization may be done for both men and women. Female sterilization includes tubal ligation (cutting and tying the fallopian tubes) and tubal cauterization (cauterizing or burning the tubes), so ova cannot pass through. Vasectomy is the male form of surgical sterilization. Vasectomy involves cutting the vas deferens, thereby preventing sperm from being ejaculated in the semen. Although both male and female sterilizations are considered permanent, there is a slight chance of reversing each.

Nursing Interventions for Altered Function

A holistic approach addresses both physical and psychological issues related to sexual dysfunction. Each patient needs assistance to live as fully as possible, even when dysfunction is present. This is accomplished through counseling and education regarding a specific problem area, treating a specific problem if appropriate, promoting ADLs, making referrals to appropriate resources, and assisting with home management.

LEVELS OF ACTIVITIES OF DAILY LIVING

One of the nurse's responsibilities is to assist patients in achieving and maintaining a level of daily living that maximizes their potential. Nurses can be instrumental in suggesting ways to improve patients' levels of activities of daily living (ADLs) despite sexual dysfunction. For example, nurses play a key role in counseling older adults regarding sexuality and their ability to maintain active sex lives. Give guidance on modifications

such as using lubricants to counteract the effect of women's decreased lubrication and engaging in more foreplay to allow more stimulation of men so that they can more easily have erections. Also, help older adults to discover alternative forms of sexual expression, such as physical closeness and caressing, in addition to sexual intercourse.

COUNSELING

When treating a person with a nursing diagnosis of Sexual Dysfunction, direct interventions toward educating and counseling the patient and his or her partner regarding various patterns of human sexual response. Talking with and allowing the patient to describe his or her feelings will provide a clearer sense of the patient's perspective on the sexual dysfunction. In this way, you will discover what the dysfunction means to the patient and how the patient is responding to it; these perspectives will enable the development of individualized interventions.

The PLISSIT Model

One specific technique that nurses can use in working with patients with altered sexual functioning is the PLISSIT model developed by Annon (1976) and based on learning principles. The acronym stands for the following: *P*, permission giving; *LI*, limited information; *SS*, specific suggestions; and *IT*, intensive therapy (Association of Reproductive Health Professionals, 2008).

Using this approach, nurses begin with nonthreatening actions: permission giving and limited information. If the patient continues to need further therapy or has more serious problems, specific suggestions will be recommended, and, possibly, intensive therapy will be warranted. According to this model, the belief is that many sexual problems stem from lack of education, so applying learning principles may help alleviate many sexual problems. Table 42-4 gives the principles of the PLISSIT model with examples of how it may be used.

REFERRAL

Nurses may refer patients for further counseling if they deem that to be appropriate. In addition, nurses may refer patients to organizations that educate and provide support to people regarding sexuality.

Home and Community Care

Many nurses work with patients who are experiencing sexual dysfunction in ambulatory settings or with hospitalized patients preparing for discharge. Because sexual functioning is crucial for all human beings, consider the possibility of sexual dysfunction for all patients, regardless of healthcare setting. Many patients are discharged to assisted living sites or are cared for in day care facilities. A greater emphasis on case management transcends individual sites of healthcare. Inclusion of sexuality is essential to a comprehensive case management approach.

TABLE 42-4 PRINCIPLES OF THE PLISSIT MODEL*

Acronym	Definition	Example
P	Permission giving (allows patient to speak his or her mind without the nurse communicating value judgments)	The patient says, "I need to practice birth control. Too many pregnancies are tiring me out physically and emotionally. But I'm not sure if birth control is right." The nurse may reply, "Some people practice birth control, while others choose not to. It is an individual choice."
LI	Limited Information (gives/provides patient with information but not too much to be overwhelming)	After further questions, the nurse says, "Various contraceptives exist, each with advantages and disadvantages. People choose contraceptives that are best for their situation."
SS	Specific Suggestions (gives patient specific advice in an attempt to solve the patient's problems or alleviate concerns/worries)	The nurse gives specific information regarding various contraceptives: advantages, disadvantages, contraindications, side effects, effectiveness, cost, and procedures for each.
IT	Intensive Therapy (provides more in-depth, perhaps long-term treatment if problems are not solved with specific suggestions)	If the patient has had several (planned or unplanned) abortions, she may need intensive, professional help related to using a specific contraceptive; dealing with grief, guilt, self-blame, or other emotional results; fitting for a specific method.

*The PLISSIT model provides an organized approach to the patient, based on teaching–learning principles.

DISCHARGE PLANNING

Questions regarding sexual functioning are common as patients prepare to return home. Such questions are common after birth, cesarean section, hysterectomy, or other surgery. Be prepared to give guidance. Refer patients for group therapy in instances that seem appropriate.

Home visits by nurses may be appropriate to assess how well patients are doing. Nurses can reinforce specific treatment protocols prescribed for patients. In addition, they can assess how well patients are after the treatment protocols and can answer any questions that patients may have regarding the treatment. Most importantly, nurses provide support and allow patients to develop a trusting relationship. When patients are being treated for sexual problems, many personal issues often arise as well, and the supportive presence of the nurse is important for the patient's well-being.

AMBULATORY SETTINGS

Education is a prominent nursing role related to sexuality issues. Such teaching can take place in various settings. Schools, walk-in clinics, family planning offices, and malls are examples. Teaching may be as simple as creating wall posters, as informal as a one-to-one counseling session, or as formal as a video presentation.

Nurses may function independently, particularly in the area of anticipatory guidance. Be nonjudgmental, allowing patients to express their feelings, concerns, and fears. Rapport, truth, and respect should be the characteristics of such teaching. Often, nurses can clear up misconceptions and dispel myths that may be interfering with a person's sexual relationship or acceptance of his or her own sexuality.

Patients may approach nurses for information and counseling regarding family planning; therefore, nurses need a working knowledge of family planning and contraceptives. Some nurses may work in family planning clinics, where their major responsibility is assistance in family planning and contraceptive methods. Adolescents may approach school nurses for counseling. Encourage sex education. It is also appropriate for nurses to become involved at the community level. By supporting and encouraging sex education in the schools, nurses can support educating people about their own bodies and sexuality.

EVALUATION

Specific outcome criteria help to evaluate attainment of patient goals related to sexuality. These criteria may differ from criteria related to other physiologic problems where nurses can observe results in many physiologic problems. To evaluate progress toward goals related to sexuality, in most instances, the nurse must rely on the patient/couple's report of goal achievement in sexuality. Examples of possible outcome criteria for sexuality are listed below. Criteria may be similar because some goals overlap.

Goal

The patient/couple will recognize symptoms of sexual dysfunction.

POSSIBLE OUTCOME CRITERIA

- Patient describes male and female reproductive anatomy after next teaching session with the nurse.
- Within 6 months, patient/couple describes normal sexual functioning to nurse, as learned in teaching session.
- Patient identifies specific symptom experiences, including etiology and treatment, while talking with nurse in the next 6 months.

Goal

The patient will have decreased symptoms of altered sexual functioning.

PATIENT PLAN OF CARE
The Patient With Sexual Dysfunction

NURSING DIAGNOSIS

Sexual Dysfunction related to inability to conceive as manifested by altered sexual satisfaction

PATIENT GOAL

The patient/couple will restore normal sexual functioning.

PATIENT OUTCOME CRITERIA

- Patient/couple verbalizes increased satisfaction in sexual relationship within 3 months of treatment, as measured by their self-evaluation.
- Patient/couple verbalizes to healthcare provider that they are more relaxed and feeling better within 6 months.

NURSING INTERVENTION	SCIENTIFIC RATIONALE
1. Encourage couple to discuss their current patterns of sexual behaviors, with acknowledgment by the nurse that the patient's complaints are understandable.	**1.** If the partners are able to discuss their current patterns of sexual behavior and these patterns are acknowledged by the nurse as normal, the couple may feel more relaxed and less concerned about their new sexual patterns.
2. Suggest possible ways for the couple to attain and maintain a close physical relationship even without sexual intercourse if they are uncomfortable with it.	**2.** If permission is given to have close physical contact without sexual intercourse, the couple may feel more relaxed and less pressured to have unspontaneous sexual intercourse.
3. Give couple permission to "take a vacation" from infertility at times in an effort to restore their previous sexual relationship.	**3.** Permission to take a vacation from infertility may help restore some spontaneity into their sexual relationship.

EVALUATION

11/5/17: 14:00—On return to the clinic, the couple reports that implementing the suggestions for intervention has been successful in their sexual relationship.
- The couple states that the tension has lessened in their relationship.

—M. Klim, RN

POSSIBLE OUTCOME CRITERIA

- Within 6 months, patient verbalizes to nurse that symptoms are decreasing.
- Within 1 year, patient and partner report satisfaction with sexual relationship.

Goal

The patient/couple will express satisfaction with level of sexual functioning.

POSSIBLE OUTCOME CRITERIA

- Within 6 months, patient states success in using alternate method of sexual functioning.
- Within 6 months, patient reports satisfaction with level of sexual functioning.
- Within 1 year, patient's partner reports satisfaction with level of sexual relationship.

KEY CONCEPTS

- Nurses must understand the reproductive systems, sexuality, and sexual orientation because sexual health is part of a holistic approach to healthcare.
- Sexuality encompasses function of the sexual organs, individual perceptions of functioning, sexual expression, and preferences.
- Sexual activity is highly individual, with wide variations in expression.
- Reproduction depends on the establishment of the menstrual cycle in women and spermatozoa production and motility in men.
- Sexual orientation may be heterosexual, homosexual, or bisexual.
- Factors that affect sexual function include relationships; cognition and perception; culture, values, and beliefs; self-concept; previous experience; pregnancy; gender identification; environment; illness; surgery; and/or medications.

- Altered sexuality may be manifested by sexual abuse, inhibited sexual desire, impotence, ejaculatory dysfunction, orgasmic dysfunction, dyspareunia, and/or vaginismus.

- Assessment includes subjective and objective data regarding normal sexual function, risk factors, and sexual dysfunction.

- Teaching about sexuality includes self-awareness, self-examination, Kegel exercises, sex education, responsible (safer) sex, and contraceptive use.

- Nursing interventions for altered function include guidance in increasing levels of ADLs, ensuring privacy, counseling, and referral as necessary.

- Nurses function independently in areas of teaching and anticipatory guidance and refer patients with major sexual dysfunction to specialists.

PRACTICING FOR THE NCLEX

CHECK YOUR ANSWERS IN APPENDIX A.

1. Which of the following factors may influence sexual function among individuals? Select all that apply:
   a. Cognition
   b. Values and beliefs
   c. Illness
   d. Medications

2. Physical factors that may influence altered sexuality include which of the following? Select all that apply:
   a. Inhibited sexual desire
   b. Sexual abuse
   c. Dyspareunia
   d. Ejaculatory dysfunction

3. A nurse is seeing a teenage girl at an annual visit. In her assessment about the girl's sexual activity, which question would be most appropriate to ask first?
   a. "Do you ever masturbate?"
   b. "When did you begin menstruating?"
   c. "How frequently do you have sexual activity?"
   d. "Are you secure with your sexual orientation?"

4. A nurse is providing patient education to a 22-year-old male. Which of the following topics would be most appropriate to include? Select all that apply:
   a. Testicular examinations
   b. Kegel exercises
   c. Contraceptive methods
   d. Self-awareness

5. A patient with a pregnancy of 9 weeks is discussing her desire for an elective abortion with the nurse. According to the PLISSIT model of counseling, which would be the nurse's best response after giving the patient permission to discuss abortion?
   a. "It is an individual choice."
   b. "You should consider a clinic that is cost-effective for you and that is known to provide safe, supportive care."
   c. "You may want to discuss this decision, both prior to and following the procedure, with a counselor to help you through any difficult emotions."
   d. "People choose contraceptive methods that are appropriate for their situation."

REFERENCES

Albaugh, J. (2014). Female sexual dysfunction. *The International Journal of Urological Nursing, 8*(1), 38–43.

Althof, S., McMahon, C. G., Waldinger, M. D., Serefoglu, E. C., Shindel, A. W., Adaikan, P. G., et al. (2014). An update of the International Society of Sexual Medicine's Guidelines for the diagnosis and treatment of premature ejaculation (PE). *Sexual Medicine, 2*(2), 60–90.

Bahamondes, L., & Bahamondes, M. V. (2014). New and emerging contraceptives: A state-of the-art review. *International Journal of Women's Health, 6*, 221–234.

Burd, E. (2014). Updated guidelines for cervical cancer screening. *Clinical Microbiology Newsletter, 36*(13), 95–103.

American Cancer Society. (2014). Breast Awareness and Self-Exam. Retrieved May 26, 2015 from http://www.cancer.org/cancer/breastcancer/more-information/breastcancerearlydetection/breast-cancer-early-detection-acs-recs-bse

American College of Obstetricians and Gynecologists. (2013). FAQ114, Emergency Contraception. Retrieved August 17, 2014 from http://www.acog.org/Patients/FAQs/Emergency-Contraception

American Psychiatric Association. (1994). *Diagnostic criteria from DSM-IV.* Washington, DC: Author.

American Psychiatric Association. (2011). Answers to your Questions about Transgender People, Gender Identity and Gender Expression. Retrieved on July 28, 2014 from http://www.apa.org/topics/lgbt/transgender.pdf

American Psychiatric Association. (2013). Masturbation. Retrieved on July 28, 2014 from http://www.healthychildren.org/English/ages-stages/grade-school/puberty/Pages/Masturbation.aspx

Annon, J. S. (1976). *The behavioral treatment of sexual problems, Vol. 1. Brief therapy.* Philadelphia, PA: J. B. Lippincott.

Association of Reproductive Health Professionals. (2008). Talking to patients about sexuality and sexual health. Retrieved August 19, 2010, from www.arhp.org/publications-and-resources/clinical-fact-sheets/sexuality-and-sexual-health

Basson, R. (2001). Human sexual response cycles. *Journal of Marital and Sexual Therapy, 11*, 361–376.

Centers for Disease Control and Prevention. (2008). A guide to taking a sexual history. (CDC Publication: 99–8445). Retrieved August 18, 2011, from www.cdc.gov/std/see/HealthCareProviders/SexualHistory.pdf

Centers for Disease Control and Prevention. (2006–2010). Key Statistics from the National Survey of Family Growth (data are for 2006–2010). Retrieved on July 28, 2014 from http://www.cdc.gov/nchs/fastats/reproductive-health.htm

Centers for Disease Control and Prevention. (2013). Morbidity and Mortality Weekly Report (MMWR), Published June 13, 2014 Youth Risk Behavior Surveillance, United States—2013. Retrieved on July 28, 2014 from http://www.cdc.gov/mmwr/pdf/ss/ss6304.pdf

Centers for Disease Control and Prevention Resources for Serving LGBT patients. Retrieved on July 28, 2014 from http://www.cdcnpin.org/stdawareness/LGBTResources.aspx

Centers for Disease Control and Prevention. (2014a). Sexual Orientation and Health Among U.S. Adults: National Health Interview Survey, 2013. *National Health Statistics Report, 77,* July 15, 2014 Retrieved on August 11, 2014 from http://www.cdc.gov/nchs/data/nhsr/nhsr077.pdf

Centers for Disease Control and Prevention. (2014b). 2012 Sexually Transmitted Disease Surveillance. Retrieved August 25, 2014 from http://www.cdc.gov/std/stats12/default.htm

Cleland, J., Conde-Agudelo, A., Peterson, H., Hoss, J., & Tsui, A. (2012). Contraception and Health. *The Lancet, 380,* 149–156.

Corona, G., Rastrelli, G., Maseroli, E., Forti, G., & Maggi, M. (2013). Sexual function of the ageing male. *Best Practice & Research Clinical Endocrinology & Metabolism, 27,* 581–601.

Curtis, K. M. (2010). U.S. medical eligibility criteria for contraceptive use, 2010. Retrieved August 18, 2011, from www.cdc.gov/mmwr/preview/mmwrhtml/rr59e0528a1.htm

Denny, D. (2004). A chorus of transgender voice. *Journal of Sex Research, 41*(4), 410–411.

Dumoulin, C., & Hay-Smith, J. (2010). Pelvic floor muscle training versus no treatment, or inactive control treatments, for urinary incontinence in women. *Cochrane Database of Systematic Reviews,* Issue 1, Art. No.: CD005654. doi: 10.1002/14651858.CD005654.pub2

Fenway Institute. (2010). *Glossary of gender and transgender terms.* Retrieved August 18, 2011, from www.fenwayhealth.org/site/PageServer?pagename=FCHC_ins_fenway_EducPro_modules#7

Fortenberry, J. D. (2013). Puberty and adolescent sexuality. *Hormones and Behavior, 64*(2), 280–287.

Garcia, J. R., Reiber, C., Massey, S. G., & Merriwether, A. M. (2012). Hook-up culture: a review. *Review of General Psychology, 16,* 161–176.

Glina, S., Sharlip, I. D., & Hellstrom, J. G. (2013). Modifying risk factors to prevent and treat erectile dysfunction. *Journal of Sexual Medicine, 10,* 115–119.

Gray, P. B. (2013). Evolution and human sexuality. *American Journal of Physical Anthropology, 57,* 94–118.

Green, R. (2009). Gender identity disorders. In B. J. Sadock, V. A. Sadock, & P. Ruiz (Eds.), *Kaplan and Sadock's comprehensive textbook of psychiatry* (9th ed.). Philadelphia, PA: Lippincott Williams & Wilkins.

Guttmacher Institute. (2011, August). *Facts on American Teens' Sexual and Reproductive Health.* In Brief. Retrieved September 3, 2011, from www.guttmacher.org/pubs/FB-ATSRH.html

Guttmacher Institute. (2014a). *Contraceptive Use in the United States.* Retrieved July 17, 2014 from http://www.guttmacherinstitute.org/pubs/fb_contr_use.pdf

Guttmacher Institute. (2014b). *Induced Abortion in the United States. July, 2014.* Retrieved on August 24, 2014 from http://www.guttmacher.org/pubs/fb_induced_abortion.html

Guttmacher Institute. (2014c). American Teens' Sexual and Reproductive Health Fact Sheet. Retrieved on August 9, 2014 from http://www.guttmacher.org/pubs/FB-ATSRH.html

Hacker, N. F., Gambone, J. C., & Hobel, C. J. (2010). *Hacker and Moore's essentials of obstetrics and gynecology.* Philadelphia, PA: Saunders/Elsevier.

Healthy People 2020. Retrieved August 25, 2014 from http://www.healthypeople.gov/2020/topicsobjectives2020/overview.aspx?topicid=37

Heidelbaugh, J. J. (2010). Management of erectile dysfunction. *American Family Physician, 81*(3), 305–312.

Institute for Reproductive Health. (2010). *CycleBeads®.* Retrieved October 4, 2010, from www.cyclebeads.com/

Jensen, S. (2014). *Nursing health assessment: A best practice approach* (2nd ed.). Philadelphia, PA: Lippincott Williams & Wilkins.

Kaplan, H. S. (1979). *Disorders of sexual desire.* New York, NY: Simon & Schuster.

Keel, C. E., Dorsey, P. J., Acker, W., & Hellstrom, W. J. (2010). New concepts in the diagnosis and treatment of premature ejaculation. *Current Urology Reports, 11*(6), 414–420.

Kingsberg, S., & Rezaee, R. (2013). Hypoactive sexual desire in women. *Menopause: The Journal of The North American Menopause Society, 20*(12), 1284–1300.

Koyama, A., Hagopian, L., & Linden, J. (2013). Emerging options for emergency contraception. *Clinical Medicine Insights: Reproductive Health, 7,* 23–35).

Lahaie, M. A., Boyer, S. C., Amsel, R., Khalife, S., & Binik, Y. M. (2010). Vaginismus: A review of the literature on the classification/diagnosis, etiology and treatment. *Women's Health (London, England), 6*(5), 705–719.

Lamont, J. (2012). SOGC Clinical Practice Guideline. Female Sexual Health Consensus Clinical Guidelines. *Journal of Obstetrics and Gynaecology Canada, 34*(8), S1–S56.

Latif, E., & Diamond, M. (2013). Arriving at the diagnosis of female sexual dysfunction. *Fertility and Sterility, 100*(4), 898–904.

Lauver, D., & Welch, M. B. (1990). Sexual response cycle. In C. I. Fogel & D. Lauver (Eds.), *Sexual health promotion.* Philadelphia, PA: W. B. Saunders.

Mark, K., Temkin, S., & Terplan, M. (2014). Breast self-awareness – the evidence behind the euphemism. *Obstetrics and Gynecology, 123*(4), 734–736.

Martin, E., & Silverstone, P. (2013). How Much Child Sexual Abuse is "Below the Surface," and Can We Help Adults Identify it Early? *Frontiers in Psychiatry, 4,* 58. Published online Jul 15, 2013. Prepublished online May 24, 2013. doi: 10.3389/fpsyt.2013.00058.

Masters, W., & Johnson, V. (1966). *Human sexual response.* Boston, MA: Little, Brown & Co.

Masters, W., Johnson, V., & Kolodny, R. (1988). *Human sexuality* (3rd ed.). Boston, MA: Little, Brown & Co.

May, K. A., & Mahlmeister, L. R. (1994). *Comprehensive maternity nursing: Nursing process and the childbearing family* (3rd ed.). Philadelphia, PA: J. B. Lippincott.

McMahon, C. G., Jannini, E., Waldinger, M., & Rowland, D. (2013). Standard operating procedures in the disorders of orgasm and ejaculation. *Journal of Sexual Medicine, 10,* 204–229.

Narrigan, D. (2006). Gynecologic history and physical examination. In K. D. Schuiling & F. E. Likis (Eds.), *Women's gynecologic health* (pp. 101–134). Sudbury, MA: Jones & Bartlett.

National Institutes of Health. (2009). *Sexual health (general).* Retrieved October 20, 2010, from http://health.nih.gov/topic/SexualHealthGeneral/ReproductionandSexualHealth

Neilson, J. P. (2009). Pelvic floor muscle training for prevention and treatment of urinary and faecal incontinence in antenatal and postnatal women. *Obstetrics and Gynecology, 113*(3), 733–735.

Neuroscience Education Institute. (2010). *HSDD: Having the sexual dysfunction discussion.* Carlsbad, CA: NEI Press.

NANDA-Association International (NANDA-I). (2014). *Nursing diagnoses: Definitions and classification, 2015–2017.* West Sussex, England: Wiley-Blackwell.

Obamacarefacts (2014). Retrieved on August 31, 2014 from http://obamacarefacts.com/obamacare-facts.php

Ogas, O., & Gaddam, S. (2011). *A Billion Wicked Thoughts.* New York: Dutton.

Pinkerton, J., & Stanczyk, F. (2013). Clinical effects of selective estrogen receptive modulators on vulvar and vaginal atrophy. *Menopause: The Journal of the North American Menopause Society, 21*(3), 309–319.

Printz, C. (2013). HPV vaccine uptake remains low: Why some adolescents are not receiving the vaccine and what can be done about it. *Cancer, 119*(6), 2947–2948.

Ribeiro, M., Nakamura, M., Torloni, M., Scanavino, M., Sant'Ana do Amaral, M., dos Santos Puga, M. E., et al. (2014). Treatments of female sexual dysfunction symptoms during pregnancy: a systematic review of the literature. *Sexual Medicine Reviews 2,* 1–9.

Sadock, V. A. (2009). Normal human sexuality and sexual dysfunctions. In B. J. Sadock, V. A. Sadock, & P. Ruiz (Eds.), *Kaplan and Sadock's comprehensive textbook of psychiatry* (9th ed.). Philadelphia, PA: Lippincott Williams & Wilkins.

Schorge, J. O., Schaffer, J. I., Halvorson, L. M., Hoffman, B. L., Bradshaw, K. D., & Cunningham, F. G. (Eds.). (2008). *Williams gynecology.* New York, NY: McGraw-Hill Medical.

Shamloul, R., & Ghanem, H. (2013). Erectile dysfunction. *The Lancet, 381,* 153–165.

Slough, J., Hennrikus, W., & Chang, Y. (2013). Reliability of tanner staging performed by orthopedic sports medicine surgeons. *Medicine and Science in Sports and Exercise, 45*(7), 1229–1234.

Smoley, B., & Robinson, C. (2012). Natural family planning. *American Family Physician, 86*(10), 924–928.

Stewart, A., & Graham, S. (2013). Sexual risk behavior among older adults. *The Clinical Advisor, 16*(4), 28–38.

Sungur, M. Z., & Gunduz, A. (2014). A Comparison of DSM-IV-TR and DSM-5 definitions for sexual dysfunctions: Critiques and challenges. *The Journal of Sexual Medicine, 11*(2), 364–373.

U.S. Office of the Surgeon General. (2001). *The Surgeon General's call to action to promote sexual health and responsible sexual behavior.* Washington, DC: U.S. Department of Health & Human Services.

Van Lankveld, J. J., Granot, M., Schultz, W. W., Binik, Y. M., Wesselmann U., Pukall, C. F., et al. (2010). Women's sexual pain disorders. *Journal of Sex Medicine, 7*(1 Pt 2), 615–631.

Vital and Health Statistics. (2011). Teenagers in the United States: Sexual Activity, Contraceptive Use, and Childbearing, 2006–2010 National Survey of Family Growth. Series 23, Number 31. Retrieved on July 28, 2014 from http://www.cdc.gov/nchs/data/series/sr_23/sr23_031.pdf

Weber, M., Maki, M., & McDermott, M. (2014). Cognition and mood in perimenopause: A Systematic Review and Meta-Analysis. *Journal of Steroid Biochemistry and Molecular Biology, 142*, 90–98.

World Health Organization. (2006). *Defining sexual health: Report of a technical consultation on sexual health 28–31 January 2002, Geneva.* Geneva, Switzerland: Author.

World Health Organization. (2010). *Measuring sexual health: Conceptual and practical considerations and related indicators.* Geneva, Switzerland: Author.

World Health Organization. (2011). Sexual and reproductive health: Core competencies in primary care. Retrieved August 9, 2014 from http://www.who.int/reproductivehealth/publications/health_systems/9789241501002/en/

World Health Organization. (2015). Sexual health, human rights and the law. Retrieved Sep 30, 2015 from http://www.who.int/reproductivehealth/publications/sexual_health/sexual-health-human-rights-law/en/

Wylie, K., & Kenney, G. (2010). Sexual dysfunction and the ageing male. *Maturitas, 65*(1), 23–27.

Yoost, J. (2014). Understanding benefits and addressing misperceptions and barriers to intrauterine device access among populations in the United States. *Patient Preference and Adherence, 8*, 947–957. Retrieved on August 18, 2014 from http://dx.doi.org/10.2147/PPA.S45710

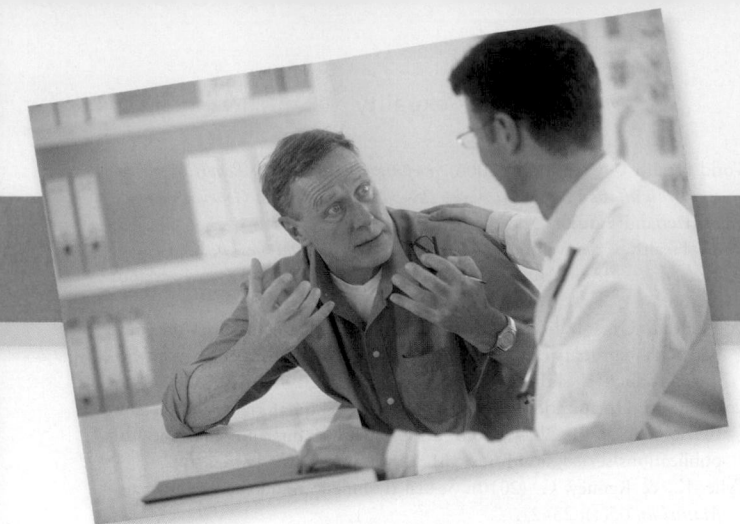

CHAPTER 43

Spiritual Health

Patricia Lisk

KEY TERMS
agnosticism
atheism
faith
holism
spiritual care
spiritual crisis
spiritual dimension
spirituality
spiritual need
spiritual well-being
theism

Case Scenario

You are a nurse working in a daytime drug rehabilitation program. One of the patients, a cocaine user, tells you that his younger brother attempted suicide by jumping from a building. The patient says that the night before the suicide attempt, the brother had called him and asked to go skiing, but the patient (on a "high") said "no." The subsequent suicide attempt was unsuccessful, and the brother is now in serious condition, paralyzed from the waist down. The patient also learned that this is his brother's second suicide attempt in a month. The patient's family had not told him of the previous attempt because he was "stoned" all the time. The patient confides that when he visited with his brother last night, "I tried to pray, but nothing would come."

Once you have completed this chapter and have incorporated concepts of spiritual health into your knowledge base, review the above scenario and reflect on the following areas of critical thinking:

1. Consider the potential underlying spiritual issues in the above scenario from the patient's point of view, that of the family, and that of the injured brother.

2. Reflect on your own spiritual perspective. How did you respond to the issues presented above? How have your ideas and responses changed since you have read and studied this chapter?

3. Construct ideas for how you would respond to this patient.

LEARNING OBJECTIVES

Upon completion of this chapter, you will be able to do the following:

1. Explore philosophic questions about life.

2. Discuss your personal spiritual journey.

3. Identify spiritual needs in self and others.

4. Identify major religious faiths and their traditions.

5. Incorporate age-appropriate spiritual assessment questions into nursing assessment.

6. Use appropriate nursing diagnoses in writing plans of care for patients with spiritual problems.

7. Plan how to use self in spiritual support.w

Spirituality has been a central aspect of nursing and nursing care since its beginnings and continues to impact nursing practice today. Spirituality was central to Florence Nightingale's thoughts, care, and practice of nursing. Early notes and annotations from Nightingale attest to the importance of spirituality in her practice and in her private life (Nightingale, 1860). Nurses have the opportunity to contribute to and participate in patients' spiritual health by promoting **spiritual well-being** and providing the climate for spiritual healing. All people have a spiritual component or dimension that they can develop; however, the way in which each person expresses spirituality depends on background, family, society, culture, and particular religion.

In terms of **spiritual care**, your own background, family, culture, and religion are integral parts of interactions with patients. For this reason, taking a step back and examining your own spirituality, values, and beliefs is essential. Often, this examination leads you to reflect on some deep philosophic questions, such as, Who am I? Why am I here? What am I doing? Why am I doing it? How can I justify these things? Reflecting on these questions helps to develop a philosophic base for clearer thinking about nursing and health. For example, what one believes about the **spiritual dimension** is reflected in one's relationships and interactions with others.

NORMAL SPIRITUAL FUNCTION

"The spiritual dimension is a quality that goes beyond religious affiliation that strives for inspiration, reverence, awe, meaning, and purpose, even for those who do not believe in any god. The spiritual dimension tries to be in harmony with the universe, strives for answers about the infinite, and comes into focus when the person faces emotional stress, physical illness, or death" (Murray & Zentner, 2001). This dimension is considered by many to be fundamental to the existence of each individual.

Although all people have the spiritual dimension within their being, not all have the same depth or intensity of it in their lives. Spirituality is the dynamic quality or essence that pervades, integrates, and transcends one's biopsychosocial nature. Spirituality is integral to man's existence, permeating all aspects of his being and giving meaning to life and life's journeys.

More specifically, *spirituality* can be defined as "a dynamic and intrinsic aspect of humanity through which persons seek ultimate meaning, purpose, and transcendence..." (Puchalski, Vitillo, Hull, & Reller, 2014, p. 646). Transcendence may be within the self or beyond the self. Self-transcendence is a process that involves deep self-examination and reflection where the individual emerges committed to living according to his or her own unique values. This process helps the individual gain clarity, purpose, and meaning to life and life events. Transcendence beyond the self involves a relationship with a higher being or power. This relationship is characterized by a deep belief and **faith** in a higher power, which gives meaning to life and life events. The relationship also provides hope for positive outcomes in this life or in the life or continuity hereafter. The terms *spirituality* and *religion* are at times used interchangeably. In fact, spirituality may or may not be related to religion and religious practices. For some, religious affiliation may strengthen spirituality through values, traditions, rituals, or beliefs in God or a higher being. For others, spirituality may not be based upon religion. Their spirituality may be related to their personal search for meaning and purpose in life.

Characteristics of Spirituality

The major characteristics of spirituality include a sense of wholeness and harmony within one's self, with others, and with God or a higher power as one defines it. People—according to their developmental level—experience and project personal security, strong identity, and a sense of hope. This does not mean that individuals are totally satisfied with life or have all the answers. As each person's life normally unfolds, situations occur that cause anxiety, helplessness, hopelessness, or confusion. Difficult situations often generate complex spiritual questions. Assisting patients with the ensuing spiritual struggle is a valid and important aspect of maintaining health and providing holistic nursing care.

HOLISM

The concept of **holism** states that each human comprises several parts—a mind, body, and soul. These parts, including the soul or the spiritual portion, are integrated into an inseparable whole that interacts within itself, with others, and with the universe. Health and well-being exist when all parts are balanced and are working in harmony with each other and the universe. An imbalance in one of these parts or interactions interferes with a person's well-being or health (Erickson, 2007).

Hence, a holistic approach to nursing and nursing care recognizes the spiritual struggle as a fundamental aspect of health and healthcare (Fig. 43-1).

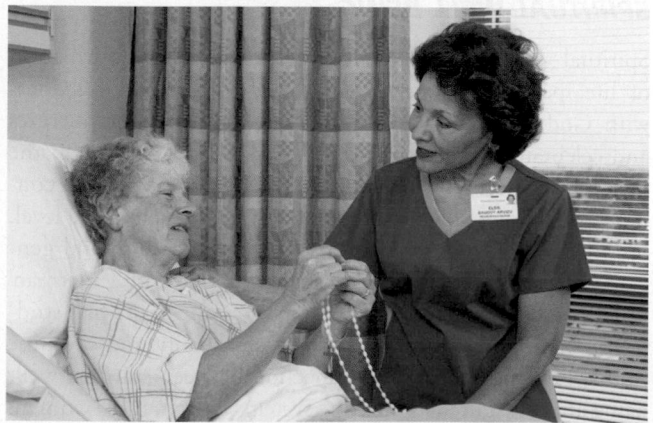

FIGURE 43-1 In spiritual care, the nurse addresses both the physical and spiritual needs of the patient.

SPIRITUAL NEED

Definitions of **spiritual need** vary according to each author's belief system. Spiritual need represents a normal expression of a person's inner being that seeks meaning in all experience as well as in a dynamic relationship with self, others, and with the supreme other as the person defines it. Spiritual needs are derived through affective experiences of faith, hope, and love and through positive experiences that serve as catalysts of synthesis and meaning. For example, a recent study of advanced cancer patients receiving palliative care revealed two major spiritual needs of patients. First, patients want to be treated and recognized as people throughout their illnesses even until death. By treating each patient with kindness, consideration, and as a person of value, nurses can meet this spiritual need. Next, the patient wishes to be kept informed and to hear the truth about his or her illness. Patients expressed that this helped to give them a sense of control over their illness and lives (Vilalta, Valls, Porta, & Viñas, 2014). Nurses are in a unique position to assist patients as they explore and seek meaning for various life experiences.

SPIRITUAL QUEST

Life may be viewed as a spiritual quest or journey, not only to answer life's philosophic questions but also to seek a higher level of consciousness or a deeper awareness of spiritual life. For example, the long recognized Twelve-Step program of Alcoholics Anonymous identifies recovery as a spiritual journey; group members practice spiritual discipline to live more meaningfully day by day. Recovery begins as members are involved in prayer and meditation, leading to higher levels of spirituality. Higher levels of spirituality lead to higher levels of personal growth, thereby enhancing the chances of a lasting recovery from an often debilitating addiction (Streifel & Servanty-Seib, 2009). Similarly, Ben-Arye et al. (2012) noted in a study of Jewish oncology patients using complementary medicine that those with a higher spiritual quest expressed higher expectations in improvement of daily function, in coping with cancer, and in lessening the side effects of chemotherapy.

SPIRITUAL WELL-BEING

Spiritual well-being is a condition marked by an affirmation of life, peace, harmony, and a sense of interconnectedness with God, self, community, and environment that nurtures and celebrates wholeness (John-Roger & Kaye, 2010). In the hierarchy of human needs, spiritual well-being appears to connote fulfillment of needs beyond the self-actualization level. Spiritual well-being has been associated with health and general well-being. Dalmida, Holstad, Diiorio, and Laderman' (2009) study of HIV-positive women was one of the first studies to show an association between spirituality and immune status. Results suggested a connection between spiritual well-being and a heightened immune system status in these women. Hirsch, Webb, and Kaslow' (2014) study of African American females revealed an association between decreased suicidal thoughts and ideations for those having greater levels of spiritual well-being. Spiritual well-being has also been shown to play a positive role in recovery from mental illness (Unterrainer, Lewis, & Fink, 2014).

Normal Spiritual Pattern

Part of a person's spiritual pattern relates to his or her values, beliefs, and faith. Beliefs may range from **atheism** (denial of God's existence) to **agnosticism** (belief that God's reality is unknown and unknowable) or to **theism** (belief that God's reality is personal, without a body, perfect in all things, and creator and sustainer of the universe). For example, Christians, Jews, and Muslims are all theists, although each group further holds distinct beliefs about God's nature and activity. Faith, however, is more than belief; it is the way that a person acts out beliefs in his or her life. It involves "one's dynamic way of making meaning" (Fowler, 1995). It is the personal expression of living out one's spiritual pattern and beliefs with confidence in something of which there is no absolute proof or tangible evidence. Thus, beliefs, faith, and values are interconnected because what one sets one's heart on, believes in, or lives out constitutes one's values. Faith is central to the way the person makes meaning in his or her life.

The expression of spirituality, often through a specific religious group, usually follows an established order of practices. These practices may range from simple meditation and relaxation to more formal worship such as church services or rituals at shrines. Many observances take place within the home, in private, or with the family. Some traditions involve special foods or ceremonies as part of the celebration of special holy days. These celebrations hold symbolic meaning and a sense of deep mystery or miracle to those who follow the religion.

Some people practice their form of spirituality daily; others formally observe only 1 or 2 holy days; still others answer a "call" to full-time service in a specific religious group. Whatever the spiritual or religious beliefs the person holds and practices, these beliefs fulfill the following needs:

- Give meaning to life, illness, other crises, and death
- Contribute a sense of security for present and future
- Guide daily living habits
- Drive acceptance or rejection of other people
- Furnish psychosocial support within a group of like-minded people
- Provide strength in meeting life's crises
- Give healing strength and support

The major world religions include Christianity, Judaism, Hinduism, Buddhism, and Islam. These religions are practiced in the United States and have many branches that arose from historical events. For example, when the ancient Roman Empire fell, the Catholic Church was divided, becoming the Eastern Orthodox Church and the Roman Catholic Church. Still later, the Roman Catholic Church split again. King Henry VIII of England formed the Anglican Church, or the Church of England, when he decided that he, rather than the Pope, should rule the church. During and after the Protestant Reformation, more Christian groups were formed, including such denominations as Lutheran and Presbyterian, and Methodists and Baptists. Judaism has three main branches: Reform, Conservative, and Orthodox. Islam also has several branches in the United States.

Today, nearly 73% of adults living in the United States report affiliation with a Christian faith, about 6% report affiliations with other religions, and about 19.6% report affiliation with no specific religion. Approximately 48% of individuals reporting affiliation with the Christian faiths are Protestant and 22% are Catholic. The remaining major faith traditions in the United States include Jewish, Buddhist, Islam, and Hindu traditions (Pew Forum on Religion and Public Life, 2012).

Most religious groups have a spiritual leader. That person may be a pastor, priest, or rabbi, who is educated in spiritual direction or pastoral counseling, or a shaman or spiritual healer, who is educated in ancient cultural traditions. Shamans and spiritual healers are found among Native Americans and many Southeast Asian groups. These leaders are often the center of the spiritual or religious community, leading worship, teaching, and healing. (A summary of the practices of major religious groups in the United States and relevant healthcare considerations can be found in Table 43-1.)

TABLE 43-1 SELECTED PRACTICES OF MAJOR RELIGIOUS GROUPS RELATED TO HEALTH

Religious Faiths	Dietary Rules	Birth Control and Abortion	Organ Transplants	Death and Dying
Observant Jews	Orthodox Jews observe Kosher dietary laws; Reform Jews usually do not observe dietary restrictions.	Orthodox Jews do not encourage birth control; abortion may be performed only to save mother's life.	Organ transplants generally are not permitted by Orthodox or Reform Jews without rabbinical consent.	Advocate use of life support without heroic measures. Believe that family or friends should be with the dying person. Require special procedures for care of the body after death
Roman Catholics	Observe fasting and abstinence from meat on certain Holy Days; hospitalized patients are excused from dietary obligations.	Birth control is prohibited except for abstinence and natural family planning. Abortion is prohibited.	Organ donation and transplantation are acceptable.	Believe that each Roman Catholic should have the anointing of the sick as well as the Eucharist and penance by a priest before death
Mainline Protestants (e.g., Baptist, Nazarene, Lutheran, Methodist, Presbyterian, Episcopal)	Use of alcohol and tobacco is forbidden by many denominations. Episcopalians may observe fasting and abstinence from meat on some days.	Birth control is generally left as a matter of personal choice. Abortion is generally discouraged, but there may be some exceptions.	Organ donation and transplantation are acceptable.	Believe that notification of clergy, scripture reading, and prayer are appropriate
Islam (Muslims)	Pork and alcohol are forbidden.	Contraception is permitted by Islamic law. Abortion is forbidden.	Donation of body parts or organs is generally not allowed. Vigilant attitude is required to avoid misuse.	Believe family should be with the dying person so that they can read the Koran and pray. Believe in special procedures for care of body after death; men wash male bodies and women wash female bodies and perform various other rituals.
Other Western Faiths *Christian Science*	Alcohol and tobacco are prohibited.	Personal choice	Donations of organs unlikely	May require that Christian Science practitioner be called
Special concerns: Normally do not seek medical care				
Jehovah's Witnesses	Use of alcohol and tobacco is discouraged.	Birth control is personal choice. Abortion is opposed.	Organ transplant is a personal decision but must be cleansed with a nonblood product.	No special practices
Church of Jesus Christ of Latter Day Saints (Mormons)	Abstinence from tobacco, alcohol, and caffeine-containing beverages such as coffee, tea, and cola	Personal choice		Notify church elder

TABLE 43-1 SELECTED PRACTICES OF MAJOR RELIGIOUS GROUPS RELATED TO
HEALTH (*Continued*)

Religious Faiths	Dietary Rules	Birth Control and Abortion	Organ Transplants	Death and Dying
	Special concerns: A sacred undergarment must be worn at all times.			
Seventh Day Adventists	Alcohol, tobacco, coffee, and tea are prohibited. Most members are vegetarians.	All of life is sacred, so generally not practiced; however, there is preference for male children, and female infant sacrifices have been known. There may be some concern that amniocentesis could be used to preference male children. Because India has a population problem, both birth control and abortion are permitted but not generally practiced. Abortion has been legal since 1972.	Personal choice	No special practices. Notify clergy
Other Eastern Faiths *Hinduism* represents a 5,000-year tradition. Its many different beliefs and practices depend on the culture and tribal unit. One medical tradition is the Ayurveda system in which illness and wellness are viewed as a state of balance. In this world view, the human being is continuous with the environment.	Wide range from complete vegetarian to restrictions on certain foods such as poultry and milk products. Traditional foods include many legumes, yogurt, and spices. There is also a belief system of "hot" and "cold" food, depending on how the body responds. Balancing tastes is also important (e.g., sour, bitter). In some places, to refuse food means that one is angry or hurt.	There is ambiguity about when life begins, so there is no clear-cut view on abortion. They are against killing or injuring humans and animals. Both birth control and abortion have been known and practiced. The practice may not reflect the faith as much as current social and political policies.	In the Hindu tradition, ancient myths often are reinterpreted to fit current circumstances. At present, there is no information available as to how this procedure is viewed; however, the wealthy may go to other countries for medical care.	Believe in reincarnation, so life never ends. Regard untimely death with fear and sorrow. The family participates in mourning rituals both before and after mortal death. At death, some place the body on the floor or the earth to facilitate the soul's journey. Cremation is the common practice; fire purifies the body, and the family gives the ashes to the holy waters.
Buddhism began in the sixth century BC in northeast India and expanded along trade routes to the South, Southeast Asia, China, and Japan and in the latter 19th century to the West. The medical system used is the Ayurveda system. The path of health is right living and thinking. There are many different Buddhist groups who follow different leaders.	Diet is an issue of balance, similar to Hindu beliefs. Alcohol and other drugs are forbidden because they can lead to moral carelessness. The laity may consume fairly heavily, however, and recent attempts at reform have not been taken seriously.	Personal choice	At present, there is no stated view about organ transplants. The principles guiding such decisions would include "all is interdependent (family, donor, healthcare people, society) and suffering" (personal communication from Ronald Nakasone, Ph.D., Institute of Buddhist Studies, Berkeley, CA).	Believe life is a temporary state as a combination of body/mental elements; thus, death is temporary and is necessary for rebirth. Family needs to be present; certain prayers need to be said by the priest. The color white means death, so the use of white by healthcare personnel may cause increased anxiety for some patients/families. Priest visits family home every day for prayers until burial. Prayers are said at certain times and up to 1 year after death and then every year.

Special concerns: Most Buddhists have no hesitation about seeking medical advice from non-Buddhist physicians. Thus, some see medical interventions, such as organ transplant, as a technologic issue only.

Source: Anles, P. (1989). Medicine and living tradition of Islam. In L. E. Sullivan (Ed.), *Healing and restoring, health and medicine in the world's religious traditions* (p. 189). New York, NY: Macmillan; Carson, V. B., & Koenig, H. G. (2008). *Spiritual dimensions of nursing practice*. West Conshohocken, PA: Templeton Press; Desai, P. N. (1989). *Health and medicine in the Hindu tradition*. New York, NY: Crossroad Publishing Company; Kitagawa, J. M. (1989). Buddhist medical history. In L. E. Sullivan (Ed.), *Healing and restoring, health and medicine in the world's religious traditions* (pp. 9–32). New York, NY: Macmillan.

Life Span Considerations

A person's level of growth and development influences his or her spiritual expression. Building on the theories of Erikson and Piaget, Fowler (1995) formulated a theory of faith development as the person's integrating center of valuing. Fowler's theory does not address the content of a person's faith, such as a specific religious belief system, but views faith as another way of knowing the world, a spiritual knowing based on a particular phase of psychological and cognitive development. The stages of faith knowing have parallels with Piaget's stages of cognitive development and Erikson's stages of psychosocial development. Table 43-2 is adapted from *Stages of Faith* (Fowler, 1995). The following discussion integrates faith stage concepts with growth and development and identifies spiritual needs arising from these stages.

NEWBORN AND INFANT

Trust in caregivers is the basis not only for development of a sense of safety, security of self in the world, and interpersonal relationships but also for faith development. Human beings' initial knowledge of the world is through relationships. If parents who are secure and have a sense of meaning and commitment meet basic trust needs, infants will sense this kinesthetically and incorporate this feeling into their "innermost being." This sense of trust will later broaden and deepen into trust in the world, the universe, and a "higher power."

TODDLER AND PRESCHOOLER

The first stage of faith development, intuitive–projective, is characterized by a continuing differentiation of self from others and an awakening of consciousness and memory. The introduction of language and gestures facilitates the child's ability to participate in some faith rituals of the family's religion. Children will respond to routines such as grace before meals, bedtime stories and prayers, special celebrations, and holy days if they are offered as a consistent, natural part of family life. Children also respond positively to those who

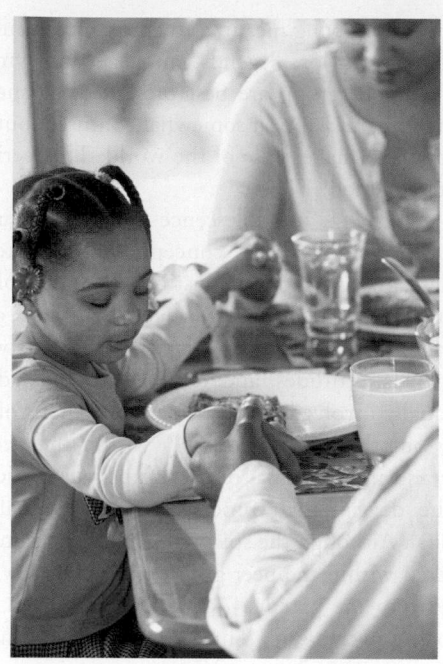

FIGURE 43-2 The preschool-age child might participate in religious rituals without having a full understanding of their meaning.

treat seriously their questions about the world, life, and death. Although children do not know about such matters rationally, they intuitively sense the deeper spiritual questions of existence (Fig. 43-2).

SCHOOL-AGE CHILD AND ADOLESCENT

Children notice the difference between themselves as individuals and others in similar or different groups. Although they are still primarily oriented to the parents' authority, children value belonging and acceptance in their own groups. They continue to be sensitive to good–bad issues, often trying to "make up" for wrongdoing in concrete, literal ways.

Children can now think in a historical perspective and see themselves as part of their family tree. The use of "story" is a

TABLE 43-2 STAGES OF HUMAN DEVELOPMENT: OPTIMAL PARALLELS

Stages (years)	Erikson	Piaget	Fowler
Infancy (0–1.5)	Trust (hope) Autonomy (will)	Sensorimotor	Undifferentiated–primal
Early childhood (2–6)	Initiative (purpose)	Intuitive/preoperational	Intuitive–projective
Childhood (7–12)	Industry (competence)	Concrete operational	Mythic–literal faith
Adolescence (13–21)	Identity (fidelity)	Formal operational	Synthetic–conventional
Young adulthood (21–35)	Intimacy (love)		Individuative–reflective faith
Adulthood (35–60)	Generativity (care)		Conjunctive faith
Maturity (60–)	Integrity (wisdom)		Universalizing faith

Source: Fowler, J. W. (1995). *Stages of faith* (2nd ed.). San Francisco, CA: Harper.

major strategy for giving meaning to experience. Childhood is the period when the lore, legends, language, and symbols of a particular religious group are best presented. Wishes, needs, facts, and fantasy may appear somewhat confused, but children are attempting to make sense of the world. This period is the mythic–literal period.

The major change in adolescence is the beginning of the ability to think abstractly, to conceptualize, and to synthesize. Adolescents ask more sophisticated, philosophic questions; test the truth; evaluate others' behavior; and note incongruities. They develop their own personal style, based on their beliefs, attitudes, and values. Although adolescents are individually involved in this personal synthesis of identity, they carry out this function mainly within the peer group. Mutuality and interpersonal relationships have major effects, making the development process both individualistic and conventional. Although the spiritual need is the same, faith is now centered within the peer group and may be synthesized differently from the parents. Authority has moved from the parents to the peer group. Thus, the name for this stage is synthetic–conventional.

ADULT AND OLDER ADULT

In the individuative–reflective stage, young adults move away from the conforming peer group and clarify boundaries of selfhood and commitment. An encounter with people or groups other than those that provided support in the previous stage often precipitates this shift. Values, beliefs, and attitudes change as a result of interacting in more diverse, pluralistic settings, which can be stressful and frightening. Some situations precipitating this shift include new jobs, international travel, advanced study or education, or new religious affiliations possibly intertwined with achieving intimate relationships, choosing careers, and starting families. The challenge during this stage is to establish one's own sense of faith and commitment based on personal experience and reflection on meaning in life (Fowler, 1995).

The middle years are fulfilled through productive activity—in Erikson's term, generativity. This time is of growth and renewed questioning, in some ways very similar to adolescence. Adults, however, deal with a broader world view rather than with group conformity. Older adults notice the polarities or extremes in life, such as young and old, rich and poor, masculine and feminine, war and peace, constructive and destructive, and self-awareness and self-denial. These tensions, enhanced or precipitated by personal and environmental situations, demand integration and resolution. This is referred to as the stage of conjunctive faith (Fowler, 1995). Most people do not achieve the final stage of faith—universalizing. Usually, only great leaders such as Mahatma Gandhi, Martin Luther King, and Mother Theresa appear to have achieved this world view. One's social perspective expands to include everyone as God's children with a more radical living-out of one's vision of the earth community. Terms such as justice, love, and compassion describe the goals of the person in the universalizing stage.

APPLY YOUR CRITICAL THINKING

While working in a long-term care facility, Mrs. Harvey, age 86 years, tells you that she knows she is nearing the end of her life. She says that she has been an occasional church attendee but feels like she would like to talk to you about faith. She asks you what you believe about a higher being and about life after death. How will you respond to her? What actions should you take?

Check your answers in Appendix B.

Cultural Considerations

An individual's culture is the specific set of beliefs, values, and assumptions that are held and passed on from generation to generation. Madeleine Leininger (1991), a noted nursing theorist, states that "culture refers to the learned, shared, and transmitted values, beliefs, norms and lifeways of a particular group that guides their thinking, decisions, and actions in patterned ways" over a span of time (p. 47). Among these beliefs and lifeways are an individual's unique religious beliefs and spiritual traditions.

Attitudes, beliefs, and values arise from one's sociocultural background. Usually, but not always, people follow the spiritual and religious traditions of their families of origin. Children learn the importance of religious practices, including moral values, from family relationships and participation in religious activities. In interfaith marriages, children may follow the practices of one parent over the other. Some parents try to instill the strengths of both religions in their offspring.

Culture and spirituality play an important role in how individuals view themselves and others with whom they interact. These concepts are also linked to an individual's health, heath beliefs, and health practices. Culture and spirituality influence how individuals understand illnesses and death and play a role in the decisions that individuals may make regarding these (Weiner, McConnell, Latella, & Ludi, 2013).

Many times, religious preference is tied to ethnic background. For example, many Italians and Irish are Roman Catholics, many Scandinavians and Germans are Lutherans, and many East Indians are Hindus. No matter what religious tradition or belief system a person follows, the inner spiritual experience remains uniquely personal and is honored and respected by the nurse. To provide culturally and spiritually competent care, nurses must be aware of their own individual feelings about their own culture and spirituality. Nurses can then explore and appreciate the unique cultural and spiritual needs of the patient. The nurse who respects and values the unique needs of the individual is poised to deliver care that is both holistic and patient centered.

FACTORS AFFECTING SPIRITUAL HEALTH

Several factors affect expression of spiritual needs. Such things include culture, gender, and previous experience.

Individual reactions vary depending on personality and past coping styles. Other factors contributing to spiritual health include appropriate religious education, a firm spiritual identity, and a dynamic and adaptable belief system. Maintaining belief systems in times of adversity or when questioned by others, recognizing the need for spiritual assistance, having empathy for others' beliefs and values, and possessing a sense of spiritual fulfillment are other factors that can lead to spiritual health and well-being.

Factors such as crises, moral issues, and separation may cause changes in spiritual health and well-being, placing individuals at risk for altered spiritual function. These factors, however, are subjective and mean different things to different people. For example, a job change may challenge one person's sense of meaning, whereas a broken relationship may influence that of another.

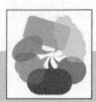 **THERAPEUTIC DIALOGUE: AFTERLIFE**

SCENE FOR THOUGHT

Jeremy Gaston is 17 years old and in the hospital for his third chemotherapy treatment for leukemia. He is lying in bed and seems very quiet when the nurse stops in during morning rounds.

LESS EFFECTIVE	MORE EFFECTIVE
Nurse: Hi, Jeremy. How are you this morning? *(Checks the central venous catheter and the medication's drip rate.)*	**Nurse:** Hi, Jeremy. How are you this morning? *(Checks the central venous catheter and the medication's drip rate.)*
Jeremy: I was just thinking about dying. *(Looks off into space.)*	**Jeremy:** I was just thinking about dying. *(Looks off into space.)*
Nurse: *(Stops to look at him in surprise, then continues checking the intravenous drip.)* What were you thinking?	**Nurse:** *(Stops to look at him in surprise, then continues checking the intravenous drip.)* What were you thinking?
Jeremy: What it was like, just in case I don't make it through this cancer.	**Jeremy:** What it was like, just in case I don't make it through this cancer.
Nurse: I thought we talked about how much better you're getting?	**Nurse:** What do you think it would be like? *(Sits down next to the bed.)*
Jeremy: *(Looks sheepish.)* Yeah, I know, but sometimes, it gets to me, all the chemo and how long it's taking and the pain. Sorry.	**Jeremy:** My father almost died from a heart attack and said he could see himself on the emergency room table with everyone working on him. He said it wasn't scary, just weird.
Nurse: You don't have to apologize, Jeremy. I know you get discouraged, but I also know you have Someone *(points up)* watching over you and caring for you. I feel that very strongly. So don't worry about dying just yet. *(Has tears in her eyes that Jeremy doesn't see.)*	**Nurse:** You've talked about this with your dad?
	Jeremy: Yeah. A few years ago. But my family isn't religious at all, so I'm not sure about the bright light or angels or anything like that. *(Sounds worried.)*
Jeremy: Okay. *(Looks off into space again.)*	**Nurse:** You sound worried about that.
Nurse: I'll let you rest now. Think good thoughts and this treatment will be over in a jiffy. *(Leaves the room.)*	**Jeremy:** I am. I'd hate to think there was nothing.
	Nurse: So you're worried there might be nothing after death but you're not sure. Is that right?
	Jeremy: Yeah.
	Nurse: You know, we've talked about pain and chemo and leukemia, but I don't think we've talked about this. What kind of help do you need now?
	Jeremy: *(Smiles.)* Maybe a philosophy course! Could we just talk a little about what you think death is?
	Nurse: Sure. *(They continue....)*

CRITICAL THINKING CHALLENGE

- From the first nurse's conversation, detect whom she was reassuring and how the patient responded.
- Analyze what the second nurse helped the patient do.
- Construct your own thoughts about an afterlife and how they affect the way you live.
- Analyze how your thoughts affect the way you care for your patients.

Gender

Spiritual expression also depends on society's and the religious group's beliefs and teachings about gender or expected behaviors for males and females. For example, in some religions that follow dietary laws, women are responsible to see that their families follow those laws. A person's organized religion may prescribe how each sex dresses and if one wears a head covering. In some cases, the spiritual leader is always a man, while other religions encourage women to assume pastoral positions.

Previous Experience

Fowler (1995) and others observed that many people direct their lives based on personally established values. If something disruptive occurs, these values may be questioned, leading to a test of faith. When one's faith and values are confronted, deeper spiritual needs can arise. During such a crisis, past coping styles or learned ways of handling situations are likely to be evident. These coping patterns can be healthy and adaptive, or they can be maladaptive. Previous life experiences in general influence responses to subsequent life experiences.

Crisis and Change

Crisis and change can also affect one's spirituality. Individuals experiencing marked changes in health status, sudden acute illnesses, or the loss of loved ones may encounter a crossroads in their spirituality or a **spiritual crisis**. Agrimson and Taft (2009) have defined a spiritual crisis as a unique form of grieving or loss, which is accompanied by profound questioning about life and its meaning. Individuals may reach a turning point in their lives that leads to significant changes in the way they view themselves or their lives. Such crisis may be related to pathophysiologic changes, required treatments, or challenging personal situations. The diagnosis of a debilitating, disfiguring, or terminal illness may lead individuals to question their belief systems. Sudden trauma, miscarriage, or stillbirth may cause a person to doubt the presence of a higher being or to challenge their faith. Some treatments required for trauma and illness lead to a sense of isolation or uncertainty. Treatments like amputations, surgery, medication administration, dietary restrictions, or other challenging procedures may generate trials and uncertainty. Personal changes that result from the death or illness of a loved one or the opposition to personal religious beliefs by significant others can lead to spiritual distress. Hospitalization can interrupt individuals' usual religious practices at a time when these are most needed, which can further compound spiritual distress and crisis.

Experiences like these may strengthen a person's spirituality or may have a detrimental effect on it. The consequences of a spiritual crisis can be either positive or negative. The outcome depends upon the individual's personal characteristics, coping mechanisms, and support given to the individual during the

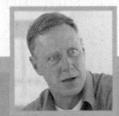

Spiritual Health PICO

Ginger is the nurse taking care of the patient from the chapter-opening scenario. While talking with the patient, she learns that he suffers from posttraumatic stress disorder (PTSD). He confesses to her that his cocaine use started when he got back from the war. However, after the incident with his brother, he wants to get help. Ginger wonders if self-reflection could be a useful tool for her patient to help work out his feelings. She turns to the Cochrane library to begin her search: *In patients with posttraumatic stress disorder, how does reflective journaling/diaries compare to no reflective journaling/diaries in improving psychological distress?*

P = patients with posttraumatic stress disorder

I = reflective journaling or diaries

C = no reflective journaling or diaries

O = improve psychological distress

The only current article that Ginger found was a systematic review that analyzed the effectiveness of journaling in an ICU setting. The study evaluated how patients and their family members used diaries as a debriefing tool during the ICU admission and stay. The review included three studies randomized control trials with 358 participants. Unfortunately, there was not any strong evidence that supported that self-reflection journals could improve psychological distress. The sampling size of the studies was too small to determine overall effectiveness, and more research is needed.

After reading the study, Ginger decides that her patient needs more help than she can provide. She contacts the rehab doctor to see if a psych referral could be considered. She also asks the patient if he wants to talk with a chaplain.

REFERENCE

Ullman, A. J., Aitken, L. M., Rattray, J., Kenardy, J., Le Brocque, R., MacGillivray, S., et al. (2014). Diaries for recovery from critical illness. *Cochrane Database of Systematic Reviews*, (12), CD010468. doi: 10.1002/14651858.CD010468.pub2.

crisis (Burke et al., 2014). Suicide is an example of an extremely negative consequence of a spiritual crisis. In contrast, a spiritual crisis can have a positive effect on an individual's life. The crisis may cause the individual to rethink and evaluate uncertainties within his or her life, realizing that crisis and uncertainty are natural parts of life. The crisis may lead introspection and a renewed commitment to one's spiritual beliefs and higher power.

Separation from Spiritual Ties

Experiences of being hospitalized or becoming a resident in an assisted living facility or long-term care facility can initially be shattering. To some extent, such individuals are isolated from personal freedoms, personal privileges, and social support systems. They may be in private rooms with unfamiliar surroundings and may feel insecure. Daily habits may change. Some people are unable to attend formal services, have the accoutrements of faith, or receive regular support from familiar groups or their faith community. This separation from spiritual ties places people at risk for altered spiritual function.

Moral Issues Regarding Therapy

Many religions view healers and the healing process as evidence of God at work in the world. Certain religious groups, however, object to some modern medical interventions. For example, Jehovah's Witnesses do not accept blood transfusions. Some Christians oppose abortion because of their belief that the soul enters the body at conception. The Amish may refuse expensive treatments for individual members because the cost would impose a severe financial hardship on the entire community. Religious teachings influence attitudes toward many other medical procedures, such as right-to-die decisions, organ transplantation, circumcision, birth control, sterilization, autopsies, and handling of the deceased. Some groups, such as Christian Scientists and Amish, have been legally exempted from immunizations; however, many medical decisions are reviewed on a case-by-case basis, depending on the patient's age and the imminence of death. The choice to treat may be difficult to make if the religious beliefs say "no" and the healthcare system says "yes." Many healthcare agencies have ethics committees to clarify and review such situations so that more adequate and informed decisions are made.

Inadequate or Inappropriate Care

When providing spiritual care, nurses must be careful neither to avoid assisting patients nor to involve themselves without the desire of the patient but to base their decisions on the cues provided by the patient. Cues occur when the patient verbally or nonverbally invites the nurse to share a deeper spiritual connection. Such behaviors may include direct requests, singing of religious hymns, chanting, or praying. Patients may state that they had planned to go to church or fast during a given time. Additional indicators may include requesting a Bible or Bible reading, requesting time alone to pray, or asking to

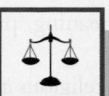

meet with their spiritual minister or leader. Careful assessment of these critical verbal and nonverbal cues guides the nurse as spiritual problems are identified and explored (Tokpah & Middleton, 2013).

In general, people receiving healthcare depend on nurses and the healthcare team. Nurses attempt to overcome this inherent dependency by being advocates for patients and by involving patients in mutual goal setting and care planning. Doing nothing, jumping in too quickly, or not looking for patient cues may result in inadequate or inappropriate spiritual care.

Nurses may avoid giving spiritual care for several reasons. Rushton (2014) notes that this may be because there is no specific definition of spirituality and the concept is often confused with religion. She also notes that nurses are at times confused about their role in providing spiritual care, noting that some nurses have limited education and training in this area.

Nurses may express insecurity in their own spiritual lives and needs and therefore feel unprepared to assist others with their spiritual needs. They may believe that spiritual needs are best addressed by a chaplain or pastoral advisor or that the environment is not conducive to spiritual care. Lastly, some nurses assign less value and importance to spiritual care, citing time limitations for this type of care as other physiologic needs take precedence (Rushton, 2014). Granstrom (1985) ALSO elaborated on these reasons when she identified five complex values issues between nurses and patients that influence the delivery of spiritual care:

- *Pluralism:* Nurses and patients embracing a wide spectrum of beliefs and creeds
- *Fear:* Related to not being able to handle situations, intruding on patient's privacy, or becoming confused in one's own belief and value system

- *Awareness of own spiritual quest:* What gives meaning, purpose, hope, and sense of love in one's own life
- *Confusion:* Confusion over differences between religious and spiritual concepts
- *Basic attitudes:* Attitudes relative to illness, aging, and suffering

As nurses confront these issues when delivering spiritual care, they need to reflect on their own philosophies and belief systems to effectively assist patients and provide adequate care. Listed below are some useful questions to assist with spiritual exploration and reflection (King & Koenig, 2009, p. 116):

- "Are you in any way a spiritual person?"
- "Do you observe a religion?"
- "Is your spirituality mainly about you personally, or is it found more in your relationship with other people?"
- "Does your spirituality help you cope with life difficulties?"
- "Does your spirituality help you cope with illness or disability?"
- "Have you ever been aware of a spiritual realm or presence?"
- "Have you ever had a very intense experience (unrelated to drugs or alcohol) in which you felt some deep new meaning in life or at one with the world or the universe?" (If you believe in God, it may have felt like an experience of God.)

By clarifying personal belief systems, nurses can effectively assist patients with their spiritual needs and care.

ALTERED SPIRITUAL FUNCTION

Verbalization of Distress

Various behaviors and expressions may be warning signs that patients are experiencing spiritual concerns. Table 43-3 is a compilation of categorizations regarding adaptive and maladaptive expressions of spiritual needs that may help examine potential spiritual distress manifested in patients or that may appear in support persons or families.

Persons suffering spiritual dysfunction may verbalize such distress or express a need for help. The manifestation may be precise: "I feel guilty because I should have realized earlier he was having a heart attack." A person may state that he or she misses Sunday church services and the beautiful music of the choir or may say, "I've never missed a service in 20 years." The manifestation may be more subjective, as in the case of the patient's rambling speech about life, death, and worth. Patients may ask nurses to pray for them or to notify a spiritual leader or chaplain of their illness.

Altered Behavior

A change in behavior may be a manifestation of spiritual dysfunction. A patient who is nervous about the outcome of a diagnostic test or who shows anger after hearing the test results

may be suffering from spiritual distress. Some people become more introspective while attempting to figure out the situation and search for facts online or in available literature. Some react emotionally, seeking information and support from friends and family. Still others suffering from spiritual distress appear not to "hear" or show outward signs of the problem; their distress may surface as sleeplessness or lack of concentration. Guilt, fear, depression, and anxiety may also be indicative of altered spiritual function.

Recall the patient in the case scenario at the beginning of the chapter. He is struggling with drug addiction and his younger brother's suicide attempts. He has tried praying over the situation but is unable to. Use the concept map (Fig. 43-3) to help the patient understand and manage his spiritual health.

ASSESSMENT

Since 2001, the Joint Commission on Accreditation of Healthcare Organizations (the Joint Commission) has set minimum standards for spiritual assessment to include the assessment of religious preferences or denominations, beliefs, and spiritual practices. The revised guidelines (2008) require that healthcare organizations identify the qualifications of persons gathering initial spiritual assessment data (Joint Commission, 2014). Nurses are in a prime position to collect these data because of their education and their initial contact with the patient. Faull, de Caestecker, Nicholson, and Black (2012) suggest that prior to assessment, nurses should be aware of their own spiritual condition. Acknowledging and recognizing select spiritual beliefs as personal will allow the nurse to discern and focus on the specific needs of the patient. Spiritual assessments may be planned using a formal questionnaire, or they may occur spontaneously as the patient provides the nurse cues regarding their spirituality. In either case, conducting a spiritual assessment is an essential aspect of maintaining health and providing holistic and sensitive nursing care. Following the assessment, if the patient has additional questions or concerns related to spirituality, the nurse may suggest follow-up with a chaplain as necessary.

Normal Pattern Identification

Several nurses have developed spiritual assessment tools. Stoll's (1979) *Guidelines for Spiritual Assessment* is an early widely recognized spiritual assessment tool. This tool is built around a definition of spirituality that encompasses religion and belief in a higher power. It identifies four areas and suggests questions for each: (a) concept of God or deity, (b) source of hope and strength, (c) religious practices and rituals, and (d) relationship between spiritual beliefs and state of health. Some questions include the following:

- Is religion or God significant to you?
- To whom do you turn when you need help?

TABLE 43-3 ADAPTIVE AND MALADAPTIVE EXPRESSIONS OF SPIRITUAL NEEDS

Needs	Adaptive Behavior/Pattern	Maladaptive Behavior/Pattern
Trust	Trusts self and own endurance Accepts that others will be able to meet needs Trusts in life Accepts life's outcomes Is open to God	Shows discomfort with self-awareness Is gullible Feels that only certain people and places are safe Expects people to be unkind and unreliable Is impatient Fears God's intentions
Forgiveness	Accepts fallibility of self and others Is nonjudgmental Views illness realistically Experiences self-forgiveness Offers to forgive others Accepts God's forgiveness Has realistic perspective on the past	Views illness as punishment Believes God is judgmental Feels that forgiveness depends on behavior Is unable to accept self Either blames self or projects blame
Love and relatedness	Expresses feelings of being loved by God/others Accepts help Is self-accepting Seeks the good in others	Feels others judge him or her Behaves self-destructively Fears dependence on others Refuses to cooperate with health regimen Worries about separation from loved ones Is self-rejecting or displays false pride and selfishness Lacks love relationship with God Feels distant/separated from God
Faith	Depends on divine wisdom/God Is motivated toward growth Expresses satisfaction with explanation of life after death Expresses need to enter into and/or understand larger drama of human history Expresses need for the symbolic, ritual Expresses need for sense of a shared faith/community	Expresses ambivalent feelings about God Lacks faith in a transcendent power/God Fears death/life after death Senses isolation from faith community Is bitter, frustrated, and/or angry with God Has unclear values, beliefs, and goals Has values conflicts Lacks commitment
Creativity and hope	Asks for information about condition Talks about condition realistically Uses time during illness constructively Seeks ways for self-expression Finds comfort in inner self rather than physical self or worldly criteria Expresses hope in the future Is open to the possibility of peace	Expresses fear of loss of control Expresses boredom Lacks vision of possible alternatives Fears therapy Despairs Cannot help self or accept self Cannot enjoy anything Has put life/major decisions on hold
Meaning and purpose	Expresses contentment with life Lives life in accordance with value system Accepts or uses suffering to understand self Expresses meaning in life/death Expresses commitment and goal orientation Has clear sense of what is important	Expresses no reason to live Finds no meaning in suffering Questions the meaning of suffering Questions the purpose of illness Cannot form goals or has unattainable goals Abuses drugs/alcohol Jokes about life after death
Grace	Is alive in the moment Senses blessing/abundance Senses mercy given beyond self from God Senses harmony/wholeness	Is anxious about the past/future Is oriented toward achievement/production Focuses on regrets/remorse Talks about doing better/trying harder Is perfectionistic

- Do you feel your faith (religion) is helpful to you? If yes, tell me how.
- Has being sick (or what has happened to you) made any difference in your feeling about God or the practice of your faith?

Later spiritual assessment tools have been built around a broader definition of spirituality as asking patients questions that focus specifically on specific religious preferences and practices may cause some patients discomfort (Timmins & Kelly, 2008). Delgado (2007), for example, suggests that the following questions would be useful during a spiritual assessment:

- Do you think of yourself as a spiritual or religious person?
- Tell me about spiritual or religious beliefs that are important to you.

SPIRITUAL HEALTH

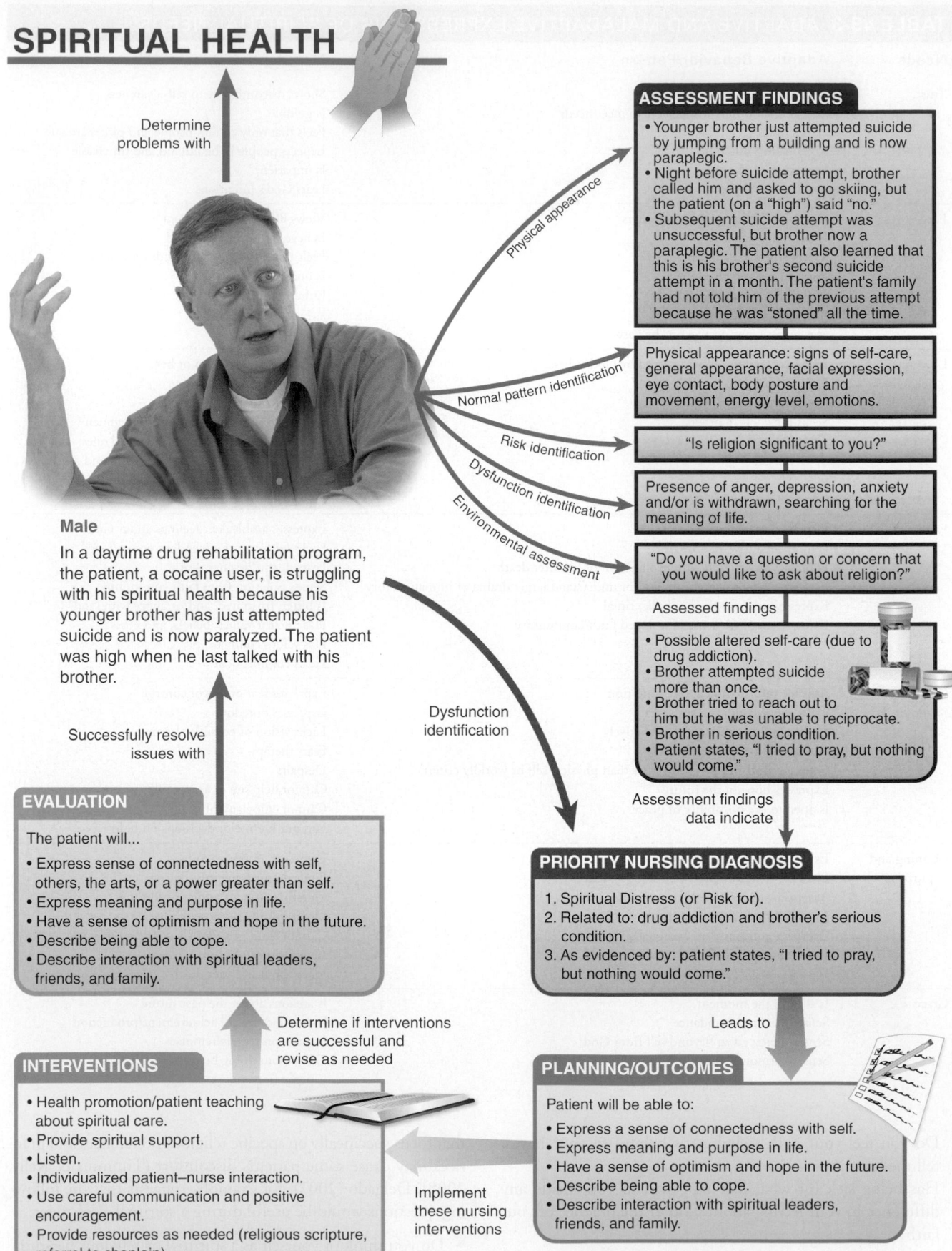

Determine
problems with

Male

In a daytime drug rehabilitation program, the patient, a cocaine user, is struggling with his spiritual health because his younger brother has just attempted suicide and is now paralyzed. The patient was high when he last talked with his brother.

Successfully resolve
issues with

Physical appearance

Normal pattern identification

Risk identification

Dysfunction identification

Environmental assessment

Dysfunction
identification

ASSESSMENT FINDINGS

- Younger brother just attempted suicide by jumping from a building and is now paraplegic.
- Night before suicide attempt, brother called him and asked to go skiing, but the patient (on a "high") said "no."
- Subsequent suicide attempt was unsuccessful, but brother now a paraplegic. The patient also learned that this is his brother's second suicide attempt in a month. The patient's family had not told him of the previous attempt because he was "stoned" all the time.

Physical appearance: signs of self-care, general appearance, facial expression, eye contact, body posture and movement, energy level, emotions.

"Is religion significant to you?"

Presence of anger, depression, anxiety and/or is withdrawn, searching for the meaning of life.

"Do you have a question or concern that you would like to ask about religion?"

Assessed findings

- Possible altered self-care (due to drug addiction).
- Brother attempted suicide more than once.
- Brother tried to reach out to him but he was unable to reciprocate.
- Brother in serious condition.
- Patient states, "I tried to pray, but nothing would come."

Assessment findings
data indicate

EVALUATION

The patient will...

- Express sense of connectedness with self, others, the arts, or a power greater than self.
- Express meaning and purpose in life.
- Have a sense of optimism and hope in the future.
- Describe being able to cope.
- Describe interaction with spiritual leaders, friends, and family.

Determine if interventions
are successful and
revise as needed

INTERVENTIONS

- Health promotion/patient teaching about spiritual care.
- Provide spiritual support.
- Listen.
- Individualized patient–nurse interaction.
- Use careful communication and positive encouragement.
- Provide resources as needed (religious scripture, referral to chaplain).

Implement
these nursing
interventions

PRIORITY NURSING DIAGNOSIS

1. Spiritual Distress (or Risk for).
2. Related to: drug addiction and brother's serious condition.
3. As evidenced by: patient states, "I tried to pray, but nothing would come."

Leads to

PLANNING/OUTCOMES

Patient will be able to:

- Express a sense of connectedness with self.
- Express meaning and purpose in life.
- Have a sense of optimism and hope in the future.
- Describe being able to cope.
- Describe interaction with spiritual leaders, friends, and family.

FIGURE 43-3 Concept map for spiritual health.

- Does the present situation (or illness) interfere with spiritual or religious activities that are important to you?
- What spiritual or religious practices do you find most comforting?
- Is there anyone you would like to see or talk to? May I assist in arranging a visit?
- Can you share your feelings with me?
- What can I do to help you at this time?

The Joint Commission (2014) also provides questions to consider during spiritual assessment. For example, "Who or what provides the patient with strength or hope?" "What is the name of the patient's clergy, ministers, chaplains, pastor, or rabbi?" "What does suffering mean to the patient?" "How does faith help the patient cope with illness?" and "What helps the patient through this healthcare experience?"

Assessment tools have been modified to address various populations. For example, Tanyi (2006) suggests different questions to assess family's spiritual needs. Some of these questions include the following:

- What gives the family meaning in their daily routines?
- What gives your family strength?
- What helps your family deal with crisis?
- Does the family have a relationship with a god/higher power, universe, or other?
- What are the family's beliefs? What do these beliefs mean to their health?

In addition to the use of assessment tools, the nurse's sensitive observation and listening can elicit other patient cues to spiritual health. Bull and Gillies (2007) note that this is especially true when working with children. Understanding a child's unique spiritual needs revolves around identifying the child's support systems as well as gaining an understanding of the home environment and the family profile. McSherry and Smith (2007) further note that children rely on prior spiritual experiences to make sense of challenging life events and crises. Listening carefully to children, carefully observing their behaviors, and using developmentally appropriate assessment techniques and tools will provide further insight into a child's spirituality.

Examples of other spiritual assessment tools, using the acronyms of FICA and HOPE, are given in Box 43-1.

Risk Identification

In one sense, all patients suffering from ill health are at risk for spiritual distress. They may be physically separated from usual sources of spiritual help, such as a faith community that maintains relationships and performs rituals of worship. They may be emotionally separated as well, especially if they lack introspection. Even for those who have spiritual strengths, the time of illness and accompanying crises increase anxiety. Certainly, patients with critical or terminal illnesses who are facing death or other profound physical changes face ultimate, meaning-in-life questions. Caldeira, Carvalho, and Vieira (2013) identify cues and characteristics that may be indicative of a patient at risk for spiritual distress. Such cues may be overt or may be subtle. Patients who are expressing anger toward God or

---

BOX 43-1   **Spiritual Assessment**

Patient Name _____ Date _____
Days in Treatment _____ Religious Preference _____
Marital Status _____ Children _____
Age _____

Spiritual Assessment
FICA

F   is for questions of *faith.* Examples of questions to ask: Do you consider yourself a spiritual person? What gives your life meaning?

I   represents the *importance* of this resource in the patient's life. Assessment questions might include the following: How often do you attend worship services? Do your beliefs largely influence your decisions with regard to your medical practices?

C   is for *community.* Are you actively involved with a church community, and do you use this as a support?

A   is for the practitioner to *address* these concerns with the patient, such as to ask, How would you like me to address these issues in your healthcare?

HOPE

H   addresses spiritual resources, such as *hope,* with direct focus on religion or spirituality.

O   represents importance of *organized* religion in their lives; the spiritual door is open.

P   represents inquiry with regard to *personal practices.*

E   is to remind the practitioner to work with the patient to discuss *end-of-life* issues, such as living wills.

Source: George Washington Institute for Spirituality and Health. (2002). *GWish.* Retrieved February 1, 2015, from http://www.gwumc.edu/gwish/clinical/fica-spiritual/fica-spiritual-history/index.cfm; *HOPE information from:* Anandarajh, G., & Hight, E. (2001). Spirituality and medical practice: Using the HOPE questions as a practical tool for spiritual assessment. *American Family Physician, 63*(1), 81–89. Retrieved January. 29, 2015, from http://www.aafp.org/afp/2001/0101/p81.html

a higher power, those who are feeling hopelessness or emptiness, or those who are withdrawn from interactions may be struggling and searching for meaning in life events. Further, spiritual distress can be expressed through unexpected questioning by the patient. For example, patients may question the meaning of life, why they have a particular illness, or why they must suffer.

Dysfunction Identification

The discovery of actual spiritual distress depends on the nurse's observation of the patient's verbal and nonverbal responses to the nursing history interview. Assist the patient in understanding that his or her nursing history is a review of the whole human being and that questions will be wide ranging, including spiritual health, as well as physical and emotional health. A patient who appears angry, anxious, depressed, or defensive when asked spiritual questions may need to hear something like, "I can see from your response that you might not have expected these questions; however, they do let you know that we are interested in how you are experiencing your current situation. Do you have a question or concern in this area?" Some patients are relieved to know that the spiritual aspect of their being is worthy of the nurse's concern. Still other patients indicate that they have spiritual concerns, but they will deal with them in their own time and way.

Identifying which spiritual need is lacking is related to the nurse's ability to listen and observe the patient carefully. The interview's content or facts combined with the assessment of nonverbal behaviors may evolve into a theme or a tone, such as distrust, judgment, isolation, or bitterness. Such themes can then be linked with spiritual needs, such as trust, forgiveness, love and relatedness, and faith.

Objective Data

Objective data can help in assessing spiritual health. Because of the qualities of the spiritual dimension, objective assessment must be verified against subjective information. Sometimes, in patients reluctant to verbalize such issues, objective data are the only clues to a difficulty.

Glean information about patients from general appearance, facial expression, eye contact, body posture and movement, sleeplessness, anxiety, crying, and inappropriate emotions. Materials such as religious articles, books, cards, and pictures also indicate the spiritual dimension, as do visitors from the church or clergy. Look for physical signs and symptoms of anxiety or distress that may provide additional evidence.

NURSING DIAGNOSES

Spiritual care diagnoses are addressed by NANDA-International (NANDA-I, 2014) under the domain Life Principle in Taxonomy II. Life Principle is described as "Principles underlying conduct, thought, and behavior about acts, customs, or institutions viewed as being true or having intrinsic worth." Under this domain are three classes: Values, Beliefs, and Values/Beliefs/Action Congruence. The Beliefs class has the concept Spiritual Well-Being, with the diagnosis of Readiness for Enhanced Spiritual Well-Being. The third class, Values/Beliefs/Action Congruence, has nine nursing diagnoses: Spiritual Distress, Risk for Spiritual Distress, Decisional Conflict (specify), Noncompliance (specify), Risk for Impaired Religiosity, Impaired Religiosity, Readiness for Enhanced Religiosity, Moral Distress, and Readiness for Enhanced Decision Making. A select few are presented in a separate table with Nursing Outcomes Classification (NOC) and Nursing Interventions Classification (NIC) considerations (Table 43-4).

 *Concept Mastery Alert*

It is important to differentiate between Impaired Religiosity and Spiritual Distress. Spiritual Distress is characterized by a disturbance in an individual person's belief system. Impaired Religiosity, however, involves challenges in exercising the beliefs of an individual's chosen faith community.

OUTCOME IDENTIFICATION AND PLANNING

After nursing diagnoses and related factors are identified, the patient and nurse plan outcomes and interventions. Goals for patients with spiritual distress or spiritual alterations should focus on providing an environment that supports usual religious practices and beliefs. Goals need to be individualized by considering the patient's history, areas of risk, evidence of dysfunction, and related objective data. Examples of outcomes for the patient with or at risk for spiritual distress include the following:

- The patient expresses a sense of connectedness with self, others, the arts, or a power greater than self.
- The patient expresses meaning and purpose in life.
- The patient has a sense of optimism and hope in the future.
- The patient discusses personal response to dying.
- The patient expresses satisfaction with life circumstances.

Goals for enhancing spiritual well-being can be very similar to those for patients in spiritual distress. The focus is on supporting the patient's strengths. The opportunity for spiritual growth may also be present as the patient explores creative ways to deal with pain and suffering. Some outcomes might include the following:

- The patient expresses hope, sense of meaning, and purpose.
- The patient describes being able to cope.
- The patient describes interaction with spiritual leaders, friends, and family.

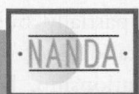

Table 43-4 SELECTED NANDA-I NURSING DIAGNOSES INVOLVING SPIRITUALITY

Nursing Dx	Related Factors	Dx Statement	NOC*	NIC†
Spiritual Distress—impaired ability to experience and integrate meaning in life through the individual's connectedness with self, others, the world, or a power greater than oneself	Self-alienation, loneliness, or social isolation; anxiety; sociocultural deprivation; thought of death of self or dying of others; pain; life changes; and chronic illness of self or others	**Spiritual Distress** R/T disconnectedness with others AEB refusing interactions with spiritual leaders, refusing interactions with friends and family, verbalizing separation from support systems, and expressing alienation	Coping; Grief Resolution; Hope; Personal Well-Being; Spiritual Health	Anticipatory Guidance; Forgiveness Facilitation; Hope Instillation; Referral; Spiritual Growth Facilitation; Spiritual Support; Values Clarification
Readiness for Enhanced Spiritual Well-Being—ability to experience and integrate meaning and purpose in life through connectedness with self, others, art, music, literature, nature, or a power greater than oneself	Health-seeking behaviors, empathy, self-care, self-awareness, desire for harmonious interconnectedness, and desire to find meaning and purpose in life	**Readiness for Enhanced Spiritual Well-Being** R/T connectedness with others AEB providing service to others; requesting interaction with spiritual leaders, friends, and family; and requesting forgiveness of others	Patient Satisfaction: Cultural Needs Fulfillment; Coping; Hope; Personal Well-Being; Spiritual Health	Hope Instillation; Referral; Spiritual Growth Facilitation; Spiritual Support

Dx, diagnosis; R/T, related to; AEB, as evidenced by.
*From: Moorhead, S., Johnson, M., Maas, M., & Swanson, E. (2014). *Iowa Outcomes Project: Nursing Outcomes Classification (NOC)* (5th ed.). St. Louis, MO: C. V. Mosby.
†From: Bulecheck, G., Butcher, H., Dochterman, J., & Wagner, C. (2014). *Iowa Intervention Project: Nursing Interventions Classification (NIC)* (4th ed.). St. Louis, MO: C. V. Mosby.
From: NANDA-International (NANDA-I). (2014). *Nursing diagnoses: Definitions and classification, 2015–2017.* West Sussex, UK: Wiley-Blackwell.

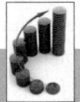

OUTCOME-BASED TEACHING PLANS

Billy Nelson, age 7 years, has been diagnosed with advanced cancer of the brain. His parents are being asked to participate in noncurative treatment plans for Billy. They are deeply distraught. They want to do what is best for their son, follow their religious beliefs, and participate knowledgeably in the decision making. Billy's parents turn to you, the nurse in the children's clinic, for advice.

OUTCOME

Family can verbalize feelings about their son's condition and how that intersects with their religious beliefs.

STRATEGIES

- Encourage the parents to explore their own feelings and beliefs.
- With the parents, evaluate Billy's level of understanding of the event.
- Encourage expression of Billy's feelings about his health using developmentally appropriate activities.
- Encourage the family to talk openly about Billy's situation and the feelings it generates, particularly in regard to their religious beliefs.
- Encourage Billy and his parents to discuss their concerns with their clergyperson.
- Support parents as they verbalize their wishes for Billy's treatment plan with healthcare providers.

EVALUATION

10/5/17: 13:00—Billy's parents effectively explored and verbalized their feelings about Billy's condition with their clergyperson.
- Billy and his parents continue to confront their anxiety and decisions in concert with healthcare providers and clergy.

—S. Roberts, RN

IMPLEMENTATION

Essential in implementing spiritual care are commitment to the nurse–patient relationship, good communication skills, trust, empathy, self-awareness, and acceptance of a broad definition of spirituality.

Although qualitative aspects play a large part in performing nursing interventions, implementation also includes continuing data collection, maintaining current documentation, and collaborating with the healthcare team. These steps are important because they ensure consistency and continuity in patient care. The provision of spiritual care is not limited to one individual nurse but requires collaboration from a team of nurses and other professionals.

The process should affirm the individual. Through effective communication, the nurse helps facilitate the patient's use of his or her own spiritual resources or helps to find someone else to assist the patient. The timing should not be forced but will be based upon patient cues and should demonstrate sensitivity and empathy from the professionals providing this care.

Health Promotion

Spiritual care is dynamic and embodies some of the basic tenets of nursing. The nurse's use of presence, therapeutic use of self, patient centeredness, intuitive sense, and the creation of a spiritually nurturing environment are integral to providing spiritual care. Such care has positive effects for patients including healing and the promotion of psychological and spiritual well-being (Ramezani, Ahmadi, Mohammadi, & Kazemnejad, 2014).

Koenig's (2009) research examines individuals in different medical and nonmedical settings, from diverse ethnic backgrounds, in differing age groups, and from various locations from the United States to countries in the East. Findings reveal that religious involvement is related to better coping with stress and related less to anxiety, depression, substance abuse, and suicide. Similarly, Park and colleagues (2013) noted a positive relationship between individuals with high religious and spiritual involvement and their overall well-being and happiness. In an earlier study, Koenig (1999) found that participation in a faith community and involvement in religious activities were positively related to good physical health. His research explores a prevention model in which faith community participation improved mental health, provided social support, and promoted positive health habits.

USE OF SELF

Spiritual care occurs within the nurse–patient relationship. This relationship does not simply consist of talking with patients. This therapeutic relationship requires the purposeful use of self to help another person grow in the ability to face reality and to discover potential solutions to problems. Spiritual care is a relationship that the nurse perceives as a valuable part of therapy and to which he or she holds a commitment.

Qualities such as trust and empathy are partially built on good communication skills and an understanding of the processes and phases of the nurse–patient relationship. For example, making oneself and one's time available to patients is necessary to build trust in the initial phase of the relationship. Through active listening, nurses can understand the perspectives of patients and be more sensitive to their needs, including spiritual needs. Without the establishment of trust and empathy in the relationship's first phase, nurses will be unable to discern deeper concerns such as meaning and purpose and connection with others or a higher power.

Being able to take part in the lives of patients is a privilege and responsibility (Fig. 43-4). Involvement in the meeting of spiritual needs is very personal for both nurses and patients and fundamental to providing holistic nursing care.

SPIRITUAL SUPPORT

Nurses need to have a broad definition of spirituality to discern the spirituality and spiritual needs of others. By being knowledgeable about other spiritual and religious expressions while remaining nonjudgmental and supportive, the nurse empowers the patient to explore difficult questions and find answers that are uniquely suited to his life situation. Each patient varies in respect to expression of spiritual needs and in the level or depth of spiritual care that may be required. Therefore, nurses need to remain available and sensitive to this variability in order to offer spiritually appropriate nursing care.

Faull et al. (2012) note that the use of therapeutic communication is integral in spiritual assessment and care. Using effective communication skills helps the nurse and other care providers build trust and foster connections with the patient. Effective communication encourages patient choice and patient-centered care. Active listening helps the nurse focus on what the patient is saying—and, just as important, what the patient has not said. By focusing on the patient's unique spirituality and by avoiding personal witness and evangelism during spiritual distress, the nurse supports and respects the patient's personal beliefs and spiritual needs. Nurses should not attempt

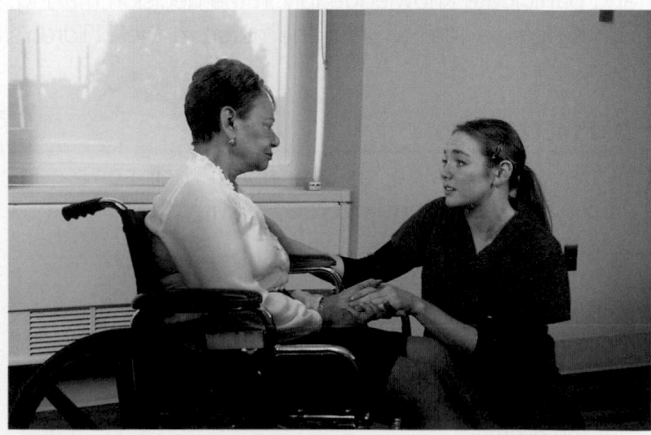

FIGURE 43-4 Being with the patient when she needs someone is an important aspect of spiritual care.

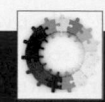

COLLABORATING WITH THE HEALTHCARE TEAM
Requesting Spiritual Care Consult for Patient's Concern About Blood Transfusion

As a nurse on surgical unit, you administer blood products frequently. Your patient today, 28-year-old MaryAnn Jones, has a hematocrit of 22, and her physicians are recommending a blood transfusion. She is refusing because "it seems wrong to mix someone's blood with my own." The medical team and nursing team have explained the risk/benefit of transfusion for her situation; however, she has yet to decide what to do. An order for a spiritual care consult is requested by the previous shift registered nurse after talking it over with MaryAnn. They arrive on the unit and meet with you prior to meeting with the patient and are requesting more information.

SITUATION: MaryAnn has a low blood count, and her doctors are recommending a transfusion of red blood cells.

BACKGROUND: She was admitted 6 days ago, and this is her first hospitalization and surgery. She is unsure if she wants to proceed with their recommendations because she says "it seems wrong to mix someone's blood with my own." She identifies herself as a spiritual but not religious person and did not designate a religious preference on admit. The medical and nursing teams have discussed the risk versus benefit of a transfusion, but she says she feels too "overwhelmed" to make a decision.

ASSESSMENT: By MaryAnn's own report, she is overwhelmed with being hospitalized and doesn't feel able to make a decision at this point. She has mentioned that "it seems wrong" to mix one person's blood with another, though she has not elaborated on this.

RECOMMENDATION: I would like to ask for you to speak with MaryAnn and help her sort out her feelings to give her the support to make an informed decision.

CRITICAL THINKING QUESTIONS
- How might a spiritual care consult help MaryAnn versus a discussion with her physicians and nurses?
- What topics might be discussed during a spiritual care consult?

---

to change faith that patients already possess but instead should build on patients' faith. If faith is removed, patients will lose hope; without hope and the will to live, many people are beyond the help of the most potent medical powers.

SUPPORT OF SPIRITUAL PRACTICES

Information regarding the patient's spiritual needs and religious preference is obtained during assessment. To facilitate meeting spiritual needs or specific religious practices, become familiar with the various religious groups within the community. Pay attention to special religious considerations such as beliefs about birth, death, sacraments, diet, holy days, and holy objects. For example, dietary practices reflect dietary laws (e.g., no pork or beef) as well as celebration of holy days by fasting or feasting. If the food required is so specialized that the healthcare facility's dietary department cannot accommodate the patient's needs, the family may ask to bring in their own food. Refer back to Table 43-1, which gives a brief overview of the major religious groups' practices related to health.

In general, patients have the right to practice personal spiritual expressions in private, such as reading Holy Scriptures, praying, or meditating while in the hospital. In some cases, the nurse may share in these activities; in other cases, the nurse may arrange for a pastoral visit or inform the patient of other available resources. When a patient wears special amulets or garments on areas exposed for tests, treatments, or surgery, the circumstances

may call for a special consultation with the patient, family, or spiritual leader rather than the nurse routinely removing them.

If the spiritual leader or healer plans to visit, prepare the patient's room and religious articles appropriately. If the sacraments or other rituals are to be performed, make sure the bedside stand or table is clear and available.

Nursing Interventions for Altered Spiritual Function

When implementing spiritual care, prioritize emergency patient needs. For example, basic survival needs, such as maintaining an airway, take priority over growth needs that have to do with self-actualization. However, if the patient has found no meaning in suffering, is experiencing hopelessness, or is unable to take part in his or her faith community, the spiritual dimension becomes a central need. The patient may have regained physical strength, but the spirit remains unfulfilled. Interventions include anticipatory guidance, counseling, crisis intervention, emotional support, forgiveness facilitation, grief work, guided imagery, relaxation, and instillation of hope (NANDA-I, 2009).

LISTENING AND SUPPORTING

Active listening with empathy and sensitivity is one of the most valuable nursing interventions. Through purposeful listening, the patient defines personal spiritual questions and directs the most useful type of support. De Silva and Henricson (2013) note that touch or physical contact may express caring and foster hope and connection with the patient. The use of touch may involve simply holding or touching the hand of a distressed patient. In some cases, connecting or support may require stepping beyond the physical realm into the spiritual realm with the patient. Nurses may be asked to participate in common practices of prayer and meditation with patients and their families. Prayer and meditation aid the patient in physical relaxation connection with the inner self and higher power. Since prayer and meditation are highly personal, some patients may wish for the nurse to participate with them while others may not. Discerning this preference and need is an important element in a complete spiritual assessment.

The following situation, adapted from Frye and Long (1985), illustrates the intervention of listening and support as an integral part of providing spiritual care.

Robert, the son of a practicing physician and the eldest of four children, was a junior medical student. He was a handsome, popular young man with a keen, satirical sense of humor. Robert was scheduled to be at his first family practice clinic, but he didn't make it. Traffic was heavy on the freeway, and Robert found himself between a truck and a semitrailer with cars on either side. He tried to swerve into an adjacent lane and rear-ended a large truck. The impact propelled him off and under his motorcycle, resulting in instant unconsciousness. When he arrived at the emergency room, the outlook was grim.

The next 5 months were a battle. Fluctuating intracranial pressures with complications, pervading depression, and thoughts of suicide haunted him. Having deeply religious parents and a strong background in religious education, Robert seemed to have the spiritual strengths to deal with this crisis … until one day when the depth of his loneliness and doubt surfaced.

His nurse approached him, suspecting that he needed permission to doubt previous convictions. As a result, there was an outpouring of questions: Where was God when he needed Him? Why had God let him down?

Many conversations followed with Robert's mother, nurses, doctor, therapists, and chaplain. Family, friends, and staff supported Robert in his questions. Robert identified with the biblical story of Job and began to talk of his hope.

As part of denial of his former convictions, Robert frequently requested pain medication during the day to help him sleep. He stated, "I just don't want to be awake." After listening carefully, the nurse confronted him, asking him if he was truly in pain or was trying to escape from the realities of his situation. She supported him as they began to work together on a different approach.

REFERRAL

Being comfortable listening to a patient's spiritual needs and hearing religious requests is important. If the patient or family members ask for prayer or scripture reading and you are comfortable doing that, try to identify the special focus or topic before beginning. When the patient and family appear to have no religious tradition, ask to assist them in a quiet, reflective moment. Respond to any patient or family requests to see personal clergy or the hospital chaplain. When necessary, initiate a referral to see one. Nurses and chaplains are often viewed as allies in providing spiritual care for patients. Nurses make every effort to meet the spiritual needs of patients, but with numerous demands and responsibilities in today's healthcare system, nurses are often hampered from comprehensively meeting the patient's spiritual needs (Ronaldson, Hayes, Aggar, Green, Carey, 2012). Here, referral to a chaplain can be a viable option to assist with meeting patients' spiritual needs.

Nurses refer patients and their families to the chaplain for various reasons. Weinberger-Litman and colleagues (2010) noted that nurses frequently refer to the chaplain patients who are having difficulty resolving issues in the healthcare setting and need to talk about these feelings and emotions. Nurses refer patients who are dying and in need of spiritual care at the end of life. Additionally, the families or loved ones of patients who have died or are near death are frequently referred for spiritual care. The chaplain may perform end-of-life religious rituals because families and patients are often in need emotional and spiritual support during this difficult time and find comfort in these sacred activities. Nurses who are uncertain of a given faith community's beliefs and traditions may refer patients to the chaplain for support and care. Pastoral care departments can be resources for finding representatives of other religious groups who can assist the families and patients in need.

AGE-SPECIFIC INTERVENTIONS

Newborn and Infant

Hospitalization and illness potentially disrupt an infant's basic trust in parents. Parents play an instrumental role in the lives of infants and newborns; thus, attention given to recognizing the needs of parents can in turn assist in meeting infant needs. Nurses have the responsibility of meeting the needs of both the babies and their families. Hospitalization and illness can lead to questioning, intense emotions as parents search for meaning in the experiences. Supporting the spiritual needs of parents by listening, offering comfort and encouragement, and promoting stability also in turn helps to meet the infant's needs. Nurses can support and encourage parents to be present and involved in the caring process with infants.

Toddler and Preschooler

According to Ferrell and Coyle (2010), preschoolers and toddlers use very concrete terms when talking about their spirituality. Responding to these concrete questions and comments while carrying out established routines are important considerations when caring for toddlers and preschoolers. Supporting families as they carry out rituals of faith is an important aspect of spiritual care. If the family is unavailable, the nurse can carry out these rituals for them. For example, bedtime may be a difficult transition time for children at this age, especially while in hospital. Offering to assist the child with established family faith traditions, rituals, or prayers is often comforting and supportive.

Young children are very sensitive to good–bad issues. Do not tell them that painful or scary treatments are in any way a punishment. Affirm that the children, although ill or hospitalized, are still loved by their parents, the nurse, God, Jesus, or whoever is appropriate according to the family's faith.

School-Age Child and Adolescent

Bull and Gillies (2007) note that children value supportive relationships that provide a sense of comfort and strength and ones that recognize the importance of their spiritual needs. Nurses can provide such support to families by carrying out familiar religious rituals in the healthcare setting. For children, clarifying fact and fantasy when it comes to all medical interventions and procedures allays anxiety and provides support. Often, a "story" about a similar situation will aid in this reality-orienting process for a child. Local libraries frequently have books that describe children's trips to health clinics or the hospital. Again, children must not associate illness and hospitalization with wrongdoing and punishment, which would increase their anxiety and fear. Acceptance and clarification of the experiences are the effective modes to offer meaning to children.

Religious beliefs change as children move into adolescence as a result of maturation and the development of more global thinking. Adolescents move from their trusted dependent beliefs of childhood to a stage of searching for identity in life and spirituality (Haley, 2014). In contrast to younger children, adolescents are less likely to believe in a completely literal translation of the Holy Bible. Children are more likely to report that they believe in God because of what their parents tell them, whereas adolescents rely more on rational or logical thinking when determining their faith. Adolescents are capable of conceptualizing personal relationships with God. In times of illness, they may question the meaning of the experience, trying to integrate it into their lives, much as adults would do under similar circumstances. These issues are often discerned during a nursing history and assessment. Encouraging adolescents to express their feelings verbally or in writing may help them during these times. Adolescents may wish to write letters to God, to their parents, or to other significant individuals in their lives as a way of exploring and integrating thoughts during challenging and difficult times (Haley, 2014). Follow-up on the data or involvement of the hospital chaplain or with the adolescent's spiritual counselor may be helpful.

Developing a personal style and interacting with peers remain priorities even during illness for adolescents. Involve the adolescent's peers by encouraging them to remain available through visits, cards, telephone, or the Internet. If a long-term illness, accident, or some other severe condition is involved, other networks of support might be useful, such as the school or church. Youth groups can serve as communication links for hospitalized adolescents. Peers may also need the opportunity to explore their own responses to illness to work through their feelings about life. Youth leaders or hospital chaplains can be resources for this kind of experience.

Adult and Older Adult

Young adults clarify personal beliefs and commitments based on experience and relationships. Their faith challenge is to establish and reflect on personal faith and life's meaning. Nurses can be available to listen, support, and validate feelings and experiences. They can help patients explore the meaning in life or meaning in death. Young adults may have the need for spiritual mentoring. Nurses can remain open and support patients as they explore possibilities about who might fulfill this role in their lives. Remaining supportive of each patient's family and social network is key because these relationships give meaning to the patient's life.

During the middle years, adults become more concerned with a broader world view and polarities. Resolution of these polarities lies in being able to see and live with life's paradoxes and being open to diversity, not threatened by it. In some ways, these individuals have much to offer others. For example, a young adult nurse might gain personally by spending time with an adult working through a paradox of health and illness. By being available to listen, support, and reflect with the patient, the nurse can better understand the patient's struggle. By accepting the possibility of mutuality in the relationship, the nurse has the opportunity to give new meaning and hope to the patient. Risking mutuality demonstrates true respect and care, which, in turn, enhances both patient and nurse (Fowler, 1995).

As with other age groups, listening and support are essential as older adults deal with health and illness. Older adults used several religious or spiritual interventions with health professionals and also in isolation (Griffin, Salman, Lee, & Fitzpatrick, 2008). Interventions that were effective included being involved in family activities, serving others, and recalling positive thoughts and memories. Most older adults studied reported participating in conventional religious practices such as worship and prayer either alone or in groups. Since these activities, traditions, and rituals are meaningful to older adults, encouraging participation in these or a reconnection with these activities can be beneficial. One example might be encouraging the use of prayer, a practice that major world religions incorporate into their spirituality. For many, prayer is an essential practice and spiritual connection. Prayer does not depend on physical capabilities. However, as infirmity increases, older adults may be less able than in previous years to participate and pray in their faith communities. At this point, nurses may facilitate connections with people or groups in the community who can either visit regularly or assist with transportation. Such connections provide meaning and hope for older persons because some faith rituals are satisfactorily performed only in group settings.

SPECIAL POPULATIONS

The above is a general review of spiritual care needs along the lifespan continuum, but there are many special groups of patients who may have unique needs depending upon the type of illness, phase of illness, or setting of care. There are differences in the spiritual concerns of persons with acute illness, persons with chronic illness, persons living with depression, or persons who are facing loss or death (Faull et al., 2012; Magyar-Russell et al., 2014; Unterrainer et al., 2014; White, 2013). For example, persons living with a mental illness often have spiritual questions because the mental illness can be in a form expressed in terms of religious delusions or hallucinations. Healthcare providers, including nurses, may avoid spiritual issues for fear of supporting the symptoms of the mental illness. In some cases, this has led to a lack of consistent assessment of spiritual needs and spiritual care. Bonelli and Koenig (2013) note that religious and spiritual involvement is correlated with better mental health in individuals suffering from depression and substance abuse, further emphasizing the importance of spiritual care for all individuals.

Home and Community Care

Assessing and planning for spiritual care constitutes an ongoing process. Settings that encourage this process most consistently are usually those in which nurses and patients can establish relationships over time. Examples may be in a clinic with the nurse as case manager, in a long-term care facility with the nurse as team leader, or in a community hospice program with the nurse making regular visits. In acute care settings, nurses most certainly can become aware of patients' spiritual needs and begin to address them. The most important part of that care, however, will be the discharge summary and a plan of care that identifies areas of spiritual distress. In this way, follow-up care can be more holistic.

Some patients want nurses to prearrange visits from pastors, priests, or other members of the religious community after their return home or transfer to another healthcare facility. In some areas of the United States, faith communities have developed various health ministries. One of these, called congregation care nursing, parish nursing, or faith community nursing, is considered a specialty area of practice, recognized by the American Association of Nursing and having its own standards of practice. Parish nurses work in churches across the country providing health promotion and health screening activities to individuals in the community. Parish nurses view patients holistically addressing spiritual issues as well as health issues that arise for individuals in their faith community. At a time when medical and healthcare costs are on the rise, parish nurses from churches across the United States are stepping up to address and fill patient needs (Yeaworth & Sailors, 2014).(Box 43-2). Patients need not be church members to be included in faith community care. For example, as relationships develop with community agencies, healthcare chaplains, and discharge planners, patients can be referred by geographic area. However, that referral should be mutual, with patients' permission.

BOX 43-2   Parish Nursing

Goal
To promote the health of a faith community and the community by working with the ministry team

Models
(Hickman, 2011)
- Congregation-based, volunteer/unpaid
- Congregation-based, paid
- Institutional
- Consortium model, paid

Roles
(Hickman, 2011)

The congregational nurse practitioner, parish nurse, faith community nurse, or congregational care nurse serves in the following roles to provide holistic spiritually based care:
- Models integration of faith and health
  - Assesses congregational needs and assets
  - Identifies opportunities to promote congregational knowledge of the integration of faith and health
- Serves as a personal health counselor
  - Provides health counseling and health education in conjunction with spiritual support
  - Encourages expression of faith beliefs and supports during times of distress or crisis
  - Works with church staff to plan health promotion education and health-related activities

- Serves as a health educator
  - Plans educational opportunities based upon congregational needs assessment
  - Prepares and delivers educational opportunities addressing congregational needs
  - Assesses effectiveness of training on congregational outcomes and attendance
  - Is a health resource to congregation and ministerial staff
- Provides volunteer training
  - Provides training to eligible professionals and members within in the congregation
  - Encourages and assists volunteers when appropriate to meet health needs of the congregation
- Assists with support group development
  - Assesses congregational needs for support groups
  - Leads or supports volunteers leading groups
  - Makes referrals as appropriate to community support
- Acts as a referral agent
  - Identifies appropriate community resources for parishioner and makes referrals as needed
  - Documents referrals
  - Networks with area parish nurses
- Acts as a patient health advocate
  - Educates and assists individuals and families when making decisions regarding medical services and healthcare needs
  - Promotes participation of parishioners in activities that foster health, well-being, and overall health status

Much healing and spiritual growth can occur without professional assistance because some patients find ways to meet their spiritual needs independently. Therefore, a sensitive and nonintrusive attitude on the nurse's part is crucial; nurses cannot force patients to deal with spiritual issues or to assume religious beliefs. Spiritual health is one area that cannot be put onto a specific "road map" or trajectory. However, assisting patients to reconnect to their faith community or to utilize the resources of a faith community has health benefits.

EVALUATION

Specific outcome criteria are the evaluative tools for measuring goal attainment for patients in spiritual distress. Examples of outcome criteria are listed in the following sections and use "Robert" (see the Listening and Supporting section) as an example. Outcome criteria need to be specifically tailored to each patient so that the criteria will uniquely measure that patient's attainment of goals.

PATIENT PLAN OF CARE
The Patient With Spiritual Distress*

NURSING DIAGNOSIS

Spiritual Distress related to crisis of illness as evidenced by loss of meaning in life, suicidal thoughts, and overuse of pain medication

PATIENT GOAL

Patient will express increased understanding and acceptance of current life situation.

PATIENT OUTCOME CRITERIA

- Patient verbalizes feelings of despair, anger, and fear after 3 weeks.
- Patient identifies support provided by staff, family, and friends during periods of questioning and despair after 5 weeks.
- Patient will identify some alternative coping mechanisms other than requesting pain medications after 10 weeks.

NURSING INTERVENTION	SCIENTIFIC RATIONALE
1. Offer patient opportunity for one-on-one nurse–patient relationship. Actively listen to the patient. Allow expression of negative feelings.	**1.** Initiating a one-on-one relationship establishes a climate of acceptance and builds trust and safety.
2. Plan and coordinate a multidisciplinary team conference including the chaplain. Facilitate a care planning conference involving the social support network including family and friends.	**2.** Initiating a multidisciplinary social network of conferences facilitates a sense of acceptance, love, and belonging.
3. Explore past coping mechanisms including use of music, scripture, prayer, and relaxation techniques. Help patient identify times when he or she can use various alternative strategies.	**3.** Building on past positive coping mechanisms enhances a sense of self-control and self-esteem.
4. Use the "life review" technique focusing on faith/spiritual development. Help patient explore ways to use this experience in a unique way such as sharing in a group or with medical students or other healthcare professional students.	**4.** By focusing on personal faith/spirit, the patient can gain new insights into his or her relationship with God and can sense hope and the potential for creativity or self-actualization.

*Refers to the situation of Robert in the Listening and Supporting section.

EVALUATION

12/12/17: 12:00—Patient expresses feelings of despair, anger, and fear after 3 weeks.
- Patient identifies support provided by staff, family, and friends during periods of questioning and despair after 5 weeks.
- Patient identifies and uses alternative coping mechanisms thereby decreasing the amount of pain medication required after 10 weeks.

—M. Klim, RN

Goal

The patient will express acceptance of current life situation and satisfaction with the meaning and purpose of illness, suffering, and death.

POSSIBLE OUTCOME CRITERIA

- Patient exhibits feelings of despair, anger, and fear during the first few days.
- Patient identifies support provided by staff, family, and friends during periods of questioning and despair.

Goal

The patient will participate in spiritual practices that are personally supportive and express satisfaction with spiritual condition.

POSSIBLE OUTCOME CRITERIA

- Within the first month, patient asks to speak to a spiritual advisor.
- Patient demonstrates spiritual practices such as prayer or reading of religious/spiritual texts within the second month.
- Patient expresses satisfaction with being able to maintain relationships with his or her faith community within second month.

KEY CONCEPTS

- Spirituality, like the role of philosophy, is to help people ask the right questions and develop a view of life rather than answer the questions.
- The spiritual dimension is the essence of a person and is expressed in the need to seek meaning in experiences and to make a spiritual journey through life.
- Spiritual well-being is the condition in which a person is at peace with God, self, community, and environment.
- Fowler's stages of faith have parallels to Piaget's stages of cognitive development and Erikson's stages of psychosocial development.
- Nurses may provide inadequate or inappropriate care if they have not fully addressed their own spirituality and spiritual well-being and if they hesitate to encourage the patient to speak of personal spirituality.
- Altered spiritual function may be expressed verbally or through various altered behaviors.
- Every patient has the right to practice his or her spirituality according to personal preference. The nurse should not be judgmental but should assist the patient in fulfilling those needs.
- Nursing interventions include use of self, spiritual support, support of religious practices, listening and supporting, and referral.

PRACTICING FOR THE NCLEX

CHECK YOUR ANSWERS IN APPENDIX A.

1. A teen has recently survived a car accident in which his friend was killed. The nurse assigns the nursing diagnosis of Spiritual Distress. Which of the following statements would best support this diagnosis?
   a. "I need some time alone; can't we do this later?"
   b. "Why did I have to survive?"
   c. "I just want to sleep!"
   d. "I don't want those pills!"

2. An elderly woman has recently become a resident in a skilled nursing facility as a result of her worsening health conditions. Which of the following may lead to impaired spiritual health? Select all that apply:
   a. Anger at treatment regimen
   b. Lack of concentration and short-term memory
   c. Lack of transportation to usual meditation group
   d. Fear about living in a new environment

3. A Catholic patient is anxious related to her hospitalization. The nurse attending to her is Buddhist. Which statement is most appropriate for the nurse to make?
   a. "I have to give pain medications to another patient, so I'll leave you alone to pray."
   b. "I can't pray with you; we believe in different Gods."
   c. "Do you have a Bible or book of Psalms that I can read to you?"
   d. "Don't worry; many patients are anxious about being in the hospital."

4. A nurse is developing outcome criteria for a patient's plan of care regarding the patient with spiritual distress. Which of the following is an appropriate criterion?
   a. Patient verbalizes feelings.
   b. Patient identifies support provided by family.
   c. Patient expresses increased understanding and acceptance of current situation.
   d. Patient expresses satisfaction with tie to faith community within 1 month.

5. A nurse is caring for a patient with terminal lung cancer. Which of the following would indicate potential risk for spiritual distress? Select all that apply:
   a. Patient has had many visitors while hospitalized.
   b. Patient formerly sang in the local choir, quitting due to shortness of breath.
   c. Patient is a member of a church group and attends regular mass.
   d. Disease prognosis is terminal with projected mortality within 3 months.

REFERENCES

Agrimson, L., & Taft, L. (2009). Spiritual crisis: A concept analysis. *Journal of Advanced Nursing, 65*(2), 454–461.

American Nursing Diagnosis Association International (NANDA-I). (2014). *Nursing diagnoses: Definitions and classification, 2015–2017.* West Sussex, UK: Wiley-Blackwell.

Anandarajh, G., & Hight, E. (2001). Spirituality and medical practice: Using the HOPE questions as a practical tool for spiritual assessment. *American Family Physician, 63*(1), 81–89. Retrieved January 29, 2015, from http://www.aafp.org/afp/2001/0101/p81.html

Anles, P. (1989). Medicine and living tradition of Islam. In L. E. Sullivan (Ed.), *Healing and restoring, health and medicine in the world's religious traditions* (p. 189). New York, NY: Macmillan.

Bonelli, R., & Koenig, H. (2013). Mental disorders, religion and spirituality 1990–2010: A systematic evidenced-based review. *Journal of Religious and Health, 52,* 657–673. doi 10.1007/s10943-013-9691-4

Bull, A., & Gillies, M. (2007). Spiritual needs of children with complex healthcare needs in hospital. *Paediatric Nursing, 19*(9), 34–38.

Burke, L., Neimeyer, R., Holland, J., Dennard, S.,Olliver, L., & Shear, K. (2014). Inventory of complicated spiritual grief: Development and validation of a new measure. *Death Studies,* (38), 239–250. doi: 10.1080/07481187.2013.810098

Caldeira, S., Carvalho, E., & Vieira, M. (2013). Spiritual distress-proposing a new definition and defining characteristics. *International Journal of Nursing Knowledge, 24*(2), 77–84.

Dalmida, S., Holstad, M., Diiorio, C., & Laderman, G. (2009). Spiritual well-being, depressive symptoms, and immune status among women living with HIV/AIDS. *Women & Health, 49*(2), 119–143.

Delgado, C. (2007). Meeting client's spiritual needs. *Nursing Clinics of North America, 42,* 279–293.

Desai, P. N. (1989). *Health and medicine in the Hindu tradition.* New York, NY: Crossroad Publishing Company.

de Silva, J., & Henricson, M. (2013). Promotion of hope in patients cared for in an intensive care unit in Indonesia. *Nordic Journal of Nursing Research & Clinical Studies, 33*(1), 4–8.

Erickson, H. (2007). Philosophy and theory of holism. *Nursing Clinics of North America, 42*(2), 139–163.

Faull, C., de Caestecker, S., Nicholson, A., & Black, F., Eds. (2012). *Handbook of palliative care* (3rd ed.). Hoboken, NJ: John Wiley & Sons, Inc.

Ferrell, B., & Coyle, N. (2010). *Textbook of palliative nursing* (3rd ed.). New York, NY: Oxford University Press.

Fowler, J. W. (1995). *Stages of faith* (2nd ed.). San Francisco, CA: Harper.

Frye, B., & Long, L. (1985). Spiritual counseling approaches following brain injury. *Rehabilitation Nursing, 10,* 14–16.

George Washington Institute for Spirituality and Health. (2002). *GWish* (2), 100–102. Retrieved February 1, 2015, from http://www.gwumc.edu/gwish/clinical/fica-spiritual/fica-spiritual-history/index.cfm

Granstrom, S. L. (1985). Spiritual care of oncology client. *Topics in Clinical Nursing, 7*(1), 39–45.

Griffin, M., Salman, A., Lee, Y., & Fitzpatrick, J. (2008). A beginning look at spiritual practices of older adults. *Gerontologic Care, 25*(2), 100–102.

Haley, J. (2014). How do adolescents develop faith and how can nurses/nurse practitioners help? *Journal of Christian Nursing, 31*(2), 120–126.

Hickman, S. (2011) *Fast facts for the faith community nurse: Implementing fcn/parish in a nutshell.* New York, NY: Springer Publishing Company, LLC.

Hirsch, J., Webb, J., & Kaslow, N. (2014). Daily hassles and suicide ideation in African-American female suicide attempters: Moderating effect of spiritual wellbeing, *Mental Health, Religion & Culture, 17*:5, 529–541, doi: 10.1080/13674676.2013.858682

John-Roger, & Kaye, P. (2010). Living the spiritual principles of health and well-being. Los Angeles, CA: Mandeville Press.

Joint Commission. (2014). *Spiritual assessment* (revised November 24, 2008). Retrieved July 15, 2014, from www.jointcommission.org/standards_information/jcfaqdetails.aspx?StandardsFaqId=290&ProgramId=1

King, M., & Koenig, H. (2009). *Conceptualizing spirituality for medical research and health service provision.* BMC Health Services Research, 9:116, doi: 10.1186/1472-6963-9-116

Kitagawa, J. M. (1989). Buddhist medical history. In L. E. Sullivan (Ed.), *Healing and restoring, health and medicine in the world's religious traditions* (pp. 9–32). New York, NY: Macmillan.

Koenig, H. G. (1999). *The healing power of faith.* New York, NY: Simon & Schuster.

Koenig, H. G. (2009). Research on religion, spirituality, and mental health: A review. *Canadian Journal of Psychiatry, 54*(5), 283–291.

Leininger, M. (1991). *Culture care diversity and universality: A theory of nursing.* New York, NY: National League for Nursing Press.

Magyar-Russell, G., Brown, I., Edara, I., Smith, T., Marine, J., & Ziegelstein, R. (2014). In search of serenity: religious struggle among patients hospitalized for suspected acute coronary syndrome. *Journal of Religious and Health, 53,* 562–578. doi: 10.1007/s10943-013-9713-2

McSherry, W., & Smith, J. (2007). How do children express their spiritual needs? *Paediatric Nursing, 39*(3), 17–20.

Murray, R. B., & Zentner, J. P. (2001). *Health promotion strategies throughout the lifespan* (7th ed.). Englewood Cliffs, NJ: Prentice Hall.

Nightingale, F. (1860). *Notes on nursing: What it is and what it is not.* New York, NY: D. Appleton & Co. Retrieved from http://digital.library.upenn.edu/women/nightingale/nursing/nursing.htmlNorth

Pew Forum on Religion and Public Life. (2012). Nones on the rise: One-in-five adults have no religious affiliation. Retrieved July 6, 2014, from http://www.pewforum.org/files/2012/10/NonesOnTheRise-full.pdf

Park, N., Lee, B., Sun, F., Klemmack, D., Roff, L., & Koenig, H. (2013). Typologies of religiousness/spirituality: Implications for health and well-being. *Journal of Religion and Health, 52*(3), 828–839.

Puchalski, C., Vitillo, R., Hull, S., & Reller, N. (2014). Improving the spiritual dimension of whole person care: Reaching national and international consensus. *Journal of Palliative Medicine, 17*(6), 642–656.

Ramezani, M., Ahmadi, F., Mohammadi, E., & Kazemnejad, A. (2014). Spiritual care in nursing: A concept analysis. *International Nursing Review, 61*(2), 211–219.

Ronaldson, S., Hayes, L., Aggar, C., Green, J., & Carey, M. (2012). Spirituality and spiritual caring: Nurses' perspectives and practice in palliative and acute care environments. *Journal of Clinical Nursing, 21,* 2126–2135. doi: 10.1111/j.1365-2702.2012.04180.x

Rushton, L. (2014). What are the barriers to spiritual care in a hospital setting? *British Journal of Nursing, 23*(7), 370–374.

Stoll, R. I. (1979). Guidelines for spiritual assessment. *American Journal of Nursing, 79,* 1574–1577.

Streifel, C., & Servanty-Seib, H. (2009). Recovering from alcohol and other drug dependency: Loss and spirituality in a 12-step context. *Alcoholism Treatment Quarterly, 27,* 184–198. DOI: 10.1080/07347320902785558

Tanyi, R. A. (2006). Spirituality and family nursing: Spiritual assessment and interventions for families. *Journal of Advanced Nursing, 53*(3), 287–294.

Timmins, F., & Kelly, J. (2008). Spiritual assessment in intensive and cardiac care nursing. *Nursing in Critical Care, 13*(3), 124–131.

Tokpah, M., & Middleton, L. (2013). Psychiatric nurses' understanding of the spiritual dimension of holistic psychiatric nursing practice in South Africa: A phenomenological study. *African Journal of Nursing and Midwifery, 15*(1)81–94.

Unterrainer, H., Lewis, A., & Fink, A. (2014). Religious/spiritual well-being, personality and mental health: A review of results and conceptual issues. *Journal of Religious and Health, 53.* doi: 10.1007/s10943-012-9642-5

Vilalta, A, Valls, J., Porta, J., & Viñas, J. (2014).Evaluation of spiritual needs of patients with advanced cancer in a palliative care unit. *Journal of Palliative Medicine, 17*(5), 592–600.

Weinberger-Litman, S., Muncie, M., Flannelly, L., & Flannelly, K. (2010). When do nurses refer patients to professional chaplains? *Holistic Nursing Practice, 24*(1), 44–48.

Weiner, L., McConnell, D., Latella, L., & Ludi, E. (2013). Cultural and religious considerations in pediatric palliative care. *Palliative and Supportive Care, 11,* 47–67.

White, M. (2013). Spirituality self-care effects on quality of life for patients diagnosed with chronic illness. *Self-Care, Dependent-Care and Nursing, 20*(1), 23.

Yeaworth, R. & Sailors, R. (2014). Faith community nursing: Real cost savings. *Journal of Christian Nursing, 31*(3), 178–183.

Appendix A

Answers with Rationales for Practicing for the NCLEX Questions

Chapter 1

1. **d.** Advanced beginner is identified as being the first 5 years after graduation from nursing school and is described as seeing situations in parts to seeing them more conceptually, or as a whole. Competency occurs 5 to 10 years after graduation, and the nurse is no longer outside the situation observing but is directly involved. The expert nurse has an enormous background of experience, intuitive grasp of each situation, and accurately targets the problem without unnecessary consideration of a large range of alternative diagnoses and solutions. The novice nurse moves from relying on abstract principles to using concrete experiences.

2. **a, b, d.** Collaboration, performance appraisal, and quality of care are all elements of professional performance. Other elements include education, collegiality, ethics, research, and use of resources. Standards of care designate professional nursing responsibilities such as assessment, diagnosis, outcome identification, planning, implementation, and evaluation.

3. **a.** The **nurse practice act** of each state defines the practice of nursing within that area. The board of nursing in each state sets requirements for licensure. Scope of practice is established at the state level in the nurse practice act, not by schools of nursing or Commission for Nursing Education Accreditation. Reciprocity involves meeting licensure requirements in a state other than the state where there is current licensure. As long as the nurse maintains licensure, the licensure exam does not need to be retaken.

4. **a, b.** The nurse should use her knowledge of the sciences to make safe judgments on the patient's behalf. The nurse should also communicate the patient's needs in written and oral form. Administering the drug does not utilize professional judgment and is not appropriate for this patient; the nurse is not advocating for the well-being of the patient. Complaining to peers does not exhibit collegiality with the healthcare team.

5. **a.** Sleep is part of the foundation of Maslow's hierarchy, included in physiologic need. Safety (fall risk), love and belonging (family, friends, social support), and self-esteem (lack of confidence in self-care abilities) are later considerations according to this model.

Chapter 2

1. **a.** Holism acknowledges and respects the interaction of a person's mind, body, and spirit within the environment; thus, it cannot be fully understood if examined solely in pieces apart from their environment. High-level wellness recognizes health as an ongoing process toward a person's highest potential of functioning. To achieve high-level wellness requires first the choice to assume responsibility for the quality of your life; this patient does not display this quality in his current condition. The clinical model interprets health narrowly as the absence of signs and symptoms of disease or injury; therefore, the opposite of health is disease. This patient is reporting physical effects of his current situation, not necessarily a disease process. In the health belief model, a relation exists between a person's beliefs and actions. Factors that influence those beliefs include personal expectations in relation to health and illness, earlier experiences with health and illness, sociocultural context, age, and developmental state.

2. **a, b, c.** Statement A affirms the patient's role in maintaining her own health and validates her ability to take control, addressing her self-concept. Statement B allows the patient to participate in self-care to increase her independence and control, and thus self-worth. Statement C aims to establish self-awareness in the patient to increase participation and a feeling of control over planning for discharge. Statement D relays information for discharge but does not address the patient's engagement, self-worth, or self-concept and thus may not attain the desired level of self-care.

3. **a.** This statement describes demoralization and the precontemplation phase. Contemplation is described by stalling. Preparation involves planning and going public with the desire to change. Termination is complete confidence or "permanent maintenance."

4. **b, c.** The nurse should ask about all complementary and alternative medicine (CAM) therapies and document appropriately in order to determine interactive effects and potential sequelae. Asking only about prescribed medications ignores the reference to CAM supplements and additional therapies that the patient may be using. Referring to CAM supplements and other non-Western treatments as "non–evidence based" confers judgment and bias, contributing to poor reporting of CAM therapies by patients and increasing the risk of interactions with medical treatments.

5. **a, b, c, d.** All of these actions would enhance knowledge and understanding of CAM practices, including current research related to the CAM modality.

Chapter 3

1. **b, c.** Economic and political determinants of health underlie these health outcomes. Educational factors are not discussed in this scenario. Healthcare services only account for 10% to 20% of the overall health status of individuals and communities.

2. **b. Community-based nursing care** can be defined as nursing care directed toward a specific group or population within the community and may be provided for individuals and groups as described previously. The level of care can be primary, secondary, or tertiary. **Community-based healthcare** is the design, delivery, and evaluation of healthcare services developed in partnership with communities. Primary care combines health promotion and prevention of disease. **Secondary prevention** is done with the purpose of identifying and detecting disease in its earliest stages, commonly through screening.

3. **c.** Fragmentation of service often results as patients move from one system of care to the next (or when a government agency or program is not able to address communities' needs because the issues are so complex). Fragmentation may proliferate as different specialists prescribe different medications and require follow-up visits. Such lack of care coordination can confuse and upset the patient and family as well as compound the patient's health problems. Other terms are not discussed in this chapter as healthcare phenomena.

4. **a, b, d.** Statement A illustrates collaboration, statement B exemplifies facilitation, and statement D describes negotiation. Collaboration, facilitation, and negotiation are elements of nursing discharge planning elements. Providing paperwork at the time of discharge does not display planning or attention to patient needs.

5. **a, b, c, d.** All of these statements should be noted. Statements A and B are barriers to independence. Statement C displays an adequate environment for wheelchair access and safe mobility on the stairs. Statement D provides additional information on the person's values and avocations, possibly providing an opportunity for self-actualizing activity in the face of recent health challenges.

Chapter 4

1. **a.** The tool "Asking Why 5 Times" is used in root cause analysis. Just culture refers to a process of error review that focuses on system issues as well as individual responsibility. CMS outcomes include mortality and infection rates and come from tracking patient data. Bundles of care are grouped interventions that improve outcomes.

2. **c.** CMS adjusts hospital reimbursement based on adherence to guidelines for processes and outcomes of care and patient satisfaction. Although ensuring "never events" never occur is a goal of healthcare, it is not the basis for value-based purchasing (VBP). Conducting root cause analysis of errors and determining cost of care are not related to VBP.

3. **d.** Nurses are uniquely prepared to help keep patients safe, and their presence at the bedside 24 hours every day puts them in a position to monitor for and intervene as needed for safety. Nurses work collaboratively with physicians to achieve patient safety. Safe care is not necessarily of the highest quality. Although patient satisfaction with care is important, it does not mean care is necessarily safe.

4. **b.** The nationally recognized bundle of care is the most important to include. Although information from another hospital might be helpful, if it doesn't include the bundle, it is not sufficient. Websites directed toward the public likely don't have enough information for a policy. Typically, references for professional work should be dated within the last 5 years.

5. **d.** Latent errors are those due to systems issues; active errors are those attributable to an individual. The effects of latent errors may be apparent immediately and may certainly cause significant harm to patients.

Chapter 5

1. **a, b, c, d.** Culture is learned from other people (not innate), changes at variable rates, uses one's own culture as the correct standard, and is related to the socioecologic context in which it is embedded. Culture is not necessarily logical or reasonable to the outside observer and varies on the level of the individual (not a prescribed set of traits).

2. **a, b, d.** Accurate nursing assessments require that the nurse minimize ethnocentric tendencies and maximize cultural sensitivity. Patient assessments that consider the patient's perspective are most likely to yield diagnoses and interventions appropriate to the patient. Trained interpreters are important because interpretation of behavior goes beyond translation of words, thus family members should not be used. Assigning behaviors to a specific category is the definition of a stereotype, and such preconceived descriptors may lead to incorrect assessments and inappropriate and potentially harmful or unethical interventions.

3. **c.** Rituals are common, observable expressions of culture, particularly used in times of stress and uncertainty. Ethnicity refers to self-conscious, past-oriented form of identity, and meaning depends on who is using it. Skin color and other biologic markers are not necessarily associated with belief

systems and may be a detrimental assumption if associated with negative beliefs or actions, as in racism. Language is not indicative of cultural beliefs, and meaning can be modified depending on cultural background or understanding. Verbal language also only accounts for one third of social interaction and may not accurately depict cultural beliefs.

4. **c.** Trained interpreters assist in behavioral and language translation; interpreters should be provided when requested and at any time when plans for care are being established. Attempting to act in the patient's best interest may result in incongruence between the nurse's interpretation of the patient's best interest and the patient's actual beliefs. The use of a bilingual family member may limit behavioral interpretation needed for healthcare assessment and interventions. Key informants may be valuable in providing cultural insight; however, in the hospital or clinic setting, the most useful key informants are bicultural trained interpreters.

5. **a, b, c, d.** Subcultural identity adheres to a holistic belief system that differs from that of the larger population or maintains beliefs and standards that are unique to a particular social capacity, such as an occupational group. Like ethnic identity, subcultural identity can be a source of social support. The subculture of poverty has been disproven by demonstrating that broad societal mechanisms maintain people in poverty rather than a cultural practice.

Chapter 6

1. **a, b, c, d.** Giving advice, changing the subject, being moralistic, and giving false reassurance are all components of nontherapeutic communication. Open-ended questions are a therapeutic technique.

2. **d.** Active, achieving adults may find it difficult to suddenly need assistance from nurses and may struggle with role transition during hospitalization. Empathy relates to the ability to perceive, reason, and communicate understanding of the other person's feelings. A comfortable sense of self refers to the nurse's ability to be self-aware of biases, communication styles, and values; not relevant in the patient's behavior. Intimacy versus isolation is part of Erikson theory of self-concept; though appropriate for the age, it does not address this specific behavior.

3. **c.** Limit setting is a key factor in working effectively with children and adolescents. Although considered a therapeutic technique, silence may not be appropriate with this patient. False reassurance should be avoided with all patients, particularly pediatric patients and those who are developing trust. An informal contract would not be appropriate based only on the patient experiencing a developmental delay.

4. **c.** Assisting the patient's sister in compiling a list of questions should be done first to clarify patient and family needs and does not interfere with the physician–patient relationship. While discussing the case and advocating for the family with the physician and social work are important steps, these would not be the first action. Admitting problems with the healthcare system can undermine confidence in the system and is not the best option in patient advocacy.

5. **b.** Voicing concerns about discussions of patient information in nonprivate areas states the nurse's ethical concerns and violation of the Patients' Bill of Rights. Alternative options do not address violation of the Patient's Bill of Rights directly to the providers.

Chapter 7

1. **a, b, c, d.** All questions posed should be considered in evaluating values in relation to the professional nursing role.

2. **c.** Socialization during mealtime is the value that is described by the patient's statement and subsequent withdrawal related to not being able to eat. Independence and individuality are not reflected by the statement or setting. The patient's role within the family may be affected but is not the best answer for this setting. Human nature describes the way in which people interpret the world around them; it is not relevant in this scenario.

3. **a, b, c, d.** All of the statements should be considered in resolving value conflicts and establishing a therapeutic relationship between the nurse and patient.

4. **d.** Justice would be in question because the patient is not willing to receive medical therapies to support the transplanted liver after another patient died waiting to receive the same organ. Beneficence would be in question because this describes whether it is in the best interest of the patient; a transplant would be the only course of treatment for severe overdose of Tylenol and would be in the patient's best interest. Nonmaleficence is the principle to not do harm. Autonomy is the patient's ability to consent and participate in his or her own care. This patient was not able to consent related to her physical and mental health state at the time of admission.

5. **b.** Breach of duty is the failure to conform to the standard of practice, thus creating a risk for a person that a reasonable person would have foreseen. The nurse may be accused of breach of duty whenever reasonably accepted standards of nursing care are not met, such as failure to observe and monitor a patient's condition. Fraud is purposeful misrepresentation of self or an act that may cause harm to a person or property, such as qualifications. Negligence by commission is doing something that a reasonably prudent person would not do; this example is negligence by omission. A nurse may be sued for battery if he or she fails to obtain consent for a procedure or allows the patient to refuse a therapy.

Chapter 8

1. **a, b, c, e.** Evidence-based practice (EBP) is based on outcome studies, recognizes that pathophysiologic reasoning and personal experience are not sufficient, and involves the incorporation of individual clinical expertise with the best available external evidence from systematic research. The goal of EBP is to provide the highest quality individualized care based on thorough assessment, history taking, sound research evidence, clinical proficiency, and information from the patient on values and care preferences to ensure favorable outcomes. EBP standardizes practice and methods

based on research, thus discouraging facilities to follow a single practitioner's recommendations.

2. **b, c, d.** Institutional review boards evaluate these elements as well as the ability to withdraw from the investigation at any time, self-determination, anonymity, confidentiality, and fair treatment. Study subjects must be informed of the risks and benefits of a study and voluntarily consent.

3. **d.** Nursing research includes clinical practice problems, modes of patient care, nursing education, and administration.

4. **d.** Translation of research forms the foundation for evidence-based protocols and interventions that increase the quality of nursing care and improve patient outcomes. Qualitative and quantitative data collection are methods used in nursing research. Disseminating research results can be done in various ways but does not necessarily include evaluating effects on patient outcomes. Classifying nursing phenomena is a priority for nursing research but is not described by bundle implementation.

5. **c.** Review of existing literature is the first step of conducting research, followed by developing a theoretical framework, formulating a problem statement or hypothesis, proceeding with the study, and disseminating findings.

Chapter 9

1. **c.** Psychomotor learning refers to the muscular movements learned to perform new skills and procedures. This type of knowledge is easiest to measure because it can be physically demonstrated. Cognitive learning refers to rational thought and may involve learning facts, reaching conclusions, solving problems, making decisions, or using critical thinking skills. Affective learning changes beliefs, attitudes, or values. Sensitivity and emotional climate influence all types of learning but are especially important in the affective domain.

2. **a, b, c, d.** All patient education practices are evident in this scenario. Patient education should aim to include these as well as holistic consideration of the whole person rather than focusing on just specific content.

3. **d.** The patient's emotional state is the most important element in this scenario; the patient may be too anxious or depressed to learn or unable to concentrate since she has just received a new diagnosis. Physical weakness, pain, discomfort, and fatigue can affect attention span and decrease learning and would be an additional concern, although not the priority. Educational goals for children, adolescents, and adults differ, and patients require different teaching styles at different ages. Cognitive status should also be considered because patients with dementia, short-term memory deficits, or altered mental status may be unable to retain information or learn new skills. It may be necessary to identify another person (caregiver/family member) to teach. This is not an element included in the scenario and thus is not a priority.

4. **c.** This statement best encompasses the numerous issues that the patient is dealing with and acknowledges that these

may impact her ability to adhere to a complex healthcare regimen. Statement A shows judgment on the part of the nurse and does not take into consideration the numerous factors that are affecting the patient's health and well-being. Statement B relates to the nurse's feelings, rather than the patient, which is not therapeutic. Statement D shows analysis that is starting to look at factors related to the patient's behavior but only describes culture as a factor and continues to refer to the behavior as noncompliance, which infers judgment.

5. **b.** Ineffective Therapeutic Regimen Management is the most appropriate nursing diagnosis. It is described as the failure to incorporate treatment regimens into daily routines; failure to take action to reduce risk factors; or makes choices in daily living ineffective for meeting health goals. Ineffective Health Maintenance, in contrast, describes a lack of adaptive behaviors to environmental changes, lack of knowledge of health practices, lack of interest, inability to take responsibility for meeting basic health practices, or impaired personal support systems. Health-seeking Behavior would be indicated if the patient were looking to maximize current health status and prevent disease. Deficient Knowledge is not appropriate because the patient can state why diet modification is important, illustrating understanding.

Chapter 10

1. **b, d.** Approximately 52% of household incomes for adults 65 years or older are under $35,000. Most older women live alone because their life expectancy is higher than for men. The number of older adults is increasing. Most older adults are married or widowed.

2. **d.** Validation therapy is a type of interpersonal interaction in which the health professional attempts to understand and validate the patient's current needs. Reality orientation is appropriate with reversible confusional states such as delirium but often causes agitation or anger in patients with latter stages of irreversible confusion. Sensory stimulation should be minimized to decrease confusion. Assistance with self-care does not facilitate cognition.

3. **d.** Benzodiazepines increase the risk for falls in elderly patients. History of falls, impaired mobility, and environmental hazards are risk factors for all patients, not unique to the elderly population.

4. **a, b, c, d.** All interventions listed would be appropriate for someone with a high risk for skin breakdown.

5. a. Ineffective coping would be most related to failure to thrive. Loneliness, impaired sleep pattern, and impaired self-perception may all affect health but are not as directly related to failure to thrive.

Chapter 11

1. **a, d.** Primary sources of information are attained from the patient themselves (i.e., physical assessment and patient report of symptoms). Secondary sources include family members and the health record.

2. **b.** Assessment should be the first step in the nursing process. Calling the physician, an intervention, is necessary, but only after performing an assessment. Administering medications would also be an intervention, as would moving the patient back to bed.

3. **d.** Evaluation commonly refers to rating, grading, and judging. In the evaluation phase, nurses discover why the patient plan of care was a success or failure. Assessment involves confirming a proposed nursing diagnosis with the patient using objective and subjective data. Planning phase involves identifying goals and intervention strategies that will reduce identified problems. The planning phase involves preparing an **initial** patient plan of care, which directs the activities of the nursing staff in the provision of patient care. Implementation is the actual initiation of the plan, evaluation of response to the plan, and recording of nursing actions and patient response to these actions.

4. **b.** Critical thinking is needed in situations that bring nursing judgment into play; those situations that are not addressed clearly by physician orders or by a changing patient condition. The nursing process is the broad description of the theoretical structure of preparation and action of patient care. The nurse practice act details the practice ethics for a registered nurse (RN). Medical simulation is a method of developing critical thinking skills via creating acute or changing patient scenarios in the safe practice environment of a learning laboratory.

5. **b.** Patient 2 should be seen first for the new-onset hematuria. Although Patient 1 is admitted for respiratory distress, there is no current oxygenation need or change in condition. Patient 3 may have immediate needs related to nicotine withdrawal but is not the most acute patient. Patient 4 should be seen shortly because he is a fall risk and has had a change in mental status but is not the most acute patient of the four.

Chapter 12

1. **b.** Statement B targets an existing problem that has already been identified and attempts to determine changes in the status of the problem. Statements A, C, and D do not address the current problem and are beyond the scope of the focus assessment.

2. **c.** "Identifying activities that exacerbate symptoms" is an example of data collection or assessment. Defining patient goals is an example of outcome identification. Evaluation of current home regimen is an evaluation rather than an assessment. Applying oxygen is an example of Implementation.

3. **c.** Subjective data contain symptoms that are supplied by the patient or family and are obtained via interview. Laboratory studies, direct observation, and descriptions in the health record of signs are examples of objective data.

4. **a, b, c.** These three statements assess the functional health patterns of Nutrition–Metabolism, Coping–Stress Tolerance, and Sleep–Rest. Statement D focuses on past symptoms in relation to the current admission adhering to a medical model or review of body systems. Vital signs are objective data collected in adherence to a head-to-toe model to first gauge the current state of health.

5. **b, d.** Introduction of self, including position, and observing behavior and self-perceptions are both elements of the introductory phase. The introductory phase is the second phase following the preparatory phase. Focus on goals and goal attainment are included in the maintenance phase.

Chapter 13

1. **b, d, e.** Nursing diagnoses describe human responses and include descriptors and risk factors for health problems. Nursing diagnoses also identify relationships between health problems and contributing factors. A medical diagnosis describes a disease or pathology. Collaborative health problems include actual and potential complications addressed by both the medical and nursing teams. Nursing diagnoses may have legal implications based on licensure-defined scope of practice and appropriate treatment for the patient independent from those prescribed by physicians.

2. **b.** The nursing diagnosis correctly incorporates the three parts of diagnostic label, related factors, and defining characteristics. Statement A lacks sufficient evidence (daily bowel movements) to identify constipation as a current problem. Statement C lacks related factors. Statement D lacks defining characteristics and does not give sufficient evidence for ineffective coping as a current problem.

3. **a.** Data synthesis or cue clustering should be done first after attaining subjective and objective data. Comparing data with norms or cluster interpretation should follow cue clustering. Assigning a nursing diagnosis should be done next. Validation of a diagnosis is done using research and/or experience with similar patient problems. This would be done after assigning a diagnosis and prior to formulating the complete diagnostic statement.

4. **b.** This statement correctly establishes a nursing diagnosis appropriate to the patient problem, relates to contributing factors, and describes evidence that is congruent. Statement A is incorrect because it assumes the patient is incontinent, which can, but does not necessarily, occur with confusion and UTI. Statement C does not provide evidence that is sufficient, particularly for a patient experiencing acute mental status changes. Statement D incorrectly defines contributing factors because the acute mental status changes are a result of the urinary tract infection, not vice versa.

5. **c.** This nursing diagnosis includes the appropriate term "risk" and identifies a risk factor for Ineffective Breast-Feeding. Statement A lacks the correct diagnostic label as accepted by NANDA-I. Statement B reverses the diagnostic label, and cues in the "related to" statement lack validation. Statement D reverses the diagnostic label and uses "potential" instead of the accepted term "risk for."

Chapter 14

1. **a, c.** Outcome identification individualizes care to the patient and plans care that is realistic and measurable. The nursing process identifies potential health problems, but this is not a characteristic unique to outcome identification. Outcome identification allows for support people to be involved rather than prevents it.

2. **d.** Wound care should be the priority based on the life-threatening situation of a hemorrhage. Pain may be the patient's first priority but would be less important than extensive bleeding. Diminished lung sounds and hypoactive bowel sounds, although abnormal, are not unusual in a recent postoperative patient and could be addressed once the patient is stable.

3. **a, b, c.** Statements A through C appropriately identify outcomes for the described patient scenario. Statement D includes criteria for outcome.

4. **d.** Statement includes all elements of specific, measurable, realistic outcome criteria. Statement A lacks circumstances and criteria. Statement B lacks subject and criteria. Statement C lacks specific time.

5. **a, b, d.** Plans of care should include nursing diagnosis, patient goal, patient outcome criteria, nursing interventions, scientific rationale, and evaluation. A critical or clinical pathway may be included depending on the diagnosis and the organization. The nursing diagnosis, patient outcome criteria, and pathway are correct. "Encourage ambulation frequently" is not a correct nursing intervention because it lacks a time frame and how the action will be carried out. "No shortness of breath with incentive spirometry therapy" is not a correct patient goal because it does not include behavioral verbs.

Chapter 15

1. **a, b, d.** Patient condition; new information from reassessment; time and resource availability for nursing interventions; feedback from the patient, family, and healthcare staff; and the nurse's experience are all elements of priority setting. Modification of the plan of care may occur after setting priorities if these differ from those outlined previously in the plan of care.

2. **d.** Example of interpersonal intervention. Providing hygiene assistance is a technical intervention. Providing education and supervision are cognitive interventions.

3. **b.** Process evaluation focuses on nurse performance and whether the nursing care provided was appropriate and competent. Structure evaluation focuses on the attributes of the setting where healthcare is provided. Outcome evaluation focuses on the patient and patient's function and can only take place once standards have been developed. Functional evaluation is not a type of evaluation.

4. **d.** The plan of care must be modified because it is not a priority for the patient to feed herself when she is unable to tolerate oral intake. The goal would be completely met if the patient could state the appropriate parameters and measure and monitor her intake.

5. **a, d.** Peer review is evaluation and judgment of a nurse's performance by other nurses. The Joint Commission performs external review and establishes standards to ensure that nurses and institutions function within specified criteria. The Joint Commission also requires continuous monitoring by departments of nursing. Management audit is not a standard evaluation mechanism in nursing. The American Nurses Association develops standards of behaviors for evaluating nursing care and performance but does not directly perform evaluation of nurses.

Chapter 16

1. **d.** Documentation of the nursing process within this record provides essential data related to assessment, interventions, and goals. Clear, accurate, and up-to-date patient documentation is a cornerstone for safe care delivery providing flow of information between providers of care. If a patient record or portions of it are unavailable or inaccurate, a vital line of communication is blocked. Medicare and Medicaid stopped reimbursement in 2008 for some hospital-acquired complications, including pressure ulcers. The admission assessment is not an issue of lack of documentation.

2. **a, b, c, d.** All characteristics mentioned in statements A through D improve nursing documentation, patient safety, and tracking of patient care.

3. **c.** Disclosure of protected health information is at issue when patient cases are discussed in public. Patient education on privacy protection, patient recourse if privacy protections are violated, and limiting use of information to accomplish the intended purpose are also aspects of HIPAA but are not discussed in this scenario.

4. **d.** A recommendation is missing from this SBAR, answering the question of "What should we do to correct the problem?" Situation, Background, and Assessment are all included in the scenario.

5. **d.** Double-check of all high-risk infusions should be performed by both the off-going and oncoming nurses. Acute changes or interventions (e.g., neurologic status) may be indicated by patient status but are not relevant for this patient scenario. A complete list of medications is not needed since this is available as part of the patient's medical record. Similarly, a complete past medical history is not needed and is available in the patient's chart.

Chapter 17

1. **a, c.** A focused health assessment should be limited to the patient's problems: pain and circulation to affected leg. Psychological, spiritual, and social elements are included in a comprehensive health assessment.

2. **a, b, c, d.** Reason for seeking healthcare, past surgical history, perception of health status, and significant spiritual practices are all part of the health history interview. Auscultation of lung sounds is attaining objective data as part of the physical examination.

3. **d.** The four basic techniques of physical examination are inspection, palpation, percussion, and auscultation.

Interview is a technique of acquiring subjective information. Resonance is the degree to which sound propagates on percussion. Objective data are acquired through the entire physical examination; interview, subjective data, and closure are not techniques of physical examination.

4. **b, c, e.** The assessment identifies receptive aphasia, orientation only to self (×1), and impairment of cranial nerve VII. Expressive aphasia would affect patient ability to communicate effectively, but the patient would be able to understand and follow directions. Accommodation relates to pupillary reflex to adjust to close and distant objects.

5. **a, b, d.** Clubbing of the nail bed indicates chronic hypoxia, crackles in the lungs indicates air passing through fluid, and pitting in dependent extremities such as the ankles indicates fluid accumulation in the tissues. Vesicular breath sounds are a normal respiratory finding heard over all areas of the lung except major airways.

6. **b.** Tactile fremitus or bronchophony is determined by having the patient say "99." In egophony, the patient states "ee" and the sound translates as "ay" if consolidation or atelectasis is present. Excursion measures chest expansion during respiration. A pleural friction rub is an adventitious lung sound created by two pleural surfaces rubbing together, such as in pleuritis.

7. **a.** Striae are streaks caused by rapid or prolonged stretching of the skin; ascites, pregnancy, and weight gain or loss are common causes. Scaphoid (boat-shaped or hollowed) abdominal shape is not seen with ascites, which creates a protuberant or distended and firm abdomen. Visible peristalsis is seen in thin patients only, not those with protuberant abdomens. Borborygmi or bowel sounds are a normal finding not related to ascites.

8. **a, b, c, d.** Decreased sensation related to epidural pain medication or disease process places the patient at risk for pressure-related skin breakdown and injury related to falling. Sensation and pain relief should be determined based on relief by dermatomes around and distal to the epidural placement. Documentation should be completed following assessment of lower extremity sensation including the inability to sense stimuli and the affected location of the body.

9. **a, c, d.** Teenagers should be examined unaccompanied by a parent regardless of the type of assessment. Assessment of the genitalia at any age should focus on health promotion and self-examination. Examination should be done by both the patient and nurse in order to solidify self-examination techniques. Utilizing simple games for distraction is a technique used with school-age children and is not appropriate for adolescent patients.

10. **b.** Summarizing findings and concerns with the patient validates your impressions and clarifies any misunderstandings. It also involves the patient in their own plan of care. Acquiring secondary data to verify health problems should be done prior to conducting the health assessment. Discussing the patient's history with other providers is appropriate if information is pertinent to the patient's case

at this time but should be done either prior to or following the assessment, not during. Interventions may be applied once the assessment and planning phases are complete.

Chapter 18

1. **a, d.** Elderly adults may have temperatures less than 36.4°C (97.6°F) because baseline body temperature may drop as an individual ages. Temperature is also lowest in the early morning. Stress of hospitalization would increase body temperature. Menopausal state would explain intermittently increased temperature, and postmenopausal state only indicates that mean temperature norms would be the same for men and women; this does not explain a lowered temperature.

2. **c.** The temporal artery or forehead is the most appropriate site for infants because it is easy and well tolerated. Temperatures measured in the ear are at risk for poor measurement technique resulting in errors in measurement and have been found to have a high degree of variance when compared with oral temperatures. Rectal temperatures are highly invasive and may be falsely high if fecal material is present. Oral temperature assessment is not prudent or safe for infants, young children, unconscious or delirious patients, or patients with seizure disorders.

3. **b.** The apical pulse provides the most accurate assessment of the pulse rate and is the preferred site when the peripheral pulses are difficult to assess or the pulse rhythm is irregular. Correct technique includes placing the diaphragm of the stethoscope at the fifth (not third) intercostal space at the midclavicular line and counting for a full 60 seconds. The first pulsation should be counted as "zero," and S_1 and S_2 should be counted as one beat.

4. **b.** Opioid medications used to alleviate pain in surgery and postoperatively may be related to a decreased respiratory rate. This should be noted as a safety risk for the patient and closely monitored. Male gender may be related to a decreased respiratory rate but is not most indicated in this scenario with a respiratory rate of 10 breaths per minute. Stress and pain would both increase, rather than decrease, the respiratory rate of the patient.

5. **d. Wheezing** is a high-pitched musical sound usually heard on expiration but may be heard on inspiration. It is associated with partial obstruction of the bronchi or bronchioles, as in asthma. **Stridor** is a harsh inspiratory sound that may be compared to crowing. It may indicate an upper airway obstruction. It is commonly heard in children with croup or after aspiration of a foreign object. **Unlabored breathing** reflects a normal breathing pattern, but this child shows "marked trouble breathing." **Exertional dyspnea** describes respirations that require excessive effort during activity.

6. **b.** In order to measure blood pressure on this patient, the lower extremities must be used. Use of the upper arms may obstruct the arteriovenous fistula (used for hemodialysis) or impede circulation, leading to lymphedema on the side with the mastectomy. Thigh measurement is preferable, using an appropriate size of cuff and placing the patient in a supine position. When an appropriately sized cuff is used, blood pressure measurements should vary only

slightly from readings measured in the upper extremity (unless the patient has peripheral vascular disease). Using a cuff that is too small will result in falsely high readings. The left ankle is more appropriate to calculate an ankle brachial index (ABI) to determine if it is safe to use compression therapy for venous ulcers. Lower arm blood pressures should use auscultation of the radial artery but would not be appropriate in this patient.

7. **a, b, c.** The first three statements are accurate patient education regarding safety and orthostatic hypotension. Statement D does not promote patient safety or address the cause of orthostatic hypotension, which is most likely fluid volume deficit in a postoperative patient.

8. **d.** The nurse should support the arm level with the fourth intercostal space. If the patient's arm rests on the arm of the chair, or below heart level, the result will be a falsely high reading. Failure to support the arm causes the patient to contract the arm muscles, elevating the blood pressure. Blood pressure may be taken in any position, but attention should be to maintain the position of the arm at the level of the heart.

9. **a.** First position the patient, then place fingertips in the groove at the base of the thumb, and count for 30 seconds and multiply by two, if the pulse is regular. Use the Doppler if the pulse is not easily palpable by first applying gel to the probe or radial site.

10. **c.** The best nursing action is to wait to assess respirations until the child is not crying. Noting the pattern and rate when crying does not indicate normal function, although thorough documentation is beneficial to provide context. Calling the physician with the current respiratory pattern and rate is not advised because this does not reflect the normal condition or current trend. Measuring the respiratory rate before the temperature is advised before the child is upset. In this scenario, the child is already upset, so this advice would not be pertinent.

Chapter 19

1. **a.** Sepsis is an infection that manifests with systemic or widespread microbial destruction of tissues, often accompanied by high fever or hypotension. Infectious disease refers to pathologic events that result from the invasion and multiplication of microorganisms in a host. Opportunistic infections do not occur in individuals with properly functioning immune systems; there is not enough evidence to support this choice. Nosocomial infections are those that occur in the setting of the hospital; there is not enough evidence to support this choice.

2. **d.** Droplet transmission occurs when mucous membranes of the nose, mouth, or conjunctiva are exposed to secretions of an infected person who is coughing, sneezing, or talking. Contact transmission describes body surface to body surface contact causing the physical transfer of organisms between the infected or colonized person and a susceptible host. Vehicle transmission involves transfer of microorganisms via contaminated items such as food,

water, drugs, or blood. Airborne transmission occurs when fine particles are suspended in the air for a long time or when dust particles contain pathogens.

3. **c.** Gowns should be worn for all types of transmission-based precautions; gloves and a mask with eye shield (or goggles) are needed when contamination from respiratory secretions is possible. A respirator is used only with diagnosed or suspected airborne diseases such as tuberculosis.

4. **a, b, c, d.** All infections listed are common healthcare-associated infections and are cited by the Institute for Healthcare Improvement as preventable using specified interventions.

5. **a, b, c.** Hand hygiene should be performed at the beginning and end of the shift; before and between contact with patients; before and after contact with dressings, wounds, specimens, or bedclothes; before performing any invasive procedure; before administering medication; after contact with patient secretion or excretion; before and after using the bathroom; after sneezing, coughing, or blowing your nose; after removing gloves; and before eating. Alcohol-based gel should not be used with *Clostridium difficile* and Norovirus, when hands are visibly soiled, or when the patient has diarrhea.

6. **c.** Answer c is the definition of standard precautions, broader than universal precautions and medical asepsis. Universal precautions are only part of this; decreasing the risk of transmission of bloodborne pathogens. Medical asepsis or "clean technique" are measures taken to control and reduce the number of pathogens present. Measures include hand hygiene, gloving, gowning, and disinfecting. Protective isolation is used to prevent infection for people whose body defenses are known to be compromised, such as neutropenic patients as a result of chemotherapy or other immunosuppression.

7. **b.** Personal protective equipment should be removed with the most contaminated items (gloves) removed first. Hands should be washed, then remove goggles or a face shield using only the headband or ear pieces. The gown should be removed next, grasping from the inside and rolling into a ball. Then, mask should be removed and hands washed again.

8. **d.** Inspecting the sterile kit for package integrity is the most important step because it ensures that a sterile field can be established. All other techniques are correct but occur later in the process to maintain sterility.

9. **c.** Slipping the gloved hand inside the second gloved cuff assists the dominant hand in applying the glove while maintaining sterility. Inserting the dominant hand and extending the cuff would follow. Unfolding the cuff of the nondominant hand's glove and adjusting fit, keeping the hands above the waist, would be next.

10. **a.** The chain of infection details the passage of infections pathogens from the source, portal of exit, mode of transmission, and portal of entry to susceptible host. Hepatitis A is transmitted via fecal–oral contact, usually with contaminated food from infected human to stool, via contact or vehicle transmission with food to the gastrointestinal tract of a susceptible host.

Chapter 20

1. **c.** A fundamental rule of safe medication administration is, "Never administer an unfamiliar medication." Thus, the medication should be looked up either in a drug handbook or using a computer database to evaluate dosing, expected therapeutic effects, possible adverse actions and interactions with other medications, and whether the drug is appropriate for this patient. It is not sufficient to delay or refuse treatment based on lack of understanding of the medication. It is within the nurse's scope of practice to determine whether the medication is appropriate to administer at this time if it adheres to the physician's orders.

2. **d.** Assessment should always be done first before applying nursing interventions, including administering medications. Once it is determined that the order is appropriate for this level of pain, the nurse could administer the dose, document the administration, and then assess the effects of the medication (approximately 30 minutes after for PO [oral] medications).

3. **c.** The most appropriate action would be to call the physician and discuss the nurse's concerns that this medication is not appropriate for the patient's condition. If the nurse is dissatisfied with the provider's response and still believes that the order is inappropriate, he or she may notify the supervisor and decline to administer the medication. It is not suitable to administer the medication and then follow up with the physician or monitor the patient because the nurse is ultimately responsible for the patient's safety in relation to the medications administered.

4. **c.** All patients have the right to refuse medications and other therapies. The nurse has the duty to explain the purpose of the medication. If a patient then refuses the medication, attempt to clarify the patient's concern about the medication and notify the provider of the patient's refusal along with his or her concerns. Crushing the medication and slipping it into applesauce or food is unethical in relation to the patient's right to refuse. Charting the medication as not given does not give the patient the opportunity to take the prescribed medications and does not address the patient's concerns. Asking the patient why she has been refusing should be done after discussing the purpose of the medication.

5. **b.** Constipation is a common side effect of morphine administration. Minor adverse effects are called side effects and are usually harmless but can be uncomfortable if untreated. Tolerance refers to a decreased response to a medication, thus requiring a larger dosage. Allergic reactions result from an immunologic response to a medication and may range from hives and itching to anaphylactic reaction, requiring immediate medical intervention.

6. **a, b, c, d.** Patient identity was not confirmed using two identifiers (name, birth date, medical record number). The medication was not checked against the order or labeled when it was brought into the patient's room.

Documentation may be done, but there is no assurance that the medication was actually taken because it was left on the dinner tray. It can be assumed that the pill was appropriate for oral administration for the patient since she had a dinner tray, but this also should be checked against the order.

7. **a, b, c.** An incident report should be filed because this error occurred as a result of an improperly functioning system (i.e., the medication dispensing device released the wrong type of intravenous [IV] fluid bag). All errors should be reported to prevent future errors from occurring. Medication errors also require the physician to be notified and are best discussed with the patient, even if no harm has occurred. To not tell anyone is inappropriate because the system defects will not be corrected and the same error is likely to occur again.

8. **a, c, d.** Prior to administration of oral potassium, the nurse should check the medication administration record, ability to swallow and current diet order, and most recent potassium level. Venous access is not necessary for PO medication administration, although is a valuable assessment piece when administering IV medications.

9. **a, d.** For a subcutaneous injection, the needle should be ½ to $\frac{5}{8}$ inches and 26 to 30 gauge with a 0.5-mL syringe for this medication. A longer needle with a larger gauge should be used for intramuscular injections (1 to 3 inches long and 19 to 23 gauge).

10. **c.** A 2-year-old should receive a flu vaccine as an intramuscular injection in the vastus lateralis because of the volume. The deltoid may be used for this age, but only with volumes up to 0.5 mL. Z-track method may be used but is not essential since the medication is not especially irritating to the subcutaneous tissue. A short needle, not more than 1 inch, is recommended for the vastus lateralis site in children.

Chapter 21

1. **a, b, c, d.** All statements are advantages to having a dedicated IV team.

2. **c.** Isotonic fluids are used to expand the intravascular compartment and thus increase circulating volume. Because these solutions do not alter serum osmolarity, interstitial and intracellular compartments remain unchanged and would be most appropriate for the patient with hypovolemia. **Hypotonic** solutions lower serum osmolarity, causing body fluids to shift out of the blood vessels and into the cells and interstitial space. Thus, hypotonic fluids are administered when a patient needs cellular hydration. **Hypertonic** solutions are considered high risk and usually only are administered in critical care units. They would significantly pull fluid from the cells and the interstitial tissues into the vascular space, increasing serum osmolarity. **Total parenteral nutrition** (TPN) is a hypertonic solution containing 20% to 50% dextrose, proteins, vitamins, and minerals that is administered into the venous system.

TPN is indicated when there is interference with nutrient absorption from the gastrointestinal tract or when complete bowel rest is necessary for healing.

3. **c.** When connecting an intermittent IV line, the nurse should first wipe the needleless connector for 15 seconds with mechanical friction prior to establishing access. Flushing with 3 mL of normal saline (NaCl) using pulsing, positive pressure is then done to check line patency. Flushing with diluted heparin is not indicated with a peripheral line.

4. **d.** Peripherally inserted central catheter (PICC) lines are placed peripherally but deliver medications and solutions centrally and are used for patients who require intermediate- to long-term venous access. Peripheral lines are for short-term therapy only and should not be used for blood draws because they may damage the small vessels into which they are inserted. Midline catheters are more durable than standard peripheral catheters but may not be suited for TPN, hyperosmolar infusions, or vesicant therapy. They should also not be routinely used for blood drawing. Dialysis access is a specialty access that should only be utilized by specialized nurses and not for routine blood draws.

5. **c, d.** Chemotherapy and other vesicants should be administered via a central line; both Hickman (tunneled) catheters and PICC lines are examples of this type of line. Peripherals and midlines are inserted into vessels that are too small to prevent damage to the vessel when vesicant drugs are infused.

6. **d.** Catheter breakage and retained fragment of the catheter can result in embolism to the heart or pulmonary artery. Infiltration is leakage of fluid into the subcutaneous tissue due to a catheter slipping outside of the vein. Vesicants are caustic drugs that damage tissue when leakage occurs outside of the vein. Air embolism occurs when air enters the circulatory system. A complication that is more common when centrally placed catheters are used is air entry due to the change in intrathoracic pressure during respiration.

7. **a, c, d.** An IV house is recommended to protect the site from bumping and tugging. An electronic infusion device (EID) or IV pump should be used because continuous infusions in this population could be lethal if infused too quickly. Due to the difficulty of finding veins of adequate size, the metacarpal or great saphenous veins may be used along with the cephalic or dorsalis pedis. Tourniquets are not always indicated in older adults because dependent positioning of the arm may be sufficient to fill the veins.

8. **b.** Cyclic infusion of TPN is done to promote independence of activities of daily living (ADLs) during the daytime. TPN does not need to be given only in 12-hour shifts and may be done continuously at the beginning of therapy. Metabolism is not improved with sleeping or decreased patient activity. Fluid overload is not related to intake of oral fluids and concurrent TPN therapy but rather to too rapid infusion of TPN, particularly in patients with congestive heart failure or renal insufficiency.

9. **d.** The first step after detecting a possible blood transfusion reaction is to stop the infusion since reactions are dose related with the amount of blood received. Notifying the physician of a possible blood reaction would be appropriate after the infusion is stopped and the patient has been fully assessed. Providing patient education about future reaction prevention is important, but only after the immediate reaction has been addressed and the patient is stabilized. Placing a nonrebreather mask on the patient with supplemental oxygen may be needed in some transfusion reactions but is not indicated with only an itchy rash.

10. **c.** RhoGAM is the commercial name for antibodies directed against the Rh factor and is given after the first miscarriage, abortion, or pregnancy to prevent hemolytic reaction in the fetus. Not enough information related to fluid status is given in this scenario to evaluate whether a reduced infusion rate is appropriate. Antihistamine drugs are administered to patients with a history of mild transfusion reaction but are not appropriate for mismatched mother/fetus Rh factor. Blood administration is not contraindicated in pregnant patients with a history of mismatched Rh factor in a fetus.

Chapter 22

1. **b.** A breast biopsy is an example of a diagnostic procedure to confirm a suspected diagnosis. Explorative surgery (e.g., laparotomy) confirms the type and extent of a disease process. Curative surgery (e.g., appendectomy, kidney transplant) removes diseased or damaged body organs or structures, which may be replaced with donated or artificial organs. Palliative surgery (e.g., tumor debulking or feeding tube placement) alleviates pain or other disease symptoms but does not cure the underlying disease.

2. **a, c, d.** Decreased or hypoactive bowel tones following surgery are related to decreased oral intake and physical activity as well as the general anesthetic and opioid pain medications received. Diabetes does not result in gastroparesis or decreased peristalsis (bowel activity) specifically following surgery.

3. **d.** Paralytic ileus is a condition in which the bowel becomes distended and partially paralyzed, resulting in significantly decreased bowel function. This condition is possibly a result of bowel manipulation during surgery and is commonly associated with gastrointestinal surgery. Pain, constipation, and fluid volume deficit are all effects of surgical procedures but are not necessarily complications.

4. **b.** Self-concept is closely related to physical appearance, and the impact of the surgery depends on the patient's perception of his or her value or image. Emotional support may be needed to help the patient overcome minor or major changes. Cognition may be related to medications, unfamiliar surroundings, sensory overload, electrolyte imbalances, pain, anxiety, or sleep deprivation. However, this patient's statements are appropriate for the situation and do not reflect decreased orientation or alertness.

Coping may be impaired related to the physical alterations that this patient has experienced, although it is difficult to tell immediately following surgery and discussion of self-concept is the root cause of the need for coping behaviors. Relationships and roles may also change following surgery but are more long-term effects. Again, self-concept is the root cause that may impact the patient's ability to relate to others as she has in the past.

5. **c.** The nurse's role in informed consent is to witness the patient's signature on the consent document and is part of the patient's medical record before the procedure begins. If the patient is unsure or indicates lack of understanding, the surgeon should be notified so that more information can be provided. Statements A and B describe tasks that are out of scope for the RN (reviewing or explaining complications and procedural specifics). Statement D does not fulfill the nurse's duties around informed consent and puts the patient at risk for a procedure of which they are not fully educated.

6. **c.** Procedural pause is a final oral verification involving all team members in the operating room. The team reviews that the correct patient is in the room and positioned correctly and that the site/procedure is agreed upon before the incision is made. Preoperative teaching should occur prior to arriving in the OR. The patient is then given anesthesia and skin prep to prevent infection at the incision site.

7. **a, b, c, d.** All statements are correct procedures to maintain sterility in the operating room.

8. **b, c, d.** Pain management, renal function, and neurologic function are priorities in the postanesthesia care unit period (as are respiratory function, cardiac function, and conditions of incisional dressings). These systems indicate physical response to analgesia, sedation, and fluid loss (usually related to bleeding). Bowel function is less of a concern immediately following surgery because the patient is not alert enough to take in food.

9. **d.** Deep vein thrombosis (DVT) or venous thromboembolus (VTE) are complications resulting from immobility and venous stasis that lead to blood clots forming in the lower extremities. These are usually first suspected based on patient's report of lower leg pain, redness, and swelling. Positioning during surgery would not produce these findings 3 days later. Wound infection would be localized at the surgical site (shoulder). Atelectasis is collapse of the alveoli in the lungs impairing gas exchange and would not result in lower extremity pain or swelling.

10. **a.** Rings and watches are removed prior to the surgical hand scrub, because jewelry can be a reservoir for pathogens. Likewise, artificial nails and nail polish are contraindicated for OR personnel because artificial or polished nails are more likely to harbor pathogens. Hand hygiene in the form of a surgical scrub is done at the beginning of every case and when any break in sterility occurs, not just when one starts work.

Chapter 23

1. **d.** Restraint application is not an appropriate method for reducing fall risk and may cause more injury to the patient. Injury control interventions are centered at three primary levels: the individual level (e.g., providing education about safety hazards and prevention strategies); the design phase, using engineering and environmental controls (active or passive safety features that can prevent injury from product or equipment use); and the regulatory level, creating, monitoring, and enforcing regulations to ensure safe products and environments. Reminding the patient to use the call light would be individual education, placing the mattress on the floor would be environmental or design prevention, and developing an organizational policy for monitoring would be at the regulatory level of injury prevention.

2. **g.** Sentinel events or other serious safety events are required to be reported to regulatory agencies such as the Joint Commission and to state health agencies. The Occupational Safety and Health Administration (OSHA) establishes regulations for safety in the physical work environment, such as air quality, ergonomics (body positioning during work maneuvers), prevention of infection transmission from used and uncapped needles that pierce the skin of a healthcare worker, and prevention of exposure to toxic substances. The Institute of Medicine (IOM) has published reports on healthcare errors and has been integral in developing a culture of safety in healthcare. The Joint Commission publishes annual patient safety goals for healthcare facilities and credentials healthcare facilities contingent on their attention to these goals. Based on these recommendations, healthcare facilities develop policies and procedures for patient care and standard work to minimize hazards. State health agencies regulate safety and quality for facilities as well as professional standards of practice for nurses and other healthcare professions.

3. **a, c, d.** Advancing age entails loss in physical function and usually in acuity of sensory–perceptual function (e.g., impaired vision). Older adults may have impaired eyesight and hearing and decreased proprioception to maintain balance and sensitivity to touch. The ability to thermoregulate may become impaired; older adults are at higher risk than younger adults for hypothermia and heat stroke. Reflex responses slow, and the musculoskeletal system can lose flexibility and strength. Various conditions, such as arthritis, osteoporosis, or heart failure, can limit the ability to endure sustained physical activity. Medications taken to control conditions such as high blood pressure or Parkinson disease may result in orthostatic hypotension and increase the potential for falling. Alcohol impairment is not unique to older adults.

4. **a, b, c, d.** All of the listed safety hazards are relevant to nursing work environments. Other occupational hazards may include noise, hazardous dusts (e.g., asbestos, lead, coal) and chemicals, heights, dangerous machines,

biologically infectious agents, and violence. Other dangers result when employers or workers do not follow safety precautions, such as wearing protective gear and following safe work practices.

5. **a, b, d.** Documentation of an error in an incident report should completely describe all aspects of the event that occurred. Specifically, the report should include the accident, patient assessment, and interventions provided for the patient. The report is used for internal review to improve the system to prevent similar errors and cannot be subpoenaed by a court of law. This document remains confidential and is not part of the patient's medical record; thus, the incident should not be detailed in the nursing notes or other areas of the patient chart.

6. **a.** Environmental safety hazards include patient care devices such as catheters, surgical drains, or sequential compression devices. All other statements are appropriate surgical discharge education but are not related to environmental safety.

7. **a, d.** For a patient managing deficits following a stroke, neurologic and musculoskeletal system assessments would be a priority. Cardiovascular assessment is not indicated because the cardiovascular capacity is not directly impacted by this diagnosis. Skin assessment may provide important clues to the patient's history of accidents or injuries but would not indicate new risk following a stroke.

8. **a, c.** Appropriate goals for this stroke patient are to identify high-risk settings (e.g., drinking thin liquids) and to demonstrate appropriate safety habits (chin tuck). Avoiding drinking liquids is not appropriate at this stage. Compensation for a vision cut is not related to risk for aspiration.

9. **a, d.** Restraints are only clinically justified in selected instances to prevent irreparable harm associated with pulling out therapeutic devices or when endangering self or others. Risk for falls does not indicate restraint use because restraints have not been shown to reduce fall or injury rates and may actually increase incidence of unintended negative consequences. Impulsive behavior and confusion are not indicators for restraints because restraints may increase agitation and injury.

10. **c.** Determining which patients are in immediate danger is the priority for nurses in case of a fire (assessment of the situation). Giving patients wet washcloths, closing windows, and evacuating patients are all interventions that should be done once assessment of risk is complete.

Chapter 24

1. **d.** Oral care should be done daily and as needed to manage oral mucosa integrity and secretions. Dentures should be removed and brushed or soaked in special cleanser. Failure to remove dentures may lead to bacterial or fungal colonization between the palate and dentures. The patient should be positioned in the high Fowler's or side-lying position; Trendelenburg refers to supine with head lower than feet.

Never place fingers in the unconscious patient's mouth because the patient may respond to oral stimulus by biting down.

2. **a, b, d.** Placing the basin and washcloth on the nonaffected side of the body assists the patient in being able to bath himself. Assisting the patient to the bedside commode for toileting maximizes the patient's ability to void as independently as possible. Specialized utensils may be acquired so that this patient may be able to feed himself without assistance. Performing oral care, although important to do daily, does not promote independence in self-care.

3. **a.** Assessment should be done first according to the nursing process. Providing nail care is an intervention. Developing a plan of care is the planning phase. Evaluating support on discharge is the evaluation phase.

4. **b.** The patient receiving chemotherapy may lack energy related to a fluid/electrolyte imbalance from severe vomiting and diarrhea. This patient may also be fatigued from the treatment and the resultant effects to red blood cell counts, which carry oxygen to the cells. Preference for bathing weekly does not present the most critical barrier to self-care. The stroke patient represents minimal risk because there are no cognitive or motor impairments. The surgical patient with moderate pain does not have the largest risk for poor self-care.

5. **c.** This question is open-ended and allows for the patient to define her feelings and values. Other options are incorrect because they present judgment, elicit yes/no responses, and do not provide the opportunity for the patient to guide her own care.

6. **b, c.** Ineffective coping and powerlessness are nursing diagnoses related to psychological risk factors for self-care deficit. Caregiver role strain is not pertinent in this scenario because the spouse has already passed away. Impaired skin integrity is a consequence of failure to thrive but not a contributing factor.

7. **a.** Female patients should always be washed from front to back to avoid contamination of the vagina or urethra with microorganisms from the anus. Because such contamination can cause infection, this is the priority for this patient. Temperature extremes should be avoided, but this is not the most appropriate issue for this patient. All folds between the legs and labia should be cleansed thoroughly, but this is not the priority. Unconscious patients should be turned on their sides during mouth care to avoid aspiration; risk of aspiration is not heightened during perineal care.

8. **d.** The simplest of these ADLs is feeding, which is retained longer according to Katz Index of ADLs. Loss of self-care is a natural part of aging and proceeds in an orderly fashion with more complex activities, such as dressing, bathing, and toileting, being lost first.

9. **a, b, d.** External factors include proximity of shops, ability to prepare food, and a support network. Motivation or will to participate in self-care activities is an internal resource.

10. **b, d.** In the morbidly obese patient, skinfolds and areas of friction are especially prone to skin breakdown and fungal infections. Under the pannus and between the thighs are

two of the places in which skin breakdown is more likely to occur in this population. Elevating the heels from the bed is appropriate for any patient at risk for skin breakdown and not unique to bariatric patients. Nasal cannulas may lead to skin breakdown behind the ears; however, this option is not an intervention but rather an assessment.

Chapter 25

1. **b, d.** Locking the wheels will prevent unexpected movements and result in injury of the nurse or patient. Using mechanical aids (e.g., transfer belts, mechanical lifts, slide boards, body mobilizers) will decrease stress of movement for the patient and nurse, thus reducing risk of injury. Using other motions rather than lifting allows the nurse's body weight to assist with power. This prevents injury only with the nurse, not the patient. Pivoting the entire body similarly prevents back strain and injury in the nurse but is ineffective in preventing patient falls or ensuring patient safety.

2. **c.** Instructing the patient to bend legs and place feet flat on the bed allows the patient to assist by pushing legs against the bed. Explanation of procedure also reduces anxiety and increases cooperation. Placing feet in a broad stance lowers the nurse's center of gravity and would be the next step. Placing arms under the shoulders and thighs supports the heaviest parts of the patient's body and would be the third step. Elevating the head of the bed and replacing pillows, after the move is complete, is the final step to provide for patient comfort and safety.

3. **a, b, c, d.** Assessments of comfort, ability to follow directions, patient's weight, and limitations of equipment are all important assessments to perform prior to beginning the transfer process.

4. **d.** Diagnosis of malnutrition and advanced age puts this patient at risk for skin breakdown; elbow protectors reduce mattress pressure and remove elbow friction when the patient moves in bed. A trapeze allows a patient to raise his or her trunk from the bed but would not be the most appropriate intervention for this patient. A bed cradle keeps the pressure of linen off the feet but is not indicated simply related to age or malnutrition. A hand roll keeps hands in functional positions, preventing finger contractures, but there is no indication of contractures in this description.

5. **c.** Risk for self-care deficits is most appropriate in the environment of unilateral weakness. Activity intolerance involves insufficient energy to complete required activities. This patient may have the energy but not the physical ability. Disuse syndrome would be more indicated if there was immobility from hemiparesis or flaccidity; weakness alone would not support this diagnosis. Impaired skin integrity is not indicated from the description provided.

6. **b.** Elevating the foot wound will decrease edema and possibly subsequent pain. Although bed rest decreases metabolic needs, this is not an indication for immobility. A balance must be found between activity and the patient's energy; bed rest is not ordered solely to prevent mobility due to weakness. Although you would want to place a patient on limited activity to prevent mobilization of a DVT once it has developed, bed rest also elevates the risk for DVT formation.

7. **a, d.** Babinski reflex and tonic neck are subcortical reflexes that are present in newborns and subside as higher brain function matures and exerts an inhibitory influence. Limited hip flexion may be a sign of hip dysplasia and would be an abnormal finding, although it is commonly checked during the first year. Foot drop is a contracture in which the foot is fixed in plantar flexion due to immobility. It would be an abnormal finding, particularly in an infant of this age.

8. **c.** Pain medication is a risk factor for falls, particularly within the first 24 hours following surgery. A history of dizziness would not necessarily imply current fall risk. Depression is not relevant in this scenario. Confusion would be a risk factor, particularly in a new environment like the hospital, but is not indicated in this scenario nor common for a 26-year-old.

9. **d.** Trendelenburg position would increase perfusion to important organs, particularly the brain. Semi-Fowler's is a semi-sitting position with the head elevated 30 to 40 degrees. It improves cardiac output, promotes ventilation, and eases eating but would further decrease perfusion to the brain and upper torso. Sims' position is semi-prone with the weight distributed toward the hip and shoulder; it would not be appropriate for a patient who is hypotensive. Lithotomy position has the patient supine with the hips flexed and calves/heels parallel to the floor and is used mainly for vaginal/rectal examinations.

10. **d.** The nurse should stop movement if the patient reports any pain or resistance. Assessment is an important first step but should be done after the range of motion (ROM) is stopped. Continuing slow ROM could potentially increase damage to the joint if the cause is not determined first. Documentation should be done but later after the assessment and subsequent interventions are performed.

Chapter 26

1. **d.** Lack of surfactant, a substance that decreases surface tension and permits alveolar expansion, is an issue in premature babies. Functioning alveoli, which make breathing effective, are present at approximately 24 to 25 weeks. Bronchospasm and ineffective cough are not associated with premature infant respiratory development.

2. **c.** Clubbing is a phenomena thought to be related to long-term tissue hypoxia causing the release of a substance that dilates the vessels of the fingertips. Clubbing is seen in such diseases as lung cancer, cystic fibrosis, lung abscesses, and chronic obstructive pulmonary disease (COPD). Cyanosis is bluish skin discoloration caused by hemoglobin that is less saturated with oxygen. Dyspnea describes labored breathing and breathlessness. Arthritis is commonly present in the fingers and may cause enlarged joints but is unrelated to COPD.

3. **c.** A spacer attachment and patient education would sustain the patient's independence in medication administration and provide the appropriate dosing of the metered-dose inhaler (MDI). The spacer effectively holds the aerosolized medication until the patient is ready to inhale. Additional puffs do not necessarily increase the amount that the patient receives and it will be hard to interpret how much is actually obtained. The nurse administering the MDI may allow for accurate dosing but undermines patient independence and misses an educational opportunity for future dosing. Administering oxygen does not address the problem of ineffective MDI administration and is not necessarily indicated in this scenario.

4. **c.** A patient who is adequately oxygenated could have his supplementary oxygen reduced. Masks typically deliver more oxygen than nasal cannula; because the patient is well oxygenated, additional oxygen is not needed, so neither a mask nor an increase in the oxygen flow rate is needed.

5. **b.** Ineffective airway clearance is when a patient is unable to clear secretions or obstructions from the respiratory tract or clear the airway, as evidenced by adventitious lung sounds. Ineffective breathing pattern is the state in which a patient's inspiratory or expiratory pattern does not provide adequate ventilation. With impaired gas exchange, there must be evidence that there is an excess or deficit in oxygen absorption or carbon dioxide elimination usually validated by the arterial blood gas. Although deep breathing may be impaired, there is no evidence to support this conclusion. Increased respiratory rate and reported difficulty breathing could be related to any of these nursing diagnoses.

6. **c, d.** It is important for the nurse to ask the patient about tobacco use and smoking cessation on every visit, especially when the visit is focused on health promotion. Positive encouragement is reinforcing, and it often takes more than one attempt to successfully quit. Pursed lip breathing is used by patients with obstructive air disease to reduce the amount of air trapped in the lungs. Oxygen use and care is a priority when the patient has been prescribed oxygen therapy.

7. **a, d.** Safety considerations when using oxygen include fire prevention to keep flames, heat, or sparks away from the oxygen source. If the connections are not tight, the correct concentration of oxygen may not be delivered, causing serious health consequences in some patients. The nurse may want to discuss current evidence about COPD and talk with the spouse about the impact of COPD on the family, including role changes after the safety issues have been addressed.

8. **c, b, a, d.** The patient is first prepared for the procedure by explaining the procedure and positioning to prevent aspiration of secretions. The nurse considers the sequence of the procedure using principles of sterile technique. The cup should be filled prior to placing gloves because the saline is usually poured from a clean container. The gloves are placed next, and the nondominant hand is then contaminated when the catheter is connected to the clean suction tubing. The nurse uses the sterile hand holding the catheter for suctioning the patient.

9. **d.** The tracheostomy ties secure the tube into the tracheostomy hole in the patient by tying it from one side, around the neck, and to the other side. If the tube is not secured and the patient coughs, the pressure can force the tube out, and the airway can collapse or be compromised. A tracheostomy button is used to test the patient's ability to breathe normally; it must be properly applied. If the cuff is inflated, the tube must never be plugged. Saline lavage is an outdated practice in which saline is inserted during suctioning. This practice can cause a significant drop in oxygenation and is not recommended, particularly in pediatric populations.

10. **a, d, b, c.** The incentive spirometer can be confusing to some patients as they may expect to blow into the device; explain that it works by "sucking in" rather than blowing out. The goal is to get the patient to breathe more deeply and ventilate better. Explain that bigger breaths in help expand the lungs; the goal amount of inhalation can be increased as improvements are made. The mouth must be sealed around the mouthpiece during deep inhalation; it can be released during exhalation. It is normal for proper use of the incentive spirometer to induce coughing in the patient with atelectasis or impaired gas exchange.

Chapter 27

1. **d.** Dysrhythmia is an abnormal conduction through the heart muscle and is the result of a high potassium value, among other factors. Mitral regurgitation is an incompetence of the mitral valve, allowing blood to flow backward as well as forward. Myocardial infarction (MI) or a heart attack is ischemia or loss of oxygenated blood flow to part of the myocardial muscle. Low cardiac output is simply minimal outflow of blood, possibly related to poorly functioning cardiac muscle or conductivity problems resulting in ineffective pumping mechanism.

2. **a, b, c.** Hypertension, hyperlipidemia, and cigarette smoking are all risk factors for atherosclerosis. Depression is not a known contributor to atherosclerosis.

3. **a.** Quitting smoking would be the priority modification to decrease risk of cardiovascular sequelae. Anticoagulant medications are not indicated by this scenario alone. Reducing salt intake would be an appropriate lifestyle modification but would not be a priority over quitting smoking. Decreasing fluid consumption may indirectly decrease blood pressure but would not be recommended as a long-term lifestyle modification.

4. **b.** Right-sided heart failure is characterized by fluid overload best seen in edema, elevated blood pressure and heart rate, and jugular venous distension (JVD). Endocarditis, an inflammation of the cardiac muscle, is described as chest pain; elevated heart rate could be related to cardiac output or pain. Atrial fibrillation, an irregularly irregular heart rate, would not produce edema or JVD. The patient is not said to be postoperative, thus postoperative fluid overload would not be indicated.

5. **a.** Risk for decreased cardiac output describes a person who is at high risk for experiencing inadequate blood pumped by the heart to meet the metabolic demands of the body. Self-care deficit and activity intolerance may increase the risk of cardiac complications but are not indicated simply by a diagnosis of diabetes mellitus. Infection would not be indicated, although risk for infection would be elevated in the environment of hyperglycemia if diabetes is not well controlled.

6. **a.** Low blood pressure and elevated heart rate suggest bleeding and puts the patient at risk for ineffective tissue perfusion. Activity intolerance may occur after delivery, but the degree of low blood pressure and elevation in heart rate suggest something more significant is happening. Although infection might increase pulse, a drop in blood pressure would not be expected unless the patient was developing sepsis. There is no evidence in the scenario for ineffective childbearing process.

7. **a, d.** Knowledge of treatment regimen and electrolyte imbalance would be most indicated for a patient with end-stage renal disease (ESRD). Respiratory status: ventilation would not be indicated, although fluid overload could lead to impaired respiratory status: gas exchange. Urinary continence would not necessarily be affected by ESRD.

8. **b.** Antiembolism stockings should be removed every 8 hours. Toes should remain warm, and no obvious constriction or excoriation should be noted. Applying sequential compression devices (SCDs) would not address poor circulation from constriction of stockings. Calf-pumping exercises are useful to prevent DVT but would not address the tissue perfusion. Anticoagulation medication would not be appropriate because the issue is poor-fitting antiembolism stockings. A DVT would present with pain, warmth, and swelling at the affected site.

9. **c.** The most appropriate answer is to assess the nature of the pain per the nursing process. Pain medication would not be appropriate since it may mask the signs of chest pain. The second answer would assume that anxiety is the root cause without assessment. It would also be premature to call a code before an assessment is done.

10. **c.** The head of the bed should be lowered first to prepare to start cardiopulmonary resuscitation (CPR). It is inappropriate for the first responder to leave the room to retrieve the crash cart. It is not possible to begin CPR while the patient is still upright. It is also not appropriate to remove furniture from the room as the first responder to a code.

Chapter 28

1. **b.** Respiratory acidosis. The pH is less than 7.35, making it an acidosis. The $PaCO_2$ is high, which indicates an excess of the respiratory gas carbon dioxide. The HCO_3^- is normal, indicating that the kidneys have not yet had time to compensate for the acidosis. The patient is also hypoxemic, as indicated by the low oxygen level.

2. **a.** The fluid has leaked from the intravascular space into the interstitial fluid compartment, causing the tissues to swell. If the fluid excess were intracellular, the patient would experience symptoms related to brain cell adaptation, such as mental status changes and seizures.

3. **a, c.** Potassium and fluids are lost in the emesis and diarrhea. Peripheral edema is present with fluid excess. Diaphoresis is a symptom that may lead to volume deficit.

4. **b.** The patient with a low blood pressure and dizziness is experiencing a critical drop in blood pressure and symptoms related to poor cerebral perfusion. This may be a life-threatening situation and requires an acute intervention.

5. **b.** Serious problems can develop quickly since the total blood volume of an infant or newborn is much smaller. Although A, C, and D are important, teaching about safety and acute situations is most important.

6. **a, b, c, d.** The patient is instructed to "push fluids" or "force fluids," with a goal for each shift or day. Intake and output, along with daily weights, are important assessments. The serum Na^+ is expected to be elevated because of water losses, concentrating the sodium level.

7. **c.** The patient is having acute symptoms of fluid volume excess. An increased dose of diuretics may be necessary. Rest periods would be recommended, but the problem will not be resolved unless accurate treatment is sought. There are no data to support nutritional supplements or increased potassium as a recommendation.

8. **a.** Rinsing the mouth can decrease thirst but will not count in the intake because the patient spits out the fluid before swallowing. The alcohol in many mouthwashes can have a drying effect. Fluids are offered in small cups to avoid the temptation to drink too much at one time. Sugared candy and gum increases oral tonicity and can cause even further thirst 15 to 30 minutes later.

9. **d.** Serum K^+, Ca^{++}, and Mg^{++} are measured to evaluate the levels and provide replacement if needed. Although the healthcare provider order is needed, this answer does not provide the patient with information important to learning. The nurse should be able to answer the question using sound rationale. Protein values are measured with a separate blood test.

10. **a, b, c, d.** After the age of 25 years, the number of nephrons in the kidney decreases. There are decreases in kidney mass, blood flow, and glomerular filtration rate. All of these factors place the elderly at risk for fluid and electrolyte imbalances.

Chapter 29

1. **b.** Vitamin D actively assists in calcium absorption; osteoporosis is defined as a reduction in bone mass and is commonly related to chronic insufficient calcium intake; thus, increasing calcium intake is necessary. Iron is not indicated for osteoporosis but is more appropriate treatment for a low red blood cell (RBC) count and low hemoglobin. Vitamin K is indicated for formation of prothrombin and other clotting factors; B-complex vitamins assist in various carbohydrate, protein, and glycogen metabolism (B_1, B_2, B_3, folic acid) and formation of RBCs (B_{12}). Fluoride maintains bone/tooth structure but is not directly related to osteoporosis.

2. **b, c.** Alcohol's toxic effect on the intestinal mucosa can impair the normal absorption of nutrients. Chronic alcohol use can cause irreversible changes to the liver cells, affecting the liver's role in metabolic pathways.

3. **a.** The diet for pregnant women should include substantial increases in calories, protein, calcium, folic acid, and iron. Lactating women do not need to increase iron, older adults do not need a high-protein diet, and newborns do not need dietary supplements.

4. **a, b, d.** Meat is an excellent source of protein, B-complex vitamins, iron, and zinc. Vegetables provide vitamins A and C, folate, magnesium, and iron. Enriched breads and cereals are good sources of thiamine, iron, niacin, and riboflavin. Milk contains little iron.

5. **a, b, c.** These are true statements. It is not appropriate to discontinue the vitamins and parenteral nutrition based on oral intake because absorption and metabolism are impaired.

6. **a, b, c, d.** All are important considerations related to nutrition and food availability, particularly for elderly patients.

7. **b.** Calcium is important in the conversion of prothrombin to thrombin and other steps of the coagulation process as well as nerve impulse transmission via the formation of acetylcholine and contraction/relaxation of muscles, most notably the heart muscle. Increase in bone fractures and delayed fracture healing are also common in osteoporosis.

8. **a.** Spinach, kale, chard, and broccoli are all high in vitamin K, which decreases the effectiveness of the anticoagulant Coumadin. Leg pain and swelling would be symptoms of a DVT or clot. Dietary intake of vitamin K should be consistent while on Coumadin; adoption of a new diet indicates the time of highest risk. Bleeding gums indicate anticoagulation, normal levels of iron indicate no blood loss, and an international normalized ratio (INR) of 2.6 is therapeutic while on Coumadin.

9. **b.** Prealbumin has a half-life of 2 days and accurately assesses protein synthesis and nitrogen balance. It is considered a very sensitive and specific marker for nutritional status. Low albumin indicates a more chronic nutritional problem since the half-life is about 18 days. Low albumin may also be related to overhydration. Elevated white blood cell count may indicate infection not directly related to nutritional status. Low white blood cell count may be exhibited in severe nutritional depletion. Elevated cholesterol does not indicate malnutrition.

10. **a.** Maintaining the head of the bed at 30 to 45 degrees in Fowler's position at all times when feedings are infusing and 30 minutes after completion of intermittent or continuous feedings minimizes the risk of aspiration. Gastric residual volumes (GRVs) are not correlated with gastric emptying and aspiration and thus cannot be relied on to protect patients. Blood glucose monitoring is not indicated in relation to aspiration.

Chapter 30

1. **a, b, c, d.** The 23-year-old would be at risk because of decreased nutrition, which may lead to abnormal skin changes and decreased immune function. The 45-year-old would be at risk for skin breakdown due to moisture particularly between skinfolds; infection (as evidenced by fever) may also directly affect the skin surface. The 61-year-old would be at risk because of recent surgery and immunosuppression to prevent organ rejection. The 72-year-old with heart failure would be at risk due to edema and decrease oxygenation of tissues.

2. **c.** The site is healing appropriately; the stoma should be beefy, red, and moist because it is created from intestinal wall. Infection would be displayed by purulent drainage or odor. Maceration at the site could be from stool coming in contact with the surrounding skin, but surrounding skin is intact. Evidence of the wafer being too tight would be poor perfusion to the stoma resulting in a dusky color or cool temperature.

3. **c.** Pressure would be the biggest risk for this patient because he or she would not be able to move at all or be turned to prevent pressure ulcers. Friction and shear are related to movement in bed, which is not possible due to the therapy that this patient is receiving. Option D would not be relevant.

4. **d.** This wound would be unstageable because the base of the wound is not visible. Stage I is defined by red, non-blanchable but unbroken skin. Stage II is a partial-thickness loss of dermis presenting a shallow open ulcer with a red-pink wound bed. Stage III is full-thickness tissue loss, and slough may be present but does not obscure the depth of tissue loss.

5. **a, b.** Oxygenation and blood flow are decreased to the extremities and thus to the wound bed in diabetic patients. Smoking and obesity, if present, may impair wound healing but they are not indicated in this scenario.

6. **c, d.** Granulation describes the new formation of tissue in the wound bed during the proliferation phase; it is beefy and granular and consists of a matrix of collagen embedded with macrophages, fibroblasts, and capillary buds. Dehiscence describes a total or partial disruption in wound edges, mostly commonly used to describe surgical incisions in which the skin has separated but underlying subcutaneous tissue has not parted. A fistula is an abnormal tube-like passageway that forms between two organs or from one organ to outside the body. These can be the result of poor wound healing after tissue injury. A hematoma is a localized collection of blood and appears as a swelling or mass underneath the skin surface, often with a bluish color.

7. **a, b.** Appropriate interventions for this patient would be to secure a pressure relief surface for the bed and to turn the patient every 2 hours to prevent worsening or new pressure ulcer development. Silver dressings are antimicrobial, used for infected wounds; there is no indication that this wound is infected. Debridement is the removal of foreign material or dead tissue from a wound to discourage the growth of microorganisms and to promote wound healing.

8. **a, b, c, d.** All areas would be recommended to check in a full head-to-toe skin check, usually conducted on admission. These areas represent potential skin breakdown due to friction with the bed sheets (elbows) and medical devices (nasal cannula tubing, TED hose, urinary catheter).

9. **b.** Irrigating an abdominal wound would be the most appropriate choice for sterile gloves. Emptying wound suction or other surgical drains would only require clean

gloves. Clean glove are necessary when applying dry dressings; however, a moist or wet-to-dry dressing would require sterile gloves. Applying dressings to a coccygeal ulcer would not require sterile gloves due to the contaminated location.

10. **c.** After emptying the drain, the bulb should be recompressed to establish suction. The proper order of steps is as follows: (1) expose the suction device, (2) examine the tube and container, (3) open the plug on the reservoir, (4) measure the drainage in a calibrated container, (5) clean the drainage spout with an antiseptic swab, and (6) compress the reservoir to establish suction.

Chapter 31

1. **a, b, c.** This infant is at increased risk for illness related to the early age (statement A) and being formula, not breast, fed (statement B). Newborns may also display illness subtly as lethargy, poor feeding, or restlessness (statement C). Vaccinations are timed to cover developing immunocompetence, but an infant of this age is minimally able to receive vaccinations.

2. **a, c, d.** Elderly patients are at increased risk due to chronic disease, medications/therapies that may further impair natural responses to infection, and decreased natural defenses (intact skin/mucous membranes, body pH) and impaired function (swallowing, urinary retention, immune response). Shrinking thymus impairs humoral immune response; thyroid is unrelated to immune response.

3. **a, b, c, d.** All are examples of hospital-acquired infections (HAIs) that are under increasing surveillance by regulatory and accrediting agencies and have been identified as preventable. HAIs may also occur in any level of healthcare, including long-term care facilities, jails, and residential facilities.

4. **a, c, d.** These questions would be important in determining risk for infection and exposure to infectious illness. Question B relates more to risk for infection in a healthy individual.

5. **b.** The prodromal phase is characterized by nonspecific symptoms such as nausea, fever, weakness, aches, or pains. The incubation period is the time between the pathogen's entrance and appearance of symptoms. Acute phase of illness occurs when specific symptoms appear. The convalescent period describes when body systems return to normal and appetite and energy return; antibodies begin to appear in the person's blood.

6. **a, b, c.** Purulent or foul-smelling drainage, increased white blood cell count, and increased localized or systemic temperature are all symptoms of infection. Difficulty breathing is not indicated in limb infection.

7. **d.** Bacteremia or septicemia (sepsis) are systemic infections in which an infection is disseminated to other organs via the bloodstream. An opportunistic infection is any infection that takes advantage on an immunocompromised host due to existing disease, malnutrition, or medications. A nosocomial infection is one that is associated with healthcare delivery (HAI). Neutropenia is a significant risk for developing infections and is defined by an absolute neutrophil count of less than 1,000 cells/mm³.

8. **a.** An opportunistic infection is any infection that takes advantage on an immunocompromised host due to existing disease, malnutrition, or medications. Colonization refers to the introduction of microorganisms onto a body surface where they grow and multiply but do not invade the body or result in an immune response. Neutropenia is a significant risk for developing infections and is defined by an absolute neutrophil count of less than 1,000 cells/mm³. Immunodeficiency is used to describe the immune system's ability to produce memory cells and antibodies or to activate T lymphocytes. AIDS and cancer can cause this condition.

9. **c.** Avoiding flowers and fresh fruit will help to eliminate pathogens from the environment, which could introduce infection to the patient. The patient should also be placed in a private room, visitors should be limited, and the door should be kept closed. Invasive procedures, including injections, shaving, and rectal temperatures, should be avoided. Good hygiene is paramount, but flossing should be avoided because it may cause bleeding.

10. **d.** The proper procedure for collecting a wound sample is as follows: (1) remove soiled dressing, (2) insert culture swab into wound, (3) crush ampule of medium, (4) secure specimen in plastic bag, and (5) apply clean dressing.

Chapter 32

1. **c.** The tubules are passageways that permit urine to flow to the renal pelvis and then to the ureters, selectively reabsorbing or secreting substances from the urine to maintain fluid and electrolyte balance. Bowman capsule surrounds the glomerulus (a network of blood vessels), where urine formation begins. The small intestine reabsorbs some water and ions but is not part of the nephron and is not as selective in reabsorption.

2. **c.** Emptying of the bladder or voiding (micturition) occurs when the external bladder sphincter relaxes, abdominal muscles contract, and pelvic floor muscles relax. Detrusor muscles are the three layers of muscle in the body of the bladder itself; bladder fullness is not micturition. Sympathetic impulses stimulate the internal sphincter, keeping urine in the bladder.

3. **a.** Cloudy urine represents pus in the urine. Dark amber color may be related to urine volume and when occurring alone does not indicate an infection. Odor may be caused by concentration, time prior to emptying container, and certain medications or foods. Sediment may occur when urine is sitting unemptied in a device.

4. **a.** Postoperative patients have decreased fluid volume due to limited intake and loss of body fluid. Stress of surgery also increases the release of antidiuretic hormone, which decreases urine output. Urinary frequency alters the intervals in voiding but not the volume. A pregnant patient may have increased frequency but should not have decreased volume, particularly if not vomiting frequently. CVA patients may experience continence difficulty but should not exhibit decreased urinary volume.

5. **d.** Incontinence is not normal or an inevitable part of aging, although aging is a risk factor and is twice as likely in women. Newborns should void 30 to 40 times per day. Nighttime incontinence is normal until about 7 years of age. Nocturia is voiding during normal sleeping hours and is not abnormal.

6. **e.** Polyuria in hyperglycemia, anuria in ESRD, hematuria in a urinary tract infection, and urinary retention in a thoracic spinal cord injury are all expected findings.

7. **b.** Assessment of sensations of fullness and distention is the first step in the nursing process. A bladder ultrasound is an appropriate diagnostic tool following physical assessment. Encouraging oral intake and assisting the patient to the bathroom are interventions and should be done following assessments.

8. **d.** Stress incontinence is the sudden, involuntary loss of small amounts of urine that accompanies a sudden increase in intra-abdominal pressure such as during coughing, sneezing, laughing, lifting, and jumping. Urge incontinence is involuntary loss of urine after perceiving the need to urinate; inability to hold urine until reaching the bathroom. Functional urinary incontinence involves the inability of a person with normal bladder control to reach the bathroom in time to void. Environmental barriers, disorientation, or physical limitations may contribute. Reflex urinary incontinence is involuntary loss of urine at predictable intervals when a specific bladder volume is reached. Examples include neurologic impairment, CVA, or brain tumor.

9. **a, b.** Timed and prompted voiding schedules are effective with cognitively impaired older adults. Encouraging a patient to avoid bladder irritants is not the best choice since the patient presents with an altered mental status. Medications to improve bowel function are not indicated. Requesting an order for a urinary catheter is not indicated based on altered mental status and incontinence and could increase the risk of a UTI.

10. **d.** Indwelling catheters are indicated for recurrent urinary retention not relieved by intermittent catheterization, surgical procedures with general anesthetic for 1 to 2 days, and incontinence with pressure ulcers. Impaired mobility is not an indication without other factors present.

Chapter 33

1. **d.** Fecal incontinence is always an abnormal finding in adults. It is a normal finding in breast-fed infants to stool once every 3 days. It is not unusual that sometime during toddlerhood smearing or playing with feces will occur. Most children attain bowel control before 4 years of age and usually achieve bowel control before bladder control.

2. **a, b, c, d, e.** Postoperative use of opioids, reduced activity, and fear of pain inhibit normal bowel motility, as does bowel manipulation during surgery. Supine position may also decrease the urge to defecate. Lack of privacy may lead to the patient feeling psychologically uncomfortable defecating and thus ignoring the urge to defecate.

3. **a.** Antibiotics can promote diarrhea by irritating the gastrointestinal mucosa or by inhibiting the growth of normal intestinal flora. When normal flora is altered, *Clostridium difficile* can proliferate and release toxins. Dietary supplements would not cause diarrhea. Opioids could lead to constipation rather than diarrhea because they decrease gastrointestinal motility. Diuretics are unrelated to overactive bowel function, although high doses may lead to constipation.

4. **b.** Positive guaiac indicates blood in the stool and is an abnormal finding. Borborygmi are the normal sounds of gastrointestinal peristalsis. Hollow tympany is the normal sound on percussion over the left upper quadrant (stomach); dull sound or tympany over other quadrants would be abnormal. A convex, symmetric abdominal shape is expected; hollow, distended or asymmetric would be an abnormal finding.

5. **c.** After applying a smear of stool, close the slide cover and wait 3 to 5 minutes, then open the reverse side flap and apply two drops of Hemoccult developing solution onto each window and one onto the control window. Documentation of the result would be the final step.

6. **b.** Perceived constipation describes a self-diagnosis of constipation (not supported by nursing assessment). A patient may act on this perception through abuse of laxatives, enemas, and suppositories to ensure daily bowel movement. A nursing diagnosis of constipation would be supported by the following nursing assessments: decreased bowel tones, lack of flatus, and distended/firm/tender abdomen. Deficient Fluid Volume would be related to large losses of fluid through diarrhea (altered bowel function). Anxiety could lead to diarrhea, not constipation.

7. **c.** Promoting ambulation will assist with the return of gastric motility related to general anesthesia and can begin the earliest. High-fiber foods would be appropriate once bowel function has returned. Warm, not cold, liquids could also promote gastrointestinal motility.

8. **b.** Ensuring accurate placement of the nasogastric tube is essential prior to connecting to suction or administering medications. Irrigation should occur after medication administration.

9. **a, b, d.** The wafer should be tight to the stoma without restricting blood flow. Leakage of acidic bowel contents onto surrounding skin can cause irritation and skin breakdown. Bleeding may occur in small amounts because stoma tissues are fragile. Stomas should be a healthy pink. Dusky or pale color suggests inadequate circulation and should be reported.

10. **a.** New colostomies often affect body image, but continued inability to look at the site by the time of discharge presents barriers to self-care. Colostomy bags should be emptied when one-third full, and a "beefy" red stoma is normal. Some abdominal discomfort is not unusual but should not affect discharge.

Chapter 34

1. **b.** Sleep deprivation is prolonged periods of time without sleep. Disturbed sleep patterns are characterized by complaints of difficulty falling asleep, awakening, dissatisfaction, and statements of fatigue. Coping may be indicated if the patient has normal sleep patterns but desires sleep as a method of avoidance. Activity intolerance is not evident in this statement.

2. **d.** Apneic and other chronically sleep deprived patients may have more pronounced sedation due to medications effects. Apneic periods for more than 10 seconds are a normal finding for a patient with obstructive sleep apnea (OSA). During transfer, a patient would be disturbed and not likely apneic at that time. Continuous monitoring of patients with OSA should be done to capture saturation levels while asleep. Patients with OSA commonly have elevated blood pressure; this blood pressure is not the most concerning finding.

3. **d.** A pain assessment should be done first to determine if pain is the stimuli disturbing the patient's sleep.

4. **a.** The amount of sleep/rest may vary with developmental stage. Relationships, nutrition, alcohol, and shift work are factors in acquiring sleep/rest, not in amount needed.

5. **d.** A 1-year-old pediatric patient should exhibit normal circadian rhythms. People living alone without regular occupational or social contact are at risk for disturbed circadian rhythms. Variable night shift work and travel across time zones can impair the sleep–wake cycle.

Chapter 35

1. **a, b, c.** A pain assessment should include definition of pain location, intensity, quality, temporal pattern, and associated characteristics. Statements A, B, and C describe intensity, quality, and temporal pattern. Statement D looks at interventions, and although appropriate at a later point, this is not part of the pain assessment.

2. **d.** Allodynia describes a pain sensation produced by an innocuous stimulus such as light touch. This is an example of dynamic nervous system plasticity or adaptation after pain, in this case due to nerve inflammation. Hyperalgesia is enhanced pain sensation produced by a noxious stimulus. Neural plasticity is a broader term for nervous system adaptation after pain but is not specific to this scenario. Nociception is pain sensation; receptors are found within the skin, blood vessels, subcutaneous tissue, muscle, fascia, periosteum, viscera, joints, and other structures.

3. **b, c.** Increased blood pressure, heart rate, respiratory rate, and metabolic responses are all physiologic responses to pain. Facial grimacing, guarding, vocalizations, and muscle tension are other verbal and nonverbal responses. Decreased urinary output, although a fight-or-flight mechanism, is not generally linked to increases in pain levels.

4. **a.** Pain evokes emotional responses that may be expressed as depression, anger, fear, anxiety, sadness, excitement, denial, or regression. Although it is important to determine the cause of such behavior and rule out confusion, this is not appropriate for the scenario. This behavior, although seemingly erratic, does not indicate a psychiatric history. The patient may be struggling to cope with her pain, but there is not enough information to know what her current pain level is; based on the comments, it should be assumed that it is not well controlled.

5. **a, b.** Cold compresses reduce inflammation, blood flow, and edema. Massage relaxes muscles and reduces tension. Menthol products are a common over-the-counter intervention to reduce pain and inflammation but would be considered a pharmacologic intervention. Lidocaine patches are an effective pharmacologic intervention; the patch is commonly placed at the pain site.

6. **a.** Respiratory depression (respiratory rate less than 12 breaths per minute) with opioid use is easily observed and treated with an opioid antagonist. Respiratory depression is also uncommon when using patient-controlled analgesia since the opioid drug is self-administered. A pain scale rating of 3/10 is not abnormal following surgery. Moderate hypotension as described is not uncommon following surgery due to fluid loss and opioid administration. Lethargy following surgery is also not uncommon but should be monitored regularly.

7. **b.** Statement B treats the patient's nonverbal cues for pain and validates the family's concerns for the patient. Relieving pain, even if it hastens death, is the ethical and moral obligation of the professional nurse. It is not euthanasia or assisted suicide. Statement A addresses risk factors associated with opioid administration but is not reason to withhold pain medication for this patient. Statement C analyzes the nurse's reaction to the request but is in opposition to the American Nurses Association's position on proper care for a dying patient and may be considered abandonment. The nurses must fulfill a professional obligation regardless of personal values. Statement D describes nonverbal cues of pain; it is appropriate to treat nonverbal or nurse-assessed pain levels.

8. **d.** Pain relief is best managed using prevention rather than waiting until the pain becomes severe to treat. Statements A, B, and C reflect important information but are not the best guidance in correct opioid use.

9. **b.** The IV route provides the fastest relief for acute pain. Other options for pain relief may be used to provide longer lasting and good relief for severe pain, but the IV morphine should be used first to immediately decrease the patient's pain level.

10. **b.** Japanese culture is one example of a culture that highly values stoicism and high levels of pain tolerance, especially from men. A low rating on the pain scale does not necessarily mean that the patient has a high tolerance level or that he is not currently experiencing pain.

It should also not be assumed that this patient does not understand the pain scale. The best response from the nurse would be to assess nonverbal indicators of pain and treat accordingly.

Chapter 36

1. **a, d.** Overstimulation may heighten cognitive dysfunction and may be caused by a new environment, particularly in geriatric populations. Helplessness and loss of self-esteem may lead to depression and withdrawal. Sensory reception may be affected by loss of peripheral vision on the left.

2. **b.** Pain control will help the patient be better able to focus on other sensory inputs. Lengthy explanations add to sensory overstimulation and should not be used with patients experiencing sensory perception dysfunction. Lights should be dimmed to decrease sensory overstimulation. Roommates and their visitors should be quiet as they create more noise and the patient may misinterpret overheard conversations, thus contributing to sensory dysfunction.

3. **a, b, d.** Understanding of contributing factors, avoiding injury, and achievement or maintenance of self-care is desired. Sensoristasis is the optimal level of arousal; a nursing goal should be to achieve sensoristasis rather than minimizing it.

4. **b.** Pain can alter an individual's ability to cope and perceive. Assessment is the first step in the nursing process. Cleaning the glasses may be important to minimize altered sensory perception, and a bed alarm may be indicated intervention based on the patient's confusion, but both would be done following an assessment. Agitation is not stated as an issue at this time.

5. **e.** A nursing assistant can encourage independence while providing a safe setting for ADLs and can assist with sensory aids through touch. The nurse should first assess the patient's gait and safety prior to ambulation. Safety should take precedence over independence in mobilization, and assistance should be available when out of bed. Lights should be dim to decrease sensory overstimulation, but night-lights should remain on to assist with safety; this would not be appropriate use of delegation.

Chapter 37

1. **a, b, c, d, e.** Impaired blood flow to the brain, inadequate or impaired use of glucose, low sodium levels, impaired rest or sleep, and infectious processes all may be related to impaired cognition.

2. **a, b, c.** Delirium is characterized by acute onset of mental impairment including confusion and reduced level of consciousness. Aging, dementia, and drug/alcohol use are also predisposing factors.

3. **a.** Expressive aphasia is described by good comprehension but difficulty verbalizing and writing one's own thoughts. Anomia more specifically describes difficulty with word finding. Dysarthria is motor control deficit resulting in physical inability to pronounce words correctly, which may lead to slurred speech and heavy or unclear sounds;

understanding is not impaired. Receptive aphasia is speech that is well articulated but with impaired comprehension and feedback resulting in talking but not making sense. Global aphasia results from extensive damage, and patients have no functional skills in any language modality and poor comprehension.

4. **c.** Leaving the bed low and locked will best provide a safe environment for the patient with cognitive impairment. Posting a sign may not be appropriate for a confused patient. A large clock may help with orientation to surroundings but is not the best answer because safety would be a priority. Limiting visitors and loud stimuli may decrease confusion but would not ultimately keep the patient safest.

5. **a, c, d.** Preparing family members for discharge with resources and techniques to best manage the well-being of this patient is a priority. It is not appropriate to delay discharge based on the information given.

Chapter 38

1. **d.** Self-perception is based on several dimensions: self-knowledge, self-expectation, social self, and self-evaluation. Self-esteem and role performance are elements of normal self-concept patterns.

2. **c.** Disturbed body image is defined by verbalization of feelings or perceptions that reflect an altered view of one's body in appearance, structure, or function. Behaviors of avoidance, monitoring, or acknowledgement of one's body are also common clinical cues related to disturbed body image. Impaired coping and powerlessness are not the most directly indicated nursing diagnoses. Anticipatory grieving is not appropriate because the patient has already experienced the surgical change and is not making these statements prior to the surgery.

3. **b.** According to the nursing process, assessment should be done first; thus, asking for more information is most appropriate. Recommending counseling is an intervention. This is not a developmentally appropriate method of coping with body and role changes of adolescence. Physiologic changes do not identify the issues of self-concept; evaluation should be done last according to the nursing process.

4. **a, b.** Social support/coping influence self-concept and may impact a patient's ability to manage a new health regimen. Self-efficacy is the degree of confidence a person has about his or her ability to perform specific activities. Education about evaluation is not indicated, and role ambiguity is not noted as an issue.

5. **c.** To break a cycle of poor self-concept and negative self-evaluation, realistic self-evaluation and identification of positive attributes are needed. Risk identification is part of assessment. Classification of developmental level is not indicated. Assessing stressors is not an intervention.

Chapter 39

1. **b.** Change in family relationships and/or functioning may be expressed by inability to make decisions, lack of acceptance of ideas/actions, and inappropriate direction of energy; this patient is also the financial supporter for the family.

2. **a, c.** Caregiver health status is compromised with physical or emotional difficulty in caring for the patient, as is evident in a lack of sleep. Changes in work or leisure activities related to patient's dependency also indicate impact and strain on the caregiver's role.

3. **a.** Sexual intimacy is an aspect of family structures. Culture and chronic/acute illness are factors that affect family function, not an aspect of family function. Role strain is an example of manifestations of altered family function. Parental role is an aspect of family social relationship assessment, not an aspect of family function itself.

4. **a.** Gathering more information to identify contributing factors would be a priority before developing solutions. Referring to counseling may assist in coping but does not directly address the cause of the isolation (e.g., limited mobility).

5. **e.** Statement E describes a nonfamily household even though the individual may belong to a larger extended family. Blended (stepfamily), cohabited, communal, and commuter families are all appropriate examples of family.

Chapter 40

1. **c.** Dysfunctional Grieving describes unsuccessful use of intellectual and emotional responses by which individuals attempt to work through the process of modifying self-concept based on the perception of loss. Characteristics include difficulty expressing loss, interference with life functioning, and labile affect. Anticipatory Grieving does not reflect the time period following the son's death. There is not enough information to conclude that there is either Ineffective Health Maintenance or Impaired Family Processes.

2. **b.** Religious and ethnic beliefs and customs should be observed as much as possible in the grief process and caring for the deceased. Assessment of these aspects is a priority according to the nursing process and should also be done prior to interventions or evaluation. Gaining closure through viewing the body is a Western construct of mourning and may not be appropriate for this family. Other interventions and evaluation should follow assessment.

3. **a, c.** Helping to mobilize a support system and establish coping behaviors used in the past are appropriate interventions for the Shock Phase. Encouraging the expression of diverse feelings and providing role models are appropriate for the Protest Phase of the Grief Cycle Model.

4. **d.** Palliative care is the "active total care for those patients whose diseases are no longer curable and the focus of the treatment is to achieve the best possible quality of care for patients and their families." It may be used from as early as diagnosis, may be used together with curative treatments, and may occur in the hospital.

5. **a.** Nutrient and metabolic needs are decreased in active stages of dying. Placing a feeding tube would not be appropriate in an actively dying patient since this is a surgical procedure. Ordering desirable foods may be appropriate for dying patients; however, this patient is unresponsive. Gastromotility is decreased in the dying process, but this is

not the best answer since the patient is unable to eat due to her lack of responsiveness; nausea is not the primary concern.

Chapter 41

1. **b.** Allostasis is described in the definition above. Homeostasis refers to the automatic, coordinated, self-regulating process to maintain a steady state rather than appropriate adaptation to change. Coping is a process to manage stress, including but not limited to physiologic management. Adaptation is a person's capacity to flourish and survive; an outcome of coping.

2. **b.** Immunosuppression is associated with chronic stress. Blood glucose would not be elevated related to chronic stress. Dilated pupils and rapid respiratory rate are signs of acute stressors.

3. **c.** Adequate exercise and diet are lifestyle changes that help to release tension and promote healthy management of stress. This mother has already verbalized active stressors and expressed her feelings. Crisis intervention resources are not appropriate at this time.

4. **d.** Ineffective Coping is characterized by inability to meet basic needs and a high illness rate. Defensive Coping does not involve physical illness. Caregiver Role Strain is not appropriate because the situation does not describe a caregiver relationship at this time. Chronic Sorrow is not appropriate based on the amount of time elapsed since the significant other's death.

5. **a, b, c, d.** All questions are appropriate in eliciting coping and adaptation behaviors.

Chapter 42

1. **a, b, c, d.** Sexual function can be influenced by numerous factors, including relationships, cognition and perception, culture, values, beliefs, self-concept, previous experience, pregnancy, gender identification, environment, illness, surgery, and/or medications.

2. **c, d.** Dyspareunia is painful intercourse, which occurs regularly in 1% to 2% of women and occasionally in up to 15%. Ejaculatory dysfunction, either premature ejaculation or the inability to ejaculate, physically alters a man's ability to feel confident during sexual acts. Inhibited sexual desire and sexual abuse both may influence altered sexuality but are not physically motivated.

3. **b.** The most appropriate question to ask first would be "When did you begin menstruating?" This question begins with objective information and allows the patient to establish a rapport with the nurse prior to moving into more sensitive topics. Question A implies judgment. Question C is objective but too sensitive to begin with. Question D may be appropriate once further information is gathered.

4. **a, c, d.** Testicular examinations are the best hope for early detection of testicular cancer, which has a high prevalence among young males 15 to 35 years of age. Contraception is important to discuss with male and female patients alike. Self-awareness is important for all patients in order to understand their anatomy and stimulants that may help them develop healthy sexual relationships. Kegel exercises

are pelvic floor exercises used for women to increase tone, resulting in improved bladder control, relief from constipation, postpartum recovery, and sexual performance.

5. **d.** Statement D provides limited information and supports the patient's decision, appropriate for the second step of PLISSIT. Statement A reaffirms permission giving (step 1). Statement B provides specific suggestions (step 3). Statement C recommends intensive therapy (step 4).

Chapter 43

1. **b.** Evidence of survivor guilt is related to spiritual distress. Requesting time alone may indicate effective coping or spiritual well-being. Using sleep as a coping mechanism may be ineffective but does not indicate spiritual distress. Refusing medications or refusing to participate in the therapeutic regimen is evidence of noncompliance, not spiritual distress.

2. **c.** Lack of transportation to attend a spiritual group could cause impaired spiritual health. Anger, lack of concentration

or memory, and fear describe manifestations of altered spiritual function.

3. **c.** Statement C best displays understanding of the patient's spiritual needs by the nurse, despite differing beliefs. Statement A shows avoidance and a lack of attention to the importance of spiritual care. Statement B shows fear and a lack of comfort with spiritual care. Statement D fails to address the patient's need for spirituality for coping.

4. **d.** Outcome criteria phrasing should be specific, measurable, and include a time frame. Other statements lack time frames or reflect broad patient goals.

5. **b, d.** Illness that forces a patient to change his or her way of living may lead to spiritual distress. A terminal diagnosis also may lead the patient to question meaning in life and end of life beliefs. Many visitors indicate social support and reinforce spirituality. Membership in a group, particularly a religious or spiritual group, indicates both social support and a strong faith-based belief system that may assist in coping.

Appendix B

Apply Your Critical Thinking Answers

Chapter 1

Nursing professional organizations offer nurses opportunities to join voices and make a difference on a larger scale. Many organizations set standards for the practice of nurses in that field; being a member allows you to have a say in those standards. Nursing journals, conferences, educational opportunities, and networking are additional benefits. Of course, membership costs money; many organizations have a student rate. The American Nurses Association is the organization for all nurses; numerous specialty organizations address the needs of particular areas of nursing—for example, oncology, critical care, emergency, pediatrics. Check out organization websites and find an organization that fits your needs. Active membership is professionally and personally rewarding and can provide career opportunities.

Chapter 2

You need to understand from Sue what her perspective is on allopathic versus complementary and alternative medicine (CAM) treatments. Talking to her about integrative medicine in which she can incorporate the most beneficial parts of treatment modalities is important. As more oncologists integrate chemotherapy with other CAM therapies, the oncologist would be a primary resource for Sue. It is important to keep your interactions with Sue nonjudgmental but clear and accurate.

Chapter 3

The hospital discharge planner works with patients early during their hospital stay to begin planning for leaving the hospital. The discharge planner may be a social worker or nurse. Options for Mrs. Ellis might include returning to home, living with her children, or entering a nursing facility for a short time. Community resources might include senior centers, home meal delivery services, and home health nursing organizations that might provide registered nurse or nursing assistant care. With strong support systems, no stairs, and a bathroom prepared with handrails, Mrs. Ellis has many resources already in place. Her mental status, good appetite, and progress in physical therapy suggest she is doing well physically. Her forgetfulness and limited financial resources might be areas of concern. Programs that assist elders with financing prescription drugs

can be investigated. Connecting with church supports might be sufficient to allow Mrs. Ellis to return to her own home and maintain her independence.

Chapter 4

Patient safety is the utmost priority. Even though the patient does not appear to be harmed, an incident report should be filed for several reasons. First, adverse effects may show up later, and an incident report on file can help determine what happened. Second, the error may be due to a systems issue that needs to be corrected to prevent further similar errors in the future. Perhaps most importantly, as professionals, nurses are accountable for their actions. Covering up a mistake is a serious breach of professional ethics. Even without harm to the patient, covering up a mistake may lead to disciplinary action, including loss of employment and possibly loss of licensure. If nurses do not act with honesty and integrity, the profession of nursing is at risk.

Chapter 5

1. Refer to the definition of *culture*: "Culture is a learned, patterned behavioral response acquired over time that includes implicit versus explicit beliefs, attitudes, values, customs, norms, taboos, arts, and life ways accepted by a community of individuals. Culture is primarily learned and transmitted in the family and other social organizations, is shared by the majority of the group, includes an individualized worldview, guides decision making, and facilitates self-worth and self-esteem." With this in mind, this family's beliefs, attitudes and values about asthma, the cause and contributing factors, medication, interactions with health professionals, and other issues may be implicit. Implicit means that they may not be aware of their views and how they differ from those of the providers. Therefore, questions such as "Do you have any cultural beliefs that might impact your health?" would probably not be helpful. Rather, examples of "high-yield" questions include the following:

"What do you think makes your asthma better or worse?"
"What do you call your condition, and in your opinion, what causes it?"

"In your country, how are children with asthma cared for, and was this true for you when you were young?"

"When in the refugee camp, how was your asthma treated and what made it better?"

"How did asthma impact your life at home and in the refugee camp, and how does it now impact your life?"

"What do people in your community at home say about asthma and how to make it better?"

"What do you hope for with regard to your health?"

2. Write about your assumptions related to people with limited English proficiency who became refugees due to war and subsequently lived in a refugee camp. Visualize how this couple may appear at your first meeting, and write down your involuntary responses and assumptions based on their physical appearance. If they make little eye contact, what is your involuntary response? Describe your involuntary reaction to the idea of explaining a complex disease such as asthma via an interpreter.

3. Prior to the interview, use online resources to learn about the country, cultural groups, traditions, religions, economy, basic health data, and recent history. Ask key informants such as interpreters for cultural and historical information.

4. Subsequent open-ended questions are based on these answers and use the patient's words to encourage the patient to expand on his or her thoughts.

5. This answer will be based on the individual's cultural perspective and may include responses related to disease origin, health and healing approaches, diet, religion, decision making, interaction with health professionals, traditions, and other areas.

Chapter 6

Gather information from other healthcare colleagues on what has worked for them. This situation can be frustrating for you as the nurse. Talk with family about any behaviors they have found effective with Mr. Snyder. You remember that patient-directed eye gaze, head nodding, smiling, forward-leaning, and affective touch are frequently used effective communication behaviors. Collaborate with speech therapy and any plans they may introduce, such as picture boards to prompt speech. As a nurse, you will develop your own personal style of affective touch. Indicators for determining the effectiveness of your communication with this nonverbal patient could include the patient's eye gaze; head nodding, both affirmatively and negatively; and smiling. Any behaviors that work particularly well should be shared with the team in order to provide effective continuity of care for Mr. Snyder.

Chapter 7

Truthfulness, confidentiality, and privacy are ethical concerns involved in Mr. Washington's request to you. Patients have a right to decline treatment advice, but there are risks associated with doing so. Smoking with an oxygen tank present is dangerous. You need to assess whether the patient understands the consequences of his behavior. This dilemma can relate to the patient's safety. Assessing his knowledge will help you individualize your approach.

If the patient denies the need to remedy a dangerous situation, you have a difficult decision to make. As a nurse, you need to understand your scope of practice and your competency to intervene in a way that promotes well-being. It is best to be honest with Mr. Washington, explaining that you are unable to promise to keep his smoking a secret. Suggest that he be honest with both his physician and his daughter.

Chapter 8

Focusing your question more specifically will help you define the information you want to search for. Some examples to assist you include:

● List main topics and alternate terms from your PICO question that can be used for your search
● List your inclusion criteria—gender, age, year of publication, language
● List terms that you may want to exclude in your search
● List where you plan to search—for example, EBM Reviews, Medline, CINAHL, PubMed

You can share the information you have found with your instructor and, after consultation with the instructor, you can make a plan for how to effectively share your findings with your patient.

Chapter 9

Mrs. Babbitt seems motivated to learn, but you must assess her baseline knowledge about medications, attitude about taking medications, daily routine, cognitive abilities, literacy level, ability to hear and see (to read medication labels), and psychomotor ability to remove medications from their containers.

Start teaching as soon as possible. When you give Mrs. Babbitt her medications, say each drug name and explain what each does. A day or two before discharge, sit down with Mrs. Babbitt (and hopefully a close family member) to give written and verbal information regarding each medication. In consultation with Mrs. Babbitt and her family, develop a medication calendar of when to take medications.

Confusion can occur when the drug regimen is complex. Have both Mrs. Babbitt and her family members restate each medication, dose, purpose, and any special considerations. Provide positive reinforcement for correct answers. Inquire as to the plan for medication administration after discharge (e.g., using a medication administration set, checking off on written schedule). Follow-up by the primary health provider or a home health nurse may be indicated if Mrs. Babbitt does not demonstrate mastery before discharge.

Chapter 10

Assess the history of the bladder infection, including how long it has been resolved, what medications Ms. Bennet was taking, and what her diet has included. Determine how long the diarrhea has been going on and how frequently it occurs during the day. Examine the perineal area for inflammation of the perineal skin, how extensive it is, and whether the skin is still intact. Explain that antibiotics used to treat the bladder infection may kill off the normal flora of the intestinal tract leading to overgrowth of yeast spores. What Ms. Bennet is experiencing may well be a yeast infection, which can lead to diarrhea and inflamed skin.

Replacing the normal flora of the intestines will relieve the yeast overgrowth. This can be enhanced by eating yogurt and other probiotic foods. As the normal gut organisms are regenerated, the yeast will be brought back into balance and normal bowel function will return. In the meantime, keep the perineal skin clean after every bowel movement and protect it with use of protective emollients. The care provider may also prescribe yeast infection medications, topically and/or orally. Encourage adequate oral intake. The goal of care is to maintain normal nutrition and fluid balance and to protect the integrity of the perineal skin.

Chapter 11

(This chapter does not have an Apply Your Critical Thinking feature.)

Chapter 12

Primary sources of information are those collected directly from the patient: the patient's health history (including his complaints and past medical history), physical examination findings, and his perception of ability to cope with life stressors. Secondary sources are laboratory tests, such as complete blood count (CBC) and chest x-ray results, description from family members, and the physical therapy report.

Chapter 13

It is normal to feel less confident managing complex nursing diagnoses such as Ineffective Role Performance, especially when you are a new nurse. The first step is validating this nursing diagnosis and assessing Mr. Mason's feelings about it. Meet with him at the beginning of your shift, saying "I read your chart yesterday to better understand your situation so we can individualize your care. You certainly have had a lot going on since your accident. It may have required some adjustments in what both you and your wife do to manage the household. How has it been for you?" Mr. Mason may want to discuss it or he may not. He may not be ready to actively deal with his feeling at this time. Many complex nursing diagnoses require collaboration with other team members such as social work or a mental health professional. Listen to Mr. Mason, validate his readiness to address the problem, and make appropriate referrals.

Chapter 14

The highest priority for this patient is Impaired Physical Mobility. He is in the skilled nursing facility to regain mobility after his hip replacement, and mobility outcomes must be accomplished before he can go home. Constipation is a side effect of his decreased mobility, so hopefully once he is more active his problem with constipation will resolve. Collect additional information on his pain level and use of pain medication. Adequate pain management is essential for him to

actively participate in physical therapy. In addition, his use of opioid medication during this postoperative period may be contributing to his constipation. Another area to explore is his emotional state because this can impact his recovery. He states that his daughter was unwilling to take care of him, and he states frustration with not being able to care for himself. Ineffective Coping might be another nursing diagnosis to add to his plan of care.

Chapter 15

Audits are tools to evaluate whether the unit is meeting required outcome measures. Standards can be established by outside agencies such as the department of health (DOH) or the Joint Commission. Often meeting and documenting compliance with such standards are necessary for accreditation or to receive reimbursement. Participation in an audit is an opportunity for professional development, and it helps a nurse be aware of and appreciate many factors that influence the care patients receive. Consistently meeting standards helps ensure that all patients will receive the best care possible.

Chapter 16

All efforts must be maintained to protect the patient's confidentiality. Failure to do so violates HIPAA and has serious consequences for the nurse and the healthcare facility. The nurse may wish to talk to the boyfriend and urge him to share the information about his health status with the cousin if he has not already done so. The nurse also may wish to discuss the matter with a supervisor for strategies on how to deal with this problem.

Chapter 17

Subjective data are back pain for the last 7 months, description of the pain as incapacitating, report of doing nothing but watching television and reading, report of medication not working, and pain rated as 7/10. Objective data are the fact that he has been out of work and receiving disability, the vital sign measurements, and a distant and unexpressive demeanor. In this situation, the subjective data are more important. His vital signs are normal, but chronic pain does not cause an increase in blood pressure, pulse, or respiration rate as accompanies acute pain. The pain problem is causing restrictions on the patient's lifestyle. The nurse must accept the reports of pain and work to treat it, even though objective values may be normal.

Chapter 18

Assessing blood pressure in the basal state provides the most accurate data. Stress, increased activity, and anxiety can elevate blood pressure. The medical assistant should delay blood pressure measurement until Ms. George has a chance to calm down. The assistant should not apply the cuff nor listen with a stethoscope over Ms. George's clothes because hearing will be impaired. Also, blood pressure should not be monitored in the arm in which the intravenous (IV) line is infusing. The arm should be supported to avoid a falsely high reading, and the assistant should be close enough to the gauge to read it accurately. It appears from the photograph that the cuff is loosely wrapped around the arm and the head of the stethoscope is not placed over the brachial artery.

Chapter 19

Because influenza is transmitted via the airborne route, it is likely that other family members, including the other children, will contract it. Children are infectious as long as influenza symptoms are present. Instruct the mother to keep the child home from day care/school and isolated from friends during this time. Also stress the need for good handwashing, which is always important. Reinforce hygiene measures including proper disposal of any tissues or secretions. Additionally, encourage the mother not to let the children and other family members share dishes and personal care items; doing so will reduce the risk of transmission. Influenza vaccine should be encouraged, especially for high-risk patients (e.g., the elderly, those with respiratory disease).

Chapter 20

To calculate the dose to administer, use the formula:

$$\frac{\text{dose on hand}}{\text{quantity on hand}} = \frac{\text{dose desired}}{\text{quantity desired}}$$

$$\frac{10,000 \text{ units}}{1 \text{ mL}} = \frac{7,500 \text{ units}}{X}$$

$$10,000X = 7,500$$

$$X = 0.75 \text{ mL}$$

Because the heparin is to be administered subcutaneously, use a short, ½-inch needle. You can use a small gauge (25 to 27) because the medication is not thick and can easily go through a needle with a small diameter. The size of the syringe should be 1 mL so that visualization of 0.75 mL dose will be clear. A tuberculin syringe would be appropriate in this situation.

Many agencies require that heparin be administered in the abdomen away from vascular areas, which might cause more bruising. More research needs to be done to confirm this practice because some studies show no difference in bruising when arm or thigh sites are used. Additional precautions used for heparin injections to prevent bruising include no aspiration and not rubbing the site after injecting the medication.

Chapter 21

IV controller rate: To calculate the number of milliliters per hour, divide the total volume by the number of hours for the infusion (3,000/24 = 125 mL/hour).

Gravity infusion—macrodrip: Use the formula to obtain the drops per minute:

$$\text{Drop/min} = \frac{\text{Total volume infused} \times \text{drop factor}}{\text{Total time for infusion in minutes}}$$

$$\frac{3,000 \times 20}{24 \text{ h} \times 60} = \frac{60,000}{1,440} = 41.7 \text{ or } 42 \text{ drops/min}$$

An easier method of calculation is to reduce the amount to an hourly rate first (3,000/24 hours = 125/60 minutes). Working with smaller numbers can be less confusing.

$$\frac{125 \text{ mL} \times 20 \text{ drops/mL}}{60 \text{ min}}$$

By reducing to lowest terms, you divide 125 by 3 and arrive at the same answer of 41.7 drops per minute.

Gravity infusion—microdrip: Because the drop factor for a microdrip is 60 and the number of minutes in an hour is 60, you are multiplying and dividing by the same number. When using a microdrip, the number of drops per minute is the same as the number of milliliters per hour, so simply calculate the hourly infusion rate.

Chapter 22

When interpreting postoperative vital signs, evaluate these data in terms of trends, looking for decreasing blood pressure and increasing pulse rate to promptly detect shock. Mr. Johnson's vital signs show some fluctuations but generally remain close to baseline values. Increased blood pressure and pulse rate may indicate pain if this upward trend continues.

Other important assessments to regularly monitor include airway patency and quality of respirations, level of consciousness and recovery from anesthetic agent, amount and quality of drainage on dressing or from drains, urinary output, and level of pain.

Chapter 23

Restraints are not always the best way to maintain a patient's safety. In acute care agencies, restraints may be applied, but a physician's order must be obtained per the facility's policy. Protocols should be in place for the appropriate use and monitoring of restraints to prevent injury. Assess circulatory and neurovascular status frequently. Consider other options, such as having a family member sit with the patient or using a sitter if a family member is unavailable. Make an effort to detect the cause of Mr. Rau's acute confusion to direct treatment at resolving the underlying cause.

Chapter 24

Mrs. Ramirez needs much assistance with bathing due to her mobility and cognitive deficits. A shower using a shower chair seems most appropriate at this point, especially with Mrs. Ramirez's history of falls. First, take Mrs. Ramirez to the toilet, encouraging her to void and defecate. Confused patients sometimes need prompting for elimination and can be incontinent in the shower when bladder and bowel are full. Verbally keep her informed of what you are doing and encourage as much participation as possible. Give positive feedback for attempts to participate in self-care. Keep Mrs. Ramirez warm by wrapping her in a bath blanket since older adults can easily become hypothermic. Use mild soap and gently cleanse and inspect all skin surfaces for breakdown or injury. Wash Mrs. Ramirez's hair, using a cream rinse if her hair is tangled or matted.

Pat Mrs. Ramirez dry, especially in areas of skinfolds where moisture can accumulate and cause skin maceration and fungal infections. When you return to Mrs. Ramirez's room, dry and comb her hair and provide care for her teeth.

Chapter 25

From the data provided, the most important concern before getting Mrs. Jones up is whether she is volume depleted. Data that support this concern are a blood pressure below baseline and a low urine output (less than 30 mL/hour). Fluid volume deficits will cause postural or orthostatic hypotension, which can result in dizziness and possible syncope when arising. The medications she is receiving for pain and nausea could further contribute to hypotension. Before getting Mrs. Jones up, take a postural blood pressure and pulse reading. If Mrs. Jones is orthostatic, her blood pressure will drop and her pulse will rise when she sits on the edge of the bed. She also may complain of dizziness, diaphoresis, and generalized weakness. If the postural drop is significant (a systolic blood pressure drop of 25 mm Hg or greater with a pulse increase), you may need to give her extra fluids. If Mrs. Jones is not orthostatic, get her up slowly, elevating the head of the bed to prevent putting extra pressure on her incision. Make sure she is adequately medicated for pain by using her patient-controlled analgesia (PCA) before ambulation. Mrs. Jones requires standby assistance; a transfer belt is not usually required for postoperative patients with no prior mobility problems. Organize her IV fluids, PCA, and urinary catheter so that they are not in the way during ambulation. Assess Mrs. Jones frequently during ambulation to detect signs of activity intolerance quickly.

Chapter 26

During the first postoperative day of care, Mr. Jacob needs aggressive respiratory interventions to prevent atelectasis. Data that indicate that atelectasis may already be present include elevated temperature; shallow, slow respirations; and diminished breath sounds with crackles. Limited mobility after surgery, pain and the fear of pain when breathing deeply, and diminished respirations from the opiates used to manage pain all contribute to postoperative atelectasis. To reverse atelectasis and promote optimal oxygenation, it is important to get Mr. Jacob up and moving. Encourage deep breathing, and perhaps see if you can get an order for an incentive spirometer. Supplemental oxygen is usually not given until O_2 saturation falls below 93%.

Chapter 27

As part of your role as the visiting nurse, you are evaluating the patient's recovery from the heart attack. It is normal for the patient to experience discomfort from the surgery. Assess the wound for redness, drainage, or swelling that may indicate infection. Take Mr. Brown's vital signs, and note any temperature elevation. Encourage Mr. Brown to take his pain medication as needed, and report any increases in pain.

Over time, the pain should resolve. The patient should immediately report any heart pain that might indicate another heart attack or angina. Risk reduction is another focus of your visit. Provide positive feedback for his attempts at diet revision and walking. Encourage other health promotion activities such as proper use of medications to reduce the risk of another heart attack and control blood pressure. Reinforce care of incisions to prevent infection. Discuss causes of stress and ways to control it, such as listening to music, talking, or relaxing. In closing the visit, provide praise for all that Mr. and Mrs. Brown have done, review symptoms to report, and leave opportunities for health promotion.

Chapter 28

Express your concern for Ms. Simpson's discomfort, and explain the rationale for the fluid restriction. Then offer her sugar-free candy or gum. Allow her to rinse her mouth with a sip of water. Tell her to swish it around in her mouth and then spit it out before she swallows the fluid. Also, perform frequent oral care. Ms. Simpson may use mouthwashes, but be sure that they are alcohol free since alcohol has a drying effect. Moisten her lips with a water-soluble lubricant to prevent drying and cracking.

Chapter 29

The Isocal has to be diluted with water to obtain a half-strength solution. For a can containing 240 mL, you should add 240 mL of water. Only prepare one can of Isocal at a time. You do not want large volumes of tube feeding hanging for a long time—warm formula can support microbial growth. Although aspiration is less likely with a gastrostomy tube than with a nasogastric (NG) tube, tube placement is important to assess before starting feeding. Quickly inject air into the tube, listening over the gastric area for a swoosh or aspirate gastric contents from the tube. Position Gina in a semi- or high-Fowler's position to prevent gastric reflux and possible aspiration.

Chapter 30

Assess Ms. Nelson's feet, looking for injuries such as blisters, cuts, and abrasions. Examine areas for inflammation, infection, burns, edema, or other problems. Identify what Ms. Nelson understands about foot care and have her explain how she performs it. Caution her about the need for careful foot care in order to maintain skin integrity. Explain the importance of wearing socks and good fitting shoes at all times to prevent injury. Injury can occur without her knowledge because of her decreased sensation. Explain that using an emery board on skin will traumatize it, possibly causing breakdown that will then have difficulty healing. Enlisting Ms. Nelson as an active participant in preventing foot trauma or injury is essential—sharing some of the negative consequences of poor foot care may help. Encourage her to seek professional care for her feet if needed and to call the clinic at any time with questions about her feet and skin.

Chapter 31

Risk factors that increase the likelihood of infection include abdominal surgery, which breaks skin integrity; abdominal incision and pain level, which promote shallow respirations; reluctance to move, which promotes shallow breathing and increases the likelihood of atelectasis (which can cause a respiratory infection); history of asthma, which indicates a chronic respiratory problem; and age, which decreases the natural defense mechanisms to fight infection.

The most important factor that supports infection is a high fever (38°C). Low-grade fevers often occur postoperatively due to stress and inflammation, but when high fevers are present, infection should be ruled out, especially in light of Mr. Foscarelli's risk factors for respiratory infection. Elevated respiratory rate, shallow breathing, and a productive cough support this. Pulse rate is elevated due to the increased metabolic rate. Diminished breath sounds might indicate atelectasis (alveolar collapse), and rhonchi indicate secretions in the bronchioles, which can occur with respiratory infections such as pneumonia.

Mr. Foscarelli's primary care provider will probably order a white blood cell count with a differential, looking for an elevated leukocyte count and a shift to the left to confirm infection. A sputum culture and sensitivity will be obtained (before giving antibiotics) to identify the organism and determine appropriate antibiotic therapy. Because the culture results are not available for 48 hours, a Gram stain is usually done to help guide early antibiotic therapy. A chest x-ray will also be ordered.

Chapter 32

Answer to first Apply Your Critical Thinking feature in Chapter 32:

An amount of 100 mL is not an adequate volume for a void. A person usually has the urge to void when 250 to 400 mL are in the bladder. This volume stretches the detrusor muscle, which stimulates the parasympathetic nervous system and alerts the brain that the bladder is full. When an indwelling catheter has been in place for an extended period, the bladder may lose tone, contributing to urinary retention. Because the color of Mr. Phillips's urine is light yellow, he is not volume depleted. If during the past before 6 hours he has only voided 100 mL (less than 20 mL/hour), he is not emptying his bladder completely, which could lead to urinary tract infection (UTI). Bladder ultrasound or in-and-out catheterization can evaluate postvoid residual volumes.

Answer to second Apply Your Critical Thinking feature in Chapter 32:

Report Mr. Sanchez's change in status to his physician. Acute confusion has many different causes in older adults but commonly results from UTI. The indwelling Foley catheter and the following data also support this tentative diagnosis for Mr. Sanchez: low-grade fever (older adults often do not have a high temperature with infection), low urine output, and cloudy sediment in urine. Some agencies allow you to obtain a urine culture and sensitivity for suspected UTIs, but a physician must then sign this order.

Chapter 33

Irrigate the NG tube with normal saline as per physician orders. The absence of bowel sounds 2 days postoperatively is normal but indicates that the NG tube should remain in place to prevent abdominal distention. Absence of NG drainage indicates that the tube is probably plugged, especially because the gastric drainage was viscous and contained mucus. Complaints of nausea also support the conclusion that the NG tube is not functioning properly. If after irrigating the NG tube it still is not draining, reposition the tube by advancing it 1 inch. Know that this action is contraindicated if the patient has had gastric surgery. If the NG tube still does not drain, notify the physician.

Chapter 34

Although Mrs. Wilson has come to you for help with her sleep difficulties, it is likely that her husband has the most serious problem. Loud snoring is a symptom of sleep apnea, which warrants a full medical evaluation. Suggest to Mrs. Wilson that she ask her husband to come in for an examination and a possible referral to a sleep clinic. Hypnotics can be used as a short-term method to induce sleep, but these pharmacologic agents usually affect sleep quality. Trying nonpharmacologic methods first is a better way to try to improve sleep.

Chapter 35

First complete a comprehensive pain assessment, including checking his eMAR to determine what pain medications he has received in the past 24 hours. Mr. Ward needs his pain well managed to be able to actively participate in physical therapy to regain enough mobility to be safely discharged. It is also important that his pain be managed on oral medications because he cannot go home on IV morphine. He should have received Percocet before the PCA was discontinued. If he did not, it is likely that his pain is out of control, and he may require the IV morphine. Because the onset of Percocet is between 15 and 30 minutes, and the peak effect of the medication is within 1 hour, the best choice is 2 Percocet now with a reassessment of pain 15 minutes prior to the physical therapy appointment. Explain that it will be important to control his pain on oral medication before discharge. Also it will be important to monitor the total amount of acetaminophen he is receiving, including the round-the-clock Tylenol and the acetaminophen in the Percocet PRN. Limit acetaminophen to 4 g/24 hours to avoid liver toxicity.

Chapter 36

Discuss with Mr. Myer when he first noticed this blurring of his central vision. Identify whether he has peripheral vision and can move about safely. Do not just assume that he is confused. Mr. Myer may have developed some degenerative changes in the retina's macular area that are distorting his sensory input. Help him to clarify his limited vision versus confusion. Reassurance and reassessment of his vision may be very helpful.

Chapter 37

Assess specifically whether Mr. Moran is oriented to person, place, and time. Complete the neurologic assessment (level of consciousness [LOC] reflexes, sensory, and motor function), noting any significant changes from previous readings. Assess Mr. Moran's ability to understand simple directions and willingness to comply with requests (such as staying in bed). You may want to assess his normal alcohol intake because withdrawal from alcohol can cause delirium.

Try to speak calmly to him, listening to his concerns. Use touch and good communication skills. If he appears disoriented, explain where he is and what happened. Explain why the IV is in place. Keep his call light within reach, and hopefully move him to a room close to the nursing station, where he can be constantly observed. Inquire if he has family who might be able to come sit with him. If the confusion continues and he poses a risk to himself or others, a sitter may need to be employed to stay with him. Medications are contraindicated in this situation because of the head trauma.

Chapter 38

To begin with, assess Boden's height and weight to determine the ratio in terms of norms for his age. Determine whether there is a big discrepancy and whether you should refer them on to a dietitian. Explore with Boden what his feelings are about gym, the other children, and how he might be able to manage them. Having his father become involved with the situation might be useful so that Boden can understand that his father understands his feelings and helps him work through them. Bringing both parents into Boden's support system can help him feel less alone.

Boden and his parents may want to talk the situation over with the gym coach and school counselor. This problem with gym attendance is common for middle and high school boys so they may be able to offer some insights into what is occurring within the gym and with the interactions with other classmates.

Chapter 39

Young children frequently fall and injure themselves. Your assessment reveals some data, however, that may indicate child abuse (i.e., the child's stoic nature, avoidance of eye contact, multiple bruises). Try to ascertain as much information as possible from the mother, asking her to outline how the incident occurred. Speak with the boyfriend separately for his description of the incident. Compare the individual descriptions for consistency. Closely observe nonverbal behaviors during the interview. If after the interviews you suspect child abuse, you are required by law to report your suspicions to child protective authorities. The law requires all healthcare workers to report any incident of suspected abuse so that a follow-up investigation may occur.

Chapter 40

Paulie's mother is in shock. Her son's death was completely unexpected and just occurred. Help mobilize support for her and her husband. Do not falsely reassure them that all will be well. Recognize and honor any display of grief. Provide for their physical safety by making sure that they have a ride home from the hospital.

Chapter 41

The symptoms are due to stimulation of the sympathetic nervous system as a response to stress. Stress response is affected by how the individual interprets stimuli. Your concern about the test is heightened by the fact that you did poorly on the first test and probably need to do well now to obtain the grade you desire in the course. Using some relaxation techniques (e.g., slow breathing, focusing) may help decrease your anxiety. Overall, take good care of yourself. Sleeping and eating properly before an exam will help you think clearly as you ponder the correct answers to the test questions. If test anxiety is an ongoing problem, use available resources (such as a learning center or counseling center) to develop strategies that will help ensure your success.

Chapter 42

Start by expressing that the question is good and that you are glad they felt comfortable enough to approach you. Ask each student to discuss why he or she thinks a person can or cannot get pregnant during menstruation. Then give students the correct answer, explaining why it is correct. Assess the need for additional sex information, provide pamphlets, and see if other members of the class might like to participate in an informal discussion about sexuality. If the students seem receptive, you might encourage them to participate in the planning process. Explain when you will be in the health office if they (or their friends) have questions.

Chapter 43

Because faith is highly personal, you need to reflect the question back to her rather than answer about your personal experience. Rather than wanting to know the details about you, she may be seeking someone to listen to her concerns. Explore with her the kind of help you can assist her with. If this facility has a chaplain, ask her if she would like to visit with that person. If there is a particular church or religious group that she prefers, offer to make contact for her.

Appendix C

Abbreviations Commonly Used in Documentation

Abbreviation	Meaning
ā	before
abd	abdomen
ac	before meals
ADLs	activities of daily living
amp.	ampule
ant.	anterior
AP	anterior–posterior
ax.	axillary
b.i.d.	twice a day
BP	blood pressure
BR	bed rest; bathroom
BRP	bathroom privileges
C	Centigrade
c̄	with
caps	capsule
CVP	central venous pressure
c/o	complains of
drsg	dressing
ext	external
F	Fahrenheit
fx.	fracture, fractional
gm	gram
gtt	Drop; drip
h	hour
HOB	head of bed
hx	history
I & O	intake and output
IM	intramuscular

Abbreviation	Meaning
IV	intravenous
kg	kilogram
KVO	keep vein open
L	left; liter
lat	lateral
MAE	moves all extremities
mg	milligram
ml, mL	milliliter
NAD	no apparent distress
NG	nasogastric
noc	night
NPO	nothing by mouth
OOB	out of bed
oz	ounce
p̄	after
p.c.	after meals
post	Posterior; after
prep	preparation
prn	when necessary
q	every
q, 2 (3, 4, etc.) hours	every 2 (3, 4, etc.) hours
R/O	rule out
ROM	range of motion
s̄	without
SBA	stand by assistance
SL	sublingual
SOB	shortness of breath
sol, soln	solution

Abbreviation	Meaning
spec	specimen
S/P	status post
sp. gr.	specific gravity
stat	immediately
tab	tablet
t.i.d.	three times a day
TKO	to keep open
TO	telephone order
TPN	total parenteral nutrition
TPR	temperature, pulse, respiration
tsp	teaspoon
TWE	tap water enema
VO	verbal order
VS	vital signs
VSS	vital signs stable
W/C	wheelchair
WNL	within normal limits

Selected Abbreviations Used for Specific Descriptions

Abbreviation	Meaning
AKA	above-knee amputation
ASCVD	arteriosclerotic cardiovascular disease
ASHD	arteriosclerotic heart disease
BKA	below-knee amputation
ca	cancer
CCU	critical care unit
chest clear to A & P	chest clear to auscultation and percussion
CMS	circulation movement sensation
CNS	central nervous system; clinical nurse specialist
D5W	5% dextrose in water
DJD	degenerative joint disease
DOE	dyspnea on exertion
DTs	delirium tremens
ED	Emergency department
FUO	fever of unknown origin
GB	gallbladder
GI	gastrointestinal
GYN	gynecology
H_2O_2	hydrogen peroxide
HA	hyperalimentation; headache
HEENT	head, ear, eye, nose, throat

Abbreviation	Meaning
HF	heart failure (also CHF, congestive heart failure)
HPI	history of present illness
ICU	intensive care unit
I & D	incision and drainage
L & D	labor and delivery
LLE	left lower extremity
LLQ	left lower quadrant
LOC	level of consciousness
LMP	last menstrual period
LUE	left upper extremity
LUQ	left upper quadrant
MI	myocardial infarction
Neuro	neurology; neurosurgery
NS	normal saline
NWB	non-weight bearing
O.D.	overdose
ORIF	open reduction internal fixation
Ortho	orthopedics
OT	occupational therapy
PACU	postanesthesia care unit
PE	physical examination; pulmonary embolism; pulmonary edema
PERRLA	pupils equal, round, and react to light and accommodation
PID	pelvic inflammatory disease
PM & R	physical medicine and rehabilitation
Psych	psychology; psychiatric
PT	physical therapy
RL (or LR)	Ringer's lactate; lactated Ringer's
RLE	right lower extremity
RLQ	right lower quadrant
RT	respiratory therapy
RUE	right upper extremity
RUQ	right upper quadrant
Rx	prescription
STSG	split-thickness skin graft
Surg	surgery, surgical
T & A	tonsillectomy and adenoidectomy
THR, TJR, TKR	total hip replacement; total joint replacement; total knee replacement

Abbreviation	Meaning
URI	upper respiratory infection
UTI	urinary tract infection
vag	vaginal
VD	venereal disease
WNWD	well nourished, well developed
Selected Abbreviations Related to Common Diagnostic Tests	
BE	barium enema
B.M.R.	basal metabolism rate
Ca^{++}	calcium
CT	computed tomography
CBC	complete blood count
Cl^-	chloride
C & S	culture and sensitivity
Dx	diagnosis
ECG, EKG	electrocardiogram
EEG	electroencephalogram
FBS	fasting blood sugar
hct	hematocrit
Hgb	hemoglobin
IVP	intravenous pyelogram
K^+	potassium
LP	lumbar puncture
MRI	magnetic resonance imaging
Na^+	sodium
RBC	red blood cell
UA	urinalysis
UGI	upper gastrointestinal x-ray
WBC	white blood cell

Abbreviation	Meaning
Commonly Used Symbols	
>	greater than
<	less than
=	equal to
≈	approximately equal to
≤	less than or equal to
≥	equal to or greater than
↑	increased
↓	decreased
♀	female
♂	male
°	degree
#	number or pound
×	times
@	at
+	positive
–	negative
±	positive or negative
F_1	first filial generation
F_2	second filial generation
PaO_2	partial pressure of arterial oxygen
$PaCO_2$	partial pressure of arterial carbon dioxide
:	ratio
∴	therefore
%	percent
2°	secondary/due to
Δ	change

Glossary

A

Abrasion: Wound in which skin or mucous membranes are rubbed or scraped away

Abscess: A localized collection of white blood cells and cellular debris (pus) that appears swollen and inflamed

Absorption: The process by which a medication enters the bloodstream

Abuse: Nonaccidental use of force resulting in physical, sexual, emotional, or involve threats or intimidation, or economic deprivation

Accessory muscles: Scalene and sternomastoid muscles of the neck and shoulders

Accommodation: Test that engages a patient to look at a close object and then look at a distant object to see whether patient's pupils constrict to focus on the close object and dilate to see the distant object

Acid: Any substance capable of releasing hydrogen ions in solution

Active euthanasia: Physician- or nurse-caused death that deliberately hastens a person's death and may be considered murder in many states

Active transport: Movement of substances across a cell membrane against an electrochemical gradient

Activity intolerance: Physical inability to withstand activity

Actual nursing diagnosis: An existing human response to a health problem the nurse identifies that is amenable to nursing intervention

Acupuncture: Component of traditional Chinese medicine based on the principle of inserting very fine needles into various areas of the body to stimulate the meridians and promote harmony within the system

Acute pain: Pain that lasts less than 6 months

Adaptation: Process by which a person changes to conform to the environment

Addiction: A maladaptive or compulsive use of a substance for effects that are not therapeutic

Adherence: The extent to which health behavior reflects a health plan constructed and agreed to by the patient as a partner

Adjuvant: Medication added to a regime, often in pain management, to increase therapeutic effects (e.g., antidepressant used in addition to opioid to manage chronic pain)

Advanced care planning: The process of thinking about, talking about, and planning for healthcare and end-of-life care

Advance directive: Written document (e.g., living will) that states in advance a patient's desires about the types of healthcare he or she wishes to receive should the patient become unable to decide

Advanced practice nurse: Nurse who has advanced degrees and certification (e.g., nurse practitioner)

Adverse drug effect: Any effect other than the therapeutic effect

Advocacy: Communicating and acting on behalf of another person's welfare, especially a patient in the healthcare system; keeping the patient informed about treatment and nursing care

Aerobic exercise: Exercise that requires oxygen for energy and involves elevation of heart rate for an extended period

Aesthetics/spirituality: Communion with families that strives to accomplish knowledge of health through the arts, exploration of alternative and complementary therapies, and experience of self-awareness, faith, hope, and love

Afebrile: State of normal body temperature in a patient

Affective: Refers to emotional reactions or feelings

Agnosticism: Belief that God's reality is unknown and unknowable

Agranulocytes: Mononuclear cells that lack digestive enzymes

Air embolism: Air bubble in the vascular space that may obstruct circulation

Allodynia: Enhanced sensation of pain produced by an innocuous stimulus, such as a light touch

Allopathic medicine: Traditional Western medicine

Allostasis: Capacity of physiologic systems to maintain stability through change

Allostatic load: Wear and tear on the body, which grows over time as the individual is exposed to repeated or chronic stress

Alopecia: Hair loss

Altered family function: Manifestations that include structural, functional, developmental, and systems changes in a family

Alveoli: Spherical, saclike epithelial structures in the lungs through which gas exchange occurs

American Nurses Association: Professional nursing organization concerned with all aspects of professional nursing provides standards and leadership for the profession comprised of individual state nursing associations and also has nursing specialty bodies representing all nursing practice areas

Anaerobes: Organisms requiring reduced oxygen for growth often associated with serious infections

Anaerobic exercise: Exercise in which muscles cannot extract enough oxygen, and anaerobic pathways are used to provide additional energy for a short time; useful in endurance training

Anaphylactic reaction: A severe allergic reaction that requires immediate medical intervention because it can be fatal

Andragogy: Adult learning theory

Anesthesiologist: Physician who specializes in anesthesia administration

Angina: Pain and discomfort about the heart, characteristic of myocardial ischemia; severe pain felt in the anterior chest, shoulder, left arm, neck, and jaw

Anions: Negatively charged ions

Anomia: Problems with word retrieval

Anonymity: Protection of a research participant in such a way that the participant cannot be linked to the information provided

Anorexia: Loss of appetite

Anorexia nervosa: Eating disorder in which the person refuses to eat from fear of becoming overweight, even with normal or less than ideal body weight

Antagonism: Interaction of chemicals by which drug effects decrease

Antagonist: Pharmacologic agent that binds with a receptor but does not produce a physiologic response or block the effect of an agonist

Anterior-posterior (AP) diameter: Distance between the sternum and vertebral column, drawn as a straight line through the thorax

Antibodies: Circulate in the bloodstream and interact with antigens they encounter; also called immunoglobulins

Anticipatory grief: Pattern of psychological and physiologic responses a person makes to the impending loss (real or imagined) of a significant person, object, belief, or relationship

Anticipatory guidance: Information given to a patient about a situation before it occurs so the patient can develop problem solving and coping strategies

Antigens: Substances that provoke irritation or damage to the body tissues and induce the formation of antibodies

Antiseptic: Agent that stops or slows the growth of microorganisms on living tissue, commonly used for handwashing, skin preparation, and wound packing or irrigation

Anuria: Formation and excretion of less than 100 mL of urine in 24 hours

Aphasia: Communication disorder that may affect speech, reading, and writing

Apnea: Absence of respiration; a potentially serious sleep disorder in which breathing repeatedly stops and starts; may be obstructive or central in origin

Appraisal: The process of interpreting a situation and determining if it is a stress

Approximated: Lightly pulled together

Arterial blood gas (ABG): Laboratory test that provides more specific information concerning patient's acid–base status and response to oxygen therapy

Arterial oxygen saturation (SpO₂): Percent of hemoglobin saturated with oxygen; measured by pulse oximeter

Arthroscopy: Direct visualization of a joint by insertion of a scope

Articulation: Enunciation of words and sentences

Ascites: Accumulation of serous fluid in the peritoneum

Asepsis: Absence of disease-producing microorganisms

Asphyxiation: Lack of oxygen, leading to cell death

Assault: Threat of touching a person without his or her consent

Assessment: First phase of the nursing process in which data are gathered to identify actual or potential health problems

Assisted suicide: Providing the patient with a means to end life, but not the direct action that results in death

Ataxia: Impaired muscle coordination

Athetosis: Movement characterized by slow, irregular, twisting motions

Atelectasis: Collapse of alveoli

Atheism: Denial of God's existence

Atrophy: Wasting away of an organ, muscle, or body tissue

Attention: Ability to concentrate on and take in specific sensory stimuli

Attitude: A person's dispositions toward an object or situation; can be a mental or emotional mind-set and positive or negative

Audiometer: Device in hearing tests that uses headphones capable of transmitting sounds of different frequencies

Audit: Review of records

Auscultation: Technique of listening to body sounds with a stethoscope

Auscultatory gap: Absence of audible sounds during blood pressure measurement that may cause inaccurate readings

Automaticity: Heart's capability of generating its own electrical impulse, which is then conducted through specialized conduction fibers

Autonomy: Degree of discretion and independence a practitioner has

B

Bacteremia: Presence of bacteria in the blood

Bactericidal: Able to kill bacteria

Bacteriostatic: Able to inhibit the growth of bacteria

Bariatric equipment: Depending on the patient's weight, may be required to hold the increased weight and accommodate larger size, as well as provide additional support

Baroreceptors: Stretch receptors located in major arteries and veins that monitor vascular volume

Basal metabolism: Amount of energy required to carry out involuntary activities at rest

Base (or alkali): Any substance that can combine with and decrease hydrogen ions in solution; alkali

Batch charting: Waiting until the end of the shift to record events on several patients

Battery: Unlawful touching of a person's body without his or her consent

Behaviors: Observable actions

Beliefs: Ideas that a person accepts as true

Beneficence: Doing or promoting good, the basis for all healthcare

Bereavement: Response to the death of a significant person

Binders: Large bandages used to support a body part or to hold a dressing in place

Biofeedback: A technique in which the patient learns voluntary control over autonomic functions

Bioterrorism: The use of biologic agents to compromise safety and to cause fear

Bisexual: Relating to both men and women sexually

Bladder ultrasound (BUS): A noninvasive technology that can estimate the volume of urine in the bladder

Blended family: Two parents with unrelated children who are being raised together

Blood pressure: Force the blood exerts against the walls of the blood vessels

Body image: Feelings about one's body

Body mechanics: Positioning or moving the body to prevent or to correct problems related to activity or immobilization

Borborygmi: Loud, rumbling sounds produced by the normal movement of gas through the intestines, referred to as "stomach growling"

Botanicals (Herbs): Plant species with medicinal properties

Bradycardia: Abnormally slow heart rate (usually less than 60 beats per minute in adults)

Bradypnea: Abnormally slow respiratory rate (usually less than 10 breaths per minute in adults)

Brain death: Irreversible cessation of heart and lung functions or an irreversible loss of all functions of the entire brain

Bronchial breath sounds: Loud, high-pitched sounds, with a hollow quality often compared to the sound of air blowing through a pipe

Bronchioles: Narrow airways that conduct air into alveolar ducts and alveoli

Bronchospasm: Narrowing of the bronchioles caused by tightening of the smooth muscles in the airways

Bruits: Sounds heard with auscultation; due to turbulent blood flow, such as occurs in partially obstructed blood vessels, tight or floppy heart valves, or dialysis fistulas

Buccal: Pertaining to the inside cheek

Buffers: Compounds that help stabilize the pH of a solution by neutralizing added acid or base

Bundle: A combination of patient care elements that can be consistently implemented to reduce harm

Burns: Injuries caused by exposure to thermal, chemical, electrical, or radioactive energy

C

Calorie (kilocalorie): Unit of heat, commonly used to describe the energy value of food

Capacity: Mental or physical ability to make healthcare decisions

Capillary refill time: Simple test of circulatory status that uses the nailbeds

Capnography: Displaying the results of end-tidal carbon dioxide monitoring in a graphic display

Capnometry: Displaying results of end-tidal carbon dioxide monitoring in a numeric display

Carbohydrates: Food group containing simple and complex sugars composed of carbon, hydrogen, and oxygen

Cardiac biomarkers: Proteins that are released from cells when tissue damage occurs

Cardiac output: The amount of blood pumped by the heart each minute

Care plan conference: Meeting to discuss revisions to the plan of care and coordination of care

Caries: Cavities in the tooth enamel

Carriers: Person from whom a microorganism can be cultured but who shows no sign of a disease

Case management: Professional approach to providing care in which one provider coordinates a patient's services

Catheter-associated urinary tract infection (CAUTI): A urinary tract infection that develops when an indwelling urinary catheter is in place greater than 2 days prior to the onset of infection

Catheter-related bloodstream infection (CRBSI): A bloodstream infection due to an invasive vascular device.

Cations: Positively charged ions

Celibacy: Abstention from sexual intercourse

Centers for Medicare and Medicaid Services (CMS): A federal organization that pays for healthcare for low-income and elderly people and tracks healthcare outcomes

Central sensitization: Nociceptive nerve signals triggered by inflammation or nerve injury bombard the central nervous system from the periphery

Central venous catheter: Catheter whose tip is placed in the superior vena cava or at the entrance of the right atrium

Certified registered nurse anesthetist (CRNA): Professional with specialized education and skills in the administration of general or regional anesthesia anesthetic agents and in monitoring patients during surgical and other procedures

Cerumen: Earwax

Charge nurse: Nurse responsible for the functioning of a nursing unit for a particular work shift

Charting by exception (CBE): Charting in which the nurse documents only those findings that fall outside the standard of care and norms the institution has developed

Chemical name: The name for a medication based on its molecular structure

Chorea: Spontaneous, brief, involuntary muscle twitching of the limbs or facial muscles

Chronic illness: Ongoing or constant physical or mental disease

Chronic pain: Pain that lasts more than 6 months

Circadian rhythms: Regular occurrence of certain phenomena in cycles of about 24 hours

Circle of confidentiality: Those who have access to a patient's information like the people in a nursing unit who have responsibility for the patient as well as the family, unless the patient objects

Circulating nurse: Nurse who manages patient care in the operating room environment and protects the patient's safety and health needs

Circulation, movement, and sensation (CMS): Areas evaluated when an acute problem with a limb is possible

Civil law: The body of law that deals with relationships between private individuals

Climacteric: Menopause

Clinical experience: Use of knowledge, critical thinking, and past performance to solve problems

Clinical nurse specialist: Registered nurse who holds a master's degree in a nursing specialty and has advanced clinical experience

Clinical pathways: Models for ensuring quality of care, providing direction about major interventions to perform for a specific condition

Clinical reasoning: Use of critical thinking to question why the patient has an abnormal finding

Clitoris: Small, erectile organ located just above the urinary meatus in females; plays a key role in female orgasm

***Clostridium difficile* (*C. diff*):** Organism that causes a severe gastrointestinal infection resulting in frequent loose and often bloody bowel movements; the most common cause of hospital-acquired diarrhea in the United States

Clubbing: Swelling in the nails that flattens the profile angle to 180 degrees or less

Cluster: Patient data combined into meaningful patterns

Cochrane Database of Systematic Reviews (CDSR): Database containing systematic reviews and protocols (reviews still in progress) of the effects of healthcare interventions

Cognition: Thinking and awareness; system by which sensory input, past experiences, and emotions are integrated and made meaningful

Cognitive: Rational thought, what one generally considers "thinking"

Cognitive reframing: A coping skill that helps one to alter or reframe one's perception of an event and helps us overcome catastrophic thinking about an event

Cohabited family: People living together without the formal or legal bond of marriage

Collaboration: Actions taken in coordination with other professionals

Collaborative health problems: Problems based on medical diagnoses, medically ordered treatments, or other related problems that require interdependent standards and activities to be addressed

Colloid: Fluids that contain proteins or starch molecules

Colonization: State in which a microorganism is present but no immune reaction or tissue destruction occurs

Colonoscopy: An endoscopic procedure that can visualize the colon up to the ileocecal valve

Colostomy: Opening of a part of the colon onto the abdominal skin surface

Coma: Abnormally deep stupor occurring in illness or as a result of injury; external stimuli fail to arouse the patient

Commode: Portable chair with a toilet seat and a waste receptacle beneath that can be emptied so a patient who cannot walk to the bathroom can manage toileting

Communal family: Related and unrelated people with common goals and beliefs who share a household

Communicable disease: Disease transmissible between hosts

Communicable period: The time frame during which a disease can be passed from one person to another

Communication: Interchange of information

Communication channel: Medium through which a message is sent (e.g., television, writing, speaking)

Community: Social group whose members may or may not share common geographic boundaries but who interact because of common interests or shared values to meet their needs within a larger society

Community-based healthcare: Healthcare directed toward a specific group within the community

Community-based no code order: Document that requires the signatures of the primary physician or nurse practitioner and the patient or legal surrogate and allows emergency medical personnel, if called, to provide care and support to patient and family without resuscitation

Community-based nursing care: Nursing care directed toward a specific group or population within the community; may be provided for individuals or groups

Community resources: Economic stability, social and health supports, and cultural norms

Comparative effectiveness research (CER): A systematic research design comparing the effectiveness of different interventions

Compassion fatigue: When nurses continue to care for their patients, in addition to their families and significant others, but become unable to care for themselves

Competency: Ability to understand rights and responsibilities

Complement system: Series of proteins found in the bloodstream that enhances phagocytosis of microbes, helps in lysis of bacterial cell walls, and encourages the inflammatory response

Complementary and alternative medicine (CAM): Those practices that do not form part of the dominant system for managing health and disease

Complete proteins: Proteins that contain sufficient amounts of essential amino acids to maintain body tissues and to promote body growth

Compliance: (1) Adherence to recommended plan; (2) Measure of the lung's "stretchiness"

Comprehension: Capacity for understanding and reasoning

Comprehensive health assessment: Assessment that encompasses the physical, psychological, social, and spiritual dimensions of living

Compromised Family Coping: State in which a usually supportive primary person is providing insufficient, ineffective, or modified support, comfort, assistance, or encouragement that the patient may need to manage or to master adaptive tasks related to his or her health challenge

Computer-based personal record (CPR): Record of a patient's health saved on and easily accessed by computer system

Computerized physician (provider) order entry (CPOE): Allows authorized providers to enter all orders directly into the computer, electronically communicating orders to the laboratory, pharmacy, and nursing personnel

Concentrative meditation: Activity involving a person's focusing on a specific internal object or an external object to tune and train the mind, leading to greater efficiency in everyday life

Concept map: A graphical tool for organizing and representing knowledge

Conceptual framework: Formal explanation that links concepts and emphasizes relationships among them

Condom catheter: Noninvasive urinary collection device for incontinent male patients; consists of a thin, flexible sheath placed over the penis and attached to tubing and a collection bag

Confidentiality: Practice of keeping patient information private

Consciousness: State of awareness and full responsiveness to stimuli

Constipation: Infrequent, sometimes painful passage of hard, dry stool

Consults: Ordering by a physician of a specialist or a health team member to provide expert opinions or specialized care for a patient

Continuity of care: Provision of uninterrupted service as a patient moves between settings

Contractility: Force of contraction

Contracture: Shortening of a muscle and loss of joint mobility from fibrotic changes in the tissues surrounding the joint

Controlled substances: Drugs that are considered to have either limited medical use or high potential for abuse or addiction

Coordination: Care for a patient and family that requires development of plans of care that maximize the person's ability to remain in a safe environment

Coping: Problem-solving process a person uses to manage stress

Coping mechanisms: Efforts used to manage stress

Core temperature: Internal body temperature

Crackles: Adventitious breath sound

Crepitus: Grating feeling and pain that accompany problems with the temporal mandibular joint

Crime: Violation of the law punishable by the state

Criminal law: A type of public law that deals with the public's safety and welfare

Critical thinking: Purposeful process that is disciplined, active, multidimensional, reasonable, rational, and reflective to arrive at insight and draw conclusions

Crystalloid: Fluids that are clear

Cues: Pieces of data, subjective or objective, about a patient

Cultural diversity: Plurality of ideas and opinions for behavior to which people are exposed, adding to the texture and complexity of a society

Cultural relativity: Principle that meaning is created by one's culture and truth is culture-specific; the same experience may carry different meanings to people of different cultures

Culturally competent nursing: Nursing that has the "attitudes, knowledge, and skills necessary to provide quality care to diverse populations" American Association of Colleges in Nursing (2014, p. 1). *Cultural Competency in Baccalaureate Nursing Education.* Retrieved from http://www.aacn.nche. edu/education-resources/cultural-competency

Culture: (1) A society's behavior and institutions; (2) Growth of microorganisms in a specialized medium under precise conditions

Culture change: Dynamic in which a culture evolves as people come into contact with new beliefs and ideas

Culture shock: Failure to comprehend the culture in which one is living

Cyanosis: Grayish, bluish, or purplish skin tone

Cycling: Interruption of an intravenous infusion for a period of time

Cystectomy: A urinary diversion procedure in which the bladder is surgically removed

Cystocele: The protrusion or herniation of the bladder into the vaginal canal

D

Dangling: Preliminary step to ambulation, especially for patients who may be unable to ambulate initially, which involves sitting on the side of the bed with the legs dependent

Death: Cessation of heart-lung function, or of whole-brain function, or of higher-brain function

Debridement: Removal of foreign material or dying tissue from a wound

Decode: Process of understanding a message

Deep tissue injury (DTI): Purple or maroon localized area of discolored intact skin or blood-filled blister due to damage of underlying soft tissue from pressure and/or shear that is unstageable

Deep vein thrombosis (DVT): A thrombus originating in the large veins of the legs because of the relatively low velocity of blood flow there

Defecation reflex: Involuntary response of intestinal contraction and anal sphincter relaxation to rectal distention

Dehiscence: Accidental separation of wound edges, especially a surgical wound

Delegation: Transferring to a competent person the authority to perform a selected nursing task in a selected situation

Delirium: Reversible disorder of cognition; confusion

Delusions: Beliefs that are not based in reality and that reflects an unconscious need or fear

Dementia: Cognitive impairment as the result of irreversible organic changes in brain cell function

Denuded: Tissue that has lost the epithelial layer of skin

Dependent variable: Variable (or item of interest that varies) that is the outcome; hypothesized to depend on or be caused by another variable

Dermatitis: An inflammation of the skin

Dermatome: The band of skin innervated by the sensory root of a single spinal nerve

Dermis: Layer of skin beneath the epidermis; composed of dense connective fibers, blood vessels, nerves, hair follicles, and glands

Desquamation: Process in which the thin, outermost layer of the epidermis (the stratum corneum or horny layer) is continuously shed

Detrusor muscle: Smooth muscle of the urinary bladder

Development: Process of ongoing change throughout a person's life

Developmental stages: Points in life when old responsibilities are discarded and new ones are assumed

Developmental tasks: Psychomotor, psychosocial, or cognitive skills attained at certain stages of life that are prerequisites for successive skill development

Diagnostic reasoning: The process of gathering and clustering data to draw inferences and propose diagnoses

Diagnostic reasoning process: Skills used to make nursing diagnoses

Diaphragmatic excursion: Percussion of the posterior diaphragm and measurement of the difference between complete exhalation and full inhalation

Diarrhea: Frequent evacuation of watery stools

Diastole: Period of rest in the cardiac cycle, when the ventricles are not contracting and the coronary arteries are filling with blood

Diastolic blood pressure: Pressure in the blood vessels during cardiac ventricular relaxation

Diffusion: Movement of molecules from an area of higher concentration to one of lower concentration

Digestion: Mechanical and chemical processes necessary to convert food to an absorbable state

Disabled Family Coping: Behavior of a significant person (family member or other primary person) that disables his or her own and the patient's capacities to effectively address tasks essential to either person's adaptation to the health challenge

Disaccharide: Simple sugar

Discharge planning: Process of coordinating, planning, and arranging for the transition from one healthcare setting to another

Disease: State of disharmony of mind, body, emotions, and spirit

Disease prevention activities: Avoidance behaviors that seek to prevent specific diseases or conditions

Disinfectant: Chemical used to kill microorganisms on lifeless objects

Distention: Condition of being stretched or inflated

Distribution: Process by which a drug passes from the circulation of the blood and lymphatic system across cell membranes to a specified tissue

Diuresis: Formation and excretion of large amounts of urine

Diuretic: Medications administered to remove body fluid by increasing urine output

Do not resuscitate (DNR) orders: Orders not to provide resuscitation in the event of cardiopulmonary arrest

Documentation: Written communication of patient information and care

Drug: Substance that alters physiologic function with the potential for affecting health

Drug incompatibility: When an intravenous drug precipitates from solutions, or becomes chemically inactive, if mixed with other medications

Durable power of attorney for healthcare: Advance directive that allows a person to designate another to make decisions if the patient becomes incapacitated and cannot make independent decisions

Dying: End-of-life process in which the lungs become less efficient for gas diffusion and oxygenation, the heart and blood vessels become inadequate to maintain circulation and to perfuse tissues, and the brain ceases to regulate vital centers

Dysarthria: Disorders affecting either single or combined motor control of the muscles of speech

Dysfunctional grief: Grief that falls outside normal parameters; may manifest as absence of, delayed, exaggerated, or prolonged grief

Dyspareunia: Painful sexual intercourse

Dysphagia: Inability to swallow

Dyspnea: Breathing that requires marked effort

Dysrhythmia: Abnormality in heart rhythm

Dystonia: Similar to athetosis but usually involves larger areas of the body

Dysuria: Painful voiding

E

Edema: Accumulation of fluid in the interstitial tissues

Elder Abuse and Mistreatment: Nonaccidental use of force resulting in physical, sexual, or emotional harm, or involving threats, intimidation, abandonment, or economic deprivation

Electrical shock: Interruption of body functions due to electrical current

Electrolytes: Chemical compounds that dissociate into ions when in solution; usually refers to extracellular sodium, potassium, and chloride

Electronic infusion device (EID): A drip chamber

Electronic medication administration record (eMAR): Interfaces medication orders with pharmacy dispensing and allows direct computer charting of medication administration

Elimination: Act of voiding or expelling waste material from the bowels

Empathy: Ability to understand how another person sees a situation, while maintaining objectivity

Encoding: Process of translating the purpose of a communication into a message that can be sent

End-tidal CO$_2$ (EtCO$_2$): Carbon dioxide measured at the end of exhalation (end-tidal); is a sensitive indicator of adequacy of ventilation

Endocardium: The innermost layer of the heart

Endogenous (autogenous) opioids: Chemical substances with an opioid effect produced by the body

Endotoxin: Potent substances released by bacteria into the blood that can cause shock

Endurance: Ability to withstand physical or other stressors over time

Enema: Insertion of fluid into the rectum and colon

Enhanced Family Coping: Family member's desire and readiness to use adaptive behaviors in response to the patient's health challenge

Enuresis: Involuntary voiding with underlying pathophysiologic origin after the age that bladder control is usually achieved; nocturnal enuresis is bedwetting

Environment: Context in which a person lives; includes social and inanimate characteristics

Epicardium: The outer layer of the heart

Epidermis: Thin, avascular, outermost skin layer

Epithelialization: Process in which epidermal cells, which appear pink in color, reproduce and migrate across the surface of the partial-thickness wound

Erectile dysfunction (ED): Impotence

Erythema: Redness, usually from irritation or inflammation

Ethics: Professional standards of behavior related to right and wrong

Ethnicity or ethnic identity: Shared cultural characteristics that symbolize a common group origin

Ethnocentrism: Use of one's own culture to judge the beliefs, behaviors, attitudes, and values of people of another culture

Eupnea: Normal respiratory rhythm and depth

Evaluation: Judgment of the effectiveness of nursing care in achieving patient goals

Evidence-based practice: Approach to healthcare that realizes that pathophysiologic reasoning and personal experience are necessary, but not sufficient, for making decisions and emphasizes decision making based on the best available evidence

Evisceration: Protrusion of internal organs through an open wound

Excretion: Process by which a drug or urine is eliminated from the body

Exogenous opioids: Opiate-like substances administered to the patient

Expressive aphasia: Communication disorder in which the patient understands and follows directions but cannot verbally and effectively communicate with the nurse

Expressive meditation: Meditation with whirling, shaking, or dancing

Extended-spectrum beta lactamases (ESBLs): Enzymes that give bacteria immunity to both penicillin and cephalosporin antibiotics

Extended family: Family structure that includes grandparents, aunts, uncles, and cousins

Extracellular fluid (ECF): Body fluid outside the cells; mainly interstitial fluid and plasma

Extravasation: When IV solutions inadvertently leak into the subcutaneous tissues

F

Facilitator: Coordinator of education, advocacy, spiritual communion, and case management

Faith: Belief held; a relational phenomena

Falls: Collapses, dropping down, or toppling

Family: Basic human social unit; membership is based on mutual commitment, heredity, or legal arrangements

Family-centered care: Caring for the patient and family as a unit

Fatigue: A subjective state of weariness; lack of energy

Fats: Lipid organic substances composed of carbon, hydrogen, and oxygen

Fecal impaction: The accumulation of hardened feces in the rectum

Fecal occult blood test (FOBT): Evaluates stool for blood that is not apparent upon visual examination

Feedback: In communication, the sender and receiver use one another's reactions to produce further messages

Fiber: Component of food that adds bulk to the diet and is not broken down by digestion

Fidelity: Being faithful to one's commitments and promises

Filtration: Passage of a solution through a semipermeable membrane from a region of higher pressure to a region of lower pressure

Financial resources: Allocation and expenditure of money

Fistula: Abnormal tubelike passage between organs or between an organ and the body surface, often as the result of poor wound healing

Flaccidity: Without muscle tone or resistance; decreased muscle tone

Flatus: Gas in the gastrointestinal tract

Flow sheet: Form for charting routine nursing assessments or procedures often in a chart or table format.

FOCUS system: Documentation system that organizes data entry around data (D), action (A), and response (R). The FOCUS can be a problem area but does not need to be. An entry can be positive growth or learning

Focused health assessment: Assessment based on the patient's problems; components include performing a general survey, taking vital signs, and assessing specific areas that relate to the problem

Foot drop: Temporary or permanent plantar flexion due to weakness or paralysis

Foreground questions: Those questions specific to a particular patient asked as part of use of the PICO model in nursing research

Foreplay: Sexual activity before sexual intercourse

Foreskin: Loose skin at the head of the penis, removed during circumcision; prepuce

Fraction of inspired oxygen concentration (FIO₂): The percentage of oxygen being inhaled; increased with oxygen administration

Friction: Occurs when two surfaces rub together

Functional health assessment: Assessment that evaluates the effects of the mind, body, and environment in relation to a person's ability to perform the tasks of daily living

Functional health patterns: A framework for collecting and organizing nursing assessment data to ascertain the patient's strengths and any actual or potential dysfunctional patterns

Futility: Situation in which interventions are unlikely to result in desirable state

G

Gait: Character of one's walk

Gallops: Auscultation of S3 and S4 heart sounds that is clearest at the apex when the patient is positioned on the left side

Gastric lavage: Irrigation of the stomach

Gastric residual volumes (GRVs): Volume aspirated from the stomach as a way to assess tolerance of enteral feeding

Gavage: Liquid instilled into the stomach through a nasogastric tube

General anesthetic: Agent used to induce complete loss of sensation and consciousness

General survey: Apparent state of health, level of consciousness, and signs of distress in a patient

General systems theory: A systems framework that assumes all systems must be goal directed; a system is more than the sum of its parts; a system is ever-changing and any change in one part affects the whole; boundaries are implicit and in human systems are open and dynamic

Generic name: A medication's name that is not owned by a company and is given by the United States Adopted Names Council; it is the drug's official name throughout its lifetime

Genetics: Characteristics determined by the DNA code inherited from biologic mother and father

Gingiva: Oral mucosa

Glasgow Coma Scale: Standardized assessment tool used when serial assessments are done for high-risk patients (e.g., brain tumor, after brain surgery, after a cerebral vascular accident)

Glycogenesis: Anabolic process or glycogen storage; formation of glycogen from glucose

Goal: Aim or expected end to which the nurse and patient work together

Granulation tissue: Soft, pink, highly vascularized connective tissue formed during wound repair

Granulocytes: Polymorphonuclear white blood cells: neutrophils, eosinophils, and basophils

Grief: Psychological and physiologic response after the loss of a significant person, object, belief, or relationship

Ground: To connect electricity between an electrical conductor and the ground or earth

Growth: Progressive increase in physical size or psychosocial development

Guaiac: Test to reveal the presence of blood in feces; also called hemoccult

H

Halitosis: Mouth odor

Hallucinations: False sensory perceptions: seeing, hearing, smelling, feeling, or tasting objects that are not there

Hand hygiene: Handwashing with soap and water or cleansing the hands with a water-less alcohol-based cleanser to prevent the spread of infection

Handoff: Transfer of care for a patient from one health provider to another

Health: (1) State of well-being and optimal functioning; (2) Interactive process between the person and the internal and external environment

Health and wellness coaching: A collaborative partnership between the nurse as a professional coach and the patient/healing partner to assist the patient to identify their own health goals and how to best achieve them

Health determinants: Social, economic, political, and educational health factors and trends that can promote positive healthcare in a community

Health disparity: A "particular type of *health difference that is* closely linked with social or economic disadvantage" (National Partnership for Action to End Health Disparities. (2014). *Health Equity & Disparities*. Retrieved from http://minorityhealth.hhs.gov/npa/templates/browse.aspx?lvl=1&lvlid=34)

Health equity: "Attainment of the highest level of health for all people" (National Partnership for Action to End Health Disparities. (2014). Retrieved from http://minorityhealth.hhs.gov/npa/templates/browse.aspx?lvl=1&lvlid=34)

Health history (or interview): Goal-directed conversation between nurse and patient

Health Insurance Portability and Accountability Act (HIPAA): Legislation introduced to protect personal health information (PHI)

Health literacy: Ability to read and understand healthcare information

Health-maintenance activities: Behaviors that a person in stable health uses to maintain or improve that state over time

Health promotion: Lifestyle choices to prevent illness that strive toward high-level wellness

Health promotion activities: Health behaviors that enhance a person's level of health

Health protection activities: Environmental or regulatory measures that seek to protect the health of a community or large population

Healthcare-associated infection (HAI): A term that encompasses infections contracted in all healthcare settings and is now used in place of the older term, nosocomial infection, which refers only to hospital-acquired infection

Healthy communities/healthy cities: Wellness programs, existing in integrated healthcare systems, that nurses often manage

Hematoma: Localized accumulation of blood in a body tissue, organ, or space as a result of broken blood vessel

Hematuria: Presence of blood in urine

Hemolysis: Red blood cell destruction

Hemolytic transfusion reaction: When a donor's blood is incompatible with the recipient's blood, hemolysis occurs as the antibodies in the recipient's blood quickly react to the donor's blood cells; symptoms are immediate and include facial flushing, fever, chills, headache, low back pain, tachycardia, dyspnea, hypotension, and blood in the urine

Hemoptysis: Expectoration of blood

Hemorrhoids: Enlarged or varicose veins in the anal canal

Herbs (Botanicals): Plant species with medicinal properties

Herbal medications: Plant species with medicinal properties used to treat illness and disease

Heterosexual: Person who relates sexually to a member of the opposite sex

High-level wellness: Way of living in which a person strives toward the highest potential in physical, mental, emotional, and spiritual health

Holism: Seeing the universe—and the patient—as a system of connected parts rather than a sum of isolated parts

Holistic healthcare: Concept that emphasizes humanism, choices, self-care activities, and a peer relationship between healthcare provider and patient

Holistic interventions: Activities for the interrelated needs of body, mind, emotions, and spirit

Home healthcare: Healthcare services provided at home

Homeostasis: State of balance in the body, including the balance of body fluids and their chemical constituents

Homosexual: Person who relates sexually to a member of the same sex

Hospice: Family-focused health service that provides care for terminally ill patients

Human needs: Any physiologic or psychological factors necessary for a healthy existence

Human patient simulator: A life-sized mannequin with a sophisticated computer interface, which presents clinical scenarios that evolve based on decisions a user makes

Hydronephrosis: Distention of the kidney pelvis with urine secondary to the increased resistance caused by obstruction to normal urine flow

Hygiene: Observance of health rules as related to self-care activities (bathing, dressing, feeding, and toileting)

Hyperalgesia: Enhanced sensation of pain produced by a noxious stimulus

Hypercapnia: Abnormally high carbon dioxide in the blood

Hyperosmolar: One compartment contains a greater concentration of a dissolved substance (hyperosmolar) than the other compartment (hypoosmolar)

Hypertension: Abnormally high blood pressure

Hypertonic: Of greater concentration than in body fluids

Hyperventilation: Breathing in excess of metabolic demands, resulting in removal of too much carbon dioxide from the blood; indicated by decreased $PaCO_2$

Hypnotics: Medications that induce or maintain sleep

Hypoosmolar: One compartment contains a lesser concentration of a dissolved substance (hypoosmolar) than the other compartment (hyperosmolar)

Hypopnea: Shallow breathing

Hypotension: Abnormally low blood pressure

Hypothalamic-pituitary-adrenal (HPA) axis: The complex interaction of the hypothalamus, pituitary, and adrenal glands to regulate stress

Hypothesis: Statement that predicts the relationships between the variables under study

Hypotonic: Of lower concentration than in body fluids

Hypoventilation: Breathing insufficient to meet metabolic demands and adequately remove carbon dioxide from the blood indicated by elevated $PaCO_2$

Hypoxemia: Below normal amount of oxygen in the blood

Hypoxia: Decreased amount of oxygen available to the tissues

Iatrogenic illness: Disease that results from treatment and may be traced to overuse and adverse responses to medication, in addition to abuse of prescription medications

Identity: Awareness of self as separate and distinct from others

Ileostomy: Opening of the ileum onto the abdominal skin surface via a stoma

Illness: The impairment of the normal state of a person that interrupts or modifies the body's performance

Imagery: Focusing the mind on a series of images for self-awareness, relaxation, and healing

Immunity: Protection or exemption from an organism or disease

Implementation: Action phase of the nursing process in which nursing care is provided

Implicit bias: An extension of implicit cultural perspectives that is frequent and long-lasting, functioning at an unconscious level and impacting one's views, conduct, and recall of events

Impotence: Inability to attain or maintain an erection long enough to have satisfactory sexual intercourse

Incapacity: Mental or physical inability to make healthcare decisions

Incident: Unusual happening to a patient or visitor at a healthcare facility

Incident report: A report filed that documents an accident or injury occurring in the hospital

Incision: A type of acute wound created intentionally as part of surgical treatment

Incomplete proteins: Proteins that do not contain enough amino acids to independently maintain life, build tissue, or promote growth:

Independent variable: Variable that causes or affects the dependent variable

Induration: Firmness of skin and subcutaneous tissue when palpated from the surface

Infarction: Dead tissue resulting from ischemia due to lack of circulation

Infections: States of contamination from disease-producing germs

Infectious disease: Process resulting from infection that produces manifestations such as fever, leukocytosis, inflammation, or tissue damage

Infiltration: Abnormal or accidental seepage or deposition of a substance into the tissues; accidental administration of IV fluids into subcutaneous tissues that occurs when the needle or catheter becomes dislodged from the vein

Inflammation: An immune response of the body causing increased local blood flow and migration of WBCs to fight infection or injury

Informed consent: Legal document giving permission for surgical or diagnostic procedure signed by patient or legal guardian; before signing, the physician has explained all aspects of the procedure, including risks

Inquiry: Thoughtful questioning and drawing conclusions

Insomnia: Difficulty sleeping; may be characterized by trouble falling or staying asleep or by waking too early

Inspection: Systematic visual examination of the patient

Institute for Healthcare Improvement: An organization that focuses on safety of patients and that has developed a number of bundles of care to achieve that goal

Institute of Medicine: A professional organization that has identified six aims of 21st century healthcare: that all healthcare should be safe, effective, patient-centered, timely, efficient, and equitable

Integrative healthcare (IHC): Cross-disciplinary reality and progressive acceptance of a broader aspect of care

Integrative medicine: Complementary or alternative medicine or those practices that do not form part of the dominant system for managing health and disease

Interferon: Protein produced by the body cells on exposure to viruses that retards viral replication

Intermittent catheterization: In-and-out catheterization performed on a routine, scheduled basis for a particular patient

Intermittent claudication: Limb pain caused by poor blood flow

Interpersonal skills: Skills that determine a person's ability to relate happily and productively with others

Intersex: People born with "ambiguous genitalia," in which it is difficult to determine sex

Interstitial fluid: Fluid between the cells

Interviewing: Communication technique in which the nurse questions the patient in a goal-directed conversation

Intracellular fluid (ICF): Portion of body fluid contained within the cells

Intradermal: Involving administration of a medication into the dermis located just beneath the skin surface

Intramuscular: Involving administration of a medication into the muscle layer beneath the dermis and subcutaneous tissue

Intraoperative phase: Time that starts when the patient is transferred to the operating room bed and ends with transfer to the postanesthetic area

Intraosseous access: Access with a large-bore rigid needle inserted into the medullary cavity of a long bone for the administration of emergency fluid, medication, or blood if adequate venous access is not available

Intravascular fluid: Fluid inside the blood and lymphatic vessels

Intravenous (IV): Involving administration of fluid or medication within a vein

Intravenous (IV) therapy: Infusion of fluid into a vein to treat or to prevent fluid and electrolyte or nutritional imbalances may be used to deliver medications or blood products

Intuition: Use of insight, instincts, and clinical experience to make judgments

Ions: Charged particles formed by the dissociation of electrolytes in a solution

Ischemia: Insufficient blood supply to a body part due to obstruction of circulation

Isolation: Techniques used to prevent or to limit the spread of infection

Isometric exercise: Exercise involving muscle contraction without a change in muscle length (often occurs against resistance)

Isotonic: Osmotic concentration equal to that of body fluids

Isotonic exercise: Dynamic form of exercise in which there is constant muscle tension, muscle contraction, and active movement

J

Jaundice: Yellowish tone to the skin that is also observed in liver disease

Judgment: Process of reasoning; ability to process incoming stimuli and to determine meanings that encompass many aspects of a situation

Just culture: An approach to error evaluation that examines the nature of the error to assist in determining the appropriate response to the individual who made the error

Justice: Principle of fairness basis of the obligation to treat all patients equally and fairly

K

Key informants: Persons who know and will discuss certain aspects of their culture with someone outside that culture

Korotkoff sounds: Sounds heard during auscultation that indicate the systolic and diastolic blood pressure

Kyphosis: Thoracic abnormality that includes an exaggerated convex curve of the spine

L

Laceration: Wound caused by tearing of body tissue

Laws: Standards of human conduct established and enforced by the authority of an organized society through its government

Leadership: Ability to influence others to strive for a vision or goal or to change

Learning: Multidimensional process of acquiring knowledge that depends on symbols, language, classifications, concepts, and other concrete operations along with abstract functions

Learning styles: How students learn best

Leukocytosis: Increase in production of white blood cells

Levels of healthcare: Include primary (health promotion, education, protection, and screening), secondary (emergency care, acute and critical care, diagnosis, and treatment), and tertiary (emergency care, acute and critical care, diagnosis, and treatment)

Liability: Responsibility for one's actions an obligation one is bound to perform

Libel: False communication by means of print that results in injury to a person's reputation

Licensed practical nurse: Person licensed by a state after completing a state-approved nursing program to provide technical nursing care under the direct supervision of a registered nurse

Lift team: Trained, physically fit individuals competent in transfer techniques and well trained on any special equipment who work together to accomplish safe transfers

Limited English proficiency (LEP): A term used to describe individuals with limited ability to speak, read, or write English

Literature review: Process of selecting published materials about the concepts to be examined in a research study

Living will: Written evidence of a patient's preferences regarding treatment options

Local anesthetic: Depresses superficial peripheral nerves and blocks conduction of pain impulses from their site of origin

Loneliness: Loss of important relationships or lack of company

Lordosis: Commonly known as "swayback," in which the lumbar region curves inward and the sacral region curves outward

Loss: Experience of parting with an object, person, belief, or relationship that one values and the sadness that follows the loss requires a reorganization of one or more aspects of the person's life

Low literacy: Limited ability to comprehend written materials

M

Macerated: Softened tissue due to excessive moisture

Macronutrients: Carbohydrates, proteins and fats; used by the body in large amounts

Malignant hyperthermia: Severe body temperature elevation after administration of certain anesthetics

Malpractice: Professional misconduct, causing harm or injury to a person from lack of experience, skill, knowledge, or judgment

Maslow's hierarchy of human needs: Theory that states that all humans are born with instinctive needs, grouped into five categories, and arranged in order of importance from those essential to physical survival to those necessary to develop a person's fullest potential

Masturbation: Autostimulation of the genitals

Meaningful use: Effective use of the electronic health record including access for patients and use of the record to inform clinical decision making

Meconium: First feces of a newborn

Medical Adhesive-Related Skin Injury (MARSI): Damage to skin due to reaction to tape or adhesive products or from their improper removal

Medical asepsis: Measures taken to control and to reduce the number of pathogens present; also known as "clean technique"; measures include handwashing, gloving, gowning, and disinfecting to help contain microbial growth

Medical diagnosis: Identified disease or pathologic process; treatment focuses on correcting or preventing specific pathology of specific organs or body systems

Medication: Drug given for its therapeutic effects

Medication reconciliation (medication verification): Important safety procedure during patient handoffs, including new and intermittent clinic visits, emergency room visits, hospital admission, transfers between hospital units, and discharge from one healthcare facility to another or to home, between healthcare providers or agencies

Meditation: Deep personal thought and reflection

Memory: Ability to recall a thought at least once and usually again

Menarche: First menstrual period

Menopause: Permanent cessation of menstruation

Menstruation: Monthly vaginal bleeding due to sloughing of uterine lining

Meta-analyses: Systematic reviews that combine results from several studies using qualitative statistics

Metabolic syndrome (syndrome X): A genetic metabolic disorder characterized by diabetes, hypertension, atherosclerosis, centrally distributed obesity, and elevated blood lipids

Metabolism: (1) Chemical reactions in the cells that produce heat as a byproduct; (2) Breakdown of a drug (usually in the liver) to an inactive form

Metacommunication: Meanings beyond the literal level of communication, such as the roles of the communicators and the context in which communication is taking place

Methods: Procedure a researcher follows to gather and analyze data

Micronutrients: Vitamins and minerals; used by the body in small quantities

Micturition: Urination

Milliequivalent (mEq): Unit used to give the concentration of an electrolyte in solution; commonly expressed as mEq/L

Minimum inhibitory concentration (MIC): Quantifies the minimal amount of the drug that is necessary to inhibit microbial growth in the laboratory

Minority: Smaller segment of society

Mobility: Acts of movement like walking, driving, shopping, and exercise

Moderate sedation: Sometimes referred to as procedural sedation or conscious sedation, involves the use of IV sedation administered during a surgical or diagnostic procedure to alter the patient's conscious state, thereby allaying fear and anxiety

Moisture-associated skin damage (MASD): Skin damage caused by inflammation and erosion from prolonged exposure to various sources of moisture, including urine or stool, perspiration, wound exudate, mucus, or saliva

Monosaccharide: Simple sugar

Monounsaturated fatty acid (MUFA): "Unsaturated" double bond that forms between two side-by-side carbon atoms when an unsaturated fat has a single hydrogen atom missing from each of two carbon atoms

Mood: Emotional state or outlook

Moral courage: The ability to surmount fear and act to protect patient's rights and values

Morality: The set of beliefs about the standards of right and wrong that help a person determine the correct or permissible action in a given situation

Motivation: Something that provides drive or incentive

Mourning: Behavior after the death of a significant other, which varies among cultures

Multidrug-resistant organisms (MDROs): Organisms that have developed resistance to multiple antibiotics

Multigenerational families: Several generations living together in one residence

Multimodal therapy: Uses two or more analgesics with different mechanisms of action to maximize pain relief and diminish side effects

Murmur: Vibrating sound that results from turbulent blood flow through the heart

Myocardial infarction (heart attack): Ischemia of heart muscle and death of portions of the heart muscle from decreased blood flow through the coronary arteries

Myocardium: Layer of cardiac muscle that forms the walls of the heart

N

Narcolepsy: Sleep disorder characterized by sudden, uncontrollable episodes of sleep

Needleless connectors: Available to provide access to secondary ports on IV tubing or for flushing access; provide an alternative to needles to reduce the risk of injury from contaminated sharps during IV procedures

Negative pressure wound therapy (NPWT): A wound management system that applies negative pressure to a wound to decrease excess moisture and increase perfusion to the wound bed promoting wound healing; sometimes referred to as vacuum-assisted closure, or VAC

Negligence: Failure to do something that a reasonably prudent person would do, or doing something that a reasonably prudent person would not do

Networking: System of meeting and establishing contacts with colleagues who share common interests

Neural plasticity: Nervous system adaptation after pain

Neuropathic pain: Pain caused by nerve damage

Neutropenia: Decrease in the neutrophils in the blood, the white blood cells responsible for quick response to invasion by infectious organisms

Never events: Hospital-acquired complications deemed reasonably preventable through the use of evidence-based guidelines and not reimbursable by Medicare and Medicaid

No code order: Order not to provide resuscitation in the event of a cardiopulmonary arrest

Nociception: The normal processing of painful stimuli described in terms of a four-step process that occurs when acute pain becomes a conscious event

Nociceptive pain: Occurs in tissues other than the nervous system and is transmitted via intact nociceptors during normal pain transmission

Nociceptor: Free nerve endings that sense and respond to potentially noxious thermal, electrical, mechanical, or chemical stimuli

Nocturia: Voiding during normal sleeping hours

Noncompliance: Failure to adhere to a recommended plan

Nonmaleficence: Principle of avoidance of doing harm

Nontraditional families: Families that do not fit the description of nuclear family

Nonverbal communication: Messages sent without words (e.g., gestures, facial expressions, postures, silence)

Normal flora: Microorganisms commonly found in a body location that ordinarily cause no harm

Nosocomial infection: Infection acquired during receipt of healthcare

Nuclear family: Traditionally includes a married man and woman and their children

Nurse administrator: Nurse who supervises the organization of nursing care to ensure overall safety and quality

Nurse anesthetist (CRNA): Nurse who specializes and is certified in the administration of anesthesia

Nurse educator: Nurse responsible for nursing and healthcare education in various settings

Nurse executive: Top administrative nursing position in an organization; also known as chief nursing officer

Nurse midwife: Nurse with advanced education and certification in the care of women during pregnancy and childbirth

Nurse practice act: State guideline that governs the practice of professional nursing

Nurse practitioner: Nurse with advanced education and certification who may practice independently in various settings

Nurse researcher: Nurse responsible for continued development of nursing knowledge and improvement of practice through research

Nursing: Profession that involves diagnosis and treatment of human responses to actual or potential health problems

Nursing audit: Any review completed by a nurse of a patient's care or records to evaluate whether established standards were met

Nursing competencies for community-based care: Monitoring, treatment, teaching, prioritizing, intervention, and planning skills that nurses should possess to meet the epidemiologic and demographic needs of a community

Nursing diagnosis: Actual, potential, or possible health problem identified by the nurse that is amenable to nursing intervention

Nursing informatics: Combination of computer science, information science, and nursing science designed to assist in the management and processing of nursing data to support nursing practice and care delivery

Nursing interventions: Any treatment the nurse performs to enhance patient outcomes based on clinical judgment and knowledge

Nursing intervention classification (NIC): System of organizing nursing interventions in a three-level taxonomy consisting of domains, classes, and interventions and developed by a research team at the University of Iowa College of Nursing

Nursing judgment: Knowledge, experience, critical thinking, and clinical reasoning

Nursing monitor: Review by a nurse of a patient's care or records to determine the extent to which the care or records meet established standards; also called nursing audit

Nursing outcome classification (NOC): System of organizing desired patient outcomes according to categories, classes, labels, outcome indicators, and measurement activities for outcomes

Nursing process: Systematic approach to providing nursing care using assessment, diagnosis, outcome identification, planning, implementation, and evaluation

Nursing research: Research that focuses on establishing a scientific base for the practice of nursing

Nursing theory: Explanation or description of nursing issues that defines and predicts nursing practice

Nutrients: Food containing elements for normal body functioning

Nutrition: Process by which living things take in and use food materials; study of diet

Nystagmus: Involuntary, rhythmic oscillations of the eyes

O

Obese: Body mass index (BMI) over 30 kg/m² or more

Obesity: Weight more than 20% over ideal body weight

Objective data: Observable, measurable information that can be validated or verified

Observation: Art of noticing patient cues

Oliguria: Formation and excretion of less than 500 mL of urine in 24 hours

Ophthalmoscope: Instrument for examining the interior of the eye

Opportunistic infections: Infections that do not result in disease in individuals with properly functioning immune systems

Opportunistic organisms: Organisms that invade the tissues when the body's defenses are suppressed

Orgasm: Climax phase of the human sexual response cycle; men experience expulsive contractions of the entire length of the urethra, and women experience contractions in the outer third of the vagina and labia minora, as well as uterine contractions

Orientation: The basic process by which people know their location in the dimensions of time and place

Osmolality: Concentration of solutes in a solution, expressed as milliosmols per kilogram

Osmolarity: Concentration of solutes in a solution expressed as milliosmols per liter

Osmosis: Movement of a fluid through a semipermeable membrane from a region of lower to higher solute concentration

Osmotic pressure: Pressure exerted by nondiffusible particles in a solution across a semipermeable membrane; tends to hold fluid within its container and is opposed by hydrostatic pressure

Osteoarthritis: Degeneration of the articular surface of weight-bearing joints

Otoscope: Instrument for examining the ear

Outcome: A measurable statement of expectations

Outcome and Assessment Information Set (OASIS): A system that accurately measures the patient's status at various specified points during an episode of care, thus providing the basis for measuring patient outcomes; mandated by Medicaid and Medicare for home care agencies

Outcome criteria: Specific, measurable, realistic statement of goal attainment

Outcome identification: Formulation of goals and measurable outcomes that provides the basis for evaluation

Overactive bladder: Frequency and urgency to urinate occurring together

Overweight: Body mass index (BMI) between 25 and 29.9 kg/m²

Oxygen saturation: Amount of oxygen in the blood

P

Pain management: Ability and strategy to deal with pain

Palliative care: Specialized care for people with serious illness that emphasizes symptom management and improved quality of life

Pallor: Skin color that may appear pale with hypoxia and anemia

Palpation: Use of the sense of touch to ascertain the size, shape, and configuration of underlying body structures

Pannus: A large protuberant abdominal skin fold

Paradoxical blood pressure: Significant decrease in systolic blood pressure with inspiration

Paralytic ileus: Condition in which the bowel is temporarily paralyzed and distention occurs

Paraplegia: Decreased motor and sensory function to the legs

Parasomnias: Group of disorders (e.g., sleepwalking, enuresis) involving autonomic and motor activity associated with partial arousal from sleep

Parenteral: Medications given by injection or infusion

Parenteral nutrition: Nutritional elements supplied through an intravenous route, usually into a central vein

Partial pressure of carbon dioxide (PCO$_2$): The pressure exerted by carbon dioxide gas on surrounding structures; may be measured in the alveolus (PACO$_2$), artery (PaCO$_2$), or vein (PvCO$_2$)

Partial pressure of oxygen (PAO$_2$): The pressure exerted by oxygen gas on surrounding structures; may be measured in the alveolus (PAO$_2$), artery (PaO$_2$), or vein (PvO$_2$)

Partially complete proteins: Proteins that contain sufficient amounts of amino acids to maintain life but do not promote growth

Pathogenicity: An organism's ability to harm and to cause disease

Pathogens: Microorganisms that can harm humans

Patient: Person requiring the services of a healthcare provider

Patient education: Interactive, collaborative process between nurse and patient to progress toward the patient's goal of assuming responsibility for his or her health and self-care

Pedagogy: Teaching as applied to children or adolescent learners

Pediculosis: Infestation with lice

Peer review: Evaluation and judgment of performance by other nurses

Perceiving: Process of receiving and interpreting sensory stimuli that function as a basis for understanding, knowing, or learning

Perceptions: Views of oneself and the world, influenced by culture, religion, family, experiences, expectations, and knowledge

Percussion: Examination by tapping the body surface with the fingertips and evaluating the sounds obtained

Perfusion: Passing of blood through an area

Peripherally inserted central catheter (PICC): Long-line catheter made of soft silicone or Silastic material that is placed peripherally but delivers medications and solutions centrally

Peristalsis: Motility and movement of the intestines

Periwound: Around the wound edges

Person: Human being; recipient of nursing care

Persistent (chronic) pain: An abnormal pain signaling process with origins that can occur both peripherally and centrally

Personal health information (PHI): Confidential documents and records regarding a patient's care

Personal values: Beliefs a person considers highly important and are learned through interactions with social systems

Personal protective equipment (PPE): Techniques or equipment that prevents the transfer of pathogens from one person to another; also referred to as "barriers"

Pharmacodynamics: Study of the physiologic and biochemical effects of a drug on the body

Pharmacokinetics: Study of how a medication changes as it passes through the body and undergoes absorption, distribution, metabolism, and excretion

Phlebitis: Inflammation or infection of a vein, manifested by redness, swelling, and tenderness along the course of the vein

Phonation: Process by which humans create vocal sounds

Physical dependence: A physiologic adaptation that is characterized by the development of withdrawal symptoms such as diaphoresis, anxiety, tachycardia, or nausea when an opioid drug is stopped abruptly

Physical examination: Use of the techniques of inspection, palpation, percussion, and auscultation to obtain information about the structure and function of body parts

PIE charting: System of documentation that incorporates the plan of care into the progress notes and is structured according to problem (P), intervention (I), and evaluation (E)

Plasticity: The ability of nerve cells to change through new experiences and function well into adulthood

Plan of care: Plan generated at admission and revised to reflect changes in the patient's condition

Planning: Management function of deciding what to do, when, where, how, by whom, and with what resources

Plaque: Substance that forms and hardens on the teeth and is composed primarily of bacteria and saliva

Point of care documentation: Documentation that takes place as care occurs

Point of maximal impulse: Visible pulsation with ventricular contraction as the left side of the heart strikes the anterior chest wall

Poisoning: Ingesting, inhaling, or absorbing potentially hazardous substances

Pollution: Substances in air, water, or land that are potentially harmful to health

Polysaccharide: Complex sugar

Polysomnography: Polygraph recordings of electrophysiologic changes in brain waves (electroencephalogram), eye movements (electrooculogram), and muscles (electromyogram)

Polyunsaturated fatty acid (PUFA): Two or more carbonto-carbon double bonds when an unsaturated fat has a single hydrogen atom missing from each of two carbon atoms

Polyuria: Formation and excretion of large amounts of urine in the absence of a concurrent increase in fluid intake

Positional IV: Term used when position changes cause the needle bevel or catheter to rest against a vein wall

Possible nursing diagnosis: Health problem amenable to nursing intervention that requires additional data collection and validation before it can be confirmed or deleted as a nursing diagnosis

Postanesthesia care unit (PACU): Designated area of the hospital or ambulatory care facility where immediate postoperative care is usually given

Postoperative phase: Phase that begins with transfer to the surgical recovery area and ends with recovery

Postural (orthostatic) hypotension: A fall in blood pressure associated with a change in position from supine to sitting or standing

Prehypertension: Blood pressure between 120/80 and 139/89 for adults of any age

Premature closure: Selecting a diagnosis before analyzing pertinent information

Premature ejaculation: Condition in which the man cannot delay ejaculation long enough for the woman to reach orgasm, or for satisfactory sexual intercourse to occur

Preoperative phase: Phase that begins with the decision to have surgery and ends with transfer to the operating room bed

Prepuce: Loose skin at the head of the penis; foreskin

Prescription: Directive written by a physician or other person legally permitted to do so (e.g., nurse practitioner)

Pressure ulcer (bedsore): Result of the impeding of capillary blood flow to the skin or underlying tissue

Primary data: Information that includes vital signs, height, and weight gathered directly from the patient during the initial stage of the assessment to obtain a general overview of the patient's status

Primary source: The patient

Prions: Organisms that cause a rapidly progressing neurodegenerative disease affecting both animals and humans that is untreatable and always fatal

Priority: Nursing problem that takes on a position of prominence

Privacy: Patient confidentiality

Problem solving: Systematic process that involves identifying and analyzing the problem, determining and weighing the possible solutions, choosing and implementing a solution, and evaluating the results

Problem statement: Key step in the research process that identifies the direction a project will take

Procedural pause or "time-out": A pause prior to an invasive procedure (e.g., central line placement) to ensure proper patient and procedural site

Professional ethics: Values held by a disciplinary group deemed as having generalizable standards of conduct to be upheld in all situations

Professional nurse: Nurse possessing the baccalaureate degree in nursing

Proprioception: Awareness of the position and movements of body parts in space, sensed by sensory nerve terminals in muscles, tendons, and the labyrinth of the ear

Proteins: Organic compounds composed of polymers of amino acids connected by peptide bonds

Proxy directive: Advance directive that allows a person to designate another to make decisions if the patient becomes incapacitated and cannot make decisions independently

Psychomotor: Relating to muscle movements resulting from a mental process

Psychosomatic: Indicative that the mind or emotions cause illness and that the mind and body are so interrelated that they act on each other intimately, directly, and inseparably

Puberty: Period of life in which the sex organs mature, secondary sex characteristics appear, and reproduction becomes possible

Pulse deficit: Mathematical difference between apical and radial pulse

Pulse oximetry: Noninvasive means for approximating oxygenation that uses infrared light and a sensor attached to the patient's finger or earlobe to determine the percentage of hemoglobin that has combined with oxygen

Pulse pressure: Mathematical difference between systolic and diastolic blood pressure

Purulent: Producing or containing pus

Pyuria: Presence of pus in urine

Q

Qi: Vital energy source or life force

Qualifier: Description of the parameter for achieving a goal

Qualitative research: Involves the systematic collection and analysis of subjective materials, using procedures in which there tends to be a minimum of researcher-imposed control

Quality: The excellence or superiority of something; often viewed on a continuum, from poor quality to high quality

Quality and Safety Education for Nurses (QSEN): A project designed to provide a framework for the knowledge, skills, and attitudes necessary for future nurses

Quality assurance memos: Reports used to assess patterns of errors and the need to change the procedures involved

Quality improvement programs: Mechanisms for healthcare organizations to assess and improve care

Quantitative research: Involves the systematic collection of numeric information, usually under conditions of considerable control, and analysis of findings using statistical procedures

R

Race: Group defined by biologic characteristics

RACE: A mnemonic device that helps employees remember how to prioritize actions during a fire; stands for rescue, alarm, confine, evacuate

Racism: Oppression and exploitation of people of a different skin color or ethnic origin

Range of motion (ROM): Extent to which a person can move joints and muscles

Reality orientation: Nursing technique to help restore the patient's awareness of reality

Receptive aphasia: Disorder in which patients cannot understand simple directions

Receptive meditation: Activity that focuses on the deep interconnection between mind and body

Reflection: Identifying the main emotional themes contained in a communication and directing them back to the patient for the purpose of verifying and checking feelings that are being heard

Reflective meditation: Activity in which the person chooses a theme, question, or topic of reflection to gain insight into significant questions or concepts related to philosophy or spirituality. The focus is on the person's query; he or she returns to it as the object of attention

Regional anesthetic: Agent used to induce loss of sensation in a selected body area

Reporting: Sharing of patient information by two or more healthcare professionals

Res ipsa loquitur: "The thing speaks for itself" invoked when it is impossible to prove who was at fault when a patient's injury results from negligence

Research design: Overall plan for collecting and analyzing data

Resilience: Being able to recover from an adverse event

Resistance: Adaptability to adversity; ability to buffer the potentially negative health effects of life stress

Resonance: Echoing of sound through passages

Resident Assessment Instrument (RAI): A federally mandated tool for assessment in long-term care settings designed to provide thorough and systematic appraisal of residents

Respiration: Exchange of carbon dioxide for oxygen in lungs and in tissues

Respiratory excursion: Normal chest expansion during inspiration; usually symmetric, indicating equal expansion of both lungs

Respondeat superior: "Let the master answer"; doctrine in which a facility is held liable for an employee's negligence

Rest: Physical and emotional state of decreased muscle and cognitive activity

Restatement: Content portion of communication, in which the nurse, after listening carefully to the patient, repeats the content of the message back to the patient, to verify understanding

Restraint: Device that prevents a patient from moving or gaining normal access to a body part

Resuscitation: Act of reviving after apparent death or unconsciousness

Reticular activating system (RAS): Part of the brain responsible for bringing together information from the cerebellum and other brain parts as well as from the sense organs

Retraction: Backward or inward movement of an organ or part

Return demonstration: Observing a patient's performance of a new skill; this tool is valuable for evaluating psychomotor learning

Risk nursing diagnosis: State of being at risk for the development of a health problem amenable to nursing intervention

Rituals: Common and observable expressions of culture

Role: Expected function and behavior

Role ambiguity: Occurs when the person lacks knowledge of role expectations, which fosters anxiety and confusion

Role conflict: Occurs when a person's expectations concerning his or her role differ from the reality

Role-playing: Acting out feelings or knowledge

Role strain: Occurs when the person perceives himself or herself as inadequate or unsuited for a role

Roles and relationships: Expected function and behavior that define interaction with others

Root cause analysis (RCA): A process used to determine the underlying cause of an event

S

Safety: The avoidance or prevention of adverse outcomes for patients

Safety science: The study of safety knowledge and technology to prevent harm to patients

Safety zones: Safe places for children to stand or sit when a potentially dangerous activity is under way

Sandwich generation: Term used to describe adult children facing the dilemma of meeting their own generativity needs while assisting the older generation (their parents) and the younger generation (their children)

Sanguineous: Pertaining to or containing blood

Saturated fats: Chemically, two hydrogen atoms attached to each of the carbon atoms in the carbon atom chain

SBAR: Situation-Background-Assessment-Recommendation: a technique providing a framework for communication between members of the healthcare team about a patient's condition

Schizophrenia: Serious, persistent brain disease that is characterized by distortion of reality and difficulty processing information

Scientific rationale: Reason for a nursing intervention that is supported by clinical research

Scoliosis: Lateral curvature of a portion of the spine

Scrub person: Wears a sterile gown, mask, headgear, gloves, disposable shoe covers, and eye protection, and provides the surgeon with required instruments, sponges, drains, and other equipment, anticipating what will be needed throughout surgery

Secondary data: Sources of data other than the patient, such as the chart

Secondary sources: Family, significant others, other healthcare professionals, health records, and literature review

Self: A person's unique dimensions, potentials, and purposes

Self-actualization: Process of developing one's maximum potential and managing one's life confidently

Self-awareness: Knowing and caring for oneself recognizing one's strengths and limitations

Self-care: A person's ability to perform primary care functions in the four areas of bathing, feeding, toileting, and dressing without the help of others

Self-care deficit: An impaired ability to perform or complete activities of daily living

Self-concept: Mental image of oneself

Self-efficacy: A person's belief that he or she is capable of doing something

Self-esteem: Evaluation and judgment of one's worth

Self-evaluation: Conscious assessment of the self

Self-expectation: The self a person wants to be

Self-knowledge: Basic understanding of oneself

Self-perception: A person's awareness or identification of self the filtering process of evaluating events and entering them into the subconscious

Sensation (sensory) information: Telling a patient what he or she will see, hear, smell, taste, or feel in a particular situation

Sensoristasis: State of optimal sensory input, which differs for each person

Sensory deprivation: Lack of meaningful sensory stimuli; monotonous input or interference with the processing of information; leads to behavioral changes ranging from boredom to psychosis

Sensory overload: State of arousal in which a person cannot manage the intensity or quantity of incoming sensory stimuli

Sensory perception: The ability to receive sensory input and transform the inputs through various physiologic processes into meaningful information

Sentinel event: Safety error in which hospitals are required to report serious safety events to regulatory agencies and state health agencies

Sepsis: Poisoning of body tissues; usually refers to bloodborne organisms or their toxic products

Serosanguineous: Containing serum and blood

Sequential compression devices (SCDs): Devices that sequentially compress veins in the legs to promote venous return

Serous: Thin, watery, serum-like

Sexuality: Person's characteristics and perceptions concerning sexual expression

Sexually transmitted infection (STI): An infection transmitted through both heterosexual and homosexual encounters

Shear: Tissue damaging force that occurs when tissue layers move on each other, causing blood vessels in subcutaneous tissue to stretch and become damaged

Shift to the left: An increase in the number of immature white blood cells indicating infection

Shock: Severe circulatory insufficiency

Side rails: Safety bars that assist patients in turning and serve as a reminder not to inadvertently roll out of bed; used on beds, stretchers, and similar equipment

Sigmoidoscopy: Diagnostic examination of the rectum and sigmoid colon

Simulation: Education strategy that allows learners to act out or verbalize what they would do in a situation

Single-parent families: Families consisting of one parent and a child or children

Skin integrity: Completeness or purity of the skin

Skin staples: Type of wound healing device made of stainless steel that decreases the risk of infection and reduces tissue handling because they allow faster wound closure

Skin turgor: Tension or rigidity of skin

Slander: False communication by spoken word that results in injury to a person's reputation

Sleep: Readily reversible state of altered consciousness in which awareness and responsiveness to the environment are decreased

Sleep apnea: Condition in which, at least five times an hour, the patient stops breathing for 10 seconds or more during sleep

Sleep deficiency: An inadequate amount of, or mistimed, sleep

Sleep-disordered breathing (SDB): A cluster of disorders associated with difficulty breathing and sleeping at the same time

Sleep health: Sleep of adequate duration occurring at appropriate times of the day with sustained alertness during waking hours

Sleep latency: Time it takes one to get to sleep after going to bed

Sleep loss: Lack of sufficient sleep

Sleep sufficiency: Also called sleep health, is sleep of adequate duration occurring at appropriate times of the day with sustained alertness during waking hours

Sleepiness: Refers to an urge of varying intensity to go to sleep

Small-bore feeding tubes: Flexible tubes of small diameter designed for comfort during tube feeding

Smart pump: An enhanced electronic infusion device that has an embedded computer software program to ensure patient safety

SOAP note: Method of organizing charting entries so that each entry includes subjective, objective, assessment, and planning information

Social isolation: State in which a person's desire for interpersonal relationships is perceived as unattainable; negative feelings of being alone

Social self: One's behavior and interaction with others in social situations

Socialization: Process in which a person is familiarized with the ways of a specific culture or group

Somatic pain: Pain that originates in bone, skin, and soft tissue and is often well localized

Somnambulism: Sleepwalking

Spasticity: Sudden, involuntary increase in muscle tone or contractions due to central nervous system lesions

Specificity: Organism's attraction to a specific host, which may include humans

Spinal dorsal horn: Site in the spinal cord where complex processing of messages occurs; one of the most important areas for pain modulation

Spiritual care: Mutual, potentially healing or integrating process in which the patient's spiritual needs are met

Spiritual crisis: A unique form of grieving or loss, which is accompanied by profound questioning about life and its meaning

Spiritual dimension: Quality beyond religious affiliation that strives for inspiration, reverence, awe, meaning, and purpose, even for those who do not believe in any god

Spiritual need: Normal expression of a person's inner being that seeks meaning in all experience and a dynamic relationship with self, others, and the supreme other as the person defines it

Spiritual well-being: Condition marked by an affirmation of life and a sense of unity with God, self, community, and environment

Spirituality: Sacred or holy matters that belong to or relate to a god or church

Splinting: Use of a pillow to immobilize a wound when a patient has had abdominal or thoracic surgery

Standard Precautions: The latest CDC isolation system that combines the major features of Universal Precautions (blood-borne transmissions) and Body Substance Isolation (moist body substances transmission), thus protecting against blood and body-fluid transmission of potentially infective agents

Standards of care: Comprise the expected level of performance or practice as established by guidelines, authority, or custom

Stereotypes: Preconceived beliefs about a person or people

Sterilization: (1) Destruction of all bacteria, spores, fungi, and viruses on an item, accomplished by heat, chemicals, or gas; (2) Rendered unable to reproduce biologically

Stethoscope: Device that collects and transmits sound, selects frequencies, and screens out extraneous sound

Stoma: Artificially created opening of bowel on the abdominal skin surface

Stress: State of arousal of mind and body in response to demands made on the person

Stressor: Stimulus or event that requires coping or adaptation

Stridor: A harsh inspiratory sound due to obstruction that may be compared to crowing

Stroke: Cerebrovascular accident (CVA); involves a sudden onset of hemorrhage, blood clots, or other vascular lesions, causing damage to the brain

Stroke volume: Amount of blood ejected from each cardiac ventricle with each heart contraction

Subculture: Beliefs held by a portion (e.g., occupational or age group) of the larger population

Subcutaneous: Pertaining to the layer of tissue under the dermis

Subcutaneous tissue: Underlies the skin; consists primarily of fat and connective tissues that support the skin

Subjective data: Symptoms or covert cues that include the patient's feelings and statements about his or her health problems

Sublingual: Under the tongue

Suffering: An emotional response to increased pain, associated with events that threaten a person's intactness

Suffocation: Oxygen deprivation

Sundown syndrome: State of disorientation and agitation that occurs at night in institutionalized patients who are oriented during the day.

Superinfection: a secondary infection that occurs when antibiotics, immunosuppression, or cancer treatment destroys normal flora

Suppository: Medication inserted into the rectum or vagina

Surgical asepsis: Refers to "sterile technique" in which an object is free of all microorganisms to prevent the introduction or spread of pathogens from the environment into the patient; employed when a body cavity is entered with an object that may damage the mucous membranes, when surgical procedures are performed, and when the patient's immune system is already compromised

Surrogate decision maker: Person identified to act on a patient's behalf when the patient is an infant, young child, mentally handicapped or incapacitated, or in a persistent vegetative state or coma and does not have the capacity to participate in decision making about healthcare

Surgical verification: A protocol developed to prevent wrong-patient, wrong-site surgery

Suture: Material used to stitch together the edges of traumatic or surgical wounds

Syncope: A temporary loss of consciousness or fainting spell that may signal decreased perfusion to the brain

Synergism: Medication interaction that increases a drug's effects

Systematic reviews: Use of explicit methods to identify, select, and critically evaluate relevant research

Systemic inflammatory response syndrome (SIRS): Global, generalized inflammatory response of many or all major organ systems triggered by tissue injury or infection

Systole: Period of contraction of the ventricles

Systolic blood pressure: Pressure in the blood vessels during cardiac ventricular contraction

T

Tachycardia: Abnormally rapid heart rate, usually above 100 beats per minute in an adult

Tachypnea: Abnormally rapid respiratory rate, usually more than 20 breaths per minute in an adult

Tactile fremitus: Sensation felt by a hand placed on a part of the body (as the chest) that vibrates during speech

Tartar: Plaque that remains and hardens on the teeth, which cannot be removed by simple brushing

Taxonomy: Classification system to organize information

Teach-back: A method of teaching in which the patient verbalizes information that he or she has learned

TeamSTEPPS™: Team Strategies and Tools to Enhance Performance and Patient Safety; a safety curriculum designed to improve patient outcomes by cultivating teamwork among healthcare providers

Telehealth: An interactive system that allows communication to happen simultaneously between a patient's home and the clinical medical setting

Teratogenic: Drugs known to cause birth defects

Terminal sedation: Infrequently used method of pain management, not considered euthanasia, provided in response to a dying person's persistent and unremitting pain and suffering; it provides analgesia that produces light sedation even though this is likely to hasten death somewhat secondary to resulting immobility

Tetraplegia: Paralysis of the arms and the legs and all muscle movement below the level of injury; also referred to as quadraplegia

Theism: Belief in God

Theory: A set of interrelated constructs or propositions that attempts to present or explain some phenomenon systematically

Therapeutic communication: Interactions that help a person express feelings and work out problems

Therapeutic effects: A medication's desired and intentional effects

Therapeutic touch: A healing meditation in which the practitioner assesses and treats the patient's energy field and attempts to redirect any obstructed, disordered, or depleted areas

Thrombophlebitis: Blood clot that accompanies vein inflammation

Thrombus: Blood clot in a blood vessel

Tidal volume: Amount of air moving in and out with each breath

Tolerance: Occurs when a patient receives a drug, such as an opioid, continuously over an extended period of time and a neuroadaptive response occurs, requiring a larger dose of the drug to produce the same effect

Tonicity: Fluid's effect on cell size

Tort: Wrong committed against a person or property; subject to action in a civil court

Total parenteral nutrition (TPN): Administration of hypertonic solutions containing dextrose, proteins, vitamins, and minerals to provide for nutritional deficits

Trace elements: Subgroup of minerals found in small amounts in food

Tracheostomy: Permanent or temporary opening into the trachea through the neck

Trade or brand name: Medication name used by a pharmaceutical company for a 17-year period during which it has the exclusive rights to make and sell the drug

Traditional Chinese Medicine (TCM): Complete healing system that includes acupuncture, massage, herbal treatments, nutrition, moxibustion, movement such as Qi gong, and meditation

Trans fatty acids: Unsaturated fat molecules with an unusual configuration around the double carbon bond(s)

Transcultural nursing: Synthesis of anthropology and nursing that focuses on the cultural dimension of care and recognizes that a person's cultural background influences and determines both health and illness

Transcutaneous electrical nerve stimulation (TENS): Mild electrical impulse to an area or over the pain zone and controlled by the patient

Transdermal: Topical medication that is released through the epidermis and dermis to the blood

Transfusion: Introduction of whole blood or blood components (packed red cells, plasma, platelets) directly into a patient's circulatory system

Transfusion-related acute lung injury (TRALI): An adverse response to a blood transfusion thought to occur when donor plasma contains an antibody against the recipient's leukocyte-specific antigen

Transient ischemic attack (TIA): Temporary cerebral ischemia due to transient interruption in blood supply

Transgendered: Someone who appears as, may have had surgery for, or desires to be a member of the opposite sex

Transsexual: Person who psychologically sees himself or herself as a member of the opposite sex

Tremor: A rhythmic, repetitive movement that can occur at rest or when movement is initiated

Tunneling: A narrow channel or pathway that extends from a wound

U

Undermining: Wound edges not attached to wound bed

Underweight: Body mass index (BMI) below the ideal BMI of 20 to 25 kg/m^2

Unit dose: A prescribed amount of medication dispensed at a specified time

Unsaturated fats: Fats with a single hydrogen atom missing from each of two side-by-side carbon atoms

Urgency: The subjective feeling of needing to void immediately

Urinal: Metal or plastic receptacle into which the penis can be placed to facilitate urinating without spilling

Urinary incontinence: Involuntary loss of urine from the bladder

Urinary retention: Inability to empty the bladder of urine

V

Vaccination: The process of injecting weakened or killed organisms into a person, stimulating antibody production to prevent a specific infection

Vaginismus: Involuntary contraction of the muscles around the vaginal orifice, which makes sexual intercourse painful or impossible

Validation: Reexamining information to check its accuracy

Valsalva's maneuver: The combination taking a deep breath against a closed glottis (to move the diaphragm down), contracting the abdominal muscles (to increase intra-abdominal pressure), and contracting the pelvic floor muscles (to push the feces downward) to defecate

Values: Personal standards for decision making

Value system: Enduring set of personal principles and rules

Variables: Property that varies from another

Variance: Deviation that alters an expected outcome or date of discharge

Venipuncture: Insertion of a needle or catheter into a vein

Ventilation: Movement of air in and out of the lungs; breathing

Veracity: Principle of telling the truth, essential to the integrity of the patient-provider relationship

Verbal communication: Spoken word; an exchange using the elements of language

Vesicular breath sounds: Sounds described as soft and breezy, with inspiration markedly longer than expiration, normally heard over all areas of the lung except over or near the major airways

Virulence: Vigor with which an organism can grow and multiply

Visceral: A type of nociceptive pain that originates internally and is the result of stretching, distention, inflammation, or damage to the hollow and solid organs

Vesicant: Highly irritating medication that can cause extensive tissue damage when it leaks into the subcutaneous tissues; examples are chemotherapy and solutions with high or low pH

Vitamins: Organic compounds that do not supply energy but are necessary to the body in small amounts for growth, development, maintenance, and reproduction

Vulnerability: The inability to adapt to adversity

W

Wellness: Dynamic balance among the physical, psychological, social, and spiritual aspects of a person's life

Wellness nursing diagnosis: Diagnostic statement that describes the human response to levels of wellness in an individual, family, or community that have a potential for enhancement to a higher state

Wheezing: Adventitious breath sound

World view: Unquestioned framework or predominant set of assumptions through which people view life

Written communication: Means to document and convey information to others; the writer's selection and organization of words that is legible and comprehensible to the reader

X

Xerostomia: Dry mouth

Y

Yang: Aspect considered more active, dynamic, and representative of male energy

Yin: Aspect that represents the Qi of the Earth and considered representative of female energy

Index